Library of Congress Cataloging-in-Publication Data

Ball, Jane.
  Principles of pediatric nursing : caring for children / Jane W. Ball,
Ruth C. Bindler, and Kay J. Cowen.—5th ed.
     p. ; cm.
  Rev. ed. of: Pediatric nursing : caring for children / [edited by]
Jane W. Ball, Ruth C. Bindler. 4th ed. © 2008.
  Includes bibliographical references and index.
  ISBN-13: 978-0-13-211175-1 (alk. paper)
  ISBN-10: 0-13-211175-6 (alk. paper)
  1. Pediatric nursing. I. Bindler, Ruth McGillis. II. Cowen, Kay J.
III. Ball, Jane. Pediatric nursing. IV. Title.
  [DNLM: 1. Pediatric Nursing—methods. 2. Child. 3. Infant.
4. Nursing Assessment—methods. WY 159]
  RJ245.P4414 2012
  618.92'00231—dc22

                                          2010046060

Publisher: Julie Levin Alexander
Assistant to Publisher: Regina Bruno
Executive Acquisitions Editor: Kim Mortimer
Editorial Assistant: Marion Gottlieb
Director of Marketing: David Gesell
Marketing Manager: Phoenix Harvey
Marketing Specialist: Michael Sirinides
Development Editor: Kim Wyatt
Development, Supplements: Molly Ward
Managing Editor, Production: Patrick Walsh
Production Editor: Lynn Steines, S4Carlisle Publishing Services
Production Liaison: Anne Garcia
Media Product Manager: Travis Moses-Westphal
Senior Editor for Media: Sarah Wrocklage
Media Project Managers: Rachel Collett and Leslie Brado
Manufacturing Manager: Ilene Sanford
Art Director: Kristine Carney
Cover Design: Janice Bielawa
Interior Design: Rachael Cronin
Chapter Opener Image: Gustav Klimt/Superstock, Inc.
Composition: S4Carlisle Publishing Services
Printer/Binder: Courier/Kendallville
Cover Printer: Lehigh-Phoenix Color/Hagerstown

Notice: Care has been taken to confirm the accuracy of
information presented in this book. The authors, editors, and the
publisher, however, cannot accept any responsibility for errors or
omissions or for consequences from application of the
information in this book and make no warranty, express or
implied, with respect to its contents.
    The authors and publisher have exerted every effort to ensure
that drug selections and dosages set forth in this text are in accord
with current recommendations and practice at time of
publication. However, in view of ongoing research, changes in
government regulations, and the constant flow of information
relating to drug therapy and reactions, the reader is urged to
check the package inserts of all drugs for any change in
indications or dosage and for added warning and precautions.
This is particularly important when the recommended agent is a
new and/or infrequently employed drug.

www.pearsonhighered.com

10 9 8 7 6 5 4 3
ISBN-13: 978-0-13-211175-1
ISBN-10: 0-13-211175-6

Creating a Floor-Ready Nurse

W9-BBA-780

Instructor Resources—Redefined!

INTRODUCING
Pearson Nursing Class Preparation Resources

- **New and Unique! Correlation to Today's Nursing Standards!**
  - Correlation guides link book and supplement content to nursing standards such as the *2010 ANA Scope and Standards of Practice*, QSEN, National Patient Safety Goals, *AACN Essentials of Baccalaureate Education* and more!

- **New and Unique! Pearson Nursing Lecture Series**
  - Highly visual, fully narrated and animated, these short lectures focus on topics that are traditionally difficult to teach and difficult for students to grasp
  - All lectures accompanied by case studies and classroom response questions for greater interactivity within even the largest classroom
  - Useful as lecture tools, remediation material, homework assignments and more!

- **Additional instructor resources!**
  - Find assets such as **videos, animations, lecture starters, classroom and clinical activities** and more!
  - **Add selected resources** to presentations that can be shown online or exported to PowerPoint™ or HTML pages
  - Organized by topic and **fully searchable** by type and keyword
  - **Upload your own resources** to keep everything in one place
  - **Rate resources** and view other instructor ratings!

- **Pearson Nursing Question Bank**
  - Even **more** accessible with both pencil and paper and online delivery options
  - **All NCLEX®-style** questions
  - **All New!** Approximately 30% of questions now in alternate-item format!
  - **Complete rationales** for both correct and incorrect answers mapped to learning outcomes

Book-specific resources also available to instructors including:
- Online Instructor's Manual and Resource Guide with detailed lecture outlines and activities organized by learning outcome
- Comprehensive PowerPoint™ presentations integrating lecture notes° and images
- Image library
- Classroom Response Questions
- Online course management systems complete with instructor tools and student activities

WITHDRAWN

mynursinglab
- Saves instructor time by providing quality feedback, ongoing formative assessments, and customized remediation for students
- **New!** Select *Real Nursing Simulation* scenarios
- Includes select set of *Real Nursing Skill 2.0* videos
- Available with *Pearson's Interactive e-Text*
  - Integrated media and website links
  - Full search capability and note-taking functionality
  - Customizable organization

REAL NURSING SIMULATIONS
- 25 simulation scenarios that span the nursing curriculum
- Consistent format includes learning objectives, case flow, set-up instructions, debriefing questions and more!
- Companion online course cartridge with student pre- and post-simulation activities, videos, skill checklists and reflective discussion questions

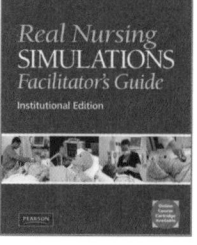

Real Nursing SIMULATIONS *Facilitator's Guide* Institutional Edition

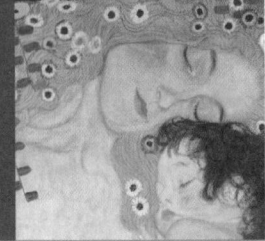

Brief Table of Contents

PRINCIPLES OF PEDIATRIC NURSING
Caring for Children
Fifth Edition

Jane W. Ball, RN, CPNP, DrPH
Consultant
Trauma System Development
Gaithersburg, Maryland

Ruth C. Bindler, RNC, PhD
Professor
Washington State University
    College of Nursing
Spokane, Washington

Kay J. Cowen, RNC, MSN
Clinical Professor
University of North Carolina at
    Greensboro School of Nursing
Greensboro, North Carolina

Pearson
Boston Columbus Indianapolis New York San Francisco
Amsterdam Cape Town Dubai London Madrid Milan Munich
Delhi Mexico City São Paulo Sydney Hong Kong Seoul

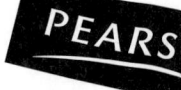

Dedication

We dedicate this book to:

- Our families who are ever supportive and understanding about our passion for children and writing,
- Our mentors, colleagues, and students who inspire us to apply our knowledge and challenge our thinking,
- The children, adolescents, and families with whom we work and who foster our philosophy of pediatric nursing.

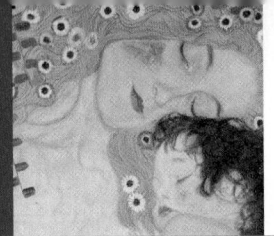

About the Authors

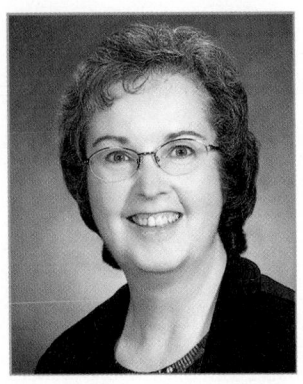

Jane W. Ball graduated from the Johns Hopkins Hospital School of Nursing, and subsequently received a BS from the Johns Hopkins University. She worked in the surgical, emergency, and outpatient units of the Johns Hopkins Children's Medical and Surgical Center, first as a staff nurse and then as a pediatric nurse practitioner, beginning her career as a pediatric nurse and advocate for children's health needs. Jane obtained both a master of public health and a doctor of public health degree from the Johns Hopkins University Bloomberg School of Public Health with a focus on maternal and child health. After graduation she became the chief of child health services for the Commonwealth of Pennsylvania Department of Health. In this capacity she oversaw the state-funded well-child clinics and explored ways to improve education for the state's community health nurses. After relocating to Texas, she joined the faculty at the University of Texas at Arlington School of Nursing to teach community pediatrics to registered nurses returning to school for a BSN. During this time she became involved in writing her first textbook, *Mosby's Guide to*

Physical Examination, which is currently in its seventh edition. After relocating to the Washington, DC, area, she joined Children's National Medical Center to manage a federal project to teach instructors of emergency medical technicians from all states about the special care children need during an emergency. Exposure to the shortcomings of the emergency medical services system in the late 1980s with regard to pediatric care was a career-changing event. With federal funding, she developed educational curricula for emergency medical technicians and emergency nurses to help them provide improved care for children. A textbook entitled *Pediatric Emergencies, A Manual for Prehospital Providers* was developed from these educational ventures. For 15 years she managed the federally funded Emergency Medical Services for Children's National Resource Center. As executive director, Dr. Ball directed the provision of consultation and resource development for state health agencies, health professionals, families, and advocates about successful methods to improve the health care system so that children get optimal emergency care in all health care settings. Having left that position, she devotes more time to writing and serves as a consultant to the American College of Surgeons, supporting state trauma system development. In 2010, Dr. Ball received the Distinguished Alumna Award from the Johns Hopkins University.

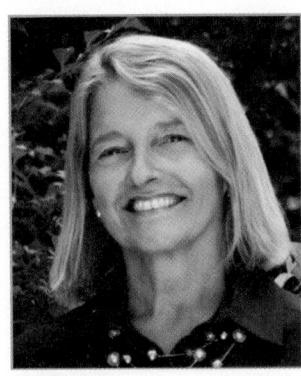

Ruth C. McGillis Bindler received her BSN from Cornell University—New York Hospital School of Nursing. She worked in oncology nursing at Memorial-Sloan Kettering Cancer Center in New York, and then moved to Wisconsin and became a public health nurse in Dane County, Wisconsin. Thus began her commitment to work with children as she visited children and their families at home, and served as a school nurse for several elementary, middle, and high schools. Due to this interest in child health care needs, she earned her MS in child development from the University of Wisconsin. A move to Washington State was accompanied by a new job as a faculty member at the Intercollegiate Center for Nursing Education in Spokane. Dr. Bindler has been fortunate to be involved for over 35 years in the growth of this nursing education consortium, which is a combination of public and private universities and

colleges and is now the Washington State University (WSU) College of Nursing. Ruth obtained a PhD in human nutrition at WSU. She has taught theory and clinical courses in child health nursing, cultural diversity and health, graduate research, pharmacology, and assessment, as well as serving as lead faculty for child health nursing. She is presently professor and associate dean for the college's graduate programs. Her first professional book, *Pediatric Medications*, was published in 1981, and she has continued to publish articles and books in the areas of pediatric medications and pediatric health. Research efforts are focused in the area of childhood obesity, type 2 diabetes, metabolic syndrome, and cardiometabolic risk factors in children. Ethnic diversity and interprofessional collaboration have been additional themes in her work. Dr. Bindler believes that her role as a faculty member has enabled her to learn continually, foster the development of students in nursing, lead and mentor junior faculty into the teaching role, and participate fully in the profession of nursing. In addition to teaching, research, publication, and leadership, she enhances her life by professional and community service, and by activities with her family.

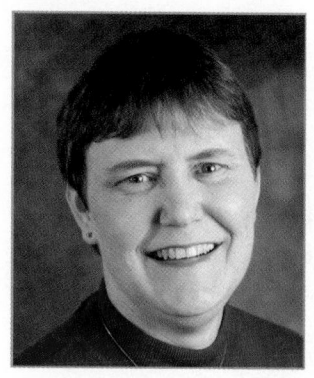

Kay J. Cowen received her BSN from East Carolina University in Greenville, North Carolina, and began her career as a staff nurse on the pediatric unit of North Carolina Baptist Hospital in Winston-Salem. She developed a special interest in the psychosocial needs of hospitalized children and preparing them for hospitalization. This led to the focus of her master's thesis at the University of North Carolina at Greensboro (UNCG) where she received a master of science in nursing education degree with a focus in maternal child nursing.

Mrs. Cowen began her teaching career in 1984 at UNCG where she continues today as clinical professor in the Parent Child Department. Her primary responsibilities include coordinating the pediatric nursing course, teaching classroom content, and supervising a clinical group of students. Mrs. Cowen shared her passion for the psychosocial care of children and the needs of their families through her first experience as an author in the chapter "Hospital Care for Children" in Jackson & Saunders' *Child Health Nursing: A Comprehensive Approach to the Care of Children and Their Families* published in 1993.

In the classroom, Mrs. Cowen realized that students learn through a variety of teaching strategies and became especially interested in the strategy of gaming. She led a research study to evaluate the effectiveness of gaming in the classroom and subsequently continues to incorporate gaming in her teaching. In the clinical setting, Mrs. Cowen teaches her students the skills needed to care for patients and the importance of family-centered care, focusing on not only the physical needs of the child but also the psychosocial needs of the child and family.

During her teaching career, Mrs. Cowen has continued to work part time as a staff nurse: first on the pediatric unit of Moses Cone Hospital in Greensboro and then at Brenner Children's Hospital in Winston-Salem. In 2006 she became the part-time pediatric nurse educator in Brenner's Family Resource Center. Through this role she is able to extend her love of teaching to children and families.

Through her role as an author, Mrs. Cowen is able to extend her dedication to pediatric nursing and nursing education. She is married and the mother of two college-age sons.

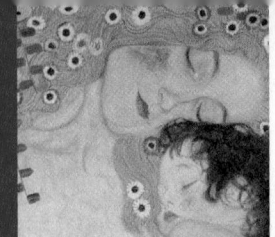

Thank You!

We are grateful to all the nurses, both clinicians and educators, who reviewed the manuscript of this text. Their insights, suggestions, and eye for detail helped us prepare a more relevant, useful, and current book, reflective of the present time and of the essential components of learning in the field of child health nursing.

Ann Acona, Kent State University

Kim Adams, Forsyth Technical Community College

Mike Aldridge, University of Texas at Austin School of Nursing

Monique Alston-Davis, Montgomery College

Traci Arney, Asthma Athletics CEO, Banner Children's Hospital

Johnett Benson-Soros, Kent State University at Ashtabula

Sharen Brady, Weber State University

Carissa Carie, Medical University of South Carolina

Dawn Chapelle, National Institutes of Health

Teresa Chase, University of Kentucky College of Nursing

Jennifer Compere, Brenner Children's Hospital, Winston-Salem

Marilyn Cox, Children's Medical Center Dallas

Kari Crawford, Levine Children's Hospital, Charlotte

Joseph De Santis, University of Miami School of Nursing and Health Studies

Ann Earhart, Clinical Nurse Specialist, Mesa, Arizona

Pat B. Egland, City University of New York, Borough of Manhattan Community College

Tonsha Emerson, East Mississippi Community College

Lori Sholders Farmer, Advanced Practice Nurse in Genetics, Distance Education Instructor, University of North Carolina at Pembroke

Betty Freund, College of Nursing, Kent State University

Julie Garcia, University of Texas Health Science Center at San Antonio

Vicki Grubbs, Eastern Kentucky University

Amy Zlomek Hedden, California State University, Bakersfield

Karen Joris, Lorain County Community College

Robin E. Koch, Piedmont Virginia Community College

Sarah Kulinski, Lenoir Rhyne University

Patricia A. Kuster, Samuel Merritt University

Meredith Lahl, Pediatric Nurse Practitioner, Cleveland Clinic

Mikki Meadows-Oliver, Yale University School of Nursing

Cheryl Mele, Drexel University

Earlene Merrill, Coppin State University

Sara Mitchell, Georgia Baptist College of Nursing of Mercer University

Mary Ellen Mitchell-Rosen, Nova Southeastern University

Maureen E. O'Brien, Marquette University College of Nursing

Brenda Pavill, University of North Carolina Wilmington

Marisue Rayno, Luzerne County Community College

Katherine Roberts, Lamar University

T. Kim Rodehorst, UNMC-College of Nursing

Cheryl Shaffer, Suffolk County Community College

Sue Solecki, Drexel University

Lisa D. South, East Mississippi Community College

Joanna Spahis, Children's Medical Center Dallas

Daphnee Stewart, Georgia Baptist College of Nursing, Mercer University

Marie H. Thomas, Forsyth Technical Community College

Maureen Tippen, University of Michigan–Flint

Debbie Treolar, East Mississippi Community College

Diane K. Van Os, Westminster College

Terri L. Walker, Oklahoma City Community College

Rosie Wilbon, East Mississippi Community College

Cynthia Williams, Oklahoma City Community College

Donna Wilsker, Lamar University

Ronda M. Wood, Long Beach City College

Contributor

Linda D. Ward, MN, ARNP
Clinical Assistant Professor
Washington State University College of Nursing
Spokane, Washington
Chapter 3: Genetic and Genomic Influences

Preface

Health care and health care delivery systems are changing dramatically. Pediatric nurses must respond to and integrate these changes into their practice. In addition, pediatric nursing presents unique challenges and issues in the changing health care scene. Student nurses must learn what helps them to provide safe, effective, and excellent care today, while integrating new knowledge and skills needed as nursing practice continues to develop and respond to health care needs. Students must learn how to think and apply information as new knowledge becomes available. "As the student uses knowledge in situations of practice, new understanding is gained as well as knowing how, when, and why it is relevant in particular situations. . . . We call this teaching for a sense of salience."*

Faculty are responsible for selecting patient care assignments that assist the student to apply knowledge in the clinical setting, as well as various pedagogies to assist the student to focus on the patient experience. We have integrated these concepts and others in this text from the Carnegie Report by offering a variety of critical thinking and clinical reasoning questions, patient care scenarios, research and evidence-based practice features, and support for teaching with current information technology in mind.

Preparation for Nursing Excellence

The goal of the fifth edition of this textbook is to provide core pediatric nursing knowledge that prepares students for excellence in nursing, and to offer the tools of scholarship and critical thinking needed to apply this learning in the future. Students must learn to question, evaluate the research evidence available, apply pertinent information in clinical settings, and constantly adapt to growing knowledge and an evolving health care system.

This textbook reflects a multitude of approaches to learning that can be helpful to all students. We acknowledge that many students learn pediatric nursing in a very short time period. Therefore, the approaches in this textbook are designed to assist students to assess the child's needs, take into account population-based practice, and make care decisions based on the standards of pediatric nursing practice.

Realities of Pediatric Nursing

Pediatric nursing occurs in many acute care and community health care settings, such as hospitals, homes, schools, and health centers. Many procedures are performed in short-stay units, and long-term care is often provided at home for children with complex health conditions. Families are often the providers of care and case managers for these children. Technological advances are resulting in earlier diagnoses and new therapies; these technological approaches are integrated whenever pertinent throughout the textbook.

Pediatric nursing care is provided within the context of a rapidly changing society. An examination of the major morbidities and mortalities of childhood guided the revision of material and topics throughout the text. Specific chapters focus on the family, health promotion across the life span, pediatric nutrition, and care for chronic conditions. A chapter addressing cultural influences on health care provides guidance for students caring for children in our growing intercultural society. A chapter on genetics has been added to help students recognize the impact of genetics and genomics knowledge on pediatric nursing. Current social challenges for children have guided the further development of a chapter on societal and environmental influences on child health.

Many graduating nurses practice in acute care facilities, and this textbook continues to emphasize the information necessary to prepare students for working in hospitals. In addition, the information provided in this textbook will enable graduates to assume positions in ambulatory care facilities, home health nursing, schools, and a variety of other settings. Effective communication methods, principles of working with families, and knowledge of pathophysiologic, psychologic, developmental, and environmental factors found in this book can all be applied in a wide variety of settings.

In keeping with the pressures and demands on student time to learn and read, the textbook was redesigned to be more compact and focus on essential content. The companion website is used to provide some supplemental content, case studies, and care planning exercises to enhance learning.

Another major change in our society involves access to information and reliance on the Internet. Nurses must learn to obtain information and then analyze and judge the quality of information they find. Increasingly, nurses need experience with information technology and management. In this edition, margin tabs send the student online to obtain the latest information available on many topics. Nurses must also assist children and family members to use the Internet wisely to help them in making health care decisions, so the student is assisted to make practice decisions based on scholarship and evidence-based research.

Organization and Integrated Themes

We have organized *Principles of Pediatric Nursing: Caring for Children*, fifth edition, to present important information on growth and development, family-centered care, culture, genetics, physical assessment, health promotion, nutrition, health issues in today's world, and children's responses to illness and injury. This information is needed to care for children in the many health care settings where pediatric nursing care is provided. Following the foundational chapters, this book is organized by body systems to

---

*Benner, P., Sutphen, M., Leonard, V., & Day, L. (2010). *Educating nurses: A call for radical transformation* (p. 94). San Francisco, CA: Jossey-Bass.

facilitate the student's ability to locate information, focus studying, and prepare for clinical experiences with children and families. The organizational framework also eliminates redundancy, so that the student uses time efficiently.

In addition to the significant revisions made to all chapters to update clinical information and resources, we added one new chapter—Chapter 3: Genetic and Genomic Influences—to reflect the emerging information about the impact of genetics on the health conditions occurring in children. Such content is cited in "Clinical Prevention and Population Health" in *The Essentials of Baccalaureate Education for Professional Nursing Practice* (American Association of Colleges of Nursing, 2008).

The **Bindler-Ball Child Healthcare Model** is used to illustrate the important core value that all children need health promotion and health maintenance interventions, no matter where they seek health care or what health conditions they may be experiencing.

The nursing process is used as the framework for nursing care. **Nursing Management** is the major heading, with subheadings of **Nursing Assessment and Diagnosis, Planning and Implementation,** and **Evaluation.** When it is appropriate to focus on care in a specific setting, Hospital-Based Care, Discharge Planning, and Community Care are separated into sections. We feature nursing care plans throughout the text to help students approach care from the nursing process perspective. Additional nursing care plans are provided on the companion website. **Nursing Care Plans** include nursing intervention classifications (NIC) and nursing outcome classifications (NOC), as well as nursing diagnoses, goals, interventions, and rationale.

Several major concepts are integrated throughout the textbook to encourage the student to think creatively and critically about nursing care. These major themes are interwoven throughout the text through the features and supplements.

- **Nursing care** is the critical and central core of this textbook. Nursing assessment and management are emphasized in all sections of the book, with nurses shown providing care in a variety of settings.

- **Collaborative care** descriptions of the diagnostic and therapeutic care for various health conditions reflects the interprofessional team role of nurses with other health professionals (e.g., physicians, physical therapists, mental health counselors, pharmacists, and others) as described in *The Essentials of Baccalaureate Education for Professional Nursing Practice* (American Association of Colleges of Nursing, 2008).

- **Clinical reasoning and problem-solving principles** are integrated in the organization, pedagogy, writing style, evidence-based practice features, research boxes, clinical judgment boxes, exercises on the companion website, and art captions. Students practice clinical reasoning and critical thinking in their everyday lives, but need help to apply these concepts to the practice of nursing. This book and the accompanying learning materials help students understand how their normal curiosity and problem-solving ability can be applied to pediatric nursing.

- **Communication** is one of the most important skills that students need to learn. Effective communication with children is challenging because they communicate differently, according to their developmental levels. Family members have communication needs in addition to those of their children. This book integrates communication skills by applied examples that help the student to communicate effectively with children and their families.

- **Family and patient education** about health care is an integral part of the pediatric nurse's responsibilities. Since hospitalizations are short and families increasingly care for children at home, information about health care needs and procedures has become even more important.

- **Developing cultural competence** is critical for all nurses in the increasingly diverse community of today's world. Students have all met people from different ethnic and cultural groups, but they need help to understand, respect, and integrate differing beliefs, practices, and health care needs when providing care.

- **Growth and development considerations and physical assessment** are central to the effective practice of pediatric nursing. A separate chapter is devoted to each area, Chapter 4 and Chapter 5, respectively. In addition, both topics are integrated where appropriate in narrative, growth and development boxes, figures, captions, and on the companion website.

- **Health promotion** is an important focus of nursing care for children with acute and chronic health conditions. Four chapters focus on health promotion. One provides an overview of concepts related to health promotion. Three chapters address health promotion principles for children of different ages. In addition, health promotion boxes help illustrate opportunities for health promotion for children with health conditions.

- **Community care** is an increasing part of nursing responsibilities. To assist students in transferring knowledge to caring for children in community settings, information is provided in the nursing management sections of chapters. In addition, an entire chapter is devoted to nursing care in the community and directly addresses the nurse's roles in several community settings.

These themes and others are interwoven in the narrative of most chapters and are reflected in the art, as well as in the supplements that students can use to augment their learning.

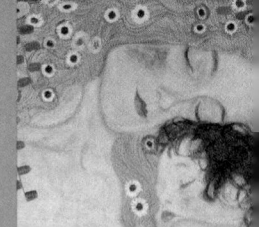

Features to Help You Use This Textbook Successfully

Instructors and students alike value the in-text learning aids that we include in our textbooks to help meet the challenges of pediatric nursing. The following guide will help you use the features and resources from Principles of Pediatric Nursing: Caring for Children, fifth edition, to be successful in the classroom, in the clinical setting, on the NCLEX-RN(r) examination, and in nursing practice.

Case Scenarios and photos at the beginning of each chapter engage you with a child's real-life experience with a specific health challenge. Questions at the end of each scenario highlight nursing considerations. Additional information appears throughout the chapter to help build knowledge.

Key Terms are introduced at the beginning of each chapter, with page numbers showing where each term first appears in the chapter, designated in bold type.

Learning Outcomes identify measurable objectives based on topics covered in each chapter.

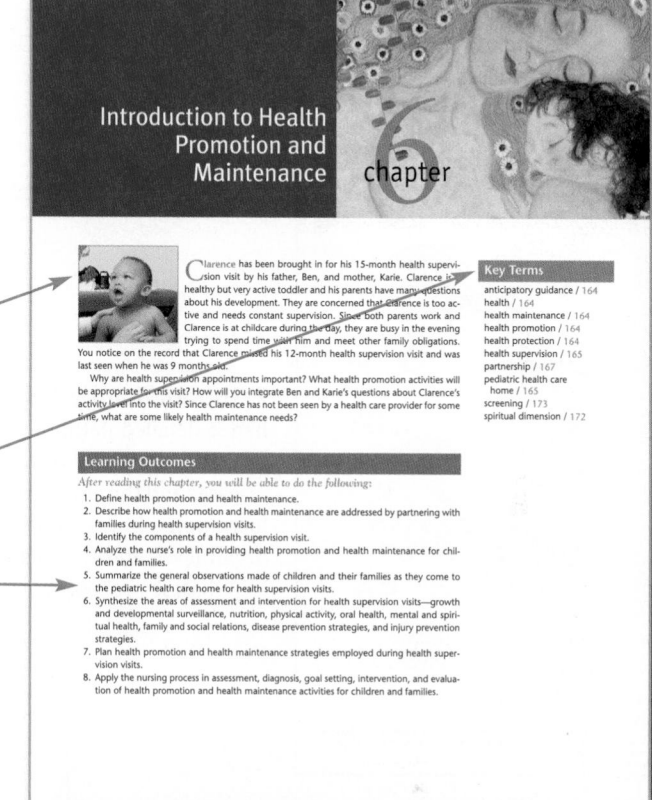

Introduction to Health Promotion and Maintenance 6 chapter

Clarence has been brought in for his 15-month health supervision visit by his father, Ben, and mother, Karie. Clarence is healthy but very active toddler and his parents have many questions about his development. They are concerned that Clarence is too active and needs constant supervision. Since both parents work and Clarence is at childcare during the day, they are busy in the evening trying to spend time with him and meet other family obligations. You notice on the record that Clarence missed his 12-month health supervision visit and was last seen when he was 9 months old.

Why are health supervision appointments important? What health promotion activities will be appropriate for this visit? How will you integrate Ben and Karie's questions about Clarence's activity level into the visit? Since Clarence has not been seen by a health care provider for some time, what are some likely health maintenance needs?

Key Terms

anticipatory guidance / 164
health / 164
health maintenance / 164
health promotion / 164
health protection / 164
health supervision / 165
partnership / 167
pediatric health care home / 165
screening / 173
spiritual dimension / 172

Learning Outcomes

After reading this chapter, you will be able to do the following:

1. Define health promotion and health maintenance.
2. Describe how health promotion and health maintenance are addressed by partnering with families during health supervision visits.
3. Identify the components of a health supervision visit.
4. Analyze the nurse's role in providing health promotion and health maintenance for children and families.
5. Summarize the general observations made of children and their families as they come to the pediatric health care home for health supervision visits.
6. Synthesize the areas of assessment and intervention for health supervision visits—growth and developmental surveillance, nutrition, physical activity, oral health, mental and spiritual health, family and social relations, disease prevention strategies, and injury prevention strategies.
7. Plan health promotion and health maintenance strategies employed during health supervision visits.
8. Apply the nursing process in assessment, diagnosis, goal setting, intervention, and evaluation of health promotion and health maintenance activities for children and families.

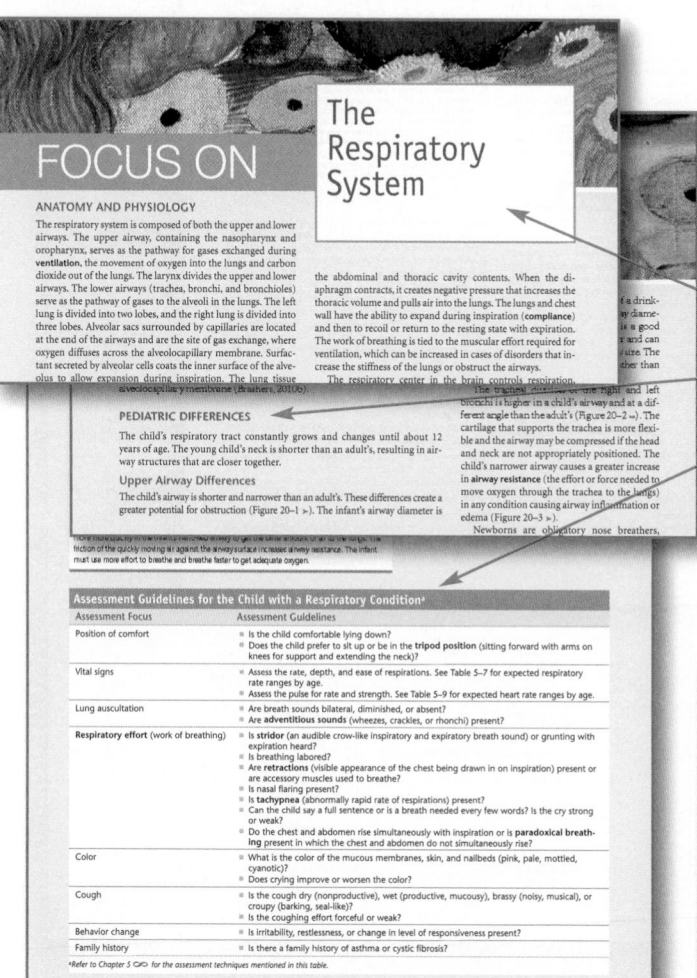

FOCUS ON The Respiratory System

ANATOMY AND PHYSIOLOGY

The respiratory system is composed of both the upper and lower airways. The upper airway, containing the nasopharynx and oropharynx, serves as the pathway for gases exchanged during **ventilation**, the movement of oxygen into the lungs and carbon dioxide out of the lungs. The larynx divides the upper and lower airways. The lower airways (trachea, bronchi, and bronchioles) serve as the pathway of gases to the alveoli in the lungs. The left lung is divided into two lobes, and the right lung is divided into three lobes. Alveolar sacs surrounded by capillaries are located at the end of the airways and are the site of gas exchange, where oxygen diffuses across the alveolocapillary membrane. Surfactant secreted by alveolar cells coats the inner surface of the alveolus to allow expansion during inspiration. The lung tissue alveolocapillary membrane (Brashers, 2010b).

the abdominal and thoracic cavity contents. When the diaphragm contracts, it creates negative pressure that increases the thoracic volume and pulls air into the lungs. The lungs and chest wall have the ability to expand during inspiration (**compliance**) and then to recoil or return to the resting state with expiration. The work of breathing is tied to the muscular effort required for ventilation, which can be increased in cases of disorders that increase the stiffness of the lungs or obstruct the airways.

The respiratory center in the brain controls respiration. [...] drink-[...] diame-[...] is a good [...] and can [...] lung. The [...] other than [...]

The [...] distance are right and left bronchi is higher in a child's airway and at a different angle than the adult's (Figure 20–2 ►). The cartilage that supports the trachea is more flexible and the airway may be compressed if the head and neck are not appropriately positioned. The child's narrower airway causes a greater increase in **airway resistance** (the effort or force needed to move oxygen through the trachea to the lungs) in any condition causing airway inflammation or edema (Figure 20–3 ►).

Newborns are obligatory nose breathers,

PEDIATRIC DIFFERENCES

The child's respiratory tract constantly grows and changes until about 12 years of age. The young child's neck is shorter than an adult's, resulting in airway structures that are closer together.

Upper Airway Differences

The child's airway is shorter and narrower than an adult's. These differences create a greater potential for obstruction (Figure 20–1 ►). The infant's airway diameter is

[...] more molecules to the nearby narrowed airway to get the same amount of air in the lungs. [...] friction of the quickly moving air against the airway surface increases airway resistance. The infant must use more effort to breathe and breathe faster to get adequate oxygen.

Assessment Guidelines for the Child with a Respiratory Condition*

Assessment Focus	Assessment Guidelines
Position of comfort	▪ Is the child comfortable lying down? ▪ Does the child prefer to sit up or be in the **tripod position** (sitting forward with arms on knees for support and extending the neck)?
Vital signs	▪ Assess the rate, depth, and ease of respirations. See Table 5–7 for expected respiratory rate ranges by age. ▪ Assess the pulse for rate and strength. See Table 5–9 for expected heart rate ranges by age.
Lung auscultation	▪ Are breath sounds bilateral, diminished, or absent? ▪ Are **adventitious sounds** (wheezes, crackles, or rhonchi) present?
Respiratory effort (work of breathing)	▪ Is **stridor** (an audible crow-like inspiratory and expiratory breath sound) or grunting with expiration heard? ▪ Is breathing labored? ▪ Are **retractions** (visible appearance of the chest being drawn in on inspiration) present or are accessory muscles used to breathe? ▪ Is nasal flaring present? ▪ Is **tachypnea** (abnormally rapid rate of respirations) present? Is the cry strong or weak? ▪ Can the child say a full sentence or is a breath needed every few words? Is the cry strong or weak? ▪ Do the chest and abdomen rise simultaneously with inspiration or is **paradoxical breathing** present in which the chest and abdomen do not simultaneously rise?
Color	▪ What is the color of the mucous membranes, skin, and nailbeds (pink, pale, mottled, cyanotic)? ▪ Does crying improve or worsen the color?
Cough	▪ Is the cough dry (nonproductive), wet (productive, mucousy), brassy (noisy, musical), or croupy (barking, seal-like)? ▪ Is the coughing effort forceful or weak?
Behavior change	▪ Is irritability, restlessness, or change in level of responsiveness present?
Family history	▪ Is there a family history of asthma or cystic fibrosis?

*Refer to Chapter 5 for the assessment techniques mentioned in this table.

A **Focus On** section appears at the beginning of each systems chapter as a reference to use while reading the chapter. Each Focus On section includes the following features:

- **Anatomy and Physiology** provides a quick review of the system.
- **Pediatric Differences** will help you recognize physical and mental differences in children at various ages.
- The **Assessment Guidelines table** in each of the systems chapters provides an overview of the key aspects of an integrated assessment within the body system.
- **Diagnostic Tests and Laboratory Procedures** offer information related to the specific system to assist in clinical application.

TABLE 20–1	Diagnostic and Laboratory Procedures/Tests for the Respiratory System*
Diagnostic Procedures	Laboratory Tests
Bronchoscopy	Arterial blood gas analysis
Chest radiograph	Cultures
Polysomnography (sleep study)	Neonatal screening for cystic fibrosis
Pulse oximetry	Protein-purified derivative (PPD), the Mantoux test
Spirometry (pulmonary function tests)	Sweat chloride test
Sweat chloride test	

*See Appendices C and D ⟶ for information about these diagnostic procedures and tests.

This chapter explores several factors in the child's respiratory system that create ongoing threats to respiratory function and overall health. Most respiratory problems in children produce mild symptoms, last a short time, and can be managed at home. Other respiratory problems are chronic and potentially life threatening. Respiratory conditions are the most common cause of hospitalization in children between 1 and 9 years of age, and a leading cause in children between 10 and 19 years of age (National Center for Health Statistics 2008). See Chapter 19 ⟶ for

Respiratory problems may result from structural problems, functional problems, or a combination of both. Structural problems involve alterations in the size and shape of parts of the respiratory tract. Functional problems involve alterations in gas exchange and threats to the process of ventilation due to irritation by large particles and chemicals or infection. Alterations in other organ systems, especially the immune and neurologic systems, may also threaten respiratory function. Try to

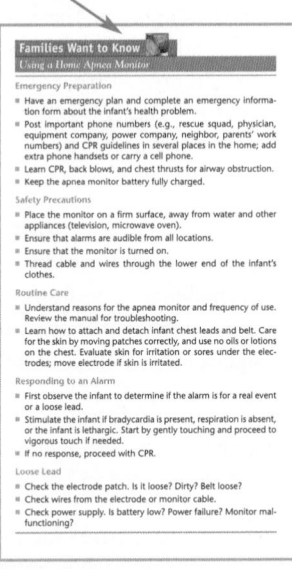

As Children Grow boxes illustrate the anatomic and physiologic differences between children and adults. This visual feature will help you consider developmental differences when working with children in different age groups.

Families Want to Know boxes apply the concepts of family-centered nursing care by offering teaching in formats directly applicable when working with families.

Pathophysiology Illustrated boxes enhance detailed pathophysiology in the text by offering a visual of the cause of various diseases and the effect on children. These illustrations show conditions at a cellular or organ level, and may also portray step-by-step disease processes.

NEW

Health Promotion speed bumps appear in the text to help you recognize opportunities for health promotion for children with health conditions.

NEW

Clinical Judgment speed bumps appear in the text to help hone critical thinking and clinical reasoning skills by presenting a brief scenario and asking for the appropriate response in that situation.

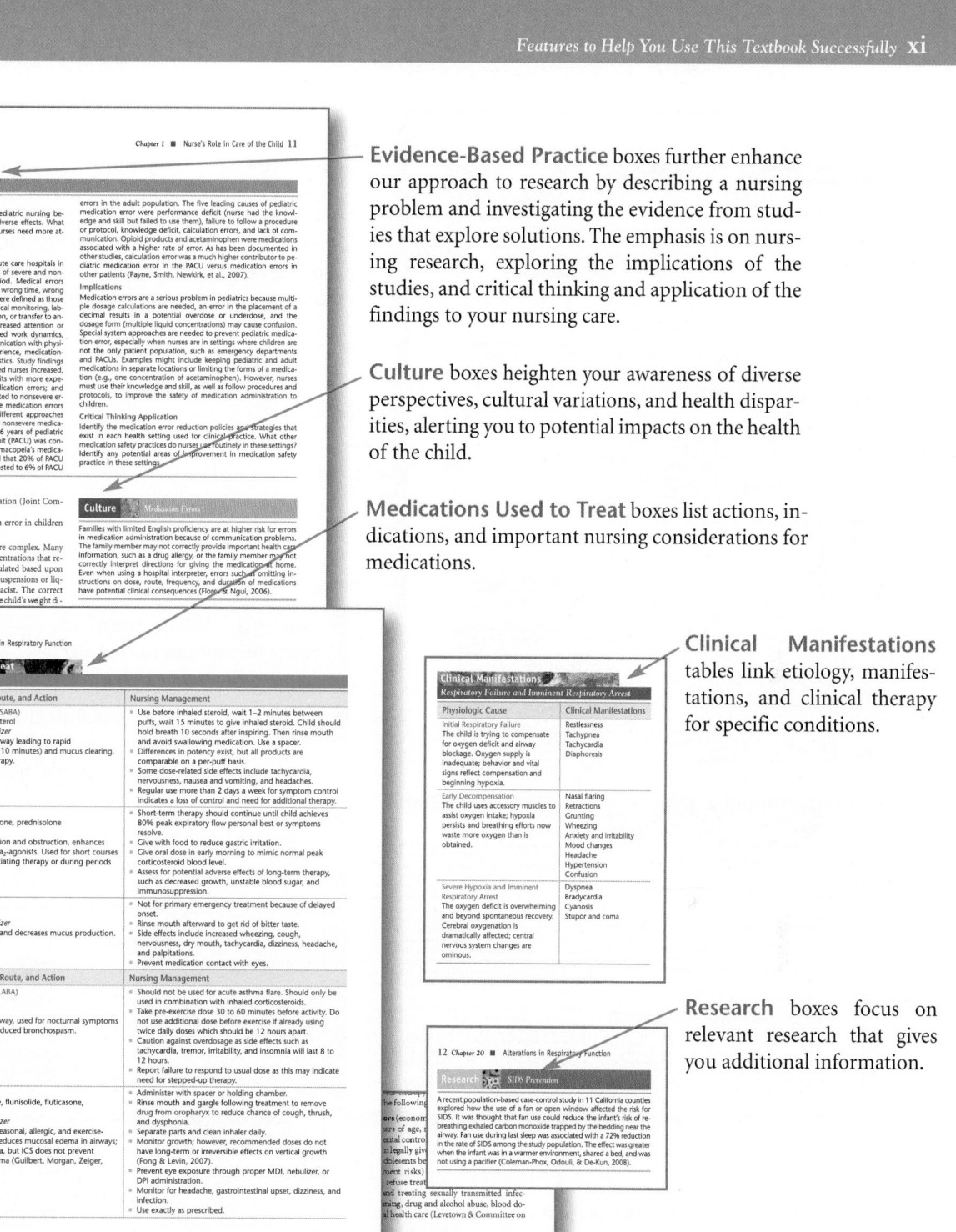

Evidence-Based Practice boxes further enhance our approach to research by describing a nursing problem and investigating the evidence from studies that explore solutions. The emphasis is on nursing research, exploring the implications of the studies, and critical thinking and application of the findings to your nursing care.

Culture boxes heighten your awareness of diverse perspectives, cultural variations, and health disparities, alerting you to potential impacts on the health of the child.

Medications Used to Treat boxes list actions, indications, and important nursing considerations for medications.

Clinical Manifestations tables link etiology, manifestations, and clinical therapy for specific conditions.

Research boxes focus on relevant research that gives you additional information.

Growth and Development boxes highlight nursing care at specific stages of development.

Law and Ethics boxes highlight the many issues that nurses face related to pediatric nursing, preparing you for the clinical setting.

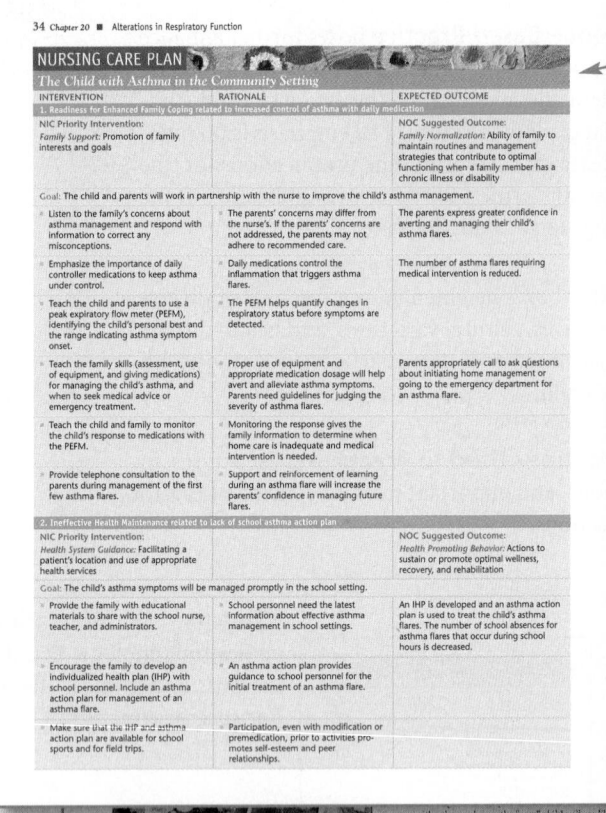

Nursing Care Plans, which are presented in every chapter that includes health conditions, illustrate the conceptual approach that nurses need in caring for children, including assessment, NANDA nursing diagnoses, goals, plans, and interventions.

Nursing Alerts warn of safety precautions to consider in providing care.

Clinical Tips, which are embedded throughout the book, are "pearls" from clinical nurse experts.

Complementary Therapy boxes present approaches other than traditional medical prescriptions that may be used by children and their families to prevent or treat disease. These boxes include research, when possible, to support or refute the efficacy of the modalities. In addition, these boxes highlight the necessity to gather information from families when planning care.

The **companion website margin tabs** in each chapter offer extra resources that enhance learning and provide an application beyond the textbook experience.

Each chapter ends with **Chapter Highlights**, which outline the main points of the chapter, and **Clinical Reasoning in Action**, a recap of the opening scenario with questions to help you apply concepts learned in the chapter.

At the end of each chapter, you will also find a list of current **References**, and directions to the companion website for additional resources.

We have continued our tradition of providing excellent visuals to enhance student learning by including dozens of new photographs. In addition, **Critical Thinking Highlights** often appear with photos, encouraging application of knowledge.

---

46 Chapter 20 ■ Alterations in Respiratory Function

- Parietal pleura (outer lining)
- Air in pleural space
- Visceral pleura (inner lining)
- Partially collapsed lung

FIGURE 20–17 ▶ A, A pneumothorax is air in the pleural space that causes a lung to collapse. Whether the air results from an open injury or from bursting of alveoli due to a blunt injury, it is important to focus on airway management and maintain lung inflation. B, Tension pneumothorax. Note the collapsed lung on the patient's right side and the deviation of the child's heart and trachea to the right side of the chest.
Note: B, Courtesy of Dorothy I. Bulas, M.D., Professor of Radiology and Pediatrics, Children's National Medical Center, Washington, DC.

Chapter Highlights

- Respiratory conditions are a leading cause of hospitalization for all children between 1 and 19 years of age.
- The child's airway is shorter and narrower than an adult's, increasing the risk for obstruction. The lungs have no muscles; diaphragm and intercostal muscles power ventilation.
- Foreign body aspiration is a major health problem for infants and toddlers, often related to their increasing mobility and tendency to put small objects such as food and toy parts in their mouth.
- Impending respiratory failure in infants and children causes worsening respiratory distress, irritability, lethargy, pallor or cyanosis, diaphoresis, and increased respiratory signs such as dyspnea, tachypnea, nasal flaring, grunting, and retractions.
- Apparent life-threatening event (ALTE) is an episode of apnea accompanied by a color change (e.g., cyanosis or pallor), muscle tone, choking, or gagging in an infant less than 12 months of age.
- Obstructive sleep apnea syndrome (OSAS) in children is commonly caused by enlarged tonsils and adenoids. Children snore loudly and have labored breathing during sleep.
- Sudden infant death syndrome (SIDS) is a leading cause of death in infants. Onset of the fatal episode occurs during sleep and remains unexplained after a thorough investigation, including an autopsy, a review of the circumstances of death, and clinical history.
- Laryngotracheobronchitis (LTB) is a viral croup syndrome with a gradual upper respiratory illness, hoarseness, tachypnea, inspiratory stridor, and a seal-like barking cough. Fever may or may not be present.
- Epiglottitis is a potentially life-threatening airway obstruction caused by bacterial invasion of the laryngeal soft tissue causing inflammation and edema of the epiglottis and surrounding tissues. Classic signs include dysphonia, dysphagia, drooling, and distressed respiratory effort.
- Respiratory syncytial virus (RSV) is the most common cause of bronchiolitis, a lower respiratory tract infection that causes inflammation and obstruction of the bronchioles.
- Symptoms of pneumonia in infants and children include elevated temperature, rales, crackles, wheezes, cough, dyspnea, tachypnea, restlessness, and decreased breath sounds if consolidation occurs.
- Children under 2 years are at increased risk for developing active tuberculosis, including tubercular meningitis and disseminated TB.
- An asthma flare or episode results from inflammation and a stimulus causing excessive mucous formation, mucosal swelling, and airway muscle contraction, leading to airway obstruction.
- Chronic lung disease or bronchopulmonary dysplasia (BPD) usually develops in neonates with a birth weight of 1000 g or less. Treatment with oxygen and positive pressure ventilation causes inflammation and damages the bronchioles, resulting in fibrosis, edema of the bronchioles, and smooth muscle hypertrophy.
- In cystic fibrosis, defective chloride-ion transport across the exocrine and epithelial cell walls results in an abnormal accu-

---

Chapter 20 ■ Alterations in Respiratory Function 597

mulation of viscous, dehydrated mucus that affects the respiratory, gastrointestinal, and reproductive systems.
- Signs of smoke inhalation injury in children include burns of the face and neck, singed nasal hairs, soot around the mouth or nose, and hoarseness with stridor or voice change.

- A pneumothorax may become life threatening when air leaking into the chest cavity during inspiration cannot escape during expiration, increasing compression. Venous blood return to the heart is impaired as the mediastinum shifts toward the unaffected lung.

Clinical Reasoning in Action

Recall Shaun, the 13-year-old from the opening scenario. He is in the hospital for infection management and aggressive respiratory therapy. Because he has cystic fibrosis and infectious organisms in his lungs, he is in a single room. He is not permitted to interact with the other children on his unit. Shaun uses a mask when he leaves his room and the nursing unit. He is not feeling ill and welcomes company and distractions. His mother and sister are only able to visit after work. This is an optimal time to continue teaching Shaun to manage his condition.

1. What is Shaun's developmental stage, and what information and self-care skills should be included in a teaching plan for Shaun to correspond to that stage?

2. What information should be reviewed with Shaun about his condition and the treatments needed to keep it from progressing?

3. What signs should Shaun learn to recognize that might indicate a new infection?

4. What approaches might be taken to help Shaun schedule his treatments around school and recreational activities that might increase adherence to the schedule?

See Pearson Nursing Student Resources for possible responses.

Pearson Nursing Student Resources
Find additional review materials at
nursing.pearsonhighered.com
Prepare for success with NCLEX®-style practice questions, interactive assignments and activities, web links, animations and videos, and more!

References

Adams, S. M., Good, M. W., & Defranco, G. M. (2009). Sudden infant death syndrome. *American Family Physician, 79*(10), 870–874.
Allergy and Asthma Network. (2010). *Medications at school.* Retrieved from http://www.aanma.org/advocacy/meds-at-school/
Al-Saif, S., Alvard, R., Manfreda, J., Kwatkowski, K., Cates, D., Qurashi, M., & Rigatto, H. (2008). A randomized controlled trial of theophylline versus CO₂ inhalation for treating apnea of prematurity. *Journal of Pediatrics, 153*(4), 513–518.
American Academy of Allergy, Asthma, and Immunology (AAAAI). (2009). *Peak flow meter.* Retrieved from http://www.aaaai.org/
American Academy of Pediatrics (AAP). (2009). *Red book: 2009 Report of the Committee on Infectious Diseases* (28th ed.). Elk Grove Village, IL: Author.
American Academy of Pediatrics (AAP) Subcommittee on Diagnosis and Management of Bronchiolitis. (2006). Diagnosis and management of bronchiolitis. *Pediatrics, 118*(4), 1774–1793.
American Academy of Pediatrics (AAP), Task Force on Sudden Infant Death Syndrome. (2005). The changing concept of sudden infant death syndrome: Diagnostic coding shifts, controversies regarding the sleeping environment, and new variables to consider in reducing risk. *Pediatrics, 116*(5), 1245–1255.
Antoon, A. Y., & Donovan, M. K. (2007). Burn injuries. In R. M. Kliegman, R. E. Behrman, H. B. Jenson, & B. F. Stanton, *Nelson textbook of pediatrics* (18th ed., pp. 450–458). Philadelphia: Elsevier Saunders.
Arnold, L. D. (2006). Ingested and aspirated foreign bodies: Making sure what went in comes out. *Contemporary Pediatrics, 23*(11), 32–44.
Askin, D. F., & Diehl-Jones, W. (2009). Pathogenesis and prevention of chronic lung disease in the neonate. *Critical Care Nursing Clinics of North America, 21*, 11–25.
Ayala, G. X., Miller, D., Zagami, E., Riddle, C., Willis, S., & King, D. (2006). Asthma in middle schools: What students have to say about their asthma. *Journal of School Health, 76*(6), 208–214.
Baker, L. K., & Denyes, M. J. (2008). Predictors of self-care in adolescents with cystic fibrosis: A test of Orem's theories of self-care and self-care deficit. *Journal of Pediatric Nursing, 23*(1), 37–48.
Banasiak, N. C. (2007). Childhood asthma: Part two: Management update. *Journal of Pediatric Health Care, 21*(3), 184–191.
Baraldi, E., & Filippone, M. (2007). Chronic lung diseases after premature birth. *New England Journal of Medicine, 357*(19), 1946–1955.
Bell, E. (2006). Pulmonary pharmacotherapy options changing for cystic fibrosis patients. *Infectious Diseases in Children, 19*(10), 12–13.

Chapter 1 ■ Nurse's Role in Care of the Child 13

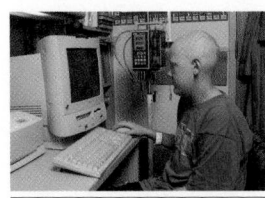

FIGURE 1–10 ▶ Marvin, a 15-year-old boy with acute nonlymphocytic leukemia, has definite opinions about his treatment, but his parents disagree. **At what age can children make an informed decision about whether to accept or refuse treatment?**

Informed Consent

Informed consent is a formal authorization by the child's parent or guardian allowing an invasive procedure to be performed or for participation in research. The physician is legally responsible for obtaining informed consent. In the case of research, the investigative researcher may formally designate a person to obtain informed consent. The nurse should verify that informed con-

Law & Ethics *Legal Advice*

Obtain legal advice for complex family issues related to guardianship, divorced parents disagreeing over care, or a caregiver who is not the legal guardian. Each agency should have designated legal experts or consultants for provision of such legal advice.

does not have legal authority to sign consent. Proxy consent can be granted in writing by the parent to another adult so that children can obtain health care when needed. In an emergency, treatment to preserve life or limb does not require consent if it cannot be immediately obtained (Emanuel, 2007).

Child Participation in Health Care Decisions

Children are considered to have the cognitive capacity to make medical decisions when they can understand that a decision must be made, they are able to receive and process information about the decision to be made, and they are able to state an opinion using the presented information (Van Norman, 2008). Children under 18 or 21 years of age (the age of majority), depending on state law, are considered minor children and need their parents' consent for therapy. Adolescents can legally give informed consent in the following special circumstances:

- **Emancipated minors** (economically self-supporting adolescents under 18 years of age, no longer living at home and not subject to parental control), including minor parents of

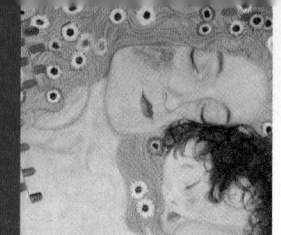

Acknowledgments

It is both exciting and challenging to have the opportunity to write a textbook. It is inspiring to observe the evolution of pediatric nursing practice, and to encourage nursing students to share the excitement and enthusiasm we feel for working with children and their families. Although each edition carries its own unique set of challenges and circumstances, it continues to be a privilege to contribute to the education of the new generation of student nurses.

This edition has undergone significant changes and integrates some new features developed in collaboration with Pearson Nursing. Our third edition editor, Maura Connor, supported the vision for development and enhancement of this textbook that matched our own. Our present editor, Kim Mortimer, worked closely with us so that our views of pediatric nursing could be conveyed effectively to students and faculty. The vice president and publisher, Julie Alexander, enthusiastically supported this venture, and has supported us in decisions regarding changes, updates, and features for the text.

Our developmental editor, Kim Wyatt, has worked with us on several publications and is a tireless proponent for the approach, philosophy, and conceptual framework underlying the text. She explained our goals to others, and worked endlessly to enhance and organize the materials we provided. This effort could not have succeeded without her.

George Dodson again provided us with fresh new photography to help illustrate current nursing concepts. We are grateful to the families and many health care facilities that have permitted us to capture the images used in photographs throughout the book. Our special thanks go to the Shriners Hospital for Children and Sacred Heart Children's Hospital, both in Washington, and to the Washington State University College of Nursing that permitted us to capture our most recent images.

We would like to acknowledge the contributions of Linda Ward, a nurse leader who contributed the Genetic and Genomic Influences chapter.

We thank Anne Garcia, production editor; Patrick Walsh, production managing editor; and Phoenix Harvey, senior marketing manager, for their expertise and valuable contributions. Our thanks also go to Maria Guglielmo and Kristine Carney, art directors, for creating the fresh textbook design. New media editors Travis Moses-Westphal and Sarah Wrocklage helped bring our media ideas to fruition, and Molly Ward and Elisabeth Tinsley helped round out the supplement team. At S4Carlisle Publishing Services, we thank Lynn Steines for coordinating production, and Joan Lyon for her copyediting skills. The authors and Prentice Hall Health would also like to thank those who have enhanced the learning and teaching package for this text by contributing to the resources that accompany it.

Finally, our families once again have supported us tirelessly through the revision process. They sacrificed by allowing us to work on the book when we could have been with them. Yet, they show others the book with pride. We could not have accomplished this without their love and patience.

Jane W. Ball

Ruth C. Bindler

Kay J. Cowen

Special Features

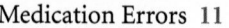

Culture

Pathophysiology Illustrated

Families Want to Know

Growth & Development

Nursing Care Plan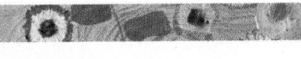

Research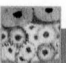

Contents

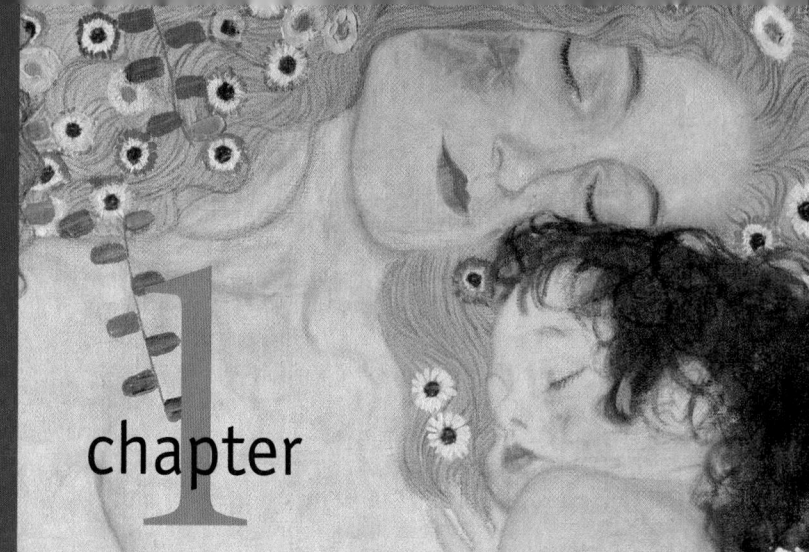

Nurse's Role in Care of the Child
Hospital, Community, and Home

chapter 1

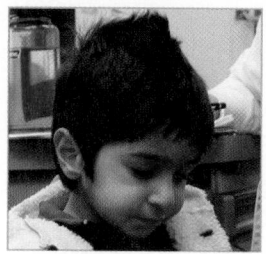

Manny is a 3-year-old boy who has a seizure disorder that until a week ago was controlled by medication. He and his family receive their routine health care from the mobile care van that visits their neighborhood each week. A pediatric nurse and pediatrician collaborate with the neurologist in the health center by providing Manny's health care and monitoring his developmental progress.

When Manny had a seizure last week, his phenytoin blood level was slightly lower than the therapeutic range. His parents report that they give Manny his medicine daily as prescribed. He might need a higher dosage of the same medication because he has grown, or maybe he needs a different medication. Because of the recent seizure, an electroencephalogram is ordered to identify any change in the electrical pattern of his brain. Other laboratory tests are also ordered, following the health center's clinical practice guideline for children with seizure disorders.

Over the past 2 years, Manny's family and the pediatric nurse have worked together to ensure that Manny is treated as a healthy child with a chronic condition. The nurse has helped his parents to obtain information about his condition, to understand the action of his medication, and to take appropriate action when he has a seizure. Think about the role of the nurse in working with children who have seizures. In how many different settings could you find nurses providing care to these children?

Key Terms

advance directives / 14
advocacy / 4
assent / 13
case management / 4
clinical practice guideline / 5
confidentiality / 14
continuity of care / 4
critical thinking / 5
emancipated minors / 13
ethics / 15
evidence-based practice / 5
family-centered care / 6
futility / 15
infant mortality / 6
informed consent / 13
mature minors / 13
moral dilemma / 15
morbidity / 8
quality improvement / 12
risk management / 11

Learning Outcomes

After reading this chapter, you will be able to do the following:

1. Describe the continuum of pediatric health care.
2. Compare the roles of nurses in child health care.
3. Analyze the current societal influences on pediatric health care and nursing practice.
4. Report the most common causes of child mortality and reasons for hospitalization by age group.
5. Contrast the policies for obtaining informed consent of minors to policies for adults.
6. Examine three unique pediatric legal and ethical issues in pediatric nursing practice.

■ PEDIATRIC HEALTH CARE OVERVIEW

Nurses provide care to healthy children, as well as to those with illnesses, injuries, and chronic conditions such as seizures, in a wide variety of settings. Nurses contribute to the health and welfare of children as they monitor their growth and development, and help them to adapt to and manage their health conditions. Fortunately, most children are healthy, experiencing only occasional short-term health problems, and nurses have the opportunity to help children and families to prevent disease and promote a healthy lifestyle. However, children with special health care needs require frequent contact with the health care system to achieve and maintain their optimal level of health.

Pediatric health care occurs along a continuum that reflects not only the various settings of care, but also the complexity and range of care needed by individual children and their families.

For example, all children need health promotion and health maintenance services, but some children will need care for chronic conditions, acute illnesses and injuries, and even end-of-life care. See Figure 1–1 ➤ for the model of pediatric health care upon which this text is based.

The range of health care settings where pediatric nurses work includes the following:

- The hospital, including pediatric wards, intensive care units, newborn nursery, emergency department, radiology, and specialty clinics
- Physician offices, clinics, and health care centers
- The child's home
- Rehabilitation centers and residential treatment centers
- Schools, childcare centers, and camps
- The community

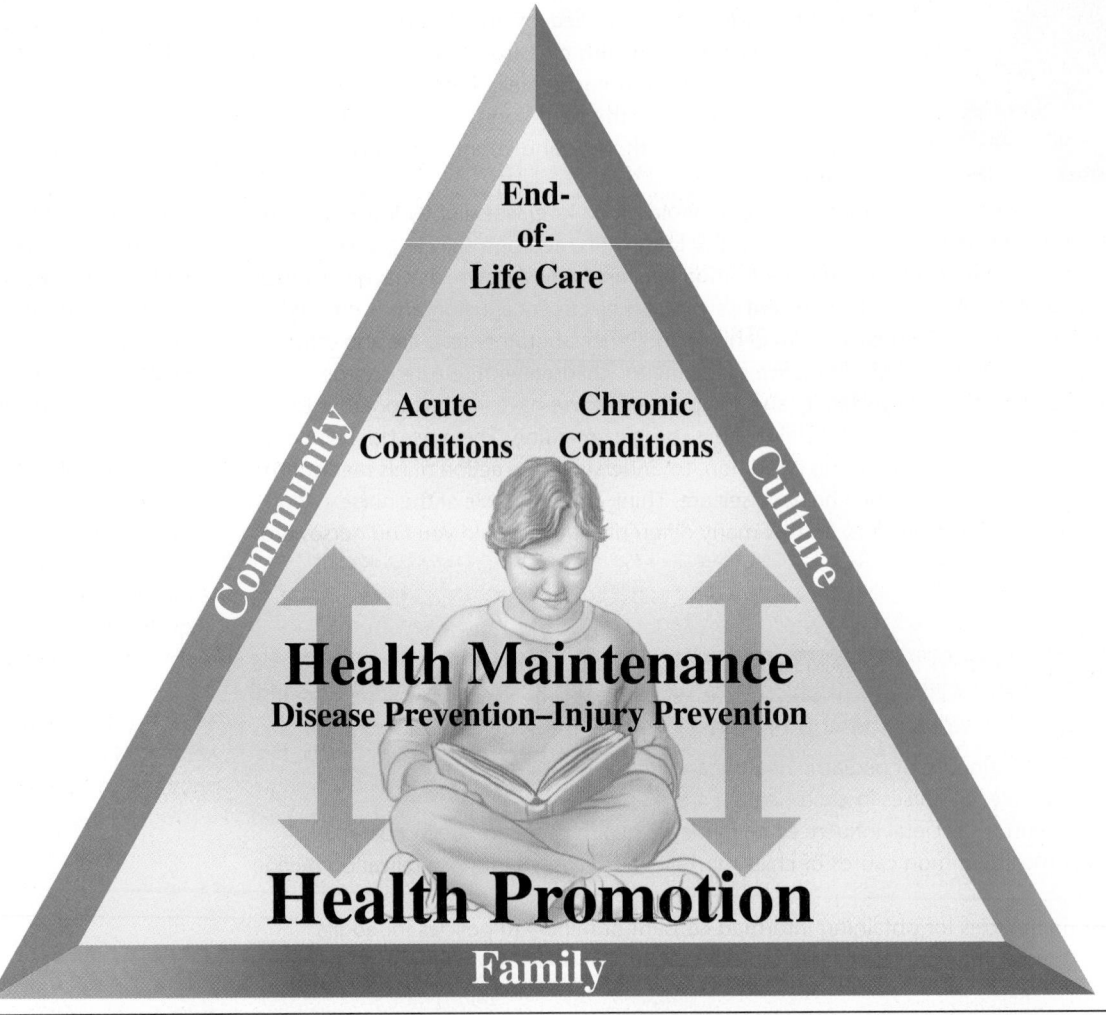

FIGURE 1–1 ➤ The Bindler-Ball Continuum of Pediatric Health Care for Children and Their Families The outer bars represent the family, cultural, and community influence on the care that the child receives, either through the services sought by the family or the services provided in the community. Cultural influences include the family's decision to seek health care and follow recommendations, as well as the health care provider's cultural competence in caring for a child and family.

The inner categories represent the different types of health care needed by children. All children need health promotion and health maintenance services, represented by the base of the triangle. Notice the wave and arrows representing the upward and downward movement between the levels of care as the child's condition changes.

Children may be healthy with episodic acute illnesses and injuries. Some children develop a chronic condition for which specialized health care is needed. A child's chronic condition may be well controlled, but acute episodes (such as with asthma) or other illnesses and injuries may occur. This child also needs health promotion and health maintenance services. A few children develop a life-threatening illness and ultimately need end-of-life care. A healthy child can also experience a catastrophic injury that causes death. The family then needs supportive end-of-life care.

Nurses play a significant role in the provision of health care for children. Their responsibilities vary in the different clinical settings as they collaborate with other health care providers, such as physicians, social workers, pharmacists, optometrists, psychologists, dentists, nutritionists, speech therapists, and physical and occupational therapists.

Assessment, nursing care interventions, and patient education are universal roles for nurses regardless of the setting in which they work. This chapter defines the various roles for the nursing care of children and reviews concepts important to pediatric nursing.

ROLE OF THE NURSE IN PEDIATRICS

Pediatric nursing, using a family-centered care approach, focuses on protecting children of newborn age through young adulthood from illness and injury; assisting them to attain optimal levels of health, regardless of health problems; alleviating suffering through the diagnosis and treatment of the child's response; and advocating for the care of children and their families (American Nurses Association, 2008). The nursing roles in caring for children and their families include direct care, patient education, advocacy, and case management.

Nurses who specialize in pediatrics apply foundational knowledge learned during their nursing education such as the nursing process, anatomy and physiology, physical assessment, health care condition recognition and management, and the full range of nursing skills. Pediatric nurses then add additional competencies related to the care of children and their families. The special knowledge and skills that nurses caring for children must acquire and apply are listed in Box 1–1.

Direct Nursing Care

The primary role of pediatric nurses is to provide direct nursing care to children and their families. The nursing process provides the framework for delivery of direct pediatric nursing care. The nurse assesses the child, identifies the health concerns, and lists the nursing diagnoses describing the responses of the child and family to those health concerns in the nursing care plan. The nurse then implements and evaluates nursing care. This care is designed to meet the physical and emotional needs of the child and family. It is tailored to the child's developmental stage, giving the child additional responsibility for self-care with increasing age. Planned care is offered in a sensitive manner, compatible with the child's and family's cultural beliefs in collaboration with the family, using family-centered care principles (see Chapter 2 ∞).

Nurses play an important role in minimizing the psychologic and physical distress experienced by children and their families. Providing support to children and their families is one component of direct nursing care. This often involves listening to the concerns of children and parents, being present during stressful or emotional experiences, and implementing strategies to help children and family members cope (see Chapter 2 ∞). Nurses can help families by suggesting ways to support their children in all health care settings, including the home.

The Society of Pediatric Nurses has identified these standards for the generalist pediatric nurse:

- An understanding of the unique anatomical, physiological, and developmental differences among neonates, infants, children, adolescents, and young adults in transition;
- The ability to care for children in the context of their families;
- A sensitivity to cultural issues, especially those related to how the family and health care providers tend to children's healthcare needs;
- The ability to communicate effectively with children, families, and other health care providers, and appropriate educational agency staff;
- The provision of safety assurance and injury prevention to children and their families;
- The ability to promote children's health in the context of their families;
- The assessment of the unique growth and development needs of children who have chronic conditions and their families;
- The provision for the exceptional needs of children with episodic injuries or illnesses;
- An understanding of the economic, social, and political influences outside the family that have an impact on children's health and development and family functioning.

Note: From Pediatric Nursing: Scope and standards of practice *(p. 17). Copyright © 2008 by American Nurses Association. Reprinted with permission. All rights reserved.*

Patient Education

The education of children and their families improves treatment results. In pediatric nursing, patient education may be challenging, because nurses work with children at various levels of understanding. Rather than giving simple facts, the goal of patient education is to help the child and family to make informed choices about health and healthy behaviors.

As patient educators, nurses help children adapt to the hospital setting and prepare them for procedures (Figure 1–2 ➤). Most hospitals encourage a parent to stay with the child and to provide much of the direct and supportive care. Nurses teach parents to watch for important signs and responses to therapies, to increase the child's comfort, and even to provide advanced care. Taking an active role prepares the parent to assume total responsibility for care after the child leaves the hospital.

Planning and preparation, as well as an understanding of the child's developmental level, are needed to effectively educate children and parents. An assessment of the child's and family's knowledge about the condition or health practices, their past experiences, and their attitudes and beliefs is a starting point for education. The nurse needs to think about strategies and resources available to help the child and family learn about the health condition. Education can be evaluated during future visits of children receiving ongoing health promotion and health maintenance care and of those with a chronic condition that requires home management.

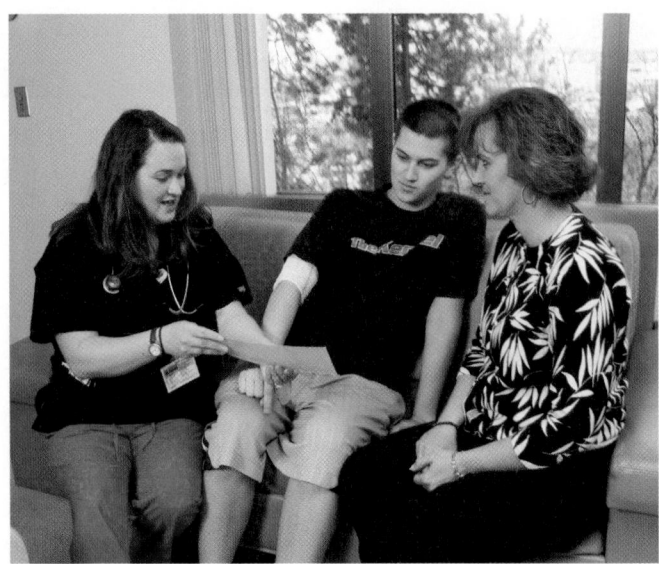

FIGURE 1–2 ➤ Explaining procedures can reduce the patient's and family's fears and anxieties about what to expect as well as teach procedures and proper home care.

Culture · Literacy and Communication

Many parents cannot read above a fifth-grade level. Some tips for developing patient education materials at an appropriate reading level include the following:

■ Use short familiar words with one or two syllables in short sentences.

■ Substitute simple language that defines a medical term rather than using the term.

■ Use graphics when possible.

■ Use active voice rather than passive voice.

■ Use "must" to express a requirement.

■ Divide the content into small sections and use headers.

■ Use lists and tables to simplify content.

Patient Advocacy

Advocacy—acting to safeguard and advance the interests of another—is directed at enabling the child and family to adjust to the changes in the child's health in their own way. To be an effective advocate, the nurse must be aware of the needs of the child and family, the family's resources, and the health care services available in the community. The nurse can then assist the family and the child to make informed choices about these services and to act in the child's best interests.

As advocates, nurses often serve on committees to ensure that the policies and resources of health care agencies meet the psychosocial needs of children and their families. The nurse must also protect the child and family by taking appropriate actions related to any incidents of incompetent, unethical, or illegal practices by any member of the health care team.

Case Management

What happens when a child has significant health problems? Can one nurse handle it all? When a child has a significant chronic health condition, health care professionals (physicians, nurses, social workers, physical and occupational therapists, and other specialists) often create an interdisciplinary plan to meet the child's medical, nursing, developmental, educational, and psychosocial needs. Because nurses spend time with the child and family while providing nursing care, they often know more than other health care professionals about the family's wishes and resources. As a member of the interdisciplinary team, the nurse can serve as the family's advocate to ensure that the care plan considers the family's wishes and contains appropriate services. A nurse may become the child's case manager, coordinating the implementation of the interdisciplinary care plan. Sometimes the parent or a social worker becomes the case manager.

Case management is a process of coordinating the delivery of health care services in a manner that focuses on both quality and cost outcomes. This is often a collaborative practice with other health care providers that promotes **continuity of care**, an interdisciplinary process of facilitating a patient's transition between and among settings based on changing needs and available resources. The nurse case manager has control over the use of health care resources that are considered appropriate for the patient's condition and links the child and family to these services. The goal is to help the child and family have the best health care outcome and decrease fragmentation of care, while controlling the cost of health care services. Case management may be used for care of the patient when hospitalized as well as for long-term care of chronic conditions.

Discharge planning is a form of case management. Good discharge planning promotes a smooth, rapid, and safe transition into the community and improves the results of treatment begun in the hospital. To be a discharge planner, the nurse needs to know about community medical resources, home care agencies qualified to care for children, educational interventions, and services reimbursed by the child's health plan or other financial resources.

Research

Research is conducted to determine effective methods for treating a child's health condition or providing care. Innovations in care are evaluated to determine if practice is improved. Research provides a scientific basis for nursing practice. This research is also used in developing evidence-based practice guidelines specific to the health care facility. Pediatric nurses are also responsible for keeping current with new pediatric research findings and identifying when changes in practice are needed.

As a clinical pediatric research nurse, it is important to safeguard the child while maintaining the integrity of the research study protocol (McCabe & Lawrence, 2007). The nurse in this role needs to understand the research process and have experience carrying out a protocol. Pediatric nurses can also help identify research questions, assist with the design of research studies, and collect data.

■ NURSING PROCESS IN PEDIATRIC CARE

Pediatric nurses use the nursing process to identify and solve problems and to plan patient care, the same process used for other patients. Consider how the five steps of the nursing process relate to children:

- *Assessment* involves collecting patient and family data and performing physical examinations in all health care settings. The nurse analyzes and synthesizes data to make a judgment about the patient's problems.
- *Nursing diagnoses* describe the health promotion and health patterns that nurses can identify and manage by developing a plan for specific nursing actions. The North American Nursing Diagnosis Association (NANDA) has established the standard language for these nursing diagnoses. Each nursing diagnosis has defining characteristics, related factors or risk factors, nursing intervention classifications (NIC), and nursing outcome classifications (NOC).
- *Nursing care plans* are based on goals that will improve the child's or family's healthy or dysfunctional health patterns. The nurse creates a nursing care plan for the child and family or customizes standard care plans for specific diagnoses that may be used in a hospital or home health agency. Standard care plans are customized based on data collected from the child's assessment and an evaluation of the child's response to care. The family (and the child, when old enough) and the nurse should agree with the care plan goals.
- *Implementation* is performing the interventions or specific action steps outlined in the nursing care plan.
- *Evaluation* is the use of specific objective and subjective measures (often called outcome measures or criteria) to measure the progress of the child and family in reaching the goals defined in the nursing care plan. As the child's condition improves and goals are attained, the nursing care plan is modified with new goals and nursing actions based on data from ongoing assessments.

Critical Thinking

Critical thinking—an individualized, creative thought or reasoning process—is used by nurses to solve problems associated with patient care. The critical thinking process involves identifying the specific problem or issue that needs to be addressed or the nursing goal to be achieved. The nurse then analyzes information from multiple sources (e.g., the child, family, health facility, community, experts, and published literature) to make judgments about appropriate actions for safe clinical practice (Mundy & Denham, 2008).

Evidence-Based Practice

Evidence-based practice (EBP) is a problem-solving approach that integrates the best research evidence with a health professional's clinical expertise and the patient's values or preferences. The use of EBP improves patient outcomes and can help reduce costs of health care (Melnyk, Fineout-Overholt, Hockenberry, et al., 2007). EBP is one strategy to keep nursing practice current and to promote positive outcomes for children and their families. It has also become an important strategy for health care institutions focusing on patient safety and quality of care.

The EBP process involves five steps (Long, Burkett, & McGee, 2009):

1. Ask and clearly describe the specific clinical question.
2. Collect the most relevant and best evidence from well-designed studies.
3. Critically review, synthesize, and analyze the evidence.
4. Integrate the evidence with your clinical experience and the patient's preferences and values, leading to a decision to maintain or change nursing practice.
5. Evaluate the nursing practice change resulting from the EBP process.

Teams of health care providers from multiple disciplines, including nurses, may collaborate on EBP clinical questions to develop a clinical practice guideline or clinical pathway. A **clinical practice guideline** (clinical pathway) is a comprehensive evidence-based interdisciplinary care plan developed to describe optimal care for a specific health condition. It describes the sequence and timing of effective interventions that should reduce costs and result in expected patient outcomes (Kurtin & Stucky, 2009). Clinical practice guidelines promote patient safety and uniformity in care so that patient outcomes and health professional performance can be measured. Many clinical practice guidelines are developed by federal agencies or national organizations. One example is the pediatric asthma guidelines developed by the National Asthma Education Program. See the companion website for a web link to this guideline.

■ SETTINGS FOR PEDIATRIC NURSING CARE

Pediatric nurses function in a variety of settings within the hospital. Acute care may be provided in the emergency department, observation or short-stay unit, postanesthesia unit, intensive care unit, general pediatric inpatient unit, and various outpatient clinics. In rehabilitation centers, nurses provide inpatient and ambulatory care to help restore children to an optimal state and plan for discharge management of chronic conditions. Pediatric nurses working with children and families on a general pediatric hospital unit promote health improvement in the following ways:

- Gathering data and assessing the health of children and their families
- Providing ordered medical therapies
- Providing nursing care in a manner that preserves as many of the child's and family's normal routines as possible while maintaining the family unit
- Working with the family and health care team to develop an individualized health care plan and a discharge plan, or to implement a clinical practice guideline

The hospital stay is part of a care continuum that allows children to complete therapy at home, at school, or in other community settings. Pediatric nurses assist families to transition from the acute hospital setting to the home or other facility, such as a rehabilitation center or long-term care facility. Managing the child's transition from acute care to another setting involves discharge planning that integrates interdisciplinary care plans and collaboration with a broad range of health care professionals. The nurse may assist the family of a child with significant health problems to prepare for the child's return home and to develop an emergency care plan in case the child has an unexpected health care crisis. See Chapter 11 ∞ for more information on caring for children in the hospital setting.

Pediatric nurses also work in several community health care settings such as physician offices, health centers, specialty care clinics, home health agencies, and schools. See Chapter 10 ∞ for more information about nursing care in community settings.

■ CONTEMPORARY CLIMATE FOR PEDIATRIC NURSING CARE

In 2007, more than 82.4 million children under the age of 20 years lived in the United States. They accounted for 27.3% of the population (U.S. Census Bureau, 2009). (See Figure 1–3 ➤ for a distribution of the population by age group.) The racial and ethnic diversity of children in the United States continues to increase and is currently estimated as follows (Federal Interagency Forum on Child and Family Statistics, 2009):

- White, non-Hispanic—56%
- Black, non-Hispanic—15%
- Hispanic—22%
- Asian—4%
- All other races—5%

Culturally Sensitive Care

The U.S. population has a varied mix of cultural groups, with ever-increasing diversity. More than 37% of all children less than 18 years of age are from families of minority populations (U.S. Census Bureau, 2009). By the year 2021, it is expected that the proportion of children who are of Hispanic origin will increase to one child in every four (Federal Interagency Forum on Child and Family Statistics, 2009). It is also important to recognize the diversity among the non-Hispanic White population as they

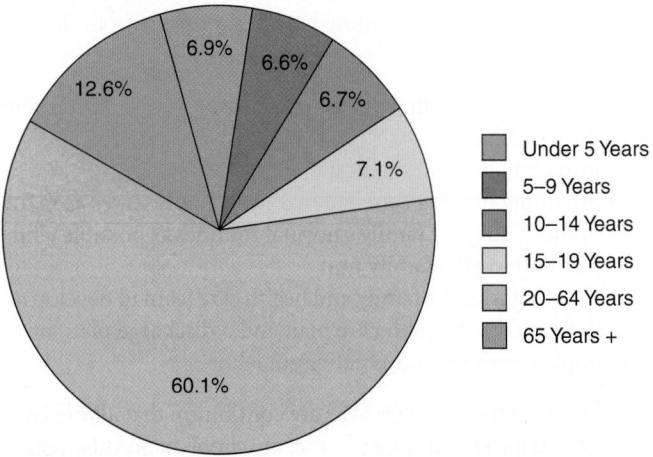

FIGURE 1–3 ➤ The population of children less than age 20 years was estimated in 2007 to account for 27.3% of the population in the United States.

Data from: U.S. Census Bureau. (2009). Population. Statistical Abstract of the United States. Retrieved from http://www.census.gov/prod/www/abs/stattab2006_2009.html

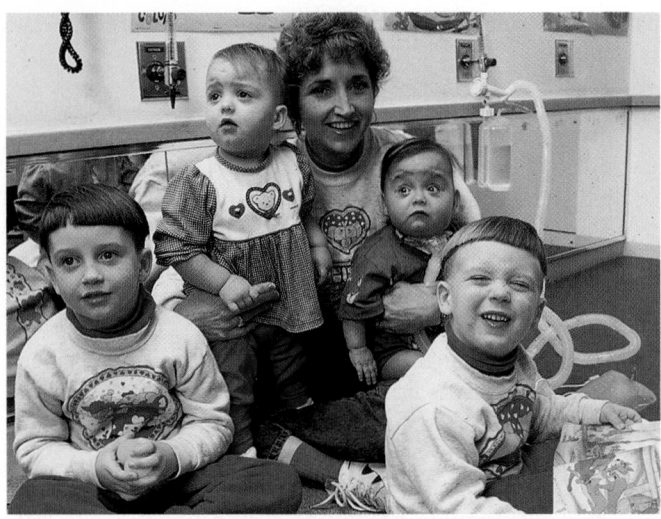

FIGURE 1–4 ➤ Many facilities now encourage family visitation for children with health problems that require long-term hospitalization. Extended family visits enable parents to learn about the child's care, and provide siblings with opportunities to interact with the hospitalized child.

represent many cultural groups, such as immigrants from former Soviet bloc countries. See Chapter 2 ∞ for more information on culture.

Family-Centered Care

Recognizing the family as the constant influence and support in a child's life is the foundation for developing a trusting relationship with families. The family is the principal caregiver and support for the child, and the family is important in helping the child recover from an illness or injury (Figure 1–4 ➤). The effort to address and meet the emotional, social, and developmental needs of children and families seeking health care in all settings is a concept known as **family-centered care**. Families are often considered partners in care, learning about children's conditions and participating in decisions regarding their care. Thus, families gain greater confidence and competence in caring for their children who have health care problems. The key elements of family-centered care are described in Chapter 2 ∞.

■ PEDIATRIC HEALTH STATISTICS

Mortality

Children have different health care problems than adults, and the problems may be related to stage of development or other factors. The **infant mortality** (death in infants less than 12 months of age) rate was 6.69 deaths per 1,000 live births in the United States in 2006. See Figure 1–5 ➤ for the leading causes of infant mortality in 2006 compared to 1996. The mortality rate for Black infants is more than twice the rate of Whites (Heron, Hoyert, Murphy, et al., 2009). The leading causes of infant mortality vary according to the age of the infant. For example, the leading causes of death in the neonatal period (birth to 28 days of age) are short gestation, low birth weight, and congenital malformations. The leading causes of mortality in the postneonatal period (between 1 and 12 months of age) are sudden infant

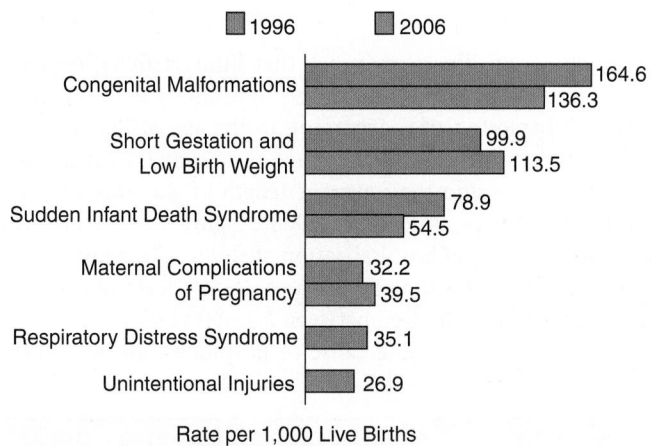

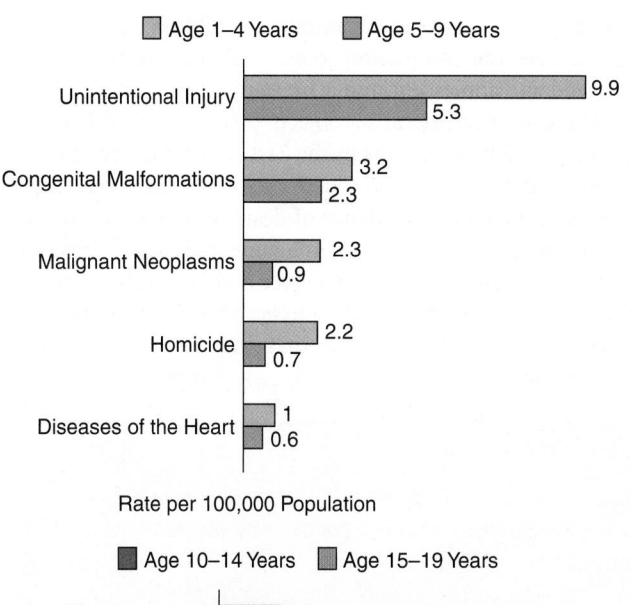

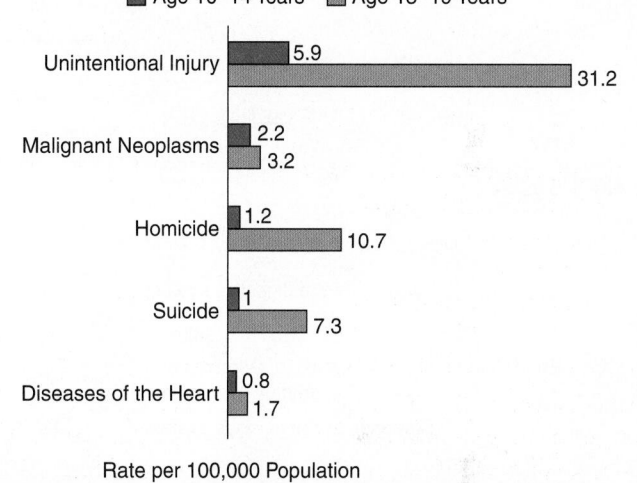

FIGURE 1–5 ➤ Comparison of the five leading causes of infant mortality by rate in 2006 and 1996. What could account for the dramatic reduction in the rate of sudden infant death syndrome over the 10 years? See Chapter 20 ∞ to find the answer.

Data from: Heron, M., Hoyert, D. L., Murphy, S. L., Xu, J., Kochanek, K. D., & Tejada-Vera, B. (2009). Deaths: Final data for 2006. National Vital Statistics Reports, 57(14), 1–135; MacDorman, M. F., & Atkinson, J. O. (1998). Infant mortality statistics from the 1996 period: linked birth/infant death data set. Monthly Vital Statistics Report, 46(12 Suppl), 20. Retrieved from http://www.cdc.gov/nchs/data/mvsr/supp/mv46_12s.pdf

death syndrome and congenital malformations (National Center for Health Statistics, 2009).

The most common cause of death for children between 1 and 19 years of age is unintentional injury. Congenital malformations, cancer, and diseases of the heart are the most common medical causes of death. Figure 1–6 ➤ shows the age-specific mortality rates for the five leading causes of death by age group.

Although unintentional injury is the leading cause of death, it is disturbing that intentional injury (homicide and suicide) is a major cause of death for our nation's children. The major causes of unintentional injury mortality in childhood include motor vehicle (passengers and pedestrians), other land transport, drowning, fires and burns, and suffocation. Table 1–1 illustrates the leading causes of injury deaths by age group. Many injury prevention programs have been implemented by state health departments, health care facilities, and national

FIGURE 1–6 ➤ Age-specific death rates per 100,000 children in the United States in 2006. A, Death rates for children between 1 and 9 years of age. B, Death rates for children between 10 and 19 years of age. The leading cause of death in children in all age groups was unintentional injury. Why do you think that is? Which type of injury has the highest rate of death? Drowning? Fires and burns? Motor vehicle crashes? See Table 1–1 for the answer.

Data from: Heron, M., Hoyert, D. L., Murphy, S. L., Xu, J., Kochanek, K. D., & Tejada-Vera, B. (2009). Deaths: Final data for 2006. National Vital Statistics Reports, 57(14), 1–135.

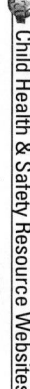

Child Health & Safety Resource Websites

TABLE 1–1 Five Leading Causes of Injury Death by Age Group, 2006

	Ranking				
Age Group	First	Second	Third	Fourth	Fifth
Under 1 year	Suffocation	Homicide, unspecified cause	Motor vehicle	Homicide, specified cause	Drowning
1 to 4 years	Motor vehicle	Drowning	Fire, burns	Homicide, unspecified cause	Suffocation
5 to 9 years	Motor vehicle	Drowning	Fire, burns	Homicide, firearm	Other land transport
10 to 14 years	Motor vehicle	Homicide, firearm	Suicide, suffocation	Drowning	Other land transport
15 to 19 years	Motor vehicle	Homicide, firearm	Poisoning	Suicide, firearm	Suicide, suffocation

Data from: National Center for Health Statistics. (2009). National Vital Statistics System. Retrieved August 17, 2009, from http://webappa.cdc.gov/sasweb/ncipc/leadcaus10.html
Shading indicates intentional injuries.

organizations to reduce the number of children who die unnecessarily. See the companion website for organizations focused on child and adolescent injury prevention.

The U.S. government set objectives to improve the health of children and young adults in the 21st century in the report entitled *Healthy People 2020.* These national health objectives focus on reducing the incidence of death and disability from the major causes of death shown in Figures 1–5 and 1–6, as well as Table 1–1. *Healthy People 2020* over-arching goals are listed in Box 1–2. Often federal funding in grants is linked to the development of programs aimed at reducing the number of deaths from these factors in specific high-risk groups.

Morbidity

Morbidity is an illness or injury that limits activity, requires medical attention or hospitalization, or results in a chronic condition. Morbidity varies according to the age of the child. In 2006, children under 15 years of age accounted for 7% of hospital discharges and their average length of stay was 4.8 days (DeFrances, Lucas, Buie, et al., 2008). Figure 1–7 ➤ compares the leading causes of hospitalization of children by age group in 1999 and 2006. Respiratory diseases are the leading cause of hospitalization in children between 1 and 9 years of age. Mental disorders are a leading cause of hospitalization in adoles-

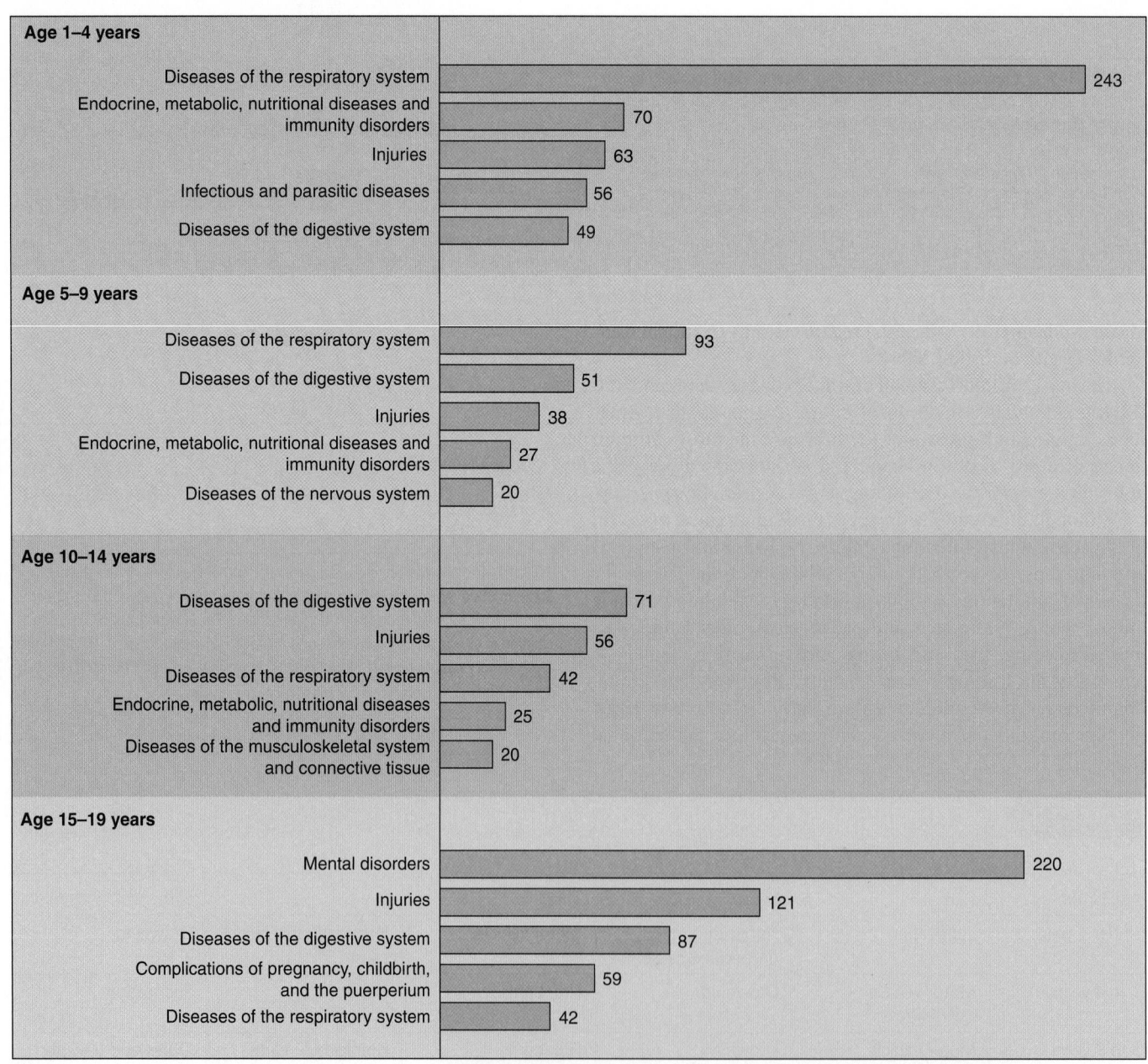

FIGURE 1–7 ➤ The leading causes of hospitalization in the United States in 2006 were much the same as those in 1999 in those 21 years of age and younger, but the number of hospital discharges (in 1,000s) changed for some causes. What do you think might account for the rise in hospital discharges for mental disorders? What do you think the current hospital discharge numbers are today?

Data from: National Center for Health Statistics. (2009). National hospital discharge survey. Unpublished data; National Center for Health Statistics. (1999). National hospital discharge survey. Unpublished data.

BOX
1–2

Healthy People 2020
Over-Arching Goals

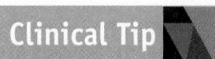

Goal 1: Attain high quality, longer lives free of disease, disability, injury, and premature death.

Goal 2: Achieve health equity, eliminate disparities, and improve the health of all groups.

Goal 3: Create social and physical environments that promote good health for all.

Goal 4: Promote quality of life, healthy development, and healthy behaviors across all life stages.

From: U.S. Department of Health and Human Services. (2010). Healthy People 2020. Retrieved from http://www.healthypeople.gov

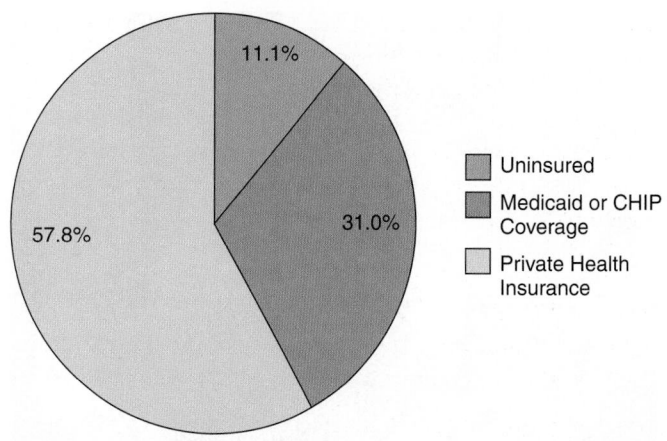

FIGURE 1–8 ➤ In the United States, how is health care of children paid for? These data from 2005 show that our taxes support 31% of the costs. What can you do to help? Something as simple as counseling parents about injury prevention and providing immunizations while a child is under care for other problems can prevent potential health problems. Part of good nursing care is supporting the well-being of the child in addition to caring for the presenting problem.

Data from: Rhoades, J. A. (2006). Health insurance status of children in America, 1996–2005: Estimates for the U.S. civilian noninstitutionalized population under age 18 (Statistical Brief No. 131). Rockville, MD: Agency for Healthcare Research and Quality. Retrieved from http://www.meps .ahrq.gov/mepsweb/data_files/publications/st131/stat131.pdf

cents between 15 and 21 years. Complications of pregnancy and childbirth are also among the leading causes of hospitalization in adolescents between 15 and 21 years of age (National Center for Health Statistics, 2009). What do you think could account for the increase in hospital discharges for mental disorders in adolescents from 15 to 21 years? See Chapter 6 ∞.

■ HEALTH CARE ISSUES

Health Care Financing

Not all children in the United States have access to health care. In 2005, 8.2 million children, or 11.1% of those below 18 years of age, had no health insurance. Approximately 28 million children are enrolled in Medicaid (Inglehart, 2007). At some point in 2008, 7.4 million children were enrolled in the Children's Health Insurance Program (Centers for Medicare and Medicaid Services, 2009c). Hispanic or Latino children were the group with the highest rate of no health insurance and the highest rate of public insurance (Rhoades, 2006). See Figure 1–8 ➤ for the distribution of children's health insurance status.

Clinical Tip

The federal poverty rate is used to determine eligibility for many health and welfare services. The rate is a sliding scale based on the number of persons in the family, and it is updated annually. For example, the poverty rate for a family of four in 2009 was $22,050, making the children eligible for Medicaid (Centers for Medicare and Medicaid Services, 2009a).

Law & Ethics *Children's Health Insurance Program*

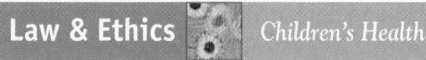

Congress created the Children's Health Insurance Program (CHIP) in 1997 and reauthorized it in 2009 to provide health insurance for children when their family's income is too high to qualify for Medicaid but inadequate to pay for private insurance coverage. States may enroll children in families at up to 300% of the federal poverty level ($66,105 for a family of four) (Centers for Medicare and Medicaid Services, 2009b).

Despite having health care coverage, more than 20% of children experience breaks in public and private health insurance coverage that jeopardize consistent care for chronic conditions and preventive health services (Cassedy, Fairbrother, & Newacheck, 2008). Low-income immigrant children are more likely to be uninsured than other children from low-income families, and public policy makes many ineligible for CHIP (Yu, Huang, & Kogan, 2008).

Despite the availability of CHIP, many eligible children are not enrolled. There may be various reasons why families have not enrolled their eligible children:

- They may believe they are not qualified.
- Some may have difficulty with the application procedure and required documentation.
- Others may lack the skills to negotiate the system to get coverage.

Nurses can play an important role in encouraging families to investigate their eligibility for the program. Obtain current guidelines in your state about eligibility requirements and coverage benefits. For example, some states require a monthly premium or co-pay for health care visits.

Health Care Technology

Research and technology have enabled many children with congenital anomalies and low birth weights to survive, with and without chronic conditions. Lifesaving technology has also created such burdens as high costs of health care and stresses on the functioning of the child's family. Technologic advances have resulted in the design of portable medical and infusion therapy equipment for home care. Many children are dependent upon or assisted by technology for physiologic functions. Some

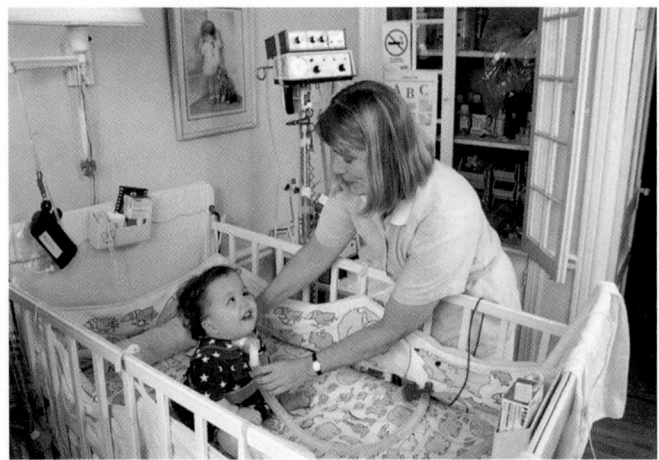

FIGURE 1–9 ➤ It is often desirable from a family and cost perspective to provide health care in the home, and technologic advances have made this possible. But is it less costly to provide care in the home for a child with technology assistance? Are the parents' out-of-pocket expenses for medical supplies considered? What about a parent's need to discontinue employment to care for the child? What is the emotional strain on families who care for their child 24 hours a day, 7 days a week? What support is needed by these families to continue providing this level of care at home? See Chapters 10 and 12 ∞ for answers.

families have regained control over their lives by creating intensive care units in their homes (Figure 1–9 ➤). For example, approximately 11% of children with special health care needs use medical equipment, such as ventilators, feeding tubes, intravenous or central lines and their associated pumps, cardiorespiratory monitors, peritoneal dialysis, and pacemakers (Health Resources and Services Administration, Maternal and Child Health Bureau, 2008). See Chapter 12 ∞. Generators are often used in case of power outages, and emergency transport and helicopter landing sites may be identified.

■ LEGAL CONCEPTS AND RESPONSIBILITIES

Regulation of Nursing Practice

Nurses are accountable for their professional actions, and each state regulates nursing practice with a nurse practice act. A state's nurse practice act defines the legal roles and responsibilities of nurses. As professionals, nurses set standards for education and practice that conform to state regulations. Standards for nursing education are modified as the science of nursing progresses. Nurses in professional organizations develop standards of nursing practice. The standards of pediatric nursing practice, jointly developed by the American Nurses Association, the Society of Pediatric Nurses, and the National Association of Pediatric Nurse Practitioners (2008), describe the expectations for patient care and professional performance. See Box 1–3.

Accountability and Risk Management

Accountability

The family entrusts the child's care to the health care team. Family members expect this team to provide good medical and

---

Professional Practice Standards for Pediatric Nursing Practice

Standards of Care for the Pediatric Nurse Include:

■ Collection of comprehensive data pertinent to the patient's health or the situation

■ Analysis of the assessment data to determine diagnoses or health-care issues

■ Identification of expected outcomes for a plan of care individualized to the child, family, and situation

■ Development of a plan of care that prescribes strategies and alternatives to attain expected outcomes

■ Implementation of the identified plan of care

■ Evaluation of progress toward attainment of outcomes.

Standards of Performance for the Pediatric Nurse Include:

■ Systematic enhancement of the quality and effectiveness of nursing care

■ Evaluation of own nursing practice in relation to professional practice standards and guidelines, relevant statutes, rules, and regulations

■ Attainment of knowledge and competency that reflects current nursing practice

■ Interaction with and contribution to the professional development of peers and colleagues

■ Collaboration with the child, family, and others in the conduct of nursing practice

■ Integration of ethical considerations and processes in all areas of practice

■ Integration of research findings into practice and, where appropriate, participation in the generation of new knowledge

■ Consideration of factors related to safety, effectiveness, cost and impact on practice in planning and delivering patient care

■ Provision of leadership in the professional practice setting and the profession

■ Advocacy for the pediatric client and family

From Pediatric Nursing: Scope and standards of practice. *Copyright © 2008 by American Nurses Association. Reprinted with permission. All rights reserved.*

---

nursing care and to avoid mistakes that cause harm. Nurses are personally accountable for adhering to the pediatric nursing standards of patient care and practice performance outlined in Box 1–3.

Patient Safety

Children are at risk for medical error as are all other patients; however, some aspects of pediatric care increase the risk for medical error. For example, most pediatric medications require dosage calculation to match the child's size. Children may be less able to tolerate a medication's adverse effects because of their developing renal, immune, and hepatic physiology (Sandlin, 2008). Many medical errors within hospitals are "systems errors," such as medication prescription and dispensing errors, rather than being the error of a single individual. (See Evidence-Based Practice: Medication Errors.) The Joint Commission has identified patient safety, including safe medication administration, as an important responsibility with

Evidence-Based Practice

Medication Errors

Problem

Medication error is a significant problem in pediatric nursing because children are at higher risk for serious adverse effects. What characteristics of medication errors involving nurses need more attention by hospital patient safety programs?

Evidence

A study, involving 279 nursing units in 146 acute care hospitals in the United States, investigated the antecedents of severe and nonsevere medication errors over a 6-month period. Medical errors were defined as the wrong dose, wrong patient, wrong time, wrong drug, wrong route, or omission. Severe errors were defined as those needing increased nursing observation or technical monitoring, laboratory or radiologic testing, medical intervention, or transfer to another unit. Nonsevere errors did not need increased attention or interventions. Antecedents investigated included work dynamics, percentage of RNs among nursing staff, communication with physicians, nursing expertise, education level, experience, medication-related support services, and patient characteristics. Study findings revealed that as the percentage of BSN-prepared nurses increased, severe medication errors decreased; nursing units with more experienced nurses reported more nonsevere medication errors; and medication support services were positively related to nonsevere errors. Results indicate that severe and nonsevere medication errors might have different antecedents, and thus different approaches may be needed to prevent or reduce severe and nonsevere medication errors (Chang & Mark, 2009). A study of 6 years of pediatric medication errors in the postanesthesia care unit (PACU) was conducted using data from the United States Pharmacopeia's medication error reporting program. Findings revealed that 20% of PACU pediatric medication errors were harmful, contrasted to 6% of PACU errors in the adult population. The five leading causes of pediatric medication error were performance deficit (nurse had the knowledge and skill but failed to use them), failure to follow a procedure or protocol, knowledge deficit, calculation errors, and lack of communication. Opioid products and acetaminophen were medications associated with a higher rate of error. As has been documented in other studies, calculation error was a much higher contributor to pediatric medication error in the PACU versus medication errors in other patients (Payne, Smith, Newkirk, et al., 2007).

Implications

Medication errors are a serious problem in pediatrics because multiple dosage calculations are needed, an error in the placement of a decimal results in a potential overdose or underdose, and the dosage form (multiple liquid concentrations) may cause confusion. Special system approaches are needed to prevent pediatric medication error, especially when nurses are in settings where children are not the only patient population, such as emergency departments and PACUs. Examples might include keeping pediatric and adult medications in separate locations or limiting the forms of a medication (e.g., one concentration of acetaminophen). However, nurses must use their knowledge and skill, as well as follow procedures and protocols, to improve the safety of medication administration to children.

Critical Thinking Application

Identify the medication error reduction policies and strategies that exist in each health setting used for clinical practice. What other medication safety practices do nurses use routinely in these settings? Identify any potential areas of improvement in medication safety practice in these settings.

---

requirements that must be met for accreditation (Joint Commission, 2009).

Reasons for the higher rate of medication error in children may include the following:

- Medication dosage calculations are more complex. Many adult medications are produced in concentrations that require dilution, or dosages must be calculated based upon the child's weight. Children often need suspensions or liquid preparations prepared by a pharmacist. The correct daily dose must be calculated based on the child's weight divided by doses per day, and the amount of liquid preparation for each individual dose must also be calculated. Errors in these mathematical calculations are common.
- A misplaced decimal when calculating a medication dosage can result in an overdose that can harm the child. Critically ill and injured children do not have the reserves to deal with an overdose of medication like a healthy older child or adult.
- Prescribed medications are sometimes not yet approved for use in children by the U.S. Food and Drug Administration, so the appropriate pediatric dose and adverse effects are unknown.
- Young children cannot communicate well regarding the adverse effects of medication.

Culture *Medication Errors*

Families with limited English proficiency are at higher risk for errors in medication administration because of communication problems. The family member may not correctly provide important health care information, such as a drug allergy, or the family member may not correctly interpret directions for giving the medication at home. Even when using a hospital interpreter, errors such as omitting instructions on dose, route, frequency, and duration of medications have potential clinical consequences (Flores & Ngui, 2006).

Clinical Judgment

Think about problems that could be associated with the administration of acetaminophen in the home setting due to the many liquid concentrations, different dosage tablets or capsules, and presence of the medication in combination with other drugs. What information should you discuss with parents when acetaminophen is recommended for use at home?

Risk Management

Health care facilities are challenged to promote optimal patient care and to reduce liability by implementing strategies to reduce medical errors in all child patients. **Risk management** is a process

System Strategies to Reduce Pediatric Medication Errors

- The child should be weighed in kilograms in all health care settings, and the weight in kilograms should be the standard weight used for prescriptions.

- Every prescription should include the child's weight and age, as well as the calculated dose and mg/kg dose. Unit dose dispensing systems should be used. The administration rate for all IV medications should be specified.

- A zero should not be used after a whole number (e.g., 5.0 could be misread as 50) because this can potentially result in a 10-fold dosage increase. A leading zero should be used before a decimal point when the dose is less than a whole unit.

- Have separate areas to prepare and store pediatric and adult medications, such as in the pharmacy or a busy emergency department.

- Capital letters can be used to help distinguish between medications with similar sounding names (e.g., DOBUTamine and DOPamine). Such medications with similar sounding names should not be stored close together.

- Prescriptions should be typed or written legibly with printed letters. A computerized physician order system enables the prescriber to check for drug interactions and allergies.

- Bar coding may be used for patient identification and medication administration.

Note: Data from: Sandlin, D. (2008). Pediatric medication error prevention. Journal of PeriAnesthesia Nursing, 23(4), 279–281; The Joint Commission. (2008). Sentinel event alert: Preventing pediatric medication errors. Retrieved from http://www.jointcommission.org/SentinelEvents/SentinelEventAlert/sea_39.htm

established by a health care institution to identify, evaluate, and reduce the risk of injury to patients, staff, and visitors, and thus reduce the institution's liability. This involves the study of causes of medical errors within a health care institution and implementing system changes to prevent future errors similar to those studied. Several strategies developed to reduce medication errors in children are listed in Box 1–4.

Quality improvement is the continuous study of systems, processes of care, and services and using that information to improve health care processes, services, and patient outcomes. Nurses participate in the development of institutional policies and standards of nursing practice. Hospitals and home health agencies encourage the development of diagnosis-specific nursing care plans and interdisciplinary clinical practice guidelines that serve as minimal institutional standards of care.

Clinical Tip

Policy and procedure manuals should be current and have evidence incorporated to provide guidance on nursing procedures, use of technology, patient education, and evaluation of interventions to promote patient safety. Nurses often participate as committee members in the development and revision of these policy and procedure manuals.

Law & Ethics  *The Patient's Record*

The patient's record is a legal document that is admissible evidence in court. Information in the patient's record must be legibly written in objective terms or appropriately recorded in the electronic medical record. When recording a patient's response to therapy, the nurse must include physiologic responses and exact quotes. The date, time, and nurse's signature and title are required.

During the development of institutional standards of care, indicators of effective care by pediatric nurses and other providers are identified. These indicators may measure either the process of care, the institution's systems, or the expected outcome of care for a specific patient condition. Patient records are regularly reviewed to identify deviations from the institutional standards or clinical practice guidelines. When deviations from expected processes and outcomes are identified, opportunities to improve the system or processes of care provision are explored with all care providers. Recommendations for the revision of institutional standards to further improve care by nurses and other health providers in the institution often result.

Documentation of nursing care is an essential part of risk management and quality improvement. If a patient record is subpoenaed, documented care is considered the only care provided, regardless of the quality of undocumented care. The patient assessment, the nursing care plan, and the child's responses to medical therapies and nursing care, including the regularly scheduled evaluation of the patient's progress toward nursing goals, must all be documented accurately and sequentially. Nurses must also report any untoward incidents that could inhibit the patient's recovery.

■ LEGAL AND ETHICAL ISSUES IN PEDIATRIC CARE

Marvin, a 15-year-old boy with acute nonlymphocytic leukemia, has come out of remission with an acute onset of fever, joint pain, and petechiae (Figure 1–10 ➤). A hematopoietic stem cell (bone marrow) transplant is one of his therapeutic options. Although Marvin has agreed to a transplant if a suitable donor is found, he does not want to be resuscitated and placed on life support equipment should he have a cardiac arrest. Marvin has experienced all the burdens of therapy up to this point. He has talked extensively with the hospital chaplain and social worker and feels comfortable with his decision. His parents want an all-out effort to sustain his life until a donor is located.

Marvin's case illustrates the legal and ethical dilemmas in caring for children, especially since he has the ability to understand and make reasonable decisions. At what age can children make an informed decision about whether to accept or refuse treatment? What happens when the parents and child have conflicting opinions about treatment? How are ethical decisions resolved?

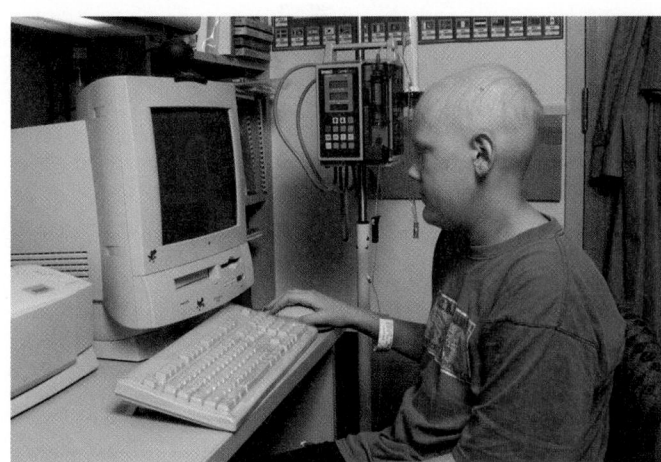

FIGURE 1–10 ➤ Marvin, a 15-year-old boy with acute nonlymphocytic leukemia, has definite opinions about his treatment, but his parents disagree. At what age can children make an informed decision about whether to accept or refuse treatment?

Informed Consent

Informed consent is a formal authorization by the child's parent or guardian allowing an invasive procedure to be performed or for participation in research. The physician is legally responsible for obtaining informed consent. In the case of research, the investigative researcher may formally designate a person to obtain informed consent. The nurse should verify that informed consent has been obtained prior to any procedure or research participation, alert physicians to the need for informed consent, serve as a witness for informed consent, and respond to questions asked by parents and children.

Consent must be given voluntarily and prior to the procedure or research. Parents, as the legal custodians of minor children, are customarily requested to give informed consent on behalf of a child. Both children and parents must understand that they have the right to refuse treatment at any time.

When parents are divorced and have joint custody, in most cases either may give informed consent. When parents are divorced and one parent has custody, some states limit the parental rights to give informed consent to the parent with custody. Obtain information about your state law regarding custody and who can provide informed consent for health care procedures and treatments.

Many children live in homes with a parent and other adult (stepparent, cohabiting unmarried adult, or grandparent) who

 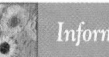
 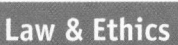
does not have legal authority to sign consent. Proxy consent can be granted in writing by the parent to another adult so that children can obtain health care when needed. In an emergency, treatment to preserve life or limb does not require consent if it cannot be immediately obtained (Emanuel, 2007).

Child Participation in Health Care Decisions

Children are considered to have the cognitive capacity to make medical decisions when they can understand that a decision must be made, they are able to receive and process information about the decision to be made, and they are able to state an opinion using the presented information (Van Norman, 2008). Children under 18 or 21 years of age (the age of majority), depending on state law, are considered minor children and need their parents' consent for therapy. Adolescents can legally give informed consent in the following special circumstances:

- **Emancipated minors** (economically self-supporting adolescents under 18 years of age, no longer living at home and not subject to parental control), including minor parents of a child patient, can legally give informed consent.
- **Mature minors** (adolescents between 14 and 18 years able to understand treatment risks) may give independent consent to receive or refuse treatment for limited conditions, such as testing and treating sexually transmitted infections, family planning, drug and alcohol abuse, blood donation, and mental health care (Levetown & Committee on Bioethics, 2008).

Make an effort to more actively involve a child in treatment decisions as reasoning skills develop. **Assent** is the voluntary agreement to accept treatment or to participate in a research project. To give assent the child needs a basic understanding of what will be done and what is required for participation. The child must also know that he or she can say no (dissent). Assess the child's developmental level to determine how much of a role the child should have in the decision-making process. Parents may prefer that their child be involved in decision making (Coyne, 2006). Adolescents may seek joint decision making with parents (Miller & Nelson, 2006). Their parents, however, make final decisions regarding the treatment or research participation. The child's dissent to participate in research should be respected.

Child's Rights versus Parents' Rights

Parents or guardians have absolute authority to make choices about their child's health care except in the following cases:

- When the child and parents do not agree on major treatment options
- When the parents' choice of treatment does not permit life-saving treatment for the child
- When there is a potential conflict of interest between the child and parents, such as with suspected child abuse or neglect

In cases when the child and parents do not agree on major treatment options, negotiation and compromise may be tried as a first step to avoid destruction of the family relationships. Medical consultation may be sought to identify other treatment options that might be acceptable to both the child and parents. An ethics committee usually becomes involved to help resolve the issue. In some cases, the court may be requested to appoint a proxy decision maker for the child or to determine that the child is capable of making a major treatment decision.

Confidentiality

The Health Insurance Portability and Accountability Act (HIPAA), P.L. 104-191, was enacted by Congress in 1996. One goal of the law is to protect the privacy of citizens by establishing standards for the management of confidential electronic medical information. Health care organizations have developed policies to prevent the inappropriate disclosure of protected health information. Patients have the right to determine who can have access to their health information. Violating confidentiality guidelines puts the nurse at risk for liability and legal action (U.S. Department of Health and Human Services, 2009).

Confidentiality is an agreement between a patient and a provider that information discussed during the health care encounter will not be shared without the patient's permission. Adolescents often do not want their parents informed about sensitive conditions. Their concerns about confidentiality influence if and when they seek health care (Campbell, 2006). When

Culture · *Religious Beliefs*

Jehovah's Witnesses oppose transfusions of blood products for themselves and their children because they believe transfusions are equivalent to the oral intake of blood, which is morally and spiritually wrong according to their interpretation of the Bible (Leviticus 17:13–14). A Jehovah's Witness who receives a transfusion believes he or she has committed a sin and may have forfeited everlasting life. Most health care facilities have policies to address the care of these children. Every effort is made to avoid the use of blood products with alternative therapies, except when a blood product will be lifesaving. Then a judicial order is sought.

Families Want to Know
Adolescents and Confidentiality

Adolescents need a safe and confidential environment to discuss health care issues so they will seek health care when needed. Ways to promote confidentiality include the following actions:

- Enable adolescents and parents to talk separately to the health care provider about their concerns.
- Ensure privacy when collecting an adolescent's medical history or discussing sensitive issues. Create a comfortable atmosphere and environment to encourage adolescents to discuss concerns about their health.
- Display and offer educational materials on confidentiality to adolescents and parents.
- Discuss how confidentiality is protected between health professionals and the adolescent, as well as the parents, at the beginning of the health care visit. Discuss situations in which you are limited in providing confidentiality.
- Obtain the phone number or other contact information to enable health professionals to contact the adolescent.
- Make sure clinic literature is small enough to fit discreetly into a purse or wallet.

the child is an emancipated or mature minor, many states permit health care providers to provide contraception, treatment for sexually transmitted infections including HIV, pregnancy and prenatal care, as well as mental health and substance abuse care without informing the child's parents (Someshwar & Nield, 2009). State laws vary, so obtain information about your state's law regarding confidentiality for emancipated minors. If the state law does not require the consent of the parent for the listed conditions, the consenting minor controls the health care decisions, as well as the parent's access to the health information related to that care. However, the issue of minors giving consent is complicated because the parents are responsible for the financial costs of the health care services. In some cases parents may get indirect information from health insurance bills. See Families Want to Know for ways to promote confidentiality.

Patient Self-Determination Act

The federal Patient Self-Determination Act directs health care institutions to inform hospitalized patients about their rights, which include making **advance directives** (writing a living will or authorizing a durable power of attorney for health care decisions on the patient's behalf). An adolescent with a serious or life-limiting condition, such as Marvin on page 12, has a strong and legitimate interest in expressing an opinion about aggressive therapy. The adolescent and parents should be encouraged to talk and reach a joint therapy decision. If the parents and adolescent are unable to agree, the legal issues become complex. Adolescent decisions to forgo life-prolonging treatment have been upheld in some courts of law (Levetown & Committee on Bioethics, 2008).

Do-not-attempt-resuscitation (or allow natural death) orders have become more common for children with terminal illnesses in which no further aggressive treatments are desired. To ensure that no resuscitation measures are initiated by any emergency care provider when the child has a life-threatening event, state health policies must be developed (Berkowitz & Morrison, 2007). See Chapter 13 ∞ for issues related to palliative and end-of-life care.

Ethical Issues

Ethics is the philosophic study of morality, and the analysis of moral problems and moral judgments. It is an inquiry into the justification of particular actions. Ethical issues may arise from a **moral dilemma**, a conflict involving individual beliefs, social values, and ethical principles. Each side of the conflict may possibly support different courses of action (e.g., performing or refraining from performing a therapy). Ethics has become a prominent discipline because of significant developments in medical care and research.

Emotions play a significant role in the development of ethical dilemmas. Parents want to protect the child, and they have their vision of what is good for the child. Health care professionals have different values than families because of their culture and life experiences. Value differences may also exist between members of the health care team caring for the child. Regardless, all health professionals want the child to benefit from care provided.

Nurses may face ethical dilemmas when providing pediatric care. They witness parents struggling to decide among treatment options. Pediatric nurses have a responsibility to become knowledgeable about the moral and legal rights of their patients and families and to protect and support those rights. Work with parents to form a therapeutic alliance, and attempt to prevent conflicts when the values of the family and health professionals do not match. Find out what is important to the parents in the care of their child. They may be able to describe what they wish to avoid having happen to their child, and this could become a starting point for discussion about the child's care with health professionals.

Clinical Tip

No matter what decision parents make about their child's care, they need to be reassured that they are trying to do what they think is best for their child.

Health care facilities have an ethics committee to resolve conflicts about treatment decisions between health professionals and the child and family, or to resolve a dispute between health professionals about the care to provide a child. The ethics committee resolves the conflict or dispute by performing an individual case consultation. A health care provider or the family can request a consultation.

Withholding or Withdrawing Medical Treatment

Infant John, at 5 days of age, has a birth weight of 1200 grams, acute respiratory distress, and a severe intraventricular hemorrhage. See Figure 1–11 ➤. His physicians are seeking his parents' consent for surgical placement of a ventriculoperitoneal shunt. Regardless of intensive medical care and planned surgical intervention, the infant is expected to have a severe disability. The in-

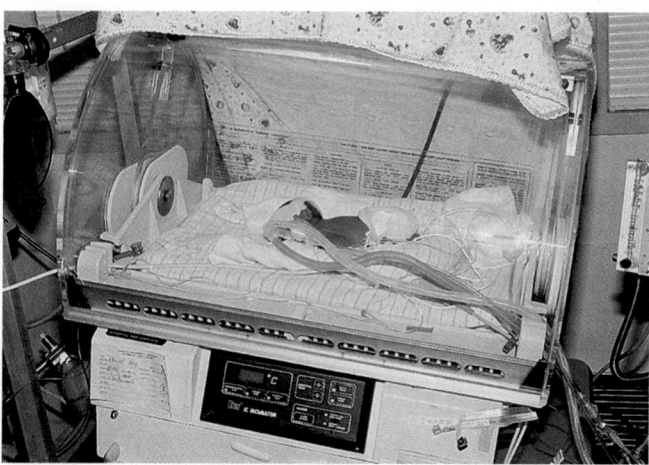

FIGURE 1–11 ➤ Due to technological advances that sustain life, parents must sometimes face difficult decisions. If an infant is certain to have severe disabilities, at what point should they decide to withhold or withdraw treatment?
Courtesy of Carol Harrigan, RNC, MSN, NNP.

fant's condition is critical, and it is not certain how well he will respond to surgery. The parents, after much consideration and discussions with their family and pastor, have requested that comfort measures only be provided. They want life-sustaining treatment to be withheld, because they believe the additional procedures will cause excessive suffering for the infant, especially when the outcome is uncertain.

The Child Abuse and Treatment Act of 1984, also known as the Baby Doe Regulations, defines withholding of medically indicated treatment as child abuse, except when care is futile (Curtin, 2008). This act was enacted to protect the rights of newborns with severe defects. **Futility** is a situation in which treatments do not provide a clear clinical benefit. Physicians are not obligated to offer interventions that cause extreme pain and suffering when there is no or limited potential benefit.

Parents are participants in the decisions made about care for infants with severe disabilities, and they are entitled to full information about the risks and benefits of a procedure as well as the child's long-term prognosis. Factors important to parents in making their decision include clear information on the seriousness of the child's condition and prognosis, the child's potential quality of life, the degree of pain and suffering, a trusting relationship with the physician, and physician recommendations (Kendall & Guo, 2008; Racine & Shevell, 2009). Conflict may arise when parents choose to withhold therapy or request aggressive therapy when the health care providers' recommendations differ. An ethical consultation may be needed to resolve conflicts.

Genetic Testing of Children

With advances in genetics research, it is now possible to conduct genetic testing of infants for the presence of carrier status. It is also possible to conduct presymptomatic testing for a specific condition, such as Huntington disease or Duchenne muscular dystrophy, or the predisposition to develop a condition, such as breast cancer or colon cancer (Twomey, Bove, & Cassidy, 2008). See Chapter 3 ∞ for additional information about ethical issues associated with genetic testing.

Organ Transplantation Issues

The death of a child can benefit several other children through organ transplantation, and organ transplantation has become an accepted therapeutic option for some life-threatening conditions. The limited supply of organs has created numerous ethical issues. Which patients on the waiting list should receive the organs available? Should a patient with multiple congenital anomalies, disabilities, or abnormal chromosomes be eligible for a transplant? Should families be permitted to pay donor families for organs? Should the family's ability to pay for an organ transplant give a child higher priority for an organ? Should a patient receive a second organ transplant, replacing an organ deteriorating because of rejection? Should parents conceive another child hoping that the new baby is a potential stem cell donor for a child with an illness? If so, what pressures does this place on both children as they grow older? Each institution performing organ transplants develops guidelines for ethical decision making regarding these questions.

Partnering with Families

The topics discussed in this chapter reflect the current challenges children and their families face in the health care system—access to health care, specific disease and injury risks, and ethical and legal concerns. A nurse in collaboration with parents and children is essential every step of the way:

- Obtaining informed consent and assent
- Respecting that the parent is the expert with regard to the child's care
- Acknowledging and supporting cultural values in the provision of care
- Preparing parents to assume ongoing complex health care responsibilities for their child

Developing relationships with children and families is challenging, exciting, and ultimately gratifying for nurses who choose to specialize in pediatrics.

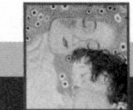

Chapter Highlights

- Roles of nurses in caring for children include direct patient care, patient education, patient advocacy, case management, and research.
- Nurses care for children in many different settings: emergency department, radiology, inpatient units, critical care units, postanesthesia units, outpatient clinics, schools, childcare centers, physician offices, community health centers, rehabilitation centers, and the home.
- Family-centered care is a method designed to meet the emotional, social, and developmental needs of children and families needing health care.
- Nurses must identify culturally relevant facts about their patients to provide appropriate and competent care to an increasingly diverse population.
- Unintentional injury is the leading cause of death for children between 1 and 19 years of age.
- One national effort to decrease the number of children who do not have health insurance coverage is the Children's Health Insurance Program (CHIP).
- Documentation of nursing care is essential for risk management and quality improvement. Be sure to include the patient assessment, the nursing care plan, the child's responses to medical therapies and nursing care, and a regular evaluation of the child's progress in meeting nursing goals.

- Informed consent is the formal preauthorization for an invasive procedure or participation in research. Parents typically give informed consent for children under 18 years of age unless the child is an emancipated minor, a self-supporting adolescent not subject to parental control.
- Children should be actively involved in decisions about their care as their decision-making abilities develop. Even though they cannot provide informed consent, children should receive information about a research project and be asked their opinion about participation.
- Because adolescents fear disclosure of confidential information, they may avoid seeking health care. It is important to tell adolescents when confidentiality cannot be maintained, such as when a reportable disease must be reported to a public health agency.
- Adolescents with a potentially life-limiting health condition should be encouraged to talk with their parents and to make joint decisions about future care.
- A formalized ethical decision-making process may assist health care providers and families in making important decisions about withholding, withdrawing, or limiting a child's therapy.

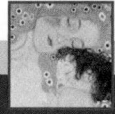

Clinical Reasoning in Action

Recall 3-year-old Manny, at the beginning of the chapter, who has a seizure disorder. He receives his care in a mobile van sent to his community by the local children's hospital. Manny has a regular source of care because his family income qualifies him for the state's Child Health Insurance Program (CHIP).

1. Explain the standards of pediatric nursing care as they relate to caring for Manny and his family.
2. Identify at least four different settings in which a child with a seizure disorder could receive health care.

3. List three specific injury prevention messages for a child of Manny's age that should be provided to Manny's parents to reduce his risk for morbidity and mortality.
4. List specific steps that should be used in the health care setting to ensure that an error is avoided when prescribing Manny's seizure medication.

See Pearson Nursing Student Resources for possible responses.

Pearson Nursing Student Resources

Find additional review materials at
nursing.pearsonhighered.com
Prepare for success with NCLEX®-style practice questions, interactive assignments and activities, web links, animations and videos, and more!

References

American Nurses Association, Society of Pediatric Nurses, & National Association of Pediatric Nurse Practitioners. (2008). *Pediatric nursing: Scope and standards of practice.* Silver Spring, MD: NursesBooks.org

Berkowitz, I., & Morrison, W. (2007). Do not attempt resuscitation orders in pediatrics. *Pediatric Clinics of North America, 54,* 757–771.

Campbell, A. T. (2006). Consent, competence, and confidentiality related to psychiatric conditions in adolescent medicine practice. *Adolescent Medicine Clinics, 17,* 25–47.

Cassedy, A., Fairbrother, G., & Newacheck, P. (2008). The impact of insurance instability on children's access, utilization, and satisfaction with health care. *Ambulatory Pediatrics, 8*(5), 321–328.

Centers for Medicare and Medicaid Services. (2009a). *2009 poverty level guidelines.* Retrieved from http://www.cms.hhs.gov/MedicaidEligibility/Downloads/POV09Combo.pdf

Centers for Medicare and Medicaid Services. (2009b). *Child Health Insurance Program Reauthorization Act of 2009.* Retrieved from http://www.cms.hhs.gov/CHIPRA/

Centers for Medicare and Medicaid Services. (2009c). *National CHIP Policy.* Retrieved from http://www.cms.hhs.gov/NationalCHIPPolicy/

Chang, Y., & Mark, B. A. (2009). Antecedents of severe and nonsevere medication errors. *Journal of Nursing Scholarship, 41*(1), 70–78.

Coyne, I. (2006). Consultation with children in hospital: Children, parents' and nurses' perspectives. *Journal of Clinical Nursing, 15*(1), 61–71.

Curtin, L. (2008). The Babies Doe: Finding middle ground. *American Nurse Today, 3*(1), 7–10.

DeFrances, C. J., Lucas, C. A., Buie, V. C., & Golosinskiy, A. (2008). *2006 National Hospital Discharge Survey* (National Health Statistics Report No. 5). Hyattsville, MD: National Center for Health Statistics. Retrieved from http://www.cdc.gov/nchs/data/nhsr/nhsr005.pdf

Emanuel, E. J. (2007). Bioethics in the practice of medicine. In L. Goldman & D. Ausiello (Eds.), *Cecil medicine* (23rd ed.). Philadelphia: Saunders Elsevier.

Federal Interagency Forum on Child and Family Statistics. (2009). *America's children: Key national indicators of well-being 2009.* Retrieved from http://www.childstats.gov/americaschildren/index.asp

Flores, G., & Ngui, E. (2006). Racial/ethnic disparities and patient safety. *Pediatric Clinics of North America, 53,* 1197–1215.

Health Resources and Services Administration, Maternal and Child Health Bureau. (2008). *The national survey of children with special healthcare needs chartbook 2005–2006.* Retrieved from http://mchb.hrsa.gov/cshcn05

Heron, M., Hoyert, D. L., Murphy, S. L., Xu, J., Kochanek, K. D., & Tejada-Vera, B. (2009).

Deaths: Final data for 2006. *National Vital Statistics Reports, 57*(14), 1–135.

Inglehart, J. K. (2007). Insuring all children—the new political imperative. *New England Journal of Medicine, 357*(1), 70–76.

Joint Commission. (2008). *Sentinel event alert: Preventing pediatric medication errors.* Retrieved from http://www.jointcommission.org/SentinelEvents/SentinelEventAlert/sea_39.htm

Joint Commission. (2009). *Hospital national patient safety goals.* Retrieved from http://www.jointcommission.org/NR/rdonlyres/31666E86-E7F4-423E-9BE8-F05BD1CB0AA8/0/HAP_NPSG.pdf

Kendall, A., & Guo, W. (2008). Evidence-based neonatal bereavement care. *Newborn & Infant Nursing Reviews, 8*(3), 131–135.

Knox, C. A., & Burkhart, P. V. (2007). Issues related to children participating in clinical research. *Journal of Pediatric Nursing, 22*(4), 310–318.

Kurtin, P., & Stucky, E. (2009). Standardize to excellence: Improving the quality and safety of care with clinical pathways. *Pediatric Clinics of North America, 56,* 893–904.

Levetown, M., & Committee on Bioethics. (2008). Communicating with children and families: From everyday interactions to skill in conveying distressing information. *Pediatrics, 121*(5), 21441–21442.

Long, L. E., Burkett, K., & McGee, S. (2009). Promotion of safe outcomes: Incorporating evidence into policies and procedures. *Nursing Clinics of North America, 44,* 57–70.

MacDorman, M. F., & Atkinson, J. O. (1998). Infant mortality statistics from the 1996 period: linked birth/infant death data set. *Monthly Vital Statistics Report, 46*(12 Suppl), 20. Retrieved from http://www.cdc.gov/nchs/data/mvsr/supp/mv46_12s.pdf

McCabe, M., & Lawrence, C. A. C. (2007). The clinical research nurse. *American Journal of Nursing, 107*(9), 13.

Melnyk, B. M., Fineout-Overholt, E., Hockenberry, M., Huth, M., Jamerson, P., Latta, L., et al. (2007). Improving healthcare and outcomes for high-risk children and teens: Formation of the National Consortium for Pediatric and Adolescent Evidence-Based Practice. *Pediatric Nursing, 33*(6), 525–529.

Miller, V. A., & Nelson, R. M. (2006). A developmental approach to child assent for nontherapeutic research. *Journal of Pediatrics, 149,* S25–S30.

Mundy, K., & Denham, S. (2008). Nurse educators—still challenged by critical thinking. *Teaching and Learning in Nursing, 3,* 94–99.

National Center for Health Statistics. (2009). *Health United States, 2008 with chartbook* (pp. 48–50). Hyattstown, MD: Author. Retrieved from http://www.cdc.gov/nchs/data/hus/hus08.pdf

Payne, C. H., Smith, C. R., Newkirk, L. E., & Hicks, R. W. (2007). Pediatric medication errors in the postanesthesia care unit: Analysis of MEDMARX data. *AORN Journal, 85*(4), 731–740.

Racine, E., & Shevell, M. I. (2009). Ethics in neonatal neurology: When is enough, enough? *Pediatric Neurology, 40*(3), 147–155.

Rhoades, J. A. (2006). *Health insurance status of children in America, 1996–2005: Estimates for the U.S. civilian noninstitutionalized population under age 18* (Statistical Brief No. 131). Rockville, MD: Agency for Healthcare Research and Quality. Retrieved from http://www.meps.ahrq.gov/mepsweb/data_files/publications/st131/stat131.pdf

Sandlin, D. (2008). Pediatric medication error prevention. *Journal of PeriAnesthesia Nursing, 23*(4), 279–281.

Someshwar, J., & Nield, L. S. (2009). Adolescent confidentiality: Where are the boundaries? *Consultant for Pediatricians, 8*(5), 182–183.

Twomey, J. G., Bove, C., & Cassidy, D. (2008). Presymptomatic genetic testing in children for neurofibromatosis 2. *Journal of Pediatric Nursing, 23*(3), 183–194.

U.S. Census Bureau. (2009). Population. *Statistical Abstract of the United States.* Retrieved from http://www.census.gov/prod/www/abs/stattab2006_2009.html

U.S. Department of Health and Human Services. (2010). *Healthy People 2020.* Retrieved from http://www.healthypeople.gov

U.S. Department of Health and Human Services. (2009). *Health information privacy.* Retrieved from http://www.hhs.gov/ocr/privacy/

Van Norman, G. A. (2008). Ethical issues in informed consent. *Perioperative Nursing Clinics, 3,* 213–221.

Yu, S. M., Huang, Z. J., & Kogan, M. D. (2008). State-level health care access and use among children in US immigrant families. *American Journal of Public Health, 98*(11), 1996–2003.

Family-Centered Care and Cultural Considerations

chapter 2

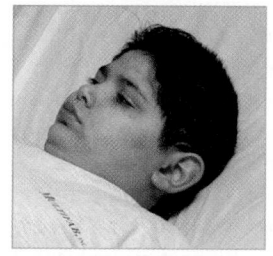

Casey, a 16-year-old, is recuperating from injuries sustained in a motor vehicle crash in which he was the passenger. He was not wearing a seatbelt and experienced a brain injury after striking the windshield. His cognitive and motor functions are impaired. Following a 7-day acute care hospital stay, he was moved to an inpatient rehabilitation hospital where he has been for the past 5 days. He is much more responsive to stimuli and to family members 12 days after his injury. Physical therapy is provided twice a day to promote range of motion and muscle tone and to prevent contractures. Plans are being made to discharge him home with outpatient rehabilitation care within the next 5 days. A case manager will be assigned to coordinate his health care services.

Casey lives with his mother, two half-brothers (10 and 6 years old), and stepfather. Both his mother and stepfather are employed full time and are trying to determine how to manage care for Casey once he returns home. Casey's grandparents live nearby and may provide some support to the family. Because Spanish is the language spoken primarily by the family, teaching materials are provided in both Spanish and English.

What family supports will Casey need as he continues his rehabilitation from the brain injury? What family and cultural assessment information is needed to effectively plan nursing care for this adolescent and his family? Does this family have strengths and coping strategies that will help them adapt to Casey's disability?

Key Terms

adoption / 32
acculturation / 39
alternative therapy / 44
assimilation / 39
complementary therapy / 44
coping / 35
culture / 38
discipline / 28
ecomap / 37
ethnicity / 39
faith-based belief / 42
family / 20
family-centered care / 20
family strengths / 36
foster care / 31
genogram / 37
joint custody / 24
legal guardianship / 32
limit setting / 26
parenting / 26
punishment / 28
race / 39
religion / 42
resilience / 36
spirituality / 42
stereotyping / 39

Learning Outcomes

After reading this chapter, you will be able to do the following:

1. Describe key concepts of family-centered care.
2. Identify characteristics of different types of families.
3. Contrast four different parenting styles and analyze their impact on child personality development.
4. Explain the effects of major family changes on children.
5. List the categories of family strengths that help families develop and cope with stressors.
6. Identify family support services that might be available in a community.
7. Summarize the advantages of using a family or cultural assessment tool.
8. Develop a family-centered nursing care plan for the child and family.
9. Examine the role of the nurse in promoting cultural competence.
10. Describe cultural influences on the family's beliefs about health, illness, and treatments.
11. Discuss nursing interventions for providing culturally sensitive and competent care to the child and family.

■ FAMILY AND FAMILY ROLES

The U.S. Census Bureau defines a **family** as two or more individuals who are joined together by marriage, birth, or adoption and live together (U.S. Census Bureau, 2008). More broadly, however, a family may be a self-identified group of two or more persons joined together by shared resources and emotional closeness, whether or not they are related by blood, marriage, or adoption, or even living in the same household. The family as defined by its members is likely to be dynamic, because membership often changes over time. For example, second marriages often integrate children into a newly formed family, and spouses of married children are integrated into an existing family while the newly married couple begins a new family. Family members may live in different cities, states, or even countries. So, there is no *typical* family.

Generally, family members depend upon each other for emotional, physical, and economic support. Families are guided by a common set of values or beliefs about the worth and importance of certain ideas and traditions. These values often bind family members together, and these values are greatly influenced by external factors including cultural background, social norms, education, environmental influences, socioeconomic status, and beliefs held by peers, coworkers, political and community leaders, and other individuals outside the family unit. Because of the influence of these external factors, a family's values may change considerably over the years, or members within a family may hold values that conflict with those of other family members.

Roles of the family include the following:

- Caring, nurturing, and educating children
- Maintaining the continuity of society by transmitting the family's knowledge, customs, values, and beliefs to children
- Receiving and giving love
- Preparing children to become productive members of society
- Meeting the needs of its members
- Serving as a buffer between its members and environmental and societal demands while advocating or addressing the interests and needs of the individual family members

Individual family members take on certain social and gender roles and hold a designated status within the family based on the values and beliefs that bind extended families together. These values and beliefs may evolve from the family's cultural values and practices, social norms, education, and other influences to which parents were exposed during childhood, adolescence, and early adult years. Parental roles, including childrearing practices and beliefs, are usually learned through a socialization process during childhood and adolescence.

Parents have important roles that involve childrearing and the long-term care of children until they reach adulthood. Depending upon their other roles in society, parents work to successfully nurture and rear children, helping them to meet role expectations. Parents must also meet the needs of the family unit and provide economic support for the family. Children also learn specific roles through a socialization process. Parents set expectations of behavior with discipline and modeling of appropriate behavior.

Ideally the family is a child's source of strength and support, the major constant in the child's life. Families are intimately involved in their children's physical and psychological well-being, and they play a vital role in the health promotion and health maintenance of their children. By respecting the family's role, strengths, and experiences with the health care system, nurses have an opportunity to develop an effective partnership with the child and family as they make health care decisions that promote the child's health. This partnership between nurses and families is known as family-centered care.

■ FAMILY-CENTERED CARE

Family-centered care is a philosophy of health care in which a mutually beneficial partnership develops between families and the nurse, and also other health professionals. In this way the priorities and needs of the family are addressed when the family seeks health care for the child. Each party respects the knowledge, skills, experience, and cultural beliefs that the other brings to the health care encounter. This is in contrast to family-focused care, in which the role of the health professional is that of an expert who directs care, tells the family what to do, and intervenes on behalf of the family.

History of Family-Centered Care

Family-centered care became integral to the nursing care of children when it was recognized that families had a significant role in promoting the psychosocial and developmental needs of children in the hospital. When parents were initially allowed to stay with hospitalized children, nurses and other health professionals noticed that children were quieter, happier, and recovering sooner. Research confirmed that children and parents had decreased anxiety when the parents were allowed to be present during painful procedures (Egemen, Ikizoglu, Karapinar, et al., 2006). Eventually "rooming in" became a standard for hospital credentialing. See Chapter 11 ∞ for additional information related to the hospitalized child.

Research | *Parental Presence During Procedures*

Increasingly, parents are permitted to be present during medical procedures performed on their children. Resistance to parental presence has been based on the fear that parents would delay or interfere with the procedure, distract or increase the anxiety of the health professionals performing the procedure, and increase parental anxiety. Studies have investigated parental presence in various situations involving medical procedures, such as venipuncture, lumbar puncture, laceration repair, resuscitation, and induction of anesthesia (Arai, Ito, Kandatsu, et al., 2007; Egemen et al., 2006; Jones, Qazi, & Young, 2007; Maxton, 2008). In most cases, parents are less anxious and the ability of health professionals to perform procedures is not affected (Dingeman, Mitchell, Meyer, et al., 2007; O'Malley, Brown, & Krug and the Committee on Pediatric Emergency Medicine, 2008).

Defining Family Video

Institute for Family-Centered Care Website

Gradually health care providers recognized that parental presence during certain medical procedures, and sometimes resuscitation, was also beneficial to children and their families (Piira, Sugiura, Champion, et al., 2005; Sacchetti, Paston, & Carraccio, 2005). Parents are now recognized as partners in their child's care, not as visitors in the health care setting. Parents serve on hospital advisory committees and help educate health professionals about how to improve family-centered care (Dokken & Ahmann, 2006) (Figure 2–1 ➤).

Nurses have long embraced the family-centered care philosophy. This philosophy is becoming more widely accepted by other health professionals, including pediatricians and emergency room physicians (American Academy of Pediatrics, 2006). The Society of Pediatric Nurses and the American Nurses Association have developed nursing practice guidelines for family-centered care. See Table 2–1.

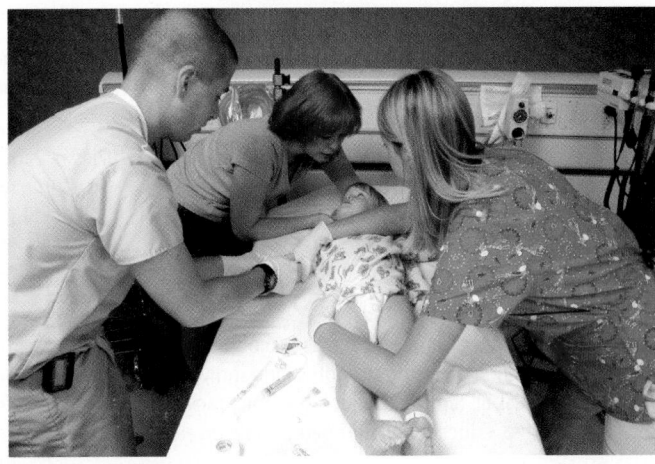

FIGURE 2–1 ➤ A health facility policy that permits a parent to be present during a procedure performed on a child is an example of a family-centered care policy. The parent plays an important role in providing security and comfort to this child who is having blood drawn.

TABLE 2–1	**Elements of Family-Centered Care and Recommendations for Nursing Practice**
Elements	Nursing Practice Recommendations
The Family at the Center: Incorporate into policy and practice the recognition that the family is the constant in a child's life, while the service systems and support personnel within those systems fluctuate, and that the illness or injury of a child affects all members of the family system.	• Establish a therapeutic relationship with the family. • Perform a comprehensive family assessment in collaboration with the family, identifying both strengths and needs. • Use the family assessment when working with the family to plan, implement, and evaluate care, considering the impact of the child's illness or injury on the entire family, with special attention to the siblings. • Provide siblings with information about their sibling's illness/injury at an appropriate developmental level and answer questions honestly. • Promote sibling visitation in hospital settings and participation in home care activities. • Identify extended family members who should receive information and be included in the educational process.
Family-Professional Collaboration: Facilitate family-professional collaboration at all levels of hospital, home, and community care for: • Care of an individual child • Program development, implementation, evaluation, and evolution • Policy formation	• Develop provider-family relationships that are guided by goals and expectations of both the family and the provider. • Ensure that parents are integral and critical collaborators in the decision-making process about their child's care. Involve children and adolescents in the decision-making process as appropriate for their cognitive and emotional development. • Ensure that parents have 24-hour access to their children and facilitate their participation in the child's care. • Provide parents with the option to stay with their child during procedures and tests, and provide ways for the parent to support the child during the procedure. • Provide comfort and hygiene facilities for families who spend long hours at the facility or travel great distances. • Promote the family's development of expertise in the special care of their child, fostering family independence and empowerment. • Incorporate parents and children into the quality assessment/improvement process. • Integrate family members into institutional and community advisory groups and in policy development.

(continued)

TABLE 2–1	Elements of Family-Centered Care and Recommendations for Nursing Practice (*continued*)
Elements	Nursing Practice Recommendations
Family-Professional Communication: Exchange complete and unbiased information between families and professionals in a supportive manner at all times.	• Provide information about the child's problem, prognosis, and needs in a manner that respects the child and family as individuals and promotes two-way dialogue. • Encourage the family to share information about the child and the illness/injury so that care planning and decisions are made in the most informed and collaborative manner.
Cultural Diversity of Families: Incorporate into policy and practice the recognition and honoring of cultural diversity, strengths, and individuality within and across all families, including ethnic, racial, spiritual, social, economic, educational, and geographic diversity.	• Practice family-centered care in a culturally competent manner with respect and sensitivity for the wide range of families with diverse values and beliefs. • Seek to understand the family's beliefs and practices related to race, culture, and ethnicity when developing relationships and collaborating in the child's health care. • Seek to understand and respect the family's religious/spiritual beliefs and practices and integrate these into the child's care, as the family desires. • Assist the family to address care issues related to socioeconomic status, insurance status, geography, and access to health care. • Integrate training programs on diversity, cultural understanding, and culturally competent care into staff development programs.
Coping Differences and Support: Recognize and respect different methods of coping. Implement comprehensive policies and programs that provide families with the developmental, educational, emotional, spiritual, environmental, and financial supports needed to meet their diverse needs.	• Assess the strengths and weaknesses of the family's coping strategies and their resiliency factors and characteristics. Identify maladaptive coping mechanisms and assist the family to augment their coping efforts. • Assess and support the family's needs and desires for support and assist the family in accessing and accepting assistance from support networks as needed or desired.
Family-Centered Peer Support: Encourage and facilitate family-to-family support and networking.	• Educate parents about parent-to-parent and family support resources and assist them to access such resources in the institution and community. • Provide access to psychoeducational groups that might be useful to parents, siblings, or ill/injured children.
Specialized Service and Support Systems: Ensure that hospital, home, and community service and support systems for children needing specialized health and developmental care and their families are flexible, accessible, and comprehensive in responding to diverse family-identified needs.	• Provide collaborative, flexible, accessible, comprehensive, and coordinated services to children and their families. • Provide comprehensive case management/care coordination for children and families with ongoing care needs. • Along with families, take an active role in advocating for the needs of ill and injured children.
Holistic Perspective of Family-Centered Care: Appreciate families as families and children as children, recognizing that they possess a wider range of strengths, concerns, emotions, and aspirations beyond their need for specialized health and developmental services and support.	• Encourage attention to the normal developmental needs and developmental tasks of the entire family unit and individual family members. • Encourage and facilitate the development of individual and family identities beyond a focus on illness or injury. • Facilitate "normalization" as valued and desired by the family.

Promoting Family-Centered Care

Collaborating with families in the provision of health care is essential to promote the best outcome when caring for children. Families have important knowledge to share about their child, their child's health condition, and how their child responds to various actions and events. They also need access to information that will make it possible for them to fully participate in planning and decision making. Parents have a role in developing an effective collaborative relationship with nurses and other health professionals. Parents often become experts in their

Clinical Tip

Some health care facilities are developing family resource centers to provide consumer information and support (Figure 2–2 ➤). In most cases, the resource center is a consumer-oriented health library with staffing, but peer support services may also be coordinated through the center. Families can be supported to access useful information that helps them become informed participants in decision making about their child's care. In addition, the family resource center may serve as a place for family members to read, rest, and reflect (Institute for Family-Centered Care, 2009).

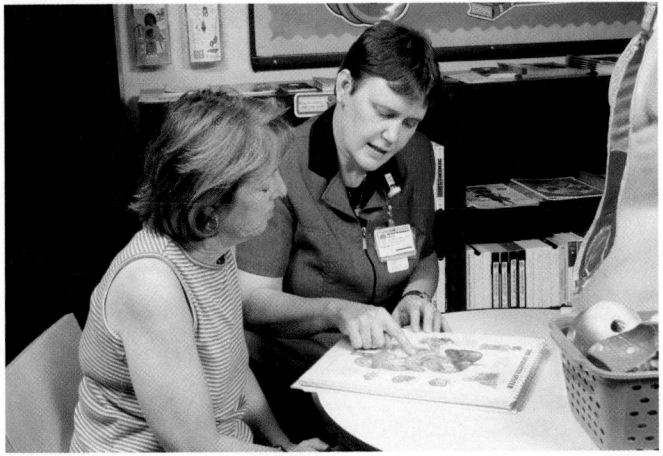

FIGURE 2–2 ➤ The family resource center provides an opportunity for family members to obtain more information about their child's illness from the pediatric nurse educator. This nurse uses pictures from a chart to explain a child's illness to the parent.

child's health condition and learn to advocate for their child. They also must learn to communicate effectively with the health professionals caring for their child, and in the process develop a trusting relationship.

Beyond the provision of nursing care itself, children and parents can participate in the development of policies and guidelines for family-centered care in all types of health care settings. Their experiences while receiving care in the health care setting may reveal valuable insights. Considering parents' perspectives can be critical for staff and hospital administrators to provide quality patient care and achieve successful patient satisfaction. Parents who exhibit leadership qualities can be empowered to serve on advisory boards or councils, representing the family and community perspective.

Parents can also serve a valuable role in family-to-family support networks as mentors to new families entering the health care system for a new chronic condition. Parents may help raise awareness about specific health care issues, serve as advocates for public policy issues, and assist with fundraising activities. Guidelines for working with families as advisors and tools for assessing the family-centered policies in various health care settings are available from the Institute for Family-Centered Care.

It is important to consider how a health care setting's written policies, procedures, and literature for families refer to families and what attitudes these materials convey. Words like *policies, allowed,* and *not permitted* imply that hospital personnel have authority over families in matters concerning their children. Words like *guidelines, working together,* and *welcome* communicate an openness and appreciation for families in the care of their children.

Clinical Judgment

When providing care to children, recall that the family is central to all health care interventions with parents and child as the partners in care. Families need to sense that the nurse cares about them and respects them as an integral part of the child's life. What are some actions by the nurse that indicate a sense of caring for both the child and the family?

■ FAMILY COMPOSITION

Families are diverse in structure, roles, and relationships. Various types of families—both those considered traditional and nontraditional—exist in contemporary American society. This section identifies common types of family structure.

Nuclear Family

In the nuclear family, children live with both biological parents, and no other relatives or persons live in the household. One parent may stay home to rear the children while one parent works, but more commonly, both parents are employed by choice or necessity. Two-income families must address important issues such as childcare arrangements, household chores, and how to ensure quality family time. Important nursing considerations include:

- Respecting a parent who stays home to rear the children while appreciating the value of childrearing
- Helping parents to develop strategies to ensure that the child's health promotion needs are met, such as a nutritious diet with appropriate calories and adequate physical exercise

Blended or Reconstituted Family

The blended or reconstituted nuclear family includes two parents with biological children from a previous marriage or relationship who marry or cohabit. This family structure has become increasingly common because of high rates of divorce and remarriage. Potential advantages to the children may include better financial support and a new supportive role model. Stressors that can cause challenges in forming a cohesive family unit may include lack of a clear role for or acceptance of the stepparent, financial stresses when two families must be supported by stepparents, and communication problems. Parents in the blended family also may have difficulties overcoming differences in parenting styles, discipline strategies, and values. Important nursing considerations include directing families to resources that may help reduce the potential conflicts associated with different parenting styles, discipline, and manipulative behaviors by children that can develop with the blended family. See the discussion on pages 30–31 regarding stepparenting.

Another type of blended family is two parents with adoptive or foster children, sometimes including biological children. See the discussion beginning on page 31 regarding foster care and adoption.

Extended Family

Extended families exist when one parent or a couple shares expenses as well as household and childrearing responsibilities with grandparents, the sibling of a parent, or other relatives. Families may reside together to share housing expenses and childcare. However, in many cases, the child may reside with the grandparent and one parent because of issues associated with unemployment, parental separation, parental death, or parental substance abuse. Grandparents may raise children due to the inability of parents to care for children. In 2008, 54% (1.5 million) of children who did not live with either parent lived with grandparents

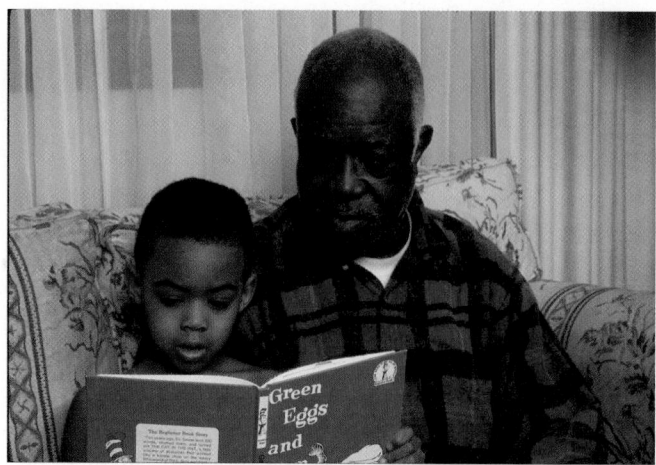

FIGURE 2–3 ➤ This child lives with his mother and grandparents following the divorce of his parents. The special attention provided by his grandfather is helping him to adapt to the change in his family, and it enables the mother to work, feeling confident that her son is safely cared for before and after school.

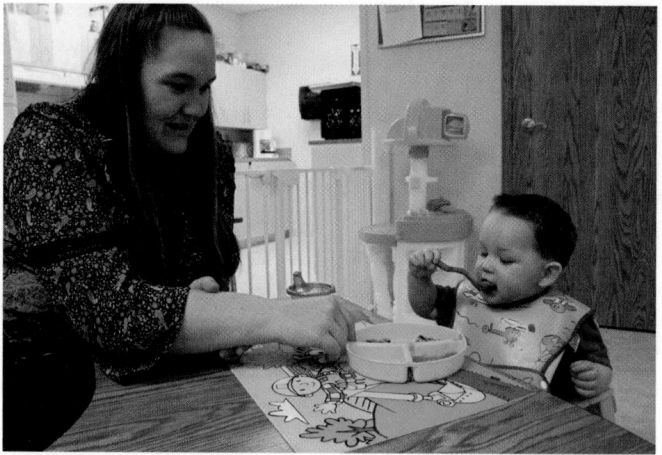

FIGURE 2–4 ➤ Adolescents who are single parents face challenges balancing school, personal time, and care of the infant.

(Childstats.gov, 2009). Grandparents endure emotional, physical, and financial stresses when taking on the childrearing role of one or more grandchildren (Figure 2–3 ➤).

Another example of an extended family is the extended relative network family in which two nuclear families of primary relatives or unmarried relatives live in close proximity to each other. The family shares a social support network in which chores, goods, and services are exchanged. This type of family model is common in the Latino community.

Single-Parent Family

The family of a single parent is formed when the mother or father is widowed, divorced, abandoned, or separated. According to 2007 data, 25% of children under 18 years of age lived in single-parent families (Kreider & Elliott, 2009). Although the majority of children who live with a single parent reside with their mother, the number of children residing with their father has increased significantly over the past several years (Clark, 2008).

Single-parent families often face difficulties because the sole parent may lack social and emotional support, need assistance with childrearing issues, and face financial strain. Single-parent families experience higher rates of poverty. In 2007, 9% of children living with their married parents lived at the poverty level, compared to 43% who lived with only their mother (Childstats.gov, 2009). Depending upon social support and family resources, the single parent may be stressed from working to support the family, managing household responsibilities, serving as both mother and father, and attempting to have a personal life. Single mothers are often impoverished due to lack of child support, inequitable pay for work performed, work skill deficiencies, and cutbacks in social welfare programs. An important nursing consideration for working with single parents is to assess their strengths and needs in providing care to the child, such as after-school and backup childcare arrangements that enable the parent to fulfill work commitments (Figure 2–4 ➤).

Determine if the child has access to all resources available to support growth and development, such as school breakfast and lunch programs that provide nutritional support.

Binuclear Family

In a postdivorce family the biological children can be members of two nuclear households, with co-parenting by the father and the mother. The children alternate between the two homes, spending varying amounts of time with both parents in a situation called co-parenting, usually involving joint custody. **Joint custody** is a legal situation in which both parents have equal responsibility and legal rights, regardless of where the children live. The binuclear family is a model for effective communication. It enables both biological parents to be involved in a child's upbringing and provides additional support and role models from extended family members. Special nursing considerations in this family type involve ensuring that health promotion guidance and education for care of the child with an acute or chronic condition are communicated effectively to both biological parents.

Heterosexual Cohabiting Family

In this family type, a heterosexual couple that may or may not have children lives together outside of marriage. This may include never-married individuals as well as divorced or widowed persons. Biological children may result from the relationship, or in some cases children of one parent are present and help form a blended type of cohabiting family. In 2008, 6% of all children in the United States lived with a cohabiting parent or parents (Childstats.gov, 2009). An important nursing consideration for children who live in informal stepfamilies is that the nonbiological parent has no legal authority to seek emergency medical care for the child. However, in the case of a true emergency that could result in loss of life or diminished functioning, health professionals are obligated to provide care and obtain consent as soon as possible afterward. The nonbiological parent also may not have any knowledge of the child's medical history.

Gay or Lesbian Family

A gay or lesbian family involves two adults of the same sex who live together as married or domestic partners with or without children, or a gay or lesbian single parent rearing a child. Children in these families may be from a previous heterosexual union, or be born to or adopted by one or both members of the same-sex couple. A biological child may be born to one of the partners through artificial insemination or through a surrogate mother. It is estimated that 96% of all U.S. counties have at least one gay or lesbian couple with children under 18 years in the household (Pawelski, Perrin, Foy, et al., 2006).

Children who are adopted or born into lesbian and gay families are highly valued, as with heterosexual families (Figure 2–5 ➤). Small studies that have evaluated children reared by same-sex couples found no significant differences in childrearing or in the children's adjustment from children reared in other types of families. These children have been found to do as well emotionally, behaviorally, and psychosocially as those born into heterosexual families (Pawelski et al., 2006).

Nursing Alert

It is important to identify the biological or adoptive parent, or a caregiver's legal documentation proving the right to medical decision making, when obtaining consent for the child's health care.

Children in homosexual families sometimes have only one biological or adoptive legal parent. The other partner is the co-parent and has no legal parental status in the majority of states. Several states do allow second-parent adoption for same-sex couples (Evan B. Donaldson Adoption Institute, 2008). Co-parent adoption helps maintain the child's rights to a continuing relationship if the legal parent dies or becomes incapacitated, or if the parents separate. Either parent could then provide consent

for health care and make other important decisions on behalf of the child. Financial support of the child is more assured if one parent dies or parents separate. Nursing considerations for this type of family involve respect for the relationship between partners and recognition of the nurturing capacity in these families.

■ FAMILY FUNCTIONING

Transition to Parenthood

Choosing to become a parent is a major life change for adults. Couples experience significant family and cultural pressure to have a child. Mothers may be eager to have a child, but be concerned about fulfilling all of the expectations of others (father, the baby, other children, her parents, close friends, and employer). Fathers anticipate increased responsibility and are concerned about their ability to provide adequate support for the family.

At the time of birth the parents experience stresses and challenges along with feelings of pride and excitement. Mothers and fathers both make adjustments to their lifestyles to give priority to parenting. The baby is dependent for total care 24 hours a day, and this often results in sleep deprivation, irritability, less personal time, and less time for the couple's relationship. In addition, the family often experiences a change in financial status.

Several factors influence how well the parents adjust to their new role. Social support provided to the mother, especially by the father, is important for the mother's adjustment. Marital happiness during pregnancy is an important adjustment factor for both parents. Infants with significant health conditions or those with difficult temperaments can cause extra stress for the parents and affect their adjustment to the parenting role.

With the birth of the first child, mothers and fathers both have challenges related to renegotiating their employment to accommodate family and childcare time. Fathers are sometimes additionally challenged to develop closeness with the infant and to learn how to care for the infant, especially when they may not have had role models or any childcare experience. Most parents find that caring for infants and children takes more time than anticipated.

Nurses can help parents through this important transition by listening to the challenges they describe during the infant's first health visits. Encourage fathers as well as mothers to attend and participate in health promotion visits with the health care

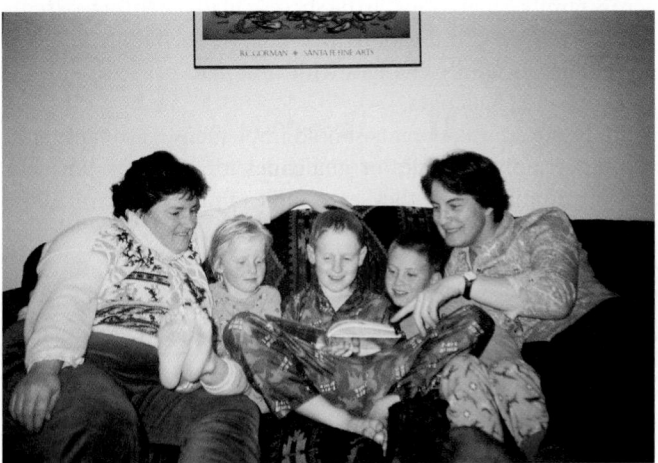

FIGURE 2–5 ➤ No evidence exists to indicate that children raised in a homosexual family are at any greater developmental or dysfunction risk than a child raised in a heterosexual family (Pawelski et al., 2006). These parents are as dedicated as heterosexual families to promoting the growth and development of their children.

Law & Ethics   *Medical and Family Leave Act*

Eligible parents of newborns and adopted children are entitled to 12 weeks of unpaid leave during any 12-month period initially authorized under the federal Family and Medical Leave Act of 1993. Vacation or sick leave may often be used to pay for time away from work. This act also applies if a child, spouse, or parent of the employee develops a serious health condition. The employee is entitled to return to the previous position or an equivalent position with all the same pay, benefits, and other conditions (U.S. Department of Labor, 2009).

provider so that positive parenting can be supported. Answer questions and offer ideas to address described problems that the parents may be too tired to solve on their own. Help them recognize that frustrations and feelings they have regarding the challenges of infant care are normal and expected. Encourage both parents to become active in caring for the infant and to gain comfort in that care. Help each parent find activities that they enjoy with regard to infant care to encourage interaction and bonding with the infant.

Parental Influences on the Child

The qualities of family relationships and of family behaviors are important aspects of family strengths and family functioning. Positive family relationships are characterized by parent–child warmth and supportiveness. Warm parent–child relationships can buffer children from stress and promote positive cognitive and social outcomes. Parents who are warm and place high demands on their children for appropriate behavior have children who tend to be content, self-reliant, self-controlled, and open to learning in school.

Mothers and fathers each contribute to the psychological, emotional, and social health and development of their children. Both parents provide affection, nurturing, and comfort. They teach children life skills and healthy lifestyles. Fathers play an important role in the sexual identity and gender role development of their children. They also promote the social competence, academic achievement, and problem-solving abilities of their children (American Academy of Pediatrics, 2004).

Family Size

The size of the family influences the amount of attention given to children. In small families, parents often have more time to give attention to the children, to encourage achievement, to meet family expectations, and to support involvement in community activities. Children in larger families are encouraged to be cooperative so that the family group functions well. The child usually receives less personal attention from the parents and must often turn to others in the family for support. Family finances may be more limited. Children may adopt a specialized family role to gain recognition, such as the "responsible one," "the clown," or "the black sheep."

Sibling Relationships

Siblings are the first peers of a child and often have a lifelong relationship lasting up to 70 or more years. Siblings, especially those of the same gender, who are closer in age tend to have a closer relationship because they often share many common experiences through childhood and adolescence. In general, for children who are more widely spaced in age, the parents have greater influence than siblings. However, the older sibling may be a strong role model for younger siblings.

Sibling rivalry exists between children at times in all families. Children learn to share, compete, and compromise with their siblings. Some siblings take on roles such as protector, problem solver, friend, and supporter for dealing with issues in the family and in the environment. Some siblings learn to work well together to maintain privacy or to form a coalition for negotiating

with the parents. An older sibling helps reinforce rules and roles in the family by prompting and inhibiting certain patterns of behavior in the younger siblings. However, one sibling may test the waters by breaking a previously implicit rule to determine what rule flexibility is allowed in the family.

Children develop different personalities because of a need to establish a distinct identity for themselves and be seen as unique in the family. Siblings may share some experiences, but they are often exposed to different environmental experiences that help shape their personalities (Craig & Dunn, 2007).

First-born children do have some advantages, such as more favorable treatment in the family. First-born children have slightly higher IQs and greater achievement in school and in their careers (Craig & Dunn, 2007). Their intellectual development may be enhanced through experiences of teaching their younger siblings.

■ PARENTING

The family is an important component in the lives of all children, and it plays an essential role in fostering the development of infants, children, and youth. A significant concept in families is that of parenting. **Parenting** is a leadership role in the family in which children are guided to learn acceptable behaviors, beliefs, morals, and rituals of the family and to become socially responsible contributing members of society. The manner in which children are parented, in combination with their individual personality traits and characteristics, influences their developmental outcomes.

Parents have responsibility for providing stability to children with a nurturing, safe, and structured environment. The child needs to have physical and emotional space to grow and develop. This space enables the child to personally find the relationship balance between closeness and distance, as well as safety and risk. Parents also provide their children with the values, beliefs, rituals, and behaviors learned and transmitted across family generations. To be successful in parenting, parents must have a certain flexibility that enables the family to adapt and adjust to family changes with time and other significant stressors and challenges.

To be successful, parents should implement reasonable **limit setting** (established rules or guidelines for behavior) on children's autonomy while they learn values and self-control. At the

Culture *Family Structure and Roles*

A family's structure and roles are largely dependent upon cultural influence. For example, culture may determine who has authority (head of household) and is the primary decision maker for other members of the family. Sometimes the decision maker role varies by the type of decisions to be made. For example, in some cultures such as Hispanic, decisions regarding the health care of children are primarily the responsibility of the female, whereas other decisions are male dominated. Family dominance patterns may be *patriarchal*, as may be seen in Appalachian cultures; *matriarchal*, as may be seen in African American cultures; or more *egalitarian*, as may be seen in European American cultures.

TABLE 2–2	**Characteristics of Significant Parenting Attributes**	
Parenting Attribute	Parental Warmth	Parental Control
High level	Warm, nurturing Express affection and smile at children frequently Limit criticism, punishment Express approval of child	Restrictive control of behavior Survey and enforce compliance with rules Encourage children to fulfill their responsibilities May limit freedom of expression
Low level	Cool, hostile Quick to criticize or punish Ignore children Rarely express affection or approval Rejection may be seen	Permissive, minimally controlling Make fewer demands Fewer restrictions on behavior or expression of emotion Permit freedom in exploring environment

same time, parents need to foster the child's curiosity, initiative, and sense of competence. Parents use different styles to parent their children. Parental warmth and control are two major factors that are important in the development of children. Parental warmth refers to the amount of affection and approval displayed. Parental control refers to how restrictive the parents are regarding rules. See Table 2–2 for the characteristics associated with parental warmth and control.

Diana Baumrind identified three parenting styles (*authoritarian*, *authoritative*, and *permissive*) and described the influences each style has on children. This proposed classification is still useful in identifying parenting behavior (Baumrind, 2005), as is another parenting style, called *indifferent*, that exists in some families (Craig & Dunn, 2007). Although families generally exhibit one style, they may vary their style for certain situations. See Table 2–3 for characteristics or parenting styles by levels of warmth and control.

Authoritarian Parents

Authoritarian parents tend to be punitive and adhere to rigid rules, or be more dictatorial. Parents who use this style might say, "Because I'm your parent, that's why," "A rule is a rule," or "Just do what I say." While this style sets firm limits, those limits or rules are not negotiable or open to any discussion. Parents expect family beliefs and principles to be accepted without question. Children have no opportunity to participate in the family decision-making process. Children with authoritarian parents do not develop the skills to examine why a certain behavior is desirable or how their actions might influence others.

Authoritative Parents

Authoritative parents use firm control to set limits, but they establish an atmosphere with open discussion, or are more democratic. Limits for behavior are clear and reasonable, but the child

TABLE 2–3	**Parenting Styles by Level of Warmth and Control**		
Parenting Style	Warmth/Control	Behavior of Parent	Child Outcomes
Authoritarian	High control Low warmth	Highly controlling, issues commands and expects them to be obeyed Little communication with the child Inflexible rules Permits little independence	No negotiation skills No ability to direct and initiate own activities Frustrated in efforts to achieve autonomy May become fearful, withdrawn, and unassertive Girls often passive and dependent during adolescence Boys often rebellious and aggressive
Authoritative	Moderately high control High warmth	Sets reasonable limits on behavior Accepts and encourages growing autonomy of the child Open communication with the child Flexible rules	More willingly accepts restrictions Tends to be more self-reliant, self-controlled, and socially competent Higher self-esteem Better school performance
Permissive	Low control High warmth	Few or no restraints Unconditional love Communication flows from child to parent Much freedom and little guidance No limit setting	May become rebellious, aggressive, socially inept, self-indulgent, or impulsive May be creative, active, and outgoing
Indifferent	Low control Low warmth	No limit setting Lacks affection for the child Focused on stress in own life May show hostility toward or neglect of the child	May show a high expression of destructive impulses and delinquent behavior

From Craig/Dunn, Understanding human development, *"Parenting Styles by Level of Warmth and Control" p. 230. © 2007 Pearson Education, Inc. Reproduced by permission of Pearson Education, Inc.*

is encouraged to talk about why certain behaviors occurred and how the situations might be handled differently another time. Parents provide explanations about inappropriate behaviors at the child's level of understanding. Children are allowed to express their opinions and objections, and some flexibility is permitted when appropriate. However, parents make it clear that they are the ultimate authority for decisions. Children with authoritative parents develop a sense of social responsibility since they converse about their responsibilities and approaches.

Permissive Parents

Permissive parents show a great deal of warmth, but set few controls or restraints on the child's behavior. Parents are so intent on showing unconditional love that they fail in performing some important parenting functions. Children are allowed to regulate their own behavior. Discipline is inconsistent, and parents may threaten punishment but not follow through. Both extremes result in excessive permissiveness, and the child does not learn socially acceptable limits of behavior. When the parents do not impose any controls on the child, the child ends up controlling the parents.

Indifferent Parents

Parents may be indifferent because of disinterest or because their lives are busy and stress-filled, leaving little time or energy for their children. Children who experience this style of parenting often have the worst outcomes, such as destructive impulses and delinquent behavior. If the parents are also hostile, the child often develops delinquent behavior (Craig & Dunn, 2007).

Parent Adaptability

Parents who are able to adapt their behavior to meet the needs of children at different developmental stages are also more effective. Parenting styles may change as the child grows older. For example, parents may use negotiation to help the child develop problem-solving skills and learn how to compromise and get along with others. This enables the child to have more self-control and self-responsibility over time. Parents and some children can develop shared goals and jointly participate in decision making, whereas other children require constant negotiation for decision making. See Families Want to Know: Guidelines for Promoting Acceptable Behavior in Children.

Assessing Parenting Styles

Nurses can assess parenting styles by asking families how they handle situations that require limit setting. The nurse in all settings is often in a position to discuss parenting styles and to offer suggestions for managing certain types of child behaviors that are frustrating to the family. Keep in mind that all children are different and parents often must vary their parenting styles for different children in the family. For example, the child's temperament is often tied to his or her behavioral style. (See Chapter 4 ∞ for more information on child temperament.) One child may need very clear limits set with discussion and reinforcement, whereas a sibling may immediately respond to the parents' limit setting without a need for discussion. Also see Culture: Influences on Parenting.

Families Want to Know
Guidelines for Promoting Acceptable Behavior in Children

- Set realistic expectations and directions for behavior based upon the child's age and understanding; consistently enforce the expected directions and behaviors.
- Focus on promoting appropriate and desirable behaviors in the child:
  - Model or suggest appropriate behavior,
  - Review expected behavior for special situations, such as a family party, going to the movies, or other social events,
  - Help the child distinguish between inside and outside voice and behaviors, and
  - Praise or reward the child for using appropriate behaviors.
- Tell the child about his or her inappropriate behavior as soon as it begins and offer guidelines for behavior change or provide a distraction.
- When reprimanding the child, focus on the behavior rather than stating that the child is bad. Explain how the behavior is inappropriate; how it makes you, as the parent, and any other person involved feel. Avoid ridicule or accusation that can take the form of shame or criticism. These actions can have an impact on the child's self-esteem if repeated often enough.
- Be alert for situations when the child could potentially misbehave, such as when tired or overexcited. Use a distraction to control or calm the child.
- Help children gain self-control with friendly reminders (e.g., count to three, as soon as the clothes are on the doll, as soon as you finish the game) regarding the timing for transition to the next event of the day, such as bedtime, putting the toys away, or washing hands before dinner.
- Discuss reasons and social rules for expected behaviors when the child is old enough to understand.

Discipline and Limit Setting

Discipline is a method for teaching the rules that govern behavior or conduct. **Punishment** is the action taken to enforce the rules when the child misbehaves. Parenting styles play an important role in the type of discipline and punishment used with children. When clear limits are set and consistently maintained, as with authoritative parenting, punishment may be needed less often. Limit setting and firm control of those limits are important discipline methods used so children learn to what extent they can safely and independently operate within the environment. Firm limits also help children to feel secure because they are reassured by consistency and the sense of protection per-

Culture   *Influences on Parenting*

Some cultural influences on parenting are associated with chosen lifestyle. For example, living in a predominantly ethnic neighborhood makes it possible to participate in special events that help teach the child about the culture. Parents use the community for social contacts that help to reinforce patterns of parenting and to establish behavioral expectations of their children. Frequent contact or living with the extended family helps the child learn family and ethnic traditions, behaviors, and values. Children may be sent to faith-based schools that foster values important to the family.

ceived by the limits. Punishment helps children learn that there are consequences for misbehavior, and that other individuals may be affected by that behavior. This helps children develop a sense of responsibility for their behavior.

Parents use various strategies for the discipline and punishment of children. Factors that affect what type of discipline is used are related to sex of the child, education level and age of the parents, family income, and culture. In addition, the type of misbehavior and the location in which it occurs affects the type of discipline used (Socolar, Savage, & Evans, 2007).

Clinical Tip

Nurses have an important educational role in helping parents to identify an appropriate discipline method and to take an authoritative role with their children. Encourage and educate parents about the need to be in charge, to set the rules, and to stand by them so that children learn how to behave.

Common strategies used with children include (Hicks-Pass, 2009; Regalado, Sareen, Inkelas, et al., 2004; Slade & Wissow, 2004; Socolar et al., 2007):

- Reasoning—explaining why a behavior or action is inappropriate or describing how limit setting is important. By reasoning, parents can help the child to understand why certain behaviors are wrong. Similarly, parents can share personal stories and fables to help children understand social and moral values or to better understand acceptable behavior.
- Behavior modification—giving positive rewards or reinforcement for good behavior or consistently ignoring inappropriate behavior to minimize the behavior. This encourages children to behave in specified ways.
- Experiencing consequences—allowing the child to learn important lessons associated with misbehavior, such as taking away a toy, using a time-out, withdrawing privileges, and providing no dessert if the child misses dinner or does not eat nutritious foods (Figure 2–6 ➤).
- Corporal punishment—spanking or inflicting pain with a paddle, whip, or other object. Although this is one of the most widely used techniques for punishing children, it is not recommended because it teaches children that violence is acceptable. If parents are out of control or in a rage, the child may be seriously injured.
- Scolding or yelling—use of harsh language directed at the child.

See Chapters 7 through 9 ∞ for age-specific discipline strategies.

Clinical Tip

Time-out is a punishment method of placing the child in a location away from toys and attention as a consequence of misbehavior. The general rule for the length of time-out is 1 minute per year of age.

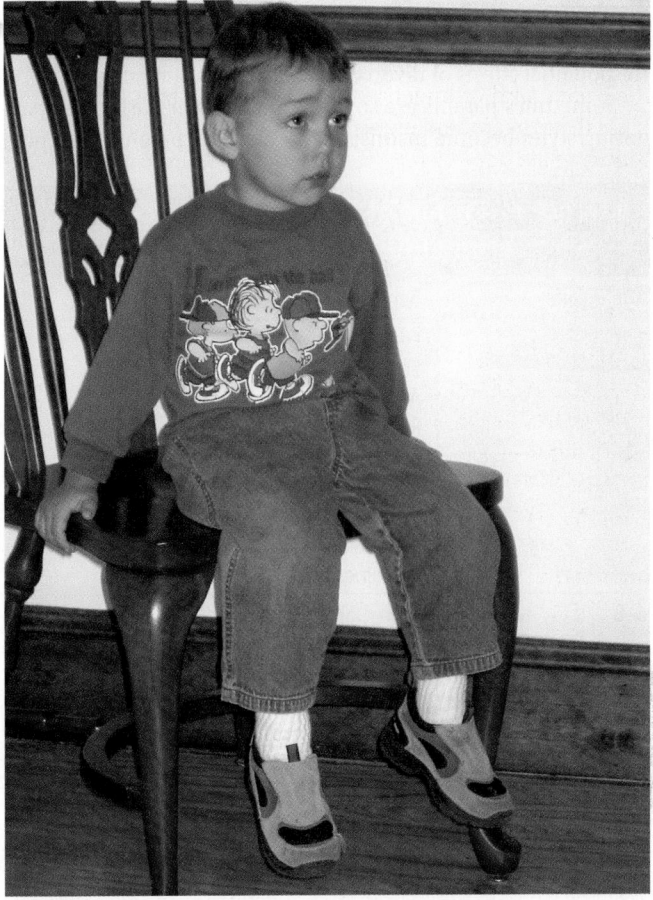

FIGURE 2–6 ➤ One effective discipline method is to remove the child to an isolated area where no interaction with children and adults can occur and no toys are present. This is used to demonstrate that there is a consequence to misbehavior. For older children, consider the loss of phone, computer, or other privileges.

■ SPECIAL FAMILY CONSIDERATIONS

Divorce and Its Effects on Children

The divorce rate in the United States is estimated to be around 50% of all marriages. Each year, an additional 1 million children are affected by divorce (Portnoy, 2006). Children are affected in many ways when the family breaks apart, even if the divorce was preceded by periods of stress and tension in the home. Many children believe they are at fault for the separation and divorce, having said or done something to make the parent leave. When one parent leaves, the children may feel abandoned and divorced by that parent. They may also fear being abandoned by the remaining parent. Children may become engaged in the disputes of parents, and they experience conflicts of loyalty when parents fight for their affection.

In divorces involving a lot of conflict and hostility, the children may have increased problems with adjustment. When children must make a lot of changes in their lives in addition to the parents' separation (new home, different school), their adjustment is made more difficult as their sense of order is upset. Predictable routines have changed and children may test limits to see if they still apply. The more changes they must make in the period immediately after the divorce, the more challenging is their adjustment. The disruption associated with divorce is also linked to academic and behavior problems among children (Portnoy, 2006). See Table 2–4 for potential effects of divorce on children of different ages.

Sometimes parents are so stressed that their customary parenting styles become inconsistent. They may be unable to pro-

TABLE 2–4	Potential Effects of Divorce on Children of Different Ages
Age (Years)	Behavior*
3–5	Fear, anxiety, worry Sorrow and grief Anger Regression Searching and questioning Temper tantrums Increased crankiness and aggression Self-blame Loneliness, unhappiness, depression
6–8	Worry, anxiety, depression Fantasy Self-blame Inability to concentrate on schoolwork Regression Confusion Grief Anger and aggression Resentment Behavioral problems at school and home
9–10	Anger Anxiety and depression Grief Manipulation of parents Withdrawal from friends and activities Resentment Behavioral problems at school and home
11–13	Panic Fear Depression Guilt Risk taking Fear of loneliness and abandonment Denial
14–17	Struggle with morality Loneliness Anger Fear Depression Guilt Truancy, use of drugs and alcohol Sexual acting out

This table lists some of the behaviors that could potentially be seen with different age groups and is not all-inclusive. Many other behaviors could be present as well, depending on the individual child.

Source: Data from Wallerstein, J. S., & Blakeslee, S. (2004). What about the kids? Raising your children before, during, and after divorce. New York: Hyperion; Douglas, E. (2006). The effects of divorce on children. University of New Hampshire Cooperative Extension. Retrieved from http://ceinfo.unh.edu; Craig, G. J., & Dunn, W. L. (2007). Understanding human development. Upper Saddle River, NJ: Pearson/Prentice Hall.

vide the warmth, affection, and support that the children need during this time. Battles over custody, child support, property division, and visitation rights all cause more distress for the children.

Nurses can assist families experiencing divorce by inquiring about the circumstances and changes that the child is experiencing. Talk with parents about the child's fears of abandonment and concerns, reminding parents that even infants and toddlers can sense tensions in the home. Remind parents about the need to keep children out of the middle of confrontations, and to maintain limits of acceptable behavior. Encourage parents to avoid saying negative statements about the other parent, and encourage them to make every effort to maintain the relationship with the children. Help parents recognize their children's needs for love and security during this difficult period.

The quality of the relationship between the divorced parents has an important impact on the future relationships their children have with them as adults. Children do better when both parents remain involved with their children and cooperate with each other after divorce (American Academy of Child and Adolescent Psychiatry, 2008).

Fathers who do not live with their children but live nearby are more likely to have involvement with their children if they have a good relationship with the child's mother, financial resources, and work experience. The relationship between father and child may be improved when the father can interact with the child in a conflict-free environment. See Families Want to Know: Promoting Relationships with Parents Following Separation and Divorce.

Stepparenting

When divorced or widowed parents remarry, the child may respond with ambivalence, divided loyalty, anger, or uncertainty. Parents should anticipate how the child and the entire family will respond to changes in lifestyles, routines, and interaction patterns and address them early in the formation of the new family relationship. When a stepparent joins a ready-made family, opportunities for improved emotional and financial support of the child can result, but the development of a new cohesive family requires many adjustments by all family members.

Families Want to Know
Promoting Relationships with Parents Following Separation and Divorce

Guidelines that may help to reduce conflict and to foster maintenance of a close relationship between the child and each parent include the following:

■ Develop a way to stay in touch with the child even when apart, such as phone calls, text messages, faxes, or e-mail.

■ Encourage a liberal visitation schedule so that each parent has time to be a normal parent. Overnight stays rather than a few hours at a time allow for more normal interactions.

■ When parents have difficulty minimizing conflict in front of the child, transition the child to the other parent after school or childcare, or from a friend's home. This keeps the child from feeling responsible for the conflict.

Blending two families often results in the need to identify or negotiate new customs, traditions, rituals, and routines for the family. Children may fear or experience losses such as a close relationship with the noncustodial parent, neighborhood friends (if a move was required), contact with grandparents, and family traditions. Discussions with children about their feelings may help the new family develop plans that ease the transition.

Stepparents must adjust to the habits and personality of the child and then work to gain trust and acceptance. If the child has not accepted the divorce or loss of a biological parent, the stepparent faces more challenges in developing a trusting, affectionate, and respectful relationship. Sharing in childrearing decisions and responsibilities is an important task for stepparents, but their roles and the role of the joint or noncustodial parent need to be discussed and negotiated.

Stepparents are additional parents, not replacement parents. The stepparent and the child need to adjust to each other. The stepparent should try to establish a position in the child's life that is different from that of the missing biological parent, rather than competing with the biological parent. Stepmothers often have more challenges than stepfathers adjusting to their new role. This may be because they spend more time with the children.

In most stepparent families, discipline is a challenge. Family members must agree upon standards of behavior, as well as the type of discipline and who carries it out; these guidelines need to be consistently maintained. Discipline by a stepparent is difficult until a bond develops between the stepparent and stepchild. The development of this bond cannot be forced. Time and honest communication are needed to gain the child's trust.

Clinical Tip

Identify the parent who can legally provide consent for medical treatment when there has been a divorce and potentially a remarriage. In some states the noncustodial parent cannot give consent. The stepparent cannot give consent unless the custodial parent grants written permission. Stepparents or other family members may also not know the child's medical history. Identify the legal framework for informed consent with regard to these children so that care is provided in an appropriate and responsible manner.

Contact with the biological parent often continues through custody arrangements, financial support, and visitation. Children may actually move between two households, adding to the complexity and stressors in their lives. They may have divided loyalties between the two sets of parents. Power conflicts may emerge if the biological parents do not make efforts to cooperate in parenting decisions. When parents agree to work together for the child's benefit, a parenting coalition between all parents in the two families can reduce the conflicts and tensions that can emerge.

■ FOSTER CARE

Foster care is the provision of protection and shelter for a child in an approved living situation away from the family of origin. It is legally coordinated by the state's child welfare system. The goal of foster care is to ensure the safety and well-being of vulnerable children. As of September 30, 2006, approximately 510,000 children were in foster care. The average length of stay was approximately 28 months; however, some children were in foster care shorter or longer times. Of these children, 40% were White non-Hispanic, 32% were Black non-Hispanic, and 19% were Hispanic (U.S. Department of Health and Human Services, 2008a).

During 2006, 303,000 children entered foster care and 289,000 exited. Of those children exiting foster care, 53% were united with their parent or primary caregiver, 11% were placed with another relative, and 17% were adopted (U.S. Department of Health and Human Services, 2008a).

Children enter the foster care system for many reasons. The primary reason is child abuse and neglect. Other reasons, but to a much lesser extent, include a parent's inability to care for the child because of drug addiction or health issues (Whenan, Oxlad, & Lushington, 2009). Each state has guidelines regarding qualifications and standards for foster care parents and the process for becoming a foster parent. In an effort to ensure that the child is placed in a safe and nurturing environment, state guidelines used to investigate the home often include an interview with the interested adults to check for readiness to be a foster parent, health of all family members, legal background checks, and safety of the residence. Foster parents are also required to have initial training and annual continuing education.

Foster parents may be relatives (kinship care) or unrelated families with whom the child has a strong emotional bond. However, many children needing foster care are placed in extended families because there are fewer suitable nonkinship family foster homes. Although there are psychological benefits in keeping the child within the extended family, especially for helping the child learn and understand cultural and family values, the kinship foster parents have more challenges than other foster parents. They may be older or in poorer health, have less income, and have less education. Kinship foster parents may receive less funding than licensed foster care parents. In addition, they tend to receive less supervision and family service support than in nonkinship foster care (Raphel, 2008).

Foster Parenting

Foster parenting is very demanding. Foster parents must provide for the daily needs of children, support them emotionally, and provide appropriate responses to their behaviors; however, they may not feel they are prepared to do so (Whenan et al., 2009). Foster parents provide transportation to medical and mental health counseling appointments, coordinate visits with birth parents and caseworkers, and advocate for the child in school settings. When the child has complex problems or needs, the challenge of caring for the foster child is even greater. Foster parents receive some funding to care for children, but it is often inadequate for the child's needs, so the family subsidizes the child's care from their own funds. Faced with the challenges of inadequate financial support and lack of respect and trust from the social worker, many foster parents become frustrated and stop serving in this role within a year (Chipungu & Bent-Goodley, 2004). When the child must be moved to a different foster family, this may further exacerbate the ongoing stress that the individual child experiences in the foster care system.

Much of the child's adjustment rests with the stability of the family and available resources. Even though foster care is intended to be a temporary short placement—until the child can be returned home or an adoptive home is found—placed children may actually reside with the foster family for a lengthy time, sometimes for years. For children who have come from an environment that has been unstable, abusive, or neglectful, the foster care home can be supportive to the child's health status, development, and academic achievement.

Foster parents caring for children need to provide continuity, consistency, and predictability. Foster parents should be able to provide an environment that enhances the development of the child, and be able to recognize cultural differences and the influence the environment has on the child (Chipungu & Bent-Goodley, 2004). It is essential that foster parents provide a nurturing environment for these children and show love and affection toward them. Developmentally appropriate activities are essential to foster the child's long-term physical and emotional development.

Health Status of Foster Children

Children in foster care often have complex health problems and chronic illness. They are also more likely to have developmental delays, behavioral and psychiatric disorders, as well as academic difficulty (Whenan et al., 2009). Efforts to ensure that children receive appropriate health care while in foster care are challenged by various barriers, such as lack of coordination between health care providers and social workers. Lack of preventive care for foster children may result because of fragmentation in caregiving systems, loss of medical records, and foster parents who simply do not know how to obtain the services the foster child needs (Schneiderman, 2006).

Every child entering foster care should receive an initial health screening, followed by a more comprehensive health assessment within a month. Findings and recommendations from the health assessment and additional health evaluations should be incorporated into the child's social service case plan. Nurses can play an important role in partnering with foster parents to arrange for and obtain the services needed by the child. Foster parents need to be supported in their efforts to care for these children, helping them to develop self-esteem and resilience.

Transition to Permanent Placement

Although many children are reunited with birth parents, other children cannot be. The Adoption and Safe Families Act of 1997

Law & Ethics — *Foster Care Independence Act*

The Foster Care Independence Act of 1999 (P.L. 106-169) requires states to provide youth 18 to 21 years of age with services to help them make the transition to self-sufficiency—training and education with services to help them gain employment, mentors for personal and emotional support, as well as financial, housing, counseling, and other supports and services (U.S. Department of Health and Human Services, 2009a).

(P.L. 105-89) led to significant changes in child welfare, including the development of a process to evaluate the performance of care providers (Strijker, Knorth, & Knot-Dickscheit, 2008). Timelines were shortened for decision making about permanent placement of children, and incentives were established for states to encourage adoption. States were given guidelines regarding when reasonable efforts to reunite children with birth parents are no longer necessary, and when action is required in certain circumstances to terminate parental rights. Kinship foster care was formally recognized. **Legal guardianship** (a permanent placement option for the child, often with relatives, in which parental rights are not terminated) was established as an alternative to **adoption** (a legal relationship between the child and parents not related by birth in which the adoptive parents assume all legal and financial responsibility for the child). Long-term foster care was eliminated as a permanent placement option in nonkinship care, but it could continue for kinship foster care to promote stability for the involved children (Adoption.com, 2010).

For those children with kinship foster care, adoption is often not perceived as the best option. Legal guardianship enables the child to retain legal connections with the birth family and relationships with the extended family. The guardian assumes limited financial liability for the child's care. Legal guardianship can be reversed at a future point in time if the birth parents petition the court.

■ ADOPTION

Motivations for adoption of a child vary with the families seeking adoption. In some cases, couples have infertility problems and are unable to have a biological child. In a family that already has biological children, the reasons could include the following:

- A desire to provide a home to a child who needs one or to have a larger family without additional biological children
- Fertility issues requiring invasive medical procedures that are too extensive, expensive, or psychologically overwhelming for a subsequent pregnancy
- Adoption of a foster child with whom the family has established strong bonds
- Adoption by a family relative or stepparent

The supply of healthy infants available for adoption is much smaller than the number of families who want to adopt. Most children in the United States available for adoption are older children, often of minority populations or of mixed races, and those with special health care needs. In 2008, the number of children waiting to be adopted was 130,000, down from 134,000 in 2002 (U.S. Department of Health and Human Services, 2008b). Because most families choosing to adopt prefer to have an infant, many children have been adopted from foreign nations. Since 1995, the nations that have provided the largest number of orphans for adoption in the United States include mainland China, Russia, Guatemala, and South Korea (U.S. Department of State, 2007). Adopted children account for approximately 2% of all children in the United States (U.S. Department of Health and Human Services, 2009b).

Legal Aspects of Adoption

Adoption is controlled by individual state law. Adoption may be arranged through an authorized agency, such as a licensed social service agency. Some adoptions are arranged through independent agencies in collaboration with physicians, lawyers, nurses, and members of the clergy. State laws require any family who wants to adopt a child to undergo a home study, a process in which parents are interviewed about a large number of topics and issues and are provided education and guidelines to prepare for the adoption. The National Adoption Information Clearinghouse provides information about state adoption laws.

Birth mothers and birth fathers are each required to relinquish legal rights to a child before an adoption can occur. The legal period between the child's birth and when the birth mother relinquishes legal rights varies by state. Efforts are made to ensure that the birth mother is not coerced into relinquishing legal rights to the child immediately after birth. In an open adoption, the birth mother and adoptive parents often have contact with each other prior to the birth and have jointly planned potential future contacts between the child and biological mother. In some adoptions, birth mothers write a letter to the child that is given to the child at an appropriate age.

Preparation for Adoption

Adopting parents often benefit from preadoption counseling, which may help provide the support and reassurance needed about parenting and the adoptive process, and help them make connections with support groups or other families with adopted children. Parents may wonder about their ability to love and parent the child, and may have concerns about the responses of relatives, other children, and friends, especially if the child is from a different ethnic or racial group. Children already present in the family need to be reassured that they will not be displaced by the new child. Families need information about the child's understanding of what adoption means and guidance to help inform the child about being adopted.

Responses by Adopted Children

Children vary in their understanding and response to adoption by age (Borchers & Committee on Early Childhood, Adoption, and Dependent Care, American Academy of Pediatrics, 2003):

- Children under 3 years of age do not recognize a difference between being adopted into a family versus being a biological child in the family.
- Starting at about 3 years of age, children like to hear about their adoption story and they begin to ask what adoption means. Children adopted at this age may experience the separation from their other family and relatives. They are aware of physical differences between themselves and the adoptive family when they are of a different race or ethnic group. They may be fearful of abandonment by the adoptive family.
- By 5 years of age, adopted children begin to recognize they are different from most of their peers who were not adopted.

Some children develop a feeling of responsibility for their biological parents' decision not to keep them.

- School-age children may fantasize about their biological family and what their life might have been like if they were not adopted. Their self-esteem may be affected if they think there was a flaw in them that was the reason their biological parents gave them up for adoption.
- Adolescents may continue to fantasize about the "ideal" biological family and try out identities similar to what they know or imagine about their biological parents. They may also become angry that their own life experience is different from societal norms. Adoption issues continue into young adulthood as the individual deals with aspects of loss or rejection by the birth family and attempts to determine an identity (Cox & Lieberthal, 2005). They may seek information about their biological family through a reunion registry. See Families Want to Know: Informing the Child About Adoption.

Children who are older when adopted must also make the commitment to the family relationship. They often have a memory of parents and other caregivers, so developing a close relationship with the adoptive parents takes more time. It may also be more challenging for the adoptive parents to develop as strong an emotional bond to the older child as occurs when an infant is adopted. Even when a serious commitment has been made to adopt an older child, adjustment of the family and child may be difficult for everyone. Counseling may be helpful to some families during the transition process.

International Adoptions

Over 150,000 families in the United States have adopted children from another country since 1989 and that number continues to increase. Many of these children have spent time in orphanages and are at increased risk for developmental and emotional problems (McGuinness & Dyer, 2006). Internationally adopted children often need special health care services. Nurses work with families that have adopted children from other countries to provide a comprehensive evaluation of the child to detect potential developmental problems and health conditions as soon as the child is brought into the country.

Emotional and psychological problems may be the result of long-term institutionalization in an orphanage, such as inconsistency in interpersonal development and delayed developmental milestones. The child and family may need counseling and support to help the child adjust to being part of a family. The initial response of the child who has been in an orphanage to the new parents may be crying or turning away. Children need a transition period of several months to adjust to a different daily routine and to bond with the parents. Exposing the child to large numbers of family members or to busy environments may be stressful to the child. The nurse may become involved in providing counseling to the family trying to integrate the adopted child into the family's life and routine (Figure 2–7 ➤). As the child grows, efforts to help the child understand the cultural birth heritage are also important.

Adoption Resource Websites

Families Want to Know

Informing the Child About Adoption

Most parents have anxiety about when and how to tell the child that he or she was adopted. There is no perfect age to tell the child about the adoption, so consider the child's age and developmental stage when sharing information.

■ Some authorities believe the child should be told at such a young age that the child will always know that he or she is adopted. This may be especially important when the child is of a different ethnic or racial group, or has very different physical characteristics than the parents.

■ The terms *adoption, adopted, birth family,* or *biologic family* should be part of the family's natural conversation (Borchers et al., 2003).

■ Decide when you and the child are most ready to introduce the topic of adoption—such as when a discussion of babies and where they come from occurs. However, avoid waiting for "just the right moment" because children may wonder what other information has not yet been shared.

■ Make sure the child is told before a third party is likely to say something. The chances of this happening increase as the child enters school.

■ Tell the child in a matter-of-fact manner about the adoption. Let the child know how much he or she was wanted and that some personal qualities of the child made the selection special. Avoid phrases such as "given up" for adoption. A more positive phrase to use is that the biologic family made an adoption plan in the best interest of the child's future.

■ Make sure the child understands that his or her place in the family is permanent. The adoptive family's commitment to the child should be repeated frequently.

■ Be willing to honestly discuss the child's biological family and the adoption process so the child feels comfortable asking questions. More discussion about adoption will be needed as the child grows older, especially when the child begins to ask at about 5 to 6 years of age why he or she was not wanted by the biological parents. Anticipate that the child will grieve about the loss of the birth parents.

■ As the child grows older and asks for more information about the birth parents, provide what information is known and try to help the child deal with information that is difficult to hear. Help the child decide what information to share with strangers, friends, and extended family members.

■ Recognize that the adolescent may fantasize about the birth parents and want to find them. Listening to the adolescent's concerns and providing support during this challenging time of development is important.

■ FAMILY THEORIES

Families must be understood in their own context. It is important to understand each family's strengths and uniqueness and how the family and its members respond to the complex and often conflicting demands for time and attention.

Family social system theories are helpful in understanding family functioning, environment–family interchange, family changes over time, and family response to health and illness. A brief review of family theories provides a context about family functioning that can assist with planning nursing care and developing future partnerships with families and their children.

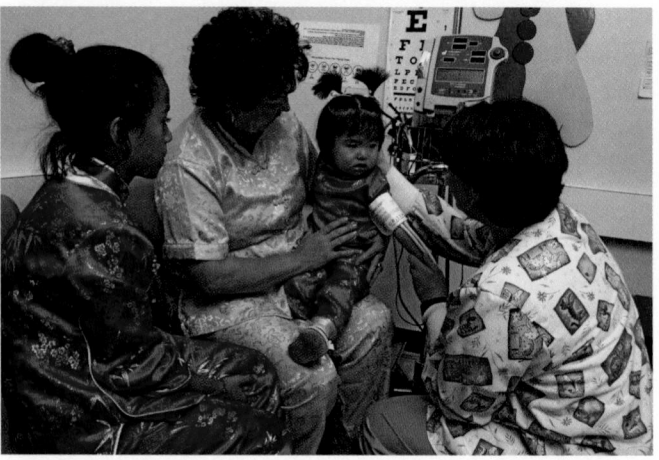

FIGURE 2–7 ➤ Adopted children who are of mixed race or a different ethnic group than the parents may cause a few additional challenges for the adoptive parents. Family members may be less supportive of the adoption initially. Because the children may have different physical characteristics, the family may capture more attention than it wishes. The family needs to learn to appreciate the different cultures represented in the newly formed family.

Each family has structure and functions to help it maintain stability while responding continuously to various stresses and strains within the family and in the family's interactions and functioning within the community. Families develop and modify their responses and functioning over time to adapt or be tolerant of family, community, and environmental changes. Family processes include the behaviors and strategies that help to regulate space, time, energy, and other aspects of family functioning to promote family stability, growth, and control.

Family Development Theory

Family development theories use a framework to categorize a family's progression over time according to specific, typical stages in family life. These are predictable stages in the life cycle of every family, but they follow no rigid pattern. Duvall's (1977) eight stages in the family life cycle of a traditional nuclear family have been used as the foundation for contemporary models of the family life cycle that describe the developmental processes and role expectations for different family types. Table 2–5 lists the eight stages of Duvall's family life cycle to illustrate important developmental transitions that occur at some point in most families.

Life cycle stages have been developed for the more contemporary blended families, dual-career families, and others. Although each family is unique, the members experience fairly predictable, similar, and consistent changes (Friedman, Bowden, & Jones, 2003). Developmental tasks, goals, or challenging issues for the family in each stage have been defined for different family types.

Nurses can assess families by their developmental stage, how well they are fulfilling the tasks of that stage, and the availability of resources to accomplish developmental tasks. The stages provide a method for anticipating transitions and potential stressors with family role changes that occur at different points along the developmental continuum for different family types. By un-

TABLE 2–5	Eight-Stage Family Life Cycle
Stages	Characteristics
Stage I	Beginning family, newly married couples*
Stage II	Childbearing family (oldest child is an infant through 30 months of age)
Stage III	Families with preschool children (oldest child is between 2.5 and 6 years of age)
Stage IV	Families with school-age children (oldest child is between 6 and 13 years of age)
Stage V	Families with teenagers (oldest child is between 13 and 20 years of age)
Stage VI	Families launching young adults (all children leave home)
Stage VII	Middle-aged parents (empty nest through retirement)
Stage VIII	Family in retirement and old age (retirement to death of both spouses)

*Keep in mind that this was the norm at the time the model was developed, but today families form through many different types of relationships.
Adapted from: Duvall, E. M. (1977). Marriage and family development (5th ed.). Philadelphia: Lippincott; Duvall, E. M., & Miller, B. C. (1985). Marriage and family development (6th ed.). New York: Harper Row; Friedman, M. M., Bowden, V. R., & Jones, E. G. (2003). Family nursing: Research, theory, and practice (5th ed.). Upper Saddle River, NJ: Prentice Hall; Gedaly-Duff, V., Heims, M. L., & Nielsen, A. E. (2009). Family child health nursing. In J. R. Kaakinen, V. Gedaly-Duff, D. P. Coehlo, & S. M. H. Hanson, Family health care nursing (4th ed., pp. 332–378). Philadelphia: F. A. Davis.

derstanding the family's developmental stage, the nurse can analyze the family growth and health promotion needs and identify developmental transitions and potential stressors. This enables the nurse to identify the types of teaching and anticipatory guidance that might be needed.

Family Systems Theory

Family systems theory, in which there is interaction between the components (family members) of the system (family) and between the system and the environment, was developed by Murray Bowen in the mid-1970s (Friedman et al., 2003). A family is a living social system, consisting of a small group of individuals who are closely interrelated and interdependent while collaborating to attain family functions and goals. In short, the family is more than the sum of its members (Hanson & Kaakinen, 2009; Kaakinen & Hanson, 2004). In family systems theory, due to the amount of interrelationship and interdependence in the family, any change or stressor experienced by one or more family members affects the entire family and causes disruption. Families are adaptable, and can change interactions and behaviors associated with the disruption in response to positive feedback.

From a systems perspective, the family may or may not exchange materials, energy, and information with its physical, social, and cultural environments. An *open family* seeks information and resources, and actively interacts with the community to solve problems. A *closed family* views change and offered support as a threat, and resistance to outside influences is a strategy the family uses to maintain control. These attributes have an effect on the capacity of the family to adapt—to modify behavior and change as the situation demands (Hanson & Kaakinen, 2009; Kaakinen & Hanson, 2004).

Family systems theory encourages nurses to see the child and parents as participating members of a whole family (Hanson & Kaakinen, 2009). It encourages looking at the processes within the family and the relationships between subsystems (spouse, parent–child, and siblings) and suprasystems (the community within which it is embedded). Stress and crises motivate the family to mobilize its resources and to begin problem solving.

Using this perspective, the nurse can assess the effects of illness or injury on the entire family system and the reciprocal effects of the family on the illness or injury. Assessing how open or closed the family is to information and resources is important in planning nursing care. Open families will be more receptive to referrals and interventions from health professionals. The nurse will need to work with the closed family to establish trust and acceptance before the family is receptive to ideas and interventions proposed.

Family Stress Theory

Family stress theory focuses on the family's response to unexpected or unplanned events. These events are generally stressful and can be very disruptive for the family (Hanson & Kaakinen, 2009). Most families have developed coping strategies to deal with routine stressors (e.g., completion of household chores, homework). Nonroutine stressors (such as surgery or the birth of a child) and unexpected events (accidents or emergency room visits) are often more stressful because the family has not had time to review resources and prepare a response.

Families experience many stressors as an inevitable part of life. Some stressors are positive, such as the birth of a child that leads to transitions within the family. Other stressors are unexpected and not considered positive, such as learning that a child has a serious health condition. Many families live in a stressed state due to inadequate finances, health care concerns, relationship challenges, and other pressures.

No one theory is sufficient for viewing the needs and behaviors of all families. The theories previously described herein continue to evolve as researchers identify new or broadened explanations for behaviors, so it is difficult to attach one specific theorist to each family theory. When assessing families, you may find it useful to consider more than one of these theories to help you understand the full set of behaviors associated with individual families and to plan effective nursing interventions.

■ FAMILY ASSESSMENT

Nurses need to be able to assess family strengths and support mechanisms, to identify strategies for **coping** (the use of learned behavioral and cognitive strategies to manage or relieve perceived stress), and to determine when families have overextended their resources and need additional support. In some cases, nurses can provide the additional support needed. At other times, referral to other health professionals is appropriate to address the family's needs.

Children and families live within a variety of settings and interact with those settings in ways that directly or indirectly influence behaviors and learning. Because of these environmental influences on the family, it is important to consider the relationship of the family with the social networks within the community.

Family Stressors

A child's illness or injury affects every member of the family. Such a stressor demands a response from the family members that can change the way they interact with each other and with other people. Nurses need to identify and assess how families respond to the stress of illness or injury of a child or other family members because of the potential hardships it causes the entire family.

Family Strengths

Family strengths are the positive relationships and processes that support and protect families and family members during times of adversity and change. Nurses can use family strengths as an effective tool in problem solving within the family (Wright & Leahey, 2009). Four types of strengths that enable families to develop, adapt to change, and cope with challenges (Tarko & Reed, 2004) include:

- Individual or family traits, such as optimism or resilience
- Individual or family assets, such as finances
- Individual or family capabilities, skills, and competencies, such as problem solving
- Another quality less permanent than a trait or asset, such as motivation

An important focus for family assessment prior to planning nursing interventions is to identify the family's **resilience**, its capacity to develop strengths and abilities, to "bounce back" from the stress and challenges. When a family can control and deal with events satisfactorily, the family members gain a sense of competence, making them more resilient, in contrast to families who are overwhelmed by traumatic experiences. Characteristics of a resilient family include the following (Benard, 2007):

- Social competence, involving cultural flexibility, empathy, and caring
- Developing competence in communication skills
- Problem solving that involves planning, help seeking, and critical and creative thinking that enables them to make decisions
- Maintaining family flexibility and adapting to changing circumstances, while maintaining a commitment to the family as a unit
- Having a sense of purpose and belief in a positive outcome (can set goals, have optimism and faith)
- Connectedness and maintenance of supportive relationships outside the family

Most families have the capacity for resilience. However, they often need nursing support to help family members learn new skills, make adaptations, and gain confidence in their abilities to manage the challenges they face. Potential resources to foster re-

- **Communication skills**—the ability of family members to listen, gather information, and discuss their concerns in an honest and open manner
- **Shared family values and beliefs**—the family's common perceptions of reality and willingness to have hope and to appreciate that change is possible; family celebrations; family traditions
- **Intrafamily support**—the provision of support and reinforcement by extended family members to promote family cohesion and an atmosphere of belonging; family time and routines
- **Self-care abilities**—the family's ability to take responsibility for health problems and the demonstrated willingness of individual members to take good care of themselves
- **Problem-solving skills**—the family's use of negotiation in problem solving, using everyday experiences as resources, and focusing on the present rather than past events or disappointments; effective utilization of health care resources
- **Community linkages**—maintenance of active linkages with the community; reaching out to others in the social network including extended family and friends

silience include religious faith, finances, social support, physical health, family flexibility, and family coping mechanisms. Families with diminished resources will be more susceptible to disruption because of a health care crisis or event. Nurses need to help families identify their strengths and areas for improvement that will lead to increased resiliency.

Functional families use their strengths and a variety of coping strategies to successfully reduce stress. See Box 2–1 for family strengths that promote resilience and coping. Coping strategies of dysfunctional families include denial of family problems, exploitation of a family member, use of threats or withdrawal of affection and support, dominance and submissive patterns, and family substance abuse.

Nurses can use recognition of family strengths to develop rapport with the family. One approach is to help family members recognize that the strengths they have used in prior life experiences can apply to the current health care experience. Focus on family competence and acknowledge and validate family members' emotions. The more a family recognizes its strengths in managing the child's health problem, the more likely that family will become an effective partner in the process.

Collecting Data for Family Assessment

To obtain an accurate and concise family assessment, the nurse needs to establish a trusting relationship with the child and family. Identify the parent's and the child's greatest concern, and expect these concerns to be different. It is important to acknowledge these multiple concerns and demonstrate respect for the diversity of the family. The goal is to obtain family information that will be helpful in planning nursing interventions that will help the family care for the child and improve the child's outcomes while valuing each person within the family.

Information about the family is collected continuously during the health care process, through interviews, observations of the family interactions, reports from other health care providers or agencies working with the family, and family assessment tools. Family assessment data that are important to collect include the following:

- Name, age, sex, and family relationship of all people residing in the household
- Family type, structure, roles, and values
- Cultural associations, including cultural norms and customs related to childrearing and infant feeding
- Faith-based affiliations
- Support systems network, including extended family, friends, and community associations
- Communication patterns, including language barriers
- Environmental data—place of residence, condition of housing, number of persons living in the residence, sleeping arrangements, play areas, and neighborhood characteristics

See Chapter 5 ∞ for suggested data to collect about the psychosocial history and daily living patterns. Observation of the home and family members is recommended in some cases to obtain valuable information about family functioning.

Family Assessment Tools

Family assessment tools can be used to gather additional information about the family's functioning and can place particular focus on family stresses, coping strategies, and family strengths. Information about the way the family functions in nurturing its members, problem solving, and communicating may help iden-

tify strategies that are potentially more effective for management of the child's health care. They enable the nurse to work more effectively, such as collaborating with the family in planning for health maintenance and health promotion strategies.

Genogram

Information about family structure can be illustrated on a **genogram** (a pedigree that incorporates information about the family members' significant life events, health, and illness status over at least three generations). A genogram is used most often to focus on the health history of a family, although additional identifying features such as social class, occupation, place of residence, religion, and ethnicity may be added for the family assessment process. (See Chapter 3 ∞ for an example of a genogram.)

Family Ecomap

An **ecomap** illustrates the family's relationships and interactions with the social networks in the community, enabling the nurse and other health care providers to visualize the family's social network. By having the family participate in preparation of the ecomap, it is possible to have some information about how the family perceives or receives social support, as well as the strength of family relationships with significant other persons and organizations. The ecomap provides an opportunity to identify the community resources being used by the family and to highlight any potential community resources that may help promote the family's health. See Figure 2–8 ➤ for a sample ecomap for Casey's family from the chapter opener.

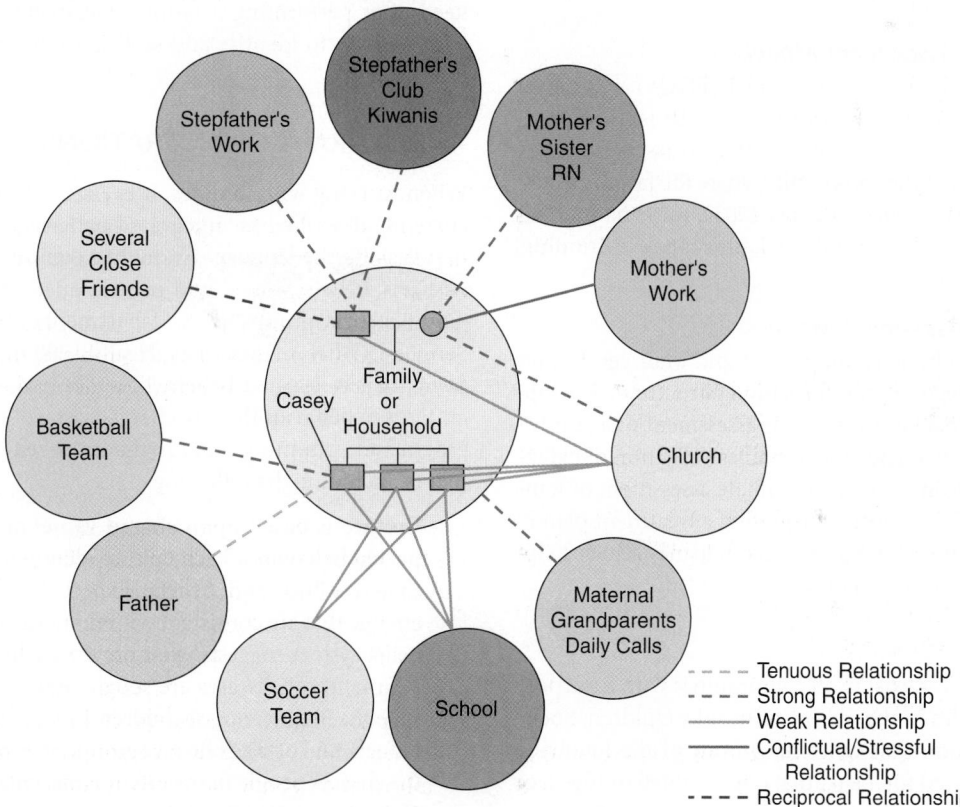

Ecomap of Casey's Family

----- Tenuous Relationship
- - - Strong Relationship
——— Weak Relationship
——— Conflictual/Stressful Relationship
- - - Reciprocal Relationship

FIGURE 2–8 ➤ An ecomap illustrates the family's relationships and interactions with groups and individuals in the immediate external environment.

Family APGAR

The Family APGAR is a quick five-item questionnaire that may be used as an initial screening tool for family assessment. The five family concepts measured include family adaptability, partnership, growth, affection, and resolve. The questionnaire can be administered quickly to family members over 10 years of age. Ask all family members to complete a separate copy of the questionnaire to gain a picture of the family's perspective on family functioning.

Home Observation for Measurement of the Environment (HOME)

The HOME Inventory is an assessment tool developed to measure the quality and quantity of stimulation and support available to the child in the home environment (Caldwell & Bradley, 1984). Four age-specific scales are available (birth to 3 years, 3 to 6 years, 6 to 10 years, and 10 to 15 years). Examples of subscales within each age-specific scale include parental responsivity, acceptance of the child, the physical environment, learning materials, variety in experience, and parental involvement. Data are collected during an informal, low-stress interview and observation over 45 to 90 minutes in the home setting. The child's primary caregiver and the child must be present and awake during the interview because observation of their interaction is an essential part of the assessment. The intent is to allow family members to act normally. Assessment of the home environment will help to identify factors that promote the child's growth and development, such as items in the home that can be used for toys and strategies for interacting with the child to promote learning.

Visit the companion website to find more information about the HOME Inventory and other models.

Friedman Family Assessment Model

The Friedman Family Assessment Model (FFAM) was developed by Marilyn Friedman to assist nurses with family assessment. This tool provides a method for nurses to assess the entire family in the context of the community where the family resides (Tarko & Reed, 2004; Friedman et al., 2003). Information collected contains data about a family's relationships, functioning, strengths, and problems.

Calgary Family Assessment Model

This tool, developed by Lorraine Wright and Maureen Leahey (2009), has three categories of information (structural, developmental, and functional family data) for assessment of a family's strengths and problems. The model enables collection of extensive family information, and it can facilitate assessment of family challenges, such as problems integrating a treatment plan in family routines. A family genogram or ecomap may also be helpful in completing the assessment.

Family Support Services

Family support services exist in all communities with a purpose of supporting families in the rearing of healthy children. Social support is information that can result in one of the following outcomes: feeling cared for, belief that one is valued or loved, or sense of belonging to a reciprocal network (American Academy of Pediatrics Task Force on the Family, 2003). Many factors stress families trying to provide for their children's needs, including divorced or single parenting, both parents being in the workforce, more time each day that parents and children are separated, and families separated from extended families and natural support systems. Families may also be stressed by economic factors, poor living conditions, or even homelessness. See Chapter 17 ∞. Many communities have worked to develop programs to support the health and development of children and to promote positive family relationships. Examples of these family support services include the following:

- Head Start and Early Head Start
- Before- and after-school programs for children of working parents
- School-based health and counseling services
- Play groups for preschool children
- Peer support groups
- Social service programs offered by the faith community
- Home visiting programs for high-risk children and parents
- Job skills training, adult education, and literacy programs
- Crisis care and respite care programs

Many of these family support services work to promote positive family relationships, parental competencies, and behaviors that contribute to the health and development of the children and family. Most programs are designed with the premise that no family is entirely self-sufficient and most can benefit from some external support.

Think about the formal and informal family support services in your community. Nurses play an important role in helping to link families to the types of community support services they need after performing a family assessment and collaborating with families to identify and seek assistance most beneficial to their needs.

■ CULTURAL CONSIDERATIONS

When working with families, it is essential to consider **culture**, currently described as "integrated patterns of human behavior that include the language, thoughts, communications, actions, customs, beliefs, values, and institutions of racial, ethnic, religious, or social groups" (U.S. Department of Health and Human Services: Office of Minority Health, 2005). Culture develops from socially learned beliefs, lifestyles, values, and integrated patterns of behavior that are characteristic of the family, cultural group, and community and is characterized by certain key elements, including the following:

- **Culture is based upon shared values and beliefs, and expected behaviors.** Each culture identifies and articulates its shared values and beliefs. Expected behaviors and roles emerge that are consistent with those values and beliefs. This belief system suggests what preventive health measures and treatment for diseases are sought and accepted. It may also state the importance of children, of the family, of other individuals, and of the collective group, all of which can influence the choices people in the culture make regarding health.
- **Culture is learned and dynamic.** A child is born into a culture and starts learning the beliefs and practices of the

Family Assessment Tool Websites

group from birth. Children who are members of two cultural groups, such as African and immigrant, learn about both groups as they grow and develop. Immigrants may face challenges when integrating the rules of the dominant culture. Children who have family members from two or more cultural groups integrate parts of the world view from each group. Therefore, although culture is connected with groups, each individual's manifestation of his or her cultural background will be unique. Culture evolves and adapts as new members are born into or join the group, and as the surrounding social and physical environments change. For example, as first-generation immigrants enter a new country, they generally closely follow the cultural patterns of their native lands. As their children grow, the youth maintain some of the family cultural patterns but begin to incorporate some of the new culture.

- **Culture is integrated into life and uses symbols.** Culture is integrated through social institutions such as schools, churches, mosques, synagogues, friendships, families, and occupation. This provides a variety of opportunities for learning about one's culture. The sense of integration may be disrupted or harder to maintain as individuals move frequently and as cultures intertwine with each other. Symbols are an important way that many cultures communicate with each other and with the outside world. Language, dress, music, tools, and nonverbal gestures are symbols used to display and transmit the culture (Figure 2–9 ➤).

Race refers to a group of people who share biological similarities such as skin color, bone structure, and genetic traits. Examples of races include White (sometimes called Caucasian or European American), Black (sometimes called African American in the United States), Hispanic, Natives (such as Native Americans, Alaskan Native, Hawaiian Native, and First Nation people of Canada), and Asian.

Ethnicity describes a "cultural group's sense of identification associated with the group's common social and cultural heritage" (Spector, 2009, p. 349). Examples of ethnic groups include Hmong, Jews, and Irish Americans. Even the mainstream or majority groups usually identify with an ethnic group. Some beliefs and practices are common among certain ethnic groups, but it is important to avoid **stereotyping** individuals, assuming that all members of a group have the same characteristics. The nurse should assess the child and family to see which characteristics common to a group are possessed by them rather than assume that because individuals identify themselves as a specific ethnicity they must practice certain customs.

Acculturation refers to the process of modifying one's culture to fit within the new or dominant culture. **Assimilation** is related to acculturation and is described as adopting and incorporating traits of the new culture within one's practice (Spector, 2009). Acculturation frequently occurs when people leave their country of origin and immigrate to a new country. Often acculturation is associated with improved health status and health behaviors, especially if the immigration is associated with improved socioeconomic status, which leads to better nutrition and access to health care. This is frequently true for people who immigrate to the United States from a developing country. On the other hand, health sometimes declines with acculturation. For example, obesity is a problem that is growing rapidly within the United States and particularly among immigrant populations.

Cultural Assessment

In addition to the family assessment tools referred to on pages 37–38, there are several tools that can be used for cultural assessment of the family. See Table 2–6.

Nurses must also consider contexts, such as the person's family, culture, work, community, history, and environment. The person must be in a state of balance within all personal and contextual parts. Illness occurs as a result of imbalance of one or all parts of the person (mind, body, spirit).

Cultural Practices That Influence Health Care

Family Roles and Organization

A family's organization and the roles played by individual family members are largely dependent upon cultural influence. For example, culture may determine who has authority (head of household) and is the primary decision maker for other members of the family. Nurses should be alert for roles and functions in families. Teaching may need to be directed to those responsible for decision making in order to effectively promote the child's health.

Culture also defines gender roles, as well as the roles of the elderly and of extended family. In some cultures, major decisions for the family, including a child's health care, involve input from grandparents and other extended family members (Figure 2–10 ➤). Grandparents may even assume responsibility for care of the children in the family. In these cases, nurses must direct teaching for health promotion and demonstration for treatment procedures to the grandparent.

Family goals are also determined by cultural values and practices, as are family member roles and childrearing practices and beliefs. In some families, children are expected to take on responsibilities early and may be expected to take on tasks such as management of their own chronic disease and nutritional

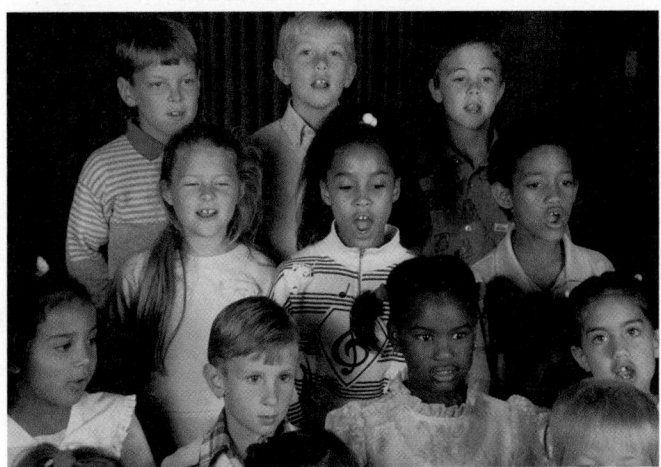

FIGURE 2–9 ➤ No longer are communities limited to one culture. The children in this multicultural choir are representative of the changes in demographics in the United States and Canada. Even though they may differ in cultural background, a common thread is found in their religious preference.

TABLE 2–6	**Cultural Assessment Models**		
Theorist	Model	Description	Components/Concepts
Dr. Madeleine Leininger	Sunrise Enabler	A guide that can be used to examine a variety of influences on care and culture.	• Cultural values and lifeways • Political and legal factors • Economic factors • Educational factors • Kinship and social factors • Religious and philosophical factors • Technological factors (Leininger, 2006, pp. 24–25)
Dr. Larry Purnell	Model for Cultural Competence	Twelve major concepts that are common to all cultures and can be assessed to provide important information about an individual child and family (Purnell & Paulanka, 2008).	• Overview, inhabited localities, and topography • Communications • Family roles and organization • Workforce issues • Biocultural ecology • High-risk health behaviors • Nutrition • Pregnancy and childbearing practices • Death rituals • Spirituality • Health care practices • Health care practitioners (Purnell & Palunka, 2008, p. 20)
Dr. Joyce Newman Giger and Dr. Ruth Davidhizar	Transcultural Assessment Model	The client is the center of care and culturally unique. Knowledge of the cultural heritage, beliefs, attitudes, and behaviors of the client is required to provide culturally competent care. This model is based on six phenomena that nurses must assess.	• Communication • Space • Social organization • Time • Environmental control • Biological variations (Giger & Davidhizar, 2008, p. 7)
Dr. Rachel Spector	HEALTH Traditions Model	Predicated on the concept of holistic health and describes practices that can be used to maintain, protect, and restore health. Health is a complex, interrelated, and balanced state of the physical, mental, and spiritual.	• Physical—all physical aspects, such as anatomical organs, gender, age, nutrition, genetic inheritance, body chemistry, and physical condition • Mental—cognitive processes, such as memories, thoughts, and knowledge of such emotional processes as feelings, self-esteem, and defenses • Spiritual—both positive and negative learned spiritual practices and teachings, dreams, stories, and symbols; protecting forces; and metaphysical or innate forces (Spector 2009, p. 77)

Data from: Giger, J. N., & Davidhizar, R. E. (2008). *Transcultural nursing: Assessment & intervention* (5th ed.). St. Louis, MO: Mosby Elsevier; *Leininger, M. (2006). Culture care diversity and universality theory and evolution of the ethno-nursing method. In M. M. Leininger & M. R. McFarland (Eds.),* Culture care diversity and universality: A worldwide nursing theory *(2nd ed., pp. 1–41). Boston: Jones and Bartlett; Purnell, L. D., & Paulanka, B. J. (2008).* Transcultural health care: A culturally competent approach *(3rd ed.). Philadelphia: F. A. Davis. Spector, R. E. (2009).* Cultural diversity in health and illness *(7th ed.). Upper Saddle River, NJ: Pearson Prentice Hall.*

intake. In other families, children are given long periods to grow up and are not expected to manage health care needs. Examples of childrearing practices common to particular cultures are listed in Table 2–7. Realize that the practices listed are common in these cultures, but not necessarily practiced by all members of that culture.

Communication

Communication is the method by which members of cultural groups share information and preserve their beliefs, values, norms, and practices. Information is transmitted through both verbal and nonverbal methods. Verbal communication consists of spoken or written words, including tone and level of voice, language, verbal style and dialect, and written material.

Obviously, verbal communication is improved when a health care provider speaks the same language as the patient and family. Children are most likely to speak both the language of the parents and the health care providers and may appear to be likely interpreters. However, it is recommended that children never be used to interpret in health care situations due to the confidentiality needs of both parent and child. Additionally, if children are used as interpreters, it can create an imbalance in power that could adversely affect parental authority. Signs, posted literature, and brochures should be available in the languages of the children and families served. Even when children speak the language of the health care providers, written material must be provided at a level that the family can read and understand.

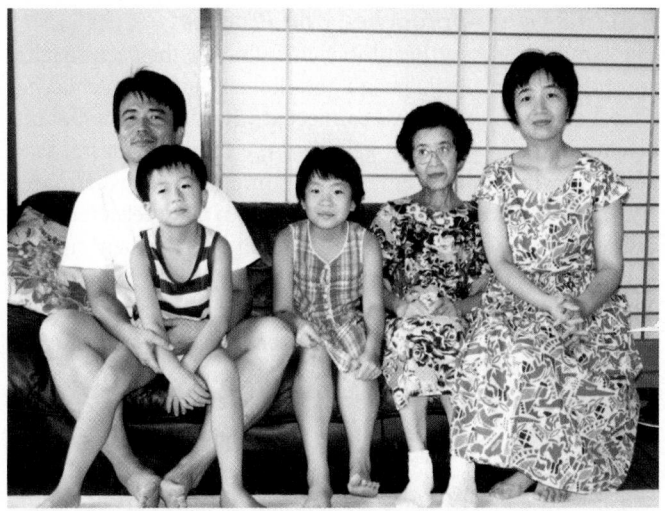

FIGURE 2–10 ➤ Many cultures value the input of grandparents and other elders in the family or group. For example, in this multigenerational family, the grandmother's guidance is highly valued and significantly influences the family's childrearing practices.

Language can also affect health literacy skills, as a large number of instructions are given in writing, including prescriptions and directions on medication bottles, signs hanging in health facilities, consent forms for procedures and surgery, insurance forms, directions for techniques or procedures, future appointment dates, and health promotion materials. Verify what the child and family can read and whether alternative methods should be used. Nurses can verbally give the information and provide paper and pencil so the family can take notes in their own language. Translation services should be available in all health care settings, including the pharmacy, the appointment desk, and for phone calls, in order to ensure access to services for all children and families served.

Nonverbal communication refers to body language such as posture, gestures, facial expressions, eye contact, and touch, as well as the use of silence. The nurse's use of nonverbal communication may hinder or help communication. Gestures and body language may be misunderstood or misinterpreted. For example, eye contact has different meanings among cultures. Silence is considered a sign of respect in some cultures. Watch

TABLE 2–7	Childrearing Practices of Selected Cultures
Culture	Childrearing Practices
African American	Grandmothers play an important role in the care of children. Extended family is very important Children are expected to demonstrate respectfulness, conformity to rules, obedience, and good behavior.
Amish	There is an average of seven children per family. Childrearing is regarded as the highest priority for parents. Grandparents often provide care to children. Children are expected to continue with the Amish tradition. Children are expected to follow the rules as prescribed by the church district.
Appalachian	Large families are common. Strict parenting practices and physical punishment are common. Grandparents frequently provide care to children.
Arab	The father is typically the disciplinarian. The child's character is considered a reflection of the family's influence. Children are expected to respect their elders and to have good behavior. Adolescents are expected to do well in their studies. Discipline may include physical punishment and shaming.
Chinese	The family may lavish resources on the child. Children typically depend on the family for all needs and may not be expected to earn their own money as adolescents. Male children are often more valued than female children. Children may be taught to avoid displaying their emotions/feelings. Children are expected to assist parents in the home (chores). High educational achievement is expected.
Mexican	Children are closely protected and are not encouraged to leave the home. Extended family members frequently live close by. Children are expected to demonstrate respect for parents and elder family members. Discipline may include physical punishment. Education is a priority.
Navajo Indian	Large families are important Grandmothers are important decision makers in the family Children are allowed to make decisions about their care.

Data from Purnell, L. D., & Paulanka, B. J. (2008). Transcultural health care: A culturally competent approach *(3rd ed.). Philadelphia: F. A. Davis.*

for patterns in various cultures and alter your approach to be more congruent.

Touch is another form of nonverbal communication. The appropriateness of touch varies by culture. Adults commonly feel that it is acceptable to touch children of all ages, but this may not be accurate. Look for responses from the child and family to touch. Nurses must touch children to weigh them, take blood pressures, and give immunizations, but this does not mean that close touch is appropriate at all times.

Clinical Tip

Speaking and reading may not occur in the same language. For example, an immigrant may read and speak fluently in a primary language and speak but not read the language of the new country. The immigrant's child may read and speak the language of the present country and speak but not read the native language of the family. Always ask about both reading and speaking preferences.

Time Orientation

Cultures have specific values and meanings regarding time orientation. Cultural groups may place emphasis on the events of the past, those events that occur in the present, or those that will occur in the future. Children reflect the time orientation of their families and of the cultures in which they live. Time is also influenced by development so that young children sometimes do not understand the use of clocks, the importance ascribed to being "on time," or other time orientations.

Time also refers to punctuality regarding schedules and appointments. In the United States and Canada, the predominant culture respects being on time and considers time valuable and not to be wasted. Other cultures may not emphasize the concern for time. This may be manifested by a family's inability to follow timed medication schedules or treatments, or to show up as scheduled for an appointment. In these cases, it is not intended as a sign of disrespect.

Nutrition

Nutritional practices begin even before birth as many cultural groups have beliefs that determine foods that are healthy to eat or should be avoided during pregnancy. Nutritional habits and patterns vary among cultures and are related to both religious practices and health beliefs. Certain cultures and religions have restrictions on or prescriptions about specific foods and preparation methods.

Additionally, some cultures value large size or may associate a healthy child with being "large." Other cultures value slimness and look down upon overweight individuals. Both of these views influence family eating patterns and expectations for the child; the child's self-esteem can therefore be influenced. Nutrition may also be essential to the culture's practices for health promotion and care during illness. Health problems associated with specific cultures may require dietary changes. Recognize that nutrition can be closely related to environmental situations. Families with few resources may not be able to obtain cultural foods due to access or financial issues. Nutrition plays a powerful role in maintaining health, so resources for nutritious and desired foods may be needed.

Health Beliefs, Approaches, and Practices

The family members' health beliefs influence their approaches and practices regarding health and illness. The young child has a view of health and illness connected with developmental understanding and gradually takes on the family's cultural view while growing older. Additionally, some families, when faced with a life-threatening illness of their child, may seek alternative health practices that are not considered part of their cultural heritage. This is especially true if the family becomes frustrated with traditional biomedical treatments that are unable to cure their child. See Table 2–8 for examples of health practices common to specific cultures. Nurses and other health care professionals should learn about the family's belief system and integrate all types of care that the family wishes as long as there is no danger to the child.

Faith-based belief and practice is an integral part of culture for some families. Views of religion and spirituality can shape their approaches and responses to a child's illness and guide practices to maintain health. Religious beliefs may influence the family's explanation of the cause of a child's illness, their perception of the severity of the illness, and choices of treatments for the illness, and can offer solace to the family and child. For these reasons, it is important to determine the influence of religion and spirituality within the family.

Faith and spirituality can be a source of great comfort and support for children who are ill and their families. Conversely, conflicts may arise between the family's religion or spirituality and biomedical care for the child. For example, the family's pursuit of specific religious therapies can serve as a barrier to biomedical care, because some parents may believe that their spiritual practices can substitute for medical treatment of the child. **Religion**, commonly referred to as **faith-based belief**, is an organized system of shared beliefs regarding the significance of the nature, cause, and purpose of life and of the universe. Religion is usually centered on the belief in or the worshipping of a supernatural or supreme being (such as God or Allah). **Spirituality** refers to the individual's experience and own interpretation of his or her relationship with a supreme being. Children in general are more open than adults to their spirituality because they have not yet been exposed to cultural pressures. Spirituality helps children to establish their values and beliefs (Hufton, 2006).

Specific differences in beliefs between families and health care providers are common in the following areas: help-seeking behaviors, causes of diseases or illnesses, death and dying, caretaking and caregiving, and childrearing practices.

These elements in differing degrees influence the cultural beliefs and values of an ethnic group, making the group unique. Misunderstandings may occur when the health care professional and the family come from different cultural groups. In addition, past experiences with health care may have made the family angry or suspicious of providers. Nurses must be able to recognize, respect, and respond to ethnic diversity in a way that leads to a mutually desirable outcome. The nurse must identify culturally relevant facts about the patient to provide culturally appropriate and competent care. For example, some cultural groups practice complementary and alternative therapies that are unknown to the nurse (see page 45). While some of these therapies are beneficial or cause

TABLE 2–8	Health Practices of Selected Cultures	
Culture	Health Practices	
African American	Religious healing (laying on hands) Talismans (amulets or lucky charms) Herbal remedies/oils Use of healers: "Old woman" healers	Voodoo healers Shamans Spiritualists Root doctors

Asian American	Acupuncture/acupressure
	Coin rubbing
	Cupping
	Herbs
	Hot and cold foods
	Massage
	Meditation
	Moxibustion (heat therapy)
	Qigong (combines meditation, movement,
	  and regulation of breathing)
		Restoring energy between yin and yang
		Tai chi
		Tiger balm
		Use of healers:
		  Physicians
		  Herbalists
		  Acupuncturists

European American	Healing rituals
	Dietary modifications
	Exercise
	Traditional medicine
		Amulets
		Use of healers:
		  Traditional health care providers:
		    physicians, nurses, and nurse practitioners

Hispanic or
Latin American
	Hot and cold foods
	Herbs
	Massage
	Prayers
	Religious medals
		Use of healers:
		  Curanderos/curanderas
		  Yerberos or jerberos (herbalists)
		  Brujos/brujas (witches)
		  Espiritistas (spiritualists)
		  Sobadores

Native American	Ceremony
	Counseling
	Herbs and plants
	Healing touch/acupressure
	Medicine bundle
	Singing
	Pipe ceremony
	Drumming and chanting (prayer)
		Smudging
		Sun dance
		Sweat lodge (purification ceremony)
		Vision quest (a powerful ceremony)
		Use of healers:
		  Medicine men or women
		  Shamans

Source: Data from Andrews, M. M., & Boyle, J. S. (2008). Transcultural concepts in nursing care (5th ed.). Philadelphia: Lippincott Williams & Wilkins; Giger, J. N., & Davidhizar, R. E. (2008). Transcultural nursing: Assessment & intervention (5th ed.). St. Louis, MO: Mosby Elsevier; Huebscher, R., & Shuler, P. A. (2004). Natural, alternative, and complementary health care practices. St. Louis, MO: Mosby; Fontaine, K. L. (2005). Complementary & alternative therapies for nursing practices (2nd ed.). Upper Saddle River, NJ: Prentice Hall; Spector, R. E. (2009). Cultural diversity in health and illness (7th ed.). Upper Saddle River, NJ: Pearson Prentice Hall.

no harm, others may interact with prescribed medications and cause harm.

Clinical Tip

Avoid imposing your personal cultural values on the children and families in your care. By learning about the values of the different ethnic groups in the community—religious beliefs that have an impact on health care practices, beliefs about common illnesses, and specific healing practices—you can develop an individualized nursing care plan for each child and family.

A collaborative relationship among the family and the health care team that addresses cultural values and respects diversity is essential in providing optimal family-centered care (Gance-Cleveland, 2006). The nurse should also consider the potential that an extended family member may need to be consulted regarding the treatment plan for the child, especially if the child spends a lot of time with extended family members.

Nurses demonstrate appropriate strategies to delivering culturally sensitive care when they develop techniques in assessing the influence of culture on the child and family and incorporate that information into an individualized plan of care. When the family's cultural values are incorporated into the care plan, the family is more likely to accept and adhere to the recommended care, especially in the home care setting.

Culturally competent nurses find effective ways to work with the family to determine how they can incorporate prescribed therapies with their health care practices. Ensure that the child

Culture  *Traditional Health Care Providers*

When appropriate, collaborate with the family to determine the role traditional health care providers and other practitioners, such as folk healers and spiritualists, will have in the care of the child. Encourage collaboration and communication between practitioners to ensure continuity of care.

and family understand the problem or illness, treatment, and health promotion activities. Apply culturally sensitive techniques when dispelling any cultural myths.

Nurses can also collaborate with a multidisciplinary team including social workers and language specialists to assist the family in receiving assistance with barriers to care such as transportation, financial issues, remote access, and others.

■ COMPLEMENTARY AND ALTERNATIVE MODALITIES

Complementary and alternative modalities (CAM) are defined as a group of diverse medical and health care systems, practices, and products that are not presently considered to be part of conventional medicine (NCCAM, 2009a).

- **Complementary therapy** is a product or treatment used together with conventional medicine, for example, the use of massage therapy along with pain medication in a child.
- **Alternative therapy** is a product or treatment used in place of conventional medicine. Examples include the use of herbal medicines instead of conventional cancer therapies.

CAM use among specific cultural groups has been in practice for thousands of years. The use of CAM in the United States is widespread and is found in all cultural groups. Four out of 10 adults used CAM in 2007. While 12% of children (1 in 9) used CAM in the prior 12 months, the percentage was higher when their parents used CAM (Barnes, Bloom, & Nahin, 2007). Parents may choose to use CAM because the therapies conform to their beliefs and values regarding health and life (Kemper, Vohra, Walls, et al., 2008).

The NCCAM (2009a) classifies CAM into five categories: whole medical systems, mind–body interventions, biologically based therapies, manipulative and body-based methods, and energy therapies. Some examples of CAM used in children are provided in Table 2–9.

Safety Issues Concerning CAM Therapies

The misleading claims of usefulness, dosing safety of some products, and lack of manufacturing standards of natural products are just a few of the issues raised with the use of herbs and natural products. Parents often believe that herbs and natural products are less likely to be harmful than prescribed medications, failing to recognize that safety concerns exist. However, "natural" is not the same as safe, and many CAM products have not been evaluated for use in children. Examples of problems that may occur with the use of CAM include:

- Interaction with prescribed medications (interferes with metabolism of medication or increases the effect of the prescribed medication, like an overdose)
- Side effect or allergic reaction directly associated with the product
- Substitution of the product for a prescribed medication that is potentially lifesaving
- Toxic effects because of contaminants or other additives in the product, or if the plant used for the herb was incorrectly identified

Some CAM can be encouraged for use in children with conventional medical therapies. The following CAM therapies have demonstrated effectiveness (Ernst, 2006):

- Acupuncture for nausea and vomiting
- Biofeedback or massage for constipation
- Biofeedback or hypnotherapy for headache
- Hypnotherapy for irritable bowel syndrome

Other CAM therapies are used effectively for relaxation and pain management, such as guided imagery, deep breathing exercises, and meditation.

CAM practices must be assessed for safety, including positive and negative benefits, cost, efficacy, and clinical usefulness. To date, limited research has been conducted on the safety and effectiveness of CAM for children. Parents may not share information about the use of CAM because they do not think these therapies are relevant or of interest to the health care provider. Several professional organizations, including the Society of Pediatric Nurses and the American Academy of Pediatrics, have affirmed that children and families should be educated about the benefits and risks of CAM, while being respectful of the family's desires to use these therapies. All health care providers must become knowledgeable about the broad range of CAM therapies to help families understand potential benefits and risks to the child (Asher, 2007; Kemper et al., 2008). See Families Want to Know: CAM Therapies.

Nursing Alert

The Society of Pediatric Nurses has affirmed that nurses must educate children and families about the benefits and risks of complementary and alternative medicine (CAM) (Asher, 2007). All health care providers must become knowledgeable about CAM and the people who are providing these therapies to be able to balance risks and benefits to the child (Kemper & Cohen, 2004). The use of CAM in the care of children must be addressed because of the limited research with this age group and developmental variations that may influence efficacy and safety.

Families Want to Know

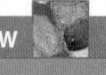

CAM *Therapies*

Once the nurse has been informed about CAM therapies used, potential side effects and risks can be considered, such as interactions between an herb and a prescribed medication. Partner with the family to promote the following safe practices for CAM use (NCCAM, 2009b):

- Ensure that your child has received an accurate diagnosis from a licensed health care provider and that CAM use does not replace or delay conventional medical care.
- If you decide to use CAM for your child, do not increase the dose or length of treatment beyond what is recommended. More is not necessarily better.
- If your child experiences an effect from a CAM therapy that concerns you, contact your child's health care provider.
- Store herbal and other dietary supplements out of the sight and reach of children.

TABLE 2–9	Common Types of Complementary and Alternative Modalities		
Therapy	Description	Potential Use in Children	Nursing Implications
Aromatherapy	Essential oils (extracts or essences) from flowers, herbs, and trees provide strong pleasant odors to promote relaxation, health, and well-being.	The family may use candles or oils to promote a child's pain relief or to encourage the child's relaxation. Use of aromatherapy in the hospital may reduce nausea due to hospital odors.	Few side effects when used as directed; however, allergies to oils may worsen symptoms in a child with asthma and other pulmonary disorders. Caution these families to avoid aromatherapy.
Dietary supplements	A product (other than tobacco) is taken by mouth that contains an ingredient intended to supplement the diet, such as vitamins, minerals, herbs or other botanicals, amino acids, and substances such as enzymes, organ tissues, and metabolites. Dietary supplements come in many forms, such as extracts, tablets, capsules, liquids, and powders. They have special labeling requirements.	Many parents administer daily multiple vitamins to their children. Adolescents may use creatine to improve body image or athletic performance (Kemper et al., 2008). Echinacea is an herb that is frequently used to treat a cold.	Assess the family's use of dietary supplements for the child. Determine potential interactions between supplements and prescribed medications. Teach parents about safe dosages and safe storage of vitamins and other dietary supplements for children.
Massage	Therapists press, rub, and manipulate muscle and soft tissues to enhance function of those tissues and promote relaxation, well-being, and relief of pain.	Massage has been found to be beneficial for reducing the symptoms of asthma, insomnia, colic, cystic fibrosis, and juvenile rheumatoid arthritis. It is used in NICUs to promote growth of preterm infants (Kemper et al., 2008).	Assess the child for benefits of massage. Potential contraindications to massage therapy may include bleeding disorders, fractures, and an open or healing wound.
Therapeutic touch	In therapeutic touch the healing force of the therapist affects the patient's recovery. Healing is promoted when the body's energies are in balance. By passing their hands over the patient, without touching the patient, healers can identify energy imbalances.	The family may enlist a spiritualist or other practitioner to perform therapeutic touch on their child to promote pain relief or a quicker recovery.	Assess the benefits of therapeutic touch on the child (e.g., pain relief). Partner with the family to establish other methods of pain relief if therapeutic touch is not effective.
Faith-based therapies	Spiritual healing, including prayer, is the most prevalent complementary therapy in the United States (Kemper et al., 2008). Other faith-based therapies may include faith healing, laying on hands, meditation, and anointing.	Families may include a variety of faith-based therapies depending on the child's condition. Spiritual health may help improve quality of care, decrease anxiety, and increase positive feelings, such as hope, optimism, and freedom from regret.	Provide the child and family a private environment for faith-based practices. Assess for benefits of the therapies. Partner with the family to determine if alternative methods of therapy are needed.

Source: Data from: National Center for Complementary and Alternative Medicine. (2009). What is complementary and alternative medicine (CAM)? *Retrieved, from http://www.nccam.nih.gov/health/whatiscam; National Cancer Institute. (2009a). Spirituality in cancer care. Retrieved from http://www.cancer.gov/cancertopics/pdq/ supportivecare/spirituality/Patient/; Kemper, K. J., Vohra, S., Walls, R., and the Task Force on Complementary and Alternative Medicine, the Provisional Section on Complementary, Holistic, and Integrative Medicine. (2008). The use of complementary and alternative medicine in pediatrics.* Pediatrics, 122(6), 1374–1386.

NURSING MANAGEMENT

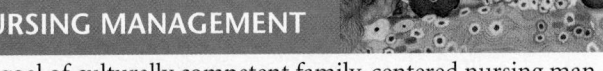

The goal of culturally competent family-centered nursing management is to assess and help families recognize their strengths and resiliency. This information can then be used in collaboratively planning the nursing care with the child and family.

Nursing Assessment and Diagnoses

The presence of a newly acquired disability, such as has occurred in Casey's family, adds a dimension of developmental risk. The child and family members may respond with either psychological or behavioral problems, or they may respond in a more positive manner.

Collect the psychosocial history and daily living patterns data from the family and child. Assessment of the culturally diverse child and family includes determining the family's health care practices such as health traditions, health beliefs, health-seeking behaviors, health care practitioner, and religion or spirituality.

Select the appropriate family assessment tool to collect information that can help evaluate the family's strengths and resources. Analyze the information collected and focus on key information that will help develop a plan of care for the child and family. Follow these steps:

- Determine how this condition influences family functioning.
- Identify how all of the family members have responded to the child's acute condition and disability.
- Obtain information about how the family is considering management of the child's care at home.
- Determine if other family issues or stressors must be integrated into the plan of care.
- Identify the family's expectations of different health professionals and facilities to help manage the child's care.
- Prepare an ecomap and genogram.

Examples of nursing diagnoses that may result from the family and home assessment include:

- Compromised Family Coping related to multiple simultaneous stressors
- Interrupted Family Processes related to child with a significant disability requiring alteration in family functioning
- Risk for Caregiver Role Strain related to child with a newly acquired disability and the associated financial burden
- Impaired Social Interaction (Parents and Child) related to lack of family or respite support

Planning and Implementation

Like all families, Casey's family needs support to increase resources and coping behaviors so they can successfully manage the multiple stressors of daily living along with a child's chronic condition.

Establishing a therapeutic relationship with the family is an important intervention. This relationship should be characterized by empathy and trust, as well as the development of mutually identified goals for the child's care. To help families develop resiliency, focus on family competence and strengths. Acknowledge and validate their emotions. Provide information in a clear, timely, and sensitive manner. Ask questions that help direct the family's thinking rather than providing them with all of the answers. Teach families to identify solutions until they are able to independently problem solve. Linkage with other families who have faced similar situations may be helpful.

Assist the family to begin planning for ongoing care using family-centered principles:

- Identify the primary decision maker for the child's health care.

- Discuss the family's goals for managing the child's care in the home setting.
- Consider how the family's strengths and previous problem-solving experiences can be integrated into the intervention.
- Consider the family's ethnic and religious background in developing intervention recommendations. Assist the child and family to determine how they can incorporate prescribed therapies with their health care practices. Ensure that the child and family understand the child's illness, treatment, or health promotion. Apply culturally sensitive techniques when dispelling any cultural myths.
- Ask questions in a respectful and nonjudgmental manner to help identify a family's use of CAM, encouraging the parent to share the information.
- Offer the family one or more potential interventions rather than trying to force one intervention. Be open to modifying the intervention or devising an alternative intervention to better match the family's lifestyle or cultural preferences.
- Identify the type of support or assistance the family would like to have.
- Identify potential resources in the community that match the child's and the family's needs for support. Collaborate with the family to discuss those resources and to select those that are acceptable to the family.
- Make sure the family has a care coordinator, especially when a family member seems to be unable to assume the case management role initially. Assist families in obtaining resources through such actions as role rehearsal, providing instructions and support when making an initial call, or connecting with another family support person who can help with resource linkage.
- Refer families with moderate or severe dysfunction to community resources for social support and counseling as appropriate.

Evaluation

Expected outcomes of nursing care include:

- Collaboration of the child and family with an assigned case manager so that interventions are implemented as recommended by the nurse and health care team
- Appropriate care provided by the family to the child with an acquired disability

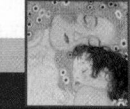

Chapter Highlights

- A family is composed of individuals who are joined together by marriage, blood, adoption, or residence in the same household, sharing resources and emotional closeness. Family membership often changes over time.

- Family-centered care is the development of a mutually beneficial partnership between families and the nurse, and also other health professionals. Each party respects the knowledge, skills, and experience that the other brings to the health care encounter. Partnering with families in the provision of health care is essential to promote the best outcome when caring for children.

- Various family composition models are common in today's society, including nuclear families, extended families, blended or reconstituted families, single-parent families, binuclear families, heterosexual cohabiting families, and gay and lesbian families.
- Health-related events may cause unexpected stresses for the parents, such as changed relationships with their parents, changes regarding employment, and lifestyle changes.
- Positive family relationships are characterized by parent–child warmth and supportiveness, and these traits help buffer children from stress while promoting positive social and cognitive outcomes.
- Parenting is a leadership role in the family in which children are guided to learn acceptable behaviors, beliefs, morals, and rituals of the family, and to become socially responsible contributing members of society.
- Discipline is a method for teaching the rules that govern behavior or conduct. Punishment is the action taken to enforce the rules when a child misbehaves.
- The quality of the relationship between the divorced parents has an important impact on their future relationships with their children. Better maintenance of family and kinship ties results when divorced parents are able to minimize the conflict and continue sharing parenting.
- Stepparenting that involves the blending of two families leads to the need to identify and renegotiate new customs, traditions, rituals, and routines for the family. A child must adjust to the stepparent, and vice versa.
- The goal of foster care is to ensure the safety and well-being of vulnerable children by placing them in an approved living situation, away from the family of origin, that is legally coordinated by the state's child welfare system.
- Adoption is a legal relationship between a child and parents not related by birth in which the parents assume legal and financial responsibility for the child. Many children are adopted from foreign nations.
- Family social systems theories help in understanding the family functioning, environment–family interchange, family changes over time, and family response to health and illness.
- Resilience is the family's capacity to develop strengths and abilities to bounce back from the stresses and challenges faced, and to eliminate or minimize negative outcomes.
- Family strengths are the relationships and processes that support and protect families and family members during times of adversity and change. These strengths enable families to develop, adapt to change, and cope with challenges.
- Family assessment tools are used to gather information about the family's functioning with regard to characteristics such as nurturing its members, problem solving, and communication. Information gathered helps the nurse work more effectively with the family in meeting the child's health care needs.
- Culture is a significant determinant of an individual's beliefs, behavior, and response to health and illness. Parental beliefs and behaviors can either promote the child's health care or impede preventive care, delay or complicate medical care, or result in the use of ineffective or harmful remedies.
- Complementary and alternative modalities (CAM) are defined as diverse medical and health care systems, practices, and products that are not presently considered to be part of conventional medicine.
- Cultural barriers to health care include lack of cultural awareness and sensitivity in health care providers, health-seeking behaviors, perceptions of health and illness, how health information is communicated, socioeconomic factors, and inadequate access.
- Cultural competence refers to the ability of the nurse to understand and respond effectively to the cultural needs of the child and family.

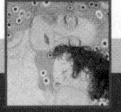

Clinical Reasoning in Action

Think about Casey and his family from the beginning of the chapter. Casey's family is coping with his initial survival of a serious brain injury, and facing a long rehabilitation process. The family is just now recognizing that life as they have known it is changing.

Casey is totally dependent for care including bathing, toileting, feeding, and mobilizing. Although he is expected to regain self-care abilities, the impact of the injury on his cognitive ability and future functioning is unknown.

Casey's extended family has provided support to the family during the past 12 days, but the level of support in the future weeks will decrease because of other family obligations. Casey's mother has already initiated a leave of absence from work so she can care for him when he returns home; however, this will mean the family has reduced income during that time period. Casey's younger brothers have been able to visit him, and they are very anxious because Casey cannot talk with them. They have been trying to avoid bothering their mother and father during this time, but they are wondering when life will be more normal and they can again participate in their usual after-school activities.

1. What information about the family strengths, needs, and resilience can be identified from the chapter-opening scenario, the ecomap on page 37, and the previous information?

2. What additional information would be helpful to know about family strengths and needs prior to developing a nursing care plan?

3. Based on your assessment of the family and challenges facing them, list at least one nursing diagnosis (additional to those listed on page 46) that addresses issues important for planning nursing care for Casey and his family.

4. Describe the use of family-centered care principles in planning Casey's nursing care in collaboration with the family.

See Pearson Nursing Student Resources for possible responses.

Pearson Nursing Student Resources

Find additional review materials at
nursing.pearsonhighered.com
Prepare for success with NCLEX®-style practice questions, interactive assignments and activities, web links, animations and videos, and more!

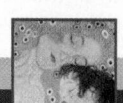

References

Adoption.com. (2010). *Summary of the Adoption and Safe Families Act of 1997.* Retrieved, from http://library.adoption.com/articles/summary-of-the-adoption-and-safe-families-act-of-1997.html

American Academy of Child and Adolescent Psychiatry. (2008). *Children and divorce.* Retrieved, from http://www.aacap.org/cs/root/facts_for_families/children_and_divorce

American Academy of Pediatrics. (2004). Fathers and pediatricians: Enhancing men's roles in the care and development of their children. *Pediatrics, 113*(5), 1406–1411.

American Academy of Pediatrics, Committee on Pediatric Emergency Medicine; American College of Family Physicians, Pediatric Emergency Medicine Committee. (2006). Patient- and family-centered care and the role of the emergency physician providing care to a child in the emergency department. *Pediatrics, 118*(5), 2242–2244.

American Academy of Pediatrics Task Force on the Family. (2003). Family pediatrics: Report of the Task Force on the Family. *Pediatrics, 111*(6), 1541–1571.

Arai, Y.-C. P., Ito, H., Kandatsu, N., Kurokawa, S., Kinugasa, S., & Komatsu, T. (2007). Parental presence during induction enhances the effect of oral midazolam on emergence behavior of children undergoing general anesthesia. *Acta Anaesthesiologica Scandinavica, 51,* 858–861.

Asher, C. (2007). Position statement on complementary and alternative medicine in pediatrics. *Journal of Pediatric Nursing, 22*(2), 159–161.

Barnes, P. A., Bloom, B., & Nahin, R. L. (2007). Complementary and alternative medicine use among adults and children: United States, 2007. *National Health Statistics Reports, 12,* 1–24.

Baumrind, D. (2005). Patterns of parental authority and adolescent autonomy. *New Directions for Child and Adolescent Development, 108,* 61–69.

Benard, B. (2007). *The foundations of the resiliency framework: From research to practice.* Retrieved from http://www.resiliency.com/htm/research.htm

Borchers and Committee on Early Childhood, Adoption, and Dependent Care, American Academy of Pediatrics. (2003). Families and adoption: The pediatrician's role in supporting communication. *Pediatrics, 112*(6), 1437–1441.

Caldwell, B. M., & Bradley, R. H. (1984). *The Home Observation for Measurement of the Environment.* Little Rock: University of Arkansas.

Childstats.gov. (2009). *America's children: Key national indicators of well-being, 2009.* Retrieved from http://www.childstats.gov/americaschildren/famsoc1.asp

Chipungu, S. S., & Bent-Goodley, T. B. (2004). Meeting the challenges of contemporary foster care. *The Future of Children, 14*(1), 75–93.

Clark, M. J. (2008). Care of families. In M. J. Clark, *Community health nursing: Advocacy for population health* (5th ed., pp. 317–348). Upper Saddle River, NJ: Pearson Prentice Hall.

Cox, S. S., & Lieberthal, J. (2005). Intercountry adoption: Young adult issues and transition to adulthood. *Pediatric Clinics of North America, 52,* 1495–1506.

Craig, G. J., & Dunn, W. L. (2007). *Understanding human development.* Upper Saddle River, NJ: Pearson Prentice Hall.

Dingeman, R. S., Mitchell, E. A., Meyer, E. C., & Curley, M. A. Q. (2007). Parent presence during complex invasive procedures and cardiopulmonary resuscitation: A systematic review of the literature. *Pediatrics, 120,* 842–854.

Dokken, D., & Ahmann, E. (2006). The many roles of family members in "family-centered care"—Part 1. *Pediatric Nursing, 32*(6), 562–565.

Douglas, E. (2006). *The effects of divorce on children.* University of New Hampshire Cooperative Extension. Retrieved from http://ceinfo.unh.edu

Duvall, E. M. (1977). *Marriage and family development* (5th ed.). New York: Harper & Row.

Duvall, E. M., & Miller, B. L. (1985). *Marriage and family development* (6th ed.). New York: Harper & Row.

Egemen, A., Ikizoglu, T., Karapinar, B., Cosar, H., & Karapinar, D. (2006). Parental presence during invasive procedures and resuscitation: Attitudes of health professionals in Turkey. *Pediatric Emergency Care, 22*(4), 230–234.

Ernst, E. (2006). Complementary and alternative medicine for children: A good or a bad thing? *Archives of Diseases in Childhood, 91*(2), 96–97.

Evan B. Donaldson Adoption Institute. (2008). *Expanding resources for waiting children II: Eliminating legal and practice barriers to gay and lesbian adoption from foster care. Policy & practice perspective.* Retrieved from http://www.adoptioninstitute.org/publications/2008_09_Expanding_Resources_Legal.pdf

Friedman, M. M., Bowden, V. R., & Jones, E. G. (2003). *Family nursing: Research, theory, and practice* (5th ed.). Upper Saddle River, NJ: Prentice Hall.

Gance-Cleveland, B. (2006). Decreasing health disparities. *Journal for Specialists in Pediatric Nursing, 11*(1), 72–76.

Gedaly-Duff, V., Heims, M. L., & Nielsen, A. E. (2009). Family child health nursing. In J. R. Kaakinen, V. Gedaly-Duff, D. P. Coehlo, & M. H. Hanson, *Family health care nursing* (4th ed., pp. 332–378). Philadelphia: F. A. Davis.

Giger, J. N., & Davidhizar, R. E. (2008). *Transcultural nursing: Assessment & intervention* (5th ed.). St. Louis, MO: Mosby Elsevier.

Hanson, S. M. H., & Kaakinen, J. R. (2009). Theoretical foundations for family nursing. In J. R. Kaakinen, V. Gedaly-Duff, D. P. Coehlo, & S. M. H. Hanson (Eds.), *Family health care nursing* (4th ed., pp. 332–378. Philadelphia: F. A. Davis.

Hicks-Pass, S. (2009). Corporal punishment in America today: Spare the rod, spoil the child? Systematic review of the literature. *Best Practices in Mental Health, 5*(2), 71–88.

Hufton, E. (2006). Parting gifts: the spiritual needs of children. *Journal of Child Health Care, 10*(3), 240–250.

Institute for Family-Centered Care. (2009). *Patient and family resource centers.* Retrieved, from http://www.familycenteredcare.org/advance/topics/pafam-resource.html

Jones, M., Qazi, M., & Young, K. D. (2007). Ethnic differences in parent preference to be present for painful medical procedures. *Pediatrics, 116*(2), 191–197.

Kaakinen, J. R., & Hanson, S. M. H. (2004). Theoretical foundations for family health nursing practice. In P. J. Bomar (Ed.), *Promoting health in families* (3rd ed., pp. 93–113). Philadelphia: Saunders.

Kemper, K. J., & Cohen, M. (2004). Ethics meet complementary and alternative medicine: New light on old principles. *Contemporary Pediatrics, 21*(3), 61–72.

Kemper, K. J., Vohra, S., Walls, R., and the Task Force on Complementary and Alternative Medicine, the Provisional Section on Complementary, Holistic, and Integrative Medicine. (2008). The use of complementary and alternative medicine in pediatrics. *Pediatrics, 122*(6), 1374–1386.

Kreider, R. M., & Elliott, D. B. (2009). America's families and living arrangements: 2007. *Current Population Reports.* Washington, DC: U.S. Census Bureau.

Leininger, M. (2006). Culture care diversity and universality theory and evolution of the ethnonursing method. In M. M. Leininger & M. R. McFarland (Eds.), *Culture care diversity and universality: A worldwide nursing theory* (2nd ed., pp. 1–41) Boston: Jones and Bartlett.

Lewandowski, L. A., & Tesler, M. D. (Eds.). (2003). *Family-centered care: Putting it into action. The SPN/ANA guide to family-centered care.* Washington, DC: American Nurses Association.

Maxton, F. J. C. (2008). Parental presence during resuscitation in the PICU: the parents' experience. Sharing and surviving the resuscitation: a phenomenological study. *Journal of Clinical Nursing, 17,* 3168–3176.

McGuinness, T. M., & Dyer, J. G. (2006). International adoption as a natural experiment. *Journal of Pediatric Nursing, 21*(4), 276–288.

National Center for Complementary and Alternative Medicine (NCCAM). (2009a). *What is complementary and alternative medicine (CAM)?* Retrieved from http://www.nccam.nih.gov/health/whatiscam/

National Center for Complementary and Alternative Medicine (NCCAM). (2009b). *CAM use in children.* Retrieved from http://www.nccam.nih.gov/health/children

O'Malley, P. J., Brown, K., & Krug, S. E. and the Committee on Pediatric Emergency Medicine (2008). Patient- and family-centered care of children in the emergency department. *Pediatrics, 122*(2), e511–e521.

Pawelski, J. G., Perrin, E. D., Foy, J. M., Crawford, J., Del Monte, M., Kaufman, M., et al. (2006). The effects of marriage, civil union, and domestic partnership laws on the health and well-being of children. *Pediatrics, 118*(1), 349–364.

Piira, T., Sugiura, T., Champion, G. D., Donnelly, N., & Cole, A. S. J. (2005). The role of parental presence in the context of children's medical procedures: A systematic review. *Child: Care, Health & Development, 31*(2), 233–243.

Portnoy, S. M. (2006). The psychology of divorce: A lawyer's primer, Part 2: The effects of divorce on children. *American Journal of Family Law, 21*(4), 126–134.

Purnell, L. D., & Paulanka, B. J. (2008). *Transcultural health care: A culturally competent approach* (3rd ed.). Philadelphia: F. A. Davis.

Raphel, S. (2008). Kinship care and the situation for grandparents. *Journal of Child and Adolescent Psychiatric Nursing, 21*(2), 118–120.

Regalado, M., Sareen, H., Inkelas, M., Wissow, L. S., & Halfon, N. (2004). Parents' discipline of young children: Results from the national survey of early childhood health. *Pediatrics, 113*(6), 1952–1958.

Sacchetti, A., Paston, C., & Carraccio, C. (2005). Family members do not disrupt care when present during invasive procedures. *Academic Emergency Medicine, 12*(5), 477–479.

Schneiderman, J. U. (2006). Innovative pediatric nursing role: Public health nurses in child welfare. *Pediatric Nursing, 32*(4), 317–321.

Slade, E. P., & Wissow, L. S. (2004). Spanking in early childhood and later behavior problems: A prospective study of infants and young toddlers. *Pediatrics, 113*(5), 1321–1330.

Socolar, R. R. S., Savage, E., & Evans, H. (2007). A longitudinal study of parental discipline of young children. *Southern Medical Journal, 100*(5), 472–477.

Spector, R. E. (2009). *Cultural diversity in health and illness* (7th ed.). Upper Saddle River, NJ: Pearson Prentice Hall.

Strijker, J., Knorth, E. J., & Knot-Dickscheit, J. (2008). Placement history of foster children: A study of placement history and outcomes in long-term family foster care. *Child Welfare, 87*(5), 107–124.

Tarko, M. A., & Reed, K. (2004). Family assessment and intervention. In P. J. Bomar (Ed.), *Promoting health in families* (3rd ed., pp. 274–298). Philadelphia: Saunders.

U.S. Census Bureau. (2008). *Current Population Survey (CPS)—Definitions and explanations.* Retrieved from http://www.census.gov/population/www/cps/cpsdef.html

U.S. Department of Health and Human Services. (2008a). *The AFCARS Report.* Retrieved, from http://www.acf.hhs.gov/programs/cb/stats_research/afcars/tar/report14.htm

U.S. Department of Health and Human Services. (2008b). *Trends in foster care and adoption—FY 2002–FY 2007.* Retrieved from http://www.acf.hhs.gov/programs/cb/stats_research/afcars/trends_02-07.pdf

U.S. Department of Health and Human Services. (2009a). *Foster Care Independence Act of 1999.* Retrieved from http://www.acf.hhs.gov/programs/cb/laws_policies/cblaws/public_law/pl106_169/pl106_169.htm

U.S. Department of Health and Human Services. (2009b). *Adoption USA: A chartbook based on the 2007 national survey of adoptive parents.* Retrieved from http://aspe.hhs.gov/hsp/09/NSAP/chartbook/chartbook.cfm?id=1

U.S. Department of Health and Human Services: Office of Minority Health. (2005). *What is cultural competency?* Retrieved, from http://www.omhrc.gov/templates/browse.aspx?lvl=2&lvlid=11

U.S. Department of Labor. (2009). *Fact Sheet No. 28: The Family and Medical Leave Act of 1993.* Retrieved from http://www.dol.gov/esa/whd/regs/compliance/whdfs28.pdf

U.S. Department of State. (2007). *Immigrant visas issued to orphans coming to the U.S.* Retrieved from http://www.travel.state.gov/family/adoption/stats/stats_451.html#

Wallerstein, J. S., & Blakeslee, S. (2004). *What about the kids? Raising your children before, during, and after divorce.* New York: Hyperion.

Whenan, R., Oxlad, M., & Lushington, K. (2009). Factors associated with foster carer well-being, satisfaction, and intention to continue providing out-of-home care. *Children and Youth Services Review, 31,* 752–760.

Wright, L., & Leahey, M. (2009). *Nurses and families: A guide to family assessment and intervention* (5th ed.). Philadelphia: F. A. Davis.

Genetic and Genomic Influences

chapter 3

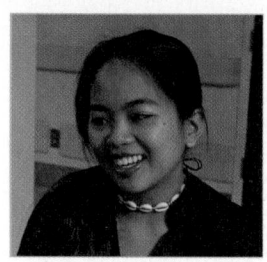

Sarah Hart is a mature 17-year-old who arrives alone at the clinic for a sports physical. Sarah was raised by her mother, Diane, and does not know her father. Sarah appears anxious and tells the nurse about her concerns. Sarah has memories of her mother's father dying from Huntington disease when she was 8 years old, and she has recently begun researching information. She knows that Huntington disease is inherited in an autosomal dominant pattern with symptoms often manifesting by age 40 years and that symptoms often begin earlier with succeeding generations. Sarah also knows there is no treatment or cure for Huntington disease. Diane will not discuss her father's death or the inheritance issues with Sarah even though they have a very close relationship. Sarah states that her mother is a free spirit and always "lives in the moment." Sarah, on the other hand, has told the nurse that she is concerned about whether she should save money, attend college, pursue a career, get married, have children, or just live in the moment herself, travel, and take on no responsibilities. Sarah would like to be tested to see if she has the altered gene and will develop Huntington disease, but her mother strongly objects. Diane is not interested in knowing if she has the altered gene. If Sarah were found to have the dominant gene that causes Huntington disease, it could be inferred that her mother also has the gene.

Does the nurse have enough knowledge about genetics to evaluate Sarah's knowledge and also to provide reinforcement of information and guidance to Sarah? Is Sarah able to give informed consent for genetic testing or is she too young to make a decision? Where can the nurse refer Sarah to find the answers to her questions in order to make an informed decision? If Sarah tests positive for the altered gene, will she blame her mother? How will a positive finding impact their roles and relationship?

Learning Outcomes

After completing this chapter, you will be able to:

1. Explain the role of genetic and genomic concepts in health promotion, disease prevention, screening, diagnostics, selection of treatment, and monitoring of treatment effectiveness.
2. Elicit a minimum three-generation family health history and construct a pedigree using standardized symbols and terminology.
3. Incorporate knowledge of genetic and genomic influences and risk factors into physical assessment.
4. Identify children or families who might benefit from genetic information and services.
5. Recognize when to make a referral to a genetics professional.
6. Integrate basic genetic and genomic concepts into care planning and child and family education.
7. Understand implications of genome science on the nursing role with particular attention to ethical, legal, and social issues.
8. Discuss the significance of recent advances in human genetics and genomics and their impact on health care delivery.

Key Terms

alleles / 55
aneuploidy / 54
anticipation / 60
association / 66
autosome / 53
carrier / 58
cell / 53
consanguinity / 65
consultand / 63
copy number variation / 56
crossing over / 53
cytogenetics / 62
dominant / 57
dysmorphology / 64
epigenetic / 51
gamete / 53
gene / 55
gene expression / 51
genetic disease / 51
genome / 51
genome-wide association
 study / 56
genomics / 51
genotype / 55
heterozygous / 55
homologous chromosomes / 53
homozygous / 55
human genome / 53
independent assortment / 53
inversion / 54
karyotype / 53
major anomaly / 64
meiosis / 53
microarray analysis / 62
minor anomaly / 64
mitosis / 53
monosomic (monosomy) / 54
mosaicism / 54
multifactorial / 56

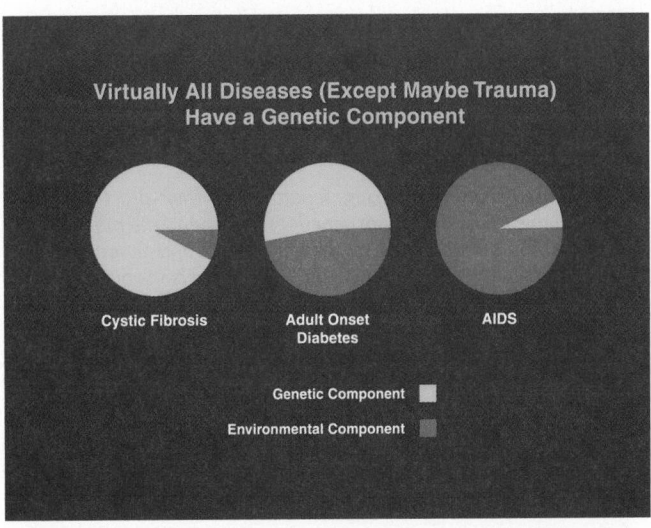

FIGURE 3–1 ➤ Although the causes for nearly all diseases and health conditions have both genetic and environmental components, the relative contribution of genetic and environmental influences varies widely. At one end of the spectrum lie "traditional" genetic diseases, such as cystic fibrosis (CF). Although CF is caused by a gene alteration, its morbidity and mortality vary according to environmental effects such as medical management. On the other hand, AIDS is an infectious disease that will not occur without environmental exposure to the HIV virus. Still, there are genetic alterations that cause some people to be resistant to HIV infection. In type 2 diabetes, the genetic and environmental contributions are fairly equivalent.

Source: Reprinted with permission of Francis Collins, M.D., Ph.D., Director, National Human Genome Research Institute, National Institutes of Health.

■ PARTNERING WITH FAMILIES: MEETING THE STANDARD OF GENETIC NURSING CARE DELIVERY

Completion of the Human Genome Project in 2003 heralded the dawn of the genomic era of health care. It has long been known that some diseases occur due to specific gene defects and therefore are often inherited. **Genetic diseases** have traditionally been thought of as inherited diseases, and while "typical" genetic diseases have enormous health consequences for affected individuals and families, they have relatively little public health impact. The Human Genome Project decoded human deoxyribonucleic acid (DNA), revealing the sequence of its 3 billion nucleotides or "letters." Research associated with the Human Genome Project has revealed virtually all diseases to have a genetic component. The human **genome** is the entire DNA sequence of an individual, and the study of **genomics** takes a holistic view of gene function. Human genomics is the study of all DNA in the human genome, including gene interactions with each other and with environmental, psychosocial, and cultural factors. While essentially all diseases and health conditions have both genetic and environmental components, the genetic contribution to various diseases varies widely (Figure 3–1 ➤).

DNA is central to our state of health because of its role in determining gene structure and gene function. There are about 23,000 genes in the human genome, and each gene directs the formation of one or more proteins. Proteins include enzymes, cell receptors, ion channels, structural molecules, antibodies, and other molecules necessary for biological function. Good health is dependent on both normal gene structure and normal gene function. Normal gene structure is necessary so that the proteins encoded by the gene have the correct amino acid sequence. Normal gene function means that genes are expressed (i.e., translated and transcribed to make protein products) at the appropriate time and in appropriate amounts to support normal physiological function. **Gene expression**, which is affected by all manner of environmental and **epigenetic** effects, is therefore just as important as gene structure. Genetic abnormalities may cause too much or too little of a specific protein, or perhaps a dysfunctional protein, to be formed, and increased risk for disease can result. Both traditional genetic disorders and common complex diseases such as heart disease, stroke, diabetes, and cancer are now known to be related to gene structure and function. Research has uncovered many of the genetic and environmental factors that increase risk for disease, leading to development of new treatments that range in scope from promoting healthy lifestyles to specific genetic therapies. Knowl-

edge gained from human genome research is changing all aspects of health care, including health promotion and disease prevention, screening, treatment, and monitoring of treatment effectiveness.

Nurses must be prepared to deliver genetically competent care in many health care settings to individuals, families, communities, and populations. Nurses in newborn nurseries and mother–baby units may be the first to suspect a newborn has a genetic condition. Pediatric nurses often care for children with genetic conditions, who may require frequent hospitalization. Nurses in general and specialty clinics must be prepared to help asymptomatic individuals and families who are increasingly seeking information about their risk for an inherited disease or condition. Parents who order direct-to-consumer genetic tests may bring questions about their results to nurses. For these and other reasons, nurses must achieve genetic and genomic literacy in order to deliver competent care in the genomic era.

The translation of genetic and genomic knowledge to clinical care requires nurses to integrate new genetic knowledge into their nursing practice. This expectation has been formally established by the American Nurses Association (ANA) and the International Society of Nurses in Genetics (ISONG) in a joint statement, *Genetics/Genomics Nursing: Scope and Standards of Practice*. This document outlines the levels of genetic knowledge required of all registered nurses, including basic and advanced practice nurses in general practice as well as those who specialize in genetics nursing (Box 3–1). In addition, a set of essential competencies in genetics and genomics has been defined and

BOX 3–1 ANA/ISONG Scope and Standards of Genetics/Genomics Nursing

The ANA/ISONG statement on the scope and standards of genetics and genomic nursing practice is as follows:

All licensed registered nurses, regardless of their practice setting, have a role in the delivery of genetics services and the management of genetic information. Nurses require genetics and genomics knowledge to identify, refer, support, and care for persons affected by, or at risk for manifesting or transmitting conditions or diseases with a genetic component. As the public becomes more aware of the genetic contribution to health and disease, nurses in all areas of practice are being asked to address basic genetics- and genomics-related questions and service needs.

endorsed by nearly 50 nursing organizations. These competencies represent the minimal level of genetic and genomic competency expected of every registered nurse across all practice settings (Consensus Panel, 2009). Examples of nursing activities that reflect genetic and genomic competence include:

- Identifying risk for disease by collecting a family history and drawing a three-generation pedigree
- Helping individuals and families to understand the implications and limitations of genetic testing
- Administering gene-based therapies
- Providing nondirective counseling to assist families who have questions or concerns about their reproductive risks
- Recognizing dysmorphic features that may indicate a genetic condition in a newborn
- Anticipating variable responses among individuals to "standard" medication doses, due to pharmacogenetic effects
- Ensuring the delivery of genetically competent care for the child and family, for example, ensuring that a child about to start thiopurine treatment has completed pharmacogenetic testing
- Helping individuals and families to identify credible sources of genetic information
- Applying concepts of health promotion and health maintenance to assist children and families at increased risk to develop common chronic conditions, such as heart disease, to make informed lifestyle choices
- Partnering with families affected by genetic conditions, including providing advocacy, supporting the child's and family's decisions, teaching, making appropriate referrals, clarifying information, and providing further information about available resources and services
- Partnering with the community to educate the public about genetics
- Supporting legislation to protect genetic information and to protect those with genetic conditions from discrimination
- Applying knowledge of the ethical, legal, and social implications of genetic information

Through informed application of fundamental genetic and genomic concepts, nurses can significantly improve the nursing care provided to children and their families. In fact, understanding and applying these concepts is an essential part of child and family nursing.

Impact of Genetic Advances on Health Promotion and Health Maintenance

Health promotion and health maintenance for children and their families are foundational for all nursing care (see Chapters 6 through 9 ∞). The genomic era offers a promise of personalized health care based on an individual's or a population's risk for disease, which varies according to the set of genes they inherited and a multitude of environmental factors. Although some people may be aware that they carry an altered gene associated with a specific disease, most individuals do not know details of their genetic makeup or how their genetic inheritance influences their future health. This is particularly true for common conditions such as heart disease and diabetes, where risk varies with inheritance of a number of altered genes and is modified by lifestyle factors such as diet and physical activity. Having specific knowledge about one's genetic makeup and associated increased risk for disease provides a basis for health screening and may provide motivation for people to maintain a healthy lifestyle. Imagine, then, if people knew their statistical risks for inheriting or developing disease, based on their specific genotype. Health promotion and health maintenance teaching and nursing interventions would be targeted to individuals according to their disease risk. Children and families may experience increased motivation to adhere to lifestyle choices and health screenings that are personalized according to their disease risk. Personalized health care is a major goal in the genomic era.

With knowledge of genetic conditions, the pediatric nurse can ensure health teaching and early detection of complications from genetic conditions with emphasis on primary and secondary care interventions. For example:

- Nurses should ensure informed consent for newborn screening and provide teaching and support to families whose infants have positive screens.
- Nurses should stress to all teenage girls the importance of folic acid (see Chapter 9 ∞) whether they consider themselves sexually active or not. Folic acid supplementation around the time of conception is demonstrated to significantly reduce the incidence of neural tube defects, a relatively common birth defect.
- A child who screens positive for scoliosis (see Chapter 29 ∞) should be assessed for axillary freckling and café au lait spots, due to the relationship between scoliosis and neurofibromatosis.
- Screening for Marfan syndrome (see Chapter 21 ∞) should be a part of all sports physicals, due to the lethal cardiovascular complication of aortic dilation. This can be accomplished by assessing for common characteristics such as myopia, scoliosis, tall stature, long fingers and thumbs, a hollow chest, and an arm span greater than the height.
- Nurses should both teach and support families regarding any specific interventions necessary to avoid complications in

BOX 3–2	**Using the People-First Approach**

The nurse must incorporate a person-first philosophy and use genetic terminology that is sensitive to the maintenance of an individual's positive self-image. When communicating genetic concerns to children, families, other health care providers, or the public, take care to use words that do not reflect value.

Use the term **wild type gene** or *expected gene* or *unaltered gene* (rather than "normal" gene) and *altered gene* or *disease-producing gene* (rather than "mutated" or "abnormal" gene).

Name the diagnosis rather than apply the label. For example, newborn Sammy, who exhibits Down syndrome, should not be identified as the "Down baby" but as Sammy who has Down syndrome. And describe Sally as having (a diagnosis of) autism, not as being autistic.

Also, the term *developmental disability* is preferred (rather than "mental retardation").

Adapted from: Snow, K. People First Language *at http://www.disabilityisnatural.com*

children with genetic conditions. Examples are the importance for children with phenylketonuria (PKU) to maintain a phenylalanine-free diet for life, and the need to maintain children with sickle cell disease (see Chapter 23 ∞) on penicillin.

• When caring for the child with Down syndrome (see Chapter 28 ∞), the pediatric nurse can help the parents shift from the more expected and traditional focus of disease management to health promotion and protection, by teaching parents about the established guidelines for exams and screenings specific to children with Down syndrome.

Early diagnosis and early intervention with health-promoting care that is specific to a genetic diagnosis allows children affected with genetic alterations to achieve maximal function, better health, and improved quality of life. The pediatric nurse must be able to identify both community-based and genetic-based resources that are available to assist the child or adolescent and the family with strategies to support both health promotion and health maintenance activities. See Box 3–2.

■ GENETIC BASICS

A basic knowledge of the cell, DNA, cell division, chromosomes, and genes is essential to deliver the genetic standard of care to children, adolescents, and their families.

The **cell** is the basic unit of life and the working unit of all living systems. Life starts as a single cell, but the developed human body is made up of trillions of cells. These cells share common features such as a nucleus that contains 46 chromosomes and **organelles** such as mitochondria. Cells are specialized in appearance and function, according to their location. For example, pancreatic cells function much differently than nerve cells.

All human cells, except red blood cells, contain a complete set of DNA molecules, which are long sequences of nucleotides. A nucleotide is a base with an attached sugar and phosphate group. Four different bases, designated A, C, T, and G, make up DNA. The order, or sequence, of these bases provides exact instructions

for protein building. The entire DNA in a human cell is referred to as the **human genome** and represents the complete set of inheritance for an individual. Most of the DNA is organized into chromosomes, which are contained in the cell nucleus. A small amount of DNA is found in the mitochondria, which will be discussed later in this section. Each person's genome is unique, with the exception of monozygotic twins who are derived from the same fertilized ovum and therefore share identical DNA.

Each cell nucleus contains about 6 feet of DNA that is tightly wound and packaged into 23 pairs of chromosomes, making a complete set of 46 chromosomes. The set includes 22 pairs of **autosomes**, which are by tradition numbered according to size, with chromosome 1 being the largest and chromosome 22 the smallest. There are two copies of each autosome, one inherited from the mother and the other from the father. Copies of a chromosome pair are called **homologous chromosomes**. The 23rd chromosome pair, the **sex chromosomes**, determine an individual's gender. A female has two copies of the X chromosome (one copy inherited from each parent), and a male has one X chromosome (inherited from his mother) and one Y chromosome (inherited from his father). The structure and number of chromosomes can be shown by preparing a **karyotype**, or picture of an individual's chromosomes (Figure 3–2 ➤). The sperm and ova represent exceptions to the 23-pair rule, because each contains only a single chromosome from each homologous pair.

Cell Division

Mitosis and meiosis are the two types of cell division in human cells. **Mitosis** takes place in somatic or tissue cells of the body, allowing the formation of new cells. Cell division by mitosis results in two cells called daughter cells that are genetically identical to the original cell and to each other. Mitosis is responsible for rapid human growth in early life and also replaces cells lost daily from skin surfaces and the lining of gastrointestinal and respiratory tracts.

Meiosis is also known as reduction cell division. Meiosis occurs only in the reproductive cells of the testes and ovaries and results in the formation of sperm and oocytes (**gametes**). Meiosis is similar to mitosis in that it is a form of cell division; however, through a series of complex mechanisms, the amount of genetic material is reduced to half. Each gamete contains a single copy of each of the 22 autosomes, plus a single sex chromosome. This is critical to ensure that when the two gametes combine during fertilization, the correct total number of chromosomes (46) is present in the offspring's cells. The other purpose of meiosis is to make new combinations of genetic material through processes of crossing over and independent assortment. New combinations are necessary to promote diversity in the human population. **Crossing over** results from an exchange or shuffling of material between homologous chromosomes inherited from the father and mother. This exchange results in new intact chromosomes that represent a patchwork of maternal and paternal genetic material. Only the Y chromosome does not have the ability to cross over, since it lacks a homologous mate. **Independent assortment** means that chromosome pairs segregate randomly into one or another gamete, further enhancing the genetic diversity that is possible at fertilization.

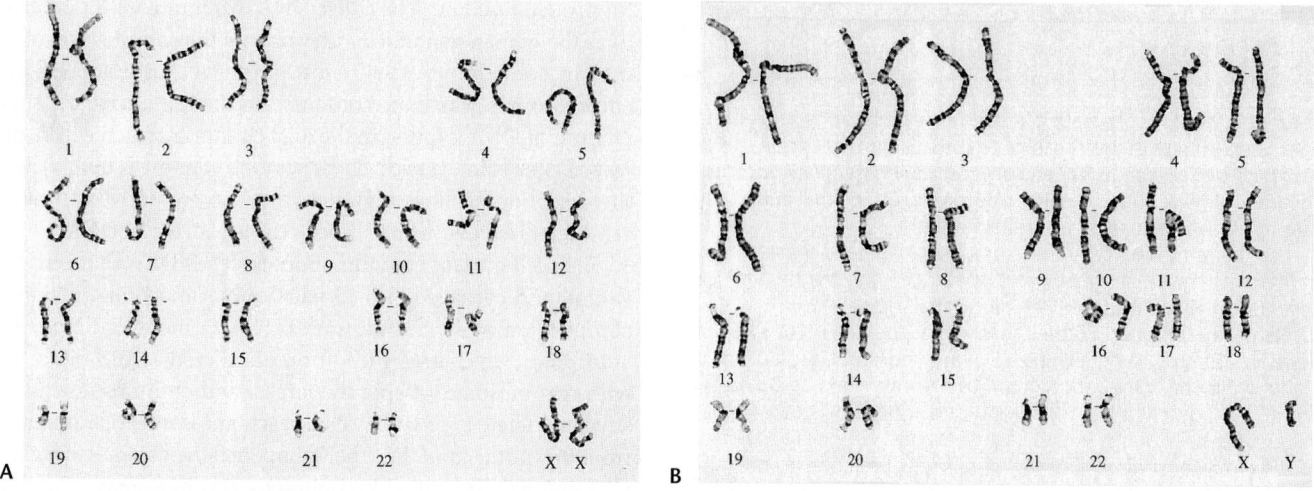

FIGURE 3–2 ➤ A karyotype is a picture of an individual's chromosomes. It depicts the number and structure of the 22 pairs of autosomes and the sex chromosomes. A, Female. B, Male.

Source: Courtesy of the Greenwood Genetic Center, Greenwood, SC.

Chromosomal Alterations

Alterations in chromosomes sometimes occur during cell division (meiosis or mitosis) and are classified as alterations in either chromosome number or chromosome structure. The clinical consequences of both types of alterations vary according to the amount of DNA involved.

Alterations in Chromosome Number

An increase or decrease in chromosome number is called **aneuploidy**. Aneuploidy is the result of an error during cell division, most often when **nondisjunction** occurs during meiosis. With nondisjunction, paired homologous chromosomes do not separate before migrating into egg or sperm cells. This creates a gamete with either two copies or no copies of a particular chromosome. When such a gamete is fertilized by a normal gamete with all 23 chromosomes, a **zygote** that is **monosomic** (missing one member of a chromosome pair) or **trisomic** (having three homologous chromosomes instead of the usual two) results.

In general, humans do not tolerate either extra or missing DNA very well. Most monosomic or trisomic conceptions result in early pregnancy loss. For example, Turner syndrome is the only monosomic condition that is compatible with life. Trisomies involving chromosomes with small numbers of genes may result in live births. Examples are trisomy 13 (Patau syndrome), trisomy 18 (Edwards syndrome), and trisomy 21 (Down syndrome). Each of these aneuploidies produces clinical features that vary according to the chromosome that is duplicated. It is not a coincidence that the three nonlethal trisomic conditions involve duplication of chromosomes containing the smallest number of genes (Nussbaum, McInnes, & Willard, 2007).

Mosaicism   Monosomy and/or trisomy can also occur during mitosis, resulting in an individual with two, or occasionally more, separate cell lines with different chromosomal makeup. This is known as **mosaicism**. The earlier in development the error occurs, the more cells that will be abnormal. The converse is also true. The degree to which a person is affected by this chro-

mosomal error varies. For example, individuals with mosaic Turner syndrome may show varying degrees of infertility or short stature, and an individual with mosaic Down syndrome may have a higher intelligence level than children whose every cell has three copies of chromosome 21.

Structural Chromosomal Alterations

Inversion   A chromosomal **inversion** occurs when a chromosome breaks in two places and the piece between the breaks turns end for end and reattaches within the same chromosome. An inversion changes the DNA sequence for that portion of the chromosome. Inversion often results in *balanced* rearrangements, because the amount of DNA in the chromosome remains normal. The clinical consequences of an inversion depend on how much chromosomal material is involved and where the inversion occurs. An inversion within the gene that codes for factor VIII, a clotting factor, is an important cause of hemophilia A.

Deletion and Duplication   Chromosomal alterations sometimes occur when unequal crossing over or abnormal segregation causes a chromosome to have a missing segment (deletion) or an additional segment (duplication) of genetic material. These are called *unbalanced* rearrangements. Conditions associated with unbalanced rearrangements may be incompatible with life or cause altered physical and/or mental development. An example is cri du chat syndrome, caused by a large deletion on chromosome 5. Children with cri du chat have developmental delays, low-set ears, and a peculiar cry during infancy that sounds like a cat mewing (Nussbaum et al., 2007).

Translocation   **Translocation** occurs when two, usually nonhomologous, chromosomes exchange segments of DNA. A translocation that results in a correct amount of chromosomal material but a new arrangement is a *balanced translocation*. The individual who has a balanced rearrangement has all of the chromosomal material present and therefore does not usually have any physical or mental disabilities. However, individuals with a balanced translocation are at high risk to produce gametes with unbalanced rearrangements. This leads to increased risk of pregnancy loss or having children with mental and/or physical disabilities due to missing or extra genetic material. A common *unbalanced translocation* is responsible for 3–5% of children diagnosed with Down syndrome (Ranweiler, 2009). When a child with Down syndrome is born, it is important to conduct a chromosome study to determine if the cause is nondisjunction or translocation. Translocation, while unrelated to maternal age, carries a significantly greater recurrence risk with subsequent pregnancies (Ranweiler, 2009).

Genes

In addition to understanding chromosomal alterations, the nurse must have knowledge of genes—what they are, their function, and the consequences of gene alterations. The nurse must understand the inheritance of gene alterations in order to design appropriate nursing interventions and teach the child, adolescent, and family at risk for or with a known genetic condition. Also, as genetic influences on common chronic disease are better understood, knowledge of gene function and inheritance has become increasingly relevant in health promotion and health maintenance.

A **gene** is a small segment of the nucleotide sequence of a chromosome that can be identified with a particular function, most commonly protein production. Each chromosome contains numerous genes arranged in a linear order. All genes that reside on autosomes (i.e., chromosomes 1 through 22) come in pairs, with one copy on each homologous chromosome. Because each gene copy is inherited from a different parent, differences in their nucleotide sequence likely exist; these different forms or versions of genes are called **alleles**. An individual who has two functionally identical alleles of a gene is said to be **homozygous** (*homo* = same) for that gene. An individual who has two different alleles of the gene is said to be **heterozygous** (*hetero* = different). As previously discussed, genes on the sex chromosomes of males are unpaired, since the X and Y chromosomes contain different genes.

Genes have a specific location on a designated chromosome; this is called the *genetic locus.* Gene mapping has documented the locus for most human genes. For example, it is known that the Huntington gene is located at the tip of chromosome 4, whereas the gene associated with cystic fibrosis is on chromosome 7.

Genes are described as *altered* or *mutated* when a change has taken place in their nucleotide sequence. Such a change may or may not result in an altered protein product; a gene alteration that does not change the protein product is called a silent mutation. Other changes in nucleotide sequence, perhaps at a locus some distance from the gene itself, may affect gene expression, or a gene's activity in making protein. Smaller, non-DNA molecules are also involved in gene expression; these epigenetic effects can cause genes to be overexpressed (making more than expected protein product), underexpressed (making less than expected), or expressed at a time in development when the gene is normally inactive. The observable, outward expression of an individual's entire physical, biochemical, and physiologic makeup, as determined by the person's genotype and environmental factors, is referred to as **phenotype**. Phenotype may be expressed as physical appearance such as curly or straight hair or physiologic function, for example, signs or symptoms of a disease.

Function and Distribution of Genes

It is believed that only about 2% of the human genome is actually represented by genes (Pierce, 2008). The vast majority of human DNA does not encode proteins. In humans, protein-coding DNA is organized into about 23,000 genes; each individual's particular set of genes represents his or her **genotype**. These 23,000 genes are responsible for encoding the more than 300,000 proteins that carry out all the functions in the human body (Pierce, Fakhari, Works, et al., 2007). Proteins are highly specialized and perform virtually all cellular functions. They form structures, transmit messages between cells, fight infection, direct genes to turn on or off, metabolize nutrients and drugs, and sense light, taste, and smell. Gene activity in making proteins can change moment to moment in response to thousands of intra- and extracellular signals. An example is the mechanism that stimulates cells to produce insulin after eating a candy bar. After eating, a gene on chromosome 11 directs pancreatic cells to produce, modify, and secrete insulin. Although the gene for producing insulin is present in all nucleated cells of the body, it is only functional in insulin-secreting pancreatic cells.

Mitochondrial Genes

Chromosomes in the cell nucleus are not the only site where genes reside. Mitochondria (organelles involved in energy metabolism, or the "powerhouse" of the cell) also contain a small amount of DNA identified as mitochondrial DNA (mtDNA). There are 37 genes on mitochondrial DNA (DiMauro, 2007). Mitochondria are the sites for energy production, and cells requiring large amounts of energy contain more mitochondria than other cells. Because ova have many mitochondria and sperm do not (most mitochondria are located in the tail of the sperm that detaches at fertilization), mtDNA is inherited from the mother in a *matrilineal* pattern. This creates a unique pattern of inheritance. A female with a mutation of a mitochondrial gene will pass that mutation to all of her children, whereas an affected male will not pass the mtDNA mutation to any of his children (Nussbaum et al., 2007). Clinical manifestations occurring as a result of mitochondrial gene alterations primarily affect high-energy tissues such as skeletal muscle, brain, and heart muscle (DiMauro, 2007).

Human Genetic Variation

The Human Genome Project and other genetic studies have shown that humans are remarkably similar to each other at the DNA level. On average, any two humans vary in only 0.1% of their nucleotide sequence. Perhaps 90% of human variation can be attributed to single nucleotide (or "single letter") changes in DNA sequence. DNA sequencing of hundreds of individuals around the globe has shown that these single nucleotide changes occur at about 17 million sites (or loci) across the genome (Genome Statistics, 2009); the rest of the genome is identical in 99% of individuals. That means most of human genetic variation can be attributed to variation at these 17 million loci. These single letter variations are called **single nucleotide polymorphisms** or SNPs (pronounced "snips"). Most SNPs are benign, although collectively they account for most phenotypic variation in appearance and risk for disease. By convention, SNPs known to be associated with disease are considered to be mutations and are often called point mutations, indicating the single nucleotide cause. SNPs have been mapped to the human genome, and the resulting SNP maps are of enormous value to researchers. For example, scientists exploring the genetic contribution to type 2 diabetes mellitus are comparing SNP patterns in large numbers of individuals with and without the disease to uncover genetic variations associated with this common multifactorial disease. Such **genome-wide association studies** (GWAS) are uncovering the genetic contribution to common chronic conditions that cause most of the disease burden in developed countries.

In recent years, DNA research has identified **copy number variation** as an additional source of human genetic variation. In some individuals, stretches of DNA of variable size (up to 3 million bases) are replicated one or more times. These DNA segments appear to be fairly common and can contain entire genes, resulting in more than expected gene product. In some cases, copy number variation has been associated with disease (Zhang, Gu, Hurles, et al., 2009).

Gene Alterations and Disease

An alteration in the DNA sequence of a gene may cause a defective protein to be formed, which may have clinical significance. Gene alterations can be inherited or they can be acquired. Mutations inherited from one or both parents (hereditary mutations) are also known as germline mutations, because the mutation exists in the reproductive cells or gametes. Consequently, the DNA in every cell of that offspring will have the gene alteration, which can then be transmitted to following generations.

The second kind of gene alteration is an acquired, or somatic mutation. Acquired mutations can occur in the DNA of cells of an individual at any time throughout a lifetime. They result from errors during cell division (mitosis) or environmental influences such as radiation, toxins, or viral infections. Acquired mutations are also called sporadic or *de novo* mutations. Most cases of cancer, for example, are due to somatic mutations. Somatic mutations are not directly inherited.

Single-gene alterations are responsible for approximately 6,000 hereditary diseases such as cystic fibrosis, Duchenne muscular dystrophy, and phenylketonuria. Each of these disorders is relatively rare, although collectively they affect 1 of every 300 newborns (Centers for Disease Control and Prevention [CDC], n.d.). Although they are of enormous consequence to affected families, they constitute a relatively small portion of the total public health burden.

Genes vary enormously in size, but all are very long, containing tens or even hundreds of thousands of base pairs. Consequently, mutations can occur at multiple different loci within a gene and result in a wide variety of signs and symptoms. For example, the cystic fibrosis transmembrane conductance regulator

(CFTR) gene on chromosome 7 encodes a protein that forms a chloride channel. More than 1,400 different CFTR mutations that disrupt the chloride channel have been identified. Over 1,000 of those mutations cause cystic fibrosis, but others are associated with milder disorders such as absence of the vas deferens, pancreatitis, and rhinosinusitis (CFTR, 2009).

Alterations as small as a single nucleotide are known to cause disease. Sickle cell anemia is such a disorder: a single A-for-T substitution in the HBB gene causes an incorrect amino acid (valine) to be inserted at a site in the protein product (β-globin) normally occupied by a different amino acid (glutamic acid). The altered β-globin protein is then incorporated into hemoglobin molecules. Under conditions of low oxygen tension, the altered β-globin causes red blood cells to assume an abnormal, sickle-like shape. This leads to vascular occlusion and hemolytic anemia (Steinberg, 2008).

In other situations, multiple gene alterations combine with environmental factors and lead to disease or health conditions. These conditions are called **multifactorial**. Most common chronic disorders, including hypertension, heart disease, type 2 diabetes, and most cancers, are multifactorial, as are several birth defects. Alterations in regulatory genes may also occur. Regulatory elements are stretches of DNA sequence, usually located away from a gene, that control gene expression or activity in making proteins. They include gene promoters, enhancers, silencers, and other control mechanisms and are important in maintaining homeostasis (Nussbaum et al., 2007). Mutation of a regulatory gene might lead to the loss of expression of a gene, unexpected expression in a tissue in which it is usually silent, or a change in the time when a gene is expressed. Smaller, non-DNA molecules are also known to affect gene function; these epigenetic factors are of great interest in genetics research.

Gene Alterations That Decrease Risk of Disease

Although gene mutations are commonly associated with disease, they can also be helpful and decrease the risk of disease. For example, having a single copy of some genes known to cause autosomal recessive disorders may confer some protection against disease. Individuals with a single altered sickle cell disease (SCD) gene have protection against malaria. Another protective gene alteration involves a deletion in the CCR5 gene, which encodes a cell receptor to which the HIV virus binds. Persons who have two copies of the altered CCR5 gene are almost completely resistant to infection with HIV type 1, and those who are heterozygous for the deletion (have one copy of the altered gene) progress much slower from the stage of HIV infection to AIDS (Piacentini, Biasin, Fenizia, et al., 2008). As genome research continues, more beneficial gene alterations are being identified. For example, genome-wide association studies (GWAS) have uncovered gene alterations that seem to be protective against type 2 diabetes and other disorders (Florez, 2008).

■ PRINCIPLES OF INHERITANCE

Knowledge of inheritance prepares the nurse to offer and reinforce genetic information to children, adolescents, and their families. Genetic knowledge may be important in assisting patients with care management and reproductive decision making. Basic underlying principles of inheritance that nurses can apply to inheritance risk assessment and teaching include: (1) nearly all genes are paired, (2) only one gene of each pair is transmitted (passed on) from each parent to an offspring, and (3) one copy of each gene in the offspring comes from the mother and the other copy comes from the father. Understanding of Mendelian patterns of inheritance is based on these principles.

Classic Mendelian Patterns of Inheritance

Conditions that are caused by a mutation or alteration of a single gene are known as monogenic or single-gene disorders. More than 6,000 known single-gene disorders have been catalogued, with detailed information posted to a searchable public database, the Online Mendelian Inheritance in Man (OMIM) (2009). Single-gene disorders are known as Mendelian disorders, because they are predictably passed on from generation to generation following Mendel's laws of inheritance (CDC, n.d.). Monogenic disorders that occur due to a mutation on an autosome (chromosome numbers 1 through 22) are inherited in either an autosomal dominant or autosomal recessive pattern. Disorders due to a mutation on one of the sex chromosomes are inherited in an X-linked, or occasionally Y-linked, pattern. See Table 3–1.

Dominant Versus Recessive Disorders

For some disorders, the presence of a single altered gene allele is enough to cause disease; these disorders are said to be **dominant**. An individual who is heterozygous for a dominant disorder will therefore have (or express) the disorder, despite the presence of the one functioning allele. Other disorders occur only when both alleles of a gene pair are altered. In these **recessive** disorders, the gene product produced from a single unaltered gene is enough to perform the expected function and maintain homeostasis (Nussbaum et al., 2007). Because most human genes reside on autosomes, the most common inheritance patterns are therefore called autosomal dominant or autosomal recessive.

Autosomal Dominant

More than half of the known Mendelian conditions are autosomal dominant (AD). Examples include neurofibromatosis, achondroplasia (dwarfism), Marfan syndrome, Huntington disease, and familial hypercholesterolemia. By definition, AD disorders involve altered genes on autosomes rather than the sex chromosomes X and Y. Disease occurs in AD disorders despite the presence of one unaltered gene, and most individuals with AD disorders are heterozygous for the disease-producing gene. Homozygous dominant conditions can occur, but they are

TABLE 3–1	Selected Genetic Conditions Inherited in a Mendelian Pattern	
Genetic Condition	Description	Inheritance Pattern
Achondroplasia	Abnormal bone growth resulting in short stature	Autosomal dominant More than 80% of cases represent a new mutation
Beta-thalassemia major	Reduced synthesis of hemoglobin beta chain resulting in anemia	Autosomal recessive
Cystic fibrosis	Complex multisystem disease leading to end-stage lung disease	Autosomal recessive
Duchenne muscular dystrophy	Progressive disease leading to atrophy of skeletal and/or cardiac muscle	X-linked recessive
Fragile X syndrome	Minimal-to-moderate developmental disability due to trinucleotide repeat expansion	X-linked recessive Anticipation is demonstrated
Gaucher disease	Several subtypes, but all are lipid storage diseases due to enzyme deficiency	Autosomal recessive
Hemophilia A	Bleeding disorder due to deficient factor VIII clotting activity	X-linked recessive About 30% of cases represent a new mutation
Marfan syndrome	Connective tissue disorder with cardiovascular, ocular, and skeletal involvement	Autosomal dominant 25% represent a new mutation
Neurofibromatosis (NF-1)	Variable expression with café au lait spots and benign cutaneous and subcutaneous neurofibromas	Autosomal dominant 50% of cases represent a new mutation
Phenylketonuria (PKU)	Enzyme deficiency results in accumulation of phenylalanine, inhibiting brain and cognitive development	Autosomal recessive
Sickle cell disease	Abnormal hemoglobin causes vaso-occlusive events and chronic anemia	Autosomal recessive
Tay-Sachs disease	Fatal neurodegenerative disorder of lipid accumulation due to enzyme deficiency	Autosomal recessive

Information adapted from GeneTests. Retrieved December 3, 2009, from http://www.ncbi.nlm.nih.gov/sites/GeneTests/?db=GeneTests

generally much more severe or lethal and frequently result in early pregnancy loss. For example, the child who is born homozygous for achondroplasia (short stature; short-limbed dwarfism) is much more severely affected than a heterozygous child and usually will not survive early infancy.

Inheritance Risk in Autosomal Dominant Conditions

Because the gene alteration in AD conditions occurs on an autosome rather than a sex chromosome, both males and females have an equal chance of being affected. There is a 50% chance that an affected parent will pass the altered disease-producing gene on to a child. Nurses must remember and teach families that each pregnancy is an independent event with a 50% chance of an affected child, no matter how many of a couple's previous children inherited the altered gene. Family histories will often reflect this 50% inheritance rate as well as both males and females being affected. An affected child always has an affected parent, who in turn also has an affected parent. See Box 3–3. Exceptions to this inheritance pattern occur when the condition is due to a spontaneous new mutation, as discussed later in this chapter.

Autosomal Recessive

Autosomal recessive (AR) conditions occur when both copies of the same gene in an individual are altered. Generally, AR conditions are more severe and have an earlier onset than conditions with other patterns of inheritance. Examples of AR conditions include cystic fibrosis, sickle cell anemia, Tay-Sachs disease, and most inborn errors of metabolism. Like autosomal dominant disorders, AR conditions involve genes on one of the 22 autosomes. A condition is called "recessive" when two copies of the altered gene are needed to express the condition. A child born with a recessive condition has therefore inherited one altered gene from each parent. Both parents are **carriers** of the condition. Usually carriers do not exhibit signs or symptoms (Nussbaum et al., 2007). There are, however, exceptions to this general rule, with sickle cell anemia (SCA) being an example. Although individuals with a single copy of the sickle cell gene are usually asymptomatic, they can develop symptoms in situations of extremely low oxygenation such as high altitudes. The heterozygous state for SCA (known as sickle cell trait) actually affords some evolutionary benefit, as a single copy of the SCA gene provides some resistance to malaria. Individuals whose ancestors are from malaria-endemic areas are therefore more likely to carry the sickle cell gene. See Culture: Ethnic or Population Groups and Autosomal Recessive Inheritance. Because carrier status usually confers no symptoms, parents are often unaware of their carrier status until they have an affected child.

Inheritance Risk in Autosomal Recessive Conditions

Because AR conditions do not involve genetic material on the sex chromosomes, males and females have an equal chance of inheriting the altered genes and exhibiting the condition. When both parents are carriers of an autosomal recessive gene alteration, each pregnancy presents the same inheritance risks. Each child born to carrier parents has a 25% chance of inheriting two copies of the altered gene and having the condition, a 50% chance of inheriting only one altered gene copy and being a carrier, and a 25% chance of inheriting both unaltered genes and thus neither being affected nor being a carrier. Remembering that each pregnancy is an independent event, these probability percentages remain constant with each pregnancy, no matter how many affected or unaffected children a family already has. This is often a difficult concept for parents to grasp, and the nurse should carefully evaluate the parent's level of understanding of this important detail about inheritance. See Box 3–4.

The transmission percentages stated previously apply when both parents are carriers of an autosomal recessive condition. Percentages will change if only one parent is a carrier, or if a parent is homozygous for the condition. The nurse must be able to teach a parent about these simple inheritance percentages.

X-Linked

X-linked conditions are the result of an altered gene on the X chromosome. Examples include hemophilia A and Duchenne muscular dystrophy. Recall that the sex chromosomes are unevenly represented in males and females. Males, with their single X chromosome, have just one copy of each gene that resides on the X chromosome. Any altered X gene will consequently be expressed in males, because an unaltered allele is not present for

---

BOX 3–3 Autosomal Dominant Mendelian Inheritance Characteristics

When gathering a family history, the nurse should assess for any of the following characteristics of autosomal dominant inheritance:

1. Both males and females are affected.
2. Males and females are usually affected in equal numbers.
3. An affected child will have an affected parent and/or all generations will have an affected individual (appearing as a vertical pattern of affected individuals on the family pedigree).
4. Unaffected children of an affected parent will have unaffected offspring.
5. A significant proportion of isolated cases are due to a new mutation.

BOX 3–4 Autosomal Recessive Mendelian Inheritance Characteristics

When gathering a family history, the nurse should assess for any of the following characteristics of autosomal recessive inheritance:

1. Both males and females are affected.
2. Males and females are usually affected in equal numbers.
3. An affected child will have an unaffected parent but may have affected siblings (appearing as a horizontal pattern of affected individuals on the family pedigree).
4. The condition may appear to skip a generation.
5. The parents of the affected child may be consanguineous (close blood relatives).
6. The family may be descendants of an ethnic group that is known to have a more frequent occurrence of a certain genetic condition.

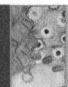

Culture *Ethnic or Population Groups and Autosomal Recessive Inheritance*

Because the prevalence of autosomal recessive conditions varies around the globe, certain recessive genetic conditions are more common in particular ethnic populations. This is one reason nurses should ask about the country of origin of an individual's ancestors when collecting a family history. In populations where individuals tend to marry within their own community, autosomal recessive conditions are especially common. This is known as the "founder effect." For example, Ellis-van Creveld syndrome, an inherited condition in which polydactyly (an extra finger) occurs, is commonly found among the Old Order Amish population of Pennsylvania.

Common examples of disorders that occur more commonly in specific populations are as follows.

Ashkenazi Jewish—Tay-Sachs Disease, Gaucher Disease

Tay-Sachs disease is approximately 100 times more common in infants of Ashkenazi Jewish ancestry (central-eastern Europe) than in non-Jewish populations (Tay-Sachs Disease, 2009). The carrier rate for Gaucher disease is as high as 1 in 18 in the Ashkenazi Jewish population, compared to 1 in 100 in the general population (Pastores & Hughes, 2008).

Turkish, Irish, East Asian Populations, Pennsylvania Amish—Phenylketonuria (PKU)

Carrier rates as high as 1 in 26 have been found in Turkish populations. The PKU gene is rare in African and Ashkenazi Jewish populations.

Mediterranean (Italians, Greeks), Middle Eastern, Central and Southeast Asian, Indian, Far East, African—ß-Thalassemia

High gene frequency of β-thalassemias in these populations is most likely related to selective pressure from malaria. The highest incidences are reported in Cyprus and Sardinia (with 12–14% carrier rates) and southeast Asia.

Northern European—Cystic Fibrosis (CF)

CF is the most common life-limiting autosomal recessive condition in individuals with Northern European ancestors. Carrier rates of about 1 in 28 have been found among Caucasians in North America.

Sub-Saharan African, Mediterranean, Middle Eastern, Indian, Caribbean, and Populations from Parts of Central and South America—Sickle Cell Disease

The prevalence of sickle cell trait is 8–10% among African Americans. Approximately one in every 250 to 600 African American infants born in the United States has sickle cell disease (Vichinsky & Schlis, 2006).

BOX 3–5 **X-Linked Mendelian Inheritance Characteristics**

When gathering a family history, the nurse should assess for any of the following characteristics of X-linked inheritance:

1. More males will be affected than females; rarely seen in females.
2. An affected male will have all carrier daughters.
3. There is no male-to-male inheritance.
4. Affected males are related by carrier females.
5. Females may report varying milder symptoms of the condition.
6. A new sporadic case could occur due to a new mutation.

to his sons, because only Y chromosomes are transmitted from fathers to sons. See Box 3–5.

X Inactivation Early in embryonic life, within a week of fertilization, one of the X chromosomes inherited by females is inactivated. This process results in equalizing the expression of X-linked genes in the two sexes. Each female receives an X chromosome from her mother (maternal X) and one from her father (paternal X). The inactivation of either the maternal or paternal X chromosome is random. However, once that X has been inactivated in any given cell, all of the cell's descendants (through mitosis) contain the same inactive X chromosome. Therefore, females are mosaic for X-linked genes; some cells will express genes from the maternal X chromosome, whereas other cells will express genes from the paternal X. Females who inherit altered genes on an X chromosome therefore show variable expression, because the gene alteration will be present in only some cells. Expression of symptoms can vary from extremely mild to a full manifestation of the condition. For example, female carriers of the X-linked recessive condition hemophilia A may exhibit prolonged bleeding times, and carriers of Duchenne muscular dystrophy may exhibit muscle weakness (Nussbaum et al., 2007).

Y-Linked Disorders

Because the Y chromosome has very few genes, alterations on the Y chromosome are not often associated with health problems. A single gene (SRY) on the Y chromosome produces a protein that initiates testicular development during embryogenesis. Other genes are associated with male fertility, and alterations in those genes account for a significant portion of male infertility (Noordam & Repping, 2006).

Variability in Classic Mendelian Patterns of Inheritance

In addition to classic Mendelian inheritance patterns, nurses must be prepared to help families understand several other concepts that affect risk for inheriting a genetic disorder. These concepts include the following common variations in traditional Mendelian patterns of inheritance.

Penetrance

Penetrance is the probability that a gene will be expressed phenotypically. It is an "all or none" concept in that a gene is considered to be penetrant if it is expressed to any degree.

"backup." Females have two copies of each X gene, and the unaltered gene generally compensates for an altered allele, making the female a carrier.

Inheritance Risk in X-Linked Conditions In families with X-linked disorders, a pattern of maternal transmission is seen. Females who are carriers of X-linked conditions have a 50% chance of passing the altered gene to their offspring. Any daughter who receives the altered gene is likely to receive an unaltered X chromosome from her father and therefore be a carrier like her mother. Sons of carrier mothers, however, have no backup X chromosome. Therefore, a son who inherits the altered X will display the condition and go on to pass that altered X to each of his daughters, who will then be carriers of the altered gene. A male can never transmit an altered gene on the X chromosome

Penetrance can be measured in the following way. In a certain group of individuals with the same genotype, what percentage of them will exhibit any signs or symptoms of the condition? If the number is less than 100%, then that condition is said to show *reduced* or *incomplete penetrance* (Nussbaum et al., 2007). For example, both achondroplasia and Huntington disease exhibit 100% penetrance because every individual with one copy of the altered gene will exhibit signs and symptoms of the disease.

Variable Expressivity

The term *expressivity* is used to describe the degree to which a phenotype is expressed. When people with the same genetic makeup (genotype) exhibit signs or symptoms with varying degrees of severity, the phenotype is described as showing *variable expression* (Nussbaum et al., 2007). Variable expression is common in the autosomal dominant condition neurofibromatosis (NF-1). Although neurofibromatosis has 100% penetrance, members of the same affected family often exhibit variation in degree of signs or symptoms.

New Mutation

When there is no previous family history of a condition, the disease may be caused by a spontaneous new mutation. A new mutation is said to be sporadic or *de novo*. Mutation rates have been estimated for a number of inherited disorders and vary over a thousand-fold due to a number of factors, only some of which are understood (Arnheim & Calabrese, 2009). Diseases with high new mutation rates include neurofibromatosis (NF-1), achondroplasia (dwarfism), Duchenne muscular dystrophy, and hemophilia A and B. A number of new mutations have been associated with advanced parental age, both maternal (consider the well-known association between aneuploidies and maternal age) and paternal (Arnheim & Calabrese, 2009). Determining whether a genetic condition is due to an inherited or a *de novo* mutation has important implications in calculating a family's recurrence risk.

Anticipation

Anticipation is said to occur when successive generations in a family exhibit earlier onset of symptoms and more severe signs and symptoms of certain diseases. Anticipation occurs in disorders characterized by unstable repeat expansions, which are DNA sequences that consist of repeating units of three or more nucleotides, for example CAGCAG . . . CAG. Repeat units have a tendency to expand, or accumulate repeats, during meiosis, especially during spermatogenesis. As a result, the number of repeats tends to increase in successive generations. More than a dozen diseases, usually neurological in nature, result from unstable repeat expansions. These include Huntington disease, fragile X syndrome, and myotonic dystrophy (Nussbaum et al., 2007).

Imprinting

The expression of some genetic conditions varies depending on whether the altered gene is inherited from the mother or the father. This differential gene expression is due to genomic imprinting. Imprinting takes place before gametes are formed, when certain genes are chemically marked as having maternal or paternal origin. After conception, the imprint controls gene expression so that only one allele, either maternal or paternal, is expressed. If the unsilenced (active) allele carries a mutation, disease may result. A well-studied example of imprinting involves a deletion in a gene on chromosome 15 that causes two very different disorders depending on whether the altered gene comes from the mother or the father. Prader-Willi syndrome, characterized by hypotonia in infancy, excessive eating habits leading to obesity, and mild-to-moderate developmental disability, is due to a deletion on chromosome 15 that is inherited from the father. Angelman syndrome is due to a similar deletion in the same gene on chromosome 15, but it is inherited from the mother. The clinical presentation is very different. Individuals with Angelman syndrome have severe developmental disability, a jerky gait, seizures, and a happy, sociable disposition (Gurrieri & Accadia, 2009).

Uniparental Disomy

In cases of uniparental disomy, the child inherits both copies of a chromosome pair (or homologous parts of a chromosome pair) from the same parent instead of one copy from each parent. If there are no altered genes on these chromosomes, the child may not be affected by this event. However, if the chromosomes contain an altered gene for an autosomal recessive disease, the child will receive both altered genes and express the disease. For instance, if a child inherits two altered copies of chromosome 7 from a mother who is a carrier for cystic fibrosis, the child will then exhibit signs and symptoms of cystic fibrosis.

Multifactorial Inheritance

Most inheritable traits, such as eye and skin color, are polygenic. That is, they occur as a result of variations on several genes. Most diseases and health conditions are polygenic as well, and the expression of those altered genes is often modified by environmental influences. These are called multifactorial conditions and include many birth defects such as cleft lip and palate, pediatric conditions such as autism and asthma, and adult-onset conditions such as cancer and heart disease. Because the term *polygenic* does not imply the influence of the environment, the term *multifactorial* is the preferred terminology. The relative contribution of genetic and environmental influences varies across disorders.

Multifactorial conditions aggregate in families but do not follow the characteristic Mendelian patterns of inheritance seen with single-gene conditions. Recurrence risk varies among multifactorial conditions, but is usually less than that of Mendelian conditions. Recurrence risk is calculated from population studies and expressed as a percentage. For some disorders, recurrence risk is not easily predicted. Recurrence risk is higher when more than one family member is affected. For cleft lip, recurrence risk in a family with one affected child is 3% but increases to 8% with the birth of a second affected child. Recurrence risk can also increase with increased severity of the defect. The recurrence risk for cleft lip in a family with one child with unilateral cleft lip is 4%, and the recurrence risk for cleft lip in a family with one child with a bilateral cleft lip and palate is 8% (Nussbaum et al., 2007). See Table 3–2.

TABLE 3–2	Common Birth Defects and Conditions with a Multifactorial Cause
Neural Tube Defects	A neural tube defect (NTD) is a condition that occurs early during fetal development with incomplete closure of the neural tube. Severity of the disorder varies, depending on which part of the tube does not close. Anencephaly, meningomyelocele, and spina bifida are examples of NTD. Recurrence risk is increased in families with an affected child, but that risk can be modified by maternal dietary folic acid supplementation (Nussbaum et al., 2007).
Congenital Heart Defects	Most congenital heart defects are thought to be of multifactorial cause. A number of genes have been associated with patent ductus arteriosus, atrial or ventricular septal defects, and other heart defects (Pierpont, Basson, Benson, et al., 2007). Families with one affected child face a recurrence risk that varies with the condition but is generally relatively low, from 2–5% (Nussbaum et al., 2007).
Cleft Lip and Palate	Cleft lip and/or palate (CL/P) occurs due to failure of bony fusion early in gestation. While rare gene mutations can cause CL/P, most cases are thought to be multifactorial. Maternal smoking and a number of gene variations have been associated with CL/P (Nussbaum et al., 2007).
Autism Spectrum Disorder	Although the etiology of autism spectrum disorder remains poorly understood, most experts believe it to be multifactorial. Twin studies suggest a strong genetic component, with 60–92% concordance between identical twins. A number of environmental influences have been suspected to influence the development of autism as well, including environmental exposures, food intolerances, and specific perinatal events (Inglese & Elder, 2009).

COLLABORATIVE CARE

Many health professionals work together in the screening, diagnosis, identification, and treatment of genetic disorders. The goals of collaborative care are early diagnosis through assessment and testing, development of an effective treatment plan combined with psychosocial support to enhance coping, and referral to a genetic specialist when needed.

Diagnostic Procedures

Genetic testing is available for both chromosomal and gene-based alterations, and the field of genetic testing is changing rapidly. New methodologies and broader applications of older techniques have greatly expanded the number of conditions for which genetic testing is available. Increasingly, genetic testing is offered directly to consumers, who receive limited counseling about test results. Patients and families often have unreliable sources for information related to genetic testing. They can easily form misconceptions about the types of genetic tests available and what information those tests are able and not able to

---

BOX 3–6   What Is a Genetic Test?

A genetic test involves the analysis of chromosomes, DNA, RNA, genes, or gene products (e.g., enzymes and other proteins) to detect variations related to disease or health. Whether a laboratory method is considered a genetic test also depends on the intended use, claim, or purpose of a test. For example, amino acid analysis to detect metabolic disorders such as PKU is considered a genetic test, but the use of this same analysis to monitor general nutritional status is not (U.S. Department of Health and Human Services, 2008).

---

provide. For example, a test for cystic fibrosis may be reported as negative, but the significance of that finding relies on how many of the multiple CF-causing mutations were included in the test. The pediatric nurse needs knowledge of available genetic tests and their implications in order to assist patients and their families as they weigh choices regarding genetic testing. See Box 3–6.

Recommendations for Genetic Testing Genetic tests are useful to diagnose disease, predict risk of future disease, inform reproductive decision making, and manage patient care. Guidelines regarding who should be tested and when to test are available for some genetic conditions. However, new knowledge accumulates rapidly, and recommendations for practice often lag behind research findings by several years.

Categories of Genetic Tests Genetic tests have been used for some time to detect heritable conditions that are passed from generation to generation. There are several categories of genetic testing, each with a unique purpose. See Table 3–3. Genetic testing utilizes a variety of methods and may analyze DNA, products of DNA, or other substances that indicate a genetic defect. DNA can be analyzed on a number of levels, from karyotyping an entire set of chromosomes to examining a specific gene for a mutation. Tests of DNA products (RNA or proteins) are sometimes done to measure gene function or expression. Some genetic tests measure metabolites that accumulate when individuals lack a specific enzyme due to a gene mutation.

It is especially important for the pediatric nurse to understand the difference between screening tests, which are used in populations to find individuals at risk for a disorder, and diagnostic tests, which are required to make a diagnosis. Newborn screening is carried out on most newborns in developed countries and provides a means to identify children who may have a genetic disease such as a metabolic disease, sickle cell disease, or congenital hypothyroidism. Many of these disorders are exceedingly rare. In recent years, a laboratory technique called tandem mass spectrometry has allowed greatly expanded newborn screening with little increase in laboratory cost. Issues around expanded newborn screening are of considerable interest, in part due to issues of follow-up. Even the most specific of screening tests will result in false-positive results, which must be followed up with a diagnostic test. The cost of follow-up testing is significant both in terms of parental anxiety and financial burden (Gurian, Kinnamon, Henry, et al., 2006). See Chapter 7 ∞ for further description of newborn screening.

Diagnostic tests are performed to confirm a diagnosis in a symptomatic child or adult. Diagnostic tests may be ordered

TABLE 3–3	Categories of Genetic Tests
Type of Test	Description
Diagnostic testing	Used to establish a diagnosis of a genetic disorder in an individual who is symptomatic or has had a positive screening test.
Prenatal testing	Testing to identify a fetus with a genetic disease or condition. Some prenatal testing is offered routinely; other testing may be initiated due to family history or maternal factors.
Newborn screening	Testing of a newborn to identify the presence of a condition that requires immediate initiation of treatment to prevent death or disability.
Preimplantation testing	Following in vitro fertilization (IVF), testing to identify embryos with a particular genetic condition.
Carrier testing	Testing in an asymptomatic individual to identify carrier status for a genetic condition.
Predictive testing	• Offered usually to asymptomatic individuals to detect genetic conditions that occur later in life. May be presymptomatic or predispositional. • *Presymptomatic testing* detects mutations that, if present, are likely or certain to eventually cause symptoms (an example is Huntington disease). • *Predispositional testing* detects mutations that increase the likelihood that symptoms will develop (such as BRCA 1 and 2).

Source: Adapted from Constantin, C. M., Faucett, A., & Lubin, J. M. (2005). A primer on genetic testing. Journal of Midwifery and Women's Health, 50, 197–204. Copyright Elsevier, 2005.

when a child is suspected of having a specific disorder based on clinical presentation or screening test results. Diagnostic testing is sometimes carried out prenatally to identify genetic disease such as a trisomy in a fetus.

Diagnosing Chromosomal Alterations Cytogenetics, or the study of chromosomes, describes the microscopic examination of chromosomes to reveal large alterations such as additions, deletions, breaks, and rearrangements or rejoinings (translocations). Prenatally, amniocentesis and chorionic villi sampling (CVS) can be undertaken to provide specimens for cytogenetic examination. After a child is born, chromosomal diagnostic examination can be accomplished with a blood, skin, or buccal cell sample. Cytogenetic testing includes karyotyping, as described earlier in this chapter, as well as molecular cytogenetic techniques, which are capable of detecting DNA variations too small to be seen on a karyotype.

Diagnosing Gene Alterations Recent advances in molecular genetic technology along with the mapping of the human genome have resulted in tremendous expansion of available genetic testing. Genetic testing is currently available for over 1,800 diseases, with new tests constantly being added (GeneTests, 2009). DNA-based tests involve sophisticated new technology that permits the detection of even single nucleotide variations in DNA sequence. These tests can be performed on blood, bone marrow, amniotic fluid, fibroblast cells of the skin, or buccal cells from the mouth. Genetic testing can examine DNA (to determine specific nucleotide sequence), RNA (to measure gene expression), or proteins (to analyze gene products). Tests commonly require several days to weeks, or occasionally several months are required before results are reported.

Genes are very long DNA sequences, made up of hundreds of thousands of nucleotides (or base pairs). Alterations at various sites along a gene may alter its function and cause disease. As an example, the CFTR gene (which in an altered form causes cystic fibrosis) is 230,000 base pairs long, and over 1,600 different CFTR mutations have been identified (Cystic Fibrosis Mutation Database, 2007). Most CFTR mutations are rare, and the most common (named delta F508) causes about 70% of cystic fibrosis. Although DNA testing is capable of detecting any of these alterations in DNA sequence, it is not feasible to test for them all. Currently available CFTR tests detect from about 23 to 98 different mutations. Depending on which test is selected, 85–98% of altered genes can be detected (Genzyme Genetics, n.d.; Moskowitz, Chmiel, Sternen, et al., 2008). Therefore, a "negative" CF test must be interpreted with caution and an eye on how many mutations were included in the test. This is just one of the limitations of genetic testing that nurses must understand in order to provide genetically competent care. See The Role of the Nurse in Genetic Testing later in this chapter.

Tests of gene expression are available as well. For example, **microarray analysis** can detect levels of messenger RNA in cells, which indicates which genes are "turned on" or being expressed. Microarray analysis is especially useful to examine tumor cells (U.S. Department of Health and Human Services, 2008).

Other genetic tests examine gene products, rather than the makeup of the gene itself. One example is a biochemical test for PKU. PKU is caused by an alteration in the gene encoding the enzyme phenylalanine hydroxylase (PAH). However, the PKU test actually measures phenylalanine levels, which are markedly elevated in individuals with PAH deficiency. Many of these biochemical tests have been in use for years.

Quality and Accuracy of Genetic Tests

Genetic nurses express concern that genetic tests are becoming available very quickly without regulation of the companies offering them. The quality, accuracy, and reliability of genetic test results are not measured against any common standard. Of particular concern is the growing popularity of direct-to-consumer marketing of genetic testing, which is increasingly accessible and affordable and allows individuals to access genetic testing without consulting a health care provider. In most cases little or no education is provided for the individual undergoing testing, nor is counseling or follow-up uniformly provided. Individuals often make hard and irrevocable life-altering decisions after receiving test results, so accuracy and reliability, along with professional counseling, are essential (Lea, 2008).

Law & Ethics · *ELSI*

Since its inception, the National Human Genome Research Institute has designated a percent of its budget to examining the ethical, legal, and social implications (ELSI) of genetic and genomic information. Genetic testing raises many questions that have been addressed by ELSI. Genetic exceptionalism, the idea that genetic information should be treated differently than other health information, continues to be a subject of great interest and little consensus. Proponents of genetic exceptionalism point out that genetic information is unique and deserving of special consideration and protection because it is predictive, is potentially stigmatizing, and may reveal information about family members other than the patient undergoing testing. The contrasting view points out that other information is also predictive (consider blood cholesterol and risk for cardiovascular disease) and stigmatizing (for example, information about sexually transmitted infections).

Federal health privacy protection, as mandated under the federal Health Insurance Portability and Accountability Act (HIPAA) privacy rule, does not afford special protection to genetic information, treating it as being no more sensitive than other health-related information. However, the majority of states have enacted legislation that takes the exceptionalist view, providing protection against discrimination based on genetic information and penalties for violating genetic privacy (U.S. Department of Health and Human Services, 2008). Public fear of genetic discrimination, however, is high. In one study, fewer than 25% of individuals said they would trust their employer or insurance company with genetic information (Genetics and Public Policy Center, 2007). A public health concern is that individuals might be reluctant to seek potentially beneficial genetic testing based on concerns around the confidentiality, privacy, and security of that information (U.S. Department of Health and Human Services, 2008). For example, an individual may have health coverage for a genetic test but be unwilling to submit the claim due to concerns about the insurance company "owning" the information in the test result. Federal legislation to prohibit discrimination based on genetic information in health insurance and employment (the Genetic Information Nondiscrimination Act, or GINA) was implemented in November 2009.

NURSING MANAGEMENT

By simply integrating genetic and genomic concepts into assessment, observation, and history gathering, the pediatric nurse can improve the standard of care delivered and have a positive impact on the child and family. The pediatric nurse does not need to be a genetic expert, but baseline knowledge and heightened awareness of genetic and genomic issues will support appropriate assessment and referral to genetic specialists as needed.

Family Risk Assessment

Genetic Family History

While gathering a family history, the nurse must look for genetic information that might indicate the need for referral to a genetic specialist. Examples that would indicate a family may benefit from a genetic referral include a family history of conditions known or suspected to be genetic, several family members with the same condition, developmental disability or learning difficulties, dysmorphic features or congenital anomalies, neonatal or pediatric death of unknown cause, recurrent miscarriage, or established genetic carrier status (Gaff, Emery, & Metcalfe, 2007).

Family History Initiative Website

Pedigrees

Pediatric nurses and all other health professionals should know how to collect a three-generation family history, record the history in a pedigree, and "think genetic." A **pedigree** is a graphic representation or diagram of a family's medical history and genetic relationships (Figure 3–3 ➤). A standard format and nomenclature for pedigrees, which includes multiple symbols (Figure 3–4 ➤), has been adopted (Bennett, French, Resta, et al., 2008). A pedigree is constructed around a designated "index" patient, called the **proband** (if he or she is affected with the genetic disorder of interest) or **consultand** (if he or she seeks genetic counseling without being known to have the disorder). A finished pedigree provides a clear, visual representation of a

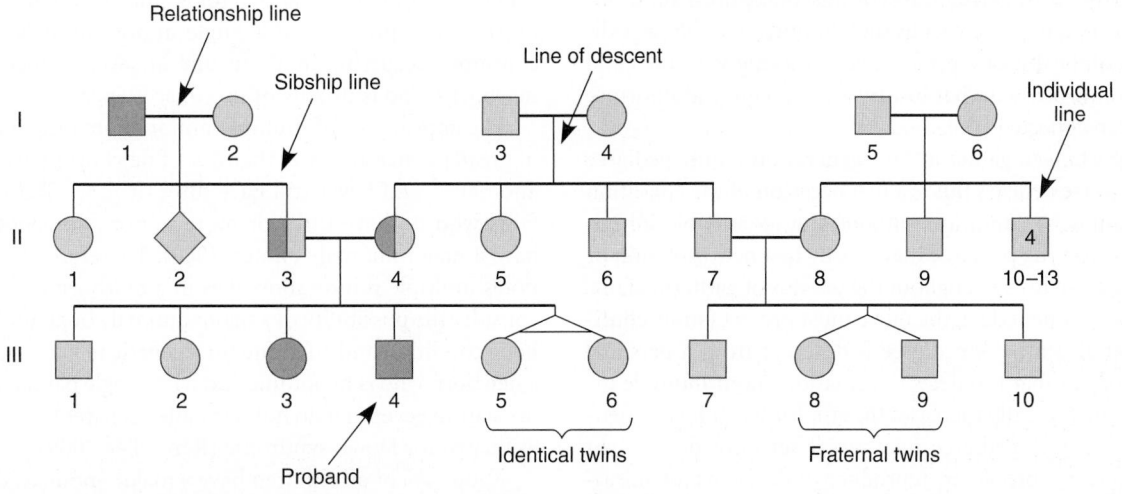

FIGURE 3–3 ➤ Sample three-generation pedigree.

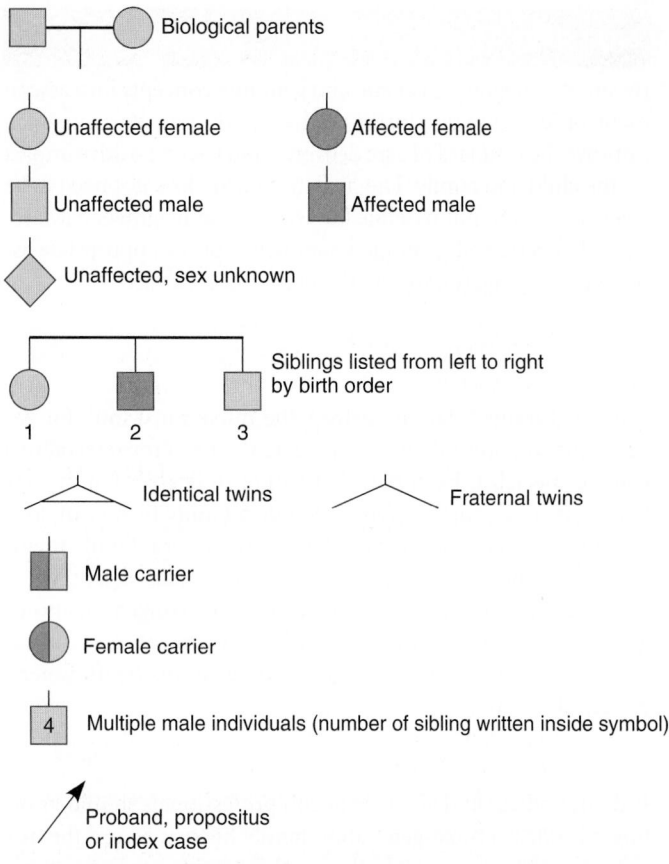

FIGURE 3–4 ➤ Selected standardized symbols for use in drawing a pedigree.

family's medical data and biological relationships at a glance. A pedigree identifies affected individuals in the immediate and extended family and can identify family members who might benefit from a genetic consultation. A pedigree can also illustrate patterns of inheritance and clusters of multifactorial conditions. On the basis of the pedigree, genetic referral and/or reproductive risk teaching for the individual and family can occur. The visual nature of a pedigree enhances a family's learning and can be used to clarify misunderstandings or misconceptions about inheritance. If completed correctly and comprehensively, a pedigree allows all health care professionals working with the child or family to quickly see what history and background information has been collected (Box 3–7).

It is important to gather a three-generation family pedigree even if the nurse believes this is a first occasion of the condition within a family. A condition without any identifiable inheritance pattern on the pedigree may be due to a new mutation or variable expressivity. Throughout the process of gathering family history assessment data, the nurse must protect family confidentiality at all times. A pedigree is different from a personal health history in that it reflects information about multiple individuals, which greatly increases the risk for harm if confidentiality is broken. A pedigree may reveal sensitive details that include infertility problems, reproductive decisions, or misassigned paternity that may not be known by a current partner or other family members. Other sensitive issues include pregnancies conceived by technology, a history of suicides, drug or alcohol abuse, and same-sex relationships. See Box 3–8.

Challenges inherent in recalling the family history include the parents' inability to remember conditions that have been surgically repaired and then forgotten. Parents may fail to report conditions thought not to be genetic or that have been attributed incorrectly to other causes. Also, parents may be reluctant to reveal sensitive information, particularly information unknown to other family members.

Families are encouraged to collect and record their own family history in a form that can be shared within the family as well as with health care providers. The U.S. Surgeon General's Family History Initiative is a national campaign to promote the collection of family histories, providing a web-based program that allows individuals to easily record their information.

Genetic Physical Assessment

The pediatric nurse in any health care setting should also "think genetic" when performing physical assessment (see Chapter 5 ∞). An early finding by the nurse will provide the child and family with an opportunity for a genetic referral and more specialized health care.

Major and Minor Anomalies **Dysmorphology** refers to the study of human congenital defects or abnormalities of body structure that begin before birth. Traditionally, congenital anomalies have been included under the umbrella of genetic disorders whether they occur due to a gene alteration or another cause of abnormal embryonic or fetal development. Dysmorphic anomalies can occur anywhere in the body, but are perhaps most often associated with facial features. As a routine part of patient assessment, the nurse should screen for both minor and major anomalies. A **minor anomaly** or malformation is an unusual morphologic feature that in itself is of no serious medical or cosmetic concern to the individual or family. Some minor anomalies are merely family traits or are present in certain ethnic groups. Minor anomalies include such traits as wide-set eyes, single palmar creases, café au lait patches, low anterior hairline, preauricular (in front of the ears) pits and tags, broad face, or mild proportionate short stature. Examples of variations associated with ethnic origin include upward-slanting eyes or prominent epicanthal folds among individuals of Asian descent. The presence of a single minor anomaly is relatively common, occurring in about one in seven otherwise normal newborns, and is usually of no consequence.

The appearance of multiple minor anomalies in an infant is of greater concern. Fewer than 1% of newborns have two minor anomalies, and fewer still have three or more. But of those infants who do have three or more minor anomalies, 90% also have a major anomaly (Jones, 2006). Therefore, the nurse who notes multiple minor anomalies in a newborn or child should consider the possibility of a major anomaly or an underlying genetic condition and advocate for a genetic referral. For example, a newborn who is hypotonic and has a single palmar crease with up-slanting eyes that do not resemble his parent's eyes should be evaluated for Down syndrome (Ranweiler, 2009).

About 3% of all children have a **major anomaly**, defined as a serious structural defect present at birth that may have severe medical or cosmetic consequences, interfere with normal functioning of body systems, lead to a lifelong disability, or even cause an early death. Congenital heart defects, cleft lip and/or

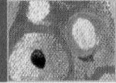

BOX 3–7 Steps in Drawing a Pedigree

I. Organization
1. Begin recording data in the middle of the sheet of paper (to allow enough room for both the maternal and paternal sides of the family).
2. Use only standard pedigree symbols (see Figure 3–4).
3. Place the male individual in a couple on the left of the relationship line; the paternal side of the family will also be on the left side of the paper.

II. Determining Family Relationships
1. Determine relationships within the family by asking questions such as:
   • Do you have a partner or are you married?
   • How many biological brothers and sisters do you have?
   • How many children do you have? Are they with the same partner?
   • Do all the children have the same biological father?
   • Do your siblings share the same mother and father as you?
2. Referring to "the baby's father or mother" can be helpful until the relationship between parents is established.
3. Referring to a "union" if marriage does not exist can also help communication.

III. Who Should or Should Not Be Included
1. To ensure accuracy, the pedigree should include the parents, offspring, siblings, aunts, uncles, grandparents, and first cousins of the individual seeking counseling.
2. Detailed information about the spouses of the proband's family can be omitted unless there is a history of some kind of disorder or condition.
3. Eliminating persons or information that does not contribute any valuable information can help keep the pedigree small and more manageable.

IV. Recording the Family History
1. It may be useful to determine the approximate size of the family, to plan spacing on paper.
2. Begin the drawing with the proband (the person who is seeking counseling or is affected with the genetic condition). Mark the proband with an arrow.

3. Then add the symbols for the brothers and sisters of the proband and an individual line for each. Connect the individual lines with a sibship line and add a line of descent, the relationship line for the parents, and symbols for parents of the proband.
4. Repeat this step for children of the proband and children of the proband's siblings.
5. Continue with symbols for all immediate relatives of the proband's parents and grandparents. Record the ethnicity of the first generation at the top of the page.
6. Mark each symbol to designate relevant information (see Figure 3–4).
7. Create a key to contain all information relevant to interpretation of the pedigree.
8. The pedigree should include at least three generations.
   • Mark each generation with a Roman numeral along the left side of the paper with the first generation marker (I) at the top.
   • Each person in a generation should fall along the same imaginary horizontal line.
9. The pedigree should include:
   • Half-siblings, pregnancy losses, stillbirths, previous marriages, and adopted children
   • The reason for taking the pedigree (e.g., developmental disability, dysmorphology)
   • The name of the family historian (person relaying the information)

V. Other
1. **Consanguinity** may be suspected if the historian repeatedly gives the same last name on both sides of the family. Ask if any relatives in the family have ever had a child together.

VI. Completing the Pedigree
1. When completed, the pedigree should be dated and signed with the name, credentials, and position of the person drawing it.

Data from Bennett, R. L. (2010). The practical guide to the genetic family history (2nd ed.). Copyright © 2010 John Wiley & Sons. Reproduced with permission of John Wiley & Sons, Inc.

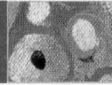

BOX 3–8 Specific Facts and Health Information to Include/Indicate in a Pedigree

■ First name of proband or consultand
■ First names or initials of relatives
■ Age or year of birth
■ Age or year of death
■ Cause of death
■ Age at diagnosis
■ Full siblings distinguished from half siblings
■ Relevant health information including medical conditions
■ Any current pregnancy with gestational age (LMP) or estimated date of delivery (EDD)
■ Infertility versus no children by choice
■ Pregnancy complications with gestational ages noted (e.g., 6 weeks, 32 weeks):
   • Miscarriage or spontaneous abortion (SAB)
   • Stillbirth (SB)

   • Pregnancy termination (TOP)
   • Ectopic pregnancy (ECT)
■ Ethnic background/country of origin for each grandparent
■ Consanguinity
■ Date pedigree taken or updated
■ Reason for taking pedigree
■ Historian (person relaying family history information)
■ Name and credentials of person who took pedigree
■ Key or legend (symbols or acronyms used on the chart)

Source: Bennett, R. L. (2010). The practical guide to the genetic family history (2nd ed.). Hoboken, NJ: Wiley-Blackwell. Reproduced with permission of John Wiley & Sons, Inc.

palate, myelomeningocele, duodenal atresia, and craniosynostosis are considered major anomalies, as is developmental disability (Jones, 2006). Some major anomalies are present at birth but are not apparent, such as deafness, various skeletal dysplasias, and some types of congenital heart defects.

A **syndrome** is a collection of multiple anomalies, major or minor, that occurs in a consistent pattern and has a common cause. For example, Down syndrome is the cause of a variety of anomalies that can appear in multiple body systems, including the eyes, ears, hair, mouth and tongue, heart, and brain. An **association** is a group of abnormalities of unknown cause that occur together more often than is expected by chance (Nussbaum et al., 2007).

The nurse can identify clues to genetic problems by examining the child and considering the physical characteristics of the parents and other family members (Table 3–4). Nurses may even ask to look at family photographs and examine them for common dysmorphic features and family traits. Several standardized craniofacial measurements have been defined, and tables are available displaying normal values according to age, so that dysmorphic facial features are more easily identified (Figure 3–5 ➤). By making a genetic referral, the pediatric nurse can make a difference in the child's state of health.

The Role of the Nurse in Genetic Testing

Many people have misconceptions about genetic testing. Nurses play an important role in teaching parents and children about the implications and limitations of genetic tests to ensure that they make informed decisions. The nurse should promote communication, autonomy, and privacy when helping families. Rec-

TABLE 3–4	Selected Dysmorphic Physical Assessment Findings*	
Skull	Asymmetric head/face	Fontanels too large or small
	Brachycephaly (short, broad head shape) (See Figure 27–15 ∞.)	Frontal bossing (prominent central forehead)
		Microcephaly or macrocephaly
	Craniosynostosis (premature closing of skull sutures)	Micrognathia (small jaw)
	Flattened or prominent occiput	Prognathism (projection of jaw beyond that of the forehead)
Extremities	Abnormally positioned feet	Hypoplastic (very small) or absent nails
	Arachnodactyly (long fingers or toes)	Hypotonia (diminished muscle tone)
	Brachydactyly (short fingers or toes)	Loose joints
	Camptodactyly (permanent flexion of fingers or toes)	Polydactyly (extra fingers and/or toes)
	Clinodactyly (curved fingers or toes, most often the fifth finger)	Rocker bottom feet
		Single transverse palmar crease (See Figure 5–46 ∞.)
	Edema of the hands or feet	Syndactyly (webbing between fingers and toes)
	Extremely long/thin or short extremities	
Ears	Ear tags or pits	Hearing loss
	Ears that are posteriorly rotated	Low-set or malformed ears
Hair	Excessive body hair	Large section of white hair in otherwise pigmented hair
	Unusual hairline or hair distribution	Sparse or brittle hair
Eyes	Blue sclera	Extreme myopia (nearsightedness)
	Different colored eyes	Hypertelorism (widely spaced eyes)
	Down-slanting eyes	Hypotelorism (closely spaced eyes)
	Epicanthal folds inconsistent with ethnicity (See Figure 5–14 ∞.)	Short palpebral fissures (distance between inner and outer canthus of eyes)
	Extreme hyperopia (farsightedness)	Up-slanting eyes (See Figure 5–15 ∞.)
Skin	Axillary freckling (See Figure 27–16 ∞.)	Hirsutism (excessive hair)
	Café au lait spots (See Figure 27–16 ∞.)	Hyperelastic skin
	Excessive skin	Leaf-shaped white markings
	Extremely loose or thin skin	Syndactyly (webbing between fingers and toes)
Mouth	Cleft lip with or without cleft palate (See Figure 25–3 ∞.)	Early loss of teeth
		Late eruption of teeth
	Large or small tongue	Smooth or abnormal philtrum
	Misshapen, missing, or extra teeth	Thin upper lip
Other	Abdominal wall defect	Seizures
	Ambiguous genitalia	Short, webbed neck
	Cryptorchidism (undescended testicle)	Single umbilical artery
	Hernia (inguinal or umbilical)	Small or widely spaced nipples
	Hypospadias	Multiple fractures
	Hypogonadism	Unusual cry (catlike/mewing, hoarse, weak)
	Obesity	Unusually tall or short stature
	Scoliosis	Webbed neck

This list is not all-inclusive, but is meant to increase the nurse's awareness of assessment findings that may be significant and require a referral to a genetic specialist.

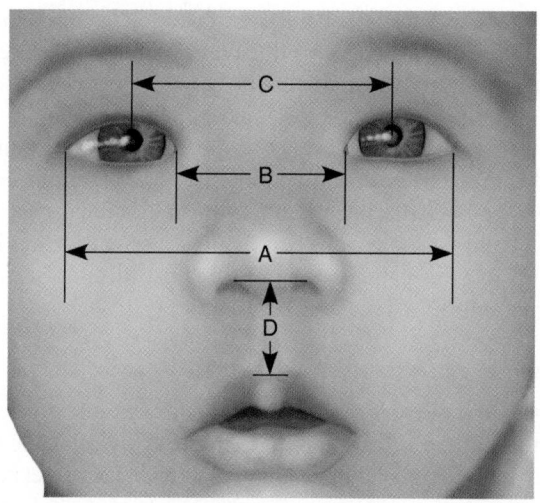

FIGURE 3–5 ➤ Classic facial measurements for genetic assessment with a focus on facial features. A, Outer intercanthal distance. B, Intercanthal distance. C, Interpupillary distance. D, Philtrum length.

ognizing that genetic testing affects families, and not just individuals, the nurse should use a family perspective when assisting parents and children who are making decisions about genetic testing (Twomey, 2006). All voices should be heard, and each family member's decision should be respected, whether it is to participate in genetic testing or to decline. Not all family members will want to know their genetic risks. The pediatric nurse has a responsibility to ensure autonomy, and a nondirective approach is critical. Nurses must take care to avoid imposing their own values or personal opinions onto patients and families. Finally, as with all aspects of delivering genetic nursing care, privacy and confidentiality are paramount.

Genetic Testing Issues of Minors In order to support, advocate for, and educate children, adolescents, and their families, the pediatric nurse must have knowledge of the issues related to genetic testing of minor children. Parents may request genetic testing for their minor children and not foresee the consequences associated with a positive finding.

The primary focus of genetic testing in children is to promote the child's well-being. Guidelines generally recommend that genetic testing in children only be conducted if the results would affect medical management soon after testing (Cameron & Muller, 2009). In most instances, predictive genetic testing for adult-onset diseases such as Huntington disease and certain cancers is deferred until a child reaches age 18 years. Exceptions are made for conditions that cause morbidity at a young age or for which specific health promotion, screening, or treatment is indicated. Although various genetic and medical associations have published guidelines regarding genetic testing in minors, timelines for genetic testing are not standardized (Borry, Goffin, Nys, et al., 2008).

Communication with the child and family about genetic testing should include an assessment of the positive and negative outcomes of the test. Are there existing treatments for the condition being tested? What are the potential psychological issues associated with a positive or negative test? Who will be affected by the test results? Will the test results be shared with

extended family members? The nurse has an important role in educating adolescents and parents in issues around genetic testing to ensure that they are making informed decisions. The nurse should also consider the decision-making ability of the child. There is little consensus regarding the age at which children may be able to take part in a decision-making process involving genetic testing, and it is imperative for the nurse to be an advocate for the child.

Nurses should help families to clearly understand why a genetic test is being done. In general, four reasons have been suggested to consider genetic testing of minors. The first is if the testing offers an immediate medical benefit for the child in terms of disease prevention or early treatment. An example is testing for familial adenomatous polyposis (FAP), a genetic disease in which removal of the colon during adolescence is often required to prevent colon cancer. In recent years, the availability of genomic testing for common chronic disease risk has blurred the issues around genetic testing in minors. Consider a child who is tested and found to have a genetic predisposition to type 2 diabetes. Typically, the disease risk is moderately elevated—perhaps two to three times the population risk. Does knowledge of that genetic test have immediate medical benefit for the child? Does the potential benefit outweigh any harm that may accompany the knowledge? Issues such as these are of great interest in genomic medicine but clear guidelines have yet to be established (Haga & Terry, 2009).

A second kind of situation occurs when an adolescent is facing a reproductive decision of his or her own. If the adolescent has a family history of a genetic condition, he or she may be interested in genetic testing that offers no specific medical benefit to that adolescent other than family planning. Recall Sarah, the young woman in the opening scenario who wanted to be tested for Huntington disease. Might genetic testing affect her reproductive decisions?

A third situation occurs when a parent or child requests genetic testing for a condition for future planning in the absence of any immediate benefit. This situation may arise with adult-onset inherited disorders. For example, an older child who has a relative with familial (early-onset) Alzheimer disease may wish confirmation of whether he or she carries the altered gene, in order to plan for a life career or to make relationship decisions such as marriage. Parents sometimes request predictive or carrier testing for their children who are well below reproductive age. In the genetics community, there is widespread consensus that predictive genetic testing for minors should not be performed in the absence of targeted preventive, surveillance, or treatment interventions (Borry et al., 2008).

Finally, a family member may request genetic testing for a child when the test results are entirely for the benefit of another family member, with no direct benefit to the child. This may occur during DNA linkage studies, in which multiple blood samples from both affected and unaffected individuals within a family must be analyzed and compared in order to produce a recognized DNA pattern for diagnosing a genetic condition in that particular family.

The pediatric nurse must be aware of these potential situations and know that decisions to perform genetic tests on children and adolescents are not made easily. Unless the potential benefits of testing outweigh the potential harms to the child, a genetic test is not justified and should be postponed until the child is capable of making an informed decision. That time often comes when an adolescent is making reproductive decisions. Recognizing the difficult issues and lack of consensus around genetic testing in children and minors, the genetics community is calling for standardized practice recommendations to guide clinical decision making (Borry, Nys, & Dierickx, 2007).

Ensuring Informed Consent for Genetic Testing The pediatric nurse is responsible for alerting children and their families of their right to make an informed decision prior to *any* genetic testing with consideration of the special circumstances arising from the family, culture, and community life. All genetic testing should be voluntary, and it is the nurse's responsibility to ensure that the consent process includes discussion of the risks and benefits of the test, including any physical or psychological harm, as well as potential societal injury due to stigmatization or discrimination. The nurse should be aware that health insurance policies may not cover genetic testing, which is often very expensive. Even if the insurance benefit will cover the test, many individuals are fearful of discrimination based on genetic test results that are included in their medical record. The pediatric nurse should inform the child and the family of their right to know who will have access to the genetic test results.

Ensuring Confidentiality and Privacy for Genetic Testing Issues of confidentiality and privacy are of particular concern when genetic information is involved. Results of genetic tests can be far reaching and have the potential, despite recent implementation of legal protection, to affect employment and insurance options. Will the results affect the child's or parents' ability to obtain and/or maintain insurance coverage? Can an employer refuse to hire or promote an individual because of genetic testing results? Can genetic information be released to the courts, military, schools, or adoption agencies? Would a child with a known gene alteration for Huntington disease be offered a college scholarship for the best law school? The technology that has made genetic testing possible has far outpaced the ability of health policy makers and legislators to put in place systems to protect genetic information.

Psychosocial Issues Pediatric nurses must be prepared to assist children and families to manage anxiety around genetic testing. Uncertainty and stress associated with making a decision to undertake genetic testing may extend into weeks or even months before results are available. That stress may be increased or relieved once test results are known. Although receiving favorable test results may decrease anxiety for the family or individual anxiety, potential problems do occur and the pediatric nurse must be prepared to address them. Concerns about carrier status may interfere with development of intimacy and interpersonal relationships. A positive test result may lead to feelings of unworthiness and self-image disturbance. Survivor guilt may affect children with negative results if their siblings are positive. Younger children may blame themselves, thinking they did or said something to cause the gene alteration. The adolescent carrying a gene alteration for a late-onset disease may have an increased tendency for risky behaviors. The adolescent who has inherited an altered disease-producing gene may foster deep resentment toward the parent who carries the altered gene. Parental guilt may exist for passing the altered gene to the child. Finally, parent–child bonds may be altered if parents become either overprotective or overly permissive. The parent and other family members may unconsciously form lowered expectations for the child or adolescent. Nurses must use counseling interventions to assist patients to process, adjust to, and use genetic information (ANA/ISONG, 2007).

Planning and Implementation

The pediatric nurse is responsible for comprehensively delivering the standard of care to children and families, while being aware of limitations of his or her own knowledge and expertise. In addition to the continuous integration of genetic aspects into the nurse's assessment of family history and physical assessment, the nurse is also responsible for providing genomically competent care that may include initiating referrals to genetic specialists (Consensus Panel, 2009).

Genetic Referrals and Counseling

After gathering assessment data that incorporate genetic concepts, the pediatric nurse is able to partner with children and their families by initiating a referral to genetic specialists if there are indicators for a genetic referral (Box 3–9). The nurse should provide the family with information about the advantages of a referral to a genetic specialist, and the disadvantages of not following through with the referral. The nurse should inform the child and family that a genetic referral can provide information and answer questions they may have concerning genetic health. Families should be encouraged to address all their concerns with the genetic specialist, who will be able to answer questions regarding genetic condi-

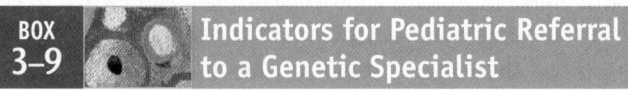

BOX 3–9 Indicators for Pediatric Referral to a Genetic Specialist

- If the child or family reports a known or "believed" genetic condition in the family
- Single major or multiple minor congenital anomalies
- Dysmorphic features that are not familial
- Developmental delay or regression
- A known or suspected metabolic disorder
- Speech problems
- Learning disability
- Failure to thrive
- Delays in physical growth, unusual body proportions, or low muscle tone
- Abnormal or delayed development of secondary sex characteristics or sex organs
- Short or extremely tall stature
- Blindness or cataracts in infants or children
- Deafness
- Hypotonia in an infant or child
- Seizures in newborns or infants
- Skin lesions such as café au lait spots

tions, inheritance, availability of treatment, as well as economic, insurance, and future implications of genetic conditions.

Those who are concerned about genetic disease may benefit from a genetic consultation whether or not genetic testing is available for that condition. Many people seek information and coping strategies as much as they do test results. Referral of a child with a suspected genetic problem to a geneticist, genetic clinical nurse specialist, or genetic clinic is an expected nursing responsibility in the same way as referrals to a dietitian or a social worker. When in doubt, the pediatric nurse should contact the advanced practice genetic clinical nurse, genetic counselor, or geneticist to discuss concerns.

Family Preparation for Genetic Referrals and Genetic Counseling

Not knowing what to expect from a genetic referral is common, and fear of the unknown may cause anxiety for both the child and family. In order to facilitate a genetic referral to genetic specialists, the pediatric nurse should educate the child and family so they know what to expect during as well as after a genetic evaluation.

Usually before the first genetic evaluation visit, the parents will be contacted to provide a detailed medical and family history and to make an appointment for genetic consultation. The parent should be prepared to give as exact a family history as possible so that a detailed three-generation pedigree can be constructed. The parents should be informed that a genetic consultation can last several hours. During the appointment, a genetic clinical nurse, genetic counselor, and/or physician will perform an initial interview with the parents and their child. A geneticist will examine the child and possibly the parent(s) in order to establish an accurate diagnosis. Tests may be ordered. These may include chromosome analysis, DNA-based testing, radiographs, biopsy, biochemical tests, developmental testing, or linkage studies. After the exam and the completion of any applicable testing, the geneticist or genetic counselor will discuss the findings with the parents and/or child and make recommendations. The discussion will include the natural history of the condition, the inheritance patterns, the current preventive or treatment options, and the risks to the child or family. The visit will also include opportunities for questions and answers as well as the assessment and evaluation of the family's understanding. It is typical for the information retention of a family facing a new genetic diagnosis to be very low. This makes it imperative for the nurse to reinforce genetic concepts at a later time when the individual or family is ready (Skirton, 2006).

As the visit concludes, the child and parents can expect that appropriate referrals will be made, available services will be discussed, and a follow-up visit may be scheduled. A summary of the information is usually sent to the family. The child's health care provider will receive a report if requested by the individual or parents.

Genetic health care providers present the individual and the family with information to promote informed decisions. They are also sensitive to the importance of protecting the individual's autonomy. A challenge during any visit to a genetic specialist is in providing nondirective counseling. Families should be permitted to make decisions that are not influenced by any biases or values from the nurse, counselor, or geneticist. Many families are accustomed to practitioners and nurses providing direction and guidance in their decision making, and families may be uncomfortable with the nondirectional approach of the nurse. They may believe that the nurse or health care provider is withholding very bad news. The nurse should discuss the positives and negatives of each decision and present as many options as possible through the use of therapeutic listening and communication skills.

Family Teaching

The pediatric nurse must be aware of available genetic resources and participate in education about genetic disorders as well as health promotion and prevention. Informing children and their families of what to expect from a genetic referral as well as clarifying and reinforcing information obtained during a genetic referral or genetic test results is also important.

Cultural and religious beliefs and values of the individual and family must be assessed by the nurse prior to teaching. Gene alterations may be viewed as uncontrollable, as occurring secondary to cultural beliefs such as a stranger looking at the infant, or as a "punishment." A family's readiness to learn can be influenced by cultural or religious beliefs and values. Obtaining educational materials in the primary language of the child or family will help facilitate the teaching–learning experience.

The nurse must be aware of common inheritance misconceptions such as a parent's belief that with a 25% recurrence risk, after one child is affected the next three children will be unaffected, or with a 50% recurrence risk every other child will be affected. The recurrence risk *for each pregnancy* should be continually stressed by the nurse. Families often believe that certain family members have inherited a genetic condition because they look like or "take after" a relative with a genetic condition. When new gene alterations or mutations are discussed, families will often exhibit surprise because no one else in the family has the condition so they perceive that the trait or condition cannot possibly be inherited. Helping families to understand these genetic concepts is fundamental to delivering competent genetic nursing care (Twomey, 2006).

Psychosocial Care In order to meet the psychosocial needs of the child and family, the nurse should identify their expectations and needs as well as their cultural, spiritual, value, and belief systems. Denial of a genetic diagnosis is common, and nurses must be aware of the family's state of acceptance. Nurses must often help alleviate anxiety or guilt in the child or family. Anxiety of the unknown is common when awaiting diagnosis or test results, but individuals also experience anxiety from not understanding the future implications of a confirmed genetic disease. Guilt may be associated with knowledge of a genetic condition being in a family. It is important for the nurse to reassure parents that the genetic condition is not the result of something they did or did not do during pregnancy. The nurse should encourage open discussions and the expression of fears and concerns. Guilt and shame are common as a family deals with the loss of the expectation and dream of a healthy child, grandchild, niece, or nephew. Reinforce to parents that genetic alterations are caused by changes within a gene and not by superstitions related to sin or other cultural beliefs. As mothers, fathers, and extended family members provide continuous care for the individual with a genetic condition, depression can result. Depression also can occur in the individual with the condition. The nurse must maintain awareness of the possibility of depression and be proactive in obtaining support for the individual or family (Skirton, 2006). See Chapter 28 ∞.

The nurse also is responsible for assessing the family's coping mechanisms as well as available family, spiritual, cultural, and community support systems. Genetic conditions can cause a permanent strain on family dynamics and relationships. The pediatric nurse may need to help the child and family reaffirm self-worth and value. If seen in an academic setting, parents and children may feel they are part of a "production line" even though they are present for a very private problem (Skirton, 2006). Nurses must be sensitive to these perceptions, provide open communication, and encourage discussion of feelings. Growth and development can be altered by actual or potential genetic disorders. Especially unique is the potential or actual inheritance of a late-onset condition such as Huntington disease, as discussed in the chapter-opening scenario. Like Sarah, the adolescent with this altered gene may not meet any of the developmental tasks in moving toward adulthood. Should the adolescent attend college or worry about the future? The pediatric nurse must identify the impact of genetic knowledge on activities of daily living but also movement through developmental milestones. Both individual and family strengths need to be identified (Twomey, 2006). See Chapter 2 ∞.

The nurse can refer the individual or family to a support group. However, it is important to have permission from the child or family if the nurse is providing a support group with their names and contact information. Electronic sources of genetic information abound and are unregulated; many of them are proprietary, offering expensive genetic testing that may have little scientific basis. Nurses should help families to both select and evaluate credible websites and online discussion groups.

Another key role for the nurse is to help families with the often difficult task of communicating genetic information such as inheritance patterns to extended family members. Cultural values of autonomy and privacy are affected when a person must consider whether to communicate genetic information to extended family members who may also carry the altered gene. Family members often have difficulty understanding that some genetic conditions have variable expressivity. Members of the

extended family often are shocked and feel a profound sense of guilt that they carry the gene alteration that has caused their loved one to have a genetic condition.

Managing Care Through Advocacy Careful self-assessment of feelings is essential for the nurse. The pediatric nurse must continually advocate for the child and family and support their decisions even if the decisions contradict the nurse's own ideals and morals. Coping with genetic revelations and making genetic-related treatment decisions are difficult activities for everyone. The nurse must remember that families will need resources and support, and also help in gathering information about reproductive options.

Evaluation

Expected outcomes of delivering nursing care with a genetic focus include:

- The child and family will make informed and voluntary decisions related to genetic health issues.
- The child and family will accurately identify:
  - Basic genetic concepts and simple inheritance risk probabilities
  - What to expect from a genetic referral
  - The influence of genetic factors in health promotion and health maintenance
  - Social, legal, and ethical issues related to genetic testing

■ VISIONS FOR THE FUTURE

Nurses are often the primary caregivers that children and their families turn to for information, guidance, and clarification of ideas. This nursing role is essential not only in providing direct nursing care but also as a member of the community. As more information about the genetic revolution is available to consumers—in areas such as **pharmacogenomics**, gene transfer, ethics, genetic engineering, and stem cell research—the role of nurses not only remains vital but also grows enormously. For example, research in pharmacogenetics is leading to prescribing medications based on an individual's genomic profile. As that testing becomes the standard of care, the nurse's role in ensuring the testing is completed and in interpreting results to families expands. Nurses must remain educated, informed, knowledgeable, and ready to discuss trends and changes with children, adolescents, and their families.

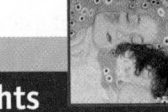

Chapter Highlights

- Nurses are responsible for basic genetic knowledge and delivering the expected standard of genetic nursing care.
- Genetic concepts can be applied to health promotion and health maintenance.

- When cell division does not occur as expected, chromosomal alterations in autosomes or sex chromosomes can result.
- Mosaicism may cause varied clinical manifestations of chromosomal alterations.

- Large chromosomal alterations can be seen in a karyotype.
- Protein-directing genes are important to life and functioning as a human being because proteins are highly specialized and perform a variety of functions within the cell.
- Different forms of a gene that occupy the same place on a pair of chromosomes are alleles.
- An individual may be identified as heterozygous or homozygous for a single gene.
- Some gene alterations cause disease, and some protect individuals from disease.
- Mitochondrial gene alterations are inherited from the mother and are primarily involved in high-energy organs such as skeletal muscles, brain, and heart muscle.
- Knowledge of the principles of inheritance allows the nurse not only to offer and reinforce genetic information to children, adolescents, and their families but also to assist them in managing their care and in making reproductive decisions.

- Multifactorial conditions do not follow Mendelian inheritance patterns.
- Basic genetic nursing care involves family risk assessment through a detailed family history, drawing a three-generation pedigree, and integrating genetic concepts into physical assessment.
- Basic genetic nursing involves initiating a referral to genetic specialists.
- Genetic health care providers present the individual and the family with information to promote informed decisions.
- There are several types of genetic tests available, all with special considerations related to the genetic testing of minors.
- The nurse must be aware of the social, ethical, cultural, and spiritual issues related to the delivery of genetic nursing care.

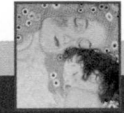

Clinical Reasoning in Action

Recall 17-year-old Sarah from the chapter opening scenario. While at the sports clinic for a routine physical, she questions the nurse about the likelihood that she will acquire Huntington disease. Huntington disease is a progressive disorder of motor, cognitive, and psychiatric disturbances. Symptoms typically present between age 35 and 44 years, with a median survival time of 15 to 18 years after onset.

Sarah's mother, Diane, is of western European Caucasian descent. Sarah's knowledge about her father is limited. She knows that he is a third-generation Filipino American but has no medical information on him or his extended family.

Sarah's grandmother on her mother's side has three sisters and two brothers. The two brothers died of myocardial infarctions at the ages of 37 and 55 years, respectively. Sarah's maternal grandfather had no brothers but two sisters. Her maternal grandfather died at age 62 years of Huntington disease. The sisters are alive and well and have no medical problems.

Diane has two brothers and two sisters. She is the youngest of the siblings. Her oldest brother, Ken, was diagnosed 10 years ago with Huntington disease at age 41 years. Ken has two daughters

ages 21 and 25 years. Sarah is very close to these cousins and she knows that they have no medical problems beyond seasonal allergies and migraine headaches. Diane's other brother, Brian (age 38 years), has recently had bouts of depression and has noticed slight difficulties in coordination and involuntary movements. Brian and his wife Sally adopted a son, Dave, with Down syndrome, and he is 19 years old. Sarah's brother is age 12 years and does not have any medical problems.

1. What further data would you gather from Sarah before referring her to a genetic specialist?
2. What are the signs and symptoms of Huntington disease? The prognosis? Is it linked to any ethnic group?
3. Create a family pedigree for Sarah based on the family information she has provided. What does the pedigree reveal, and what nursing actions would you plan for Sarah?
4. Should Sarah be tested at this time? Give a rationale for your answer.

See Pearson Nursing Student Resources for possible responses.

Pearson Nursing Student Resources

**Find additional review materials at
nursing.pearsonhighered.com**

Prepare for success with NCLEX®-style practice questions, interactive assignments and activities, web links, animations and videos, and more!

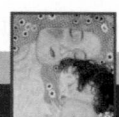

References

American Nurses Association (ANA) & International Society of Nurses in Genetics (ISONG). (2007). *Genetics/genomics nursing: Scope and standards of practice.* Silver Spring, MD: NursesBooks .org

Arnheim, N., & Calabrese, P. (2009). Understanding what determines the frequency and pattern of human germline mutations. *Nature Reviews Genetics, 10,* 478–488.

Bennett, R. L. (2010). *The practical guide to the genetic family history* (2nd ed.). Hoboken, NJ: Wiley-Blackwell.

Bennett, R. L., French, K. S., Resta, R. G., & Doyle, D. L. (2008). Standardized human pedigree nomenclature: Update and assessment of the recommendations of the National Society of Genetic Counselors. *Journal of Genetic Counseling, 17*(5), 424–433.

Borry, P., Goffin, T., Nys, H., & Dierickx, K. (2008). Predictive genetic testing in minors for adult-onset genetic diseases. *Mount Sinai Journal of Medicine, 75,* 287–296.

Borry, P., Nys, H., & Dierickx, K. (2007). Carrier testing in minors: Conflicting views. *Nature Reviews Genetics, 11,* 828.

Cameron, L. D., & Muller, C. (2009). Psychosocial aspects of genetic testing. *Current Opinion in Psychiatry, 22,* 218–223.

Centers for Disease Control and Prevention (CDC). (n.d.). *Single gene disorders and disability (SGDD).* Retrieved from http://www.cdc.gov/ ncbddd/single_gene/default.htm

CFTR. (2009). Retrieved from http://ghr.nlm.nih .gov/gene=cftr

Consensus Panel on Genetic/Genomic Nursing Competencies. (2009). *Essentials of genetic and genomic nursing: Competencies, curricula guidelines, and outcome indicators* (2nd ed.). Silver Spring, MD: American Nurses Association.

Cystic Fibrosis Mutation Database. (2007). Retrieved from http://www.genet.sickkids.on.ca/ cftr/StatisticsPage.html

DiMauro, S. (2007). Mitochondrial DNA medicine. *Bioscience Reports, 27,* 5–9.

Florez, J. C. (2008). The genetics of type 2 diabetes: A realistic appraisal in 2008. *Journal of Clinical Endocrinology and Metabolism, 93*(12), 4633–4642.

Gaff, C., Emery, J., & Metcalfe, S. A. (2007). Family genetics. *Australian Family Physician, 36*(10), 802–805.

GeneTests. (2009). Retrieved from http://www .genetests.org

Genetics and Public Policy Center. (2007). *U.S. public opinion on uses of genetic information and genetic discrimination.* Retrieved from http:// www.dnapolicy.org/resources/GINAPublic_ Opinion_Genetic_Information_Discrimination .pdf

Genome Statistics: Assembly and Genebuild. (2009). Retrieved from http://www.ensembl.org/ Homo_sapiens/Info/StatsTable

Genzyme Genetics. (n.d.). *Cystic fibrosis (CF) gene sequencing.* Retrieved from http://www .genzymegenetics.com/about/news/gene_p_ news_cfgenesequencing.asp

Gurian, E. A., Kinnamon, D. D., Henry, J. J., & Waisbren, S. E. (2006). Expanded newborn screening for biochemical disorders: The effect of a false-positive result. *Pediatrics, 117*(6), 1915–1921.

Gurrieri, F., & Accadia, M. (2009). Genetic imprinting: The paradigm of Prader-Willi and Angelman syndromes. *Endocrine Development, 14,* 20–28.

Haga, S. B., & Terry, S. F. (2009). Ensuring the safe use of genomic medicine in children. *Clinical Pediatrics, 48*(7), 703–708.

Inglese, M. D., & Elder, J. H. (2009). Caring for children with autism spectrum disorder, Part I: Prevalence, etiology, and core features. *Journal of Pediatric Nursing, 24*(1), 41–48.

Jones, K. L. (2006). *Smith's recognizable patterns of human malformations* (6th ed.). Philadelphia: Saunders.

Lea, D. H. (2008). Genetic and genomic healthcare: Ethical issues of importance to nurses. *Online Journal of Issues in Nursing, 13*(1), 6.

Moskowitz, S. M., Chmiel, J. F., Sternen, D. L., Cheng, E., & Cutting, G. R. (2008). *CFTR-related disorders.* Retrieved from http://www.ncbi.nlm .nih.gov/bookshelf/br.fcgi?book=gene&part= cf#cf.T11

Noordam, M. J., & Repping, S. (2006). The human Y chromosome: A masculine chromosome. *Current Opinions in Genetics and Development, 16,* 225–232.

Nussbaum, R. L., McInnes, R. R., & Willard, H. F. (2007). *Thompson & Thompson genetics in medicine* (7th ed.). Philadelphia: Saunders.

Online Mendelian Inheritance in Man (OMIM). (2009). Baltimore: McKusick-Nathans Institute for Genetics Medicine, Johns Hopkins University; Bethesda, MD: National Center for Biotechnology Information Library of Medicine. Retrieved from http://www.ncbi.nlm.nih.gov/sites/entrez? db=OMIM

Pastores, G. M., & Hughes, D. A. (2008). *Gaucher disease.* Retrieved from http://www.ncbi.nlm.nih .gov/bookshelf/br.fcgi?book=gene&part= gaucher

Piacentini, L., Biasin, M., Fenizia, C., & Clerici, M. (2008). Genetic correlates of protection against HIV infection: The ally within. *Journal of Internal Medicine, 265*(1), 110–124.

Pierce, B. A. (2008). *Genetics: A conceptual approach* (3rd ed.). New York: W. H. Freeman and Company.

Pierce, J. D., Fakhari, M., Works, K. V., Pierce, J. T., & Clancy, R. L. (2007). Understanding proteomics. *Nursing and Health Science, 9,* 54–60.

Pierpont, M. E., Basson, C. T., Benson, D. W., Gelb, B. D., Giglia, T. M., Goldmuntz, E., et al. (Congenital Cardiac Defects Committee, Council on Cardiovascular Disease in the Young). (2007). Genetic basis for congenital heart defects: Current knowledge. *Circulation, 115,* 3015–3038.

Ranweiler, R. (2009). Assessment and care of the newborn with Down syndrome. *Advances in Neonatal Care, 9*(2), 17–24.

Skirton, H. (2006). Parental experience of a pediatric genetic referral. *MCN. The American Journal of Maternal Child Nursing, 31,* 178–184.

Snow, K. (n.d.). *People first language.* Retrieved from http://www.disabilityisnatural.com

Steinberg, M. H. (2008). Sickle cell anemia, the first molecular disease: Overview of molecular etiology, pathophysiology, and therapeutic approaches. *Scientific World Journal, 8,* 1295–1324.

Tay-Sachs Disease. (2009). Retrieved from http:// www.ncbi.nlm.nih.gov/entrez/dispomim .cgi?id=272800

Twomey, J. G. (2006). Issues in genetic testing of children. *MCN, American Journal of Maternal Child Nursing, 31*(3), 156–163.

U.S. Department of Health and Human Services. (2008). *United States system of oversight of genetic testing: A response to the charge of the Secretary of Health and Human Services. Report of the Secretary's Advisory Committee on Genetics, Health, and Society (SACGHS).* Retrieved from http:// oba.od.nih.gov/oba/SACGHS/reports/ SACGHS_oversight_report.pdf

Vichinsky, E., & Schlis, K. (2006). *Sickle cell disease.* Retrieved from http://www.ncbi.nlm.nih.gov/ bookshelf/br.fcgi?book=gene&part=sickle

Zhang, F., Gu, W., Hurles, M. E., & Lupski, J. R. (2009). Copy number variation in human health, disease and evolution. *Annual Reviews of Genomics and Human Genetics, 10,* 451–481.

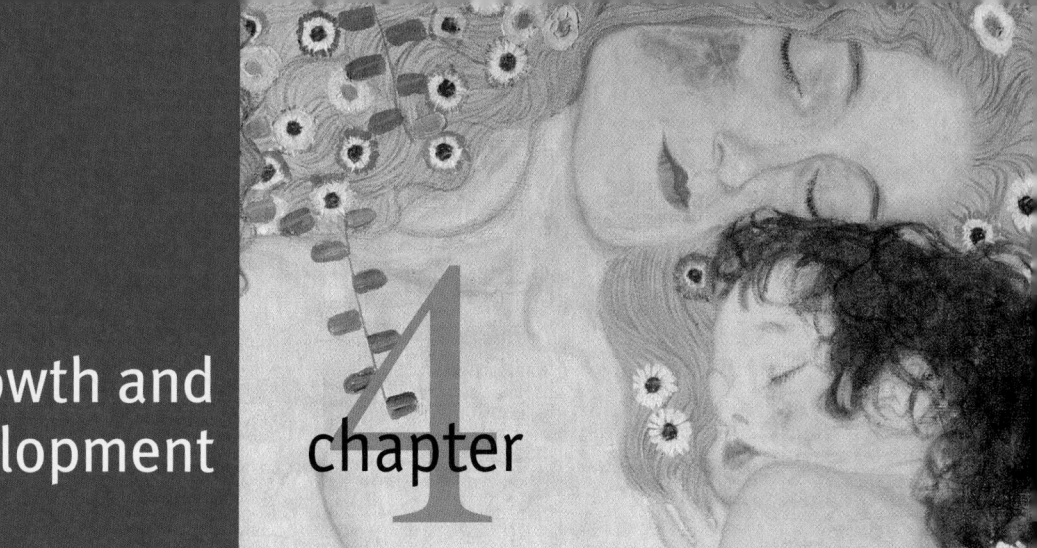

Growth and Development chapter 4

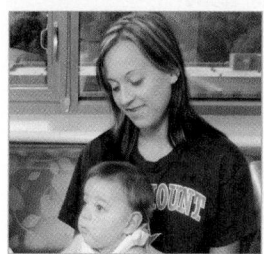

Yolanda and Pepe Gomez are the parents of Sergio, who was born at 29 weeks gestation. Sergio is their first child, and all appeared to be going well in the pregnancy until Yolanda went into labor. The family had no significant history of congenital conditions or premature births. Sergio was born after a short labor and weighed 1250 grams (2.75 pounds). Although he did well initially, Sergio soon developed respiratory distress syndrome, and was placed on a ventilator in the neonatal intensive care unit. He required parenteral feedings but as he grew and improved, he was able to start gavage feedings of his mother's breast milk, and finally learned to breastfeed. Sergio was discharged from the hospital in stable condition at 2 months of age. He is now 6 months, and other than two respiratory illnesses, he has continued to grow and develop without additional health problems. The nurse in the pediatric health care home monitors Sergio monthly, performing developmental assessments, monitoring his visual and hearing responses, and providing ideas for his parents about how to best promote his development. How can the nurse best facilitate Sergio's continued developmental progression? What do the parents need to know about prematurity and how to best support their son?

Learning Outcomes

After reading this chapter, you will be able to do the following:

1. Describe major theories of development as formulated by Freud, Erikson, Piaget, Kohlberg, social learning theorists, and behaviorists.
2. Plan nursing interventions for children that are appropriate for the child's developmental state, based on theoretical frameworks.
3. Explain contemporary developmental approaches such as temperament theory, ecologic theory, and the resilience framework.
4. Recognize major developmental milestones for infants, toddlers, preschoolers, school-age children, and adolescents.
5. Synthesize information from several theoretical approaches to plan assessments of the child's growth and developmental milestones.
6. Describe the role of play in the growth and development of children.
7. Use data collected during developmental assessments to plan activities that promote development of children and adolescents.

■ INTRODUCTION

Children develop as they interact with their surroundings. They learn skills at different ages, but the order in which they learn them is universal. Development is affected by factors such as nutrition and cultural practices, as well as the social situation in the country or neighborhood. While Sergio will develop in a unique manner influenced by his genetic makeup, his early treatment for prematurity, his life experiences, the interaction between these factors, and certain principles of development can assist his parents and the nurse in fostering positive adaptations for him.

In this chapter, you will learn general principles of growth and development and will explore several theories related to childhood development, as well as their nursing applications. Each age group, from infancy through adolescence, is described in detail. Developmental milestones, physical and cognitive characteristics, play patterns, communication strategies, and conditions that interfere with usual developmental progression are presented. This information will help you provide developmentally appropriate care for children in each age group and in a variety of situations. You can apply these concepts to all children, including special situations such as the one described in the opening scenario. This chapter serves as a review of growth and development as well as an analysis and application of growth and development theories directly applicable in nursing. The information here will lead you directly to Chapters 6 through 9 ∞ where growth and development knowledge is applied to plan health promotion and maintenance visits with children and adolescents.

■ PRINCIPLES OF GROWTH AND DEVELOPMENT

It is essential to understand the concepts of growth and development when learning to care for children. A skilled pediatric nurse integrates knowledge of physical growth and psychosocial development into each child health care encounter. **Growth** refers to an increase in physical size. Growth represents quantitative changes such as height, weight, blood pressure, and number of words in the child's vocabulary. **Development** refers to an increase in capability or function. Developmental skills unfold in a complex manner as a relationship between the child's innate, unfolding capabilities and the stimuli and support provided in the environment. Developmental skills, such as the ability to sit without support or to throw a ball overhand, unfold over time in a complex manner influenced by the relationship between the child's innate capabilities and the stimuli and support provided by the environment. The quantitative and qualitative changes in body organ functioning, ability to communicate, and performance of motor skills during developmental progression are key components in the process of planning pediatric health care.

Each child displays a unique maturational pattern during the process of development. Although the exact age at which skills emerge differs, the sequence or order of skill performance is uniform among children. Skill development proceeds according to two processes: from the head downward and from the center of the body out to the extremities. Development that proceeds from the head downward through the body and toward the feet is called

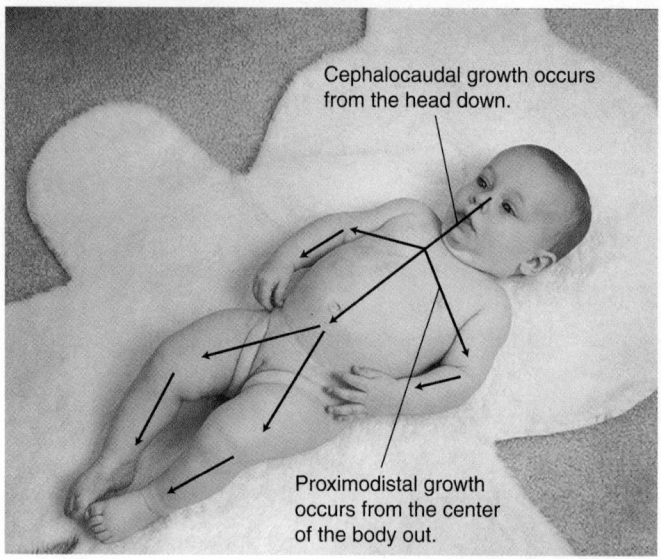

FIGURE 4–1 ➤ In normal cephalocaudal growth, the child gains control of the head and neck before the trunk and limbs. In normal proximodistal growth, the child controls arm movements before hand movements. For example, the child reaches for objects before being able to grasp them. Children gain control of their hands before their fingers; that is, they can hold things with the entire hand before they can pick something up with just their fingers.

cephalocaudal development (Figure 4–1 ➤). For example, at birth, an infant's head is much larger proportionately than the trunk or extremities. Similarly, infants learn to hold up their heads before sitting, and to sit before standing. Skills such as walking that involve the legs and feet develop last in infancy. Development that proceeds from the center of the body outward to the extremities is called **proximodistal development** (see Figure 4–1). For example, infants are first able to control the trunk, then the arms; only later are fine motor movements of the fingers possible. Pediatric nurses use these concepts of predictable and sequential developmental direction to analyze the infant's and child's present state and to assist parents to plan ways to encourage and support the next emerging developmental abilities.

During the childhood years, extraordinary changes occur in all aspects of development. Physical size, motor skills, cognitive ability, language, sensory ability, and psychosocial patterns all undergo major transformations. Nurses study normal patterns of development so they can perform thorough pediatric assessments and identify children who demonstrate slow or abnormal development. These assessments can guide the nurse in planning interventions for the child and family, such as referring the child for a diagnostic evaluation or rehabilitation, or teaching the parents how to provide adequate stimulation for the child. When development is proceeding normally, the nurse uses the knowledge of usual patterns to plan teaching approaches based on the child's cognitive and language ability, to offer appropriate toys and activities during illness, and to respond therapeutically during interactions with the child.

■ MAJOR THEORIES OF DEVELOPMENT

Child development is a complex process. Many theorists have attempted to organize their observations of behavior into a description of principles or a set of stages. Each theory focuses on a particular facet of development. Most developmental theorists separate children into age groups by common characteristics. See Box 4–1 and Table 4–1.

Freud's Theory of Psychosexual Development

Theoretical Framework

The psychoanalytic techniques used by Freud led him to believe that early childhood experiences form the unconscious motivation for actions in later life. He developed a theory that sexual energy is centered in specific parts of the body at certain ages. Unresolved conflict and unmet needs at a certain stage lead to a fixation of development at that stage (Craig & Dunn, 2010).

Freud viewed the personality as a structure with three parts: the *id*, the basic sexual energy that is present at birth and drives the individual to seek pleasure; the *ego*, the realistic part of the person, which develops during infancy and searches for acceptable methods of meeting impulses; and the *superego*, the moral and ethical system, which develops in childhood and contains a set of values and conscience (Craig & Dunn, 2010). The ego diverts impulses and protects itself from excess anxiety by use of **defense mechanisms**, which are unconscious techniques that distort reality to protect the self from excessive anxiety (Table 4–2).

Stages

Oral (Birth to 1 Year)   The infant derives pleasure largely from the mouth, with sucking and eating as primary desires.

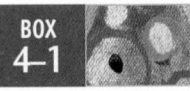

BOX 4-1   Developmental Age Groups

Infancy—Birth to 12 months. Includes infants or babies up to 1 year of age who require a high level of care in daily activities.

Toddlerhood—1 to 3 years. Characterized by increased motor ability and independent behavior.

Preschool—3 to 6 years. The preschooler refines gross and fine motor ability and language skills and often participates in a preschool learning program.

School age—6 to 12 years. Begins with entry into a school system and is characterized by growing intellectual skills, physical ability, and independence.

Adolescence—12 to 18 years. Begins with entry into the teen years. Mature cognitive thought, formation of identity, and influence of peers are important characteristics of adolescence.

Anal (1 to 3 Years)   The young child's pleasure is centered in the anal area, with control over body secretions as a prime force in behavior.

Phallic (3 to 6 Years)   Sexual energy becomes centered in the genitalia as the child works out relationships with parents of the same and opposite sexes.

Latency (6 to 12 Years)   Sexual energy is at rest in the passage between earlier stages and adolescence.

TABLE 4–1   Major Developmental Theorists

Theorist	Years of Life	Background
Sigmund Freud	1856–1939	Freud was a physician in Vienna, Austria. His work with adults who were experiencing a variety of nervous disorders led Freud to develop the approach called psychoanalysis, which explored the driving forces of the unconscious mind.
Erik Erikson	1902–1994	Erikson studied Freud's theory of psychoanalysis under Freud's daughter, Anna, but later established his own developmental theory emphasizing the psychosocial nature of individuals. Erikson's theory is one of the few that addresses development over the entire life span.
Jean Piaget	1896–1980	Piaget was a 20th-century Swiss scientist who watched his own three children carefully and wrote detailed journals of their behaviors and verbalizations. He studied the intellectual abilities of children, focusing on child psychology and its application to education.
Lawrence Kohlberg	1927–1987	Kohlberg used Piaget's cognitive stage theory as the basis for his theory of moral development. He worked with children in his native Germany and in many other countries, including Kenya, Taiwan, and Mexico.
Albert Bandura	b. 1925	Bandura is a Canadian who has conducted psychologic research at Stanford University for many years. He believes that children learn from their social environment, particularly by modeling the observed behaviors of others.
John Watson	1878–1958	Watson was an American scientist who applied the work of animal behaviorists, such as Ivan Pavlov and B. F. Skinner, to children.
Urie Bronfenbrenner	1917–2005	Bronfenbrenner established the ecologic theory of development and served as a professor at Cornell University. He viewed the child as interacting with the environment at different levels, or systems. This revolutionary approach emphasizes the series of mutual interactions between the child and the various systems.
Stella Chess and Alexander Thomas Chess (1914–2007); Thomas (1914–2003)		Chess and Thomas were psychiatrists who began the New York Longitudinal Study in 1956 with 141 children, which they expanded in 1961 with 95 additional children. Most of these individuals are still being assessed periodically as adults. Their research identified characteristics of personality and provides a basis for the ongoing study of temperament (Chess & Thomas, 1995).

TABLE 4–2	Common Defense Mechanisms Used by Children	
Defense Mechanism	Definition	Example
Regression	Return to an earlier behavior	A previously toilet-trained child becomes incontinent when separated from parents during a hospitalization.
Repression	Involuntary forgetting of uncomfortable situations	An abused child cannot consciously recall episodes of abuse.
Rationalization	An attempt to make unacceptable feelings acceptable	A child explains hitting another because "he took my toy."
Fantasy	A creation of the mind to help deal with unacceptable fear	A hospitalized child who is weak pretends to be Superman.

Genital (12 Years to Adulthood) Mature sexuality is achieved as physical growth is completed and relationships with others occur.

Nursing Application

Freud's theory has been criticized for several reasons—he developed a theory of childhood based on his work with adults, primarily women who sought help in dealing with emotional issues; he viewed males as dominant; and he ignored the effects of culture and other experiences. However, some parts of his theory can be applied in nursing. Freud emphasized the importance of meeting the needs of each stage in order to move successfully into future developmental stages. The crisis of illness can interfere with normal developmental processes and add challenges for the nurse who is striving to meet an ill child's needs. For example, the importance of sucking in infancy guides the nurse to provide a pacifier for the infant who cannot have oral fluids. The preschool child's concern about sexuality guides the nurse to provide privacy and clear explanations during any procedures involving the genital area. It may be necessary to teach parents that masturbation by the young child is normal and to help parents deal with it through distraction or refocusing. The adolescent's focus on relationships suggests that the nurse should include questions about significant friends during history taking. Table 4–3 summarizes ways in which the nurse can apply these theoretical concepts to the care of children.

Erikson's Theory of Psychosocial Development

Theoretical Framework

Erikson's theory establishes psychosocial stages during eight periods of human life. For each stage, Erikson identified a crisis, that is, a particular challenge that exists for healthy personality development to occur (Erikson, 1963, 1968). The word *crisis* in this context refers to normal maturational social needs rather than to a single critical event. Each developmental crisis has two possible outcomes: When needs are met, the consequence is healthy and the individual moves on to future stages with particular strengths. When needs are not met, an unhealthy outcome occurs that will influence future social relationships.

Stages

Trust Versus Mistrust (Birth to 1 Year) The task of the first year of life is to establish trust in the people providing care. Trust is fostered by provision of food, clean clothing, touch, and comfort. If basic needs are not met, the infant will eventually learn to mistrust others.

Autonomy Versus Shame and Doubt (1 to 3 Years) The toddler's sense of autonomy or independence is shown by controlling body excretions, saying no when asked to do something, and directing motor activity. Children who are consistently criticized for expressions of autonomy or for lack of control—for example, during toilet training—will develop a sense of shame about themselves and doubt in their abilities (Figure 4–2 ➤).

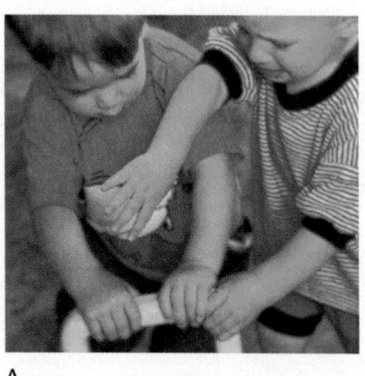
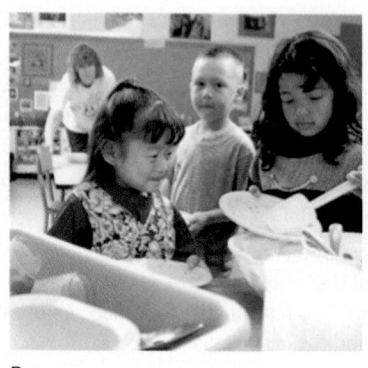
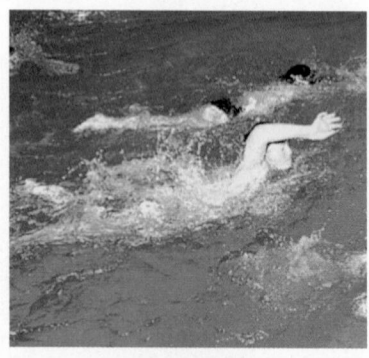

A   B   C

FIGURE 4–2 ➤ Erikson's Psychosocial Stages. A, The toddler shows *autonomy* by exerting control over toys and activities. B, Preschoolers demonstrate *initiative* by planning and carrying out activities. C, School-age children excel at *industry* when they take pride in accomplishments, such as those achieved in sporting activities.

Age Group	Developmental Stages	Nursing Applications
Infant (birth to 1 year)	Oral stage (Freud): The baby obtains pleasure and comfort through the mouth.	When a baby is NPO, offer a pacifier if not contraindicated. After painful procedures, offer a baby a bottle or pacifier or have the mother breastfeed.
	Trust versus mistrust stage (Erikson): The baby establishes a sense of trust when basic needs are met.	Hold the hospitalized baby often. Offer comfort after painful procedures. Meet the baby's needs for food and hygiene. Encourage parents to room in. Manage pain effectively with use of pain medications and other measures.
	Sensorimotor stage (Piaget): The baby learns from movement and sensory input.	Use crib mobiles, manipulative toys, wall murals, and bright colors to provide interesting stimuli and comfort. Use toys to distract the baby during procedures and assessments.
Toddler (1–3 years)	Anal stage (Freud): The child derives gratification from control over body excretions.	Ask about toilet training and the child's rituals and words for elimination during the admission history. Continue the child's normal patterns of elimination in the hospital. Do not begin toilet training during illness or hospitalization. Accept regression in toileting during illness or hospitalization. Have potty chairs available in the hospital and childcare centers. Allow self-feeding opportunities.
	Autonomy versus shame and doubt stage (Erikson): The child is increasingly independent in many spheres of life.	Encourage the child to remove and put on own clothes, brush teeth, or assist with hygiene. **(1)** If restraint for a procedure is necessary, proceed quickly, providing explanations and comfort.
	Sensorimotor stage (end); preoperational stage (beginning) (Piaget): The child shows increasing curiosity and explorative behavior. Language skills improve.	Ensure safe surroundings to allow opportunities to manipulate objects. Name objects and give simple explanations.
Preschooler (3–6 years)	Phallic stage (Freud): The child initially identifies with the parent of the opposite sex but by the end of this stage has identified with the same-sex parent.	Be alert for children who appear more comfortable with male or female nurses, and attempt to accommodate them. Encourage parental involvement in care. Plan for playtime and offer a variety of materials from which to choose.
	Initiative versus guilt stage (Erikson): The child likes to initiate play activities.	Offer medical equipment for play to lessen anxiety about strange objects. **(2)** Assess children's concerns as expressed through their drawings. Accept the child's choices and expressions of feelings.
	Preoperational stage (Piaget): The child is increasingly verbal but has some limitations in thought processes. Causality is often confused, so the child may feel responsible for causing an illness.	Offer explanations about all procedures and treatments. Clearly explain that the child is not responsible for causing the illness.

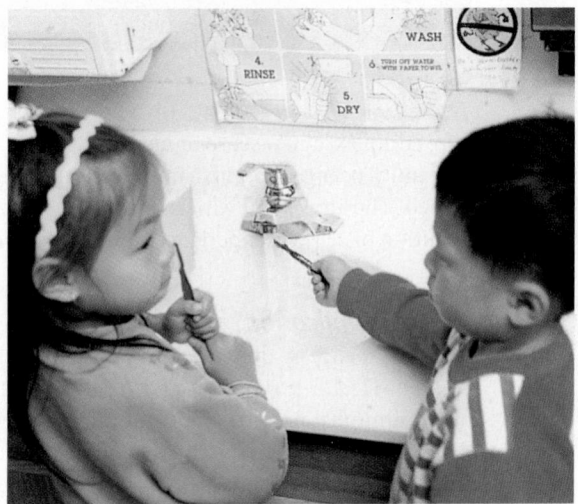

(1)

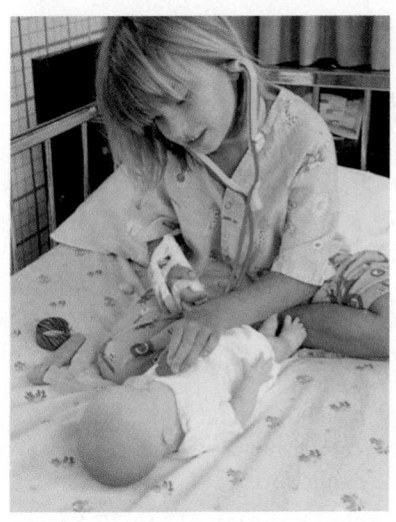

(2)

(continued)

TABLE 4–3	Nursing Applications of Theories of Freud, Erikson, and Piaget	*(continued)*
Age Group	Developmental Stages	Nursing Applications
School age (6–12 years)	Latency stage (Freud): The child places importance on privacy and understanding the body. Industry versus inferiority stage (Erikson): The child gains a sense of self-worth from involvement in activities. Concrete operational stage (Piaget): The child is capable of mature thought when allowed to manipulate and see objects.	Provide gowns, covers, and underwear. Knock on door before entering. Explain treatments and procedures. Encourage the child to continue school work while hospitalized. Encourage the child to bring favorite pastimes to the hospital. **(3)** Help the child adjust to limitations on favorite activities. Give clear instructions about details of treatment. Show the child equipment that will be used in treatment.
Adolescent (12–18 years)	Genital stage (Freud): The adolescent's focus is on genital function and relationships. Identity versus role confusion stage (Erikson): The adolescent's search for self-identity leads to independence from parents and reliance on peers. Formal operational stage (Piaget): The adolescent is capable of mature, abstract thought.	Ensure access to gynecologic care for adolescent girls. Provide information on sexuality. Ensure privacy during health care. Have brochures and videos available for teaching about sexuality. Provide a separate recreation room for teens who are hospitalized. **(4)** Take the health history and perform examinations without parents present. Introduce the adolescent to other teens with the same health condition. Give clear and complete information about health care and treatments. Offer both written and verbal instructions. Continue to provide education about the disease to the adolescent with a chronic illness, as mature thought now leads to greater understanding.

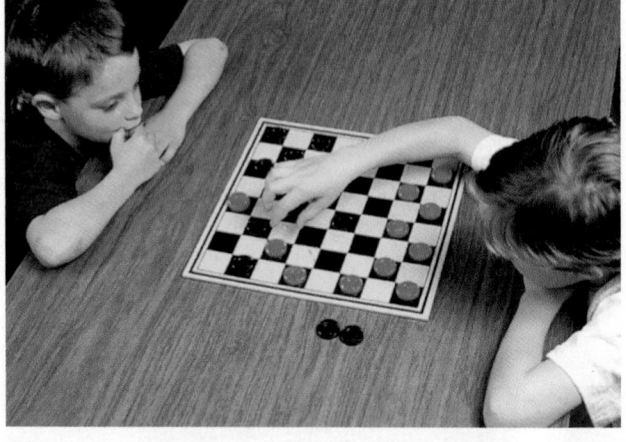

(3)

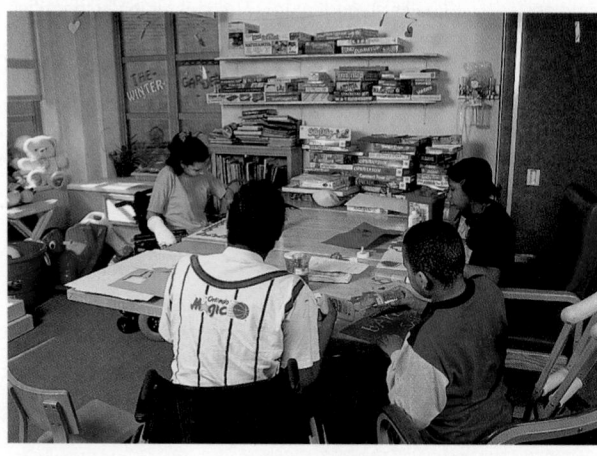

(4)

Initiative Versus Guilt (3 to 6 Years) The young child initiates new activities and considers new ideas. This interest in exploring the world creates a child who is involved and busy. Constant criticism, however, leads to feelings of guilt and a lack of purpose.

Industry Versus Inferiority (6 to 12 Years) The middle years of childhood are characterized by development of new interests and by involvement in activities. The child takes pride in accomplishments in sports, school, home, and community. If the child cannot accomplish what is expected, however, the result will be a sense of inferiority.

Identity Versus Role Confusion (12 to 18 Years) In adolescence, as the body matures and thought processes become more complex, a new sense of identity or self is established. The self, family, peer group, and community are all examined and redefined. The adolescent who is unable to establish a meaningful definition of self will experience confusion in one or more roles of life.

Nursing Application

Erikson's theory is directly applicable to the nursing care of children. Health promotion and health maintenance visits in the community provide opportunities for helping caregivers meet children's needs. Parents benefit from learning what the child's developmental tasks are at each stage and from discussing ideas about how to encourage healthy psychosocial development. Such discussions may also highlight parental concerns and provide a forum for reassurance about normal developmental characteristics.

The child's usual support from family, peers, and others is interrupted by hospitalization. The challenge of hospitalization also adds a situational crisis to the normal developmental crisis a child is experiencing. Although the nurse may meet many of the hospitalized child's needs, continued parental involvement is necessary both during and after hospitalization to ensure progression through expected developmental stages (see Table 4–3). Asking parents about the child's developmental progression offers clues to activities and provides information about the child's psychosocial needs during hospitalization.

Piaget's Theory of Cognitive Development

Theoretical Framework

Based on his observations and work with children, Piaget formulated a theory of cognitive (or intellectual) development. He believed that the child's view of the world is influenced largely by age and maturational ability. Given nurturing experiences, the child's ability to learn matures naturally (Ginsberg & Opper, 1988; Piaget, 1972; Zirkle, 2005; Bremner, Bryant, & Mareschal, 2006). The child incorporates new experiences via **assimilation** and changes to deal with these experiences by the process of **accommodation**. An example of assimilation occurs when the infant uses reflexes to suck on objects that touch the lips. With more experiences the infant accommodates by realizing that not all objects are pleasant to suck; cognitive structures change to integrate and learn from the experiences of sucking.

Stages

Sensorimotor (Birth to 2 Years)   Infants learn about the world by input obtained through the senses and by their motor activity. Six substages are characteristic of this stage.

Use of Reflexes (Birth to 1 Month)   The infant begins life with a set of reflexes such as sucking, rooting, and grasping. By using these reflexes, the infant receives stimulation via touch, sound, smell, and vision. The reflexes thus pave the way for the first learning to occur.

Primary Circular Reactions (1 to 4 Months)   Once the infant responds reflexively, the pleasure gained from that response causes repetition of the behavior. For example, if a toy grasped reflexively makes noise and is interesting to watch, the infant will grasp it again (Figure 4–3A ➤).

Secondary Circular Reactions (4 to 8 Months)   Awareness of the environment grows as the infant begins to connect cause and effect. The sounds of bottle preparation will lead to excited behavior. If an object is partially hidden, the infant will attempt to uncover and retrieve it.

Coordination of Secondary Schemes (8 to 12 Months)   Intentional behavior is observed as the infant uses learned behavior to obtain objects, create sounds, or engage in other pleasurable activity. **Object permanence** (the knowledge that something continues to exist even when out of sight) begins when the infant remembers where a hidden object is likely to be found; it is no longer "out of sight, out of mind." However, the concept of object permanence is not fully developed. The infant knows the parent well, objects to new people, and seems very worried when the parent leaves. Other caretakers may be rejected as the infant does not understand that the parent will return. This phase of "stranger anxiety" is quite common and heralds the infant's growing recognition of and desire to be cared for by the parent.

Tertiary Circular Reactions (12 to 18 Months)   Curiosity, experimentation, and exploration predominate as the toddler tries out actions to learn results. Objects are turned in every direction, placed in the mouth, used for banging, and inserted in containers as their qualities and uses are explored (Figure 4–3B).

Mental Combinations (18 to 24 Months)   Language provides a new tool for the toddler to use in understanding the world. Language enables the child to think about events and objects before or after they occur. Object permanence is now fully developed as the child actively searches for objects in various locations and out of view. The child who has had successful separations from the

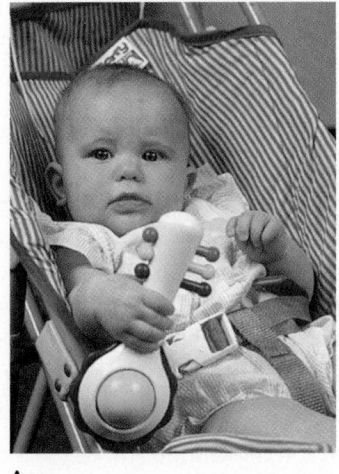 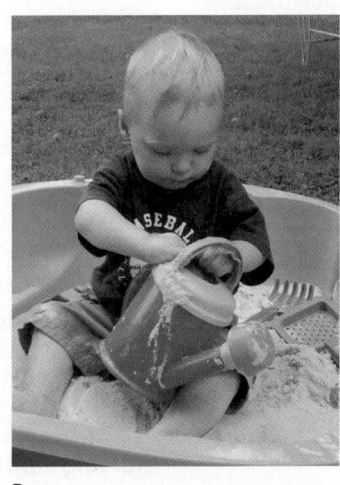 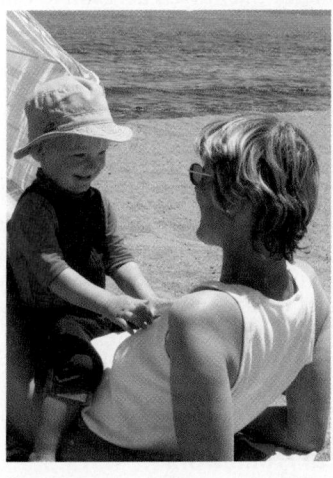

A   B   C

FIGURE 4–3 ➤ Piaget's Cognitive Stages. A, A young infant displays *primary circular reactions* when a reflexive response, such as shaking a rattle, results in pleasure and is repeated. B, As the infant becomes a toddler, *tertiary circular reactions* are demonstrated when the child experiments with objects by turning them, placing them in the mouth, and banging them. C, Toddlers and preschoolers demonstrate *mental combinations* as they increasingly use language to describe and understand their worlds.

parents followed by return, such as hours spent in another's home or childcare center, begins to understand that the missing parent will return (Figure 4–3C).

Preoperational (2 to 7 Years)   The young child thinks by using words as symbols, but logic is not well developed. During the *preconceptual substage* (2 to 4 years), vocabulary and comprehension increase greatly, but the child shows **egocentrism** (that is, an inability to see things from the perspective of another). In the *intuitive substage* (4 to 7 years), the child relies on **transductive reasoning** (that is, drawing conclusions from one general fact to another). For example, if a child disobeys a parent and then falls and breaks an arm that day, the child may ascribe the broken arm to bad behavior. Cause-and-effect relationships are often unrealistic or a result of **magical thinking** (the belief that events occur because of thoughts or wishes). Additional characteristics noted in the thought of preschoolers include **centration**, or the ability to consider only one aspect of a situation at a time, and **animism**, or ascribing life to inanimate objects because they move, make noise, or have certain other qualities.

Concrete Operational (7 to 11 Years)   Transductive reasoning has given way to a more accurate understanding of cause and effect. The child can reason quite well if concrete objects are used in teaching or experimentation. The concept of **conservation** (that matter does not change when its form is altered) is learned at this age.

Formal Operational (11 Years to Adulthood)   Fully mature intellectual thought has now been attained. The adolescent can think abstractly about objects or concepts and consider different alternatives or outcomes.

Nursing Application

Piaget's theory is essential to pediatric nursing. The nurse must understand a child's thought processes in order to design stimulating activities and meaningful, appropriate teaching plans. Health teaching is tailored to understanding of cognitive stages. For example, understanding a child's concept of time suggests to the nurse how far in advance to prepare that child for procedures. Similarly, the nurse's decision to offer manipulative toys, read stories, draw pictures, or give the child reading material to explain health care measures depends on the child's cognitive stage of development (see Table 4–3).

 Health Promotion

Refer back to the opening scenario and 6-month-old Sergio. How can you encourage his motor development? What play activities will you plan for Sergio that his parents can introduce at home? What kind of toys are most appropriate? Suggest some that will foster his development.

Kohlberg's Theory of Moral Development

Theoretical Framework

Lawrence Kohlberg's focus was on a particular type of cognitive development concerned with moral decisions. He presented stories involving moral dilemmas to children and adults and asked them to solve the dilemmas. Kohlberg then analyzed the motives

Research   *Cognitive Theories*

All developmental theories are simply that—theories. A theory is developed to explain a collection of observations or facts and to predict future occurrences. No theory can explain all of reality, and all have some strengths and some weaknesses. Although Piaget's theory of cognitive development provides a useful framework to examine and understand the thought process of young children, like all theories, it is not perfect. He developed the theory mainly by observation of his own three children. It may lack some applicability in cross-cultural contexts, and it does not explain the importance of social contexts in learning. Two other important cognitive theories help to expand the work of Piaget and may provide assistance for nurses planning to teach young children:

1. Lev Vygotsky (1896–1934) agreed with Piaget's theory of the child's cognition. However, he believed that children are embedded in social contexts that influence learning. As parents and others guide and assist children, they learn tasks that were impossible for them to master alone. He also viewed the social structure of language as essential to development of thought (Santrock, 2009; Vygotsky, 1962).
2. Information processing is another theory about cognitive development that views attention and memory as the most important parts of learning, rather than the structures described by Piaget. Infants tend to habituate or become bored with the same stimuli and therefore are more attentive to, and learn from, new stimuli that are introduced to them. Both long-term and short-term memory are important to learning. The older child actively engages in strategies to assist with memorization, thereby playing an active part in learning (Meltzoff & Gopnick, 1997; Santrock, 2009).

people expressed when making decisions about the best course to take. Based on the explanations given, Kohlberg established three levels of moral reasoning. Although he provided age guidelines, he stated that they are approximate and that many people never reach the highest (postconventional) stage of development (Santrock, 2009).

Kohlberg's work has been criticized for insensitivity to cultural differences in moral reasoning, lack of consideration of the family in moral development, an emphasis on moral reasoning rather than actual actions, and sexual bias. However, it remains a useful framework to help understand moral decision making.

Stages

Preconventional (4 to 7 Years)   Decisions are based on the desire to please others and to avoid punishment.

Conventional (7 to 11 Years)   Conscience or an internal set of standards becomes important. Rules are important and must be followed to please other people and "be good."

Postconventional (12 Years and Older)   The individual has internalized ethical standards on which to base decisions. Social responsibility is recognized. The value in each of two differing moral approaches can be considered and a decision made.

Nursing Application

Decision making is required in many areas of health care. Children can be assisted to make decisions about health care and to consider alternatives when available. The nurse should keep in mind that young children may agree to participate in research simply because they want to comply with adults and appear co-operative. Guidelines for child participation in research are available (see Chapter 1 ∞).

Parents can be provided with information so that they can assist their children in moral judgments. Encourage talking with a child or adolescent about how a given decision was made. Parents can then add information and help the child learn to integrate more factors into decision making. Talking about the process is important in helping children progress to higher stages of moral development. Focusing on the feelings of others, using positive discipline techniques, and clearly identifying positive and negative behaviors are important.

Social Learning Theory

Theoretical Framework

Bandura, a contemporary psychologist, believes that children learn attitudes, beliefs, customs, and values through their social contacts with adults and other children. Children imitate (or model) the behavior they see; if the behavior is positively reinforced, they tend to repeat it. However, Bandura also believes that people can consciously choose how to act, such as deciding to handle problems by talking rather than using violence. The external environment (the behavior of others) and the child's internal processes are both key elements in the behaviors the child manifests (Bandura, 1986, 1997a).

Bandura believes that an important determinant of behavior is **self-efficacy**, or the expectation that someone can produce a desired outcome. For example, if adolescents believe they can avoid use of drugs or alcohol, they are more likely to do so. A child who has confidence in his or her ability to exercise regularly or lose weight has a greater chance of success with these behav-

ior changes. Parents who have confidence in their ability to care adequately for their infants are more likely to do so (Bandura, 1997b). See Evidence-Based Practice: Self-Efficacy below.

Nursing Application

The importance of modeling behavior can readily be applied in health care. Children are more likely to cooperate if they see adults or other children performing a task willingly. A frightened child may watch another child perform vision screening or have blood drawn and then decide to allow the procedure to take place. Contact with positive role models is useful when teaching children and adolescents self-care for chronic diseases such as diabetes. Positive reinforcement should be given for desired performance.

Nurses can utilize the concept of self-efficacy to increase the chance of success with lifestyle behavior changes. For example, encouraging youth who are trying to quit smoking, providing them with role models, and pointing out parental successes with their children all demonstrate methods of fostering self-efficacy.

Behaviorism

Theoretical Framework

John Watson studied the research of Pavlov and Skinner, who demonstrated that actions are determined by responses from the environment. Pavlov and, later, Skinner worked with animals, presenting a stimulus such as food and pairing it with another stimulus such as a ringing bell. Eventually the animal being fed began to salivate when the bell rang. As Skinner and then Watson began to apply these concepts to children, they showed that behaviors can be elicited by positive reinforcement, such as a food treat, or extinguished by negative reinforcement,

---

Evidence-Based Practice
Self-Efficacy

Problem

How can nurses use the concept of self-efficacy when planning interventions for children and families?

Evidence

A federally funded study sought to measure the effectiveness of a preventive parent training program among low-income families with small children. The weekly sessions involved viewing a videotape and discussing positive and negative parenting skills observed. The researchers compared characteristics of the parents who chose to attend the sessions, including a measure of parental self-efficacy, or belief that they could manage a range of tasks and situations in caring for their young children. Parents with lower self-efficacy scores were significantly more likely to enroll in and attend the parenting training sessions (Garvey, Julion, Fogg, et al., 2006).

Mothers who have a greater degree of self-efficacy about ability to breastfeed are significantly more likely to begin and to continue breastfeeding. A Breastfeeding Self-Efficacy Scale has been developed to identify risk and protective factors that influence the self-efficacy of new mothers. Educational level, support from other women, quality of postpartum care, maternal anxiety, and plans made for feeding method all influence the breastfeeding self-efficacy scores of women (Dennis, 2006).

A program that was designed using self-efficacy theory and creating opportunities for personal empowerment among adolescents

resulted in improved healthy lifestyle choices and lower depression and anxiety (Melnyk, Jacobsen, Kelly, et al., 2009).

Implications

In addition to providing information about health behaviors, nurses need to integrate methods to increase self-efficacy in teaching projects with families. Assessments should be designed to identify self-efficacy of parents and children around health topics of interest. When planning interventions to encourage health behaviors in children and adolescents, assess the youth's belief that the new behaviors are important and that they can be adopted. Include interventions that demonstrate that others have adopted the health behaviors, and plan approaches to enhance the child's belief in ability to change.

Critical Thinking Application

Plan a teaching project about the importance of physical activity for presentation to a group of 12-year-olds. What approaches will enhance the self-efficacy of the children? How would interventions to enhance self-efficacy differ for young elementary schoolchildren compared to those in middle or high school? What theoretical approaches discussed earlier in this chapter help you to understand the cognitive abilities of children at various ages and suggest ways to influence their self-efficacy?

such as scolding or withdrawal of attention. Watson believed that he could make a child into anyone he desired—from a professional to a thief or beggar—simply by reinforcing behavior in certain ways (Santrock, 2009).

Nursing Application

Behaviorism has been criticized for its simplicity and its denial of the inherent capability of persons to respond willfully to events in the environment. This theory does, however, have some use in health care. When particular behaviors are desired, health care providers can establish positive reinforcement to encourage these behaviors. Using behavioral techniques, nurses may influence behavior of children who misbehave or teach skills to children who are physically challenged. Parents often use reinforcement in toilet training and other skills learned in childhood. Indeed, combining behaviorism with social learning theory can be beneficial. For example, children might have desired activities, such as tooth brushing, modeled by an adult or older child (social learning theory), and be rewarded (behaviorism) for carrying out the activity on a regular basis.

Ecologic Theory

Theoretical Framework

You may have noticed that there is controversy among theorists concerning the relative importance of heredity versus environment—or nature versus nurture—in human development. **Nature** refers to the genetic or hereditary capability of an individual. **Nurture** refers to the effects of the environment on a person's performance (Box 4–2). Piaget believed in the importance of internal cognitive structures that unfold at their appointed times, given any environment that provides basic opportunities. He emphasized the strength of nature. The behaviorist John Watson, however, believed that behaviors are primarily shaped by environmental responses; he thus stressed the predominance of nurture. Contemporary developmental theories increasingly recognize the interaction of nature and nurture in determining the child's development.

The **ecologic theory** of development was formulated by Urie Bronfenbrenner to explain the child's unique relationship in all of life's settings, from close to remote (Bronfenbrenner, 1986, 2005; Bronfenbrenner, McClelland, Ceci, et al., 1996). The theory has been applied to research and clinical practice that views the importance of the child's settings on health behaviors (Wiium & Wold, 2009; Power, Bindler, Goetz, et al., 2010; Trickett, 2009). Ecologic theory emphasizes the presence of mutual interactions between the child and these various settings. Neither nature nor nurture is considered of more importance. Bronfenbrenner believed each child brings a unique set of

BOX 4–2 Nature Versus Nurture

Does nature or nurture have primary importance in the theories of Erikson, Kohlberg, Freud, and social learning? Think about whether each of the theories emphasizes the role of heredity (nature) or the role of the environment (nurture) in influencing the development of children.

genes—and specific attributes such as age, gender, health, and other characteristics—to his or her interactions with the environment. The child then interacts in many settings at different levels or systems (Figure 4–4 ➤).

Levels or Systems

Microsystem This level is defined as the daily, consistent, close relationships such as home, childcare, school, friends, and neighbors. For the child with a chronic illness requiring regular care, the health care providers may even be part of the microsystem. In the ecologic model, the child influences each of these settings in addition to being influenced by them, with reciprocal interactions. Consider Sergio's microsystems, which have involved the hospital, his family, and now other care providers. What stability is needed now to foster his ability to develop and form relationships with his family?

Mesosystem This level includes relationships of microsystems with one another. For example, two microsystems for most children are the home and the school. The relationships between these microsystems are shown by parents' involvement in their children's school. This involvement, in turn, influences the effects of the home and school settings on the children.

Exosystem This level is composed of those settings that influence the child even though the child is not in close daily contact with the system. Examples include the parents' jobs and the governing board of the local school district. Although the child may not go to the parents' workplaces, he or she can be influenced by policies related to health care, sick leave, inflexible work hours, overtime, travel, or even the mood of the boss (through its impact on the parent). The child's needs may influence a parent to give up a certain job or to work harder to obtain money for the child's education. Likewise, when a local school board votes to ban certain books or to finance a field trip, the child is influenced by these decisions; the child, in turn, can help establish an atmosphere that will guide future school board decisions.

Macrosystem This level includes the beliefs, values, and behaviors expressed in the child's environment. Culture is a powerful influence in the macrosystem, as is the political system. For instance, a democratic system creates different beliefs, values, and even eating practices than an anarchic system.

Chronosystem This final level brings the perspective of time to the previous settings. The time period during which the child grows up influences views of health and illness. For example, the experiences of children with influenza in the 19th versus 20th centuries were quite different.

Nursing Application

Nurses use ecologic theory when they assess the child's settings to identify influences on development. Table 4–4 provides an assessment tool based on this theory. Interventions are planned to enhance the strengths of the child's settings and to improve on areas that are not supportive. Ask yourself the following questions:

- How does the child influence each system?
- How is the child influenced by each system?
- What interventions should be planned for the child?

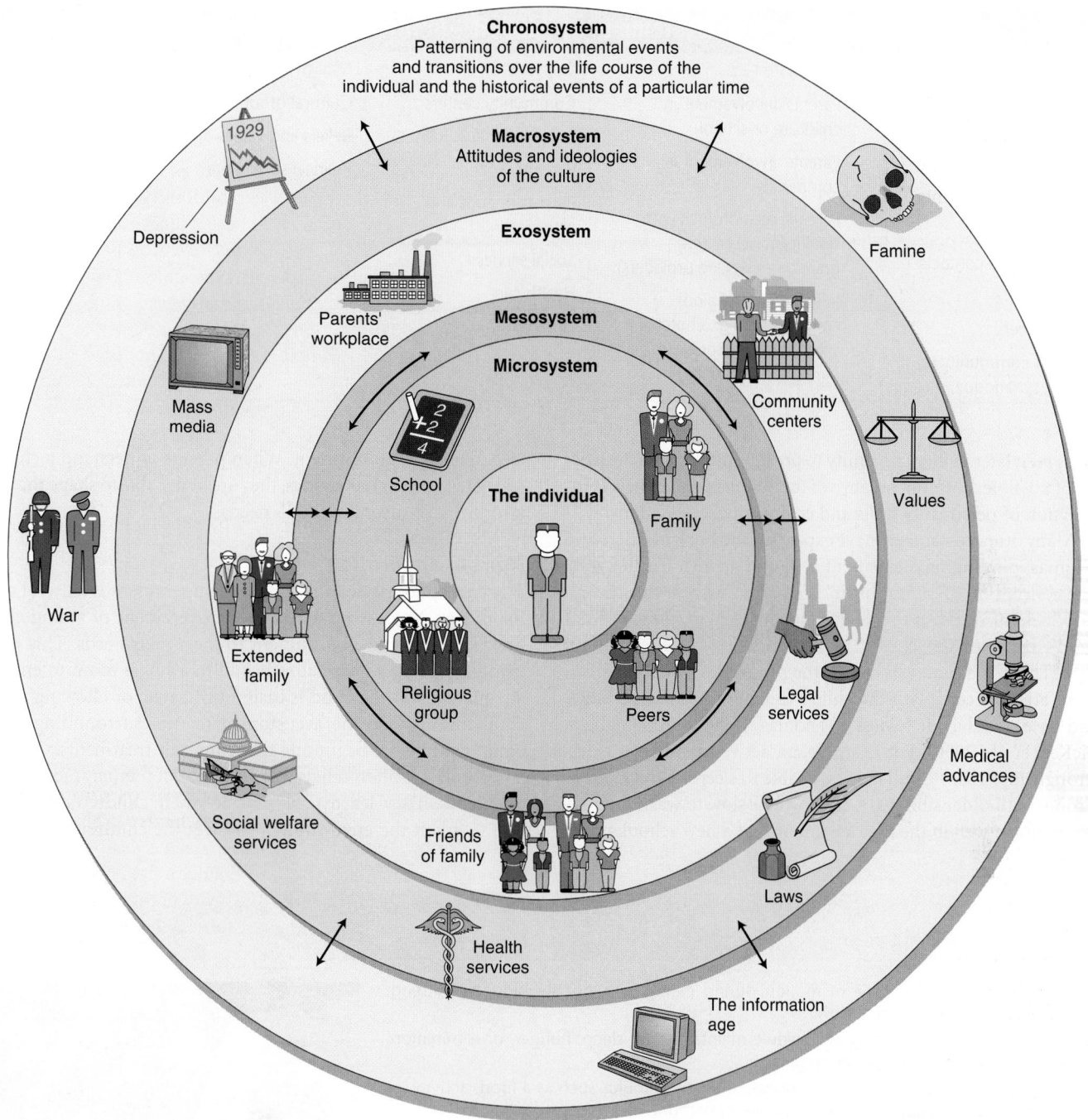

FIGURE 4–4 ➤ Bronfenbrenner's ecologic theory of development views the individual as interacting within five levels or systems.

Note: Redrawn from Santrock, J. W. (2005). Life span development. Madison, WI: Brown & Benchmark. Based on Bronfenbrenner's (1979, 1986) works in "Contexts of child rearing: Problems and prospects." American Psychologist, 34, 844–850; and "Ecology of the family as a context for human development: Research perspectives." Developmental Psychology, 22, 723–742.

Temperament Theory

Theoretical Framework

In contrast to behaviorists such as Watson or maturational theorists such as Piaget, Chess and Thomas (1995, 1996) recognized the innate qualities of personality that each individual brings to the events of daily life. They, like Bronfenbrenner, viewed the child as an individual who both influences and is influenced by the environment. However, Chess and Thomas focused on one specific aspect of development—the wide spectrum of behav-

iors possible in children, identifying nine parameters of response to daily events (Box 4–3). Infants generally display clusters of responses, which Chess and Thomas classified into three major personality types (Box 4–4). Although most children do not demonstrate all behaviors described for a particular type, they usually show a grouping indicative of one personality type (Chess & Thomas, 1995, 1996).

Longitudinal research has demonstrated that personality characteristics displayed during infancy are often consistent with

TABLE 4–4	**Assessment of Ecologic Systems in Childhood—Bronfenbrenner**			
Microsystems	Mesosystems	Exosystems	Macrosystems	Chronosystems
Parents	Parents' involvement in childcare or school	Community centers	Cultural group membership	Child's age
Significant others in close contact	Parents' involvement in community	Local political influences	Beliefs and values of group	Parents' ages
Childcare arrangements	Parents' relationships with significant others (e.g., grandparents, care providers)	Parents' work	Political structure	
School		Parents' friends and activities		
Neighborhood contacts		Social services		
Clubs	Influences of religious community (e.g., church, synagogue, mosque) or parents and school	Health care		
Friends, peers		Libraries		
Religious community (e.g., church, synagogue, mosque)				

those seen later in life. The ability to predict future characteristics is not possible, however, because of the complex and dynamic interaction of personality traits and environmental reactions.

Many other researchers have expanded the work of Chess and Thomas, developing assessment tools for temperament types. The concept of "goodness of fit" is an outgrowth of this theory. Goodness of fit refers to whether parents' expectations of their child's behavior are consistent with the child's temperament type. There is a "good fit" when the properties of the environment are in accord with the child's capabilities, characteristics, and style of behavior (Chess & Thomas, 1999; Rettew, Stanger, McKee, et al., 2006). For example, an active infant who reacts strongly to verbal stimuli may be unable to sleep when placed in a room with older siblings. A child who is slow to warm up may not perform well in the first few months at a new school, much

to parents' disappointment. When parents understand a child's temperament characteristics, they are better able to shape the environment to meet the child's needs.

Nursing Application

The concept of personality type or temperament is a useful one for nurses. Nurses can assess the temperament of young children and alter the environment to meet their needs. This may involve moving a hospitalized child to a single room to ensure adequate rest if the child is easily stimulated, or allowing a shy child time to become accustomed to new surroundings and equipment before beginning procedures or treatments.

Parents are often relieved to learn about temperament characteristics. They learn to appreciate their children's qualities and to adapt the environment to meet the children's needs. A

BOX 4–3   **Nine Parameters of Personality—Chess and Thomas**

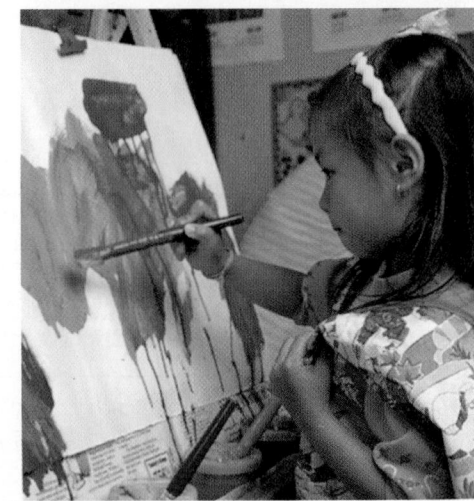

1. **Activity level.** The degree of motion during eating, playing, sleeping, or bathing. Scored as high, medium, or low.
2. **Rhythmicity.** The regularity of schedule maintained for sleep, hunger, or elimination. Scored as regular, variable, or irregular.
3. **Approach or withdrawal.** The response to a new stimulus such as a food, activity, or person. Scored as approachable, variable, or withdrawn.
4. **Adaptability.** The degree of adaptation to new situations. Scored as adaptive, variable, or nonadaptive.
5. **Threshold of responsiveness.** The intensity of stimulation needed to elicit a response to sensory input, objects in the environment, or people. Scored as high, medium, or low.
6. **Intensity of reaction.** The degree of response to situations. Scored as positive, variable, or negative.
7. **Quality of mood.** The predominant mood during daily activity and in response to stimuli. Scored as positive, variable, or negative.
8. **Distractibility.** The ability of environmental stimuli to interfere with the child's activity. Scored as distractible, variable, or nondistractible.
9. **Attention span and persistence.** The amount of time devoted to activities (compared with other children of the same age) and the degree of ability to stick with an activity in spite of obstacles. Scored as persistent, variable, or nonpersistent.

Note: Adapted from Chess, S., & Thomas, A. (1996). Temperament: Theory and practice. *Philadelphia: Brunner/Mazel Publishers.*

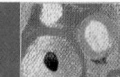 **Patterns of Temperament—Chess and Thomas**

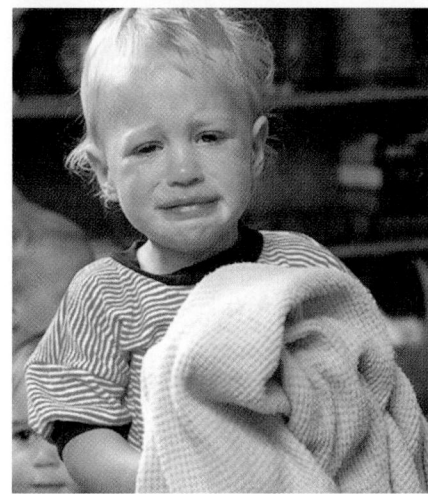

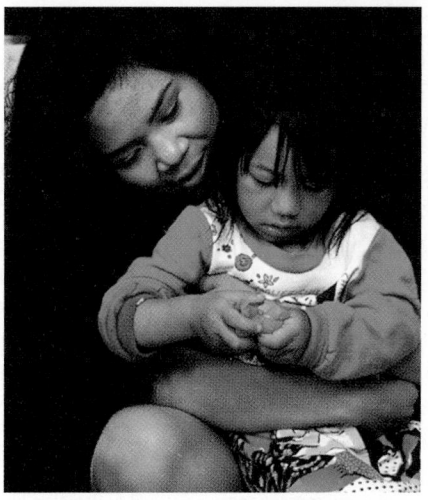

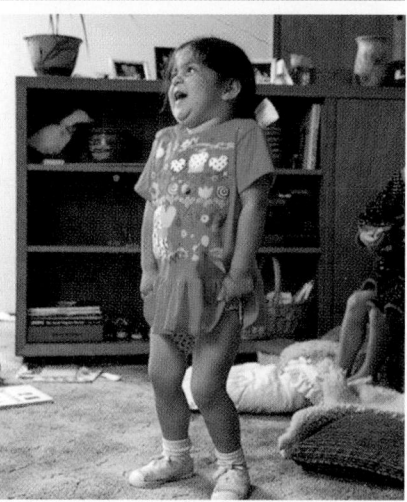

The "difficult" child displays irregular schedules for eating, sleeping, and elimination; adapts slowly to new situations and persons; and displays a predominantly negative mood. Intense reactions to the environment are common. About 10% of children in the New York Longitudinal Study displayed this personality type.

The "slow-to-warm-up" child has reactions of mild intensity and slow adaptability to new situations. The child displays initial withdrawal followed by gradual, quiet, and slow interaction with the environment. About 15% of children in the New York Longitudinal Study displayed this personality type.

The "easy" child is generally moderate in activity; shows regularity in patterns of eating, sleeping, and elimination; and is usually positive in mood and when subjected to new stimuli. The easy child adapts to new situations and is able to accept rules and work well with others. About 40% of children in the New York Longitudinal Study displayed this personality type. The remaining 35% of children studied showed some characteristics of each personality type.

Note: Adapted from Chess, S., & Thomas, A. (1996). Temperament: Theory and practice. *Philadelphia: Brunner/Mazel Publishers.*

burden of guilt can also be lifted from parents who feel that they are responsible for their child's actions. The nurse can teach parents ways of enhancing goodness of fit between the child's personality and the environment (Table 4–5). See further suggestions for helping parents understand temperament during health promotion and health maintenance visits in Chapters 6 through 9 ∞.

TABLE 4–5	Ways to Improve Goodness of Fit Between Parent and Child
Child's Behavior	Parent's Activity
Extremely active	Plan periods of active play several times in a day. Have restful periods before bedtime to foster sleep.
Shy	Allow time to adapt at own pace to new people and situations.
Easily stimulated	Have a quiet room for sleeping as an infant. Have a quiet room for homework as a school-age child.
Short attention span	Provide projects that can be completed in a short period. Gradually encourage longer periods at activities.

Resiliency Theory

Theoretical Framework

Why do some children coming from similar backgrounds have such different behavioral outcomes? The resiliency model is a theory that examines both the individual's characteristics as well as the interaction of these characteristics with the environment. **Resilience** is the ability to function with healthy responses, even with significant stress and adversity (Henderson, Benard, & Sharp-Light, 2007). In this model, the individual or family members experience a crisis that provides a source of stress, and the family interprets or deals with the crisis based on resources available. Families and individuals have **protective factors** that provide strength and assistance in dealing with crises, and **risk factors** that promote or contribute to their challenges. Risk and protective factors can be identified in children, in their families, and in their communities (see Chapter 17 ∞ for further description of the interplay of social and environmental factors with individual characteristics). A crisis for a young child might be a transfer to a new childcare provider. Protective factors could involve past positive experiences with new people, an "easy" temperament, and awareness of the new childcare provider about adaptation needs of young children to new experiences. Risk factors for a similar child might be repeated moves to new care providers, limited close relationships with adults, and a "slow-to-warm-up" temperament.

TABLE 4–6	Components of Resiliency Model		
Component	Meaning	Example
A = Crisis event or health challenge	Nature of health care challenge	Parent leaving home
V = Vulnerability; risk factors	Stresses and risks related to dealing with the health challenge	Prior abandonment; financial instability; child's developmental understanding of abandonment
T = Typology	Family methods of functioning	Reliance on extended family; parent alcoholism
B = Protective factors	Strengths for dealing with challenge	Child's desire to succeed in school; positive role modeling of maternal grandparents
C = Appraisal	Family's interpretation of crisis event	Abandonment by loved one; inability to trust others
PS = Problem-solving or coping techniques	Skills that help family work toward solution	Use of community resources; acceptance of school and community counselors; child's involvement in classroom activities
X = Response	Positive or negative response to tension created by the health challenge	Remaining parent using counseling available; child identifying with a teacher in school; establishment of sense of mutual interdependence among remaining family members

Data from: Ahern, N. R. (2006). Adolescent resilience: An evolutionary concept analysis. Journal of Pediatric Nursing, 21, *175–185.*

Once confronted by stress or a crisis, the child and family first experience the **adjustment phase**, characterized by disorganization and unsuccessful attempts at meeting the crisis. In the **adaptation phase**, the child and family meet the challenge and use resources to deal with the crisis (Ahern, 2006). Adaptation may lead to increasing resilience as well when the child and family learn about new resources and inner strengths and develop the ability to deal more effectively with future crises. The model and examples are described in Table 4–6.

Nursing Application

Nurses gather information about the individual characteristics, prior life experiences, and environmental factors that act as protective and risk factors for children. Box 4–5 lists questions that can be helpful as the nurse gathers information from a child or family members. Nurses then use concepts of resiliency theory in planning interventions for children and families. Nursing strategies can target risk factors, such as encouraging family behaviors to ensure gun safety in families with firearms by teaching about use of gun trigger locks and locked gun cabinets. In addition, protective factors can be emphasized, such as encouraging holding and verbalization to parents of infants to provide an environment that meets needs for trust establishment and speech development.

■ INFLUENCES ON DEVELOPMENT

As we have seen, both nature and nurture are important in determining individual patterns of development. The interaction of these two forces can explain differences in time frames for acquisition of developmental skills, personality variations between identical twins, and other unique characteristics of individuals. Genetic and environmental factors interact and contribute to individual differences in child development. Several of these influences are discussed next.

Genetic inheritance plays an important part in the child's potential and the unfolding of developmental milestones. Each

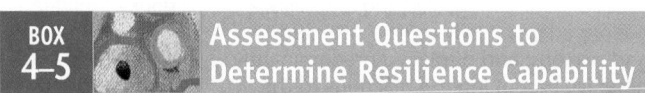

BOX 4–5 Assessment Questions to Determine Resilience Capability

Questions to Determine Risk Factors
■ Describe the event that occurred and what it has been like for your family.
■ What other stressors do you have in your family right now?
■ Are there financial worries?
■ Are there things you think and worry about late at night?
■ Describe your job, your friends.
■ Describe your typical day.
■ Describe your neighborhood.
■ Do you have friends, people to call in emergencies?

Questions to Determine Protective Factors
■ What gives you strength?
■ How do you deal with this stress?
■ What do you think you do well in your family?
■ Who do you call when you need help?
■ Do you have a computer? Internet access?
■ Are you religious? Spiritual?
■ Do you exercise regularly?
■ How do you spend free time?

child inherits 23 chromosomes from the mother's egg and 23 from the father's sperm, resulting in a unique individual with 46 chromosomes. Two of these are **sex chromosomes**, and determine the child's gender; the rest are called **autosomal chromosomes**, and govern all remaining characteristics. Every chromosome carries many genes that determine physical characteristics, intellectual potential, personality type, and other traits. Children are born with the potential for certain features; however, their interaction with the environment influences how and to what extent particular traits are manifested. For example, a child may have the potential for a high level of intellectual performance, but because he or she lives in an unstimulating environment, that potential is never reached. See Chapter 3 ∞ for a further description of the influences of genetics upon development.

Some Asian cultures calculate age from the time of conception. This practice acknowledges the profound influence of the prenatal period. Nurses work closely with pregnant families to encourage safe health practices. One example of prenatal influence is that of nutrition. The mother's nutrition and general state of health play a part in pregnancy outcome. Poor nutrition can lead to low-birth-weight infants and infants with compromised neurologic performance, slow development, or impaired immune status with resultant high disease rates. Low maternal stores of iron can result in anemia in the infant (American Academy of Pediatrics, 2009). Maternal smoking is associated with low-birth-weight infants. Ingestion of alcoholic beverages, including beer and wine, during pregnancy may lead to fetal alcohol syndrome or fetal alcohol effects. See Chapter 28 ∞ for a detailed description and a photo of this condition. Substance abuse by the mother may result in neonatal addiction, convulsions, hyperirritability, poor social responsiveness, and other neurologic disturbances of the infant, as well as changes in neurobehavioral and cognitive function of children (Huizink & Mulder, 2006). See Chapter 27 ∞ for a discussion of neonatal withdrawal syndrome.

Even prescription or nonprescription drugs may adversely affect the fetus. This was brought to general attention with the drug thalidomide, commonly used in Europe to treat nausea during the 1950s. This drug resulted in the birth of infants with limb abnormalities to women who used the drug during pregnancy. Differences in physiology related to gastric emptying, renal clearance, drug distribution, and other factors contribute to variations in pharmacokinetics during pregnancy. Drugs can cause teratogenesis (abnormal development of the fetus) or mutagenesis (permanent changes in the fetus's genetic material) (Kyle, 2006; Nguyen, Sharma, & McIntyre, 2009). Certain drugs can cause bleeding, stained teeth, impaired hearing, or other defects in the infant. The U.S. Food and Drug Administration (FDA) has established risk categories for drugs in pregnancy.

Some maternal illnesses are harmful to the developing fetus. An example is rubella (German measles), which is rarely a serious disease for adults but can cause deafness, vision defects, heart defects, and mental retardation in the fetus if it is acquired by a pregnant woman. Some illnesses, such as certain influenza infections, are serious in pregnant women, and can lead to the death of the woman or loss of the fetus. A fetus can also acquire diseases, such as acquired immunodeficiency syndrome (AIDS) and human immunodeficiency virus (HIV) infection or hepatitis B, from the mother.

Radiation, chemicals, and other environmental hazards may adversely affect a fetus when the mother is exposed to these influences during her pregnancy. The best outcomes for infants occur when mothers eat well; exercise regularly; seek early prenatal care; refrain from use of drugs, alcohol, tobacco, and excessive caffeine; and follow general principles of good health.

An environmental factor that is extremely important in the development of children is the profile of family characteristics. The family is an important component in the lives of all children, and plays an essential role in fostering the development of

youth. A significant concept in families is that of parenting. How children are parented interacts with their individual characteristics to influence risk and protective factors, personality characteristics, and developmental outcomes. Chapter 2 ∞ discusses types of families, frameworks used to understand families, the roles of families in fostering the development of children, and types of parenting styles.

The families into which children are born influence them profoundly. Children are supported in different ways and acquire different world views depending on such factors as whether they have one or two parents or stepparents, whether one or both parents work, how many siblings are present, and whether an extended family is close. Note should be made of variations in family structure such as single parent, adoptive parents, homosexual parents, extended family, and stepparents.

Culture is another factor that influences child development, through traditional practices and due to genetic variations among some ethnic groups. The traditional customs of the many cultural groups represented in North America influence the development of the children in these groups. Nutritional practices of various ethnic groups may influence the rate of growth for infants. In addition, development may be influenced by childrearing practices. For example, the Native American practice of carrying infants on boards often delays walking when it is measured against the norm for walking on some developmental tests. Children who are carried by straddling the mother's hips or back for extended periods have a low incidence of developmental dysplasia of the hip since this keeps their hips in an abducted position. It is important for nurses to take cultural practices into account when performing developmental screening; some tests may not be culturally sensitive and can inaccurately label a child as delayed when the pattern of development is simply different in the group, perhaps due to childrearing practices in the family. In these cases there is no lasting delay in any milestone, but variation in acquiring skills may occur. In addition, certain ethnic or racial groups are more prone to develop certain diseases due to genetic variation. Examples include Hispanics who have a high incidence of diabetes, African Americans who more commonly have sickle cell disease, and northern European Americans who have a higher incidence of phenylketonuria.

All cultural groups have rules regarding patterns of social interaction. Schedules of language acquisition are determined by the number of languages spoken and the amount of speech in the home. The particular social roles assumed by men and women in the culture affect school activities and ultimately career choices.

Culture *Reaching Developmental Milestones*

In traditional Native American families, children are allowed to unfold and develop naturally at their own pace. Children thus wean and toilet train themselves with little interference or pressure from parents. The nurse should be sensitive to the childrearing practices of the family and support them in these culturally accepted practices, rather than imposing a more structured approach to developmental milestones.

Attitudes toward touching and other methods of encouraging developmental skills vary among cultures. Chapter 2 ∞ discusses the influences of family and special situations such as adoption on child development. Chapter 10 ∞ includes further description of other factors that influence child development such as school and childcare, community services, and additional community and family factors.

■ INFANT (BIRTH TO 1 YEAR)

Can you imagine tripling your present weight in a single year? Or becoming proficient in understanding fundamental words in a new language and even speaking a few? These and many more accomplishments take place in the first year of life. Starting as a mainly reflexive creature, the infant can walk and communicate by the year's end. Never again in life is development so rapid and profound (Figure 4–5 ➤).

Physical Growth and Development

The first year of life is one of rapid change for the infant. The birth weight usually doubles by about 5 months and triples by the end of the first year (Figure 4–6 ➤). Height increases by approximately 1 foot during this year. Teeth begin to erupt at about 6 months, and by the end of the first year the infant has six to eight deciduous teeth (see Chapter 5 ∞). Physical growth is closely associated with type and quality of feeding. See Chapter 14 ∞ for a discussion of nutrition in infancy.

Body organs and systems, although not fully mature at 1 year of age, function differently than they did at birth. Kidney and liver maturation helps the 1-year-old excrete drugs or other toxic substances more readily than in the first weeks of life. The changing body proportions mirror changes in developing internal organs. Maturation of the nervous system is demonstrated by increased control over body movements, enabling the infant to sit, stand, and walk. Sensory function also increases as the infant begins to discriminate visual images, sounds, and tastes (Table 4–7). See Chapter 7 ∞ for a detailed list of the developmental milestones of the infant.

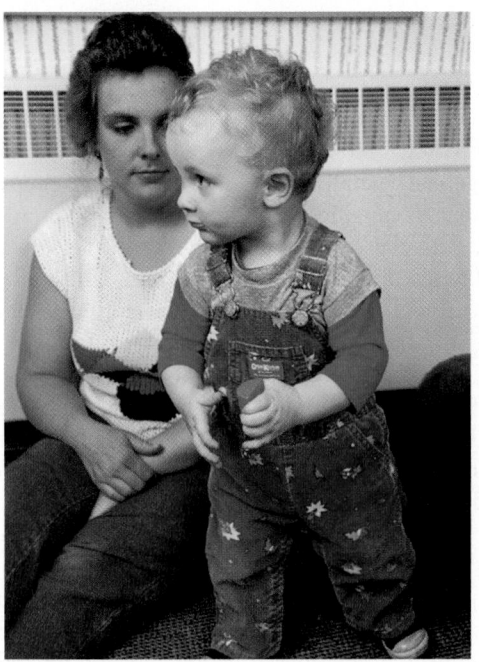

FIGURE 4–5 ➤ A 12-month-old child has tripled his birth weight, is learning to walk, and is beginning to talk.

Cognitive Development

The brain continues to increase in complexity during the first year. Most of the growth involves maturation of cells, with only a small increase in cell number. This growth of the brain is accompanied by development of its functions. One has only to compare the behavior of an infant shortly after birth with that of a 1-year-old to understand the incredible maturation of brain function. The newborn's eyes widen in response to sound; the 1-year-old turns to the sound and recognizes its significance. The 2-month-old cries and coos; the 1-year-old says a few words and understands many more. The 6-week-old grasps a rattle for the first time; the 1-year-old reaches for toys and self-feeds.

The infant's behaviors provide clues about thought processes. Piaget's work outlines the infant's actions in a set of

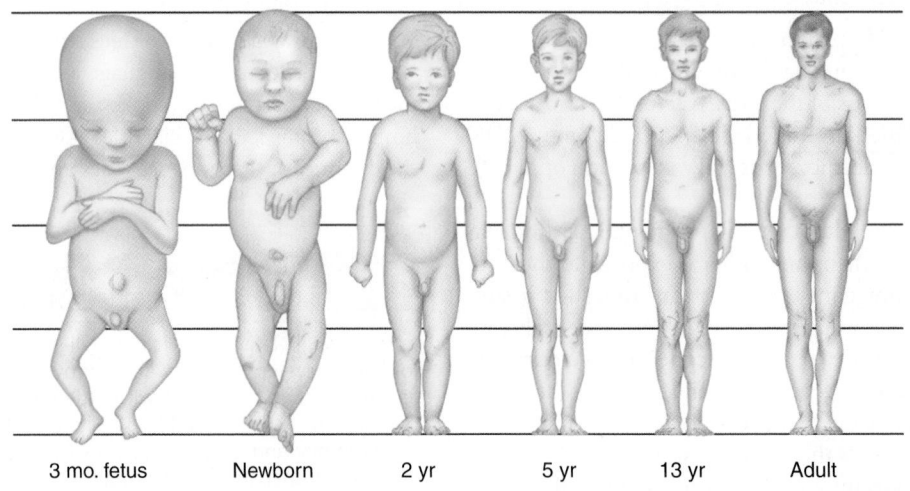

| 3 mo. fetus | Newborn | 2 yr | 5 yr | 13 yr | Adult |

FIGURE 4–6 ➤ Body proportions at various ages.

TABLE 4–7	**Growth and Development Milestones During Infancy**			
Age	Physical Growth	Fine Motor Ability	Gross Motor Ability	Sensory Ability
Birth to 1 month	Gains 5–7 oz (140–200 g)/ week Grows 1.5 cm (1/2 in.) in first month Head circumference increases 1.5 cm (1/2 in.)/ month	Holds hand in fist **(1)** Draws arms and legs to body when crying	Inborn reflexes such as startle and rooting are predominant activity May lift head briefly if prone **(2)** Alerts to high-pitched voices Comforts with touch **(3)**	Prefers to look at faces and black-and-white geometric designs Follows objects in line of vision **(4)**

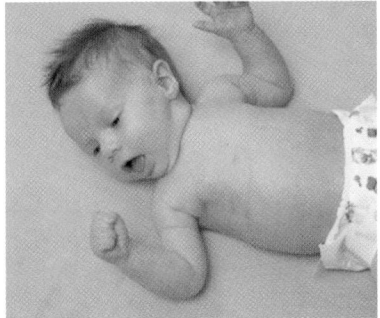

(1) Holds hand in fist

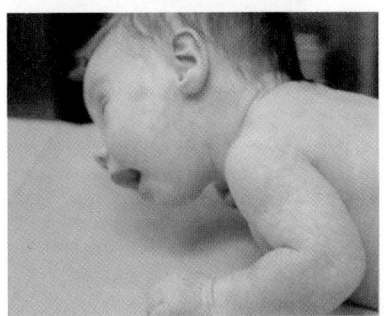

(2) May lift head

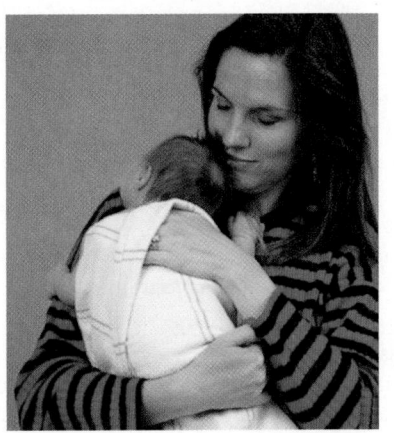

(3) Comforts with touch

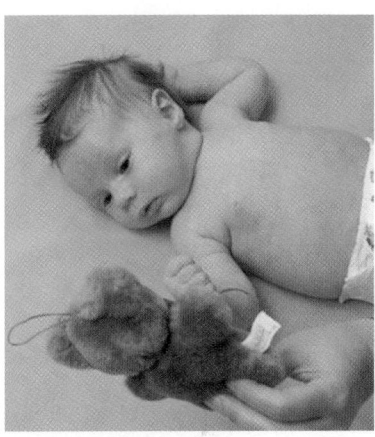

(4) Follows objects

2–4 months	Gains 5–7 oz (140–200 g)/ week Grows 1.5 cm (1/2 in.)/ month Head circumference increases 1.5 cm (1/2 in.)/ month Posterior fontanel closes Ingests 120 mL/kg/24 hr (2 oz/lb/24 hr)	Holds rattle when placed in hand **(5)** Looks at and plays with own fingers Brings hands to midline	Moro reflex fading in strength Can turn from side to back and then return **(6)** Decrease in head lag when pulled to sitting; sits with head held in midline with some bobbing When prone, holds head and supports weight on forearms **(7)**	Follows objects 180 degrees Turns head to look for voices and sounds

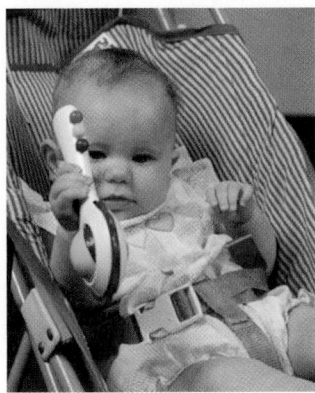

(5) Holds rattle

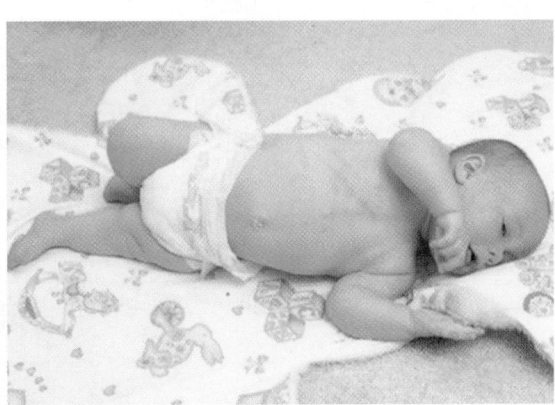

(6) Can turn from side to back

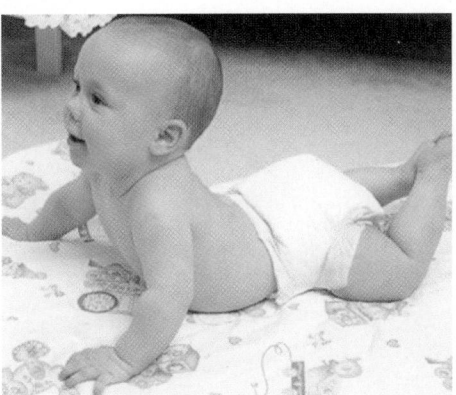

(7) Holds head up and supports weight with arms

(continued)

TABLE 4–7	Growth and Development Milestones During Infancy			(continued)
Age	Physical Growth	Fine Motor Ability	Gross Motor Ability	Sensory Ability
4–6 months	Gains 5–7 oz (140–200 g)/week Doubles birth weight at 5–6 months Grows 1.5 cm (1/2 in.)/month Head circumference increases 1.5 cm (1/2 in.)/month Teeth may begin erupting by 6 months Ingests 100 mL/kg/24 hr (1 1/2 oz/lb/24 hr)	Grasps rattles and other objects at will; drops them to pick up another offered object **(8)** Mouths objects Holds feet and pulls to mouth Holds bottle Grasps with whole hand (palmar grasp) Manipulates objects **(9)**	Head held steady when sitting No head lag when pulled to sitting Turns from abdomen to back by 4 months and then back to abdomen by 6 months When held standing, supports much of own weight **(10)**	Examines complex visual images Watches the course of a falling object Responds readily to sounds

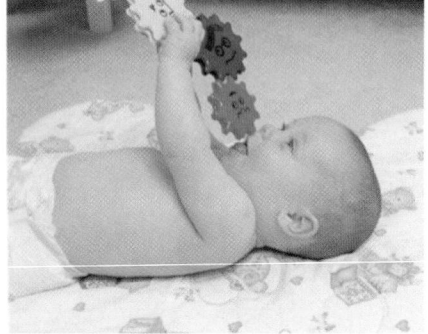
(8) Grasps objects at will

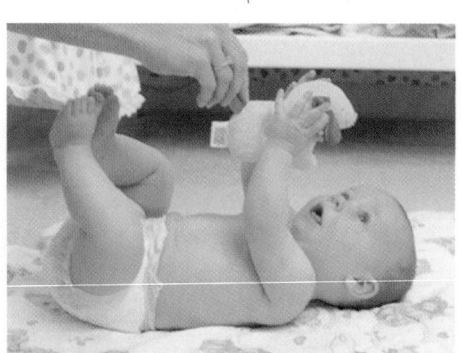
(9) Manipulates objects

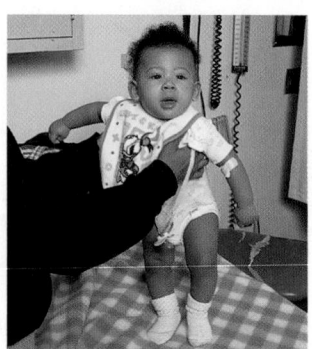
(10) Supports most of weight when held standing

| 6–8 months | Gains 3–5 oz (85–140 g)/week
Grows 1 cm (3/8 in.)/month
Growth rate slower than first 6 months | Bangs objects held in hands
Transfers objects from one hand to the other
Beginning pincer grasp at times | Most inborn reflexes extinguished
Sits alone steadily without support by 8 months **(11)**
Likes to bounce on legs when held in standing position | Recognizes own name and responds by looking and smiling
Enjoys small and complex objects at play |

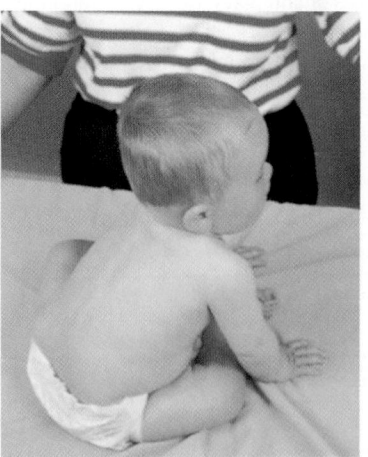
(11) Sits alone without support

TABLE 4–7	Growth and Development Milestones During Infancy *(continued)*			
Age	Physical Growth	Fine Motor Ability	Gross Motor Ability	Sensory Ability
8–10 months	Gains 3–5 oz (85–140 g)/ week Grows 1 cm (3/8 in.)/month	Picks up small objects **(12)** Uses pincer grasp well **(13)**	Crawls or pulls whole body along floor by arms **(14)** Creeps by using hands and knees to keep trunk off floor Pulls self to standing and sitting by 10 months Recovers balance when sitting	Understands words such as "no" and "cracker" May say one word in addition to "mama" and "dada" Recognizes sound without difficulty

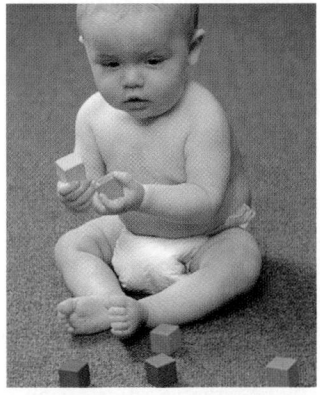
(12) Picks up small objects

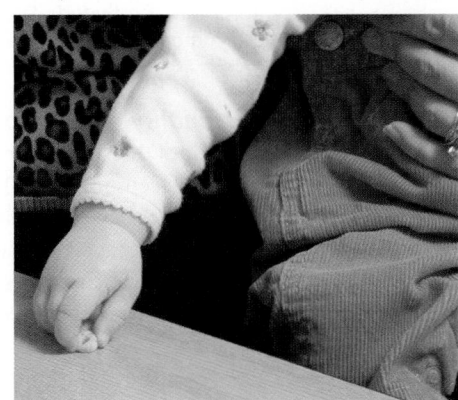
(13) Uses pincer grasp well

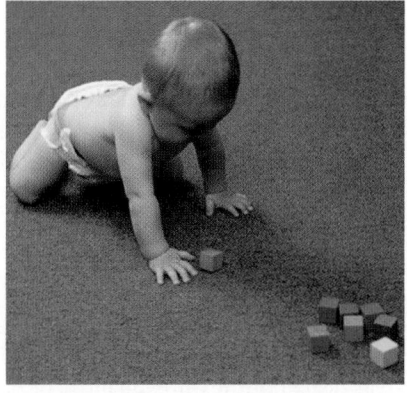
(14) Crawls or pulls body by arms

10–12 months	Gains 3–5 oz (85–140 g)/ week Grows 1 cm (3/8 in.)/month Head circumference equals chest circumference Triples birth weight by 1 year	May hold crayon or pencil and make mark on paper Places objects into containers through holes **(15)**	Stands alone **(16)** Walks holding onto furniture Sits down from standing **(17)**	Plays peek-a-boo and patty cake

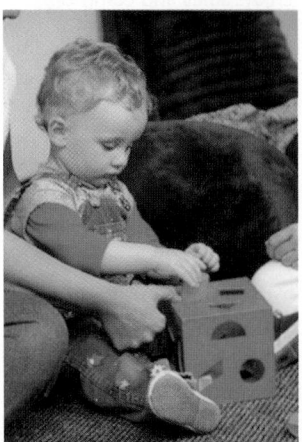
(15) Places objects in container through holes

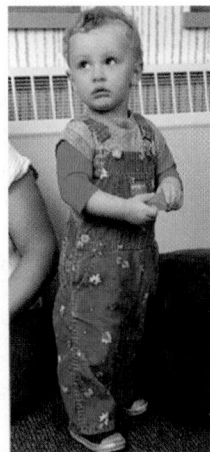
(16) Stands alone

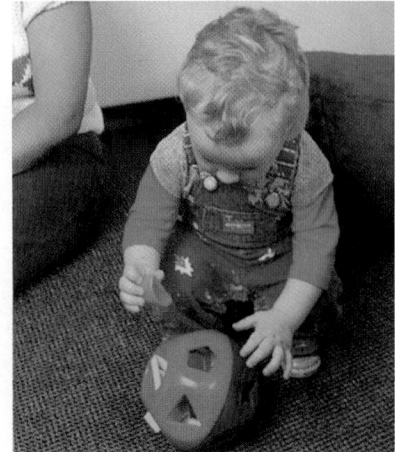
(17) Sits down from standing

rapidly progressing changes in the first year of life. The infant receives stimulation through sight, sound, and feeling, which the maturing brain interprets. This input from the environment interacts with internal cognitive abilities to enhance cognitive functioning.

Psychosocial Development

The infant relies on interactions with primary care providers to meet needs and then establishes a sense of trust in other adults and in children. As trust develops, the infant becomes comfortable in interactions with a widening array of people.

Play

An 8-month-old infant is sitting on the floor, grasping blocks and banging them on the floor. When a parent walks by, the infant laughs and waves hands and feet wildly (Figure 4–7 ➤). The infant plays primarily alone with toys (**solitary play**) but enjoys the presence of adults or other children. Physical capabilities enable the infant to move toward and reach for objects of interest.

Cognitive ability is reflected in manipulation of the blocks to create different sounds. Social interaction enhances play. The presence of a parent or other person increases interest in surroundings and teaches the infant different ways to play.

The play of infants begins in a reflexive manner. When infants move extremities or grasp objects, they experience the foundations of play. They gain pleasure from the feel and sound of these activities, and gradually perform them purposefully. For example, when a parent places a rattle in the hand of a 6-week-old infant, the infant grasps it reflexively. As the hands move randomly, the rattle makes an enjoyable sound. The infant learns to move the rattle to create the sound and then finally to grasp the toy at will to play with it.

The next phase of infant play focuses on manipulative behavior. The infant examines toys closely, looking at them, touching them, and placing them in the mouth. The infant learns a great deal about texture, qualities of objects, and all aspects of the surroundings. At the same time, interaction with others becomes an important part of play. The social nature of play is obvious as the infant plays with other children and adults.

Toward the end of the first year, the infant's ability to move in space enlarges the sphere of play. Once infants crawl or walk, they can get to new places, find new toys, discover forgotten objects, or seek out other people for interaction. Play is a reflection of every aspect of development, as well as a method for enhancing learning and maturation (Table 4–8).

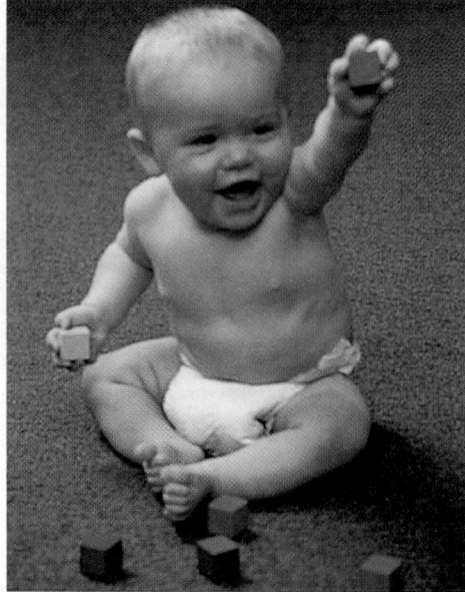

FIGURE 4–7 ➤ Garrett shows us that an 8-month-old child can play with blocks, demonstrating physical, cognitive, and social capabilities. Notice also his ability to sit well and engagement with his environment.

Complementary Therapy
Infant Massage

Infant massage has been used for communicating with and soothing infants in many cultures throughout history, but it is not traditionally used within most families in the United States and Canada. It has many benefits both for infants and parents and can be taught to families who are interested. Some of the benefits for babies include improved sleep, soothability, decreased stress hormones, and positive parent–child interaction (Underdown, Barlow, Chung, et al., 2006). Premature infants are particularly benefited by this intervention. Massage periods of 10–15 minutes daily can be encouraged and facilitated. Such episodes will enhance bonding and attachment between parents and infant.

Personality and Temperament

Why does one infant frequently awaken at night crying while another sleeps for 8 to 10 hours undisturbed? Why does one infant smile much of the time and react positively to interactions while another is withdrawn around unfamiliar people and frequently frowns and cries? Such differences in responses to the environment are believed to be inborn characteristics of temperament. Infants are born with a tendency to react in certain ways to noise and to interact differently with people. They may display varying degrees of regularity in activities of eating and sleeping, and manifest a capacity for concentrating on tasks for different amounts of time (see Table 4–5).

Nursing assessment identifies personality characteristics of the infant that the nurse can share with the parents. With this information, the parents can appreciate more fully the uniqueness of their infant and design experiences to meet the infant's needs. Parents can learn to modify the environment to promote adaptation. For example, an infant who does not adapt easily to new situations may cry, withdraw, or develop another way of coping when adjusting to new people or places. Parents might be advised to use one or two baby-sitters rather than engaging new sitters frequently. If the infant is easily distracted when eating, parents can feed the infant in a quiet setting to encourage a focus on eating. Although the infant's temperament is unchanged, the ability to fit with the environment is enhanced.

Communication

Even at a few weeks of age, infants communicate and engage in two-way interaction, and express comfort by soft sounds, cuddling, and eye contact. The infant displays discomfort by thrashing the extremities, arching the back, and crying vigorously. From these rudimentary skills, communication ability continues to develop until the infant speaks several words at the end of the first year of life (see Table 4–8). Nonverbal methods continue to be a primary method of communication between parent and child.

Nurses assess communication to identify possible abnormalities or developmental delays. Language ability may be assessed with the Denver II Developmental Test and other specialized language screening tools (see Chapter 6 ∞). Normal infants and toddlers understand (**receptive speech**) more words than they can speak (**expressive speech**). Abnormalities may be caused by a hearing deficit, developmental delay, or lack of

TABLE 4–8	Psychosocial Development During Infancy	
Age	Play and Toys	Communication
Birth–3 months	Prefers visual stimuli of mobiles, black-and-white patterns, mirrors Auditory stimuli are music boxes, tape players, soft voices Responds to rocking and cuddling Moves legs and arms while adult sings and talks Likes varying stimuli—different rooms, sounds, visual images	Coos Babbles Cries
3–6 months	Prefers noise-making objects that are easily grasped like rattles Enjoys stuffed animals and soft toys with contrasting colors	Vocalizes during play and with familiar people Laughs Cries less Squeals and makes pleasure sounds Babbles multisyllabically (mamamamama)
6–9 months	Likes teething toys Increasingly desires social interaction with adults and other children Soft toys that can be manipulated and mouthed are favorites	Increases vowel and consonant sounds Links syllables together Uses speechlike rhythm when vocalizing with others
9–12 months	Enjoys large blocks, toys that pop apart and go back together, nesting cups and other objects Laughs at surprise toys like jack-in-the-box Plays interactive games like peek-a-boo Uses push-and-pull toys	Understands "no" and other simple commands Says "dada" and "mama" to identify parents Learns one or two other words Receptive speech surpasses expressive speech

verbal stimulation from caretakers. Further assessment may be required to pinpoint the cause of the abnormality.

Nursing interventions focus on providing a stimulating and comforting environment. Parents are encouraged to speak to infants and teach words. Hospital nurses should include the infant's known words when providing care, and provide nonverbal support by hugging and holding. Consider the family's cultural patterns for communications and development.

■ TODDLER (1 TO 3 YEARS)

Toddlerhood is sometimes called the first adolescence. An infant only months before, this child from 1 to 3 years is now displaying independence and negativism. Pride in newfound accomplishments emerges.

Physical Growth and Development

The rate of growth slows during the second year of life. Parents may become concerned because the child has a limited food intake. They need reassurance that this is normal. See Chapter 14 ∞ for further discussion of nutrition in toddlerhood. By age 2 years, the birth weight has usually quadrupled and the child is about one-half of the adult height. Body proportions begin to change, with legs longer and head smaller in proportion to body size than during infancy (see Figure 4–6). The toddler has a "pot-bellied" appearance and stands with feet apart to provide a wide base of

support. By approximately 33 months, eruption of deciduous teeth is complete, with 20 teeth present.

Gross motor activity develops rapidly (Table 4–9), as the toddler progresses from walking to running, kicking, and riding a tricycle (Figure 4–8 ➤). As physical maturation occurs, the toddler develops the ability to control elimination patterns. See Chapter 8 ∞ for more information about development of the toddler.

Cognitive Development

During the toddler years, the child moves from the sensorimotor to the preoperational stage of development. The early use of language awakens in the 1-year-old the ability to think about objects or people when they are absent. Object permanence is well developed.

At about 2 years of age, the increasing use of words as symbols enables the toddler to use preoperational thought. Rudimentary problem solving, creative thought, and an understanding of cause-and-effect relationships are now possible.

Psychosocial Development

The toddler is soundly rooted in a trusting relationship and feels more comfortable in asserting autonomy and separating the self from primary care providers. It will be important to become an autonomous person while learning the patterns that promote interactions with adults and children.

TABLE 4–9	Growth and Development Milestones During Toddlerhood			
Age	Physical Growth	Fine Motor Ability	Gross Motor Ability	Sensory Ability
1–2 years	Gains 8 oz (227 g) or more per month Grows 3.5–5 in. (9–12 cm) during this year Anterior fontanel closes	By end of second year, builds a tower of four blocks **(1)** Scribbles on paper **(2)** Can undress self **(3)** Throws a ball	Runs Shows growing ability to walk and finally walks with ease Walks up and down stairs a few months after learning to walk with ease **(5)** Likes push-and-pull toys	Visual acuity 20/50
2–3 years	Gains 1.4–2.3 kg (3–5 lb)/year Grows 5–6.5 cm (2–2.5 in.)/year	Draws a circle and other rudimentary forms Learns to pour Learning to dress self **(4)**	Jumps Kicks ball **(6)** Throws ball overhand	

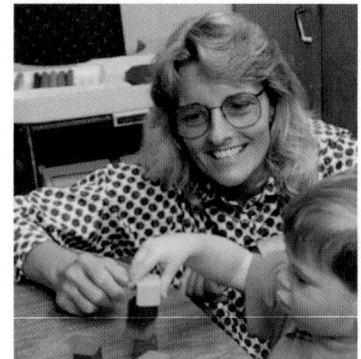

(1) By end of second year, builds tower of four blocks

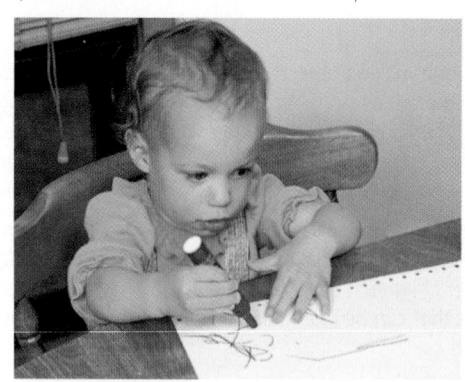

(2) Scribbles on paper

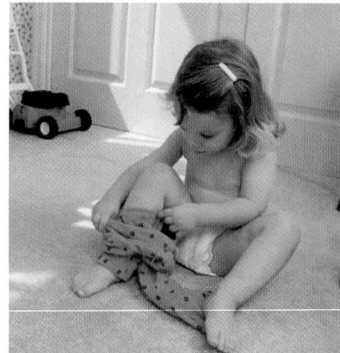

(3) Can undress self

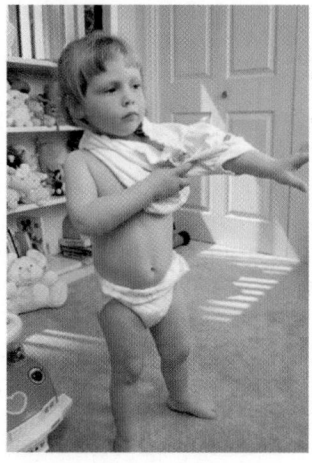

(4) Learning to dress self

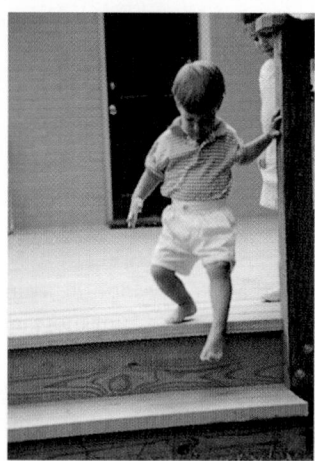

(5) Walks up and down stairs

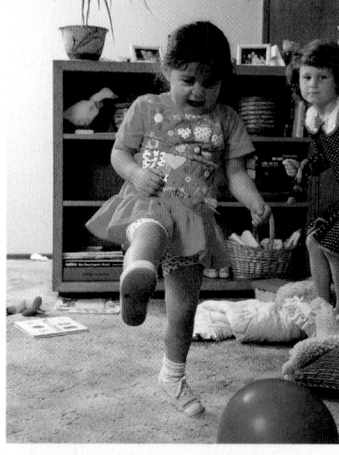

(6) Jumps and kicks ball

Play

Many changes in play patterns occur between infancy and toddlerhood. Developing motor skills enable toddlers to bang pegs into a pounding board with a hammer. The social nature of toddler play is also readily seen. Toddlers find the company of other children pleasurable, even though socially interactive play may not occur (Figure 4–9 ➤). Two toddlers tend to play with similar objects side by side, occasionally trading toys and words. This is called **parallel play**. This playtime with other children assists toddlers to develop social skills. Toddlers engage in play activities they have seen at home, such as pounding with a hammer and talking on the phone. This imitative behavior helps them to learn new actions and skills (Figure 4–10 ➤).

Physical skills are manifested in play as toddlers push and pull objects, climb in and out and up and down, run, ride a Big Wheel, turn the pages of books, and scribble with a pen. Both gross motor and fine motor abilities are enhanced during this age period.

Cognitive understanding enables the toddler to manipulate objects and learn about their qualities. Stacking blocks and placing rings on a building tower teach spatial relationships and other lessons that provide a foundation for future learning. Various kinds of play objects should be provided for the toddler to

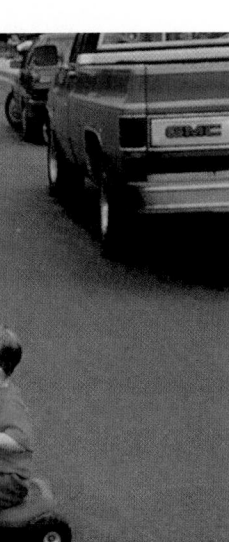

FIGURE 4–8 ➤ This toddler has learned to ride a Big Wheel, which he is doing right into the street. Toddlers must be closely watched to prevent injury. What other characteristics of toddlerhood can you identify? Notice the boy's short legs and arms, which are typical in toddlerhood.

meet play needs. These play needs can easily be met whether the child is hospitalized or at home (Table 4–10).

Personality and Temperament

The toddler retains most of the temperamental characteristics identified during infancy, but may demonstrate some changes. The normal developmental progression of toddlerhood also plays a part in responses. For example, the infant who previously responded positively to stimuli, such as a new baby-sitter, may appear more negative in toddlerhood. The increasing independence characteristic of this age is shown by the toddler's use

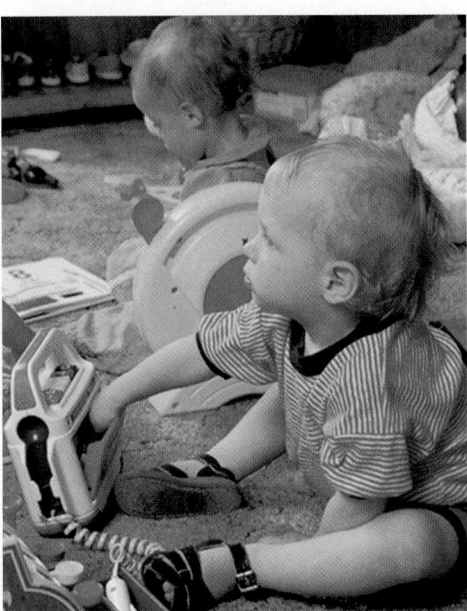

FIGURE 4–9 ➤ Mobility enlarges the sphere of play, allowing the child to seek new toys and spaces and to seek out people for interaction. Which psychosocial, cognitive, and motor skills do you see taking place in this photograph?

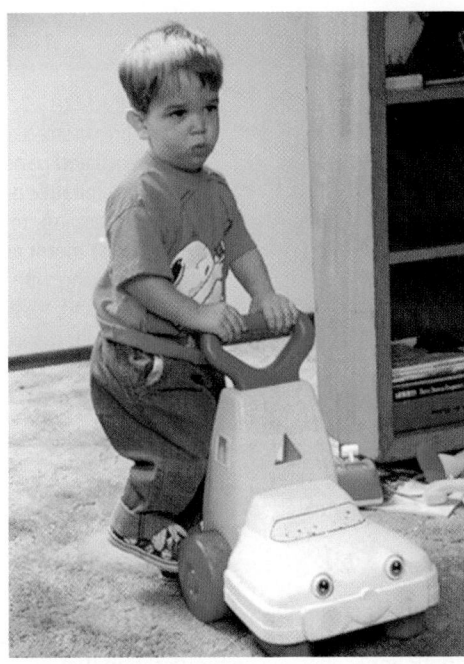

FIGURE 4–10 ➤ Imitative play such as pushing and pulling a vacuum allows the toddler to develop gross and fine motor skills. What are the benefits to the toddler from imitating behaviors of adults?

of the word *no*. The parent and child constantly adapt their responses to each other and learn anew how to communicate with each other.

Communication

Because of the phenomenal growth of language skills during the toddler period, adults should communicate frequently with children in this age group. Toddlers imitate words and speech intonations, as well as the social interactions they observe.

At the beginning of toddlerhood, the child may use four to six words in addition to "mama" and "dada." Receptive speech (the ability to understand words) far outpaces expressive speech. By the end of toddlerhood, however, the 3-year-old has a vocabulary of almost 1,000 words and uses short sentences.

Communication occurs in many ways, some of which are nonverbal. Toddler communication includes pointing, pulling an adult over to a room or object, and speaking in **expressive jargon** (using unintelligible words with normal speech intonations as if truly communicating in words). Another communication method occurs when the toddler cries, pounds feet, displays a temper tantrum, or uses other means to illustrate dismay. These powerful communication methods can upset parents, who often need suggestions for handling them. It is best to verbalize the feelings shown by the toddler, for example, by saying, "You must be very upset that you cannot have that candy. When you stop crying you can come out of your room," and then to ignore further negative behavior. The toddler's search for autonomy and independence creates a need for such behavior. Sometimes an upset toddler responds well to holding, rocking, and stroking.

Parents and nurses can promote a toddler's communication by speaking frequently, naming objects, explaining procedures in simple terms, expressing feelings that the toddler seems to be

TABLE 4–10 Psychosocial Development During Toddlerhood

Age	Play and Toys	Communication
1–3 years 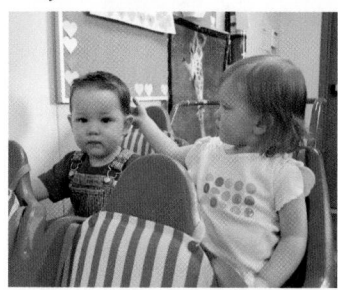	Refines fine motor skills by use of cloth books, large pencil and paper, wooden puzzles Facilitates imitative behavior by playing kitchen, grocery shopping, toy telephone Learns gross motor activities by riding Big Wheel tricycle, playing with soft ball and bat, molding water and sand, tossing ball or bean bag Cognitive skills develop by educational television shows, music, stories and books	Increasingly enjoys talking Exponential growth of vocabulary, especially when spoken and read to Needs to release stress by pounding board, frequent gross motor activities, and occasional temper tantrums Likes contact with other children and learns interpersonal skills

Families Want to Know
Communicating with a Toddler

Procedures such as drawing blood, getting immunizations, or even having ears checked can be frightening for a toddler. Parents and nurses can both apply effective communication that minimizes the trauma caused by such procedures. Share these tips with parents:

■ Avoid telling toddlers about the procedure too far in advance. They do not have an understanding of time and can become quite anxious. Telling them just before the procedure begins is most appropriate.

■ Use simple terminology. "We need to get a little blood from your arm. It will help us to find out if you are getting better." If the parent is willing, say, "Your Mom will hold your arm still so we can do it quickly." Approach positively and confidently.

■ Give short, clear instructions. Do not give choices if none exist. Offer a choice of two alternatives when possible. "Would you like apple juice or grape juice after you drink this medicine?"

■ Tell the toddler what you are doing; name objects.

■ Allow the toddler to cry. Acknowledge that it must be frightening and that you understand. Encourage parents to allow the child to cry out during a procedure or other frightening event.

■ If in a hospital, perform the procedure in a treatment room so that the toddler's bed and room are a safe haven.

■ Be sure the toddler is restrained, with the joints above and below the procedure immobilized so the procedure can be quickly accomplished with the least trauma.

■ Use a Band-Aid to cover up the site. This can reassure the toddler that the body is still intact.

■ Allow the toddler to choose a reward such as a sticker after the procedure.

■ Praise the toddler for cooperation and acknowledge that you know this was difficult.

■ Comfort the toddler by rocking, offering a favorite drink, playing music, and holding. If parents are present, they can offer the comfort needed.

displaying, and encouraging speech. The toddler from a bilingual home is at an optimal age to learn two languages. If the parents do not speak English, the toddler will benefit from a childcare experience because both languages can then be learned.

The nurse who understands the communication skills of toddlers is able to assess expressive and receptive language and communicate effectively, thereby promoting positive health care experiences for these children. Parents often need ideas of strategies for communication with the young child. See Families Want to Know: Communicating with a Toddler.

■ PRESCHOOL CHILD (3 TO 6 YEARS)

The preschool years are a time of new initiative and independence. Most children are in a childcare center or school for part of the day and learn a great deal from this social contact. Language skills are well developed, and the child is able to understand and speak clearly. Endless projects characterize the world of busy preschoolers. They may work with play dough to form animals, then cut out and paste paper, then draw and color (Figure 4–11 ➤).

Physical Growth and Development

Preschoolers grow slowly and steadily, with most growth taking place in long bones of the arms and legs. The short, chubby toddler gradually gives way to a slender, long-legged preschooler (Table 4–11).

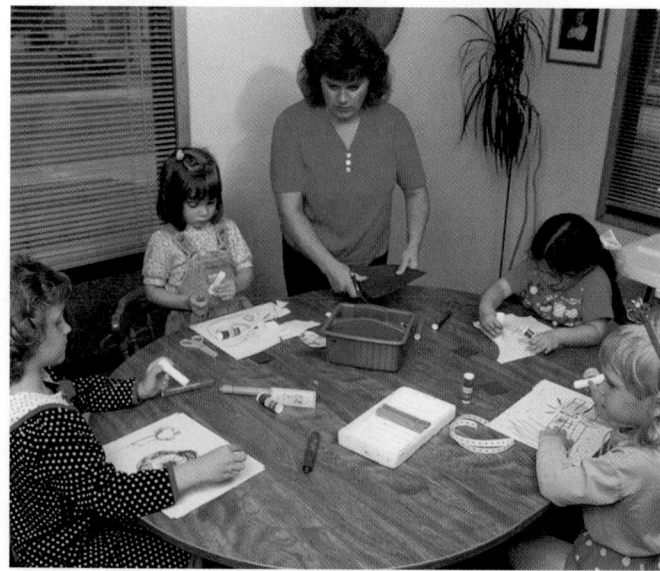

FIGURE 4–11 ➤ Preschoolers have well-developed language, motor, and social skills, and they can work creatively together on an art project, as this group is doing at an in-home childcare center.

TABLE 4–11 Growth and Development Milestones During the Preschool Years

Physical Growth		Fine Motor Ability

Physical Growth

Gains 1.5–2.5 kg (3–5 lb)/year   Grows 4–6 cm (1 1/2–2 1/2 in.)/year

Fine Motor Ability

Uses scissors **(1)**
Draws circle, square, cross **(2)**
Draws at least a six-part person
Enjoys art projects such as pasting, stringing beads, using clay
Learns to tie shoes at end of preschool years **(3)**
Buttons clothes **(4)**
Brushes teeth **(5)**
Uses fork, knife, spoon

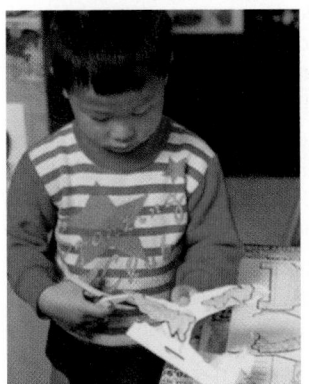

(1) Uses scissors

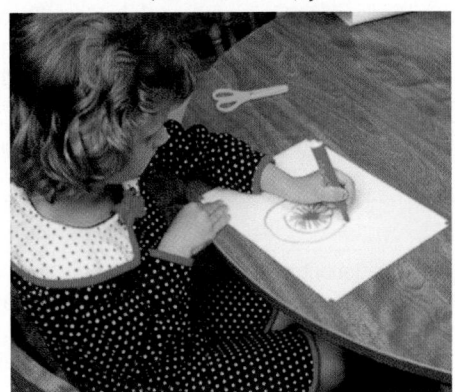

(2) Draws circle, square, cross

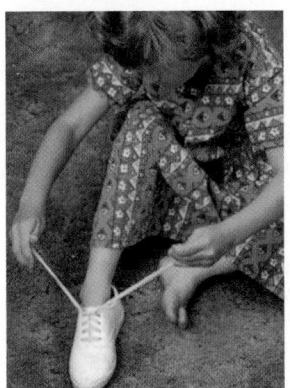

(3) Ties shoes

(4) Buttons clothes

(5) Brushes teeth

Gross Motor Ability

Throws a ball overhand
Climbs well **(6)**
Rides tricycle **(7)**

Sensory Ability

Visual acuity continues to improve
Can focus on and learn letters and numbers **(8)**

Fine Motor Ability

Eats three meals with snacks
Uses spoon, fork, knife

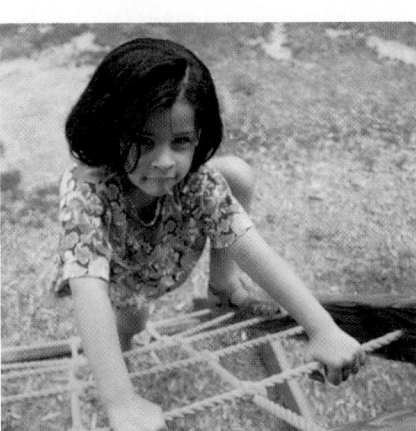

(6) Climbs well

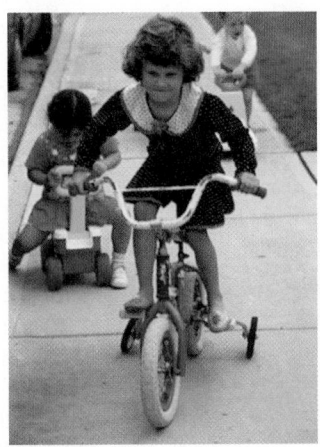

(7) Rides tricycle or bicycle with training wheels

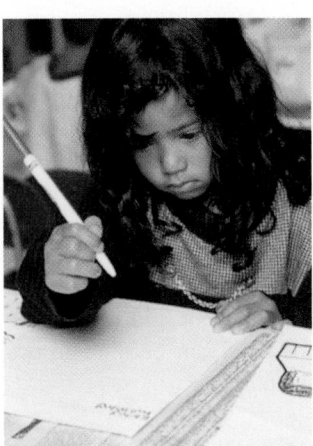

(8) Learns letters and numbers

TABLE 4–12 **Characteristics of Thought Identified by Piaget**

Characteristic	Definition	Development Stage	Nursing Implications
Object permanence	Ability to understand that when something is out of sight it still exists	Sensorimotor period, especially in coordination of secondary schemes substage from 8–12 months	Before development of object permanence, babies will not look for toys or other objects out of sight; as the concept is developing they are concerned when a parent leaves since they are not certain the parent will return.
Egocentrism	Ability to see things only from one's own point of view	Preoperational thought	Peers or others who have gone through an experience will not impress the preschooler; teaching should focus on what an experience will be like to the child.
Transductive reasoning	Connecting two events in a cause-effect relationship simply because they occur together in time	Preoperational thought	Ask the child what he or she thinks caused an occurrence; ask how the two events are connected; correct misconceptions to lessen the child's guilt.
Centration	Focusing only on one particular aspect of a situation	Preoperational thought	Listen to the child's comments and deal with concerns in order to present new concepts to the child.
Animism	Giving lifelike qualities to nonliving things	Preoperational thought	Ask preschool children to describe how a machine works, or how the trees move. Provide opportunities to learn about machines that may move and make noises (intravenous pumps, magnetic resonance imaging) to decrease fears.
Magical thinking	The belief that events occur because of one's thoughts or actions	Preoperational thought	Ask young children how they became ill, or what caused a parent's or sibling's illness. Correct misconceptions when the child blames self for causing problems by wishing someone ill or having bad behavior.
Conservation	Knowledge that matter is not changed when its form is altered	Concrete operational thought	Before conservation of thought is reached, the child may think that gender can be changed when hair is cut, or that the leg under a cast is broken in separate pieces. Ask perceptions and clarify misconceptions.

Physical skills continue to develop. The preschooler runs with ease, holds a bat, and throws balls of various types. Writing ability increases, and the preschooler enjoys drawing and learning to write a few letters. See Chapter 8 ∞ for a detailed list of developmental milestones during the preschool period.

The preschool period is a good time to encourage good dental habits. Children can begin to brush their own teeth with parental supervision and help to reach all tooth surfaces. Parents should floss children's teeth, give fluoride as ordered if the water supply is not fluoridated, and schedule the first dental visit so the child can become accustomed to the routine of periodic dental care.

Cognitive Development

The preschooler exhibits characteristics of preoperational thought. Symbols or words are used to represent objects and people, enabling the young child to think about them. This is a milestone in intellectual development; however, the preschooler still has some limitations in thought (Table 4–12).

The preschooler's thought processes are important to understand in order to plan appropriate teaching for health care and development of health habits.

Psychosocial Development

The preschooler is more independent in establishing relationships with others. The child interacts closely with children and adults as well as planning and carrying out activities.

Play

The preschooler has begun to play in a new way. Toddlers simply play side by side with friends, each engaging in his or her own activities; preschoolers interact with others during play. One child cuts out colored paper while her friend glues it on paper in a design. This new type of interaction is called **associative play** (Figure 4–12 ➤). The child life therapist in hospital settings recognizes the therapeutic value of play in planning activities for children that enable them to work through feelings about procedures and separation, as well as facilitating

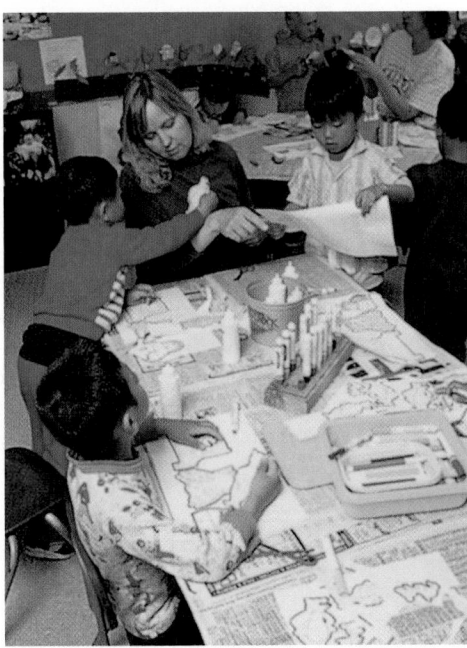

FIGURE 4–12 ➤ These preschoolers are participating in associative play, which means they can interact. One child is cutting out shapes, and the other is gluing them in place.

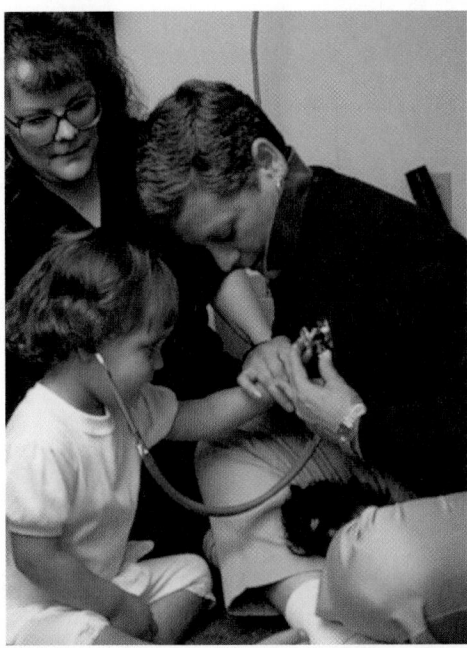

FIGURE 4–13 ➤ Jasmine is participating in dramatic play with a nurse while her mother looks on. In dramatic play, the child uses props to play out the drama of human life. It can be an excellent way for a nurse to assess the developmental level of children while talking to them. Notice that the child and the nurse are on the floor at the same level and the atmosphere is informal. Why is it important to be at the same level as the child?

the normal developmental need for interaction with other children (see Chapter 11 ∞).

In addition to this social dimension of play, other aspects of play also differ. The preschooler enjoys large motor activities such as swinging, riding a tricycle, and throwing a ball. Increasing manual dexterity is demonstrated in greater complexity of drawings and manipulation of blocks and modeling. These changes necessitate planning of playtime to include appropriate activities. Preschool programs and child life departments in hospitals help meet this important need.

Materials provided for play can be simple but should guide activities in which the child engages. Because fine motor activities are popular, paper, pens, scissors, glue, and a variety of other such objects should be available. The child can use them to create important images such as pictures of people, hospital beds, or friends. A collection of dolls, furniture, and clothing can be manipulated to represent parents and children, nurses and physicians, teachers, or other significant people. Because fantasy life is so powerful at this age, the preschooler readily uses props to engage in **dramatic play**, that is, living out the drama of human life (Figure 4–13 ➤).

The nurse can use playtime to assess the preschooler's developmental level, knowledge about health care, and emotions related to health care experiences. Observations about objects chosen for play, content of dramatic play, and pictures drawn can provide important assessment data. The nurse can also use play periods to teach the child about health care procedures and offer an outlet for expression of emotions (Table 4–13). Further information about play for hospitalized children is found in Chapter 11 ∞ . Play therapy for children with psychological alterations is described in Chapter 28 ∞ .

Personality and Temperament

Characteristics of personality observed in infancy tend to persist over time. The preschooler may need assistance as these characteristics are expressed in the new situations of preschool or nursery school. An excessively active child, for example, will need gentle, consistent handling to adjust to the structure of a classroom. Encourage parents to visit preschool programs to choose the one that would best foster growth in their child. Some preschoolers enjoy the structured learning of a program that focuses on cognitive skills, whereas others are happier and more open to learning in a small group that provides much time for free play. Nurses can help parents to identify their child's personality or temperament characteristics and to find the best environment for growth.

Communication

Language skills blossom during the preschool years. The vocabulary grows to over 2,000 words, and children speak in complete sentences of several words and use all parts of speech. They practice these newfound language skills by endlessly talking and asking questions.

The sophisticated speech of preschoolers mirrors the development occurring in their minds and helps them to learn about the world around them. However, this speech can be quite deceptive. Although preschoolers use many words, their grasp of meaning is usually literal and may not match that of adults. These literal interpretations have important implications for health care providers. For example, the preschooler who is told she will be "put to sleep" for surgery may think of a pet recently

TABLE 4–13 Psychosocial Development During Preschool Years

Age	Play and Toys	Communication
3–6 years 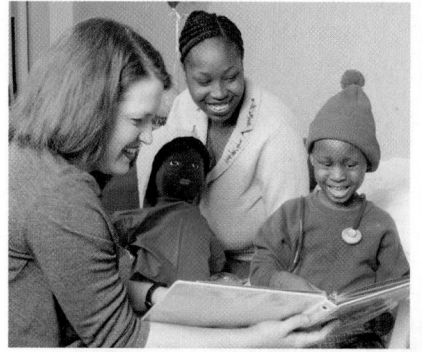	Associative play is facilitated by simple games, puzzles, nursery rhymes, songs Dramatic play is fostered by dolls and doll clothes, play houses and hospitals, dress-up clothes, puppets Stress is relieved by pens, paper, glue, scissors Cognitive growth is fostered by educational television shows, music, stories and books	All parts of speech are developed and used, occasionally incorrectly Communicates with a widening array of people Play with other children is a favorite activity Health professionals can: • Verbalize and explain procedures to children • Use drawings and stories to explain care • Use accurate names for body functions • Allow the child to talk, ask questions, and make choices

euthanized; the child who is told that a dye will be injected for a diagnostic test may think he is going to die; mention of "a little stick" in the arm can cause images of tree branches rather than of a simple immunization.

The child may also have difficulty focusing on the content of a conversation. The preschooler is egocentric and may be unable to move from individual thoughts to those the nurse is proposing, as the following conversation illustrates:

Nurse: I'd like to tell you about the operation that you will have tomorrow.

Sharisse: OK. Did you know my brother just got a new squirt gun?

Nurse: That's nice. Now, first thing in the morning you will wake up early and your foot will be scrubbed with a special soap.

Sharisse: The gun can spurt for about 40 feet—you have to pump it up.

Nurse: We'll talk about that later. Let me tell you about your operation now. After your foot is scrubbed, the nurse will measure your blood pressure and temperature and feel the pulse in your arm. Do you remember my doing those things today?

Sharisse: Yes. And I got a sticker when I came into the hospital today, too. Do you know that my Mom is going to stay here tonight?

During this interchange, Sharisse engages in **collective monologue**, in which separate conversations occur even though each person waits for the other to speak. Though waiting for the nurse to speak, Sharisse is not generally responding to the nurse's content but is instead focusing on content from her own mind. The nurse needs to respond to Sharisse's content and then reinsert more facts about the preparations for surgery.

Concrete visual aids such as pictures of a child undergoing the same procedure or a book to read together enhance teaching by meeting the child's developmental needs. Handling medical equipment such as intravenous bags and stethoscopes increases interest and helps the child to focus. Teaching may have to be done in several short sessions rather than one long session.

Some general approaches are:

• Allow time for the child to integrate explanations.
• Verbalize frequently to the child.
• Use drawings and stories to explain care.
• Use accurate names for body functions.
• Allow choices.

■ SCHOOL-AGE CHILD (6 TO 12 YEARS)

Errol, 10 years old, arrives home from school shortly after 3 p.m. each day. He immediately calls his friends and goes to visit one of them. They are building models of cars and collecting baseball cards. Endless hours are spent on these projects and on discussions of events at school that day (Figure 4–14 ➤).

Nine-year-old Karen practices soccer two afternoons a week and plays in games each weekend. She also is learning to play the flute and spends her free time at home practicing (see Figure 4–14 ➤). Although practice time is not her favorite part of music, Karen enjoys the performances and wants to play well in front of her friends and teacher. Her parents now allow her to ride her bike unaccompanied to the store or to a friend's house.

These two school-age children demonstrate common characteristics of their age group. They are in a stage of industry in which it is important to the child to perform useful work. Meaningful activities take on great importance and are usually carried out in the company of peers. A sense of achievement in these activities is important to develop self-esteem and to prevent a sense of inferiority or poor self-worth.

Physical Growth and Development

School age is the last period in which girls and boys are close in size and body proportions. As the long bones continue to grow, leg length increases (see Figure 4–6). Fat gives way to muscle, and the child appears leaner. Jaw proportions change as the first deciduous tooth is lost at 6 years and permanent teeth begin to erupt. Body organs and the immune system mature, resulting in fewer illnesses among school-age children. Medications are less likely to cause serious side effects, because they can be metabo-

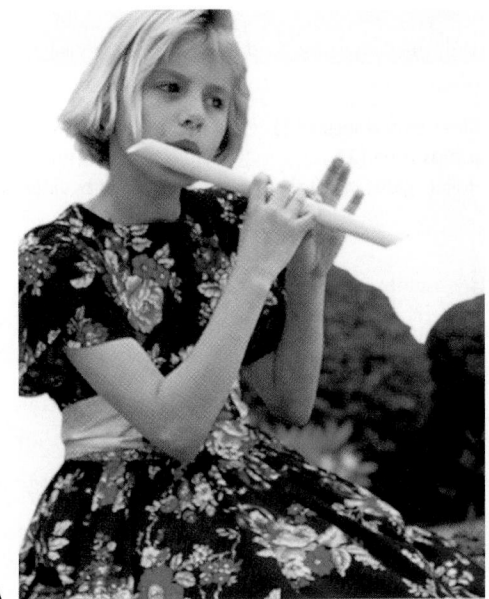

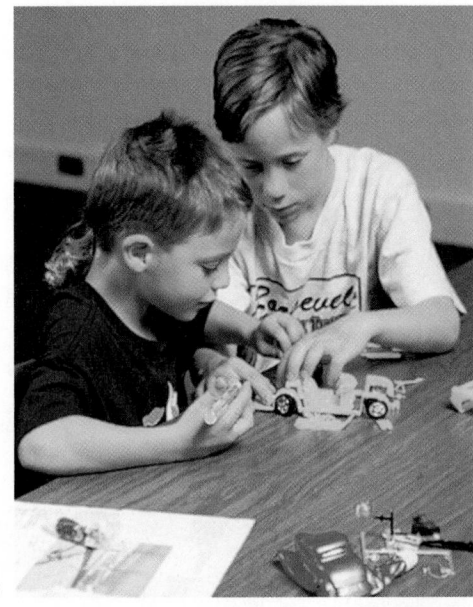

A   B

FIGURE 4–14 ➤ A, School-age children may take part in activities that require practice. This is a consideration when children are hospitalized and unable to practice or perform. Why? B, School-age children enjoy spending time with others the same age on projects and discussing the activities of the day. This is an important consideration when they are in an acute care setting. When you are in the clinical setting, look for examples of this type of interaction taking place.

lized more easily. The urinary system can adjust to changes in fluid status. Physical skills are also refined as children begin to play sports, and fine motor skills are well developed through school activities (Figure 4–15 ➤ and Table 4–14).

Although it is commonly believed that the start of adolescence (age 12 years) heralds a growth spurt, the rapid increases in size commonly occur during school age. Girls may begin a growth spurt as early as 9 or 10 years and boys a year or so later (Figure 4–16 ➤). Nutritional needs increase dramatically with this spurt.

The loss of the first deciduous teeth and the eruption of permanent teeth usually occur at about age 6 years, or at the beginning of the school-age period. Of the 32 permanent teeth, 22 to 26 erupt by age 12 years and the remaining molars follow during the teenage years (see Figure 4–15). The school-age child should be closely monitored to ensure that brushing and flossing are adequate, that fluoride is taken if the water supply is not fluoridated, that dental care is obtained to provide for examination of teeth and alignment, and that loose teeth are identified before surgery or other events that may lead to loss of a tooth.

Cognitive Development

The child enters the stage of concrete operational thought at about 7 years. This stage enables school-age children to consider alternative solutions and solve problems. However, school-age children continue to rely on concrete experiences and materials to form their thought content.

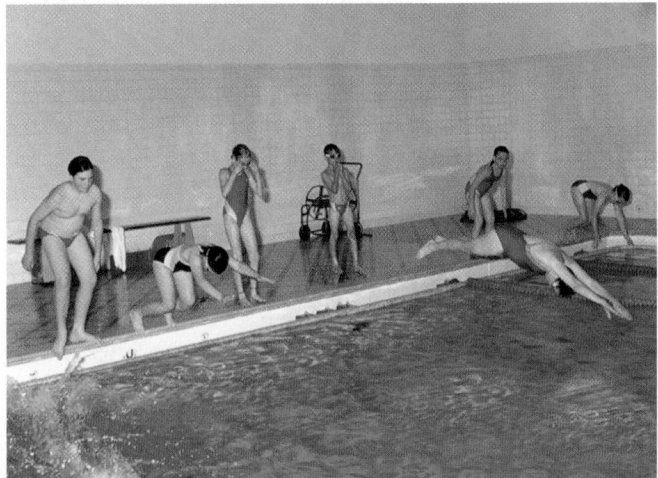

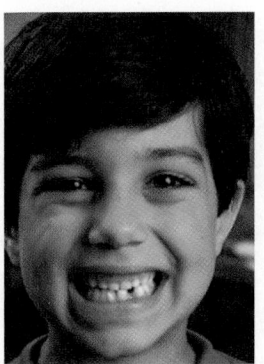

FIGURE 4–15 ➤ School-age girls and boys enjoy participating in sports. They begin to lose fat while developing their muscles, so they appear leaner than at earlier ages. Front teeth are lost around age 6 years. The family may have rituals associated with the loss of teeth that could affect the child's behavior if he loses a tooth while in the hospital.

TABLE 4–14 Growth and Development Milestones During the School-Age Years

Physical Growth	Fine Motor Ability	Gross Motor Ability	Sensory Ability
Gains 1.4–2.2 kg (3–5 lb)/year Grows 4–6 cm (1 1/2–2 1/2 in.)/year	Enjoys craft projects Plays card and board games	Rides two-wheeler **(1)** Jumps rope **(2)** Roller skates or ice skates	Can read Able to concentrate for longer periods on activities by filtering out surrounding sounds **(3)**

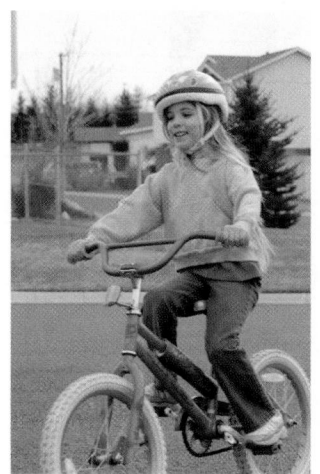 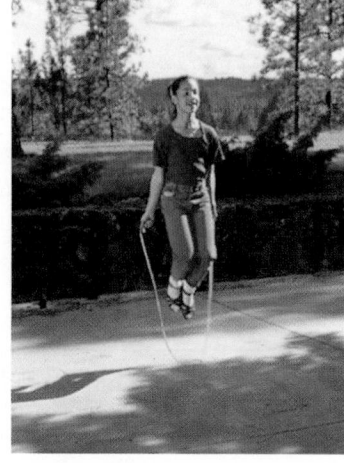 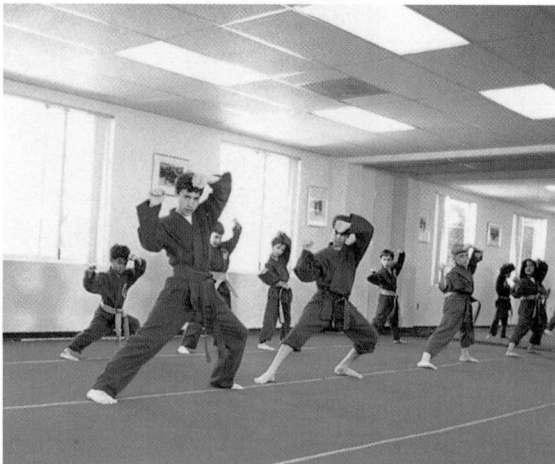

(1) Rides two-wheeler   *(2) Jumps rope*   *(3) Concentrates on activities for longer periods*

During the school-age years, the child learns the concept of conservation (that matter is not changed when its form is altered). At earlier ages, a child believes that when water is poured from a short, wide glass into a tall, thin glass, there is more water in the taller glass. The school-age child recognizes that although it may look like the taller glass holds more water, the quantity is the same. The concept of conservation is helpful when the nurse explains medical treatments. The school-age child understands that an incision will heal, that a cast will be removed, and that an arm will look the same as before once the intravenous infusion is removed.

Psychosocial Development

The school-age child has many friends and cooperatively interacts with others to accomplish tasks. The child develops a sense of accomplishment from activities and relationships.

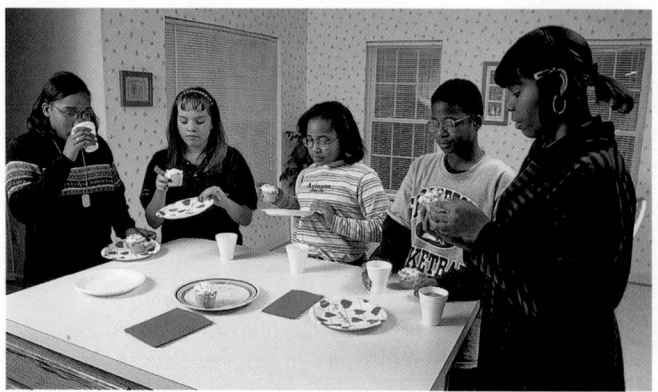

FIGURE 4–16 ➤ Because girls have a growth spurt earlier than boys, girls often are taller than boys of the same age. Remember what it was like at your first dance?

Play

When the preschool teacher tries to organize a game of baseball, both the teacher and the children become frustrated. Not only are the children physically unable to hold a bat and hit a ball, but they seem to have no understanding of the rules of the game and do not want to wait for their turn at bat. By 6 years of age, however, children have acquired the physical ability to hold the bat properly and may occasionally hit the ball. School-age children also understand that everyone has a role—the pitcher, the catcher, the batter, the outfielders. They cooperate with one another to form a team, are eager to learn the rules of the game, and want to ensure that these rules are followed exactly (Table 4–15).

The characteristics of play exhibited by the school-age child are cooperation with others and the ability to play a part in order to contribute to a unified whole. This type of play is called **cooperative play**. The concrete nature of cognitive thought leads to a reliance on rules to provide structure and security. Children have an increasing desire to spend much of their playtime with friends, which demonstrates the social component of play. Play is an extremely important method of learning and living for the school-age child. Active physical play has decreased in recent years as television viewing and playing of computer games have increased, leading to poor nutritional status and a high rate of overweight among children. See Chapter 14 ∞ for further discussion of nutrition and physical activity in children.

When a child is hospitalized, the separation from playmates can lead to feelings of sadness and purposelessness. School-age children often feel better when placed in multibed units with other children. Games can be devised even when a child uses a wheelchair (Figure 4–17 ➤). Normal, rewarding parts of play

TABLE 4–15 Psychosocial Development During the School-Age Years

Age	Activities	Communication
6–12 years 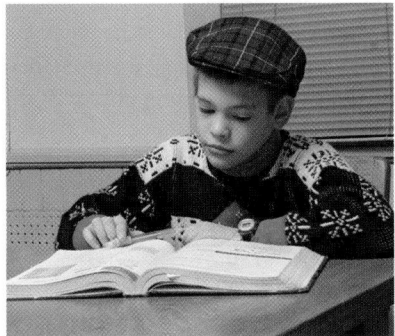	Gross motor development is fostered by ball sports, skating, dance lessons, water and snow skiing/boarding, biking A sense of industry is fostered by playing a musical instrument, gathering collections, starting hobbies, playing board and video games Cognitive growth is facilitated by reading, crafts, word puzzles, school work	Mature use of language Ability to converse and discuss topics for increasing lengths of time Spends many hours at school and with friends in sports or other activities Health professionals can: • Assess child's knowledge before teaching • Allow the child to select rewards following procedures • Teach techniques such as counting or visualization to manage difficult situations • Include both parent and child in health care decisions

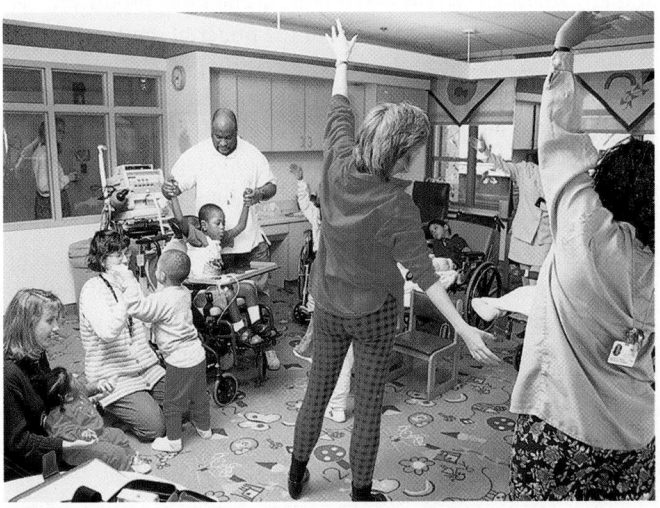

FIGURE 4–17 ➤ The nurse can help the child and family accept and adjust to new circumstances. Encouraging the child who uses a wheelchair to participate in group activities can help build confidence in physical skills. Positive self-esteem, goal attainment, personal satisfaction, and general health are the continued benefits.

should be integrated into care. Many children enjoy music played through earphones or on CD players. Friends should be encouraged to visit or call a hospitalized child. Discharge planning for the child who has had a cast or brace applied should address the activities in which the child can participate and those the child must avoid. Reinforce the importance of playing games with friends.

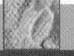
Complementary Therapy
Music Therapy

Most children are accustomed to listening to music via earphones or earbuds. They should be encouraged to bring their favorite music to the hospital as a form of stress reduction. Music may reduce the need for sedation during diagnostic tests or other medical procedures. Music has also been effective when integrated into treatment programs for children with developmental delay, severe illness, or family stress (Evans, Tsao, & Zeltzer, 2008; Wetherick, 2009).

Personality and Temperament

The enduring aspects of temperament continue to be manifested during the school years. The child classified as "difficult" at an earlier age may now have trouble in the classroom. Advise parents to provide a quiet setting for homework and to reward the child for concentration. For example, after homework is completed, the child may watch a television show. Creative efforts and alternative methods of learning should be valued. Encourage parents to see their children as individuals who may not all learn in the same way. The "slow-to-warm-up" child may need encouragement to try new activities and to share experiences with others, whereas the "easy" child will readily adapt to new schools, people, and experiences.

Communication

During the school-age years, the child should learn how to correct any lingering pronunciation or grammatical errors. Vocabulary increases, and the child learns about parts of speech in school. School-age children enjoy writing and can be encouraged to keep a journal of their experiences while in the hospital as a method of dealing with anxiety. The literal translation of words characteristic of preschoolers is uncommon among school-age children. An increasing array of electronic equipment is used to communicate with friends. School-age children often have cell phones, used for conversation or texting, as well as computers, and even linked video games. These techniques can be used to teach and engage school-age children such as using texting to remind them of upcoming health appointments or encouraging healthy behaviors.

Some communication strategies helpful with the school-age child include:

• Provide concrete examples of pictures or materials to accompany verbal descriptions. Include technological approaches such as web sites and video teaching.
• Assess knowledge before planning the instruction.
• Allow the child to select rewards following procedures.
• Teach techniques such as counting or visualization to manage difficult situations.
• Include the child in history gathering and health discussions with the parent.

Sexuality

Although children become aware of sexual differences between genders during preschool years, they deal much more consciously with sexuality during school age. As children mature physically, they need information about their body changes so that they can develop a healthy self-image and an understanding of the relationships between their bodies and sexuality. Children become interested in sexual issues and are often exposed to erroneous information on television shows, in magazines, or from friends and siblings. Schools and families need to use opportunities to teach school-age children factual information about sex and to foster healthy concepts of self and others. It is advisable to ask occasional questions about sexual issues to learn how much the child knows and to provide correct information when answers demonstrate confusion. Appropriate and inappropriate touch should be discussed, with lists of trusted people who can be approached (teachers, clergy, school counselors, family members, neighbors) to discuss any episodes with which the child feels uncomfortable. Recognize that even these trusted people can be implicated in inappropriate episodes, so encourage the child to go to more than one person, an important approach if the child is uncomfortable about a relationship with any individual.

■ ADOLESCENT (12 TO 18 YEARS)

Adolescence is a time of passage signaling the end of childhood and the beginning of adulthood. Although adolescents differ in behaviors and accomplishments, they are in a period of identity formation. If a healthy identity and sense of self-worth are not developed in this period, role confusion and purposeless struggling will ensue. The adolescents in your care will represent various degrees of identity formation, and each will offer unique challenges.

Physical Growth and Development

The physical changes ending in **puberty**, or sexual maturity, begin near the end of the school-age period. The prepubescent period is marked by a growth spurt at an average age of 10 years for girls and 13 years for boys, although there is considerable variation among children (see Figure 4–16). The increase in height and weight is generally remarkable and is completed in 2 to 3 years (Table 4–16). The growth spurt in girls is accompanied by an increase in breast size and growth of pubic hair. Menstruation occurs last and signals achievement of puberty. In boys, the growth spurt is accompanied by growth in size of the penis and testes and by growth of pubic hair. Deepening of the voice and growth of facial hair occur later, at the time of puberty. See Chapter 5 ∞ for a description of the pubertal stages.

During adolescence, children grow stronger and more muscular and establish characteristic male and female patterns of fat distribution. The apocrine and eccrine glands mature, leading to increased sweating and a distinct odor to perspiration. All body organs are now fully mature, enabling the adolescent to take adult doses of medications.

The physical and emotional changes of adolescence occur with great variability, so difference from maturation of peers is common. The adolescent must incorporate the new body and its functions, and retain a healthy sense of self in relationship to peers. The formation of self-identity is a psychological

TABLE 4–16	Growth and Development Milestones During Adolescence		
Physical Growth	Fine Motor Ability	Gross Motor Ability	Sensory Ability
Variation in age of growth spurt During growth spurt, girls gain 7–25 kg (15–55 lb) and grow 2.5–20 cm (2–8 in.); boys gain approximately 7–29.5 kg (15–65 lb) and grow 11–30 cm (4 1/2–12 in.)	Skills are well developed **(1)**	New sports activities attempted and muscle development continues **(2)** Some lack of coordination common during growth spurt	Fully developed

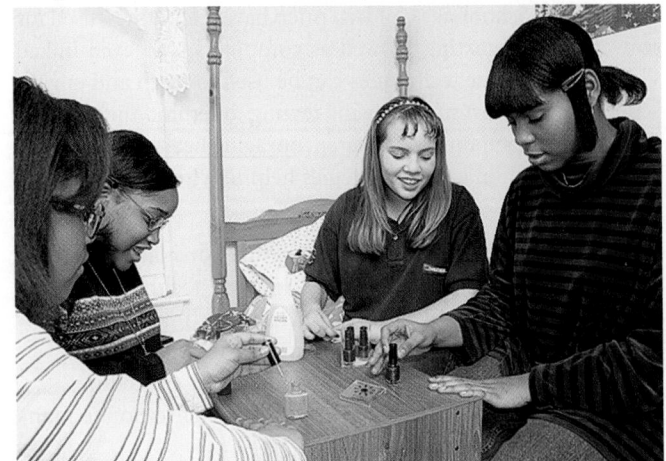

(1) Motor skills are well developed

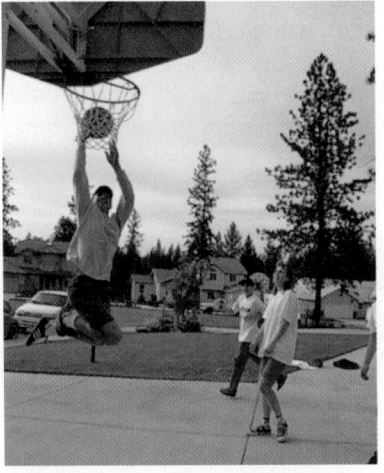

(2) New sports activities attempted

process but is necessarily closely connected with the body changes occurring.

Cognitive Development

Adolescence marks the beginning of Piaget's last stage of cognitive development, the stage of formal operational thought. The adolescent no longer depends on concrete experiences as the basis of thought but develops the ability to reason abstractly. Such concepts as justice, truth, beauty, and power can be understood. The adolescent revels in this newfound ability and spends a great deal of time thinking, reading, and talking about abstract concepts.

The ability to think and act independently leads many adolescents to rebel against parental authority. Through these actions, adolescents seek to establish their own identity and values.

Psychosocial Development

The adolescent is mature in relationships with others. The key aspect that the teen is working on during relationships and activities is to establish a meaningful identity.

Activities

Maturity leads to new activities. Adolescents may drive, ride buses, or bike independently. They are less dependent on parents for transportation and spend more time with friends. Activities include participation in sports and extracurricular school activities, as well as "hanging out" and attending movies or concerts with friends (Table 4–17). The peer group becomes the focus of activities (Figure 4–18 ➤), regardless of the teen's interests. Peers are important in establishing identity and providing meaning. Although same-sex interactions predominate, boy–girl relationships are more common than at earlier stages. Adolescents thus participate in and learn from social interactions fundamental to adult relationships.

Research — *Youth Risk Behavior Surveillance*

The federal government administers questionnaires to a large cross-section of youth annually to monitor their behaviors related to risk behavior. The Youth Risk Behavior Surveillance (YRBS) system gathers data about six high-priority areas: unintentional and intentional injury, tobacco use, alcohol and other drug use, sexual behavior, dietary behavior, and physical inactivity. Visit the *Morbidity and Mortality Weekly Report* website to search for a recent YRBS report. How can nurses use this information to plan appropriate interventions for populations of adolescents?

Personality and Temperament

Characteristics of temperament manifested during childhood usually remain stable in the teenage years. For instance, the adolescent who was a calm, scheduled infant and child often demonstrates initiative to regulate study times and other routines. Similarly, the adolescent who was an easily stimulated infant may now have a messy room, a harried schedule with assignments always completed late, and an interest in many activities. It is also common for an adolescent who was an easy child to become more difficult because of the psychologic changes of adolescence and the need to assert independence.

Similar to the child's earlier ages, the nurse's role may be to inform parents of different personality types and to help them support the teen's uniqueness while providing necessary structure and feedback. Nurses can help parents to understand their teen's personality type and to work with the adolescent to meet expectations of teachers and others in authority.

Communication

All parts of speech are used and understood by the adolescent. Colloquialisms and slang are commonly used with the peer group. The adolescent often studies a foreign language in school,

TABLE 4–17 Psychosocial Development During Adolescence

Age	Activities	Communication
12–18 years	Sports—ball games, gymnastics, water and snow skiing/boarding, swimming, school sports School activities—drama, yearbook, class office, club participation Quiet activities—reading, school work, television, computer, video games, texting, music	Increasing communication and time with peer group—movies, dances, driving, eating out, attending sports events Applying abstract thought and analysis in conversations at home and school

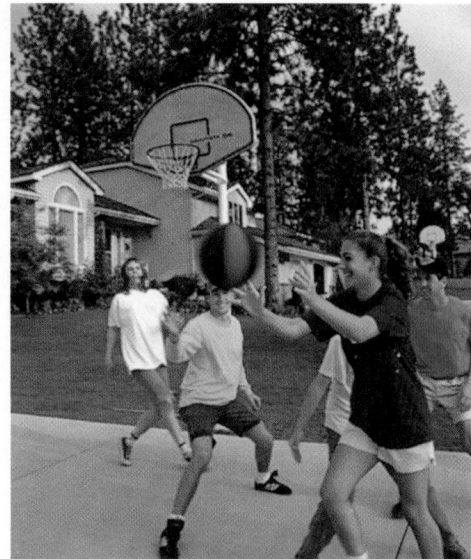

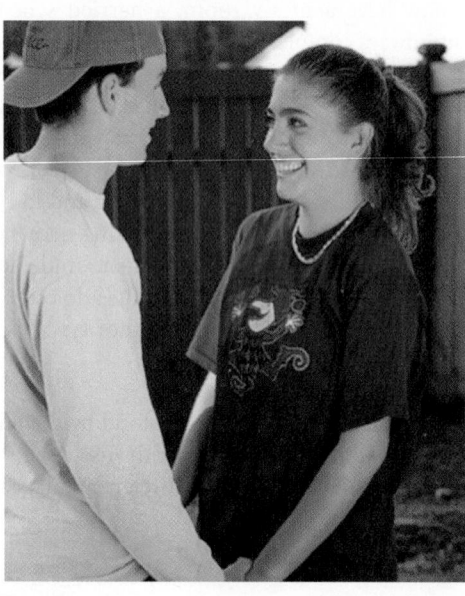

FIGURE 4–18 ➤ Social interaction between children of the same and opposite sex is as important inside the acute care setting as it is outside. A, Teenagers enjoy playing together. B, Emotional relationships form during adolescence.

having the ability to understand and analyze grammar and sentence structure. Communication by technological means is an important part of socialization in developed countries today. Social networking via websites, texting using phones, and other methods form a large part of many adolescents' days.

The adolescent increasingly leaves the home base and establishes close ties with peers. These relationships become the basis for identity formation. There is generally a period of stress or crisis before a strong identity can emerge. The adolescent may try out new roles by learning a new sport or other skills, experimenting with drugs or alcohol, wearing different styles of clothing, or trying other activities. It is important to provide positive role models and a variety of experiences to help the adolescent make wise choices.

The adolescent also has a need to leave the past, to be different, and to change from former patterns to establish a self-identity. Rules that are repeated constantly and dogmatically will probably be broken in the adolescent's quest for self-awareness. This poses difficulties when the adolescent has a health problem, such as diabetes or a heart problem, that requires ongoing care. Introducing the adolescent to other teens who manage the same problem appropriately is usually more successful than telling the adolescent what to do.

Privacy should be ensured during the taking of health histories or interventions with teens. Even if a parent is present for part of a history or examination, the adolescent should be given the opportunity to relay information or ask questions alone with the health care provider. The adolescent should be given a choice of whether to have a parent present during an examination or while care is provided. Most information shared by an adolescent is confidential. Some states mandate disclosure of certain information to parents such as an adolescent's desire for an abortion. In these cases, the adolescent should be informed of what will be disclosed to the parent. See Chapter 1 ∞ for further information about the legal implications of care for adolescents.

Setting up teen rooms (recreation rooms for use only by adolescents) or separate adolescent units in hospitals can provide necessary peer support during hospitalization. Frequently used technology such as computers, televisions, and videos can be available. Most adolescents are not pleased when placed on a unit or in a room with young children. Choices should be allowed when possible, and include preference for evening or morning bathing, the type of clothes to wear while hospitalized, timing of treatments, and visitation guidelines. Use of negotiations and agreements with adolescents may increase adherence with health care recommendations. Firmness, gentleness, choices, and respect must be balanced during care of adolescent patients.

Some specific communication strategies that help with the adolescent include:

- Provide written and verbal explanations.
- Direct history and explanations to the teen alone; then include the parent.
- Allow for safe exploration of topics by suggesting that the teen is similar to other teens. ("Many teens with diabetes have questions about. . . . How about you?")
- Arrange meetings for discussions with other teens.

Sexuality

With maturation of the body and increased secretion of hormones, the adolescent achieves sexual maturity. This complex process involves a growing interest in sexuality and romantic or sexual relationships, a recognition of the influences of society and family, and identity formation. The early adolescent progresses from dances and other social events with members of the opposite sex to the late adolescent who is mature sexually and may have regular sexual encounters. About one-half of all high school students in the United States have had intercourse, and 35% are currently sexually active at a given time; however, only 62% of these youths used a condom at their last sexual encounter, putting this age group at high risk of acquiring sexually transmitted infections (Centers for Disease Control and Prevention, 2008).

Teenagers need information about their bodies and emerging sexuality. To make informed decisions about their behavior, teenagers should understand the interests and forces they experience. Including sex education in school classes and health care encounters is important. Information on methods to prevent sexually transmitted infections is given, with most school districts now providing some teaching on HIV. Far more common risks to teens, however, are diseases such as gonorrhea, herpes, and hepatitis. Health histories should include questions on sexual activity, sexually transmitted infections, and birth control use and understanding. Most hospitals routinely perform pregnancy screening on adolescent girls before elective procedures.

Adolescents will benefit from clear information about sexuality, an opportunity to develop relationships with adolescents in various settings, an open atmosphere at home and school where problems and issues can be discussed, and previous experience in problem solving and self-decision making. Sexual issues should be among topics that adolescents can discuss openly in a variety of settings. Alternatives and support for their decisions should be available.

Some adolescents identify with a sexual minority group such as lesbian, gay, bisexual, or transgendered. They are at particular risk of being stigmatized and harassed by other youth or adults. They are more likely to suffer a variety of problems such as isolation, rejection by significant others, violence, suicide, and taking sexual risks (Van Leeuwen, Boyle, Salomonsen-Sautel, et al., 2006). Nurses are instrumental in helping these youths by providing information for them and their parents, integrating sexual minority content into sexual education curricula, and providing referrals for health and social care when needed. Nurses must examine their own beliefs and communication styles to provide culturally competent care. They can promote trust and acceptance among youth and in the general school community. See Chapter 17 ∞ for further information about the health issues related to homosexuality and other sexual minority practices.

Chapter Highlights

- Development unfolds in a predictable pattern, but at different rates dependent on the particular characteristics and experiences of each child.
- Major theories of development encompass the psychosexual (Freud), psychosocial (Erikson), cognitive (Piaget), moral (Kohlberg), social learning (Bandura), and behavioral (Skinner and Watson) components of individuals.
- The ecologic theory of Bronfenbrenner and the temperament theory of Chess and Thomas emphasize the interactions of the individual within the environment.
- Resiliency theory examines risk and protective factors that hinder or help children and families when dealing with developmental and life crises.
- Influences on the developmental process include one's genetic potential and a series of environmental influences unique to each family and individual.
- Infancy spans the time from 1 month to 1 year, and is marked by rapid physical growth, mastery of basic fine and gross motor skills, and beginning cognitive and language skills.
- Toddlers range in age from 1 to 3 years, and become increasingly mobile and communicative. They master control over excretion and are known for exerting their own opinions and wishes to parents. Injury prevention and toilet training are specific parental teaching needs.
- Preschool years range from 3 to 6 and are marked by increasing social skills. Most preschool children attend childcare programs and learn to play with other children. Continued mastery of physical coordination and language occur.
- School age spans the years from 6 to 12, when children mature in many areas. They show slow, steady growth until reaching puberty between 9 and 12 years, when a growth spurt marks increased height and weight, as well as sexual maturation. School-age children play cooperatively with other children and participate in various school and community activities.
- Adolescence occurs from about 12 years of age through the teen years. Adolescents establish their own identities distinct from parents and other adults. They are mature physically and cognitively. The peer group exerts the major influence at this age.
- The nurse is involved in assessing development at each stage, and in providing anticipatory guidance to families to foster optimal development.

Clinical Reasoning in Action

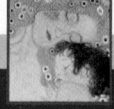

Consider Sergio, who was introduced in the chapter-opening scenario. He is now 6 months of age and growing well. His mother has altered her work schedule to stay with him each day; she works for a few hours in the evening when her husband is home. One pair of grandparents live about 30 miles away and visit frequently. The family has medical insurance but has had to budget carefully to pay household bills since Yolanda is working less and they have expenses connected with Sergio's care.

Since they have no other children and have limited experience with children, Pepe and Yolanda, Sergio's parents, have all the needs of new parents. Due to prematurity, Sergio has additional needs for developmental surveillance and parental education.

Some developmental milestones that the nurse observes about Sergio include:

- Personal social—smiles, watches his own hand
- Fine motor—hands meet at midline, regards and watches small objects, and has begun to grasp a rattle
- Language—turns to sounds and voices, squeals and makes a variety of other sounds

- Gross motor—holds head steady when in sitting position; holds head and chest up using arms when prone

1. Sergio and his parents have many challenges and yet possess many strengths. Using the theory of resilience, list the infant and family risks and protective factors.
2. The parents note that Sergio has recently learned the sound of his bottle being prepared and gets visibly excited. What cognitive substage does this represent in Piaget's cognitive framework? Is this the substage you would expect for him?
3. Analyze Sergio's developmental milestones. Consult the list of expected milestones in this chapter. What skills will Sergio learn next? What specific suggestions do you have for his parents as they seek to encourage his development?
4. You are the nurse in the clinic where Sergio receives health care. Briefly outline the physical growth, developmental progression, and family assessments that you expect for him.

See Pearson Nursing Student Resources for possible responses.

Pearson Nursing Student Resources

Find additional review materials at
nursing.pearsonhighered.com

Prepare for success with NCLEX®-style practice questions, interactive assignments and activities, web links, animations and videos, and more!

References

Ahern, N. R. (2006). Adolescent resilience: An evolutionary concept analysis. *Journal of Pediatric Nursing, 21,* 175–185.

American Academy of Pediatrics. (2009). *Pediatric nutrition handbook* (6th ed.). Elk Grove Village, IL: Author.

Bandura, A. (1986). *Social foundations of thought and actions: A social cognitive theory.* Englewood Cliffs, NJ: Prentice Hall.

Bandura, A. (1997a). *Self efficacy in changing societies.* New York: Cambridge University Press.

Bandura, A. (1997b). *Self efficacy: The exercise of control.* New York: W. H. Freeman.

Bremner, A. J., Bryant, P. E., & Mareschal, D. (2006). Object-centered spatial reference in 4-month-old infants. *Infant Behavioral Development, 29*(1), 1–10.

Bronfenbrenner, U. (1986). Ecology of the family as a context for human development: Research perspectives. *Developmental Psychology, 22,* 723–742.

Bronfenbrenner, U. (Ed.). (2005). *Making human beings human: Bioecological perspectives on human development.* Thousand Oaks, CA: Sage Publications.

Bronfenbrenner, U., McClelland, P. D., Ceci, S. J., Moen, P., & Wethington, E. (1996). *The state of Americans.* New York: Free Press.

Centers for Disease Control and Prevention. (2008). Youth Risk Behavior Surveillance—United States, 2007. *Morbidity and Mortality Weekly Report, 57*(SS-4), 1–136.

Chess, S., & Thomas, A. (1995). *Temperament in clinical practice.* New York: Guilford Press.

Chess, S., & Thomas, A. (1996). *Temperament: Theory and practice.* Philadelphia: Brunner/Mazel.

Chess, S., & Thomas, A. (1999). *Goodness of fit: Clinical applications from infancy through adult life.* Philadelphia: Brunner/Mazel.

Craig, G. J., & Dunn, W. L. (2010). *Understanding human development* (2nd ed.). Upper Saddle River, NJ: Pearson Prentice Hall.

Dennis, C. L. (2006). Identifying predictors of breastfeeding self-efficacy in the immediate postpartum period. *Research in Nursing and Health, 28,* 256–268.

Erikson, E. (1963). *Childhood and society.* New York: W.W. Norton.

Erikson, E. (1968). *Identity: Youth and crisis.* New York: W.W. Norton.

Evans, S., Tsao, J. C., & Zeltzer, L. K. (2008). Complementary and alternative medicine for acute procedural pain in children. *Alternative Therapeutic Health Medicine, 14*(5), 52–56.

Garvey, C., Julion, W., Fogg, L., Kratovil, A., & Gross, D. (2006). Measuring participation in a prevention trial with parents of young children. *Research in Nursing & Health, 29,* 212–222.

Ginsberg, H., & Opper, S. (1988). *Piaget's theory of intellectual development* (3rd ed.). Paramus, NJ: Prentice Hall.

Henderson, N., Benard, B., & Sharp-Light, M. (2007). *Resiliency in action.* Ojai, CA: Resiliency in Action, Inc.

Huizink, A. C., & Mulder, E. J. (2006). Maternal smoking, drinking, or cannabis use during pregnancy and neurobehavioral and cognitive functioning in human offspring. *Neuroscience and Biobehavior Review, 30,* 24–41.

Kyle, P. M. (2006). Drugs and the fetus. *Current Opinion in Obstetrics and Gynecology, 18*(2), 93–99.

Melnyk, B. M., Jacobsen, D., Kelly, S., O'Haver, J., Small, L., & Mays, M. Z. (2009). Improving the mental health, healthy lifestyle, and physical health

of Hispanic adolescents: Random controlled pilot study. *Journal of School Health, 79*(12), 575–584.

Meltzoff, A., & Gopnick, A. (1997). *Words, thoughts, and theories.* Cambridge, MA: MIT Press.

Nguyen, H. T., Sharma, V., & McIntyre, R. S. (2009). Teratogenesis associated with antipolar agents. *Advanced Therapeutics, 26*(3), 281–294.

Piaget, J. (1972). *The child's conception of the world.* Totowa, NJ: Littlefield, Adams.

Power, T., Bindler, R., Goetz, S., & Daratha, K. (2010). Interventions for youth health: Youth, family and teacher perspectives. *Journal of School Health, 80,* 13–19.

Rettew, D. C., Stanger, C., McKee, L., Doyle, A., & Judziak, J. J. (2006). Interactions between child and parent temperament and child behavior problems. *Comprehensive Psychiatry, 47,* 412–420.

Santrock, J. (2009). *Life-span development* (12th ed.). Boston: McGraw-Hill.

Trickett, E. J. (2009). Multilevel community-based culturally situated interventions and community impact: An ecological perspective. *American Journal of Community Psychology, 43*(3–4), 257–266.

Underdown, A., Barlow, J., Chung, V., & Stewart-Brown, S. (2006). Massage intervention for promoting mental and physical health in infants aged under 6 months. Cochrane Review, Issue 4, No. CD005038.

Van Leeuwen, J. M., Boyle, S., Salomonsen-Sautel, S., Baker, D. N., Garcia, J. T., Hoffman, A., & Hopfer, C. J. (2006). Lesbian, gay, and bisexual homeless youth: An eight-city public health perspective. *Child Welfare, 85*(2), 151–170.

Vygotsky, L. (1962). *Thought and language.* Cambridge, MA: MIT Press.

Wetherick, D. (2009). Music in the family: Music making and music therapy with young children and their families. *Journal of Family Health Care, 19*(2), 56–58.

Wiium, N., & Wold, B. (2009). An ecological system approach to adolescent smoking behavior. *Journal of Youth and Adolescence, 38*(10), 1351–1363.

Zirkle, D. L. (2005). *Think First for Kids (TFFK): A longitudinal analysis of a school-based injury prevention curriculum* (Doctoral dissertation). University of San Diego.

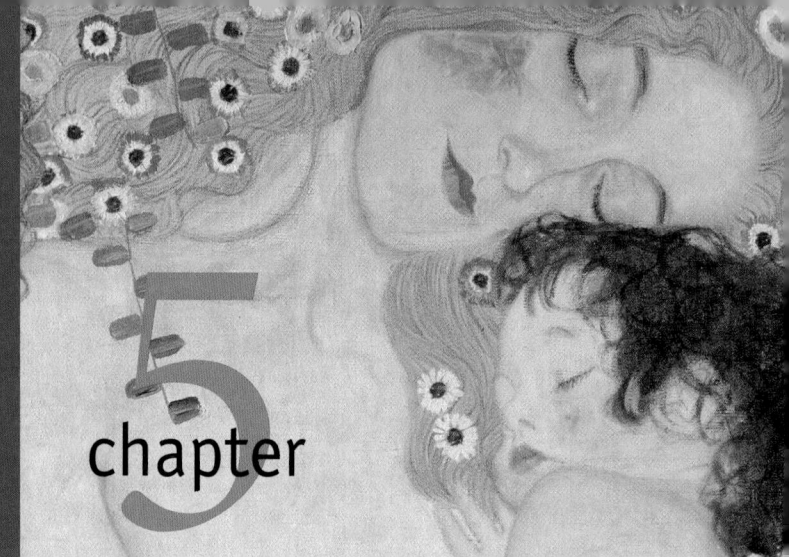

Pediatric Assessment   chapter 5

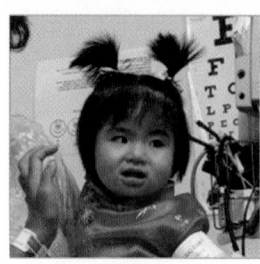

Two-year-old Jasmine was recently adopted into the Porter family. She has been brought to the health clinic for internationally adopted children by her new mother and sister for a comprehensive health assessment. Until 3 weeks ago, Jasmine was living in a center for children eligible for adoption in her native China. She speaks no English and she is very fearful of new and different situations. Mrs. Porter is anxious to have Jasmine evaluated to identify any health promotion or special health care issues that need to be addressed, such as development, growth, nutrition, immunizations, and health conditions. Jasmine had many immunizations before leaving China, and she has never had a major illness or injury. Limited information is available about her biological parents and their health. Mrs. Porter thinks Jasmine seems small for her age, and she is also concerned that she may have an ear infection. Jasmine's appetite has not been good for the past day, and she has been cranky. She has a slight fever.

The patient history and physical examination provide a structure and sequence for collecting and analyzing relevant assessment data. The initial physical examination findings provide the baseline for monitoring Jasmine's future growth and development and response to care for any identified health problems. Analysis of the assessment data enables you to form nursing diagnoses and to develop a nursing care plan to guide the nursing care that Jasmine will receive.

Do examination techniques vary for children of different ages? How does the nurse encourage the toddler and young child to cooperate with the examination?

Key Terms

apical impulse / 140
auscultation / 116
bradypnea / 137
bronchophony / 139
clubbing / 151
coloboma / 124
crepitus / 138
edema / 120
egophony / 139
hypertelorism / 124
induration / 120
inspection / 116
nasal flaring / 130
palpation / 116
percussion / 116
retractions / 137
stadiometer / 118
stridor / 139
sutures / 122
tachypnea / 137
tactile fremitus / 138
vocal resonance / 139
wheezing / 139
whispered pectoriloquy / 139

Learning Outcomes

After reading this chapter, you will be able to do the following:

1. Describe the elements of a health history for an infant and child at different ages.
2. Apply communication strategies to improve the quality of historical data collected.
3. Describe strategies to gain cooperation of a young child for assessment.
4. Demonstrate the differences in sequence of the physical assessment for infants, children, and adolescents.
5. Modify physical assessment techniques according to the age and developmental stage of the child.
6. Determine the sexual maturity rating of males and females based upon physical signs of secondary sexual characteristics present.
7. Analyze findings from the assessment of multiple systems and identify signs indicating the presence of a health condition.

How do examination techniques vary by the age of the child? How does the nurse encourage infants and toddlers to cooperate with the examination? This chapter provides an overview of pediatric assessment, including history taking and examination techniques geared to the unique needs of pediatric patients. Strategies for obtaining the child's history are presented first. The remainder of the chapter then outlines a systematic process for physical examination of the child.

■ ANATOMIC AND PHYSIOLOGIC CHARACTERISTICS OF INFANTS AND CHILDREN

Children and infants are not only smaller than adults, but also significantly different physiologically. Knowledge of pediatric anatomic and physiologic differences will aid in recognizing normal variations found during the physical examination. It also assists with understanding the different physiologic re-

sponses children have to illness and injury. Figure 5–1 ➤ provides an overview of important anatomic and physiologic differences between children and adults.

Obtaining the Child's History

Communication Strategies

What makes communication effective? What does it mean when a parent or caretaker will not look you in the eye when speaking with you? What types of cues indicate that a parent may be withholding historical information?

The health history interview is a very personal conversation with a parent, caretaker, or adolescent during which private concerns and feelings are shared. Try to ensure that this exchange of information is effective, with the parent or the child and the nurse understanding each other. Effective communication is difficult to accomplish because parents and children often do not correctly interpret what the nurse says, just as the nurse may

As Children Grow
Anatomic and Physiologic Characteristics

Body surface area large for weight, making infants susceptible to hypothermia.

Anterior fontanel and open sutures palpable up to about 18 months. Posterior fontanel closes between 2 and 3 months.

Tongue large relative to small nasal and oral airway passages.

Short, narrow trachea in children under 5 years makes them susceptible to foreign body obstruction.

Until late school age and adolescence, cardiac output is rate dependent not stroke volume dependent, making heart rate more rapid.

Abdomen offers poor protection for the liver and spleen, making them susceptible to trauma.

Until 12 to 18 months of age, kidneys do not concentrate urine effectively and do not exert optimal control over electrolyte secretion and absorption.

Until later school age, proportion of body weight in water is larger, with more water in extracellular spaces. Daily water exchange rate is much higher.

All brain cells present at birth; myelinization and further development of nerve fibers occur during first year.

Head proportionately larger, making child susceptible to head injury.

Higher metabolic rate, higher oxygen needs, higher caloric needs.

Until puberty, percentage of cartilage in ribs is higher, making them more flexible and compliant.

Until about 10 years, there is a faster respiratory rate, fewer and smaller alveoli, and less lung volume. Tidal volume is proportional to weight (7 to 10 mL/kg).

Up to about 4 or 5 years, diaphragm is primary breathing muscle. CO_2 is not effectively expired when child is distressed, making child susceptible to metabolic acidosis.

Until puberty, bones are soft and more easily bent and fractured.

Muscles lack tone, power, and coordination during infancy. Muscles are 25% of weight in infants versus 40% in adults.

Blood volume is weight dependent: 80 mL/kg.

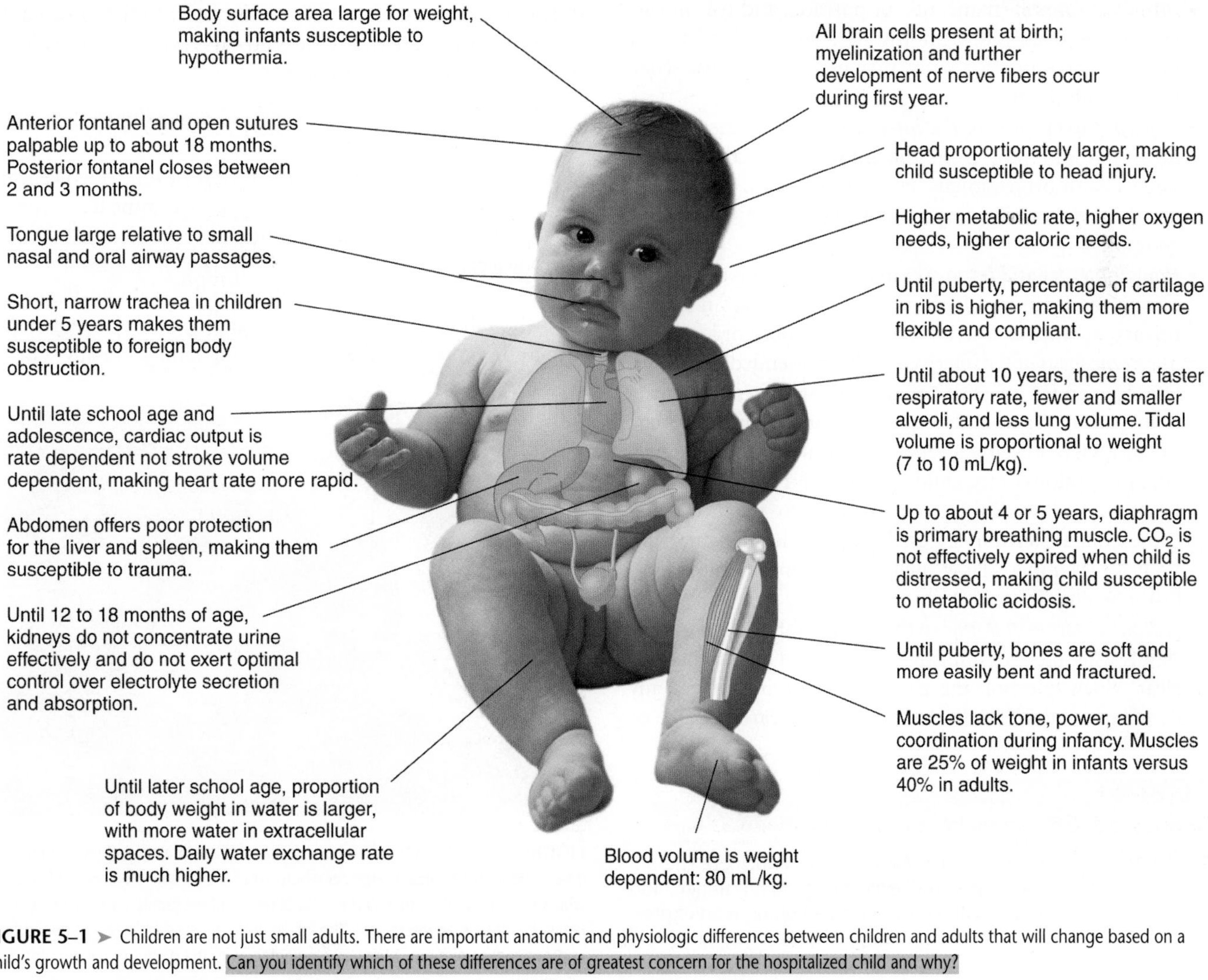

FIGURE 5–1 ➤ Children are not just small adults. There are important anatomic and physiologic differences between children and adults that will change based on a child's growth and development. Can you identify which of these differences are of greatest concern for the hospitalized child and why?

Assure the parents and the child that the information provided during the assessment is protected under the Health Insurance Portability and Accountability Act (HIPAA), a federal law that requires written consent to be provided before health information can be shared with health care providers outside the facility. To ensure confidentiality of information for parents, avoid using a family member as an interpreter for history taking.

not understand completely what the parent or child says. Interpretation of information is based on a person's life experiences, culture, and education.

Strategies to Build a Rapport with the Family

When beginning the history, make sure the parents understand the purpose of the interview and that the information will be used appropriately. To develop rapport, demonstrate interest in and concern for the child and family during the interview. This rapport forms the foundation for the collaborative relationship between the nurse and parent that will provide the best nursing care for the child. The following strategies help to establish rapport with the child's family during the nursing history:

- *Introduce yourself* (name, title or position, and role in caring for the child). To demonstrate respect, ask all family members present what name they prefer you to use when talking with them.
- *Explain the purpose of the interview* and why the nursing history is different from the information collected by other health professionals. For example, "The nurses will use this information to plan nursing care best suited for your child."
- *Provide privacy* and remove as many distractions as possible during the interview. If the patient's room does not offer privacy, attempt to find a vacant patient room or lounge.
- *Direct the focus of the interview* with open-ended questions. Use close-ended questions or directing statements to clarify information. Open-ended questions are useful to initiate the interview, develop a rapport, and understand the parent's perceptions of the child's problem; for example, "What problems led to Roberto's admission to the hospital?" Close-ended questions are used to obtain detailed information; for example, "How high was Tommy's temperature this morning?"
- *Ask one question at a time* so that the parent or child understands what piece of information is desired and so that it is clear which question the parent is answering. "Does any member of your family have diabetes, heart disease, or

Some cultural groups, particularly Asians, try to anticipate the answers you want to hear, or say "Yes" even if they do not understand the question. This is done in an effort to please you or as an expression of politeness. Remember to phrase your questions in a neutral manner.

sickle cell anemia?" is a multiple question. Ask about each disease separately to ensure the most accurate response.

- *Involve the child in the interview* by asking age-appropriate questions. Young children can be asked "What is your doll's name?" or "Where does it hurt?" Demonstrating an interest in the child initiates development of rapport with both child and parents. Ask older children and teens questions about their illness or injury. Offer them an opportunity to privately discuss their major concerns when their parents are not present.
- *Be honest with the child* when answering questions or when giving information about what will happen. Children need to learn that they can trust their nurse.
- *Choose the language style* that is best understood by the parent and child. Commonly used phrases can have different meanings to persons in various regions of the country or to different ethnic groups. To improve communication, ask for frequent feedback from the parents or child to ensure that their interpretation of phrases is accurate.
- *Use an interpreter to improve communication* when not fluent in the family's primary language (Figure 5–2 ▶).

Careful Listening

Complete attention is necessary to "hear" and accurately interpret information the parents and child give during the nursing history. Carefully *listen* to the information provided by the parent, as well as how it is expressed, and *observe behavior* during the interaction.

- Does the parent hesitate or avoid answering certain questions?
- Pay attention to the parent's attitude or tone of voice when the child's problems are discussed. Determine if it is consistent with the seriousness of the child's problem. The tone of voice can reveal anxiety, anger, or lack of concern.
- Be alert to any underlying themes. For example, the parent who talks about the child's diagnosis, but repeatedly refers to the impact of the illness on the family's finances or on

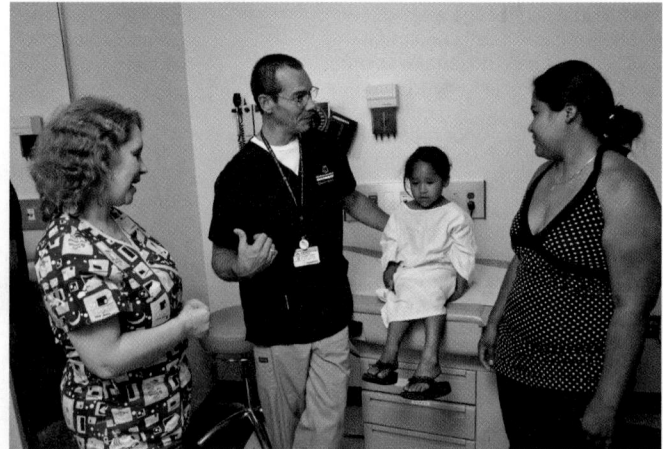

FIGURE 5–2 ➤ Most hospitals have designated interpreters that you should use. If not, find a professional interpreter whom you have identified beforehand and who knows medical terms and the cultural norms of the family. Avoid using a family member as an interpreter. The interpreter (center) should be positioned to improve communication. Maintain eye contact with the parent or patient, not the interpreter.

Certain cultures, such as some Asian and Native American groups, consider the use of silence during conversations as respectful. The nurse should avoid interruption of silence and allow the person time to reflect and formulate responses when communicating. In other cultures, silence may be noticed when the issue discussed is painful or sensitive. Be compassionate and recognize that parents and children will talk when they are ready (Seidel, Ball, Dains, et al., 2010).

Prolonged eye contact may be avoided by some cultural groups, such as persons of Native American, African American, Hindu, Hmong, Japanese, or Chinese heritage, because it is considered impolite, aggressive, or a sign of disrespect. Other cultures, such as persons of Arabic, European, and Russian heritage, seek eye contact and some may look for a response or impact regarding what is said (Purnell, 2009).

meeting the needs of other family members, is requesting that these issues be addressed.

- Observe the parent's *nonverbal behavior* (posture, gestures, body movements, eye contact, and facial expression) for consistency with the words and tone of voice used. Is the parent interested in and appropriately concerned about the child's condition? Behaviors such as sitting up straight, making eye contact (if culturally acceptable), and appearing apprehensive reflect appropriate concern for the child. Physical withdrawal, failure to make eye contact, or a happy expression could be inconsistent with the child's serious condition.

Subtle nonverbal and verbal cues often indicate that the parent has not provided complete information about the child's problem. Observe for behaviors such as avoiding eye contact, change in voice pitch, or hesitation when responding to a question. Being supportive and asking clarifying questions encourage further description or the expression of information that is difficult for the parent or child to share; for example, "It sounds like that was a very difficult experience. How did Latasha react?"

Encourage parents to share information, even if it is private or sensitive, especially when it influences nursing care planning. Often parents avoid sharing some information because they want to make a good impression, or they do not understand the value of the missing information. If parents hesitate to share information, briefly explain why the question was asked—for example, to make their child's hospital experience more pleasant or to begin planning for the child's discharge and home care.

In some cases the parent becomes too agitated, upset, or angry to continue responding to questions. When the information is not needed immediately, move on to another portion of the history to determine whether the parent is able to respond to other questions. Depending on the parent's emotional status, it may be more appropriate to collect the remaining historical data later.

Data to Be Collected

Collect and organize the child's health, medical, and personal-social history to plan the child's nursing care. Health status, psychosocial, and developmental data are organized to help develop the nursing diagnoses and the nursing care plan.

Patient Information   Obtain the child's name and nickname, age, sex, and ethnic origin. The child's birth date, race, religion, address, and phone number can be obtained from the admission form. Ask the parent for an emergency contact address and phone number, as well as work and cell phone numbers. Record the person providing the patient history and that person's relationship to the patient.

Physiologic Data   Collect information about the child's health problems and diseases chronologically in a format similar to the traditional medical history.

Chief Complaint   Identify the child's primary problem or reason for hospital admission or visit to a health care setting, stated in the parent's or child's exact words.

History of the Present Illness or Injury   Obtain a detailed description of the current health problem to include characteristics listed in Table 5–1. Each problem is described separately with the same level of detail.

Past History   Collect a more detailed description of the child's prior health problems, including all major past illnesses and injuries. A detailed and complete birth history is obtained when the child's present problem may be related to the birth history (Table 5–2). Record the child's age at the time of each major illness or injury, and remember to include common communicable diseases, surgeries, and hospitalizations. If any transfusions (blood or blood products) have been given in the past, identify the circumstances, type of transfusion, and any reaction. Obtain information about each specific diagnosis, treatment, outcome, complication, or residual problem, and the child's reaction to the event.

Current Health Status   Obtain a detailed description of the child's typical health status.

- **Health Maintenance**—child's primary care provider, dentist, and other health care providers, and when each was last visited.

TABLE 5–1	History of Present Illness or Injury
Characteristic	Defining Variables
Onset	Sudden or gradual, previous episodes, date and time began
Type of symptom	Pain, itching, cough, vomiting, runny nose, diarrhea, rash, etc.
Location	Generalized or localized—anatomically precise
Duration	Continuous or episodic, length of episodes
Severity	Effect on daily activities; e.g., interrupted sleep, decreased appetite, too fatigued for usual activities
Influencing factors	What relieves or aggravates symptoms, what precipitated the problem, recent exposure to infection or allergen
Past evaluation for problem	Laboratory studies, physician's office or hospital where done, results of past examinations
Previous and current treatment	Prescribed and over-the-counter drugs used, complementary therapies or other treatments used (heat, ice, rest), response to treatments

TABLE 5–2	**Birth History**
Prenatal Condition	• Mother's age, health during pregnancy, prenatal care, weight gained, special diet, expected date of birth • Details of illnesses, radiograph or sonogram findings, hospitalizations, medications, complications, and their timing during pregnancy • Prior obstetric history
Intrapartum—Description of Birth	• Site of birth (hospital, home, birthing center) • Labor induced or spontaneous, rupture of membranes, length of labor • Vaginal or cesarean birth, forceps or suction used, vertex or breech position • Length of pregnancy, single or multiple birth
Condition of Baby at Birth	• Weight, Apgar score, cried immediately • Need for incubator, resuscitation, oxygen, ventilator • Any abnormalities detected, meconium staining
Postnatal Condition	• Difficulties in the nursery—feeding, respiratory difficulties, jaundice, cyanosis, rashes, seizures • Length of hospital stay, special nursery, home with mother • Breast- or bottle-fed, weight lost/gained in hospital • Medical care needed in first week—readmission to hospital

• **Medications**—prescribed and over-the-counter medications taken daily, frequently, or for home management of fever, colds, coughs, cuts, and rashes. Ask about the use of plants, herbs, teas, or other complementary therapies.

• **Allergies**—to food, medication, animals, insect bites, or other exposures, and the type of reaction (e.g., respiratory difficulty, rash, hives, itching).

• **Immunizations**—review dates immunizations were received, and any unexpected reactions. See Chapter 16 ∞.

• **Safety Measures Used**—car seat restraint, window guards, medication storage, sports protective gear, smoke detectors, bicycle helmet, firearm storage, and others.

• **Activities and Exercise**—physical mobility and limitations, adaptive equipment used; play and/or sports activities.

• **Nutrition**—formula-fed or breastfed; if breastfed, for how long; type and amount of daily formula intake; when solid foods were introduced; enrollment in the WIC (Women, Infants, and Children) Program; eating and snacking habits, variety of foods consumed, "junk foods" eaten, appetite.

• **Sleep**—length and timing of naps and nighttime sleep; nightmares or night terrors, other sleep disturbances; where the child sleeps, and bedtime rituals.

Family History Obtain a list of the major familial and hereditary diseases in three generations of family members, including the parents, grandparents, aunts, uncles, cousins, child, and siblings. Collect information about the health status and ethnic background of each parent, and ask if they are related to each other. Label the generations and make a key for relevant diseases. Record information in either a pedigree or a narrative format; see Chapter 3 ∞ for information on how to create a pedigree. Specific diseases to ask about are listed in Table 5–3.

Review of Systems Collect a comprehensive overview of the child's health using the guidelines in Table 5–4. Additional signs and symptoms associated with the child's condition may be identified, as well as other problems that may have no direct re-

lationship to the child's significant health problem. Such problems could potentially impact nursing care or home care. For example, asking about allergies could reveal that the child has a latex allergy. The nurse would then need to ensure that the child is not exposed to latex and be prepared for allergic reactions. For each problem, obtain the treatment, outcomes, residual problems, and age at time of onset.

TABLE 5–3	**Familial or Hereditary Diseases**
Infectious diseases	Tuberculosis, HIV, hepatitis, varicella, herpes
Heart disease	Heart defects, myocardial infarctions, hypertension, dyslipidemia, sudden childhood deaths
Allergic disorders	Eczema, hay fever
Eye disorders	Glaucoma, cataracts, vision loss
Ear disorders	Hearing loss
Hematologic disorders	Sickle cell disease, thalassemia, G6PD deficiency, leukemia, hemophilia
Lung disorders	Cystic fibrosis, asthma
Cancer	Type, early age of onset
Endocrine disorders	Diabetes mellitus type 1 and 2, hypothyroidism, hyperthyroidism, Turner syndrome
Mental disorders	Mental retardation, epilepsy, psychiatric disorders
Musculoskeletal disorders	Arthritis, muscular dystrophy, scoliosis, spina bifida
Gastrointestinal disorders	Ulcers, colitis, celiac disease, kidney disease
Metabolic disorders	Phenylketonuria, galactosemia, maple syrup urine disease, Tay-Sachs disease
Problem pregnancies	Repeated miscarriages, stillbirths
Learning problems	Attention deficit disorder, Down syndrome

TABLE 5-4	Review of Systems
Body Systems	Examples of Problems to Identify
General	General growth pattern, overall health status, ability to keep up with other children or tires easily with feeding or activity, fever, sleep patterns
	Allergies, type of reaction (hives, rash, respiratory difficulty, swelling, nausea), seasonal or with each exposure
Skin and lymph	Rashes, dry skin, itching, changes in skin color or texture, tendency for bruising, swollen or tender lymph glands
Hair and nails	Hair loss, changes in color or texture, use of dye or chemicals on hair
	Abnormalities of nail growth or color
Head	Headaches
Eyes	Vision problems, squinting, crossed eyes, lazy eye, wears glasses, eye infections, redness, tearing, burning, rubbing, swelling eyelids
Ears	Ear infections, frequent discharge from ears, or tubes in ears
	Hearing loss (no response to loud noises or questions, inattentiveness, was hearing test ever done?), hearing aids or cochlear implant
Nose and sinuses	Nosebleeds, nasal congestion, colds with runny nose, sinus pain or infections
	Nasal obstruction, difficulty breathing, snoring at night
Mouth and throat	Mouth breathing, difficulty swallowing, drooling, sore throats, strep infections, mouth odor
	Tooth eruption, cavities, braces
	Voice change, hoarseness, speech problems
Cardiac and hematologic	Heart murmur, anemia, hypertension, cyanosis, edema, rheumatic fever, chest pain
Chest and respiratory	Trouble breathing, choking episodes, cough, wheezing, cyanosis, bronchiolitis, bronchitis, exposure to tuberculosis, other infections
Gastrointestinal	Bowel movements, regularity or frequency, color, consistency, discomfort, constipation or diarrhea, abdominal pain, bleeding from rectum, flatulence, encopresis
	Nausea, vomiting, usual appetite
Urinary	Frequency, urgency, dysuria, dribbling, strength of urinary stream
	Toilet trained—age when day and night dryness was attained, enuresis
Reproductive	For pubescent children
Female	Menses onset, amount, duration, frequency, discomfort, problems; vaginal discharge, breast development
Male	Puberty onset, emissions, erections, pain or discharge from penis, swelling or pain in testicles
Both	Sexual activity, use of contraception, sexually transmitted infections
Musculoskeletal	Weakness, clumsiness, poor coordination, balance, tremors, abnormal gait, painful muscles or joints, swelling or redness of joints, fractures, scoliosis
Neurologic	Brain or head injuries, delayed speech and vocabulary development, problems with articulation
	Seizures, fainting spells, dizziness, numbness
	Learning problems, attention span, hyperactivity, memory problems

Psychosocial Information Obtain information about family composition to establish a socioeconomic and sociologic context for planning the child's care in the hospital and at home.

- **Family composition**—family members living in the home, their relationship to the child, marital status of parents or other family structure, and people helping to care for the child.
- **Financial resources**—household members employed, family income, health insurance, State Child Health Insurance Program (SCHIP), food stamps, or Temporary Assistance for Needy Families (TANF).

- **Home environment**—housing description (condition, safe play area); city or well water; sanitation; and availability of electricity, heat, and refrigeration.
- **Community environment**—neighborhood description, safety, playgrounds, transportation, access to shopping; school or childcare arrangements.
- **Family or lifestyle changes**—for example, unemployment, relocations, divorce; how the child and family members have coped.

Newborns The psychosocial history for parents of newborns should focus on readiness to care for the infant at home. Inquire about support for the parent in the initial postpartum period, safe transport, and a home environment that provides heat, refrigeration, and safe water supplies.

Children Information about the child's daily routines, psychosocial information, and other living patterns should focus on issues that may have an impact on the quality of daily living (Box 5–1).

Adolescents The psychosocial history for adolescents should focus on critical areas in their lives that may contribute to a less than optimal environment for normal growth and development. See the companion website for questions that should be asked about key topics that are included in the HEEADSSS screening tool (Goldenring & Rosen, 2004):

- Home environment
- Education/employment, Eating
- Activities
- Drugs (substance abuse)
- Sexuality, Suicidal thoughts, Safety from injury and violence

Developmental Status Information about the child's motor, cognitive, language, and social development will help when planning nursing care. Ask the parent about the child's milestones and current fine and gross motor skills. Obtain the age at which the child first used words appropriately and the current words used or language ability. For children in school, ask about academic performance to assess cognitive development. Ask the parent about the child's manner of interaction with other children, family members, and strangers. Guidelines for a nursing assessment of development can be found in Chapter 4 ∞.

■ DEVELOPMENTAL APPROACH TO THE EXAMINATION

The sequence and approach to the examination varies by age, but the techniques are the same for all ages (Box 5–2). Provide a comfortable atmosphere for the examination with privacy so that modesty is respected. Explain the procedures as you begin to perform them. In young children, a foot-to-head sequence is often used so that the least distressing parts of the examination are completed first. In older cooperative children, the head-to-toe approach is generally used.

Newborns and Infants Under 6 Months of Age

Infants are among the easiest children to examine, as they do not resist the examination procedure. Keep the parent present to provide security to the infant. Provide physical comfort during the examination by feeding, using a pacifier, cuddling, or changing the diaper to keep the infant calm and quiet. Distraction such as rocking or clicking noises may help when the infant begins to get distressed. Observe the infant for general level of activity, overall mood, and responsiveness to handling.

Keep the sequence of the examination flexible to take advantage of times the infant is quiet or asleep to listen to the lungs, heart, and abdominal sounds. If the infant continues to be quiet or can be quieted with a pacifier, palpate the abdomen while the muscles are relaxed. The remainder of the examination can proceed in a head-to-toe sequence. Portions of the examination that are likely to disturb the infant, such as the hip assessment, should be performed at the end.

Infants Over 6 Months of Age

Because of developing separation and stranger anxiety, it is often best to keep the older infant with the parent. The infant and

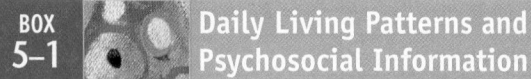

BOX 5–1 Daily Living Patterns and Psychosocial Information

Role Relationships
Family relationships/alterations in family process
Social and peer interactions: e.g., childcare, preschool, organized sports, school activities

Self-Perception/Self-Concept
Personal identity and role identity
Self-esteem, body image, presence of nonvisible disorder such as brain injury

Coping/Stress Tolerance
Temperament
Coping behaviors
Discipline
Any substance abuse

Values and Beliefs
Part of a spiritual group or faith community
Any foods, beverages, or medical interventions prohibited according to spiritual beliefs; special food preparation
Personal values/beliefs

Home Care Provided for Child's Condition
Resources needed/available; respite care available
Knowledge and skills of parents, other family members

Sensory/Perceptual Problems
Any sensory loss (vision, hearing, cognitive, or motor) and adaptations made

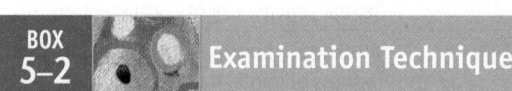

BOX 5–2 Examination Techniques

Following are the specific examination techniques:

- **Inspection.** Purposeful observation of the child's physical features and behaviors. Physical feature characteristics include size, shape, color, movement, position, and location. Detection of odors is also a part of inspection.
- **Palpation.** Using touch to identify characteristics of the skin, internal organs, and masses. Characteristics include texture, moistness, tenderness, temperature, position, shape, consistency, and mobility of masses and organs. The palmar surface of the fingers and fingerpads helps determine position, size, consistency, and masses. The ulnar surface of the hand is best to detect vibrations.
- **Auscultation.** Listening to sounds produced by the airway, lungs, stomach, heart, and blood vessels to identify their characteristics. Auscultation is usually performed with a stethoscope to enhance the sounds heard.
- **Percussion.** Striking the surface of the body, either directly or indirectly, to set up vibrations that reveal the density of underlying tissues and borders of internal organs.

toddler can be examined on the parent's lap and then held against the parent's chest for some steps, such as the ear examination. The infant will not object to having clothing removed, but make sure the room is warm for the infant's comfort. Observe the infant's general level of activity, mood, and responsiveness to handling by the parent.

Smile and talk soothingly to the infant during the procedure. Use toys to distract the older infant. Use a pacifier or bottle to quiet the child when necessary. Because the infant may be fearful of being touched by a stranger, begin with the feet and hands before moving to the trunk. However, take advantage of opportunities presented when the infant is sleeping or quiet to listen to the heart, lungs, and abdomen.

Toddlers

Toddlers may be active, curious, shy, cautious, or slow to warm up. Because of stranger anxiety, keep toddlers with their parents, often examining them on the parent's lap. It is possible to create a flat surface for the abdominal and genital examination by sitting knee to knee with the parent. For invasive procedures (ear, eye, and mouth exam) the parent can hold the child closely to the chest with legs between the parent's legs. The cranial nerve assessment or developmental assessment can be used as a method to gain cooperation for other procedures. Much of the neurologic and musculoskeletal assessment can be conducted by observing the child play and walk around in the examining room.

Tell the child what you will do at each step of the examination, using a confident voice that expects cooperation rather than asking. When a choice is possible, let the child have some control. For example, let the toddler choose which ear to examine first or to stand or sit for a certain part of the examination. Let the child hold a security object if it helps. Attempt to reduce the child's anxiety by demonstrating the use of instruments on the parent or security object. Begin the examination by touching the feet and then moving gradually toward the body and head. Instruments to examine the ears, eyes, and mouth are usually viewed as the most fearful and should be used at the end of the examination.

Preschoolers

Assess the willingness of the child to be separated from the parent. Younger children often prefer to be examined on the parent's lap, whereas older children are comfortable on the examining table. Most children are willing to undress, but leave the underpants on until conducting the genital examination. Most children in this age group are cooperative during the physical examination. Some children prefer to have the head, eyes, ears, and mouth examined first; others prefer to postpone them to the end.

Allow the child to touch and play with the equipment. Give simple explanations about the assessment procedures, and offer choice where there is one during the examination. Use distraction to gain the child's cooperation during the examination, such as asking the child to count, name colors, or talk about a favorite activity. Give positive feedback when the child cooperates.

School-Age Children

School-age children willingly cooperate during the examination and sit on the examining table. Anticipate the development of modesty in school-age children and offer a patient gown to cover the underwear. Let the older school-age child determine if the examination will be conducted in privacy or with the parent or siblings present.

A head-to-toe sequence can be used in this age group. Demonstrate how the instruments are used and let the child handle them if desired. As you perform the examination, tell the child what you are doing and why. Offer as many choices as possible to help the child feel empowered. The examination is a good opportunity to teach the child about how the body works, such as by letting the child listen to heart and breath sounds.

Adolescents

Protect the adolescent's modesty before and during the examination. Provide a private place to undress and put on the patient gown, and keep body parts covered when not being assessed. Examine the adolescent in a head-to-toe sequence as done for adults. Perform the examination in private without parent or siblings unless the adolescent specifically requests the parent's presence. Provide a chaperone when the parent or accompanying adult is not present during the examination.

Adolescents often have lots of concerns regarding their developing bodies. When appropriate, provide reassurance about the normal progression of secondary sexual characteristic development and what further changes to expect.

■ GENERAL APPRAISAL

The examination begins upon first meeting the child. Observe the child's general appearance and behavior. The child should appear well nourished and well developed. Infants and young children are often fearful and seek reassurance from their parents. The child may resist interacting with the nurse until rapport is established.

Observe the behavior and tone of voice used by the parent when he or she is talking to the child. Is the child encouraged to speak? Is the child appropriately reassured or supported by the parent? The child should feel secure with the parent and perceive permission to interact with the nurse.

Take the child's temperature, heart rate, respiratory rate, and blood pressure. (See the *Clinical Skills Manual.*)

Anthropometric Measurements

Equipment Needed

Tape measure

Measure the child's weight, length or height, and head circumference, if appropriate. Accurate assessment of growth throughout childhood is important for several reasons: to ensure health, to identify the impact of a disease on the child, and for medication dosage calculation. Plot height, weight, and head circumference measurements on appropriate growth charts for the child's age and sex to assess trends in growth. See Appendix A ∞.

Infants and Toddlers

Length   Measure the length of all children under age 2 years in supine position, even when they are able to stand independently. Growth charts for children under age 2 years are based on length rather than height, so a length measurement is important for accurate assessment of growth.

Use a measuring board and place the infant's head against the top of the board. Ask the parent or an assistant to hold the infant's head in the midline while you gently push down on the knees until the legs are straight. Position the heels of the feet against the footboard and record the length to the nearest 0.5 cm or 1/4 inch (Figure 5–3 ➤). Repeat the measurement for accuracy and average the readings if a difference is found between the two readings.

Weight   Infants are weighed with all clothing removed on a platform scale (Figure 5–4 ➤), either in a supine or sitting posi-

tion, depending on their age. Keep a diaper close at hand in case the baby voids while unclothed. Check the balance of the scale before placing the infant on it, and put a paper cover on the scale. Distract the infant, and take the reading when the infant stops moving. Place a hand close to the chest without touching the infant to prevent the infant from falling. Record the weight in the nearest 10 g or 1/2 oz.

Head Circumference   Head circumference is measured at regular intervals until age 2 to 3 years because the brain grows rapidly and achieves 80% of adult size by age 2 years. Use a disposable paper tape, but take care to prevent the paper from cutting the infant. Wrap the tape around the head at the supraorbital prominence, above the ears, and around the occipital prominence, the point of largest circumference of the head (Figure 5–5 ➤). Record the circumference in the nearest 0.5 cm or 1/8 inch. Repeat the measurement to confirm the reading. A larger-than-normal head is associated with hydrocephalus, and a smaller-than-normal head suggests microcephaly.

Preschoolers and School-Age Children

Height   After the age of 2 to 3 years, a **stadiometer**, a height measuring device attached to the wall, is used to improve the accuracy of the height measurement (Figure 5–6 ➤). With the child's shoes removed, have the child stand straight with the back to the wall. The head should be held erect and in the midline position. The head, shoulders, buttocks, and heels should touch the wall. Move the headpiece down to touch the crown. Measure the height reading to the nearest 0.5 cm or 1/4 inch.

Weight   Measure the child's weight on a standing scale. Check the balance of the scale before use. Weigh young children in their underclothes. Weigh older children in their street clothes with coats, other heavy clothing, and shoes removed. Record the weight to the nearest 0.1 kg or 1/4 lb.

Body Mass Index   The body mass index (BMI) is a formula (weight in kilograms/meters^2 of height) used to assess total body

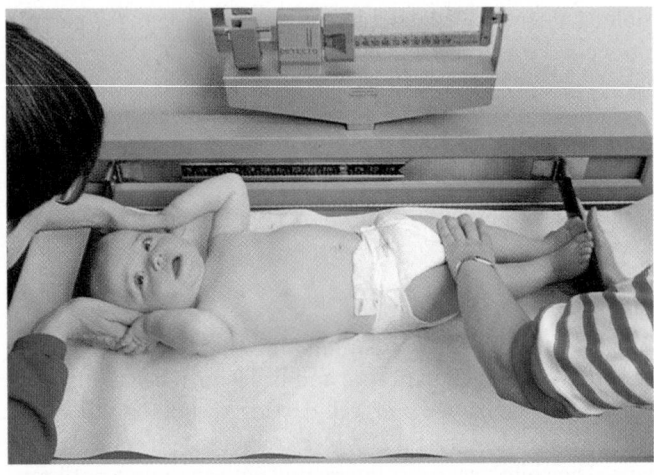

FIGURE 5–3 ➤ Measuring infant length.

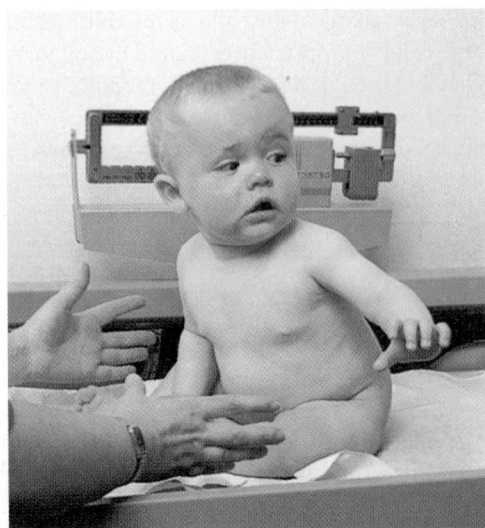

FIGURE 5–4 ➤ Measuring infant weight.

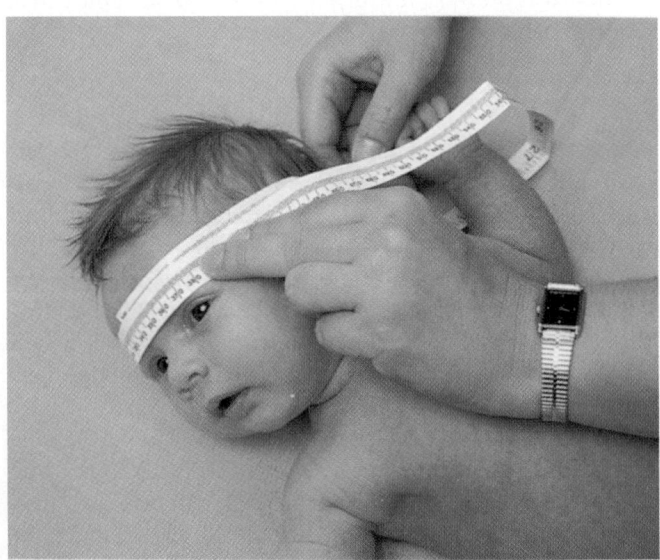

FIGURE 5–5 ➤ Measuring head circumference.

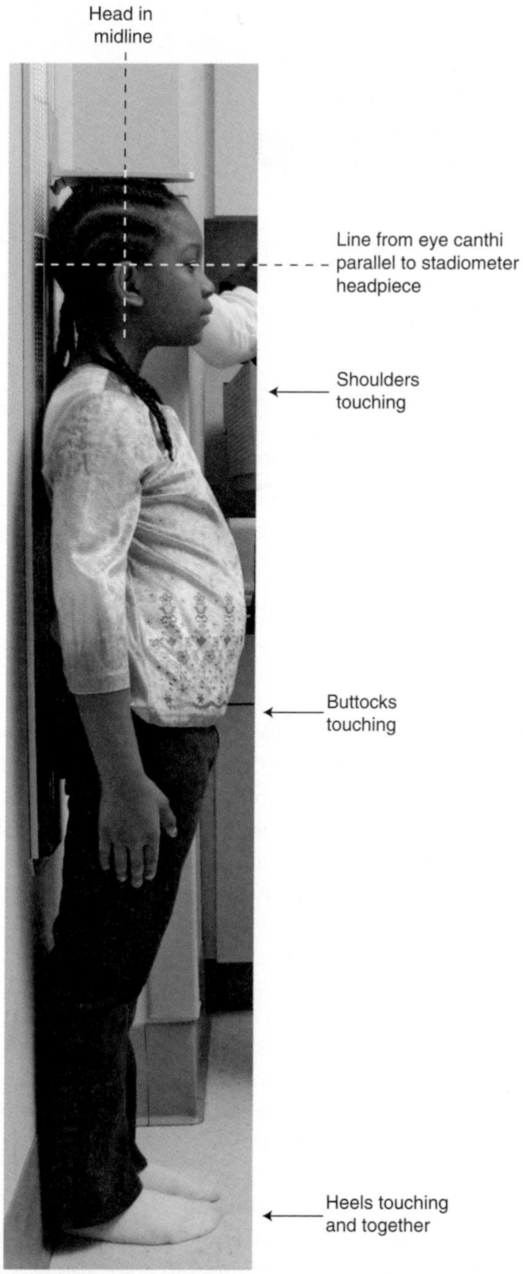

Head in
midline

Line from eye canthi
parallel to stadiometer
headpiece

Shoulders
touching

Buttocks
touching

Heels touching
and together

FIGURE 5–6 ➤ Measuring child height with a stadiometer.

fat and nutritional status. Once the weight and height of children have been measured, the body mass index can be calculated and plotted on the growth curve. See Chapter 14 ∞ for the formula to calculate the BMI, or visit the Centers for Disease Control and Prevention (CDC) website and enter the child's height and weight for an automatic calculation of the BMI.

Clinical Tip

See the companion website for links to special growth curves for children with Down syndrome, children with Turner syndrome, and children adopted from other countries.

■ ASSESSING SKIN AND HAIR CHARACTERISTICS

Examination of the skin requires good lighting to detect variations in skin color and to identify lesions. Daylight is preferred when available. Rather than inspecting the child's entire skin surface at one time, examine the skin simultaneously with other body systems as each region of the body is exposed.

Equipment Needed

Gloves

The Skin

Inspection

Use gloves to inspect the child's skin for color and the presence of imperfections, elevations, or other lesions.

Skin Color   The color of the child's skin usually has an even distribution. Check for color variations—such as increased or decreased pigmentation, pallor, mottling, bruises, erythema, cyanosis, or jaundice—that may be associated with local or generalized conditions. Some variations in skin color are common and normal, such as freckles found in the White population and Mongolian spots found on dark-skinned infants (Figure 5–7 ➤). The skin of healthy infants and toddlers may have a yellow tone due to an excess ingestion of yellow vegetables.

Bruises are common on the knees, shins, and lower arms as children stumble and fall. Bruises are uncommon in infants under 9 months of age before walking (Kaczor, Pierce, Makoroff, et al., 2006). Bruises on other parts of the body, especially in various stages of healing, should raise a suspicion of child abuse.

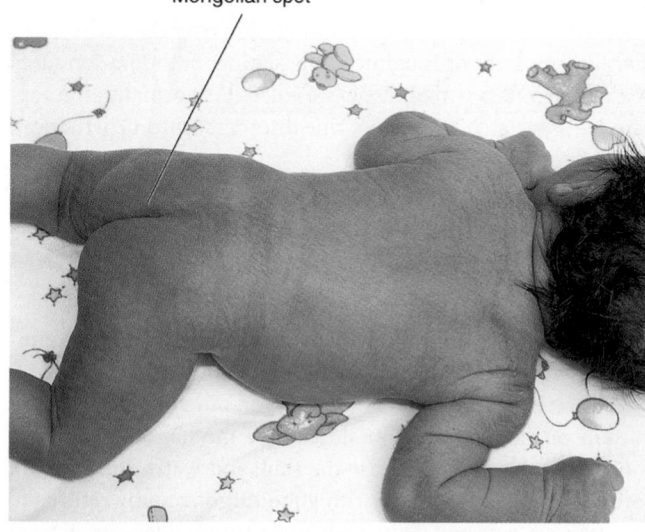

Mongolian spot

FIGURE 5–7 ➤ Mongolian spots are large patches of bluish-colored skin with wavy borders and irregular shapes often seen in the sacral area of the back. They are a normal occurrence in a large majority of Native American, Asian, Black, and Hispanic infants, but are sometimes incorrectly thought to be bruises. Mongolian spots usually fade during the first few years of life and disappear by puberty. Mongolian spots covering extensive areas of the posterior and anterior trunk and extremities may be a sign of an inborn error of metabolism (Ashrafi, Shabanian, Mohammadi, et al., 2006).

The palms of the hands and soles of the feet are often lighter than the rest of the skin surface in children with dark skin. In addition, their lips may normally appear slightly bluish.

See Chapter 17 ∞ for other potential indicators of child abuse. Bruises often go through various color changes as the body re-absorbs blood over several days. The transition of color often progresses through reddish blue, brownish blue, brownish green, greenish yellow, and yellow-brown before returning to normal skin color. Note any tattoos or body piercings.

Skin Tone When a skin color abnormality is suspected, inspect the buccal mucosa and tongue to confirm the color change. This is especially important in children with darker skin because the mucous membranes are usually pink, regardless of skin color. Press the gums lightly for 1 to 2 seconds. Any residual color, such as that seen in jaundice or cyanosis, is more easily detected in blanched skin. Jaundice may also be noticed in the sclerae of the eyes. Generalized cyanosis is associated with respiratory and car-diac disorders. Jaundice is associated with liver disorders.

Palpation

Lightly touch or stroke the skin's surface to evaluate the char-acteristics below. Follow standard precautions by wearing gloves when palpating mucous membranes, open wounds, and lesions.

Temperature The child's skin normally feels warm to the touch when placing the wrist or dorsum of the hand against the child's skin. Excessively warm skin may indicate the presence of fever or inflammation, whereas abnormally cool skin may be a sign of shock or cold exposure.

Texture Children have soft, smooth skin over the entire body. Identify any areas of roughness, thickening, or **induration** (area of extra firmness with a distinct border). Abnormalities in tex-ture are associated with endocrine disorders, chronic irritation, and inflammation.

Moistness The child's skin is normally dry to the touch. The skin may feel slightly damp when the child has been exercising or crying. Excessive sweating without exertion may be associ-ated with a fever or an uncorrected congenital heart defect.

Resilience (Turgor) The child's skin is taut, elastic, and mo-bile because of the balanced distribution of intracellular and ex-tracellular fluids. To evaluate skin turgor, pinch a small amount of skin on the abdomen or dorsum of the hand between the thumb and forefinger, release the skin, and watch the speed of recoil (Figure 5–8 ►). Skin with good turgor rapidly returns to its previous contour. Skin with poor turgor tents or it takes longer to resume its previous contour. Poor skin turgor is com-monly associated with dehydration.

If **edema**, an accumulation of excess fluid in the interstitial spaces, is present, the skin feels doughy or boggy. To test for the degree of edema present, the examiner presses for 5 seconds against a bone beneath the area of puffy skin, releases the pres-sure, and observes how rapidly the indentation disappears. If the

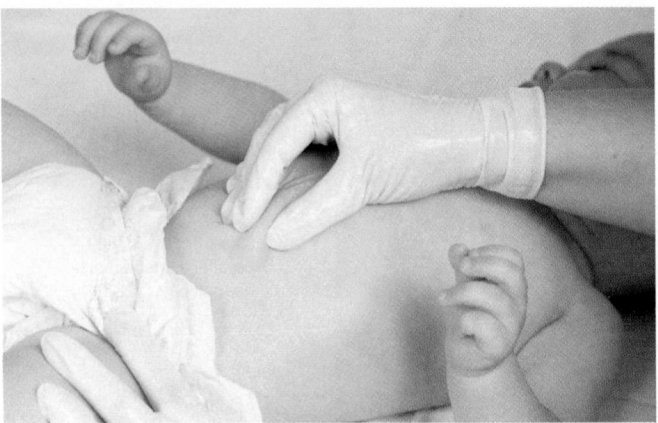

FIGURE 5–8 ► Tenting of the skin associated with poor skin turgor. Assess skin turgor on the abdomen, forearm, or thigh. Skin with normal turgor is elastic and will quickly return to a flat position.

indentation rapidly disappears, the edema is "nonpitting." Slow disappearance of the indentation indicates "pitting" edema, which is commonly associated with kidney or heart disorders.

Capillary Refill Time

See Figure 5–9A and B ► for the technique used to assess capil-lary refill time, a method for evaluating the adequacy of tissue perfusion (oxygen circulating to the tissues). The capillary refill time is normally less than 2 seconds. When the time is prolonged to 3 or 4 seconds, suggesting that tissue perfusion is inadequate, immediately assess the child for shock or a physical constriction such as a cast or bandage that is too tight.

Skin Lesions

Skin lesions usually indicate an abnormal skin condition. Char-acteristics such as location, size, type of lesion, pattern, and discharge, if present, provide clues about the cause of the condi-tion. Inspect and palpate the isolated or generalized skin color abnormalities, elevations, lesions, or injuries to describe all characteristics present.

Primary lesions (such as macules, papules, and vesicles) are often the skin's initial response to injury or infection. Mongolian spots and freckles are normal findings that are also classified as primary lesions. Figure 5–10 ► describes common primary le-sions. *Secondary lesions* (such as scars, ulcers, and fissures) are the result of irritation, infection, and delayed healing of primary lesions (see Chapter 31 ∞).

Common patterns of skin lesions are described as follows:

- *Annular* circular, begins in center and spreads to periphery (e.g., ringworm). When annular lesions run together, they are polycyclic.
- *Linear* in a row or stripe (e.g., poison ivy).
- *Herpetiform* grouped or clustered (e.g., herpes or chicken-pox).
- *Reticulated* networked or lace-like (e.g., parvovirus B19).

Inspection of the Hair

Inspect the scalp hair for color, distribution, and cleanliness. The hair shafts should be evenly colored, shiny, and either curly or

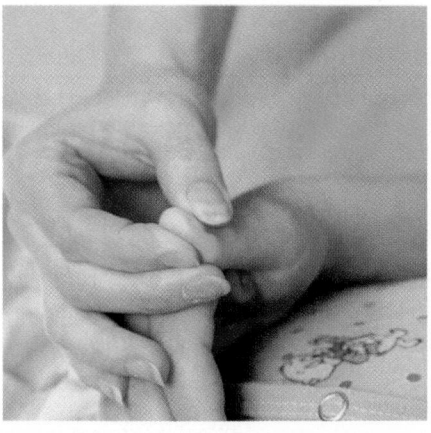 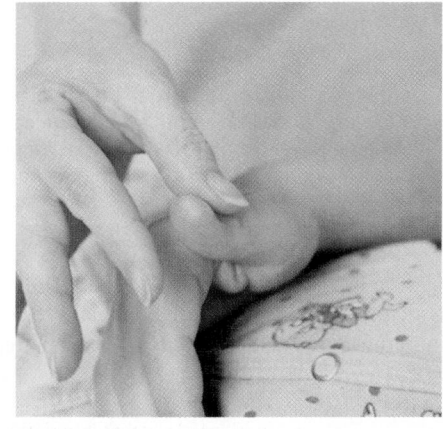

A **B**

FIGURE 5–9 ➤ Capillary refill technique: A, Pinch the end of a finger until the skin is blanched. B, Quickly release the finger and watch the blood return to the veins. Count the seconds it takes for the color to return or veins to fill. Slow color return or vein filling time could be related to shock or constriction due to a tight bandage or cast.

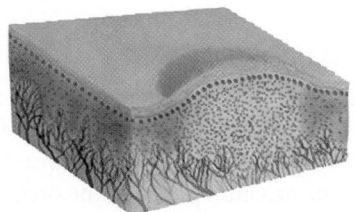

Lesion Name: Papule
Description: Elevated, firm, diameter less than 1 cm (1/2 in.)
Example: Warts, pigmented nevi

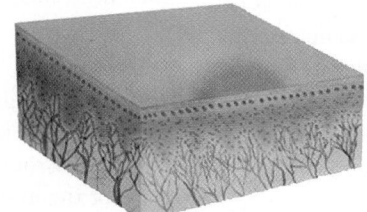

Lesion Name: Macule
Description: Flat, nonpalpable, diameter less than 1 cm (1/2 in.)
Example: Freckle, rubella, rubeola, petechiae

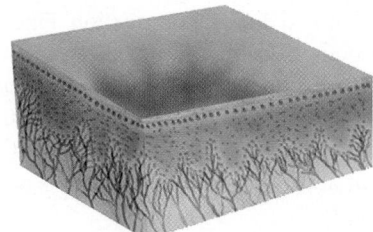

Lesion Name: Patch
Description: Macule diameter greater than 1 cm (1/2 in.)
Example: Vitiligo, Mongolian spot

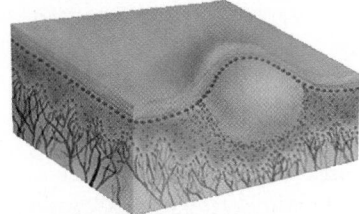

Lesion Name: Pustule
Description: Vesicle filled with purulent fluid
Example: Impetigo, acne

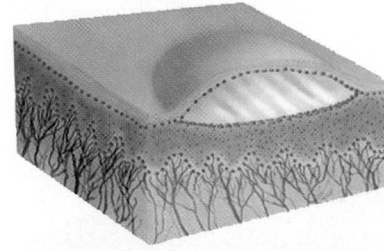

Lesion Name: Vesicle
Description: Elevated, filled with fluid, diameter less than 1 cm (1/2 in.)
Example: Early chickenpox, herpes simplex

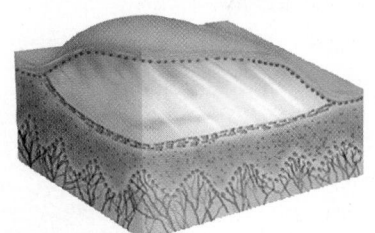

Lesion Name: Bulla
Description: Vesicle, diameter greater than 1 cm (1/2 in.)
Example: Burn blister

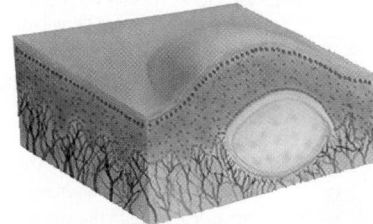

Lesion Name: Nodule
Description: Elevated, firm, deeper in dermis than papule, diameter 1–2 cm (1/2 in.–1 in.)
Example: Erythema nodosum

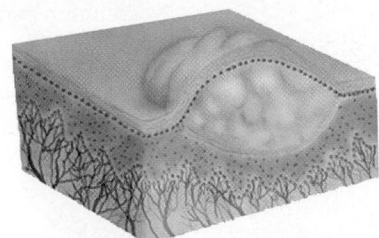

Lesion Name: Tumor
Description: Elevated, solid, diameter greater than 2 cm (1 in.)
Example: Neoplasm, hemangioma

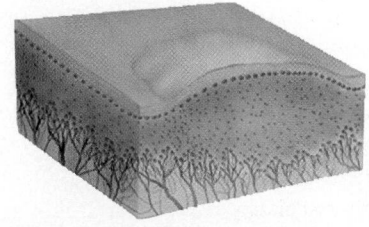

Lesion Name: Wheal
Description: Irregular elevated solid area of edematous skin
Example: Urticaria, insect bite

FIGURE 5–10 ➤ Common primary skin lesions and associated conditions.

Culture *Hair Characteristics*

Hair varies by genetic origin. Children of African origin often have hair that can appear curly, wavy, or coiled, and this hair more easily breaks. Children of Asian origin have hair that is coarse and straight. Children of Caucasian origin have hair with fine to medium coarseness that is straight or wavy.

Growth & Development *Pubic Hair Development*

Pubic hair begins to develop in children between 8 and 12 years of age, and axillary hair develops about 6 months later. Facial hair is noted in boys shortly after axillary hair develops.

---

straight. Variation in hair color not caused by coloring or bleaching can be associated with a nutritional deficiency. Normally, hair is distributed evenly over the scalp. Investigate areas of hair loss. Hair loss in a child may result from tight braids or skin lesions such as ringworm (see Chapter 31 ∞). Notice any unusual hair growth patterns. An unusually low hairline on the neck or forehead may be associated with a congenital disorder such as hypothyroidism.

Children are frequently exposed to head lice. Inspect the individual hair shafts for small nits (lice eggs) that adhere to the hair (see Chapter 31 ∞). None should be present.

Observe the distribution of body hair as other skin surfaces are exposed during examination. Fine hair covers most areas of the body. Body hair in unexpected places should be noted. For example, a tuft of hair at the base of the spine may indicate a pilonidal cyst. It is important to note the age at which pubic and axillary hair develops in the child. See Chapter 31 ∞. Development at an unusually young age is associated with precocious puberty.

Palpation of the Hair

Palpate the hair shafts for texture. Hair should feel soft or silky with fine or thick shafts. Endocrine conditions such as hypothyroidism may result in coarse, brittle hair. Part the hair in various spots over the head to inspect and palpate the scalp for crusting or other lesions. If scalp lesions are present, describe them using the characteristics in Figure 5–10 or Table 31–2 ∞.

■ ASSESSING THE HEAD FOR SKULL CHARACTERISTICS AND FACIAL FEATURES

What can cause a child's head or face to be asymmetric? How does a normal fontanel feel? What does an unusually large or small head suggest in an infant?

Inspection of the Head and Face

During early childhood the skull's sutures permit expansion for brain growth (Figure 5–11 ➤). Infants and young children normally have a rounded skull with a prominent occipital area. The shape of the head changes during childhood, and the occipital

As Children Grow
Skull Development

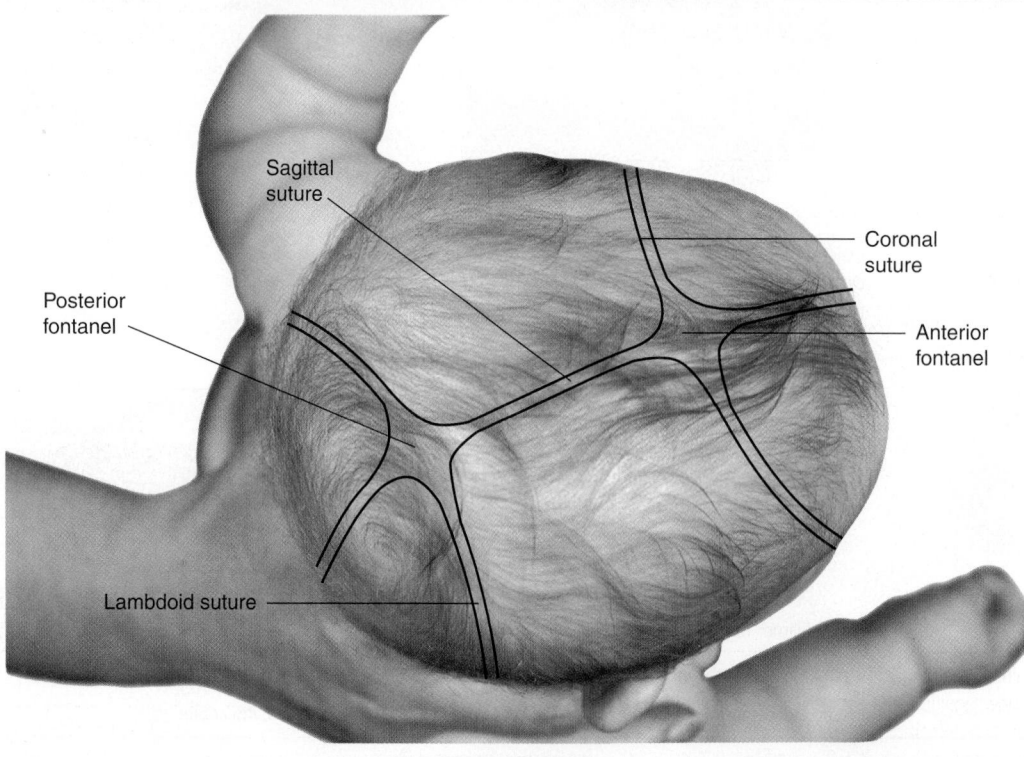

Sagittal suture

Coronal suture

Posterior fontanel

Anterior fontanel

Lambdoid suture

FIGURE 5–11 ➤ The **sutures** are fibrous connections between the bones of the skull that have not yet ossified. The fontanels are formed at the intersection of these sutures where bone has not yet formed. Fontanels are covered by tough membranous tissue that protects the brain. The posterior fontanel closes between 2 and 3 months. The anterior fontanel and sutures are palpable up to the age of 18 months. The suture lines of the skull are seldom palpated after 2 years of age. After that time, the sutures rarely separate.

area becomes less prominent. An abnormal skull shape can result from premature closure of the sutures.

Clinical Tip

Children who were low-birth-weight infants often have a flat, elongated skull because the soft skull bones were flattened by the weight of the head early in infancy. Head flattening is also associated with the recommended sleeping position for infants—on their back. See Chapter 27 ∞.

Inspect the child's face for symmetry during several facial expressions such as resting, smiling, talking, and crying (Figure 5–12 ➤). Significant asymmetry may result from paralysis of trigeminal or facial nerves (cranial nerves V or VII), in utero positioning, and swelling from infection, allergy, or trauma.

Next inspect the face for unusual facial features such as coarseness, wide eye spacing, or disproportionate size. Tremors, tics, and twitching of facial muscles are often associated with seizures.

Palpation of the Skull

Palpate the skull in infants and young children to assess the sutures and fontanels and to detect soft bones.

Sutures

Use your fingerpads to palpate each suture line. The edge of each bone in the suture line can be felt, but normally there is no separation of the two bones. If additional bone edges are felt, it may indicate a skull fracture.

Fontanels

At the intersection of the sutures, palpate the anterior and posterior fontanels. The fontanel should feel flat and firm inside the bony edges. The anterior fontanel is normally smaller than

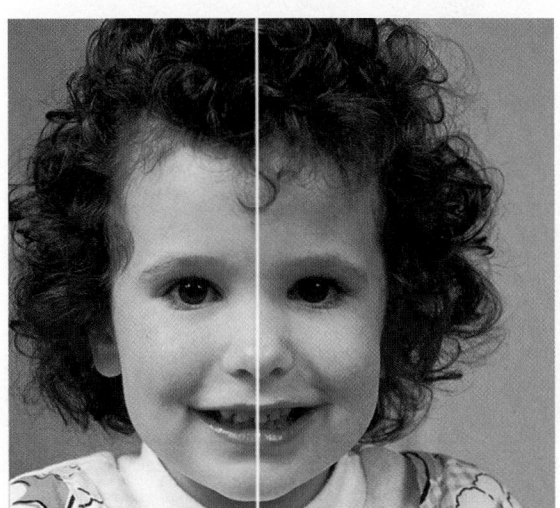

FIGURE 5–12 ➤ Draw an imaginary line down the middle of the face over the nose and compare the features on each side. Significant asymmetry may be caused by paralysis of cranial nerve V or VII, in utero positioning, and swelling from infection, allergy, or trauma.

Culture   *Touching the Head*

The head is a sacred part of the body to Southeast Asians. Ask for permission before touching the infant's head to palpate the sutures and fontanels (Purnell, 2009, p. 383).

5 cm (2 in.) in diameter at 6 months of age and then becomes progressively smaller. It closes between 12 and 18 months of age. The posterior fontanel closes between 2 and 3 months of age.

A tense fontanel, bulging above the margin of the skull, is an indication of increased intracranial pressure. A soft fontanel, sunken below the margin of the skull, is associated with dehydration.

▣ ASSESSING EYE STRUCTURES, FUNCTION, AND VISION

What is the red reflex and what does it indicate? How is eye muscle balance tested? Is it normal for a child's visual acuity to be different at certain ages?

Equipment Needed

Ophthalmoscope
Vision chart
Penlight
Small toy
Index card or paper cup

Inspection

External Eye Structures

The function of the external and internal eye structures and related cranial nerves makes vision possible. Inspect the external eye structures, including the eyeballs, eyelids, and eye muscles (Figure 5–13 ➤). Test the function of cranial nerves II, III, IV, and VI, which innervate the eye structures (see page 157).

Eye Size and Spacing Inspect the eyes and surrounding tissues simultaneously when examining facial features. The eyes should be the same size but not unusually large or small.

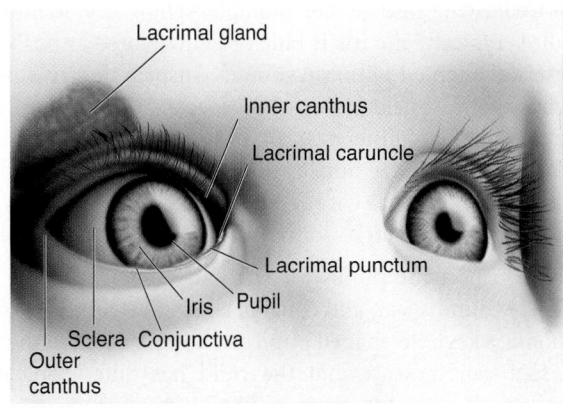

FIGURE 5–13 ➤ External structures of the eye. Notice that the light reflex is at the same location on each eye.

Observe for eye bulging, which can be identified by retracted eyelids, or for a sunken appearance. Bulging may be associated with a tumor, and a sunken appearance may reflect dehydration.

Next inspect the eyes to see if they appear appropriately spaced from each other. **Hypertelorism**, or widely spaced eyes, can be a normal variation in children.

Eyelids and Eyelashes Inspect the eyelids for color, size, position, mobility, and condition of the eyelashes. Eyelids should be the same color as surrounding facial skin and free of swelling or inflammation along the edges. Sebaceous glands that look like yellow striations are often present near the hair follicles.

Inspect the conjunctivae lining the eyelids by pulling down the lower lid and then everting the upper lid. The conjunctivae should be pink and glossy. The lacrimal punctum, the opening for the lacrimal gland on each lid, is located near the medial canthus. No redness or excess tearing should be present.

Clinical Tip

Children of Asian descent often have an extra fold of skin, known as the epicanthal fold, covering all or part of the medial canthus of the eye.

When the eyes are open, inspect the level at which the upper and lower lids cross the eye. Each lid normally covers part of the iris but not any portion of the pupil. The lids should also close completely over the iris and cornea. *Ptosis*, drooping of the eyelid that covers some of the pupil, is often associated with injury to the oculomotor nerve, cranial nerve III. *Sunset sign*, in which the sclera is seen between the upper lid and the iris, may indicate retracted eyelids or hydrocephalus.

Inspect the eyes for the palpebral slant (Figure 5–14 ➤). The eyelids of most people open horizontally. An upward slant is a normal finding in Asian children; however, children with Down syndrome also often have an upward slant (Figure 5–15 ➤). A downward slant is seen in some children as a normal variation.

Eye Color Inspect the color of each sclera, iris, and bulbar conjunctiva. The sclera is normally white or ivory in darker-skinned children. Sclerae of another color suggest the presence of an underlying disease. For example, yellow sclerae indicate jaundice. Typically the iris is blue or light colored at birth and becomes pigmented within 6 months. Inspect the iris for the presence of Brushfield spots, white specks in a linear pattern around the iris circumference, which are often associated with Down syndrome. The bulbar conjunctivae, which cover the sclera to the edge of the cornea, are normally clear. Redness can indicate eyestrain, allergies, or irritation.

Pupils Inspect the pupils for size and shape. Normally the pupils are round, clear, and equal in size. Some children have a **coloboma**, a keyhole-shaped pupil caused by a notch in the iris. This sign can indicate that the child has other congenital anomalies.

To test the pupillary response to light, shine a bright light into one eye. A brisk constriction of both the pupil exposed to direct

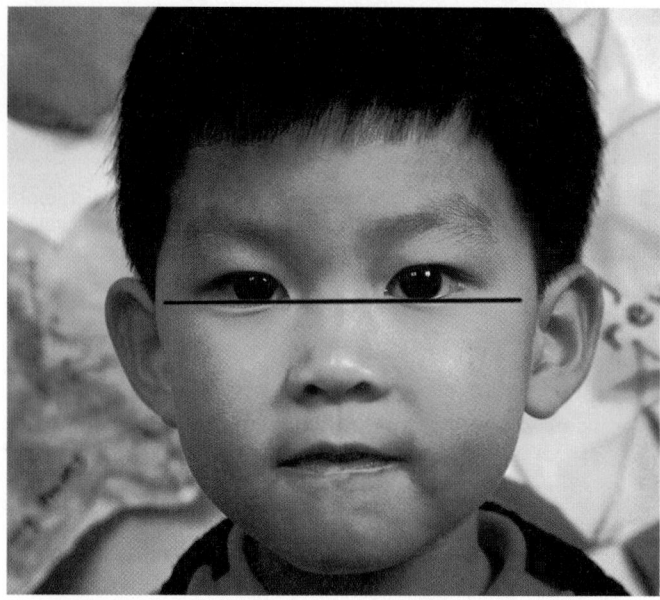

FIGURE 5–14 ➤ Draw an imaginary line across the medial canthi and extend it to each side of the face to identify the slant of the palpebral fissures. When the line crosses the lateral canthi, the palpebral fissures are horizontal and no slant is present. When the lateral canthi fall above the imaginary line, the eyes have an upward slant. A downward slant is present when the lateral canthi fall below the imaginary line. Epicanthal folds are present when an extra fold of skin partially or completely covers the caruncles in the medial canthi. Which type of slant does this child have?

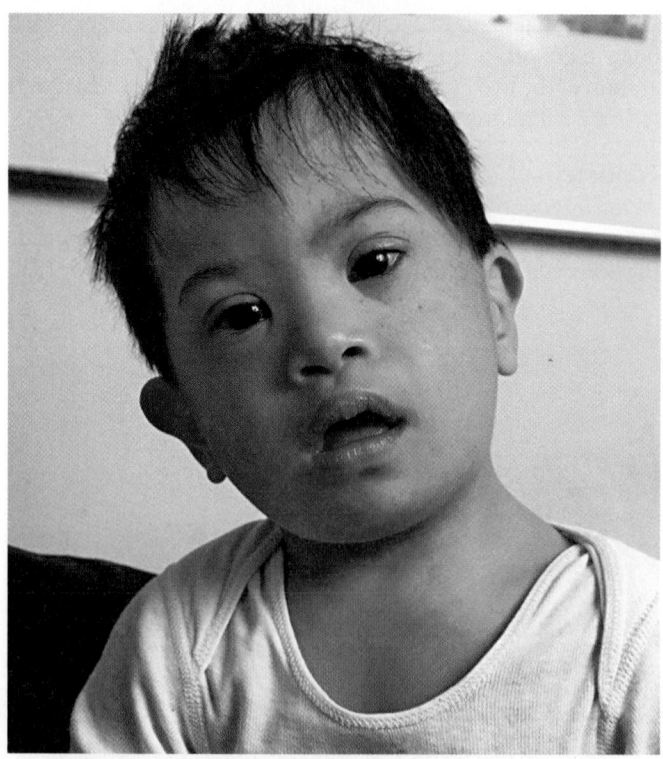

FIGURE 5–15 ➤ The eyes of this boy with Down syndrome show an upward slant.

light and the other pupil is a normal finding. To test pupillary response to accommodation, ask the child to look first at an object held near to the face and then at a distant picture on the wall. The expected response is pupil constriction with near objects and pupil dilation with distant objects. These procedures test the optic nerve, cranial nerve II.

Assessment of the Eye Muscles

It is important to detect strabismus, or crossed eyes, because, if uncorrected, visual impairment can result. The evaluation of extraocular movements, the corneal light reflex, and the cover–uncover test are used to detect a muscle imbalance.

Extraocular Movements   Seat the child at eye level to evaluate the extraocular movements. Hold a toy or penlight 30 cm (12 in.) from the child's eyes and move it through the six cardinal fields of gaze as shown in Figure 5–16 ➤. Test a young infant's ability to follow an object from side to side. The child's head may need to be held still until fine motor eye movement develops. Both eyes should move together, tracking the object. This procedure tests the oculomotor, trochlear, and abducens nerves (cranial nerves III, IV, and VI).

Corneal Light Reflex   To test the corneal light reflex, shine a light on the child's nose, midway between the eyes. Identify the location where the light is reflected on each eye. The light reflection is normally symmetric at the same spot on each cornea. An asymmetric corneal light reflex indicates strabismus (see Figure 5–13).

Cover–Uncover Test   The cover–uncover test can be used to test for eye muscle weakness in older, cooperative children, usually at about 4 or 5 years. See Figure 5–17 ➤ for the technique. Because the eyes work together, no obvious movement of either eye is expected. Unexpected movement of one eye indicates a muscle imbalance.

Internal Eye Structures

The funduscopic examination allows inspection of the internal eye structures—the retina, optic disc, arteries and veins, and

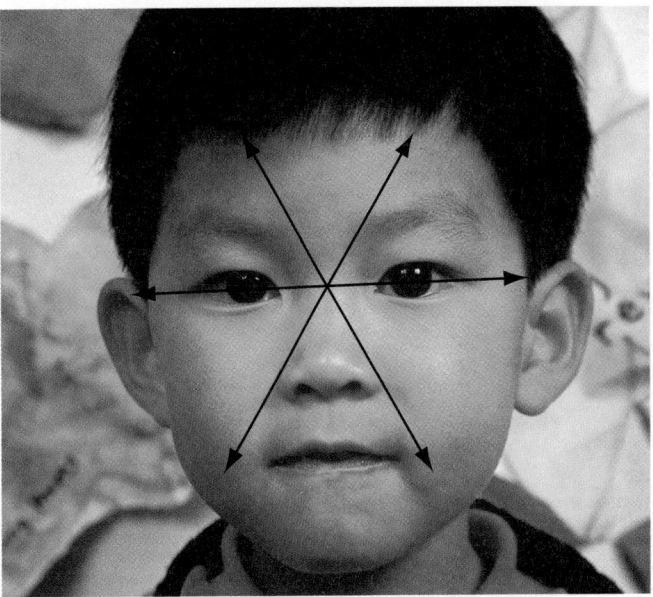

FIGURE 5–16 ➤ Begin the eye muscle examination with inspection of the extraocular movements. Have the child sit at your eye level. Hold a toy or penlight about 30 cm (12 in.) from the child's eyes and move it through the six cardinal fields of gaze. Both eyes should move together, tracking the object. This procedure tests cranial nerves III, IV, and VI.

macula (Figure 5–18 ➤). The ophthalmoscope is a complex instrument and requires practice to master. The examination is difficult to perform on uncooperative children; it is most often performed by experienced examiners.

Darken the room so the child's pupils dilate. Explain the procedure to the child to gain cooperation. Have a picture on the wall or have the parent hold a toy for the child to stare at so that the child's eye will not have to be forcibly held open.

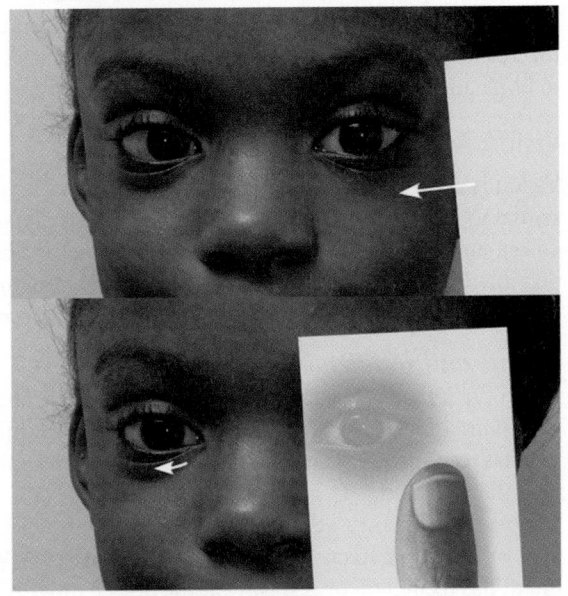

A Right, uncovered eye is weaker

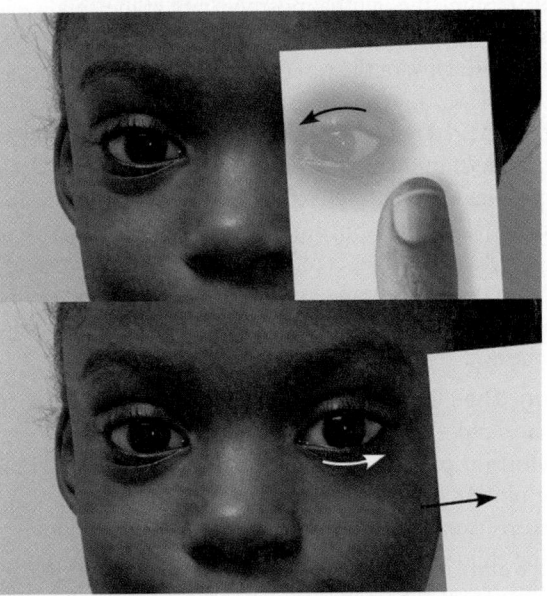

B Left, covered eye is weaker

FIGURE 5–17 ➤ Cover–uncover test. With the child at your eye level, ask the child to look at a picture on the wall. A, As you cover one eye with an index card or paper cup, simultaneously observe for any movement of the uncovered eye. If it jumps to fixate on the picture, the uncovered eye has a muscle weakness. B, As you remove the cover from the eye, simultaneously observe the covered eye for any movement to fixate on the picture. If the eye has a muscle weakness, it drifts to a relaxed position once covered.

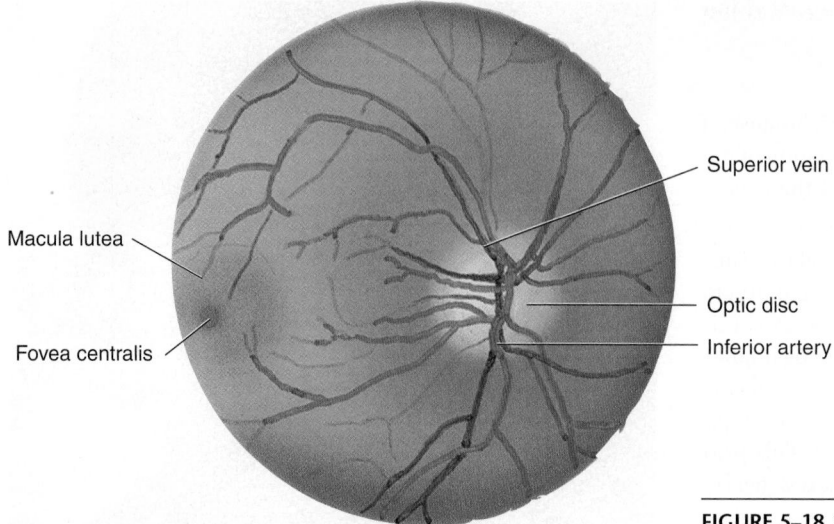

Macula lutea

Fovea centralis

Superior vein

Optic disc

Inferior artery

Retina

FIGURE 5–18 ➤ Normal fundus (retina). Only a small portion is seen at a time with the ophthalmoscope.

Using the Ophthalmoscope The ophthalmoscope has a lens-and-mirror system and a bright light for inspecting the structures of the internal eye. Different lens powers are arranged on the rotating disk of the ophthalmic head. This system permits compensation for vision differences between the child and examiner. The black-numbered plus lenses magnify images, and the red-numbered minus lenses reduce image size. The lens power can be changed by rotating the disk with the forefinger.

Turn the ophthalmoscope on and set the lens power at zero. Keep a forefinger on the disk to change the lens power as needed. Look through the lens of the ophthalmoscope, stabilizing it by resting the top against your eyebrow and the handle against your cheek. Place a hand on the child's head for stabilization.

Red Reflex Shine the ophthalmoscope light at the child's eye from a distance of 30 cm (12 in.). The first image seen is the red reflex, the reddish glow of the vascular retina, as the light travels through the cornea, aqueous humor, lens, and vitreous humor to the retina. The red reflexes should be an orange-red glow that is symmetric and uniform (Prentiss & Dorfman, 2008). Black spots or opacities within the red reflex are abnormal and may indicate congenital cataracts, hemorrhage, or corneal scars. If a white reflex is seen, the light is reflecting off a white abnormality, such as a retinoblastoma tumor (McLaughlin & Levin, 2006). The red reflex can also be tested by shining a small flashlight into the eye.

Visualizing the Internal Eye Structures Slowly move closer to the child. Deeper levels of the vitreous humor are inspected before the pink retina details come into view. The retina is a deeper pink in dark-skinned children. A blood vessel is the first structure usually seen on the retina. Continue moving closer to the child's eye and adjust the plus or minus lenses to focus on this blood vessel. Retinal arteries appear smaller and brighter red than veins. The blood vessels branch to spread and cover the retina.

Inspect and follow the branching of the blood vessels toward the nose until they merge into the optic disc. The optic disc

Clinical Tip

Keep the red reflex in view to make sure your head and the ophthalmoscope move as one unit. If you lose the red reflex when moving closer to the child, move back, find the red reflex, and start again.

margin is usually sharply defined, round, and yellow to creamy pink. Blurring of the disc margins or bulging of the optic disc is a sign of increased intracranial pressure. Use the diameter of the optic disc to identify the location of other landmarks on the retina.

The macula is located approximately 2 disc diameters lateral to the optic disc. To see the macula, ask the child to look at the light. It appears as a yellow dot surrounded by deep pink. The macula is inspected last because the bright light causes the child to blink and look away.

Vision Assessment

Vision is an important sense for learning, and assessment is essential to detect any serious problems. Vision is evaluated using an age-appropriate vision test, but no simple method exists. It is possible to assess vision in infants and children by observing their behavior in response to certain maneuvers and during play.

Infants and Toddlers

When the infant's eyes are open, test the blink reflex by moving your hand quickly toward the infant's eyes. A quick blink is the normal response. Absence of the blink reflex can indicate that the infant is blind.

To test an infant's ability to visually track an object, hold a light or toy about 15 cm (6 in.) from the infant's eyes. When the infant has fixated on or is staring at the object, move it slowly to each side. The infant should follow the object with the eyes and by moving the head.

Once an infant has developed skills to reach for and then pick up objects, observe play behavior to evaluate vision. The ability to easily find and pick up small toys is a good indicator of vision in children under 3 years of age.

Standardized Vision Charts

Standardized vision charts may be used to test vision when the child can understand directions and can cooperate, usually at about 3 or 4 years of age. The HOTV chart, Snellen E chart, and the Picture chart are used to test visual acuity of preschool-age children just as the Snellen Letter chart is used for school-age children and adolescents. For all standardized vision charts, make sure the child is the appropriate distance from the chart, usually 10 or 20 feet. Cover one eye with a paper cup or index card so each eye is evaluated separately before testing them together. The *Clinical Skills Manual* describes the use of these charts.

Clinical Tip

Indications for further evaluation include visual acuity of 20/40 or less in either eye by 3 to 5 years of age, visual acuity of 20/30 or less in either eye by 6 years of age, or a difference in vision of 2 lines or more on the Snellen eye chart between the eyes, even within the passing range (Doshi & Rodriguez, 2007).

■ ASSESSING THE EAR STRUCTURES AND HEARING

What is the significance of low-set ears? Why is otitis media the most common ear problem during early childhood? What play activities can be used to test hearing in young children?

Equipment Needed

Otoscope
Noisemakers (bell, rattle, tissue paper)
Tuning fork, 500–1000 Hz

Inspection

External Ear Structures

The position and characteristics of the pinna, the external ear, are inspected as a continuation of the head and eye examination. The pinna is considered "low set" when the top lies completely below an imaginary line drawn through the medial and lateral canthi of the eye toward the ear. Low-set ears are often associated with congenital renal disorders (Figure 5–19 ➤).

Inspect the pinna for any malformation. The pinna should be completely formed, with an open auditory canal. Next, inspect the tissue around the pinna for abnormalities. A pit or hole in front of the pinna may indicate the presence of a sinus. If one of the pinna protrudes outward, there may be swelling behind the ear, a sign of infection in the mastoid process of the skull's temporal bone.

Inspect the external auditory canal for any discharge. A foul-smelling, purulent discharge may indicate the presence of a foreign body or infection in the external canal. Clear fluid or a blood-tinged discharge may indicate a cerebrospinal fluid leak caused by a basilar skull fracture.

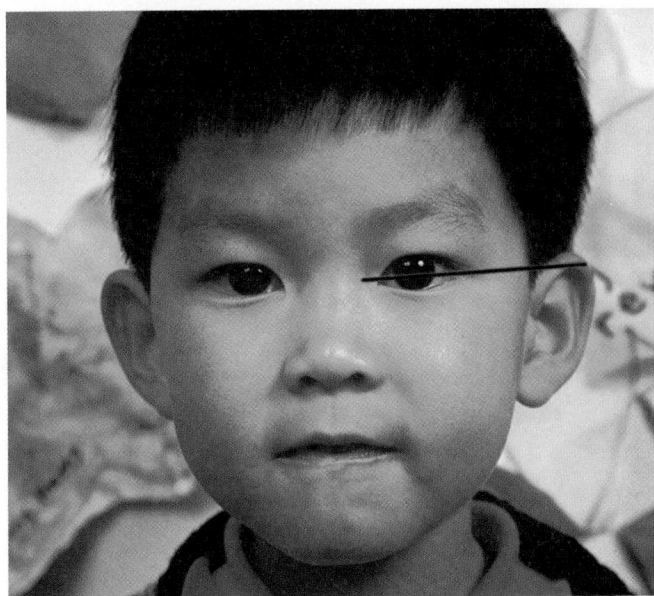

FIGURE 5–19 ➤ To detect the correct placement of the external ears, draw an imaginary line through the medial and lateral canthi of the eye toward the ear. This line normally passes through the upper portion of the pinna. The pinna is considered "low set" when the top lies completely below the imaginary line. Low-set ears are often associated with renal disorders. Is this a normal ear placement? (Yes, it is.)

Tympanic Membrane

Examination of the tympanic membrane is important in infants and young children because they are prone to acute otitis media, a middle ear infection. The eustachian tubes are shorter, wider, and more horizontally positioned in infants and young children than in older children and adults. This positioning enables bacteria to move from the pharynx, up the eustachian tube, and into the middle ear, causing an infection. See Figure 19–2 ∞.

Using the Otoscope

The otoscope, an instrument with a magnifying lens, bright light, and speculum, is used to examine the internal auditory canal and tympanic membrane. Infants and young children often resist having their ears inspected with the otoscope because of past painful experiences. This is one reason to delay the otoscopic examination until portions of the assessment requiring cooperation are completed. Use simple explanations to prepare the child. Let the child play with the otoscope or demonstrate how it is used on the parent or a doll. Figure 5–20 ➤ illustrates one method for restraining an uncooperative child.

Clinical Tip

Choose the largest ear speculum that fits into the auditory canal to form a seal for testing the movement of the tympanic membrane. A large speculum is also less likely to injure the auditory canal if the child moves suddenly.

To begin the otoscopic examination, hold the handle of the otoscope in the palm of your hand. If using a pneumatic squeeze

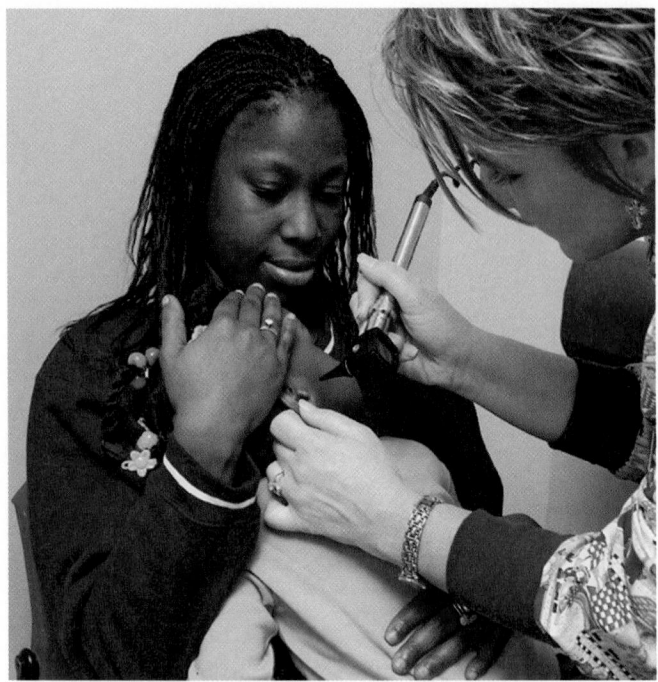

FIGURE 5–20 ➤ To restrain an uncooperative child, position the child on the parent's lap with the child's chest and head held firmly by the parent against the parent's chest. Keep your hands free to hold the otoscope and position the external ear.

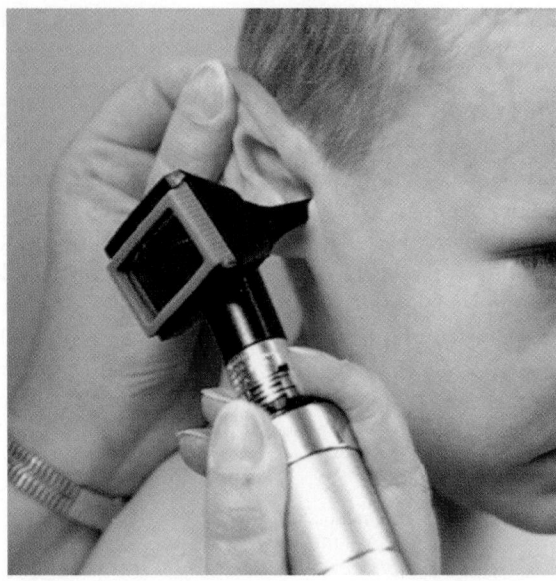

FIGURE 5–21 ➤ To straighten the auditory canal: Pull the pinna back and up for children over 3 years of age; pull the pinna down and back for children under 3 years of age.

by cerumen or a foreign body, warm water irrigation can be used to clean the canal.

Nursing Alert

Never irrigate the ear canal if any discharge is present, as the tympanic membrane may be ruptured. Water could enter the middle ear and potentially worsen the infection.

bulb, hold it between the index finger and the handle. Hold the otoscope in the hand closest to the child's face. When the child is cooperative, rest the back of that hand against the child's head to stabilize it. Use the other hand to pull the pinna toward the back of the head and either up or down. Pulling the pinna straightens the auditory canal and improves inspection of the tympanic membrane (Figure 5–21 ➤).

Slowly insert the speculum into the auditory canal, inspecting the walls for signs of irritation, discharge, or a foreign body. The walls of the auditory canal are normally pink, and some cerumen is present. Children often put beads, peas, or other small objects into their ears. If the auditory canal is obstructed

The tympanic membrane, which separates the outer ear from the middle ear, is usually pearly gray and translucent. It reflects light, and the bones (ossicles) in the middle ear are normally visible (Figure 5–22 ➤). When the pneumatic attachment is squeezed, the tympanic membrane normally moves in and out in response to the positive and negative pressure applied. Table 5–5

TABLE 5–5	Unexpected Findings on Examination of the Tympanic Membrane and Its Associated Condition	
Characteristics of Tympanic Membrane	Tympanic Membrane Unexpected Findings	Associated Conditions
Color	Redness	Infection in middle ear
	Slight redness	Prolonged crying
	Amber	Serous fluid in middle ear
	Deep red or blue	Blood in middle ear
Light reflex	Absent	Bulging tympanic membrane, infection in middle ear
	Distorted, loss of triangular shape	Retracted tympanic membrane, serous fluid in middle ear
Bony landmarks	Extra prominent	Retracted tympanic membrane, serous fluid in middle ear
Movement	No movement	Infection or fluid in middle ear
	Excess movement	Healed perforation

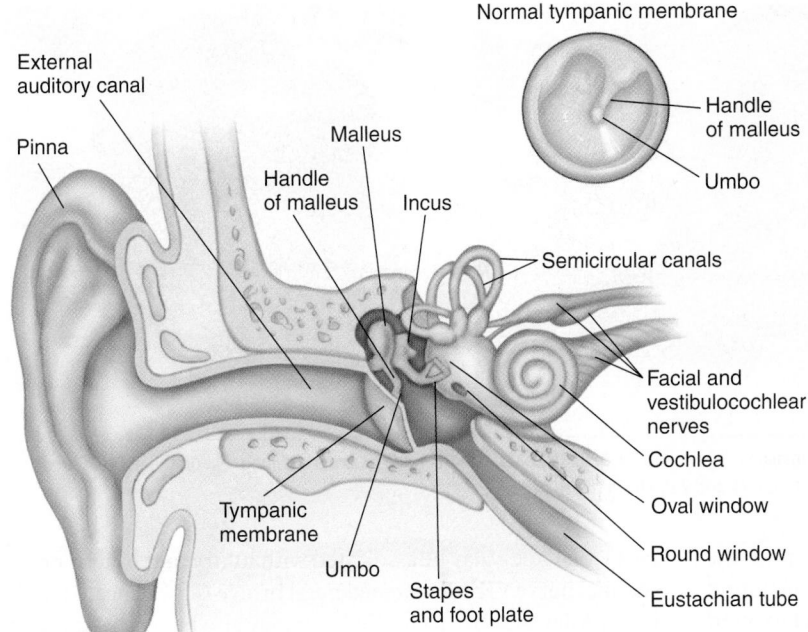

Normal tympanic membrane

External auditory canal

Pinna

Malleus

Handle of malleus

Incus

Handle of malleus

Umbo

Semicircular canals

Facial and vestibulocochlear nerves

Cochlea

Oval window

Round window

Eustachian tube

Tympanic membrane

Umbo

Stapes and foot plate

FIGURE 5–22 ➤ Cross-section of the ear. The tympanic membrane normally has a triangular light reflex with the base on the nasal side pointing toward the center. The bony landmarks, the umbo and handle of malleus, are seen through the tympanic membrane.

lists the abnormal findings of a tympanic membrane examination and their associated conditions.

Hearing Assessment

Hearing is essential for normal speech development and learning. Hearing loss may occur at any time during early childhood as the result of birth trauma, frequent acute otitis media, meningitis, or antibiotics that damage cranial nerve VIII. Hearing loss may also be associated with congenital anomalies and genetic syndromes. The hearing of newborns is evaluated at birth. Hearing is also evaluated throughout childhood.

Evaluate hearing by inspection of the child's responses to various auditory stimuli using age-appropriate methods. Use hearing and speech articulation milestones as an initial hearing screen. When a hearing deficiency is suspected after screening, refer the child for audiometry or tympanometry to obtain the most accurate evaluation of hearing. See the *Clinical Skills Manual.*

Infants and Toddlers

Select noisemakers with different frequencies, such as a rattle, bell, and tissue paper that will attract the young child's attention.

Growth & Development *Hearing Loss Indicators*

Indicators of hearing loss in an infant:

- No startle reaction to loud noises
- Does not turn toward sounds by 4 months of age
- Babbles as a young infant but stops babbling and does not develop speech sounds after 6 months of age

Indicators of hearing loss in a young child:

- No speech by 2 years of age
- Speech sounds are not distinct at appropriate ages

Ask the parent or an assistant to entertain the infant with a quiet toy, such as a teddy bear. Stand behind the infant, about 60 cm (2 feet) away from the infant's ear but outside the infant's field of vision, and make a soft sound with the noisemaker. Have the parent or assistant observe the child for any of the following responses when the noisemaker is used: widening the eyes, briefly stopping all activity to listen, or turning the head toward the sound. Repeat the test in the other ear and with the other noisemakers. See Chapter 19 ∞ for more details on hearing testing.

Preschool and Older Children

Use whispered words to evaluate the hearing of children over 3 years of age. Position your head about 30 cm (12 in.) away from the child's ear, but out of the range of vision so the child cannot read your lips. Use words easily recognized by the child, such as *Mickey Mouse, hot dog,* and *Popsicle,* and ask the child to repeat the words. Repeat the test with different words in the opposite ear. The child should correctly repeat the whispered words.

Clinical Tip

When the child will not cooperate with hearing evaluation by repeating whispered words, whisper directions for the child to point to different parts of the body. For example, "Show me your eyes" and "Point to your mouth." Children should point to the correct body part each time.

Bone and Air Conduction of Sound

Use a tuning fork to evaluate the hearing of school-age children who can follow directions. Hold the handle of the tuning fork and lightly tap or stroke the tines to begin the vibration. Avoid touching the vibrating tines, which will dampen the sound. Bone conduction is tested by placing the handle of the tuning fork on the child's skull. Air conduction is tested by holding the vibrating tines close to the child's ear (Figure 5–23 ➤).

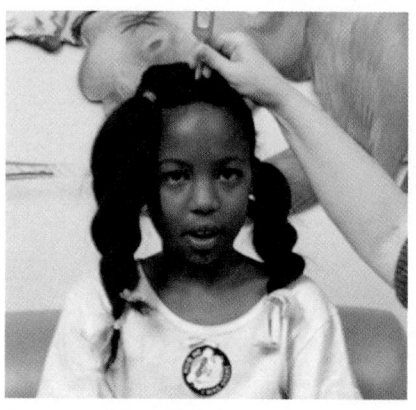
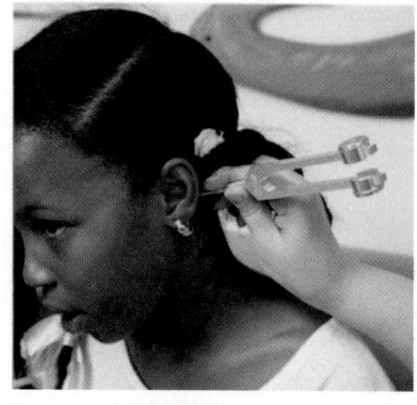
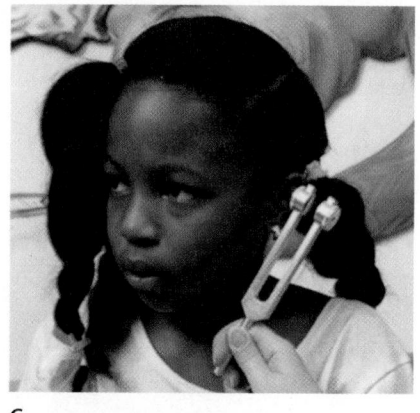

A   B   C

FIGURE 5–23 ➤ A, Weber test. Place a vibrating tuning fork on the midline of the child's head. B, Rinne test, step 1. Place a vibrating tuning fork on the mastoid process. C, Rinne test, step 2. Reposition the still-vibrating tines between 2.5 and 5 cm (1 and 2 in.) from the ear.

Weber Test Place the vibrating tuning fork on top of the child's skull in the midline. Ask the child to say where the sound is heard best, either in both ears equally or in one ear. The sound should be heard equally in both ears.

Rinne Test Place the vibrating tuning fork handle on the mastoid process behind an ear. Ask the child to say when the sound is no longer heard. Immediately move the tuning fork so that the vibrating tines are held about 2.5 to 5 cm (1 to 2 in.) from the same ear. Again, ask the child to indicate when the sound is no longer heard. The child normally hears the air-conducted sound twice as long as the bone-conducted sound. Repeat the Rinne test on the other ear.

When the sound is heard longer by bone conduction than air conduction, the affected ear may have conductive hearing loss. When sound is heard longer by air conduction than bone conduction, but less than twice as long, the affected ear may have sensorineural hearing loss.

■ ASSESSING THE NOSE AND SINUSES FOR AIRWAY PATENCY AND DISCHARGE

What is the most common cause of nasal obstruction in children? What does nasal flaring indicate? What signs indicate that a foreign body might be lodged in the nose?

Equipment Needed

Otoscope with nasal speculum
Penlight

External Nose

The external nose characteristics and placement on the face are examined simultaneously with the facial features.

Inspection

Inspect the external nose for size, shape, symmetry, and midline placement on the face. The nose should be proportional in size to other facial features and positioned in the middle of the face. The nasolabial folds are normally symmetric. Asymmetry of the nasolabial folds may be associated with injury to the facial nerve (cranial nerve VII). A flattened nasal bridge is the expected finding in Asian and Black children, but may also be seen in children with Down syndrome. A saddle-shaped nose occurs with hypertelorism or it may be a familial characteristic.

See below for the assessment of smell.

Palpation

When a deformity is noted, gently palpate the nose to detect any pain or break in contour. No tenderness or masses are expected. Pain and a contour deviation are usually the result of trauma.

Nasal Patency The child's airway must be patent to ensure adequate oxygenation. To test for nasal patency, occlude one nostril and observe the child's effort to breathe through the open nostril with the mouth closed. Repeat the procedure with the other nostril. Breathing should be noiseless and effortless. **Nasal flaring,** an effort the child makes to widen the airway, is a sign of increased respiratory effort or respiratory distress and should not be present.

If the child struggles to breathe, a nasal obstruction may be present. Nasal obstruction may be caused by a foreign body, congenital defect, dry mucus, discharge, polyp, or trauma. Newborns may have respiratory distress because of choanal atresia, a congenital membranous or bony obstruction between the nose and the nasopharynx. Young children commonly place objects up their nose, and unilateral nasal flaring is a sign of such an obstruction.

Assessment of Smell

The olfactory nerve (cranial nerve I) can be tested in school-age children and adolescents. When testing smell, choose scents the child will easily recognize such as orange, chocolate, and mint. When the child's eyes are closed, occlude one nostril and hold

| Growth & Development | | *Mouth Breathing* |

An infant under 6 months of age will not automatically open the mouth to breathe when the nose is occluded, such as by mucus.

the scent under the nose. Ask the child to take a deep sniff and identify the scent. Alternate odors between the nares. The child can normally identify common scents.

Internal Nose

Inspection

Inspect the internal nose for color of the mucous membranes and the presence of any discharge, swelling, lesions, or other abnormalities. Use a bright light, such as an otoscope light or penlight. For infants and young children, push the tip of the nose upward and shine the light at the end of the nose. The nasal speculum of the otoscope can be used in older children (Figure 5–24 ➤). Avoid touching the septum of the nose with the speculum. Injury to the septum can cause a nosebleed.

Mucous Membranes The mucous membranes should be dark pink and glistening. A film of clear discharge may also be present. Turbinates, if visible, should be the same color as the mucous membranes and have a firm consistency. When the turbinates are pale or bluish gray, the child may have allergies. A *polyp*, a rounded mass projecting from the turbinate, is also associated with allergies.

Nasal Septum Inspect the nasal septum, which should be straight without perforations, bleeding, or crusting. Crusting will be noted over the site of a nosebleed.

Discharge Observe for the presence of nasal discharge, noting if the drainage is from one or both nares. Nasal discharge is not a normal finding unless the child is crying. Discharge may be watery, mucoid, purulent, or bloody, depending on the condition present. A foul-smelling discharge in only one nostril is often associated with a foreign body. Table 5–6 lists conditions associated with nasal discharge.

Inspection of the Sinuses

The maxillary and ethmoid sinuses develop during early childhood (Figure 5–25 ➤). Sinus infections can occasionally occur in young children. Suspect a sinus problem when the child has a headache or pain and swelling around one or both eyes.

Inspect the face for any puffiness and swelling around one or both eyes; normally neither is present. To palpate over the maxillary sinuses, press up under both zygomatic arches with the thumbs. To palpate the ethmoid sinuses, press up against the bone above both eyes with the thumbs. No swelling or tenderness is expected. Tenderness may indicate sinusitis.

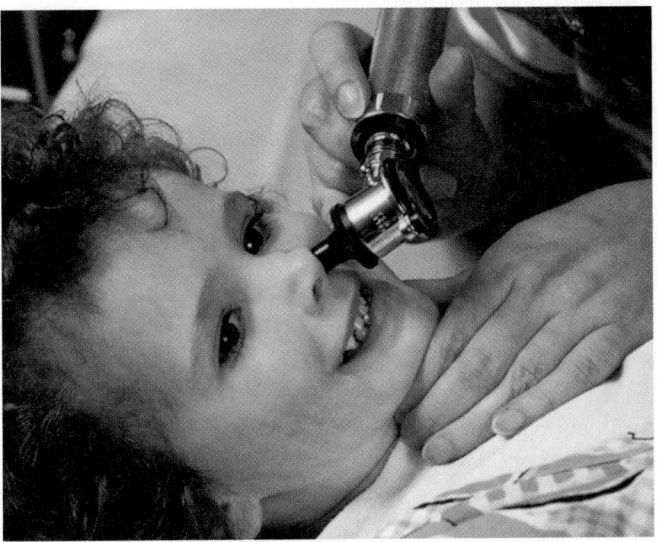

FIGURE 5–24 ➤ Technique for examining nose.

As Children Grow
Sinus Development

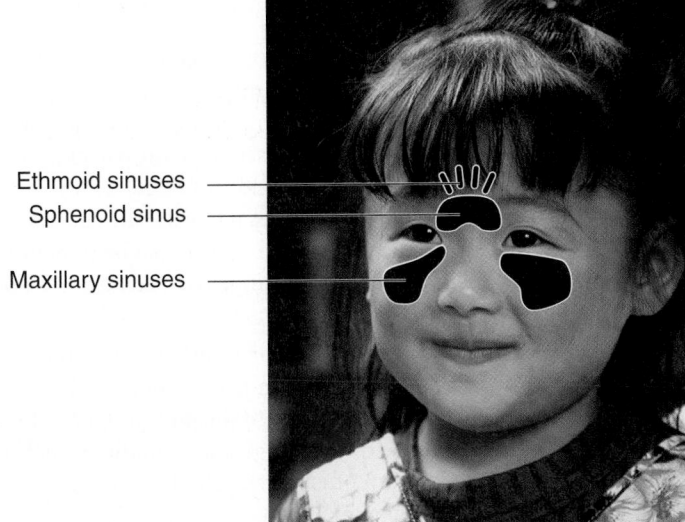

Ethmoid sinuses
Sphenoid sinus
Maxillary sinuses

FIGURE 5–25 ➤ Sinuses grow and develop during childhood. Maxillary sinuses can be identified in 1-year-old children. Ethmoid sinuses have developed in children by 6 years of age. Sinus problems occur infrequently in children under 7 years.

TABLE 5-6	Nasal Discharge Characteristics and Associated Conditions
Discharge Description	Associated Condition
Watery	
Clear, bilateral	Allergy
Serous, unilateral	Spinal fluid from a basilar skull fracture
Mucoid or purulent	
Bilateral	Upper respiratory infection
Unilateral	Foreign body
Bloody	Nosebleed, trauma

■ ASSESSING THE MOUTH AND THROAT FOR COLOR, FUNCTION, AND SIGNS OF ABNORMAL CONDITIONS

What is the best site to evaluate cyanosis in children? What is the expected sequence of tooth eruption? How is it determined that the tongue has adequate movement for all speech sounds? How can the throat be inspected without causing the child to gag?

Equipment Needed

Tongue blade
Penlight
Gloves

The Mouth

Inspection

Young children often need coaxing and simple explanations before they will cooperate with the mouth and throat examination. Most children readily show their teeth. If the child clenches the teeth and resists opening the mouth, the teeth can be gently separated with a tongue blade. Wear gloves when examining the mouth. See Figure 5–26 ➤ for mouth structure to examine.

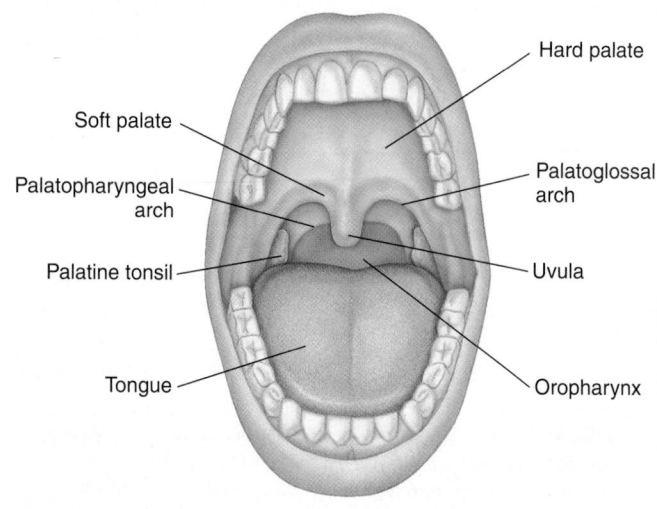

FIGURE 5–26 ➤ The structures of the mouth.

Labels: Hard palate, Soft palate, Palatoglossal arch, Palatopharyngeal arch, Palatine tonsil, Uvula, Tongue, Oropharynx

Lips Inspect the lips for color, shape, symmetry, moisture, and lesions. The lips are normally symmetric without drying, cracking, or other lesions. Lip color is normally pink in White children and more bluish in darker-skinned children. Pale, cyanotic, or cherry-red lips indicate poor tissue perfusion caused by various conditions. Note any clefts or edema.

Teeth Inspect and count the child's teeth. The timing of tooth eruption is often genetically determined, but there is a regular sequence of tooth eruption. Figure 5–27 ➤ presents the typical sequence of tooth eruption for both deciduous and permanent teeth.

Inspect the condition of the teeth, look for loose teeth, and note any spaces where teeth are missing. Compare empty tooth spaces with the child's developmental stage of tooth eruption. Once the permanent teeth have erupted, none should be missing. Teeth are normally white, without a flattened, mottled, or pitted appearance. Discolorations on the crown of a tooth may indicate caries. Discolorations on the tooth surface may be associated with some medications and fluorosis. See Chapter 19 ∞ .

Mouth Odors During inspection of the teeth, be alert to any abnormal odors that may indicate problems such as diabetic ketoacidosis, infection, or poor hygiene. Be alert for alcohol odors in older children that could signal substance abuse.

Gums Inspect the gums for color and adherence to the teeth. The gums are normally pink, with a stippled or dotted appearance. Use a tongue blade to help visualize the gums around the upper and lower molars. No raised or receding gum areas should be apparent around the teeth. When inflammation, swelling, or bleeding is observed, palpate the gums to detect tenderness. Inflammation and tenderness are associated with infection, some seizure medications, and poor nutrition.

Buccal Mucosa Inspect the mucous membrane lining the cheeks for color and moisture. The mucous membrane is usually pink, but patches of hyperpigmentation are commonly seen in darker-skinned children. The Stensen duct, the parotid gland opening, is opposite the upper second molar bilaterally. Normally pink, the duct opening becomes red when the child is infected with mumps. Small pink sucking pads can be present in infants. No areas of redness, swelling, or ulcerative lesions should be present.

Tongue Inspect the tongue for color, moistness, size, tremors, and lesions. The child's tongue is normally pink and moist, without a coating, and it fits easily into the mouth. A protuberant tongue is associated with various genetic conditions, such as Down syndrome. A pattern of gray, irregular borders that form a design (geographic tongue) is often normal, but it may be associated with fever, allergies, or drug reactions. Tremors are

As Children Grow
Sequence of Tooth Eruption and Shedding

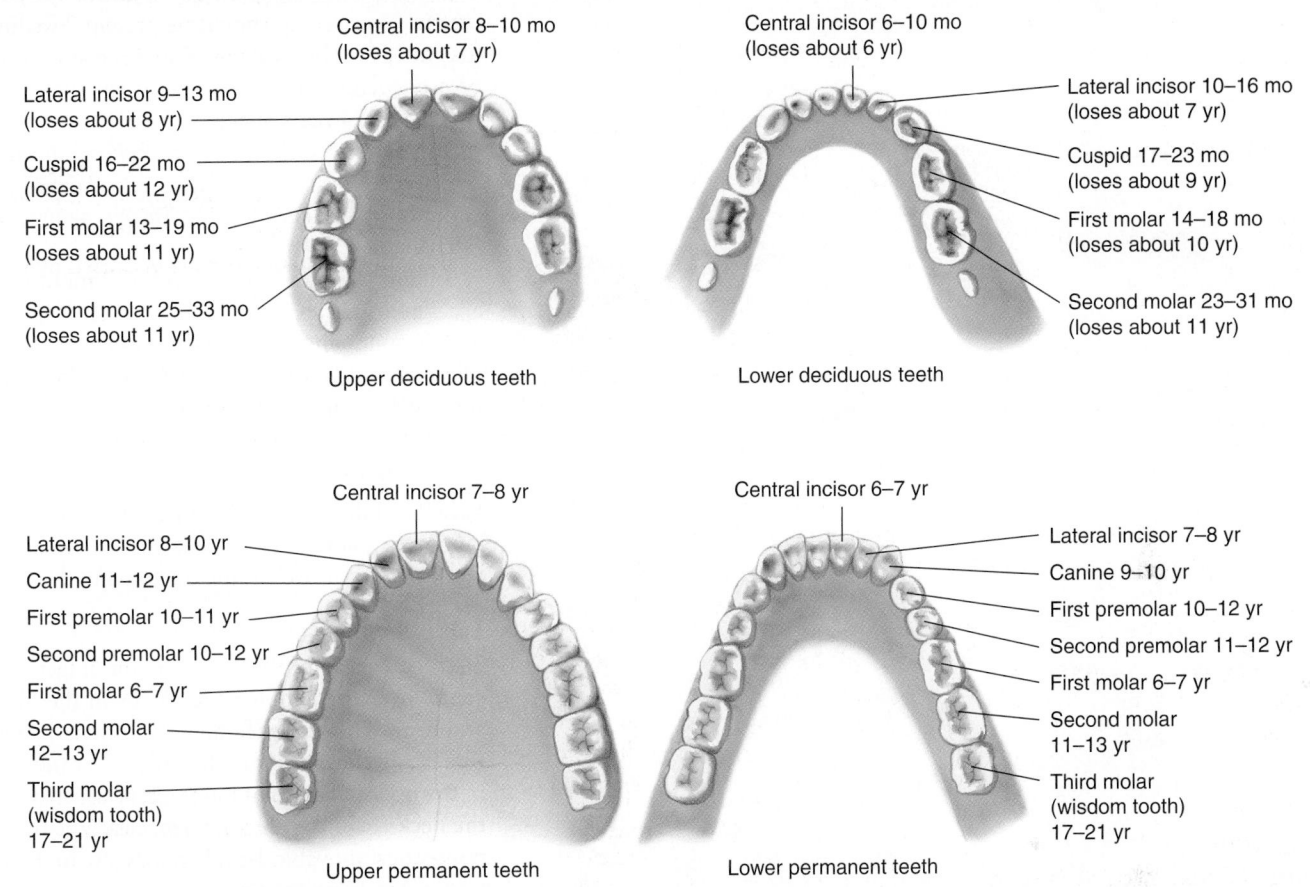

Lateral incisor 9–13 mo
(loses about 8 yr)

Central incisor 8–10 mo
(loses about 7 yr)

Cuspid 16–22 mo
(loses about 12 yr)

First molar 13–19 mo
(loses about 11 yr)

Second molar 25–33 mo
(loses about 11 yr)

Upper deciduous teeth

Central incisor 6–10 mo
(loses about 6 yr)

Lateral incisor 10–16 mo
(loses about 7 yr)

Cuspid 17–23 mo
(loses about 9 yr)

First molar 14–18 mo
(loses about 10 yr)

Second molar 23–31 mo
(loses about 11 yr)

Lower deciduous teeth

Central incisor 7–8 yr

Lateral incisor 8–10 yr
Canine 11–12 yr
First premolar 10–11 yr
Second premolar 10–12 yr
First molar 6–7 yr
Second molar 12–13 yr
Third molar (wisdom tooth) 17–21 yr

Upper permanent teeth

Central incisor 6–7 yr

Lateral incisor 7–8 yr
Canine 9–10 yr
First premolar 10–12 yr
Second premolar 11–12 yr
First molar 6–7 yr
Second molar 11–13 yr
Third molar (wisdom tooth) 17–21 yr

Lower permanent teeth

FIGURE 5–27 ➤ Typical sequence for the eruption of both the deciduous and permanent teeth. Notice that bottom teeth erupt first for each kind of tooth: incisors, cuspids, and molars. Teeth are shed or lost in the same pattern.

abnormal. A white adherent coating on an infant's tongue may be caused by thrush, a *Candida* infection (see Chapter 31 ∞).

Observe the mobility of the tongue. Ask the child to touch the gums above the upper teeth with the tongue, adequate movement to clearly enunciate all speech sounds. Ask the child to stick out the tongue and lift it so the underside of the tongue and the floor of the mouth can be inspected for distended veins.

Palate Inspect the hard and soft palate to detect any clefts or masses or an unusually high arch. The palate is normally pink, with a dome-shaped arch and no cleft. The uvula hangs freely from the soft palate. Newborns often have Epstein pearls, white papules in the midline of the palate that disappear in a few weeks. A high-arched palate can be associated with sucking difficulties in young infants.

Palpation
Palpate any masses seen in the mouth to determine their characteristics, such as size, shape, firmness, and tenderness. No masses should be found.

Tongue To assess the tongue's strength, while simultaneously testing the hypoglossal nerve (cranial nerve XII), place the index finger against the child's cheek and ask the child to push against your finger with the tongue. Some pressure against the finger is normally felt.

Palate To palpate the palate, insert the little finger, with the fingerpad upward, into the mouth. While the infant sucks against your finger, palpate the entire palate. This procedure also tests the strength of the sucking reflex, innervated by the hypoglossal nerve (cranial nerve XII). No clefts should be palpated.

The Throat
Inspection
Inspect the throat for color, swelling, lesions, and the condition of the tonsils. Ask the child to open the mouth wide and stick out the tongue. A penlight is used to illuminate the throat. A tongue blade can be used, if needed, to visualize the posterior pharynx. The throat is normally pink without lesions, drainage, or swelling. The epiglottis lies behind the tongue and is normally pink like the rest of the buccal mucosa. Swelling or bulging in the posterior pharynx may be associated with a peritonsillar abscess (see Chapter 19 ∞). The gag reflex is rarely tested in children.

Pathophysiology Illustrated
Stages of Tonsil Inflammation

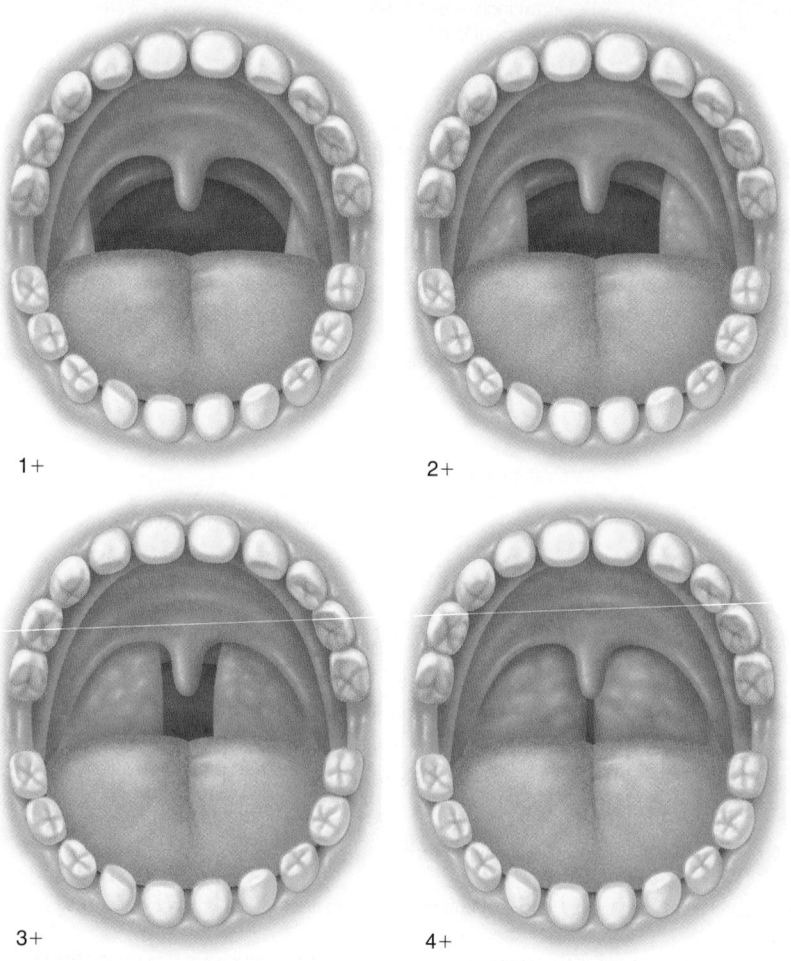

1+   2+

3+   4+

FIGURE 5–28 ➤ Tonsil size can be graded from +1 to +4 in relation to how much of the airway is obstructed. Tonsil size of +1 or +2 is normal. Tonsil size of +3 is common with infections such as strep throat. Tonsils that "kiss" or nearly touch each other (+4) significantly reduce the size of the airway.

Clinical Tip

Moistening the tongue blade may decrease the child's tendency to gag.

Tonsils   During childhood the tonsils are large in proportion to the size of the pharynx because lymphoid tissue grows fastest in early childhood. The tonsils should be pink without exudate, but *crypts* (fissures) may be present as a result of prior infections. The size of the tonsils can be graded as indicated in Figure 5–28 ➤.

■ ASSESSING THE NECK FOR CHARACTERISTICS, RANGE OF MOTION, AND LYMPH NODES

What does it mean when a child's head is tilted to one side? By what age should an infant be able to control his or her head? What does a lymph node feel like?

Inspection of the Neck

Inspect the neck for size, symmetry, swelling, and any abnormalities. A short neck with skin folds is normal for infants. The neck is normally symmetric. No swelling should be present. Swelling may be caused by local infections such as mumps or a congenital defect. The neck lengthens between 3 and 4 years of age.

Inspect the child's neck for *webbing*, an extra skin fold on each side of the neck. Webbing is commonly associated with Turner syndrome (see Chapter 30 ∞).

Infants develop head control by 2 months of age. By this age an infant can lift the head up and look around when lying on the stomach. A lack of head control can result from neurologic injury, such as an anoxic episode.

Palpation of the Neck

Face the child and use your fingerpads to simultaneously palpate both sides of the neck for lymph nodes, as well as the trachea and thyroid.

Lymph Nodes

To palpate the lymph nodes, slide your fingerpads gently over the lymph node chains in the head and neck. The sequence for lymph node palpation is as follows: around the ears, under the jaw, in the occipital area, and in the cervical chain of the neck (Figure 5–29 ➤). Firm, clearly defined, nontender, movable lymph nodes up to 1 cm (1/2 in.) in diameter are common in young children. Enlarged, firm, warm, tender lymph nodes indicate a local infection.

Trachea

Palpate the trachea to determine its position and to detect the presence of any masses. The trachea is normally in the midline of the neck. It is difficult to palpate in the short necks of children under age 3 years. To palpate the trachea, place your thumb and forefinger on each side of the child's trachea near the chin and slowly slide them down the trachea. Any shift to the right or left of midline may indicate a tumor or a collapsed lung.

Thyroid

As the fingers slide over the trachea in the lower neck, attempt to feel the isthmus of the thyroid, a band of glandular tissue crossing over the trachea. The lobes of the thyroid wrap behind the trachea and are normally covered by the sternocleidomastoid muscle. Because of the anatomic position of the thyroid, its lobes are not usually palpable in the child unless they are enlarged.

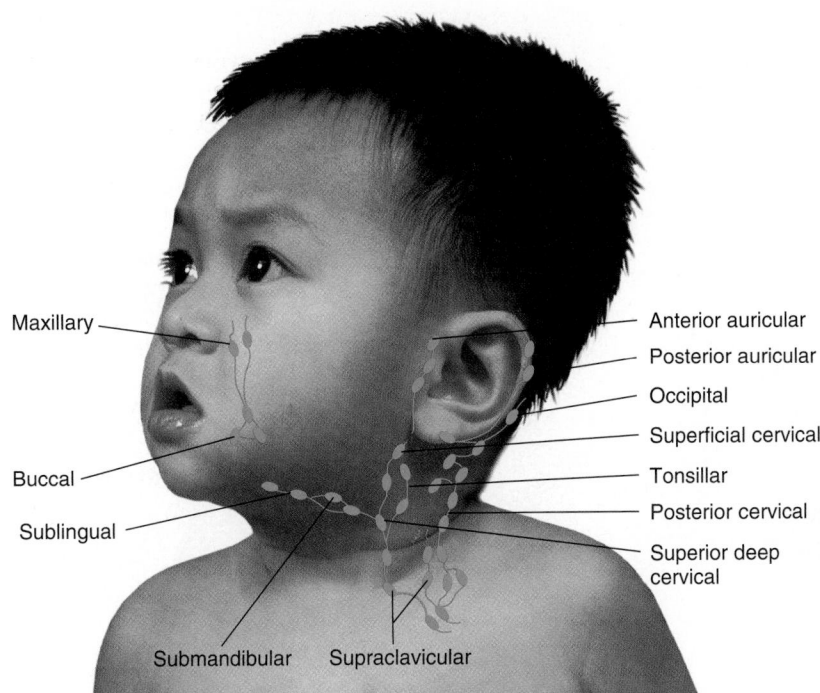

Maxillary

Buccal

Sublingual

Submandibular   Supraclavicular

Anterior auricular

Posterior auricular

Occipital

Superficial cervical

Tonsillar

Posterior cervical

Superior deep cervical

FIGURE 5–29 ➤ The neck is palpated for enlarged lymph nodes around the ears, under the jaw, in the occipital area, and in the cervical chain of the neck.

Range of Motion Assessment

To test the neck's range of motion, ask the child to touch the chin to each shoulder and to the chest and then to look at the ceiling. Move a light or toy in all four directions when assessing infants. Children should freely move the neck and head in all four directions without pain.

When the child is unable to move the head voluntarily in all directions, passively move the child's neck through the expected range of motion. Limited horizontal range of motion may be a sign of *torticollis*, persistent head tilting. Torticollis results from a birth injury to the sternocleidomastoid muscle or from unilateral vision or hearing impairment. Pain with flexion of the neck toward the chest (Brudzinski sign) may indicate meningitis. See Chapter 27 ∞.

■ ASSESSING THE CHEST FOR SHAPE, MOVEMENT, RESPIRATORY EFFORT, AND LUNG FUNCTION

What terms are used to describe the location of specific sounds heard when auscultating the chest? What are retractions and what do they indicate? How can normal and adventitious breath sounds be distinguished when auscultating the lungs?

Examination of the chest includes the following procedures: inspecting the size and shape of the chest, palpating chest movement that occurs during respiration, observing the breathing effort, and auscultating breath sounds.

Equipment Needed

Stethoscope

Inspection of the Chest

Position the child on the parent's lap or on the examining table with all clothing above the waist removed to inspect the chest. The thoracic muscles and subcutaneous tissue are less developed in children than in adolescents and adults, so the chest wall is thinner. As a result the rib cage is more prominent.

Topographic Landmarks

The chest skeleton provides most of the landmarks used to describe the location of findings during examination of the chest, lungs, and heart. The intercostal spaces between the ribs are the horizontal markers. The sternum and spine are the vertical landmarks (Figure 5–30 ➤). Vertical landmarks are described in Figure 5–31 ➤. When both a horizontal and a vertical landmark are used, the location of findings can be precisely described on the right or left side of the patient's chest. For example, a finding can be located in the third intercostal space 3 cm (1 in.) from the sternal line.

Size and Shape of the Chest

Inspect the chest for any irregularities in shape. Children less than 2 years of age have a rounded chest as the anteroposterior and lateral diameters are approximately equal. The chest becomes more oval as the lateral diameter becomes greater than the anteroposterior diameter. A rounded chest in an older child may be due to a chronic obstructive lung condition such as asthma or cystic fibrosis.

An abnormal chest shape may be the result of a structural deformity (Figure 5–32 ➤). If the sternum protrudes, increasing the anteroposterior diameter, pigeon chest (pectus carinatum) may be present. If the lower portion of the sternum is depressed, decreasing the anteroposterior diameter, funnel chest (pectus

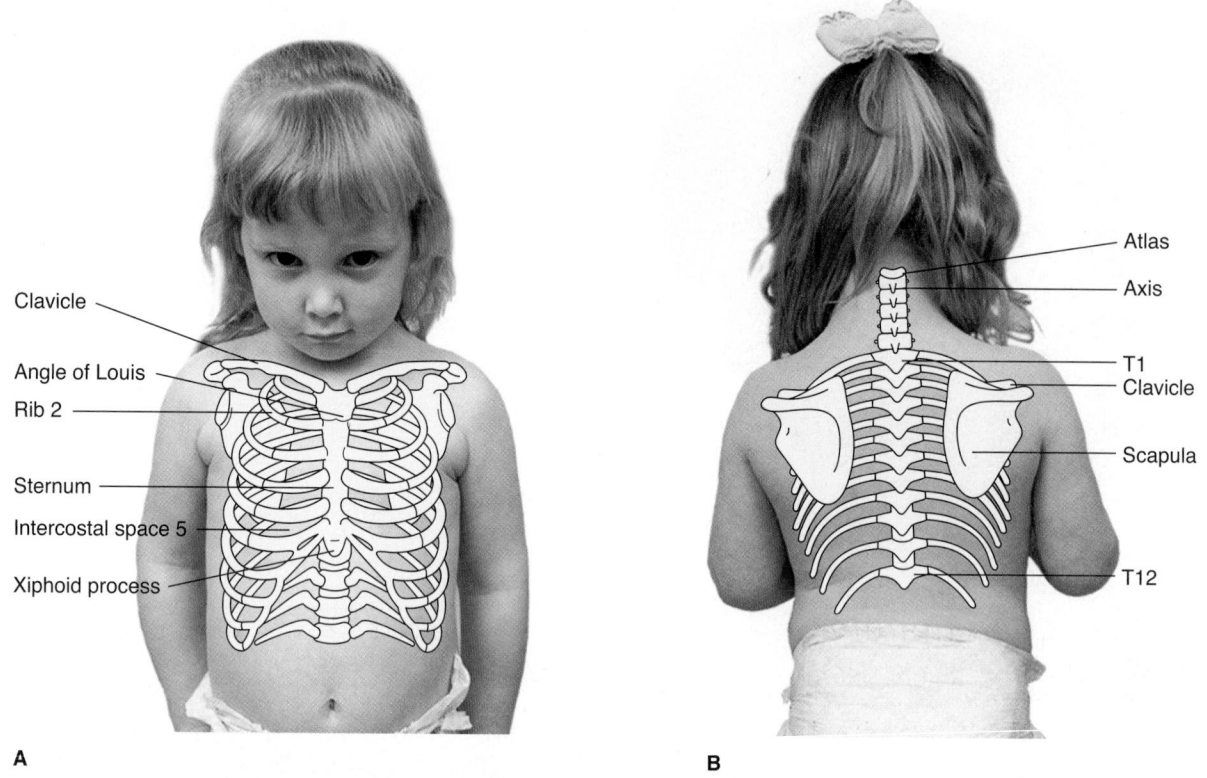

A

B

FIGURE 5–30 ➤ Intercostal spaces and ribs are numbered to describe the location of findings. A, To determine the rib number on the anterior chest, palpate down from the top of the sternum until a horizontal ridge, the angle of Louis, is felt. Directly to the right and left of that ridge is the second rib. The second intercostal space is immediately below the second rib. Ribs 3–12 and the corresponding intercostal spaces can be counted as the fingers move toward the abdomen. B, To determine the rib number on the posterior chest, find the protruding spinal process of the seventh cervical vertebra at the shoulder level. The next spinal process belongs to the first thoracic vertebra, which attaches to the first rib.

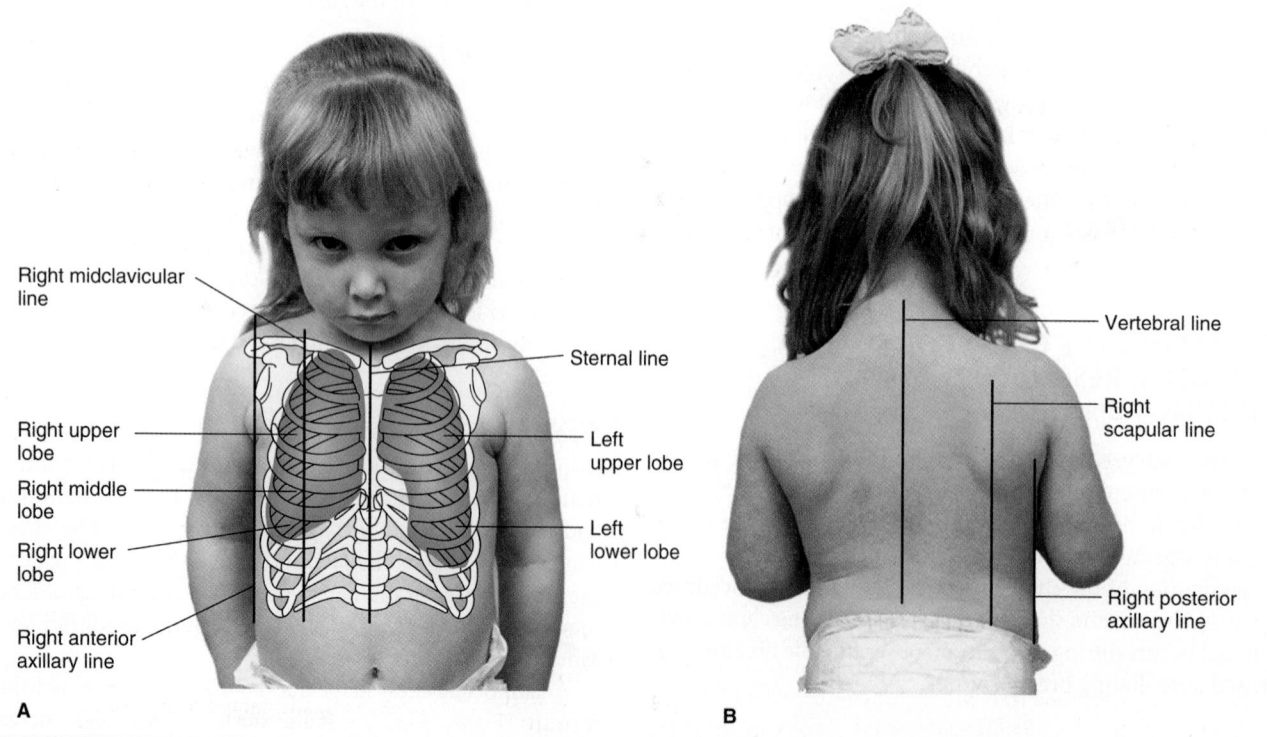

A

B

FIGURE 5–31 ➤ The middle of the sternum and spine are the vertical landmarks used to describe the anatomic location of findings. Other imaginary lines are parallel to these two vertical landmarks. The midclavicular line is from the middle of the clavicle. The anterior axillary line is from the anterior axillary fold. The midaxillary line is from the middle of the axilla. The posterior axillary line is from the posterior axillary fold. The scapular line is from the middle of the scapula. A, Anterior chest. B, Posterior chest.

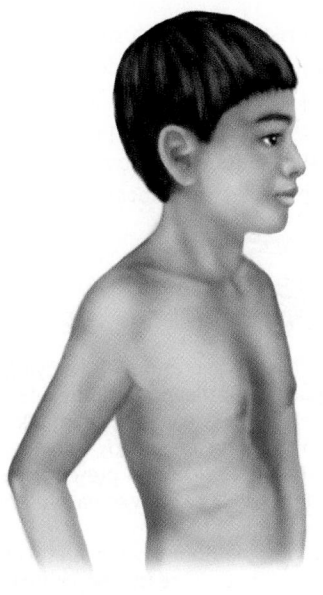
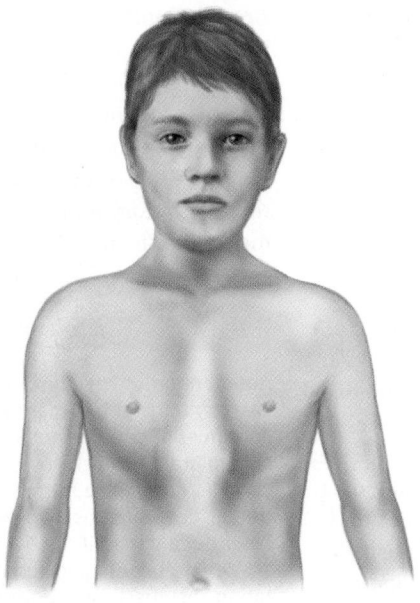

A   **B**

FIGURE 5–32 ➤ Two types of abnormal chest shape. A, Funnel chest (pectus excavatum). B, Pigeon chest (pectus carinatum).

excavatum) may be present. Scoliosis, curvature of the spine, causes a lateral deviation of the chest. See Chapter 29 ∞.

Chest Movement and Respiratory Effort

Inspect for simultaneous chest expansion and abdominal rise. Chest movement is normally symmetric bilaterally, rising with inspiration and falling with expiration. The chest movement of infants and young children is less pronounced than the abdominal movement. The diaphragm is the primary breathing muscle in infants and children less than age 6 years. The thoracic muscles are less developed and serve as accessory muscles in cases of respiratory distress. As the thoracic muscles develop, they become primarily responsible for ventilation. On inspiration the chest and abdomen should rise simultaneously. Asymmetric chest rise is associated with a collapsed lung. **Retractions**, depression of sections of the chest wall with each inspiration, are seen when the accessory muscles are used for breathing in cases of respiratory distress.

Respiratory Rate

Because young children use the diaphragm as the primary breathing muscle, observe or feel the rise and fall of the abdomen to count the respiratory rate in children under age 6 years. Table 5–7 gives the normal respiratory rates for each age group. Make every effort to count the respiratory rate when the child is quiet. **Tachypnea**, an elevated respiratory rate, occurs in

Growth & Development *Respiratory Rate*

Infants and children have a faster respiratory rate than adults because of a higher metabolic rate and oxygen requirement. Young children are also unable to increase the depth of respirations because the intercostal muscles are inadequately developed to lift the chest wall and increase intrathoracic volume (Ralston, Hazinski, Zaritsky, et al., 2006, p. 40).

TABLE 5–7	Normal Respiratory Rate Ranges for Each Age Group
Age	Respiratory Rate Per Minute
Newborn	30–55
1 year	25–40
3 years	20–30
6 years	16–22
10 years	16–20
17 years	12–20

response to excitement, fear, respiratory distress, fever, and other conditions that increase oxygen needs. A sustained respiratory rate at a value higher than normal is an important sign in respiratory distress. Children may develop hypoxemia if treatment is not started. **Bradypnea**, an abnormally slow respiratory rate, occurs in response to respiratory failure.

Clinical Tip

To get the most accurate reading of a newborn's or young infant's respiratory rate, wait until the baby is sleeping or quietly resting. Use the stethoscope to auscultate the rate or place your hand on the abdomen. Count the number of breaths for an entire minute, because newborns and young infants can have irregular respirations.

Palpation of the Chest

Palpation is used to evaluate chest movement, respiratory effort, deformities of the chest wall, and tactile fremitus.

Chest Wall

To palpate the chest motion with respiration, place your palms and outspread fingers on each side of the child's chest. Confirm the bilateral symmetry of chest motion. Use fingerpads to palpate any depressions, bulges, or unusual chest wall shape that might indicate abnormal findings such as tenderness, cysts, other growths, crepitus, or fractures. None should be found. **Crepitus**, a crinkly sensation palpated on the chest surface, is caused by air escaping into the subcutaneous tissues. It often indicates a serious injury to the upper or lower airway. Crepitus may also be felt near a fracture.

Tactile Fremitus

Crying and talking produce vibrations that can be palpated on the chest, known as **tactile fremitus**. Place the palms of your hands on each side of the chest to evaluate the quality and distribution of these vibrations. Ask the child to repeat a series of words or numbers, such as *Mickey Mouse* or *ice cream*. As the child repeats the words, move your hands systematically over the anterior and posterior chest, comparing the quality of findings side to side. The vibration or tingling sensation is normally palpated over the entire chest. Decreased sensations indicate that air is trapped in the lungs, as occurs with asthma. Increased sensations indicate lung consolidation, as occurs with pneumonia.

Auscultation of the Chest

Auscultate the chest with a stethoscope to assess the quality and characteristics of breath sounds and to identify abnormal breath sounds. Use an infant or pediatric stethoscope when available to help localize any unexpected breath sounds. Use the stethoscope's diaphragm because it transmits the high-pitched breath sounds better.

Breath Sounds

Evaluate the quality and characteristics of breath sounds over the entire chest, comparing sounds between the sides. Select a routine sequence for auscultating the entire chest so assessment of all lobes of the lungs will be consistently performed. Figure 5–33 ➤ shows one suggested sequence. Listen to an entire inspiratory and expiratory phase at each location before moving to the next site.

Clinical Tip ◣

Auscultation of breath sounds is difficult when an infant is crying. First, try to quiet the infant with a pacifier, bottle, or toy. If the infant continues to cry, all is not lost. At the end of each cry the infant takes a deep breath, which you can use to assess breath sounds, vocal resonance, and tactile fremitus. Encourage toddlers and preschoolers to take deep breaths by providing a pinwheel to blow or have them blow out a penlight.

When encouraging the child to breathe normally while auscultating the chest, use suggestive language to increase cooperation. "You certainly are good at breathing slowly. Have you been practicing?" The child will often deepen and slow the breathing pattern as you give praise and draw attention to it.

Three types of normal breath sounds are usually heard when the chest is auscultated. *Vesicular breath sounds* are low-pitched, swishing, soft, short expiratory sounds. They are usually heard in older children but not in infants and young children. *Bronchovesicular breath sounds* are medium-pitched, hollow, blowing sounds heard equally on inspiration and expiration in all age groups. The location of these sounds on the chest is related to the

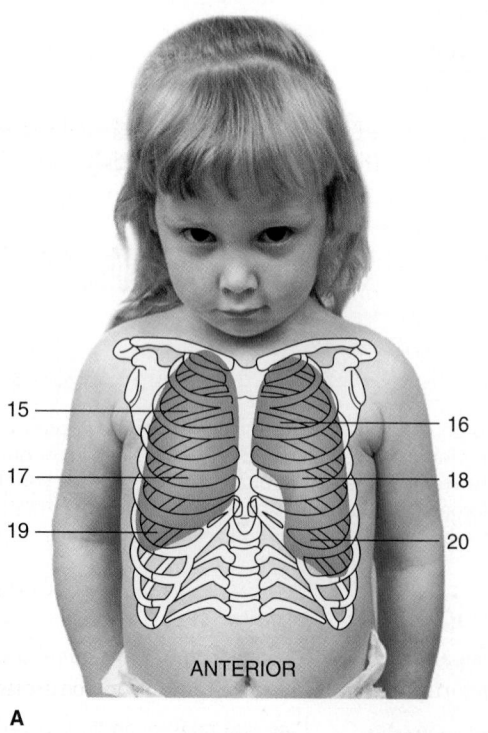

A ANTERIOR

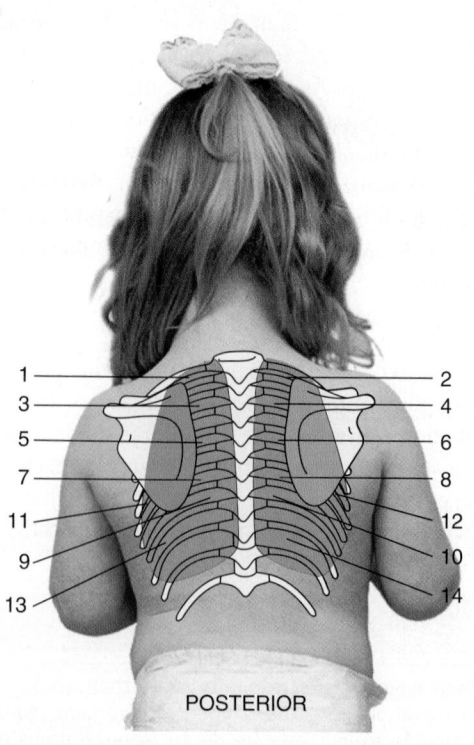

B POSTERIOR

FIGURE 5–33 ➤ One example of a sequence for auscultation of the chest. A, Anterior. B, Posterior.

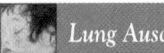

Infants and young children have a thin chest wall because of immature muscle development. The breath sounds of one lung are heard over the entire chest. It takes practice to accurately identify absent or diminished breath sounds in infants and young children. Because the distance between the lungs is greatest at the apices and midaxillary areas in young children, these sites are best for identifying absent or diminished breath sounds. Carefully auscultate, comparing the quality of breath sounds heard bilaterally.

child's developmental status. *Bronchial/tracheal breath sounds* are hollow and higher pitched than vesicular breath sounds.

Breath sounds normally have equal intensity, pitch, and rhythm bilaterally. Absent or diminished breath sounds generally indicate a partial or total obstruction, such as from a foreign body or mucus, that does not permit airflow.

Vocal Resonance

Auscultate the chest to evaluate **vocal resonance**, the transmission of voice sounds. Have the child repeat a series of words, such as *hot dog, apple,* or *Popsicle.* Use the stethoscope to auscultate the chest, comparing the quality of sounds from side to side and over the entire chest. Voice sounds, with words and syllables muffled and indistinct, are normally heard throughout the chest.

If voice sounds are absent or more muffled than usual, an airway obstruction condition such as asthma may be present. When a lung consolidation, such as from pneumonia, is present, the quality of vocal resonance changes in characteristic ways. These abnormal characteristics are called whispered pectoriloquy, bronchophony, and egophony. **Whispered pectoriloquy** is present when syllables are heard distinctly in a whisper. **Bronchophony** is the increased intensity and clarity of sounds while the words remain indistinct. **Egophony** is the transmission of the "eee" sound as a nasal "ay" sound.

Abnormal Breath Sounds

Abnormal breath sounds, also called *adventitious sounds*, generally indicate disease. Examples of abnormal breath sounds are crackles, rhonchi, and friction rubs. To further assess abnormal breath sounds, the examiner determines their location, if present during inspiration or expiration, and whether they change or disappear when the child coughs or shifts position. It takes practice to routinely identify these adventitious sounds. Table 5–8 describes adventitious sounds.

Other Abnormal Sounds

Observing the quality of the voice and other audible sounds is also important during an examination of the lungs. **Stridor** is a noise resulting from air moving through a narrowed trachea and larynx; it is associated with croup. **Wheezing** is a noise resulting from the passage of air through mucus or fluids in a narrowed lower airway with sounds as described for sibilant rhonchi. It is associated with asthma. A *cough* is a reflexive clearing of the airway associated with an allergy or respiratory infection. Hoarseness is associated with inflammation of the larynx.

Percussion of the Chest

Percussion is a method sometimes used to assess the resonance of the lungs and the size and density of underlying organs, such as the heart and liver. Radiograph examination is now used more commonly for these evaluations.

■ ASSESSING THE BREASTS

What does breast tissue feel like? Do boys have breast development during puberty?

Inspection of the Breasts

The nipples of prepubertal boys and girls are symmetrically located near the midclavicular line at the fourth to sixth ribs. The areola is normally round and more darkly pigmented than the surrounding skin. Inspect the anterior chest for other dark spots that may indicate supernumerary nipples, which are small, undeveloped nipples and areolae that may be mistaken for moles. Their presence may be associated with congenital renal or cardiac anomalies.

See page 148 for pubertal development.

Palpation of the Breasts

Palpate the developing breasts of adolescent females for abnormal masses or hard nodules while the patient is supine. Use a concentric pattern covering all quadrants of each breast including the axilla, all around the areola, and then around the nipple. Breast tissue normally feels dense, firm, and elastic.

The majority of boys have unilateral or bilateral breast enlargement during adolescence called gynecomastia. It is often most noticeable around 14 years of age and commonly disappears by the time of full sexual maturity. Palpate the tissue to differentiate actual breast tissue from fatty tissue in the pectoral area, and to detect any masses.

TABLE 5–8	Description of Selected Adventitious Sounds and Their Cause	
Type	Description	Cause
Fine crackles	High-pitched, discrete, noncontinuous sound heard at end of inspiration *(Rub pieces of hair together beside your ear to duplicate the sound.)*	Air passing through watery secretions in the smaller airways (alveoli and bronchioles)
Sibilant rhonchi (*Wheezing*)	Musical, squeaking, or hissing noise heard during inspiration or expiration, but generally louder on expiration	Bronchospasm or an anatomic narrowing of the trachea, bronchi, or bronchioles
Sonorous rhonchi (coarse crackles)	Coarse, low-pitched sound like a snore, heard during inspiration or expiration; may clear with coughing	Air passing through thick secretions that partially obstruct the larger bronchi and trachea

■ ASSESSING THE HEART FOR HEART SOUNDS AND FUNCTION

What is the point of maximum intensity and where is it located? What is the normal heart rate for infants and children? What is the difference between heart sounds and murmurs?

Equipment Needed

Stethoscope
Sphygmomanometer

Inspection of the Precordium

Begin the heart examination by inspecting the *precordium,* or anterior chest. Place the child in a reclining or semi-Fowler position, either on the parent's lap or on the examining table. Inspect the shape and symmetry of the anterior chest from the front and side views. The rib cage is normally symmetric. Bulging of the left side of the chest wall may indicate an enlarged heart.

Observe for any chest movement associated with the heart's contraction. The **apical impulse,** sometimes called the point of maximum intensity, is located where the left ventricle taps the chest wall during contraction. The apical impulse can normally be seen in thin children. A *heave,* an obvious lifting of the chest wall during contraction, may indicate an enlarged heart.

Palpation of the Precordium

Place the entire palmar surface of the fingers together on the chest wall to palpate the precordium. Systematically palpate the entire precordium to detect any pulsations, heaves, or vibrations. Palpating with minimal pressure increases the chance of detecting abnormal findings.

Apical Impulse

The apical impulse is normally felt as a slight tap against one fingertip. Use the topographic landmarks of the chest to describe its location (see Figures 5–30 and 5–31). Any other sensation palpated is usually abnormal.

Abnormal Sensations

A *lift* is the sensation of the heart lifting up against the chest wall. It may be associated with an enlarged heart or a heart contracting with extra force. A *thrill* is a rushing vibration that feels like a cat's purr. It is caused by turbulent blood flow from a defective heart valve and a heart murmur. If present, the thrill is palpated in the right or left second intercostal space. To describe a thrill's location, use the topographic landmarks of the chest (see Figures 5–30 and 5–31) and estimate the diameter of the thrill palpated.

Growth & Development *Apical Impulse*

The location of the apical impulse changes as the child's rib cage grows. In children under 7 years old, it is located in the fourth intercostal space just medial to the left midclavicular line. In children over 7 years old, it is located in the fifth intercostal space at the left midclavicular line.

Percussion of the Heart Borders

Percussion of the heart borders is rarely performed during physical examination. The borders of the heart are better identified by radiologic examination.

Auscultation of the Heart

Auscultation is used to count the apical pulse, to assess the characteristics of the heart sounds, and to detect abnormal heart sounds. Use the bell of the stethoscope to detect these lower pitched sounds.

To completely assess heart sounds, auscultate the heart with the child in both sitting and reclining positions. Differences in heart sounds caused by a change in the child's position or by a change in the position of the heart near the chest wall can then be detected. If differences in heart sounds are detected with a position change, place the child in the left lateral recumbent position and auscultate again.

Heart Rate and Rhythm

The apical heart rate can be counted at the site of the apical impulse, either by palpation or by auscultation. Count the apical rate for 1 minute in infants and in children who have an irregular rhythm. The brachial or radial pulse rate should be the same as the auscultated apical heart rate. Table 5–9 gives normal heart rates in children of different ages.

Listen carefully to the heart rate rhythm. Children often have a normal cycle of irregular rhythm associated with respiration called sinus arrhythmia. With *sinus arrhythmia* the child's heart rate is faster on inspiration and slower on expiration. When any rhythm irregularity is detected, ask the child to take a breath and hold it for a few seconds while you listen to the heart rate. The rhythm should become regular. Other rhythm irregularities are abnormal.

Growth & Development *Heart Rate*

The child's heart rate varies with age, decreasing as the child grows older. The heart rate also increases in response to exercise, excitement, anxiety, and fever. Such stresses increase the child's metabolic rate, creating a simultaneous need for more oxygen. Children respond to the need for more oxygen by increasing their heart rate, a response called sinus tachycardia.

TABLE 5–9	Normal Heart Rates for Children of Different Ages	
Age	Heart Rate Range (beats/min)	Average Heart Rate (beats/min)
Newborns	100–170	120
Infants to 2 years	80–130	110
2–6 years	70–120	100
6–10 years	60–110	90
10–16 years	60–100	80

Differentiation of Heart Sounds

Heart sounds result from the closure of the valves and vibration or turbulence of blood produced by that valve closure. Two primary sounds, S_1 and S_2, are heard when the chest is auscultated.

S_1, the first heart sound, is produced by closure of the tricuspid and mitral valves when the ventricular contraction begins. The two valves close almost simultaneously, so only one sound is normally heard.

Clinical Tip

Palpate the carotid pulse when auscultating the heart to distinguish between the two heart sounds. The heart sound heard simultaneously with the pulsation is S_1.

S_2, the second heart sound, is produced by the closure of the aortic and pulmonic valves. Once blood has reached the pulmonic and aortic arteries, the valves close to prevent leakage back into the ventricles during diastole. The timing of the valve closure varies with respirations. Sometimes S_2 is heard as a single sound and at other times as a split sound, that is, two sounds heard a fraction of a second apart.

Sound is easily transmitted in liquid, and it travels best in the direction of blood flow. Auscultate heart sounds at specific areas on the chest wall in the direction of blood flow, just beyond the valve (Figure 5–34 ➤). The sounds produced by the heart valves or blood turbulence are heard throughout the chest in thin infants and children. Both S_1 and S_2 can be heard in all listening areas.

Auscultate heart sounds for quality (distinct versus muffled) and intensity (loud versus weak). First, distinguish between S_1 and S_2 in each listening area. Heart sounds are usually distinct and crisp in children because of their thin chest wall. Muffling or indistinct sounds may indicate a heart defect or congestive heart failure. Document the area where heart sounds are heard the best. Table 5–10 and Figure 5–34 review the location where each sound is normally best heard for assessment of quality and intensity. If the child has a potential murmur, auscultate the heart in the sitting, reclining, and standing positions to see if differences are noted by position change.

TABLE 5–10	Identification of the Listening Sites for Auscultation of the Quality and Intensity of Heart Sounds	
Heart Sound	Locations Best Heard	Where Heard Softly
S_1	Apex of the heart	Base of the heart
	Tricuspid area	Aortic area
	Mitral area	Pulmonic area
S_2	Base of the heart	Apex of the heart
	Aortic area	Tricuspid area
	Pulmonic area	Mitral area
Physiologic splitting	Pulmonic area	
S_3	Mitral area	

Splitting of the Heart Sounds

After distinguishing the first and second heart sounds, try to detect *physiologic splitting*. A split S_2 is more apparent during inspiration when the child takes a deep breath. More blood returns to the right ventricle, causing the pulmonic valve to close a fraction of a second later than the aortic valve. To detect physiologic splitting, auscultate over the pulmonic area while the child breathes normally and then while the child takes a deep breath. Splitting is normally more easily detected after a deep breath. The splitting returns to a single sound with regular breathing. If splitting does not vary with respiration, it is called *fixed splitting*. This is an abnormal finding associated with an atrial septal defect.

Third Heart Sound

A third heart sound, S_3, is occasionally heard in children as a normal finding. S_3 is caused when blood rushes through the mitral valve and splashes into the left ventricle. It is heard in diastole, just after S_2. It is distinguished from a split S_2 because it is louder in the mitral area than in the pulmonic area.

Murmurs

Occasionally abnormal heart sounds are auscultated. These sounds are produced by turbulence of blood passing through a

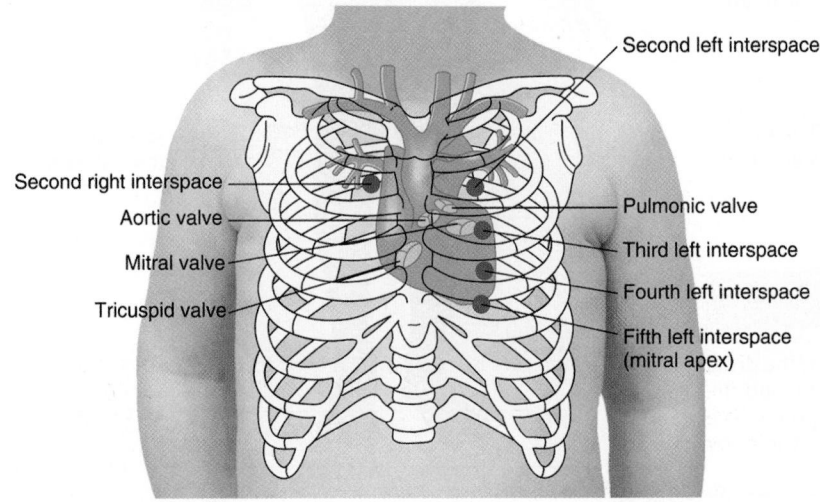

Second left interspace

Second right interspace
Aortic valve
Mitral valve
Tricuspid valve

Pulmonic valve
Third left interspace
Fourth left interspace
Fifth left interspace (mitral apex)

FIGURE 5–34 ➤ Sound travels in the direction of blood flow. Rather than listen for heart sounds over each heart valve, auscultate heart sounds at specific areas on the chest wall away from the valve itself. These areas are named for the valve producing the sound. *Aortic*: Second right intercostal space near the sternum. *Pulmonic*: Second left intercostal space near the sternum. *Tricuspid*: Fifth right or left intercostal space near the sternum. *Mitral* (apical): In infants—third or fourth intercostal space, just left of the left midclavicular line. In children—fifth intercostal space at the left midclavicular line.

defective valve, great vessel, or other heart structure. Some murmurs are benign or innocent whereas others indicate pathology. An experienced examiner must be consulted to distinguish between murmurs.

To hear murmurs in children takes practice. Often, murmurs must be very loud to be detected. For softer murmurs, normal heart sounds must be distinguished before a murmur or an extra sound is recognized. Once a murmur is detected, define the characteristics of the extra sound.

Murmurs are classified by the following characteristics:

- **Intensity.** How loud is it? Can a thrill also be palpated?
- **Location.** Where is the murmur the loudest? Identify the listening area and precise topographic landmarks. Is the child sitting or lying down?
- **Radiation.** Is the sound transmitted over a larger area of the chest, to the axilla, or to the back?
- **Timing.** Is the murmur heard best after S_1 or S_2? Is it heard during the entire phase between S_1 and S_2?
- **Quality.** Describe what the murmur sounds like—for example, machine-like, musical, or blowing.

Following are guidelines for grading the intensity of a murmur:

Intensity	Description
Grade I	Barely heard in a quiet room
Grade II	Quiet, but clearly heard
Grade III	Moderately loud, no thrill palpated
Grade IV	Loud, a thrill is usually palpated
Grade V	Very loud, a thrill is easily palpated
Grade VI	Heard without the stethoscope in direct contact with the chest wall

Venous Hum

Auscultate for a venous hum over the supraclavicular fossa above the middle of the clavicle or over the upper anterior chest with the bell of the stethoscope. A venous hum is heard as a continuous low-pitched hum throughout the cardiac cycle. It may be loudest during diastole or when the child stands, and it does not change with respirations. It may be quieted by having the child turn the neck. A venous hum may be associated with anemia, but it has no pathological significance.

Completing the Heart Examination

To complete the assessment of cardiac function, palpate the pulses, measure the blood pressure, and evaluate signs from other systems.

 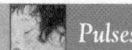

Infants have a low systolic blood pressure, and detecting the distal pulses is often difficult. Use the brachial artery in the arms and the popliteal or femoral artery in the legs to evaluate the pulses. The radial and distal tibial pulses are normally palpated easily in older children.

Palpation of the Pulses

Palpate the characteristics of the pulses in the extremities to assess the circulation. The technique and sites for palpating the pulse are the same as those used for adults (Figure 5–35 ➤). Evaluate the pulsation for rate, regularity of rhythm, and strength in each extremity and compare your findings bilaterally. The femoral and brachial pulses are the most important pulses to evaluate.

Palpate the femoral arteries and compare their strength with the strength of the brachial pulse. The femoral pulsations are equally as strong or stronger than the brachial pulsations. A weaker femoral pulse is associated with coarctation of the aorta.

Blood Pressure

Assessment of blood pressure is important to detect conditions of hypertension or hypovolemic shock. The child should be seated and quiet for 3 to 5 minutes before the blood pressure is taken. See the *Clinical Skills Manual* for the technique to obtain the blood pressure in children. The systolic reading is the onset

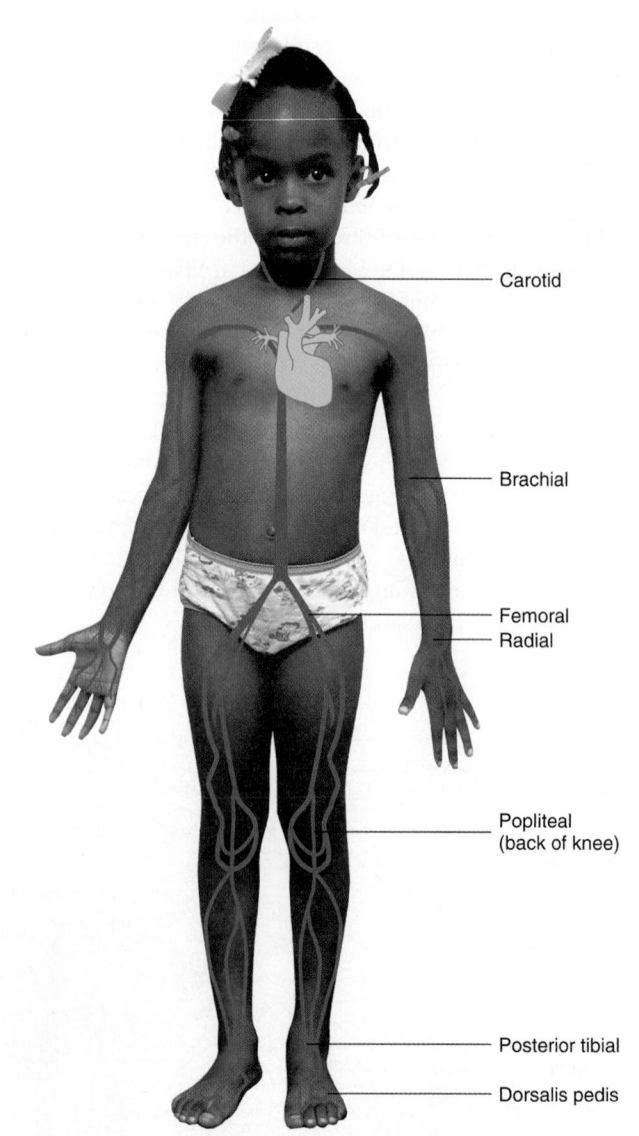

Carotid

Brachial

Femoral
Radial

Popliteal
(back of knee)

Posterior tibial

Dorsalis pedis

FIGURE 5–35 ➤ The sites used to assess the pulses in children.

of Korotkoff sounds. The diastolic reading is the fifth Korotkoff sound. If sounds are heard to 0 mmHg, the diastolic reading is the muffling of sound at the fourth Korotkoff sound in children and adolescents (Schell, 2006).

Compare the systolic and diastolic readings with the standard blood pressure values by age, sex, and height percentile in Appendix B ∞. Use the child's height percentile for age and sex from the standard growth curves to determine the expected blood pressure for the child. A blood pressure value at the 50th percentile for the child's age, sex, and height is considered the midpoint of the normal range. A reading above the 95th percentile indicates hypertension.

Nursing Alert

In any child in which there is a concern about a heart condition, obtain a blood pressure reading in both an arm and a leg and compare the readings. The blood pressure in the leg should be the same or up to 10 mmHg higher than the arm reading. If the reading in the leg is lower than the arm, coarctation of the aorta may be present.

Other Signs

To assess the heart and tissue perfusion, consider other signs, including skin color, capillary refill, and respiratory distress. The mucous membranes are usually pink. Cyanosis is most commonly associated with a congenital heart defect in children. Capillary refill is normally less than 2 seconds, indicating good circulation and perfusion of the tissues. Signs of respiratory distress, such as tachypnea, flaring, and retractions, may be associated with the child's attempts to compensate for hypoxemia caused by a congenital heart defect.

■ ASSESSING THE ABDOMEN FOR SHAPE, BOWEL SOUNDS, AND UNDERLYING ORGANS

What does a sunken abdomen indicate? How frequently should bowel sounds be heard in children? What do the various percussion tones indicate? What does a rigid abdomen indicate?

Topographic Landmarks of the Abdomen

The location of underlying organs and structures of the abdomen must be considered when the abdomen is examined. The abdomen is commonly divided by imaginary lines into quadrants for the purpose of identifying underlying structures (Figure 5–36 ➤).

Clinical Tip

Perform inspection and auscultation before palpation and percussion because touching the abdomen may change the characteristics of bowel sounds.

Equipment Needed

Stethoscope

Inspection of the Abdomen

Begin the examination of the abdomen by inspecting the shape and contour, condition of the umbilicus and rectus muscle, and abdominal movement. Inspect the child's abdomen from the front and side with good lighting. Note any creases, striae, or scars.

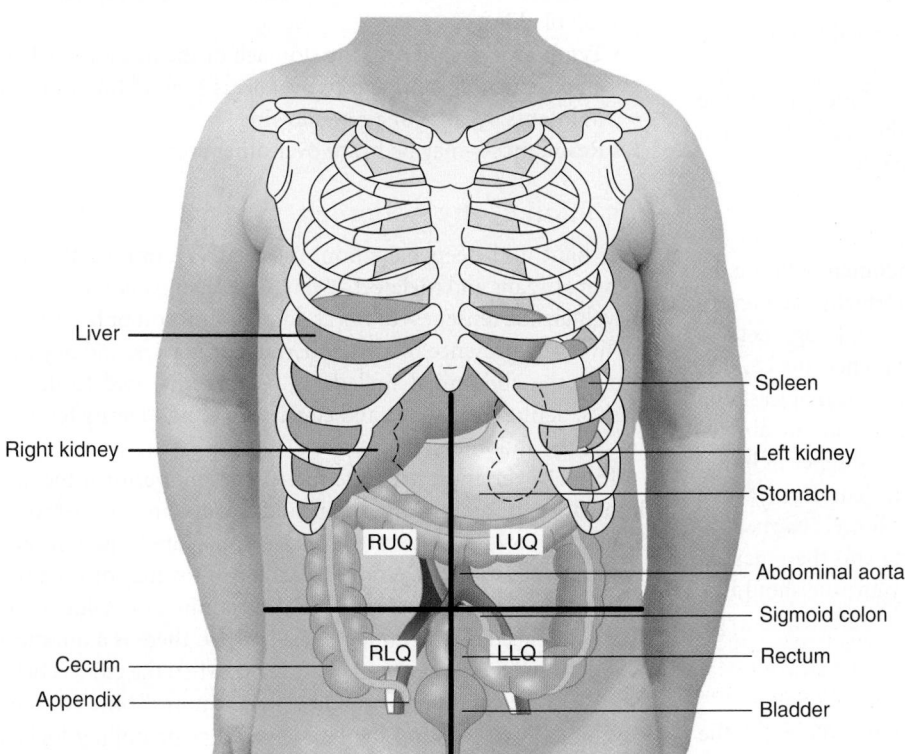

FIGURE 5–36 ➤ Topographic landmarks of the abdomen. The abdomen is commonly divided by imaginary lines into quadrants for the purposes of identifying underlying structures.

Shape

Inspect the shape of the abdomen to identify an abnormal contour. The child's abdomen is normally symmetric and rounded or flat when the child is supine. A scaphoid or sunken abdomen is abnormal and may indicate dehydration.

Umbilicus

Observe the newborn's umbilical stump for color, bleeding, odor, and drainage. The stump becomes black, dry, and hard within a couple of days after birth. The stump normally falls off between 7 and 14 days after birth. After the stump falls off, inspect the umbilicus for complete healing. Continued drainage may indicate an infection or a granuloma.

Inspect the umbilicus in older infants and toddlers. Children in these age groups often have an umbilical hernia, a protrusion of abdominal contents through an open umbilical muscle ring.

Rectus Muscle

Inspect the abdominal wall for any depression or bulging at midline above or below the umbilicus, indicating separation of the rectus abdominis muscles. The depression may be up to 5 cm (2 in.) wide. Measure the width of the separation to monitor change over time. As abdominal muscle strength develops, the separation usually becomes less prominent. However, the splitting may persist if congenital muscle weakness is present.

Abdominal Movement

Infants and children up to 6 years of age breathe with the diaphragm. The abdomen rises with inspiration and falls with expiration, simultaneously with the chest rise and fall. When the abdomen does not rise as expected, peritonitis may be present.

Other abdominal movements such as peristaltic waves are abnormal. *Peristaltic waves* are visible rhythmic contractions of the intestinal wall smooth muscle, which move food through the digestive tract. Their presence generally indicates an intestinal obstruction, such as pyloric stenosis (see Chapter 25 ∞).

Auscultation of the Abdomen

To evaluate bowel sounds, auscultate the abdomen with the diaphragm of the stethoscope. Bowel sounds normally occur every 10 to 30 seconds. They have a high-pitched, tinkling, metallic quality. Loud gurgling (*borborygmi*) is heard when the child is hungry. Listen in each quadrant long enough to hear at least one bowel sound. Before determining that bowel sounds are absent, auscultate at least 5 minutes in each quadrant. Absence of bowel sounds may indicate peritonitis or a paralytic ileus. Hyperactive bowel sounds may indicate gastroenteritis or a bowel obstruction.

Next auscultate over the abdominal aorta and the renal arteries for a vascular hum or murmur. No murmur should be heard. A murmur may indicate a narrowed or defective artery.

Percussion of the Abdomen

Use indirect percussion when the child is supine to identify the borders of the liver, spleen, bladder, and any masses. To perform

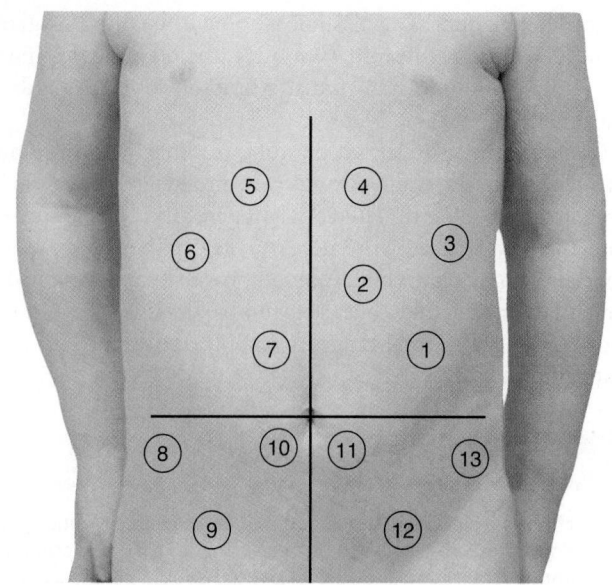

FIGURE 5–37 ➤ Sequence for indirect percussion of the abdomen.

indirect percussion, lay your middle finger of the nondominant hand on the child's abdomen. Keep your other fingers off the abdomen. With a spring-like motion, use the fingertip of the other hand to tap the finger in contact with the abdomen. Choose a sequence to systematically percuss the entire abdomen (Figure 5–37 ➤).

Different tones are expected when the abdomen is percussed related to the underlying structures. The expected pattern of percussion tones over the abdomen is as follows:

- **Dullness**—found over organs such as the liver, spleen, and full bladder
- **Tympany**—found over the stomach or the intestines when an obstruction is present or over areas beyond the stomach in infants because of air swallowing
- **Resonance**—may be heard over other areas

Palpation of the Abdomen

Both light and deep palpation are used to examine the abdomen's organs and to detect any masses. *Light palpation* is used to evaluate the tenseness of the abdomen (how soft or hard it is), the liver, the presence of any tenderness or masses, and any defects in the abdominal wall. *Deep palpation* is used to detect masses, define their shape and consistency, and identify tenderness in the abdomen.

To make the most accurate interpretation, perform the abdominal examination when the child is calm and cooperative. Organs and other masses are more easily palpated when the abdominal wall is relaxed. A bottle, pacifier, or toy may distract the child and improve cooperation for the examination. Older children often need distraction, especially when there is a question of abdominal tenderness and guarding or when the child is ticklish. Have the child perform a task that requires some concentration, such as pressing the hands together or pulling locked hands apart.

Use suggestive words to help the child relax so you can palpate the abdomen. "How soft will your tummy get when my hand feels it? Does it get softer than this? Yes. See, it softens as you breathe out. Will it also be softer here?" In this way, the child learns to relax the abdomen and is challenged to do it better.

To begin palpation, position the child supine with knees flexed. Infants and toddlers often feel more secure lying supine across both the parent's and the examiner's laps. Stand beside the child and place warmed fingertips across the child's abdomen. Palpate with the edge of the fingers, not just the fingerpads, and palpate in a sequence to examine the entire abdomen. Watch the child's face during palpation for a grimace or constriction of the pupils, which indicates pain.

Clinical Tip

When children are ticklish, some special approaches are needed to gain their cooperation. Use a firm touch and do not pretend to tickle the child at any point in the examination. Alternatively, put the child's hand on the abdomen and place your hand over the child's. Let your fingertips slide over to touch the abdomen. The child has a sense of being in control, and you may be able to palpate directly.

Light Palpation

For light palpation, use a superficial, gentle touch that slightly depresses the abdomen. Usually the abdomen feels soft and no tenderness is detected. Palpate any bulging along the abdominal wall, especially along the rectus muscle and umbilical ring. If an umbilical hernia is present, measure the diameter of the muscle ring, rather than the protrusion. The muscle ring normally becomes smaller and closes by 4 years of age.

To palpate the lower liver edge, place the fingerpads in the right midclavicular line at the level of the umbilicus. Lightly palpate and move the fingers toward the costal margin with each expiration. As the liver edge descends with inspiration, a flat, narrow ridge is usually felt. Measure the distance of the liver edge from the right costal margin at the right midclavicular line. The liver edge is normally palpated 2 to 3 cm (1 in.) below the right costal margin in infants and toddlers, but it may not be palpable in older children. If the liver edge is more than 3 cm (1 in.) below the right costal margin, the liver is enlarged, possibly due to congestive heart failure or hepatic disease.

Deep Palpation

To perform deep palpation, press the fingers of one hand (for small children) or two hands (for older children) more deeply into the abdomen. Because the abdominal muscles are most relaxed when the child takes a deep breath, ask the child to take regular deep breaths when palpating each area of the abdomen. The spleen tip may be felt at the left costal margin in the midclavicular line when the child takes a deep breath. If the spleen is more easily palpated below the left costal margin, it is enlarged. The kidneys are in a deep layer of abdominal muscles and

intestines, and thus are rarely palpated except in newborns. If a kidney is actually palpated, an abnormal mass may be present.

Nursing Alert

If an enlarged kidney or mass is detected, do not continue to palpate. Pressure on the mass may release cancerous cells.

Occasionally other masses, both normal and abnormal, can be palpated in the abdomen. A tubular mass commonly palpated in the lower left or right quadrant is often an intestine filled with feces. A distended bladder is often palpated as a firm, central, dome-shaped mass above the symphysis pubis in young children. Any fixed mass that moves laterally, pulsates, or is located along the vertebral column may be a neoplasm.

Assessment of the Inguinal Area

The inguinal area is inspected and palpated during the abdominal examination to detect enlarged lymph nodes or masses. The femoral pulse, a part of the heart examination, may be assessed simultaneously with the abdominal examination.

Inspection

Inspect the inguinal area for any change in contour, comparing sides. A small bulge noted over the femoral canal in girls may be associated with a femoral hernia. A bulging in the inguinal area in boys may be associated with an inguinal hernia.

Palpation

Palpate the inguinal area for lymph nodes and other masses. Small lymph nodes, less than 1 cm (1/2 in.) in diameter, are often present in the inguinal area because of minor injuries on the legs. Any tenderness, heat, or inflammation in these palpated lymph nodes could be associated with a local infection.

■ ASSESSING THE GENITAL AND PERINEAL AREAS FOR EXTERNAL STRUCTURAL ABNORMALITIES

What can a vaginal discharge indicate in a preadolescent girl? Is swelling in a newborn's scrotum normal? Where should the urethral meatus be located on the penis?

Equipment Needed

Gloves
Lubricant
Penlight

Preparation of Children for the Examination

Examination of the genitalia and perineal area can cause stress in children because they sense their privacy has been invaded. To make young children feel more secure, position them on the parent's lap with their legs spread apart. Children can also be positioned on the examining table with their knees flexed and the legs spread apart like a frog.

In younger children the genital and perineal examination is performed immediately after assessment of the abdomen. The genitals and perineum may be examined last in older children and adolescents.

Female Genitalia

Inspection

Inspect the external genitalia of girls for color, size, and symmetry of the mons pubis, labia, urethra, and vaginal opening (Figure 5–38 ➤). At that time, determine the stage of pubertal maturation. Simultaneously, look for any abnormal findings such as swelling, inflammation, masses, lacerations, or discharge.

Clinical Tip

Preschool-age children are often taught that strangers are not permitted to touch their "private parts." When a child this age actively resists examination of the genital area, ask the parent to tell the child you have permission to look at and touch these parts of the body. Some children develop modesty during the preschool period. Briefly explain what you need to examine and why. Then calmly and efficiently examine the child.

Mons Pubis   Inspect the mons pubis for pubic hair and its characteristics. Preadolescent girls have no pubic hair. See page 149 for guidelines to assess the stage of pubic hair development.

Labia   The labia minora are usually thin and pale in preadolescent girls but become dark pink and moist after puberty. In young infants the labia minora may be fused and cover the structures in the vestibule. These adhesions often need to be separated.

Hymen   Use the thumb and forefinger of one gloved hand to separate the labia minora for viewing structures in the vestibule. The hymen is just inside the vaginal opening. In preadolescents

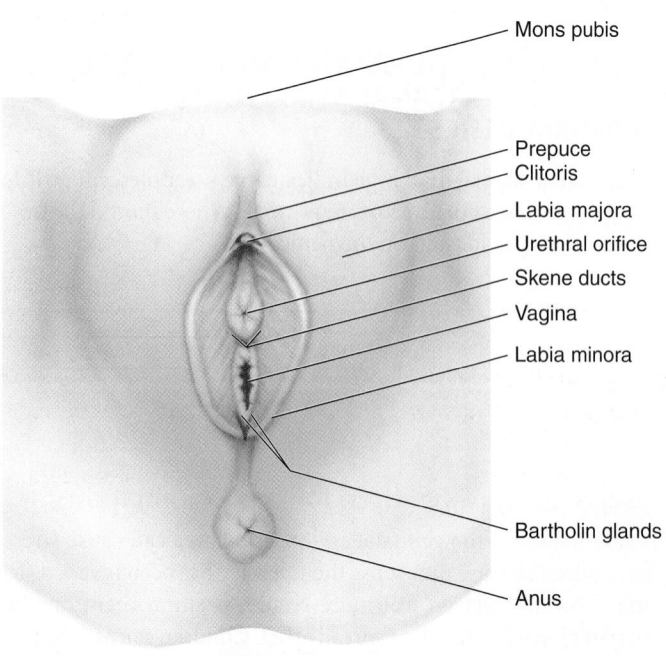

- Mons pubis
- Prepuce
- Clitoris
- Labia majora
- Urethral orifice
- Skene ducts
- Vagina
- Labia minora
- Bartholin glands
- Anus

FIGURE 5–38 ➤ Anatomic structures of the female genital and perineal area.

Growth & Development *Genital Structure*

The full-term newborn's external genital structures are strongly influenced by maternal hormones. The labia majora are swollen and the labia minora may be more prominent. The clitoris is usually covered by the labia. A white mucoid vaginal discharge, sometimes mixed with blood, may be seen for a couple of weeks after birth (Seidel et al., 2010). As the hormonal influence decreases over a few weeks, these structures attain normal size.

it is usually a thin membrane with a crescent-shaped opening. The vaginal opening is usually about 1 cm (1/2 in.) in adolescents when the hymen is intact. Sexually active adolescents may have a vaginal opening with irregular edges.

Urethral and Vaginal Openings   Inspect the vestibule for lesions. No lesions or signs of inflammation are expected around the urethral or vaginal opening. Redness and excoriation are often associated with an irritant such as bubble bath.

Vaginal Discharge   Preadolescent girls do not normally have a vaginal discharge. Adolescents often have a clear discharge without a foul odor. Menses generally begin approximately 2 years after breast-bud development. A foul-smelling discharge in preschool-age children may be associated with a foreign body. Various organisms may cause a vaginal infection in older children.

Nursing Alert

Signs of sexual abuse in young children include bruising or swelling of the vulva, foul-smelling vaginal discharge, enlarged opening of the vagina, and rash or sores in the perineal area.

An internal vaginal examination is indicated when abnormal findings, such as a vaginal discharge or trauma to the external structures, are noted. Only an experienced examiner should perform the vaginal examination of the child.

Palpation

Palpate the vaginal opening with a finger of your free gloved hand. The Bartholin and Skene glands are not usually palpable. Palpation of these glands in preadolescent children indicates enlargement because of an infection such as gonorrhea.

Male Genitalia

Inspection

Inspect the male genitalia for the structural and pubertal development of the penis, scrotum, and testicles. Place boys in the tailor position, seated with their legs crossed in front of them. This position puts pressure on the abdominal wall to push the testicles into the scrotum. See page 149 for guidelines to assess the staging of pubic hair and external genital development.

Penis   Inspect the penis for size, foreskin, hygiene, and position of the urethral meatus. The length of the nonerect penis in the newborn is normally 2 to 3 cm (1 in.). The penis enlarges in length and breadth during puberty. The penis is normally

Growth & Development *Foreskin Separation*

The foreskin is usually not completely separated from the glans at birth. Separation is normally completed by 3 to 6 years of age. A foreskin opening large enough for a good urinary stream is normal, even when the foreskin does not fully retract.

straight. A downward bowing of the penis may be caused by a *chordee*, a fibrous band of tissue associated with hypospadias.

When the penis is circumcised, the glans penis is exposed. To inspect the glans penis of an uncircumcised boy, ask the child or parent to pull the foreskin back. Alternatively, the examiner may retract the foreskin. The foreskin of children over 6 years of age normally retracts past the corona easily. If the foreskin is tight and cannot be retracted, phimosis is present.

Nursing Alert

When the boy's foreskin does not easily retract, do not forcefully pull it back. Force may result in torn tissues that heal with adhesions between the foreskin and the glans (Horner, 2007). Preputial adhesions are normal in infants and young boys, and usually resolve on their own.

The glans penis is normally clean and smooth without inflammation or ulceration. The urethral meatus is a slit-shaped opening near the tip of the glans. No discharge should be present. A round, pinpoint urethral meatus may indicate meatal stenosis. Location of the urethral meatus at another site on the penis is abnormal, indicating *hypospadias* (meatus is located on the ventral or undersurface of the penile shaft between the perineum to the tip of the glans) or *epispadias* (meatus is located on the dorsal surface of the penile shaft) (see Chapter 26 ∞). Inspect the urinary stream. The stream is normally strong without dribbling. Erythema and edema of the glans (balanitis) may result from infection or trauma. In the uncircumcised penis, purulent discharge and an edematous foreskin may be seen.

Scrotum Inspect the scrotum for size, symmetry, presence of the testicles, and any abnormalities. The scrotum is normally loose and pendulous with rugae, or wrinkles. The scrotum of infants often appears large in comparison to the penis. A small, undeveloped scrotum that has no rugae indicates that the testicles are undescended. Enlargement or swelling of the scrotum is abnormal. It may indicate an inguinal hernia, hydrocele, torsion of the spermatic cord, or testicular inflammation. A deep cleft in the scrotum may indicate ambiguous genitalia.

Palpation

Make sure your hands are warm and have the boy sit with legs crossed to avoid stimulating the cremasteric reflex that causes the testicles to retract. Palpate the shaft of the penis for nodules and masses. None should be present.

Testicles Palpate the scrotum for the presence of the testicles. Place your index finger and thumb over both inguinal canals on each side of the penis to keep the testicles from retracting into the abdomen (Figure 5–39 ➤).

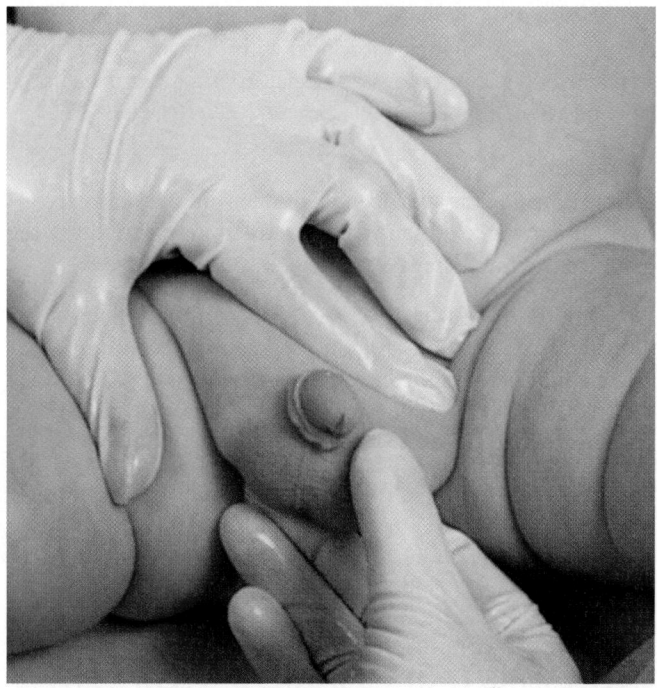

FIGURE 5–39 ➤ Palpating the scrotum for descended testicles and spermatic cords. Note the position of the index finger over the inguinal canal.

Gently palpate each testicle with only enough pressure to identify the shape and size. The testicles are normally smooth and equal in size. They are approximately 1 to 1.5 cm (1/2 in.) in diameter until puberty, when they increase in size. A hard, enlarged, painless testicle may indicate a tumor.

If a testicle is not palpated in the scrotum, the inguinal canal should be palpated for a soft mass. When the testicle is found in the inguinal canal, an experienced examiner should try to move it to the scrotum to palpate the size and shape. The testicle is descendible when it can be moved into the scrotum. An undescended testicle is one that does not descend into the scrotum or cannot be palpated in the inguinal canal.

Scrotum Palpate the length of the spermatic cord between the thumb and forefinger from the testicle to the inguinal canal. It normally feels solid and smooth. No tenderness is expected. When bulging or swelling of the scrotum is present, palpate the scrotum to identify the characteristics of the mass. Try to determine whether the mass is unilateral or bilateral and attempt to reduce the mass by pushing it back through the external inguinal ring. A mass that decreases may indicate an inguinal hernia. A mass that does not decrease may indicate a hydrocele or an incarcerated hernia. To distinguish between a hydrocele and an incarcerated hernia, place a bright penlight under the scrotum and look for a red glow or transillumination through the scrotum. A hydrocele transilluminates; a hernia does not.

Anus and Rectum

Inspection

Inspect the anus for sphincter control and any abnormal findings such as inflammation, fissures, or lesions. The external sphincter is usually closed. Inflammation and scratch marks around the anus may be associated with pinworms. A protrusion from the rectum may be associated with a rectal wall prolapse or a hemorrhoid.

Palpation

Lightly touching the anal opening should stimulate an anal contraction or "wink." Absence of a contraction may indicate the presence of a lower spinal cord lesion.

Patency of the Anus   Passage of meconium by newborns indicates a patent anus. When passage of meconium is delayed, a lubricated catheter can be inserted 1 cm (1/2 in.) into the anus. Resistance in passage of the catheter may indicate an obstruction.

Rectal Examination   A rectal examination is not routinely performed on children. It is indicated for symptoms of intra-abdominal, rectal, bowel, or stool abnormalities. Only an experienced examiner should perform a rectal examination.

■ ASSESSMENT OF PUBERTAL DEVELOPMENT AND SEXUAL MATURATION

What is the first stage of breast development in girls? What is the first stage of pubertal development in boys? How is the stage of pubertal development determined in boys and girls?

The age of onset of secondary sexual characteristics can vary with race and ethnicity, environmental conditions, geographic location, and nutrition.

Females

Inspect the child's breasts while the child is sitting. Breast development in girls usually precedes other pubertal changes; however, pubic hair may occur first, or breast development and pubic hair may occur simultaneously (Biro, Huang, Daniels, et al., 2008). Figure 5–40 ➤ shows the Tanner stages of breast development. Breast budding, usually the first stage of pubertal development, typically occurs between 8 and 14 years of age. Black girls have a significantly earlier age for the onset of puberty (reaching Tanner stage 2 for breast or pubic hair development) than White girls (Biro, Huang, Crawford, et al., 2006). A girl's breasts may develop at different rates and appear asymmetric.

The presence, amount, and distribution of pubic hair is an indication of the sexual maturation stage in the girl. Preadolescent girls have no pubic hair. Initial pubic hair is lightly pigmented, sparse, and straight. Pubic hair development progresses in consistent stages for all girls. Figure 5–41 ➤ illustrates the normal stages of female pubic hair development. The presence of pubic hair before 8 years of age is unusual.

Males

Initial signs of puberty onset in males are enlargement of the testicles and thinning of the scrotum. This is followed by straight, downy pubic hair starting at the base of the penis 6 months later. The hair becomes darker, dense, and curly, extending over the

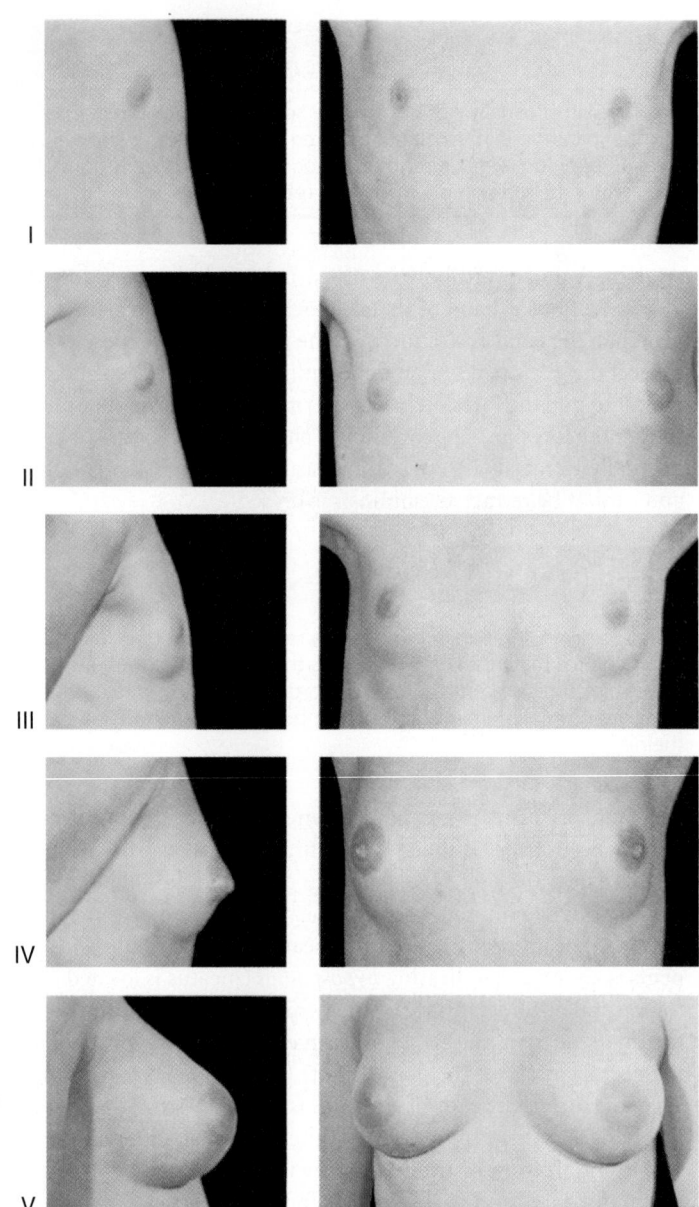

FIGURE 5–40 ➤ The Tanner stages of breast development.
Used with permission from Van Wieringen et al. (1971). Growth diagrams 1965 Netherlands. Groningen: Wolters-Noordhof.

pubic area in a diamond pattern by the completion of puberty. The presence of testicular enlargement before 9 years of age (precocious puberty) is uncommon (Kaplowitz, 2008). Delayed onset of testicular enlargement after 14 years of age needs evaluation. Penile enlargement generally follows testicular enlargement about 1 year later in genitalia Tanner stage 3. Stages of pubic hair development follow a standard pattern, as seen in Figure 5–42 ➤.

Sexual Maturity Rating

The sexual maturity rating (SMR) is an average of the breast and pubic hair Tanner stages in females and of the genital and pubic hair Tanner stages in males. The rating is the number between 2 and 5, as stage 1 is prepubertal. The SMR is then related to other

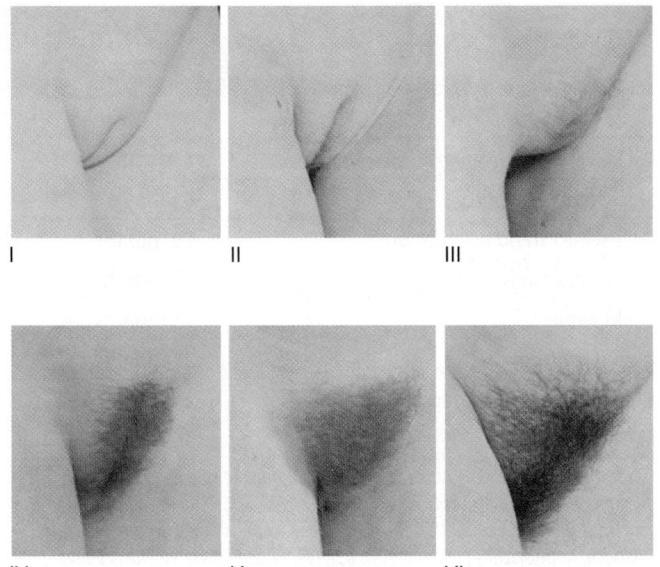

I II III

IV V VI

FIGURE 5–41 ➤ The Tanner stages of female pubic hair development with sexual maturation. In stage 2, soft downy hair along the labia majora is an indication that sexual maturation is beginning. Hair grows progressively coarse and curly as development proceeds.

Used with permission from Van Wieringen et al. (1971). Growth diagrams 1965 Netherlands. Groningen: Wolters-Noordhof.

physiologic events that happen during puberty. Compare the stage of the child's secondary sexual characteristics with information in Figure 5–43 ➤.

In females, menarche generally occurs in SMR 4 or breast stage 3 to 4. The peak height velocity usually occurs before menarche at a mean age of 11.5 years. In males, ejaculation usually occurs at SMR 3, with semen noted between SMR 3 and 4. The peak height velocity usually occurs in SMR 4 or genital stage 4 to 5, at about 13.5 years of age.

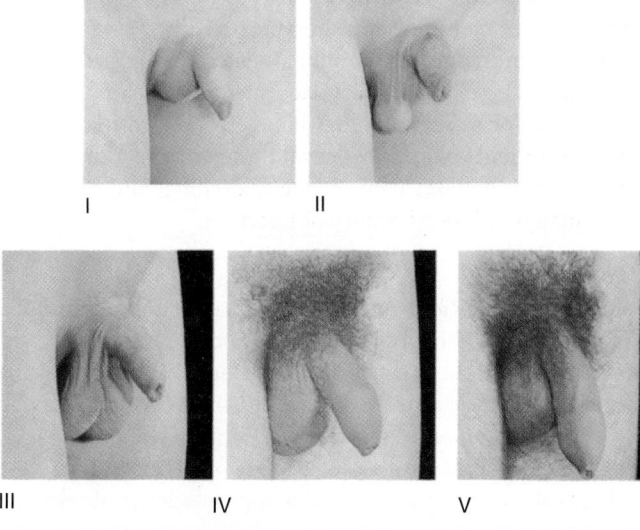

I II

III IV V

FIGURE 5–42 ➤ The Tanner stages of male pubic hair and external genital development with sexual maturation.

Used with permission from Van Wieringen et al. (1971). Growth diagrams 1965 Netherlands. Groningen: Wolters-Noordhof.

■ ASSESSING THE MUSCULOSKELETAL SYSTEM FOR BONE AND JOINT STRUCTURE, MOVEMENT, AND MUSCLE STRENGTH

What do extra skin folds on an arm or leg indicate? What condition does a rib hump indicate? At what age is it normal for children to be knock-kneed or bowlegged?

Bones, Muscles, and Joints

Inspection

Inspect and compare the arms and then the legs for differences in alignment, contour, skin folds, length, and deformities. The

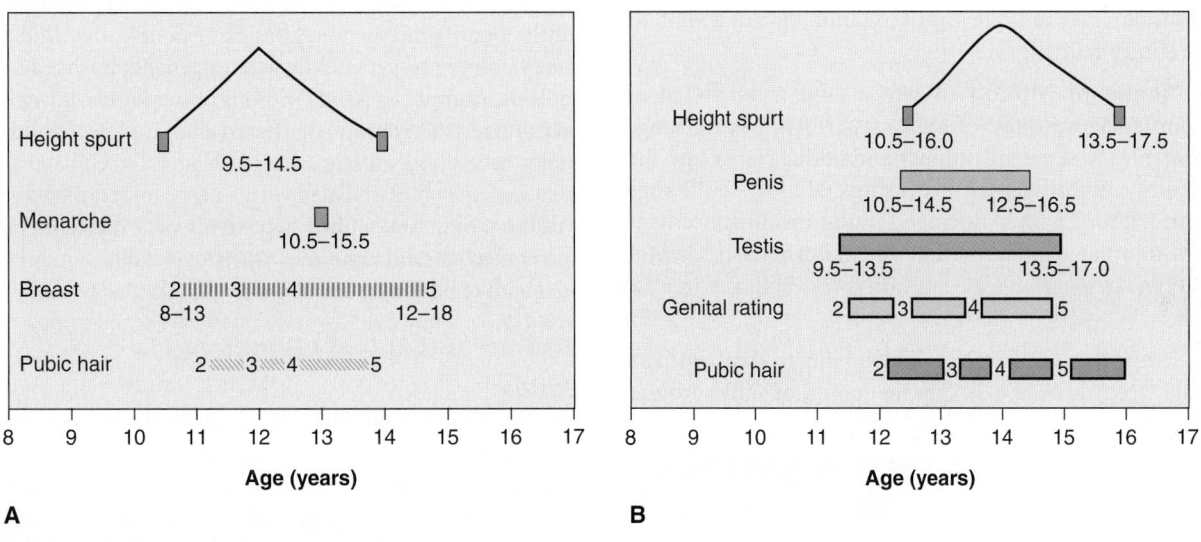

A **B**

FIGURE 5–43 ➤ Sexual maturity rating—approximate timing of developmental changes. The numbers indicate stages of development. Range of ages during which some changes occur is indicated by the inclusive numbers below them. A, Females. B, Males.

Reproduced from Archives of Disease in Childhood, Marshall, W. A., & Tanner, J. M., "Variations in Patterns of Pubertal Changes in Girls," vol. 44, p. 291; "Variations in Patterns of Pubertal Changes in Boys," vol. 45, p. 13; Copyright © 1969 with permission from BMJ Publishing Group Ltd.

extremities normally have equal length, circumference, and numbers of skin folds bilaterally. Extra skin folds and a larger circumference may indicate a shorter extremity.

Inspect and compare the joints bilaterally for size, discoloration, and ease of voluntary movement. Joints are normally the same color as surrounding skin, with no sign of swelling. Children should voluntarily flex and extend joints during normal activities without pain. Redness, swelling, and pain with movement may indicate injury or infection.

Palpation

Palpate the bones and muscles in each extremity for muscle tone, masses, or tenderness. Muscles normally feel firm, and bony masses are not normally present. Doughy muscles may indicate poor muscle tone. Rigid muscles, or hypertonia, may be associated with an active seizure or cerebral palsy. A mass over a long bone may indicate a recent fracture or a bone tumor.

Palpate each joint and surrounding muscles to detect any swelling, masses, heat, or tenderness. None is expected when the joint is palpated. Tenderness, heat, swelling, and redness can result from injury or a chronic joint inflammation such as juvenile rheumatoid arthritis.

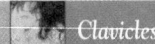

Growth & Development *Clavicles*

Palpate the clavicles of the newborn from the sternum to the shoulder. These bones are often fractured during delivery. A mass and crepitus may indicate a fracture.

Range of Motion and Muscle Strength Assessment

Active Range of Motion   Observe the child during typical play activities, such as reaching for objects, climbing, and walking, to assess range of motion of all major joints. Children spontaneously move their joints through the full normal range of motion with play activities when no pain is present. Limited range of motion may indicate injury, inflammation of a joint, or a muscle abnormality.

Passive Range of Motion   When a joint is suspected of having limited active range of motion, perform passive range of motion. Flex and extend, abduct and adduct, or rotate the affected joint cautiously to avoid causing extra pain. Full range of motion without pain is normal. Limitations in movement may indicate injury, inflammation, or malformation. Greater passive than active range of motion may indicate muscle weakness.

Muscle Strength   Observe the child's ability to climb onto an examining table, throw a ball, clap the hands, or move around

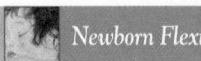

Growth & Development *Newborn Flexion*

Newborns typically have a limited extension of the hips, knees, and elbows, resulting from their flexed fetal position. When the newborn's arms and legs are extended and released, the extremities rapidly return to their flexed fetal position.

TABLE 5–11   Selected Gross Motor Milestones for Age

Gross Motor Milestones	Age Attained
Rolls over from prone to supine position	7 months
Sits without support	6 months
Pulls self to standing position	10 months
Creeps or crawls	10 months
Walks alone	15 months
Climbs on furniture	24 months
Walks up stairs, one step at a time	24 months
Rides tricycle	36 months

Data from: Zitelli, B. J., & Davis, H. W. (2007). Atlas of pediatric physical diagnosis (5th ed.). St. Louis, MO: Elsevier Mosby; Feigelman, S. (2007a). The first year. In R. M. Kliegman, R. E. Behrman, H. B. Jenson, & B. F. Stanton, Nelson textbook of pediatrics (18th ed., pp. 43–48). Philadelphia: Saunders Elsevier; Feigelman, S. (2007b). The second year. In R. M. Kliegman, R. E. Behrman, H. B. Jenson, & B. F. Stanton, Nelson textbook of pediatrics (18th ed., pp. 48–54). Philadelphia: Saunders Elsevier.

on the bed. The child's ability to perform age-appropriate play activities indicates good muscle tone and strength. Attainment of age-appropriate motor development is another indicator of good muscle strength (Table 5–11).

Clinical Tip

To check the shoulder muscle strength in a newborn, hold the infant upright with your hands under the infant's arms. An infant who is held lightly will normally not slip through the hands. Muscle weakness is present when the infant slides through the hands (Seidel et al., 2010).

To assess the strength of specific muscles in the extremities, engage the child in some games. Compare muscle strength bilaterally to identify muscle weakness. For example, the child squeezes the examiner's fingers tightly with each hand; pushes against and pulls the examiner's hands with his or her hands, lower legs, and feet; and resists extension of a flexed elbow or knee. Children normally have good muscle strength bilaterally. Unilateral muscle weakness may be associated with a nerve injury. Bilateral muscle weakness may result from hypoxemia or a congenital disorder such as Down syndrome. Asymmetrical weakness may be associated with conditions such as cerebral palsy.

Posture and Spinal Alignment

Posture

Inspect the child's posture when standing from a front, side, and back view. The shoulders and hips are normally level. The head is held erect without a tilt, and the shoulder contour is symmetric. After beginning to walk, young children often have a pot-bellied stance because of lumbar lordosis. The spine has normal thoracic convex and lumbar concave curves after 6 years of age. Table 5–12 shows normal posture and spinal curvature development.

TABLE 5-12	**Normal Development of Posture and Spinal Curves**			
2–3 months	6–8 months	10–15 months	Toddler	School-age child
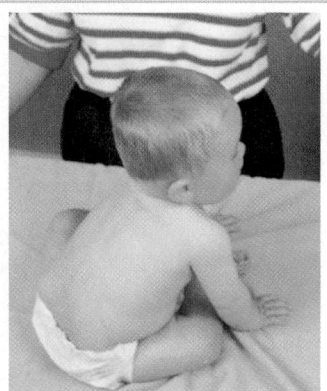	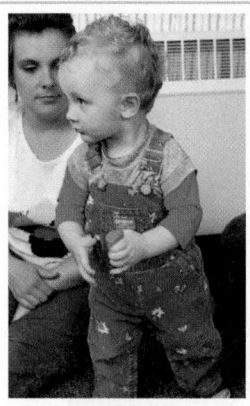	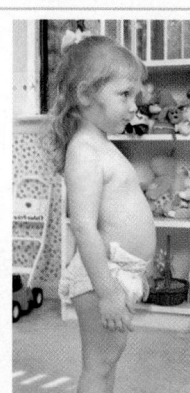	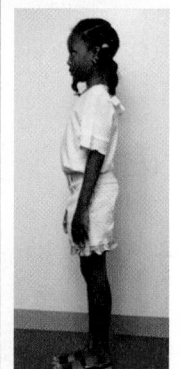	
Holds head erect when held upright; thoracic kyphosis when sitting.	Sits without support; spine is straight.	Walks independently; straight spine.	Protruding abdomen; lumbar lordosis.	Height of shoulders and hips is level; balanced thoracic convex and lumbar concave curves.

Spinal Alignment

Assess the school-age child and adolescent for *scoliosis*, a lateral spine curvature. Stand behind the child, observing the height of the shoulders and hips (Figure 5–44 ➤). Ask the child to bend forward slowly at the waist, with arms extended toward the floor. No lateral curve should be present in either position. The ribs normally stay flat bilaterally. The lumbar concave curve should flatten with forward flexion (Figure 5–45 ➤). A lateral curve to the spine or a one-sided rib hump is an indication of scoliosis (see Chapter 29 ∞).

Inspection of the Upper Extremities

Arms

The alignment of the arms is normally straight, with a minimal angle at the elbows, where the bones articulate.

Hands

Count the fingers. Extra finger digits (*polydactyly*) or webbed fingers (*syndactyly*) are abnormal. Inspect the creases on the palmar surface of each hand. Multiple creases across the palm are normal. A single transverse palmar crease that crosses the entire palm of the hand is associated with Down syndrome (Figure 5–46 ➤).

Nails

Inspect the nails for size, shape, and color. Nails are normally convex, smooth, and pink. **Clubbing**, widening of the nailbed with an increased angle between the proximal nail fold and nail, is abnormal (see Figure 21–7 ∞). Clubbing is associated with chronic respiratory and cardiac conditions.

Inspection of the Lower Extremities

Hips

Assess the hips of newborns and young infants for dislocation or subluxation. The skin folds on the upper legs are inspected first.

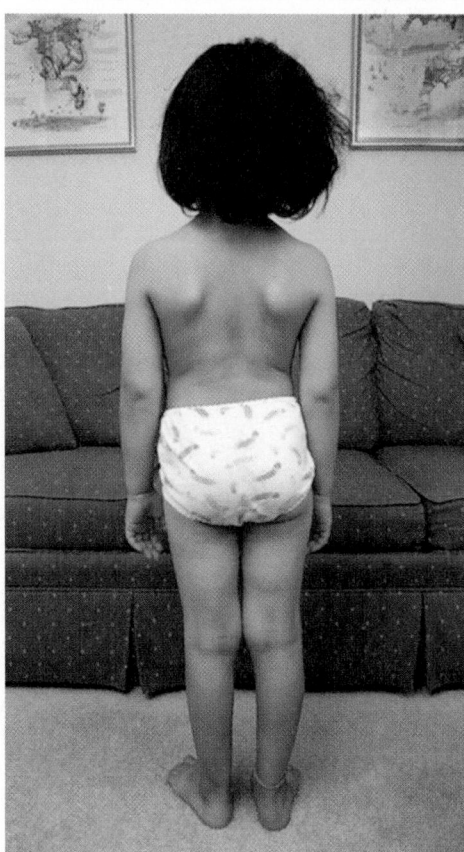

FIGURE 5–44 ➤ Does this child have legs of different lengths or scoliosis? Look at the level of the iliac crests and shoulders to see if they are level. See the more prominent crease at the waist on the right side? (This child could have scoliosis.)

The same number of skin folds should be present on each leg. Uneven skin folds may indicate a hip dislocation or difference in leg length. Then check for a difference in knee height symmetry (Allis sign) (Figure 5–47 ➤). The Ortolani–Barlow maneuver is

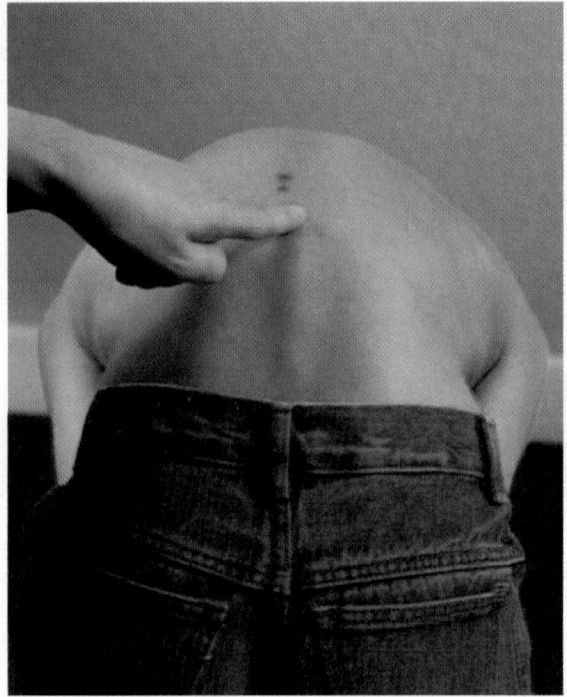

FIGURE 5–45 ➤ Inspection of the spine for scoliosis. Ask the child to slowly bend forward at the waist, with arms extended toward the floor. Run your forefinger down the spinal processes, palpating each vertebra for a change in alignment. A lateral curve to the spine or a one-sided rib hump is an indication of scoliosis.

used to assess an infant's hips for dislocation or subluxation (Figure 5–48 ➤). This maneuver should be performed by a trained health care practitioner.

Ask the child to stand on one leg and then the other. The iliac crests should stay level. If the iliac crest opposite the weight-bearing leg appears lower, the hip the child is standing on may be dislocated.

Legs

With the child standing, inspect the alignment of the legs. After a child is 4 years of age, the alignment of the long bones is straight, with minimal angle at the knees and feet where the bones articulate. Assess alignment of the lower extremities in infants and toddlers to ensure that normal changes are occurring. To evaluate the toddler with bowlegs, have the child stand on a firm surface. Measure the distance between the knees when the child's ankles are together. No more than 3.5 cm (1.5 in.) between the knees is normal. See Figure 5–49 ➤ for assessment of knock-knees.

Feet

Inspect the feet for alignment, the presence of all toes, and any deformities. The weight-bearing line of the feet is usually in alignment with the legs. Many newborns have a flexible forefoot inversion (metatarsus adductus) that results from uterine positioning. Any fixed deformity is abnormal.

Inspect the feet for the presence of an arch when the child is standing. Children up to 3 years of age normally have a fat pad

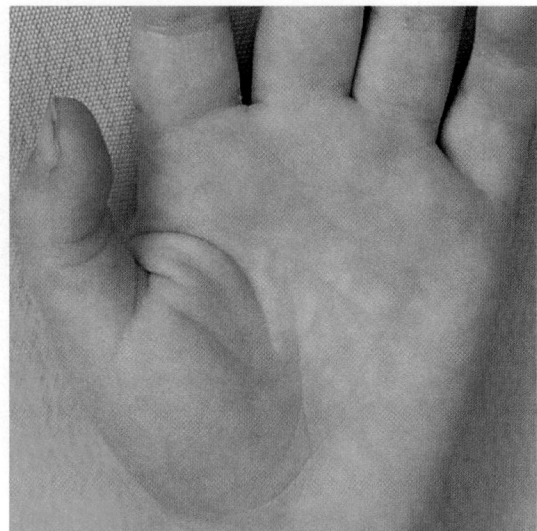

A

B

FIGURE 5–46 ➤ A, Normal palmar creases. B, Transverse palmar crease associated with Down syndrome.
Reprinted from Zitelli, B. J., & Davis, H. W. (Eds.)). Atlas of pediatric physical diagnosis (3rd ed.). St. Louis, MO: Mosby–Year Book © 1997, with permission from Elsevier.

over the arch, giving the appearance of flat feet. Older children normally have a longitudinal arch. The arch is usually seen when the child stands on tiptoe or is sitting. Inspect the nails of the feet as for the hands.

Growth & Development *Tibial Torsion*

Infants are often born with a twisting of the tibia caused by positioning in utero (tibial torsion). The infant's toes turn in as a result of the tibial torsion. Toddlers go through a skeletal alignment sequence of bowlegs (genu varum) and knock-knees (genu valgum) before the legs assume a straight alignment.

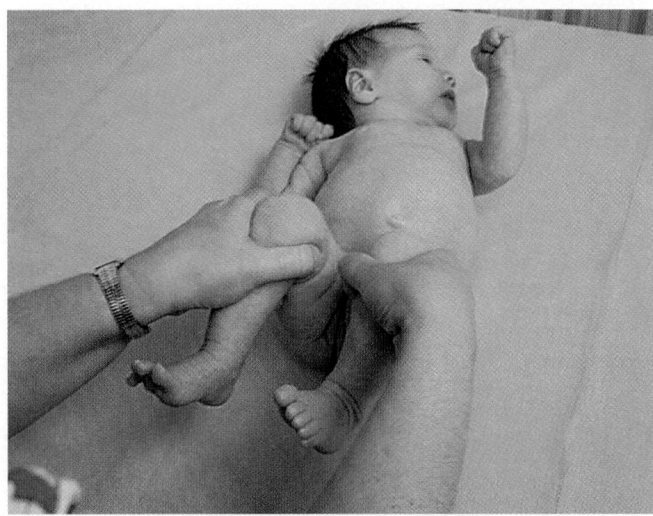

FIGURE 5–47 ➤ Flex the infant's hips and knees so the heels are as close to the buttocks as possible. Place the feet flat on the examining table. The knees are usually the same height. A difference in knee height (Allis sign) is an indicator of hip dislocation.

Courtesy of Dee Corbett, RN, Children's National Medical Center, Washington, DC.

■ ASSESSING THE NERVOUS SYSTEM FOR COGNITIVE FUNCTION, BALANCE, COORDINATION, CRANIAL NERVE FUNCTION, SENSATION, AND REFLEXES

What aspects of developmental information are useful for assessment of cognitive function? How are the infant's and child's levels of consciousness evaluated? How are cranial nerves assessed in infants? At what age does a Babinski response become abnormal?

Clinical Tip

The neurologic examination provides an opportunity to develop rapport with the child. Many of the procedures can be presented as games that young children enjoy. You can assess cognitive function by how well the child follows directions for the game. As the assessment proceeds, the child develops trust and is more likely to cooperate with examination of other systems.

Cognitive Function

Observe the child's behavior, facial expressions, gestures, communication skills, activity level, and level of consciousness to assess cognitive functioning. Match the neurologic examination to the child's stage of development. For example, cognitive function is evaluated much differently in infants than in older children because infants cannot use words to communicate.

Equipment Needed

Reflex hammer
Cotton balls
Penlight
Tongue blades

Behavior

The behavior of infants and children during the assessment indicates their alertness. Infants and toddlers are curious but seek

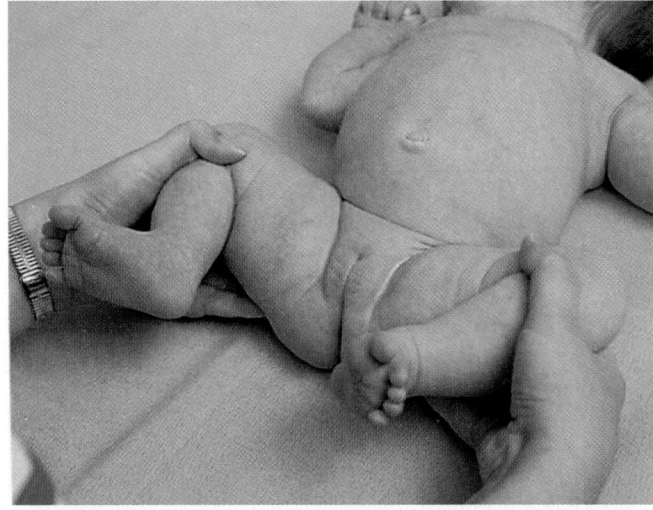

B

FIGURE 5–48 ➤ Ortolani–Barlow maneuver. A, Place the infant on his or her back and flex the hips and knees at a 90° angle. Place a hand over each knee with the thumb over the inner thigh and the first two fingers over the upper margin of the femur. Move the infant's knees together until they touch, and then put downward pressure on one femur at a time to see if the hips easily slip out of their joints or dislocate. B, Slowly abduct the hips, moving each knee toward the examining table. Keep pressure on the hip joints with the fingers in a lever-type motion. Equal hip abduction, with the knees nearly touching the examining table, is normal. Any resistance to abduction or a clunk felt on palpation can be an indication of a congenital hip dislocation.

the security of the parent, either by clinging or by making frequent eye contact. Older children are often anxious and watch all of the examiner's actions. Lack of interest in assessment or treatment procedures may indicate a serious illness. Excessive activity or an unusually short attention span may be associated with an attention deficit hyperactivity disorder.

Communication Skills

Speech, language development, and social skills provide good clues to cognitive functioning. Listen to speech articulation and

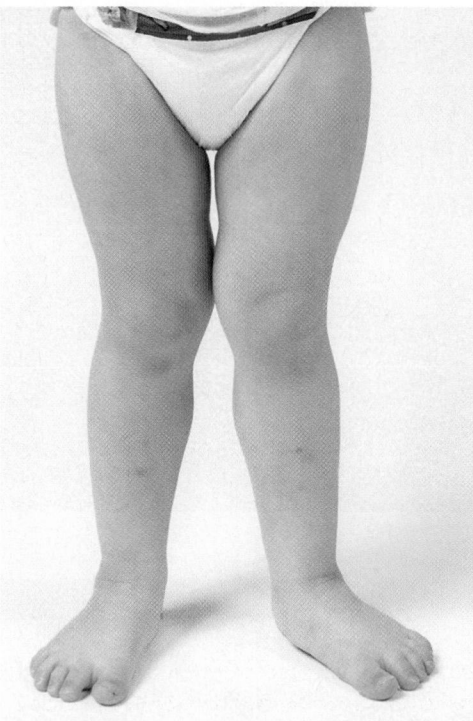

FIGURE 5–49 ➤ To evaluate the child with knock-knees, have the child stand on a firm surface. Measure the distance between the ankles when the child stands with the knees together. The normal distance is not more than 5 cm (2 in.) between the ankles.

words used, comparing the child's performance with standards of social development and speech articulation for the child's age (Table 5–13). Toddlers can normally follow simple directions such as "Show me your mouth." By 3 years of age the child's speech should be easily understood. Delay in language and social skill development may be associated with developmental disability.

Memory

Immediate, recent, and remote memory can be tested in children starting at approximately 4 years of age. To evaluate recent memory, ask the child to remember a special name or object.

Growth & Development *Memory Testing*

Test immediate memory by asking the child to repeat a series of words or numbers, such as the names of Disney or Sesame Street characters. Children can remember more words or numbers with age.

Age	Recall Ability
4 years	3 words or numbers
5 years	4 words or numbers
6 years	5 words or numbers

Then 5 to 10 minutes later during the examination, have the child recall the name or object. To evaluate remote memory, ask the child to repeat his or her address or birth date or a nursery rhyme. By 5 or 6 years of age, children are normally able to recall this information without difficulty.

Level of Consciousness

When approaching the infant or child, observe his or her level of consciousness and activity, including facial expressions, gestures, and interaction. Children are normally alert, and sleeping children arouse easily. The child who cannot be awakened is unconscious. A lowered level of consciousness may be associated with a number of neurologic conditions such as a head injury, seizure, infection, or brain tumor.

Cerebellar Function

Observe the young child at play to assess coordination and balance. Development of fine motor skills in infants and preschool children provides clues to cerebellar function.

Balance

Observe the child's balance during play activities such as walking, standing on one foot, and hopping (Table 5–14). The Romberg procedure can also be used to test balance in children over 3 years of age (Figure 5–50 ➤). Once balance and other motor skills are attained, children do not normally stumble or fall when tested. Poor balance may indicate cerebellar dysfunction or an inner ear disturbance.

TABLE 5–13 Expected Language Development for Age

Language Milestones	Age Attained
Babbles speech-like sounds, including *p, b,* and *m.*	3–4 months
Says 1 to 2 words like "mama," "dada," and "bye-bye."	12 months
Increases words each month, 2-word combinations (e.g., "Where baby?" and "Want cookie").	1–2 years
Uses 2- to 3-word sentences to ask for things or talk about things, large vocabulary, speech understood by family members.	2–3 years
Sentences may have 4 or more words, speech understood by most people.	3–4 years
Says most sounds correctly except a few like *l, s, r, v, z, ch, sh,* and *th.* Tells stories and uses same grammar as rest of family.	4–5 years

Data from: American Speech and Language Association. (2009). How does your child hear and talk? Retrieved from
http://www.asha.org/public/speech/development/chart.htm

TABLE 5–14	Expected Balance Development for Age
Balance Milestones	Age Attained
Stands without support briefly	12 months
Walks alone well	15 months
Walks backward	2 years
Balances on 1 foot for 5 seconds	4 years
Hops on 1 foot, heel-toe walking	5 years
Heel-toe walking backward	6 years

TABLE 5–15	Expected Fine Motor Development for Age
Fine Motor Milestones	Age Attained
Transfers objects between hands	5–6 months
Thumb finger pincer grasp	10 months
Feeds self with spoon	15 months
Scribbles with crayon or pencil	18 months
Builds two-block tower	18 months
Builds six-block tower	24 months

Data from: Zitelli, B. J., & Davis, H. W. (2007). Atlas of pediatric physical diagnosis (5th ed.). St. Louis, MO: Elsevier Mosby; Feigelman, S. (2007a). The first year. In R. M. Kliegman, R. E. Behrman, H. B. Jenson, & B. F. Stanton, Nelson textbook of pediatrics (18th ed., pp. 43–48). Philadelphia: Saunders Elsevier; Feigelman, S. (2007b). The second year. In R. M. Kliegman, R. E. Behrman, H. B. Jenson, & B. F. Stanton, Nelson textbook of pediatrics (18th ed., pp. 48–54). Philadelphia: Saunders Elsevier.

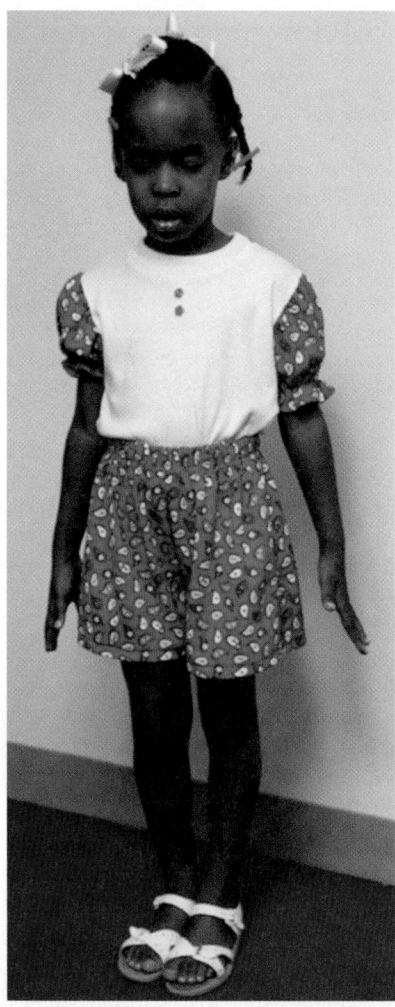

FIGURE 5–50 ➤ Romberg procedure. Ask the child to stand with feet together and eyes closed. Protect the child from falling by standing close. Preschool-age children may extend their arms to maintain balance, but older children can normally stand with their arms at their sides. Leaning or falling to one side is abnormal and indicates poor balance.

Coordination

Tests of coordination assess the smoothness and accuracy of movement. Development of fine motor skills can be used to assess coordination in young children (Table 5–15). After 6 years of age the tests for adults (finger-to-nose, finger-to-finger, heel-to-shin, and alternating motion) can be used (Figure 5–51 ➤). The child usually responds enthusiastically when these tests are presented as games. Jerky movements or inaccurate pointing (past pointing) indicate poor coordination, which can be associated with delayed development or a cerebellar lesion.

Gait

A normal gait requires intact bones and joints, muscle strength, coordination, and balance. Inspect the child when walking from both a front and a rear view. The iliac crests are normally level during walking, and no limp is expected. A limp may indicate injury or joint disease. Staggering or falling may indicate cerebellar ataxia. *Scissoring*, in which the thighs tend to cross forward over each other with each step, may be associated with cerebral palsy or other spastic conditions. Persistent walking on the toes may indicate a possible neurologic dysfunction.

Growth & Development 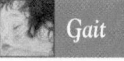 *Gait*

Gait is related to the motor development of the child. Toddlers beginning to walk have a wide-based gait and limited balance. With practice the toddler's balance improves and the gait develops a narrower base.

Cranial Nerve Function

To assess the cranial nerves in infants and young children, modify the procedures used to assess school-age children and adults (Table 5–16). Abnormalities of cranial nerves may be associated with compression of an individual nerve, head injury, or infections.

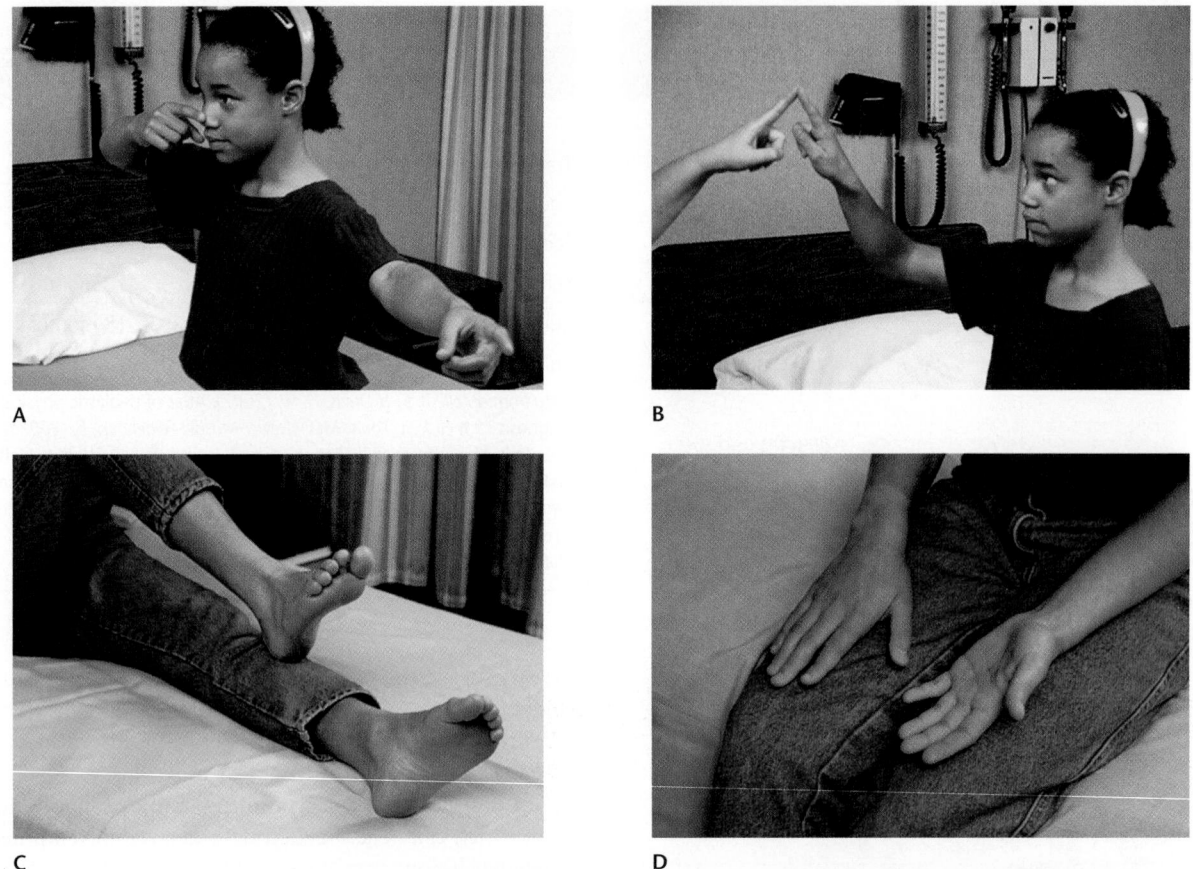

FIGURE 5–51 ➤ Tests of coordination. A, Finger-to-nose test. Ask the child to close the eyes and touch his or her nose, alternating the index fingers of the hands. B, Finger-to-finger test. Ask the child to alternately touch his or her nose and your index finger with his or her index finger. Move your hand to several positions within the child's reach to test pointing accuracy. Repeat the test with the child's other hand. C, Heel-to-shin test. Ask the child to rub his or her leg from the knee to the ankle with the heel of the other foot. Repeat the test with the other foot. This test is normally performed without hesitation or inappropriate placement of the foot. D, Rapid alternating motion test. Ask the child to rapidly rotate his or her wrist so the palm and dorsum of the hand alternately pat the thigh. Repeat the test with the other hand. Hesitating movements are abnormal. Mirroring movements of the hand not being tested indicate a delay in coordination skill refinement.

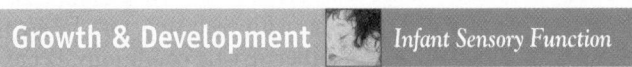
Growth & Development · *Infant Sensory Function*

An infant's sensory function is not routinely assessed. Withdrawal responses to painful procedures indicate normal sensory function.

Sensory Function

To assess sensory function, compare the responses of the body to various types of stimulation. Bilaterally equal responses are normal. Loss of sensation may indicate a brain or spinal cord lesion.

Superficial Tactile Sensation

Stroke the skin on the lower leg or arm with a cotton ball or a finger while the child's eyes are closed. Cooperative children over 2 years of age can normally point to the location touched.

Superficial Pain Sensation

Break a tongue blade to get a sharp point. After asking the child to close the eyes, touch the child in various places on each arm and leg, alternating the sharp and rounded ends of the tongue blade. A paper clip may also be used. Children over 4 years of age can normally distinguish between a sharp and dull sensation each time. To improve the child's accuracy with the test, let the child practice telling you the difference between the sharp and dull stimulation.

An inability to identify superficial touch and pain sensation may indicate sensory loss. Identify the extent of sensory loss, such as all areas below the knee. Other sensory function tests (temperature, vibratory, deep pressure pain, and position sense) are performed when sensory loss is found. Refer to other texts for a description of these procedures.

■ INFANT PRIMITIVE REFLEXES

Evaluate the movement and posture of newborns and young infants by the Moro, palmar grasp, plantar grasp, placing, stepping, and tonic neck primitive reflexes (Table 5–17). These reflexes appear and disappear at expected intervals in the first few months of life as the central nervous system develops. Movements are normally equal bilaterally. An asymmetric response may indicate a serious neurologic problem on the less responsive side.

TABLE 5–16	Age-Specific Procedures for Assessment of Cranial Nerves in Infants and Children
Cranial Nerve[a]	Assessment Procedure and Normal Findings[b]
I. Olfactory	Infant: Not tested. Child: Not routinely tested. Give familiar odors to child to smell, one naris at a time. *Identifies odors such as orange, peanut butter, and chocolate.*
II. Optic	Infant: Shine a bright light in the eyes. *A quick blink reflex and dorsal head flexion indicates light perception.* Child: Test vision and visual fields if cooperative. *Visual acuity appropriate for age.*
III. Oculomotor IV. Trochlear VI. Abducens	Infant: Shine a penlight at the eyes and move it side to side. *Focuses on and tracks the light to each side.* Child: Move an object through the six cardinal points of gaze. *Tracks object through all fields of gaze.* All ages: Inspect eyelids for drooping. Inspect pupillary response to light. *Eyelids do not droop and pupils are equal sized and briskly respond to light.*
V. Trigeminal	Infant: Stimulate the rooting and sucking reflex. *Turns head toward stimulation at side of mouth (if hungry) and sucking has good strength and pattern.* Child: Observe the child chewing a cracker. Touch forehead and cheeks with a cotton ball when eyes are closed. *Bilateral jaw strength is good. Child pushes cotton ball away.*
VII. Facial	All ages: Observe facial expressions when crying, smiling, frowning, etc. *Facial features stay symmetric bilaterally.*
VIII. Acoustic	Infant: Produce a loud sound near the head. *Blinks in response to sound, moves head toward sound or freezes position.* Child: Use a noisemaker near each ear or whisper words to be repeated. *Turns head toward sound and repeats words correctly.*
IX. Glossopharyngeal X. Vagus	Infant: Observe swallowing during feeding. *Good swallowing pattern.* All ages: Elicit gag reflex (not routinely tested). *Gags with stimulation.*
XI. Spinal accessory	Infant: Not tested. Child: Ask child to raise the shoulders and turn the head side to side against resistance. *Good strength in neck and shoulders.*
XII. Hypoglossal	Infant: Observe feeding. *Sucking and swallowing are coordinated.* Child: Tell the child to stick out the tongue. Listen to speech. *Tongue is midline with no tremors. Words are clearly articulated.*

[a]*Bracketed nerves are tested together.*
[b]*Italic indicates normal findings.*

Superficial and Deep Tendon Reflexes

Evaluate the superficial and deep tendon reflexes to assess the function of specific segments of the spine.

Superficial Reflexes

Assess superficial reflexes by stroking a specific area of the body. The plantar reflex, testing spine levels L4 to S2, is routinely evaluated in children (Figure 5–52 ➤). To assess the cremasteric reflex in boys, stroke the inner thigh of each leg, testing spine levels T12, L1, and L2. The testicle and scrotum on the stroked side normally rise.

Deep Tendon Reflexes

To assess the deep tendon reflexes, tap a tendon near specific joints with a reflex hammer (or with the index finger for infants), comparing responses bilaterally. See Table 5–18 for scoring of deep tendon reflex response. The biceps, triceps, brachioradialis, patellar, and Achilles reflexes are commonly evaluated in children. Inspect for movement in the associated joint and palpate the strength of the expected muscle contraction (Table 5–19). Responses are normally symmetric bilaterally. The absence of a response is associated with decreased muscle tone and strength. Hyperactive responses are associated with muscle spasticity.

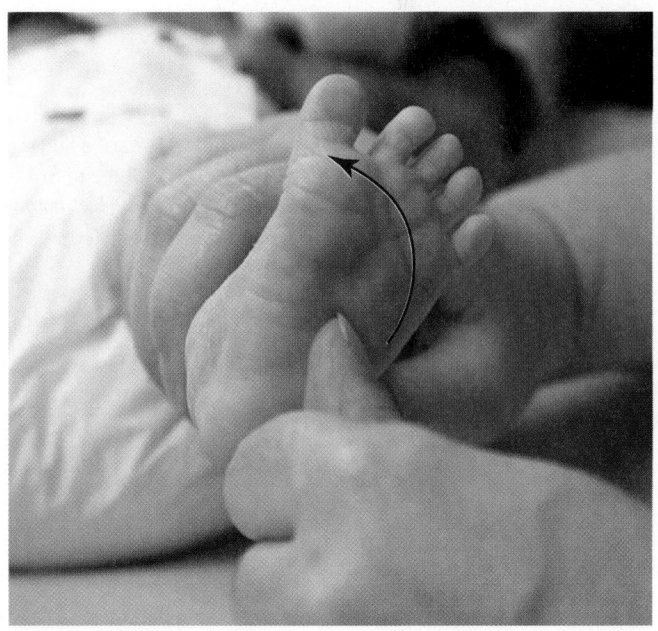

FIGURE 5–52 ➤ To assess the plantar reflex, stroke the bottom of the infant's or child's foot from the heel, along the lateral sole of the foot and across the ball of the foot. Watch the toes for plantar flexion or the Babinski response, fanning and dorsiflexion of the big toe. The Babinski response is normal in children under 2 years of age. Plantar flexion of the toes is the normal response in older children. A Babinski response in children over 2 years of age can indicate neurologic disease.

TABLE 5–17	Techniques for Assessing Selected Primitive Reflexes, with Normal Findings and Their Expected Age of Occurrence	
Primitive Reflex	**Technique and Normal Findings[a]**	**Normal Appearance and Disappearance**
Moro 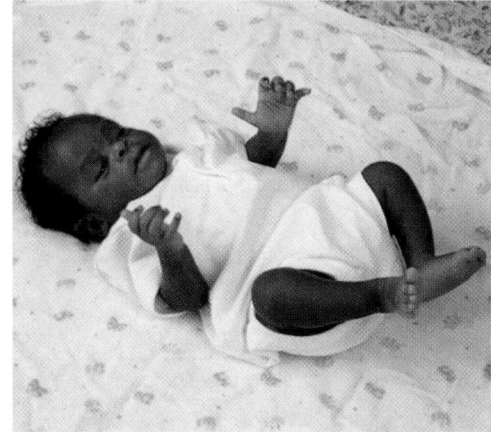	Startle the infant with a sudden noise or change in position. *The arms extend and the fingers form a C as they spread. The arms slowly move together as in a hug. The legs may make a similar motion.*	Present at birth. Decreases in strength by 4 months of age. Disappears by 6 months of age.
Palmar grasp 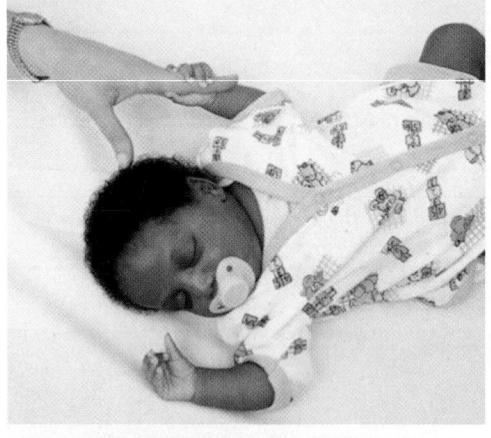	Place a finger across the infant's palm and avoid touching the thumb. *A strong grip around the finger is normal.*	Present at birth. Disappears by 3 months of age.
Plantar grasp 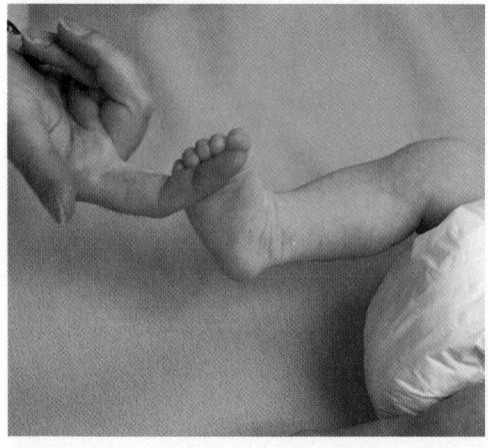	Place a finger across the foot at the base of the toes. *The toes normally curl as if gripping the finger.*	Present at birth. Disappears at about 8 months of age.

TABLE 5–17	Techniques for Assessing Selected Primitive Reflexes, with Normal Findings and Their Expected Age of Occurrence *(continued)*	
Primitive Reflex	Technique and Normal Findings[a]	Normal Appearance and Disappearance
Placing 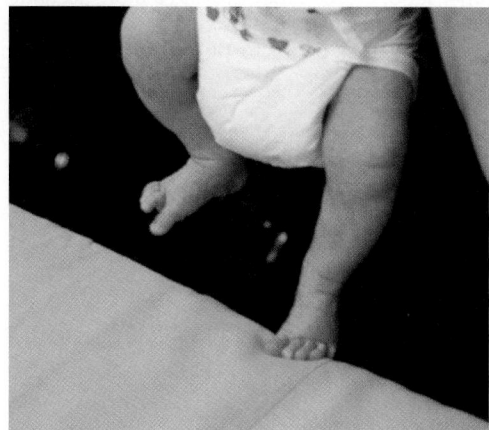	Hold the infant erect and touch the top of one foot with the edge of a table or chair. *The infant normally lifts the foot, as if to step up onto the surface.*	Present within days of birth. Disappears at various times.
Stepping 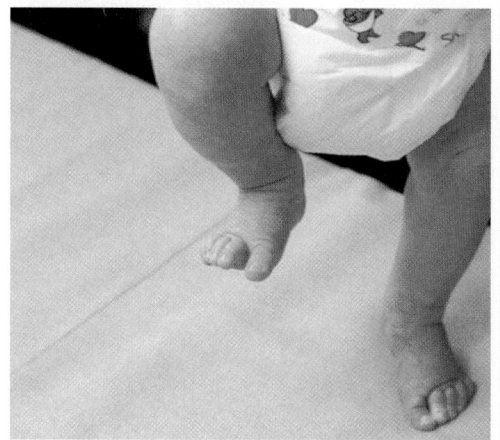	Hold the infant erect and touch the bottom of one foot on the surface of a table or chair. *The feet lift in an alternating pattern as if to walk.*	Present at birth. Disappears between 4 and 8 weeks of age.
Tonic neck 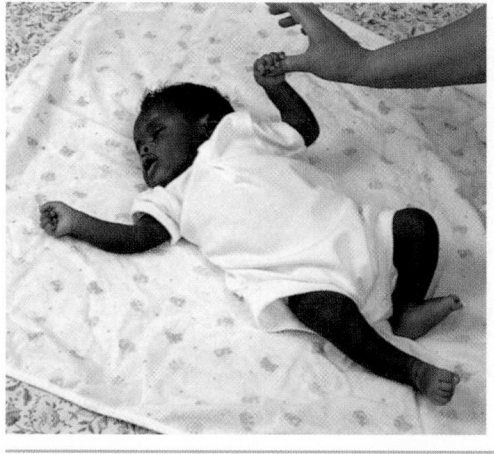	Place the infant in a supine position and, when relaxed, turn the head to one side. Repeat by turning the head to the opposite side. *The arm and leg on the face side normally extend and the opposite arm and leg flex, as if to assume a fencing position.*	Appears about 2 months of age. Decreases by 4 months of age. Disappears no later than 6 months of age. This reflex must disappear before the infant can roll over.

[a]*Italic indicates normal findings.*

	TABLE 5–18	Numeric Scoring of Deep Tendon Reflex Responses

Grade	Response Interpretation
0	No response
1+	Slow, minimal response
2+	Expected response, active
3+	More active or pronounced than expected
4+	Hyperactive, clonus may be present

Clinical Tip

The best response to deep tendon reflex testing is achieved when the child is relaxed or distracted. Children often anticipate the knee jerk and either tighten up or exaggerate the response. Making the child focus on another set of muscles may provide a more accurate response. When testing the reflexes on the lower legs, have the child press his or her hands together or try to pull them apart when gripped together.

	TABLE 5–19	Assessment of Deep Tendon Reflexes and the Spinal Segment Tested with Each

Deep Tendon Reflex	Technique and Normal Findings[a]	Spine Segment Tested
Biceps	Flex the child's arm at the elbow, and place your thumb over the biceps tendon in the antecubital fossa. Tap your thumb. *Elbow flexes as the biceps muscle contracts.*	C5 and C6
Triceps	With the child's arm flexed, tap the triceps tendon above the elbow. *Elbow extends as the triceps muscle contracts.*	C6, C7, and C8
Brachioradialis	Lay the child's arm with the thumb upright over your arm. Tap the brachioradial tendon 2.5 cm (1 in.) above the wrist. *Forearm pronates (palm facing downward) and elbow flexes.*	C5 and C6
Patellar	Flex the child's knees, and when the legs are relaxed, tap the patellar tendon just below the knee. *Knee extends (knee jerk) as the quadriceps muscle contracts.*	L2, L3, and L4

TABLE 5–19	Assessment of Deep Tendon Reflexes and the Spinal Segment Tested with Each *(continued)*	
Deep Tendon Reflex	Technique and Normal Findings[a]	Spine Segment Tested
Achilles 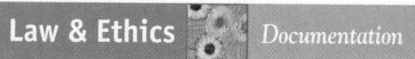	While the child's legs are flexed, support the foot and tap the Achilles tendon. *Plantar flexion (ankle jerk) as the gastrocnemius muscle contracts.*	S1 and S2

[a]*Italic indicates normal findings.*

ANALYZING DATA FROM THE PHYSICAL EXAMINATION

Once the physical examination has been completed, group any abnormal findings for each system with those of other systems. Use clinical judgment to identify common patterns of physiologic responses associated with health conditions. Individual abnormal physiologic responses are also the basis of many nursing diagnoses.

Let's return to the vignette at the beginning of the chapter. Your thorough physical assessment of Jasmine has revealed a child that appears well nourished. Her weight and height when plotted on the growth curve both fall along the 5th percentile. Her head circumference is at the 10th percentile. She has a temperature of 38°C (100.4°F). Her right tympanic membrane is red and has no light reflex and no visible landmarks, and it does not move with positive or negative pressure. Her mucous membranes are moist and skin turgor is good. Based upon these findings, you would be able to select nursing diagnoses appropriate for a child with acute otitis media and being newly adopted into this family. Examples would be the following:

- Acute Pain related to infection and pressure in middle ear
- Readiness for Enhanced Parenting related to newly available information about the child's health status
- Readiness for Enhanced Family Processes related to the parents' ability to support the integration of the adopted child into the family

These nursing diagnoses will help direct your nursing care for this child and family.

Chapter Highlights

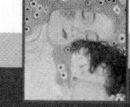

- Establish a rapport with the family and use careful listening techniques to collect historical information about the child's health status.
- Collection of historical data includes the chief complaint, history of the present illness or injury, past history, current health status, review of systems, and family history. In addition, psychosocial and developmental data are collected.
- The physical examination sequence includes assessment of the following:
  - Skin and hair
  - Head, eyes, ears, nose, and mouth structures and function
  - Neck
  - Chest and lungs
  - Breasts
  - Heart, pulses, and blood pressure
  - Abdomen
  - Inguinal area
  - Genitalia and perineal areas
  - Musculoskeletal system
  - Nervous system
- Assessment sequences vary by the age of the child and the child's cooperation with the procedures.
- Clinical judgment is used to identify common patterns of physiologic responses associated with medical conditions.
- The physiologic responses and family and child responses to health conditions become the basis for many nursing diagnoses.

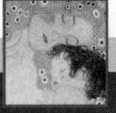

Clinical Reasoning in Action

Recall Jasmine from the opening scenario. She has recently been adopted from China by the Porter family. When Jasmine's length, weight, and head circumference are plotted on a growth curve, she is found to be in the 5th percentile for length and weight, and the 10th percentile for head circumference.

1. What behaviors would you look for that might indicate that Jasmine is beginning to develop a relationship with Mrs. Porter?
2. What actions could you take during the physical examination to develop rapport with Jasmine and to reduce her anxiety?

3. What are the important physical findings of an ear infection in a child like Jasmine who has been crying during the examination?
4. What is your interpretation of Jasmine's current growth status? Outline a plan to monitor her future growth.

See Pearson Nursing Student Resources for possible responses.

Pearson Nursing Student Resources

Find additional review materials at
nursing.pearsonhighered.com
Prepare for success with NCLEX®-style practice questions, interactive assignments and activities, web links, animations and videos, and more!

References

American Speech and Language Association. (2009). *How does your child hear and talk?* Retrieved from http://www.asha.org/public/speech/development/chart.htm

Ashrafi, M. R., Shabanian, R., Mohammadi, M., & Kavusi, S. (2006). Extensive Mongolian spots: A clinical sign merits special attention. *Pediatric Neurology, 34*(2), 143–145.

Biro, F. M., Huang, B., Crawford, P. B., Lucky, A. W., Striegel-Moore, R., et al. (2006). Pubertal correlates in Black and White girls. *Journal of Pediatrics, 148*(2), 234–240.

Biro, F. M., Huang, H., Daniels, S. R., & Lucky, A. W. (2008). Pubarche as well as thelarche may be a marker for the onset of puberty. *Journal of Pediatric and Adolescent Gynecology, 21*, 323–328.

Doshi, N., & Rodriguez, M. L. F. (2007). Amblyopia. *American Family Physician, 75*, 361–367.

Feigelman, S. (2007a). The first year. In R. M. Kliegman, R. E. Behrman, H. B. Jenson, & B. F. Stanton,

Nelson textbook of pediatrics (18th ed., pp. 43–48). Philadelphia: Elsevier Saunders.

Feigelman, S. (2007b). The second year. In R. M. Kliegman, R. E. Behrman, H. B. Jenson, & B. F. Stanton, *Nelson textbook of pediatrics* (18th ed., pp. 48–54). Philadelphia: Elsevier Saunders.

Goldenring, J. M., & Rosen, D. S. (2004). Getting into adolescent heads: An essential update. *Contemporary Pediatrics, 21*(1), 64–90.

Horner, G. (2007). Genitourinary assessment: An integral part of the complete physical examination. *Journal of Pediatric Health Care, 21*(3), 162–170.

Kaczor, K., Pierce, M. C., Makoroff, K., & Corey, T. S. (2006). Bruising and physical child abuse. *Clinical Pediatric Emergency Medicine, 7*, 153–160.

Kaplowitz, P. B. (2008). Link between body fat and the timing of puberty. *Pediatrics, 121*(Suppl 3), S208–S217.

McLaughlin, C., & Levin, A. V. (2006). The red reflex. *Pediatric Emergency Care, 22*(2), 137–140.

Prentiss, K. A., & Dorfman, D. H. (2008). Pediatric ophthalmology in the emergency department. *Emergency Medical Clinics of North America, 26*, 181–198.

Purnell, L. D. (2009). *Guide to culturally competent care* (2nd ed.). Philadelphia: F.A. Davis.

Ralston, M., Hazinski, M. F., Zaritsky, A. L., Schexnayder, S. M., & Kleinman, M. E. (Eds.). (2006). *Pediatric advanced life support provider manual.* Dallas, TX: American Heart Association.

Schell, K. A. (2006). Evidence-based practice: Noninvasive blood pressure measurement in children. *Pediatric Nursing, 32*(3), 263–267.

Seidel, H. M., Ball, J. W., Dains, J., Flynn, J. A., Solomon, B. S., & Stewart, R. W. (2011). *Mosby's guide to physical examination* (7th ed.). St. Louis, MO: Elsevier Mosby.

Zitelli, B. J., & Davis, H. W. (2007). *Atlas of pediatric physical diagnosis* (5th ed.). St. Louis, MO: Elsevier Mosby.

Introduction to Health Promotion and Maintenance

chapter 6

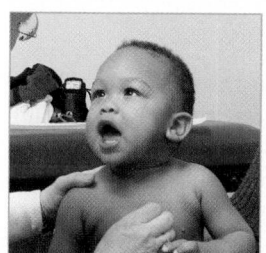

Clarence has been brought in for his 15-month health supervision visit by his father, Ben, and mother, Karie. Clarence is a healthy but very active toddler and his parents have many questions about his development. They are concerned that Clarence is too active and needs constant supervision. Since both parents work and Clarence is at child care during the day, they are busy in the evening trying to spend time with him and meet other family obligations. You notice on the record that Clarence missed his 12-month health supervision visit and was last seen when he was 9 months old.

Why are health supervision appointments important? What health promotion activities will be appropriate for this visit? How will you integrate Ben and Karie's questions about Clarence's activity level into the visit? Since Clarence has not been seen by a health care provider for some time, what are some likely health maintenance needs?

Key Terms

anticipatory guidance / 164
health / 164
health maintenance / 164
health promotion / 164
health protection / 164
health supervision / 165
partnership / 166
pediatric health care
  home / 165
screening / 173
spiritual dimension / 172

Learning Outcomes

After reading this chapter, you will be able to do the following:

1. Define health promotion and health maintenance.
2. Describe how health promotion and health maintenance are addressed by collaborating with families during health supervision visits.
3. Identify the components of a health supervision visit.
4. Analyze the nurse's role in providing health promotion and health maintenance for children and families.
5. Summarize the general observations made of children and their families as they come to the pediatric health care home for health supervision visits.
6. Synthesize the areas of assessment and intervention for health supervision visits—growth and developmental surveillance, nutrition, physical activity, oral health, mental and spiritual health, family and social relations, disease prevention strategies, and injury prevention strategies.
7. Plan health promotion and health maintenance strategies employed during health supervision visits.
8. Apply the nursing process in assessment, diagnosis, goal setting, intervention, and evaluation of health promotion and health maintenance activities for children and families.

A major goal of *Healthy People 2010* and *2020* is to help individuals of all ages increase life expectancy and improve their quality of life (*Healthy People 2020,* 2010). The concepts of health promotion and health maintenance provide for nursing interventions that contribute to meeting this goal. Many students in health professions begin their studies with a strong interest in care of ill individuals. However, as time progresses, they learn that "well" people also need care. They need teaching to improve diet, reduce stress, and obtain immunizations. They may seek information about how to exercise properly or ensure a safe environment for their children. These examples of care and teaching are components of health promotion and maintenance.

Nursing is a holistic profession that examines and works with all aspects of individuals' lives, and has a strong focus on family and community as well. Nurses therefore are uniquely positioned to provide health promotion and health maintenance activities. In fact, these activities should be a part of each encounter with families.

Health supervision visits are specifically designed to provide an overview of the child's health status and are a primary time when health promotion and health maintenance occur. However, the pediatric nurse applies health promotion and health maintenance in all settings in which children are served—well-child clinics, schools, mobile vans, physician and nurse practitioner offices, and hospitals. The nurse must possess a comprehensive background on all aspects of childcare and an understanding of child growth and development (see Chapter 4 ∞). The family's role in children's health is critical (see Chapter 2 ∞). The impact of contemporary influences on children provides an essential context to realistic nursing care planning (see Chapter 17 ∞). Finally, a thorough understanding of the health care conditions that affect children is needed so that health promotion and maintenance can be integrated within the framework of comprehensive health care.

What is the difference between health promotion and health maintenance? When should nurses engage in activities that focus on health? How can these activities be integrated into health supervision visits for the infant and young child? How do nurses collaborate with other health care professionals to offer comprehensive health services in settings accessible to parents and young children? These questions will be explored in this chapter, along with specific activities that target families with infants and young children.

■ GENERAL CONCEPTS

In order to understand health promotion and health maintenance, it is important to develop a definition of health. The World Health Organization defines **health** as a state of complete physical, mental, and social well-being and not merely the absence of disease and infirmity (World Health Organization, 2001, 2010). Others view the quality of "complete well-being" as impossible to attain, and have further developed the concept to apply to persons with various health conditions. Health in this expanded view is dynamic, changing, and unfolding; it is the realization of a state of actualization or potential (Pender, Murdaugh, & Parsons, 2006). Therefore, even individuals with chronic disease are viewed as healthy if they successfully adapt to their conditions. The basic human right of health is necessary for development of societies, and the responsibility for ensuring health rests collectively with individuals and society.

Health promotion refers to activities that increase well-being and enhance wellness or health (Pender et al., 2006). These activities lead to actualization of positive health potential for all individuals, even those with chronic or acute conditions. Health promotion enables people to increase control over and to improve their health, using a wide range of social and environmental interventions (World Health Organization, 2010). For example, nurses provide information and resources in order to:

- Enhance nutrition at each developmental stage
- Integrate physical activity into the child's daily events
- Provide adequate housing
- Promote oral health
- Foster positive personality development

Health promotion assists people to have increased control over their health, make healthy choices, and improve health (World Health Organization, 2009). Improved health requires positive health policy, supportive environments, strong communities, improved health services, and personal skills that promote health (World Health Organization, 2009). Nurses engage in health promotion by supporting policies that promote health in institutions where they are employed, and by partnering with children and families to promote family strengths and decision making in the areas of lifestyles, social development, nutrition, coping, and family interactions. Nurses provide **anticipatory guidance** for families when they understand the child's upcoming developmental stages and teach families how to provide an environment to assist in meeting each stage's milestones. Examples of application of this are found in Chapters 7, 8, and 9 ∞.

Health maintenance (or **health protection**) refers to activities that preserve an individual's present state of health and that prevent disease or injury occurrence. Examples of these activities include developmental screening or surveillance to identify early deviations from normal development, providing immunizations to prevent illnesses, and teaching about common childhood safety hazards. Health maintenance activities are often preventive in nature. Prevention levels are identified as primary prevention, secondary prevention, and tertiary prevention (Table 6–1).

Although health promotion and health maintenance activities are closely linked and often overlap, there are some differences. Health maintenance focuses on known potential health risks and seeks to prevent them or identify them early so that intervention can occur. Health promotion looks at the strengths and goals of individuals, families, and populations, and seeks to use them to assist in reaching higher levels of wellness. It involves partnerships with the family as health goals are set, and with other health professionals and resources to provide for meeting the goals (Figure 6–1 ➤). Apply both health promotion and health maintenance concepts when providing health care, recognizing that the concepts overlap. Health promotion and health maintenance are integrated into health care visits for children, with the care provider applying knowledge of health promotion and maintenance concepts. These activities commonly take place at "well child" or health supervision visits.

TABLE 6–1	Levels of Preventive Health Maintenance Activities	
Level	Description	Example of Nursing Actions
Primary prevention	Activities that decrease opportunity for illness or injury	Giving immunizations Teaching about car safety seats
Secondary prevention	Early diagnosis and treatment of a condition to lessen its severity	Developmental screening Vision and hearing screening
Tertiary prevention	Restoration to optimum function	Rehabilitation activities for child after a car crash

Adapted from Murray, Zentner, & Yakimo, 2009.

Health supervision is the provision of services that focus on disease and injury prevention (health maintenance), growth and developmental surveillance, and health promotion at key intervals during the child's life. What health promotion and health maintenance activities are parts of health supervision visits? How can these activities be integrated into all settings where care is provided for children? What are the recommended times for health visits to occur and what care is provided at certain times? How can you organize a health supervision visit to accomplish goals of the family and health professionals? These and other questions will be answered in this section and the section that follows on nursing management.

Children all need a medical home or **pediatric health care home**, a site of comprehensive health care by a pediatric health care professional, in order to ensure optimal health (NAPNAP, 2009). Accessible, continuous, and coordinated health supervision is provided at this site during the developmental years (Schoenbaum & Abrams, 2006). (See Chapter 1 ∞ for further description of a medical home or pediatric health care home.) Accessibility refers to both financial and geographic access; continuous indicates that the care is ongoing with consistent care providers; coordination refers to the need for communication among health professionals to provide for the needs of the child. When a family has an established partnership with a care provider, comprehensive, family-centered health services can be presented based on the family's risks and protective factors. These services may be provided at physician offices, community health clinics, and in the home, schools, childcare centers, shelters, or mobile vans (Figure 6–2 ➤). National guidelines for preventive health services have been developed for infants, children, and adolescents by the U.S. Department of Health and Human Services, the American Academy of Pediatrics (AAP), and the American Medical Association. The National Association of Pediatric Nurse Practitioners supports the list of comprehensive services of a pediatric health care home identified by the AAP.

The health supervision visit is individualized to the family and child. Standardized screenings and examinations are included, and time is provided for the family's specific concerns and questions about the child's health. Nurses play an integral

Law & Ethics — *Pediatric Health Care Home*

The American Academy of Pediatrics and the National Association of Pediatric Nurse Practitioners agree that a pediatric health care home should offer:

- Family-centered care
- Compassionate, developmentally appropriate and culturally competent care
- Sharing of unbiased and clear information
- Provision of primary care to include acute and chronic care, breast-feeding promotion, immunizations, growth and development, screenings, health care supervision, anticipatory guidance about health, nutrition, safety, and parenting and psychosocial issues
- Continuously accessible care
- Continuity of care
- Referral to specialists and community care as needed
- Referral to early intervention and childcare
- Coordination of services and collaboration among professionals
- Maintenance of a comprehensive central record
- Provision of developmentally appropriate and culturally competent care

(Pan, 2006; NAPNAP, 2009)

National Preventive Health Guidelines Websites

Health Promotion and Health Maintenance Overlap

Health Promotion	Overlap	Health Maintenance
• Nutrition to meet all RDAs and enhance health and well-being, with emphasis on whole grains, fruits, vegetables.	• Nutrition that provides for growth and energy needs also helps prevent chronic diseases.	• Nutrition to prevent obesity or growth retardation.
• Activities to promote self-concept formation including body image and decision-making skills.	• Integrating positive activities will both promote self-image and decrease potential for injury.	• Limiting television viewing to decrease exposure to violence which may lead to disturbed sleep and aggressive behaviors.

FIGURE 6–1 ➤ Health promotion and health maintenance overlap. While the focus and goals for health promotion and health maintenance differ, there is often overlap in nursing activities and expected outcomes, as demonstrated in these examples.

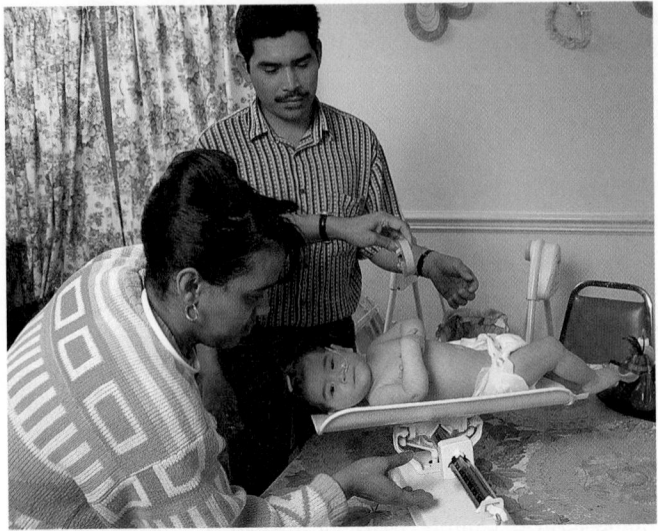

A

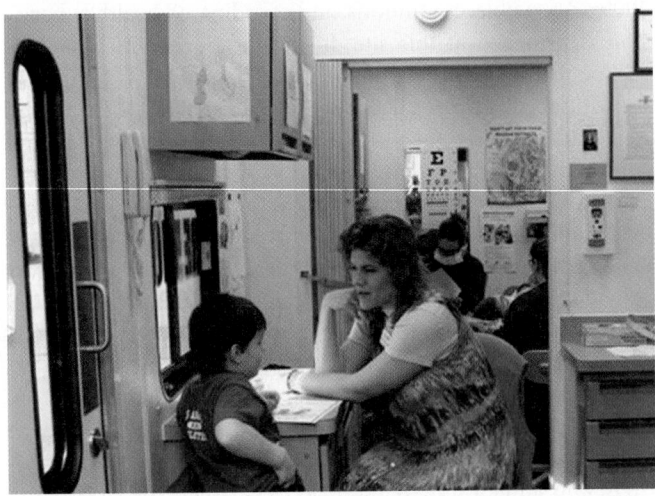

B

FIGURE 6–2 ➤ A, The nurse is providing a health supervision visit in the child's home after discharge from the hospital for an acute illness. B, A nurse is providing information to a child visiting a mobile health care van.

part in these comprehensive visits and they partner with other health care providers to accomplish health supervision.

A tracking system in the pediatric health care home site helps to identify appropriate health supervision activities for each child at every visit. Electronic health records are increasingly used to list appropriate topics for visits at specific ages and to schedule families for appointments. If a child misses a visit, the family should be contacted and encouraged to make an appointment for the recommended care. Recognizing that not all families get into their pediatric health care home for each visit, every health visit, including an episodic illness visit or care for a chronic illness, is an opportunity to complete health promotion and health maintenance activities. For example, immunizations may be given during a visit for an acute condition such as otitis media (ear infection) if the child has missed a prior health supervision visit. When you see children in hospitals, emergency rooms, or other settings, ask about their pediatric health care home, and when the last visit occurred. Identify children who

need basic health supervision services and provide services or refer families to other resources to meet their needs.

Nurses play an important role in managing health supervision visits. Depending on the setting, the advanced practice nurse may provide all services or support other care providers by obtaining an updated health history, screening for diseases and other conditions, conducting a developmental assessment, and providing immunizations, anticipatory guidance, and health education. Nurses in all settings are instrumental in identifying children who need health supervision and are not obtaining recommended care (Figure 6–3 ➤).

Although health supervision visits can address many health-related topics, a limited time generally exists in which to engage a child or family. The nurse needs to direct the encounters and have some ideas for pertinent agendas. *Bright Futures*, an initiative of the United States Maternal and Child Health Bureau and the American Academy of Pediatrics, promotes the foundational belief that each child deserves to be healthy and that the community, health professional, family, and child must partner together to achieve this goal. A series of *Bright Futures* booklets on health supervision, nutrition, physical activity, and mental health provide guidance about how the nurse can manage health supervision visits. The following six concepts should be integrated into child health care:

1. The care provider *builds effective partnerships* with the family. A **partnership** is a relationship in which participants join together to ensure health care delivery in a way that recognizes each partner's critical roles and contributions in promoting health and preventing illness. The partners in child health include the child, the family, health professionals, and the community.
2. The nurse *fosters family-centered communication* by showing interest in the child and family, and effectively conveying information and understanding.
3. The nurse *focuses on health promotion and health maintenance topics during visits,* recognizing that families may not initiate these discussions.
4. The nurse *manages time well* to enable health promotion topics to be addressed during visits. This includes reviewing the child's health record and selecting topics pertinent for the child's age and the family's situation.
5. The nurse *educates the family during "teachable moments."* Large teaching plans are not always needed; children and families often learn best when presented with small bits of information based on parents' questions or your observations.
6. The nurse *becomes an advocate for child health issues.* When an issue arises as you care for a child, seek additional data from various sources, talk with others, and strategize how the problem could be solved (Hagan, Shaw, & Duncan, 2008).

■ COMPONENTS OF HEALTH PROMOTION AND MAINTENANCE VISITS

The nurse identifies and isolates pertinent topics for health promotion and health maintenance during health supervision visits. The nurse applies knowledge of areas that need to be addressed with an infant or child of a particular age, and then makes general

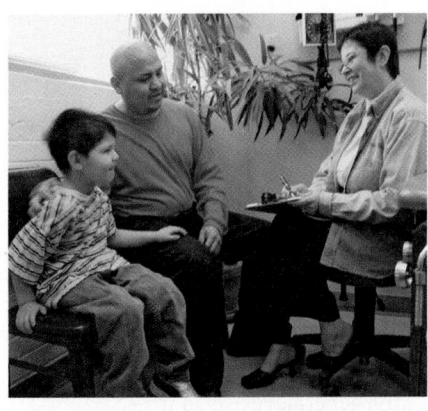
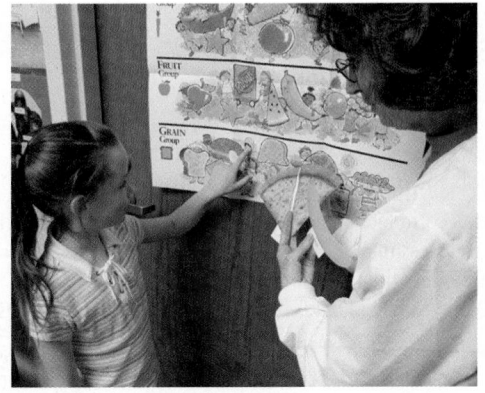
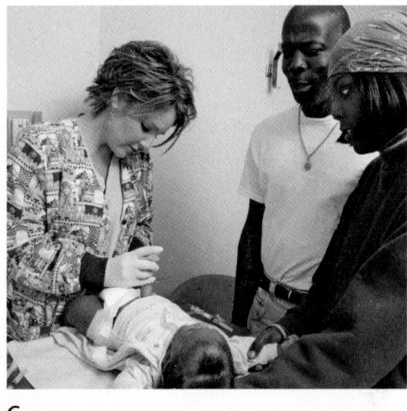

A   B   C

FIGURE 6–3 ➤ The nurse plays many roles in providing health promotion and health maintenance for children. A, Data are collected from the time a nurse calls the child and family to the examination room and during the history-taking phase. The nurse asks questions while observing the child's behaviors and the relationship between parent and child. The nurse also performs screening tests, including blood pressure, tuberculosis, vision and hearing, and developmental screening. B, Interventions that include teaching may take place. C, A nurse may administer immunizations as parents watch and assist by holding the child. Nurses also play important roles in teaching families information to enhance health.

observations of the child and family to guide additional topics. Although categories to consider vary depending on the child's age, the family's particular needs, and community resources, some common topics generally require attention. Start with the topics described in the following text, integrating general observations as the visit progresses, and address additional areas as needed.

Contact with the Family

Health care providers work with families in diverse settings and must adapt approaches and interventions dependent on the needs of these families. Prospective parents sometimes interview potential health care providers while pregnant with a child in order to choose the pediatric health care home that will best meet their needs and approaches to child health. In other situations, parents choose the most convenient setting or a facility that is included in their health insurance coverage. Some families remain with one care provider for years, while others have multiple providers.

Whatever the individual situation, the nurse recognizes that all contacts with family members are a vital link to the child. They are a time to learn about the development of the child, to observe interactions among family members, and to implement effective nursing interventions. Telephone calls, face-to-face meetings, e-mail contacts, and brief encounters all serve to provide a mutual interaction with the goal of ensuring child health. Consider Clarence's parents, who are described in the opening scenario. They have questions about Clarence's activity level and will likely be receptive to nursing interventions that help them meet parenting challenges.

General Observations

As a pediatric nurse, you will make *general observations* of infants and their families in your encounters. Be observant during the health supervision visit, and you will have many opportunities to assess the family. General observations begin as you call the family in and welcome them to the facility. They continue as you weigh and measure the infant or child, and throughout the visit. Observe the physical contact between the child and other family members, the developmental tasks displayed by the child, and parental level of stress or ease in conducting childcare activities.

Growth and Developmental Surveillance

Growth and developmental surveillance provides important clues about the child's condition and environment. In order to evaluate growth, the nurse calculates the child's height, weight, and body mass index at each health supervision visit, and places the results on percentile charts (see Chapters 5 and 14, and Appendix A ∞). Parents are given the information in written form and it is interpreted for them. Physical assessment is performed to be sure the child is growing as expected and has no abnormal or unexplained physical findings (see Chapter 5 ∞). Developmental surveillance is a flexible, continuous process of skilled observations that also provides data about the child's capabilities, allows for early identification of any neurological problems, and helps to verify that the home environment is stimulating. Early development is important to later health and it must be evaluated consistently and systematically during health care visits (Fine & Mayer, 2006; King, Tandon, Macias, et al., 2010). Information may be collected from several sources; for instance, a questionnaire that the parent completes, trigger questions asked during the interview, or observation of the child during the visit. Interview parents to identify any developmental concerns they may have about the child or adolescent. When talking with parents, review physical, social, and communication milestones for infants, young children, older children, or adolescents. Detailed milestones for each age group are found in Chapter 4 ∞.

Development is a fragile process determined by both innate conditions and environmental influences. Developmental screening of all children using a regular and organized approach is needed, since about 16% of children have some type of developmental delay or disability (Earls & Hay, 2006). Standardized developmental questionnaires are effective for developmental surveillance of most children, especially when time for health supervision visits is limited (Commonwealth Fund, 2008) (see Tables 6–2 and 6–3). Screening tests should be administered at the 9-, 18-, and 24- or 30-month

TABLE 6–2	Developmental Surveillance Questionnaires
Questionnaire	Guidelines for Administration
Parent's Evaluation of Developmental Status[a] (birth to 8 years)	Consists of 10 questions for parents to answer in interview; based on research about parents' concerns. Requires less than 5 minutes to complete. English and Spanish forms are available.
Prescreening Development Questionnaire (birth to 6 years)	Parents complete an age-specific form. Helps identify children who need Denver II (PDQ and Revised-PDQ)[b] assessment. Requires less than 10 minutes to complete. PDQ is available in English, Spanish, and French versions; R-PDQ in English only.
Ages and Stages Questionnaire[c] (4–48 months)	Questionnaires for 11 specific ages, with 10–15 items each in areas of fine motor, gross motor, communication, adaptive, personal, and social skills. Parents try each activity with the child. Requires less than 10 minutes to complete. English and Spanish versions are available.
Child Development Inventories[d] (3–72 months)	Consists of 60 yes-no descriptions for three separate instruments to identify children with developmental difficulties. Requires about 10 minutes to complete.

[a]*Frances P. Glascoe, Ellsworth & Vandermeer Press Ltd, P.O. Box 68164, Nashville, TN 37206.*
[b]*Denver Developmental Material, Inc., P.O. Box 371075, Denver, CO 80237-5075.*
[c]*Brookes Publishing Co., P.O. Box 10624, Baltimore, MD 21285-0625.*
[d]*Behavior Science Systems, Box 580274, Minneapolis, MN 55458.*

visits (Council on Children with Disabilities, 2006). A commonly used test is the Denver II, which can be applied as a developmental chart, like a growth curve, to monitor the child's developmental progress (see Figures 6–4 and 6–5 ➤).

To perform developmental screening with the Denver II or any other standardized screening tools, make sure all directions are followed:

- Choose the proper test for the child's age and desired information.
- Read directions thoroughly or utilize specific training tools available.
- Practice as needed until proficient with the test.

- Calculate the infant's or child's age correctly, especially if premature.
- Attempt to develop rapport with the infant or child to get the best performance.
- Follow directions for administration of items; in some cases, parents can be asked if a child demonstrates specific skills at home, especially if the child is not willing to perform an item during testing.
- Note the child's behavior and cooperativeness during the screening process.
- Analyze the findings using the test instructions to make the correct interpretation.

TABLE 6–3	Developmental Screening Tests for Infants and Young Children
Screening Test	Guidelines for Administration
Denver II[a] (birth to 6 years)	Consists of observation of the child in four domains: personal social, fine motor-adaptive, language, and gross motor. Requires 30 minutes to complete. A training video is available.
Bayley Infant Neurodevelopmental Screener (BINST)[b] (3–24 months)	Consists of observation of the child with 10–13 items for each of six age-specific scales to assess neurological processes, neurodevelopmental skills, and developmental accomplishments. Requires 10–15 minutes to complete.
McCarthy Scales of Children's Abilities[b] (2.5–8.5 years)	Consists of observation of the child in domains of motor, verbal, perceptual-performance, quantitative, general cognition, and memory. Requires 45 minutes to complete.
Denver Articulation Screening Exam (DASE)[a] (2.5–6 years)	Consists of observation of the child's articulation of 30 sound elements and intelligibility. Requires 5 minutes to complete.
Early Language Milestone Scale—2 (ELM)[c] (birth to 36 months)	Consists of observation of the child to assess auditory expressive, auditory receptive, and visual components of speech. Requires 5–10 minutes to complete.

[a]*Denver Development Materials, Inc., P.O. Box 371075, Denver, CO 80237-5075.*
[b]*Harcourt Assessment: The Psychological Corporation, 19500 Bulverde Rd., San Antonio, TX 78259.*
[c]*PRO-ED, Inc., 8700 Shoal Creek Blvd., Austin, TX 78758-6897.*

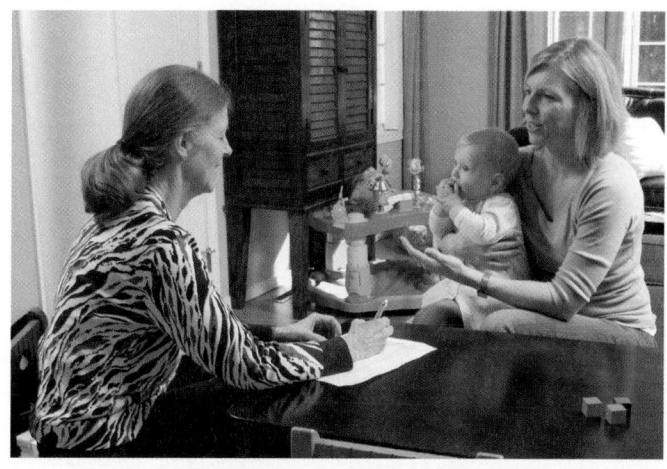

A

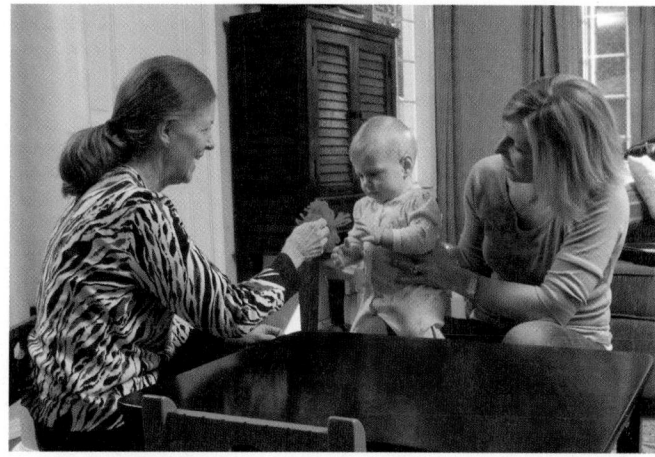

B

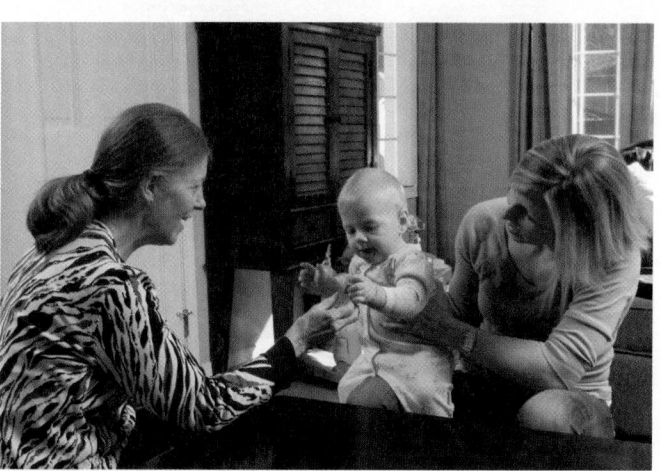

C

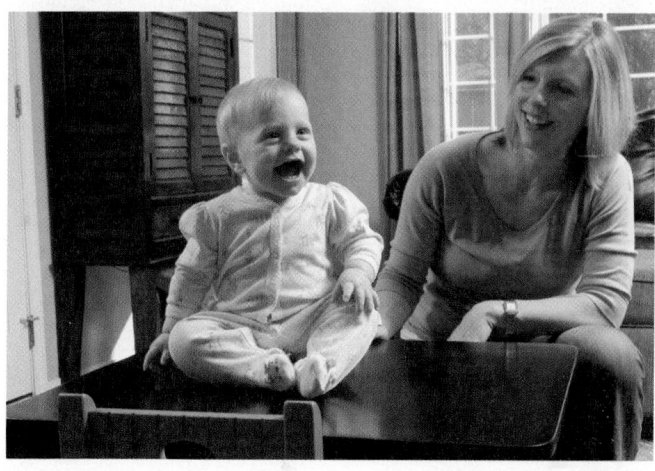

D

FIGURE 6–4 ➤ Follow all directions for performing the Denver II assessment and for interpreting responses. Use the kit provided with the test to ensure accuracy of results. For example, yarn is provided to test the infant's ability to follow an object, blocks of a uniform size test fine motor coordination, and pictures on the score sheet are used to test language abilities. Develop rapport with the child and approach the assessment as fun. This often helps the child participate more actively during the entire Denver II assessment. A, The nurse making a home visit asks the mother about personal-social tasks the child has accomplished, such as feeding self and waving bye-bye. The girl, who is 6 months of age, is tested for performance of the following age-appropriate behaviors: B, Looking for yarn and following 180 degrees. C, Banging two cubes. D, Sitting without support.

> **Clinical Tip**

A series of developmental screening tests are available to rate the interaction between caregiver and child. Developed by nurses, the Nursing Child Assessment Satellite Training (NCAST) teaches how to administer screenings of parent–child feeding and teaching interactions.

Failure to perform an item in a single domain does not mean the child has failed the test. The child should be reevaluated at a future visit. Schedule the appointment at a time of day when the child is awake and rested. Failure of multiple items within one domain or across multiple domains is of greatest concern. When poor development patterns in one or more domains are revealed, referral for diagnostic developmental assessment is needed.

Parents are key participants in their children's developmental screening. They often recognize problems not observed in brief health care encounters. Enable them to ask questions and state their observations of the child, provide them with expected developmental tasks and ways to stimulate development, and encourage them to write down observations to form the basis for developmental screening during health care visits (Council on Children with Disabilities, 2006).

Nutrition

Nutrition evaluation is a vital part of each health supervision visit. It makes important contributions to general health and fosters growth and development. Include observations and screening relevant to nutritional intake at each health supervision visit. Eating proper foods for age and activity ensures that children have the energy for proper growth, physical activity, cognition, and immune function. Nutrition is closely linked to both health promotion and health maintenance. See Chapter 14 ∞ for detailed nutritional assessment

Nursing Child Assessment Satellite Training (NCAST) Website

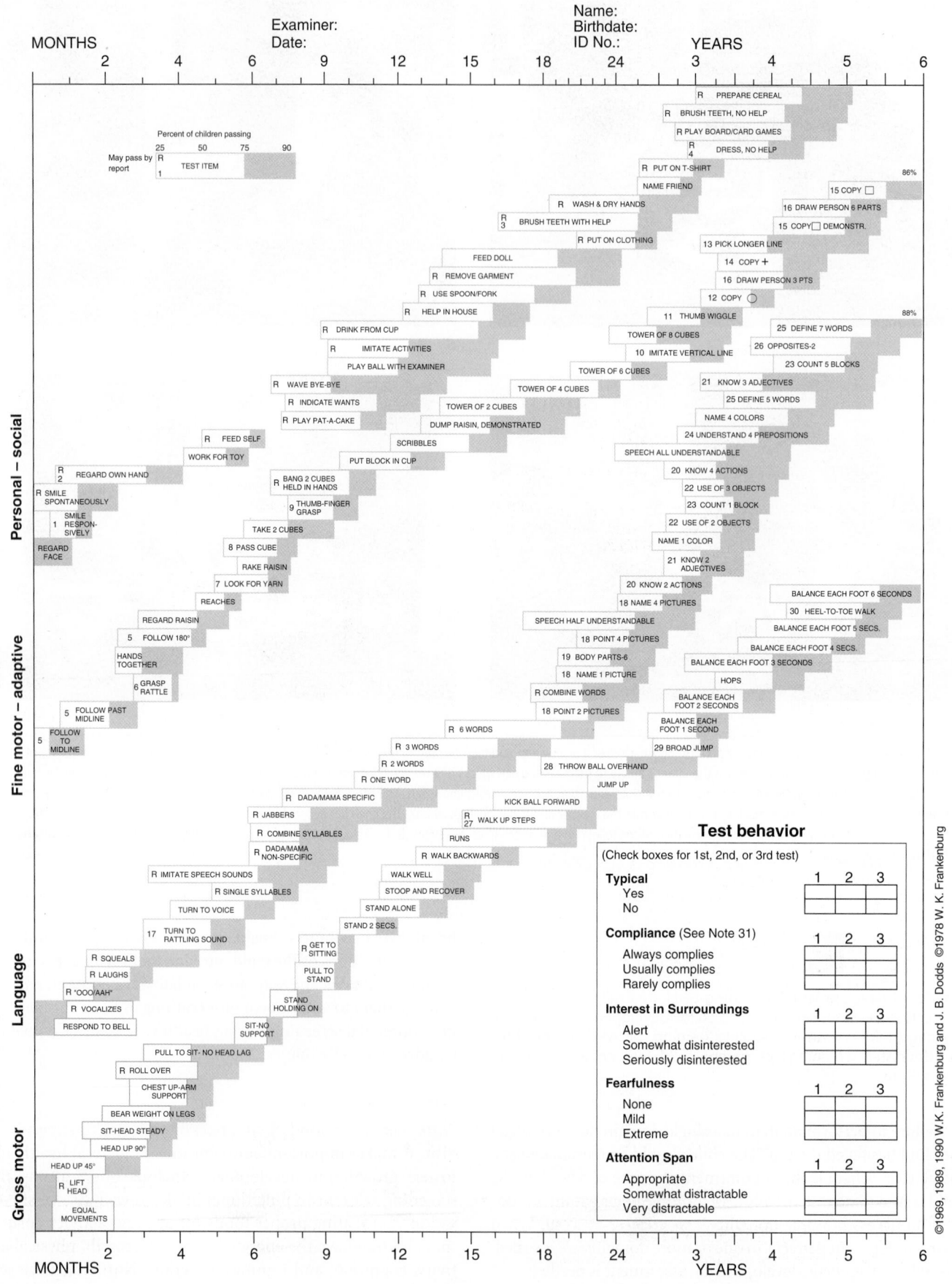

FIGURE 6–5A ➤ Denver II.

DIRECTIONS FOR ADMINISTRATION

1. Try to get child to smile by smiling, talking, or waving. Do not touch him/her.
2. Child must stare at hand several seconds.
3. Parent may help guide toothbrush and put toothpaste on brush.
4. Child does not have to be able to tie shoes or button/zip in the back.
5. Move yarn slowly in an arc from one side to the other, about 8" above child's face.
6. Pass if child grasps rattle when it is touched to the backs or tips of fingers.
7. Pass if child tries to see where yarn went. Yarn should be dropped quickly from sight from tester's hand without arm movement.
8. Child must transfer cube from hand to hand without help of body, mouth, or table.
9. Pass if child picks up raisin with any part of thumb and finger.
10. Line can vary only 30 degrees or less from tester's line.
11. Make a fist with thumb pointing upward and wiggle only the thumb. Pass if child imitates and does not move any fingers other than the thumb.

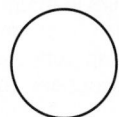 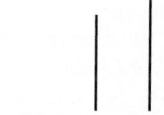 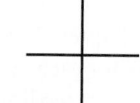 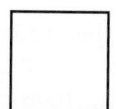

12. Pass any enclosed form. Fail continuous round motions.
13. Which line is longer? (Not bigger.) Turn paper upside down and repeat (pass 3 of 3 or 5 of 6).
14. Pass any lines crossing near midpoint.
15. Have child copy first. If failed, demonstrate.

When giving items 12, 14, and 15, do not name the forms. Do not demonstrate 12 and 14.
16. When scoring, each pair (2 arms, 2 legs, etc.) counts as one part.
17. Place one cube in cup and shake gently near child's ear, but out of sight. Repeat for other ear.
18. Point to picture and have child name it. (No credit is given for sounds only.)
If less than 4 pictures are named correctly, have child point to picture as each is named by tester.

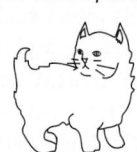 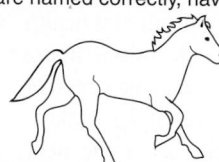 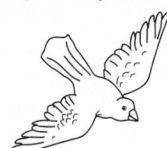 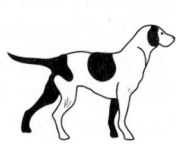 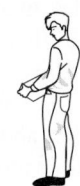

19. Using doll, tell child: Show me the nose, eyes, ears, mouth, hands, feet, tummy, hair. Pass 6 of 8.
20. Using pictures, ask child: Which one flies?... says meow?... talks?... barks?... gallops? Pass 2 of 5, 4 of 5.
21. Ask child: What do you do when you are cold?... tired?... hungry? Pass 2 of 3, 3 of 3.
22. Ask child: What do you do with a cup? What is a chair used for? What is a pencil used for? Action words must be included in answers.
23. Pass if child correctly places <u>and</u> says how many blocks are on paper. (1, 5).
24. Tell child: Put block **on** table; **under** table: **in front of** me, **behind** me. Pass 4 of 4. (Do not help child by pointing, moving head or eyes.)
25. Ask child: What is a ball?... lake?... desk?... house?... banana?... curtain?... fence?... ceiling? Pass if defined in terms of use, shape, what it is made of, or general category (such as banana is fruit, not just yellow). Pass 5 of 8, 7 of 8.
26. Ask child: If a horse is big, a mouse is _____? If fire is hot, ice is _____? If sun shines during the day, the moon shines during the _____? Pass 2 of 3.
27. Child may use wall or rail only, not person. May not crawl.
28. Child must throw ball overhand 3 feet to within arm's reach of tester.
29. Child must perform standing broad jump over width of test sheet (8 1/2 inches).
30. Tell child to walk forward, ⊂⊃⊂⊃⊂⊃ → heel within 1 inch of toe. Tester may demonstrate. Child must walk 4 consecutive steps.
31. In the second year, half of normal children are non-compliant.

OBSERVATIONS:

FIGURE 6–5B ➤ Directions for administration of Denver II. *(continued)*
© 1969, 1989, 1990, W. K. Frankenburg and J. B. Dodds. © 1978 W. K. Frankenburg.

Culture  *Developmental Testing*

Be alert that children who have recently come from other countries and even some born in this country who live in families from minority ethnic groups may have difficulty with some items on developmental tests. For example, children who are not skilled in the English language may not understand some instructions or be able to answer questions about definitions of words. If an item such as "wave good-bye" or "plays patty-cake" represents a practice not common in another culture, the child may not have had exposure to the skill. Be alert for cultural variations, allow the child time to learn a developmental skill, and retest at future visits.

recommendations, and this chapter as well as Chapters 7, 8, and 9 ∞ for specific nutritional questions to ask for each age group. Find out what questions parents have about feeding their children. Integrate the special nutritional needs of children with chronic conditions. Use the information gathered to provide both health promotion and health maintenance interventions.

Physical Activity

Physical activity provides many physical and psychological health benefits. However, there is growing disparity between recommendations and reality among most of our children. Research by the Centers for Disease Control and Prevention (CDC) has identified that about 23% of children from 9 to 13 years report no free-time physical activity. When schools do not offer daily physical education, many children have no regular activity. Participation in physical activity declines as youth get older, and females are considerably less active than males (CDC, 2006a, 2006b). Inquire about activities the child prefers and the amount of time for activity during the day. As the child grows older, insert questions about sedentary activities such as number of hours spent watching television or playing computer games. Find out if the child plays sports at school or in the community. Ask about activities in a typical day to measure amount of activity. Once the nurse gathers data about physical activity, interventions are implemented to enhance activity patterns.

Oral Health

While *oral health* may seem to require the knowledge of a specialist, many implications relate to general health care. Oral health is important because teeth assist in language development, impacted or infected teeth lead to systemic illness, and teeth are related to positive self-image formation. Dental caries is the most common chronic disease of children. Many youth in the United States are affected by tooth decay and pain that interfere with activities of daily living such as eating, sleeping, attending school, and speaking (Dye, Tan, Smith, et al., 2007). The nurse applies health promotion to dental health by teaching about oral care and access to dental visits. Health maintenance activities relate to prevention of caries and illness related to dental disease.

▲ Health Promotion

Dental Health

Over one-half of children from homes with low incomes have not received dental care in the last year; about 14% of them have unmet dental care needs. One-third of families who have difficulty paying for food or rent do not receive any preventive dental visits. Hispanic children are even more likely to have no or inadequate dental care. Low educational level of parents, and functional impairment of the child are additional risk factors for unmet dental needs (Kenney, McFeeters, & Yee, 2005; CDC, 2006c). All children in the Medicaid program are eligible for dental coverage in the Early and Periodic Screening, Diagnostic, and Treatment Services (EPSDT). Private and public clinics in many communities provide low-cost or free care for families with limited financial resources. What resources are available in your state and community? (See Chapter 1 for further descriptions about available programs.)

Mental and Spiritual Health

Mental and spiritual health are important concepts to address in health promotion and maintenance visits. Parents can be encouraged to keep a record of mental health issues to bring to health supervision visits. This helps them understand that the health care professional is willing to partner with them to assist in dealing with mental health. Suggest topics such as child and parental mood, child temperament, stresses and ways that family members manage stress, or sleep patterns (Center for Mental Health Services, n.d.). Make notes in the record as a reminder of questions to ask at the next visit (Jellinek, Patel, & Froehle, 2002). The child and family are both observed for appropriateness of affect and mood. Be alert for signs of depression, stress, anxiety, and child abuse/neglect. The nurse establishes both health promotion and health maintenance goals related to child and family mental health. Health promotion goals relate to adequate resources to meet family challenges, protective factors such as involvement in extended family and the community. Teaching stress reduction techniques such as meditation, relaxation, and imagery, as well as providing resources for yoga or other techniques, is helpful. Health maintenance goals relate to prevention of mental health problems. Examples include providing resources when domestic violence occurs, or referring cases of suspected child abuse or neglect. The **spiritual dimension** is a connection with a greater power than that in the self, and guides a person to strive for inspiration, respect, meaning, and purpose in life (Murray, Zentner, & Yakimo, 2009). Spiritual health is seen in the large context as those entities that provide meaning in life. For some, this may be membership in a faith-based group; for others, it may be feeling part of a society with a purpose of greater good, or setting goals for the future. Ask about the family's meaningful activities. Provide links to faith-based groups as needed.

The *relationships* that a child establishes with others begin at birth. The first and most important set of relationships develops with the family. The mother, father, siblings, and perhaps extended family are the contexts in which the baby learns to relate with others. With growth the world widens to encompass other children, friends of the family, peers, school, and the larger community network. In the opening scenario, Clarence spends time each day in childcare. The nurse should inquire about important relationships for Clarence and his parents in that setting. Analyzing the child's relationships at all ages provides important clues to social interactions. From the moment the family is called in from a waiting area, be alert for clues to family interactions. Who is present at the visit, and what roles and interactions can be observed? Likewise, other social interactions are important to evaluate. Does the young infant interact in an age-appropriate manner with the health care provider or other children in the area? Ask the parents questions about family and social interactions. Once assessment has taken place, establish goals and interventions related to family and social relationships.

Disease Prevention Strategies

Disease prevention strategies focus mainly on health maintenance, or prevention of disease. Some health disruptions can be detected early and treatment for the condition can begin. **Screening** is a procedure used to detect the possible presence of a health condition before symptoms are apparent. It is usually conducted on large groups of individuals at risk for a condition and represents the secondary level of prevention (Figure 6–6 ➤). Examples include developmental screening (described earlier in this chapter), blood pressure screening, and vision/hearing screening. Most screening tests are not diagnostic by themselves but are followed by further diagnostic tests if the screening result is positive. Once a screening test identifies the existence of a health condition, early intervention can begin, with the goal of reducing the severity or complications of the condition.

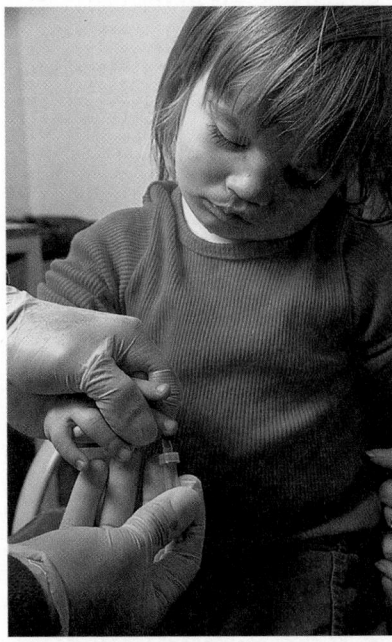

FIGURE 6–6 ➤ This 18-month-old toddler is having a blood screening test to detect iron deficiency anemia. Children are often screened for adequate levels of iron in later infancy and during toddlerhood.

Another way to prevent diseases is to immunize children against common communicable diseases. See Chapter 16 ∞ for the complete list of childhood immunizations and schedules for administration; see Chapters 7, 8, and 9 ∞ for the most commonly administered immunizations at specific ages.

Clinical Judgment

What immunizations are likely needed by Clarence, described in the opening scenario? Recall that Clarence is 15 months of age. (Consult Chapters 8 and 16.)

Injury Prevention Strategies

Most childhood mortality and hospitalization is related to injury (see Chapter 1 ∞). Therefore, it is important for the nurse to integrate *injury prevention* strategies in all health supervision visits. The family is constantly challenged to maintain a safe environment as the child grows older, reaches more advanced developmental levels, is exposed to a widening world outside of the family, and has less supervision. Safety teaching should be integrated with developmental progression. Asking parents to bring their questions about safety to each visit can be a good starting point for discussion. The nurse considers knowledge about the child's age and information from the health supervision visit to plan health maintenance interventions related to injury. Teaching is performed, resources are made available, and parents and children who have experienced injury are invited to present their experiences.

Some common universal injury prevention topics include car safety, pedestrian safety, sports injury prevention, poison prevention, and child abuse prevention.

NURSING MANAGEMENT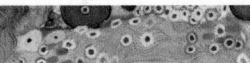

Nursing Assessment and Diagnosis

During health supervision visits, a mental portrait of a child and family should be drawn. Observe the parent–child interaction in the waiting room and all throughout the examination. If siblings are present, watch for interactions among all family members. Observe the affect and mood of the child and parents. Nursing assessment of the child and family at each visit for health supervision then focuses on the following:

- Interviewing the family and child to update the health history, to ask about the child's developmental or educational progress, and to identify dietary habits, physical activity, and safety practices
- Eliciting questions and concerns that the parent or child may have
- Conducting developmental surveillance assessments, including review of questionnaires completed by the parent in the waiting room
- Performing age-appropriate screening tests (Table 6–4)
- Performing a physical assessment

Following a thorough assessment, the nurse derives nursing diagnoses that are pertinent for the child's health status and that

American Academy of Pediatrics
DEDICATED TO THE HEALTH OF ALL CHILDREN™

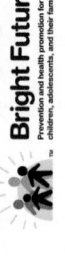

Bright Futures
Prevention and health promotion for infants, children, adolescents, and their families™

| TABLE 6–4 | Recommendations for Preventive Pediatric Health Care, Committee on Practice and Ambulatory Medicine, American Academy of Pediatrics, United States |

Recommendations for Preventive Pediatric Health Care

Each child and family is unique; therefore, these **Recommendations for Preventive Pediatric Health Care** are designed for the care of children who are receiving competent parenting, have no manifestations of any important health problems, and are growing and developing in satisfactory fashion. **Additional visits may become necessary** if circumstances suggest variations from normal.

Developmental, psychosocial, and chronic disease issues for children and adolescents may require frequent counseling and treatment visits separate from preventive care visits.

These guidelines represent a consensus by the American Academy of Pediatrics (AAP) and Bright Futures. The AAP continues to emphasize the great importance of **continuity of care** in comprehensive health supervision and the need to avoid **fragmentation of care.**

The recommendations in this statement do not indicate an exclusive course of treatment or standard of medical care. Variations, taking into account individual circumstances, may be appropriate.

Copyright © 2008 by the American Academy of Pediatrics.

No part of this statement may be reproduced in any form or by any means without prior written permission from the American Academy of Pediatrics except for one copy for personal use.

[Large landscape preventive-care schedule table spanning Infancy, Early Childhood, Middle Childhood, and Adolescence age columns with rows for History, Measurements, Sensory Screening, Developmental/Behavioral Assessment, Physical Examination, Procedures, Oral Health, and Anticipatory Guidance. Legend: ● = to be performed, ★ = risk assessment to be performed, with appropriate action to follow, if positive; range during which a service may be provided, with the symbol indicating the preferred age.]

consider the family's needs. Nursing diagnoses are developed jointly with the family as an essential component of the partnership between nurse and family. Examples of nursing diagnoses for an 18-month-old child for regular health supervision and immunizations may include the following:

- Imbalanced Nutrition: More than Body Requirements related to lack of basic nutritional knowledge
- Risk for Poisoning related to lack of proper precautions with increased mobility to reach and climb
- Health-Seeking Behaviors related to needed immunizations
- Risk for Impaired Parenting related to mother's plans to return to full-time work

Planning and Implementation

Nursing management for health supervision visits begins with collaborative planning with the family. They share their concerns and questions, and the nurse also lists procedures and discussion topics to be addressed. (See Families Want to Know: Health Supervision Visits.) These may include providing immunizations, offering anticipatory guidance about discipline, educating parents and children about healthy behaviors, addressing health promotion regarding nutrition, suggesting ways to prevent disease and injury, and providing referrals for follow-up care. For more information about the recommended schedule for immunizations and the nurse's role in ensuring full immunization status for children, refer to Chapter 16 ∞.

Most parents want to know how to contribute to their child's growth and development, and need linkages to additional community resources to foster child development (Fine & Mayer, 2006). Discussions at the conclusion of the health supervision assessments should focus on building family strengths by promoting the development of competence, confidence, and self-esteem in the growing child. Offering health promotion activities such as these provides a positive ending for the visit. Inquire about the family stresses and strengths in order to plan with them to provide for the child's health promotion.

Although health supervision most likely takes place in an office or clinic setting, nursing management for health supervision

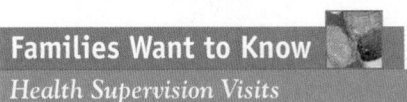

Families Want to Know
Health Supervision Visits

Focus groups with parents were conducted to learn parental views about health supervision visits with their children. Parents wanted reassurance about the child's behaviors and wanted an opportunity to discuss health with a professional. An ongoing relationship with one professional was important. Parents requested additional information on development and child behaviors, and additional ways to communicate with health care providers (Radecki, Olson, Frintner, et al., 2009). Nurses should:

- Ask what the parent priorities are at each health care visit.
- Provide handouts and information on the child's expected developmental achievements.
- Discuss child behaviors such as sleep, discipline, and other parent concerns.
- Integrate communication methods such as phone calls and Internet contact into the care setting.

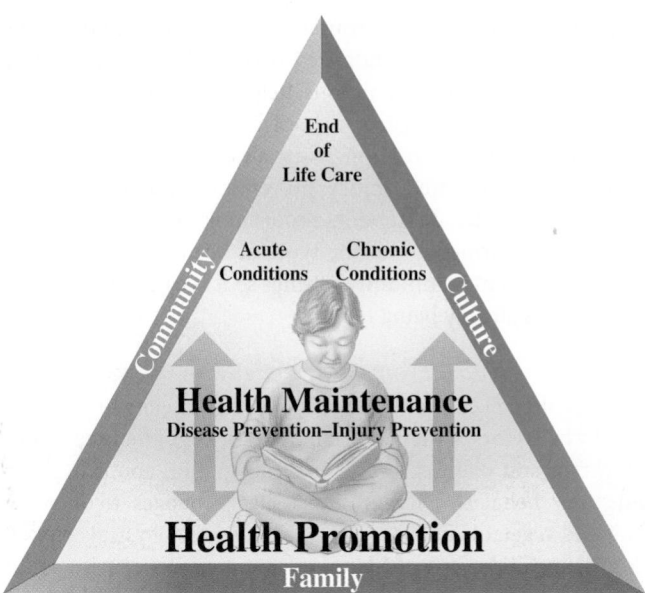

FIGURE 6–7 ➤ Health promotion and maintenance are foundational to all pediatric health care. They are integrated into every health care visit, whether for health supervision, or acute and chronic conditions.

can occur in any setting. The nurse recognizes that health promotion and health maintenance activities are key to any nurse–family relationship. Health promotion and maintenance are constant and foundational aspects of all pediatric care. This approach to health care closely reflects a partnership with families and is essential to every health care encounter (Figure 6–7 ➤).

Clinical Judgment

The pediatric nurse should apply concepts of health promotion and maintenance in all health care settings. If the child is seen in an emergency room for treatment of a fracture, what questions should the nurse ask about immunization status and safety issues? If the nurse sees a child with a chronic disorder of cerebral palsy in the outpatient clinic at an orthopedic hospital, what health promotion and health maintenance services should be integrated?

Provide Anticipatory Guidance

Anticipatory guidance involves prediction of the upcoming developmental tasks or needs of a child and gears teaching to those needs. It provides the family with information on what to expect during the child's current and next stage of development. Topics for each visit should include age-appropriate information about healthy habits, illness and injury prevention, poison prevention, nutrition, oral health, and sexuality. Use health promotional guidance to help the child and family develop strategies that support and enhance social development, family relationships, parental health, community interactions, self-responsibility, and school or vocational achievement.

Because the time for each visit is limited, build upon the parents' current knowledge and care practices, and start with a topic about which they express interest. Time can be used to focus on anticipatory guidance to introduce new information, to reinforce what the family is doing well, and to clear up any poorly understood concepts.

Take advantage of other sources of information in the community to enhance the guidance provided. For example, state and local SAFE KIDS coalitions help inform families about injury-prevention strategies. School health programs such as the National Fire Prevention Association's "Risk Watch" may educate children about injury prevention, and other school programs may educate students about smoking and drug avoidance. Keep informed about the types of health education provided in different community settings so it is easier to reinforce the concepts already being taught.

Encourage Health Promotion Activities

Families often need health education and counseling to promote healthy behaviors in their own child. Examples of focused health education and counseling may be information about limiting sedentary behaviors, integrating dietary changes to increase fruit and vegetable intake, and increasing daily physical activity. Counseling in the case of Clarence (see opening scenario) could focus on childcare arrangements, management of his high level of activity, and the management of potential behavior problems. Collaborate with Clarence's parents to learn about their concerns and how they want to improve their parenting.

Patient education and counseling are most effective when the family understands the relationship between a behavior change and the resulting health outcome. When identifying that a family would benefit from a change in health behavior, consider the family members' perceptions about the health change, consider the barriers and benefits to change, and plan interventions to enhance the possibility for change.

Steps in promoting patient education and counseling include:

- Clarifying learning needs of child and family
- Setting a limited agenda
- Prioritizing needs with the family
- Selecting a teaching strategy (explaining, showing, providing resources, questioning, practicing, giving feedback)
- Evaluating effectiveness (Hagan et al., 2008)

Perform Health Supervision Interventions

After all of the information from the interviews, physical assessment, and screening tests is collected and analyzed, specific health and developmental achievements should be summarized for the parents and child. Immunizations are provided as appropriate. Anticipatory guidance may be offered at various points during the health supervision visit.

When a child is found to be at risk for a health condition, integrate health maintenance interventions to lessen the possibility of disease or injury. If an actual health problem is detected, follow-up care must be arranged. The child may need to return for another visit to the primary care provider for further evaluation, or referral to another provider may be needed. The nurse needs to learn about all of the available community resources to make appropriate referrals. The range of such services may include the following:

- Hospital and community-based health care specialists from many disciplines (e.g., dentists, physicians, physical therapists, speech therapists, nutritionists, social workers)
- Community-based programs (e.g., childcare centers, developmental stimulation programs, home visitor programs, early intervention programs, mental health centers, diagnostic and evaluation centers, schools, family support centers, food and nutrition referral centers, public health clinics, churches, and other organizations that support families and children)

Evaluation

Expected outcomes of nursing care include the following:

- The child and family collaborate in a partnership with the health care provider in joint problem solving and decision making regarding the management of the child's health care needs after appropriate education and counseling.
- The child and family prepare for future health supervision visits by identifying questions or concerns they want to discuss.

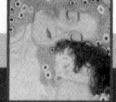

Chapter Highlights

- Health is a dynamic state of physical, mental, and social well-being and is the objective of health promotion and health maintenance activities.
- Health supervision visits are health care encounters designed to provide assessment, screening, developmental surveillance, immunizations, and health information.
- Partners in providing health supervision are the child, family, health professional, and community.
- Families are best educated in "teachable moments" with small bits of information.
- Developmental surveillance is an essential part of health supervision that provides for observations of children's fine and gross motor skills, language, and psychosocial behavior milestones.

- Nutrition, physical activity, and oral health are essential topics during health supervision visits.
- Mental health and spiritual status, as well as the relationships of the child within the family and larger community, are assessed at each health supervision visit.
- The nurse establishes diagnoses based on a thorough assessment of the child and family during health care visits.
- The nurse establishes goals for visits collaboratively with families, and plans interventions to meet goals.
- Health promotion and health maintenance interventions are essential components of all child health care, even during periods of acute or chronic illness.

Clinical Reasoning in Action

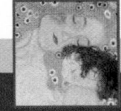

Recall the parents of 15-month-old Clarence. They are working parents who are overwhelmed by their son's activity level. They express concern about how to spend time with and ensure safety for Clarence, while having some time to spend with each other.

1. Describe the physical activity skills that you expect to observe in a 15-month-old. Is Clarence typical of this age child?
2. Plan the assessment techniques you will apply to learn more about Clarence's physical activity and social interactions.

3. Clarence's parents are concerned about providing a safe environment for him. List the most important safety precautions that should be taken in the home and during car trips to promote his safety.
4. Plan several interventions that will assist his parents in planning their time so that they have time to spend with Clarence every day and also have some time alone to rest each week.

See Pearson Nursing Student Resources for possible responses.

Pearson Nursing Student Resources

Find additional review materials at
nursing.pearsonhighered.com

Prepare for success with NCLEX®-style practice questions, interactive assignments and activities, web links, animations and videos, and more!

References

Center for Mental Health Services. (n.d.). *Caring for every child's mental health campaign.* Retrieved from http://mentalhealth.samhsa.gov/child/

Centers for Disease Control and Prevention (CDC). (2006a). *Healthy youth! Health topics: Physical activity.* Retrieved from http://www.cdc.gov/HealthyYouth/physicalactivity/facts.htm

Centers for Disease Control and Prevention (CDC). (2006b). Youth Risk Behavior Surveillance—United States, 2005. *Morbidity and Mortality Weekly Report, 55*(SS-5), 1–108.

Centers for Disease Control and Prevention (CDC). (2006c). *Dental visits.* Retrieved from http://www.cdc.gov.nohss/guideDV.htm

Commonwealth Fund. (2008). *Pediatric developmental screening: Understanding and selecting screening instruments.* New York: Author.

Council on Children with Disabilities, Section on Developmental Pediatrics, Bright Futures Steering Committee and Medical Home Initiatives for Children with Special Needs Project Advisory Committee. (2006). Identifying infants and young children with developmental disorders in the medical home: An algorithm for developmental surveillance and screening. *Pediatrics, 118*, 405–420.

Dye, B. A., Tan, S., Smith, V., Lewis, B. G., Barker, L. K., Thornton-Evans, G., et al. (2007). Trends in oral health status: United States, 1988–1994 and 1999–2004. U.S. Department of Health and Human Services, National Center for Health Statistics. *Vital and Health Statistics, 11*(248), 1–104.

Earls, M. F., & Hay, S. S. (2006). Setting the stage for success: Implementation of developmental and behavioral screening and surveillance in primary care practice—The North Carolina Assuring Better Child Health and Development (ABCD) Project. *Pediatrics, 118*, 183–188.

Fine, A., & Mayer, R. (2006). *Beyond referral: Pediatric care linkages to improve developmental health.* New York: The Commonwealth Fund. Publication No. 976.

Hagan, J. G., Shaw, J. S., & Duncan, P. M. (Eds.). (2008). *Bright futures: Guidelines for health supervision of infants, children, and adolescents* (3rd ed.). Elk Grove Village, IL: American Academy of Pediatrics.

Healthy People 2020. (2010). *Healthy People 2020 Goals.* Retrieved from www.healthypeople.gov

Jellinek, M., Patel, B. P., & Froehle, M. C. (Eds.). (2002). *Bright futures in practice; Mental health Vol. II, tool kit.* Arlington, VA: National Center for Education in Maternal and Child Health.

Kenney, G. M., McFeeters, J. R., & Yee, J. Y. (2005). Preventive dental care and unmet dental needs among low-income children. *American Journal of Public Health, 95*, 1360–1366.

King, T. M., Tandon, S. D., Macias, M. M., Healy, J. A., Duncan, P. M., Swigonski, N. L., et al. (2010). Implementing developmental screening and referrals: Lessons learned from a national project. *Pediatrics, 125*(2), 350–360.

Murray, R. B., Zentner, J. P., & Yakimo, R. (2009). *Health promotion strategies through the life span* (8th ed.). Upper Saddle River, NJ: Prentice Hall.

NAPNAP. (2009). NAPNAP position statement on pediatric health care/medical home: Key issues on delivery, reimbursement, and leadership. *Journal of Pediatric Health Care, 23*(3), 23A–24A.

Pan, R. J. (2006). A Jacobian future: Can everyone have a medical home? *Pediatrics, 118*, 1254–1256.

Pender, N. J., Murdaugh, C. L., & Parsons, M. A. (2006). *Health promotion in nursing practice* (5th ed.). Upper Saddle River, NJ: Prentice Hall.

Radecki, L., Olson, L. M., Frintner, M. P., Tanner, J. L., & Stein, M. T. (2009). What do families want from well-child care: Including parents in the rethinking discussion. *Pediatrics, 124*, 858–865.

Schoenbaum, S. C., & Abrams, J. (2006). *No place like home.* New York: Commonwealth Fund.

World Health Organization. (2001). *Background information about health promotion.* Retrieved from http://www.who.int/hpr/backgroundhp/

World Health Organization. (2010). *Health Promotion.* . Retrieved from http://www.who.int/topics/health_promotion/en/

WorldHealthOrganization. (2009). *Background: Social determinant of health.* Retrieved from http://www.who.int/chp/en/

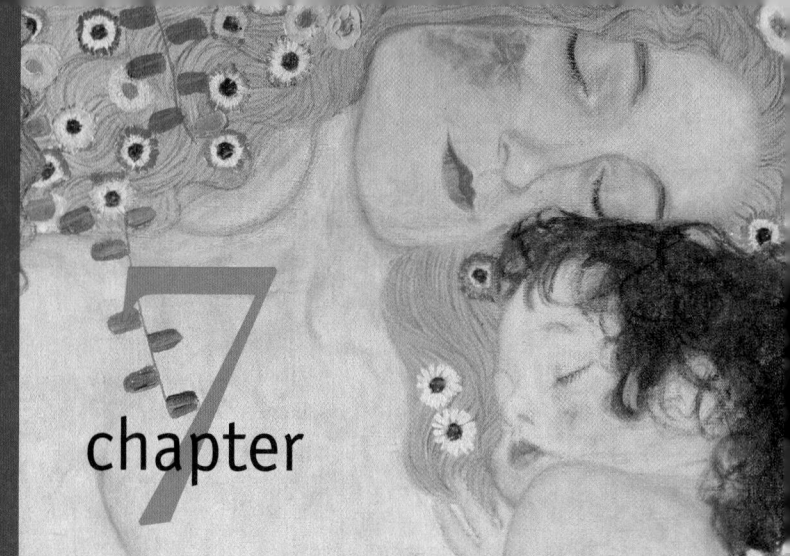

Health Promotion and Maintenance for the Newborn and Infant

chapter 7

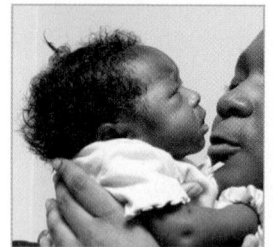

$\mathcal{S}$hannon comes to the pediatric health services clinic with her 10-day-old daughter, Rhonda. Shannon is a 22-year-old single mother who lives with her 5-year-old daughter and male partner of 2 years, who is the father of their newborn. Shannon had an uncomplicated pregnancy and birth. Rhonda was born at 37 weeks' gestation. She required phototherapy for newborn jaundice and had initial difficulties breastfeeding. Rhonda was discharged at 5 days of age in good health. The nurse weighs and measures Rhonda, and finds that she weighs 1 ounce more than her birth weight. Shannon voices concerns that Rhonda sleeps very little, cries a lot at night, and makes sleep difficult for her boyfriend, who has to get up early for work. The nurse asks Shannon how she knows when Rhonda is ready to feed. Shannon recognizes only Rhonda's crying as a feeding cue. The nurse gives Shannon information on newborn states and cues, and encourages Shannon to notice more subtle feeding cues. The nurse calls the lactation consultant and together they assess Rhonda's breastfeeding effectiveness. The lactation consultant works with Shannon on a feeding plan to ensure that breastfeeding is successful. The pediatric nurse then helps Shannon to strategize how to help Rhonda sleep for longer periods, recognizing that newborns often do not settle into a schedule until well into the second month. What ongoing assessment will Rhonda and her parents need? How can the nurse encourage shared parenting between Shannon and her boyfriend? What coordinated follow-up is required between the pediatric nurse and the lactation consultant?

Learning Outcomes

After reading this chapter, you will be able to do the following:

1. Explain the nurse's role in providing health promotion and health maintenance for the newborn, infant, and family.
2. Describe the general observations made of infants and their families as they come to the pediatric health care home for health supervision visits.
3. Identify assessment and intervention areas for health supervision visits of newborns and infants—growth and developmental surveillance, nutrition, physical activity, oral health, mental and spiritual health, family and social relations, disease prevention strategies, and injury prevention strategies.
4. Plan health promotion and maintenance strategies to employ during health supervision visits of newborns and infants.
5. Apply the nursing process in assessment, diagnosis, goal setting, intervention, and evaluation of health promotion and maintenance activities for the newborn and infant.
6. Integrate the family in newborn and infant health care, including family assessment in each health supervision visit.

■ HEALTH PROMOTION AND MAINTENANCE FOR THE NEWBORN

For a healthy woman, prenatal care, labor, and birth may be her first experience in an ongoing relationship with health care professionals. The quality of that experience is key to ensuring a continuing partnership between her and her child's health care providers.

The month following delivery is a time of huge transition for the new mother and her family. The mother is coping with not only hormonal shifts and a postpartum body but also changing roles and relationships. The nurse's role is to assess knowledge about self-care and newborn care, teach health promotion and maintenance activities, promote parental confidence in newborn caregiving, and promote a partnership among health care professionals and the family.

Contacts with the Family

The nurse who sees the expectant mother during prenatal care has the unique opportunity to help parents prepare for their new roles. The nurse listens attentively and provides information and support. During prenatal visits, parents learn to value health supervision and an active partnership with health care professionals. The nurse who interacts with the family in the prenatal period assesses risk and protective factors. Women are often receptive to altering risky behaviors in order to protect the newborn from harm. The motivation to give birth to a healthy newborn is usually strong, and the nurse can use maternal readiness for change to promote behaviors that improve maternal and newborn health.

Most obstetrical care providers encourage the expectant mother to choose her newborn's care provider prior to the baby's birth. Pediatric care providers usually welcome a short office visit, sometimes at no charge, to allow the expectant mother and care provider to assess their "fit" prior to committing to this important relationship. (See Families Want to Know: Prenatal Visit to the Pediatric Care Provider.) Many pediatric care providers have written or online information for expectant parents, explaining their professional philosophy of care as well as information about services.

The hospital length of stay for a healthy mother and newborn is short, approximately 48 hours for a vaginal birth and 72–96 hours for an uncomplicated cesarean birth. Insurance companies must provide coverage for 48 hours after vaginal and 96 hours after cesarean birth; earlier discharges should be followed by a home visit to monitor the newborn and maternal conditions (London, Ladewig, Ball, et al., 2010; U.S. Department of Labor, 2009). During the hospital stay, the nurse provides ongoing physical assessment of the mother and newborn, while providing education and anticipatory guidance to prepare the mother to care for herself and her newborn following hospital discharge.

Although it is challenging, the nurse incorporates many newborn health promotion and maintenance activities into this short stay. Starting at the moment of birth, the newborn is continuously assessed and procedures are performed to ensure newborn health. The nurse encourages bonding of newborn

---

Families Want to Know
Prenatal Visit to the Pediatric Care Provider

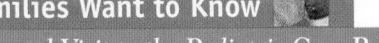

Encourage parents to visit the pediatric health care home before the baby is born. This enables the care provider to meet the family and assess for high-risk situations that will help inform care after the infant's birth, and enables the family to meet and establish trust and rapport with the care provider (Cohen & Committee, 2009). Assist parents to prepare questions and make an appointment to visit one or more providers that they are considering using.

Questions they can ask the provider include:

■ How soon after birth will the baby be examined by you? Will you report findings of your initial examination to us before hospital discharge?

■ What is your philosophy about male circumcision? Do you perform circumcision? If not, who does this procedure? Is circumcision performed in the hospital before discharge or in the office after discharge?

■ What if our baby needs intensive care? Will a transfer to another hospital or care provider be necessary?

■ When is our newborn's first office visit? Do we call for that appointment or is it made for us while we are in the hospital?

■ As our baby's provider, what can I expect from you? What is your most important job? What do you enjoy most about your work? What are the most important things you offer to new families like us?

■ As the parent of a new baby, what do you expect from me? What is my most important job?

■ What are the costs of care? Do you accept my method of payment/insurance/government assistance?

■ What are office hours? Who do we contact if we have a question or if the baby is sick outside of office hours?

■ Who covers your office when you are unavailable? Do you have partners in the office or colleagues in the community who cover for you when you are out? May I have a list of their names and phone numbers?

■ Who else answers our questions about routine baby and childcare? What is that person's training? Do you have resources to support breastfeeding mothers? Working mothers?

■ How much time is usually spent for an office visit? How much time will we have to ask questions?

■ If our child needs hospitalization, what hospital do you prefer to use? Would you be our baby's doctor, or would you refer the hospital care to someone else?

After the interview, parents can ask themselves the following questions:

■ Was I comfortable talking with this person? Did this person listen to me?

■ Did I get clear answers to my questions?

■ Do I feel that I could trust this provider with my child's care?

■ Was I comfortable in the office? Did I feel welcome? Were all staff members friendly, helpful, and competent?

■ Will this provider be a good "fit" for my family?

and parents, monitoring of physiological health, and integration of the newborn into the family unit.

For the healthy newborn, early contacts include procedures such as first bath, umbilical cord care (Figure 7–1 ➤), vitamin K and hepatitis B injections, and eye prophylaxis; a comprehensive physical assessment (see Chapter 5 ∞ for details); screening procedures such as hearing, metabolic, and maternal syphilis screenings (American Academy of Pediatrics [AAP], 2004; Joint Committee on Infant Hearing, 2007; Katbamna, Crumpton, & Patel, 2008); and observations of newborn feeding and of parent–newborn bonding. See Medications Used to Treat Newborns on the next page.

Clinical Tip

Administration of medications can be stressful for the newborn and parents.

- Administer eye prophylaxis before, or at a different time than, the vitamin K injection. The newborn may cry during the vitamin K injection, making it difficult to administer ophthalmic ointment.
- Administer eye prophylaxis when the newborn is calm. Allow first bonding with the parent if possible before the administration since vision of the newborn will be blurred after administration; however, the medication should be administered within the first hour after birth. Do not attempt to pry the newborn's eyes open when the newborn is crying, or when the infant is supine and facing bright overhead lights. Dim the room, swaddle or contain the newborn's limbs, and hold the newborn semi-upright. If the newborn is awake or drowsy, the eyes will usually open, allowing easier administration of the ophthalmic ointment.
- The newborn is less likely to cry during the vitamin K injection if the nurse lays the newborn on a firm surface and the parent gently holds the newborn's arms across the newborn's chest during the injection. This "containment" helps the newborn stay calm during the procedure.

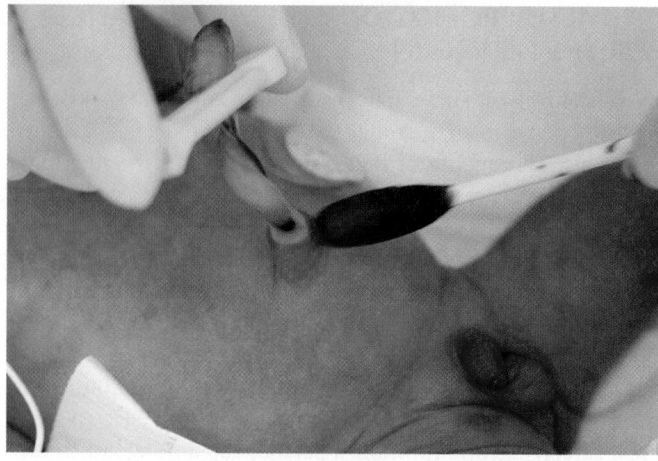

A

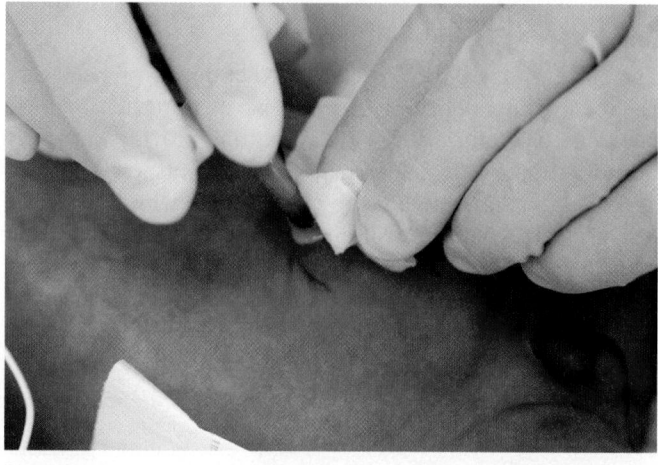

B

FIGURE 7–1 ➤ Two different methods for cord care: A, Betadine cleaning. B, Alcohol cleaning.

At discharge, the family is given an appointment for the first visit in the office or clinic setting; a physician, nurse practitioner, or nurse assessment is recommended at 3–5 days of age, with subsequent follow-up visits for newborns at risk for hyperbilirubinemia or feeding problems (AAP, 2004). See Families Want to Know: Discharge Teaching for New Parents.

General Observations

At the first office visit, the nursing assessment begins with general observations of the newborn and family (Figure 7–2 ➤). This often occurs as the family is called in from the waiting area.

Welcome the family to the facility and comment on the newborn. Ask how the family is adjusting. In the first month of the newborn's life, parents are usually exhausted and experiencing stressful adjustments in their relationship with each other. The nurse gathers information in order to assess the family's needs, to invite discussion, to validate positive parenting efforts, and to promote partnership between the family and the health care team.

The nurse assesses development of **attachment behaviors** (behaviors that demonstrate an emotional connection between newborn and caregiver), parental perception of infant temperament, feeding status, safety, family integration, parental mental

Medications Used to Treat
Newborns

Medication	Prophylactic Action	Nursing Management
Vitamin K (phytonadione)	To prevent vitamin K–dependent hemorrhagic disease of the newborn.	1 mg IM is given within 1 hour of birth. Locate the accurate site on the ventrogluteal thigh.
Sterile ophthalmic ointment containing tetracycline (1%) or erythromycin (0.5%) (American Academy of Pediatrics, 2007)	As prophylaxis against ophthalmia neonatorum caused by *Chlamydia trachomatis* or *Neisseria gonorrhoeae*.	Place a 1–2 cm ribbon along the conjunctival sac of each eye within 1 hour of birth, taking care that the agent reaches all areas of the conjunctival sac.
Hepatitis B virus (HBV) immunoprophylaxis	All women should be screened for hepatitis B as part of routine prenatal care. The first hepatitis B vaccination for the newborn is preferably received prior to hospital discharge; if not received, the newborn should receive the first dose at the initial outpatient visit.	■ For babies of HBsAg-negative women, the first dose of HBV vaccine is administered during the newborn period (recommended time) or by age 2 months; second dose 1–2 months later, and third dose by age 6–18 months. ■ Babies of HBsAg-positive women must receive the HBV vaccine within 12 hours of birth AND receive one dose of hepatitis B immune globulin (HBIG) within 12 hours of birth at a second intramuscular site (opposite thigh). Check the mother's record of hepatitis screening so doses can be given within the time recommended.

Families Want to Know
Discharge Teaching for New Parents

Parents should be taught prior to hospital discharge about education materials to help ensure adequate newborn care and instructions regarding how to access health care providers for consultation. This information should also be accessible at home. Discharge teaching includes:

■ Breastfeeding technique
    or
■ Formula feeding technique
■ Umbilical cord care
■ Bathing and skin care
■ Diapering and dressing the newborn
■ Temperature assessment using a thermometer
■ Signs of newborn illness
  • Abdominal swelling
  • Blue skin coloring, especially of the face, lips, or tongue
  • Persistent coughing or choking during feedings
  • Unusually long period of crying that will not stop despite comfort measures
  • Jaundice (yellow coloring of the skin) that appears head to toe
  • Sleeping through feedings or baby that is too tired or uninterested to eat
  • Drainage or redness of umbilical cord
  • Respiratory distress
    —Fast breathing (more than 60 breaths/minute)
    —Retractions (muscles between ribs suck in with each breath)
    —Flaring of nose
    —Grunting while breathing
■ Newborn safety
  • Infant car seat use
  • Supine sleeping position

health, and parental coping mechanisms. Look again at the photo in the chapter opener and identify what attachment behaviors you see Shannon exhibiting toward the baby, Rhonda. The nurse may determine that further assessment is required—for example, if the parent states that breastfeeding is so painful she wants to switch to formula, if she is continuously depressed, if she has started smoking again, or if she cannot calm her crying baby. The nurse in the pediatric setting is aware that pediatric health is closely connected to the entire family's health.

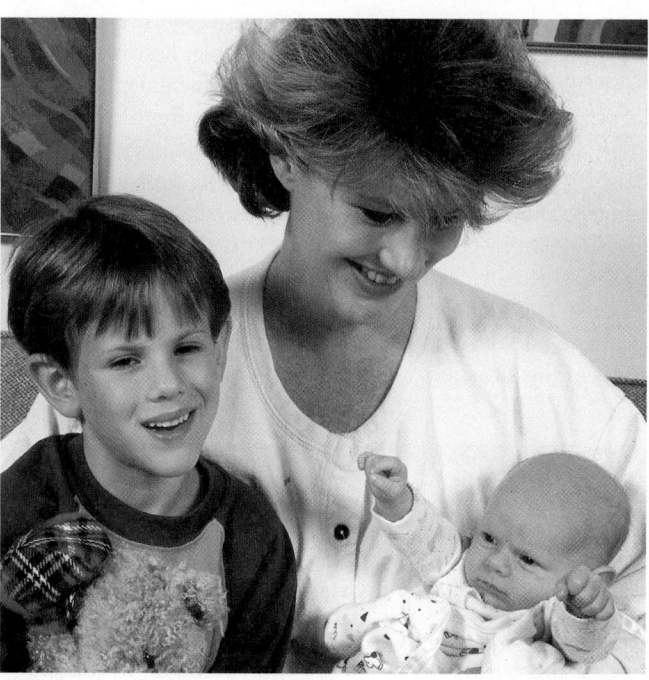

FIGURE 7–2 ➤ Observation of the newborn and family begins at first contact during the health promotion and health maintenance visit.

Many concerns require referral for parents outside the pediatric care setting; therefore, the office or clinic should have a system in place and ready access to referrals and resources for parents in need.

Clinical Judgment

When a family does not speak English fluently and is scheduled for a newborn visit, what strategies will assist in assessment and teaching of this family?

Growth and Developmental Surveillance

At this visit, the baby's current weight, length, and head circumference are measured and plotted on a growth chart (see Appendix A ∞), and a basic physical examination is performed (see Chapter 5 ∞).

In the first week of life, most babies lose about 1/10 of their birth weight. For example, a 3500-gram baby (7 pounds, 12 ounces) could lose up to 350 grams (nearly 12 ounces). Growth spurts are evident at around 7–10 days, and again between 3 and 6 weeks of age. By day 10, most babies are back to their original birth weight and gaining about 2/3 of an ounce per day. Length increases by 1–1 1/2 inches in the first month, and head circumference increases about 1 inch (AAP, 2009).

Developmental surveillance includes assessment of the baby's ability to calm when being held or spoken to, and respond to sounds by blinking, crying, quieting, or startling. The baby should be able to fixate on a human face and follow it with his or her eyes. The baby should be able to lift his or her head momentarily when placed prone, demonstrate a flexed position, and move all extremities. Most babies will sleep for 3 or 4 hours at a time and stay awake for an hour or longer (Hagan, Shaw, & Duncan, 2008).

It is normal for parents to compare their newborn's developmental skills with other children of the same age. Every baby develops according to an individual timetable; however, when a baby falls far behind, fails to reach a developmental milestone, or loses a previously acquired skill, the baby requires further evaluation. In the first month of life, signs of **developmental delay** (a delay in mastering functions such as motor coordination and behavioral skills) in a full-term infant usually merit immediate investigation by a pediatrician, a pediatric developmental specialist, a pediatric neurologist, or a multidisciplinary team of professionals. Parents require additional emotional support, clear and honest communication, and resources to cope with the stress of this situation.

TABLE 7–1	Newborn Growth and Developmental Milestones Observed in Health Promotion and Health Maintenance Visits
Growth	• Weight: Newborn may lose up to 1/10 of birth weight in the first week of life; birth weight should be reattained by day 10; weight gain is about 2/3 of an ounce per day thereafter • Length increases by 1 to 1 1/2 inches • Head circumference increases by about 1 inch
Vision	• Focuses 8–12 inches away • Eyes wander and may cross • Prefers black-and-white or high-contrast patterns • Prefers the human face to all other patterns
Hearing	• Fully mature hearing • Recognizes some sounds • May turn toward familiar sounds and voices

Table 7–1 summarizes some growth and developmental milestones that can commonly be observed during newborn care visits.

Nutrition

Health care providers in the prenatal setting play a vital role in educating expectant mothers about the health benefits of breastfeeding and providing anticipatory guidance prior to childbirth. The nurse in the birth setting promotes breastfeeding by facilitating nursing in the first 30–60 minutes of life, and providing supportive guidance as the mother begins to develop this skill prior to discharge. Shannon, described in the opening scenario, received breastfeeding information from the nurse and the lactation specialist. Continued assessment, encouragement, and support of breastfeeding are vital to the continued success of breastfeeding mothers, as many mothers initiate breastfeeding and discontinue after a few days or weeks (American Academy of Pediatrics Committee on Nutrition, 2009). The nurse who encounters breastfeeding mothers should understand the basics of breastfeeding management (Figure 7–3 ➤). Ideally, the pediatric setting has a lactation specialist or resource person who can assess breastfeeding and problem solve with the mother. Referrals to a community lactation specialist or support group may be necessary.

In some cases, mothers choose formula feeding for a newborn. Mothers who use infant formula should feed iron-fortified

---

Growth & Development *Signs of Developmental Delay*

During the second, third, or fourth week of life, the following signs of potential developmental delay require a complete medical and developmental evaluation to determine if a disability exists and to plan interventions or future management. The pediatric nurse observes the newborn for these signs and may have opportunity to assess for problems through discussing the newborn's abilities and behaviors with the caregiver.

- Sucks poorly and feeds slowly
- Does not blink when shown a bright light
- Does not focus and follow a nearby object moving side to side
- Rarely moves arms and legs; movements are not symmetrical
- Lacks muscle tone; limbs are consistently stretched out rather than flexed
- Does not respond to loud sounds

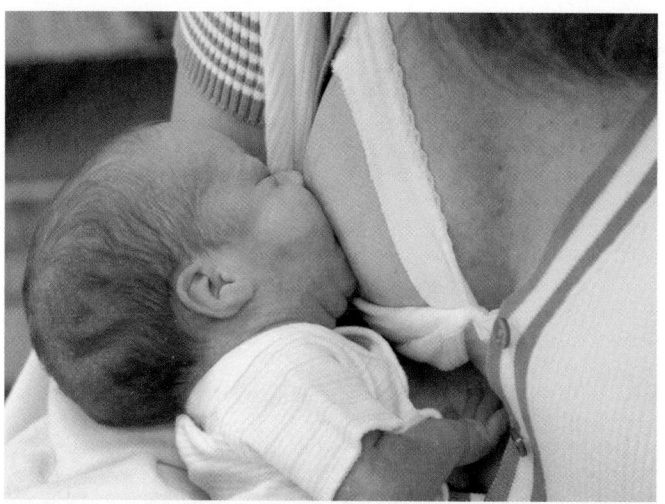

FIGURE 7–3 ➤ Breastfeeding has lifelong benefits for the mother and child and should be promoted prenatally, in the hospital, and through the first year of health promotion visits.

formula (containing 4–12 mg/L of iron) from birth to 12 months (Committee on Nutrition, 2009). This helps ensure adequate iron stores and very low rates of iron deficiency between 6 and 18 months of age. (See Chapter 14 ∞ for more information about newborn feeding.)

Physical Activity

The flexed position of the newborn demonstrates development of the flexor muscles and relaxation of the extensor muscles. This flexed position protects the newborn, conserves energy by reducing movement, and reduces heat loss (Blackburn, 2007). During the first month of life, the newborn gradually "unfolds" and the body straightens. Movements begin to change from reflexive to purposeful. By the end of the first month, the newborn should be able to:

- Bring hands to eyes and mouth
- Move head side to side when lying on abdomen
- Attempt to lift head when prone

In addition, the newborn's hands are kept in tight fists, and the reflexes are strong (see Chapter 5 ∞).

Health promotion teaching for the family includes the following activities:

- Position the baby on his or her stomach for supervised play periods. This allows the newborn to lift the head and turn it from side to side, make crawling motions, and push up on his or her arms. Allowing supervised "tummy time" is also important for prevention of flat spots on the back of the baby's head caused by constant supine positioning (Graham, 2006). Be sure to place the baby on his or her back when tired and starting to fall asleep. (See further information in Chapter 27 ∞.)
- Allow the baby free movement of arms and hands. If the baby is swaddled, allow the hands to be outside the blanket and positioned in midline. This allows flexion and extension of arms, brings hands into the line of vision, and brings hands to mouth.

- Encourage appropriate toys such as a mobile with contrasting colors and patterns; a plastic mirror; music boxes and exposure to soft music on the radio, tape recorder, or CD player; and soft toys with colors, patterns, and gentle sounds.
- Encourage switching positions when bottle-feeding. It may be most comfortable for the mother to hold the baby in a cradle position with the bottle in her right hand (or left hand if left-handed); however, switching arms encourages newborn muscle development and control on each side of the baby's body. Breastfeeding babies automatically feed from both sides. Parents who bottle-feed may need to be reminded to promote this skill in their newborn.
- Beginning at birth, prevent flat spots on the newborn's head from supine positioning by nightly alternating the head position from left to right during sleep and occasionally changing the newborn's orientation in relation to the activity at the room's doorway.

Oral Health

Ideally, pediatric oral health begins with prenatal oral health counseling for parents. If not already established, promotion of healthy oral hygiene practices and routine preventive dental care for parents establishes a foundation for a lifetime of good oral health for their children.

Protective factors for good oral health include good general health, appropriate use of fluoride in family members more than 6 months of age (either topically, in community water systems, or systemically as deemed appropriate by health care professionals), secure socioeconomic status, family intake of simple sugars occurring primarily at mealtime, and regular use of dental care in an established **dental home**, a specialized dental care provider who manages and facilitates all aspects of oral health care. Risk factors include infant's siblings with dental caries in the past 12 months, active caries present in the mother, suboptimal fluoride exposure, frequent between-meal exposure of family members to simple sugars, low socioeconomic status, no usual source of dental care, and children with special health care needs. Annual dental health care is a *Healthy People 2020* objective (*Healthy People 2010*).

Parents can help prevent tooth decay in their new baby by practicing good oral health habits from birth. In the first month of life, parents should be warned against propping the bottle in the baby's mouth while the baby falls asleep. Babies who sleep with their teeth exposed to juice, formula, or breast milk can develop early childhood caries in primary teeth, even before they emerge. (See Chapter 14 ∞ for further information on early childhood caries.)

Oral disease may be prevented if strategies are applied early enough in the child's life. The nurse should assess risk factors for dental disease, promote oral hygiene beginning in infancy, and provide anticipatory guidance to help parents ensure good oral health for their children.

Mental and Spiritual Health

Arriving at home with a newborn can be an overwhelming emotional experience for the mother, her partner, and other family members. An immediate shift in roles and responsibilities must occur within the family. In addition to meeting the newborn's needs, the new mother must also deal with meeting other family members' needs, rapidly shifting emotions, and her postpartum body. At the same time, the family is establishing a secure and healthy atmosphere for the new baby. The nurse assesses signs of a growing secure attachment between parent and child in the first month of life by making observations such as:

- Parent frequently looks at the newborn.
- Parent has specific questions and observations about the newborn's individual characteristics.
- Parent touches, massages, or gently rubs the newborn.
- Parent attempts to soothe the newborn when the newborn is upset.
- Newborn looks content.
- Newborn signals needs.
- Newborn feeds well.
- Newborn responds to parent's attempts to soothe.

Newborns begin to make their needs known to parents through verbal and nonverbal cues. Engagement cues include looking at, reaching toward, and gazing at the caretaker. Disengagement cues indicate that the baby needs to have some quiet time and include turning away, falling asleep, flailing extremities, and crying. The nurse in this chapter's opening scenario helps the mother, Shannon, to learn her baby's cues of turning toward her, rooting, and engagement as indicative of a need for feeding or attention. Babies also develop strategies for **self-regulation**, the ability to console the self.

The newborn's mental health and development is highly dependent on the mental and spiritual health of his or her primary caregiver, usually the mother. The mother who is emotionally whole and fully present in her newborn's life is best able to provide the nurturing environment necessary for optimal growth and development (Hagan et al., 2008). Assess for strengths as well as challenges, and offer resources to help the family meet their needs so that attention can be focused on the newborn (Figure 7–4 ➤).

During the health supervision visit, the nurse models behavior for parents that promotes positive infant mental health, such as handling the newborn gently, speaking in a soft voice, noticing attributes ("Look how you hold your head up today! You're really getting strong!"), and noticing likes and dislikes. The nurse strengthens parental confidence by asking the parent what the baby likes, such as, "How does he like to be carried, in your arms or up on your shoulder?" and then following the parent's advice. The nurse also promotes nurturing behavior by parents during procedures, such as allowing the parent to hold and comfort the infant while the nurse administers immunizations or draws blood.

Most women experience postpartum "blues" or temporary sadness in the first week after delivery due to hormonal shifts and sleep deprivation. This usually resolves without intervention after a few hours to several days. Postpartum depression is a more serious and debilitating postpartum mood disorder (PPMD) that occurs in 10–20% of mothers in the first year after the infant's birth (Mishina & Takayama, 2009). Screening should occur at each health visit. Necessary interventions may

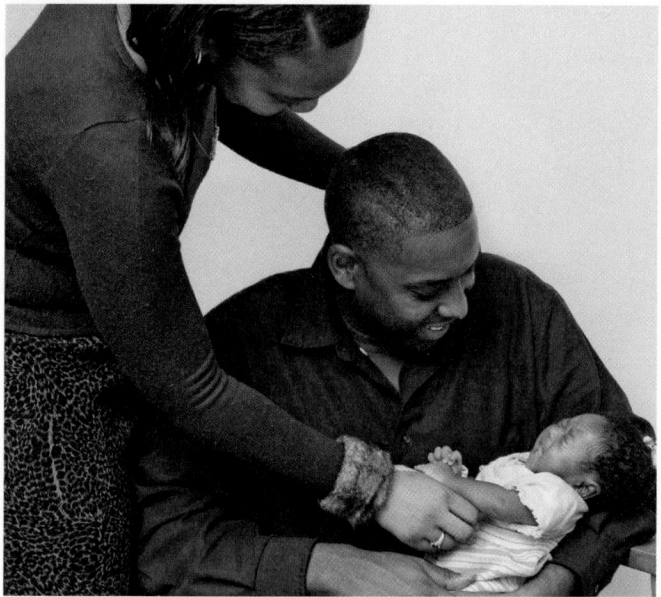

FIGURE 7–4 ➤ A healthy parent forms strong attachments to the newborn and is motivated to ensure the child's physical and mental health. What observations can you make about attachment between Rhonda and her parents?

include counseling or medication from the mother's primary care provider. Another condition, postpartum psychosis, is a serious mental health condition that is considered a psychiatric emergency.

Relationships

Family adaptation to a new baby begins in pregnancy, and evidence of initial family adaptation to pregnancy may be predictive of future parental coping (Hagan et al., 2008). The family is the primary site where the infant learns to interact with other people. Therefore, family dynamics must be examined during health supervision visits. Risks and protective factors of the family are identified during psychosocial screening (Table 7–2) (Commonwealth Fund, 2007). Observations are used to apply strategies that help parents in the relationship with the newborn.

New parents may need assistance in identifying activities that promote family health and positive parent–newborn interaction. Provide the following suggestions to parents:

- Share newborn care activities. Recognize that you may do things differently than your partner, such as the way you change a diaper or give a bath. If the baby is cared for, safe, and secure, these differences in technique do not matter.
- Compliment one another on newborn caregiving strengths, such as the mother's ability to breastfeed and the partner's ability to calm the crying baby.
- Attend health supervision visits together as much as possible.
- Be sensitive to when your partner is overstressed and overtired. Ask how you can help and then follow through with suggested activities. Sometimes listening is the most helpful thing you can do.
- Rest and take time for yourself. Make decisions about what must be done (paying bills, laundry, grocery shopping) and

TABLE 7–2 Risk and Protective Factors in Newborn and Parents	
Newborn Risk Factors	Newborn Protective Factors
Preterm birth, congenital disabilities, chronic illness	Good health
Feeding and sleep problems	Normal eating, bowel, and sleep patterns
Fussing, crying, irritability, difficulty consoling	Positive temperament
Diminished social interactions and responsiveness	Responds to parent's attention
Undernutrition, developmental delay	Normal growth and development
Parental Risk Factors	Parental Protective Factors
Baby unplanned and unwanted at birth; potential for neglect and/or rejection	Welcome baby at birth
Financial insecurity, homelessness, lack of knowledge about how to care for newborn	Meet newborn's basic needs for food, shelter, clothing, health care
Cannot promote a strong nurturing environment due to serious problems such as abusive behavior, depression, mental illness, substance abuse	Provide a strong nurturing environment
Severe marital problems, absent parent, or frequent change of partners	Parents have a strong relationship with one another, share care of newborn
Lack of parenting skills, lack of parenting self-esteem, inability to cope with multiple roles, inappropriate coping strategies	Strong self-esteem, developmental maturity, developing knowledge of infant development
History of maltreatment as a child (risk increases with positive history)	No history of maltreatment as a child

what could wait (traveling to visit grandparents, painting the house, cleaning closets). Accept help from family and friends.

- Discuss how you will raise your baby in a loving, supportive, and respectful environment.
- Discuss how you were raised and what you would like to be different in your new family. Learn about parenting strategies and try out what feels comfortable for you.
- Keep in contact with family and friends. Maintain community ties that are important to you, such as social, religious, cultural, or recreational organizations or programs.
- Leave the baby with a trusted friend or family member and take time to be alone once in awhile. Talk about something other than the baby.
- Prepare siblings for the new baby prior to the baby's arrival. Allow siblings to "help" care for the new baby in age-appropriate ways. Praise siblings for positive attention they give to the baby, and allow siblings to express their feelings about the new baby and changes in the family.
- Support one another in seeking and using community resources to strengthen parenting skills, such as classes and parenting groups.
- Cuddle, hold, and rock the baby as much as possible. Babies cannot be spoiled by too much attention.
- Take advantage of the baby's awake time to play with the baby. Singing, reading, and simply talking to the baby about what is happening around her or him provides the baby with developmental stimulation.

Disease Prevention Strategies

Disease prevention in the newborn period includes metabolic screening, hearing screening, eye examination, immunization,

prevention of environmental smoke exposure, sudden infant death syndrome (SIDS) risk reduction, formula safety, minimizing exposure to disease, and hand hygiene for the family. Monitoring of these areas ensures that the sequelae of diseases can be minimized. For example, identification of a hearing problem may lead to early intervention to maximize the infant's potential for communication development. See Table 7–3 for immunizations recommended at birth; detailed immunization recommendations can be found in Chapter 16 ∞.

Disease prevention in the first month of life includes health maintenance activities such as:

- **Prevention of secondhand smoke exposure** Encourage all parents to avoid smoking near infants, and to stop smoking so that the baby does not inhale smoke from clothing and the environment. About 25% of children live with at least one smoker. Secondhand smoke (environment tobacco smoke or ETS) contains gases and particles that are related to SIDS, acute respiratory infections, slowed lung growth, ear problems, and severe asthma in children (Centers for Disease Control and Prevention, 2010).

TABLE 7–3	Immunizations Recommended for the Newborn
Immunization	Recommendation
Hepatitis B	Before leaving hospital; for newborn with HBsAg-positive mother, must be given within 12 hours of birth
Hepatitis immune globulin	Only for newborn with HBsAg-positive mother, must be given within 12 hours of birth

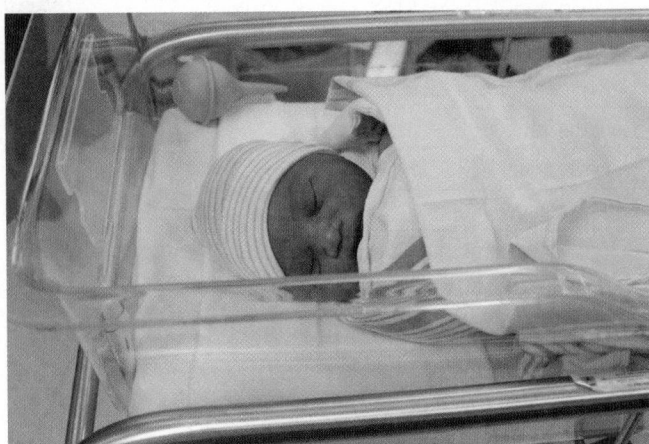

FIGURE 7–5 ➤ Parents are more likely to place newborns to sleep lying on their backs when they have seen health professionals do this in the hospital. Role model this recommended position for parents when you care for newborns.

- **SIDS risk reduction** (Figure 7–5 ➤) Sudden infant death syndrome is a devastating problem. Chapter 20 ∞ has a detailed description of the condition. Some interventions can lower the risk of SIDS. See Families Want to Know: SIDS Risk Reduction.
- **Formula safety** (see Chapter 14 ∞) When newborns are fed baby formula, parents need clear instructions about its preparation and storage. These guidelines ensure that the formula is kept free from harmful microorganisms and is prepared in the proper concentration.

Families Want to Know
SIDS Risk Reduction

Sudden infant death syndrome (SIDS) is defined as the sudden unexpected death of an infant less than 1 year of age, with onset of the fatal episode apparently occurring during sleep, that remains unexplained after a thorough investigation, including performance of a complete autopsy and review of the circumstances of death and the clinical history. SIDS is the major cause of death for infants in the United States from 1 month to 1 year of age, with most deaths occurring between 2 and 4 months (Kinney & Thach, 2009). See Chapter 20 ∞ for further information about SIDS.

Currently, there is no way to prevent SIDS, but parents and caregivers can reduce the risk of a SIDS death. Prenatal behavior and maternal health can influence the occurrence of SIDS. Parents should know the following rules for basic sleep safety to reduce the risk of SIDS:

■ Always place the baby on his or her back for sleep.

■ Use a safe crib and a firm mattress.

■ Remove all fluffy objects from the crib, such as quilts, stuffed animals, and pillows.

■ Make sure the baby's face and head stay uncovered during sleep. Use a blanket sleeper instead of blankets in the crib.

■ Avoid overheating the baby. A room temperature that is comfortable for the parent is fine for the newborn.

■ Never smoke or allow anyone to smoke around the baby. Pregnant women can lower risk by stopping smoking in pregnancy.

- **Handwashing** Handwashing is the key to preventing illness in the newborn and family members. It should be encouraged and modeled at every health promotion and health maintenance encounter. Hand hygiene products can be inserted into diaper bags so that parents always have access to cleansing products.
- **Minimizing the newborn's exposure to disease** Parents should be encouraged to avoid infant exposure to large crowds, especially in cold and influenza season; cover coughs and sneezes; and use good handwashing technique. The caregiver should be alerted if the newborn is exposed to varicella, influenza, pertussis, herpes, or other serious communicable diseases.

Injury Prevention Strategies

New parents are sometimes unaware of sources of potential injury for the newborn. Some aspects of injury prevention are pertinent to the newborn's immediate care, and other topics promote discussion and provide opportunities for anticipatory guidance. In the immediate newborn period, the nurse should assess the parents' knowledge of injury prevention strategies, and promote healthy and safe habits. Injury prevention strategies include proper and consistent use of an infant car seat, and strategies to prevent falls, burns, choking, drowning, and suffocation (Table 7–4).

Newborn safety awareness begins in the birth setting. Parents should be cautioned against laying the baby on the mother's bed instead of in the bassinet, taught to use the bulb syringe in the event that the baby spits up a large amount of fluid, and instructed to position the baby supine instead of side-lying or prone. Parents should also be oriented to procedures in place to prevent newborn abduction and to their critical role in ensuring newborn safety and security. Be sure the parents are equipped to provide the newborn a safe ride home. Refer parents to a local trained Child Passenger Safety Technician for assistance, or call 1-888-327-4236 to find a car seat inspection location. Websites are also available for car seat safety information.

Following hospital discharge, the nurse promotes safety by encouraging parents to think about the hazards that the child could encounter and how to eliminate them. In the newborn period, the parent or caregiver is uniquely responsible for ensuring that the newborn is not placed in a dangerous situation. The newborn cannot turn on a hot water faucet or run with a sharp object, but it is possible for the parent to inadvertently place the newborn in danger. The newborn is capable of twisting and rolling off any surface higher than the floor, falling out of an infant carrier seat, or drowning while left unattended for a moment in a bathtub filled with only a few inches of water.

Pediatric injuries are more likely to occur when the parents are under stress; for example, when a parent is hungry and tired (the hour before dinner), during pregnancy, during illness or death in the family, when there is tension between parents, and during changes in the environment, such as a change in the child's caregiver or the family's living environment. At these times, the parent should be particularly vigilant and closely supervise children.

TABLE 7–4	Injury Prevention Topics for Newborns
Topic	**Injury Prevention Teaching Topics**
Motor vehicle safety	• Choose an infant-only seat or a convertible seat suitable for an infant, approved by the federal Motor Vehicle Safety Standards. • Ensure the infant rides rear-facing until at least 1 year of age and more than 20 pounds. • Remember the safest place for all children to ride is in the back seat. Never place a rear-facing car safety seat in the front seat with an active passenger air bag. • Use a car safety seat every time the infant is in the car. Do not carry heavy objects that may become projectiles and cause injury in a crash. • Read and follow the manufacturer's instructions for the car safety seat and the vehicle owner's manual for installation information. • Dress the infant in clothes that allow the straps to go between the legs. Never place blankets under the baby. Buckle the baby into the seat, and place blankets over the baby. • To make sure the car safety seat is installed correctly and the baby is positioned correctly, go to a car seat inspection station. A certified Child Passenger Safety Technician will assist you. Find a list of certified CPS Technicians by state or zip code on the National Highway Traffic Safety Administration website. Find a car safety seat inspection station online or call 1-888-327-4236.
Shaken baby syndrome	Never shake a baby. Recognize that sometimes you will not be able to console your baby. Shaking a baby, even for only a few seconds, can cause serious brain damage and death. One of four shaken babies dies.
Crib	Use a safety approved crib. Slats should be no more than 2 3/8 inches apart. The mattress should be firm and fit snugly into the crib. Keep crib rails raised.
Co-sleeping	Co-sleeping with the parent is discouraged due to increased danger of suffocation and SIDS. Sleep with the baby near but not in the parental bed (AAP, 2005). The infant should never sleep in the same bed with siblings due to a significant risk of suffocation.
Baby toys	Use age-appropriate baby toys. Check toys for sharp edges or loose parts. Keep older siblings' toys out of baby's reach. Do not use toys with loops or string cords.
Drowning	Never leave the baby alone in the bathtub, even with a very small amount of water. If you must turn your back on the baby or leave the room, take the baby out of the tub. Only adults, not older children, should supervise the baby in water.
Suffocation	Keep plastic bags and wrappings away from the baby (take the plastic bag off the crib mattress). Shake baby powder into your hand first and then apply it so the baby does not inhale it. Do not allow a baby or sibling to play with a latex balloon. Keep small objects (such as safety pins, coins, small toys) out of the baby's reach. Do not attach pacifiers, medals, or other objects to the crib or to the baby's body with a string or cord. Do not put the crib near blinds, curtains, or anything with a hanging cord. Do not let the baby wear clothing with strings near the neck (such as a sweatshirt hood that ties with a cord) or a headband that could slip down and wrap around the baby's neck. Use a tight-fitting crib sheet that does not come loose when the corner is pulled.
Burns	Set the hot water heater thermostat lower than 120°F. Do not smoke or drink hot liquids while holding the baby. Do not microwave bottles of formula or breast milk due to uneven heating. Do not expose the baby to direct sunlight.
Falls	Keep a hand on the baby while dressing or diaper changing on a surface other than the floor. Never leave the baby unsupervised on any high surface such as a bed, changing table, or sofa. Always keep one hand on the baby.
Pet safety	Keep some distance between the newborn and the pet until the pet's initial reaction to the new baby is assessed. Never leave the baby unsupervised with the family dog or cat, or any animal capable of harming the newborn.
Sibling supervision	Never leave your baby alone with a young sibling. When a young child holds the baby, seat the child on a large soft surface, such as the couch, and supervise closely. Watch siblings for aggressive behavior toward the newborn, such as hitting or biting. Siblings may take on a caregiving role and imitate adults; watch for "feeding" of nonfood items or choking hazards.
Fire safety	Install working smoke detectors on every floor of the house and in every sleeping area. Have a fire escape plan from your house and practice it.
Poisoning	Post the universal phone number for U.S. poison control near your telephone: 1-888-222-1222.
Gun safety	Keep the gun unloaded and locked up. Keep the ammunition locked up separately from the gun. Consider not keeping a gun in the household due to safety hazards for family members.
In case of emergency	• Know when and how to call your pediatric care provider. • Know when it is appropriate to go to the emergency department. • Take a first aid class and learn CPR for children and adults.

Adapted from Hagan, Shaw, & Duncan, 2008.

Car Seat Safety Website

NURSING MANAGEMENT

Nursing Assessment and Diagnosis

An essential skill for the nurse in the hospital, clinic, or community setting is the ability to assess the family and newborn and identify potential health promotion and maintenance activities. Many activities are pertinent to prenatal health as well as the postpartum period. If maternal and pediatric care providers are located at different agencies, nurses must coordinate and integrate services so that the new mother and family benefit from a seamless continuum of care.

Based on nursing assessments, the nursing diagnoses form the basis for subsequent interventions. Possible nursing diagnoses for the family and newborn in the first month following birth might include:

- Anxiety (Parent) related to change in role status
- Risk for Impaired Attachment related to parental exhaustion or lack of knowledge of infant cues
- Risk for Impaired Parenting
- Effective Breast-Feeding related to basic breast-feeding knowledge
- Ineffective Breast-Feeding related to inadequate sucking by infant
- Infant Feeding Pattern, Ineffective related to newborn's inability to suck effectively
- Readiness for Enhanced Parenting related to need for information and skills for newborn care

Planning and Implementation

Newborn health maintenance and promotion begins in the prenatal period. In most cases, the expectant mother is highly motivated to engage in activities that result in a healthy newborn, and the health care team has a unique window of opportunity to promote maternal and newborn health.

In the prenatal period, the nurse's goal is to promote an optimal outcome for both mother and newborn. Comprehensive quality prenatal care is outside the scope of this text; however, important health promotion and maintenance include interventions to help ensure healthy diet and exercise; to avoid alcohol, tobacco, and drugs; and to establish or maintain a dental home. Assess the need for assistance with food, clothing, and safe housing, which entails numerous referrals and advanced skills to ensure coordinated community services. Provide anticipatory guidance regarding newborn care and safety, and assist the woman with choosing a pediatric health care provider. The nurse in the prenatal setting plays an important role in educating the woman about breastfeeding's lifelong benefits, and guiding her toward an informed infant feeding decision.

Hospital-Based Care

The hospital length of stay is short for the healthy mother and newborn. The nurse in the birth setting is responsible for assessing and implementing nursing care during a time of dramatic physiologic changes in both mother and newborn, as well as helping the new parents learn basic newborn care skills. Consistent and accurate breastfeeding information is essential to ensure con-

tinued efforts at home, and referral to a lactation specialist or support group is helpful. The nurse assesses and refers the mother to community resources as needed for domestic violence and drug, alcohol, or tobacco use. The nurse may coordinate interventions such as WIC to help ensure adequate food and nutritional support. Refer the mother to parenting classes or support groups. Through listening to the family's concerns, providing nurturing responses, respecting cultural differences, and validating parental efforts to learn parenting skills, the nurse further develops the partnership between the family and their health care providers.

Prior to discharge the newborn has blood taken for metabolic screening, has initial hearing screening, and receives the first hepatitis B vaccination. Follow-up after these interventions requires communication among multiple community agencies and the pediatric care provider to ensure that the newborn receives appropriate continuing care.

Care in the Community

In the outpatient setting, the pediatric health care team's goal is to help the parents gain knowledge and confidence in caring for the physical, intellectual, and emotional needs of their infant, and to encourage their personal growth as parents and the family's development as a unit (Hagan et al., 2008). In the first month of the newborn's life, health promotion and maintenance activities include teaching the parents how to interact with their baby to promote attachment; provide a safe sleeping environment; continue development and validation of baby care activities, especially breastfeeding; and begin to learn about the newborn's temperament in order to respond quickly and correctly to needs to promote infant mental health.

The relationship between the family and pediatric health care team must be nurtured. Time should be allowed for parents' questions. Cultural differences in perspectives must be considered. Results of screening and testing should be explained. When the nurse involves the parent in the infant's health care activities in these ways, it is more likely that parents will be cooperative and interested in promoting and maintaining their child's health.

Evaluation

Expected outcomes for the family and their infant by the end of the first month include:

- The newborn makes a successful transition from intrauterine to extrauterine life.
- Risk factors are identified in the prenatal and newborn period, and nursing assessment coordinates with medical intervention to prevent or manage complications.
- The newborn achieves expected physical and developmental milestones.
- The family begins successful integration of the newborn into the family.
- Parents demonstrate newborn care skills and beginnings of healthy attachment behaviors.
- Parents recognize the importance of health promotion and health maintenance activities and partner with health care professionals to promote and maintain the physical and mental health of their newborn and family.

■ HEALTH PROMOTION AND MAINTENANCE FOR THE INFANT

Infancy is a major life transition for the baby and parents. The infant accomplishes phenomenal physical growth and developmental milestones while the family adapts to the addition of a new member and establishes new goals for each of its existing members. Infant health supervision visits are very important to support the health of the baby and the family unit. These visits begin after the newborn period, at about 1 month of age. This is the time when parents establish an ongoing partnership with a health care provider. A medical home or pediatric health care home is identified to serve the baby's health needs. The goals of health supervision visits are to identify and address the infant's health promotion and health maintenance needs.

Facilitating breastfeeding, helping parents to understand their infant's temperament, and employing strategies to ensure adequate sleep by the baby and parents are examples of health promotion activities. Health maintenance interventions focus on disease and injury prevention, for example, administering immunizations and teaching about infant car seats.

Establishment of the relationship with a health care provider and agency is important so that trust develops and the family feels comfortable about turning to the professionals for information and guidance as the baby grows. Nurses play a vital role in welcoming new families into office and clinic settings, establishing rapport, and applying principles of communication so that trust and positive partnerships develop between providers and families. Infancy is a time when the child grows in physical, psychological, and cognitive ways; health supervision visits foster healthy growth and development. When should the infant be seen for health supervision visits? What are key components of these visits? How can the nurse best assess and intervene to ensure the infant's health and safety? These are some of the questions that will be answered in this section of the chapter.

Early Contacts with the Family

Health promotion and health maintenance occur in a series of health supervision visits during the first year of life. Schedules vary among facilities, but a common pattern includes visits at about 1 month, 2 months, 4 months, 6 months, 9 months, and 1 year of age. In addition, most children have some episodic illnesses such as gastrointestinal illness or otitis media and visit the facility at other times for treatment of these illnesses. A few children have chronic or serious health care problems during the first year, and have extensive contact with the health care home and other services.

During these first visits, assess the family for protective factors and risks. Protective factors might include the knowledge level of infant needs, support from family and friends, and the mother's good health and nutritional state during pregnancy. Risk factors could include limited financial resources, lack of preparation for the baby, transportation issues, lack of access to health care, and illness or other stress among family members (Garfield & Isacco, 2006). Knowledge of these factors will shape the nursing interventions in the first health supervision visit in

infancy. The nurse applies health promotion principles by building on strengths and fosters health maintenance by intervening to minimize risks.

General Observations

When the family comes to the clinic or office for care with an infant, general observations should begin at first contact (Figure 7–6 ➤). Welcome the family warmly to the facility and comment on the baby. Ask how the family is doing with the baby and how the adjustment is going. Be alert for signs of fatigue or depression in the parents, as these can occur when caring for an infant and can interfere with bonding and positive transition. Upon entering the examination room, it is helpful to explain the plans for the visit, such as "I will weigh and measure your baby now and show you how she is growing. Then I'll ask a few questions about her eating, sleeping, and other things. Then the nurse practitioner will be in to do Rhonda's physical examination. Do you have any questions as we start? Will you undress Rhonda now so we can weigh her accurately?"

Growth and Developmental Surveillance

Physical growth and meeting of developmental milestones provide important information about infants. The baby is measured for accurate length, weight, and head circumference (see the *Clinical Skills Manual* and Chapter 5 ∞; see Figure 7–7 ➤). The measurements should be placed on growth grids and interpreted. Parents enjoy seeing how the baby is progressing and are usually eager to learn about the child's weight gain and growth percentiles. Be alert for an infant who demonstrates a change in percentile range. For example, if the baby was in the 75th percentile for length and weight at birth, but has fallen to below the 50th percentile for weight, additional assessment will be needed about the baby's feedings. Likewise, if the head circumference is much lower or higher than the length and weight percentiles,

Infancy: A Major Life Transition Video

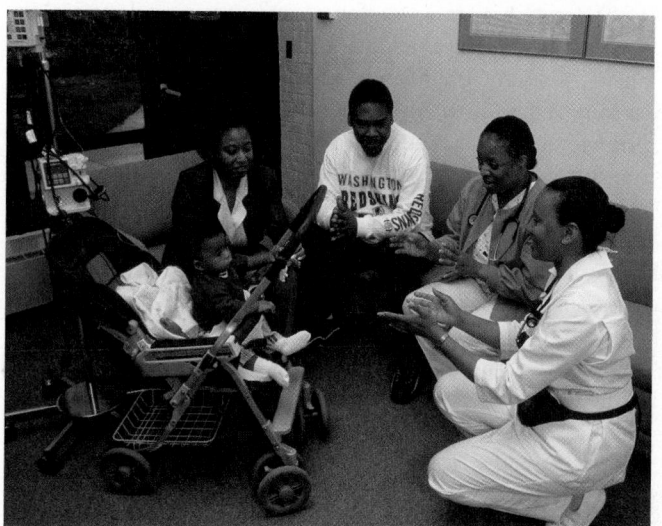

FIGURE 7–6 ➤ The nurse begins assessment of the infant's family when they are seen in the waiting room and called in for care. What observations can you make of the infant's general appearance? Developmental accomplishments? Interaction of parents with the baby?

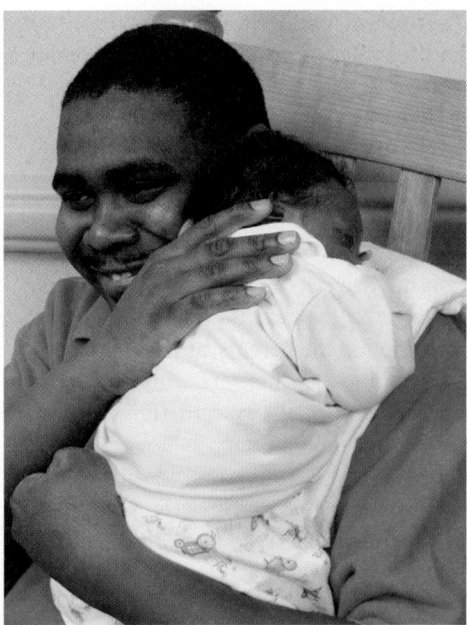

FIGURE 7–7 ➤ Interactions between the parent and infant provide clues to mental health. Do the adult and child appear comfortable with each other? Is eye contact and vocalization present? Are their bodies soft and relaxed or tense?

further neurological and developmental assessment should be done. See Chapter 14 ∞ for further information about physical measurement, and Appendix A ∞ for growth grids.

Growth measurement is followed by a physical assessment. The nurse may complete parts of the assessment, with the remainder performed by the physician, nurse practitioner, or other primary care provider. The assessment evaluates each body system, with particular attention paid to heart, skin, musculoskeletal system, abdomen, and neurological status. See Chapter 5 ∞ for a thorough discussion of physical assessment.

Developmental surveillance is integrated into each infant health care visit by observing developmental milestones in the infant (see Chapter 4 ∞ for a summary of milestones expected at different ages and see Table 7–5 for specific tasks in infancy). When there is no opportunity to directly observe a skill, ask parents about whether the infant performs the skill. In addition to direct observation, parents are usually requested to fill in a form that asks questions about common developmental tasks. Review the results and determine if additional questions should be asked. When some milestones have not been met, make an appointment for the infant to have a developmental test by a certified examiner. When a child has not been seen as often as recommended, perform a thorough developmental assessment to identify any expected milestones not yet achieved. Reinforce the need to make an appointment for the next visit and plan with the family how to remember the appointment and to ensure the family's ability to bring the child to the health care visit.

The nurse establishes health promotion and maintenance interventions related to growth and development assessment data. Anticipatory guidance related to development is a major component of health promotion. The nurse anticipates the next

Culture *Developmental Milestones*

Be alert for differences in cultural practices and beliefs that may influence developmental milestones. For example, if a child is kept on a cradleboard for much of the time, the baby may be slow in learning to crawl. This baby may progress directly to standing by furniture without demonstrating as much creeping or crawling as other infants. In addition, when parents do not have English as a primary language and the examiner uses English, common terms might be misinterpreted. Parents might not understand what is meant if you ask "Does your baby have a mobile over the crib at home?" or "Is she starting to be afraid of strangers?" How can you be alert for language differences and become sensitive to miscommunication?

milestones the infant will be meeting, and recommends ways for the parents to support the infant in progression. Some health promotion activities include:

- Teaching about food introduction that will foster growth
- Encouraging toys and activities that will assist in meeting the next developmental milestones
- Demonstrating gross and fine motor skills that the infant has achieved
- Demonstrating to parents how the child will focus on their faces and mimic their vocal sounds

Other interventions are focused on health maintenance or disease and injury prevention. Safety hazards and ways to avoid them are discussed, and parents are given brochures, websites, or videotapes to enhance injury prevention information. Can you outline additional health promotion and health maintenance interventions that relate to the infant's growth and development?

Nutrition

The importance of nutrition during the first year of life cannot be overestimated. The baby will triple his or her birth weight by 1 year of age, and has a great need for nutritional balance. From the first sips of breast milk or formula as a newborn, to eating the family meal at 1 year of age, the fast progression of nutritional intake patterns is obvious. See Chapter 14 ∞ for a thorough description of nutritional needs during infancy.

During each visit, the nurse seeks to learn what the baby is eating and whether the family has any questions or concerns related to intake (Hagan et al., 2008). Open-ended questions are a good way to begin, with more specific questions inserted after the parent's perceptions are known. Breastfeeding is encouraged and supported, with information about safe formula-feeding provided when the family has chosen that method of feeding. Once the baby is in the second half of the first year, food patterns of the family become more important; ask about feeding at childcare settings as well.

Observations from other portions of the visit can provide clues about additional questions to ask. If an infant has not gained weight as expected and has fallen into a lower channel of weight percentile, more specific analysis of intake is needed. Ask for a recall of the baby's intake in the previous day. When the baby does

TABLE 7–5	Infant Developmental Milestones Observed in Health Promotion and Health Maintenance Visits
Age	Developmental Milestones
1 month	• Responds to sound by startle or increased alertness • Follows objects and human face with eyes • Has periods of alertness and restfulness • Is comforted by touch or feeding by parent • Has symmetrical movements and generally has arms and legs flexed • Lifts head momentarily when prone
2 months	• Previous characteristics continue • Makes noises such as cooing in response to interaction with adult • Smiles • Lifts head, neck, upper chest when prone • Has increasing head control when held in sitting position
4 months	• Increasing cooing and babbling • Smiles, laughs, makes other noises during interactions • Supports self on hands when prone • Rolls front to back • Touches objects and grasps rattle placed near hand
6 months	• Uses sounds in repeated speech such as bababa, dadadada • Is interested in surroundings and toys • When pulled to sitting, has no head lag • Sits with support • Grasps objects easily and places them in mouth • Transfers objects from one hand to other • Bears weight on legs when held in standing position
9 months	• Understands simple words and uses more sounds in babbling • Responds to name • Enjoys interactive games with parent • Moves when placed on floor by crawling, creeping, or rolling repeatedly • Sits without support • Stands holding on to support • Plays with toys • Feeds self readily with fingers and tries to use cup
12 months	• Says one or more words • Imitates sounds readily • Has increasing interactions and interest in surroundings • Follows directions such as saying or waving bye • Pulls to standing, walks a few steps holding on • Has well-developed pincer grasp • Is able to drink from cup

not meet developmental milestones on schedule or is lethargic, intake may be inadequate for age. In these cases support may be needed to ensure adequate intake; a thorough description of feeding may be the first step in analyzing the problem and planning interventions. When the child's ability to take in nutrients or the parent's ability to feed the baby is questioned, an observation of a feeding might take place, either at the health care setting or during a home visit.

Additional nutritional assessment measures are used at certain points in the first year. A hematocrit or hemoglobin is generally performed between 9 and 12 months of age. Lead screening may be needed in certain population groups (see Chapter 17 ∞). Food security screening can be used when appropriate (see Chapter 14 ∞). Each visit includes nutritional teaching specific to each age group. See Table 7–6 for suggested teaching topics at these specific ages. Desired outcomes for nutrition in infancy include adequate growth, normal nutritional assessment findings, and knowledge by parents of the infant's nutritional needs.

Physical Activity

Physical activity is needed for adequate development of fine and gross motor skills in infancy. Unlike other times of life, the focus is on providing only the opportunities for activity, without a need to focus on motivation. As long as infants are meeting developmental milestones and have a stimulating environment that provides opportunity for fine and gross motor activity, they will use their motor skills, thus enhancing their performance. Time should be provided each day for the infant to reach for objects, exercise legs and arms freely, and increasingly use head control. Playing with parents or others and being surrounded by toys and other stimulating items will encourage motor behavior in all body parts. Ask the parents for a description of the baby's typical day and listen for these types of play periods.

Observe the infant's physical skills, ask questions about play periods provided, and compose a list of the family's protective factors and risk factors in this area. Table 7–7 lists risk and protective factors related to physical activity during infancy.

Based on the results of assessment and using the concept of anticipatory guidance, the nurse plans appropriate teaching for the family. Health maintenance deals with prevention of physical development delays. The nurse evaluates success of interventions by the child's progression in physical activity milestones at the next health supervision visit. Adequate parental understanding of the importance of physical activity and the means of supporting the child's activities is an important outcome of care.

Oral Health

The first teeth begin to erupt about midway during infancy. Two front teeth are common at about 6 months of age. However, even before this, parents lay the foundation for good oral health. The mother's intake during pregnancy and breastfeeding is essential to ensuring adequate availability of calcium and other nutrients that will be used as the infant's teeth develop. The nurse in child health supervision settings ensures that the baby has adequate intake of these nutrients via breastfeeding and other foods. A dietary recall of the mother's intake, as well as the infant's, is one way of assessing for nutrients. When the water supply is not fluoridated, inquire about use of fluoride drops, which are recommended after 6 months of age.

TABLE 7–6	Infant Nutrition Teaching for Health Promotion and Health Maintenance Visits
Age	Nutrition Teaching
1 month	• Support breastfeeding efforts. • Teach correct formula types and preparation if used. • Teach burping and rate of feeding information. • Suggest water during hot weather or if the family wants to use a bottle at the baby's bedtime. • Encourage families to view feedings as social interactions; emphasize the importance of holding the infant and not propping bottles.
2 months	• Continue as previously noted. • Review fluid needs of infants. • Reinforce food safety for partially used bottles of breast milk or formula. • Use warm water for heating bottles rather than a microwave to avoid burning. • Warn against feeding honey in the first year of life. • Begin cleaning of infant gums daily. • Provide information about any supplements needed (for example, iron for a premature infant, vitamin D for babies not exposed to adequate sunlight).
4 months	• Continue as previously noted. • Discuss introduction of first foods between 4 and 6 months, and surveillance for symptoms of allergy or intolerance. • Discuss changing food patterns such as increasing amounts and decreasing numbers of daily milk feedings.
6 months	• Continue as previously noted. • Reinforce proper introduction of new foods to include rice cereal, fruits, and vegetables. • Discuss any unusual food reactions observed. • Introduce a cup for drinking. • Introduce soft finger foods. • Serve juice only in a cup and limit to no more than 6 ounces daily. • Caution about common choking foods and items. • Provide information about fluoride supplements if the water supply is not fluoridated.
9 months	• Continue as previously noted. • If the mother does not continue to breastfeed, teach the family to use iron-fortified formula for the first year of life. • Encourage self-feeding of finger foods, integrating common foods for the family. • Introduce sources of protein such as tofu, cheese, mashed beans, and slivers of meats.
12 months	• Continue as previously noted. • Support the mother who wishes to continue breastfeeding beyond 1 year of age. • Encourage cups for all feedings other than breast.

Nursing Alert

Be sure that parents do not give the child excessive fluoride because it can permanently discolor the teeth. For example, this may happen if the parents administer fluoride drops each morning since their water supply has no fluoride, but then have the child at a care center several days each week where the water supply is fluoridated. Fluoride 0.25 mg is recommended for the child who is from 6 months to 3 years in communities with drinking water that contains < 0.3 ppm. Consult drug references for doses recommended at other ages.

Help the family establish healthy dental habits. The parents should wipe the infant's gums with soft moist gauze once or twice daily. This helps to clean food residues from the gums and gets the baby accustomed to having something wiping the gums, a practice that may assist when tooth brushing begins. Families are also cautioned to avoid having the baby nurse when sleeping, to avoid use of bottles in bed, and not to allow the baby to drink at will from a bottle during the day. These practices are linked to early childhood caries (see Chapter 14 ∞) and can lead to tooth decay. Nurses assess for the presence of teeth and whether

TABLE 7–7	Risk and Protective Factors Regarding Physical Activity in Infancy	
Risk Factors		Protective Factors
• Premature birth • Delayed developmental milestones • Limited stimulation by family or other care providers • Lack of knowledge by family about infant's physical activity needs • Limited community resources for families with infants		• Meets developmental milestones at expected ages • Has contact with parents, siblings, and others for significant time each day • Supportive environment with room to play safely, stimulating surroundings • Physically active family • Family knowledge about infant's physical activity needs • Community programs that promote physical activity in infants and information for families

patterns are similar to those expected (see Chapter 5 ∞). It is wise to ask if the baby has had any difficulty with teeth eruption. Many babies have increased crying and parents have disrupted sleeping during these periods. Suggest comfort measures such as offering the baby cool beverages and safe teething toys.

Mental and Spiritual Health

The baby's mental health is related to early experiences, inborn characteristics such as temperament and resilience, and relationships with caregivers. In addition, the first year of life provides opportunities for the infant to develop positive mental health; interventions during this important period can enhance the child's future mental status.

One way to evaluate mental health is to look carefully at the growth and development surveillance data that was previously described. Children who feel secure and have nurturing environments usually grow as expected and perform milestones at usual times. Slow growth and delayed development are sometimes related to a feeding disorder of infancy and early childhood (see Chapter 14 ∞). Another way to assess mental health is to observe the child and parent interacting. Does the parent hold the baby securely and does the child cuddle and settle in to the parent's arms (Figure 7–8 ➤)? Is there eye contact between parent and child? Does the parent appear comfortable in holding and comforting the baby? These interactions indicate bonding or positive attachment.

During the first year, the baby learns to identify parents; beginning at about 6 months of age, infants may cry or protest when another person holds them. This is called **stranger anxiety** and indicates expected attachment to parents. Similarly, infants in the second half of the first year of life may exhibit **separation anxiety** by inconsolable crying and other signs of distress when parents are not present. Recognize that these behaviors are normal, demonstrate healthy attachment to primary caregivers, and indicate mental health. Help parents to recognize them as expected occurrences. Provide them ideas of how to deal with this

behavior. They can remain in sight and talk to the baby during health supervision examinations, and they should be encouraged to hold and comfort the baby after painful procedures like immunizations. Once the infant has experienced that the parent leaves and returns, security in the care of others can emerge.

Another important indication of infant mental health is the ability to comfort oneself. Self-regulation is the process of dealing with feelings, learning to soothe oneself, and focusing on activities for increasing periods of time. Infants learn early how to comfort and calm themselves. Ask parents if the child sucks a finger, softly rocks, or otherwise comforts self when distressed. Some babies prefer to be alone and quiet when tired or distressed; others calm better when held, rocked, or placed in an infant swing. Help the parents to identify and reinforce the infant's methods of self-soothing, and teach swaddling and rocking techniques.

Self-regulation is needed when the infant is learning to go to sleep while tired and agitated. Infants progress into circadian rhythm at 2–3 months and begin to sleep more at night than during the day. By 6 months, the infant commonly sleeps 6 hours without waking, and returns to sleep after one nighttime feeding. A total sleep time of 12–15 hours/day is common (Murray, Zentner, & Yakimo, 2009). Nurses use health promotion principles to teach about sleep patterns in infants, and implement health maintenance when partnering with families to deal with problem sleep behaviors that lead to infant and parent fatigue. See Evidence-Based Practice: Infant Sleep.

The baby is born into a family with spiritual strengths and limitations. The nurse assesses the family and provides additional resources when needed. Although the infant is not mature enough to understand the family's spiritual framework, the atmosphere in the family that relates to nurturing, valuing children, providing a safe and secure environment, and recognizing mental balance is conveyed readily to the infant. The infant's social and psychological health is closely related to these factors. Assess the family's meaningful activities and practices and engagement in faith-based practices. Ask if they have needs or desires for referrals in the community such as to an organized religious body or other meaningful activities.

Many of the nurse's interventions are aimed at healthy mental health development in the baby. Health promotion activities focus on teaching parents the needs of infants for

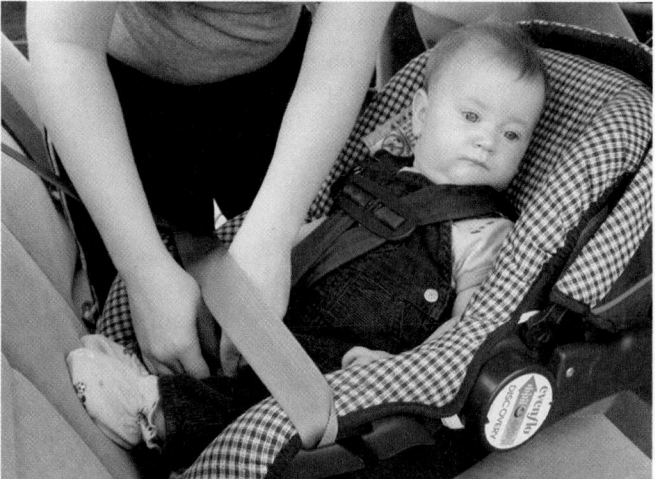

FIGURE 7–8 ➤ A young mother fastens her infant securely into a backward-facing car seat. Her installation has been evaluated by the local car seat inspector and she has been instructed in proper usage. Locate inspection stations in your community and use them to refer families to verify car seat placement.

Growth & Development *Infant Sleep Patterns*

Birth–3 months

The infant sleeps 10–16 hours daily in about five sleep periods of 30 minutes to 4 hours; sleep spans day and night hours.

3–6 months

The baby sleeps 14 hours daily with a longer sleep at night plus two to three naps daily. By 4–6 weeks, a consistent sleep pattern should emerge.

6–12 months

The baby sleeps 12–14 hours daily with a longer sleep at night plus one to two naps daily.

Source: *Adapted from Hagan, Shaw, & Duncan, 2008.*

Problem

Many babies have limited sleeping periods during the night, and their night awakenings disturb parents' sleep. Parents may have busy days and be unable to nap for adequate sleep, and thus cannot perform at a safe and productive level during the day. Parental stress and depression are associated with frequent child awakenings.

Evidence

Infant sleep is an important concern for many parents, but there is little research-based evidence about what strategies really improve infant sleep. Although parents have been advised to let the infant "cry it out" or to feed the child just before bedtime, these strategies have not been demonstrated to clearly improve sleep patterns. A group of nurse and pediatric researchers tested an intervention to assist parents in dealing with their infants' sleep problems. A 2-hour teaching session was offered to 39 families to discuss normal infant sleep and recommended comforting of the infant, followed by parental charts of infant sleep, and telephone support by the researchers. Parents were instructed to comfort their infants while leaving them in their cribs, and to increase the time between these comfort visits when the infant was crying, up to 10 minutes. Co-sleeping with the parent was discouraged. After the 16 weeks of the study, infant sleep had improved, co-sleeping had significantly decreased, breastfeeding had remained the same, and parents reported improved sleep quality, decreased fatigue, and improved mood (Hall, Clauson, Carty, et al., 2006). In another study of 1,741 children, factors associated with poor sleep included parents staying with children while they fell asleep, responding to night awakenings by feeding, holding, rocking, or bringing the child to the adult bed (Touchette, Petit, Paquet, et al., 2005). An additional study of nearly 30,000 infants and toddlers in 17 countries found that in primarily Caucasian populations a majority of children were put to sleep in their own beds or cribs whereas in Asian countries only 4% slept in their own beds (Mindell, Sadeh, Kohyama, et al., 2010).

Implications

This evidence-based practice provides implications for nursing practice. Ask parents of young newborns to record the infant sleep patterns. As the infant nears 3–4 months, patterns should demonstrate few night awakenings and feedings. Teach parents how to minimize stimulation and interaction at night, as described earlier. Provide opportunities to review results at future health supervision visits, or offer telephone or other support to parents. Consider the cultural variations that may be present and begin with a history of what the family generally considers normal sleep locations and patterns in young children.

Critical Thinking Application

What reasons might working parents have for responding eagerly and interacting with an infant who awakens at night? Do you think there are other reasons why infants awaken at night? What clues help you to decide if an infant sleep problem exists? What questions will you ask to learn about usual sleep patterns for infants in the families you see?

---

security and interaction. Suggest healthy sleep patterns and how they can be achieved (see Families Want to Know: Helping the Infant Sleep). Teach self-regulation skills so that the parents can help the infant become quiet and calm. Health maintenance seeks to identify infants with disruptions in mental health status, often manifested by growth or interaction abnormalities. When the infant has disturbed sleep patterns or difficulty calming self when upset, or the parents do not interpret infant cues related to hunger or discomfort, the nurse plans interventions to help prevent further problems. An expected outcome for these activities is the reestablishment of expected growth and development, and age-appropriate interactions of the infant with others.

Relationships

The infant's social interactions both within and outside the family display enormous growth in the first year. The family is the primary site where the infant learns to interact with other people. Therefore, family dynamics must be examined during health supervision visits. Some factors in the parents' mental health directly affect the home atmosphere and the baby's resulting health. Depression in parents or other family members is an important condition that can potentially influence the infant's health. Interactions with parents who are depressed will be altered; caretaking, both physical and emotional, can be impaired.

Another challenge to the mental health of families with depressed members is that of domestic violence, a situation in which parents or adult care providers commit violent acts toward one another. Child abuse or maltreatment may also occur in some families with infants. This problem is a serious issue that causes disturbed mental status in the baby. See Chapter 17 ∞ for a detailed description of child abuse and its effect on infants and older children. Suspected child abuse must be reported to legal authorities in order to protect children.

The nurse's role related to infant social interactions in health supervision visits is to evaluate the infant's social skills, learn what parents have noticed about the baby's temperament and how it fits with their lives, and make suggestions for positive social development. Desired outcomes for the infant include establishment of close relationships with parents and other family members, a stimulating home environment that is responsive to the baby's temperament, and developmental progression in social interactions.

Disease Prevention Strategies

Infants are prone to many infectious diseases, especially once passive immunity from the mother wanes at about 6 months of age (see Chapters 16 and 22 ∞). Recommended immunizations are administered on schedule to provide the infant protection from some diseases (Table 7–8). Further details on immunizations can be found in Chapter 16 ∞. Instruct parents about upcoming immunizations and when the baby should be seen again. Be sure the parent understands the risks and benefits of each immunization. Answer questions truthfully and have resources on hand for interested parents such as brochures and videotapes.

Helping an infant to self-regulate and be able to sleep for longer periods is often a stressful challenge for families. Parents need to have substantial sleep periods themselves in order to be refreshed and able to deal with daily life. When up several times during the night with a baby, parents may become irritable and fatigued. Question the family about the baby's sleep routine. The infant passes into light sleep several times at night and may awaken; self-regulation will assist in helping the infant get back to sleep. Suggestions helpful for the family may involve the following:

■ Place the baby to sleep in a quiet and darkened room.

■ Provide a consistent transitional object, such as a favorite blanket, each night.

■ Put the baby to bed while still awake rather than after falling asleep nursing so he or she becomes accustomed to getting to sleep without nursing.

■ Do not try to awaken the baby in NREM (quiet) sleep.

■ Establish a regular sleep routine and time; the routine may involve some cuddling and rocking time but should not be vigorous, stimulating play.

■ For the baby who has trouble going to sleep, remain in the room for a few minutes but do not establish eye contact; place a hand on the abdomen or chest or gently hold flailing arms and legs (Hagan et al., 2008).

Nursing Alert

Instruct parents to contact a health care provider if the infant has any of the following:

■ Rectal temperature ≥ 100.4°F (38.0°C)
■ Seizure
■ Skin rash, purplish spots, petechiae
■ Change in activity or behavior that makes the parent uncomfortable
■ Unusual irritability, lethargy
■ Failure to eat
■ Vomiting
■ Diarrhea
■ Dehydration
■ Cough

Data from Hagan, Shaw, & Duncan, 2008.

During each health supervision visit, the nurse performs recommended screenings and counsels the parents about why such screenings are important (Table 7–9). Vision and hearing screenings are performed at each health care encounter. Screenings for anemia and lead poisoning are added at particular times or with certain groups. Families with a history of genetic diseases such as sickle cell disease or cystic fibrosis may choose to have infant screening so that supportive care could begin early if the child has the disease. Parents benefit from teaching about common diseases and conditions of young children and measures for their prevention. Ask about environment tobacco

TABLE 7–8	Routine Immunizations Recommended During Infancy
Immunization	Age Recommended
Hepatitis B	At birth (#1) 1–2 months (#2) 6–18 months (#3)
Hepatitis A	12 months (#1) 18 months or at least 6 months after first dose (#2)
Diphtheria, tetanus, acellular pertussis	2, 4, and 6 months (three doses)
Haemophilus influenzae type b	2, 4, and 6 months (three doses; third dose is not needed if PRP-OMP [Pedvax HIB or Comvax] is used for primary series)
Inactivated poliovirus	2, 4, and 6–18 months (three doses)
Pneumococcal	2, 4, and 6 months (three doses)
Influenza	Annually from 6 months of age
Rotavirus	2, 4, and 6 months (three doses)

smoke (ETS) and encourage smoking parents to quit. Teach parents to put babies to sleep on their backs to assist in lowering the chance of SIDS. Be sure parents have a phone number to call when they have questions about conditions or whether the baby should be seen by the health care provider. Desired outcomes for disease prevention strategies include adequate management of health problems, integration of immunization and other preventive measures into infant care, and family understanding of preventive measures recommended for infants.

Injury Prevention Strategies

During the first year of life, injury becomes an increasingly common cause of mortality. (See statistics on mortality in children in Chapter 1 ∞.) Strategies must be included in each health supervision visit to lower the risk of injury. Nurses should never assume that parents understand how to insert an infant car seat (Figure 7–9 ➤) correctly or what types of toys and foods can lead to choking. Know the most common hazards at each age and teach parents methods of avoiding them (see Tables 7–10 and 7–11).

Begin the conversation by asking parents what safety hazards they are aware of in the child's environment. Use this information as the starting point for discussion. Give positive feedback for their awareness of hazards and measures they have taken to prevent them. Consider using a home assessment survey that assists parents in identifying hazards that may be present in the home. (See Chapter 2 ∞ for a description of the Home Observation for Measurement of the Environment.) When infants visit friends, relatives, or neighbors, they may be exposed to other hazardous situations. Grandparents may not have a home that is "babyproofed" and the infant could have access to electrical cords, machinery, medicines in cupboards or purses, or other hazards. Help the parents to evaluate the

TABLE 7–9	Screening During Health Promotion and Health Maintenance Visits
Age	Recommended Screening Tests
1 month	• Vision (follow objects, red reflex) • Hearing (response to sound; screening by machine if not completed in the hospital) • Physical examination with special attention to skin problems, hip dysplasia, foot position and range of motion, mouth, abdomen, cardiac abnormality, tearing of eyes, neurological (including child abuse), anthropometric measurements • Developmental milestones • Dietary screening and stool/urine pattern assessment • Review immunization record
2 months	• As previously noted
4 months	• As previously noted • Vision (add cover–uncover test for strabismus)
6 months	• As previously noted • Vision (add ability to follow object bilaterally, corneal light reflex) • Physical examination with special attention to muscle tone, extremities, appearance of first teeth, tympanic membrane, testicle descent for males
9 months	• As previously noted • Lead exposure and levels if appropriate • Anemia • Physical examination with special attention to symmetry of movement
12 months	• As previously noted • Tuberculosis test if indicated • Physical examination with special attention to condition of teeth

Adapted from Hagan, Shaw, & Duncan, 2008.

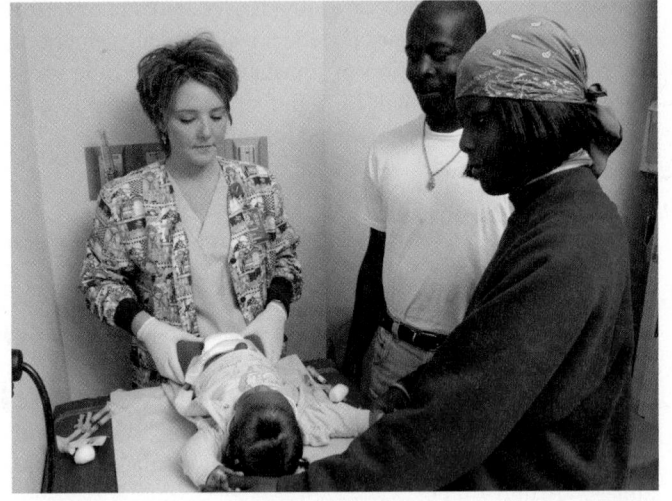

A

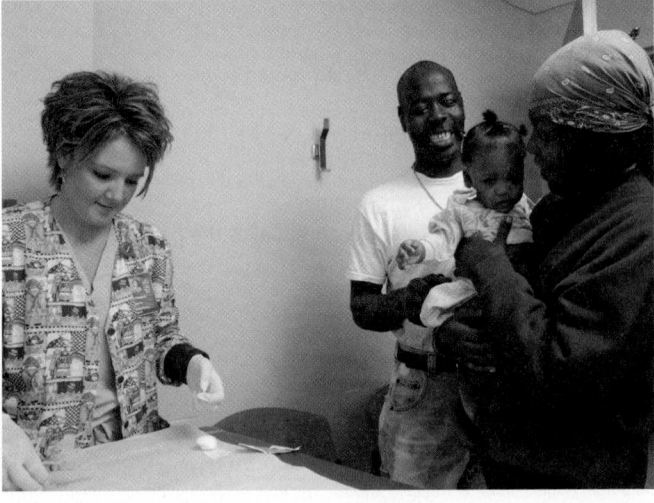

B

FIGURE 7–9 ➤ The nurse positions the baby on the edge of the examination table to isolate the vastus lateralis muscle used for immunization administration. A, The mother holds the baby's arms out of reach. B, After the immunization, the parents comfort the infant and are reassured that all is well. Instructions are given for managing side effects and scheduling the next visit.

childcare home or center. Focus on car safety since this is a frequent cause of injury for infants. Provide brochures and other types of information about recommendations. Refer every family for a car seat examination at a certified examination center. Provide resources for car seats if the family is not able to afford one. Discuss other possible safety hazards such as extensions on the parent's bicycle and use of baby strollers in areas where cars are present.

NURSING MANAGEMENT

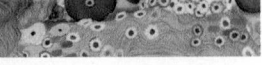

Nursing Assessment and Diagnosis

The nurse working in clinics, offices, and other settings that offer primary care for infants should be skillful in assessing health promotion and health maintenance. The infant's growth, developmental level, general physical health, and mental/social health

TABLE 7–10	Injury Prevention in Infancy	
Hazard	Development Characteristics	Preventive Measures
Falls	Mobility increases in the first year of life, progressing from squirming movements to crawling, rolling, and standing.	Do not leave the infant unsecured in an infant seat, even in the newborn period. Do not place on high surfaces such as tables or beds unless holding the child. **(1)** Once mobile by crawling, keep doors to stairways closed or use gates. Standing walkers have led to many injuries and are not recommended.
Burns	The infant is dependent on caretakers for environmental control. The second half of the first year is marked by crawling and increased mobility. Objects are explored by touching and placing in the mouth.	Check the temperature of bath water and food/liquids for drinking. Cover electrical outlets. Supervise the infant so that play with electrical cords cannot occur.
Motor vehicle crashes	The infant is dependent on caretakers for placement in the car. On impact with another motor vehicle, an infant held on a lap acts as a torpedo.	Use only approved restraint systems (according to federal Motor Vehicle Safety Standards). The seat must be used for every trip, even if very short. The seat must be properly buckled to the car's lap belt system. **(2)**
Drowning	The infant cannot swim and is unable to lift the head.	Never leave an infant alone in a bath of even 2.5 cm (1 in.) of water. Supervise when in water even when a life preserver is worn. Flotation devices such as arm inflatables are not certified life preservers.
Poisoning	The infant is dependent on caretakers to keep harmful substances out of reach.	Keep medicines out of reach. Teach proper dosage and administration of medicines to parents. Cleaning products and other harmful substances should not be stored where the infant can reach them. Remove plants from play areas. Have the poison control center number by the telephone.
Choking	The second half of infancy is marked by exploratory reaching and mouthing objects. The infant explores objects by placing them in the mouth. **(3)**	Avoid foods that commonly cause choking. Keep small toys away from infants, especially toys labeled "not intended for use by those under 3 years."
Suffocation	The young infant has minimal head control and may be unable to move if vomiting or having difficulty breathing.	Position the infant on the back for sleep. **(4)** Do not place pillows, stuffed toys, or other objects near the head. Do not use plastic in the crib. Avoid latex balloons.
Strangulation	The infant is able to get the head into railings or crib slats but cannot remove it. Curtain cords can wrap around the infant's neck when crawling.	Be sure older cribs have slats spaced 6 cm (2 3/8 in.) or less apart. The mattress must fit tightly against the crib rails. Remove all curtain cords securely out of reach.

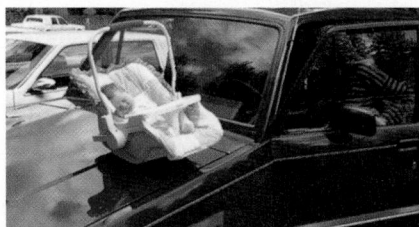

(1) Never leave an infant unsecured or on a high surface.

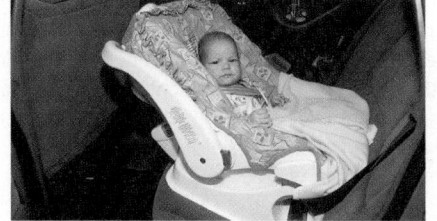

(2) Always use an approved restraint system. Place the infant in a rear-facing seat in the backseat of the car.

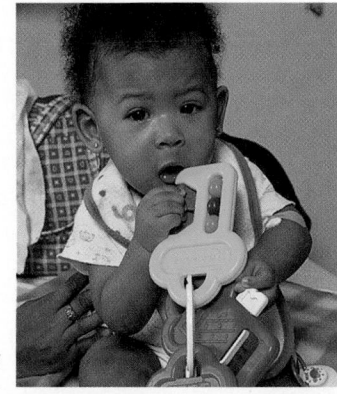

(3) The infant explores objects with his mouth.

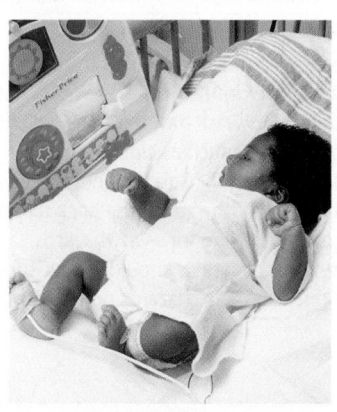

(4) Place the infant on the back for sleeping, and keep toys clear.

TABLE 7–11	Injury Prevention Topics by Age
Age	Injury Prevention Teaching Topics
1 month	• Use an infant car safety seat. • Put the baby to sleep on his or her back. • Avoid loose bedding and toys in the crib. • Avoid tobacco use in the environment. • Provide adult supervision of the baby at all times by trusted individuals. • Test bath water temperature and never leave the baby alone in the bath. • Never place the baby on a high object such as a counter, table, or bed; always keep one hand on the baby during activities like diaper changes to prevent falling. • Wash hands correctly and often. • Avoid contact with persons with communicable diseases. • Have smoke alarms and avoid fire hazards. • Learn infant CPR and airway obstruction removal. • Never shake the baby. • Have plans for emergency care.
2 months	• As previously noted. • Use only recommended playpens or cribs and keep sides up. • Avoid moldy environments. • Keep baby toys cleaned. • Avoid direct sunlight for the baby. • Keep sharp and small objects out of the baby's environment. • Keep the hot water heater lower than 120°F. • Review emergency plans with all care providers.
4 months	• As previously noted. • Get all poisonous substances out of the baby's view and reach; install locks to keep them inaccessible. • Do not use latex balloons or plastic bags near the baby.
6 months	• As previously noted. • If an infant-only car seat was used, switch to a rear-facing convertible safety seat (intended for babies up to 40 pounds) when the baby is 20 to 30 pounds or 26 inches. • Empty containers of water immediately after use; be sure pools or other bodies of water are locked and not accessible to the baby. • Use sunscreen, hat, and long sleeves when the baby is in the sun. • Keep heavy and sharp objects out of reach; check that all poisons are locked away including in homes visited; keep pet food and cosmetics out of reach. • Do not drink hot liquids or eat soup while holding the baby. • Have the poison control number by phones and programmed into cell phones. • Be alert for dangers of hot curling irons and other appliances. • Have electrical cords out of reach and not hanging down. • Have the home and environment checked for lead hazards. • Lower the infant crib mattress if still in the upper position. • Install gates and guards on stairs and windows. • Never use an infant walker.
9 months	• As previously noted. • Crawl on the floor and look for hazards at the baby's eye level. • Pad sharp corners on tables and other furniture. • Watch for tables, chairs, and other devices the baby may use for climbing to unsafe places.
12 months	• As previously noted. • Change to a forward-facing car safety seat if the baby is at least 20 pounds; install correctly and have installation checked; place in the back seat and never in the front seat with a passenger air bag. • Start teaching the child to wash hands frequently, showing how. • Provide own personal items such as clothing and blankets to childcare providers; wash often. • Change batteries in home smoke alarms and check systems. • Turn handles to the back of the stove; use back rather than front burners; watch for hot liquids. • Check the care provider setting for safety hazards. • Remember that responsible adults should always supervise your infant, not other children. • Peruse the home once again for hazards now that the child is more active, climbing, and walking.

Adapted from Hagan, Shaw, & Duncan, 2008.

are assessed. Family interactions and other settings where the infant spends time are evaluated for risks and protective factors that influence the child's development. Assess the health of siblings and patterns of integrating the infant into the rest of the family. Direct particular attention at assessment of risk for diseases and injuries. The data-gathering phase provides parents with the opportunity to ask questions and relay concerns. Further assessment may need to be directed at these areas.

Based on the assessment data, the nurse establishes nursing diagnoses that become the basis for nursing interventions. Areas of strength and need are included; often the family strengths can be used to further promote health. Some possible nursing diagnoses established during a health supervision visit of an infant might include:

- Effective Breast-Feeding related to the mother's confidence and knowledge
- Interrupted Breast-Feeding related to the mother's resumption of employment outside the home
- Compromised Family Coping related to recent role changes
- Risk for Altered Parent/Child Attachment related to anxiety associated with parenting role
- Sleep Pattern Disturbance (Infant) related to frequently changing sleep routines and cycles
- Risk for Infection (Infant) related to inadequate acquired immunity
- Risk for Injury (Infant) related to design of environment

Planning and Implementation

The nurse plays a vital role in successful health promotion and health maintenance activities. Explain to parents the procedures being performed and their purpose. Encourage them to ask questions and share their perceptions of the infant's personality, development, and other traits. This will enhance their understanding that health care involves a partnership between them and the care providers. It will lead to trust that promotes their ability to honestly share concerns. The first year of the baby's life is a key time for establishing a trusting relationship with health professionals.

Recognize the importance of data provided by simple assessments such as length and weight. Analyze all findings to learn if the child is developing as expected. Much of the visit is spent teaching parents about topics such as safety measures, providing anticipatory guidance related to development, assisting with integration of the new baby into the family, and relaying resources for support of the family in the community, Internet, or other areas. Parenting classes, childcare facilities, and family planning resources are examples of common parental needs. Perform recommended phys-

ical and developmental assessment, administer screening tests, and give immunizations. Be sure parents understand the need for tests and treatments, and relay the results of tests to them.

Nurses who work in hospitals, emergency services, and other facilities are an important link in health supervision. Ask where and how often the child is seen for care. Check immunization schedules to be sure they are up to date; administer needed vaccines. When the child is not being regularly seen, find out if the family does not understand the significance of these visits or lacks the resources to obtain them. Refer the family to resources as needed so that they can identify a pediatric health care home. Some agencies that provide health supervision are equipped to perform home visits on a regular basis or in case of special need. When nurses make regular home visits to families with many risk factors, health outcomes are improved. Seeing the family in the natural setting enables the nurse to tailor interventions to the specific situation. Nutrition, safety, and other teaching is more effective when it matches the family's needs. For example, showing how to set up a stimulating environment with safe materials, even if toys are limited, is an effective nursing strategy. Ensure that home visits are performed whenever appropriate and available, either through the pediatric health care home or through another community agency.

Before the family leaves the facility, be sure they have the next appointment scheduled. Summarize the content of the present visit, emphasizing the family's strengths and the baby's newly acquired developmental skills. Sensitively list any areas that require work in the coming weeks, such as babyproofing the home or encouraging the infant to reach for objects. Provide a journal or notebook in which the parents can record the infant's development and write down questions to ask in future visits. Suggest possible topics for the parents to learn about and provide books, brochures, and other printed material.

Evaluation

Expected outcomes of nursing care for the infant and family in health promotion and health maintenance include:

- Parents state common safety hazards at the child's present and upcoming ages.
- The infant demonstrates normal patterns of growth and progression in developmental milestones.
- The infant remains free of disease and injury.
- The infant is well adjusted, showing positive response to the environment and interactions with significant others.

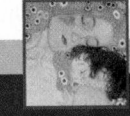

Chapter Highlights

- The first contact between the newborn infant's primary health care provider and the parents should occur prior to birth.
- A trusting relationship between the family and the care provider fosters a partnership that is influential in promoting the infant's development.
- Health supervision visits begin with careful observations of the infant and parent–child interactions.
- Surveillance of growth and development provides important clues to the well-being of the newborn and infant.
- Nutrition assessment and teaching are important to provide for the challenging nutritional needs of the first year of life.

- The early health supervision visits provide an opportunity to introduce concepts about physical activity and oral health for the infant.
- The mental health of parents influences the atmosphere in the home and the development of the newborn and infant.
- Patterns of interaction between parent and child as well as relationships with other adults and children provide the newborn and infant with strong emotional bonds that are essential to normal development.
- Disease and injury prevention strategies are integrated into each infant health care supervision visit.

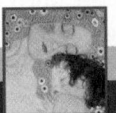

Clinical Reasoning in Action

Recall 22-year-old Shannon, who is described at the beginning of the chapter. She is a single mother with two daughters, 5-year-old Denise and 10-day-old Rhonda. Shannon lives with her male partner, who is the father of the new baby. Rhonda was born at 37 weeks' gestation, weighed 2800 g (6 lb, 3 oz) at birth, required phototherapy for newborn jaundice, and had initial difficulty breastfeeding. She was discharged from the nursery at 5 days of age.

1. What questions would the pediatric nurse and lactation consultant ask Shannon to assess the adequacy of breastfeeding at this time? What assessments of the newborn will provide clues about the adequacy of intake?

2. Consult Chapter 5 ∞ for a description of newborn reflexes. Plan a thorough newborn assessment that includes the reflexes. Why is it important to complete this neurological testing on baby Rhonda?

3. Plan a teaching session for Shannon that describes the sleep patterns of newborns. Integrate suggestions to enable Rhonda and her partner to obtain adequate rest.

4. Denise is Rhonda's 5-year-old sibling. What questions will you ask Shannon about Denise's adjustment to a new sibling?

See Pearson Nursing Student Resources for possible responses.

Pearson Nursing Student Resources

Find additional review materials at
nursing.pearsonhighered.com

Prepare for success with NCLEX®-style practice questions, interactive assignments and activities, web links, animations and videos, and more!

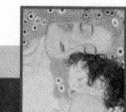

References

American Academy of Pediatrics (AAP). (2004). Hospital stay for healthy term newborns. *Pediatrics, 113*(5), 1434–1436.

American Academy of Pediatrics. (2005). The changing concept of sudden infant death syndrome: Diagnostic coding shifts, controversies regarding the sleeping environment, and new variables to consider in reducing risk. *Pediatrics, 116*(5), 1245–1255.

American Academy of Pediatrics, Committee on Fetus and Newborn & American College of Obstetricians and Gynecologists Committee on Obstetrics. (2007). Guidelines for perinatal care (6th ed.). Evanston, IL: Author.

American Academy of Pediatrics (AAP), Committee on Nutrition. (2009). *Pediatric nutrition handbook* (6th ed.). Elk Grove Village, IL: Author.

Blackburn, S. T. (2007). *Maternal, fetal, and neonatal physiology: A clinical perspective.* St. Louis, MO: Saunders.

Centers for Disease Control and Prevention. (2010). *Secondhand smoke.* Retrieved from http://www.cdc.gov/tobacco/data_statistics/fact_sheets/secondhand_smoke/

Cohen, G. J., & Committee on Psychosocial Aspects of Child and Family Health. (2009). The prenatal visit. *Pediatrics, 124*(4), 1227–1232.

Commonwealth Fund. (2007). *A practical guide for health development.* Retrieved from http://www.commonwealthfund.org

Garfield, C. F., & Isacco, A. (2006). Fathers and the well-child visit. *Pediatrics, 117*, e637–e645.

Graham, J. M. (2006). Tummy time is important. *Clinical Pediatrics, 45*(2), 119–121.

Hagan, J. G., Shaw, J. S., & Duncan, P. M. (Eds.). (2008). *Bright futures: Guidelines for health supervision of infants, children, and adolescents* (3rd ed.). Elk Grove Village, IL: American Academy of Pediatrics.

Hall, W. A., Clauson, M., Carty, E. M., Janssen, P. A., & Saunders, R. A. (2006). Effects on parents of an intervention to resolve infant behavioral sleep problems. *Pediatric Nursing, 32*, 243–250.

Healthy People 2020. (2010). Retrieved from www.healthypeople.gov

Joint Committee on Infant Hearing. (2007). Year 2007 position statement: Principles and guidelines for early detection and intervention program. *Pediatrics, 120*(4), 898–921.

Katbamna, B., Crumpton, T., & Patel, D. R. (2008). Hearing impairment in children. *Pediatric Clinics of North America, 55*(5), 1175–1188.

Kinney, H. C., & Thach, B. T. (2009). The sudden infant death syndrome. *New England Journal of Medicine, 361*(8), 795–805.

Ladewig, P. A. W., London, M. L., & Davidson, M. R. (2010). *Contemporary maternal-newborn nursing care.* Upper Saddle River, NJ: Pearson Prentice Hall.

London, M. L., Ladewig, P. A.W., Ball, J., Bindler, R. C., & Cowen, K. J. (2010). *Maternal and Child Nursing Care* (3rd ed.). Upper Saddle River, NJ: Pearson Prentice Hall.

Mindell, J. A., Sadeh, A., Kohyama, J., & How, T. H. (2010). Parental behaviors and sleep outcomes in infants and toddlers: A cross cultural comparison. *Sleep Medicine, 11*(4), 393–399.

Mishina, H., & Takayama, J. I. (2009). Screening for maternal depression in primary care pediatrics. *Current Opinion in Pediatrics, 21*(6), 789–793.

Murray, R. B., Zentner, J. P., & Yakimo, R. (2009). *Health promotion strategies through the life span* (8th ed.). Upper Saddle River, NJ: Prentice Hall.

Touchette, E., Petit, D., Paquet, J., Boivin, M., Japel, C., Tremblay, R. E., & Montplaisir, J. Y. (2005). Factors associated with fragmented sleep at night across early childhood. *Archives of Pediatrics & Adolescent Medicine, 159*, 242–249.

U.S. Department of Labor. (2009). Newborns' and mothers' health protection act. Retrieved from http://www.dol.gov/topic/health-plans/newborns.htm

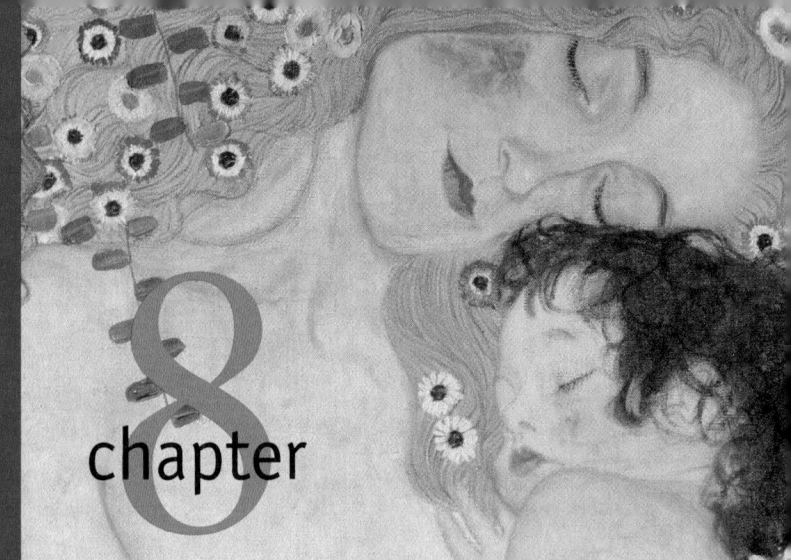

Health Promotion and Maintenance for the Toddler and Preschooler

chapter 8

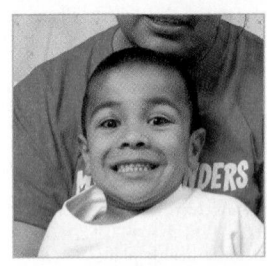

Dominic, 4 years old, visits his pediatric health care home with his mother, Sophia. Dominic has always been a healthy child. He has had all of his immunizations from infancy through toddler years. His father is serving in the military on active duty in the Middle East; he is in the middle of a 15-month deployment. Sophia has help from her mother, Hannah, to care for Dominic while she works. Hannah has moved to a house down the street in order to be close and available. Dominic attends preschool four days each week and can write his name and identify colors and letters. He has well-developed language skills. The physical examination shows that Dominic is in the 25th percentile for height and the 10th percentile for weight. He has several decaying deciduous teeth but otherwise seems to be in good health. He is energetic and talkative with clinic staff. The nurse decides to gather additional information about nutritional status, activity level, and access to dental care. Why is this information important to plan health promotion and maintenance activities for Dominic? What support does his family need at this time? What immunizations are needed during the preschool years?

Key Terms

deciduous teeth / 207
early childhood caries (ECC) / 207
kinesthesia / 206
nightmares / 209
night terrors / 209

Learning Outcomes

After reading this chapter, you will be able to do the following:

1. State components of growth and developmental surveillance needs for children of toddler and preschool ages.
2. Describe the nutrition, physical activity, and oral health needs of toddlers and preschoolers.
3. Integrate pertinent mental health care into health supervision visits for toddlers and preschoolers.
4. Synthesize data about the family and other social relationships to promote and maintain health of toddlers and preschoolers.
5. Plan assessment and interventions appropriate for health promotion and maintenance during health supervision visits of toddlers and preschoolers.
6. Apply knowledge of the major injury risks of toddlers and preschoolers to plan nursing interventions that contribute to their prevention.

░ HEALTH PROMOTION AND MAINTENANCE FOR THE TODDLER AND PRESCHOOLER

The years following infancy are challenging for parents as the child grows and acquires new developmental skills. The child progresses from the first tentative steps and words at a year of age, through the independent behaviors of toddlerhood, and into preschool age when most children attend some type of education program, have well-developed verbal communication, and acquire many gross and fine motor skills. Toddler and preschool ages are often grouped as "young childhood" since the family remains the primary system within which the child interacts, and there are many common health concerns such as nutrition, sleep, and growing independence. Facing consistent changes in development, parents rely on the pediatric health care home (medical home) for advice and information. Regular visits are recommended for 12, 15, and 18 months, and at approximately 2, 3, 4, and 5 years of age. Nurses apply concepts of anticipatory guidance during visits for health promotion and maintenance to assist parents in the transitions they face.

Health supervision visits apply the following:

1. *Assessment* is performed, using screening tests, evaluations, and observations.
2. *Education* includes anticipatory guidance about coming developmental tasks.
3. *Intervention* includes parent counseling, home visits when appropriate, and scheduling future visits.
4. *Care* is coordinated among resources serving the family (Halfon, DuPlessis, & Inkelas, 2007).

General Observations

A collaborative relationship between the family and the health care providers should already be established. If, however, the family is new to this health care home, reach out to welcome them warmly and express interest in them as individuals and parents. As families often feel uncomfortable in health care settings, it is important to establish positive rapport so they will be able to ask questions and bring up concerns about the child.

While calling the toddler in from the waiting room, recall the child just 1 year before. This young child is now able to walk in, even if with a bit of help. Watch for the child's desire for independence or signs of continuing reliance on the parent. By preschool age, the child is totally independent in walking and usually engages in conversations easily. Welcome the child warmly, and assess the preschool child's social skills and motor activities. Direct greetings or questions to the child to evaluate stranger anxiety and ability to understand simple commands or questions. What verbal skills are observed? Observe the child's general appearance, nutrition, and state of health.

Health supervision visits are adapted for older toddlers and preschoolers to include observations of parental discipline and interaction style. Be alert for the parents' understanding of your teaching and questions. Does the parent respond to the child's questions? Were age-appropriate toys or activities brought to the visit to help occupy the child while waiting? Is the child observant of the environment and alert?

Nursing Alert

Health literacy involves the parent's ability to read health-related materials, understand and communicate oral health information, and analyze important messages about health-related care (Betz, Ruccione, Meeske, et al., 2008). Inadequate health literacy can seriously affect care. Health brochures should be clear and simple, feedback after oral communication should be sought, and reinforcement of information should be a part of each encounter.

Growth and Developmental Surveillance

An essential assessment skill integrated into the visit is measurement of growth. Weight and length are measured and compared to expected patterns of growth. Once the child can stand to be measured, sometime between 2 and 3 years of age, charts for standing height rather than recumbent length are used. Body mass index (BMI) is first calculated at 2 years of age and provides information about the relationship of height and weight (see Chapter 14 ∞). Head circumference is usually measured until the child is between 1 and 2 years of age.

Growth continues to be a primary way of evaluating the child's nutritional status. It may also provide clues about conditions that have not yet been evaluated such as endocrine, cardiac, or other disorders. Depending on the results of growth measurement, the nurse may gather additional data. For a child under the 5th percentile for weight or BMI, detailed nutritional intake records should begin. Laboratory studies such as hematocrit and hemoglobin can be performed. Patterns of family growth can be examined. What size are the parents and siblings? Ask if the child has had any illness or hospitalization. For children above the 85th percentile for BMI, detailed dietary intake and physical activity history should be taken. Consult the growth grids in Appendix A ∞.

The physical assessment is performed, with some parts conducted by the nurse and others by the primary care provider such as a physician or nurse practitioner. See Chapter 5 ∞ for a thorough discussion of physical examination. The order of the examination and the approaches to the child are particularly important at this age. Leave intrusive procedures such as the ear and eye exam and visualization of genitalia until the end of the exam. Integrate techniques such as allowing the child to play with the stethoscope, "blow out" the light from the otoscope, or make a game of pushing the legs against the examiner to measure symmetry of strength (Figure 8–1 ►). Preschoolers are generally interested in their bodies, so teaching about parts of the examination is helpful. During the physical examination, ask the parents pertinent questions about development and health (Table 8–1). Consider the young child's expected developmental milestones (see Chapter 4 ∞) and ask questions related to these milestones. Developmental surveillance is integrated throughout the visit, and developmental screening or testing is performed. Ask if the child has had developmental testing done at a childcare agency or another site.

Nurses generally have in-depth knowledge of child development, through growth and development courses and pediatric nursing curricula, and are thus well positioned to address parental concerns related to child development (see Table 8–1).

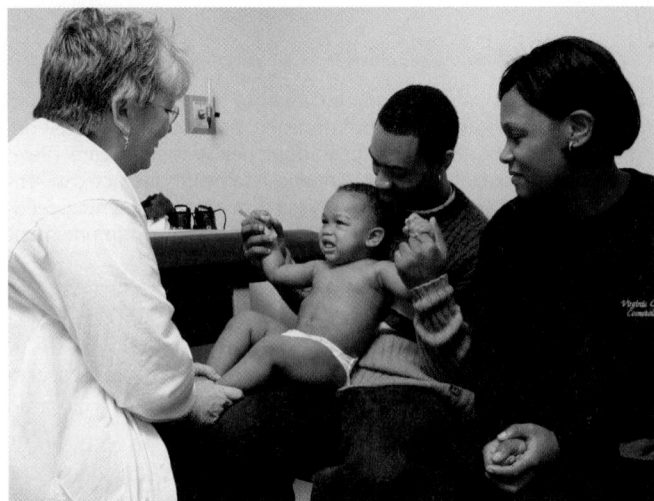

A

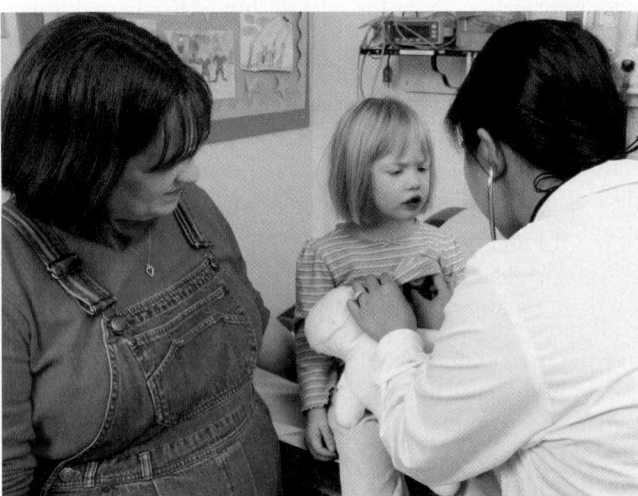

B

FIGURE 8–1 ➤ The approach to examination of the toddler or preschooler is important in order to elicit cooperation. A, The toddler may accept parts of the examination best when seated on the parent's lap such as shown in this photo of a boy with his father. B, The preschooler likes the opportunity to touch and become comfortable with equipment used, or in this case hold a doll that receives the same examinations as the child.

TABLE 8–1	Developmental Milestones Observed During Health Promotion and Health Maintenance Visits of Toddlers and Preschoolers
Age	Developmental Milestones
12 months	• Walks alone or with help • Enjoys social games and interactions • Speaks one to three words and understands simple commands • Drinks from cup and feeds self
15 months	• Walks by self, crawls or walks up stairs • Stacks two blocks • Points to one or more body parts • Is increasingly interactive • Explores environment
18 months	• Walks with ease • Pushes or pulls toy • Stacks three or more blocks • Uses spoon to eat, spilling often • Follows directions and uses 15–20 words
2–3 years	• Goes up and down steps • Kicks ball • Scribbles and draws lines on paper • Imitates words and actions of adults
3–4 years	• Jumps • Rides tricycle • Draws precise lines on paper; attempts to imitate circle, line, and cross • Always feeds self • Dresses self, though sometimes clothes are backward • Has friends and plays with others
4–5 years	• Recites rhymes and songs • States name • Draws a rudimentary person • Builds tower of blocks and bridges with blocks • Throws ball overhand

Development is the key organizing principle of early childhood health care. Developmental screening and services should be integrated within health care, childcare, and school settings, to include the multiple sites common for young children (Halfon et al., 2007). Fine and gross motor skills, communication methods and social interactions, and language skills are basic components of screening tools. See Chapter 6 ∞ for a list of commonly used tests. Nurses should verify that parents understand and can read the screening tool. Provide assistance and translators as needed.

Health promotion growth and development issues for toddlers and preschoolers are addressed at each visit. Some common examples include:

• Explaining growth patterns and what is expected in the months ahead

• Providing toys that encourage the coming developmental milestones

• Showing parents the child's developmental progression on a screening tool

Likewise, health maintenance activities are included in health supervision visits, with the primary purpose being prevention of disease and injury. Specific examples are included throughout the chapter, but some general areas addressed are:

• Connecting developmental skills with risks for injury such as drowning and car crashes

• Recognizing the possibility of infectious diseases as the child begins a childcare experience and addressing recognition and treatments for common diseases

Expected outcomes for the child include normal growth and development patterns for motor, language, and social skills; parental knowledge of stimulating activities for the child; awareness of the family about risks to growth and development; and healthy body systems for the child.

About 16% of children have a developmental disability, but less than 30% of these are identified prior to kindergarten (Wagner, Jenkins, & Smith, 2006). Developmental surveillance should be flexible and continuous so that age-appropriate screening tools are administered at intervals. Nurses are essential to establishing protocols that ensure such screening in office, home, and hospital settings.

Additionally, be alert for information that emerges during conversations at the visit and ask further questions as needed. Topics pertinent at health supervision visits of young children include sleep patterns, discipline techniques, toilet training, learning and reading practices, communication, and parental issues and questions. Many children, especially by preschool age, attend a childcare center. Ask about the experience and whether developmental skills are a focus of activity. Ask if the parent is pleased with the childcare experience or needs further resources.

Nutrition

The child's nutritional status continues to play an important part in promoting health and preventing health disruptions during toddler and preschooler years. Good nutrition fosters normal growth patterns, promotes developmental progression, and helps prevent disorders such as anemia, tooth decay, and immune dysfunction. In addition, intake of food takes on an increasingly social dimension during early childhood as children interact more with adults and other children at mealtimes.

For toddlers, questions for the family focus on introduction of foods, the child's eating patterns, and transition from breast milk or formula to other liquids. The toddler often consumes small amounts of foods, and parents consequently worry about the change in appetite. Showing the parents that the child is growing normally can help allay their anxiety about this common developmental variation. Preschoolers increasingly interact with others during food preparation and meal consumption. Questions focus on the child's likes and dislikes for particular foods, behavior at the table, health supplements, and establishment of healthy family eating patterns. Ask how often the family eats out, especially at fast food restaurants. When parents are busy and older siblings are in activities, both toddlers and preschoolers may be eating foods such as French fries or milk shakes several times weekly. Suggest alternative approaches to the busy lifestyle, such as bringing fresh fruit slices along when an older sibling is at a sporting event, keeping a cooler in the car to maintain cool items, and limiting fast food meals to no more than one or two per week. Encourage the family to set times when they all eat together, even if only a few times per week. If children help prepare this family meal, and then eat together, nutritional knowledge and intake can be positively enhanced. Obtain nutritional information about common fast food options in your community and share these with parents. Assist them to make healthy choices when eating out. When the child is in a childcare center or home, encourage the parents to find out what food is provided for the child in that setting.

During the toddler and preschool years, children are gaining much more independence about food choices and eating pat-

Many families engage in a variety of complementary practices to enhance health of their children. Dietary supplements are the most common of these and may be used to promote health or treat pediatric conditions such as attention deficit disorders or allergies. Inquire about vitamins, minerals, herbs, and other supplements to the child's diet (Rosen & Breuner, 2008; Gardiner & Riley, 2008). Provide information to answer the family's questions about complementary foods.

terns. At the same time, their eating patterns depend mainly on the family; therefore, assessment should involve the entire family unit. Parents can benefit from receiving information about nutrition in young children (Table 8–2).

Health promotion interventions include supporting breastfeeding if the mother still breastfeeds the young toddler and ensuring that preschoolers have a role in selecting foods for healthy snacks. Parental education is influential in shaping the young child's diet and should be integrated into all visits (Essery, DiMarco, Rich, et al., 2008). Teach the amounts of food that should be offered and frequency of meals. Encourage parents to make food preparation and meals a pleasant experience. See Chapter 14 ∞ for additional information about the nutritional needs of young children. An example of an important health promotion item for every family is the importance of including "five a day," or five servings of fruits and vegetables in the daily diet. Likewise, "three a day of dairy" encourages families to provide at least three servings of dairy products for children every day. Nurses and parents partner to ensure that the young child establishes healthy eating habits at home and in other daily settings. Health maintenance activities focus primarily on disease and injury prevention, with examples of feeding practices that do not include common choking foods, and limiting daily fruit juice intake to prevent dental caries and excessive caloric intake. Desired outcomes related to nutrition include meeting normal growth and development milestones, maintaining recommended weight, increasing understanding of healthy food patterns, and preventing nutrition-related disorders.

Families integrate their cultural backgrounds and past experiences into food preparation and choices. Ask what foods are common in the child's cultural group and help the family learn when to introduce each food. For example, rice may be a first food for an Asian baby, rather than rice cereal. Be sure the child also takes in adequate iron sources in the first foods offered. Tofu or bean paste may be a common protein source in some diets. A Native American child may eat fish or wild game, along with berries and roots. Ask and learn about each family's cultural patterns. Learn what you can about cultural groups in your community. Encourage the family to offer the young child their usual foods, as long as they meet needs for requirements, are prepared with minimal salt and seasoning, and are soft enough to avoid choking. Perform diet recalls and analyses to check for any specific teaching needs in all families.

TABLE 8–2	Nutrition Teaching for Health Promotion and Health Maintenance Visits
Age	**Nutrition Teaching**
1 year	• Support the mother who continues to breastfeed. • Wean the child from the bottle by substituting a cup. • If beginning to use cow milk, use whole milk. • Limit juice to 4–6 ounces daily; offer water several times daily. • Encourage safety measures—use a high chair with a strap, secure the child and use caution in grocery carts, and do not allow foods to be eaten in the car. • Provide information on choking and airway obstruction removal training. • Provide food and water safety guidelines (see Chapter 14 ∞). • Be sure all major food groups have been introduced. • Limit high-fat and high-sugar foods. • Review amounts of food commonly consumed and frequency of feedings. • Review use of fluoride if the water supply is not fluoridated.
2 years	• Ask if the mother is still breastfeeding. Support the decision to continue or to wean the child, as she desires. • Encourage total removal of the bottle if still in use. • Ensure that all foods common to the family have been offered. • Offer child-sized eating utensils. • Change to low-fat or skim milk if the family desires. • Limit milk to 2–3 servings daily. • Teach parents methods for dealing with temper tantrums over food—make food available at meal and snack times only, do not force intake, and offer a variety of foods. • Teach that the child may have days of very low intake due to slowing growth rate.
3 years	• Teach normal intake and decreasing the number of snacks. • Determine milk intake; most children are weaned from breastfeeding and drink 1% or 2% milk. • Engage the child in food preparation and pouring liquids from a small pitcher. • Recognize that food jags (periods when only 1 or 2 foods are eaten) are common. • Recognize the social nature of eating; expect the child to sit for a short period at meals with the family. • Teach that meals and snacks should not be eaten while watching television.
4 years	• Encourage involving the child in snack selection and preparation. • Start to teach food groups and the importance of nutrition for the body. • Alter intake as appropriate depending on weight and BMI. • Make dairy products consumed low or reduced fat.

Physical Activity

The toddler and preschooler consistently show gains in fine and gross motor abilities. They move around independently and have more physical activity away from the home base. They commonly visit parks, swim, attend childcare centers, and help with some household tasks. These activities are important, both because they assist the child to continue to develop motor skills, and because they limit the amount of time spent in sedentary behavior. The toddler and preschool years are an important time for setting the physical activity habits that will continue during childhood.

During toddler years, the main emphasis is on providing experiences that encourage further motor development. The child needs to walk, run, hop, push and pull objects, and throw balls. A minimum of 60 minutes per day of unstructured physical activity is needed (Centers for Disease Control and Prevention, 2008). Motor activity is a major component in all play times, and activities should engage the child's large and small muscle groups (Figure 8–2 ➤). By the preschool years, coordination becomes increasingly important. Physical activity is important for all children, including those with developmental disabilities. The preschooler learns to balance, walk on one foot, skip, and throw and catch with greater accuracy. **Kinesthesia**, or the sense of one's

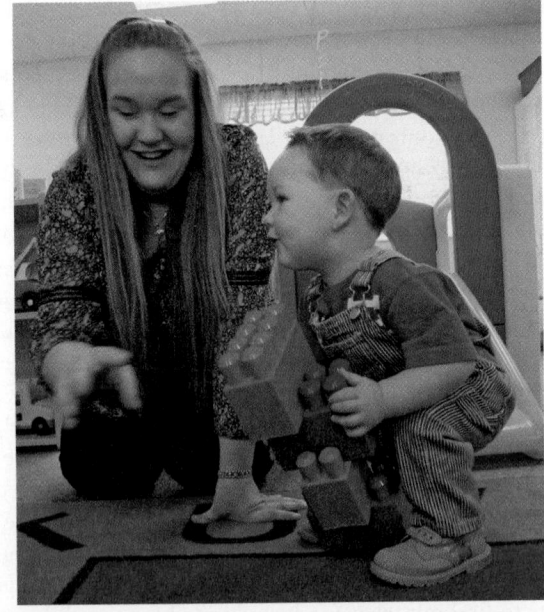

FIGURE 8–2 ➤ This toddler enjoys motor activity that uses large muscle groups. The preschooler begins to spend increasing amounts of time in coordination of both small and large muscle mass. List several physical activities that you can suggest for the parents of children in each of these age groups.

TABLE 8–3	Risk and Protective Factors Regarding Physical Activity in Toddlerhood and Preschool
Risk Factors	Protective Factors
• Limited stimulation by family or other care providers • Long work hours by parents • Parents who have little physical activity on a daily basis • Limited social time with other children • Limited access to balls, slides, balance beams, tricycles, and other materials that foster physical activity • Lack of adequate safety gear for activities • Reluctance to try new physical activity • Engagement in television or other screen activities for more than 2 hours daily • Developmental delay • Slow development of social skills • Lack of knowledge by family about child's physical activity needs • Limited community resources for childcare and physical activity • Unsafe neighborhood and lack of lawns, parks, and other facilities	• Expected developmental progression • Daily contact with other young children • Easily engaged socially with others • Eagerness to try new physical activity • Access to balls, slides, balance beams, tricycles, and other materials that foster physical activity • Availability of adequate safety gear that properly fits the child • Family members that engage in daily physical activity • Family members that spend time daily in physical activity with the child • Family understanding of motor developmental milestones and importance of physical activity in childhood • Limit of no more than 2 hours daily of television and other screen activities • Neighborhood with access to childcare that integrates physical activity • Safe neighborhood that contains lawns, parks, and other facilities

Adapted from Hagan, Shaw, & Duncan, 2008.

body position and movement, develops during these years. Eye-hand coordination improves at the same time that visual acuity matures. The social component plays an important role as children learn to engage in games and activities cooperatively with others.

The nurse applies the concept of resilience by identifying both risk and protective factors related to physical activity (Table 8–3). The assessment becomes the basis for nursing interventions, both to reinforce positive physical activity and to make recommendations for changes where needed.

Since both children and adults are commonly overweight and sedentary in today's society, emphasis on physical activity should be a part of each health supervision visit. Nurses and parents are partners in planning activities for the young child; patterns set in motion at this early age will continue into the rest of childhood and into adulthood. Suggestions for the family may include setting guidelines to limit television and other screen activities to a maximum of 2 hours daily in order to facilitate adequate physical activity time. Children should not have television and computers in their bedrooms. Suggest activities that parents can do with their children. Health promotion teaching imparts to parents the benefits of activity, such as a healthy immune and cardiovascular system, positive self-concept of the child, and the child's learning of important motor skills. Health maintenance teaching focuses on disease prevention, such as avoidance of overweight, and injury prevention, such as use of protective gear for sports.

Expected outcomes of health promotion and health supervision related to physical activity are daily inclusion of at least 60 minutes of activity into life patterns, normal developmental progression of the musculoskeletal system, growth in coordination, and appropriate balance between dietary intake and physical activity so that normal weight is maintained.

Oral Health

The early childhood years play an important part in the child's future oral health, and yet dental caries in primary teeth has increased in the 2- to 5-year-old age group (Dye, Tan, Smith, et al., 2007), from 18% in the 1988–1994 survey to 24% in the recent National Health and Nutrition Examination Survey (Centers for Disease Control and Prevention, 2009). **Early childhood caries (ECC)** is defined as one or more decayed, missing, or filled tooth surfaces in a child less than 6 years of age (Wagner & Oskouian, 2008). Other terms for this condition include "bottle mouth syndrome" or "baby bottle tooth decay." This condition is promoted by inadequate preventive care, which can include poor diet, brushing, and feeding habits, and lack of dental care. ECC is serious because young children with the condition are more likely to have continuing dental problems that can influence speech, cause pain, and delay development. Teaching prevention at an early age is key to preventing the problem.

The nurse assists the family to ensure oral health for the young child. When the first tooth erupts, and no later than 1 year of age, the child should make a first visit to the dentist. By about 2 years of age, the toddler has a full set of 20 teeth. Evaluate these teeth for condition and number. They help to maintain space for the permanent teeth, foster positive eating habits, and are needed for language development. Inquire about how the family cleans the teeth and ask them to demonstrate if the child has any dental decay. At the end of preschool, the first of these **deciduous teeth** are lost, an important developmental event for most children.

Culture   *Disparity in Dental Health*

Recent analysis of data from the National Health and Nutrition Examination Survey (NHANES) shows that no racial or ethnic group meets the *Healthy People 2010* goal of no more than 11% of children with caries in primary teeth. However, there is great disparity with about 35% of Mexican American children having primary teeth caries, 26% of non-Hispanic Blacks, and 20% of non-Hispanic Whites (Centers for Disease Control and Prevention, 2009).

Let's Move Website

Based on the results of the child's teeth assessment, observation of language skills, and answers to questions directed at parents, plan interventions that will foster maintenance of oral health, thus preventing dental disease. (See Chapter 19 ∞ for emergency treatment of dental injury.) These may include referral to low-cost dental clinics, provision of toothbrush and toothpaste, demonstration to the parents and young child about proper brushing technique, and teaching about limiting sweet snacks and drinks. Remember to positively reinforce health promotion practices such as good oral hygiene for toddlers and preschoolers who brush, visit the dentist, and are careful to limit intake of sweets. Desired outcomes for oral health are eruption of a normal set of deciduous teeth, regular dental care, nutrition and hygiene practices that foster dental health, and child and parent knowledge about oral health.

Clinical Judgment

What questions would you ask about diet and oral care to identify the reasons for Dominic's dental caries (see opening scenario)?

Mental and Spiritual Health

The family is key in fostering a positive self-image and setting the stage for the young child's mental health. Significant numbers of preschool children have mental health problems. Screening tools and observations can be used to identify children at risk and to maximize the protective factors in families. As the family is called in for the visit, begin your assessment of the family's methods of influencing mental health. Observe communication and interactions in the family and the child's ability to interact with health care providers. Ask for a description of a typical day or what the child has recently begun to do.

The child's sense of self and mental status are related to new accomplishments. Inquire about toilet training, tooth brushing, choosing clothes and getting dressed, using crayons, or other developmental tasks.

Toddlers and preschoolers use self-regulation (the ability to soothe and comfort the self) to control anger, excessive desires for objects or foods, and other socially unacceptable behaviors. In order to assist the child in developing the ability to control and regulate self, parents often use discipline techniques. Ask about how the parent deals with the child who is having a temper tantrum or showing other undesirable behaviors. Reinforce positive ways of helping the child set limits for self and make suggestions when parents need assistance (see Families Want to Know: Positive Discipline). The goal of discipline is to help the child develop a sense of right and wrong, and learn acceptable ways of dealing with other people.

Adequate sleep and rest are needed for children to master self-regulation. Most toddlers have established regular sleeping patterns with occasional night awakenings. They sleep about 10 to 12 hours at night with one or two daytime naps (Murray, Zentner, & Yakimo, 2009). Parents have usually learned to establish clear routines such as reading a story, rubbing the child's back, and then leaving the child alone. Occasionally parents who work during the day may feel guilty about putting the child to sleep. Advise them to spend quality time with the child after arriving home, and then to establish clear sleeping expectations. Transitional objects such as blankets or toys are important for the toddler and can be used during childcare experiences to provide comfort and help maintain normal routines. Some families prefer to have children sleep in the bed with parents. Advise against this pattern, but if this is the parents' decision, be sure they are aware of safety hazards such as suffocation in excessive

Families Want to Know

Positive Discipline

First, provide structure that enhances the possibility of desirable behaviors:

■ Limit rules to those that are essential. It is easier to enforce a few important rules than many that are nonessential.

■ Provide an environment where the child is mainly free to explore safely in order to avoid constant cautions. For example, have adequate play space for toddlers with limited fragile glassware in the usual daily environment. It is easier for the toddler to learn not to touch a few objects when adequate objects are provided for play.

■ Spend time interacting with the child several times each day. Praise positive behaviors frequently. Preschoolers often like to have charts with stars to record picking up toys, helping a parent, and other positive behaviors. Once a certain number of stars is reached, the child earns a reward, such as stickers or an outing with the parent.

When the child shows undesirable behaviors:

■ Use distraction as the first approach and praise the child for selecting the new activity suggested by the parent.

■ Tell the child one time that the behavior is unsatisfactory and what will happen if the behavior persists.

■ Separate the child from a setting in which behavior is undesirable. Place the child in "time-out," a separate place that is safe. Toddlers can be placed in a playpen or crib, while preschoolers are told to sit on a chair. One minute of time-out per year of age is a good length of time. Once time-out is over, provide a positive activity and move the child directly toward the activity.

When undesirable behaviors include other people, such as biting or hitting:

■ Tell the child clearly that it is not satisfactory to hurt another person.

■ Separate the child immediately from the situation and use time-out.

■ If there are repeated episodes, be sure the child is getting adequate sleep and food, has opportunities for active play that releases energy, and has positive attention from many people in the environment. Be sensitive to stresses such as a recent trauma or a new sibling.

■ Encourage the child to "use words" instead of hitting or biting. Until able to do so on his or her own, parents can model this behavior. "You feel like saying 'I am really upset that you took my toy away.' Let's use words instead of hitting so your sister knows that."

(American Academy of Pediatrics, 2007)

bedding, injury related to falling between the headboard and frame, parental smoking that could lead to fire, or parental alcohol and drug use that can lead to such sound sleep that it is possible to roll onto and suffocate the child.

The preschooler sleeps about 9 to 12 hours and may have one or no naps each day (Murray et al., 2009; Chamness, 2008). Some quiet playtime can be beneficial even for the preschooler who does not nap. At this age, some children develop awakenings at night and may need some assistance in falling back to sleep. **Nightmares** are frightening dreams that awaken the child who is often crying and upset. Parents can reassure the child, rub the child's back, provide some repeat of a bedtime routine such as reading a story, and then allow the child to settle into sleep again. It is not advisable to bring the child to the parental bed since he or she may start to awaken at night in order to continue this practice. **Night terrors** are characterized by a child who cries out and appears frightened. However, in contrast to nightmares, the child having a night terror is not fully awake and may appear disoriented. A related condition is that of sleepwalking (Chamness, 2008). Parents should quietly talk to and comfort the child, lead the sleepwalker back to bed, and allow the child to return to sleep. There is no recollection of these events the next morning.

The toddler gains more independence in many aspects of life such as mobility and speech. The control over toileting is another milestone that signals greater independence and can lead to a sense of self-control. Ask parents if the toddler has shown interest in toilet training and how they intend to work with the child to attain control over bowel and bladder. Preschoolers are generally well trained for bowel and bladder control with only occasional accidents. These accidents should be treated with understanding rather than blame in order for healthy self-concept to develop. Preschoolers are increasingly aware of gender and sexuality issues. They may ask questions about kissing, love, or their genitals. These questions should be truthfully answered, leaving the child with a positive sense of sexuality. Some exploration of genitals can occur. Children should be told simply that it is something that should occur in private, and then be offered other activities to engage them when with other people.

The family's spiritual orientation takes on additional meaning for the toddler and preschooler. They can participate in the family's faith-based practices. This enlarges their microsystem influences to include the religious group, thus reinforcing children's learning about right and wrong. The nurse assesses the family's faith-based or spiritual beliefs and provides support for the family's approach, whether it is in established religious organizations or in the family's other meaningful activities.

Health promotion activities focus on development of a healthy self-concept in the toddler and young child by helping parents to set up successful play experiences, to praise the child for successes, to use effective limit-setting techniques, and to realize and appreciate the child's unique characteristics. Health maintenance seeks to avoid poor self-image that can occur with constant criticism or expectations not in alignment with the toddler's or preschooler's developmental capabilities. Advise the family to spend time together and relax with stress-reducing activities rather than creating an environment where children are overscheduled with commitments. Further examples of family interactions that can influence the child's self-concept are provided in the following section on relationships.

Desired outcomes for the child related to mental and spiritual health include emergence of a positive self-esteem, ability to self-regulate behaviors, emergence of methods to handle daily stressors, and normal developmental progression in tasks such as toilet training and sleep.

Relationships

Family members are part of the microsystem for the toddler and preschooler; as such, they form a vital part of the child's environment. Families with members who handle stress well and have healthy lifestyle patterns offer security for the young child. When parents are stressed or depressed, the mental status of all family members can be affected. Ask how things are going for the family in general. Consider Dominic, who is described in the opening scenario. What stresses has this family experienced that might impact his relationships with others? Inquire about siblings and whether any issues of concern exist that might influence the toddler or preschooler. Illness or behavior problems in a sibling can decrease the parent's ability to deal with other children. The focus on a sibling in need can be confusing to a toddler or preschooler.

Be alert for signs of child abuse and for substance abuse in family members (see Chapter 17 ∞ for a thorough description of child abuse). Have the parents become separated or divorced? Is there a new stepparent?

During questions and observations, the nurse identifies family risk and protective factors. Reinforce strengths and provide services and referrals to deal with risks. Some strengths include:

- The family spends time together each day.
- Parents are proud of their child's accomplishments and knowledgeable about developmental progression.
- Childcare center personnel and family members interact regularly to plan consistent approaches for the toddler and preschooler.
- The teen mother of a toddler is enrolled in a high school continuation program with a childcare component.

Examples of risks to mental health include:

- The mother has been diagnosed with depression.
- An uncle in the home uses street drugs.
- The child awakens with night terrors.
- The child was recently in a serious car accident.
- A teen mother is estranged from her own family and has few goals and resources.

Toddlers continue to grow in social abilities, while preschoolers demonstrate large strides in socializing with others. Most toddlers enjoy playing with other children, although they engage in parallel play, "side by side" with other children. They also engage in play with adults for short periods, such as throwing a ball. However, preschoolers begin to engage in cooperative play activities that directly involve other children. They play "house" where one child plays the mother, and another the child. They engage in simple games where each plays a separate role. Their interactions with adults display similar maturity as they take on tasks such as setting the table for dinner, or picking up books from the floor. Social skills involve getting along with others. Young children exhibit increasing skill in language development, a primary medium for social exchange. From just a few words at 1 year, children progress to stating three-word sentences by 3 years of age. Although all parts of speech are not in place, young children certainly have the ability to make needs and thoughts known. Assessment of language skills provides a mirror into this important means of socializing.

Successful social skills involve separating from the parent at times. During toddlerhood, most children spend some time away from parents. Initially they may be fearful and display crying, but gradually they learn to adapt to the new person and place. Preschoolers need to begin developing relationships with other adults and children in order to adapt to the school setting at about 5 years of age. Ask how many people the child has contact with each week, and how he or she manages separation from the parent. Encourage parents to see separation as a skill the child is learning rather than something that is guilt-producing. When they leave the child in a secure setting, they should hug, provide a favorite object, and leave. Short periods initially will teach the child that the parent can be trusted to return. In addition, young children often have tempers and other undesirable behaviors. Assist parents in handling them successfully (see Families Want to Know: Handling Temper Tantrums).

Expected outcomes of health promotion and health maintenance activities with toddlers and preschoolers include increasing social skills with parents, siblings, and other children and adults;

successful management of temperament characteristics; adjustment to time away from the home; and improving language/communication skills.

Disease Prevention Strategies

Toddlers remain prone to many infectious diseases due to immature immune systems. By the preschool age, immune defenses are more mature and communicable diseases are less common. Some immunizations are given during this age period to complete the basic series. For children who have not had all immunizations, extra visits to catch them up to recommended levels may be needed. At the end of the preschool period, children have a complete review of the immunization record so any needed injections are given before school entry. See Table 8–4 for immunizations recommended during toddlerhood and preschool (see Chapter 16 ∞ for further information). Toddlers and preschoolers also need screening for several health conditions. Earlier visits may have failed to identify a problem due to the child's young age, so areas such as vision, hearing, and developmental milestones are always included.

Recognize that the environment is a powerful influence on children's health. Consider the presence of particular risks in rural or urban environments (Cherry, Huggins, & Gilmore, 2007). Ask if parents or others in the home smoke. Discourage this practice and describe the health implications for the child. Is the neighborhood generally safe? Are there air, water, or other toxic exposures? Ask about lead exposure in the home (see Chapter 17 ∞). How much television and other screen time is common in the home? Do older siblings play violent video

---

Families Want to Know
Handling Temper Tantrums

Temper tantrums are common in toddlers and are manifested as episodes of screaming, crying, pounding objects, kicking, and otherwise showing anger. Toddlers may be expressing frustration with something that has occurred. They have learned that they are independent individuals and have an effect by showing their dismay. Temper tantrums should gradually decrease in number as the child grows into the preschool years. Parents can learn that tantrums are normal but that techniques can assist in handling them successfully. The approaches are similar to those used when the child bites or hits. Some specific suggestions for tantrums include:

- Toddlers often become increasingly agitated and upset prior to a tantrum; hold and distract them when that occurs.
- Separate the child from others if possible (in time-out).
- Ensure that the child is safe and not throwing self against objects that could cause injury.
- Remain calm, holding the child firmly still if needed.
- Talk calmly to the child, verbalizing his or her feelings and what he or she needs to do to calm down.
- Reward the child briefly and verbally after control is gained. "It was really good that you could calm down and say you were sorry. Now let's go back to the living room." Do not give the child the item that was desired when the tantrum began.

TABLE 8–4	Immunizations Recommended for the Toddler and Preschooler
Immunization	Recommendation
Hepatitis B	Series of three doses if not previously completed
Hepatitis A	Series of two doses with first at 12 months and second at least 6 months later
Diphtheria, tetanus, acellular pertussis (Dtap)	Dose #4 in five-dose series from 15–18 months Dose #5 at 4–6 years
Haemophilus influenzae type b	Dose #3 in series if using three-dose vaccine
Inactivated poliovirus	Dose #3 given between 6 and 18 months Dose #4 given at 4–6 years
Measles, mumps, rubella	Dose #1 from 12–15 months
Varicella	Dose #1 at 12–18 months Dose #2 at 4–6 years
Pneumococcal	Dose #4 given between 12 and 15 months
Influenza	Annually from 6–23 months

See Chapter 16 ∞ and the American Academy of Pediatrics (AAP) and Centers for Disease Control and Prevention (CDC) websites for further information.

games or watch many hours of inappropriate television when the toddler or preschooler is present? Do parents watch the evening news when young children are present, including violent episodes? Do they discuss television shows with the child?

Ask if the child has had any diseases, whether common ones such as middle ear infection, or less common ones such as a serious respiratory infection. Has the child been diagnosed with a chronic disorder like cystic fibrosis or hemophilia? How has that impacted his or her general health and family functioning?

Desired outcomes for disease prevention include integration of prevention methods into the family's daily life, prompt treatment of acute diseases, and individualization of all health supervision topics for the child with a chronic condition or special health care need.

Injury Prevention Strategies

Injuries remain a common health problem for children during the toddler and preschooler years. Children's mobility, physical skills, and lack of understanding of the presence of hazards put them at particular risk. In addition, children are sometimes left to play alone for short periods and toddlers and preschoolers can quickly get into dangerous situations. Every health care visit needs to include an assessment of risks and teaching to prevent injuries. Tables 8–5 and 8–6 list injury hazards during these age periods.

Ask parents what they think the most common hazards are for the child's age and add other hazards to their awareness. Nearly 65% of child unintentional injury deaths are motor vehicle–related, with young children injured as riders, as pedestrians, or in heat- and cold-related events (Gardner & Committee on Injury, Violence and Poison Prevention, 2007), so car safety always needs reinforcing. Car seats are a key discussion item because the types of seats recommended change as the child matures. Be certain that children from 20–40 pounds:

- Use a convertible forward-facing seat with full harness that has been placed in the back seat.
- Have harness straps at or above the shoulders.

Preschoolers over 40 pounds should be placed in a belt-positioning booster seat. However, booster seats are recommended only after reaching 40 pounds and 4 years of age. The younger child who weighs more than 40 pounds should be placed in a car seat with a harness that is approved for higher heights and weights than usual seats. Once a booster seat is used, be certain that:

- The booster seat is in the back seat.
- It uses both lap and shoulder belts.
- The lap belt is positioned low and tight across the lap/upper thigh area, and the shoulder belt is snug across the chest and shoulder.

(American Academy of Pediatrics, 2009)

Recommend that parents have their car seat checked by a childcare inspector (Figure 8–3 ➤). Give them the addresses of the closest inspection stations, which you can locate by going through the National Highway Traffic Safety Administration. Check your particular state laws regulating car safety seats for children.

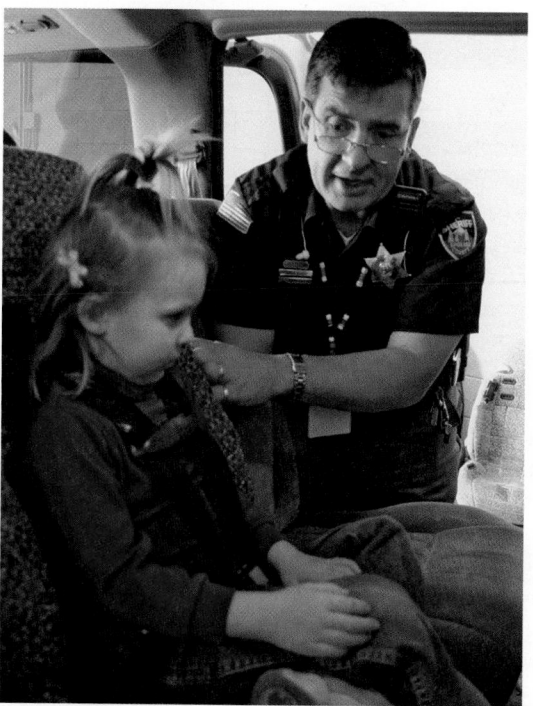

National Highway Traffic Safety Administration Website

FIGURE 8–3 ➤ The officer at this police station is certified to examine car seats for children and make recommendations for parents. He is examining a preschooler in a booster seat for proper fit and alignment. Many car seats are improperly installed or not the proper type for a specific age of child, so centers that check seats provide an important service.

Other common and serious safety hazards are falls and drowning. In addition to providing general guidelines about safety, the nurse should directly address these common injuries. Children often fall down stairs, from counters where they have been placed or have crawled, and from grocery carts. Drowning episodes occur when toddlers and preschoolers are not watched every moment while in the bathtub, near a pool or spa, or at a lake or ocean, or when they fall from boats without personal flotation devices on. All young children should begin to take swim lessons. Although this does not guarantee their safety around water, swim lessons provide a ready forum for teaching safety precautions to parents (Moran & Stanley, 2006). Children play with balls, and may follow them as they roll or are thrown into the street. Nursing interventions concentrate on relaying to parents the severity of the risk of falls, drowning, and other hazards for children. Teach them to be aware of the dangers and to avoid them, both at home and in other settings. Refer them to classes on first aid and cardiopulmonary resuscitation (CPR).

The child spends increasing time away from the parent. Childcare situations should provide the same supervision the child receives at home. Help parents to ask questions and feel confident in safety at other settings. For example, while parents may be cautious about gun safety at home, few of them inquire if a home the child is visiting has guns and how they are stored.

Preschoolers are generally interested in health and their bodies. This is a time when teaching can become directed both to the parents and to their children. Preschoolers are receptive to practicing street crossing and tricycle/bicycle riding skills. It may be helpful to have a place in the clinic or office where they can be

TABLE 8–5	Injury Prevention in Toddlerhood		
	Hazard	Developmental Characteristics	Preventive Measures
	Falls	Gross motor skills improve: The toddler is able to move chairs to counters and can climb up ladders.	Supervise the toddler closely. Provide safe climbing toys. Begin to teach acceptable places for climbing.
	Poisoning	Gross motor skills enable the toddler to climb onto chairs and then cabinets. Medicines, cosmetics, and other poisonous substances are easily reached.	Keep medicines and other poisonous material locked away. Use child-resistant containers and cupboard closures. Post the poison control center number (1-800-222-1222) by the telephone and tape on cell phones.
	Burns	The toddler is tall enough to reach the stove top. He or she can walk to the fireplace and may reach into the fire.	Keep pot handles turned inward on the stove. Do not burn fires without close supervision. Use a fire screen.
	Drowning	The toddler can walk onto docks or pool decks; may stand on or climb seats on boats; and may fall into buckets, toilets, and fish tanks and be unable to get the top of the body out.	Supervise any child near water. Swimming classes do not protect a toddler from drowning. Use child-resistant pool covers. Use approved child life jackets near water and on boats. Empty buckets when not in use.
	Motor vehicle crashes	The toddler may be able to undo a seat belt and may resist using a car seat, demonstrating characteristic negativism and autonomy.	Insist on safety seat use for all trips. Use approved safety seats only, such as a forward-facing convertible seat. The toddler is not large enough to use car seat belts.

TABLE 8–6 Injury Prevention in Preschool Years

	Hazard	Developmental Characteristics	Preventive Measures
	Motor vehicle crashes	The older preschooler independently gets into the car and puts on a seat belt. The child may forget to belt up or may do so incorrectly.	Verify that the child is belted in properly before starting the car. Keep the child in a rear-facing seat until at least 1 year of age and 20 pounds, but preferably longer, until achieving the highest weight or height recommended for the seat by the manufacturer. Forward-facing seats and booster seats are used in the back seat. The child restraint systems must be used until the child weighs at least 18 kg (40 lb) and is 57 in. tall, and can safely use regular car safety belts (generally 8–12 years of age).
	Motor vehicle/pedestrian accidents	The preschooler increasingly plays outside alone or with friends. The preschooler is unable to judge the speed of a moving car and assumes the driver knows he or she is present.	Teach the child never to go into the road. A safe, preferably enclosed, play yard is recommended. The child should be supervised by adults at all times.
	Drowning	A preschooler who has had swimming lessons may choose to go into a lake or pool.	Teach the child never to go into water without an adult. Provide supervision whenever a child is near water.
	Burns	The preschooler can understand the hazards of fire.	Teach the child to stop, drop, and roll if clothes are on fire. Practice escapes from home are useful. A visit to a fire station can reinforce learning. Teach the child how to call 911.
	Needle sticks in hospital	The preschooler can ambulate and is interested in new objects.	Keep needles out of reach. Remove them from the unit immediately after use.
	Electrical injury in hospital	The preschooler is mobile and may trip over cords and equipment or may choose to examine them.	Avoid use of electrical cords if possible. Keep equipment out of major traffic areas. Cover any electrical outlets not being used for equipment. Monitor the child closely.

taught basic skills such as hand hygiene or street crossing. Consider the time of year and geographic location and teach appropriately. Spring is often a good time to teach bicycle and water safety. Winter hazards may include woodstoves or other heating devices. See Table 8–7 for further information about toddler and preschooler hazards and safety teaching needed.

Desired outcomes for the child are integration of safe practices into car restraints and other daily activities, progression through toddlerhood and preschool with no serious injuries, prompt care for minor injuries, and increasing understanding by the child, parent, and other care providers of the common safety hazards at this age.

NURSING MANAGEMENT

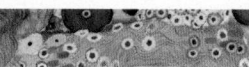

Nursing Assessment and Diagnosis

Nurses collaborate with other health care professionals such as physicians, nurse practitioners, and speech therapists to assess the health promotion and health maintenance status of young children. The toddler and preschool years are characterized by much developmental progression, and strategies need to be constantly adapted to meet the particular needs of the child and family. The parents are partners in the child's care. Every health supervision visit should address their questions and concerns,

TABLE 8–7	Disease and Injury Prevention Topics by Age
Age	Injury Prevention Teaching Topics
15 months	• Perform hand hygiene frequently (adult and toddler). • Clean toys with soap and water regularly. • Provide the child's own bedding for the childcare setting and wash weekly. • Install car safety seats correctly and have installation checked; place the child in the back seat and never in the front seat with a passenger air bag. • Empty containers of water immediately after use; be sure pools or other bodies of water are locked and not accessible. • Use sunscreen, hat, and long sleeves in the sun. • Keep heavy and sharp objects out of reach; check that all poisons are locked away including in homes visited; keep pet food and cosmetics out of reach. • Have the poison control number by phones and programmed into cell phones. • Be alert for dangers of hot curling irons and other appliances. • Have electrical cords out of reach and not hanging down. • Keep water temperature from 120–125°F. • Have the home environment checked for lead, radon, or other potential hazards. • Secure the child in shopping carts. • Do not let the child have access to alcoholic drinks. • Remember that responsible adults (not other children) should always supervise your child. • Know CPR, airway obstruction removal, and other first aid.
18 months	• As previously noted. • Bolt heavy objects that might be pulled down securely to the wall. • Be cautious of the toddler near machinery like lawn mowers or farm equipment in the yard. • Use a helmet on the child when taking him or her on the back of a bicycle. • Check batteries in home smoke alarms, carbon monoxide (CO) detectors, or radon monitors, and check the system monthly; change batteries on a scheduled basis recommended by the manufacturer. • Ask care providers about discipline methods; do not allow corporal punishment.
2–3 years	• As previously noted. • When the child is 40 pounds, switch to a belt-positioning booster seat, using the vehicle lap and shoulder belt; place in the rear seat. • Teach hand hygiene after toileting and other activities. • Clean the potty chair thoroughly. • Keep guns unloaded and locked away in a different locked place than ammunition; install trigger locks. • Teach how to cross streets. • Provide a helmet for riding tricycles. • Check playgrounds for safety hazards and hard surfaces under equipment; ensure a cushioned surface.
3–4 years	• As previously noted. • Do not let the child play unsupervised. • Know CPR, airway obstruction removal, and other first aid for the child who has become a preschooler.
4–5 years	• As previously noted. • Continue teaching safety skills to the child. • Continue supervising when near streets or water sources. • Teach safety around strangers (never go with a stranger; find a trusted person like a parent or police).

Adapted from Hagan, Shaw, & Duncan, 2008.

and they should know their observations of the child are an invaluable part of the care process. As the preschooler becomes more verbal, another partner is added to the health care team. Ask preschoolers what they want to learn, what questions they have about staying well, and other pertinent questions.

Toddlers and preschoolers are examined for growth, physical health status, and mental/social characteristics. Development is an area that many pediatricians feel ill-prepared to discuss but parents commonly want addressed. Additionally, developmental surveillance must occur at every health care visit, with standardized screening at 9, 18, and 24–30 months (Council on Children with Disabilities, 2006; Drotar, Stancin, & Dworkin,

2008). Nurses are adept at describing normal developmental milestones, evaluating children's progression, and using anticipatory guidance to address parental developmental concerns.

Based on a thorough assessment, establish nursing diagnoses that are appropriate for the young child and family. Potential nursing diagnoses established during the health supervision of a toddler or preschooler might include:

• Anxiety related to change of environment (new care provider)
• Parental Role Conflict related to lack of support from significant others

- Risk for Delayed Growth and Development related to lead exposure
- Health-Seeking Behaviors related to parental desire for safety information
- Impaired Skin Integrity related to hyperthermia (sunburn)

Planning and Implementation

Based on the established nursing diagnoses, the nurse, in collaboration with other partners, plans strategies to meet the family's needs. Explain that assessment questions are asked in order to provide a picture of the child that can be helpful in partnering with parents to plan health care. Reinforce the importance of the family coming to health supervision visits with their own list of issues. Work with other health care professionals to be sure all needs of a particular child and family are addressed.

Some teaching takes place as the examination occurs. Explain the height and weight measurements and what they mean. Relate them to questions about dietary intake and family food patterns. During the physical examination, insert information about common infections such as otitis media (middle ear infection) and share immunization information (see Table 8–8 for a list of potential teaching topics).

If the family is reluctant to ask questions, reflect on the child's development: "Many children have trouble sleeping through the night; is that the case for Cassandra? What helps her to sleep? What is it like at her bedtime?" Developmental areas such as sleep, discipline, toilet training, and expected developmental milestones should be addressed. If the parents were provided with a journal to record observations and questions in an earlier visit, ask if they have brought it with them.

TABLE 8–8	Sample Questions and Teaching Topics Pertinent to Early Childhood Visits	
Topic	Questions	Teaching
Sleep	How long does Cassandra sleep at night? Does she take naps? Does Jim ever awaken at night crying? Do you have trouble consoling him? Is your daughter able to concentrate on preschool and stay alert during the hours she is there? What concerns do you have about your son's sleep patterns?	Normal amounts of sleep at various ages Establishment of consistent sleep routines Types of sleep disruptions and their treatment
Discipline	Does Cassandra ever misbehave? When it happens, what does she typically do? How do you respond to her behavior? Have you tried using time-out when she seems out of control? How does the childcare center deal with inappropriate behavior? Do you agree with their techniques?	Consistency and limit setting Appropriate consequences for behaviors Evaluating methods of discipline Adapting methods to individual children
Toilet training	Have you thought about beginning to toilet train your toddler? How do you think you will do it? What signs have you seen that he might be ready soon? You mentioned that Cassandra has occasional accidents. How often are they and are you concerned about them? What rewards do you use when your son is successful in using the toilet? Do you have a small toilet for him to use?	Readiness cues for toilet training Introducing toilet training Positive reinforcement for children Transitions to childcare and other settings away from home
Learning/reading	Describe the things that Jim is learning now. Is he progressing as you would expect or like? How often do you read to Jim? How does he like reading with you? Have you been able to get books to keep for him at home? Do you ever visit the library together? Does your library have a story time for young children?	Providing stimulating environments for learning Importance of reading to children Importance of providing books for children to look at during playtime Pointing out letters to preschool children
Communication	What is Cassandra's language like now? Are you concerned or particularly pleased about any of her ways of communicating? How does she get along with other children in Head Start? What has she been learning about getting along with other children?	Expected language skills Social interaction with adults and other children
Parental	How is your life going right now? Do you or anyone else in your family drink more than two drinks per day, smoke, or take street drugs? How is your general mood? Are you often tired, sad, or depressed? Who helps out when you need something? Are there friends or family close to call upon? What resources that you do not have would be helpful to you (e.g., more food, counseling, other parents)?	Effects of parental substance abuse on children Need for healthy mental status to meet child's developmental needs Referrals to needed community resources to meet basic mental status needs

A key part of the visit involves health promotion activities. It is essential to apply concepts of anticipatory guidance as you address the child's approaching developmental progression. If the child will soon be toilet trained, provide information about possible approaches. If the child is learning to swim or has access to water, reinforce safety precautions near water. For the child going to a new childcare center, provide the parents with a list of questions they can ask the care provider, and tips to assist in the transition to a new setting. Teach about toys that encourage activity, such as balls, music, push toys, and tricycles. Review the diet and provide ideas for healthy meals and snacks. Emphasize the importance of daily play to healthy child development (Ginsburg & Committee on Communications, 2007).

Health maintenance activities are added to the visit as you give immunizations and screen for tuberculosis, lead, or problems with language, vision, or hearing. The focus of these activities is to prevent disease or to find it early before there are serious consequences. Whenever you find information that may indicate a problem, be sure to refer the child to the primary care provider, such as a physician or nurse practitioner. You may even recommend that the child be seen by another specialist such as a speech pathologist or dentist. Other health maintenance activities that must be part of each visit with a toddler or preschooler involve teaching about common hazards and how to avoid them. Emergency care in case of injury is also helpful information for parents, so first aid classes can be recommended.

Conclude the visit with some words of praise about the parent and the child's accomplishments. Provide the date for the next visit. List any resources that are helpful to the family, including the clinic/office contact information and emergency services.

Evaluation

Parents should occasionally be asked to evaluate the care they are receiving at the health promotion and health maintenance site. Use these comments to monitor and adjust procedures as needed. The expected outcomes for nursing care of the toddler and preschooler include:

- The child demonstrates normal patterns of growth and progression in developmental milestones.
- The child remains free of disease and injury.
- Parents relay satisfaction with the pediatric health care home.
- The child manifests positive physical, social, and emotional adjustment.

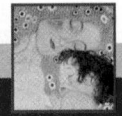

Chapter Highlights

- The toddler and preschool years are critically important times for health supervision of young children.
- Many children have developmental delays, so developmental surveillance is needed at every health care visit.
- The young child establishes eating patterns that generally last throughout childhood and adolescence; assessment and teaching are therefore critical for families.
- All children need to engage in play and obtain at least 60 minutes of physical activity every day.
- A significant number of young children develop early childhood caries, so assessment and intervention for oral care is essential for their health.

- Establishment of healthy mental and emotional patterns is important for the toddler and preschooler. Nurses provide teaching and encouragement about toilet training, discipline, sleep, and other important mental health issues.
- Disease prevention strategies involve immunization and hygiene practices for the young child.
- Injury is a major cause of death and hospitalization for toddlers and preschoolers. The nurse is influential in addressing motor vehicle safety, drowning and fall prevention, poison hazards, and other unintentional injury hazards.

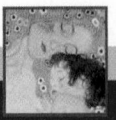

Clinical Reasoning in Action

Recall Dominic, an active 4-year-old who was described in the opening scenario. During today's visit, you learn that his mother, Sophia, is quite tired from working at a retail store about 8–9 hours daily and then caring for Dominic in the evening. The recent move of her mother, Hannah, to a house down the street to assist with care has brought her some relief. Dominic has several decaying deciduous teeth. His mother states that since he will lose them soon, she is not worried.

1. Dominic's father is serving in the military in the Middle East. What suggestions can you make to Sophia so that Dominic continues to learn about and communicate with his father during the deployment?
2. Dominic has not been seen for immunizations since early in the toddler years. List the immunizations you expect he has received and those that are likely needed at this time. Plan the history questions to learn about his immunization history.

3. Since Sophia believes that she does not need to worry about caries in the deciduous teeth, plan a teaching session that addresses the importance of even the primary teeth for good health and development of language skills. Include information about resources that provide dental care for children like Dominic.

4. Hannah has recently joined the family to assist in Dominic's care. List the changes in roles for the various family members and suggest ways that Sophia can now take care of some of her own personal needs for rest and renewal.

See Pearson Nursing Student Resources for possible responses.

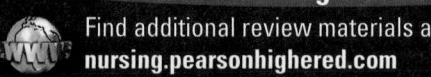

Pearson Nursing Student Resources

Find additional review materials at
nursing.pearsonhighered.com
Prepare for success with NCLEX®-style practice questions, interactive assignments and activities, web links, animations and videos, and more!

References

American Academy of Pediatrics. (2007). *Discipline.* Retrieved from http://www.aap.org

American Academy of Pediatrics. (2009). *Car safety seats: A guide for families 2009.* Retrieved from http://www.aap.org/family/carseatguide.htm

Betz, C. L., Ruccione, K., Meeske, K., Smith, K., & Change, N. (2008). Health literacy: A pediatric nursing concern. *Pediatric Nursing, 34*(3), 231–239.

Centers for Disease Control and Prevention. (2008). *How much physical activity do children need?* Retrieved from http://www.cdc.gov/physicalactivity/

Centers for Disease Control and Prevention. (2009). Quick stats: Percentage of children ages 2–4 years who ever had caries in primary teeth, by race/ethnicity and sex—National Health and Nutrition Examination Survey, United States, 1988–1994 and 1999–2004. *Morbidity and Mortality Weekly Report, 58*(2), 34.

Chamness, J. A. (2008). Taking a pediatric sleep history. *Pediatric Annals, 37*(7), 502–508.

Cherry, D. C., Huggins, B., & Gilmore, K. (2007). Children's health in the rural environment. *Pediatric Clinics of North America, 54,* 121–133.

Council on Children with Disabilities, Section on Developmental Behavioral Pediatrics, Bright Futures Steering Committee and Medical Home Initiatives for Children with Special Needs Project Advisory Committee. (2006). Identifying infants and young children with developmental disorders in the medical home: An algorithm for developmental surveillance and screening. *Pediatrics, 118*(1), 405–420.

Drotar, D., Stancin, T., & Dworkin, P. (2008). *Pediatric developmental screening: Understanding and selecting screening instruments.* Washington, DC: Commonwealth Fund.

Dye, B. A., Tan, S., Smith, V., Lewis, B. G., Barker, L. K., Thornton-Evans, G., et al. (2007). Trends in oral health status: United States, 1988–2004. National Center for Health Statistics. *Vital Health Statistics, 11*(248), 1–10.

Essery, E. V., DiMarco, N. M., Rich, S., & Nichols, D. L. (2008). Mothers of preschoolers report using less pressure in child feeding situations following a newsletter intervention. *Journal of Nutrition Education and Behavior, 40*(2), 110–115.

Gardiner, P., & Riley, D. S. (2007). Herbs to homeopathy—medicinal products for children. *Pediatric Clinics of North America, 54,* 859–874.

Gardner, H. G., & the Committee on Injury, Violence and Poison Prevention. (2007). Office-based counseling for unintentional injury prevention. *Pediatrics, 119,* 202–206.

Ginsburg, K. R., & the Committee on Communications & the Committee on Psychosocial Aspects of Child and Family Health. (2007). *Pediatrics, 119,* 182–191.

Hagan, J. F., Shaw, J. S., & Duncan, P. M. (2008). *Bright futures: Guidelines for health supervision of infants, children, and adolescents.* Elk Grove Village, IL: American Academy of Pediatrics.

Halfon, N., DuPlessis, H., & Inkelas, M. (2007). Transforming the U.S. child health system. *Health Affairs, 26,* 315–330.

Moran, K., & Stanley, T. (2006). Toddler drowning prevention: Teaching parents about water safety in conjunction with their child's in-water lessons. *International Journal of Injury Control and Safety Promotion, 13*(4), 254–256.

Murray, R. B., Zentner, J. P., & Yakimo, R. (2009). *Health promotion strategies through the life span* (8th ed.). Upper Saddle River, NJ: Prentice Hall.

Rosen, L. D., & Breuner, C. C. (2008). Primary care from infancy to adolescence. *Pediatric Clinics of North America, 54*(6), 837–858.

Wagner, J., Jenkins, B., & Smith, J. C. (2006). Nurses' utilization of parent questionnaires for developmental screening. *Pediatric Nursing, 32*(5), 409–412.

Wagner, R., & Oskouian, R. (2008). Are you missing the diagnosis of the most common chronic disease of childhood? *Contemporary Pediatrics, 25*(9), 60–79.

Health Promotion and Maintenance for the School-Age Child and Adolescent

chapter 9

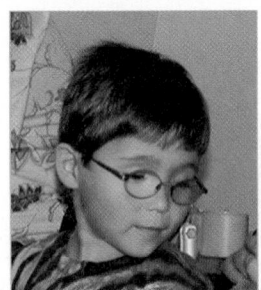

Ty is a 12-year-old boy with osteogenesis imperfecta or "brittle bone disease." The disease was diagnosed at 1 year of age when Ty experienced a severe leg fracture while learning to walk although he had his first arm fracture during infancy. Ty's parents encouraged his development and tried to protect him from risks that might lead to fractures. He had about two fractures annually during early childhood, requiring surgery several times. In spite of this, Ty showed steady gains in development. He was home schooled for several years, but about 2 years ago his family placed him in a local public school. The school and home health nurse coordinated care to provide Ty with an individualized education plan. He has excelled at school, becoming a leader among peers and an honors student. He is a class officer and performs in school plays. Ty recently had surgery to insert rods to strengthen long bones in his legs and is using a wheelchair during the healing process. His parents believe that Ty's early health care assisted him in successful disease management so that he could continue to develop his social skills. Ty regularly visits his pediatric health care home for assessment of growth, monitoring for fractures, and implementation of usual care regarding nutrition, oral health, and injury prevention. Physical activities are suggested that allow for safe exercise, so Ty joined a wheelchair basketball team and swims weekly.

Key Terms

Learning Outcomes

After reading this chapter, you will be able to do the following:

1. State components of growth and developmental surveillance needs for school-age children.
2. Describe the nutrition, physical activity, and oral health needs of school-age children.
3. Integrate pertinent mental health care into health supervision visits for school-age children.
4. Synthesize data about the family and other social relationships to promote and maintain health of school-age children.
5. Plan assessment and interventions appropriate for health promotion and maintenance during health supervision visits of school-age children.
6. Identify the major health concerns of the adolescent years.
7. Apply communication skills to interactions with adolescents and their families.
8. Apply assessment skills to plan data-gathering methods for nutrition, physical activity, and the mental health status of youth.
9. Intervene with adolescents by integrating activities to promote health and to prevent disease and injury.

Mental and Spiritual Health

The school-age years are marked by the emergence of new cognitive skills, the ability to interact cooperatively with others, and the development of self-esteem. **Self-esteem** reflects feelings of self-worth or value. **Self-concept** refers to evaluations of the self in certain specific areas, such as those related to academic achievement, athletic ability, physical appearance, and social interactions (Santrock, 2007). A child with a positive self-concept feels competent, is able to meet challenges, and applies lessons from successes and failures. Specific facets of self-concept include **body image**, the idea that one forms about one's body, and **sexuality**, the person's view of self as a sexual being. Together, self-concept and self-esteem include all of the cognitive, spiritual, sexual, and physical aspects of the individual. The child who believes in his or her ability to face good times and bad has a lowered chance of mental illness such as depression, eating disorder, and anxiety.

Many of the areas discussed already in this chapter provide clues to the child's self-concept. Are there sports or other physical activities? They may reflect a positive self-concept and body image. However, if the child is forced to do these sports by parents and feels inadequate in their performance, they may promote a negative self-concept and body image. Ask both about the child's activities and how he or she feels about them. Inquire about school performance and best friends. Is there an increasing independence and responsibility for self? Success in achieving developmental milestones leads to a positive sense of self-esteem in the child. A low sense of self-esteem is noted when the child states a disinterest in exercise, school clubs, and family activities. This can lead to loneliness, depression, and mental health problems such as eating disorders. When these feelings are noted during a health supervision visit, the nurse should recommend that the child see a counselor at school or another setting, and should recommend that parents be included in the sessions so they can best help the child.

Parents play an important part in fostering the child's self-esteem. The nurse can ask them to evaluate the child and provide suggestions about positive actions. This includes building upon and encouraging the child's abilities, allowing an increasing amount of responsibility, and asking the child about his or her own goals.

The family plays a critical part in the child's developing self-esteem and mental health. In order to understand the child, it is necessary to ask questions about and explore dynamics in the family. Several protective factors have been identified for families:

- Communication is open and clear.
- Parents use a variety of problem-solving skills.
- Members are encouraged, are appreciated, and feel understood.
- Rules and expectations are consistent and fair.
- The family is committed to each other, including spending time together.
- Religious or spiritual orientation is present.
- Social connectedness, extended family, and other support is available.
- Resilience or the ability to adapt to new situations is present (Cole, Clark, & Gable, 2007).

Ask about and observe the family's relationships when you are with them. Evaluate the effect of family interactions on children. Model respectful interchanges by listening carefully to children, as well as parents. Gently recognize children if parents answer for them or seem to put them down. Provide brochures and examples of ways to show children their importance. Encourage both parents to come to child health care visits and support the involvement of both parents in childrearing. Ask about family stressors such as job changes, financial concerns, illness, substance abuse, and domestic violence. About half of all marriages end in divorce, so be prepared to offer suggestions to deal with this situation (see Chapter 2 ∞ for a discussion of effects of divorce on children). Ask about and identify risk factors and protective factors. The child's strengths are used to assist the family functioning and will, in turn, give the child a sense of accomplishment. Some examples include:

- A child who is able to act independently can be given responsibility for parts of the home or family function, such as planning dinner two nights a week.
- A creative child can be given the task of planning books and other activities for a younger sibling.
- A child with a talent for design can be asked to set the table for dinner guests.

The school-age child is developing a sense of body image and sexuality. Look at the child's appearance and dress. Some children may have poor posture, display a sense of insecurity, and seem uncomfortable with themselves. Others may dress as if they were much older, seem sophisticated, and are clearly assuming the role identification with their gender group. Ask the parents in a private setting what observations they have about the child's body image and sexuality. Inquire about friends with whom the child seems romantically or sexually interested, and whether the parent has concerns. Questions related to sexuality will emerge during the school years. They should be answered truthfully and fully. Even children who do not ask questions usually need sex education. They may get information in school beginning in about fourth grade, but often still have misconceptions about the bodies of men and women, sexual intercourse, how babies are born, and other topics. Suggest that parents read books with their children that deal with these issues at a level the children understand. If books are available at home, children will be likely to look at them and ask questions. These books should be in the home from third grade on because many young girls may have body changes as early as 9 or 10 years of age (see Chapter 5 ∞). This can put both parent and child at ease and lead to discussion. Parents should be advised to talk with teachers to learn what is presented in school and supplement and clarify this information. Nurses often perform sexuality education in schools or work with school districts in establishing policies regarding sexuality education plans.

Suggest to parents that the Internet and other media provide information that can confuse children. Encourage them to watch movies with their children, have frank discussions related to sexuality observed, and answer questions truthfully. Children generally learn about topics such as sexual intercourse, homosexuality, and childbirth from school discussions and the media. It is better to learn from parents than from friends or the

Teen Mental and Spiritual Health Video

media. A few moments alone with parents and with children at health care visits may help to identify the concerns of each related to sexuality.

By about fourth to sixth grade, most girls have started to have prepubertal body changes and may have begun to menstruate. This provides another opening to discuss mature bodies of men and women and the transformation from childhood to greater maturity. Boys mature about 2 years later than girls. Without an event such as menstruation, parents may be less likely to start discussions with male children. Suggest that parents consciously begin conversations with boys periodically to explain changes they see in themselves and their peers. See Chapter 5 ∞ for further discussion of body changes related to puberty.

School-age children continue to develop their abilities to self-regulate activities and responses to situations. At this age, the abilities to solve problems and assume more responsibility for self are important. Encourage parents to discuss issues with the child and to seek solutions together when appropriate. The child assumes more responsibility for assisting with meal preparation and home chores, coming home alone after school, and caring for younger siblings. Encourage the parents to praise the child for assuming more family responsibilities and recognize that the child will need some guidance when taking on new tasks.

Sleep is still important for children in order to have the energy to perform well in school and other activities. They generally take charge of bedtime routines with reminders about the time to go to sleep, and they sleep through the night. Sleep time varies from 9 to 12 hours, depending on the child and his or her activity level. Busy schedules may interrupt this pattern, leading to irritability, lack of concentration, or even hyperactive behavior. Help children and families plan for healthy practices of **sleep hygiene**, or behaviors that foster a regular and sufficient sleep pattern, as well as daytime alertness (Edelman & Mandle, 2006). See Families Want to Know: Sleep Hygiene.

Families Want to Know
Sleep Hygiene

Nurses should inquire about the sleep patterns and amount of sleep that children receive. Ask if they are frequently tired or have trouble sleeping. Some simple behaviors help to promote sleep and are referred to as sleep hygiene:

- Go to bed and get up at approximately the same time each day, including weekends.
- Follow a bedtime routine to prepare for sleep.
- Recognize that we do not "make up" sleep that is "lost" by sleeping in.
- Avoid caffeine, including tea, coffee, and carbonated beverages, for several hours before sleep.
- Gradually slow down activity about an hour or two before bedtime.
- Do not watch television, play games, text on the phone, or conduct other activities in the sleep location.
- Avoid naps in the late afternoon or evening.
- Darken the room for sleep.

(Mayo Clinic, 2009; Mindell, Meltzer, Carskadon, et al., 2009)

Sleepwalking and sleep talking sometimes occur at this age, but usually decrease as the child nears adolescence. Children who have stress at home, such as parental fighting, ill family members, or inadequate food or shelter, may not get enough sleep and fall asleep at school. Ask the child if falling asleep in class is occurring, and seek additional information about family stressors. This can lead you to interventions such as recommending family counseling or referring to resources to obtain better housing or more stable food sources.

School is a major microsystem influence in the lives of children, and plays a role in self-concept and mental health formation. The child is usually ready for kindergarten when communication and cognitive skills are sufficient to support learning, the child can successfully separate from parents, experiences with other children show ability to make friends and regulate own behavior, and the child can follow rules and directions (Hagan et al., 2008). Help parents to learn the ways they can facilitate a healthy transition to school, such as ensuring good sleep and eating routines, reading with the child, showing interest in school activities, and finding a space in the home for the child's school-related work (American Academy of Pediatrics, 2007b).

Ask the child to describe a best friend; if unable to do so, isolation may be occurring. Inquire about what the three best and three worst things are about school. A child with a low self-concept often has trouble talking about and evaluating school. Find out where the child attends school, if the area is generally safe, and how the child gets to school. Encourage the parents to meet the child's teachers, to become active in school activities, and to be available to solve problems with school personnel when needed. Partner with the parents and child when interventions are needed. An office nurse may contact a school nurse when the child needs support in the school environment. This may occur if the child has become ill and missed school, has family stressors, does not get along well with a teacher, or has a condition such as attention deficit disorder. Identify the risk and protective factors in the school environment and plan interventions to support the child when risks are present. Consider the risks and strengths of children with special health care needs, such as Ty who is described in the opening scenario (Figure 9–4 ➤).

Clinical Judgment

Ty has osteogenesis imperfecta, so his bones can fracture easily. Should he be allowed to play at recess with his classmates? What are the pros and cons of playing with other children his age? He is entering the teenage years. What implications will this have for his dietary and activity needs?

Certain mental health disorders are commonly seen during the school years. One example is anxiety problems that result in worries, fears, physical symptoms, stress, and sleep disorders without significantly impairing daily functioning. However, anxiety disorders affect functioning and have more striking characteristics such as clinging, abdominal pain and headache, and refusal to attend school. Posttraumatic stress syndrome and depression may also be seen. (See Chapter 28 ∞ for further description of these disorders.) Anxiety disorder, posttraumatic stress, and depression should be referred to a mental health spe-

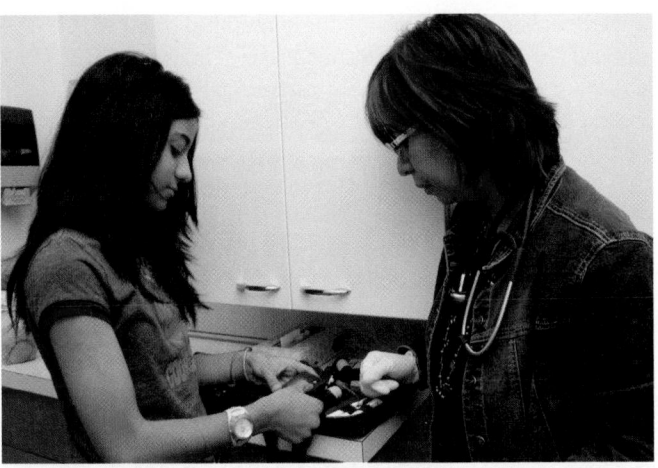

FIGURE 9–4 ➤ A student with diabetes is showing the school nurse how she programs her insulin pump. The nurse has partnered with nurses in the endocrinology office to learn about the type of pump the student is using. Such collaboration contributes to the monitoring and management of diabetes.

cialist for treatment. However, all children worry at times and this type of anxiety can be helped by learning coping skills and relaxation techniques.

Spiritual health is the ability to develop a spiritual nature, including awareness of a life purpose or meaning, a sustaining power during times of stress, a feeling of harmony with the universe, and a sense of fulfillment (Pender, Murdaugh, & Parsons, 2006; Murray, Zentner, & Yakimo, 2009). School age is a time when children learn more about the people and the world around them, and begin to find their place in that world. Connection with faith-based groups assists some children and families in defining the purpose of life, while others may do so through social activity or a strong moral sense of responsibility. Ask children what brings happiness, how they help other people, or if they are members of a church, synagogue, or mosque. If families seem to have little purpose, parents are withdrawn or depressed, or the child has difficulty answering questions about meaningful activities, suggest methods of engagement in the community. These might include providing contacts at local religious events, posting flyers about community events designed to bring unity to various cultural groups, or suggesting services needing volunteers in the community. Families who spend time together and find meaning in supporting each other nurture the spiritual health of their members. Suggest that every family plan a "family night" weekly when they play games, talk, eat, or engage in other activities together.

The nurse has an important role in fostering the mental and spiritual health of school-age children. Health promotion fosters strengths of families and children, leading to healthy self-concept and positive self-esteem. Health maintenance seeks to prevent mental health disruptions. Be alert for risk factors in families because they represent the need for intervention. Expected outcomes for health promotion and health maintenance activities with school-age children include formation of a positive sense of self-esteem and healthy body image, use of coping skills to deal with stress, sleep patterns that meet needs for rest, and a growing purpose and meaning in life.

Relationships

While the school-age child is gradually moving away from the family as the center of life, the family remains an important anchor. The previous section presented several areas in which the parents foster development. Ask also about siblings, grandparents, and other extended family members. Sometimes these persons assist in the child's formation of a self-concept. Peers are increasingly important to the school-age child's self-identity. School age is a time of cooperative engagement with others. All children need to learn how to make and maintain friendships and work with others on projects and in recreation.

Inquire about the child's best friends at school and in private, and ask parents if they are comfortable with the child's selection of friends. Find out if the parents facilitate friendships by allowing other children to come to the home and providing transportation as needed. When the child experiences a risk factor such as a move to a new town or school, role-play how to meet new children and how to make friends. If the child feels like an outcast or outsider among peers at school, explore how the family can create a safe and secure place for the child in extracurricular activities with children who have similar interests. When the child is home schooled, the family may need to plan social events and contacts after usual school hours.

Since peers are important to the school-age child, pressure begins to fit in, to appear like others, and to do what others encourage. Although such pressures are often associated with teen years, they usually begin earlier, at least by 8 or 9 years of age. Ask children what activities friends try to get them to do that they know they should not do, or if friends have tried to get them to smoke. Middle school years are the most common age for beginning to smoke, so always ask children if they have tried smoking, being careful to do this when parents are not present and the children are more likely to be honest. They may tell you about activities when parents are not in the room, such as playing with guns, drinking alcohol or other substances, or other risky behavior. It is best to ask what children do in these situations, what they want to do, and who they can turn to in order to talk about these events. Offer information about the risks connected with behaviors that are described, and suggest people such as parents, teachers, counselors, or clergy who are possible resources. If children's health is at risk, be sure to report the activity to the physician or other health care provider so it can be pursued and the children's safety can be ensured. Activities such as playing with firearms or visiting a friend whose parents are making methamphetamine, for example, place children in extreme danger.

Parents often need guidance to help them in setting limits for their school-age children. The child is becoming more independent but unacceptable behaviors must still be managed by successful discipline techniques. Some guidelines that can help families include talking calmly while expressing clearly behaviors that are unacceptable, using techniques such as natural consequences or withholding privileges, and modeling and suggesting stress relief such as physical activity (American Academy of Pediatrics, 2007a; Barkin, Scheindlin, Ip, et al., 2007).

School age is often a time when children first experience violence in relationships with others. Some children are bullied, while others are the bullies. Anger and aggression can occur, and children get in fights with each other. Ask children to describe when they last had a disagreement with someone and how the problem was solved. Suggest people like school nurses, teachers, and counselors who can help, and be sure that children feel safe in schools, neighborhoods, and homes. Ask parents how they resolve arguments between children at home and what help they need to help children learn problem-solving skills. Find out what policies the schools have in your community to assist in decreasing harassment of and by children. As you progress in your career, become active on school committees that help children learn how to solve problems peacefully and respond to episodes of violence. See Chapter 17 ∞ for further discussion of violence in children and a detailed discussion of bullying.

The child's temperament still plays a part in response to situations and the ability to self-regulate. (Refer to Chapter 4 ∞ for a detailed discussion of temperament in children.) The "difficult" child may have trouble getting to sleep or being quiet in the classroom. Have parents plan more physical activity for this child, teach the child that bedtime routines are helpful, and note that sitting near the front of the class can help with concentration. The "slow to warm up" child may need ideas about what to say when meeting new people. Parents can help this child prepare for a new school by visiting with the child, talking about it, and meeting with the teacher so that a warm welcome can occur. The "easy" child is usually adaptable in most situations and is regularly in activities. However, these children may object when other children interrupt them in conversation, fail to take turns, or otherwise "break the rules" of behavior. They might need help to understand differences in temperament in order to be more tolerant of classmates and their behaviors. Often nurses in schools address the issue of individual differences by speaking with classes or small groups of children.

Once again, the nurse takes an active role in promoting the child's health by anticipating developmental issues and preparing parents and children to deal with them. Health maintenance outcomes include preventing problems in interactions.

Disease Prevention Strategies

School-age children are generally healthy. The immune system is mature (see Chapter 22 ∞), personal hygiene practices are more mature than at earlier ages, and immunizations are usually complete. Engage school-age children in active pursuit of their own health. Teach strategies that can enhance disease prevention. Nurses in offices and schools can teach children how to effectively wash hands, how respiratory infections are transmitted, what can cause gastrointestinal illness, and how to best manage their own health problems. Ask children in your settings what topics are of most interest to them and be prepared to suggest common areas of concern such as safety, skin care, athletics, and illnesses. Children are interested in their bodies and can understand the connection between eating well and avoiding illness, maintaining normal weight and preventing type 2 diabetes, avoiding smoking to prevent cancer and other respiratory diseases, maintaining oral hygiene to promote oral health, and exercising to prevent hypertension.

School-age children are in the concrete stage of intellectual development (see Chapter 4 ∞). This means that teaching is most

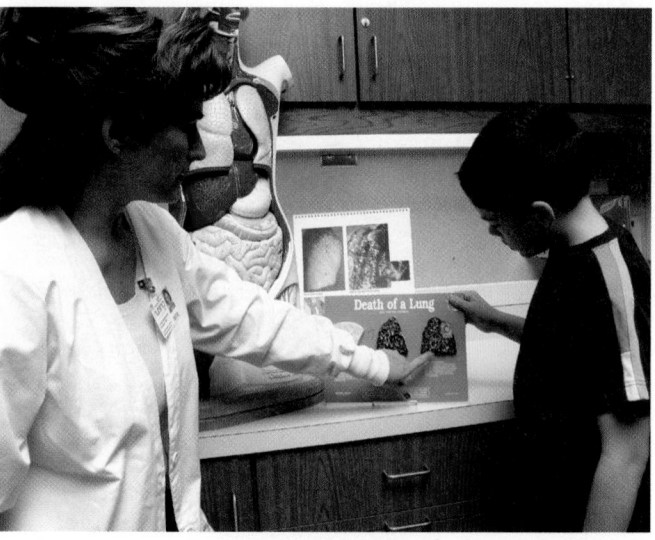

FIGURE 9–5 ➤ This boy is learning about the effects of smoking on the body through the concrete experience of examining a model of the lungs. Why does this type of hands-on technique help school-age children to learn concepts?

effective when opportunities are provided to touch, feel, and otherwise become actively engaged in learning. When teaching about smoking, provide models of lungs and have the students breathe through a straw to demonstrate the effects of airway narrowing. These concrete activities will teach them concepts more effectively than simple lecture or reading (Figure 9–5 ➤). Concepts of health promotion tend to be abstract since they deal with supporting one's highest potential for wellness. Thus, it becomes even more important to provide concrete methods of learning.

Immunizations are generally up to date for school-age children. However, some children may have missed earlier doses due to illness or missed health care visits. Evaluate the immunization record to be sure it meets all recommendations. Some of the most common immunization needs at this time are:

- Hepatitis B (whole series or a missed third dose)
- Hepatitis A (two doses if not previously administered)
- Polio and measles-mumps-rubella (if booster doses of each were not given prior to school entry)
- Tetanus-diphtheria-acellular pertussis (Tdap) at the 11–12 year visit
- Varicella if not given earlier and the child has not had the disease
- Meningococcal vaccine (MCV4) at the 11–12 year visit
- Influenza vaccine
- Certain vaccines for children at high risk, such as pneumococcal (see Chapter 16 ∞ for further information on immunizations)

Screening for health risks should occur during the visit. These include hearing and vision screening, blood pressure monitoring, hematocrit for anemia screening, urinalysis, tuberculin skin test, and in some cases screening for hyperlipidemia and lead exposure. Unusual complaints may indicate a need for further testing; examples include:

- Pain other than brief discomfort after an injury
- Headaches

- Bruising
- Lack of coordination
- Repeated infections
- Decreasing vision or hearing
- Problems or changes in school performance or behavior

Children who have an identified health problem or developmental disability may have additional needs for screening and for interventions to assist with health maintenance. For example, the child with cystic fibrosis will need information to lessen the risk of respiratory infection, and the child with diabetes may need additional blood studies. The child who has difficulty reading will need alternative approaches to teaching correct hand hygiene; demonstration with explanation may be the best approach. A family history of some diseases increases the child's risk and necessitates testing. For example, if a parent has had early cardiovascular disease (before age 55 years), a lipid profile should be performed on the child.

Inquire about any medications the child takes, including vitamins, fluoride, and nonprescription medications. Some families use complementary therapy for common conditions such as respiratory infections or gastrointestinal complaints. Complementary therapy is quite common in families where children have chronic conditions such as attention deficit hyperactivity disorder, autism, and skin conditions (Rosen & Breuner, 2007; Gardiner & Riley, 2007).

Parents should receive explanations about the screening tests performed and the results obtained. Inform them about vision and hearing results. Send home or call regarding results of blood tests when available. Be sure they understand the findings and have resources to assist in preventing or treating the specific disease in their child. Have them call with questions about health problems the child develops, and provide information about lowering the risks of diseases. Be sure that families know when to keep the child home from school (elevated temperature, active vomiting or diarrhea, coughing up brown or green mucus). Assist schools in setting guidelines for management of infectious diseases in that setting. Contact your local county and state health department for infectious disease guidelines for schools. Desired outcomes for the school-age child include prevention of infectious diseases, prompt treatment for acute infections, and careful management of existing health conditions in order to maximize health potential.

Injury Prevention Strategies

Injuries are a common cause of morbidity and mortality among school-age children, and each health maintenance encounter should include injury prevention strategies. Children have more independence and may be harmed by activities they engage in without adults, such as playing with fire or firearms. They participate in many sports and other physical activities and may suffer related injuries. Some children unfortunately suffer harm due to physical abuse or other forms of violence (see Chapter 17 ∞).

Many common injuries are preventable with the simple use of protective gear and the following safety guidelines. Over 11% of youth rarely or never wear seat belts in automobiles (CDC, 2008b). Certain groups of children are more at risk than others of not taking protective measures. Many children ride bicycles, but only a fraction of them use helmets. Strategies to make helmet use more attractive and to ensure correct wearing of helmets are needed (see Evidence-Based Practice: Bicycle Helmet Effectiveness and Use).

Identify youth engaging in risky activities and teach them safe practices. Join with schools and community groups to establish education programs. Provide information about adequate conditioning for sports in order to decrease the chance of overuse injury. Provide a variety of options for physical activity in order to maximize the opportunity for children's participation (Committee on Sports Medicine and Fitness and Council on School Health, American Academy of Pediatrics, 2006). Each visit should contain basic history questions related to injury prevention, and then pursue topics that appear to indicate problems. Once you have collected information during the visit, plan two or three health maintenance topics that seem most important for injury prevention in this family. When you have identified a history of injury in the child, collaborate with the family to plan ways to avoid repeated harm. See Table 9–2 for some common injury hazards during the school years. See Table 9–3 for injury prevention teaching.

Evidence-Based Practice
Bicycle Helmet Effectiveness and Use

Problem
About 900 children annually die of bicycle-related injuries in the United States. Although helmets can reduce injury, many times they are not worn correctly.

Evidence
A review of 22 studies on helmet use among children provides insight into which strategies are most likely to encourage use of this important safety equipment. Community-based information appeared to be the most effective method for delivery of messages, while information provided in schools was found to be slightly less successful. Provision of free helmets was also a positive factor in helmet use, and was more effective than partially subsidized helmets (Royal, Kendrick, & Coleman, 2007).

Implications
Nurses should not assume that reports of safety precautions such as wearing helmets or seat belts mean that children use these measures correctly. Ask for demonstrations and provide suggestions to improve technique as needed. Common injury causes such as car and bicycle crashes necessitate including at least these evaluations as part of health maintenance activities.

Critical Thinking Application
What are the reasons that children might not wear protective gear during sports? Are there laws in your community about wearing helmets for biking? Are helmets made available for families that might not be able to afford their purchase? How do you determine if a child is wearing a helmet correctly? Plan educational materials and programs for children who bicycle.

TABLE 9–2 **Injury Hazards of the School-Age Child**

	Hazard	Developmental Characteristics	Preventive Measures
	Motor vehicle/pedestrian/biking crashes	The child plays outside; may follow a ball into the road; rides a two-wheeler.	Teach the child safe outside play, especially near streets. Reinforce use of bike helmets and car seat belts. Teach biking safety rules and provide safe places for riding.
	Firearms	The child may have been shown the location of guns; is interested in showing them to friends.	Teach the child never to touch guns without a parent present. Guns should be kept unloaded and locked away. Guns and ammunition should be stored in different locations. Be sure guns have trigger locks.
	Burns	The child may perform experiments with flames or toxic substances.	Teach the child what to do in case of fire or if toxic substances touch the skin or eyes. Reinforce teaching about 911.
	Assault	The child may be left alone after school and may walk, bike, or take public transportation alone.	Provide telephone numbers of people to contact in case of an emergency or if the child feels lonely. Leave the child alone for brief periods initially, and evaluate the child's success in managing time. Teach the child not to accept rides from or talk to or open doors to strangers. Teach the child how to answer the phone safely. Consider a cell phone and have the child only speak on it with parents.

TABLE 9–3	Injury Prevention Topics by Age
Age	Injury Prevention Teaching
5–8 years	• Use a booster seat, properly positioned in the back seat of the car; use lap and shoulder belts. • Never place the child in a front car seat with a passenger air bag. • Be sure the child knows how to swim and works on these skills regularly. • Teach safety precautions for bicycling and other activities, including protective gear. • Protect the child with sunscreen when outside. • Check smoke alarms and keep them in proper function. • Have an escape plan in case of fire in the home. • Keep poisons, electrical appliances, and fire starters locked. • Keep firearms unloaded and locked; store ammunition in a separate locked location; have trigger locks installed on guns; keep dangerous knives locked. • Provide protective gear for bicycling and other activities and insist that it be worn. • Teach safety with strangers. • Provide a list of people a child can approach if feeling threatened by touch or other experience. • Choose care providers carefully; occasionally pick up the child earlier than expected; ask policies about discipline and do not leave the child with someone who uses corporal punishment. • Be sure the child knows emergency numbers, names, and plans. • Review carefully any hazardous event that has occurred with the child and summarize what was done correctly and how the response could be improved. • Limit screen time to 2 hours daily; do not allow violent games or viewing. • Review behavior with strangers regularly such as not getting in cars and not engaging in phone or Internet conversations.
8–10 years	• Use a car booster seat until the child sits upright against the back seat with bent knees over the edge of the seat; insist on use of lap and shoulder belts. • Do not place the child in the front seat of a car with a passenger air bag. • Do not allow the child to operate power tools or machinery. • Continue to reinforce other teaching as previously described, include the child more fully, and enlarge responsibility to the child with increasing age.
10–12 years	• Continue to reinforce teaching as previously described. • The parents and child should attend a class on cardiopulmonary resuscitation (CPR) and airway obstruction removal. • Avoid high noise levels such as when listening to music through earphones.

Adapted from Hagan et al., 2008.

Children who come home to an empty house after school are called **latchkey children**. The age at which children are ready for this responsibility varies. Parents need help to decide when the child can come home and stay alone and then plan for safety precautions for them. If children have spent increasing periods of short times alone, have displayed good judgment, and have several activities and interests that can be pursued alone, and if someone is always directly accessible, then children may be ready to spend 1 or more hours alone after school. Parents should be sure that children have a backup key or entry to the house, review the schedule for time alone, remove hazards such as firearms, review procedures for emergencies, and arrange for someone that the children can call if lonely.

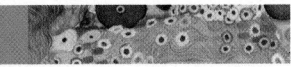

NURSING MANAGEMENT

Nursing Assessment and Diagnosis

Assessment of health promotion and health maintenance topics occurs in many settings with school-age children. They may be seen in offices or clinics, settings designed to provide such care. They may come for episodic care for a fracture or infection when health promotion and health maintenance can be easily integrated. They may be seen in the home or neighborhood center, and are frequently encountered by nurses in schools. Opportunities for assessment and intervention should be used whenever they occur. The individual child is examined, and the family, friends, school, and community are addressed. In addition, these visits provide an opportunity to identify issues early and intervene for health-related problems, including common problems that emerge or become apparent in school age. Inquire

Culture   *Use of Car Seat Belts*

There are marked differences in behaviors that influence unintentional injuries. While about 11% of children rarely or never wear a seat belt in the car, males are most at risk; almost 15% of Black males, over 14% of Hispanic males, and 13% of White males do not use seat belts (CDC, 2008b). How will you inquire about seat belt use in an open-ended manner during health promotion visits? Consider asking these questions: Where do you ride in the car? Who do you usually ride with? Are there seat belts? How often do you use them? Plan strategies to use for all children and families, especially those at high risk of not using seat belts.

about any medications the child uses and perform teaching about these as needed. Use of complementary therapy is common, involving about 33% of families. Inquire about these methods of dealing with health in the home. Common techniques involve massage, vitamins, and botanical products.

Assessment can be considered on two levels with school-age children. Individual children may be assessed for height and weight, for immunization status, and for use of protective gear during sports. Populations of children may also be assessed since school age is the first time that large numbers of children are together in certain settings. The findings from such assessments will become the basis of an **individualized approach** or a **population-based approach** to health promotion and health maintenance. For example, nurses commonly measure height and weight, and calculate BMI for *individual* children seen in a clinic. The results are shared with the family, and appropriate teaching about weight control and nutritious intake can be addressed. In other settings, nurses may measure a *classroom* of children and use the collective data to plan appropriate interventions. If 40% of children in a school are classified as overweight by BMI percentile, much emphasis should be placed on teaching about dietary intake, physical activity, and the relationship of recommended weight levels to chronic disease risk. However, if only a small number of children are overweight, interventions may not be as extensive about this topic.

Nurses perform growth assessment in school-age children, look for achievement of developmental tasks, and assess physical and mental health and social characteristics. Based on the assessment of individuals or populations of children, nursing diagnoses for children and families are established. Possible nursing diagnoses include:

- Delayed Growth and Development related to abuse
- Impaired Parenting related to lack of knowledge about child health maintenance
- Sleep Deprivation related to sleep terrors
- Risk for Violence Directed at Others related to history of witnessing family violence
- Risk for Loneliness related to long periods alone after school
- Health Seeking Behaviors related to locating swimming classes

Planning and Implementation

The nurse is instrumental in planning interventions to promote and maintain health in school-age children. These interventions may take place in offices, homes, or clinics with an individual child, or in schools and other community settings with groups of children.

When working with individuals, summarize the strengths and needs that you have identified during the visit, and ask children and family members if they concur. Plan together with them to provide the needed information for topics you all have developed. Be sure to emphasize those areas where the family excels. For example, positively reinforce use of car seat belts (see Families Want to Know: Car Safety for the School-Age Child), use of protective sports gear, and being current with immunizations. Summarize the next expected developmental tasks, such as increasing independence and growing self-responsibility for choosing snacks and

Families Want to Know
Car Safety for the School-Age Child

Recommendations include:

- For children over 40 pounds (generally 4–8 years of age), use a belt-positioning, forward-facing booster seat located in the back seat. Always use both lap and shoulder belts. Make sure the lap belt fits low and tight across the lap/upper thigh area and the shoulder belt is snug across the chest and shoulder to avoid abdominal injuries.
- Children 4 feet, 9 inches and taller can sit in a regular car seat restrained with a snug lap and shoulder belt that are correctly located across the lap and chest. Children 12 years and younger must ride in the back seat and the back seat is preferred for all children.

television shows. Then provide anticipatory guidance to assist with the child's growing independence. As peers are becoming more important, always focus some discussion on maintaining healthy social relationships through school peers, religious or community events, and sibling contacts. A combination of discussion and reading material or pertinent websites for later exploration are welcomed by most families. Provide telephone numbers of resources for questions and community contacts. Tell the parents when the next health promotion/maintenance visit is recommended. If you come in contact with school-age children for episodic care, ask when the last health maintenance visit occurred. If a child is seen for health care after a bicycling accident, the family may be receptive to teaching about safety precautions. When exposed to injuries to the skin, a review of the last tetanus booster may reveal health maintenance needs. Use every opportunity to work with individual children and insert appropriate health promotion/health maintenance topics.

When you are working with groups of children, health promotion focuses on known needs, interests, and risk areas. Nurses in school settings have used a variety of creative approaches to promote the health of youth. Nurses in schools can set up a program to train students in health topics; these students then become peer coaches or health advocates in working with other students. Another activity is evaluating the components of school health programs and making recommendations for additions as needed. Bulletin boards, community newspapers, television, and community group membership may all be as effective as teaching in school classrooms. Stress-reduction teaching should be provided on group and individual levels. Nurses can teach or assist in development of progressive relaxation, deep breathing, biofeedback, yoga, or meditation, and can help families to find relaxing activities rather than overscheduling children in multiple activities. Interventions will be most effective if they begin with an understanding of the population served.

Evaluation

Seek evaluation from parents during visits for care. Were their questions answered? Do they know where to turn for advice? Do they know when the child should be seen again for health promotion/maintenance?

The expected outcomes for nursing care of individual school-age children include:

- The child demonstrates normal patterns of growth and development.
- The child, family, and community provide a supportive and nurturing environment for the child.
- The child shows growing independence in directing his or her own health promotion activities.

Expected outcomes of nursing care for groups of children include:

- The children identify lifestyle decisions that influence their health status.
- The school and community offer resources that help to lessen risk factors related to health, and factors of disease/injury prevention.

■ HEALTH PROMOTION AND MAINTENANCE FOR THE ADOLESCENT

The line between school age and adolescence is flexible. Some 11-year-olds may have grown physically and experienced puberty; for others these changes may not occur until they are about 13 years. Likewise, cognitive and emotional maturity vary. The nurse must assess each child individually for their characteristics and related health care needs. Adolescents are often seen only sporadically for health care, even though annual visits are recommended. They are usually healthy, may not need immunizations, and consequently do not often come for health care. If adolescents seek care for a minor illness, birth control, or a sports examination, the visit should be viewed as a health supervision opportunity. Although the nurse may not perform all components of the usual visit, at least the most important parts are inserted into care. If time is limited, the nurse has to decide which topics to address during a health care visit. It is advisable to start with the topic of most interest to the teen and then add some injury prevention teaching, since injury is the greatest risk to teens.

Lifestyle behaviors are responsible for most of the preventable diseases in adults, and they typically have their origin in the adolescent years. The behaviors include sedentary lifestyle, unhealthy diet, tobacco use, alcohol use, and mental health issues. Assess for these common behaviors at all visits and insert teaching in the form of verbal information, brochures, or videos or DVDs that can be watched in the health care facility. What general principles can guide health promotion programs in adolescents? Some researchers have analyzed theory application and approaches of programs. Others have suggested key elements of programs that assist adolescents in taking on health promotion behaviors by fostering a sense of competence, promoting decision making, and increasing motivation for change toward health behaviors (Murray et al., 2009). When establishing youth programs, whether with individual adolescents or with groups, the nurse includes evaluation of the effectiveness of the plan, and uses methods to expand and sustain successful approaches.

Research — *Applying Theory to Plan for Adolescent Health*

Several theories guide health care professionals in establishing health promotion programs for adolescents. These theories provide an organized approach to planning and suggest the strategies that will be most successful, based on the person's motivation and developmental age (Murray et al., 2009). One theory commonly used in adolescent care is described here. *Social learning theory* was developed by Albert Bandura, who is described in Chapter 4 ∞ (Bandura, 1986, 1997a, 1997b; Hortz & Petosa, 2008). The key components of his theory involve **self-efficacy** (the person's belief in his or her ability to perform a behavior) and **outcome expectancy** (what the person expects to get from performing a certain behavior). Learning a new behavior occurs through **modeling**, or imitation of the behavior of someone else. Bandura believes that individuals make decisions about health behaviors based on thought about the consequences and outcomes of those behaviors. The *person's characteristics*, such as self-efficacy and outcome expectancy, interact with the external *environment* and the *behavioral choices* available. All of these components together determine health behaviors, and all can be influenced to promote health. If you were seeking to promote physical activity behaviors in adolescents, some essential components would be:

- Encouraging adolescents to believe they can perform the activity (self-efficacy)
- Pointing out the positive aspects of the behavior (outcome expectancy)
- Showing adolescents how to do the activity (modeling)
- Providing a physical setting and opportunity for performing the behavior (environment)
- Allowing trial and error, choice in time, and extent of activity (behavioral choices)

Compose a teaching plan to encourage increased physical activity for a teen using all components of the social cognitive theory. List the outcome measures or goals for the teaching, the interventions, and methods of evaluation.

General Observations

The beginning of an adolescent's visit can be an important time to gather information, just as it is with younger children. However, the observations you make will relate to the adolescent's more advanced developmental stage.

Ideally, the facility will have a waiting area designed for adolescents. Teens often dislike waiting for health care with either young children or older adults. Teen waiting areas are popular because they provide a special place, thereby relaying that the adolescent is important. Video and other popular methods can be used to impart health information while the teen waits (Figure 9–6 ➤). As you call the adolescent back for care, observe if parents or friends are present, or if the teen is alone. Young adolescents often come to the facility with parents, who then wait in the waiting room during the examination. If the teen comes in for a special problem, such as a skin lesion or other health concern, the parent may accompany the adolescent into the examination room. If someone comes with the teen, be alert that you may need to provide some private time by asking the other person to wait outside for a moment. Reassure the parents that you will talk with them about any of their concerns and questions, and provide them with an opportunity to ask questions and obtain information as well.

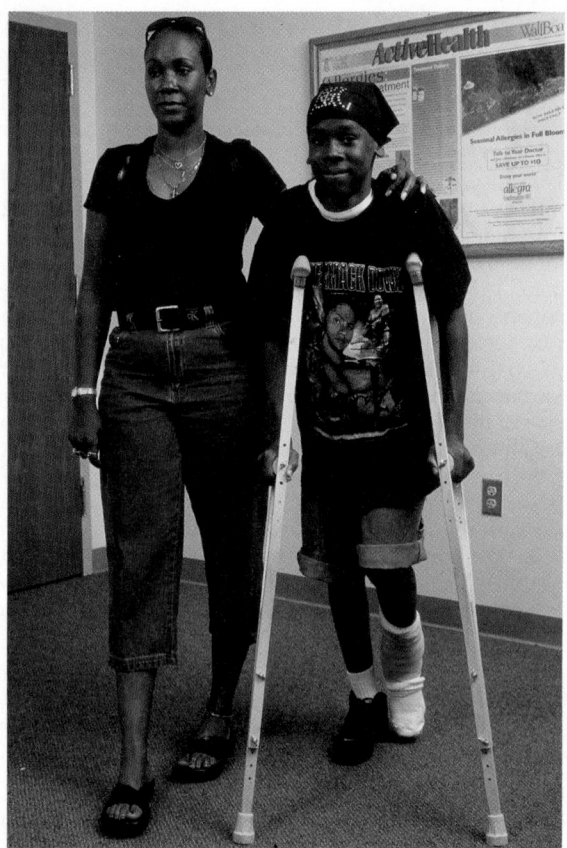

FIGURE 9–6 ➤ Parents often accompany teens with a health care problem in for the examination. Provide an opportunity to see both the teen and parent privately and integrate general health promotion and health maintenance into the visit. What questions can you ask this teen? What teaching might be needed?

Some teens are comfortable in health care settings and actively engage in conversation, whereas others are nervous and will need more explanations and reassurance as you progress with the first steps of measurement and blood pressure. By adolescence, boys and girls should be assuming more of a partnership role in their own health care. As the visit begins, greet adolescents warmly, ask what concerns and questions they have, and ask for their opinions and reactions throughout the visit. This will show that their thoughts are important and that they play an important role in guiding the health care visit. When adolescents are visiting the same office or clinic that they came to during childhood, they usually know and feel comfortable with the care providers. If the setting is new to them, explain the procedures and introduce personnel so they feel more at ease.

Growth and Developmental Surveillance

Adolescence spans several years, and growth and developmental issues vary throughout the period. For young adolescents, or those from about 12 to 13 years of age, growth measurement remains important. Many youth are still growing and use of percentile grids continues to be an important part of care. Growth should remain in the same percentile channel as during childhood, with girls reaching nearly adult height at this age, and boys still continuing to grow. Be alert for youth who

have either increased or decreased percentiles, or are above the 85th percentile or below the 5th percentile for BMI. They will need additional assessment of nutritional intake and physical activity.

By middle (14–16 years) and late (17–19 years) adolescence, adult growth is nearly achieved. This occurs earlier for girls than boys. Although measurement continues to be performed, nurses assess the BMI more carefully to be sure the height and weight indicate appropriate intake and exercise. Overweight at this age is likely to continue into adulthood, particularly if parents are overweight, so early intervention is needed to decrease this potential problem. Other youth may have eating disorders and should be referred to a specialist for care. Children from homes without sufficient financial resources may be hungry and lack adequate food of high quality. If an adolescent is thin and has little energy, consider this possibility; administer the food security questionnaire found in Chapter 14 ∞. Even the child who is overweight may live in a family with insufficient resources since foods with high fat and caloric content are often less expensive than those with greater nutrient value. For example, a dollar menu at a fast food restaurant meets hunger needs faster and with less expense than fresh fruits, vegetable, and grains. Persons who have experienced periods of hunger from inadequate food resources may overeat when food is available, a pattern that promotes weight gain (Olson, Bove, & Miller, 2007).

Few options exist for measuring the developmental competence of adolescents, but observations and questions during care provide information about the adolescent meeting developmental milestones. Key tasks for adolescents involve separating from the parents and establishing positive relationships with peers. The young teen may come to an appointment with a parent and still rely on that parent to answer some questions during the examination. However, the middle and late teen should be increasingly able to come alone, answer questions, and assume responsibility for health care decisions. Offer older teens the option of coming into the room alone, stating, "Your mom can wait here and we can come and get her later. Does that sound all right?" During your time with an adolescent, ask questions to learn about peer interactions and activities.

The adolescent receives a physical examination, often by the nurse practitioner or physician. See Chapter 5 ∞ for components of the examination. Some particular parts of the examination to include for teens are scoliosis screening; sexual maturity rating (Tanner stages); breast exam; testicular exam; sexually transmitted infections testing (among those sexually active); pelvic exam and Pap smear (for sexually active females); hematocrit for anemia annually in menstruating adolescents; hearing screening at 12, 15, and 18 years; blood pressure annually; lipid screening for those with a family history of early heart disease or other risk factors; and tuberculosis for those in high-risk areas. Most adolescents do not want parents present during the examination, but occasionally they will want a parent for something like a first pelvic examination or a blood draw. Ask them their wishes in a confidential setting so they can freely make the choice. They also may choose to have a health care provider of their own gender complete the genitourinary examination. Expected outcomes of care include screening and early identification for common health problems, normal patterns of growth, and meeting of developmental milestones.

Nutrition

The young adolescent needs a well-balanced diet to support the growth of this period, and the late adolescent requires intake that supports physical activity and provides nutrients for metabolism and to promote the immune system. While nutritional intake is important, teens often do not eat well. They may be busy and do not want to plan meals, they like to eat high-fat or sugar foods that are popular with other teens, they may diet to achieve weight loss, and some do not have enough financial resources to access proper foods.

Combine the information from the adolescent's measurements with the answers to questions about diet to identify possible areas for intervention. Find out what questions the teen has about foods, diet, maintaining desired weight, and topics like vegetarianism or supplements to enhance athletic performance. See Chapter 14 ∞ for further details about these special nutritional topics. Health promotion plans focus on practices that lead to healthy growth and development. They may include teaching about:

- Eating five servings of fruits and vegetables daily
- Including whole grain products to replace refined products whenever possible
- Applying the MyPyramid Food Guide in the daily diet
- Stressing the importance of eating three meals each day including breakfast and lunch
- Eating together as a family several times weekly, which enhances quality food intake
- Planning menus and preparing foods for balanced intake

Health maintenance plans center on those practices that prevent disease, including:

- Limiting refined sugar and high fat intake (such as soft drinks and fried foods) in order to maintain weight at the recommended level
- Including two or three servings of dairy products daily to enhance bone formation and decrease chances of osteoporosis as an adult; encourage options that are most enticing to teens such as portable yogurt and pizza with cheese
- Using resources for treatment of eating disorders if they are identified

While much of nutrition teaching should be aimed directly at the adolescent, parents are also included. They can be effective contributors to healthy intake by providing plenty of fruits and vegetables for snacks, having foods attractively prepared and ready for consumption when the teen is hungry, planning several meals together as a family each week, encouraging milk or other forms of calcium intake, and setting a good example for food intake. Help them identify the youth with an eating disorder and provide resources for intervention in these cases. Consider as well the teen with a baby. The adolescent who is pregnant or breastfeeding has even more need for nutritional teaching and may need financial resources to access sufficient food. How will you combine the growth and developmental needs of an adolescent with those of her new baby when planning teaching?

Physical Activity

Many adolescents suffer from the effects of inadequate physical activity. As children get older and enter the teenage years, physical activity decreases, particularly in girls. Only about 25% of adolescents have engaged in 60 minutes of activity on at least one day in the last seven. Activity is even less in certain groups, with 32% of females having the recommended level of activity even once in a week. Nearly 30% of teens in the 12th grade report one day of exercise weekly (CDC, 2008a). The recommendation of *Healthy People 2010* (U.S. Department of Health and Human Services, 2006) is quite moderate, stating that adolescents should get at least 20 minutes of vigorous activity 3 days weekly, while an expert panel recommends 60 minutes of moderate or vigorous physical activity daily (CDC, 2008a). At a time when teens are not very active as a group, physical education requirements in school are also decreasing. Only 23% of 12th-grade students regularly attend a PE class (CDC, 2008b). Physical activity levels must therefore be assessed at each health supervision visit or in other contacts with adolescents. Apply resilience theory and assess youth, family, and community for risk and protective factors regarding physical activity (Table 9–4).

Some youth have established regular physical activity programs, and their behaviors should be encouraged (Figure 9–7 ➤). Parents who have regular physical activity are important in influencing children, so encourage parental exercise at each pediatric health care visit. Be alert for those who exercise but have other health problems. Some athletes try to eat very little to

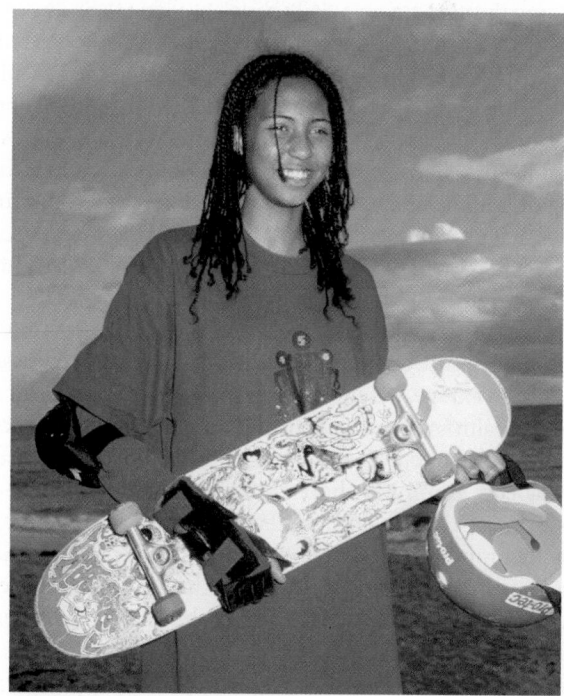

FIGURE 9–7 ➤ This teen girl is an avid "boarder." How can you encourage and praise her for this activity? What clues do you have that she is using adequate safety measures?

TABLE 9–4	Risk and Protective Factors Regarding Physical Activity in Adolescence	
Risk Factors		**Protective Factors**
• Lives in isolated setting with little opportunity for contact with other teens • Has a developmental disability that impairs physical movement • Does not like physical activity • Has a pattern and history of low activity levels • Is overweight • Does not feel competent in most sports • Limited financial resources to pay registration fees or buy protective gear for sports • Family members who have little physical activity • Parents who are not active in school sports and committees • Parents who do not like physical activity and have had low levels while their teen was growing up • Parents who have little time or facilities for exercise, or always exercise at a club out of view of their family • Lack of youth and parent knowledge about physical activity needs and benefits • Lack of neighborhood programs for physical activity promotion • Presence of neighborhood hazards and unsafe areas		• Has opportunities for participation in physical activity at home, at school, and in the community • Likes physical activity • Has exercised during all of childhood, often with parents • Knowledgeable about benefits of activity; committed to maintaining exercise patterns • Has many friends living close who participate in physical activity • Agreement between youth and parents to a 2-hour daily limit of screen time • Availability of financial and other resources for sports gear and protective equipment • Parents who participate in regular physical activity and encourage the adolescent to do so • Neighborhood and community that provide physical activity options • Public policies that maintain parks, green spaces, biking trails, and playgrounds • Available programs for adolescents with developmental disabilities or other health care needs

Adapted from Hagan et al., 2008.

remain a certain weight for wrestling, running, or other sports. Integrate nutritional teaching that includes the importance of adequate intake for sports performance. Other athletes use nutritional supplements to enhance performance. While most are not harmful, few have proven benefits and their cost is not warranted; some may actually be harmful to adolescents.

Other youth have very little physical activity and feel incompetent in performing many sports. Work with them to find at least one thing they can do on a daily basis—walking their dog in the neighborhood, riding a bike to the store, using stairs instead of elevators when possible, parking on the far side of the school lot and walking farther, swimming at a club their parents belong to or at a local YMCA or YWCA, or saving money to take lessons for something they have always dreamed of doing such as horseback riding or golf. Form interest groups at schools and community centers that provide an outlet for adolescents who cannot "make the team" for school sports. Encourage parents and adolescents to set goals together to integrate some physical activity daily.

The nurse's activities for health promotion concentrate on teaching the health and mental benefits of physical activity such as increased energy, weight control, and a feeling of control and success. Health maintenance focuses on viewing physical activity as a method to prevent disease such as cardiovascular disease and diabetes. Youth who have family members with these diseases or meet adults who have them are more likely to understand the importance of their own activity. Desired outcomes include maintenance of weight within the recommended level, daily exercise of 60 minutes, and establishment of lifetime exercise routines.

Oral Health

Continued dental care during the adolescent years can ensure oral health. The recommendations remain the same as those for young children. The adolescent should floss daily, brush twice daily with a small amount of fluoridated toothpaste, and visit a dental care provider every 6 months. By about 14 years of age, those students who do not have fluoridated water and have been taking fluoride can stop this supplement. Even the molars have been formed by that age so fluoride tablets are no longer needed. Continue to examine the condition of the teeth and the number of erupted permanent teeth present. Be alert for any unusual growths and ulcers in the mouth and refer for care as needed.

Lack of dental insurance for the adolescent is a potential concern. The teen whose family does not have dental insurance needs referrals for care to affordable resources. Dental specialists clean off plaque that has formed, apply sealants to erupting molars, examine the teeth for caries, and perform restorative care.

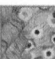

Culture *Dental Care*

An analysis of several national surveys such as the National Health and Nutrition Examination Survey (NHANES) and National Survey of Children's Health (NSCH) shows marked disparity in oral health. The major factor in disparity of dental care is poverty. While 71% of children and adolescents from families living above the poverty line have dental care, only 36% of those below the poverty line have access to dental care. Black and Hispanic youth are likely to have less access to dental services and more decayed teeth than White youth. The highest rates of families without dental insurance are foreign-born Hispanics (67% uninsured) and U.S.-born Hispanics (25% uninsured) (Liu et al., 2007). Families in rural settings are less likely to have insurance than those in urban settings.

When you work with adolescent populations from groups at high risk for lack of dental coverage or high incidence of caries, include dental assessment in health supervision visits and have resources for care readily available to carry out referrals as needed.

Certain groups are more at risk for inadequate dental care. When working with these populations, nurses can question access to care and make recommendations that foster regular checkups. Evaluate risk factors for threats to oral health such as tobacco use, particularly chewing tobacco. A risk for oral injury exists with engagement in certain sports. Ask about physical activity and if the youth engages in hockey, football, or other such sports and if a mouth guard is worn.

Some teens may wish to whiten the teeth or get orthodontia to improve their appearance. The nurse helps the youth and parents to find resources for needed or desired care. Expected outcomes are dental visits twice annually with recommended follow-up care for problems, resulting in good oral health.

Mental and Spiritual Health

Adolescents have many challenges to their mental health and need support to emerge from adolescence with mental and spiritual strengths. Mental health topics must be addressed at each health supervision opportunity to promote mental health among teens. Mental health is closely linked to developmental tasks such as growing independence, formation of close relationships with peers, becoming confident in accomplishments, and setting goals for the future. Some chronic mental health disruptions emerge during adolescence, so mental health screening is important to perform with this age group.

As during other developmental stages, the self-concept continues to evolve, influencing how the adolescent reacts to the environment. Self-regulation in the form of making decisions to govern oneself is important. Ask what the teen is proud of and has accomplished and what disappointments have occurred as well. Provide resources to deal with disappointments and give praise for the teen's accomplishments.

The adolescent's self-esteem is connected to perceptions of body image. Factors such as early or late maturation, overweight or underweight, or the role of the media can influence the teen's body image. A healthy image includes the realization that the body has positive and less positive attributes and that the individual can influence the body by healthy eating and physical activity. Be alert for the teen whose wish for a different body leads to eating disorders and excessive exercise or intake of nutritional supplements.

Sexuality involves both body changes that signal mature sexual development, and the mental concept of oneself as a sexual being. Body changes and mental concepts do not necessarily mature at the same time, and adolescents may not be ready for sexual maturity and the decisions about sexual behavior simply due to achieving sexual maturation. Most young adolescent girls have begun menstruating; by early to middle adolescence, boys are having nocturnal emissions and ejaculations. Ask teens if they have received information about puberty, body changes, and sexuality. Tell young adolescents that most teens have questions and that you will talk with them about any areas of interest, including contraception and sexually transmitted diseases. Ask adolescents directly if they have had sexual intercourse and, if so, what they are doing to protect against pregnancy and sexually transmitted infections. Provide support for adolescents who have decided not to have

sexual intercourse. Encourage them to continue this plan, telling them that sexual feelings are normal, but that decisions about sexual intercourse are their right and privilege. Ask if the adolescent has ever experienced unwanted pressure for intercourse and if there has been help and support to deal with the situation. Intimate partner violence, date rape, and other trauma signals a need for referral to a mental health specialist. See Chapter 17 ∞ for further information.

Ask teens if they have confusion about sexuality. If teens have identified as homosexual, let them know they are welcome and ask about decisions regarding sexual practices, reinforcing the need for protection against sexually transmitted infections. Provide community resources to support gay or lesbian teens so they can develop a social group in which they feel comfortable. Some adolescents are seen for health care at the time they become sexually active. Use this opportunity to reinforce and correct prior knowledge about the body and protection against pregnancy and sexually transmitted infections.

Most adolescents still need discipline or guidance from parents at certain times. Rather than maintain a constant battle over daily events, it is best if parents have just a few important rules that they rarely have to enforce. Nurses can assist parents to set useful boundaries for teens and offer resources such as parenting groups and websites for assistance.

Sleep is necessary for anyone to function safely and at a level of one's potential. Unfortunately, many youth do not get the sleep needed for healthy functioning. Although about 9 hours of sleep is needed, about 90% of teens do not get this amount of sleep, and 10% actually get less than 6 hours (Mayo Clinic, 2009). Teen growth rates and activity levels require adequate sleep for healthy functioning. Busy schedules, inability to fall asleep early from normal developmental changes, work schedules, social engagements, and waking during the night to engage in cell phone texting are examples of common adolescent behaviors that can interfere with normal sleep patterns.

The effects of sleep deprivation can be serious. Teens cannot perform to their potential in school or at work. Adolescents are often moody and difficult to communicate with when they are tired. There may be a connection between lack of sleep and substance

---

Law & Ethics *Sexuality Issues*

The nurse who works with adolescents dealing with sexuality issues may find that some teens' values are very different from the nurse's personal values. How will you react when a teen decides to have sexual intercourse or has become pregnant? Can you help the teen to make wise decisions without telling him or her what to do? It is important for adolescents to learn the significance of sexual intercourse and the meaning of close relationships. Teaching them about this early will enable them to respect others at the time they have intimate relations. Respect is also the key to working with teens. Nurses should treat them with respect, and expect them to consider options and make wise decisions. Nurses who cannot work with certain groups of teens because of moral values differing from their own have the obligation to refer the teens for care to resources where they can receive the information and services they are requesting.

abuse, and teens commonly use caffeinated beverages to stay awake. Some people tend to eat more when they are tired, and get less physical activity. One of the most serious consequences may be the danger of driving while tired; this is a common cause of accidents (Mayo Clinic, 2009).

Ask adolescents about what time they go to bed, when they awaken, and whether they are frequently tired. Provide suggestions for maintaining regular sleep schedules, avoiding caffeine products in the evening, making screen technology unavailable during sleep time, and planning a day of relaxation into every week.

School has an increasingly important influence on adolescent mental health. Peer support, meaningful activities, and a forum for learning time management and other skills are all provided by school. At the same time, some youth experience stress because of inability to fit in, worry about grades and their futures, and a violent or unsupportive school situation. Discuss the elements of school that adolescents like and those they do not like. Evaluate the presence of support in the schools. Ask the adolescent about future plans and how those are influencing choices for courses and friends in school.

Temperament or personality-type characteristics continue into adolescence, but they generally do not change from earlier years. For example, the active infant and young child is usually an active teenager. The slow-to-warm-up baby may be the adolescent who needs more time to adjust to a new school or teachers. If the adolescent or parent has trouble with personality characteristics, it may be helpful to talk about these traits, help him or her to establish a positive sense about the attributes, and discuss ways to adapt the environment as needed. For example, parents should not expect a slow-to-warm-up teen to be interested in running for a class office. Someone with irregular sleep and eating habits will find it difficult to have a job at a set time and will need to set alarms and other reminders.

Spirituality offers the adolescent comfort and support. Being a member of a teen group in a faith-based home can offer a peer group with similar values and bring meaning to life. Some adolescents reject their parent's faith and seek a different group; others seek to leave religious practices totally whereas others become more committed to them. Ask them if they have

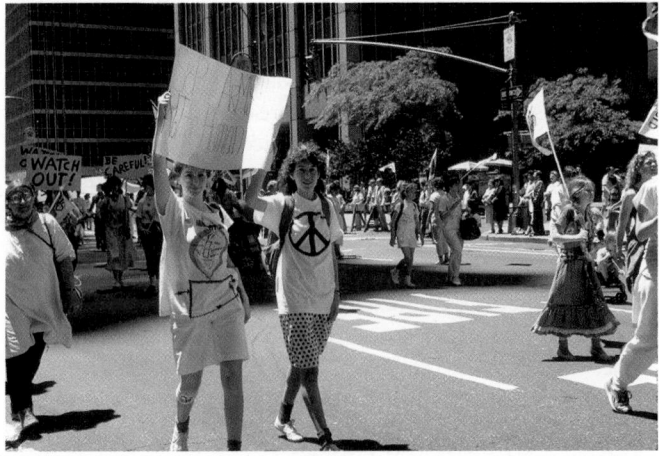

FIGURE 9–8 ➤ Teens often become associated with causes. This helps them to feel part of a social group and also provides the opportunities to examine belief systems and to make decisions about meaningful activities.

the resources they need to bring meaning to their lives; provide them if needed. Realize that participating in community food kitchens, raising money for causes, and other activities also provide meaning for many adolescents (Figure 9–8 ➤).

The nurse actively promotes the mental health of youth by understanding their developmental needs and providing information and resources. Gentle guidance and active partnership with youth help to provide the resources to ensure healthy self-concept, sexuality, and personality development. While most teenagers have many protective factors that can be identified and fostered, a few have risks that can harm mental health. It is important to identify the risks also, and to use health maintenance techniques to lessen the risk factors. Depression and substance use are two common risks to mental health. Depression is discussed in Chapter 28 ∞ and substance use in Chapter 17 ∞. See Table 9–5 to help in identification of these problems during health supervision visits.

Although health promotion and health maintenance activities commonly occur in office or clinic settings, there are many other settings where nurses work with adolescents; mental health activities are often integrated into these settings. Consider offering health promotion/maintenance wherever you might see

TABLE 9–5 **Signs of Depression and Substance Abuse**	
Depression	Substance Abuse
• History of abuse or depression in family members • Changes in behavior, school performance, sleep, and appetite • Physical complaints • Loss of interest in usual activities • Difficulty in motivating self and setting goals • Poor social skills • Feelings of worthlessness • Consideration of death or suicide	• Changes in behavior, school performance, sleep, and appetite • Accidents and other unexplained events • Lack of responsibility • Labile (changeable) mood and behavior • Inability to set goals • Hopelessness • Depression • Feelings of ambivalence • A variety of physical changes depending on the substance

Adapted from National Institutes of Health, 2009.

students. Some nontraditional settings include correctional facilities, school-based health centers, and programs for pregnant teens. Adolescents in these facilities can benefit from services to improve diet, physical activity, and lifestyle behaviors that influence mental health.

The desired outcomes for mental and spiritual health promotion and maintenance include meaningful activities in the adolescent's life, emerging independence, good choices about lifestyle behaviors, and development of successful coping skills.

Relationships

Adolescents form stronger bonds with friends than at any time earlier in development; at the same time they need their parents for guidance and reassurance as they become more independent. As teenagers strive for independence they frequently strike out at parents, test limits, and have conflicts with parents. Interactions in the family provide consistent and important ties at the same time that social interactions become a central part of life. Health promotion helps teens to form strong friendships with peers and continue to value and participate in the family. It helps parents to understand the developmental needs and their role in establishing a new type of relationship with the family's emerging young adult. Partnerships with care providers are important to help families work together to achieve these outcomes.

When adolescents are seen for health care visits, assess relationships with others. Provide time alone with both the adolescent and the parents (if they are present) so that everyone has time to talk freely and to ask questions. Some areas already discussed, such as school performance and activities, provide information about the adolescent's friends and how time is spent. Ask teens to describe their best friends and what they do together. Ask parents their opinions of the youth's friends. Inquire about the youth's roles in the family. Does the teen have jobs and responsibilities? What freedom is allowed? What are relationships like with siblings and extended family members such as grandparents and cousins? What activities are done together as a family? Are there differences in the teen's and the parents' answers to these questions? What are the teen's and parents' desires for how the family unit functions together?

Provide an opportunity alone with the teen to talk about issues such as domestic violence. Is the youth abused or is there violence between adults in the family? Are there stressors such as lack of sufficient finances, an ill parent, or a lost job? How have these occurrences affected the adolescent? Minor adjustments can be helped by discussion while some major problems will need referral to mental health specialists.

In their relationships with peers, adolescents often have many of the same issues that emerge with parents. They may have disagreements with friends or feel hurt by things that are said or done. Ask teens about how things are going with friends and what problems they have. Talk about negotiating, joining groups to form new friendships, and the importance of respecting and not making fun of others. Give them strategies for living up to their own standards even when friends are enticing them

to do other things. Suggest that having friends one can trust and who have the same ideals can be very supportive and fun in adolescent years. Expected outcomes are the formation of strong relationships both within and outside of the family, along with independence in decision making.

Disease Prevention Strategies

Teenagers typically do not have many diseases and most are minor illnesses like respiratory and gastrointestinal illness. However, some diseases occur, so nurses must always be aware of signs of potential disease. Some common health issues that are described throughout this book include:

- Acne and skin infections (see Chapter 31 ∞)
- Body piercing and tattooing (see Chapter 17 ∞)
- Sports overuse injuries (see Chapter 29 ∞)
- Constipation and diarrhea (see Chapter 25 ∞)
- Dental problems

Other observations may signal more serious health concerns and need to be referred for further evaluation. Some examples include:

- Scoliosis (see Chapter 29 ∞)
- Anemia (see Chapter 22 ∞)
- Excessive tiredness (see Chapter 24 ∞)
- Bruising (see Chapter 23 ∞)
- Sexually transmitted infections (see Chapter 26 ∞)
- Eating disorders (see Chapter 14 ∞)
- Abuse or severe bullying (see Chapter 17 ∞)

Several screening tests should be performed during health supervision visits with adolescents, including vision, hearing, smoking, depression, stress, alcohol or other substance use, blood pressure, urinalysis, sexually transmitted infection risk, and in some cases Pap smears and breast examinations. Screening tests with abnormal results require follow-up and intervention. For example, if the adolescent is anemic, iron tablets may be needed and teaching about high iron foods should be done. Vision impairment requires referral to an eye specialist. Presence of sexually transmitted infections requires teaching and medication treatment. A history of sexual activity will guide you to tests that should be included in the examination.

The adolescent should receive extensive information about ways to protect health and prevent disease. The hazardous outcomes of smoking and other tobacco use are discussed, and cessation programs are encouraged for users. Unprotected sexual activity is presented as a serious health threat. Use of sunscreens to prevent burns and future skin cancer is encouraged. Females are taught breast self-exam and males are taught testicular exam. For youth who are overweight and sedentary, the possible outcomes such as type 2 diabetes and cardiovascular disease are mentioned. Although it is not advisable to threaten or frighten an adolescent with descriptions of diseases, an understanding of the potential serious outcomes of smoking such as cancer or cardiovascular disease can be motivators for behavior change.

Nursing Alert

Sexually active teens should be screened annually for:

■ Chlamydia
■ Gonorrhea
■ Trichomoniasis
■ Human papillomavirus
■ Herpes simplex virus
■ Bacterial vaginosis

Individuals should be screened for syphilis and/or HIV/AIDS if they request testing or meet any of these criteria:

■ History of sexually transmitted infection
■ More than one sexual partner in past 6 months
■ Intravenous drug use
■ Sexual intercourse with a partner at risk
■ Sex in exchange for drugs or money
■ Homelessness
■ Males—sex with other males
■ Syphilis—residence in areas where disease is prevalent
■ HIV/AIDS—blood or blood product transfusion before 1985

All individuals from 13 to 64 years should be offered a voluntary HIV test at each health care encounter. Those at high risk of infection (<20 years and sexually active, >20 years with inconsistent use of barrier protection and a new or more than one sex partner in last 3 months) should be retested annually (Branson, 2006).

Data from: Hagan, J. F., Shaw, J. S., & Duncan, P. M. (2008). Bright futures: Guidelines for health supervision of infants, children, and adolescents (3rd ed). Elk Grove Village, IL: American Academy of Pediatrics; Branson, B. M. (2006). Revised recommendations for HIV testing in health care settings in the United States. Retrieved from http://www.cdc.gov/hiv/topics/testing/resources/slidesets/pdf/testing_healthcare.pdf

In addition to teaching to prevent disease, the nurse also administers any needed immunizations. Many adolescents have not had immunizations since about school entry time, so their record should be carefully reviewed. Some common immunizations needed by adolescents are described in the following list.

- When was the last tetanus-diphtheria booster? A booster of tetanus-diphtheria and acellular pertussis (Tdap) is now recommended at 11–12 years. If a dose of Td was given during adolescence, wait for at least 5 years, and administer one dose of Tdap.
- Was a second measles-mumps-rubella administered? A second dose may not have been routine when teens were younger so they may need it now.
- Did the teen receive hepatitis A vaccine at a younger age? If not, the vaccine series is needed now.
- Has the youth had hepatitis B vaccine series? This is important for all youth, and some may not have received it as infants.
- Did the youth have a clear history of varicella disease? If not, the vaccine is needed.
- Meningococcal vaccine (MCV4) is now recommended for all youth.
- Human papillomavirus vaccine (three-dose series) is recommended for females at 11–12 years, and for those from 13–26 years not previously immunized.
- Annual influenza vaccine is recommended for all children and adolescents.

Research *Graduated Driver Licensing*

Motor vehicle crashes are the leading cause of injury and death for youth from 16–19 years in the United States. Many states and other countries now apply graduated driver licensing policies to restrict youth driving in certain situations such as late at night, mandate certain required hours of driving with parents, and do not allow teens to drive other youth. In spite of the expansion of policies, states vary in laws and their application. A review of studies suggests that parental management of driving is important to reduce teen risky behavior, and parents can be educated to take an active role in managing their youth's driving behaviors. Applying education programs in driver licensing stations during permit and licensure acquisition shows promise for interventions (Simons-Morton & Ouimet, 2006).

The results of health screening are shared with the teen and with the parent as appropriate. Teaching and other interventions for disease prevention are examples of health maintenance activities. Expected outcomes are increasing knowledge of common diseases and methods of prevention among teen and parent, use of screening tests by the health care provider, and use of the health care home by the adolescent for treatment of diseases.

Injury Prevention Strategies

Injury is the greatest health hazard for adolescents, so injury prevention must be integrated into every health contact with youth. The major hazard is automobile crashes (see Chapter 1 ∞). Many teens learn to drive and have a license by 16 years of age. They often transport friends, get distracted by social interactions in the car, have little experience about what to do if a car slides or has mechanical problems, may drink and drive, and are often tired when driving (Figure 9–9 ➤). Driving should always be presented as a privilege and a responsibility. Because of the great risk of injury and death from car crashes, ask at each health visit if the teen drives or rides with other teens, what rules parents have established about driving, and whether the teen ever drinks and drives

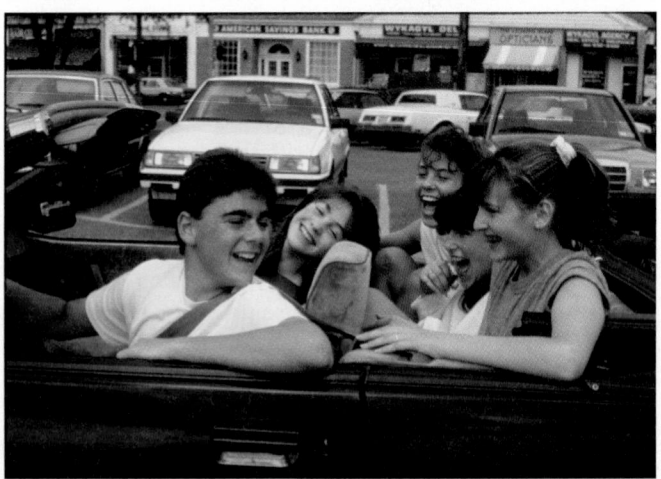

FIGURE 9–9 ➤ Adolescents often drive motorized vehicles and may be at risk for injury if not properly prepared or protected. What teaching and experience do these youth need for safe enjoyment of the experience of driving and riding with friends? Do schools in your area offer driver education classes? What are the state requirements for youth driver licensure?

or rides with someone who does. Reinforce the need to wear a lap and shoulder belt at all times and to never drink and drive.

Youth are at risk for injury with other motorized vehicles. Motorcycles, four-wheelers, boats, jet skis, and farm machinery are other sources of injury (Beer, Deboy, & Field, 2007; Cherry, Huggins, & Gilmore, 2007; Conway, McCline, & Nosel, 2007). Ask about the youth's exposure to various machines and teach about avoiding alcohol and drug use, as well as safety gear and precautions to be used. Every health visit should include other questions that help to identify a wide variety of injury hazards. Once you have asked about common causes of injury, be sure to discuss and provide written material to perform injury prevention teaching. Such measures are important health maintenance activities. See Tables 9–6 and 9–7. Desired outcomes for nursing care include absence of serious injury, the ability to state sources of risk for injury, and emergency plans for assistance when engaging in any risky activities.

NURSING MANAGEMENT

Nursing Assessment and Diagnosis

Nurses assess adolescents in a variety of settings, including offices, clinics, schools, homes, correctional facilities, extended care facilities, sports-related settings, and family planning clinics. A wide array of health concerns should be included in these assessments. They include measurement of growth; presence of any unusual findings on physical examination; lifestyle choices related to dietary intake, physical activity, and oral hygiene; assessment of mental status, family interactions, and social connections with peers; and any risky behaviors the adolescent engages in such as smoking, unprotected sexual relations, alcohol or drug use, or unsafe driving practices. The people and organizations around the adolescent such as family, school, and neighborhood are all assessed. Remember to list both risks and protective factors. The protective factors can be used during implementation to enhance the youth's resilience.

Based on a thorough assessment, you will establish nursing diagnoses that are appropriate for the adolescent and family. Some possible nursing diagnoses might be:

- Rape-Trauma Syndrome related to date rape
- Impaired Dentition related to ineffective oral hygiene
- Readiness for Enhanced Nutrition related to increasing interest in nutritional knowledge
- Disturbed Sleep Pattern related to frequently changing sleep/wake schedule
- Low Self-Esteem related to situational crisis of friends making fun of adolescent

TABLE 9–6	**Injury Prevention in Adolescence**		
	Hazard	Developmental Characteristics	Preventive Measures
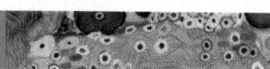	Motor vehicle crashes	Adolescents learn to drive, enjoy new independence, and often feel invulnerable.	Insist on driver's education classes. Enforce rules about safe driving. Forbid texting while driving. Seat belts should be used for every trip. Discourage drug and alcohol use. Get treatment for teenagers who are known substance abusers.
	Sporting injuries	Adolescents may participate in physically challenging sports such as soccer, gymnastics, or football. They may be allowed to drive motorboats.	Encourage use of protective sporting gear. Ensure that coaches are instructed in management of youth who receive head injuries during sports. Teach safe boating practices. Perform teaching related to hazards of drug and alcohol use, especially when using motorized equipment.
	Drowning	Adolescents overestimate endurance when swimming. They take risks diving.	Encourage swimming only with friends. Reinforce rules and teach about risks.

TABLE 9–7	Injury Prevention Topics for Adolescence
Topic	**Teaching**
Driving	• Always wear a seat and shoulder belt. • Do not drink and drive or ride with others who do. • Do not talk on a cell phone as you drive. • Do not drive when you are tired. • Drive with parents or other adults for several months in winter driving conditions if you live where there is snow, ice, or heavy rains. • Keep your car in good repair.
Sun	• Wear sunscreen. • Limit time outside, especially early in summer.
Machinery	• Learn how to correctly use power tools. • Always have someone near when you use tools or machinery.
Emergency care	• Learn first aid, CPR, and airway obstruction removal.
Water safety	• Learn to swim well. • If you supervise younger children near water, never leave them alone, even for a minute.
Fires	• Do not play with fire. • Follow guidelines to avoid igniting gasoline. • Test smoke alarms in your house every 6 months and annually change batteries.
Firearms	• Know and follow rules to keep firearms locked, with ammunition locked in a separate place. • Never take out a gun to show a friend unless your parent is also present. • Take firearm safety classes if you hunt or target shoot.
Hearing	• Avoid loud music, especially for long periods and through earphones.
Sports	• Wear protective gear recommended for your sport.
Abuse	• Report any abuse to an adult you trust. • Date with other couples whenever possible and report date rape. • Do not drink or take drugs.

Adapted from Hagan et al., 2008.

Planning and Implementation

Whatever the setting, the nurse partners with the adolescent, the parents, and other persons such as teachers or school counselors to plan appropriate goals and related interventions. Nurses work with individual adolescents in offices, schools, and other settings, and often work with groups of adolescents to perform teaching. Apply communication skills effective with teens such as listening to concerns, allowing for discussion, and bringing peers who have had experiences related to the topic being discussed.

Many of your interventions will involve teaching, so it is wise to develop a number of resources for working with teens. Consult the web resources on the companion website, and visit agencies in your community to gather appropriate materials. Teaching topics will be directed both at health promotion (providing information to enhance the adolescent's state of health) and health maintenance (sharing tips about how to avoid disease and injury). A good starting point is to have the adolescent identify a personal health goal and begin teaching there. In addition to teaching, you will provide direct care when you administer immunizations, perform vision screening, and examine the spine and posture for scoliosis.

One of the challenges during health supervision for adolescents is including the right mix of teen and parent decision making and involvement. You will again apply communication skills by tactfully allowing time for both parent and adolescent to be seen alone. Realize that you are supporting and providing information for parents, like useful discipline techniques, recognition of common parental feelings about teens, and the need for growing independence by their youth. When you provide teaching to groups of teens in schools, there may be policies about what needs to be sent home to parents. Some schools require that an outline of topics such as sexually transmitted diseases or substance use be sent home for parents to read. Parents may call you with questions about content and approach, or some may choose to attend and sit in on your presentation. This obviously requires that you partner with the school administration, teachers, parents, and others to be effective in your presentation. Collaboration with many individuals and agencies is an important skill.

Whether you see adolescents in offices or other private settings, or in schools, correction facilities, or other places with groups present, leave information about how you or another nurse or care provider can be contacted. Provide brochures, referral numbers, names, and e-mails related to the topics discussed. Encourage annual health supervision visits and suggest a variety of places to obtain this care. For example, if a youth will soon graduate from high school, find out if he or she will be working or attending college and provide links to health insurance or care providers in the new location.

Evaluation

Expected outcomes for care of adolescents and their families during health promotion and health maintenance include the following:

- Normal growth patterns and maintenance of healthy weight
- Physical activity of 60 minutes daily
- Absence of debris and plaque on dental surfaces
- Establishment of positive self-concept
- Positive relationships with peers, family members, teachers, and others
- Healthy lifestyle habits that promote prevention of disease and injury

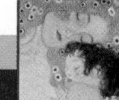

Chapter Highlights

- School-age health promotion and health maintenance visits begin with a prekindergarten examination.
- Health promotion should take place in any setting where the child is seen, even for episodic or emergency care.
- Growth measurement and developmental surveillance provide the basis for establishing risk and protective factors for an individual child.
- School-age children have increasing independence in making food choices; teaching is needed for the child and family to promote healthy choices.
- Physical activity should be included in the home and school setting for every child.
- Establishment of self-esteem and peer relationships are important for mental health of the school-age child.
- Injury prevention efforts focus on common causes of morbidity and mortality in young children, such as firearms, abuse, motor vehicle crashes, and sports-related injuries.
- The nurse integrates population-based health promotion activities into all settings where groups of children are seen; individualized approaches are used primarily in clinics and offices and focus on the particular needs of a given child.

- Health promotion and health maintenance of adolescents takes place in settings with individual youth as well as in facilities with groups of adolescents.
- Growth measurement provides useful clues about the nutrition status of teenagers. Further nutritional assessment provides information about the teen's food choices, knowledge, and nutritional intake.
- Physical activity is important for youth, but large numbers do not get adequate amounts of exercise.
- The adolescent has many mental health challenges to meet in order to emerge with a positive self-concept and body image.
- Adolescents often have conflicts with parents as they grow to become more independent individuals. Parents must learn that family roles change during the teenage years.
- Peers form a primary source of companionship, self-worth, and influence for the adolescent.
- Since they are not seen often for health care, adolescents have needs for disease and injury prevention that must be met at any health care encounter.

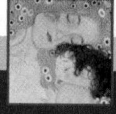

Clinical Reasoning in Action

Recall the opening scenario which described Ty, a 12-year-old boy with osteogenesis imperfecta. (Consult Chapter 29 ∞ for further information about this health condition.) Although he has a health problem, Ty still needs health promotion and health maintenance visits. They need to be adapted to consider his specific needs.

1. Ty often uses a wheelchair due to his frequent fractures and surgeries. What special dietary needs does he have? What physical activities can be encouraged? Since he swims and recently began wheelchair basketball, what safety needs does he have to prevent injuries during these activities?

2. List the mental health strengths that Ty manifests. How will you use these strengths in planning his care?
3. Plan a teaching session to explain osteogenesis imperfecta to Ty's classmates.
4. Many children with osteogenesis imperfecta have poor dental health due to the disease's effects on teeth. Plan a teaching intervention with Ty to promote good oral hygiene and oral health.

See Pearson Nursing Student Resources for possible responses.

Pearson Nursing Student Resources

Find additional review materials at
nursing.pearsonhighered.com

Prepare for success with NCLEX®-style practice questions, interactive assignments and activities, web links, animations and videos, and more!

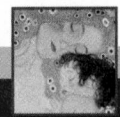

References

American Academy of Pediatrics. (2007a). *Discipline*. Retrieved from http://www.aap.org

American Academy of Pediatrics. (2007b). *Healthy children: Back to school*. Retrieved from http://www.aap.org

Bandura, A. (1986). *Social foundations of thought and actions: A social cognitive theory*. Englewood Cliffs, NJ: Prentice Hall.

Bandura, A. (1997a). *Self-efficacy in changing societies*. New York: Cambridge University.

Bandura, A. (1997b). *Self-efficacy: The exercise of control*. New York: W. H. Freeman.

Barkin, S., Scheindlin, G., Ip, E. H., Richardson, I., & Finch, S. (2007). Determinants of parental discipline practices: A national sample from primary care practices. *Clinical Pediatrics, 46*, 64–69.

Beer, S. R., Deboy, G. R., & Field, W. E. (2007). Analysis of 151 agricultural driveline-related incidents resulting in fatal and non-fatal injuries to U.S. children and adolescents under age 18 from 1970 through 2004. *Journal of Agricultural Safety and Health, 13*, 147–164.

Branson, B. M. (2006). *Revised recommendations for HIV testing in health care settings in the United States*. Retrieved from http://www.cdc.gov/hiv/topics/testing/resources/slidesets/pdf/testing_healthcare.pdf

Centers for Disease Control and Prevention (CDC). (2008a). *How much physical activity do children need?* Retrieved from http://www.cdc.gov/physicalactivity/everyone/guidelines/children/html

Centers for Disease Control and Prevention (CDC). (2008b). *Youth Risk Behavior Surveillance—2007*. *Morbidity and Mortality Weekly Report, 57*(SS-4), 1–136.

Cherry, D. C., Huggins, B., & Gilmore, K. (2007). Children's health in the rural environment. *Pediatric Clinics of North America, 54*, 121–133.

Cole, K. A., Clark, J. A., & Gable, S. (2007). Promoting family strengths. In N. Henderson (Ed.), *Resiliency in action* (pp. 199–204). Ojai, CA: Resiliency in Action.

Committee on Sports Medicine and Fitness and Council on School Health, American Academy of Pediatrics. (2006). *Active health living: Prevention of childhood obesity through increased physical activity*. Retrieved from http://www.aap.org/advocacy/releases/may06.physical activity.htm

Conway, A. E., McClune, A. J., & Nosel, P. (2007). Down on the farm: Preventing farm accidents in children. *Pediatric Nursing, 33*, 45–48.

Council on Children with Disabilities, Section on Developmental Behavioral Pediatrics, Bright Futures Steering Committee and Medical Home Initiatives for Children with Special Needs Project Advisory Committee. (2006).

Edelman, C. L., & Mandle, C. L. (2006). *Health promotion throughout the life span* (6th ed.). St. Louis, MO: Mosby.

Gardiner, P., & Riley, D. S. (2007). Herbs to homeopathy—medicinal products for children. *Pediatric Clinics of North America, 54*, 859–874.

Hagan, J. F., Shaw, J. S., & Duncan, P. M. (Eds.). (2008). *Bright futures: Guidelines for health supervision of infants, children, and adolescents* (3rd ed.). Elk Grove Village, IL: American Academy of Pediatrics.

Hortz, B., & Petosa, R. L. (2008). Social cognitive theory variables mediation of moderate exercise. *American Journal of Health Behavior, 32*, 305–314.

Liu, J., Probst, J. C., Martin, A. B., Wang, J. Y., & Salinas, C. F. (2007). Disparities in dental insurance coverage and dental care among US children: The National Survey of Children's Health. *Pediatrics, 119*, S12–S21.

Mayo Clinic. (2009). *Teen sleep: Why is your teen so tired?* Retrieved from http://www.mayoclinic.com/health/teens-health

Mindell, J. A., Meltzer, L. J., Carskadon, M. A., & Chervin, R. D. (2009). Developmental aspects of sleep hygiene: Findings from the 2004 National Sleep Foundation Sleep in America Poll. *Sleep Medicine, 10*(7), 771–779.

Murray, R. B., Zentner, J. P., & Yakimo, R. (2009). *Health promotion strategies through the life span* (8th ed.). Upper Saddle River, NJ: Prentice Hall Health.

National Institutes of Health. (2009). *Adolescent depression*. Retrieved from http://www.nlm.nih.gov/medlineplus/ency/article;001518.htm

Olson, C. M., Bove, C. F., & Miller, E. O. (2007). Growing up poor: Long-term implications for eating patterns and body weight. *Appetite, 49*, 198–207.

Pender, N. J., Murdaugh, C. L., & Parsons, M. A. (2006). *Health promotion in nursing practice* (5th ed.). Upper Saddle River, NJ: Prentice Hall.

Rosen, L. D., & Breuner, C. C. (2007). Primary care from infancy to adolescence. *Pediatric Clinics of North America, 54*, 837–858.

Royal, S. T., Kendrick, D., & Coleman, T. (2007). Promoting bicycle helmet wearing by children using non-legislative interventions: Systematic review and meta-analysis. *Injury Prevention 13*, 162–167.

Santrock, J. W. (2007). *Child development* (11th ed.). Boston: McGraw-Hill.

Simons-Morton, B., & Ouimet, M. C. (2006). Parent involvement in novice teen driving: A review of the literature. *Injury Prevention, 12*, 30–37.

U.S. Department of Health and Human Services. (2006). *Healthy People 2010: Midcourse Review*. Washington, DC: Author.

Nursing Considerations for the Child in the Community

chapter 10

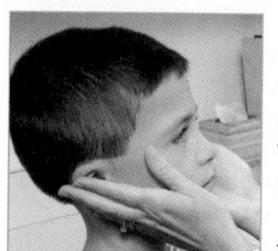

Ernesto, 7 years old, was sent by his teacher to the school nurse because he had become quiet and withdrawn. Ernesto is usually a healthy and happy child who actively participates in the classroom. When the teacher asked him what was wrong, he complained that his head and stomach were hurting.

The school nurse has seen several other children in the health office today with the same complaints. Ernesto reports that he felt fine when he arrived at school, but shortly after he started feeling achy. His throat feels scratchy and it hurts to swallow. His head aches all over. He ate breakfast this morning, and now his stomach is upset. He has not vomited. He wants to go home so he can lie down.

When the school nurse checked Ernesto's temperature, it was 38.6°C (100.5°F). She performed a quick physical assessment, including the head, eyes, ears, nose, mouth, throat, and abdomen. His eyes and ears are clear, but his throat and tonsils look inflamed. No pain is detected when lightly palpating his abdomen. The school nurse makes the decision to call Ernesto's mother to ask that he be taken home for ongoing care.

What is the role of the nurse in the school setting? How does the school nurse work with school personnel to promote the health of students? What activities might the school nurse engage in to help educate children about their health condition? How does the school nurse participate in emergency care planning to be prepared for a child with a serious acute illness or injury?

Key Terms

community assessment / 253
decontamination / 257
disaster preparedness / 255
disasters / 255
emergency preparedness / 248
epidemiologist / 254
medically fragile / 250
morbidity / 253
primary care / 244
stakeholders / 253
windshield survey / 254

Learning Outcomes

After reading this chapter, you will be able to do the following:

1. Identify the community health care settings where children receive health care services.
2. Contrast the roles of nurses in each community health care setting.
3. Develop a nursing care plan for a child in the school setting who has short-term mobility limitations.
4. Examine five ways in which nurses assist families in the home health care setting.
5. Develop a plan for emergency preparedness in a community health care setting.
6. Explain the roles of nurses in disaster preparedness.

■ COMMUNITY-BASED HEALTH CARE

Health care for children has been rapidly shifting from inpatient hospital care to community-based care over the past 15 to 20 years. Health plans and health care providers continue to explore options to provide safe, high-quality care with fewer hospitalizations or shorter stays when hospitalization is needed. Patterns of health care delivery are changing due to technologic developments and efforts to reduce health care costs. Examples include:

- Day surgery and invasive diagnostic procedures performed in outpatient surgical settings
- Short-stay or observation units in emergency departments to reduce the number of hospital admissions
- Intravenous antibiotic therapy provided in the home
- Pediatric hospice and palliative care in the home setting

The trend in out-of-hospital care has significantly increased for children with chronic health conditions and advanced disease states. Technologic advances, such as portable medical equipment, now make it possible to provide complex health care services in the home and other community settings, and this care is less costly. Home care services and other support services have been developed to assist these families. See Chapter 12 ∞ for more discussion of care for the child with a chronic illness.

However, pediatric health care in the community occurs along a continuum that covers the entire child health care system. This continuum is reflected in the Bindler and Ball Continuum of Pediatric Health (2007), including health promotion and health maintenance services; care for chronic conditions, acute illnesses, and injuries; and end-of-life care (see Chapter 1 ∞). Health care for individual children is improved when there is continuity of care and communication between health care settings.

The nurse working with families in a community setting uses knowledge of how the larger environment influences the child's health and development and the family's functioning, and integrates that information into the nursing care plan. See Chapter 4 ∞ for a discussion of the ecologic model that examines the interactions between the child and the environment, and Chapter 18 ∞ for many examples of environmental influences. Learning about the health care resources available within the child's community is important in offering families options for needed health care services.

To work effectively in the community, the nurse needs to gain experience and skills in:

- Conducting child and family assessments, working with families to plan individualized health care strategies, and implementing and evaluating nursing care strategies to match family economic, cultural, and social situations, and available resources
- Working with community agencies (schools, faith-based groups, and other community-based resources) to assess, plan strategies, and implement and evaluate approaches addressed to the health care needs of the community's children

■ COMMUNITY-BASED HEALTH CARE SETTINGS

Children receive most of their health care (health promotion and episodic health care for acute illnesses and injuries) in community settings. Depending on the community, health care resources, and age of the child, care may be received in all or only a few of the following settings:

- A *health care center* or a *physician's office* is the usual site for **primary care**, the range of health services that includes health promotion, health maintenance, episodic acute care, and health management of children with chronic conditions. See Chapters 7 through 9 ∞ for age-specific health promotion and health maintenance guidelines.
- A *public health clinic* may provide health promotion and health maintenance services. A homeless shelter may also have the capacity to offer such services.
- A *hospital outpatient center* may provide specialized services to children with chronic conditions or a full range of services similar to a health center.
- *Schools* usually provide health promotion and health maintenance services, plus first aid and emergency care as needed. School-based health centers may additionally provide counseling, health education, and care for acute conditions. Some school settings offer other services, such as preschool and after-school childcare services.
- *Childcare centers* provide first aid for emergencies and some health promotion services.
- The *home* is now a site for a child's acute condition or chronic condition management, rehabilitation, and end-of-life care when the family is supported by home health services.

The Nurse's Role in Community Settings

The nurse in any of the community settings has an important role in promoting the health and safety of the child, being a leader in setting policies in the center, and using the nursing process to help families meet the health care needs of their children. The nurse may assume the role of direct care provider, educator, advocate, or planner.

The Office or Health Care Center Setting

The nursing process is used when providing care for children in the health care center. The range of assessment responsibilities may vary by setting and by the preparation and experience of the nurse (Figure 10–1 ➤). Specific functions of the pediatric nurse in this setting include the following:

- Identifying children in need of urgent care or isolation
- Performing nursing assessments, including the health history, vital signs, growth and development, nutritional status, immunization status, and family strengths and challenges
- Conducting physical examinations
- Performing age-appropriate screening tests to detect health problems such as vision or hearing loss, anemia, and lead poisoning to ensure that the child has access to all needed health services (see Chapters 7 through 9 ∞)
- Assisting with physician examinations and diagnostic tests

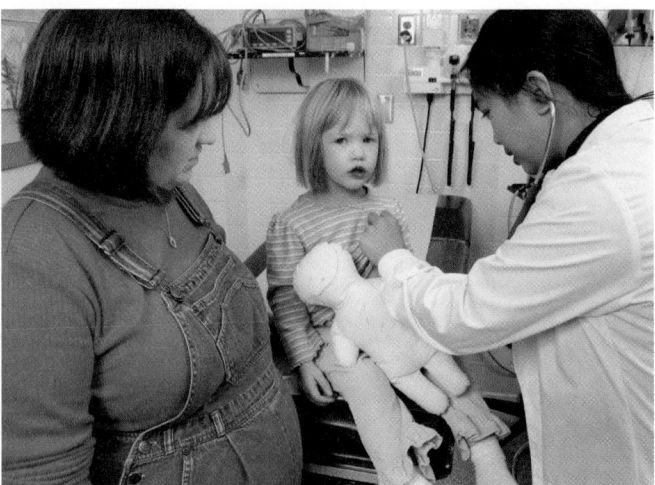

FIGURE 10–1 ➤ Nurses carefully assess children in the office setting who present with an acute illness. It is important to identify how serious the child's illness is and to monitor the child for progression of symptoms during the visit. This is also a time to gather information about the child's illness and to identify health information that will be needed for the family to care for the child at home.

- Developing nursing diagnoses and implementing a plan of care
- Providing immunizations (see Chapter 16 ∞)
- Providing information about procedures and offering reassurance
- Providing patient education for health promotion or management of the health condition
- Linking families with community resources
- Following infection control guidelines and ensuring that the health care setting is a safe environment. See the *Clinical Skills Manual* for infection control guidelines.

An important goal is to develop a positive relationship with the child and family so that optimal health care is provided. This relationship is strengthened over time during future health care visits.

Clinical Tip

The initial interaction with the child and family may set the stage for a long-term relationship since the family often returns to the same setting for health care over many years. As you approach the child and family, put aside the stressors you may be feeling. Take a few moments to play with the infant or child and to comment to the parents about one of the child's positive attributes. The parent's, and perhaps the child's, stress level will also be reduced, facilitating the beginning of a long-term partnership.

Telephone Advice

Some nurses in the office or health care setting provide telephone advice to families. They need extensive knowledge of pediatrics and excellent communication skills to listen and interpret the information given by the caller. Nurses use protocols or published manuals approved by the health facility to guide the advice given to parents, such as specific care to provide at home or the need for an urgent health care visit. The call information is documented in the child's medical record.

Identifying Severely Ill and Injured Children

Each child with an episodic illness or injury presenting to the health center must be assessed upon arrival to determine the urgency of care needed. A rapid assessment for changes in mental status, airway patency, breathing, and circulation is used to identify the child that needs immediate medical attention. The child with an urgent condition must be monitored frequently to detect any worsening of condition and need for emergency care.

Emergency Response Planning

The nurse collaborates with the physician to develop an emergency response plan for the health center. Completion of Basic Life Support and Pediatric Advanced Life Support training every 2 years is important for the nurse and physician. Nonclinical staff must be trained to recognize a child needing immediate assessment by the nurse and what their role is during an emergency. The nurse may coordinate mock drills so that all employees know how to perform their designated role when a true emergency occurs. The appropriate emergency phone numbers (poison control center, 911 or local emergency number, hospital emergency department) are posted throughout the health center. The nurse is often responsible for ensuring that all emergency care equipment, supplies, and medications are organized and readily available in a central treatment room (Box 10–1).

Educating the Child and Family

Patient education regarding injury prevention, growth and development, nutrition, and healthy lifestyles is an important nursing role. The nurse also may be responsible for selecting patient education materials for the waiting area and those specifically used to teach families about various conditions. Knowledge of the community and population served by the health center enables the nurse to select appropriate education materials.

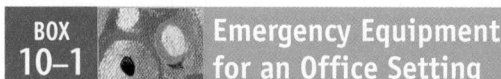

BOX 10–1 Emergency Equipment for an Office Setting

Required emergency equipment for managing a pediatric emergency in a health center includes the following in various pediatric sizes (American Academy of Pediatrics Committee on Pediatric Emergency Medicine, 2007):

- Oxygen delivery system (bag-valve masks in 450 and 1000 mL sizes, clear oxygen face masks with and without reservoir)
- Airway equipment (oral and nasopharyngeal airways, suction devices, laryngoscope handle and blades, endotracheal tubes and stylet, end-tidal CO_2 detector, nasogastric tubes)
- Pulse oximeter, peak flow meter, and a nebulizer or metered-dose inhaler with a spacer/mask
- Intravenous (IV) and intraosseous needles, IV tubing, and normal saline or lactated Ringer's IV solution
- A length-based resuscitation tape and preprinted drug dosage chart to quickly identify equipment sizes and drug dosages by the length or weight of the child
- Drugs (epinephrine 1:1000, albuterol for inhalation, activated charcoal, naloxone, and 25% dextrose)

Locate the emergency equipment in every clinical setting where you have assignments so that you can quickly take the child to it or bring the equipment to the child if an emergency occurs.

Nurses teach families to provide the condition-specific care for the child at home, and assess the need for repeated or additional education. Examples of information provided include:

- Signs that the condition is not improving as expected and when to return to the physician
- How and when to administer prescribed medications, and their potential side effects
- Modifications in diet and activity
- Other supportive care for the child's condition
- Education to help the child and family recognize the need to initiate care for a new episode of a chronic condition (e.g., asthma, sickle cell anemia, or hemophilia) that may prevent the need for a health care visit or reduce the severity of the episode

Identifying Community Resources

Nurses in the health care home are often involved in identifying community resources needed by the child and family to promote the child's health. Compiling a manual of community resources and regularly updating names and phone numbers of contacts will make it easier to provide information efficiently. Examples of community resources that might be included are early intervention programs, support groups, language and translation services, food banks, lead paint abatement services, social services, and mental health services.

Ensuring a Safe Environment for Children

The health center has many potential hazards such as equipment, cleaning supplies, needles, lancets, medications, and laboratory materials. The child must be attended at all times when in the examination area. Guidelines for infection control must be developed and implemented to reduce the transmission of infectious diseases between child patients and between the health care providers and children.

Hospital Outpatient Center

Pediatric nurses also provide care for children with acute and chronic conditions within hospital outpatient or specialty care ambulatory settings. Children may be referred to physician specialists for diagnostic workups or the long-term management of their chronic conditions. In some cases, health promotion, health maintenance, and episodic illness care are provided to children with chronic conditions in these settings. With experience, pediatric nurses working in a hospital ambulatory setting develop specialized knowledge and skill to meet the specific needs of the population of children cared for in that setting (Figure 10–2 ➤). The roles for nurses in these settings are similar to those described for the health center.

School Health Settings

Schools have a role in ensuring the physical and mental health of students because these factors are related to successful learning (American Nurses Association, 2007). School nursing is a specialized nursing practice that promotes the well-being, academic success, and lifelong achievement of students. School nurses promote normal development, health, and safety of students. They intervene with actual and potential health problems

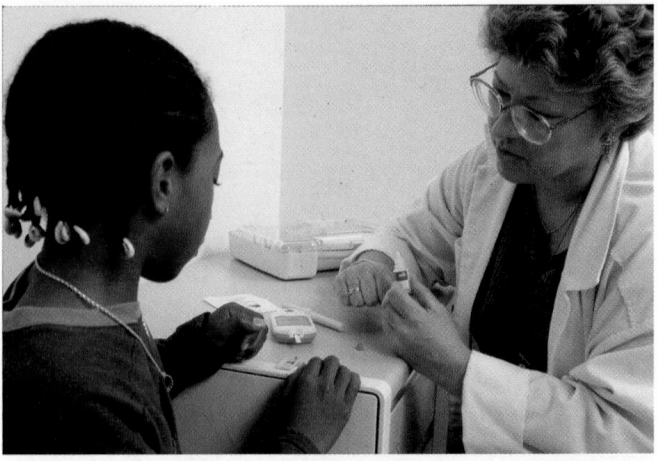

FIGURE 10–2 ➤ Nurses often assume a larger role in working with children and families with a chronic health condition in the hospital ambulatory setting. Developing a care plan and educating the family to manage type 1 diabetes is an important role of this pediatric nurse who is also a nationally certified diabetes educator.

and manage the care needed by children with complex health problems (American Nurses Association, 2007). The school nurse has seven core responsibilities (American Academy of Pediatrics Council on School Health, 2008):

- Provides direct care to students with injuries and acute illnesses, and long-term health conditions (Figure 10–3A ➤)
- Provides planning leadership for meeting health care needs of students and for responding to emergencies and disasters
- Provides screening and referral for health conditions (Figure 10–3B)
- Promotes a healthy and safe school environment by monitoring immunizations, excluding children with infectious conditions, monitoring playground equipment safety, and implementing plans for violence and bullying prevention
- Provides health education on topics such as nutrition, exercise, oral health, smoking cessation, sexually transmitted infections, adolescent pregnancy prevention, and parenting
- Serves as a leader in the development and evaluation of school health policies, such as for school health programs, wellness, disaster management, mental health intervention, and acute illness management
- Serves as a liaison between school personnel, the family, and health care professionals—for example, as a case manager for students with health problems, collaborating with the student's physician to ensure coordinated care, or participating on teams to develop individualized education plans (IEPs) and individualized health plans (IHPs)

Box 10–2 contains *Healthy People 2020* national health objectives that illustrate the breadth of school nursing.

School nurses practice independently as the only licensed health care provider in the school setting. However, each school has a physician consultant with whom the school nurse partners to discuss and update standing orders for urgent and emergency

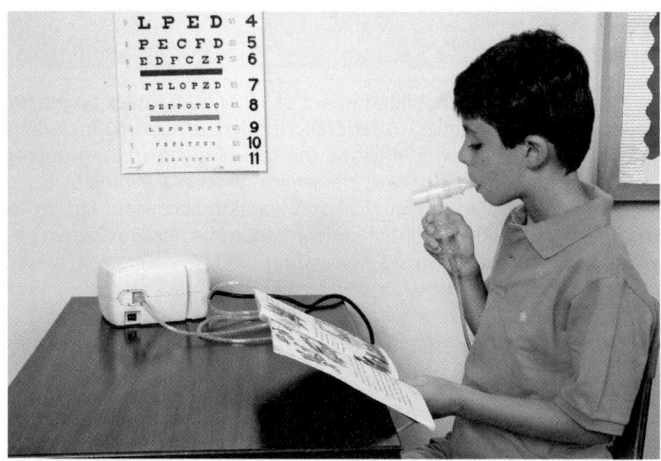

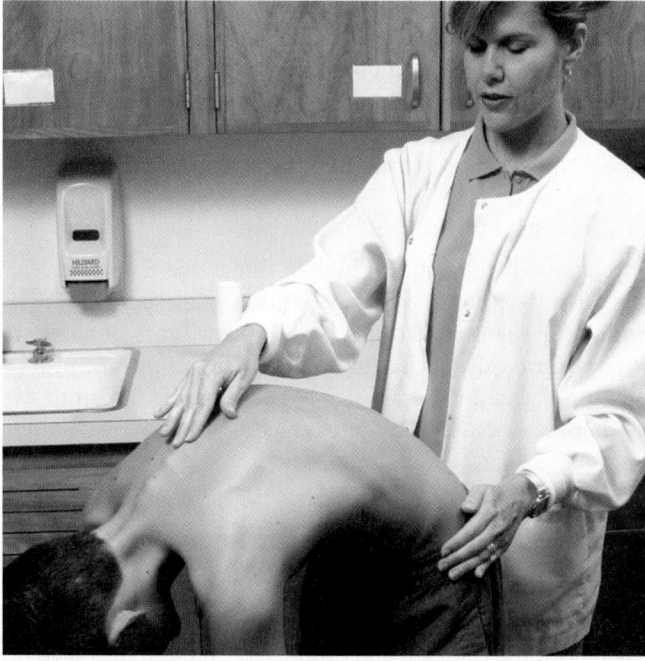

FIGURE 10–3 ➤ A, The school nurse treats this child with an asthma episode using medication in a nebulizer as directed in the child's asthma action plan. The parent should be informed about the nebulizer treatment in case the child's asthma episode continues and additional treatment is needed. B, The school nurse often performs screening for scoliosis of fifth-grade students to enable early identification and referral to the student's health care provider for care of the condition. Other screening tests (e.g., hearing and vision) are often organized so all children in a particular grade are assessed.

care for potential student health care problems. The National Association of School Nurses and other national organizations recommend a ratio of 1 nurse per 750 students, and a much lower ratio when the school setting has a large population of children with special health care needs or severe disabilities (American Academy of Pediatrics Council on School Health, 2008). Depending on the school system, some school nurses work in multiple schools and serve many more children than the recommended ratio. See the companion website for guidelines for health, mental health, and safety in school settings.

■ Increase the proportion of elementary, middle, and senior high schools that provide comprehensive school health education to prevent health problems in the following areas: unintentional injury; violence; suicide; tobacco use and addiction; alcohol or other drug use; unintended pregnancy, HIV/AIDS, and STD infection; unhealthy dietary patterns; and inadequate physical activity.

■ Increase the proportion of the nation's elementary, middle, and senior high schools that have a nurse-to-student ratio of at least 1:750.

■ Increase the proportion of elementary, middle, and senior high schools that have health education goals or objectives that address the knowledge and skills articulated in the National Health Education Standards (high school, middle, elementary).

■ Increase the proportion of public and private schools that require students to wear appropriate protective gear when engaged in school-sponsored physical activities.

■ Reduce weapon carrying by adolescents on school property.

■ Increase the percentage of schools with a school breakfast program.

■ Increase the percentage of schools that offer nutritious foods and beverages outside of school meals.

■ Increase the proportion of school-based health centers with an oral health component.

■ Increase the proportion of states and school districts that require regularly scheduled elementary school recess.

■ Increase the proportion of the nation's public and private schools that require daily physical education for all students.

■ Increase the proportion of adolescents who spend at least 50 percent of school physical education class time being physically active.

■ Increase the proportion of children and youth with disabilities who spend at least 80 percent of their time in regular education programs.

Data from: U.S. Department of Health and Human Services, Office of Disease Prevention and Health Promotion. (2010). Healthy People. *Washington, DC: Author. Retrieved from http://www.healthypeople.gov/Default.htm*

School-Based Health Centers

A school-based health center (SBHC) provides comprehensive physical, mental, and dental health services to children in a setting near the school attended. Comprehensive physical, reproductive, and mental health services plus health education are often provided by a multidisciplinary team of nurse practitioners, physicians, physician assistants, mental health providers, and other supporting staff (National Association of Pediatric Nurse Practitioners, 2009). SBHCs exist in 45 states, predominantly in urban communities. The most common diagnoses in the centers serving middle and high school students relate to reproductive health and psychosocial health issues (Scudder, Papa, & Brey, 2007). The school nurse may collaborate with a SBHC, by identifying students to receive services and then helping to implement recommended care to the student in the school setting.

Preparation for Emergencies

Every school needs a plan to ensure effective emergency care and transport for an acutely ill or injured child. The school nurse often works with the school administrators, the physician consultant,

School Health and Safety Guidelines Websites

and the local emergency medical services (EMS) agency to develop an emergency response plan for children who need transport to a local emergency department because of severe illness or injury. School nurses often train school personnel to identify an emergency that requires activation of the local EMS system and to provide first aid until the EMS providers arrive.

Because other potential emergencies can occur, such as natural and man-made disasters, and behavioral crises, each school needs an **emergency preparedness** plan, a community-based coordinated response plan for such an incident. See page 255 for more information.

Facilitating a Child's Return to School

The school nurse facilitates the child's return to the classroom following an acute illness or injury, especially when environmental adaptation is required or when a change in health status has occurred. Often an IHP must be developed or modified to meet Section 504 requirements. (See Chapter 12 ∞.) The school nurse, in collaboration with the parents, helps educate teachers and administrators about the child's special needs. Classmates may need to be prepared for a child's physical changes. Sometimes the teacher's expectations of the child need to be modified, such as a child recovering from a mild brain injury who has decreased ability to concentrate for several weeks after injury.

Clinical Judgment

How would consulting with the health care provider of a child with type 1 diabetes be of benefit in planning and advocating for the child during the school day?

 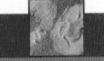

Section 504 of the Rehabilitation Act of 1973 guarantees access for children with disabilities to federally funded programs, including public schools. Section 504 allows the school nurse and a group of knowledgeable individuals to determine a child's eligibility for a student-specific plan for physical and learning accommodations to maximize the child's potential for learning in the least restrictive environment (American Nurses Association, 2007).

Children with Health Care Conditions

It is estimated that 20–30% of children have a chronic health condition, with some conditions being complex (American Nurses Association, 2007). (See Chapter 12 ∞.) Approximately 4–6% of students have daily medication administered at school, such as medications for asthma and diabetes (Clay, Farris, McCarthy, et al., 2008). Some children in the school setting require medical assistive devices such as insulin pumps or ventilators, and some other children require skilled nursing care for intermittent catheterization, tracheostomy care, and gastrostomy tube feedings. See Evidence-Based Practice: Improving School Nurse Access to Student Asthma Action Plans.

Childcare Settings

Approximately 12 million children under age 6 years receive care in out-of-home childcare settings while parents are at work (Crowley & Kulikowich, 2009). Many types of childcare arrangements exist, such as in-home care by a family member or nanny, a licensed childcare family home setting for up to five children, or a licensed childcare center for six or more children.

Evidence-Based Practice
Improving School Nurse Access to Student Asthma Action Plans

Problem

An asthma action plan describes the daily control medications, quick relief medications to take once symptoms of an asthma episode are identified, and when to call the health professional. What methods work to increase the number of children with asthma who have an asthma action plan at school?

Evidence

A pilot study explored ways to increase communication between physicians and school nurses and to empower nurses to implement an asthma education program. Participating physicians were given education on national asthma guidelines, baseline data to include in asthma action plans, a Medicaid reimbursement code for development of asthma action plans, and office support for development of plans. School nurses received similar education, support to provide asthma education in the school, and asthma action plans from participating physicians. Community organization representatives provided support to the project and facilitated communication. Study results revealed that 32 additional students (a 44% increase) had asthma action plans after the intervention (Frankowski, Keating, Rexroad, et al., 2006). Another study compared direct school nurse communication with a child's physician versus parent communication for the purpose of obtaining an asthma action plan for the child's management at school. Twenty children with asthma in grades 6 through 8 from four school districts met daily with the nurse for 2 weeks to learn correct peak flow meter technique and to

track peak flow readings. The school nurse sent this information to the parents and the child's physician with a request for an asthma action plan. The control group consisted of 20 same-aged students with asthma in the same communities but different schools. School nurses continued a standard practice of requesting asthma action plans through the control group children's parents. Significantly more asthma action plans were obtained from the physicians who were directly approached and provided with data about the child's peak flow readings (Pulcini, DeSisto, & McIntyre, 2007).

Implications

Community collaboration may be one way to improve access to and use of asthma action plans. School nurses with access to asthma action plans report using them more than 90% of the time to manage a child's asthma episode (McLaughlin, Maljanian, Kornblum, et al., 2006). Children who receive appropriate asthma management at school are more likely to return to the classroom for learning than to go home or to the emergency department.

Critical Thinking Application

During a school clinical placement, compare the estimated number of children with asthma and the number with an asthma action plan. What strategies has the school nurse used to obtain asthma action plans? How effective have the strategies been? What other strategies might increase the number of asthma action plans?

Research *Case Management*

A study of school-nurse case management of 114 children (aged 5 to 9 years) with chronic conditions such as diabetes, asthma, severe allergies, seizures, and sickle cell anemia evaluated the impact of services on academic health, and quality of life outcomes over a school year. Selected children had needs that were ongoing and interfering with their school performance. Case managers worked with children and families on a regular basis to help control symptoms and to prevent problems. Children who were case managed had improved quality of life, better skills and knowledge to manage their health condition, and greater participation in extracurricular activities (Engelke, Guttu, Warren, et al., 2008).

States establish minimum licensure requirements and guidelines for the safe operation of childcare settings that address the staff qualifications, staff-to-child ratio, staff training requirements, safe food handling, safe health practices, and environmental safety. See the companion website for guidelines for the safe operation of childcare centers.

Many states require or recommend the use of a health consultant to promote healthy and safe practices and to address the health needs of children (Crowley & Kulikowich, 2009). Nurses can assume this important consultant role by assisting in development of the childcare center's policies for health practices, teaching staff about safe health practices, and monitoring and promoting health practices in the setting. The nurse consultant can also teach staff to identify children with illnesses and to provide first aid for injured children. Head Start childcare centers are federally mandated to screen children for medical, dental, and developmental problems using licensed health consultants (Gupta, Pascoe, Blanchard, et al., 2009).

Reducing Disease Transmission

Children in childcare centers are at higher risk for infectious diseases. Children are close together in large numbers, they put things in their mouths, they may be contagious before symptoms occur, and they are susceptible to most infectious agents. The nurse can educate and work with the childcare center manager and staff to reduce disease transmission in the following ways (Mink & Yeh, 2009):

- Teaching staff when and how to perform hand hygiene, manage secretions, sanitize toys and surfaces, and manage cuts and scrapes
- Monitoring the immunization status of children and encouraging parents to get their child immunized on the recommended schedule (see Chapter 16 ∞)

Research *Nurse Consultant Effectiveness*

A study was designed to evaluate the effectiveness of nurse consultants in 111 licensed childcare centers in five California counties. The 73 childcare centers with nurse consultants were found to have a greater number and higher quality of written health and safety policies that are consistent with national standards in contrast to the 38 comparison centers. The centers with nurse consultants also improved many health and safety practices, such as emergency preparedness and handwashing (Alkon, Bernzweig, To, et al., 2009).

- Developing guidelines for the exclusion of unimmunized children when a vaccine-preventable disease occurs in the facility, and for the exclusion and return of children with various infectious conditions
- Checking each child daily for signs and symptoms of illness (e.g., behavior changes, rashes, fever, vomiting, diarrhea, and eye drainage), and caring for the sick child, reducing exposure to others until the child goes home
- Developing guidelines for diapering infants and toddlers
- Developing guidelines for food preparation

Health Promotion and Health Maintenance

Health promotion activities within a childcare center encourage the child's highest level of functioning and development, such as having activities that stimulate physical, emotional, and cognitive development as well as nutrition that fosters growth. Health maintenance activities prevent injury or disease, such as immunization monitoring, infection control, and placing infants on their back to sleep.

▲ **Health Promotion**

Nurses working with a childcare center can design and offer health education programs for the children (such as tooth brushing, hand hygiene, blowing the nose into a tissue, and coughing or sneezing into the elbow or shirt sleeve if a tissue is not available) to promote healthy habits.

Environmental Safety

Ensure that the childcare center maintains a current list of which family members may take a child from the facility, and has guidelines for verifying identity when necessary. These guidelines are important to prevent child abduction.

The nurse should inspect the childcare environment to identify hazards that could cause injury to the children. Cleaning supplies and other toxins must be stored in a locked cabinet to prevent exposure. Inspect toys used by children to ensure that there are no sharp edges or points, small parts, or pinching parts. Playground equipment should also be checked for safety (Figure 10–4 ➤).

Emergency Care Planning

As in the school setting, guidelines for assessing and identifying the child with an emergency health condition are essential. An emergency care plan must be developed to care for an acutely ill or injured child. This plan should include giving first aid, calling emergency medical services to transport the child to the emergency department, notifying the parent, and accompanying the child to the emergency department until the parent arrives.

Home Health Care Setting

Home health care is a component of the continuum of comprehensive community health care provided to children and families in their home. An estimated 500,000 children use home health services in the United States (American Academy of Pediatrics Committee on Child Health Financing, 2006). Most children receive intermittent skilled nursing visits to assess the child and to see how family members are managing the child's

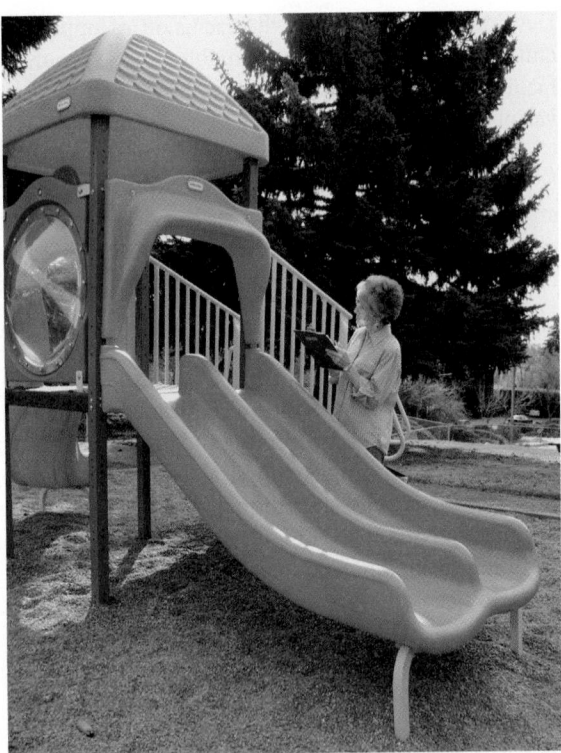

FIGURE 10–4 ➤ Assess the childcare center's environment for safety hazards. Check the area around playground equipment, making sure there are wood chips or cushioned tiles under the equipment. Inspect the playground equipment for protruding screws, loose nuts and bolts, and instability at least monthly.

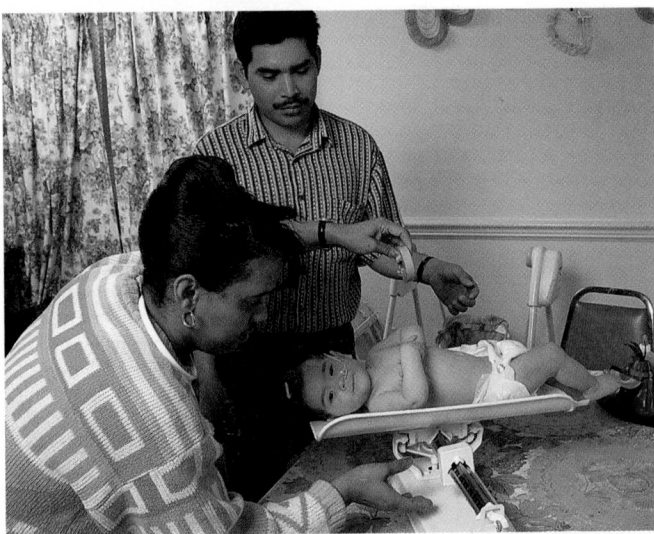

FIGURE 10–5 ➤ Nurses provide both short-term and long-term services to families in the home setting. In some cases, families need support for a short time after the child is discharged from the hospital following an acute illness. In other cases, families need assistance with complex nursing care for the child dependent on technology for survival.

health care needs. Home health services may be provided to children with complex health conditions, short-term acute conditions, and even terminal conditions. See Chapter 12 ∞ for the care of children with chronic conditions. See Chapter 13 ∞ for more information about palliative and hospice care in the home setting.

Many children needing home health care are **medically fragile**, dependent upon a medical device either for survival or prevention of further disability. Parents and other care providers without backgrounds in health care are given tremendous responsibilities to provide technology-assisted health care to their child. Technology-assisted care in the home may include any of the following: ventilators; tracheostomies; suctioning; nasogastric, gastrostomy, or parenteral feeding with feeding pumps; and intravenous fluids and medications with intravenous pumps. In some cases, families have created mini–intensive care units in their home.

The home environment is believed to be optimal for the long-term care of these children so they can participate as family members and have their growth and development promoted (Figure 10–5 ➤). The family gains some control over their lives by having the child in the home rather than coordinating visits to the child and trying to simultaneously maintain a relatively normal family life. However, the family is challenged to balance the child's fragility and life-sustaining needs with the needs of the other family members. See Chapter 12 ∞ for further discussion of support for families of children with chronic conditions.

Health insurers pay many of the costs associated with home care; however, the family may be financially burdened by paying some costs out of pocket, such as medications, supplies, and transportation. In some cases a parent must give up employment to provide care to the child and to qualify for Medicaid which is the major payer of home health services for children. Parents often feel like they have no choice about providing the ongoing care to their child (Carnevale, Alexander, Davis, et al., 2006). Health care systems (health care providers and insurers) are challenged to simultaneously address the child's illness and developmental needs while providing the support needed by these families so that children do well in their home environments.

Nurses require a variety of skills and knowledge to work in the home care setting, such as:

• Knowledge and experience in acute care practice with various medical technologies used with children. These skills enable nurses to provide direct care, teach the family and child self-care practices, and monitor the child's progress.

Culture *Assessment*

When assessing the child and family in the home, recognize when there are potential conflicts between recommended medical care and the family's preferences. Identify which family member is most influential in decisions about care provided for the child. Use open-ended questions to talk with family members and learn about the health care issue from their point of view. Ask the family to describe the issue, why it is a concern, and the impact on the lives of family members. Information gained can then be used to educate the family and to develop a nursing care plan that integrates the family's preferences for the child's care.

- An understanding of the community's health resources and health care financing mechanisms to better assist families to find the most supportive services to match the child's and family's needs.
- An understanding of the community's cultural diversity and the cultural values of the families served.
- Skills in communication and in educating family members to assume care of the child.

NURSING MANAGEMENT

Nurses in the home care setting use the nursing process to assess the child, family, and home environment. Then the nurse assists the family to manage care of a child with a chronic condition more independently while promoting the child's growth and development. A major goal of working with families in the home health care setting includes promoting or restoring the child's health while attempting to minimize the effects of the disability and illness, including terminal illness. The success of home care is also based upon effective cultural communication.

Nursing Assessment and Diagnosis

Home health care nurses assess the home, the child, and the family during intermittent skilled nursing visits. Home assessment is focused on environmental safety for the child and the resources needed for the child's care. When working with the hospital discharge planner to initiate home health care services, the nurse assesses the following aspects of the home:

- Home readiness (safe sleeping arrangements, adequate supplies, ability to meet nutritional and fluid needs, telephone access, heat, electricity, refrigeration, water supply, lack of any communicable diseases in the home, safety within the home, and safe access into and out of the home).
- Potential hazards related to the child's age, condition, and requirements for technology-assisted care (e.g., tripping hazard when extension cords used to power equipment are needed to reach electrical outlets).
- Features in the home environment that could cause an acute illness, such as using a woodstove or fireplace that could cause respiratory distress, or renovating a house built before 1960 that could expose the child to lead dust. Additionally, the nurse may identify family members who smoke.

Assessment of the child is focused on the current health status, growth, developmental progress, and social interaction with family members and health care providers (Figure 10–6 ➤). Observe for the potential of abuse and neglect as these children are at a higher risk.

Family strengths and coping abilities are evaluated using the family assessment guidelines in Chapter 2 ∞. The family is assessed for parenting skills, as well as their abilities in providing the child's needed medical procedures and monitoring the child's health status. The presence of siblings, their developmental and physical status, and their needs should also be assessed.

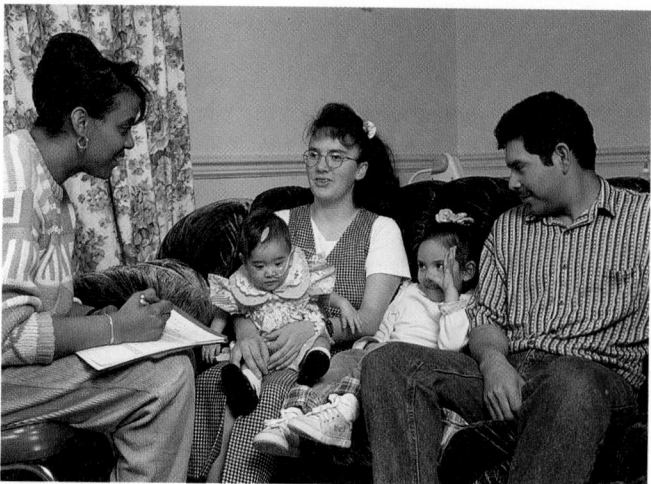

FIGURE 10–6 ➤ A visit to the home when all family members are present provides the best information for assessing caregiver readiness to care for the child being discharged from the hospital with a complex health condition.

Examples of nursing diagnoses that could apply to the family as the child transitions from the hospital to home setting include the following:

- Impaired Home Maintenance related to insufficient family organization and planning
- Impaired Adjustment (Parents) related to multiple stressors in caring for a child with a complex health condition in the home
- Ineffective therapeutic regimen management related to complexity of medical interventions
- Impaired social interaction related to therapeutic isolation

Planning and Implementation

Nursing care should focus on promoting an environment within the home for the child to develop, learn social skills, and gain a sense of identity based on family values. Nurses help families in the home setting in the following ways:

- Ensuring competent care to the child
- Educating parents about the child's condition and the physical signs and symptoms that may indicate a change in health status
- Educating parents and demonstrating methods to promote the child's development
- Linking families to community resources, including support groups, respite care, and therapeutic recreation
- Assisting families in time management skills and patient care management
- Advocating for increased insurance coverage or locating other sources of financial assistance

Collaborating with the Family

The nurse and family work in partnership in the home to promote the health of the child and of the family as a unit. It is essential for the nurse to develop a respectful and trusting relationship with the parents.

Although few families have home health care nurses in the home for extended hours, those that do lose privacy and often find it stressful to have a nonfamily member present. The home health care nurse must recognize and accept that the family has the control in the home care setting because the family employs the nurse. Every interaction is negotiated with the family, or between the family and child, if there are differences in what they want. The nurse must be flexible and able to set aside power. Conflicts may occur when differences in opinion about the child's care become apparent. Maintain open communication to learn what is important to the child and family, and then modify the nursing care plan when appropriate. House rules for such things as parking, private areas in the home, and routines may need to be negotiated, but then rules must be followed. The success of home care is also based upon effective cultural communication. For example, some Jewish families follow strict dietary guidelines that do not permit milk and meat to be mixed. The nurse needs to abide by the dietary guidelines and observe the family's food preparation practices.

Role expectations of the nurse must be clearly understood to reduce stress in the family. When nurses provide home care, it is important for a parent to be present and work in partnership with the nurse. Informed consent is needed for invasive treatments and decisions for provision of emergency care to avoid serious risk to life and limb.

The range of nursing care activities in a child's home care plan may include sensory stimulation, routines of daily living, positioning and skin care with gentle handling, respiratory care, nutrition and elimination, medications, and other supportive therapies. Other providers, such as physical therapists, speech-language therapists, occupational therapists, and social workers, may provide other health care services in collaboration with the home health care nurse. Nursing care should focus on promoting an environment within the home for the child to develop, learn social skills, and gain a sense of identity based on family values.

Supporting the Family

When home health nursing is episodic, parents of children with complex conditions often feel stressed by the constant care demands. They may be sleep deprived when caring for the child 24 hours a day and need some assistance in identifying alternative care options, such as respite care, a service that allows parents to take a short break away from the daily care (see Chapter 12 ∞ for more information). Families often need support in identifying and advocating for potential services that may be of value to their child and financial resources for which they may be eligible. The home health nurse is often valued as a resource that can provide support, educate the family about managing the child's care, and advocate for resources for the family (Koshti-Richman, 2009).

Emergency Preparedness

The nurse should help the family develop an emergency care plan for any child whose condition could worsen rapidly and become life threatening (e.g., severe congenital heart defect, tracheostomy, or apnea), or be beyond the care that the parents or home health nurse can provide. The emergency care plan should provide guidelines for when to call 911. The local ambulance company needs to be notified that a child dependent on technol-

Families Want to Know
Developing a Fire Escape Plan

Developing a fire escape plan is important when the family has one or more children with special health care needs. Important steps for families to take in developing the plan include the following:

■ Have working smoke and carbon monoxide detectors in the home and teach children what the alarm means. Make sure batteries are checked at least twice a year.

■ Draw a diagram of your house. Mark all windows and doors. Plan two routes out of every room. Think about an escape plan if the fire starts in the kitchen, bedroom, or basement.

■ Have a portable ladder to hang out of a second-floor window.

■ Figure out the best way to get infants and young children out of the house. Will you carry them? If there is more than one child who needs to be carried, how will you get them out if you are the only adult?

■ Teach preschool and school-age children to follow the escape plan by crawling, touching doors, and going to the window if the door is hot. Show children how to cover their nose and mouth to reduce smoke inhalation.

■ Prepare an alternative fire escape plan in case you are alone with the child when the fire begins.

■ Keep home exits clear of toys and debris.

■ Select a safe meeting place outside the home. Teach children not to go back inside the burning home.

ogy is cared for at home. The emergency care plan should include an essential medical history that gives the emergency care providers enough information to understand the child's health condition, to prevent delays in disease-specific treatment, and to minimize unnecessary interventions until the child's personal physician can be consulted. See the companion website for the American Academy of Pediatrics website with an emergency information form.

Families need to develop an emergency care plan for safe evacuation of the home in case of fire or other emergency. This is even more challenging when the child cannot mobilize independently and requires equipment for continued survival or quality of life. See Families Want to Know: Developing a Fire Escape Plan for information to help families develop a plan for safe evacuation of the home.

When the child is dependent upon technology, the family should notify the power company so that high priority can be given to getting resources to the home promptly after power outages. Backup generators may be needed if electrical power for life-sustaining equipment is essential. The child should also be registered for a disaster shelter that can accommodate the child's health care needs and at least one caregiver.

Evaluation

Expected outcomes of nursing care include:

- The family partners with the nurse to promote the child's health, growth, and development.
- Care of the child's medical needs is integrated into the family's routines.
- The family has an emergency care plan for the child.

Public Health Setting

Public health promotes the health of the population in a community rather than the care of individuals and has an emphasis on health promotion and disease prevention.

Community health nurses provide care to children in many public health settings, such as the following:

- *Public health clinics,* providing well-child care, immunizations, and care for other populations such as adolescents seeking family planning services or treatment for sexually transmitted diseases
- *Schools,* serving as school nurses or consultants on school health issues
- *Childcare settings,* serving as consultants for the health and safety of enrolled children
- *Homes,* providing skilled nursing care through a visiting nurses service, or by assisting high-risk families with the transition of a newborn into the family
- *Homeless shelters,* providing health promotion, health maintenance, and episodic illness care

Community health nurses take a leadership role in helping the population obtain health services through assessing community needs and resources, advocating for needed resources and services, and then developing health programs to address the needs of children and their families.

■ ASSESSMENT OF COMMUNITY NEEDS AND RESOURCES

Community Assessment

Community assessment is a process of compiling data about a community's health status and resources to develop a public health plan to address the health needs of a target population within that community. For example, the target population could be all children, a specific age group, or even a special group of children (such as those with a chronic condition). The community assessment process involves community partners, but follows the nursing process format. Information gained about the number of individuals with the health need and knowledge of existing resources helps health professionals determine if additional programs or resources are needed. An overview of the community assessment process is described, but additional resources such as a community health nursing textbook are needed to complete a full assessment.

Community assessments may be conducted for the following reasons:

- A request is made by interested community advocates or the local health department.
- Justification is needed to fund a new or expanded health care program.
- Evaluation of responses to health care programs or interventions (such as immunizations, injury prevention programs, or services targeted to new immigrants in the community) may provide the data to determine if the children with greatest needs have been appropriately targeted and are benefiting equally from the intervention.

The focus of a community assessment is on the target population, for example, ensuring that all children in the community, regardless of socioeconomic status and racial group, are considered when trying to ensure access to care or specific interventions—such as injury prevention programs, immunizations, school health services, or suicide prevention programs.

A community assessment is often initiated because one or more individuals (i.e., concerned parents, school nurse, or community leader) are concerned about a health or social issue, such as a child who is severely injured in a pedestrian crossing on the way to school. The concerned individuals partner with other **stakeholders** (all community residents, policy makers, health providers, and funders concerned with the outcome of the assessment) to investigate if this is an isolated event, or if similar incidents have happened at other locations and to identify ways to protect other children. Community partners for this investigation and community assessment may include nurses, family members, local organizations (e.g., Kiwanis, Safe Kids, parent-teacher association), the faith community, the local trauma center, an epidemiologist, elected officials, and health department representatives.

Family members, a pediatric nurse, and a school nurse are important members of the group when pediatric health issues are being addressed.

The first step in beginning a community assessment is to clearly define its purpose and scope to keep the process focused. The purpose is often associated with a specific problem that an advocate or community leader would like to have addressed by the community. Example issues could be one of the following:

- Several child pedestrians and bicyclists have been injured or killed by motor vehicles over the past 3 months in the same neighborhood.
- Two children drowned at the local lake in a boating incident.
- Three teens from a local high school have committed suicide in the past 2 months.
- The number of children who are fully immunized on school entry has decreased in the last year.

Once the purpose and scope of the assessment are determined, various factors that influence the health of a community should be considered when collecting assessment data (Clark, 2008, pp. 351–356).

- Demographic characteristics such as age composition of the community, birth statistics, age-specific and cause-specific mortality rates, racial composition, and **morbidity** (incidence and prevalence of certain diseases), as well as the immunization status of children

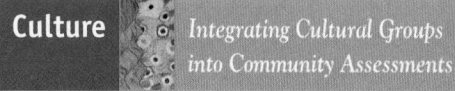

Culture *Integrating Cultural Groups into Community Assessments*

Community assessment leaders should invite community members representing different cultural groups to participate in the process. They help provide an important perspective of the community's needs and help identify culturally appropriate and culturally acceptable strategies to address the health problem.

Health Statistic Websites

- Community prospects for continuing growth or economic challenges, cohesion of the community in dealing with past health problems or crises, existing tensions between various community groups, adequacy of personal safety services, communication networks, stresses in the community, and incidence of crime, homicide, and suicide
- Type of community (rural, urban, suburban), size, climate, topographical features, housing adequacy, water supply, waste disposal, and potential hazards that could lead to a disaster
- Sociocultural characteristics such as local government and community leadership, transportation, income and education levels, employment rates, occupations, family composition, faith communities, cultural groups represented, language barriers to health care, number of homeless families and children, recreation, shopping, and social service agencies
- Behavioral characteristics such as nutrition and specific dietary patterns, use of harmful substances, exercise and recreational opportunities, and population use of safety practices
- Health services available to children in the community covered by health insurance, Medicaid, or the State Children's Health Insurance Program (SCHIP); services available to uninsured children; and barriers to health care access

Stakeholders next make plans for data collection (types of data to be gathered, sources of data, and methods for obtaining the data) and data analysis. Some of the best data to use are those calculated as rates. See Box 10–3 for commonly used rates. National, neighboring state, and state data can be compared with community data using rates to determine how similar or different the community statistics are for the health problem.

Data may be collected from many sources. For example, the Centers for Disease Control and Prevention collects state data and calculates birth rates and death rates for all types of conditions. Population data are available on the Internet from the U.S. Census. See the companion website for more resources. Other potential sources of data include a state or local trauma registry; an immunization registry; community surveys; a telephone book for numbers of health care providers and faith communi-

ties; and local health agencies for such information as the number of child abuse incidents, trauma centers for injuries requiring hospitalization, clinics for specific services, and infants served by the WIC program. Law enforcement agencies may provide information on motor vehicle crashes, assaults, or homicides. Focus groups or interviews with key community representatives may provide information on perceptions of health needs (Clark, 2008).

An **epidemiologist**, a specialist with training in the study of patterns of diseases or health risks in a population, is often responsible for analyzing the data. Data trends are analyzed over several years to determine if the identified problem is a cluster of events that is part of a larger significant pattern. For example, the timing and clustering of events, such as the number of child pedestrians and bicyclists killed or injured, provide a clue to explore recent changes in the community. Have traffic patterns changed because of construction? Does this happen every year as school sessions begin? Is it related to children enjoying spring weather after school? Once the data are collected and analyzed, the community group can then develop a plan to address the problem and have baseline data for evaluation of the planned community intervention.

Key community assets should also be identified during the data collection stage. A **windshield survey**, a walking or driving tour around a neighborhood or community for the purpose of identifying resources and characteristics of the community, often provides important information needed to plan interventions. What could be collected during a windshield survey to study child pedestrian injuries and deaths?

A community assets map can be developed to help identify the presence of some community resources such as its health care facilities, local library, grocery stores, recreation facilities, schools, and so on.

Planning and Evaluation

An intervention is planned and implemented after the collected data have been analyzed and the community health problem is more clearly described. The planning involves a collaborative effort with all the stakeholders contributing ideas, developing

---

BOX 10–3 Common Health Statistics

$$\text{Birth rate} = \frac{\text{number of births in a state in a year}}{\text{total state population (same year)}} \times 1{,}000$$

$$\text{Mortality rate} = \frac{\text{number of deaths in a state in a year}}{\text{total state population (same year)}} \times 100{,}000$$

$$\text{Age-specific mortality rate} = \frac{\text{number of deaths in children aged (e.g., 1 to 4 years) in a year}}{\text{total population of children aged 1 to 4 years (same year)}} \times 10{,}000$$

$$\text{Cause-specific mortality rate} = \frac{\text{number of deaths due to (e.g., injury) in a year}}{\text{total state population (same year)}} \times 100{,}000$$

Incidence rate = number of new cases of a disease (e.g., type 2 diabetes) in a population in a specific time period

Prevalence rate = number of children with a disease (e.g., asthma) at a point in time

strategies, considering funding sources, and ultimately promoting and advertising the plan in the community. The collaboration often includes persons with specific skill sets who can take leadership roles with different aspects of the interventions. The planning group's knowledge of the cultural beliefs, primary language, income levels, reading level, sources of community health education, and potential community partners is valuable in designing the intervention. Knowledge about potential community funding resources or barriers helps in determining potential strategies that may be approved and endorsed by community decision makers.

The plan and interventions for the health problem need to be evaluated. Data collected before the intervention can serve as one comparison for the evaluation. Evaluation should also focus on the intervention and how well the target population received it, as well as the outcome, such as reduced injuries and deaths.

■ EMERGENCY CARE PLANNING

Emergency Medical Services for Children

The EMS system is the organized community-based public health response to ensure that adults and children with acute illnesses and injuries receive emergency care and timely transport to a hospital emergency department. The EMS system at the local community level is composed of ambulance units and trained emergency medical personnel who respond to emergencies. This EMS system may be part of the fire department or a separate organization. Each local EMS service has a medical director who establishes the protocols used by emergency medical personnel when caring for ill and injured individuals. The public accesses the EMS system by placing a call to 911 or their local emergency phone number. A dispatcher then directs the ambulance unit to respond, takes information, and provides data to the caller about how to manage the ill or injured person until the emergency personnel arrive. State EMS offices set the guidelines for training and certification of emergency medical personnel, equipment to be carried on ambulances, data collection of care provided, and communication systems used. In addition, the state EMS office works closely with hospital emergency departments and trauma centers to coordinate emergency care of patients transported by the EMS system. Children have special needs during emergency care that have been integrated into the overall EMS system.

Important Pediatric Physiologic Differences

Children have different physiologic responses to emergencies because of their smaller anatomy and developing organ systems. Small children cannot communicate and describe their health problems, and they are dependent upon family members for security and recognition of the emergency. Due to differences in anatomy, pediatric-sized equipment and supplies are essential. EMS providers need education to assess the child and recognize the signs that the child's condition is a true emergency, and then to provide the appropriate medical intervention before and during transport to the hospital.

Hospitals are part of the EMS system, and their emergency departments must be prepared to treat children as well as adults.

Emergency departments need to have appropriately sized resuscitation equipment for children of all ages and well-trained emergency physicians and nurses. Educational programs like Pediatric Advanced Life Support provide opportunities for nurses and physicians to work together effectively to resuscitate a child who is critically ill or injured. In addition, clinical guidelines for a well-orchestrated response to serious trauma and medical emergencies are developed and rehearsed. Urgent care centers and smaller emergency departments need to have agreements with major medical centers to ensure that children with life-threatening injuries or illnesses can be transferred and transported to receive a more advanced level of care.

Nurses sometimes work as volunteer EMS providers in their community. Nurses also work as interfacility transport team members, providing care to critically ill children who need to be transferred by ground or air ambulance from a community hospital to a hospital with more advanced care. See Figure 10–7 ➤ to see the interconnection between the EMS system and hospitals for provision of emergency services.

Disaster Preparedness

Disasters are serious and massive events that often occur suddenly and cause extensive damage, hardship, deaths, injuries, and psychological trauma. The amount of destruction and number of people impacted often mean that a community is unable to manage the recovery process without assistance. Many types of disasters occur each year in the United States. Natural disasters may occur suddenly, and include floods, mudslides, ice storms, hurricanes, earthquakes, volcanic eruptions, tornados, and fires. Other types of disasters can occur when trains or trucks carrying toxic chemicals or nuclear waste crash or explode. Concerns of terrorism with infectious organisms, toxic chemicals, or radioactive agents have elevated the need for disaster and emergency preparedness. See Chapter 16 ∞ for information about infectious organisms used for terrorism.

State and federal agencies, hospitals, and health professionals are developing community **disaster preparedness** plans for response to natural and man-made disasters that involve multiple casualties. Special planning for the needs of infants, children, and adolescents must be integrated in these efforts. Health services are needed to treat injuries and potential illnesses caused by contaminated water or other exposures.

Growth & Development — *Disaster Planning*

Developmental considerations are important during disaster planning as young children may be unable to do the following (American Academy of Pediatrics, 2008):

- Understand what is happening or efforts to reduce the consequences of the disaster
- Figure out how to flee or take evasive action to escape danger
- Follow the instructions given to adults regarding evacuation or safe actions
- Tell others they need help
- Distinguish between reality and fantasy

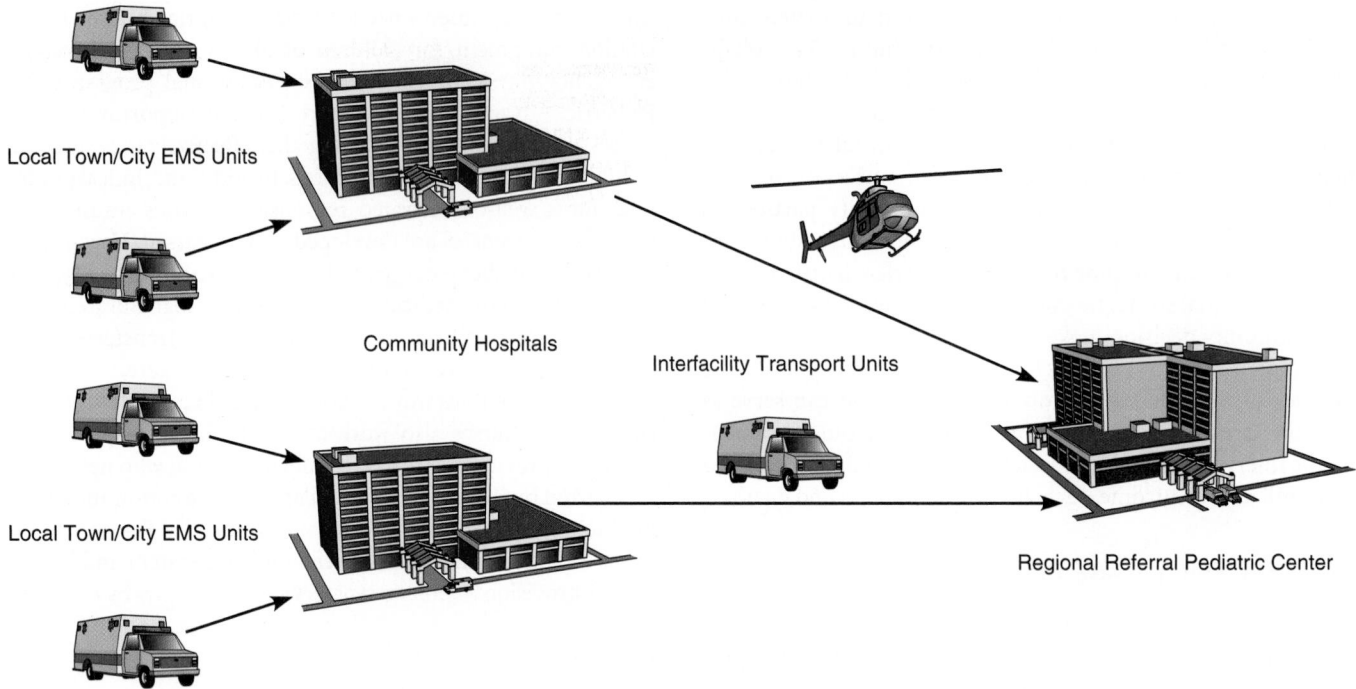

Local Town/City EMS Units

Community Hospitals

Interfacility Transport Units

Local Town/City EMS Units

Regional Referral Pediatric Center

FIGURE 10–7 ➤ The emergency medical services system is a carefully linked set of resources in the community and region that enables children with serious illnesses and injuries to get the care needed in the most appropriate hospital. The continuum of emergency care includes the child's caregiver at the scene, the communications center taking the call for help, the EMS personnel responding to the scene who provide immediate emergency care and transport the child to the emergency department, and the hospital emergency department. If the child is transported to a community emergency department, but needs more complex care, transfer to a larger hospital or trauma center is then coordinated. A team of specially trained pediatric emergency care providers often manages transfer in an ambulance, helicopter, or small plane. The goal is to get the child to the medical and specialty care resources needed to have the best chance of survival and optimal functional outcome.

Children have special vulnerabilities during a disaster. Disasters are very traumatic for children involved, and there may be immediate and delayed responses. Children may have lost their homes and personal possessions. Children may be separated from their family. Friends, pets, and family members may be injured or dead.

Nursing Roles

Nurses have an important role in disaster preparedness planning and as first responders to disasters. They also provide continuing care for individuals and families as a community emerges from the initial trauma. A primary role of nurses is to prevent disasters when possible and to assist communities with emergency preparedness for disasters. Nurses work with schools and community agencies to identify potential hazards and prevent them from causing harm.

Clinical Manifestations

Some common initial responses to a disaster include fear, anxiety, sadness, and confusion. The responses of children may be even greater if parents are also anxious or overwhelmed. The child's response depends on developmental stage, prior life experiences, and support of significant others. Some general reactions at different ages may include (Centers for Disease Control and Prevention, 2007):

- **Infancy to 6 years**—Increased crying and inconsolability, fear of separation from parents and other caregivers, clinging behaviors, and regression in developmental tasks

- **7 to 10 years**—Feelings of sadness or anger, fear the event will happen again, decreased attention span and concentration that can lead to decreased school performance, focus on details of the disastrous event, and somatic complaints

- **11 years and older**—Decreased contact with peers, fear of leaving home, increased risk-taking behaviors, increased argumentativeness, and refusal to talk about the traumatic events

Because disasters cause disruption for extended periods, the child has prolonged periods of emotional distress. These factors place the child at risk for acute stress and posttraumatic stress reactions (Markenson, Reynolds, & American Academy of Pediatrics, 2006). See Chapter 28 ∞ for more information on posttraumatic stress disorder (PTSD).

See Clinical Manifestations: Chemical and Radiologic Exposure for information on initial clinical therapy in response to exposure to various agents.

Clinical Therapy

Children's size and physiology require special management considerations when they are exposed to chemical or radiological agents used by terrorists or to toxins released during another type of exposure, such as a train crash (Figure 10–8 ➤).

The initial response to the scene of a disaster is to get the victims to fresh air and to quickly identify the level of injury or illness severity of all individuals. Emergency care and

Clinical Manifestations
Chemical and Radiologic Exposure

Type of Exposure, Potential Agents	Potential Clinical Manifestation	Initial Clinical Therapy
Chemical inhalation exposure (pulmonary agents such as chlorine and phosgene)	Burning sensation in nose, throat, and eyes Blurred vision Increased secretions Coughing, sensation of chest tightening, respiratory distress Nausea and vomiting	Get child to fresh air Decontamination with water Provide supplemental oxygen Secure the airway with an endotracheal tube and assist ventilations if needed Symptomatic care
Chemical skin and eye exposure (cryogenic liquids, acids, alkalis, corrosives, mustard gas, nitrogen mustard)	Cold injury to skin Chemical burns Erythema, blistering Eye inflammation, pain, blindness Systemic toxicity possible (respiratory distress, bradycardia or tachycardia)	Remove clothing and wash skin with soap and water Airway protection Eye irrigation Treat burns and blisters Fluid resuscitation Analgesia Other symptomatic care
Nerve agents (tabun, sarin, soman, VX, organophosphates)	Cholinergic effects include: Eyes (tearing, pupillary constriction, red conjunctiva, eye pain, blurry vision) Lacrimation, salivation, sweating, runny nose Respiratory distress due to increased respiratory secretions and bronchospasm, leading to respiratory failure Bradycardia or tachycardia (depends on agent used) Seizures, coma Muscle fasciculation, twitching, muscle weakness, paralysis	Remove clothing and wash skin and hair with soap and water Atropine or pralidoxime as an antidote Benzodiazepines for seizures Secure the airway with an endotracheal tube Provide supplemental oxygen; assist ventilation if needed Hydration Analgesia
Radiation	May be few signs and symptoms initially; nausea and vomiting Radiation sickness with intense immunosuppression Injuries from a blast	Removal of clothing and decontamination Potassium iodide Assessment of airway, breathing, and circulation if a blast injury Trauma care for injuries

Data from: Markenson, D., Reynolds, S., & American Academy of Pediatrics Committee on Pediatric Emergency Medicine and Task Force on Terrorism. (2006). The pediatrician and disaster preparedness. Pediatrics, 117(2), e340–e362; Scalzo, A. J., Lehman-Huskamp, K. L., Sinks, G. A., & Keenan, W. J. (2008). Disaster preparedness and toxic exposures in children. Clinical Pediatric Emergency Medicine, 9, 47–60; Lawrence, D. T., & Kirk, M. A. (2007). Chemical terrorism attacks: Update on antidotes. Emergency Medical Clinics of North America, 25, 567–595; Tracy, M. A. (2008). Kids and chemicals: A pediatric disaster. Journal of Emergency Nursing, 34(3), 266–267.

transportation to facilities that can provide needed care is initiated. Clinical therapy is focused on determining the type of exposure and providing immediate care to reduce the agent's effects.

Decontamination, the removal of chemicals and nerve agents from the skin, should be performed as soon as possible. Clothing is removed and the child is washed with soap and water. Eye irrigation may be needed to reduce pain and eye damage. Decontamination reduces the child's exposure to the toxin and helps protect medical personnel who will care for the child.

Antidotes such as atropine or pralidoxime may need to be administered for nerve agents. Potassium iodide may be administered for some radiation exposures. Respiratory care such as supplemental oxygen, an endotracheal tube, and assisted ventilation may be needed depending upon the exposure. Children

with exposure to blistering agents should receive burn care. Other therapies are implemented to treat the specific pathophysiology caused by the exposure.

Growth & Development *Decontamination*

Decontamination is a challenge with small children. The shower system should use lukewarm water to prevent hypothermia in the child. The shower system must be able to accommodate an adult who may be required to hold and assist an infant or young child who is unable to follow directions (Scalzo et al., 2008).

Care for children during a disaster in which health professionals must wear personal protective equipment may be challenging as young children may become fearful of these strangers and may not have supportive family members with them (Markenson et al., 2006).

As Children Grow
Response to Terrorism Agents

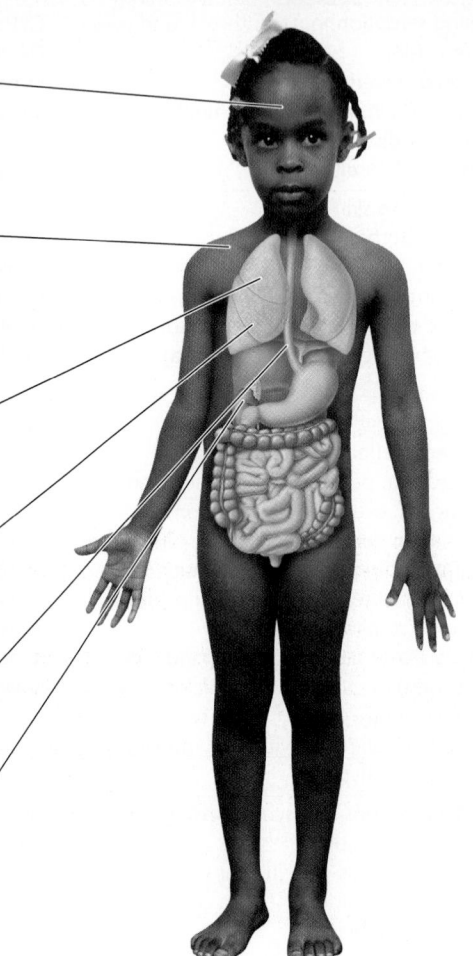

Children's developmental abilities and cognitive levels may interfere with their ability to escape danger.

Children's skin is thinner, so toxic agents falling on the skin can be absorbed more rapidly. Their increased body surface area means greater exposure to toxic agents falling on the skin.

Children breathe faster and inhale more air per weight than adults, meaning a greater exposure to aerosol toxins.

Children are shorter and have greater exposure to heavier aerosol agents that fall to the ground.

Children drink more fluids per kilogram than adults, so there is greater exposure to contaminants in water or other fluids such as milk.

Children also differ in their ability to detoxify and excrete toxic substances.

FIGURE 10–8 ➤ The child's size, physiology, and cognitive vulnerabilities lead to special considerations when the child is exposed to chemical, radiological, or biological agents by terrorism.

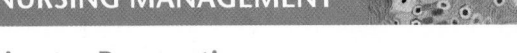

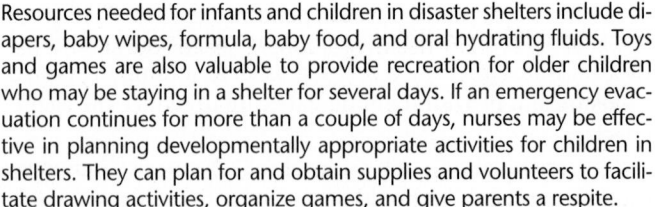

NURSING MANAGEMENT

Disaster Preparation

Pediatric nurses in schools and other community settings play a significant role in preparing families for a disaster. They can help families use developmentally appropriate information to talk with their children about disaster planning and convey information about disasters when they occur. Children need to know what to do in case of a disaster, terrorist event, or other emergency, including who should be approached for help and what actions to take when at home, at school, or elsewhere in the community (American Academy of Pediatrics, 2006).

Nurses can help the family develop a disaster plan for staying at home or for evacuation. Parents should carry phone numbers of out-of-town contacts, schools, and neighbors at all times. Having a list of medications, clothing, food, water, and other essentials is important so the family can quickly pack and respond to an evacuation order. When staying at home, families must have adequate food, water, and supplies for at least 72 hours following a major disaster. A plan for family pets

Clinical Tip

Resources needed for infants and children in disaster shelters include diapers, baby wipes, formula, baby food, and oral hydrating fluids. Toys and games are also valuable to provide recreation for older children who may be staying in a shelter for several days. If an emergency evacuation continues for more than a couple of days, nurses may be effective in planning developmentally appropriate activities for children in shelters. They can plan for and obtain supplies and volunteers to facilitate drawing activities, organize games, and give parents a respite.

should also be made. See the companion website for resources to help families with disaster planning.

Disaster Response

When a disaster occurs, nurses are often on the front line, providing emergency health care, first aid, and general public health interventions (e.g., vaccines, sanitation, food, and water). However, the child's response to psychological trauma is also addressed. With their knowledge of child and adolescent development, nurses can meet the needs of youth in disasters.

Disaster Preparedness Video

Disaster Preparedness Websites

Psychological first aid involves comforting and consoling children, protecting them from further threat or distress, providing immediate physical care, helping reunite them with loved ones, listening, and identifying those who need more help (Williams, 2006). Nurses can provide a safe place for children, away from media and unfolding traumatic events such as rescue of the dead and injured. Do not leave children unattended or permit them to leave a scene without a responsible adult. Assess for panic reactions, unexpected behaviors, and changing conditions.

Once the initial disaster is managed and children return to home or other settings, they may need extra time with their parents. Parents should attempt to reestablish daily routines for school, meals, play, and rest as soon as possible.

Encourage parents to listen and answer the child's questions about the disaster honestly and in language the child can understand. If they cannot answer a question, it is better to be honest and say so, but also reassure the child that they are trying to do everything to keep the child safe. Let young children know that a lot of adults are working hard to protect everyone. Avoid saying everything will be fine as this does not always address a child's specific concerns. Encourage older children and adolescents to discuss the disaster with family members and peers if desired.

Allow children to express their feelings about the disaster. Let them know that it is normal to be upset. Use play therapy (e.g., art, playing with action figures or dolls, and storytelling) to allow young children to express their feelings, develop a sense of mastery, and reduce their anxiety. Giving older children special tasks lets them feel that they are helping and provides a sense of control.

Help schools and other community agencies arrange for mental health specialists to assist children in exploring their feelings in safe settings. Provide grief counseling for youth who have lost peers or family members. Nurses must remain vigilant for children and families who develop PTSD (see Chapter 28 ∞). Refer individuals and families for mental health services when anxiety levels remain high or if they have difficulty performing normal life tasks.

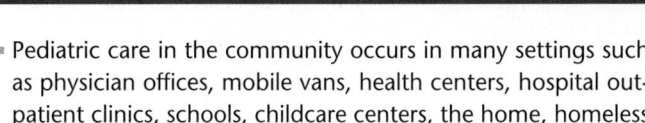

Chapter Highlights

- Pediatric care in the community occurs in many settings such as physician offices, mobile vans, health centers, hospital outpatient clinics, schools, childcare centers, the home, homeless shelters, and disaster shelters.
- Working with the child and family in the community setting requires an understanding of how the larger environment influences the child's health and development.
- Nurses working in many community health care settings develop a long-term relationship with the child and family over time that helps to promote the provision of optimal health care.
- Pediatric nurses in community settings assist with diagnostic workups and management of children with chronic health problems, including patient assessment, health education, health promotion, and linking families with community resources.
- School nursing focuses on removing or minimizing health barriers to learning so children can perform academically. Services include prevention, health promotion, health education, emergency care, and managing chronic health problems.
- Nurse consultants to childcare settings assist the administrators in the establishment of the childcare center's policies for health practices, teach staff about safe health practices, and monitor health practices.

- Home care nursing goals include promoting or restoring the health of the child while attempting to minimize the effects of the disability and illness.
- Public health promotes the health of the population in a community rather than the care of individuals, with an emphasis on health promotion and disease prevention.
- A community assessment is a process of compiling data about a community's health status and resources for the purpose of public health planning to address a population's health needs.
- The emergency medical services (EMS) system is the organized community-based public health response to ensure that children and adults with acute illnesses and injuries receive emergency care and timely transport to the hospital emergency department.
- Pediatric nurses have a significant role in working with families in preparing for a disaster. They can help families develop a disaster plan, use developmentally appropriate information to talk with children about what to do when disasters occur, provide direct care in a disaster shelter, and provide psychosocial support to families and children.

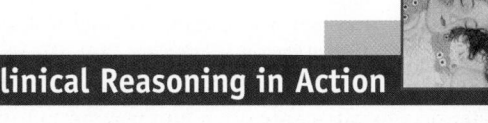

Clinical Reasoning in Action

Recall 7-year-old Ernesto at the beginning of the chapter, who visited the school nurse after becoming ill at school. Ernesto appears to have an acute illness with a sore throat and fever. He is otherwise healthy. The school nurse has called his mother to request that he go home.

1. What nursing care should be provided while Ernesto waits for his mother to come pick him up?
2. What information and recommendations should the school nurse give Ernesto's mother regarding his illness? Should he be seen by his primary health care provider?

3. Since Ernesto's health problem may be infectious, what precautions and actions should the school nurse take to protect other students?

4. What preparation should the school nurse have in place if Ernesto's condition had been an emergency?

See Pearson Nursing Student Resources for possible responses.

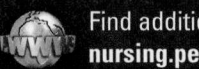

Pearson Nursing Student Resources

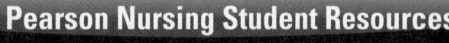

Find additional review materials at
nursing.pearsonhighered.com
Prepare for success with NCLEX®-style practice questions, interactive assignments and activities, web links, animations and videos, and more!

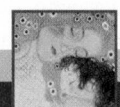

References

Alkon, A., Bernzweig, J., To, K., Wolff, M., & Mackie, J. F. (2009). Child care health consultation improves health and safety policies and practices. *Academic Pediatrics, 9*(5), 366–370.

American Academy of Pediatrics. (2008). *The youngest victims: Disaster preparedness to meet children's needs.* Retrieved from http://www.aap.org/disasters/pdf/Youngest-Victims-Final.pdf

American Academy of Pediatrics, Committee on Child Health Financing, Section on Home Care. (2006). Financing of pediatric home health care. *Pediatrics, 118*(2), 834–838.

American Academy of Pediatrics, Committee on Pediatric Emergency Medicine. (2007). Preparation for emergencies in the offices of pediatricians and pediatric primary care providers. *Pediatrics, 120*(1), 200–212.

American Academy of Pediatrics, Council on School Health. (2008). The role of the school nurse in providing school health services. *Pediatrics, 21*(5), 1052–1056.

American Nurses Association. (2007). *Assuring safe, high quality health care in pre-k through 12 educational settings.* Retrieved from http://www.nursingworld.org

Bindler, R. C., & Ball, J. W. (2007). The Bindler-Ball healthcare model: A new paradigm for health promotion. *Pediatric Nursing, 33*(2), 121–126.

Carnevale, F. A., Alexander, E., Davis, M., Rennick, J., & Troini, R. (2006). Daily living with distress and enrichment: The moral experience of families with ventilator-assisted children at home. *Pediatrics, 17*(1), e48–e60.

Centers for Disease Control and Prevention. (2007). *Maintaining a healthy state of mind: Parents and caregivers.* Retrieved from http://emergency.cdc.gov/preparedness/mind/parents/

Clark, M. J. (2008). *Community health nursing* (5th ed.). Upper Saddle River, NJ: Prentice Hall Health.

Clay, D., Farris, K., McCarthy, A. M., Kelly, M. W., & Howarth, R. (2008). Family perceptions of medication administration at school: Errors, risk factors, and consequences. *Journal of School Nursing, 24*(2), 95–102.

Crowley, A. A., & Kulikowich, J. M. (2009). Impact of training on child care health consultant knowledge and practice. *Pediatric Nursing, 35*(2), 93–100.

Engelke, M. K., Guttu, M., Warren, M. B., & Swanson, M. (2008). School nurse case management for children with chronic illness: Health, academic, and quality of life outcomes. *Journal of School Nursing, 24*(4), 205–214.

Frankowski, B. L., Keating, K., Rexroad, A., Delaney, T., McEwing, S. M., Wasko, N., et al. (2006). Community collaboration: Concurrent physician and school nurse education and cooperation increases the use of asthma action plans. *Journal of School Health, 76*(6), 303–306.

Gupta, R. S., Pascoe, J. M., Blanchard, T. C., Langkamp, D., Duncan, P. M., Gorski, P. A., & Southward, L. H. (2009). Child health in child care: A multistate survey of Head Start and non-Head Start child care directors. *Journal of Pediatric Health Care, 23*(3), 143–149.

Koshti-Richman, A. (2009). Caring for a disabled child at home: Parents' views. *Paediatric Nursing, 21*(6), 19–21.

Lawrence, D. T., & Kirk, M. A. (2007). Chemical terrorism attacks: Update on antidotes. *Emergency Medical Clinics of North America, 25*, 567–595.

Markenson, D., Reynolds, S., & American Academy of Pediatrics Committee on Pediatric Emergency Medicine and Task Force on Terrorism. (2006). The pediatrician and disaster preparedness. *Pediatrics, 117*(2), e340–e362.

McLaughlin, T., Maljanian, R., Kornblum, R., Clark, P., Simpson, J., & McCormack, K. (2006). Evaluating the availability and use of asthma action plans for school-based asthma care: A case study in Hartford, Connecticut. *Journal of School Health, 76*(6), 325–328.

Mink, C. M., & Yeh, S. (2009). Infections in child-care facilities and schools. *Pediatrics in Review, 30*(7), 259–268.

National Association of Pediatric Nurse Practitioners. (2009). NAPNAP position statement on school-based health care. *Journal of Pediatric Health Care, 23*(2), 19A–20A.

Pulcini, J., DeSisto, M. C., & McIntyre, C. L. (2007). An intervention to increase the use of asthma action plans in schools: A MASNRN study. *Journal of School Nursing, 23*(3), 170–176.

Scalzo, A. J., Lehman-Huskamp, K. L., Sinks, G. A., & Keenan, W. J. (2008). Disaster preparedness and toxic exposures in children. *Clinical Pediatric Emergency Medicine, 9*, 47–60.

Scudder, L., Papa, P., & Brey, L. C. (2007). School-based health centers: A model for improving the health of the nation's children. *Journal for Nurse Practitioners, 3*(10), 713–720.

Tracy, M. A. (2008). Kids and chemicals: A pediatric disaster. *Journal of Emergency Nursing, 34*(3), 266–267.

U.S. Department of Health and Human Services, Office of Disease Prevention and Health Promotion. (2010). *Healthy People.* Washington, DC: Author. Retrieved from http://www.healthypeople.gov/Default.htm

Williams, R. (2006). The psychological consequences for children and young people who are exposed to terrorism, war, conflict, and natural disasters. *Current Opinion in Psychiatry, 19*(4), 337–349.

The Hospitalized Child   chapter 11

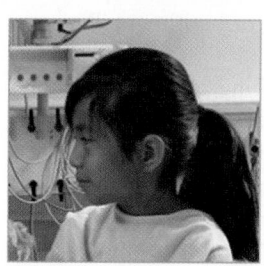

Five-year-old Tiona has a history of obstructive sleep apnea and is scheduled for a tonsillectomy and adenoidectomy (T&A) in the morning. Her mother has brought her in today for preoperative evaluation and instruction. Tiona has no other health problems. Her experience with health care is limited to well-child checkups and immunizations as well as several visits to the otolaryngologist in the past year. She has no prior hospitalizations. Tiona will return in the morning at 6:30 a.m. for surgery. She will be admitted to the pediatric short-stay hospital unit for a few hours following surgery and will then be discharged home as long as she is able to drink fluids and take oral pain medication.

How can the nurse assess what Tiona knows about the surgery? What techniques should be used to teach Tiona about the surgery? What instructions should Tiona's mother receive from the nurse in the preoperative clinic related to care prior to surgery?

Key Terms

animal-assisted activity / 282
child-life specialist / 279
dramatic play / 280
rehabilitation / 271
rooming in / 279
separation anxiety / 264
stranger anxiety / 264
therapeutic play / 280
therapeutic recreation / 283
treatment room / 272

Learning Outcomes

After reading this chapter, you will be able to do the following:

1. Contrast the child's understanding of health and illness according to the child's developmental level. 262

2. Explain the effects of and response to illness and hospitalization on children and their families. 262-63

3. Describe the child's and family's adaptation to hospitalization. 268

4. Identify nursing strategies to minimize the stressors related to hospitalization. 279

5. Examine the concept of family presence during procedures and nursing strategies to effectively prepare the family. 272

6. Summarize strategies for preparing children and families for discharge from the hospital setting. 285-286

7. Evaluate the effectiveness of teaching strategies used with the hospitalized child and the family.

Hospitalization, whether it is elective, planned in advance, or the result of an emergency or trauma, is stressful for children of all ages and their families. Because most pediatric conditions can be managed within the home and community setting, hospitalization is not always required to manage the child with an illness. However, those children who are hospitalized usually have a high level of illness acuity. (See Figure 1–7 in Chapter 1 ∞ for the most common reasons for hospitalization in children.)

Hospitalized children experience a variety of emotions as they are in an unknown environment, surrounded by strangers, unfamiliar equipment, and frightening sights and sounds. These children are subjected to unfamiliar procedures, some of which are invasive or painful, and may even require surgery. For both children and families, routines are disrupted and normal coping strategies are tested.

Nurses today are challenged to provide individualized care for the hospitalized child with complex medical conditions, acute illnesses, or injury. They must address the psychosocial and developmental concerns that accompany hospitalization. To minimize the stress of hospitalization, nurses provide support and education to children and their families before, during, and after hospitalization.

During hospitalization, nurses use a family-centered approach and work collaboratively with parents to implement various strategies that promote coping and adaptation and to prepare children for necessary procedures. Nurses also collaborate with members of a multidisciplinary team and partner with families to prepare them for discharge home or transfer to a long-term care or rehabilitation facility.

■ EFFECTS OF HOSPITALIZATION ON CHILDREN AND THEIR FAMILIES

Children's Understanding of Health and Illness

Young children have limited knowledge about the body and its relation to health and illness. They do not understand what causes them to get sick. Their understanding is based primarily on their cognitive ability at various developmental stages and on previous experiences with health care professionals. As children get older, their concept of illness becomes more sophisticated and they demonstrate an understanding of the cause of illness (Drahota & Malcarne, 2008; Myant & Williams, 2005). Table 11–1 provides a discussion of children's understanding of health and illness according to their developmental level.

Hospitalization and the accompanying medical procedures are very stressful for children, especially very young children such as toddlers and preschoolers. The child's attempts to deal with these stressors impact both the psychological and physiological well-being of the child. Infants, toddlers, and preschoolers lack the cognitive skills to understand hospitalization and are the most likely age groups to exhibit regressive behaviors. Young children have fears and anxieties related to things such as the dark, strangers, and monsters. A hospital's unfamiliar environment can exacerbate those anxieties.

TABLE 11–1	Children's Understanding of Health and Illness According to Developmental Level
Age/Stage	**Understanding**
Infant	• By approximately 6 months of age, infants have developed an awareness of themselves as separate from their mother or father. • They are unaware of the effects of illness. • They feel anxious when approached by strangers.
Toddler and Preschooler	• Toddlers and preschoolers are beginning to understand illness, but not its cause. • Preschoolers have a beginning understanding of germs but not how they are spread. • The child's concept of the body usually is limited to names and locations of some body parts. • The child's concept of internal organs and body functions is vague. • They may view illness as a form of punishment for bad behavior or something magical. • Events that occur just before the onset of the illness may be mistakenly associated with the illness.
School-Age Child	• School-age children understand how germs are spread. • Older school-age children have a more realistic understanding of the reasons for illness and are able to understand more about disease and how body organs are affected. • The school-age child's concept of body parts and function is maturing.
Adolescent	• Adolescents are increasingly aware of the physiologic, psychologic, and behavioral causes of illness and injury. • They understand that the disease may involve several causes and effects and that multiple organs or body parts may be involved. • The adolescent understands how symptoms can be related to certain organ functions in the body. • Adolescents are concerned with appearance and perceive an illness or injury in terms of its effect on their body image.

Source: Data from Drahota, A., & Malcarne, V. L. (2008). *Concepts of illness in children: A comparison between children with and without intellectual disability.* Intellectual and Developmental Disabilities, 46(1), 44–53; Koopman, H. M., Baars, R. M., Chaplin, J., & Zwinderman, K. H. (2004). *Illness through the eyes of the child: The development of children's understanding of the causes of illness.* Patient Education and Counseling, 55(3), 363–370; Myant, K. A., & Williams, J. M. (2005). *Children's concepts of health and illness: Understanding of contagious illnesses, non-contagious illnesses and injuries.* Journal of Health Psychology, 10(6), 805–819; Piko, B. F., & Bak, J. (2006). *Children's perception of health and illness: Images and lay concepts in preadolescence.* Health Education Research: Theory & Practice, 21(5), 643–653.

Significant stressors for hospitalized children of all ages include:

- Separation from parents, primary caregiver, or peers
- Loss of self-control, autonomy, and privacy
- Painful and/or invasive procedures
- Fear of bodily injury and disfigurement

Table 11–2 highlights key stressors of hospitalization for children at each developmental stage. Nursing care of the hospitalized child focuses on minimizing the child's fears, anxieties, and disruption of the child's usual routine, and supporting the family through the stressful experience. Strategies include minimizing separation anxiety, loss of control, pain related to procedures, and fear.

Research *Fear in Hospitals*

A study that examined hospital-related fears in 90 children ages 4–6 years found that 91% of the children were afraid of something. Many different types of fears were identified and were most often related to nursing interventions, fear of being a patient, and fears related to the developmental stage of the child. Other fears were related to the environment and relationships between the child and the staff. Fears mentioned most were pain, shots, sample-taking and tests, other nursing interventions, staying in the hospital, and separation from family. Nursing interventions should focus on reducing these fears (Salmela, Salanterä, & Aronen, 2009).

TABLE 11–2 Stressors of Hospitalization for Children at Various Developmental Stages

Stressors by Developmental Age	Responses	Nursing Management
Infant		
Separation anxiety Stranger anxiety Painful, invasive procedures Immobilization Sleep deprivation, sensory overload	Sleep-awake cycle disrupted Feeding routines disrupted Displays excessive irritability	Encourage parental presence. Adhere to the infant's home routine as much as possible. Use topical anesthetics or preprocedural sedation as prescribed. Promote a quiet environment and reduce excess stimuli.
Toddler		
Separation anxiety Loss of self-control Immobilization Painful, invasive procedures Bodily injury or mutilation Fear of the dark	Cries if parents leave the bedside Is frightened if forced to lie supine Wonders why parents don't come to the rescue Associates pain with punishment	Encourage parental presence. Allow parents to hold the child in their lap for examinations and procedures when possible. Allow choices when possible. Use topical anesthetics or preprocedural sedation as prescribed. Explain all procedures. Provide a night-light.
Preschooler		
Separation anxiety and fear of abandonment Loss of self-control Bodily injury or mutilation Painful, invasive procedures Fear of the dark and monsters	Displays difficulty separating reality from fantasy Fears ghosts and monsters Fears body parts will leak out when skin is not intact Fears that tubes are permanent Demonstrates withdrawal, projection, aggression, regression	Encourage parental presence. Allow choices when possible. Use topical anesthetics or preprocedural sedation as prescribed. Explain all procedures. Provide a night-light or flashlight.
School-Age Child		
Loss of control Loss of privacy and control over body functions Bodily injury Separation from family and friends Painful, invasive procedures Fear of death	Displays increased sensitivity to the environment Demonstrates detailed recall of events to self and other patients	Encourage parental participation. Allow the child choices when possible. Explain all procedures and offer reassurance. Use topical anesthetics or preprocedural sedation as prescribed. Encourage peer interaction via the Internet, phone calls, and other methods of communication.
Adolescent		
Loss of control Fear of altered body image, disfigurement, disability, and death Separation from peer group Loss of privacy and identity	Displays denial, regression, withdrawal, intellectualization, projection, displacement	Include the adolescent in the plan of care. Encourage discussion of fears and anxieties. Explain all procedures. Ask the adolescent his or her desire for parental involvement. Encourage peer interaction.

Infant

By about 6 months of age, infants have developed an awareness of themselves as separate from their mother or father. They are able to identify primary caretakers and feel anxious when in contact with strangers. Hospitalization can be a traumatic time for an infant, particularly if the parents are not staying with the child. Infants can sense the anxiety their parents are experiencing during a hospitalization.

Common stressors to the infant include painful procedures, immobilization of extremities, and the sleep deprivation caused by disruption of the infant's normal sleep patterns and routines. However, the most common stressor of hospitalization for the infant is separation from parents, which is manifested by **separation anxiety**. Bowlby identified three phases of separation anxiety exhibited in young children who were separated from their mothers for long periods of time. This theory remains an essential component of family-centered nursing care and must be incorporated as policies related to family presence are formulated (Jolley & Shields, 2009). Characteristic behaviors of children in the three phases of separation anxiety are listed in Table 11–3. Hospitalized infants and toddlers often display some of these behaviors, particularly if parents are unable to remain with the child. In addition to separation anxiety, children between 6 and 18 months of age may display **stranger anxiety** (wariness of strangers) when confronted with unfamiliar health care professionals.

Clinical Tip

Parents often feel guilty for leaving their child, especially if the child protests adamantly or cries upon return. Reassure the parents that this protest is a normal behavior and it represents healthy parent–infant attachment. Support them as they leave and provide information for them when they return about what the child's activities have been.

Because parent–infant attachment is critical to the infant's developmental achievements (see Chapter 4 ∞), the nurse

encourages the family to remain with, and be active participants in care of, the hospitalized infant. If parents are unable to remain at the hospital, support visiting the infant as often as possible.

Parents may be hesitant to touch, hold, or provide care for an infant who has tubes and wires attached. They may be afraid of hurting the child or dislodging equipment. Parents may not be aware when it is okay for them to hold their child. The nurse should advise parents when it is appropriate and assist them as needed.

Clinical Tip

Children encounter many members of the health care team, in addition to other hospital personnel, when hospitalized. Children ages 6 to 18 months perceive these people as strangers and may cry when someone new enters the room. As the child sees a person over and over again, the stranger anxiety for that person subsides. Providing consistent caregivers as much as possible will limit the number of "strangers" that the child encounters while hospitalized.

Toddler

Toddlers are the group most at risk for a stressful experience as a result of illness and hospitalization. This age group is old enough to know that their routine has been disrupted, but they do not understand why. Separation from parents is the major stressor and they protest vigorously when their parents depart. When one or both parents cannot be present, they can leave mementos to comfort the child. These might include a piece of cloth saturated with the mother's favorite perfume or father's cologne (unless the child has a respiratory condition or another contraindication for this intervention), an object belonging to the parent, or an audiotape or videotape with messages from the parents.

Clinical Tip

Nurses who work with children generally wear colorful uniforms (Figure 11–1 ➤). This eliminates the anxiety related to "white uniforms" that has existed in the past. Uniforms with familiar characters may serve as a source of comfort and distraction for the child.

The nurse encourages parents to remain present as much as possible for important rituals such as toileting, carrying out bedtime routines, and singing favorite nursery rhymes. Autonomy is the developmental task of the toddler (see Chapter 4 ∞). When possible, maintain the toddler's normal home routines for bathing and other activities. Allow the toddler to have choices when possible, such as choosing the color of Jell-O or which gown/pajamas to wear.

In addition to parental separation and schedule disruption, common stressors for the toddler include fear of pain, fear of invasive procedures, fear of change, and fear of mutilation. The parents' presence plays a large role in diminishing these fears. In addition, therapeutic play with simple explanations can diminish these fears.

TABLE 11–3	**Stages of Separation Anxiety and Expected Behaviors**
Stage	Expected Behavior
Protest	Screaming, crying Clinging to parents May resist attempts by other adults to comfort them
Despair	Sadness Quiet, appears to have "settled in" Withdrawal or compliant behavior Crying when parents return
Denial (detachment)	Lack of protest when parents leave Appearance of being happy and content with everyone Shows interest in surroundings Close relationships not established

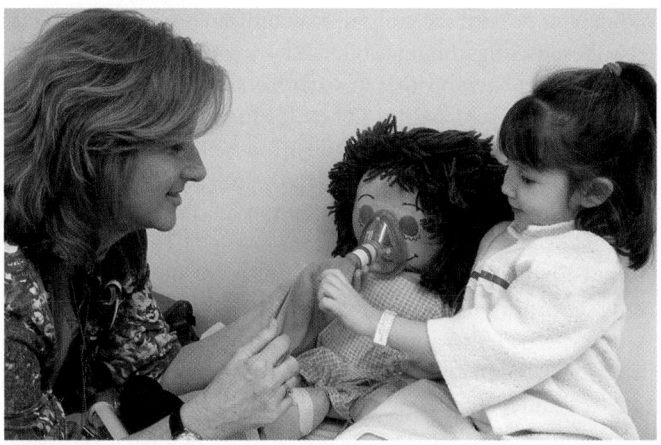

FIGURE 11–1 ➤ This pediatric nurse wears a colorful uniform to decrease anxiety associated with white uniforms.

Clinical Tip

Toddlers may present challenges to the nurse regarding cooperation with treatments and procedures, including physical assessments. To diffuse such confrontations, encourage cooperation by offering the toddler some sense of control. For example, a nurse might comment, "Once I have listened to your heart, lungs, and stomach, you can choose whether you want to ride in the wagon or be pushed in the big stroller to the playroom."

Preschooler

The greatest stressors to preschoolers are the fear of being alone, fear of the dark, fear of abandonment, fear of loss of self-control related to the body and emotions, and fear of bodily injury or mutilation. Preschoolers may also feel guilty about being sick, or they may view the illness and hospitalization as punishment.

Similar to the toddler, preschoolers desire a normal routine. Developmentally, preschoolers exhibit a sense of initiative as they explore the world around them (see Chapter 4 ∞). To promote that initiative, the nurse can encourage the preschool child's independence by offering choices such as "Do you want to take the red medicine or the purple medicine first?"

Parents should be encouraged to stay with the child if possible. For those who cannot stay, preschoolers need to know when to expect their parents to return to the hospital. Because most preschoolers lack a concept of time measurements like "2 hours," "half past four," or "3 o'clock," respond with simpler statements of time, such as "after supper" or "before breakfast." Encourage parents to make telephone calls to the preschooler if possible. Some parents are able to make calls from work, and preschoolers get a sense of security from hearing their parent's voice confirming that they will return to the hospital.

Parents often believe it is better to leave the hospital room after their child has fallen asleep so their departure will not stress the child. In fact, the opposite is true. If a child awakens to find the parent gone unexpectedly, he or she may become anxious and develop a lack of trust. Instead, encourage parents to tell their child when they need to leave and why (e.g., has to go to

work or go home). By providing honest information to the child, the parents demonstrate that they can be trusted.

School-Age Child

The school-age child relies on parents and others for support and understanding during stressful events and procedures. Although school-age children attempt to maintain their composure during painful or invasive procedures, generally they still require a great deal of support. Major sources of stress for hospitalized school-age children are loss of control related to body functions, privacy issues, fear of bodily injury, pain, and concerns related to death. School-age children may also experience separation from family as well as school friends.

School-age children understand concepts, so parents who cannot remain at the bedside are encouraged to tell the child when they will return. Parents are also encouraged to be available for telephone calls to provide support and comfort. Stressful procedures can lead to regression or other behavioral changes, although this is less likely than with younger patients. Inform the parents that this behavior is normal during stressful situations.

Developmentally, school-age children exhibit a sense of industry (see Chapter 4 ∞), taking pride in their achievements at home, at school, and in sports. To foster that sense of industry, allow these children to participate in their care as much as possible. Encourage them to continue with school work and to engage in creative outlets such as art or crafts.

Adolescent

Major stressors for hospitalized adolescents include loss of independence, control, and privacy; fear of bodily injury or changes in body image; fear of disability, pain, and even death; and separation from peers, home, and school.

Preoccupation with appearance and body image are paramount in this age group. By offering education and explanations that focus on these issues, nurses can provide significant reassurance to the adolescent. Adolescents often try to maintain independence and rigid self-control when undergoing painful and invasive procedures. Because hospitalization may increase dependence on their parents, adolescents may respond with frustration and anger.

Adolescents are in the process of establishing their identity and becoming independent of their parents' influence (see Chapter 4 ∞), so control over aspects of their care is important. Partner with the family and multidisciplinary team to ensure the adolescent is an active participant in decisions about the plan of care. Privacy and modesty are major concerns, as adolescents' physical characteristics are rapidly changing. To demonstrate respect for their feelings, knock on the door before entering and ask permission before conducting assessments or other procedures. By allowing choices in clothing, hair, and music, the nurse acknowledges the importance of the adolescent's self-image.

The peer group is a major influence in adolescents' lives. Allowing flexible visiting hours for friends helps teens maintain their social network and provides needed support. When friends are not able to visit, providing teens with Internet access offers a means of accessing their friends for support. Encouraging participation in recreation and teen lounge facilities available during hospitalization provides the adolescent with additional peer group support opportunities.

Family Responses to Hospitalization

The illness and hospitalization of a child disrupt a family's usual routines. Parental roles change when a child is being cared for by others in the hospital setting (Sarajärvi, Haapamäki, & Paavilainen, 2006). Roles may be altered as one parent remains at the hospital with the child while the other parent or siblings take on additional tasks at home. Family members may experience anxiety and fear, especially when the outcome is unknown or the reason for hospitalization is a potentially serious health condition. Parents who perceive their child is in pain find the experience difficult and require support. Family members' ability to cope can be challenged by a serious emergency, lengthy illness, chronic condition, poor prognosis, lack of family support, or lack of financial or community services. The stress on parents can be compounded by the burden of missed work, additional expenses, and concerns about feeding and caring for children at home. (See Chapter 13 ∞ for a description of nursing support for the child with a life-threatening illness or injury.) It is essential that nurses assess parental needs and attend to those needs in order to establish a trusting relationship. Needs frequently identified by parents of hospitalized children include:

- Regular information about their child's condition, prognosis, and treatment
- Help, encouragement, and support from the nursing staff
- A trusting, confidential relationship with the nursing staff (Hopia, Tomlinson, Paavilainen, et al., 2005)

Parents who have support from nursing staff have less anxiety and are better equipped to make decisions and participate in their child's care.

Nurses need to be alert to cultural patterns in the family that can influence the response to hospitalization and the family's management of the experience, such as views of health and illness and causation of illness. Cultural influences may also determine who the decision maker is in the family regarding health care practices and may provide guidelines for acceptable treatments (Spector, 2009).

Siblings' Experience

The siblings of a hospitalized child may receive little attention from the parents who are overwhelmed and anxious about their hospitalized child's health. A sibling's response depends on a variety of factors including age, family size, severity of the illness, prior experience, and information received about the illness (Gursky, 2007). Younger siblings who do not understand the causes of illness and hospitalization may feel guilty about fighting with or being mean to their brother or sister in the past. Some siblings may fear becoming ill themselves. Some may believe that they played a role in the child's illness or injury and need reassurance that they did not cause it. If the child did in some way contribute to the sibling's illness or injury, help him

or her to cope with the guilt by providing an opportunity to discuss these feelings. Siblings often have nightmares about the illness or injury their brother or sister has sustained and about the ill child dying (see Chapter 13 ∞ for further discussion of siblings' responses to the dying child).

As hospitalization causes family roles and routines to change, siblings may feel insecure and anxious. It is essential that siblings receive information about their brother's or sister's condition and hospitalization using language and concepts appropriate to their ages and developmental levels (Gursky, 2007). Providing information and support to siblings promotes coping and adaptation to a sibling's illness (Lobato, Kao, & Plante, 2006).

As appropriate, encourage siblings to visit. Such a visit is especially encouraged if the child could potentially die; this allows the sibling the opportunity to say good-bye. These visits often help to lift the spirits of the hospitalized child and assist siblings to overcome any misconceptions or negative emotions. Because children's fantasies are often worse than reality, unfounded fears may be relieved by a visit.

The nurse prepares the siblings before the visit by explaining sights and sounds likely experienced and by describing how their brother or sister will appear. If the hospitalized child acts, moves, talks, or appears different than usual, provide an explanation beforehand. Describe the hospital environment, including equipment, sounds, and smells. Using a doll, drawing pictures, or showing an actual picture of the child can help prepare the siblings. See Families Want to Know: Strategies for Working with Siblings of a Hospitalized Child.

Clinical Tip

Siblings with fever or other symptoms of infectious disease should not be allowed to visit. Inform parents/family about any specific policies related to sibling visitation.

During the visit, demonstrate how to talk to and touch the ill child and encourage the siblings to do the same. After the visit, discuss with siblings what they saw and felt, and answer any questions they may have. When siblings cannot visit, contact with the hospitalized child can be maintained by sending pictures, drawings, cards, and messages recorded on iPods, and through e-mail, instant messaging, or webcam. Collaborate with the family to determine the most appropriate and effective method of communicating if the sibling is unable to visit.

If parents are staying at the hospital with the hospitalized child, help them to establish a routine for the well siblings. For example, encourage them to call the siblings at home at a regular time each night. Allowing the siblings at home the opportunity to share their day, and to receive an update on the hospitalized child, provides a feeling of connectedness and may minimize feelings of jealousy and resentment. The phone call offers siblings a consistent link to their parents as well as the reassurance that they are important and loved.

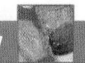

Families Want to Know
Strategies for Working with Siblings of a Hospitalized Child

The nurse working with siblings of a hospitalized child can implement the following strategies to assist the siblings in understanding:

■ Be truthful. Explain why the child is hospitalized, what the treatment involves, and how long the hospitalization is expected to last.

■ Assure siblings that they did not cause the illness and that the hospitalized child did nothing wrong. If a sibling had some involvement in or responsibility for the health crisis, referral for psychological counseling is needed.

■ Allow siblings to ask questions and discuss fears and other feelings.

■ Encourage siblings to visit if possible. Cover tubes and wires with a sheet. Wash off blood or cover bloody bandages if possible. Prepare them for any equipment, dressing, and procedures they might see, and any sounds they might hear.

■ Warn siblings if the hospitalized child is not speaking. Say something like "John can't talk now. He seems to be sleeping deeply. He may be able to hear, though, so you can touch him and talk to him."

■ Encourage siblings to express their feelings related to the disruptive effect of the child's hospitalization on family life.

Family Assessment

To support the hospitalized child and provide family-centered care, nurses develop an understanding of the family dynamics and individualize the nursing care according to the needs of the child and family. To develop a plan of care that involves all family members, the nurse assesses the impact of the child's illness or hospitalization on the family. Box 11–1 provides a list of questions to guide the nurse in determining the roles of family, knowledge of family, support systems, and effects on siblings. (See Chapter 2 ∞ for a detailed discussion on family assessment.)

Collaborate with the family to determine their resources. These resources include the coping strategies of family members, financial resources, access to health care, and availability of community services. A family with limited financial support may manage quite well because they have effective coping strategies, whereas another family with greater financial resources may have difficulty caring for an ill child if their coping strategies are ineffective. Staying with a hospitalized child can be a financial drain for parents if they must take a leave of absence from work or miss scheduled work days, or travel to the hospital. Additional expenses may include hotel rooms, meals, parking fees, and childcare for other children. Assess the family's ability to manage these additional expenses. A multidisciplinary approach to the burden of hospitalization may provide access to community resources and support for families.

The nurse also assesses the family dynamics and evaluates the quality of communication, methods of coping with stress, risk factors, and sources of strength. Collaborate with the family to identify coping mechanisms. Recognize that many children may be hospitalized far from home and their usual support systems. This creates stress for them and for their family members. Find out where family members are staying, how far they are from

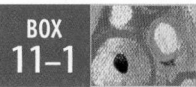

BOX 11–1 Family Assessment When the Child is Hospitalized

Family Roles
■ What changes will the child's illness create in the family?
■ Will household tasks need to be reallocated?
■ Will a burden be placed on certain family members?
■ Will one parent room in or spend a great deal of time in the hospital?
■ Will one parent or guardian be primarily responsible for communicating with other family members?

Knowledge
■ What knowledge does the family have about the child's condition and treatment? Do they need further information?
■ How quickly can discharge planning and teaching begin?

Support Systems
■ Does the family have health insurance? What percentage of costs will it cover? Will other financial support be needed? Will costs continue for ongoing care after hospitalization? If so, will existing health insurance cover those costs?
■ Are close friends or family available to provide childcare for other children, assist with family tasks, or help in other ways?
■ Are there community services such as support groups, camps for children with disabilities, education sessions, or equipment and financial resources to which the nurse can refer the family?

Siblings
■ Have siblings been informed of the ill child's condition and the expected outcome?
■ Have they been reassured that they did not cause the illness?
■ Do they understand the change in roles and family routines?
■ Are they able to visit the ill child?
■ Have their teachers been informed of the family stress?
■ If the hospitalized child's life is threatened, are the siblings involved in a therapy plan to assist them in dealing with that stress?

Culture
■ Are there any cultural beliefs that will affect the care the child receives in the hospital?

home, and what normal support systems have been disrupted. Parents use a variety of coping mechanisms in these situations, including reading, relaxation, and exercise. Additional common sources of support include friends, relatives, and pastors as well as hospital chaplains and social workers.

Examine how the family has dealt with the child's health needs if the child has been hospitalized or required home care in the past. Determine the family members' level of understanding related to the child's hospitalization and anticipated therapy. Collaborate with family members to determine their desired role in the child's care. Assess the family's needs for referral to family service agencies or other community organizations that may be required. Evaluate the need for support groups or agencies that provide medical equipment or other assistance.

Teaching the child and family, providing support, and referring them to community resources are key elements to providing family-centered care. Additional resources available for the child and family include social workers, child and family mental

Culture — *Supporting Health Practices*

Many cultural groups use a combination of Western medicine and traditional or folk medicine (Spector, 2009). This information may not be shared with nurses or physicians, both out of respect and in fear that they will be told not to use these methods. Recognizing and supporting use of traditional practices along with Western medicine can promote health and provide comfort for children and families. Ask the families about the use of traditional, complementary, or alternative therapies.

health professionals, and advanced practice nurses. Additionally, hospital programs and parent support groups are available to assist families in coping with a child's illness.

■ ADAPTATION TO HOSPITALIZATION

Hospitalization of the child may be planned or unexpected. A child may be hospitalized for any of the following reasons:

- The child develops an acute illness, or exacerbation of a chronic illness.
- The child requires diagnostic or treatment procedures or requires elective surgery.
- The child who was previously healthy suffers a serious injury, necessitating unexpected hospitalization.

Planned Hospitalization

When hospitalization is planned, children and their parents have time to prepare for the experience. (See Families Want to Know: Parental Preparation of Children for Hospitalization.) Through preadmission preparation, children and their families are introduced to the acute care setting. Assess the family's knowledge and expectations and provide information about likely experiences. A variety of approaches can be used to provide information and allay fears:

- Tours of the hospital unit or surgical area are helpful. This activity assists the child and family to become familiar with the environment they will encounter. During tours, preschoolers and school-age children are provided opportunities to see and handle items with which they will come in contact.
- The surgical team's attire is less frightening if the child has had a chance to try it on and engage in play while wearing the attire (Figure 11–2 ➤).
- Medical equipment is not as frightening when the child learns what it does and observes how it is used, for example, through demonstration on a doll (Figure 11–3 ➤).
- If a tour is not possible, photographs or a videotape can be used to demonstrate the medical setting and procedures. Puppets and skits are another effective method of explaining procedures to children.

Many hospitals offer health fairs to explain health procedures to children. During a tour, while hospitalized, or at home, the child can be exposed to books or media that explain in age-appropriate terms what to expect during various procedures. Box 11–2 lists some books that are available. (See the companion website for a more extensive list of condition-specific book

Families Want to Know — *Parental Preparation of Children for Hospitalization*

The nurse can assist the parents in preparing the child for hospitalization by suggesting the following interventions:

- Read stories to the child about the experience. Numerous books and pamphlets are available.
- Talk about going to the hospital and what it will be like. Talk about coming home.
- Encourage the child to ask questions about the hospital and surgery.
- Encourage the child to draw pictures of what the hospital will be like.
- Visit the hospital unit before hospitalization, if possible.
- Let the child touch or see equipment, if possible.
- Provide a doctor or nurse kit for the child to play with.
- Let the child dress up like a doctor or nurse, if possible.
- Plan for support via parents' presence, telephone calls, or special items of the parents that the child can keep during the stay.
- Be honest.

titles for children.) Coloring books or other methods can also be used to reinforce teaching (Figure 11–4 ➤).

Different approaches may be more effective in helping adolescents prepare for hospitalization. In addition to written materials, models, and videotapes or DVDs, adolescents also learn from talking with peers who have had similar experiences. To demonstrate respect for their sense of independence and privacy, offer adolescents an opportunity to ask questions without parents present.

Include the family in preparing the child of any age for hospitalization. Parents can be instrumental in preparing a child for hospitalization by reviewing material presented, being available to answer questions, and being truthful and supportive.

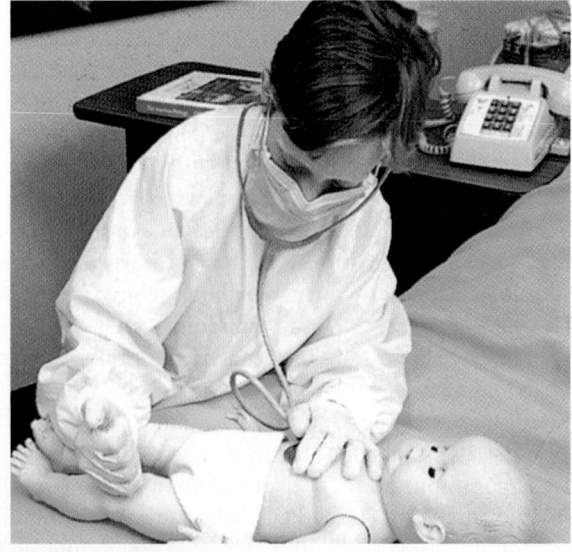

FIGURE 11–2 ➤ Allowing the child to dress up as a doctor or a nurse helps prepare the child for the hospitalization experience. This helps the child adjust to treatment, care, and the recovery process. Why? What might the child's concerns be? Can you think of any concerns that might be related to cultural background?

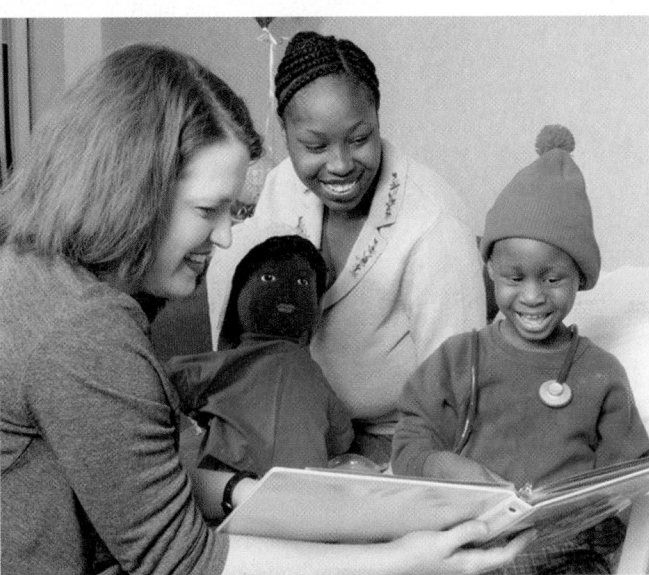

FIGURE 11–3 ➤ The child's anxiety and fear often will be reduced if the nurse explains what is going to happen and demonstrates how the procedure will be done by using a doll. Based on your experience, can you list five actions you can take to prepare a school-age child for hospitalization?

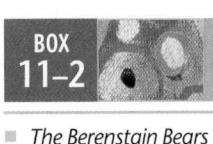

Examples of Children's Books Regarding Hospitalization

- *The Berenstain Bears Go to the Doctor,* by S. Berenstain & J. Berenstain
- *Clifford Visits the Hospital,* by N. Bridwell
- *Corduroy Goes to the Doctor,* by D. Freeman & L. McCue
- *Curious George Goes to the Hospital,* by M. Rey & H. A. Rey
- *Do I Have to Go to the Hospital? A First Look at Going to the Hospital,* by P. Thomas
- *Franklin Goes to the Hospital,* by P. Bourgeois & B. Clark
- *Going to the Hospital, First Experiences,* by M. Bates
- *Lions Aren't Scared of Shots: A Story for Children About Visiting the Doctor,* by H. J. Bennett & M. S. Weber

involve the family in the child's care. Provide the family an opportunity to express their fears and concerns. Refer to social services and parent support groups if additional support is needed.

■ NURSING CARE OF THE HOSPITALIZED CHILD

Family-centered nursing care of the hospitalized child focuses on supporting the child's and family's coping strategies to deal with the stressors of hospitalization, promoting optimal development and safety, and minimizing disruption of the child's usual routine as much as possible.

Clinical Tip

The hospital environment can pose a variety of safety risks for children, especially toddlers and preschoolers. The nurse should dispose of syringe caps, thermometer covers, gloves, and other equipment that children could chew on or swallow. Latex balloons should not be permitted due to the risk of suffocation. See Box 11–3 for age-specific safety measures.

Special Units and Types of Care

Children admitted to a hospital may be cared for in one or more of the following units: general pediatric unit, short-stay unit, outpatient unit, ambulatory surgical unit, emergency department, or pediatric intensive care unit. Hospitalized children may require surgical treatment involving preoperative and postoperative care. Children with infectious diseases require isolation precautions. Other children may require rehabilitative care to achieve or restore maximum potential.

General Pediatric Care Unit

Smaller facilities typically incorporate all pediatric care specialties in one unit or area, whereas larger medical centers and children's hospitals have separate medical units for different specialties. Specialized units may include medical and surgical units, orthopedic units, oncology units, mental health units, and units specific to developmental levels (e.g., adolescent unit). Admission to a specialized unit may be the result of an acute condition, such as pneumonia or trauma, or the result of an exacerbation of a chronic condition, such as asthma. Other

FIGURE 11–4 ➤ The nurse reads a story to reinforce teaching about the hospital to the child.

Unexpected Hospitalization

An unanticipated admission places the child at emotional risk for several reasons, including the lack of preparation for the experience, the uncertainty and unpredictability of events that follow, the unfamiliarity of the environment, and the heightened anxiety of parents. An admission for exacerbation of a disease such as cystic fibrosis or leukemia can provoke feelings of depression or hopelessness.

Assist the child and family who are not prepared for hospital admission to adapt to the experience by orienting them to their immediate environment, providing an opportunity for questions, offering truthful responses, and explaining all procedures and expectations. Discuss the anticipated plan of care for the child and

BOX 11-3 Safety Measures for the Hospitalized Child

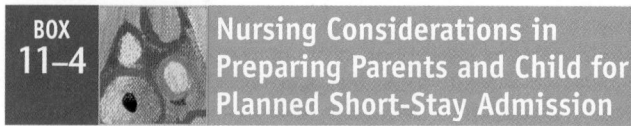

Newborn and Infant

- Use an age-appropriate crib and bedding.
- Secure equipment cords under the infant's gown or shirt.
- Do not allow the infant to chew on cords.
- Properly dispose of syringe caps and other small items that may present a choking hazard.
- Establish with parents a list of persons who may visit the child.
- Keep crib rails up when a parent is not at the bedside.

Toddler and Preschooler

- Maintain the bed in low position.
- Keep side rails up when a parent is not at the bedside.
- Do not allow the child to chew on cords.
- Keep the room clutter-free.
- Remove all unnecessary equipment from the child's room.
- Properly dispose of syringe caps and other small items that may present a choking hazard.
- Latex balloons should not be permitted due to the risk of suffocation.
- If toddlers and preschoolers are curious about hospital equipment, provide them the opportunity to explore the equipment safely and with guidance (e.g., syringes without needles, blood pressure cuffs to satisfy curiosity).
- Keep in mind that these children are naturally curious and explorative.
- Instruct family members to inform staff when they are leaving the room to ensure that the toddler or preschooler is being observed.

School-Age Child

- Instruct the child to avoid manipulating hospital equipment such as intravenous fluid pumps, patient-controlled analgesia (PCA) pumps, and oxygen gauges.
- Allow the child the opportunity to explore hospital surroundings and equipment with guidance.
- Instruct family members to inform staff when they are leaving the room to ensure that the child is being observed.

Adolescent

- Address issues such as smoking in the room and consuming alcohol since friends could possibly bring cigarettes or alcohol to the hospitalized adolescent.

BOX 11-4 Nursing Considerations in Preparing Parents and Child for Planned Short-Stay Admission

- Are there special requirements, such as no food or drink permitted or extra fluid intake requirements?
- What time and where must the child appear?
- Are any special forms, insurance numbers, or previous records needed?
- How long will the child stay in the hospital?
- Are parents expected or encouraged to be with the child or to stay in the health facility?
- Is there a chance the child may need to remain longer than expected?
- What will the child's condition be for transfer home?
- Will special equipment or care be needed?
- What symptoms can indicate problems?
- Where can the family go or who can they call in case of problems or questions?

causes for admissions include surgical procedures requiring longer than 24-hour stays and the need for inpatient treatments and services.

Nursing care for regular hospital admission includes:

- Orienting the child and family to the unit and procedures
- Adhering to the child's normal routine as much as possible, including child and family in the decision-making process
- Providing direct care to the child
- Promoting a safe environment for the child
- Promoting the child's growth and developmental needs

Short-Stay, Outpatient, and Ambulatory Surgical Units

Hospitalization stays for children have generally become short. Many procedures are performed in outpatient units, such as minor surgery (in ambulatory surgical centers), diagnostic tests (such as cardiac catheterizations), radiology studies requiring sedation, and treatments (such as chemotherapy). The child may be admitted in the morning and discharged that afternoon. In addition, children who have potentially serious illnesses may be placed on a short-stay or 23-hour observation unit for monitoring or limited treatment, after which medical staff decide either to hospitalize the child for additional treatment or, if improvement occurs, to discharge the child.

These short stays are considered beneficial primarily because they minimize disruption of family patterns and are cost-effective for the institution, health insurance company, and family. Nurses assist parents to prepare the child properly for planned admissions, monitor the child during the procedures, encourage family participation in care, and keep families well informed (Box 11–4).

Nursing care of the child in short-stay, outpatient, and ambulatory surgical units is the same as for regular hospital admission. However, time for teaching is compressed, requiring the nurse to implement teaching methods in a minimal amount of time to ensure the family understands discharge instructions. Effective teaching methods on this accelerated schedule include demonstration, videos, pamphlets with verbal review, and informal teaching sessions.

Emergency Care

When a child is brought to an emergency department, the parents are usually frightened and insecure and may even be in a state of shock. The fast pace and critical nature of the unit creates an atmosphere in which parents are hesitant to ask questions and are anxious about the outcome. Many factors can contribute to the parents' anxiety and stress (see Chapter 1 ∞):

- Unexpected nature of the situation
- Uncertainties in the emergency environment
- Necessity for quick decision making
- Need for numerous procedures, tests, and treatments
- Fear of pain

The nurse keeps both the child and the family informed about what is being done and when more news may be available. The parents and child are encouraged to remain together as much as possible. Parents who wish to remain with a child even during invasive procedures or resuscitation efforts should be allowed to do so, and this option is supported by the Emergency Nurses Association (2005). The nurse collaborates with the family members to determine their desired presence in critical situations and keeps them informed about the health care provided (see Chapter 13 ∞).

Pediatric Intensive Care Unit

The pediatric intensive care unit (PICU) provides specialized nursing care to infants and children, including children with life-threatening illnesses and injuries, acute exacerbations of chronic illness (such as status asthmaticus), or any other condition requiring advanced support and continuous monitoring.

Parents of a child in a PICU are likely to be anxious, particularly since the child's illness may be severe and the prognosis may be guarded. The unfamiliar equipment may create an atmosphere of fear or anxiety. Numerous health care professionals work in the intensive care environment, and without effective and open communication, parents may not know whom to question or even what questions to ask.

Nurses provide comprehensive care and emotional support to the child, explain the purpose of treatments and machines, help parents to hold or touch their child, and provide referral to other services if appropriate. Collaborate with the family and encourage them to write down their questions. Direct them to the appropriate source if you are unable to answer the question.

Isolation

Children who require isolation to prevent spread of infection may experience lack of stimulation due to limited contact with other children and visitors. Frequent family visits are important and should be encouraged. Family members may be reluctant to wear protective garments either out of fear of using them incorrectly or because they believe they are unnecessary. The nurse ensures that the family understands the reason for isolation and any special procedures. Having contact with and holding the child are encouraged when possible. (Standard precautions are described in the *Clinical Skills Manual.*)

Rehabilitation

Rehabilitation is the process of assisting a child with physical or mental challenges to reach full potential through therapy and education. Rehabilitation units provide children with ongoing care and support to continue recovery beyond the initial period of illness or injury (Figure 11–5 ➤). These may be separate units within a hospital or independent centers. The rehabilitation may be on an inpatient or outpatient basis. Children who experience brain injury, spinal cord injury, near drowning, or burns may require extensive rehabilitation. The rehabilitation process may be lengthy and extensive; families may need support for adapting to changes in lifestyle, income, finances, and responsibilities. Collaboration with a multidisciplinary team including parental involvement is essential. (See Chapter 12 ∞.)

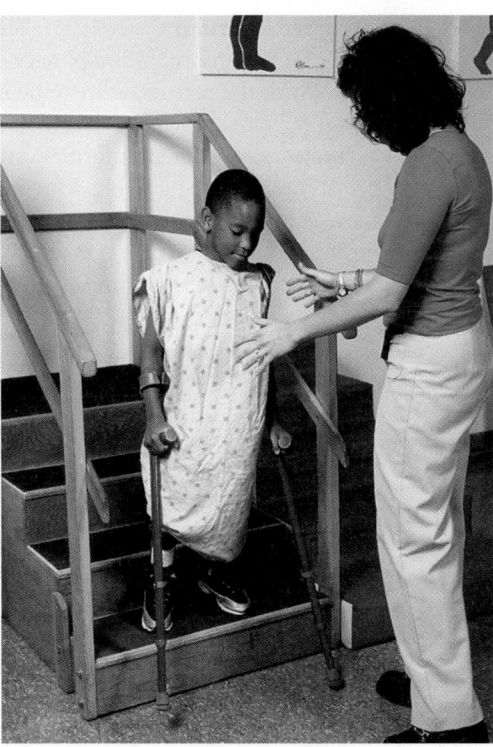

FIGURE 11–5 ➤ Rehabilitation units provide an opportunity for the child to relearn tasks like walking and climbing stairs. They provide an important transition from hospital to home and community.

Parental Involvement and Parental Presence

Family-centered care recognizes that families are essential to the child's care during illness. Integrity of the family unit is fostered through parental involvement during the child's hospital stay. Involvement provides parents with control and the feeling that they are active participants in their child's progress, and it also prepares the family for care that will be required when the child goes home. The child benefits greatly from parental presence and participation and experiences less emotional distress and anxiety if the parents are present. If the parent–child attachment remains uninterrupted, the child experiences fewer behavioral maladjustments.

Families who feel supported by nursing staff during their child's hospitalization are more confident and better equipped to cope with the crisis. They are also generally open to participating in their child's care and developing skills to provide care

---

Culture   *Support Systems*

There are many cultural influences on health beliefs and practices. For example, Mexican Americans view family as a strong support. Extended family and godparents (compadres) may want to be with a hospitalized child. The father of the child is often the spokesperson, and mothers commonly are influential in decisions regarding child health care. Hawaiian families also often wish to have many family members present with a hospitalized child, and may value playing native music and use of aromatherapy (Lassetter & Baldwin, 2005). The nurse should incorporate all people the family wishes to have present in the hospital and include them in explanations about health care.

for the child after discharge (Sarajärvi et al., 2006). The nurse should partner with the family and multidisciplinary team to determine the extent to which the parents desire to be involved in the child's care (Power & Franck, 2008; Sarajärvi et al., 2006), and to ensure that accurate and consistent information is given related to hospital care and discharge planning. Providing both emotional support and education to families enhances their ability to care for the child at home (Sarajärvi et al., 2006). See Chapter 2 ∞ for more information on family-centered care and family presence.

Preparation for Procedures

Hospitalized children may experience numerous procedures during hospitalization, from collection of urine or blood specimens to lumbar punctures and surgery. Special techniques can help the child to understand and cope with feelings about these procedures. Techniques used to prepare the child depend on developmental age, coping abilities, and previous experience.

Psychological Preparation

Preparation may begin a few moments to several days before the procedure, depending on the child's age. In providing sensitive care to the child, nurses assume that a procedure can potentially be traumatic for the child. Even providing urine in a specimen cup or undergoing radiologic examination can be frightening if the child does not understand the reason for the procedure or what to expect. When preparing the child for medication administration using techniques appropriate to the child's developmental level, the nurse ensures that the medication is safely given (Table 11–4).

Use developmentally appropriate techniques to assess the child's knowledge and feelings about the procedure. Examples include use of drawings, stories, body outline dolls, anatomically correct dolls, and conversation with the child, depending on the age of the child. When assessing the child's perception about procedures, the nurse should consider the following:

- Does the child know the purpose of the procedure?
- Has the child experienced this procedure before? Was the experience painful, frightening, or reassuring?
- What does the child think will happen? Are the child's beliefs accurate?
- Is the procedure painful?
- What techniques does the child use to gain control in challenging situations?
- Will the parents or other caregiver be present to provide support?

Culture *Use of Interpreters*

Nurses in the pediatric acute care environment frequently encounter patients and parents who do not speak English. It is imperative that nurses use appropriate interpreter services to communicate with these families. Use of children and family members to obtain patient history, to provide explanations of illness and treatment, and to obtain informed consent can lead to concerns related to accuracy of the information. In some situations, the family member providing the interpretation might actually withhold information to protect the ill child or the parents (National Center for Cultural Competence, 2010).

Clinical Tip

When a potentially painful procedure will be performed, an anesthetic cream such as EMLA, or L-M-X4, is applied before the planned procedure. This can lessen discomfort and, therefore, fear in the child. (See Chapter 15 ∞ for more information related to decreasing discomfort of painful procedures.)

When explaining a procedure and its purpose, use words that the child understands. See Table 11–5. Older children require explanations geared to their cognitive level and previous experiences. They will want to know what is happening, why, and what they can do to cope during the procedure (Table 11–6).

Clinical Tip

Procedures should never be performed in a playroom or during a play activity. The nurse acts as the child's advocate by ensuring that treatments by other health care professionals (such as blood drawing or respiratory treatments) are not performed in the playroom. Assist the child back to the treatment room or his or her own room for the procedure, and reassure the child he or she may return to the playroom after the treatment is completed.

For adolescents, provide written information, videos, DVDs, and other available media. Schedule time for questions and discussions. Allow adolescents to make choices about their own health care when possible. For example, they can be asked such questions as "Do you want your hand numbed for the IV start?" Maintain a positive attitude when preparing adolescents and reassure them that it is normal to be frightened of unknown experiences.

Physical Preparation

Physical preparation depends on the age of the child and the procedure. Preprocedural sedation may be required. If sedation is required the child will have to be NPO (nothing by mouth) for a period of time. Infants might be provided sucrose for procedures (see Chapter 15 ∞ for pain management). Procedural checklists are often used.

Performing the Procedure

Procedures on young children are generally performed in a **treatment room** (a room designated for performing treatments such as intravenous starts, blood drawing, and lumbar punctures) in order to promote the child's sense of security that the room is a "safe" and relatively pain-free site. After the procedure, the child is returned to his or her room for comfort and reassurance. A choice of reward often soothes the young child. Older children can be given the option of having a procedure performed in the treatment room or in their own hospital room. Older school-age children and adolescents may prefer to remain in their room for the procedure. See Box 11–5.

Perform procedures as quickly and efficiently as possible. If the parents wish to participate, ask them to hold the child's hand or stand close by for comfort. Utilize nursing staff instead of

TABLE 11–4 Variations in Medication Administration to Children

Route	Developmental Considerations	Techniques
Oral	Children under 5 years cannot generally swallow pills and capsules.	• Medications are usually given in liquid form (elixir, syrup, or suspension). • Avoid putting medications in a bottle of formula since it will be impossible to determine how much medication the child has taken, if some of the formula is left in the bottle. • Sometimes tablets are crushed or capsules are opened and mixed with a liquid flavoring or small amount of food. Check with the pharmacy to be sure this does not inactivate the drug. Never crush enteric-coated or timed-release medicine. • When choosing a vehicle for crushed tablets, use only one spoonful of applesauce, pudding, jelly, or similar food or 1–2 mL of liquid. • Use an oral syringe to increase accuracy.
	Children may not want to take medicine.	• Position young children upright to avoid choking and aspiration. • Give liquid medicines slowly by oral syringe (for infants) aimed at the inside of the cheek. • A preschooler may prefer to drink the medicine from a medicine cup, but the medication must first be measured using a syringe to ensure accuracy. • Have the expectation that the medicine will be taken. Let children choose the type of fluid to drink after, but do not ask if they will take their medicine now.
Rectal	Colon is small in size.	• For children under 3 years, the nurse's gloved fifth finger is used for insertion. After this age, the index finger can usually be used. • Lubricate the tip of the suppository. The nurse may need to hold the buttocks together for a few minutes to keep the medication from being expelled.
Ophthalmic and otic	Young children may be fearful of medicines placed in the eyes or ears.	• Adequate immobilization is needed to avoid injury. • The nurse's hand can be stabilized by resting the wrist on the child's head. • Explanations and therapeutic play can be used with children old enough to understand the process of administration. • Have medication at room temperature.
Topical	Skin of infants is thin and fragile.	• Only prescribed doses and medicines appropriate for young children should be used on the skin. • Covering the area or keeping the child's hands occupied may be necessary to ensure adequate contact of medication with the skin.
Intramuscular	Anatomy and physiology of children differ from that of adults.	• The gluteus maximus muscle (dorsal gluteal site) must not be used until the child has been walking for at least 1 year and has well-developed muscle mass. • The vastus lateralis (anterior thigh) site is preferred for young children because it is the largest muscle mass in children less than 3 years of age. • Amounts to be administered should be limited to no more than 1–2 mL for the ventrogluteal site, depending on muscle size. Refer to the *Clinical Skills Manual* for illustrations. • The deltoid muscle is rarely used in young children except for the small vaccine doses.
Intravenous	Veins are small and fragile.	• Careful maintenance of sites is needed. • Common infusion sites include hands and feet, although scalp veins are sometimes used in infants. • Infusion pumps require frequent monitoring.
	Fluid balance is critical.	• Syringe pumps are often used when minimal fluid is to be given over an extended period of time. • Central lines are commonly used for long-term intravenous medication therapy.

Source: Data from Bindler, R., & Howry, L. (2005). Pediatric drug guide. Upper Saddle River, NJ: Prentice Hall Health. See the Clinical Skills Manual *for further medication administration techniques.*

parents to immobilize the child as needed. The parents, or another nurse, can be designated to support the child by providing gentle touch, talking, singing, giving reassurance, or illustrating stress reduction techniques. (See Chapter 2 ∞ for more information related to parental presence during procedures.)

After the procedure, no matter how the child responded, the child should be praised. A choice of reward often soothes the young child. If the procedure is performed in a treatment room, the child is returned to his or her room for comfort and reassurance.

TABLE 11–5 Language Alternatives when Communicating with Young Children

Potentially Confusing or Ambiguous Words or Statements	Alternative Communication Choice
"We will give you some dye in your arm."	"We will put some warm medicine into your arm."
"I will give you a shot."	"I will give you some medicine through a small needle."
"This will hurt or burn."	"It might feel sore or very warm."
"The doctor will make a small cut/incision."	"The doctor will make a small opening."
"You are going to have some anesthesia."	"You will get some medicine that you breathe or get through your arm to make you sleep."
"The medicine tastes bad."	"Some children say the medicine tastes different to them."

TABLE 11–6 Assisting Children Through Procedures

Developmental Stage	Before Procedure	During Procedure
Infant	None for infant. Explain to parents the procedure, the reason for it, and their role. Allow parents the option of being present for the procedure.	Nursing staff should immobilize the infant securely and gently. Parents should not be asked to hold the child down. Perform the procedure quickly. Use touch, voice, pacifier, and bottle as distractions. Ask parents to hold, rock, and sing to the infant after the procedure.
Toddler	Give the explanation just before the procedure, since a toddler's concept of time is limited. Explain that the child did nothing wrong; the procedure is simply necessary. Allow parents the option of being present for the procedure.	Perform in the treatment room. Nursing staff should immobilize the child securely. Give short explanations and directions in a positive manner. Avoid giving choices when none are available. For example, "We are going to do this now" is better than "Is it okay to do this now?" Allow the child to cry or scream. Comfort the child after the procedure. Give the child a choice of a favorite drink or special sticker.
Preschool child	Give simple explanations of the procedure. Basic drawings may be useful. While providing supervision, allow the child to touch and play with equipment to be used if possible. Since any entry into the body is viewed as a threat, state that the child's body will remain the same, and use adhesive bandages to reassure the child that the body is intact and parts will not "fall out."	Perform in the treatment room. Nursing staff should immobilize the child securely. Give short explanations and directions in a positive manner. Encourage control by having the child count to 10 or spell his or her name. Allow the child to cry. Give positive feedback for cooperation and getting through the procedure. Encourage the child to draw afterward to explore the experience.
School-age child	Clear, thorough explanations are helpful. Use drawings, pictures, books, and contact with equipment. Teach stress reduction techniques such as deep breathing and visualization. Offer a choice of reward after the procedure is completed.	Be ready to immobilize the child if needed. Allow the child to remain in position by him- or herself if able to be still. Explain throughout the procedure what is happening. Facilitate use of stress control techniques. Praise cooperative efforts.
Adolescent	Give clear explanations orally and in writing. Teach stress reduction techniques. Explore fear of certain procedures, such as staple removal or venipuncture.	Assist the adolescent in self-control. Assist with use of stress control techniques. Explain the expected outcome and tell when results of the test will be completed.

Refer to Chapter 15 ∞ for discussion of pain management and sedation for procedures.

Preparation for Surgery

A child's surgical experience may be elective, planned in advance, or the result of an emergency or trauma. How a child responds to the experience depends on the psychological and physical preparation he or she receives. The accompanying Nursing Care Plan, beginning on page 276, provides informa-

tion related to care of the child undergoing surgery. Additional nursing diagnoses include:

- Risk for Infection and Injury related to exposure to nosocomial infection and use of preoperative medication
- Impaired Skin Integrity related to disruption of skin surface
- Risk for Constipation related to surgical procedure and anesthetics
- Risk for Fluid Volume Imbalance related to intravenous infusion and NPO status

BOX 11–5 Treatment Room

Pediatric hospitals and large medical centers generally provide treatment rooms on each unit. Smaller hospitals and community hospitals may not provide a specific treatment room designated for pediatrics; however, any room other than the child's own room is an appropriate alternative. If smaller hospitals do not have a treatment room or provide an alternative, nurses acting as a child advocate should be vigilant in encouraging the establishment of such a room to minimize the stressors the hospitalized child experiences.

- Impaired Gas Exchange related to anesthetics and pain
- Risk for Impaired Skin Integrity related to limited mobility after surgery
- Anxiety (Child and Family) related to change in health status and environments

Preoperative Care

Preoperative care of the child includes both psychosocial and physical preparation for surgery. The goal of preoperative teaching is to reduce the fear associated with the unknown and decrease stress and anxiety associated with surgery.

Psychosocial Preparation

Preoperative teaching is geared to the child's developmental level. When the child will be transferred to an intensive care unit or recovery room after surgery, a visit to the area before surgery can reduce the fear and anxiety associated with waking up in a strange environment filled with frightening sights, sounds, and smells. The use of videotapes, DVDs, puppets, body outline dolls, anatomically correct dolls, drawings, and models is encouraged to teach the child about the surgical procedure. For example, a doll was used as a teaching aid in preparing Tiona, the 5-year-old described in the opening vignette, for surgery (Figure 11–6 ➤). Playing with stethoscopes, gowns, masks, and syringes without needles also helps the child feel

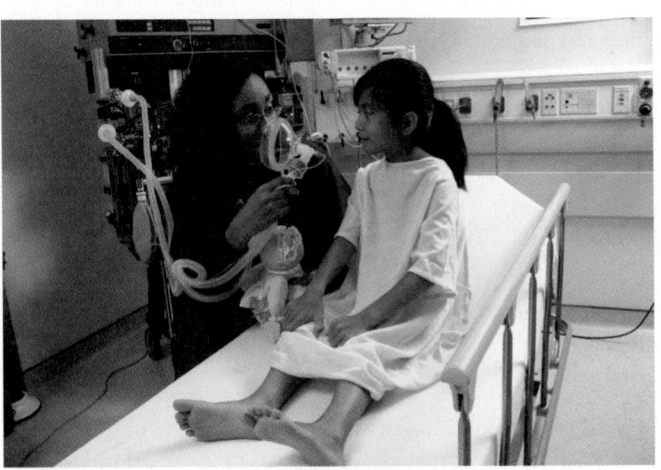

FIGURE 11–6 ➤ The nurse shows Tiona equipment that will be used during surgery to help decrease anxiety related to the unknown. What are other methods the nurse can use to teach young school-age children about surgery?

more in control (see discussion about therapeutic play later in this chapter). Children are reassured that their parents can accompany them to the operating room floor and will be waiting when they awaken from surgery. Parents should be allowed to carry infants and young toddlers to the pediatric holding area or have them ride in one parent's lap in a wheelchair. Older toddlers and preschoolers should be allowed to ride in a special wagon if possible. Special teddy bears and blankets are generally allowed in the preoperative holding area and provide comfort to the child. The nurse should make sure that the item is labeled with the child's name. Prepare family members for what to anticipate and what is expected of them. Special equipment such as intravenous setups and monitoring devices are explained. In some hospitals, only one or two immediate family members are allowed to visit the child at one time. Visitors may be required to wear special gowns, shoes, or hats, and they may be restricted to certain areas.

Parental Presence During Anesthesia Induction

Many hospitals now allow parents to be present with their child during anesthesia induction and again in the postanesthesia recovery area. Parents often want to support their child before and immediately after a surgical procedure, and their presence offers reassurance and comfort to the child. The decision to allow parents to be present during induction of anesthesia must be made on an individual basis. Nurses should be open to change in practice and realize that incorporating the option of parental presence during anesthesia induction supports the principles of family-centered care and decreases anxiety in the child (Pruitt, Johnson, Elliott, et al., 2008). The nurse explains expectations, such as surgical gown, cap, shoe covers, and the parent's role during induction. The nurse offers the parents an opportunity to ask questions and voice concerns.

Physical Preparation

Preparation for surgery may occur in designated preoperative areas. Procedures generally conducted in preoperative areas include premedication, intravenous start (if not performed following general anesthesia), and preparation of the surgical site. If urinary catheterization is necessary, it is usually not performed until the child has been anesthetized.

Preoperative procedures and guidelines vary among hospitals and outpatient surgical centers. Preoperative checklists are used in ambulatory and acute care settings to ensure proper physical preparation of patients for surgery. A sample preoperative checklist is provided in Box 11–6. Weigh the preoperative child accurately, measure vital signs, and ask about last fluid intake amount and type. Monitor urinary output. NPO status in an infant and young child is distressing to both the child and the parents. Reinforce teaching regarding necessary NPO status as needed and provide support to the child and the family. See Families Want to Know: Waiting for the Child to Go to Surgery.

Nursing management during the preoperative period includes establishing accurate baseline data, administering prescribed fluids, and performing assessments of fluid status. When an intravenous infusion is prescribed, start the infusion (see the *Clinical Skills Manual*), ensuring that the type of fluid and flow

NURSING CARE PLAN
The Child Undergoing Surgery

Intervention	Rationale	Expected Outcome
1. Nursing Diagnosis: Deficient Knowledge related to preoperative and postoperative events		
NIC Priority Intervention: *Teaching, Preoperative:* Assisting the parent and child to understand and mentally prepare for surgery and postoperative recovery		**NOC Suggested Outcome:** *Knowledge:* Extent of understanding conveyed about treatment regimen
Goal: The child and family will acquire knowledge related to the operation.		
▪ Ask questions of the parent and child about surgery.	▪ Prior knowledge and understanding can be reinforced and used to guide your presentation.	The child and family are able to verbalize details about expected preoperative and postoperative events. They ask questions that demonstrate understanding. The child demonstrates skills needed in the postoperative period.
▪ Teach about preoperative and postoperative events using appropriate developmental methods such as dolls, drawings, stories, and tours.	▪ Developmental level determines the cognitive approach that works best for teaching.	
▪ Reinforce information the family has received about the purpose of surgery.	▪ The physician may have explained the operation.	
▪ Have the child demonstrate postoperative events that pertain to his or her care such as deep breathing, putting a bandage on a doll, taping an intravenous line on a doll, and pressing the patient-controlled analgesia button.	▪ Concrete experience promotes learning.	
▪ Allow the parents and child to ask questions.	▪ Learners must have an opportunity to ask questions.	
2. Nursing Diagnosis: Anxiety related to change in health status		
NIC Priority Intervention: *Anxiety Reduction:* Minimizing apprehension, dread, foreboding, or uneasiness related to an unidentified source of anticipated danger		**NOC Suggested Outcome:** *Coping:* Actions to manage stressors that tax an individual's resources
Goal: The child and family will show decreased behavior indicating anxiety.		
▪ Question the child about expectations of hospitalization and previous experiences.	▪ Previous experiences can influence present anxiety level.	The child and family demonstrate less anxiety. They verbalize understanding and comfort in hospital routines. Parents support the child for traumatic procedures.
▪ Orient the child to the hospital setting, routines, staff, and other patients.	▪ Familiarity with the setting and people can decrease anxiety by removing unknown factors.	
▪ Institute age-appropriate play and interactions with the child.	▪ Play can increase trust level and decrease anxiety.	
▪ Explain procedures and prepare for those that might cause trauma. Encourage parents to support the child.	▪ The child is more likely to trust caregivers if they are truthful and if parents are present.	
▪ Allow the parents and child to ask questions.	▪ Questioning provides an opportunity to explain the unknown, which decreases anxiety.	

NURSING CARE PLAN

The Child Undergoing Surgery (continued)

Intervention	Rationale	Expected Outcome
3. Nursing Diagnosis: Pain related to surgical procedure		
NIC Priority Intervention: *Pain Management:* Alleviation of pain or a reduction in pain to a level of comfort that is acceptable to the patient		**NOC Suggested Outcome:** *Pain Control Behavior:* Personal actions to control pain
Goal: The child will maintain an adequate comfort level.		
■ Assess behavioral cues (e.g., crying, movement, guarding, ability to participate in activities of daily living).	■ Behavior of preverbal children provides clues to pain experience.	The child's pain is controlled as demonstrated by a low number on the pain assessment tool (behavioral or verbal).
■ Use an appropriate pain assessment tool for verbal and nonverbal children (see Chapter 15 ∞ for descriptions of a variety of pain assessment tools).	■ An age-appropriate pain assessment tool allows verbal children to quantify the amount of pain. Pain assessment tools designed for nonverbal children allow the nurse to quantify the amount of pain when the child cannot provide a self-report.	
■ Administer prescribed pain medications around the clock.	■ Opioids and nonopioid analgesics alter pain perception.	
■ Use age-appropriate nonpharmacologic methods of pain control (e.g., distraction, repositioning, massage). See Chapter 15 ∞.	■ Nonpharmacologic interventions interfere with pain perception and may decrease the child's anxiety.	
4. Nursing Diagnosis: Therapeutic Regimen Management, Effective		
NIC Priority Intervention: Facilitate family participation in the emotional and physical care of the patient		**NOC Suggested Outcome:** *Treatment regimen:* Extent of understanding conveyed about a specific treatment regimen
Goal: The child and family will verbalize self-care required at home.		
■ Provide oral and written home care instructions regarding surgical wound care, medications, activities, and diet.	■ Teaching regarding home care is necessary early in hospitalization.	The child and family demonstrate skills needed for home care following discharge. They verbalize plans for future care.
■ Provide a number to call for questions or concerns. Instruct on follow-up visits.	■ Parents need to know emergency information and that follow-up care is required.	

rate match those that are ordered and that would be expected for the weight of the child.

Of necessity, the young child who undergoes surgery usually is restricted from consuming oral foods and fluids just before, during, and for a period after surgery, thus creating a risk of fluid imbalance. The length of time the child is kept without oral intake prior to surgery varies. Recommendations from the American Society of Anesthesiologists indicate that clear liquids may be given up until 2 hours prior to surgery, breast milk until 4 hours prior to surgery, and infant formula 6 hours prior. Milk and a light meal may be consumed up until 6 hours prior to surgery (Crenshaw & Winslow, 2008). Infants will generally have very specific orders related to what time they should be made NPO for breast milk, formula, and clear liquids. These orders will depend on what time the infant is scheduled for surgery.

Families Want to Know
Waiting for the Child to Go to Surgery

Waiting for the child to go to surgery can be a very stressful time for both the family and the child. The major stressor for the infant and young child is the need to be NPO. Having a child who is upset because of hunger is very stressful for parents. Other stressors for parents include the risks of the surgery, pain the child will experience after the surgery, and concerns about the outcome. Nurses must be sensitive to the concerns of the parents and provide support to these families. If the scheduled time for surgery has passed and no one has come to transport the child to the pediatric holding area, the nurse should call the operating room and see when they expect someone to get the child for surgery. Although this takes a few minutes, it is an essential aspect of creating a trusting family-centered environment.

Preoperative Checklist

✓ Check that consent forms are witnessed and signed and in the patient's chart.
✓ Be sure the child's name band is in place.
✓ Be sure any allergies are prominently noted in the child's chart.
✓ Remove any prosthetic devices, including orthodontic appliances.
✓ Check the child's mouth for loose teeth and tongue piercings.
✓ Remove eyeglasses or contacts and jewelry.
✓ Bathe and cleanse the operative site if ordered.
✓ Put the child in a hospital gown, allowing the child to wear underwear.
✓ Check that all special tests have been completed and the results are in the child's chart.
✓ Have the child void before surgery.
✓ Keep the child NPO before surgery.
✓ Give the child prescribed medications.
✓ Transport the child safely to the operating room.

Because children beyond infancy do not usually eat or drink during the night, orders are usually written for NPO after midnight. If surgery is not scheduled for the morning, however, more specific orders should be written, especially for the toddler and preschool-age child, who will not be as tolerant of an extended NPO status. The ultimate decision on how long the child is NPO lies with the anesthesiologist and may vary depending on personal experiences and beliefs.

Infants are especially unable to conserve fluids; therefore, even a short time of NPO status for a diagnostic test may lead to imbalance. Surgery often causes fluid loss from bleeding, which can further compromise fluid balance. In addition, the child may experience third-spacing, a loss or pooling of fluid in a body space such as the abdomen, either in response to surgery or in response to the child's condition. Although decisions about the total amount of fluid required are determined by anesthesiologists during the surgery, the nurse needs an understanding of the amount of fluid generally required during the perioperative period. If a child is NPO prior to surgery and no intravenous line has been started, the child requires additional fluids during and after surgery to compensate for those not taken in during the period of fasting.

Decisions regarding the types of fluids administered before, during, and after surgery are determined based on the child's condition, length of surgery, and clinical condition. During surgery, nurses continue to administer fluids and measure fluid losses, and assess the child continuously. See Chapter 18 ∞ for fluid requirements for children.

Clinical Judgment

Sometimes, due to emergencies, planned surgeries for infants and young children may be postponed for several hours. These children are NPO and generally do not have IV access. What action should the nurse take in this case?

Postoperative Care

Postoperative care of the child includes both physical and psychologic care. In the immediate postoperative period, perform baseline monitoring of vital signs; evaluate the child's level of consciousness; evaluate for evidence of fluid loss or bleeding via dressings, vomiting, or drainage tubes; and record hourly urinary output. Maintain effective airway clearance and monitor for evidence of respiratory depression or distress (see Chapter 20 ∞). Provide comfort and pain relief. See Chapter 15 ∞ for details concerning pain management. Examine the postoperative orders and ensure that the child receives the type and amount of intravenous fluid indicated. Resumption of oral intake is dependent on the surgical procedure, the child's condition, and surgeon protocol. Once oral fluids are resumed, monitor for emesis. When the child is consuming adequate fluids, the rate of intravenous fluids is decreased or discontinued according to physician orders.

Parents are encouraged to visit with the child as soon after surgery as possible (Figure 11–7 ➤). In some facilities, after surgery, children are brought to the postoperative anesthesia care unit (PACU) or postanesthesia recovery unit (PAR), where the child recovers from anesthesia. Depending on the child's condition, he or she may be discharged home directly from an outpatient surgical procedure or transferred to a general pediatric unit or intensive care unit.

Postoperative Home Care Instructions

Routine postoperative instructions for the family of the child undergoing outpatient or 1-day-stay surgical procedures include monitoring for signs of infection, such as drainage, red-

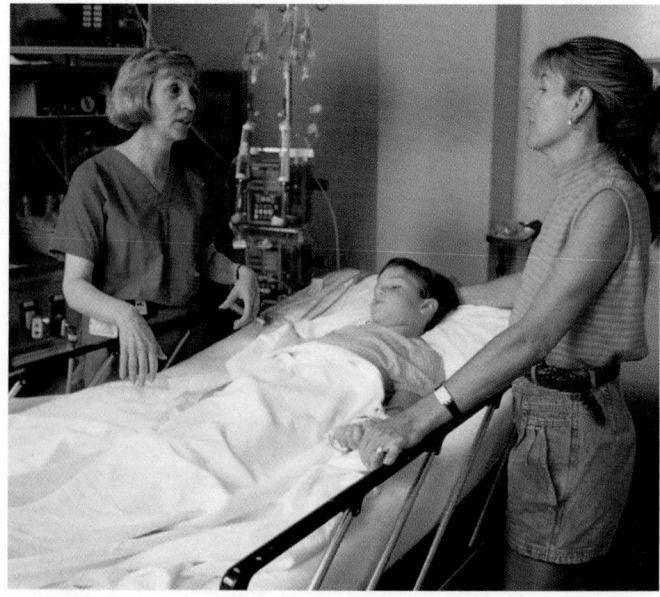

FIGURE 11–7 ➤ This child has just undergone surgery and is now in the postanesthesia care unit (PACU). Although the child's physical care is immediate and important, both the child and the family have psychosocial needs that must also be addressed. It is important to reunite the family as soon as possible after surgery.

ness, or swelling of the surgical incision; fever; and change in behavior. Instructions for follow-up visits, medications, other treatments, and wound care, as well as signs and symptoms that require medical attention, are also provided. Additional instructions are tailored according to the surgical procedure and the child's condition. The nurse ensures the family understands home care instructions through their return demonstration and verbalization of understanding.

■ STRATEGIES TO PROMOTE COPING AND NORMAL DEVELOPMENT OF THE HOSPITALIZED CHILD

During hospitalization, care of the child focuses not only on meeting physiologic needs, but also on meeting psychosocial and developmental needs. Several strategies may be used to help children adapt to the hospital environment, promote effective coping, and provide developmentally appropriate activities. These strategies include child-life programs, rooming in, therapeutic play, and therapeutic recreation.

Rooming In

The practice of **rooming in** involves a parent staying in the child's hospital room during the course of the child's hospitalization. Some hospitals provide cots, while others have special built-in beds on pediatric units. In some institutions, a parent is provided a separate room on the unit. Parents who stay at the bedside usually want to help care for their child (Power & Franck, 2008). Communication between the nurse and family is important so that the parent's desire for involvement is understood and supported.

Rooming in provides the child with the comfort and security of parental presence. Some parents may feel more comfortable staying with their child and participating in care, whereas others may experience more stress if they are missing work and are away from home and other children. Collaborate with the parents to establish a rooming-in plan that is beneficial to both the child and family. For example, parents may alternate turns staying with the child, and even grandparents, aunts and uncles, and grown siblings may be included in the plan.

Some facilities offer free or reduced-cost meals to the parent rooming in. The parent who does not receive these meals may often skip many meals due to the financial impact on an already overburdened budget related to illness and hospitalization. The nurse should be alert to parents who never leave the bedside and should make sure the parents are eating. Emphasize the importance of the child's need for a healthy parent. Social services or other departments in the hospital may be able to assist the family in obtaining meals while rooming in with the hospitalized child.

Parents rooming in with their child for an extended hospitalization can be encouraged to take advantage of facilities such as the Ronald McDonald house, or other housing available for parents, at some point during the stay as a respite for a few hours. This will provide them with an opportunity for needed rest and privacy.

Child-Life Programs

Many hospitals have child-life programs that focus on the psychosocial needs of hospitalized children. Professional child-life specialists, paraprofessionals, and volunteers staff these departments (Figure 11–8 ➤). A **child-life specialist** plans activities to provide age-appropriate play for children either in their room or in a specialized playroom. Some of the planned activities are designed to assist children in working through feelings about illness. Examples include playing with medical equipment, acting out procedures or treatments on dolls, using games to act out feelings, or drawing pictures about hospital treatments (Figure 11–9 ➤).

Both the child-life department and the nursing staff focus on the emotional needs of hospitalized children. Child-life specialists and nurses collaborate to formulate a plan to assist children with particular needs. Before engaging in activities, attention is given to the child's level of mobility, fatigue, readiness to participate, and other barriers such as pain. The nurse and child-life specialist can work together to determine appropriate methods to use to promote coping with painful procedures.

Therapeutic Play

Play is a significant component of childhood, and the stress of illness and hospitalization increases the value of play. Hospitals, however, because of the need to contain costs, may minimize

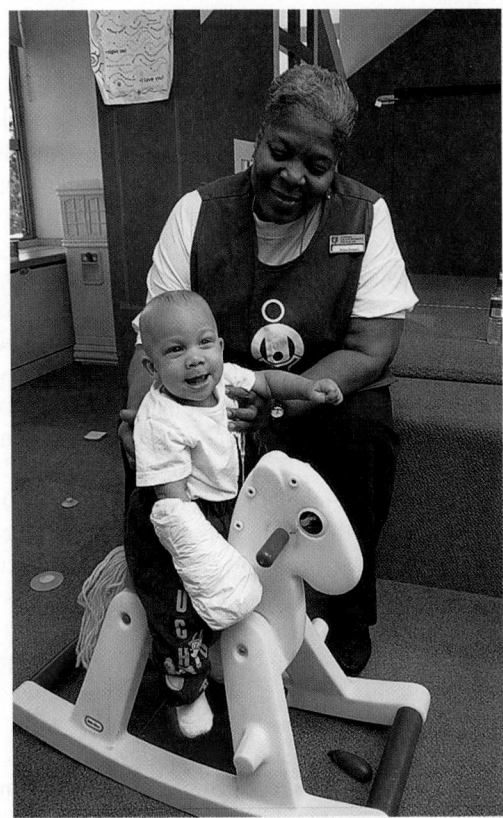

FIGURE 11–8 ➤ Volunteers such as this foster grandmother can provide stimulation and nurturing to help young children adapt to lengthy hospitalizations.

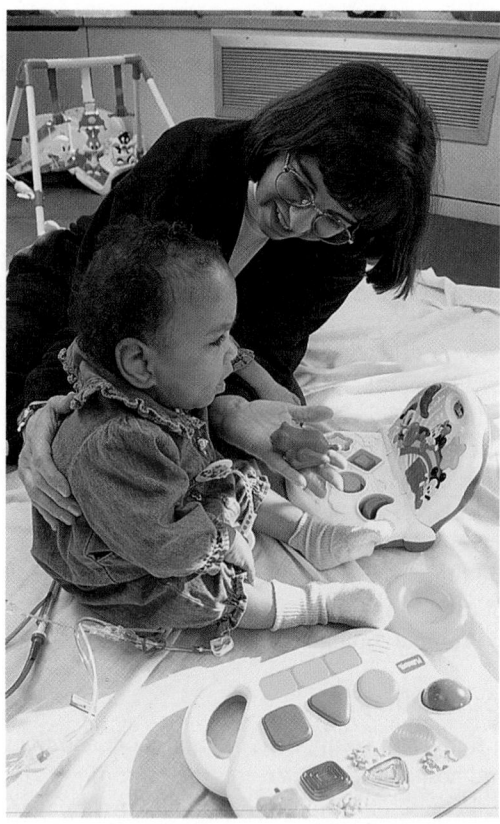

FIGURE 11–9 ➤ A child-life specialist works with children being treated for cancer. Special dolls are used to familiarize children with the procedures they undergo.

their play programs. Therefore, nurses should document the need for and benefits of play. Beyond facilitating normal development, play sessions can provide a means for the child to learn about health care, express anxieties, work through feelings, and achieve a sense of control over frightening or little-understood situations.

Play that presents an opportunity to deal with the fears, concerns, and stressors of health experiences is called **therapeutic play**. Therapeutic play has many benefits for both the child and the health professional. It allows the child an opportunity to relive, understand, and integrate fearful health care experiences. The child can achieve a sense of mastery by being in control of the occurrences during play. This helps to lower the child's stress and anxiety about the events. In addition, the health care professional can observe the child's play to learn more about the type of events that cause anxiety to the child. The child's coping methods can be observed and additional techniques offered to the child. *Play therapy* is a mental health technique used to treat children with mental health problems, rather than normal life events that have caused anxiety. This technique is discussed in Chapter 28 ∞.

Through therapeutic play, the child's knowledge of his or her illness or injury can be assessed. A common technique involves using an outline drawing of the body (Figure 11–10 ➤) or having the child draw a picture about the hospitalization. Drawings can be used to determine what the child knows and understands

about the hospitalization. In addition to assessment, drawing can be used as a nursing intervention. Demonstrate to the child on a drawing what will occur during surgery or a treatment. The child's drawings of health care experiences allow him or her to express fears and gain mastery over the situation.

Dramatic play, in which medical situations encountered are reenacted by the child, often assists the child to cope with painful treatments and intrusive procedures. Safe medical equipment such as bandages and syringes without needles, and scrubs and uniforms for dress up, are effective materials for encouraging dramatic play. Dramatic play offers an outlet for anxiety in children trying to deal with stressful and confusing situations. At the same time, these activities allow the nurse to observe and assess the child's perception of the illness and procedures. The nurse is then able to clarify any of the child's misconceptions.

A variety of techniques may be used to promote therapeutic and dramatic play (Table 11–7), depending on the child's developmental stage. The nurse can ensure that a variety of age-appropriate toys, distraction materials (stress balls, bubbles, music), and "prizes" are available (Box 11–7).

Additional techniques, such as sand or water play, may be appropriate in specific situations.

Many hospitals, particularly children's hospitals, provide playrooms on each of the units to allow children a place to play and socialize with same-age peers. These rooms are generally brightly decorated in children's themes, and provide numerous opportunities for play, such as board games, video games, supplies for painting or drawing, and age-appropriate toys for each developmental level. For younger children, families may be encouraged to bring the child's favorite age-appropriate toys from

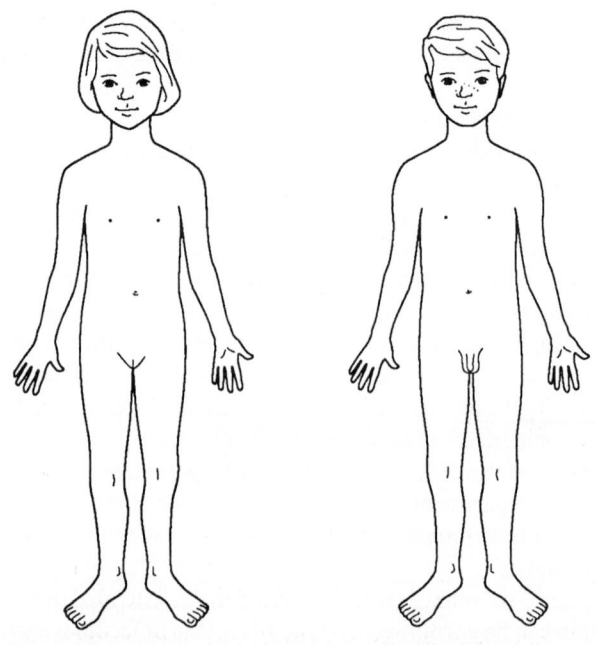

FIGURE 11–10 ➤ The nurse can use a simple gender-specific outline drawing of a child's body to encourage children to draw what they think about their medical problem. Such drawings reveal a child's interpretation, which the nurse can work with to provide enhanced teaching.

TABLE 11–7	**Therapeutic Play Techniques**	
Technique	Assessment	Interventions
Stories	Have the child make up a story about a picture. Analyze content and emotional clues in the story. Have children tell a story about an important experience in a group of other children.	Read or make up stories to explain illness, hospitalization, or other specific aspects of health care. Emotions such as fear can be included.
Drawings	Ask the child to draw a picture about being in the hospital. Consider subject matter, size and placement of items in drawings, colors used, presence or absence of physical barriers, and general emotional feeling.	Use the child's drawings or outlines of the body to explain care, procedures, or conditions. Provide an opportunity for the child to draw pictures of his or her choice or suggest topics such as a picture of the child's family or health care encounter. Ask the child to tell you about the picture. Be alert to the child's emotions. You might say "This child must be frightened by the big x-ray machine."
Music	Observe types of music chosen and effects of played music on behavior.	Encourage parents and children to bring favorite music to the hospital for stress relief. Have music playing during tests and procedures. Parents can record their voices to play for infants and young children during separations. During longer hospitalizations, children can record messages for siblings or classmates, who are then encouraged to record their responses. Playtime can include the opportunity to play instruments and sing.
Puppets	The puppets can ask questions of young children, who are often more likely to answer the puppet than a person.	Perform short skits to teach children necessary health care information. Include emotional content when appropriate.
Dramatic play	Provide dolls and medical equipment, and analyze the roles assigned to dolls by the child, the behavior demonstrated by the dolls in the child's play, and the apparent emotions. Dolls with illnesses or health problems like those of the child are especially helpful.	Provide dolls and equipment for play sessions. To ensure safety, supervise closely when actual equipment is used. Respond to emotions and behavior shown. Use dolls and equipment such as casts, nebulizer, intravenous apparatus, and stethoscope to explain care. Use dolls with problems or illnesses similar to those of the child when available. Provide toys that foster expression of emotion, such as a pounding board and indoor darts.
Pets	Provide animal-assisted activity. Watch the interaction between the child and animal.	Respond to emotions the child shows. Facilitate touch and stroking of animals.

home. For older children, there may be options for computer communication with children in other hospitals. Portable electronic gaming equipment may be available to children in isolation or those unable to come to the playroom or teen lounge. Specific interventions according to developmental level are discussed in the following text.

BOX 11–7 Prize Basket

A "prize" basket is an effective method of providing rewards and distraction to the toddler, preschooler, and even school-age child. The basket contains age-appropriate toys, games, and items that the child may choose from as a reward for participating in a procedure. For example, bubbles, stuffed animals, small dolls, coloring books, balls, and books are inexpensive (they may also be donated) items that the child can choose from. Even if the child is uncooperative, once the procedure is completed, it is important to praise the child and offer the opportunity to choose from the prize basket.

Infant

Infants require external stimuli for growth. The use of mobiles, music, mirrors, and other stimuli helps to promote stimulation and offer comfort to the infant. Parents and family are encouraged to cuddle or rock the infant and sing lullabies. Talking to the infant encourages interaction and play.

Toddler

Through play, toddlers explore the environment and learn to identify with significant people in their lives. Play is also an acceptable way for toddlers to release tensions caused by stress or aggressive impulses.

Approach toddlers slowly and make the initial approach in their parents' presence, if possible, to decrease feelings of stranger anxiety (wariness of strangers). Playing a variation of peek-a-boo or hide-and-seek using the curtain surrounding the toddler's crib or bed helps promote the realization that objects that are out of sight, such as parents, do return. The use of a familiar blanket or stuffed animal can temporarily substitute for the security of parents. The toddler can be read familiar stories.

Repetition of stories promotes a sense of stability in the unfamiliar hospital environment.

A doll is a familiar toy that can be used to re-create a stressful environment, thereby providing an opportunity for the child to express and work through feelings. Other developmentally appropriate toys for toddlers include familiar objects from home such as measuring cups or spoons, wooden puzzles, building blocks, and push-and-pull toys. Playing with safe hospital equipment (bandages, syringes without needles, and stethoscopes) helps toddlers to overcome the anxiety associated with these items. Supervise these play sessions and remove hospital equipment when you leave.

Preschooler

The nurse can intervene to reduce the stress produced by preschoolers' fears through the use of certain kinds of play. A simple outline of the body or a doll can be used to address the child's fantasies and fears of bodily harm. Playing with safe hospital equipment may help preschoolers to work through feelings such as aggression (Figure 11–11 ➤).

Preschoolers prefer crayons and coloring books, puppets, felt and magnetic boards, play dough, books, and recorded stories. Preschoolers and older children often enjoy **animal-assisted activity** (Figure 11–12 ➤). Children's hospitals and units can have visits from pets, most commonly dogs, to provide diversion and relaxation (McKenney & Johnson, 2008; Ryan, 2008).

School-Age Child

Although play begins to lose its importance in the school-age years, the nurse can still use some techniques of therapeutic play to help the hospitalized child cope with stress. Age-appropriate crafts and activities provide diversion and a sense of accomplishment. School-age children often regress devel-

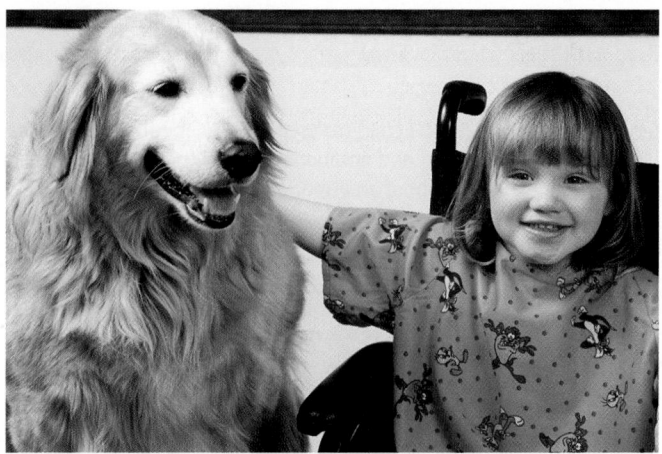

FIGURE 11–12 ➤ Hospitals may have animal-assisted activity from specially trained animals to provide comfort and distraction during health care. Both the child and the dog seem to be smiling!

opmentally during hospitalization, demonstrating behaviors characteristic of an earlier state, such as separation anxiety and fear of bodily injury. Outlines of the body and anatomically correct dolls or condition-specific dolls (Figure 11–13 ➤) can be used to illustrate the cause and treatment of the child's illness. Terms for body parts that are suitable for older children are used. Drawings provide an outlet for expression of fears and anger.

School-age children enjoy collecting and organizing objects and often ask to keep disposable equipment that has been used

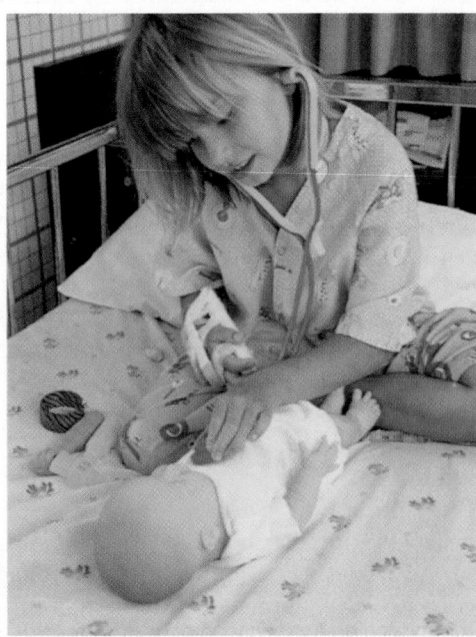

FIGURE 11–11 ➤ Age-appropriate play will help the child adjust to hospitalization and care.

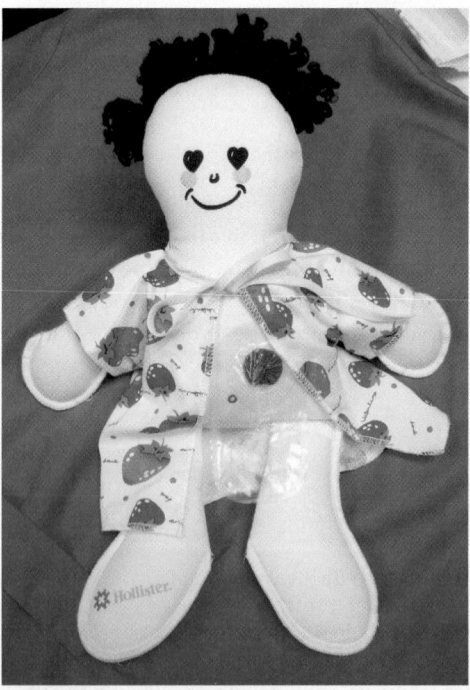

FIGURE 11–13 ➤ Having the child play with dolls, like these Shadow Buddies, that have "conditions" similar to his or her own will help the child adjust. Such play helps the child realize what activities are possible.

Used with permission from the Shadow Buddies Foundation, www.shadowbuddies.org

in their care. They may use these items later to relive the experience with their friends. Games, books, school work, crafts, tape recordings, and computers and video games provide an outlet for stress and increase self-esteem in the school-age child. The type of play used should promote a sense of mastery and achievement.

Adolescent

Many of the special play techniques used with younger children are not suitable for adolescents. However, adolescents do require a planned **therapeutic recreation** program to assist them in meeting developmental needs during hospitalization. Peers are very important to the adolescent, and the isolation of hospitalization can be difficult. Telephone contact with other teenagers and visits from friends should be encouraged. Interactions with other hospitalized teenagers at a pizza party night, playing video games, watching a movie, or participating in other activities can help adolescents feel a sense of normalcy (Figure 11–14 ➤). Physical activities that provide an outlet for stress are recommended. Even adolescents on bed rest or in wheelchairs can play a modified form of basketball. Some hospitals provide a teen room or teen lounge with age-appropriate activities such as a pool table, video games, and computers.

The independence of adolescence is interrupted by illness. Nurses can provide choices for teenagers to assist them in regaining control. Providing adolescents with options and encouraging them to choose an evening of recreational activity can promote their feelings of independence.

Strategies to Meet Educational Needs

Some hospitalizations are so short that the absence of the child or adolescent from school and peers is of minimal concern. However, if hospitalization is expected to last longer than a few

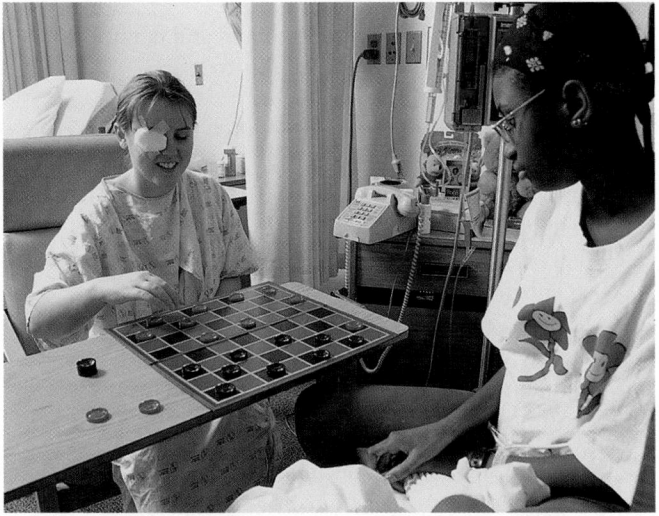

FIGURE 11–14 ➤ Having interaction with other hospitalized adolescents and maintaining contact with friends outside the hospital are very important so that the teenager does not feel alone. A friendly yet competitive checkers game helps to stimulate these teenagers and allows for self-expression. What are some of the other benefits?

days or if the child's condition will change, necessitating special school arrangements, the nurse assesses the effects of hospitalization on the child's education.

When an elective procedure occurs, collaborate with families to arrange the extended school absence with teachers. The child can then be provided with school work to complete in the hospital or at home when capable. This minimizes educational deficits and future problems for the child. Pencils, paper, comfortable work areas, computers, and quiet work times are provided to meet the child's educational needs. Telephone calls, Internet connections, and live videoconferencing with teachers can be arranged as needed. Pediatric hospitals generally provide in-house teachers. The hospital teachers collaborate with the child's school teachers to ensure the child is meeting the educational objectives to avoid deficits upon return to school.

Nurses should also consider the social aspects of school and peers. Peers can be encouraged to visit a hospitalized classmate, send cards and letters, call on the telephone, or communicate via the Internet. Classmates may even want to videotape a class session, allowing everyone the opportunity to send a message to the child. When the child returns to school, the nurse can visit the classroom to provide classmates with information about the child's medical condition or assist the child in creating his or her own presentation about the hospital experience and medical condition.

The hospital nurse may contact the child's school nurse when special arrangements are necessary for situations such as mobility challenges. For example, the child who is wearing a large cast or who requires medications or other treatments, such as tracheostomy care, may offer challenges in a traditional school setting. Refer to Chapter 10 ∞ for further discussion of caring for the child in the community.

The child with chronic health problems or requiring long-term hospitalization has additional needs with regard to school. Hospitals or rehabilitation units may have classrooms, teachers, and facilities to promote learning (Figure 11–15 ➤). Many school districts provide tutors or computer connections for students who are hospitalized or receiving home care for extended periods. Teachers can visit children at the hospital or at home. Parents are often pivotal in making arrangements to meet the child's educational needs, since they interact with the child, the school, and the health care team. Further discussion of meeting the educational needs of the child with a chronic condition is provided in Chapter 12 ∞.

Child and Family Teaching

Teaching is an essential part of the nurse's role in the care of hospitalized children and their families and begins with the initial

---

Law & Ethics *Schooling Provision*

The Joint Commission on Accreditation of Healthcare Organizations (2009) mandates provision of schooling for the child in a health care facility for an extended period.

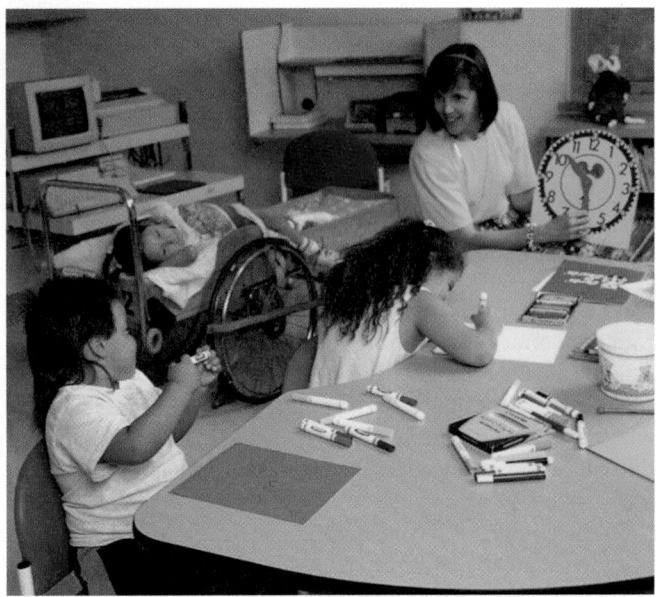

FIGURE 11–15 ➤ Shriners Hospital in Spokane, Washington, has a special classroom and teacher for children undergoing a lengthy hospital stay, enabling them to remain current with their school work. The child who falls behind other students might not fit in when he or she returns to school or might be required to repeat a grade. What are the potential consequences of these situations?

contact between the family and health care providers. Teaching may be informal, as when the nurse integrates an explanation during routine care, or structured, as when the nurse plans and implements a formal teaching program.

Nurses emphasize to the family that most teaching will occur in informal sessions rather than in formalized programs. The family should be aware of the teaching process to encourage active listening and participation. Actively involve the family in the learning process to ensure their understanding. The nurse and family work together to identify the family's learning needs and appropriate teaching method to best convey the information. Recall that different family members may be at various cognitive and anxiety levels and therefore have needs for different types of teaching. Develop a plan with both the family and other health care professionals to facilitate learning among the child and family members. Children will gain a better understanding of the illness when teaching takes into consideration their developmental level. Learning is achieved more successfully when teaching involves more than one sense (such as hearing, vision, and touch).

Teaching about the behaviors observed in hospitalized children and the strategies to deal with these behaviors is helpful for parents. For instance, provide parents of hospitalized toddlers with information on the typical behaviors of hospitalized children and the strategies to assist them. By being informed, the parents should have less anxiety and a greater capacity for involvement and support of their child during hospitalization.

Teaching directed at parents must be geared to their level of understanding. If English is not spoken or is the parents' second language, then a translator may be necessary. If translators are needed to facilitate understanding, be sure they are arranged for and available for teaching sessions.

Depending on the information to be presented, teaching may use the cognitive, psychomotor, or affective domains of learning. Teaching that includes all three domains is more effective. Explanations or reading materials, including pamphlets, booklets, videos, and models, are tailored to a level the parent can understand. The choice of tools used varies depending on the child's diagnosis and available materials.

Timing is a critical factor in teaching. Parents and children are less receptive to teaching when they are preoccupied with stress or activities. Collaborating with the parents in scheduling specific times for teaching sessions may be helpful.

Teaching Plans

Teaching plans provide structure for the creation and delivery of patient and family education. By developing a teaching plan, a nurse helps to ensure that all the necessary information is included and taught efficiently. Additionally, this written documentation of teaching allows for continuity of care between nurses and other disciplines. Multidisciplinary teaching plans provide clear communication for all health team members in the teaching process. Nurses individualize teaching plans and sessions according to the child's ability and needs. Adequate assessment of the child's strengths and abilities, along with collaboration with parents and other members of the multidisciplinary team, can assist the nurse to establish an individualized plan of the most effective teaching methods for the child.

The child's primary caretaker should be an active participant in the development and implementation of the teaching plan. The primary caretaker is most often a parent but may be a close family member (uncle, aunt, or grandparent). Prior to establishing a teaching plan the nurse should assess the child's or parent's knowledge, skills, and feelings by considering the following questions:

- What does the parent/caretaker or child know about the health issue?
- What are the expectations of the child and family?
- What is the cognitive level or ability to learn?
- Is there a desire to learn?
- What previous experiences affect the learning experience, either positively or negatively?
- What previous interventions have been the most useful for the child and family?
- What resources are available to the parents, child, and nurse that enhance understanding of the health condition?
- Are there feelings or beliefs that might interfere with the learning process?
- What complementary care does the family use, and how does this relate to the teaching plan?

The second step involves deciding what knowledge, skill, or change in attitude is desired. Outcome criteria or objectives are established with the parent and child.

Possible teaching methods and a range of approaches are explored. A variety of resources, including written materials (books, pamphlets, handouts, and stories), computer software, audiovisual presentations, and others, are available to encourage interest from the child and family. See Families Want to Know:

Families Want to Know
Standardized Teaching Plan:
Preparing the Child for Surgery

Whether the child is encountered in the clinic, preoperative admissions clinic, emergency department, or pediatric unit, the nurse should prepare the child for surgery as much as possible. Younger children should be told about a planned operation the day before the surgery. School-age children and adolescents should be told as soon as the operation is scheduled. Age-specific guidelines should be followed. (See Table 11–6: Assisting Children Through Procedures on page 274, and Nursing Care Plan: The Child Undergoing Surgery on pages 276–277.)

General Principles

- Ask the child's parents what they have told their child about the operation.
- Assess the child's perception of the operation using developmentally appropriate activities.
- Teach the child about the operation and what to expect during the pre- and postoperative period, clarifying any misconceptions.
- Reassess the child's perception of the operation.

Sample Teaching Plan for Tiona, the 5-Year-Old Girl in the Opening Scenario, Scheduled for a Tonsillectomy and Adenoidectomy

When: At the preadmissions visit the day prior to surgery

Where: In a quiet room, without distraction

How:

- Ask Tiona's mother what she has told her daughter about the surgery.
- Ask Tiona to draw a picture about going to the hospital.
- Ask Tiona why she needs the operation.
- Using a body outline doll or picture of a body outline, ask Tiona to show you what part is going to be fixed.
- Use pictures, books, dolls, and safe medical equipment to clarify misconceptions and teach Tiona about the operation and care afterward.

Standardized Teaching Plan: Preparing the Child for Surgery, and Box 11–8 for teaching methods.

Teaching for Children with Special Health Care Needs

Children who have disabilities may have special learning needs (Allen, Vessey, & Schapiro, 2010) If the child has a visual impairment or perceptual difficulty, material is presented in auditory and tactile ways. Children who have hearing deficits require visual and tactile presentations. When psychomotor skill performance is needed to assess a child with neuromuscular conditions, special aids and devices may be necessary to enable the child to hold a syringe, draw up a liquid, or perform other tasks. Children who have learning disabilities may require more frequent reinforcement and shorter teaching sessions. These children are evaluated often for comprehension in order to adjust teaching as necessary.

Children who have chronic conditions or special health care needs may have been hospitalized numerous times and have received other health care at home and in the community. They usually have adapted coping mechanisms that help them deal with the chronic illness. Nurses can talk with the child to determine what has helped in the past, provide information about what to expect during the current hospitalization, assign staff

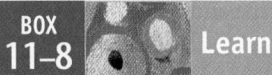

BOX 11–8 · Learning Through Senses

For children who can hear, touch, see a model or equipment, read, look at pictures, or even smell things like alcohol swabs, learning is more complete. This is particularly important for the school-age child in the stage of concrete operational thought, who must be able to manipulate materials in order to learn.

---

members who are familiar when possible, and follow each child's lead in assisting his or her coping.

Do not assume that the child with a history of numerous hospitalizations understands all activities. Each hospitalization is different. Even the most routine activities should be explained. Regularly review the updated plan of care with the parents and child. Provide the child with opportunities to ask questions and to express concerns and fears. Assess each child's individual learning needs. Older children can be asked how they best like to learn. Determine the necessity for special equipment or teaching methods.

■ PREPARATION FOR HOME CARE

Nurses play an important role in preparing the child and family for discharge home; this preparation starts early during the hospitalization. The nurse works with the social service department, home care agencies, and the family to plan for equipment, procedures, and other home care needs. Home care nurses collaborate with the hospital nurse and assist families to meet the child's health care needs.

Assessing the Child and Family in Preparation for Discharge

Preparation for the discharge process is best started upon admission to the hospital. The health care team, including the primary health care provider, nurse, social worker, and discharge planner, works with the family to ensure a smooth transition. Assess the family's ability to manage the child's care and if any special adaptation of the home environment is necessary.

When a child who has been hospitalized for an extended period is to be discharged home, the school district is contacted by the hospital teacher (if available) or social worker, and plans for education or reentry into school are made. This involves an assessment of the child by the school district and formulation of an *individualized education plan (IEP)*. The IEP may include home tutors, specialized services from persons such as physical or speech therapists, or arrangements for transport of the child with a disability to the school and provisions for special medical care as needed. An *individualized health plan (IHP)* may also be required. See Chapter 12 ∞ for a detailed discussion on IEPs and IHPs.

Some common problems that interfere with successful discharge planning include financial concerns, the family's unavailability for teaching and planning, lack of equipment, and lack of teamwork among involved health care disciplines. Nurses who assess for these potential problems from the initial contact with the child and family can intervene and assist the family to resolve them as soon as possible.

Preparing the Child and Family for Discharge

The family may need to learn physical and rehabilitative procedures for the child's care. Short-term care may be necessary until the child regains full function. In other situations, care may be required throughout the child's life. This may involve measuring vital signs or assessing blood glucose levels. For the child requiring complex long-term care, parents may need to learn about intravenous lines, medications, oxygen administration, or ventilators (Figure 11–16 ➤). See Chapter 12 for discussion of the child with a chronic condition.

Parents of children at risk for respiratory or cardiac arrest are encouraged to learn cardiopulmonary resuscitation (CPR) (refer to the *Clinical Skills Manual*). Individual sessions to teach the family CPR can be arranged. Some families require support and assistance to become providers of end-of-life care (see Chapter 13 ∞ for end-of-life care).

Not all children discharged after hospitalization will require additional care. However, these families still need support and education, as they may continue to be anxious or stressed over their child's hospitalization. Standard discharge plans for routine hospital discharge include the follow-up appointment date, phone number to call for questions, medication instructions, signs and symptoms to monitor specific to the condition, and care at home. Ensure that the family understands these instructions and has ample opportunity for questions before discharge home.

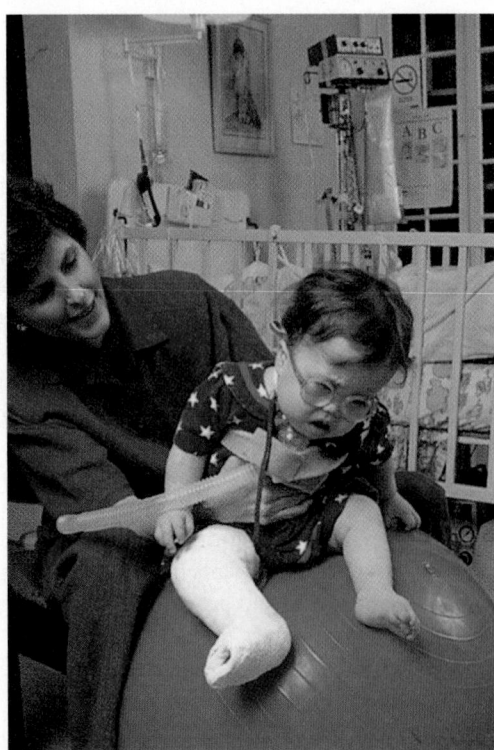

FIGURE 11–16 ➤ This child with chronic medical problems is being cared for at home. Are there any legal implications for the hospital and the nurse associated with preparing the child and family for home care?

Preparing the Child and Family for Home Health Care

Children discharged from the hospital may require short-term or long-term home health care. Children with multisystem conditions may require home care involving specialized equipment and personnel. Early planning provides the family time to investigate health insurance benefits, support services in the community, and other needs before discharge. The education provided and the parents' ability to perform care is discussed with a visiting nurse or individual who manages the home care program. See Evidence-Based Practice: Preparing Families to Provide Health Care for Children at Home.

The nurse collaborates with the social service department, home care agencies, and the family to plan for equipment, procedures, and other home care needs. Home care nurses then assume the child's care and assist families to meet the child's health care needs. See Chapter 12 ∞ for further discussion of home health care.

Preparing the Child and Family for Long-Term Care or Rehabilitation

When ill or injured children require long-term care, they are often transferred from an acute care hospital to a rehabilitation center or other long-term care facility. Like discharge planning, the rehabilitation phase of the treatment does not begin at the time of discharge from the acute care hospital but, instead, early in the hospitalization phase. The plan of care is instituted in the hospital, interventions and therapies are begun, and plans are made for continued care. A multidisciplinary team, including the nurse, social worker, and case manager, coordinates the process and collaborates with the family to ensure a transition that causes the least disruption to the child and family.

When it becomes apparent that a child will require long-term care, the health care team explores with the family the options and resources available to provide such care:

- Home care with support services such as visiting nurses and physical therapists
- A long-term care facility
- A specialized rehabilitation center that can provide care for an extended period

The nurse supports the family during the decision-making process about which option will be the most beneficial, considering the needs of the child, the financial implications, the roles and supports available to the family unit, and the resources available in the community. Guidelines to assist parents in evaluating rehabilitation centers are available from the Brain Injury Association of America (2009). Families can also be referred to the Commission on Accreditation of Rehabilitation Facilities.

Families often require assistance in determining the insurance coverage for long-term care or rehabilitation because coverage for these services may be limited. Social services can assist the family in identifying insurance resources. If a parent must take a leave of absence from work to provide care for the child, inform the parent about the coverage provided by the Family

Evidence-Based Practice

Preparing Families to Provide Health Care for Children at Home

Problem

Children are often discharged from hospitals while still requiring complicated health care procedures, so parents need to learn how to perform these procedures safely. Parents may not be able to be in the hospital consistently during the hospitalization or they may not be as involved in the child's care as would be helpful for learning the needed skills.

Evidence

A survey method was used by Sarajärvi et al. (2006) to describe support that families received during their child's illness from both the family's and the nurse's point of view. Questionnaires were collected from 344 families of children who either visited an outpatient clinic or were hospitalized during the time of the study and from 60 pediatric nurses working in these settings. Of the 344 families, 41% reported that they had been supported by the nursing staff, 21% felt they were not supported at all, and 37% did not answer. Families stated that they received support via "discussion (37%), listening (34%), information (12%) and time given to the families (11%)" (p. 207). Nurses indicated that they had provided support primarily via listening and discussion. They also indicated that they had given the most information about diagnostic testing and treatment and less about the illness itself. Some nurses reported that they had not provided any information to the families. Only one-third of the nurses felt that they had provided adequate information related to care of the child at home. Families reported the need for more support, including the need for more information about their child's illness and care at home.

A study by Weiss, Johnson, Malin, et al. (2008) evaluated readiness for discharge in 135 parents of children who were hospitalized. The parent who was the primary caregiver of the child after discharge from the hospital participated in the study. Results of this study indicated that the nurse's skill in presenting the discharge information was a significant predictor of the parents' readiness for discharge. A higher rating by the parents of the nurse's skill in discharge teaching correlated with a higher level of discharge readi-

ness. The amount of content delivered was not a significant predictor, with 90% of the parents indicating that they actually received more content than needed. Parents who had higher levels of discharge readiness also had less coping difficulty postdischarge.

Implications

For home care to be successful, informational support needed to care for the child at home is essential (Sarajärvi et al., 2006; Weiss et al., 2008). Nurses can support parents during rooming in by making them comfortable and integrating them into discussions and decisions about the child's care; they are collaborators in all of the care involved. Nurses can also view every interaction as a teachable moment and constantly include teaching whenever a parent is present. Explanations related to medications, assessments being performed, and how this will be adapted in the home situation should be included. In addition, resources including phone numbers, parent support groups, reading material, and Internet sources should be provided. The effectiveness of teaching should be evaluated prior to discharge (Weiss et al., 2008). Ask parents what care they feel comfortable with and what they need more assistance to perform. Involve them in the decision about referral to a home health care nurse or school nurse.

Critical Thinking Application

What conditions in the hospital will assist parents to feel welcome and part of the hospital routine? How can parents become a part of rounds to their own child? What questions can they be asked? How can the nurse help to explain to parents the meaning of conversations that take place near the child by health care personnel? How can you adapt your teaching plan to include integration of home care into every interaction with the parents? How can you record the teaching needs of parents so that other nurses can continue with needed information, demonstrations, and assessments? What techniques need to be part of discharge care so that parents leave with resources to get future questions answered as they take over total care of the child?

---

and Medical Leave Act of 1993 (U.S. Department of Labor, 2009). Collaborate with social services to assist the family to understand and complete the applications, if needed.

Nurses in acute care hospitals frequently coordinate services when transfer to another facility occurs. This involves providing information about the child's history, plan of care, treatment, and current status to the new facility. Forms should be available to assist the person responsible for coordinating the transfer. Provide copies of nursing and medical care plans to ensure continuity of care.

Families require support and assistance in dealing with the transfer from the acute care setting to another facility. The family may benefit from a visit to the facility before the child is transferred. Meeting the staff and becoming familiar with the environment can assist the family in preparing the child for a

new environment. The family can then provide the child with brochures, pictures, and other materials from the facility and explain what the child can anticipate experiencing upon transfer. If possible, visits from a rehabilitation center or long-term care facility nursing staff to the child before transfer can also be beneficial.

Whether the child is discharged home without the need for further care, or with the need for home health care or rehabilitative care, the nurse maintains a family-centered approach to provide the child and family with information and support during the discharge process. The nurse ensures that the family is prepared for the discharge and that any treatments and monitoring are understood by the family. Contact information is provided and any support services required are arranged before the child is discharged.

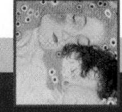

Chapter Highlights

- Hospitalization is a stressful event for all children and their families, especially when the hospitalization is unplanned and sudden.
- The understanding of children about their illnesses and hospitalizations is based on cognitive and psychosocial stage/level, and upon previous health care experiences.
- Nurses assess the impact of the child's illness or hospitalization on the family unit and provide individualized family-centered care.
- Families are always disrupted by a child's hospitalization, and various approaches can help them to understand the process and cope more successfully.
- When hospitalization is planned, both the child and parents can prepare for the experience. Nurses assist this process by teaching them what to expect.

- A teaching plan includes goals and expected outcomes, interventions needed to achieve the specified goals, and a method and time for evaluation of the expected outcomes. How the teaching plan is implemented depends on the unique characteristics of the child/family to be taught.
- The child is prepared for procedures using a variety of techniques, taking into consideration the child's developmental age, coping abilities, and previous experience.
- Strategies such as child-life programs, rooming in, therapeutic play, and therapeutic recreation help meet the psychosocial needs of the hospitalized child.
- The nurse assists the family to plan for the child's long-term health care needs and home care issues. Culturally competent care is integrated throughout all provisions of care.

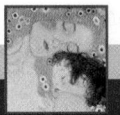

Clinical Reasoning in Action

Recall Tiona, the child described in the chapter-opening vignette. She is a 5-year-old girl who was admitted to the hospital for a tonsillectomy and adenoidectomy (T&A). Following Tiona's operation, she refused to drink liquids because it hurt when she swallowed. After receiving intravenous pain medication, Tiona realized that she could swallow without too much pain and began to eat Popsicles and drink liquids. She was then switched to oral pain medication. Later in the day, Tiona was drinking liquids well enough that she was to be discharged home.

1. What information should the nurse include in the discharge teaching plan for Tiona's mother?
2. As Tiona and her mother are preparing to leave the hospital, Tiona states "I am going to be good so I do not have to come to the hospital anymore!" How should the nurse respond?

3. Tiona's mother states that she is worried her daughter will not drink enough at home. What can the nurse suggest to Tiona's mother to encourage her to drink fluids? What symptoms of dehydration should Tiona's mother watch for over the next few days?
4. Children Tiona's age have many fears and stressors related to the hospital and surgery. How can Tiona's mother assist her daughter to express her feelings about the hospital experience once she is home?

See Pearson Nursing Student Resources for possible responses.

Pearson Nursing Student Resources

Find additional review materials at
nursing.pearsonhighered.com

Prepare for success with NCLEX®-style practice questions, interactive assignments and activities, web links, animations and videos, and more!

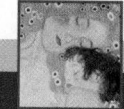

References

Allen, P. J., Vessey, J. A., & Schapiro, N. (2010). *Primary care of the child with a chronic condition* (5th ed.). St. Louis, MO: Mosby.

Bindler, R., & Howry, L. (2005). *Pediatric drug guide.* Upper Saddle River, NJ: Prentice Hall Health.

Brain Injury Association of America. (2009). *A guide to selecting and monitoring brain injury rehabilitation services.* Retrieved from http://www .biausa.org/publications/Guide.to.Selecting .Monitoring.Brain.Injury.Rehabilit.pdf

Crenshaw, J. T., & Winslow, E. H. (2008). Preoperative fasting and medication instruction: Are we improving? *AORN Journal, 88*(6), 963–976.

Drahota, A., & Malcarne, V. L. (2008). Concepts of illness in children: A comparison between children with and without intellectual disability. *Intellectual and Developmental Disabilities, 46*(1), 44–53.

Emergency Nurses Association. (2005). *Position statement: Family presence at the bedside during invasive procedures and/or resuscitation.* Retrieved from http://www.ena.org/SiteCollectionDocuments/ Position%20Statements/Family_ Presence_-_ENA_PS.pdf

Gursky, B. (2007). The effect of educational interventions with siblings of hospitalized children. *Journal of Developmental & Behavioral Pediatrics, 28*(5), 392–398.

Hopia, H., Tomlinson, P. S., Paavilainen, E., & Astedt-Kurki, P. (2005). Child in hospital: family experiences and expectations of how nurses can promote family health. *Journal of Clinical Nursing, 14*(2), 212–222.

Joint Commission on Accreditation of Healthcare Organizations. (2009). *The Joint Commission:*
2010 Accreditation Requirements Chapters: Accreditation Program: Long Term Care. Retrieved from http://www.jointcommission.org

Jolley, J., & Shields, L. (2009). The evolution of family-centered care. *Journal of Pediatric Nursing, 24*(2), 164–170.

Koopman, H. M., Baars, R. M., Chaplin, J., & Zwinderman, K. H. (2004). Illness through the eyes of the child: The development of children's understanding of the causes of illness. *Patient Education and Counseling, 55,* 363–370.

Lassetter, J. H., & Baldwin, J. H. (2005). Improving the experience of hospitalization for Hawaiian children on the mainland through cultural sensitivity to Hawaiian ways of healing. *Journal of Pediatric Nursing, 20,* 170–176.

Lobato, D., Kao, B., & Plante, W. (2006). Siblink: Meeting the needs of siblings of children with chronic illness and disability. *Brown University Child and Adolescent Behavior Letter, 22*(9) 1, 5–6.

McKenney, C., & Johnson, R. (2008). Unleash the healing power of pet therapy. *American Nurse Today, 3*(5), 29–31.

Myant, K. A., & Williams, J. M. (2005). Children's concepts of health and illness: Understanding of contagious illnesses, non-contagious illnesses and injuries. *Journal of Health Psychology, 10*(6), 805–819.

National Center for Cultural Competence. (2010). *Working with linguistically diverse populations.* Retrieved from http://www11.georgetown.edu/ research/gucchd/NCCC/features/language.html

Piko, B. F., & Bak, J. (2006). Children's perception of health and illness: Images and lay concepts in preadolescence. *Health Education Research: Theory & Practice, 21*(5), 643–653.

Power, N., & Franck, L. (2008). Parent participation in the care of hospitalized children: A systematic review. *Journal of Advanced Nursing, 62*(2), 622–641.

Pruitt, L. M., Johnson, A., Elliott, J. C., & Polley, K. (2008). Parental presence during pediatric invasive procedures. *Journal of Pediatric Health Care, 22,* 120–127.

Ryan, J. (2008). "Pet" projects: Animal-assisted therapy for young patients. *Contemporary Pediatrics, 25*(7), 88.

Salmela, M., Salanterä, S., & Aronen, E. (2009). Child-reported hospital fears in 4- to 6-year-old children. *Pediatric Nursing, 35*(5), 269–276.

Sarajärvi, A., Haapamäki, M. L., & Paavilainen, E. (2006). Emotional and informational support for families during their child's illness. *International Nursing Review, 53,* 205–210.

Spector, R. E. (2009). *Cultural diversity in health and illness* (7th ed.). Upper Saddle River, NJ: Pearson.

U.S. Department of Labor. (2009). *Fact Sheet #28: The Family and Medical Leave Act of 1993.* Retrieved from http://www.dol.gov/esa/whd/regs/ compliance/whdfs28.pdf

Weiss, M., Johnson, N. L., Malin, S., Jerofke, T., Lang, C., & Sherburne, E. (2008). Readiness for discharge in parents of hospitalized children. *Journal of Pediatric Nursing, 23*(4), 282–295.

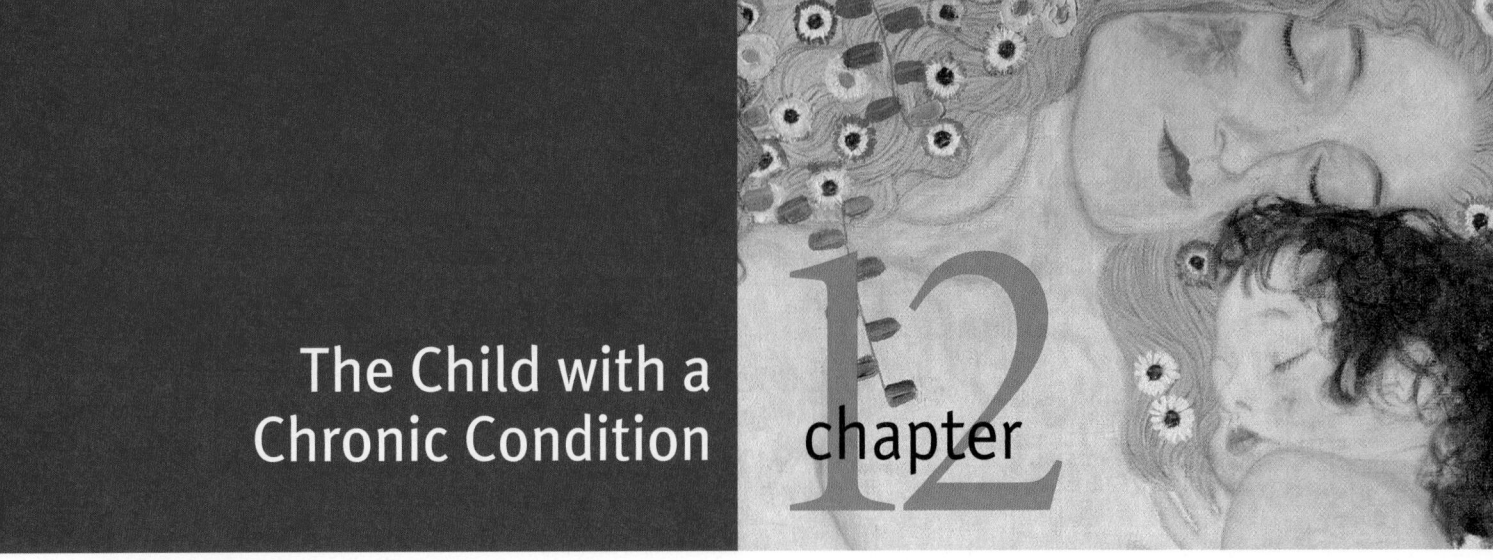

The Child with a Chronic Condition

chapter 12

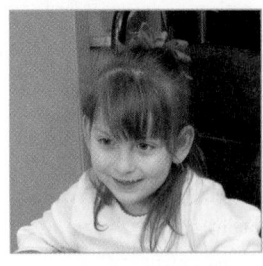

Haley is an 8-year-old girl with cerebral palsy. She had an intraventricular hemorrhage during her neonatal intensive care unit (NICU) hospitalization for very low birth weight. Haley lives with her mother and two older siblings, ages 10 and 13 years. Her parents divorced when Haley was 3 years old. She has frequent contact with her father, who she visits on weekends. Her father is supportive emotionally, physically, and financially for the care of Haley and her siblings.

Haley's mother is the full-time care provider. Routine care includes hygiene, supplemental enteral tube feedings to promote adequate nutrition in between oral feedings, range of motion (ROM) exercises, and home schooling. Haley uses her motorized wheelchair without any difficulty, and her mother has decided that she would benefit from social interaction and a structured educational environment at the local public school. Her family asks the nurse and case manager at the cerebral palsy clinic for assistance in planning Haley's entry into school.

How can the clinic nurse and case manager assist Haley and her family in this transition? What special arrangements are needed to permit a child to receive care for a chronic condition while at school? What measures can be taken to ensure an effective transition between home and school?

Learning Outcomes

After reading this chapter, you will be able to do the following:

1. Explain the causes of chronic conditions in children. 291
2. Identify the categories of chronic conditions in children. 292
3. Assess the child with a chronic condition and apply specific nursing interventions for the child at different ages. 293
4. Evaluate the family of a child with a chronic condition and analyze the impact of the child's condition on the family. 295
5. Prepare the family of the child with a chronic condition to effectively care for the child in the home. 297
6. Summarize nursing management for the child with a chronic condition to support transition to school and adult living. 299-301
7. Discuss the family's role in care coordination and case management. 305

Key Terms

accommodations / 299
care coordination / 305
caregiver burden / 295
case manager / 305
children with special health care needs (CSHCN) / 291
chronic condition / 291
chronic sorrow / 294
compassion fatigue / 308
developmental delay / 297
disability / 292
early intervention / 299
individualized education plan (IEP) / 300
individualized family service plan (IFSP) / 300
individualized health plan (IHP) / 300
individualized transition plan (ITP) / 300
medically fragile / 292
normalization / 297
respite care / 305
technology-assisted / 292

▨ GENERAL CONCEPTS

A **chronic condition** is generally thought of as one that is long term and ongoing, may or may not be considered terminal, and requires some adaptation to daily living (Coffey, 2006). Others have defined a chronic condition as one that is expected to last at least 3 months (Allen, 2010). An estimated 10 million children under the age of 18 years in the United States have special health care needs related to some type of chronic condition (Betz, 2008). Chronic conditions vary in etiology, manifestations, severity, and their effect on the child's physical, psychosocial, and cognitive development. Chronic conditions can develop from multiple causes:

- Genetic or inheritable conditions may manifest as a child's chronic condition. Examples include muscular dystrophy, hemophilia, sickle cell disease, and cystic fibrosis.
- Conditions may result from a congenital defect or insult to the infant during fetal development, such as a neural tube defect, maternal substance abuse, cleft palate, and cerebral palsy.
- Insult or injury associated with birth and care following birth (sepsis, prematurity, intraventricular hemorrhage) can lead to conditions such as bronchopulmonary dysplasia, attention deficit disorder, or vision or hearing impairment.
- Conditions can be acquired through injury or acute medical condition such as brain injury, cancer, HIV infection, drowning, and mental health problems.

In most cases, these chronic conditions become lifelong disorders. However, the impact on the affected child is variable according to the severity of the condition, the stage of growth and development when the condition occurs, and the child's and family's responses to the condition. Although some conditions require intense monitoring and technological support for survival, other conditions cause few limitations and minimal effects on quality of life. See Figure 12–1 ➤ for examples of children with visible and nonvisible disabilities.

Overview of Chronic Conditions

The wide variety of chronic health conditions experienced by children and the manifestations of these conditions impact the child's growth and development and health status in unique ways (Figure 12–1).

Chronic conditions are often defined by diagnostic categories or by functional or social limitations. Examples of these categories include the following (Allen, 2010, p. 7):

- Limitations in function that would typically be expected for the child's age and development
- Disfigurement
- Dependency on medications or a special diet for control of the condition
- Dependency on medical technology for functioning
- Need for more medical care and related services than typically used by a healthy child of the same age
- Special ongoing treatments at home or school

See Table 12–1 for examples of some chronic conditions by category.

Many children with chronic conditions have special health care needs that fall into several of these areas. In the majority of cases, the more severe the chronic condition, the greater the number of categories of special health care needs. The term **children with special health care needs (CSHCN)** is applied to

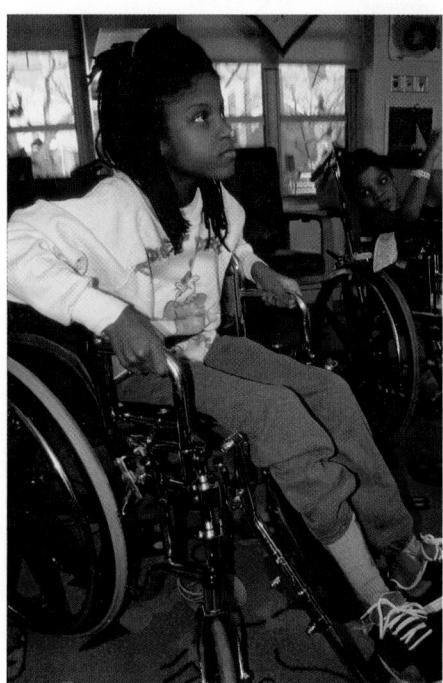

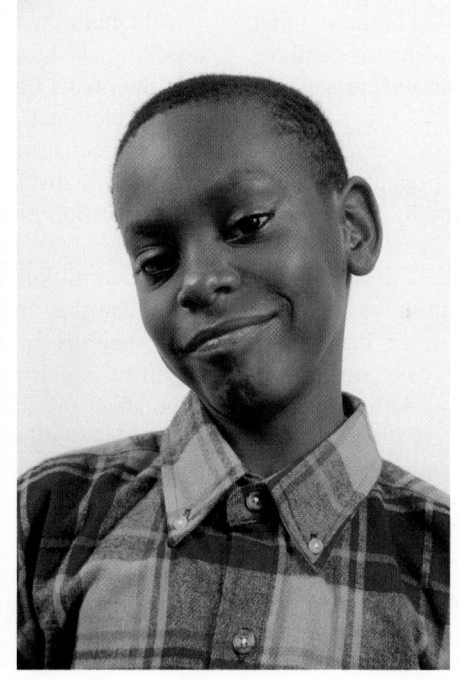

A **B**

FIGURE 12–1 ➤ A, The child who uses a wheelchair has a visible disability. B, The child with a seizure may have no visible signs of the condition unless a seizure is witnessed.

TABLE 12–1	**Examples of Chronic Conditions by Special Health Care Need Category**
Special Health Care Need Category	Chronic Health Condition Examples
Dependent on prescription medications or special diet	Diabetes mellitus, asthma, seizures, phenylketonuria, organ transplantation
Dependent on medical technology	Renal failure, bronchopulmonary dysplasia
Increased use of health care services	Cancer, sickle cell disease, cystic fibrosis
Functional limitations	Down syndrome, brain injury, autism, myelodysplasia, cerebral palsy

"those who have or are at increased risk for a chronic physical, developmental, behavioral, emotional condition and who also require health and related services of a type or amount beyond that required by children generally" (U.S. Department of Health and Human Services, Health Resources and Services Administration, Maternal and Child Health Bureau, 2008). Some of these children also have a **disability,** a limitation that interferes with a child's ability to fully participate in society, which can be related to medical impairment (chronic health condition), functional limitation (mobility, self-care, communication, or learning behavior impairment), or a mental condition that interferes with social interactions.

The prevalence of children in the United States with special health care needs increased from 12.8% in 2001 to 13.9% in 2005–2006 (Betz, 2008). Although these children represent a small percentage of the nation's children, they require significantly more health care resources than those without special health care needs, including more visits to clinics and emergency departments, dental visits, inpatient hospital days, and prescription medications. Efforts to reduce health costs have resulted in fewer hospitalizations and more care in the community for children with special health care needs (CSHCN). The proposed objectives for Healthy People 2020 include those related to health care delivery to CSHCN. The proposed objectives state that these children will have access to a medical home and that they will receive care in family-centered, comprehensive, and co-ordinated systems (U.S. Department of Health and Human Services, 2010).

The child with a life-threatening illness or a chronic condition as the result of a complex illness, prematurity, or a congenital defect may be considered **medically fragile** (Lee, Miles, & Holditch-Davis, 2006). Some of these children are **technology-assisted,** dependent on a medical device that is required to sustain life or to maintain health status (e.g., mechanical ventilators, intravenous nutrition or drugs, tracheostomy, suctioning, dialysis, oxygen, or nutritional support with tube feedings) (Figure 12–2 ➤). Other children depend on medical devices that compensate for vital body functions and require nursing care management such as urinary catheters and colostomies.

Children assisted by technology can often be cared for at home because compact portable equipment is available. Home-based equipment used for the child with a chronic condition may include ventilators, enteral feeding tubes, intravenous catheters, infusion pumps, dialysis equipment, and oxygen. With the support of home health services, many parents can learn to manage their child's care. The benefit of home health

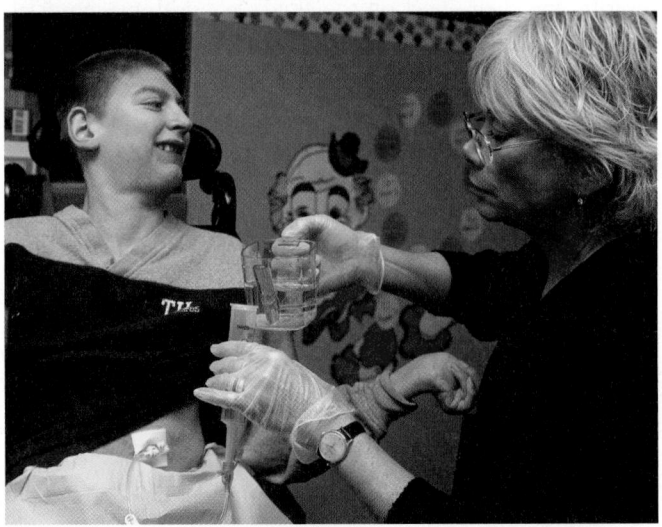

FIGURE 12–2 ➤ This child needs a gastrostomy tube to ensure adequate nutrition is obtained to support growth and promote resistance to infection.

services to the child is support of physical, emotional, and cognitive growth and development within the home care setting, in a more familiar environment.

All families with children experiencing a chronic condition need to make lifestyle adjustments, ensuring a baseline of care that maintains the child's health status and promotes growth and development. In many cases, the child has a baseline level of home management with episodic exacerbations that require the family to make sudden adjustments in family routines, such as an infection or metabolic crisis. These exacerbations often cause stress and disrupt family routines. In other cases, the chronic condition requires the family to learn and provide care that is complex and time-intensive, such as cystic fibrosis, diabetes mellitus, bronchopulmonary dysplasia, and significant cognitive impairment. These more severe chronic conditions often affect the child's physical and psychologic development. Table 12–2 outlines health care needs of these children and families and the nursing implications related to planning health services delivery.

■ THE FAMILY OF A CHILD WITH A CHRONIC CONDITION

The diagnosis of a chronic illness in a child is frequently a life-changing experience for the family. Parents experience anxiety and may have difficulty coping with the new diagnosis.

CSHCN Websites

TABLE 12–2 Health Care Needs of Children with Chronic Conditions

Health Care Need	Definition	Nursing Management
Access to care	Care includes the availability and accessibility of providers with knowledge as well as ancillary services needed by children and their families.	Assist the family in obtaining transportation assistance if required. Assist the family in identifying health care providers that provide health promotion and other services to address the child's specific health care needs.
Appropriateness of care	Services and care are delivered by individuals with expertise and experience that are developmentally and culturally appropriate for the child and family.	Support the family by outlining educational and health services needed when developing an individualized education plan (IEP) and individualized health plan (IHP).
Comprehensiveness of care	Care includes coverage of the preventive, primary, and tertiary care needs of children, and linkages with other service systems, such as education, social services, and family support systems.	Provide the family with resource contacts such as social services, family support groups, and other systems to help the family manage the child's condition. Assist the family to identify a care coordinator or to develop the skills to become the care coordinator. See page 305.
Coordination of care	Families are linked to medical care, financial health resources, and educational and community-based services; information is centralized.	Provide guidance and resources if the family decides to assume the role of care coordinator. Encourage the family to partner with the health care team to ensure continuity of care.
Continuity of care	Care is provided through a medical home or pediatric health care home; linkages between primary, specialty, therapeutic, and home care exist throughout childhood.	Facilitate communication between all the child's health care providers. Include the family and older child in all decision making.
Degree to which family-centered services are provided	The importance of the family is reflected in the way services are planned and delivered, building on individual and family strengths, and respecting the diversity of each family.	Determine the needs of the child and the family to ensure they are being addressed. Assist the family in identifying local and specialized health care providers. Recognize and respect the culture and cultural practices of the child and family.

Informing the Parents

Chronic conditions present very differently among infants and children:

- Chronic conditions may be detected at birth or early in infancy. Examples include a neural tube defect, a condition like phenylketonuria identified by newborn screening, or a complication of care provided in the NICU, such as bronchopulmonary dysplasia.
- Parents may suspect that their child has a problem and seek a diagnosis, such as in cerebral palsy when the infant does not achieve expected developmental milestones or in autism when the child does not achieve appropriate communication skills.
- Recurrent illnesses may actually be related to a chronic condition such as asthma or cystic fibrosis. Serious injury, such as a traumatic brain injury, can also cause disabilities.
- Some children may start school before their learning or behavior problems are identified.

Clinical Tip

When discussing a child's chronic condition with family, use the child's name. Avoid labeling the child with a condition, such as "diabetic child"; instead, refer to the "child with diabetes." This places the emphasis on the *child* rather than the *condition*.

The manner in which parents are informed of their child's condition and their ability to understand the information influences their ability to cope with the diagnosis. The parents' heightened anxiety level may reduce the comprehension of information heard. See Figure 12–3 ➤.

The following guidelines may be considered when the nurse helps inform parents of the diagnosis of a chronic illness or disability in their child:

- Inform parents of their child's diagnosis in person, in a private setting, and free from interruptions. Tell both parents together when possible and appropriate. Offer parents the opportunity to have a relative or friend as a support person during the discussion.

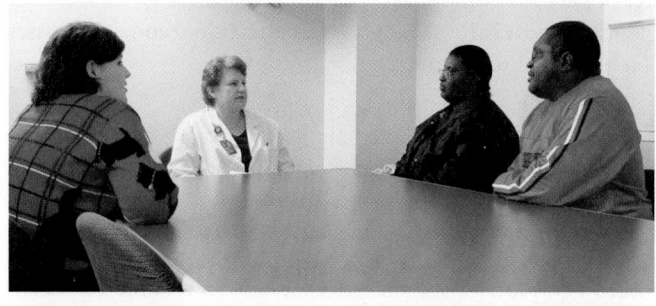

FIGURE 12–3 ➤ Inform the family about the child's chronic condition in an area with privacy, and be sure to provide adequate time for the family to initially absorb the information and then to ask questions. Offer to meet the next day to review the information and respond to additional questions.

- Present information in small amounts at a time and at the level of the parents' understanding.
- Plan and organize the information to be provided. Use simple, direct language without medical jargon. Individualize the pace of the interview and approaches taken to present the explanation, taking into consideration the family's culture and their response to the information.
- Share accurate, up-to-date information about the diagnosis, treatment options, specialty referrals, and community resources.
- Talk about the strengths and positive attributes of the child, as well as the child's limitations and characteristics due to the illness or disability.
- Evaluate the discussion with the family to assess whether the family's needs were met and to determine the type of support or additional information that should be provided.
- Plan a follow-up discussion to repeat and clarify the information provided, and to give the parents a chance to ask additional questions.

Informing the Child

Informing the child of a newly acquired chronic condition is individualized and is based on the child's developmental level and age. Input from parents regarding the best manner and time to discuss the condition with the child is useful as well. Questions the child may ask vary but often focus on the cause of the condition, how to make it better, and how it will affect daily life. Provide information tailored to the child's level of understanding and answer questions honestly. See Chapter 11 ∞.

Parental Reactions

Parents need time to comprehend and learn about the child's diagnosis and its meaning to their lives. Some parents may feel relieved that a diagnosis is finally identified after all of the concern, diagnostic testing, and uncertainty. They may feel that their concerns have been validated. For many parents, however, the information can be distressing. Initial reactions of parents to the diagnosis of a chronic illness include shock and denial. The parents may question the diagnosis and may even question the accuracy of the tests and the competency of the health care providers. Other reactions include anger, guilt (especially with an inherited illness), and a sense of hopelessness (Nuutila & Salanterä, 2006). The nurse should be empathetic and supportive of parental emotional expression.

Parents grieve for the loss of the perfect child and other losses such as the following:

- Loss of family routines and goals
- Loss of the ideal mother–child relationship
- Siblings' loss of a normal childhood
- Loss of expectations for the development and life expectancy of the child with the chronic condition
- Child's loss of a normal childhood

Parents may blame themselves or their spouse if the condition is genetic. When the child's condition results in a significant disability, the family has a daily reminder of their losses and how they differ from other families. Parents may have difficulty

bonding with an affected infant because of guilt or disappointment, because they fear that the infant will not survive, or because the infant looks or behaves differently.

Episodes of recurrent sadness are reported by parents, particularly when reminded that their child is different from healthy children (for example, when the child starts school). This sadness is a normal response to an event that is permanent, progressive, recurring, and cyclic in nature (Gordon, 2009). **Chronic sorrow** is believed to be a coping mechanism that allows parents to grieve periodically and permits them to carry on with responsibilities at other intervals (Vickers, 2006).

Siblings' Reactions

Siblings of children with a chronic condition are affected in a variety of ways, and they demonstrate emotional responses that range from negative to positive (Williams, Piamjariyakul, Graff, et al, 2010; Giallo & Gavidia-Payne, 2006). Negative responses predominate and include feelings of jealousy, resentment, anger, depression, worry, and anxiety (Williams et al, 2010;). Siblings of chronically ill children are at increased risk for behavioral problems and may demonstrate changes in mood and attention-seeking behaviors including lower self-esteem, poor peer relationships, delinquency, and poor school performance (Ballard, 2004). Siblings may fear that they will have the same disease or condition as the affected child.

Some siblings have positive responses and demonstrate emotional growth, insight, behavior improvement, increased responsibility, independence, maturity, and a tolerance for differences in others. Siblings who adjust more positively are those who are older at the time the illness occurs, have a more cohesive family, and experience positive communication with their parents (Ballard, 2004; Giallo & Gavidia-Payne, 2006). See Chapter 11 ∞ for siblings' responses to the child experiencing an illness.

Siblings of a child with a chronic condition need support from their parents to help with their coping and adjustment. Siblings who have difficulty adjusting may benefit from support groups (Houtzager, Grootenhuis, Hoekstra-Weebers, et al., 2005). Nurses should help parents to recognize that the sibling needs the following (Ballard, 2004):

- Information and reassurance about the sick child
- Reassurance about his or her own health
- Relief from guilt
- Family communication, inclusion, and emotional support

Nursing actions to help promote improved adjustment for the sibling of a child with a chronic condition include helping parents recognize the need to spend individual time with the sibling (Fanos, Fahrner, Jelveh, et al., 2004). Maintenance of family routines is helpful in promoting a sense of the normal. Help the family select appropriate ways the sibling can help care for the child with a chronic condition, while also recognizing that the sibling needs a childhood with peer interactions, physical exercise, and recreation.

Family Stressors

Having a child with a chronic condition places great demands on parents. Parents worry about the child and the care needed, both at the current time and in the future (Coffey, 2006). Stressors reported by families having a child with a chronic condition include:

- Learning as much as possible about the child's condition and expected progression in severity
- Learning about the technical aspects of care for the child and how to integrate that care into family routines
- Finding ways each family member can help with the child's care, including extended family members who may live nearby
- Communicating with health professionals and attempting to serve as a full partner in the child's care
- Identifying the most appropriate resources for the child
- Continuing employment and meeting care needs of the child
- Managing a family budget that is drained by expenses for care not covered by health insurance plans and other financial resources
- Attempting to provide siblings as normal a life as possible
- Opening the home to strangers who provide home care to the child
- Coping with episodes when the child's condition worsens and fearing that the child will die
- Working with the child to gradually assume more responsibility for self-care

Certain transitions or events are more stressful for the family because they disrupt family routines or require adaptation by the family. As mentioned, the time of diagnosis is the initial transition or event that results in changes in a family's expectations. Other times of transition that cause stress or trigger more intense feelings of sorrow include (Coffey, 2006):

- When development milestones do not occur as expected
- School entry, when the child transitions from preschool to kindergarten
- The child's 18th birthday

Some families have the strength and resilience to manage the child's health care needs and maintain family functioning. However, the burden of caring for the child with special health care needs often falls heavily on one parent, usually the mother (Coffey, 2006). This parental relationship stress may be further increased by concurrent family illnesses, a death in the family, or the presence of a family conflict. The marriage relationship is at risk for breakdown if the couple is not able to communicate, share in the care for the child and other family members, and have common expectations for the child's condition and abilities to perform self-care.

Culture   *Communication*

The family with English as a second language may experience difficulty in communicating and understanding information in English during stressful situations such as the illness of their child. An interpreter should be used during these times. Until an interpreter is available, support the family and promote a calm environment to assist in reducing the family's stress.

Caregiver Burden

Caregiver burden is the unrelenting pressure and anxiety of providing care to a child with disabilities day after day while meeting other family obligations. The parents of the child who is medically fragile must perform technical care and complicated procedures, keep records, and be vigilant in monitoring symptoms (Figure 12–4 ➤). The stressors of parents with a child who is technology-dependent vary by the child's functional status, the extent of care needed, the financial burden, the family's strengths and resiliency, and the available resources. Parents have greater personal strain and caregiver distress when the child has poor functional status and health care needs are not met (Aitken, McCarthy, Slomine, et al., 2009).

See Chapter 10 ∞ for the discussion of nursing care in the home.

Meeting family obligations can be challenging, even when a family support infrastructure exists. There is a constant struggle to keep the needs of the child and the family in balance. Mothers may be unable or not have the energy to meet their own personal needs for health care. Social isolation may be experienced by the parent who remains in the home providing care to the child who is chronically ill. Spousal support is essential to manage all the family and childcare requirements. Employment responsibilities also must be integrated into the schedule, and hours of work often must be negotiated to ensure parental coverage for the child's care.

Even when parents develop the capacity and skills to coordinate the child's medical care, the work on behalf of the child remains intensive and must be sustained long term. Administrative work, such as scheduling appointments, keeping records, developing and maintaining lists, completing health insurance claim forms, and appealing denied payments, may seem neverending. Advocacy efforts for resources and opportunities are ongoing, but should be adapted to changes in the child's condition and developmental stage. Parents need to pace themselves

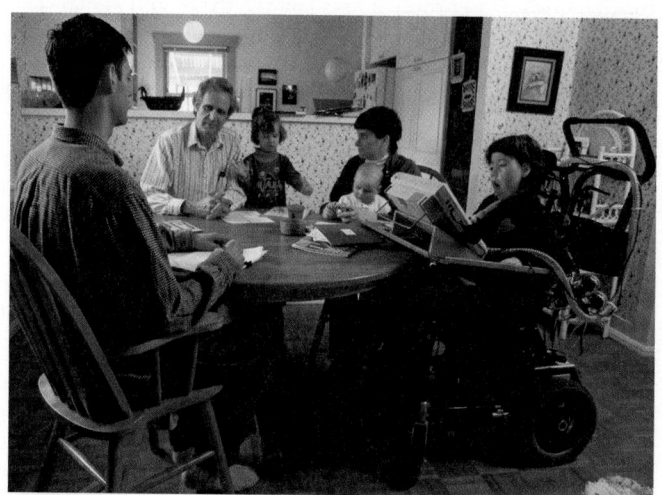

FIGURE 12–4 ➤ Daily caregiving demands of the child who is medically fragile continues 24 hours a day, 7 days a week. Parents need to identify ways to split the care of the child and other family care management. When the child lives with a single parent, additional health care resources are needed so the parent can sleep.

because there are limits on how much they can do and continue long term. Despite the challenges described, some families of children with chronic conditions are able to participate in activities with others and have meaningful relationships outside of the home (Rehm & Bradley, 2005). See Chapter 2 ∞ for family assessment and nursing interventions for family support. See Table 12–3 for nursing interventions to assist families with significant stressors.

Clinical Tip

Children with chronic illnesses and special health care needs are at increased risk for child maltreatment. Factors that increase the risk of abuse in these children include the following (Hibbard, Desch, & Committee on Child Abuse and Neglect and Council on Children with Disabilities, 2007):

■ Higher emotional, physical, economic, and social demands on the family
■ Limited social and community support
■ Failure of the child to receive medications, appropriate educational placement, and adequate medical care
■ Increased stress related to the child's behavioral characteristics (e.g., communication problems, aggressiveness)
■ Lack of adequate breaks or respite from caring for the child

Assess the family for ineffective coping and the potential for abuse. Make appropriate referrals to support services such as mental health counseling, social services, and respite.

Family Financial Issues

The economic impact of caring for a child with a chronic condition is significant. Even with good insurance coverage, the family still incurs a major financial burden. Forty percent of families in the United States who have a child with special health care needs experience a financial burden related to their child's illness (Looman, O'Conner-Von, Ferski, et al., 2009). Although health plans claim that home care of these children costs less than care in institutions, families assume responsibility for many out-of-pocket expenses. Examples of additional expenses that families pay out of pocket may include special diets, durable equipment and supplies, transportation to health care visits, respite care, and sometimes co-payment for health services. Home health nursing care may be needed if both parents continue to work or to cover the night shift so parents can sleep.

Another financial concern for the family of a child with a chronic condition in the home is the high incidence of job instability that can occur as a direct result of the child's condition. Parents may lose their employment due to excessive absences to provide care for the child or may be required to reduce hours worked to make sure the child receives adequate care. Such job instability further threatens the family's access to health insurance for the remainder of the family as well as the child with a chronic condition.

TABLE 12–3	**Nursing Interventions for Family Stressors**
Stressors	Nursing Implications
Uncertainty	Be honest in responding to the parents' questions. Serve as an advocate to ensure that information from the primary health care provider or specialists is relayed to the family.
Fear of potential loss of their child	If the death of the child is likely or uncertain, support the family and refer to social services or other support to assist the family in anticipatory grieving. Ensure that the family is kept informed about all changes in the child's condition.
Communication with health care providers	Partner with the family and serve as its advocate to ensure communication is shared between the multidisciplinary team members. Ensure the family understands all communication, and offer clarification if required. Ensure that the parents are fully informed and participate in all decision making regarding the child's care.
Deciding whom to inform about the chronic condition	Assist the family in identifying all individuals who need to know about the child's condition. Extended family members and friends can offer support and may provide assistance with care. Recommend that childcare or school officials (if school age) be informed since the child is in their care for a majority of time.
Increased out-of-pocket expenses	Partner with the family to identify cost-effective measures to reduce expenses. Refer the family to social services to determine any available financial assistance for health care services, respite care, meals, or transportation.
Social isolation and role strain	Encourage the family to participate in support groups. Parent-to-parent support groups, including online groups, can offer support and guidance. Encourage the family to take respite time from the child's care. Assist them in determining satisfactory arrangements for respite care (e.g., family member, health care or respite provider).
Dividing time between well children and the child with a chronic condition	Encourage parents to take "special time" with the siblings of the child with a chronic condition. Also encourage the family to include all members in planning family activities and to ensure that each child has an opportunity to plan activities. Identify social supports to help provide opportunities for participation in recreational or peer group activities.

Promoting Healthy Family Coping

Families often engage in a coping strategy called **normalization**. Through normalization, the family views care of the child with a chronic condition as a "normal" part of life, rather than an inconvenience or something outside of their routine. The family redefines what is normal for them by adopting a "normalcy lens" that enables them to see that their family follows some normal routines like all other families (Knafl & Santacroce, 2010).

With normalization, the parents may be able to move the child's condition to the subconscious so that it does not take a dominant place in the family's life and thoughts. They choose to focus on the normal aspects of the child and the family's life. Through normalization, families develop flexibility in management of the treatment plan, making life easier for the family (Knafl & Santacroce, 2010). Threats to sustaining normalization may include worsening of the child's health status that makes the parents more aware of the child's serious condition, changed management routines, new family additions, or other family situational changes.

Some families are unable to achieve or sustain the sense of normalization, even though it may be seen as a desired goal. In many cases these families are still adjusting to their child's condition, the child's condition may have recently changed, or another family stressor is present. In these families, the child's condition may be a major focus of family life or a source of conflict. The child could be viewed as being different from his or her peers, leading parents to modify their parenting style to accommodate their dramatically changed view of their child (Knafl & Santacroce, 2010).

Nurses can be effective in working with families by listening to the issues and offering suggestions. Often the opportunity to talk through the child's management plan will help the family consider different strategies that may be effective. The nurse

Complementary Therapy
Animal Therapy

Animal-assisted therapy has been helpful in many ways to ease stresses a child experiences with health care. Introduction of a dog into the home of a child with special health care needs may also be beneficial in helping the family with the "normalcy lens." Family members are able to express pleasure and affection to the pet, and the family may spend more time together around pet-related activities (Gasalberti, 2006). Horses have been used for many years to treat children with conditions such as cerebral palsy and muscular dystrophy. *Hippotherapy* is a type of physical therapy that uses the movement of a horse to improve the posture, balance, and motor function of the child (Lane, 2007).

may also provide linkages to community resources that may help the family.

■ CARE OF THE CHILD WITH A CHRONIC CONDITION

Developmental Considerations

The child with a chronic condition has the same developmental and emotional needs as the healthy child. The impact of the chronic condition on the child's cognitive, physical, and emotional health may lead to altered developmental achievement expectations. A **developmental delay** results when failure to achieve anticipated developmental milestones exists during specific developmental stages.

Newborn and Infant

Newborns and infants who are medically fragile are at risk for chronic conditions related to brain injury, oxygen deprivation, and respiratory problems. Newborns cared for in the NICU are exposed to an environment of bright lights and high-pitched noises that can negatively affect their development (Brandon, Ryan, & Barnes, 2007; Kellam & Bhatia, 2008; Lasky & Williams, 2009). See Figure 12–5 ➤.

Nurses should promote development and parent–infant bonding by encouraging the parents to spend time with the infant and engage in face-to-face interaction. When the newborn is stable, provide opportunities for parents to touch, soothe, and care for the infant. Provide sensory stimuli such as mobiles, soft music, and different textures for the infant to touch.

Clinical Tip ◤

Parents who become actively involved in the care of their infant in the NICU will learn to recognize and respond to their child's needs more readily (Griffin & Abraham, 2006).

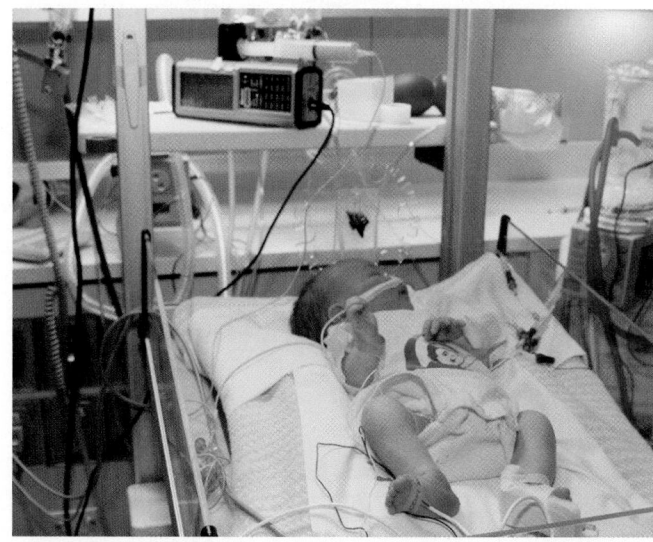

FIGURE 12–5 ➤ Development of trust may be disrupted for the infant in the NICU or hospital unit when there are multiple caregivers and experiences of painful stimuli.

Toddler

When the toddler has a chronic condition, parents may need to control and set limits on movement, play, behavior, or social interactions because of the condition. This interferes with the achievement of autonomy and development of self-control. Some parents do more by protecting the child or doing simple tasks they feel the child is incapable of accomplishing, rather than encouraging the child to learn to do things independently. The child can lose independence and lack opportunities to meet developmental tasks. See Figure 12–6 ➤.

Nurses can promote the development of toddlers with chronic conditions by offering the child choices when possible, such as which color of gown to wear or which food to eat first. Help parents recognize the toddler's capabilities and allow the child to practice and learn a skill. Identify the next most appropriate developmental tasks for the child to learn, and give the parents some strategies they can use to offer learning opportunities.

Preschooler

Preschool children recognize the association between body parts and problems associated with the chronic condition. The preschooler engages in magical thinking during this stage, and the child may believe that his or her thoughts or behaviors caused the condition. The child may also think the condition is a form of punishment. Decreased energy due to the condition may interfere with the preschooler's ability to learn about the environment, develop social relationships, gain a sense of self-confidence, and learn a sense of purpose (Vessey & Sullivan, 2010).

Nurses can promote development by explaining the purpose of treatments and procedures in terms the preschooler can un-

derstand, and by emphasizing that treatments are not punishment for any wrongdoing. Look for ways to use play so the child can learn an aspect of self-care, perform an activity, and feel a sense of accomplishment. See Chapter 11 ∞ for ways to use play in the hospital setting. Encourage social interactions with other children when possible. Give positive feedback to the child for appropriate efforts and successes.

School-Age Child

Early school-age children have an increased understanding of their condition, and they can participate in certain aspects of monitoring and care. Older school-age children begin to understand more about managing their condition and the long-term needs associated with it. They can assume more responsibility for their care such as serum glucose sampling, monitoring the condition of skin under braces, or intermittent self-catheterization.

Some children with chronic conditions have learning difficulties and other limitations that interfere with education and social competence. The child needs to gain social skills, interact with peers, master new information, learn to cope with stress, and acquire skills that lead to self-sufficiency in order to develop a sense of industry. Other children may have functional limitations (self-care, communication, mobility, stamina, and learning) that interfere with participation in school activities and prevent them from developing socially (Rehm & Bradley, 2006). Nurses can promote development of school-age children by encouraging their interaction with children in the same age group. Link the child to a peer support group to promote social interaction and to help the child recognize that others also have the same condition. When the child has an extended absence from school because of the chronic condition, encourage contact from school peers and friends through cards and computer messages, as well as the completion of school assignments. Begin to identify aspects of the child's care that the child can learn to assume under the parents' supervision. Inform families of the benefit of special camps for children with the chronic condition (when available) to promote recreation, social interaction, and learning skills of self-care.

Adolescent

Adolescence is a stage of profound physical, psychological, and physiological changes. The adolescent with a chronic condition has numerous challenges with the rapid changes in growth and sexual maturation; ongoing development of identity, body image, and self-concept; and the need to plan for vocational and health care transitions. Cognitive development and abstract thinking skills are achieved during this stage, allowing the adolescent to develop an understanding of the short-term and long-term consequences related to the condition (Figure 12–7 ➤).

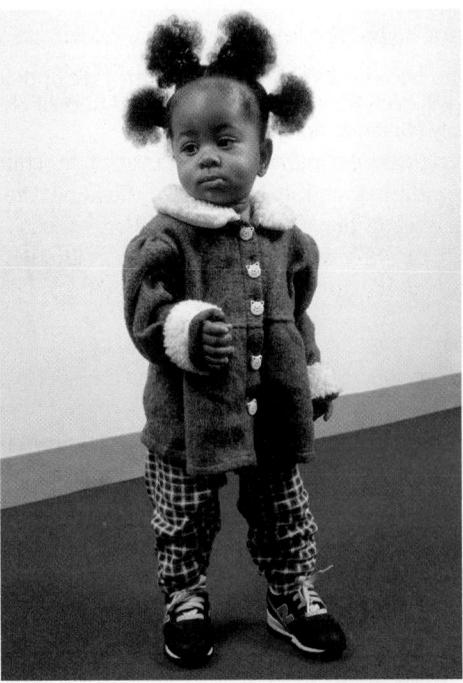

FIGURE 12–6 ➤ Toddlers may experience difficulty in adapting to constraints of the condition and treatments related to their disorder. Depending on the condition, toddlers may be unable to achieve developmental milestones such as walking, toilet training, and feeding self. Delays in speech also become apparent during this stage.

Growth & Development *Sexual Maturation*

All adolescents need education and information about sexual maturation, protected sexual activity, and sexually transmitted infections. Even though the child may have functional limitations or chronic conditions, it is important to discuss and discourage risky behaviors, such as alcohol or substance use and sexual activity.

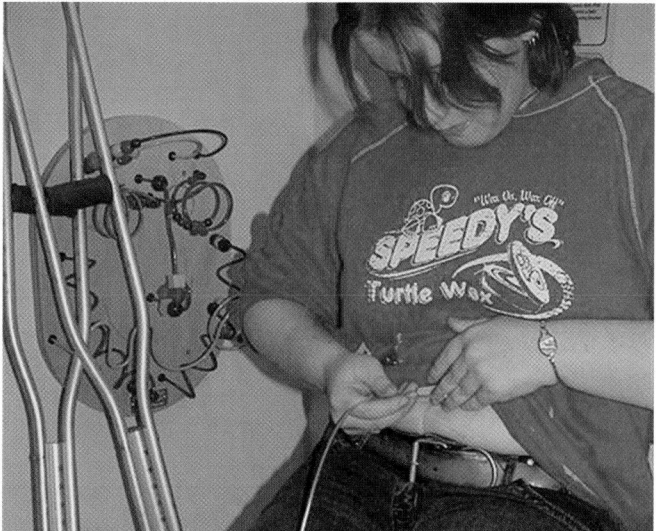

FIGURE 12–7 ➤ All adolescents need to learn how to assume responsibility for their personal care and to make good decisions about future life plans. The adolescent with a chronic condition must also learn to independently manage the health condition (such as this girl performing a self-catheterization through a stoma) and take that condition into consideration when making future life plans. This may be more challenging for adolescents that have a limited life expectancy or when parents are unable to relinquish their control and encourage the child to assume more responsibility for self-care.

The adolescent becomes more aware of differences between self and peers. Some adolescents are unable to cope with the recognizable differences between themselves and healthy peers, and they withdraw from social activities and relationships or are drawn to a peer group that may negatively influence behavior. Others may engage in risky behavior (e.g., alcohol, sexual activity, eating incorrect foods) that may be harmful to themselves or to management of their condition, just to be accepted by peers.

Nursing actions to promote development of the adolescent include patient education to help the adolescent learn about the chronic condition, the care needed to manage or control the condition, and problem solving and specific skills for integrating self-care management into daily life. Parents need to be coached to transition care over to the adolescent and to support the adolescent to make healthy decisions regarding care. Encourage the adolescent to have a safety net of friends who know enough about the chronic condition to assist if a problem occurs, such as a seizure, asthma episode, or insulin reaction. Discuss sexual maturation and the importance of protected sexual activity, and discourage risky behaviors by the adolescent.

Education and Schooling

All children, including those with chronic conditions and special health care needs, are entitled to a free education that is matched to their developmental and functional capabilities by federal law (Individuals with Disabilities Education Act and Section 504 of the Rehabilitation Act of 1973). **Early intervention,** special services for infants and toddlers who have developmental delay or are at risk for developmental delay, is provided through state and local education programs in the hopes that these children will have a lowered total cost of educational ser-

- The Rehabilitation Act, Public Law (P.L.) 93-112 of 1973, prohibited discrimination against people with a disability. Section 504 specifies that each student who has a disability is entitled to *accommodations*, services or special assistance provided in the school setting to ensure that a student with a physical or mental impairment has access to an appropriate education and is able to participate as fully as possible in school activities. Examples of accommodations might include additional time to take a test, strategies that decrease an allergic child's exposure to peanuts, or allowing the child to test his or her blood glucose. This act covers many chronic conditions not covered under other education laws. See Chapter 10 ∞ for further discussion on the nurse's role in the school setting.
- The Individuals with Disabilities Education Act (IDEA), P.L. 105-17 of 1997, and the Individuals with Disabilities Education Act of 2004, P.L. 108-446 (reauthorization of the 1997 legislation), ensure that all children with disabilities have available to them a free appropriate public education that emphasizes special education and related services designed to meet their unique needs and prepare them for employment and independent living. Every child with a disability must have a written individualized education plan (IEP), and parents have the right to question placement decisions and to due process when settling differences.

Source: Data from U.S. Department of Education. (2006a). Building the legacy: IDEA 2004. Retrieved from http://idea.ed.gov/explore/search?search_option= all&query=individuals+with+disabilities+education+act&GO.x=9&GO.y=9; Moses, M., Gilchrest, C., & Schwab, N. C. (2005). Section 504 of the Rehabilitation Act: Determining eligibility and implications for school districts. Journal of School Nursing, 21(1), 48–58; Selekman, J., & Vessey, J. A. (2010). School and the child with a chronic condition. In P. J. Allen, J. A. Vessey, & N. A. Schapiro, Primary care of the child with a chronic condition (5th ed., pp. 42–59). St. Louis, MO: Mosby.

vices (Blann, 2005). Provisions for adolescent transitional planning for adult living, including vocational training and independent living, are also included in the Individuals with Disabilities Education Act.

Attending school is an important transition for children with chronic conditions and their families. Sending the child to school has several benefits for the child and family. Children have an opportunity for socialization with children and adults beyond the immediate family (Rehm & Bradley, 2006).

Educational System Planning

Careful planning is needed when a child with special needs attends school or receives other education services. Many children have chronic medical conditions that require management during the day in the school environment, such as asthma, diabetes, and attention deficit disorder. Some children just need medications administered regularly or episodically. Other children need more extensive interventions integrated into the school day, such as blood glucose monitoring or intermittent self-catheterization. The education system is obligated to provide reasonable **accommodations** (services or special assistance provided in the school setting to ensure that a student with a physical or mental impairment has access to an appropriate education) to ensure that the child's medical needs are met during the school day. The education system's obligation is negotiated with the family in formalized plans. The school nurse is an active participant on the team that collaborates with the family to develop these formalized plans. (See Chapter 10 ∞ for more information related to the school nurse.)

- An **individualized family service plan (IFSP)** is developed for the early intervention process for infants with special health care needs and their families. The IFSP contains information about the services required to support a child's development and enhance the family's capacity to facilitate the child's development. The family and education service providers work as a team to plan, implement, and evaluate services specific to the family's unique concerns, priorities, and resources.
- An **individualized education plan (IEP)** is developed for a child with cognitive, motor, social, or communication impairments who needs special education services. The IEP is jointly planned with the school administrator, school nurse, teacher, parents, and other special support professionals as appropriate for the child's condition. The child is also included in the process when possible. The plan is developed after an assessment of the child's abilities and specific functional limitations.
- An **individualized health plan (IHP)** is developed for the child with medical conditions that need to be managed within the school setting. An IHP may be developed simultaneously with the IEP for the child with a health problem and a co-existing functional impairment. Some children only need an IHP for management of their chronic medical condition at school, such as daily medication administration or glucose monitoring and insulin injection. A physician order is required for medication administration and special treatments. Learning may be challenged when the child has frequent acute illness episodes that result in missed days of school, and the IHP often integrates methods to prevent the child from being penalized for those absences.
- An individualized Section 504 accommodation plan may be used rather than an IHP for children with physical or mental impairments. The same process is used for development of the plan.
- An **individualized transition plan (ITP)** is included in the development of an IEP for each child with a chronic disability who is 14 years or older. The ITP focuses on assisting these individuals to receive vocational training and to move successfully from the home into other community living settings as they grow older.

Parents have an important role in advocating for their child to ensure that the child receives the most appropriate educational services. School systems must provide a full range of educational services for children with special health care needs, including services that support cognitive development, self-care skills, mobility, improved communication, and social skills (Figure 12–8 ➤). Because each child's severity and combination of impairments is unique, identifying and matching the specific services for each child requires discussion and negotiation. Parents should make an effort to learn about the different types of educational services that address a child's specific disability in preparation for the IEP meeting. Parents often need a mentor or experienced parent to help with the development of the IEP the

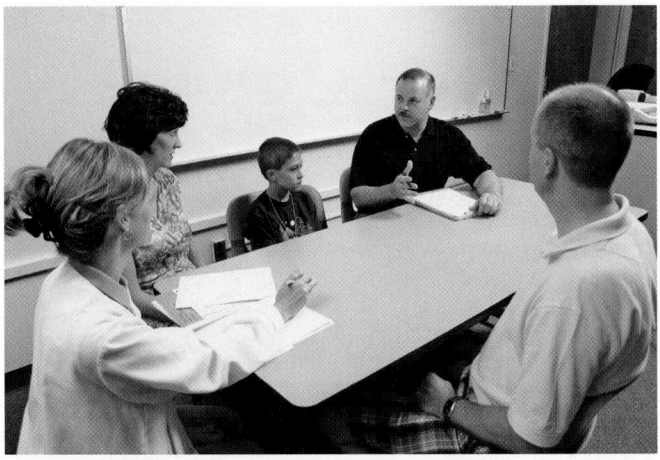

FIGURE 12–8 ➤ An annual meeting of the school administrator, teacher, school nurse, and other school personnel, as well as the parents and child, is important in identifying the educational goals for the child and the special education resources to help meet those goals for development of the child's IEP.

first few times. In this way, the parents are better prepared to participate in the educational planning and development of the child's IEP. School nurses are employees of the school system and may be limited in their advocacy role on behalf of individual students. However, school nurses are in a good position to educate the IEP team about specific interventions needed by children with medical conditions and ways to integrate those interventions into the school day. See Box 12–1 for the elements of an IEP.

The Child's Response to Entering School

Children with chronic conditions—whether they cause minimal interference in the child's daily life or significant interference, such as dependence on technology—face certain challenges in the school setting. They may for the first time recognize differences between themselves and other children, such as appearance, abilities, social skills, or special treatment needs. They may be teased and may experience social stigma for the first time (Rehm & Bradley, 2006). Some children, particularly adolescents, may attempt to hide their condition or fail to adhere to necessary recommendations, such as dietary restrictions, in order to appear like their peers.

Education for Children Who Are Medically Fragile

Children who are medically fragile or technology-assisted are also entitled to education services in the school setting. The child's need for skilled supportive nursing care must be carefully considered by the parents and the school system. Parents are often anxious about how well the child will be cared for by others during the school day. Risks for the child in the school setting include safety issues related to ventilators, tracheostomy, and medication therapy, as well as exposure to infectious diseases.

The school administration must provide the personnel, resources, and equipment needed to ensure that care and a care provider are consistently available. Modifications to the school setting for the child, such as wheelchair ramps or an elevator, may be needed. Sometimes the child is placed in a classroom with healthy children, and the teacher is expected to monitor the child

BOX 12–1 Elements of an IEP

- Student's name
- Date of meeting to develop or review the IEP
- Statement of transition service needs of the student beginning at age 14 years
- Present level of assessments and education performance, including how the child's disability affects the child's involvement and progress in a general curriculum or participation in appropriate activities
- Measurable annual goals that include benchmarks or short-term objectives in meeting the child's needs that enable the child to be involved in or progress in the general curriculum or participate in appropriate activities
- Special education and related services, supplementary aids and services, and program modifications or supports for school personnel needed to enable the child to make advancements toward attaining annual goals
- Explanation to the extent that the child will or will not participate with children who do not have disabilities
- Any specific modification in the administration of state- or district-wide assessments of achievement (e.g., oral test taking) that are needed for the child to participate in the assessment, or reasons for excluding the child from assessment of achievement
- How the child's progress toward annual goals will be measured
- How the child's parents will be regularly informed of the child's progress toward annual goals and the extent to which the child's progress is sufficient to meet goals by the end of the year

Source: Data from U.S. Department of Education. (2006b). Individualized education programs. *Retrieved from http://idea.ed.gov/explore/view/p/%2Croot%2Cdynamic%2CTopicalBrief%2C10%2C. U.S. Department of Education. (2000).* A guide to the individualized education program. *Retrieved from http://www.ed.gov/parents/needs/speced/iepguide/index.html*

with a chronic condition and provide care as needed. Health aides may be assigned to provide care for one or more children with school nurse supervision. Some children are placed in classes composed of children with special health care needs where health aides are more available to provide needed care. When the child is unable to attend school, tutoring may need to be provided at home by the school system or access provided to online education.

Nurses play a key role in assisting the family to understand that a teacher's primary responsibility is to teach, not to provide health care. The teacher is responsible for the health and safety of all children in the classroom. Parents need to have realistic expectations about the level of skilled support services that can be provided to a child who is medically fragile in a classroom. Teachers and education leaders are often challenged to meet the obligations for the child's special education services in balance with the needs of all other children in the classroom.

Homebound education is an option for these children, with resources provided through the school system. Homebound instruction provides education continuity when the child cannot attend school, and it reduces the child's stress and fatigue. This type of instruction may be used full time or for periods when the child is too ill to attend school. The benefits of providing education in the home include continuity of education when the child would otherwise be unable to attend school and reducing the child's stress and fatigue. Potential negative effects of home-

bound instruction include lack of peer and social interaction and decreased opportunity to develop social skills. Parents may also choose to home school the child. Parents who home school are responsible for the child's education and must file appropriate paperwork and follow specific guidelines. The family that chooses home schooling needs to establish a routine for the education process.

Transition to Adulthood

Improved survival rates have led to an increase in the number of adolescents with special health care needs transitioning to adulthood, many of whom have difficulty transitioning to adult health care services (Lotstein, Ghandour, Cash, et al., 2009). When their chronic condition could affect their future ability to work and live independently, customized transition planning is needed in preparation for adulthood and self-determination. A transition plan is developed in collaboration with the family based on the needs that have been identified in relation to the adolescent's goals for health care, employment, and community living. The adolescent should be involved in this process. Friends can also be involved and frequently provide valuable support to the teen in times of transition (Betz, 2007). Healthy & Ready to Work services may be particularly helpful to adolescents and families in planning for the transition to adulthood (HRTW National Resource Center, 2009). One of the proposed objectives of *Healthy People 2020* focuses on facilitation of health care transition for adolescents, including provisions of the resources available to make this transition (U.S. Department of Health and Human Services, 2010).

Clinical Judgment

Martin is a 17-year-old with sickle cell anemia. As he reaches adulthood, the need to transition from the pediatrician to an adult health care provider will arise. What factors should be taken into consideration in deciding when this health care transition should occur?

COLLABORATIVE CARE

Care of the child with a chronic condition generally requires a multidisciplinary health professional approach, including physicians, nurse practitioners, nurses, nutritionists, social workers, case workers, physical therapists, occupational therapists, and a case manager.

Hospitalization

Children with chronic disorders are more likely to be hospitalized than children without chronic disorders. Depending on the severity of the condition, frequent hospitalizations or long-term hospitalization for months or years may be required for the child with a chronic condition. The family is an integral part of the plan of care for an ill or hospitalized child. Acute hospitalization resulting from exacerbation of the child's disorder places increased demands and stressors on the child and family. The child and parent may fear worsening of the condition or even death. Hospitalization also provides an opportunity to evaluate the family's functioning and to provide additional resources that might be supportive. Refer to Chapter 11 ∞ for a discussion of nursing care of the hospitalized child.

Ethical Issues

Ethical issues often arise for children with chronic conditions or disabilities. There is an ongoing debate concerning who ultimately makes the decisions—parents or the primary health care providers—about withholding treatments, implementing treatments, and other medical care issues (see Chapter 1 ∞). Issues regarding clinical ethics related to children with chronic conditions or disabilities include the following:

- Withholding and refusal of treatment
- Advance directives (do-not-resuscitate orders) (see Chapter 13 ∞ for further discussion)
- Genetic testing and screening programs
- Sexual and reproductive rights, sterilization of adolescents with mental retardation
- Organ donation and rationing of care
- Research involving individuals with disabilities

These situations present a challenge to the family and health care providers. Most health care facilities have an ethics committee with established procedures and guidelines for addressing issues for the child with a chronic disorder or disability.

Health Promotion and Health Maintenance

Most children with a chronic condition are cared for at home with or without home nursing or other health care services, and they may rely solely on the family for their support and care. Children with chronic health conditions require regular health promotion, health screening, and health maintenance care, as well as specialized health services to assist the child and family in the condition's management. Parents need education and guidance to reduce risks for further illness and injury and to foster the child's development. The goal is to promote the child's growth and development and permit the child to have as normal a childhood as possible. The child with a chronic condition needs a medical or health care home to ensure that all the child's health care needs are met. Ideally this health care provider is located in the community where the family resides, making it more convenient for the family to obtain health care as well as care for episodic illnesses. Having a regular health care provider has many advantages for the family:

- Because the child and family are seen more frequently, a more trusting and family-centered relationship can develop. The health care provider learns about the family's strengths and coping abilities.
- The health care provider sees the child and family when things are going well and during exacerbations. This may enable the health care provider to identify strategies that help the family to better coordinate the child's care.
- When the provider is based in the same community as the child, information about community resources may be known and reduce the efforts that families need to make to identify appropriate services for the child.

An optimal health care arrangement for the child with a chronic condition exists when the medical or health care home

provider collaborates with a pediatric team or specialist that specializes in the care of children with a specific chronic condition. Pediatric specialists, advanced practice nurses, and other health care providers (e.g., physical therapists, social workers, and nutritionists) often function as a team providing coordinated care to the family and child with a chronic condition, such as spina bifida, cystic fibrosis, or cerebral palsy. These specialty teams are often found in major medical centers, requiring travel to the facility. When communication flows from the team to the child's health care provider and back to the team, new treatments can be monitored by the child's physician, and consultation can be sought if the child's health status changes.

Sometimes a pediatric specialist serves as the child's medical or health care home. Although this may seem like a good strategy for care, there are some risks that health promotion services will be minimized. It is important to ensure that regular health promotion and health maintenance services, such as immunizations, are not overlooked during the care of acute exacerbations of the chronic condition.

▲ **Health Promotion**

John, age 6, visits the pediatrician after having an asthma attack. It has been several months since he has been seen by his pediatrician. In addition to evaluation and treatment of his asthma, what else should be assessed to evaluate John's overall health and growth and development? Discuss anticipatory guidance appropriate for John and his parents.

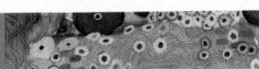
NURSING MANAGEMENT

In collaboration with the family and a multidisciplinary health care team, the nurse assists the family to manage the child's care at home; provides guidelines to promote the child's health, growth, and development; and supports the family by facilitating psychosocial adaptation.

The nurse's role in caring for the chronically ill child includes providing health supervision from infancy to transition into adulthood, collaborating with the multidisciplinary health care team, partnering with parents or caregivers to manage the child's care at home, referring the family to appropriate community services, assisting with planning for education services, promoting positive parenting behaviors and psychosocial adaptation and well-being of the child and family, and promoting growth and development of siblings.

Nursing Assessment and Diagnosis

Physiologic and Developmental Assessment

Conduct a physical assessment of the child, noting general health status and focusing on systems affected by the chronic condition. Perform a developmental assessment to help identify future developmental goals.

Family Assessment

Assess individual family members' level of understanding of the condition, treatment, and anticipated outcome of the condition. Determine the family's stage of acceptance of the child's chronic illness, and how well the child's care is integrated into family routines. Evaluate the child's home care environment to determine safety; the potential for abuse, lack of adequate care, or neglect; and opportunities to enhance care. See Nursing Care Plan: The Child with a Chronic Condition.

Planning and Implementation
The Child with a Newly Diagnosed Chronic Condition
The nurse should address the fears and concerns of the family of a child with a newly diagnosed chronic condition. Provide the condition-specific education necessary to help prepare the family for care at home and begin discharge planning. The parents'

NURSING CARE PLAN
The Child with a Chronic Condition

INTERVENTION	RATIONALE	EXPECTED OUTCOME
NIC Priority Intervention: *Individual Teaching:* Planning, implementing, and evaluating a teaching program designed to address a patient's particular need		**NOC Suggested Outcome:** *Knowledge:* Extent of understanding conveyed about the treatment regimen

Goal: The child will acquire self-care skills for lifetime management.

▪ Assess the child's developmental level and select an educational approach and self-care activities to match.	▪ Learning goals for the child must match knowledge and skill expectations appropriate for developmental stage.	The child demonstrates the proper technique in the self-care skill and is able to assume responsibility for that skill with supervision by the parent. Responsibility for self-care increases as new skills are learned.
▪ Review with the child all steps involved in the self-care skill and how to perform the skill.	▪ The child may have watched the routine used by parents many times, and asking the child to list each step helps the nurse identify extra training needed.	
▪ Use demonstration/return demonstration until the child is comfortable with procedures.	▪ Evaluation permits positive reinforcement and guidance for modification of techniques.	
▪ Help parents develop a planned sequence of self-care skills to teach the child.	▪ Parents need guidance to identify appropriate self-care skills that the child is developmentally ready to learn.	
▪ Discuss a plan for increased responsibility for self-care with the child and parents.	▪ Parents often need encouragement to transition responsibility to the child, becoming a supervisor rather than the person controlling care.	

NIC Priority Intervention: *Normalization Promotion:* Assisting parents and other family members of children with chronic illnesses or disabilities in providing normal life experiences for their children and families		**NOC Suggested Outcome:** *Family Health Status:* Overall health status and social competence of family unit

Goal: The child and family will manage the required treatments, monitoring, and medication regimen for the child's condition while maintaining family routines and functioning.

▪ Assess the child's and family's lifestyle and attempt to fit the child's care needs into those schedules.	▪ Fitting the child's care to the child's and family's lifestyle promotes adherence to the regimen and healthier family processes.	The child and family maintain important family routines and successfully manage the child's condition.
▪ Discuss the family's routines for special occasions and vacations and any activities important to the child. Identify ways to modify the child's management for these occasions and activities.	▪ It is important for the child to participate in special events with the family and peers as a normal child to promote psychological development.	

(continued)

NURSING CARE PLAN

The Child with a Chronic Condition (continued)

INTERVENTION	RATIONALE	EXPECTED OUTCOME
NIC Priority Intervention: *Resiliency Promotion:* Assisting individuals, families, and communities in development, use, and strengthening of protective factors to be used in coping with environmental and societal stressors		**NOC Suggested Outcome:** *Health-seeking Behavior:* Actions to promote optimal wellness, recovery, and rehabilitation
Goal: The child will develop a support system network.		
■ Talk with the child about how to tell friends, teachers, and other important people about the chronic condition.	■ These important people can assist the child in an emergency if they have enough information to assess the problem.	The child identifies the friends, teachers, and other important persons informed about the chronic condition who can provide support when needed.
■ Discuss ways to explain the condition to important people and how to answer questions.	■ Having an opportunity to plan and role-play the conversation will reduce the child's anxiety about condition disclosure.	
■ Role-play ways to talk about the condition with friends and teachers.	■ Sharing information about the condition helps others understand changes in lifestyle needed by the child.	
■ Encourage the child to attend peer support groups or camps specific to the child's condition.	■ Learning and support networks developed at camp can promote development of problem-solving skills that increase coping abilities.	

heightened anxiety level may reduce their comprehension of information heard.

Care of the technology-assisted child includes educating the family about equipment use and maintenance, specific tasks associated with treatment, and monitoring of the child. Ongoing assistance may be required to help families deal with financial issues, time management, and other challenges. See the chapters related to specific body systems later in this textbook for condition-specific family education and discharge planning.

Discharge Planning and Home Care Teaching

As the child with a newly diagnosed chronic condition transitions to the home, parents often feel overwhelmed with preparations for home care, the anxiety of caring for a child with

Culture *Racial and Ethnic Disparities Among CSHCN*

Children with special health care needs (CSHCN) who are of a racial/ethnic minority have more unmet health care needs than White children. A national study found that children from racial or ethnic minorities are less likely to have a personal physician (medical home) and less likely to be insured. Whereas 1 in 10 children with special health care needs overall do not have a medical home, 1 in 8 Hispanic CSHCN and 1 in 7 Black CSHCN are without one. The study also found that while 4.5% of White CSHCN were uninsured, 5.7% of Black CSHCN and 9.3% of Hispanic CSHCN had no insurance (Ngui & Flores, 2007). Efforts by health care providers and others who work with CSHCN should focus on ensuring that all of these children are insured and have a medical home to decrease the unmet health care needs among minorities.

special health care needs, and supporting the child's growth and development. Work with the parents to ensure a smooth transition from the hospital to the home environment. Assist the family in the initial discussions with the multidisciplinary team that participates in developing the child's care plan. Ensure that the family understands the role of each care provider.

Education to provide care of the child at home may be initiated by the hospital nursing staff, and then transitioned to special nurse educators or the home health nurses. Care is taken to ensure that all aspects of management are discussed with the family and that they demonstrate an understanding and ability to perform the care required.

During discharge planning the identification of a parent peer or peer support group may be helpful to provide support to the family. Parent peers who have had similar experiences may be very helpful in identifying strategies for the initial care transition in the home and additional issues that arise over time. If the family has a computer, Internet resources for information and family support should be provided.

Collaborate with the family and health care team to ensure that the child has a medical or health care home in the local community to provide health promotion and maintenance and to assist with the coordination of local community resources. Promote communication and joint planning of care between the specialty care provider and local health care provider. Nurses working in hospital specialty clinics and other community settings can help ensure that children with chronic conditions receive multidisciplinary referrals and have appointments scheduled. Social services may be called to assist the family with identifying financial resources and other community resources for home management.

Coordination of Care 🖉

Care coordination is the process of planning and integrating health care services among providers in an effort to achieve and promote good health and positive outcomes in the child (American Academy of Pediatrics, 2009; Wood, Winterbauer, Sloyer, et al., 2009). Care coordination in a medical home decreases unmet health care needs, improves family satisfaction, and decreases hospitalizations (Wood et al., 2009). A **case manager**, often a nurse or social worker, may be given responsibility to help the family with care coordination. Case managers are often paid by a health care insurer to reduce health care costs by coordinating the health care team, determining family needs, identifying financial and local support resources, and arranging for needed health care services.

Care coordination may also include helping the family modify the home to support required technology, such as mechanical ventilation or wheelchair use. Assistance may be required in purchasing or leasing specialized equipment such as ventilators or infusion pumps. The coordination plan also includes determining the potential need for home health nursing, physical therapy, or other home health services.

Families become very well educated about their child's condition and the services that would make managing the child's condition easier. Once management goals are established by the multidisciplinary team, the case manager works with the family to help in the decision-making process regarding how goals will be met. An important role is helping the family to determine cost-effective strategies to meet health care goals and to delay the time when the child reaches the cap on health insurance benefits.

Some families assume the role of care coordinator for their child. It is essential for the family to understand that care coordination is time-consuming and requires ongoing assessment and evaluation of the child's status and anticipated outcomes. Support family members in their decision to lead the care coordination process by helping the parents to become knowledgeable about the child's condition and treatment regimen. Encourage

the parents to take an active role in the treatment planning and decision-making process so that they gain confidence in their abilities. Many hospitals have workshops for parents who are managing the complex care of their children. Parent-to-parent support groups can provide advice, support, and suggestions for referrals. Review the care coordination to ensure that the child has access to the most appropriate care and resources. Provide positive feedback to the parents as their advocacy skills increase.

Suggest that the family maintain a log of the health care team members, their roles, when the child was seen and any interventions, the results of interventions, and future planned interventions or treatments. The family can use this information when communicating with the health care providers, particularly in an emergency, and it may also help eliminate unnecessary duplication of procedures.

Respite Care

Respite care is an important support service to care for the child with a chronic condition while the parents take a short break away from the daily care. Respite allows parents an opportunity for rest so they may sustain their role as a caregiver. Care may be provided by extended family, friends, or an agency and may take place in the home or an area outside of the home such as a residential setting or hospice. The length of time may vary from a few hours to several days (Eaton, 2008). An example might be skilled nursing care in a facility or the home so the family can have a weekend away. Assist the family in identifying respite care that meets the individual family's needs from the services available in the community. Many states have passed legislation for in-home family support services that include respite care. Because most respite services charge for their assistance, the family may require help in identifying respite waiver subsidies available to them. Reliable childcare and enrollment in school are other mechanisms used for families to obtain respite care. See Evidence-Based Practice: Identifying and Responding to Unmet Needs.

Clinical Tip ◥

The ARCH National Respite Network helps parents locate respite care services in their area. See the companion website for a respite service locator.

Support for the Child with a Chronic Condition

Provide the child with opportunities to express concerns about the condition and its effect on quality of life. The child who has had the chronic condition since birth or early childhood requires assistance in understanding more about the condition as cognitive development and understanding

Research — *Care Coordination for CSHCN*

Data were analyzed from the 2005–2006 National Survey of Children with Special Health Care Needs to determine the association between receiving adequate care coordination, family–provider relations, and outcomes in the child and family. Data indicated that 68.2% of the families reported receiving some type of assistance with care coordination. Of these, 59.2% indicated they received adequate help, and 40.8% indicated the assistance was inadequate. Adequate care coordination was associated with family-centered care, satisfaction with care received, and a partnership with health care professionals. Families who reported receiving adequate care coordination were less likely to have problems with specialty referrals, family financial burden, and reduction in work hours. These families also had less out-of-pocket expenses, fewer visits to the emergency room per month, and fewer missed days of school for the CSHCN than families who reported receiving inadequate assistance with care coordination (Turchi, Berhane, Bethell, et al., 2009).

Law & Ethics — *Katie Becket Act*

The Tax Equity and Fiscal Responsibility Act of 1982 (Public Law 97-248), also known as the Katie Becket Act, provides financial assistance so parents can hire trained care providers for respite care (Johnson, Kastner, & Committee/Section on Children with Disabilities, 2005).

Evidence-Based Practice
Identifying and Responding to Unmet Needs

Problem

What are the unmet needs of parents of children with complex health care conditions?

Evidence

Parents having a child with complex health care conditions have reported difficulties in obtaining the support needed to manage the child's care. Needs of families vary and depend on the diagnosis, prognosis, and specific needs of the child (Hummelinck & Pollock, 2006). Interviews with nine families (nine mothers and two fathers) having a child who had been diagnosed at least 1 year with a long-term illness helped illustrate the experiences that parents have in managing their children's health care and how health care providers affect their experiences. This study identified the specific need for health care professionals to show care toward the child. Although some parents remembered times that their child was treated with care, others recalled episodes when their child was treated in an unconcerned manner. The parents in this study also identified receiving information as an important need. While some parents reported they actually received too much information to comprehend, others reported receiving either inadequate or conflicting information (Nuutila & Salanterä, 2006).

Additional studies have focused specifically on informational needs of parents of children with chronic illness. Hummelinck and Pollock (2006) interviewed 27 parents who had varying needs for information. Although some of these parents actively sought information, resisting information was noted as a coping strategy among some of these parents. Most parents in this study perceived the information they received as inadequate. Jackson, Baird, Davis-Reynolds, et al. (2007) conducted in-depth interviews with 10 par-

ents of children with health care needs and found that they had a particular preference for how information was presented. Most preferred that information be presented one-on-one by a professional with additional written information made available to them. These parents also expressed the importance of a contact person for follow-up questions and support.

Implications

These studies revealed that families with children having special health care needs seek information, but the type of information sought varies by the type of condition, level of function, or special health care need. However, ways to promote the child's growth and development and community services that match the child's needs are required by nearly all families. Nurses are in a position to assist families by assessing their needs for information and then attempting to provide that information. The need for care and support from health care professionals was also identified as a potentially unmet need. Nurses should always treat the child and family with care and compassion. Current listings of community services and contact information of health care professionals should be provided to these families.

Critical Thinking Application

Select a specific pediatric chronic condition that usually requires parents to follow a complex routine to care for the child. What questions will you ask the family in order to learn about their perceived needs? Consider the potential supports and services such a family might need and compile a list of local resources that could be recommended to the family.

---

increase. As the child grows, collaborate with the child and family to include the child in self-care management according to cognitive and developmental level, and to participate in the decision-making process. Encourage the child to assume a role in care and management of the condition. This may include maintaining a journal, self-administering medications, or monitoring glucose levels. See Families Want to Know: Developmental Strategies for Promoting the Child's Self-Care for more information.

Support the transition of adolescents to adult health services by introducing the adolescent to members of the health care team that will eventually assume a role in providing care. Encourage the adolescent to take a more assertive role in visits with the pediatric health care team in preparation for working with a new health care team. Ensure that the adolescent understands the role each new member of the team will assume.

Complementary Therapy
CAM and Chronic Illness

Children with chronic illness are three times more likely to use complementary and alternative modalities (CAM) than children who are healthy. CAM use has increased among children with cancer, cystic fibrosis, juvenile arthritis, cerebral palsy, and inflammatory bowel disease (Tsao, Meldrum, Kim, et al., 2007; McCann & Newell, 2006). See Chapter 2 ∞ for more information related to CAM use in children.

Health Promotion

Review the next stage of expected development with parents and provide suggestions and strategies to help the child with a chronic condition achieve developmental milestones. Review the care that other children in the family are receiving to ensure that they obtain appropriate care and stimulation to promote their growth and development. Remind parents of routine health promotion and maintenance needs of all children in the family such as immunizations, dental hygiene, and any screening tests. See Chapters 6 through 9 ∞.

Discuss parenting approaches for the child with a chronic condition. Encourage a structured environment with limitations that are developmentally appropriate for the child. Assist the family as needed in providing a nurturing environment and offering praise for achievement of tasks.

Facilitate Education Service Planning

Assist the family with school entry of the child with a chronic condition. Discussions with the family can assist them in defining appropriate expectations and goals. The nurse can also communicate with school personnel about any classroom modifications required by the child, and educate teachers and other school personnel about the medical or assistive equipment used by the child. This information is then integrated into the child's individualized health plan (IHP), which may be a stand-alone plan or tied to an IEP. The school nurse can also assist the family with Section 504 planning activities by serving as

Families Want to Know
Developmental Strategies for Promoting the Child's Self-Care

When the child is cognitively able to learn about the chronic condition and begin to take some responsibility for self-care, knowledge of cognitive and psychomotor development is helpful in developing strategies to teach the child about self-care. Ideally such learning should begin early in life, but even when the condition develops at a later age, educating the child can still be based upon knowledge of the child's development. Education and assumption of self-care responsibility should be appropriately matched to the child's developmental abilities. Children who have mental impairment will need to be taught based on their cognitive abilities and not their chronological age. The ultimate goal is that the adolescent is able to assume responsibility for care and has the knowledge needed to manage problems as they occur and transition into the adult health care system when the time comes.

- Toddlers (1 to 3 years) can cooperate with the daily routines of care and assist in simple ways, such as holding an item. The toddler can also learn simple concepts such as foods allowed or not allowed. When a routine is established, the toddler learns what to expect through daily repetition.

- Preschoolers (4 to 5 years) are able to imitate some of the parent's behaviors regarding care, and they can learn simple terms that describe their condition and how they feel when the condition is not well controlled (e.g., weak and dizzy with diabetes, difficulty breathing with asthma).

  Parents can help teach the child the simple terms about the condition and have the child practice telling the information to other family members. Help the parent identify a simple task that is part of the management care routine that the child can do to help (holding the spacer during the asthma treatment, washing the hands, taking supplies out of a bag or box).

- Early school-age children (6 to 9 years) are more aware of physical feelings associated with when the condition is and is not well controlled. The child is also capable of performing some aspects of care (fingerstick for glucose monitoring, writing down the glucose reading on a log, controlling inhalation to use aerosol medication, selecting appropriate foods for a meal or snack), having seen it performed by parents repeatedly or after being taught and coached to do it well.

The parent can support the child's learning by increasing the information provided about the condition and need for treatment. Give the child an option about which self-care skill to learn first, next, and so on. The parent is then able to select skills appropriate to the child's developmental ability and teach the child to perform them. As the child demonstrates proficiency with a skill, a new skill can be added. The child can take responsibility for learned self-care skills with supervision, and the parent performs other unlearned skills.

- Late school-age children (10 to 12 years) have a greater understanding of how the body works and the impact of the chronic condition. They also have the capability of discussing some aspects of care directly with the health care provider. By 12 years of age, the child can learn to perform all the psychomotor skills associated with the condition.

  Parents can support the child in assuming more responsibility for self-care by initially providing a list of all steps in the management plan or other tools that will help with decision making (dose of insulin, adding food to the diet on days with soccer practice). Provide corrective feedback as necessary. Continue to be present to answer questions, particularly when problem solving and when decisions need to be made about care. Encourage the child to talk independently with the health care provider.

- Adolescents can, with the prior steps of preparation, become the primary manager of their daily care. They usually have the cognitive ability to solve problems and make adjustments in the care routine for special occasions or illness and to ask for help when a complex care situation develops. The adolescent should have a network of friends and family who are informed about the condition and able to assist in an emergency.

Parents should monitor the self-care provided without interfering in the adolescent's care routine unless corrective feedback is needed. Encourage the adolescent to take full responsibility for self-care management, but encourage open communication about the condition and other health care concerns. Discuss risky behaviors and the potential impact on general health, and specifically the condition. Provide support and assistance during the time the adolescent transitions to adult health care providers.

---

a liaison between the school and the child's health care team. Key health records that are needed for planning the IHP should be assembled after the family provides informed consent. Encourage the family to establish regular communication with the school personnel and school nurse.

Clinical Tip

Special accommodations for the child with disabilities may include extended test-taking times, tutors, note-takers, and the use of technological equipment to assist in the learning environment. Encourage parents to ask questions regarding computer accessibility, arrangements for tutors or note-takers, private study areas, and individualized attention.

In the case of a do-not-resuscitate (DNR) request for the child at school, encourage collaboration with school personnel, teachers, and other members of the health care team as necessary to facilitate an agreement between the school and family.

Many school systems do not have a policy that permits honoring a DNR request, and the school nurse is an important liaison in the discussion and development of the policy. Refer to Chapter 13 ∞ for further discussion of DNR requests in school.

Support the Family's Psychosocial Adjustment
A positive relationship with the health care team promotes coping in families of chronically ill children (Nuutila & Salanterä, 2006). Provide the child, parents, and siblings an opportunity to discuss how the chronic illness affects their daily lives. Listening and offering strategies to improve the organization of care, as well as the use of community and family supports, can help enhance the family's coping. Help the family see that simple chores performed by friends and extended family such as cooking meals, transporting siblings to recreational events, or picking up supplies at the supermarket can reduce stress especially during times when the child is hospitalized. Partner with the family to identify support systems, and encourage open communication

Growth & Development   *Siblings*

Siblings of children with a chronic condition may feel overwhelmingly guilty about their feelings of jealousy, shame, and anger. Inform the child that these feelings are normal and that the child is not "bad" for having these feelings.

with those systems to maintain adequate support and decrease the stressors associated with the child's illness (Coffey, 2006). Refer the family to support groups in the community or on the Internet that might offer suggestions and information. Counseling may be helpful to parents experiencing marital stress.

Identify ways to improve accessibility of services to children with chronic conditions and their families. For example, arranging transportation, finding resources closer to home, and arranging for home visits may improve accessibility.

Assist the family in providing information to the siblings about the child's disability at the appropriate developmental level so that it is tailored specifically to the siblings' level of understanding. Provide instructional materials, videos, books, pamphlets, and other information when available. Inform the parents that siblings of the child with a chronic condition may experience an array of feelings. See the discussion on page 294 regarding sibling reactions.

Emergency Preparedness

Advance planning is needed to ensure that medically fragile children who use assistive technology for survival or have the potential for life-threatening episodes have the necessary resources in the event of a disaster. The designated shelter for such children, with health professionals and electrical power for the needed equipment, should be identified and known to the family. In the meantime, battery packs for power backup should be available at all times. Additionally, parents need to arrange for durable power of attorney so that consent for emergency medical care can be available as needed. The child and parents may become separated during the disaster, or the parents may become injured and unable to care for the child.

Evaluation

Expected outcomes for care of the family of a child with a chronic condition may include:

- The child and family establish effective coping mechanisms.
- The child and family experience reduced anxiety.
- The child and family demonstrate understanding and management of the condition.
- Parenting patterns are appropriate and supportive of the child's growth and development.
- Role conflict and caregiver strain are minimized.
- Caregivers achieve adequate rest, sleep, and socialization.
- The child and family adjust to the child's chronic condition.
- The adolescent successfully transitions to adult health services and living arrangements.

■ NURSE'S REACTIONS TO CARE OF CHILDREN WITH A CHRONIC CONDITION

Nurses and other health care professionals generally describe their role in caring for families and children with chronic conditions as very rewarding. However, over time these nurses who provide care to chronically ill patients who experience pain, trauma, or suffering are at risk for emotional, spiritual, and physical fatigue (Aycock & Boyle, 2009; McMullen, 2007; Sabo, 2006). Nurses need to recognize signs of **compassion fatigue,** an emotion that comes from understanding the traumatic events experienced by families and the stress from helping or wanting to help the families. The weariness and lack of energy associated with compassion fatigue may become severe and affect the ability to function at work or home if the nurse's coping mechanisms are not effective.

Self-care activities such as exercise, meditation, recreation, maintaining a sense of humor, and social nonwork relationships are beneficial short-term personal coping strategies. Taking vacations to rest and reenergize, changing patient assignments, or transferring to a new work area are other strategies that can help the nurse balance personal mental health with the compassion needed for ongoing work with these families.

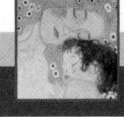

Chapter Highlights

- A chronic condition is a long-term, ongoing condition that is expected to last 3 months or more and may involve any of the following alone or in combination: functional limitations, disfigurement, dependence on technology, medications, special diet for management of the condition, and the need for more health care services than a healthy child would require.
- Approximately 10 million children in the United States have special health care needs related to a chronic condition.
- Chronic conditions can occur as a result of a genetic condition, congenital anomaly, injury during fetal development or at birth, complication of care after birth, serious infection, or significant injury.

- Children who are medically fragile are dependent on a medical device for survival or prevention of further disability.
- A developmental delay results when there is failure to achieve anticipated milestones during specific developmental stages.
- Parents may experience many of the same responses to the diagnosis of a child's chronic condition as if they had experienced the child's death, including shock, disbelief, anger, denial, and despair. Siblings of the child with a chronic illness may have feelings of jealousy, resentment, anger, depression, and guilt.
- The time of diagnosis is one of the most stressful times for families of children with chronic conditions as the parents wait

anxiously for the outcome of diagnostic procedures. Other times associated with significant stressors for the family include developmental milestones, school entry, adolescence, planning for the transition to adult health and vocational services, and planning for long-term guardianship.

- Moving the child with a chronic illness who is dependent on technology to the home setting is a life-changing decision for the family, and it must be done with collaboration between the family and the health care team.

- Caregiver burden, the ongoing pressure of caring for children with special health care needs, causes fatigue and makes it difficult for the parents to meet other family obligations.

- The financial burden of caring for a child with special health care needs is significant even when the family has health insurance.

- In an effort to cope and feel a sense of control over the family's life, the parents may use normalization, a process of focusing on those aspects of family life and routine that are similar to other families while integrating the needs of the child with a chronic condition.

- Sending the child to school has several benefits for the child and family, including socialization for the child beyond the immediate family, respite for parents, and promotion of a sense of normalization in the family.

- An individualized education plan (IEP) is developed for a child with cognitive, motor, social, or communication impairments who needs special education services in the school setting. An individualized health plan (IHP) is developed for the child with medical conditions that need to be managed within the school setting.

- Children who are medically fragile or dependent on technology are entitled to a free and appropriate education and education services in the school setting. The school administration is obligated to plan for and ensure that the personnel, resources, and equipment needed to provide care are consistently available.

- An individualized transition plan (ITP) is developed for adolescents with a chronic condition in collaboration with the family to assist in identifying appropriate support programs, living arrangements, and employment for adult life.

- The child with a chronic condition is more likely to be hospitalized than the child without a chronic condition. Sudden hospitalization resulting from exacerbation of the child's disorder places increased demands and stressors on the child and family.

- Children with chronic health conditions require regular health promotion, health screening, and health maintenance care, as well as specialized health services to assist the child and family in management of the condition.

- The role of the nurse in caring for the child with a chronic condition includes providing health supervision from infancy to transition into adulthood, collaborating with the multidisciplinary health care team, and partnering with the family to manage the child's care at home.

- Nurses who specialize in caring for children with complex chronic conditions may experience compassion fatigue as they continue their efforts to meet the ongoing needs of these families.

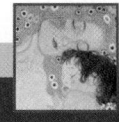

Clinical Reasoning in Action

Recall Haley, the 8-year-old child with cerebral palsy who will be attending school for the first time. Her mother believes that attending school will help promote her social development and broaden what she can learn. She also thinks that some of the special health services that Haley needs may be available in school, such as physical therapy and speech therapy. Haley's mother has asked for the clinic nurse's advice to help plan her daughter's transition to school. Haley's mother and nurse discuss the potential accommodations that Haley will need for her mobility limitations. The nurse suggests that Haley receive a full educational evaluation so her educational needs can be identified. Once the mother has signed consent, the clinic nurse prepares a summary of Haley's health history for the school nurse that can be used to develop her IEP and IHP.

1. Describe the potential signs and symptoms of cerebral palsy that might be important to consider when Haley's IEP and IHP are developed (see Chapter 27 ∞ for more information on cerebral palsy).

2. Based upon Haley's age and developmental stage, what feelings, fears, and concerns might she experience related to entering school?

3. Describe the role of the nurse as Haley's care coordinator.

4. What education does the mother need to prepare her for serving as Haley's advocate with school administrators when her IEP and IHP are developed?

See Pearson Nursing Student Resources for possible responses.

References

Aitken, M. E., McCarthy, M. L., Slomine, B. S., Ding, R., Durbin, D. R., Jaffe, K. M., . . . CHAT Study Group. (2009). Family burden after traumatic brain injury in children. *Pediatrics, 12*(1), 199–206.

Allen, P. J. (2010). The primary care provider and children with chronic conditions. In P. J. Allen, J. A. Vessey, & N. A. Schapiro, *Primary care of the child with a chronic condition* (5th ed., pp. 3–21). St. Louis, MO: Mosby.

American Academy of Pediatrics. (2009). *Tools for coordinating care.* Retrieved from http://www.medicalhomeinfo.org/tools/coordinating%20care.html

Aycock, N., & Boyle, D. (2009). Interventions to manage compassion fatigue in oncology nursing. *Clinical Journal of Oncology Nursing, 13*(2), 183–191.

Ballard, K. L. (2004). Meeting the needs of siblings of children with cancer. *Pediatric Nursing, 30*(5), 394–401.

Betz, C. L. (2007). Facilitating the transition of adolescents with developmental disabilities: Nursing practice issues and care. *Journal of Pediatric Nursing, 22*(2), 103–115.

Betz, C. L. (2008). Forthcoming issues to confront as children and youth with special health care needs grow up. *Journal of Pediatric Nursing, 23*(4), 237–240.

Blann, L. E. (2005). Early intervention for children and families with special needs. *Maternal Child Nursing, 30*(4), 263–267.

Brandon, D. H., Ryan, D. J., & Barnes, A. H. (2007). Effect of environmental changes on noise in the NICU. *Neonatal Network, 26*(4), 213–218.

Coffey, J. S. (2006). Parenting a child with chronic illness: A metasynthesis. *Pediatric Nursing, 32*(1), 51–59.

Eaton, N. (2008). "I don't know how we coped before": A study of respite care for children in the home and hospice. *Journal of Clinical Nursing, 17*(23), 3196–3204.

Fanos, J. H., Fahrner, K., Jelveh, M., King, R., & Tejeda, D. (2004). The sibling center: A pilot program for siblings of children and adolescents with a serious medical condition. *Journal of Pediatrics, 146,* 831–835.

Gasalberti, D. (2006). Alternative therapies for children and youth with special health care needs. *Journal of Pediatric Health Care, 20*(2), 133–136.

Giallo, R., & Gavidia-Payne, S. (2006). Child, parent and family factors as predictors of adjustment for siblings of children with a disability. *Journal of Intellectual Disability Research, 50*(12), 937–948.

Gordon, J. (2009). An evidence-based approach for supporting parents experiencing chronic sorrow. *Pediatric Nursing, 35*(2), 115–119.

Griffin, T., & Abraham, M. (2006). Transition to home from the newborn intensive care unit. *Journal of Perinatal Neonatal Nursing, 20*(3), 243–249.

Hibbard, R. A., Desch, L. W., & Committee on Child Abuse and Neglect and Council on Children with Disabilities. (2007). Maltreatment of children with disabilities. *Pediatrics, 119*(5), 1018–1025.

Houtzager, B. A., Grootenhuis, M. A., Hoekstra-Weebers, J. E. H. M., & Last, B. F. (2005). One month after diagnosis: Quality of life, coping and previous functioning in siblings of children with cancer. *Child: Care, Health & Development, 31*(1), 75–87.

HRTW National Resource Center. (2009). *About HRTW.* Retrieved from http://www.hrtw.org/about_us/index.html

Hummelinck, A., & Pollock, K. (2006). Parents' information needs about the treatment of their chronically ill child: A qualitative study. *Patient Education and Counseling, 62,* 228–234.

Jackson, R., Baird, W., Davis-Reynolds, L., Smith, C., Blackburn, S., & Allsebrook, J. (2007). Qualitative analysis of parents' information needs and psychosocial experiences when supporting children with health care needs. *Health Information and Libraries Journal, 25,* 31–37.

Johnson, C. P., Kastner, T. A., & Committee/Section on Children with Disabilities. (2005). Helping families raise children with special health care needs at home. *Pediatrics, 115*(2), 507–511.

Kellam, B., & Bhatia, J. (2008). Sound spectral analysis in the intensive care nursery: Measuring high-frequency sound. *Journal of Pediatric Nursing, 23*(4), 317–323.

Knafl, K. A., & Santacroce, S. J. (2010). Chronic conditions and the family. In P. J. Allen, J. A. Vessey, &

N. A. Schapiro, *Primary care of the child with a chronic condition* (5th ed., pp. 74–89). St. Louis, MO: Mosby.

Lane, K. W. (2007). Hippotherapy and the significance of complementary and alternative medicine: A Q&A with William Benda, M.D., FACEP, FAAEM. *Alternative and Complementary Therapies, 13*(5), 266–268.

Lasky, R. E., & Williams, A. L. (2009). Noise and light exposures for extremely low birth weight newborns during their stay in the neonatal intensive care unit. *Pediatrics, 123*(2), 540–546.

Lee, T. Y., Miles, M. S., & Holditch-Davis, D. (2006). Fathers' support to mothers of medically fragile infants. *Journal of Obstetric, Gynecologic, and Neonatal Nursing, 35*(1), 46–55.

Looman, W. S., O'Conner-Von, S. K., Ferski, G. J., & Hildenbrand, D. A. (2009). Financial and employment problems in families of children with special health care needs: Implications for research and practice. *Journal of Pediatric Health Care, 23*(2), 117–125.

Lotstein, D. S., Ghandour, R., Cash, A., McGuire, E., Strickland, B., & Newacheck, P. (2009). Planning for health care transitions: Results from the 2005–2006 National Survey of Children with Special Health Care Needs. *Pediatrics, 123*(1), e145–e152.

McCann, L. J., & Newell, S. J. (2006). Survey of paediatric complementary and alternative medicine use in health and chronic illness. *Archives of Disease in Childhood, 91,* 173–174.

McMullen, L. (2007). Oncology nursing and compassion fatigue: Caring until it hurts. Who is caring for the caregiver? *Oncology Nursing Forum, 34*(2), 491.

Moses, M., Gilchrest, C., & Schwab, N. C. (2005). Section 504 of the Rehabilitation Act: Determining eligibility and implications for school districts. *Journal of School Nursing, 21*(1), 48–58.

Ngui, E. M., & Flores, G. (2007). Unmet needs for specialty, dental, mental, and allied health care among children with special health care needs: Are there racial/ethnic disparities? *Journal of Health Care for the Poor and Underserved, 18*(4), 931–949.

Nuutila, L., & Salanterä, S. (2006). Children with a long-term illness: Parents' experiences of care. *Journal of Pediatric Nursing, 21*(2), 153–160.

Rehm, R. S., & Bradley, J. F. (2005). The search for social safety and comfort in families raising children with complex chronic conditions. *Journal of Family Nursing,11*(1), 59–78.

Rehm, R. S., & Bradley, J. F. (2006). Social interactions at school of children who are medically fragile and developmentally delayed. *Journal of Pediatric Nursing, 21*(4), 299–307.

Sabo, B. M. (2006). Compassion fatigue and nursing work: Can we accurately capture the consequences of caring work? *International Journal of Nursing Practice, 12,* 136–142.

Selekman, J., & Vessey, J. A. (2010). School and the child with a chronic condition. In P. J. Allen, J. A. Vessey, & N. A. Schapiro, *Primary care of the child with a chronic condition* (5th ed., pp. 42–59). St. Louis, MO: Mosby.

Tsao, J. C. I., Meldrum, M., Kim, S. C., Jacob, M. C., & Zeltzer, L. K. (2007). Treatment preferences for CAM in children with chronic pain. *Evidence Based Complementary Alternative Medicine, 4*(3), 367–374.

Turchi, R. M., Berhane, Z., Bethell, C., Pomponio, A., Antonelli, R., & Minkovitz, C. S. (2009). Care coordination for CSHCN: Associations with family–provider relations and family/child outcomes. *Pediatrics, 124,* S428–S434.

U.S. Department of Education. (2000). *A guide to the individualized education program.* Retrieved from http://www.ed.gov/parents/needs/speced/iepguide/index.htm

U.S. Department of Education. (2006a). Building the legacy: IDEA 2004. Retrieved from http://idea.ed.gov/explore/search?search_option=all&query=individuals+with+disabilities+education+act&GO.x=9&GO.y=9

U.S. Department of Education. (2006b). *Individualized education programs.* Retrieved from http://idea.ed.gov/explore/view/p/%2Croot%2Cdynamic%2CTopicalBrief%2C10%2C.

U.S. Department of Health and Human Services, Health Resources and Services Administration, Maternal and Child Health Bureau. (2008). *The National Survey of Children with Special Health Care Needs Chartbook 2005–2006.* Rockville, MD: U.S. Department of Health and Human Services.

U.S. Department of Health and Human Services. (2010). Proposed healthy people 2020 objectives. Retrieved from http://www.healthypeople.gov/hp2020/Objectives/TopicAreas.aspx

U.S. Social Security Administration. (2007). *Understanding Supplemental Security Income SSI for Children.* Retrieved from http://www.ssa.gov/ssi/text-child-ussi.htm

Vessey, J. A., & Sullivan, B. J. (2010). Chronic conditions and child development. In P. J. Allen, J. A. Vessey, & N. A. Schapiro, *Primary care of the child with a chronic condition* (5th ed., pp. 22–41). St. Louis, MO: Mosby.

Vickers, M. H. (2006). *Working and caring for a child with chronic illness: Disconnected and doing it all.* New York: Palgrave McMillan.

Williams, P. D., Piamjariyakul, U., Graff, J. C. & Stanton, A. (2010). Developmental disabilites: Effects on well siblings. *Issues in Comprehensive Pediatric Nursing, 33,* 39–55.

Wood, D., Winterbauer, N., Sloyer, P., Jobli, E., Hou, T., McCaskill, Q., & Livingood, W. (2009). A longitudinal study of a pediatric practice-based versus an agency-based model of care coordination for children and youth with special health care needs. *Maternal Child Health Journal, 13,* 667–676.

The Child with a Life-Threatening Condition and End-of-Life Care

chapter 13

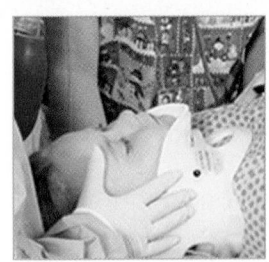

Alexa, 6 years old, was a passenger in the back seat of her parents' car when another car struck them broadside, pushing in the back passenger door. Even though Alexa was wearing a lap belt, her head struck the car window. She was unconscious at the scene, and she had a bruise across her abdomen where the lap belt restrained her. The emergency medical technicians responded and decided Alexa had injuries serious enough to transport her to the trauma center. A cervical collar was applied in case her cervical spine was also injured. Upon arrival at the trauma center, Alexa's airway, breathing, circulation, and responsiveness were assessed. She was breathing spontaneously and her heart rate was strong and regular, but more rapid than normal. Her blood pressure was appropriate for her age. Because she was still not fully responsive, an endotracheal tube was inserted and oxygen was administered. An intravenous line was started to administer lactated Ringer's solution. Alexa's abdomen was slightly distended, and she flinched and withdrew to touch when her abdomen was palpated in the left upper quadrant. She was admitted to the pediatric intensive care unit (PICU) so she could be monitored carefully for changes to her physiologic status and be provided needed treatment. Further evaluation will determine the extent of Alexa's head injury and if she has a spleen laceration or other injury in the abdomen.

What do children like Alexa face after admission to the PICU? What nursing strategies can help a critically ill or injured child cope with the experience? What stressors will families face during the child's hospitalization? What interventions could help them in this crisis?

Key Terms

air hunger / 326
brain death / 323
Cheyne-Stokes breathing / 326
coping / 313
death anxiety / 325
death imagery / 327
family crisis / 317
grief / 318
hospice / 322
life-threatening condition / 313
palliative care / 322
regression / 314
repression / 314
support systems / 314

Learning Outcomes

After reading this chapter, you will be able to do the following:

1. Summarize the child's experiences of a life-threatening illness or injury according to developmental level.
2. Describe the family's experience and reactions to having a child with a life-threatening illness or injury.
3. Identify the coping mechanisms used by the child and family in response to stress.
4. Develop a nursing care plan for the child with a life-threatening illness or injury.
5. Demonstrate assessment skills used to identify the physiologic changes that occur in the dying child.
6. Develop a nursing care plan to provide family-centered care for the dying child and family.
7. Implement strategies for bereavement support of the parents and siblings after the death of a child.
8. Describe strategies to support nurses who care for children who die.

Evaluation

Expected outcomes of nursing care include:

- A trusting relationship is developed with the child and family.
- The child is given preparation and support for procedures.
- The child's coping is promoted by family presence and therapeutic play.

■ THE PARENTS' EXPERIENCE

The uncertainty and unpredictability of a child's life-threatening illness or injury challenge a family's coping and stability. The sudden loss of the parenting role with the emergency admission of their child causes stress. Families display many different responses and coping strategies. Parents sometimes transmit their anxiety to the child, who then becomes even more anxious. Family-centered care must be provided; if the needs of the family are met, it will help ensure that the needs of the child with a life-threatening condition are met. Clear, concise communication is imperative.

The Family in Crisis

The critical care environment and the implications of a life-threatening illness or injury are far removed from the everyday experiences of most families. The unfamiliarity of the environment and the uncertainty and seriousness of the illness or injury create a **family crisis**, which occurs when the family encounters a problem that seems insurmountable and usual coping skills are not effective.

Since families have little time to prepare for the experience, a sudden admission threatens family integrity, causing enormous stress and separation from loved ones. Interruption of the unique parent–child relationship can be more stressful to parents than the physical PICU environment. Siblings are also affected; see discussion on page 321. In addition, extended family members such as grandparents must be considered. Stresses are further intensified in the case of divorce, separation, and step-parenting. Financial problems, a long distance from home to hospital, or another ill or injured family member can compound the crisis. See Chapter 2 ∞ for a discussion on family assessment and family resiliency.

Reactions to Life-Threatening Illness or Injury

When faced with a threat to their child's life, parents typically progress through stages that might include shock and disbelief, anger and guilt, deprivation and loss, anticipatory waiting, and readjustment or mourning. Some families progress through these stages in a linear fashion, while others go back and forth between stages, especially if the child's condition improves and then worsens.

Shock and Disbelief

The universal reaction to a child's life-threatening condition is shock and disbelief. As the familiar is disrupted, parents experience a loss of control, an inability to regain their bearings, and feelings of immobility. The hospital environment, emergency department, or PICU may seem unreal. The emotions parents experience initially are intensified by the physical appearance of their child (particularly after a major injury); the presence of monitors, tubing, and equipment; and the actual injury or illness. As Alexa's mother from the opening scenario stated, "I felt distanced, in a daze, in and out of it that first day after the accident."

Shock and disbelief begin in the first few moments after hearing the "news" and can last for days. The shock helps postpone the full impact of the crisis. During this period, parents search for answers and explanations about the illness or injury. Information must be repeated many times to parents, because in this stage they are often unable to assimilate information easily.

Anger and Guilt

Anger and guilt surface as parents become more aware of their child's illness or injury. Their anger may be directed toward themselves or each other because they could not protect their child. Other individuals may be blamed, such as the driver of a motor vehicle involved in the crash injuring the child. Parents may also be angry with their child. This anger may be a result of injuries the child sustained when breaking known rules such as drinking and driving, playing with matches, or riding a bike without a helmet. Lastly, the anger may not be directed at anyone specifically. Injuries caused by natural disasters such as an earthquake, flood, or hurricane provoke just as much anger as those that result from the actions of people, and they may pose a challenge to the parents' spiritual beliefs.

Parents typically react to their child's illness or injury with some degree of guilt. This reaction may be magnified in the PICU environment. The fact that the guilt usually has no basis in real events does not lessen the feeling. A question parents frequently ask at this stage is, "Why not me instead of my child?" Parents' feelings of guilt may have one of two causes:

1. *They may feel responsible for causing the illness or injury.* Statements such as, "If only I hadn't sent him to the store on his bike, this wouldn't have happened," or, from the father of a 2-year-old who nearly drowned, "Maybe if I hadn't been working, he would have been in my care and this wouldn't have happened," reflect feelings of guilt for causing or failing to prevent the injury.
2. *They may feel guilty about not noticing the onset of an illness or disregarding earlier symptoms of an illness.* The mother of a 1-year-old with meningitis repeatedly said, "I shouldn't have waited so long to take her to the doctor!"

Deprivation and Loss

As the shock associated with the child's life-threatening condition slowly recedes, new stressors emerge. Within minutes or hours, parents are deprived of their familiar role of being a parent of a healthy child and have an unexpected and unfamiliar role of being a parent of a critically ill child. The difficulty and ambivalence parents feel in releasing a part of their responsibility as the child's primary caretakers to strangers can threaten their self-esteem and self-control. If parents cannot participate in the child's care, they may feel helpless or worthless.

Anticipatory Waiting

Once the child's condition is stabilized and survival seems likely, parents often move into a period of anticipatory waiting. This stage is characterized as "life suspended in time." Parents spend a great deal of time waiting: for test results, for explanations, for their child to become conscious, or for surgery to be over. Parents may fear leaving the area because they may miss an important procedure, physician visit, or decision or change in treatment. Lack of mobility decreases the parents' ability to use typical coping mechanisms, so anxiety and the sense of powerlessness may increase. If the parents have a cell phone, write down the number and assure them that they will be called for any change in the child's condition. This allows parents to feel like they can leave at least for a few minutes. If the parents do not have a cell phone, provide a pager if available.

Parents may have a preoccupation with medical details. During this period, parents may ask questions about the long-term effects of the illness or injury on the child, about the potential for brain damage, or about the need for additional surgeries. Parents may place demands on staff and be frustrated when the child's progress is slow.

Readjustment or Mourning

The last stage that parents experience is readjustment or mourning. Readjustment is experienced as the child recovers, improves steadily, and prepares for transfer and discharge. In contrast, parents of the child who dies reenter the cycle of emotions characteristic of grief. **Grief**, an individual's feelings and behaviors in response to death or loss, is painful, individualized, and exhausting. Parents also mourn when the child remains seriously ill or unresponsive, when the outcome remains uncertain for an extended period, or when long-term care is required.

Table 13–1 lists the most important needs of parents when a child is hospitalized with a life-threatening illness or injury.

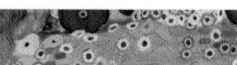

NURSING MANAGEMENT

Nursing Assessment and Diagnosis

Nurses who work with families of critically ill children have a unique opportunity to help them adapt and to promote family functioning. Begin by assessing the family's reaction to the illness, coping skills, stressors, and needs. See Chapter 2 ∞. This initial assessment provides a baseline of information for developing a care plan and strategies to meet the family's psychosocial as well as physiologic needs.

Several nursing diagnoses may apply to parents who are dealing with their child's critical illness or injury. Examples include:

- Interrupted Family Processes related to the impact of a critically ill child on the family system

TABLE 13–1	Nursing Interventions to Meet Parental Needs During Their Child's Critical Care Hospitalization
Parental Needs	Nursing Interventions
Information—the most important identified need	• Provide information and frequent updates about the child's condition. Repeat the information and provide other materials frequently because parents forget or cannot concentrate on details due to stress. • Explain about the child's condition, equipment being used, and procedures of care. • Facilitate a discussion with the physician at least daily. • Provide general information about unit policies, team members, phone numbers, and so on.
Proximity to their child	• Provide permission for the parents to remain at the bedside. • Encourage parents to touch and speak with the child, and demonstrate ways if parents are hesitant. • Work within the unit to provide open, flexible visiting hours.
Reestablishment of their parental role and control	• Implement family-centered care so parents feel recognized as important to their child's recovery and as the decision makers for the child's treatment options.
Participation in their child's care	• Encourage parents to participate in care (e.g., bathing and hair care, diaper changes, feeding, range of motion exercises, massages). • Encourage parents to help with diversional activity (e.g., reading, singing, telling stories). • Let the parents explain equipment and procedures to the child to reduce the child's fears.
Confidence in the treatment plan and caregivers	• Try to maintain continuity in staffing and health care contacts. • Demonstrate caring for the child. • Provide assurance that the child is receiving appropriate treatment and pain management.
Psychologic support	• Acknowledge that the situation is difficult. • Help parents to focus on the positive or unchanged aspects of the child's appearance. • Encourage parents to get rest and nutrition to help them maintain physical resources necessary for coping. • Provide space and privacy as needed. • Give hope—an essential component of coping. • Offer the choice of other family members to be present. • Discuss the possible responses of siblings and the long-term emotional responses of the child patient.

hospice and/or palliative care, the reluctance of the physician to relinquish control of the child's medical care to someone else, and the fact that few pediatricians have expertise related to palliative care in children (Armstrong-Dailey & Koppelman, 2007).

When a child receives palliative and/or hospice care, the family and health care providers collaborate to determine which treatments are appropriate to continue with the child's end-of-life care, such as intravenous fluids, gastrostomy feedings, and certain medications. Health plan coverage for pediatric palliative/hospice care services or alternative financial assistance is investigated.

Ethical Issues Surrounding a Child's Death

Because a child's death is so emotionally charged, many potential misunderstandings and conflicts can develop between families and health care providers. The more common ethical issues that need to be addressed include withdrawing or withholding treatment, parental treatment refusal, and do-not-resuscitate orders. See Chapter 1 ∞ for ethical decision-making principles and terminology.

Brain Death Criteria

Brain death is the irreversible cessation of all functions of the brain, including the cerebral cortex and brainstem. Brain death criteria may be used when determining if withdrawal of life-supporting equipment is appropriate or when organ transplantation is planned. See Table 13–2 for brain death criteria. Two separate examinations must be performed on the child prior to declaring brain death. The timing between the two examinations for brain death ranges from 12–48 hours depending on the age of the child (Mathers & Frankel, 2007).

Withdrawal of or Withholding Treatment

The decision to withdraw or withhold life-sustaining treatments from the dying child is very difficult and emotional for parents. Some parents feel that this is a form of abandonment, and they may feel as though they contributed to the child's death (Baergen, 2006). Withholding nutrition and hydration may be especially difficult because parents often associate food with nurturing and love, or they may fear that death will be hastened. Other treatments such as medications, mechanical ventilation, and dialysis may be withdrawn if the child's outcome is in-

evitable death and continuing treatment causes more suffering than benefit. (See Evidence-Based Practice: Improving the Quality of Pediatric End-of-Life Care.)

The nurse may feel conflicted when parents are unable to discontinue aggressive therapies that the nurse feels are extending the child's suffering. Consultation with a member of the hospital ethics committee can help clarify the issues involved and reduce the emotions associated with the conflict. An ethics committee can also assist in determining the best interest of the child (Klein, 2009).

Conflicts Regarding Parental Treatment Refusal

Parents and health care providers sometimes disagree over what, if any, medical interventions should be provided when the child is dying. Parents may refuse treatments based on religious convictions or because they wish to avoid prolonging the child's life in order to provide a peaceful death (Institute of Medicine, 2003b). Initiating highly technical, but possibly futile, interventions may cause emotional and financial stress that overwhelms parents.

Consultation with the hospital's ethics committee should be obtained to help resolve the conflict. The health care team may seek to have a surrogate legal guardian appointed in certain situations when recommended care is refused. The conflict sometimes makes it difficult for the nurse to have a supportive relationship with the parents, but proper concern for and care of the child in these cases should be provided.

Do-Not-Resuscitate Orders

Parents faced with a child's end-stage, irreversible condition may be asked to consider a do-not-resuscitate (DNR), do-not-intubate, or allow natural death (AND) order, and decide if a resuscitation attempt would be in the child's best interest. Parents must consider allowing the child to die with dignity and the possibility of causing more harm and suffering if resuscitation is implemented. Parents may feel they are "giving up" on their child and need ongoing support. When the patient is an adolescent, he or she should be involved in discussions and have a role in decision making. Provide honest information and help the family understand that the child will receive pain management, comfort care, oxygen, suctioning, and other supportive care while complying with a DNR or AND order.

End-of-Life Care Resources for Nurses

TABLE 13–2	Brain Death Criteria
Brain Functioning	Clinical Signs
Coma	Unconscious, no vocalization
Absent clinical functions of the brain	No purposeful movement No increase in heart rate with pressure on eyeballs
Absent brainstem function	Pupils midposition or dilated, nonresponsive to light No blink response to corneal stimulation No spontaneous eye movements with abrupt rotation of head or ice water irrigation in each ear No gag reflex with oropharynx stimulation or cough to tracheal stimulation No respiratory movement when removed from ventilator

Adapted from: Mathers, L. H., & Frankel, L. R. (2007). Brain death. In R. M. Kliegman, R. E. Behrman, H. B. Jenson, & B. F. Stanton, Nelson textbook of pediatrics (18th ed., pp. 411–413). Copyright © Elsevier 2007. Reprinted with permission.

Evidence-Based Practice

Improving the Quality of Pediatric End-of-Life Care

Problem

The majority of children who die because of life-limiting conditions die in the hospital setting. What are the parents' perspectives with regard to improving their child's quality of care?

Evidence

A study involving 56 parents of children who had died in the PICU 1 to 4 years previously focused on their priorities for improving end-of-life care and communication in the PICU. The six priorities identified were honest and complete information, ready access to staff, coordination of communication and care, emotional expression and support by staff as it conveys caring for the child and family, preservation of the integrity of the parent–child relationship, and faith (Meyer, Ritholz, Burns, et al., 2006).

Widger and Picot (2008) interviewed parents to evaluate their perspective of the quality of care that their dying children received in a tertiary care center. The sample consisted of parents representing 38 families of infants and children who had died between 12 and 24 months prior to the study. Parents identified communication and information most often as priority areas for improvement. Parents expressed the need for increased communication among the health care team and the need for more information about their child's condition and their child's death. Other areas for improvement included the need for increased sensitivity and empathy from the health care team and the need for follow-up following the child's death.

Implications

Knowing what parents value during this time is important for planning nursing care and multidisciplinary palliative care. Facilitating opportunities for regular communication that includes full disclosure about the child's condition by a single familiar person may help reduce the amount of conflicting information parents hear, and it may assist with decision making. Other communication options such as family conferences or office hours at the bedside may help improve communication. Ensure that family-centered care integrates values important to the family during nursing care planning and communications with them.

Critical Thinking Application

Consider the special needs of the parents of a child who has been critically injured in an automobile crash and is not expected to live. Identify the most common patterns of communication with family members in the PICU and evaluate their effectiveness in promoting family-centered care and decision making. Suggest two other communication methods that could improve communication with family members and improve the family's perception of care that their child receives.

Children with disabilities—including those with terminal illnesses—are entitled to the same education as other students. (See Chapter 12 ∞.) Children with a chronic or terminal illness may be at high risk of dying while at school. Concerns of school officials about accepting a DNR order include the effect of a student's death on classmates and liability issues. Most school districts have no policy regarding DNR orders (Hone-Warren, 2007).

Collaboration between the child, family, nurse and other health care providers, school officials, and social workers or other personnel with knowledge or expertise in DNR requests at school may lead to an agreement regarding the DNR request that respects the rights and interests of the dying child.

■ CARE OF THE DYING CHILD

Care of the dying child is challenging and requires the utmost sensitivity and compassion. Children as young as 5 years of age can sense when they are seriously ill. A child's awareness of death develops more rapidly when he or she is experiencing the progression of a disease and related medical treatment. Children with life-threatening illnesses often learn about death and their own illness from exposure to other seriously ill and dying children during hospitalization or clinic visits.

Awareness of Dying by Developmental Age

Infants and toddlers are not actually aware of death, but they are aware of and react to changes in normal routines and the behavior of parents. Toddlers may know they feel bad, but they do not understand that their physical symptoms are associated with impending death. See Figure 13–6 ➤.

Preschool children can see their bodies deteriorate and feel the effects of medications used during disease progression and treatment. Changes in self-concept occur as they perceive these body changes. They often describe their illness in terms of mutilation to their body. These physical changes may make them realize that they are dying.

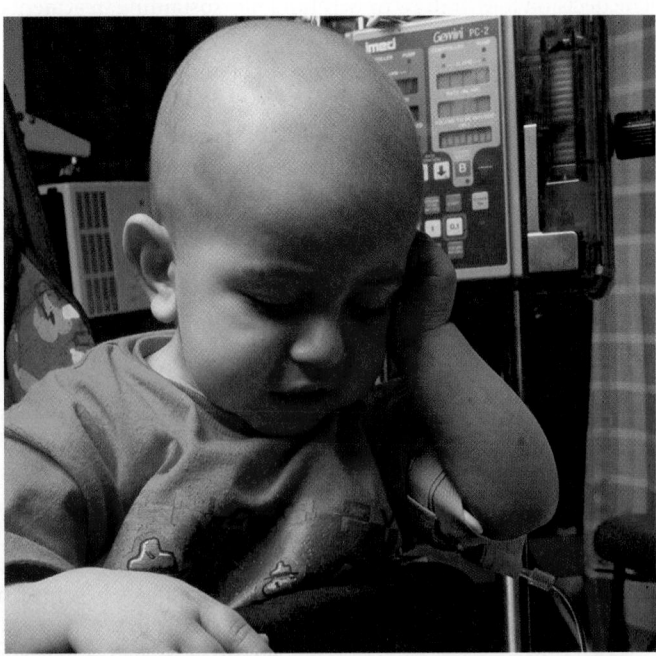

FIGURE 13–6 ➤ The toddler with a life-threatening condition recognizes that he feels bad and that routines are different. His anxiety may increase due to the concern and feelings of sadness exhibited by his parents.

School-age children also have subtle fears about body integrity and anxieties about the seriousness of their illness. This greater preoccupation with illness is considered by many professionals as the child's version of **death anxiety**, a feeling of apprehension or fear of death. Children may express death anxiety as a concern with treatments that invade the body or interfere with normal body functions.

Adolescents have a mature understanding of death, but the normal developmental milestones of adolescence add to their problems in facing a terminal illness. They are struggling to establish their own identity and plans for the future. At a time when body image is extremely important, they may be faced with the possibility of mutilation and disfigurement. Dying adolescents are often isolated from their peers during a period when peers are the most essential social group. Adolescents with terminal illnesses may be angry because they recognize their loss when the whole world is opening up to them.

Do not expect adolescents to handle feelings in the same way that adults do. Adolescents often avoid expressing anger against the family, seeking to control and direct these feelings elsewhere. They often become angry at changes in treatment procedures, lack of explanations, and threats to their independence. As death nears, the adolescent may permit comforting and support and may accept care from warm and loving family members, as long as he or she is not treated in a condescending manner.

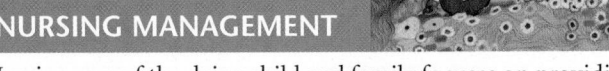

NURSING MANAGEMENT

Nursing care of the dying child and family focuses on providing family-centered support for their physical and psychosocial needs.

Nursing Assessment and Diagnosis

Assess the child's physiologic status and comfort level. Physiological changes in the dying child may be directly related to the child's disease process or injury. Signs and symptoms of approaching death are provided in Clinical Manifestations: The Dying Child on page 327. Assess the child's awareness of impending death. Examples of questions the child may ask include: What will death be like? What happens after I die? When will I be with (a deceased person to whom the child was close) again? Will my parents be all right? Will you remember me? Assess the ability of the parents to talk with the child about dying. Table 13–3 highlights children's understanding of death at different developmental stages, some of the possible behavioral responses, and nursing considerations for family education.

Assess the family for coping skills and need for social supports. Identify any cultural or spiritual traditions, rituals, and beliefs related to loss and grieving that are important to the family.

Examples of nursing diagnoses that apply to the dying child and family include the following:

- Fear (Child) related to unanswered questions and concerns of abandonment
- Death Anxiety (Child) related to impending death
- Anticipatory Grieving (Parents) related to imminent death of child

Cultural differences are important to consider when working with families dealing with the death of a loved one. Some examples of differences include the following (Dratler, Burns, & Dratler, 2006):

- African Americans often place great importance on the presence of their families and the expression of emotions. They value shared decision making between the patient and family members. Suffering as a meaningful spiritual experience is valued by many.
- Asian families often desire to protect the terminally ill from knowledge of their condition, so decisions are usually made by family members. They may prefer aggressive treatments.
- In some Filipino cultures, words are considered so powerful that talking about the patient's death is believed to make it happen. As a result, they may refuse to discuss any medical options.
- Hispanics generally believe the family should be responsible for making health care decisions. Faith is very important in times of death. Many believe death is a natural part of life, and the anniversary of a loved one's death is celebrated every year.

- Hopelessness (Parents) related to failure of therapies to prolong life

Planning and Implementation

Nursing care for the dying child and the family includes providing comfort, assisting the child in a peaceful death, assisting the child and family with coping strategies, and facilitating grief.

Physiologic Care

A major goal in care of the dying child is to promote comfort and keep the child pain-free. Provide analgesia to promote optimal pain relief. Oral, transdermal, or rectal analgesia is available for families who choose to withhold intravenous fluids. Complementary care for comfort and pain management as described in Chapter 15 ∞ can be used by the nurse and family members.

If dyspnea or air hunger occurs, elevate the head of the bed, open a window, or use a circulating fan. An opioid may be prescribed for air hunger or tachypnea as its action dilates the pulmonary vessels, reduces oxygen consumption, and decreases pulmonary congestion.

Other physiologic care includes keeping the airway clear of secretions, bathing and keeping the skin dry and intact, changing the child's position frequently, and encouraging favorite foods and liquids as tolerated. Involve the parents in physical care and encourage them to hold and comfort the child.

Clinical Tip

Some parents ask that their child not be told he or she is dying. Do you abide by their wishes when the child asks you if he or she is dying? Tell the parents that the child asked the question. Offer to set up a meeting with the health care team to discuss their fears and concerns about telling their child the truth. Offer parents words and phrases they can use to talk with their child about his or her death at a developmentally appropriate level. Some parents may prefer that the child's questions be answered honestly by another professional. A professional who has special bereavement counseling training can assist children and families with discussions.

Clinical Manifestations
The Dying Child

Body System	Clinical Manifestations
Cardiovascular system	■ The heart rate may initially increase as hypoxia develops, then the heart rate and blood pressure decrease, resulting in decreased cardiac output. ■ A change in pulse pressure and a decrease in the volume of Korotkoff sounds indicate imminent death. ■ Peripheral circulation decreases, leading to diaphoresis, clammy cool skin, and changes in skin coloring (mottled to cyanotic). Mottling is a sign of imminent death.
Respiratory system	■ Impaired cardiac function leads to pulmonary congestion, tachypnea, diminished breath sounds, and hypoxia. ■ Dyspnea; **air hunger**, the most severe form of dyspnea, may cause the child to look panicked, gasp for breath, and sit upright. ■ **Cheyne-Stokes breathing** (periods of shallow breathing alternating with apnea) is a sign of imminent death. ■ Parenteral fluids may cause edema and increased respiratory secretions, leading to shortness of breath and cough. ■ As muscles relax, secretions accumulate in the oropharynx and bronchi, causing noisy breathing as air passes through these secretions. ■ Moaning or grunting with breathing is common.
Neurological system	■ Decreased cerebral perfusion, hypoxemia, metabolic acidosis, the influences of disease-related factors, and an accumulation of toxins from renal and liver failure lead to neurological dysfunction. ■ Agitation or restlessness, withdrawal, increasing drowsiness, and confusion may occur; the child may be unconscious during the final hours. ■ The child may speak of visions (persons or objects) not visible to others. ■ Hearing and vision acuity may deteriorate. Remember that hearing is one of the last senses to diminish before death.
Musculoskeletal system	■ Extreme muscle weakness, fatigue, and difficulty with swallowing may occur. ■ The child may be unable to reposition self, toilet self, or effectively cough and clear secretions.
Renal system	■ Decreased kidney function and urine production are common. ■ Sphincters relax and incontinence can occur.
Gastrointestinal system	■ Decreased oral fluid intake and anorexia are common. ■ Sphincters relax and bowel incontinence can occur.

Communicating with the Child of His or Her Impending Death

Parents may prefer not to talk with the child about the seriousness of the illness or injury and potential for death for several reasons: a desire to protect the child from bad news, fear that the child will lose hope, or because they may feel incapable of answering the child's questions about dying. They may also fear that they will be unable to cope with their own feelings during a frank discussion about the possibility of the child's imminent death.

Even when children are not told they are dying, they know their condition is worsening. They are undergoing treatments, not feeling well, and picking up cues from their parents. Some children keep most of their thoughts about death to themselves. If they have not been told that they are dying, they may feel isolated and get the message not to discuss their condition. They may fear that the family members will abandon them emotionally. Children often avoid displaying anger, since they fear desertion more than death. They may also believe that expressing their awareness of death and their fears will place added emotional burdens on family members that could be unbearable to the family.

Provide the child with opportunities for fantasy play, drawings, and storytelling, without emphasizing or reinforcing death themes. Listen to what children tell you about themselves and their lives. **Death imagery**, references to death or death-related topics (going away, separation, funerals), may be a theme of their stories. Strategies for talking with a dying child are described in Box 13–3.

When caring for adolescents, remember that outbursts of anger are common but not personally directed at the nurse. Provide activities to help adolescents channel their feelings. Continue providing support in spite of their behavior. This approach may encourage adolescents to accept comforting without losing face. Be available to listen when the adolescent wants to talk and express feelings and frustrations. Promote friendships with other adolescents who have similar interests or problems.

Parents may not recognize the child's death anxiety because of their own fears, concerns, and feelings of helplessness. Depending on the family's cultural and religious beliefs, a chaplain or other health care professional who specializes in working with terminally ill children and families may help reduce a child's spiritual fears and promote peace and comfort among family members.

Family Support

Parents need to be present when possible during the child's actual dying as it is a pivotal event in their parent–child relationship. Their presence helps fulfill their parenting role, their last

Resources for Terminally Ill Children

TABLE 13–3	**Children's Understanding of Death and Possible Behavioral Responses**	
Understanding of Death	Potential Behaviors	Nursing Management
Infant		
Cognitive stage: sensorimotor Senses tenseness of caregivers, and altered routines Senses separation	Resists cuddling and eats less Cries excessively, clingy Sleeps more than usual	Provide a sense of security, by holding and hugging. Use a soothing voice. Try to return to usual routines.
Toddler		
Cognitive stage: preoperational No understanding of true concept of death Aware someone is missing—separation anxiety Unable to distinguish death from temporary separation or abandonment	Regresses to younger stage of development Clingy, refuses to let parent out of sight Shows distress by biting, hitting, tears Problems eating and sleeping Sleep disturbances Fearfulness	Encourage parents to hold and cuddle the toddler to help reduce the fear of separation. Follow familiar routines. Be tolerant of regressive behaviors. Talk and answer questions in terms the child will understand.
Preschooler		
Cognitive stage: preoperational Believes death is temporary Magical thinking—believes the dead person can be brought back to life Believes bad thoughts cause death Has beginning experience with death of animals and plants	Regression to earlier developmental stage, problems with bowel and bladder control, tantrums May fear going to sleep, has nightmares, afraid of the dark Crying spells Seems morbidly fascinated with death Asks many questions Complaints of abdominal pain	Listen to the child and answer questions honestly; reassure the child that his or her thoughts did not cause the death. Try to follow usual routines. Be tolerant of regressive behaviors; provide play activities. Keep memories alive with pictures and items that remind the child of the loved one. Participate in rituals (e.g., going to the cemetery, releasing helium balloons, and planting flowers).
School-Age Child		
Cognitive stage: concrete operations Has a more realistic understanding of death By 8–10 years, understands the permanence and irreversibility of death May have guilt or assume blame for the death May not realize that death can occur at any age	Crying, moody, may become more withdrawn and distant, or may deny sadness by hiding tears and acting more like adults Decreased concentration for school work, may refuse to go to school Psychosomatic complaints—stomachache or headache Angry outbursts, disruptive behaviors, aggression May try to comfort parents by taking over tasks May fear another loved person will die	Listen to the child and answer questions honestly. Return to usual routines and activities. Keep memories alive through activities such as art, music, creating a memory book, sewing a quilt, and planting a garden. Share Internet resources. Use coping support groups. Encourage the family to seek faith-based support.
Adolescent		
Cognitive stage: formal operations Intellectually capable of understanding death Recognizes all people and self must die Better understands the association between illness and death Sense of invincibility conflicts with fear of death Able to recognize effect of death on others	May have severe depression, mood swings, withdrawal from friends May feel angry or guilty Acting-out or risk-taking behavior, delinquency, suicide attempts, promiscuity, drug or alcohol use Uses abstract and philosophical reasoning Girls may seek comfort from friends Eating and sleeping problems	Be available and encourage open communication. Share your own grief and feelings with the adolescent. Keep memories alive with pictures and items that remind the teen of the loved one. Access counseling and support groups. Encourage the child to seek support from his or her faith group. Share Internet resources.

Data from: Hinds, P. S., Oakes, L. L., Hicks, J., & Anghelescu, D. L. (2005). End-of-life care for children and adolescents. Seminars in Oncologic Nursing, 21(1), 53–62; *Kirwin, K. M., & Havrin, V. (2005). Decreasing the risk of complicated bereavement and future psychiatric disorders in children.* Journal of Child and Adolescent Psychiatric Nursing, 18(2), 62–78; *Auman, M. J. (2007). Bereavement support for children.* Journal of School Nursing, 23(1), 34–39; *Korones, D. N. (2007). Pediatric palliative care.* Pediatrics in Review, 28(8), e46–e56.

BOX 13–3 Strategies for Communicating with the Dying Child

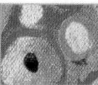

- Be receptive when the child initiates a conversation. Disruptive behavior, withdrawal, anger, hyperalert state, or sleeping more than usual may indicate the child's struggle with emotions and be an opportunity to engage the child in discussion.
- Assess how much the child knows and how much he or she wants to know. Identify any fantasies and concerns, and provide correct information. Be honest with the child when a clear question is asked.
- Allow the child to express his or her feelings and to be upset. Empathize with the child.
- Reassure the child that you will be available to listen and give support.
- Recognize that some children communicate best through nonverbal means (e.g., art, play, music, and writing). The child may be willing to talk through a puppet or a stuffed animal.
- Acknowledge that the child's life can be complete, even if it is short. Let dying children know they will always be loved and remembered.
- Empower children as much as possible in circumstances concerning their deaths. Reassure them of continued love and physical closeness.

Data from: Beale, E. A., Baile, W. F., & Aaron, J. (2005). Silence is not golden: Communicating with children dying from cancer. Journal of Clinical Oncology, 23(15), 3629–3631; Dunlop, S. (2008). The dying child: Should we tell the truth? Paediatric Nursing, 20(6), 28–31; Kersun, L. S., & Shemesh, E. (2007). Depression and anxiety in children at the end of life. Pediatric Clinics of North America, 54, 691–708; McSherry, M., Carroll, J. M., & Rourke, M. T. (2007). Psychosocial and spiritual needs of children living with a life-limiting illness. Pediatric Clinics of North America, 54, 609–629.

TABLE 13–4 Cultural Traditions in Mourning and After-Death Rites

Religious Group	Rituals You Might Observe
American Indians	• Beliefs and practices vary widely among tribes. • Seeing an owl is an omen of death.
Buddhism	• Last-rite chanting may occur at the bedside. • Cremation is common.
Catholicism	• Sacrament of the sick is common. • There is an obligation to take ordinary but not extraordinary means to prolong life. • Burial is common.
Christian Science	• No medical help is sought to prolong life. • No body parts are donated. Disposal of the body and parts is decided by the family.
Hinduism	• Death is seen as a passage; rebirth is expected. • Religious prayers are chanted before and after death. • Cremation is common. • Men and women display outward grief. • Thread tied around a wrist signifies a blessing; do not remove.
Islam	• Organ donation is acceptable. • Autopsy is acceptable only for medical or legal reasons. • The body is washed only by a Muslim of the same gender.
Jehovah's Witness	• Donation of body parts is forbidden. • Autopsy is acceptable for legal reasons. • Burial is determined by family preference.
Judaism	• Autopsy and organ donation are not acceptable. • Life support is not mandated. • The body is ritually washed, and burial occurs as soon as possible with all body parts buried together. • The mourning period lasts 7 days.
Mormonism	• If death is inevitable, promote a peaceful and dignified death. • Organ donation is an individual choice. • The body is buried in "temple clothes."
Protestantism	• Organ donation, autopsy, and burial or cremation are individual decisions. • Prolonging life may have restrictions.
Seventh Day Adventist	• Prolonging life is preferred. • Organ donation and autopsy are individual decisions. • Disposal of the body and burial are individual decisions.

Adapted from: Spector, R. E. (2009). Cultural diversity in health and illness (7th ed., pp. 141–142). Upper Saddle River, NJ: Prentice Hall Health.

time to be good parents (Woodgate, 2006). Parents also prefer to have a familiar nurse provide the care as the child is dying.

Work closely with the family when the child's death is imminent, because they will remember the experience and words spoken for the rest of their lives. Prepare the family for changes in the child's appearance and behavior. Providing the parents with a room to be alone with the child ensures privacy at this extremely personal time.

Ask the family what is important to them in the final moments and hours of their child's life and what will be important to them in the grief process. Certain religious or cultural practices may need to be planned and should be accommodated when possible. Holding the child is a universal request and should be permitted, along with touching, stroking, kissing, and talking soothingly.

Many families find that saying good-bye as a group is helpful. Families need to cry together and to tell each other how much they will miss each other. Assure them that the vigil with the child prevents the child from feeling isolated or abandoned as death approaches. The dying child should never be left alone when dying is imminent. Ask parents if there are specific rituals that they would like to participate in. See Table 13–4 for common mourning and after-death rituals.

Tissue and Organ Donation

Families may be asked about making an anatomic gift. Nurses can become better prepared to serve the family of the dying child and potential organ recipients by becoming familiar with the health care facility's criteria for organ and tissue procurement. Generally an organ procurement organization coordinator will work in collaboration with the nurses and other members of the health care team to help explain the process of organ donation and to ensure families are not coerced to make an anatomic gift (DeVeaux, 2006).

Need for Autopsy

When the exact cause of death is unclear, an autopsy may be suggested. An autopsy may be required by state law for an unnatural or unexpected death, such as suicide, homicide, or sudden infant death syndrome. When parents have a choice, they may be hesitant to consent to autopsy because it further invades the child's body. Support the family during decision making by explaining that the autopsy will likely reveal the cause of death. This information may be valuable if the death is potentially due to a genetic disorder, affecting future childbearing decisions.

Postmortem Care and Family Support

Offer ongoing support after the child dies. Questions like the following may help begin the conversation: "I am sorry for your loss. How can I help?" "What are your traditions when an infant or child dies?" "Is there someone I can call for you?" Although crying with families was once considered unprofessional, it is now recognized as an expression of caring and empathy. Nurses should feel free to express their sorrow and grief for the child and family.

Identify the family's wishes for postmortem care before performing any care. Ask before removing any jewelry or other item from the child because cultural and spiritual practices may specify that the article remain on the child after death. The nurse should follow the health care facility's guidelines for postmortem care. The child should be positioned according to guidelines or cultural/religious practices, the room should be cleaned, and medical equipment should be removed.

After the child's death, allow the family to spend as much time as they need with the child's body. Never rush family members who are saying good-bye to the child. Save all of the child's personal items—especially in the case of an infant, whose parents may have few mementos. A lock of hair from the back of the head, a hand outline or hand mold, a handprint or footprint, the infant's identification band, the child's weight and height, or a picture of the infant can be sources of comfort and remembrance for families (Figure 13–7 ➤). Ask for permission before cutting a lock of hair as some cultural and religious groups prohibit it. Seal the last clothes or patient gown worn by the child in a plastic bag to retain the child's scent. When possible, use a special remembrance box or container for this purpose. If parents refuse to take the items, give them to another family member or retain them. Document collection of the mementos and who received them in case parents ask for them at a later time (Foresman-Capuzzi, 2007).

When a newborn or young infant has died, wrap the baby in a blanket and offer the mother and other family members the opportunity to hold the baby. Parents may want to bathe and dress the infant. The family experiencing the death of a newborn may appreciate an offer to take pictures of the baby and family together, if picture taking is not prohibited by religious or cultural traditions. Some families may feel uncomfortable taking

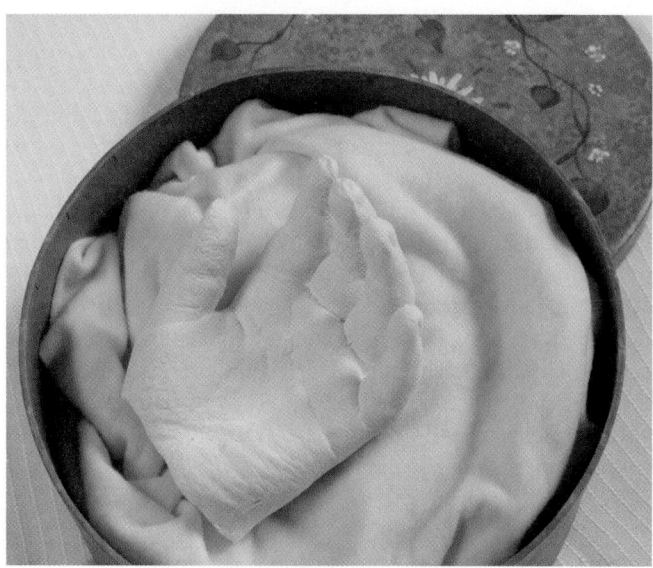

FIGURE 13–7 ➤ Nurses can provide families with a memento of the child who dies by creating a plaster cast of the child's hand, a handprint, or a footprint.

pictures and refuse the offer. The nurse should question the family about baptism or other ritual requests for the newborn, and facilitate arrangements for a religious or spiritual leader at the family's request. The mother experiencing the death of a newborn requires instructions on lactation suppression or milk donation options if she has been breastfeeding or pumping her breasts (Gale, 2006).

A bereavement folder should be provided to parents with information that includes resources available to help with a memorial service or funeral and potential sibling responses. Inform parents that certain dates, such as the day of the week the child died, the child's birthday, or family holidays, will be difficult and may trigger intense sadness. Parents may benefit from keeping a journal of their thoughts and memories, or writing letters or poems to or about their child. Many institutions have a structured program to offer support on a routine basis for families after the loss of a child. Follow-up occurs at designated time points such as the birthday, anniversary of death, 3 months, 6 months, and holidays. The follow-up is generally completed by nursing personnel who were closest to the family so that the follow-up is meaningful.

Evaluation

Expected outcomes of caring for the dying child and family may include the following:

- The child is pain-free and comfortable, and the child's physiologic needs are met.
- The cultural and spiritual needs of the dying child and family are met.
- The dying child and family receive support during the dying process.
- The family receives continued support after the child's death.

■ GRIEF AND BEREAVEMENT

Parents' Reactions

The death of one's child is probably a parent's most painful experience. Many factors influence the parents' grief responses, including their perception of the preventability of the illness or injury, the suddenness and other circumstances of the death, the nature of their attachment to the child, previous losses, spiritual or religious orientation, and culture.

Although parents progress through distinct stages of grief, as described on page 317, the timeline and nature of the grief process differ for each individual. The intense pain and shock initially felt by parents gradually give way to feelings of anger, guilt, depression, and loneliness. Very slowly, and with much support, energy returns and parents again begin to enjoy life experiences. Parents may experience friction due to differing rates and intensity of grief. Additional support may be needed to prevent a sense of loneliness and isolation.

The nurse should emphasize to parents that although the period surrounding their child's death is difficult, caring for themselves physically and mentally is important. The nurse can give parents a list of appropriate support groups, books, and articles for later use. Parents can be referred to organizations such as Compassionate Friends, First Candle, and SHARE Pregnancy and Infant Loss Support as well as to local support groups for bereaved parents or siblings. Some facilities have formal follow-up programs for bereaved parents to encourage a healthy progression through the grieving process. See the companion website for these organizations.

Sudden Death of a Child

Although many children die because of chronic illness or terminal condition, more than half of child deaths between 1 and 19 years of age are caused by unexpected injuries (Miniño, Heron, Murphy, et al., 2007; Kung, Hoyert, Xu, et al., 2008). A sudden and unexpected death that results from sudden infant death syndrome, injury, illness, suicide, or violence can place parents at risk for complicated grief (Truog, Christ, Browning, et al., 2006) because they have not had time to prepare for the child's death. Parents need support to deal with the death of the child and with their surviving children. See Families Want to Know: Strategies for Working with Parents Whose Child Dies Suddenly.

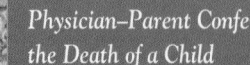

Research *Physician–Parent Conference After the Death of a Child*

A survey of 56 parents whose children had died in a PICU 4 to 15 months earlier focused on their interest in a physician–parent conference after their child's death. Only 7 of the parents had had a scheduled meeting, but 33 wanted to meet with their child's PICU physician, and the majority of those parents were willing to return to the hospital to meet. Parents wanted the content of the meeting to include information about the child's PICU treatment and cause of death, an opportunity to provide feedback to the physician about the PICU experience, and bereavement support (Meert, Eggly, Pollack, et al., 2007).

(Side margin:) Grief Support Resources

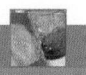

Families Want to Know
Strategies for Working with Parents Whose Child Dies Suddenly

- Provide private space with telephone access.
- Identify a spokesperson for the medical team to stay with the family and keep them informed during resuscitation efforts. Have both parents present if possible.
- During the discussion, speak plainly and directly about the condition. Assess the family's understanding of the information.
- Allow as much time as possible for the family to understand the seriousness and worsening of the child's status. Provide several updates during the resuscitation (two or three times over 15 minutes), or allow them to be present during the resuscitation. Prepare them for what is to come.
- Offer to telephone clergy, family, and friends.
- After the death, prepare the body for viewing by covering disfiguring wounds and explaining any tubes or lines that must remain because of legal or medical examiner requirements.
- Provide the time and place for the family to be with the child after death. Depending upon cultural preferences, the family may wish to bathe the child or hold and rock the child.
- Sit close and make eye contact. Let the parents know that everything possible was done for the child. If the child was not in pain or did not suffer, share that information. Share your emotions with the family. Accept whatever emotions family members express.
- Convey information to the family about the cause of death, requirements for or value of an autopsy with a sudden death, funeral preparations, and the normal grief process.
- Arrange for family follow-up to see how they are responding to the child's loss and to review autopsy findings.

Data from: Knapp, J., Mulligan-Smith, D., & Committee on Pediatric Emergency Medicine. (2005). Death of a child in the emergency department. *Pediatrics, 115*(5), 1432–1437.

Death of a Newborn or Young Infant

In 2006, 28,527 infants in the United States died either shortly after birth or during the first year of life, often because of low birth weight, severe congenital conditions, and sudden infant death syndrome (Heron, Hoyert, Murphy, et al., 2009). The death of a newborn forces parents to experience their child's entire life in a short period of time, and they are faced with overwhelming grief at a time when they anticipated the experience of joy. Unique experiences may occur with multiple births, such as the death of one or more of the infants, leading to conflicting emotions for the parents. While they mourn the death of one child, they must parent and bond with the survivor. Refer parents to a perinatal bereavement program or support group.

Siblings' Reactions

Siblings experiencing the death of a brother or sister require supportive and compassionate care. In the course of the child's illness, the siblings probably will have received less attention from parents. Siblings have reported feelings of loneliness, anxiety, anger, and jealousy during the dying process (Nolbris & Hellstrom, 2005). Depending on their developmental stage, they may fear that they caused their brother or sister to be injured or

Growth & Development *Understanding Death*

Young children will likely ask questions repeatedly, testing to see if the same responses are provided each time. Children need to understand the finality of death—that all body functions have stopped. Simple statements that can be told to children include, "Adam's heart will never beat again," "He will never get cold or hungry," and "He will never come home again."

become ill, or worry that their bad thoughts caused the illness. Nurses and other support personnel can assist the surviving children to adapt to their parent's distraction, grief, and increased protectiveness of them. The siblings need to hear that the parents' grief in no way diminishes the love felt for them.

When talking to the siblings of a child who has died, be honest and answer questions truthfully. Reassure siblings that they did not cause their brother or sister to die (unless they did contribute to the child's death) and that death was not a punishment for wrongdoing. The nurse should allow the siblings to ask questions, acknowledge the emotions they are feeling, and emphasize that it is all right for them to be sad, angry, frightened, or tearful. The nurse should use the same amount of energy and concern in acknowledging the grief of the siblings and the adults.

As appropriate and comfortable for the family, siblings should be permitted to participate in planning the child's memorial or funeral service. Being able to grieve as a family provides siblings with a sense of connectedness to parents and provides security at a vulnerable time. If siblings attend the funeral, prepare them for what to expect, such as an open casket or behaviors of mourners. The nurse can suggest designating a support person, such as a family member or close friend, who can monitor the siblings' needs while the parents attend to other matters. It is important to keep the family together as much as possible.

As with parental bereavement, sibling bereavement is a lifelong process. The nurse should encourage parents to make sure other caregivers and teachers know about the sibling's loss. Books are available for the family that might help children grieve.

■ STAFF REACTIONS TO A CHILD'S DEATH

Caring for dying children is especially stressful and demanding for health care professionals. Health professionals caring for the dying child may feel a sense of helplessness, ambivalence, and sadness because they are unable to help the child recover (Morgan, 2009). Nurses involved in long-term relationships with children experience grief when these children die. Some nurses cope by distancing themselves socially from the dying child and family to maintain composure and a professional demeanor.

Caring for the dying child may be especially difficult for nurses with young children. They tend to identify with the child, making it more difficult to recognize the dying child's anxiety

and fears because of their own personal defenses against their sense of helplessness to alter the course of the child's disease.

Nurses who work with terminally ill children and their families need special preparation to meet the needs of these individuals and to simultaneously manage personal stress. Mentorship with experienced hospice nurses, as well as additional educational experiences, may help promote professional nursing care. Nurses who work with dying children and families must learn to cope effectively with grief and develop empathy, competence, and confidence in their ability to provide more humane and effective nursing care.

Nurses working in emergency departments caring for children who die suddenly or in hospice settings and hospital units that care for terminally ill children need support systems to help balance the stresses of working with dying children. Bereavement debriefing sessions provide an opportunity for staff to discuss their feelings and concerns, manage their grief, and facilitate their coping with a child's death (Rushton, Reder, Hall, et al., 2006) (Figure 13–8 ➤). Some nurses attend funeral and memorial services when invited by the patient's family. Educational seminars on compassion fatigue may help nurses identify coping strategies for personal care (Meadors & Lamson, 2008).

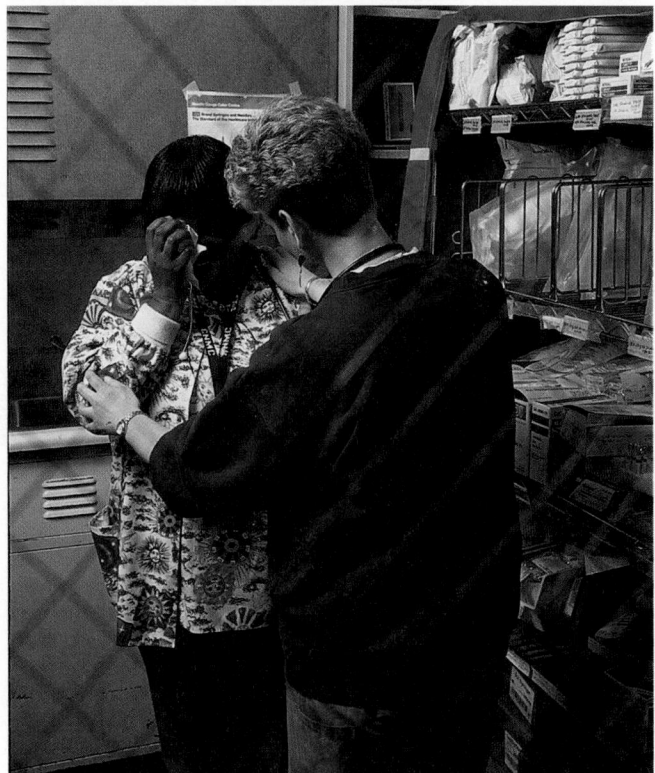

FIGURE 13–8 ➤ Nurses need to express grief in a supportive environment after a child's death. Sharing the sadness and grief or futility of resuscitation efforts with colleagues can often help nurses continue to provide supportive care to the next families who need compassionate care.

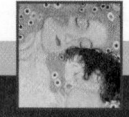

Chapter Highlights

- A life-threatening illness or injury places intense emotional and physical demands on the child and family due to the unfamiliar environment of the emergency department or intensive care unit, frightening or invasive procedures, and an uncertain outcome.

- Defense mechanisms displayed by children in stressful situations such as a life-threatening illness or injury include regression (return to an earlier behavior), denial, repression (involuntary forgetting), postponement, and bargaining.

- Nursing interventions to promote a child's psychological health include permitting parents to be present, preparing children for procedures, using play to help the child manage anxiety, and allowing the child some choices to gain a sense of control.

- Parents typically progress through the stages of shock and disbelief, anger and guilt, deprivation and loss, anticipatory waiting, and readjustment or mourning when their child has a life-threatening illness or injury.

- A family-centered approach will help meet the needs of families, minimize stress, and enhance family coping. Appropriate nursing care includes providing information and building trust, promoting family involvement (including presence during procedures and resuscitation if desired), encouraging parents to meet physical and emotional needs, facilitating effective communication, and maintaining family support systems.

- The nurse should ensure siblings receive information about their critically ill or injured brother or sister and regular messages from the parents to help them control feelings of jealousy, guilt, fear, and insecurity.

- Palliative care combines therapies to comfort and support persons with a short life expectancy, by providing therapies to improve the quality of remaining life.

- The families of dying children face many decision-making issues such as palliative and/or hospice care, advance care planning, the withholding or withdrawal of treatments, and DNR requests.

- One commonly accepted definition of death in the United States is brain death, or the irreversible cessation of all functions of the brain, including the cerebral cortex and brainstem.

- Children with life-threatening illnesses often learn about death and their own illness through exposure to other ill and dying children. Even if they have not been told they are dying, they will know their condition is worsening with extra treatments, feeling ill, and cues from their parents.

- It is essential to work closely with the family when a child's death is imminent, helping to provide the support and services most important to them in the last moments or hours of their child's life.

- The nurse caring for the dying child and family offers physiologic and psychosocial support during end-of-life care.

- Bereavement support must be provided to the family, making sure that siblings are not overlooked. Allow siblings to participate in planning the memorial service. Encourage parents to allow siblings to express their emotions.

- Caring for a dying child is difficult, and nurses need special preparation to meet the needs of the child and family while managing their own personal stress.

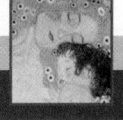

Clinical Reasoning in Action

Recall Alexa in the opening scenario. She is unconscious from hitting her head and has a serious abdominal injury following a motor vehicle crash in which she was a passenger. She is being cared for in the pediatric intensive care unit so that she can be monitored and her injuries prevented from becoming life threatening. The abdominal CT scan has revealed a spleen laceration that is bleeding, so she is being carefully monitored for hypovolemia. She has regained consciousness, but drifts off to sleep frequently. Alexa's mother is at her bedside. Her father, who was driving the car, is being evaluated at another hospital, and Alexa's 8-year-old sister Sharon is temporarily staying with a neighbor.

1. What are the developmentally appropriate nursing interventions to address Alexa's stressors related to this sudden hospitalization?
2. What physical assessment procedures are used to monitor Alexa's condition?
3. What nursing interventions should be implemented to support Alexa's family?
4. What information should be provided to Sharon to help her understand what has happened to Alexa?

See Pearson Nursing Student Resources for possible responses.

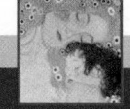

References

Aldridge, M. D. (2005). Decreasing parental stress in the pediatric intensive care unit. *Critical Care Nurse, 25*(6), 40–50.

Armstrong-Dailey, A., & Koppelman, J. (2007). Settings for pediatric palliative care in the United States. *Medical Principles and Practice, 16*(Suppl. 1), 42–43.

Auman, M. J. (2007). Bereavement support for children. *Journal of School Nursing, 23*(1), 34–39.

Baergen, R. (2006). How hopeful is too hopeful? Responding to unreasonably optimistic parents. *Pediatric Nursing, 32*(5), 482–486.

Beale, E. A., Baile, W. F., & Aaron, J. (2005). Silence is not golden: Communicating with children dying from cancer. *Journal of Clinical Oncology, 23*(15), 3629–3631.

Board, R. (2005). School-age children's perceptions of their PICU hospitalization. *Pediatric Nursing, 31*(3), 166–175.

Bowden, V. R., & Greenberg, C. S. (2009). Should family members be present when their child is being resuscitated? *Pediatric Nursing, 35*(4), 254–256.

DeVeaux, T. E. (2006). Non-heart-beating organ donation: Issues and ethics for the critical care nurse. *Journal of Vascular Nursing, 24*, 17–21.

Dratler, M. B., Burns, M. K., & Dratler, H. L. (2006). Conveying adverse news in end-of-life situations. *Gastroenterology Clinics of North America, 35*, 41–52.

Dunlop, S. (2008). The dying child: Should we tell the truth? *Paediatric Nursing, 20*(6), 28–31.

Emergency Nurses Association (ENA). (2005). *Emergency Nurses Association position statement: Family presence at the bedside during invasive procedures and cardiopulmonary resuscitation.* Retrieved from http://www.ena.org/SiteCollection Documents/Position%20Statements/ Family_Presence_-_ENA_PS.pdf

Foresman-Capuzzi, J. (2007). Grief telling: Death of a child in the emergency department. *Journal of Emergency Nursing, 33*(5), 505–508.

Gale, G. (2006). Implementing a palliative care program in a newborn intensive care unit. *Advances in Neonatal Care, 6*(1), e1–e37.

Gold, K. J., Gorenflo, D. W., Schwenk, T. L., & Bratton, S. L. (2006). Physician experience with family presence during cardiopulmonary resuscitation in children. *Pediatric Critical Care Medicine, 7*(5), 488–490.

Heron, M., Hoyert, D. L., Murphy, S. L., Xu, J., Kochanek, K. D., & Tejada-Vera, B. (2009). Deaths: Final data for 2006. *National Vital Statistics Reports, 57*(14), 1–135.

Himelstein, B. P. (2005). Palliative care in pediatrics. *Anesthesiology Clinics of North America, 23*, 837–856.

Himelstein, B. P. (2006). Palliative care for infants, children, adolescents, and their families. *Journal of Palliative Medicine, 9*(1), 163–181.

Hinds, P. S., Oakes, L. L., Hicks, J., & Anghelescu, D. L. (2005). End-of-life care for children and adolescents. *Seminars in Oncologic Nursing, 21*(1), 53–62.

Hone-Warren, M. (2007). Exploration of school administrator attitudes regarding do not resuscitate policies in the school setting. *Journal of School Nursing, 23*(2), 98–103.

Institute of Medicine. (2003a). Introduction. In M. J. Field & R. E. Behrman (Eds.), *When children die: Improving palliative and end-of-life care for children and their families* (pp. 19–40). Washington, DC: National Academies Press.

Institute of Medicine. (2003b). Patterns of childhood death in America. In M. J. Field & R. E. Behrman (Eds.), *When children die: Improving palliative and end-of-life care for children and their families* (pp. 41–71). Washington, DC: National Academies Press.

Kersun, L. S., & Shemesh, E. (2007). Depression and anxiety in children at the end of life. *Pediatric Clinics of North America, 54*, 691–708.

Kirwin, K. M., & Havrin, V. (2005). Decreasing the risk of complicated bereavement and future psychiatric disorders in children. *Journal of Child and Adolescent Psychiatric Nursing, 18*(2), 62–78.

Kissoon, N. (2006). Family presence during cardiopulmonary resuscitation: Our anxiety versus their needs. *Pediatric Critical Care Medicine, 7*(5), 488–490.

Klein, S. M. (2009). Moral distress in pediatric palliative care: A case study. *Journal of Pain and Symptom Management, 38*(1), 157–160.

Knapp, J., Mulligan-Smith, D., & Committee on Pediatric Emergency Medicine. (2005). Death of a child in the emergency department. *Pediatrics, 115*(5), 1432–1437.

Korones, D. N. (2007). Pediatric palliative care. *Pediatrics in Review, 28*(8), e46–e56.

Kung, H., Hoyert, D. L., Xu, J., & Murphy, S. L. (2008). Deaths: Final Data for 2005, *National Vital Statistics Reports, 56*(10), 11–12.

Levetown, M., & Committee on Bioethics. (2008). Communicating with children and families: From everyday interactions to skill in conveying distressing information. *Pediatrics, 121*(5), e1441–1460.

Mangurten, J., Scott, S. H., Guzzetta, C. E., Clark, A. P., Vinson, L., Sperry, J., . . . , Voelmeck, W. (2006). Effect of family presence during resuscitation and invasive procedures in a pediatric emergency department. *Journal of Emergency Nursing, 32*(3), 225–233.

Mathers, L. H., & Frankel, L. R. (2007). Brain death. In R. M. Kliegman, R. E. Behrman, H. B. Jenson, & B. F. Stanton, *Nelson Textbook of Pediatrics* (18th ed., pp. 411–413). Philadephia: Elsevier Saunders.

Mauer, S. (2008). A family affair. *Advance for Nurses, 10*(8), 33–34.

McSherry, M., Carroll, J. M., & Rourke, M. T. (2007). Psychosocial and spiritual needs of children living with a life-limiting illness. *Pediatric Clinics of North America, 54*, 609–629.

Meadors, P., & Lamson, A. (2008). Compassion fatigue and secondary traumatization: Provider self care on intensive care units for children. *Journal of Pediatric Health Care, 22*(1), 24–34.

Meert, K. L., Eggly, S., Pollack, M., Anand, K. J. S., Zimmerman, J., et al. (2007). Parents' perceptions regarding a physician-parent conference after their child's death in the pediatric intensive care unit. *Journal of Pediatrics, 151*(1), 50–55.

Meyer, E. C., Ritholz, M. D., Burns, J. P., & Truog, R. D. (2006). Improving the quality of end-of-life care in the pediatric intensive care unit: Parents' priorities and recommendations. *Pediatrics, 117*(3), 649–657.

Miniño, A. M., Heron, M. P., Murphy, S. L., & Kochanek, K. D. (2007). Deaths: Final data for 2004. *National Vital Statistics Reports, 55*(19), 21.

Morgan, D. (2009). Caring for dying children: Assessing the needs of the pediatric palliative care nurse. *Pediatric Nursing, 35*(2), 86–90.

Nolbris, M., & Hellstrom, A. L. (2005). Siblings' needs and issues when a brother or sister dies of cancer. *Journal of Pediatric Oncology Nursing, 22*(4), 227–233.

Ofoegbu, B., & Playfor, S. D. (2005). The use of physical restraints on paediatric intensive care units. *Pediatric Anesthesia, 15*, 407–411.

Rushton, C. H., Reder, E., Hall, B., Comello, K., Sellers, D. E., & Hutton, M. (2006). Interdisciplinary interventions to improve pediatric palliative care and reduce health care professional suffering. *Journal of Palliative Medicine, 9*(4), 922–933.

Schmidt, M., & Barfield, R. (2008). Visualizing meaningful assent: Interactive media design for pediatric advance care planning. *International Journal for Healthcare & Humanities, 2*(2), 1–5.

Smith, A. B., Hefley, G. C., & Anand, K. J. S. (2007). Parent bed spaces in the PICU: Effect on parental stress. *Pediatric Nursing, 33*(3), 215–221.

Snyder, B. S. (2004). Preventing treatment interference: Nurses' and parents' intervention strategies. *Pediatric Nursing, 30*(1), 31–40.

Spector, R. E. (2009). *Cultural diversity in health and illness* (7th ed., pp. 141–142). Upper Saddle River, NJ: Prentice Hall Health.

Truog, R. D., Christ, G., Browning, D. M., & Meyer, E. C. (2006). Sudden traumatic death in children: "We did everything, but your child didn't survive." *Journal of the American Medical Association, 295*(22), 2646–2654.

Ward-Begnoche, W. (2007). Posttraumatic stress symptoms in the pediatric intensive care unit. *Journal for Specialists in Pediatric Nursing, 12*(2), 84–92.

Watters, D., Sayre, M. R., & Silbergleit, R. (2005). Research conditions that qualify for emergency exception from informed consent. *Academic Emergency Medicine, 12*(11), 1041–1044.

Widger, K., & Picot, C. (2008). Parents' perceptions of the quality of pediatric and perinatal end-of-life care. *Pediatric Nursing, 34*(1), 53–58.

Woodgate, R. L. (2006). Living in a world without closure: Reality for parents who have experienced the death of a child. *Journal of Palliative Care, 22*(2), 75–83.

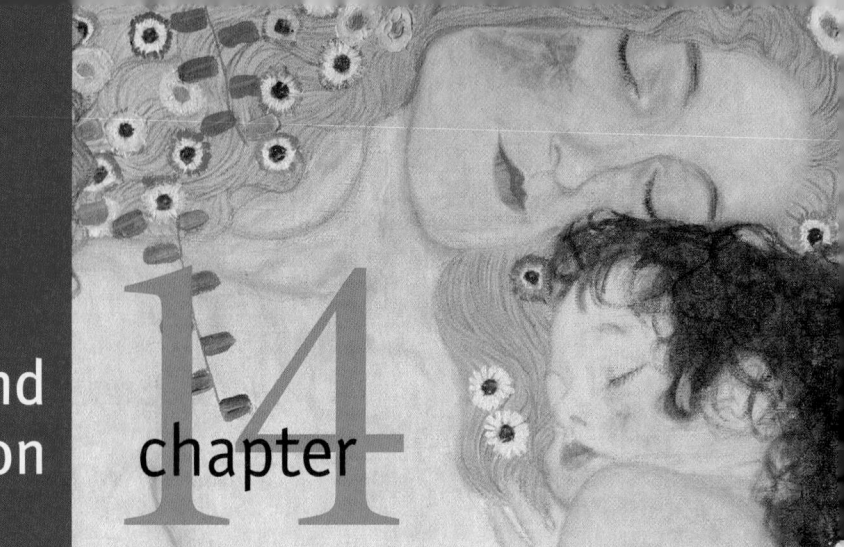

Infant, Child, and Adolescent Nutrition

14 chapter

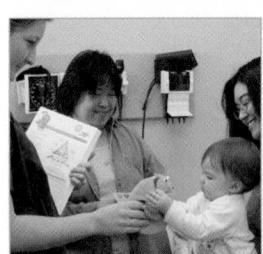

Yvonne is a 9-month-old infant who has been brought to the Women, Infants, and Children (WIC) clinic by her mother, Colleen. Her grandmother, Margarita, has also come since she will take Yvonne home by bus after the WIC appointment, and Colleen will return to work. Margarita cares for Yvonne during the day and likes to feed the baby her native Mexican dishes. Margarita speaks Spanish and demonstrates obvious pride in caring for Yvonne. The nurse weighs and measures Yvonne, takes a blood sample for hematocrit, and performs a 24-hour recall of Yvonne's intake. She learns that Yvonne breastfeeds in the morning and evening, takes an 8-ounce bottle of regular milk during the day, and eats soft table foods. What nutritional concerns are common at this age and should be addressed in the health visit? How can the nurse prepare the family for Yvonne's emerging nutritional needs?

Learning Outcomes

After reading this chapter, you will be able to do the following:

1. Summarize major nutritional concepts pertaining to the growth and development of children.
2. Describe and plan nursing interventions to meet nutritional needs for all age groups from infancy through adolescence.
3. Integrate methods of nutritional assessment into nursing care of infants, children, and adolescents.
4. Identify and explain nutritional problems of children growing up in developed countries.
5. Apply the nursing process to care for children with disordered eating.
6. Develop nursing interventions for children with nutritional disorders.

Adequate nutrition is an essential component of growth and development. The child's nutritional status begins before birth and is related to the mother's nutritional state. All children must be assessed for nutritional status, followed by teaching or other interventions to enhance health. Nurses are instrumental in giving parents information about normal nutritional needs of infants, children, and adolescents. Common techniques to assess nutrition, such as measuring growth and monitoring hematocrit, provide needed information about whether the child's intake of nutrients is adequate. How can the nurse bridge the various settings in which children's nutritional needs are met, including the home, childcare settings, schools, and hospitals? The nurse caring for Yvonne must integrate information about Colleen's knowledge of infant nutrition and the grandmother's food patterns to plan culturally appropriate interventions.

All children and their parents can benefit from information about nutritional needs, but some children have additional issues that must be considered. The nurse recognizes the special intake requirements of children with health conditions such as eating disorders, food allergies, cystic fibrosis, cerebral palsy, or diabetes. Nutrition monitoring is provided during childhood so that dietary counseling can be integrated with other teaching to promote development. The nurse helps the family prepare to meet the nutritional needs of a child who has special needs throughout childhood and in multiple settings. Some children have unique nutritional needs due to their social environments. However, parents may not be knowledgeable about their child's nutritional requirements. Perhaps the family is vegetarian and needs extra help to ensure intake of essential nutrients. If finances are limited, the family may need resources such as access to food stamps, food banks, or budget planning. The nurse considers the high rate of childhood obesity and

common nutritional deficits when applying concepts of health promotion with families. Whatever the setting in which the nurse is employed, knowledge of nutrition must be integrated within nursing care.

■ GENERAL NUTRITION CONCEPTS

Nutrition refers to taking in food and assimilating it metabolically for use by the body. It is an essential component of life and therefore an important topic to consider in discussions of child growth and development. The body requires a wide array of nutrients. **Macronutrients**, or the major building blocks of the body, are carbohydrates, proteins, and fats. Vitamins and minerals are **micronutrients**, or substances needed in small quantities for healthy body functioning. The need for nutrients is dependent on activity level, state of health and presence of disease or other stress, and age-related needs.

The **Dietary Reference Intakes (DRIs)** are a set of values established by the Food and Nutrition Board of the Institute of Medicine (2006) and the National Academy of Science that can be used to assess and plan intake for individuals of different ages. They commonly include four different values that can be considered by nursing, nutrition, and other health personnel (Table 14–1). While the DRI approach is used in the United States, other countries have developed their own approaches to dietary standards. For example, Canada uses Adequate Intake and Reference Nutrient Intake, and the United Kingdom uses Recommended Daily Nutrient Intakes. The aim of these standards is to provide a method of evaluating individual and population diets, and of planning nutrition programs and education. DRIs are generally specific to males and females in several age categories (Box 14–1). See Appendix C ∞ for a list of DRIs for children and adolescents. For more detailed explanations of recommendations,

TABLE 14–1	**Dietary Reference Intakes (DRIs)**		
Term	Definition	Use	Example
Estimated Average Requirement (EAR)	Daily intake needed to meet the requirements of 50% of a certain age and gender group.	Evaluate intake of a group; plan for intake of a group.	Compare the daily intake of vitamin C of a class of children from 24-hour recalls to this number to learn how many do not meet average requirements; plan the daily menu for a childcare center.
Recommended Dietary Allowance (RDA)	Daily intake needed to meet the requirements of most people (97–98%) of a certain age and gender group.	Set goal for daily intake.	Evaluate the dietary intake of an individual for a nutrient such as vitamin C; make recommendations to an individual for a daily menu.
Adequate Intake (AI)	Used when limited information on the needs for a vitamin is available and EAR is not available, usually because studies on its metabolism in the body are hard to carry out; rather than being based on metabolic studies, it is derived from the average intake of that nutrient by a healthy group of people.	Evaluate intake of a group; plan intake for a group.	See EAR.
Upper Intake (UI)	Upper tolerable intake level; maximum level unlikely to pose a health risk.	Limit fortification levels of foods and provide information to limit dietary supplements.	Consider intake of a fat-soluble vitamin such as vitamin A that is not readily excreted; include both food sources and supplements.

BOX 14-1 DRI Age Groups

- Pregnancy and lactation
- Birth to 6 months
- 6–12 months
- 1–3 years
- 4–8 years
- 9–13 years
- 14–18 years
- 19–30 years
- 31–50 years
- 51–70 years
- Over 70 years

MyPyramid and Alternative Pyramid Websites

consult the *Dietary Guidelines for Americans* (U.S. Department of Health and Human Services & U.S. Department of Agriculture, 2005).

Although the DRIs provide useful information when evaluating diets, their use can be time consuming. What "quick check" can be performed to provide feedback about children's daily diets? Learn the Food Guide Pyramid and hang posters of it in schools, clinics, and hospitals. Posters and instructions about personalizing the pyramid are available at the U.S. Department of Agriculture (USDA) website. The U.S. MyPyramid Food Guide provides a fast method to examine a child's intake for a day and evaluate if it meets nutrient requirements for age, gender, and activity level. See Figure 14–1 ➤ for the Food Guide Pyramid. In addition, consult the companion website for alternative pyramids for vegetarians and those from various ethnic groups, such as Hispanic and Native American, as well as Canada's Food Guide to Healthy Eating.

NUTRITIONAL NEEDS

Nutritional needs evolve during all of infancy and childhood. Nutrition supports growth and development, and influences the child's progression along the developmental path. Nutritional intake helps to maintain the child's health and fosters a state of maximal potential. Specific needs during each developmental stage are discussed in this section.

Infancy

From the first feeding of a few ounces of breast milk to a meal of soft table foods with the family at 1 year of age, the infant demonstrates an amazing ability to ingest and digest a wide variety of foods. Never again will the individual have such a high metabolic rate or high intake requirements in relation to size, or such a marked change in the types of foods eaten. Infants have an extremely fast rate of growth, since birth weight is usually doubled by about 5 months of age and tripled by 12 months. Meeting nutritional needs is challenged by the small size of the infant's stomach and the immaturity of the digestive system. The infant's great amount of physical activity also necessitates high caloric intake. Nutrient demands for protein and vitamins must be met for the cells of the nervous system and body organs to properly develop.

Breastfeeding and Formula-Feeding

The natural first food, breast milk, should be encouraged for all infants (Figure 14–2 ➤). The American Academy of Pediatrics believes that breastfeeding is the best source of nutrition for babies through the first birthday and should be encouraged by health professionals (American Academy of Pediatrics [AAP], Committee on Nutrition, 2009; AAP, Section on Breast-Feeding, 2005). The American Diabetes Association (2008) states that

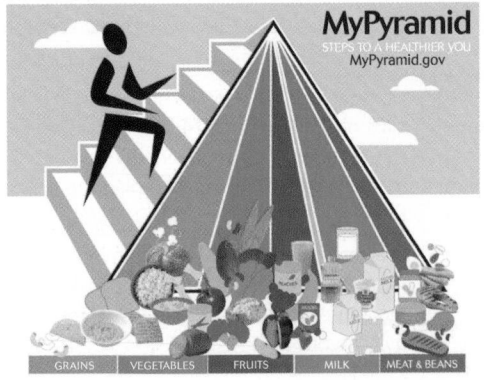

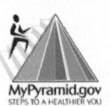

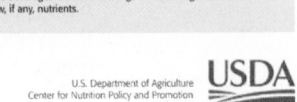

FIGURE 14–1 ➤ The MyPyramid Food Guide is used to provide teaching about amounts of foods recommended for daily intake.

U.S. Department of Agriculture and U.S. Department of Health and Human Services. (2005). http://www.mypyramid.gov/downloads/miniposter.pdf

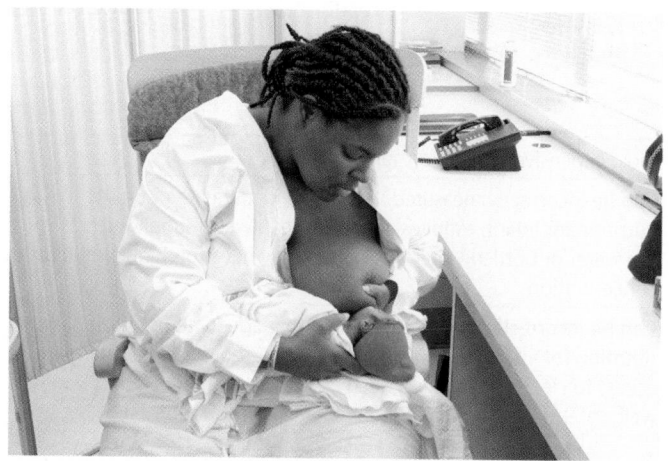

FIGURE 14–2 ➤ Breastfeeding offers many physical and emotional benefits for the infant. This new mother is learning to breastfeed her baby. How can nurses encourage mothers to have positive breastfeeding experiences?

U.S. Preventive Services Task Force Website

Families Want to Know
Infant Nutritional Supplements

1. Each infant receives a vitamin K injection after birth to promote adequate blood clotting. After this time no further vitamin K is needed, as the baby manufactures this vitamin in the gut once he or she begins eating.
2. Vitamin D is recommended at a minimum of 400 international units/day for all infants (Wagner, Greer, & Section on Breastfeeding, 2008).
3. Iron is not needed unless the infant is not taking in other sources of food with iron by 4–6 months. The baby may need an iron source earlier if the mother was anemic during pregnancy or while breastfeeding.
4. Fluoride 0.25 mg is given after 6 months of age if water is not fluoridated to a level of 0.3 parts per million (ppm) or if the baby is not drinking any water.

broad-based efforts are needed to break barriers to breastfeeding, citing that exclusive breastfeeding for 6 months, and breastfeeding with supplementary foods for at least 12 months, is the ideal feeding pattern for infants. The U.S. Preventive Services Task Force recommends breastfeeding education and behavioral counseling in 30- to 90-minute individual or group sessions with specially trained nurses or lactation specialists.

Breast milk can be the only food for the first 6 months, and should continue through 12 months of age, with addition of solid foods from 6 to 12 months. Many advantages to breastfeeding are recognized, including excellent nutritional balance, promotion of gastrointestinal function, fostering of immune defense, psychological benefits, and economic advantages. Although breast milk is the best nutritional source for infants, there may be a need for some limited supplements.

Providing breastfeeding information and instruction positively influences the number of women who decide to breastfeed and increases the number of months they choose to continue breastfeeding. Teaching can emphasize the importance of breastfeeding to the child's well-being. Lower incidence of otitis media and, later in life, less risk for type 2 diabetes, cardiovascular disease, and other chronic conditions are some benefits of breastfeeding (Centers for Disease Control and Prevention [CDC], 2009). Programs for encouraging breastfeeding should involve education and skill/problem-solving information provided by health professionals and trained supportive volunteers (Watt, McGlone, Russell, et al., 2006). Specially trained lactation consultants through the International Board of Certified Lactation Consultants can provide valuable assistance. Home visits, phone calls from hospital nursing staff, early visits after the birth to obstetric and pediatric offices, and resources such as La Leche League can provide mothers with needed breastfeeding information and problem-solving suggestions.

The nurse encourages the mother to obtain adequate nutritional intake and sufficient rest, since both are needed for successful breastfeeding. Support programs are especially helpful to mothers who have difficulty breastfeeding, feel unsure how it will fit into their family and work life, are very young, or have an infant with problems related to feeding. Supplements may be needed for some infants. Provide information about breast pumps, storing breast milk, and other information that is helpful to the family. Assist the mother to realize that six to eight wet diapers per day and adequate weight gain indicate that her infant is getting needed nutrition from breast milk. See Families Want to Know: Infant Nutritional Supplements. The mother of a hospitalized infant will need special support to continue breastfeeding. The mother should be encouraged to come to the hospital to feed her baby on the same schedule as at home. If the infant cannot breastfeed, the hospital may provide an electric pump so the mother can maintain lactation.

Some women decide not to breastfeed or are unable to do so. Some breastfeeding mothers occasionally use supplemental bottles when they are away from the infant. Nurses teach all mothers using formula about formula preparation and feeding. Three types of formula are available—ready to feed, concentrate, and powder. All are nutritionally adequate for infants. The nurse can help parents decide which preparation of formula is best suited for their infant (Table 14–2) and teach methods of preparation. Some infants, such as those with phenylketonuria or other metabolic disorders, or infants with cow milk allergy, require specialized formulas. Breastfeeding or bottle-feeding is discussed at each contact with health professionals to identify potential teaching needs.

Nursing Alert

Review type and preparation of formula at each health care visit. Concentrate or powder formula can be mixed with tap water but must be refrigerated once mixed. No water should be added to ready-to-feed formula. Formula that the baby does not drink should be discarded after use and not kept for future feedings. This minimizes the chance for bacteria to multiply and cause illness. When the family lives in older housing, caution them to run tap water for about 2 minutes before using it, and to use only cold water for formula preparation. These practices will minimize the chance that lead is leached from the older pipes in the house (see Chapter 17 ∞ for further discussion of lead poisoning). If the family has a well, the water should be tested for microorganisms before being used for the baby.

TABLE 14–2	**Advantages and Disadvantages of Formula Preparations**		
Formula Preparation	How Packaged	Advantages	Disadvantages
Ready to feed	Bottles or cans	No preparation needed	Most expensive type of formula
Concentrate	Cans of concentrated liquid	Easy to add equal amounts of formula concentrate and water directly into bottle and shake	Can be incorrectly measured, leading to inadequate or unsafe nutrition for infant; requires access to clean water supply such as city tap water or bottled water; well water may have too high a mineral concentration
Powder	Cans	Least expensive type of formula	Can be incorrectly measured, leading to inadequate or unsafe nutrition for infant; requires shaking to mix thoroughly; requires access to clean water supply such as city tap water or bottled water; well water may have too high a mineral concentration

During infancy and toddlerhood, nurses should carefully examine the patterns of breastfeeding and bottle-feeding. **Early childhood caries**, the presence of one or more decayed, lost, or filled tooth surfaces in a primary tooth from birth to 6 years of age, can occur when a young child is allowed to nurse or drink from a bottle for long periods, especially when sleeping (Figure 14–3 ➤). The milk, juice, or other fluid pools around the upper anterior teeth, salivary flow decreases, and acid buffering is decreased, resulting in tooth decay. Teach parents to avoid putting the child to bed with a bottle. Encourage pacifier use or a bottle of water instead. Mothers who breastfeed should also be cautioned to limit nursing to specific times so that milk will not pool in the infant's mouth during sleep (see also Chapters 7 ∞ and 8 ∞ for dental care in infants and young children).

Parents can be taught beginning dental care for the infant, which includes wiping the teeth off daily with a piece of moist gauze or a small infant toothbrush once the teeth erupt. Pediatric dentists advise the first dental visit within 6 months of the first tooth eruption, or no later than about 1 year of age (American Dental Association, n.d.). Have the parents select and establish contact with a dental provider during infancy.

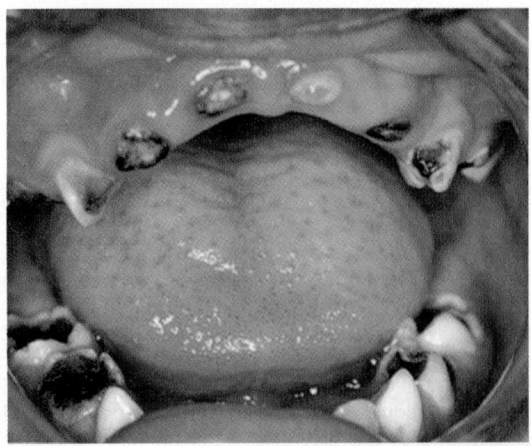

FIGURE 14–3 ➤ Early childhood caries. This child has had major tooth decay related to sleeping as an infant and toddler while sucking bottles of juice and milk.
Courtesy of Dr. Lezley McIlveen, Department of Dentistry, Children's National Medical Center, Washington, DC.

Introduction of Complementary Foods

When should foods be added to the infant's diet? The American Academy of Pediatrics recommends introducing complementary foods at 4 to 6 months (AAP, Committee on Nutrition, 2009). From 6 to 12 months, complementary foods are offered in addition to the intake of breast milk or formula, rather than replacing that essential nutrient (Hagan, Shaw, & Duncan, 2008).

By about 6 months the extrusion reflex (or tongue thrust) decreases and the infant can sit well with support. The infant develops the ability to appreciate texture and to swallow nonliquid foods, and can indicate desire for food or turn away when full.

The first complementary food added to the infant's diet is often rice cereal. The advantages of introducing cereal first are that it provides iron at an age when the infant's prenatal iron stores begin to decrease, it seldom causes an allergic reaction, and it is easy to digest. Parents should feed 1 to 2 tablespoons of cereal to the infant once or twice daily just before formula or breastfeeding. The infant may appear to spit out food at first because of normal back-and-forth tongue movement. Parents should not interpret this early feeding behavior as indicating dislike for the food. With a little practice, the infant will become adept at spoon-feeding.

Once the infant eats 1/4 cup of cereal twice daily, usually at 6 to 8 months of age, vegetables or fruits can be introduced at a rate of one new food every several days (Table 14–3). By 8 to 10 months, most fruits and vegetables have been introduced and strained meats or other protein (e.g., tofu, cheese, mashed beans) can be added to the infant's diet. Finger foods are introduced during the second half of the first year as the infant's palmar and then finger grasps develop and as teeth begin to erupt (Figure 14–4 ➤). Infants enjoy toast, O-shaped cereal, finely

Nursing Alert

Advise parents to use caution when providing finger foods to the infant. Hard foods and some soft and malleable ones slip easily into the throat and may cause choking. Avoid hot dogs, hard vegetables, candy, whole grapes, and chunks of peanut butter. Infants and other young children should always be supervised while eating. Be sure parents are familiar with techniques for airway obstruction removal and have emergency numbers clearly listed on their phones.

TABLE 14–3 Introduction of Solid Foods in Infancy	
Recommendation	Rationale
Introduce rice cereal at 4–6 months.	Rice cereal is easy to digest, has low allergenic potential, and contains iron.
Introduce fruits or vegetables at 6–8 months. Some health care providers recommend vegetable introduction before fruits.	Fruits and vegetables provide needed vitamins. Vegetables are not as sweet as fruits; introducing them first may enhance acceptability to the infant.
Introduce meats at 8–10 months.	Meats are harder to digest, have high protein load, and should not be fed until close to 1 year of age when kidney function is mature.
Use single-food prepared baby foods rather than combination meals.	Combination meals usually contain more sugar, salt, and fillers.
Introduce one new food at a time, waiting at least 3–5 days to introduce another. Delay feeding eggs, strawberries, wheat, corn, fish, and nut products until 2–3 years of age.	If a food allergy or intolerance develops, it will be easy to identify. The foods listed are those most commonly associated with food allergy.
Avoid carrots, beets, and spinach before 4 months of age. Have well water evaluated for nitrates (recommended level less than 10 mg/L).	Nitrates in these foods and in water near agricultural runoff can be converted to nitrite by young infants, causing methemoglobinemia.
Infants can be fed mashed portions of table foods such as carrots, rice, and potatoes.	This is a less expensive alternative to jars of commercially prepared baby food; it allows parents of various cultural groups to feed ethnic foods to infants.
Avoid adding sugar, salt, and spices when preparing baby foods at home.	Infants need not become accustomed to these flavors; they may get too much sodium from salt or develop gastric distress from some spices.
Avoid honey until at least 1 year of age.	Infants cannot detoxify *Clostridium botulinum* spores sometimes present in honey and can develop botulism.

sliced meats, cheese and tofu, and small pieces of cooked, softened vegetables. Avoid foods that may cause choking.

Certain foods are more commonly associated with the development of food allergies, and avoiding them in infancy may decrease allergy incidence. Recommendations for infants at risk due to a family history of allergy are to delay feeding of cow milk until 1 year; eggs until 2 years; and peanuts, nuts, fish, and shell-

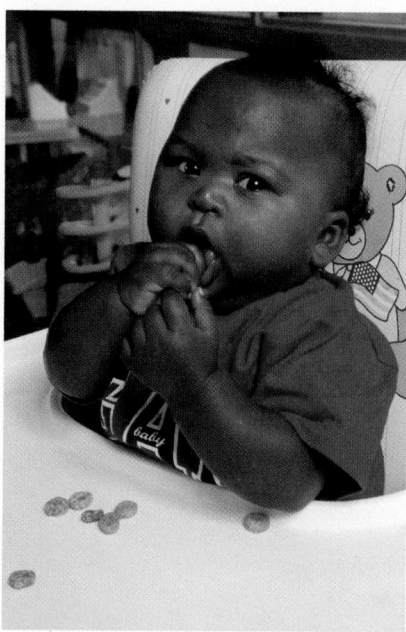

FIGURE 14–4 ➤ The infant who has developed the ability to grasp with thumb and forefinger should receive some foods that can be held in the hand.

fish until 3 years (AAP, Committee on Nutrition, 2009). See the discussion on food reactions later in this chapter for more information about food intolerance and allergy. As food and juice intake increase, formula or breastfeedings decrease in amount and frequency (Table 14–4). Nine-month-old Yvonne, introduced in the chapter-opening scenario, is learning to eat supplemental foods. Her mother needs help from the nurse to decide what foods fit into both the recommendations for her age and the ethnic patterns common in the family. She should remain on breast milk or formula until at least 1 year of age.

If breastfeeding is not chosen, or if supplemental feedings are given, only iron-fortified infant formula should be used during the first year of life. When breastfed infants are not eating foods with iron by 4 to 6 months, supplemental iron may need to be added. Careful dietary assessment and discussion of intake by the nurse at health visits helps the practitioner decide if supplemental iron is needed.

Weaning is the term used when infants give up breastfeeding or a bottle and obtain most fluids by cup. At about 8–9 months the baby should be offered a cup with assistance provided to begin learning about drinking from a cup. By about 1 year of age, infants are usually able to drink most liquids from a cup with a lid. Bottles can then be slowly withdrawn and replaced by cups. Breastfeeding may continue if the parent and infant desire, but introduction of other foods and a cup for drinking water or juice are still recommended. Infants should only be offered cups at meal and snack times so they become accustomed to drinking when thirsty rather than carrying a bottle or cup for much of the day, in order to decrease the chance for dental caries and increased calorie intake.

TABLE 14–4	Infant Nutritional Patterns
Birth to 1 month	Eats every 2–3 hours, breast or bottle Eats 2–3 ounces (60–90 mL) per feeding
2–4 months	Has coordinated suck–swallow Eats every 3–4 hours Eats 3–4 ounces (90–120 mL) per feeding
4–6 months	Begins baby food, often rice cereal, 2–3 T, twice daily Consumes breast milk or formula four or more times daily Eats 4–5 ounces (100–150 mL) per feeding
6–8 months	Eats baby food such as rice cereal, fruits, and vegetables, 2–5 T, three times daily Consumes breast milk or formula four times daily Eats 6–8 ounces (160–225 mL) per feeding
8–10 months	Enjoys soft finger foods three times daily Consumes breast milk or formula four times daily Eats 6 ounces (160 mL) per feeding
10–12 months	Eats most soft table foods with family three times daily Uses cup with or without lid Attempts to feed self with spoon, though spills often Consumes breast milk or formula four times daily Eats 6–8 ounces (160–225 mL) per feeding

Parents who want to make infant foods at home can be encouraged and instructed about how to do so. Some commercially prepared foods have unnecessary additives such as salt, sugar, and food starch, and they may be costly for some families. Parents can easily blend fruits and vegetables the family is eating before adding salt, sugar, or seasoning. Prepared foods should be used promptly and stored in the refrigerator between feedings. Foods can also be placed into ice cube trays and frozen; a cube or two can be defrosted at mealtime. Caution parents not to use honey in foods for infants, as it can lead to infant botulism.

Clinical Tip

Cow milk (including evaporated milk) can lead to bleeding and anemia, interferes with absorption of nutrients, and has a high solute load (concentration) which the immature kidneys of the infant can have difficulty excreting. Cow milk should be avoided in the first year of life.

Nursing Alert

If foods or fluids are microwaved for use with infants or children, there can be "hot spots" that lead to burning. Stirring, shaking, and checking the temperature before feeding are recommended to protect the child from burns to the mouth.

Toddlerhood

Why do parents of toddlers frequently become concerned about the small amount of food their children eat? Why do toddlers seem to survive and even thrive with minimal food intake? The toddler often displays the phenomenon of **physiologic anorexia**, caused when the extremely high metabolic demands of infancy slow to keep pace with the more moderate growth rate of toddlerhood. Although it can appear that the toddler eats nothing at times, intake over days or a week is generally sufficient and balanced enough to meet the body's demands for nutrients and energy.

Parents often need knowledge about types of foods that constitute a healthy diet. Some easy-to-prepare foods are high in salt and other additives, and can lead to exceeding the recommendation of *Healthy People 2010* and 2020 (U.S. Department of Health and Human Services, 2006; 2010) for sodium intake. Provide alternatives to hot dogs, microwave meals, or fast foods with information about easy-to-prepare sliced meats, cheese, tofu, fruits, and vegetables. Healthy snacks for young children include yogurt, cheese, milk, slices of bread with peanut butter, thinly sliced fruits, and soft vegetables.

Advise parents to offer a variety of nutritious foods several times daily (three meals and two snacks) and let the toddler make choices from the foods offered. Offer foods only at meal and snack times and have the child eat in a high chair or on a special seat at the table (Figure 14–5 ➤). Small portions are most appealing to the toddler. A general guideline for food quantity at a meal is 1 tablespoon of each food per year of age (see Table 14–5 for common serving sizes at various ages). The toddler should drink 16 to 24 ounces (1/2 to 3/4 L) of milk daily. Caution parents against giving the toddler more than 1 quart (1 L) of milk daily, since this interferes with the desire to eat other foods, leading to dietary deficiencies. Recall that the child should not be placed to bed with a bottle or allowed to carry a bottle of milk or juice around during the day, due to the risk of early childhood caries (see previous discussion in this chapter). In addition, parents should be advised to use only 100% fruit juice and to limit consumption of juice to 4 to 6 ounces daily for children ages 1 to 6 years in order to decrease the risk for overweight, dental caries, and abdominal discomfort (O'Connor, Yang, & Nicklas, 2006). Unpasteurized juice

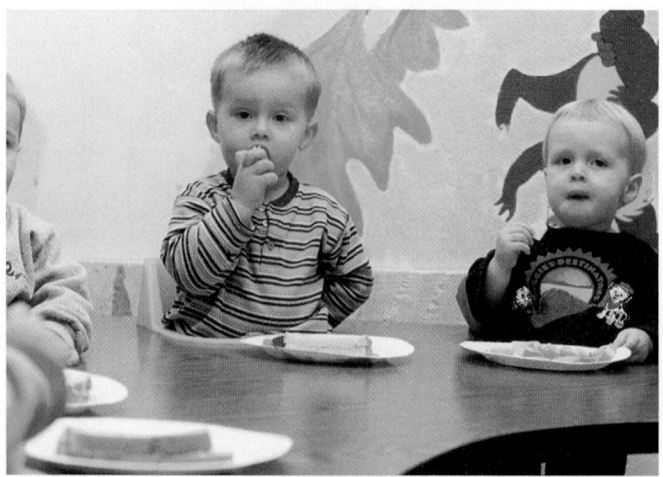

FIGURE 14–5 ➤ Toddlers should sit at a table or in a high chair to minimize the chance of choking and to foster positive eating patterns.

Growth & Development   *Toddler Feeding*

Toddlers generally eat three meals and two or three snacks daily. Toddlers can drink 2% milk starting at 2 years of age, or "follow-up" formula. A maximum of 1 L of milk daily should be consumed. Larger amounts can contribute to obesity and may interfere with the toddler's consumption of a variety of foods, leading to iron deficiency anemia. Cups are recommended for milk and other fluids; bottles should have been discontinued by this age. The child is learning to use utensils but may prefer fingers and still needs small serving sizes. Mild flavors are preferred, whereas spices and bitter tastes are generally disliked.

should never be used since it may contain pathogens, such as *Escherichia coli*, *Salmonella*, and *Cryptosporidium*, which are particularly harmful to young children (Blackburn, Mazurek, Hlavsa et al., 2006; Jain, Bidol, Austin, et al., 2009). Drinking water and eating whole fruits, which provide fiber, are healthier alternatives. Avoid eating more than one meal weekly from a fast-food restaurant due to the generally high-fat, high-sugar, and low-fiber content of such meals.

Learning how to eat with others is an important task of toddlerhood. The toddler displays characteristic autonomy or independence during mealtime. Advise parents to provide opportunities for self-feeding of food with fingers and utensils, and

TABLE 14–5 Typical Daily Intake at Various Ages

	Breakfast	Snack	Lunch	Snack	Dinner	Snack
Infant 6 months	2 T rice cereal with 2 oz (60 mL) formula	4 oz (120 mL) formula or breast milk	6 oz (180 mL) formula or breast milk	6 oz (180 mL) formula or breast milk	2 T rice cereal with 2 oz (60 mL) formula, then 6 oz (180 mL) formula or breast milk	4 oz (120 mL) formula or breast milk
12 months	1/4 to 1/2 cup (60–120 mL) apple juice 4 T rice cereal with 4 oz (120 mL) milk	3 crackers 1/2 cup (120 mL) milk	1 thin slice (1/2 oz [14 g]) of turkey 1/2 cup soft cooked carrots 1 cup (240 mL) milk	1/2 slice of cheese 1/2 cup (120 mL) milk or water	1/4 cup plain pasta 1/4 cup thin-sliced apple chunks 1/2 cup (120 mL) milk	1/2 cup yogurt
Toddler	1/4 cup (60 mL) orange juice 1/4 cup cereal with 1/2 cup (120 mL) milk 1/4 banana	5 crackers 1/2 cup (120 mL) milk	2 thin slices (1 oz [28 g]) of turkey with 1/2 slice of bread 1/2 cup cooked carrots 1 cup (240 mL) milk	1 slice cheese 1/2 cup (120 mL) juice	1/4 cup plain pasta 1/4–1/2 cup thin-sliced apple chunks 1/2 cup (120 mL) milk	1/2 cup yogurt
Preschooler	1/2 cup (120 mL) orange juice 1/3 cup cereal with 3/4 cup (180 mL) milk 1/2 banana	5 crackers 1/2 orange 1/2 cup (120 mL) milk	3 thin slices (1 1/2 oz [42 g]) of turkey with 1/2 slice bread 1/4 cup cooked carrots 3/4 cup (180 mL) milk	1 slice cheese 1/2 cup (120 mL) juice	1/4–1/2 cup plain pasta with meat sauce 1/2 cup thin-sliced apple chunks 1/2 cup (120 mL) milk	1/2 cup yogurt
School-age child	1/2 cup (120 mL) orange juice 3/4 cup cereal with 1 cup (240 mL) milk 1/2 bagel with jam		4 thin slices (2 oz [56 g]) of turkey with 1 slice bread and condiments Apple 1 cup (240 mL) milk 1 oatmeal cookie	1 1/2 cups popcorn 1 cup (240 mL) lemonade	1/2 cup pasta with meat sauce Dinner salad 1 slice garlic bread 1 cup (240 mL) milk	1 cup pudding or yogurt
Adolescent	1/2 cup (120 mL) orange juice 1 cup cereal 1 cup (240 mL) milk 1 bagel with 1 T peanut butter and jam		3 oz (84 g) meat with 2 slices of bread plus condiments Apple 1 cup (240 mL) milk 1 oatmeal cookie	3 cups popcorn 1 cup (240 mL) lemonade	1 1/2 cup pasta with meat sauce 1 slice garlic bread Salad with dressing 1 cup (240 mL) milk	1 cup pudding Fruit

Note: The young infant should be fed as often as needed rather than on a strict schedule of meals and snacks. The amounts listed for the infant are averages based on a 24-hour recommended intake.

to allow some simple choices, such as type of liquid or cup to use. Young children should eat at a table with others, not be allowed to run and play while eating, and eat at specified meal and snack times. Because social skills are developing, the hospitalized toddler may develop positive eating habits if allowed to have meals with parents or other hospitalized children. See Chapter 11 ∞ for further suggestions about management of nutrition in hospitalized children.

Preschool Age

The preschooler's diet is similar to that of the toddler, but mealtime is now a more social event. Preschoolers like the company of others while they eat, and they enjoy helping with food preparation and table setting (Figure 14–6 ➤). Involving them in these tasks can provide a forum for teaching about nutritious foods and principles of preparation such as the need for refrigeration, safety around stoves, and cleanliness. Limit visits to fast-food restaurants to about once weekly and use the opportunity to assist the child in making wise choices of nutritionally adequate foods in that setting.

Although the rate of growth is slow and steady during the preschool years, the child has periods of **food jags** (eating only a few foods for several days or weeks) and greater or lesser intake. Advise parents to assess food intake over a 1- or 2-week period rather than at each meal to obtain a more accurate impression of total intake. Food jags can be handled by providing the desired food along with other foods to foster choice. The child who chooses not to eat at snack or mealtime should not be given other foods in between. Hunger will develop and the child will become accustomed to eating when food is provided. Three meals and two or three snacks daily are the norm (see Table 14–5). Limit fruit juice to 8 to 12 ounces daily, and begin teaching the "5-a-day" program that supports having five servings of fruits/vegetables each day.

The preschool period is a good time to continue encouraging good dental habits. Children can begin to brush their own teeth with parental supervision and help to reach all tooth surfaces. See Chapter 7 ∞ for the recommended dose of fluoride when the water supply is not fluoridated. If the child has not yet visited a dentist, the first dental visit should be scheduled so the child can become accustomed to the routine of dental care.

School Age

The school-age years are a period of gradual growth when energy requirements remain at a steady level, although sometime during these years most children experience a preadolescent growth spurt. Girls may begin a growth spurt by 10 or 11 years, and boys a year or so later. Nutritional needs increase dramatically with this spurt, with large numbers of calories and increased amounts of other nutrients required (see Appendix C ∞ for Dietary Reference Intakes).

School-age children are increasingly responsible for preparing snacks, lunches, and even some other meals. These years are a good time to teach children how to choose nutritious foods and how to plan a well-balanced meal. Because school-age children operate at the concrete level of cognitive thought, nutrition teaching is best presented by using pictures, samples of foods, videotapes, handouts, and hands-on experience.

School-age children often prefer the types of foods eaten at home and may be resistant to new food items. A hospitalized child may refuse to eat, slowing the recuperative process. Encourage family members to bring favorite foods from home that meet nutritional requirements. This can be especially helpful when the hospital serves food only from the dominant cultural group. A child accustomed to a diet of rice, tofu, and vegetables may not enjoy a hospital meal of hamburger and fries. By school age, food has become strongly associated with social interaction, so it is beneficial to have children eat together or to invite family members to take the child off the unit to eat or to bring in food from home and eat with the child. Many hospitals allow children to plan a pizza night or sponsor other events to encourage eating in a social atmosphere.

Most children consume at least one meal daily in school. Although they may bring lunches to school, many children participate in the school lunch program, and perhaps the school breakfast program. Become familiar with the school district's policies in your area for providing foods, snacks, and reduced-price food to students in need. Over the past decade, many U.S. school systems have allowed vending machines for carbonated sweetened beverages and snacks to be installed. Part of the profits from these machines has enabled revenue-strapped school districts to enhance their incomes. However, schools are increasingly challenged about the presence of the machines, especially in light of the growing problem of overweight among youth. Some school districts have now limited the number of machines or the hours during which they can be used by students. Nurses are able to provide information for districts about the problems of obesity and the need for healthy foods for youth.

The loss of the first deciduous teeth and the eruption of permanent teeth usually occur at about 6 years, or at the beginning of the school-age period. Of the 32 permanent teeth, 22 to 26 teeth erupt by age 12 years, and the remaining molars follow in the teenage years. See Chapter 5 ∞ for the typical sequence of tooth eruption and Chapters 7, 8, and 9 ∞ for further information about dental needs during childhood. The school-age child should be closely monitored to ensure that brushing and

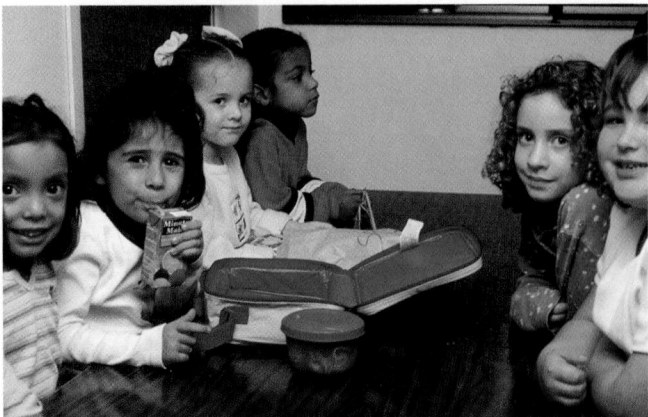

FIGURE 14–6 ➤ Preschoolers learn food habits by eating with others. Engaging them in food preparation enhances knowledge of food and promotes intake at meals.

Evidence-Based Practice
Adolescent Food Habits

Problem

Adolescents are largely independent in their food choices. They often eat "on the run" and are influenced by peers and the media. At the same time, rates of obesity are escalating upward. Nurses need to understand and apply evidence-based practice for influencing eating behaviors in adolescents.

Evidence

Adolescents frequently have poor diets but are also commonly attempting to lose weight. Unhealthy weight loss strategies involve cutting out meals and choosing less healthy foods. Persistent use of unhealthy weight control strategies was associated with lower intakes of calcium and vegetables among over 2,000 adolescents (Larson, Neumark-Sztainer, & Story, 2009). In another study by several nurses in North Carolina, 10 adolescents made significantly healthier choices from a fast-food menu after a short nutrition education session that focused on the food pyramid and food categories (Allen, Taylor, & Kuiper, 2007).

Implications

Although adolescent nutritional intake is an important health concern, there is a limited body of knowledge to guide the health professional. Findings of importance are that adolescent weight control patterns may expose them to poor eating patterns. Barriers to adolescent healthy eating include availability of unhealthy snacks, and the media messages about food consumption. Adolescents seeking to control weight may use unhealthy strategies that lead to dietary deficiencies.

Critical Thinking Application

1. What developmental stages of the adolescent provide both challenges to healthy eating and the ability to make wise food choices?
2. Construct a list of questions about food patterns that will help you identify risk and protective factors of adolescents seeking to control their weight.
3. Visit a local high school and then travel 1/2 mile in each direction from the school. Record the number of fast-food restaurants, billboards about foods, and any other food-related resources or media. Watch 2 hours of television at 3–5 p.m., when adolescents frequently arrive home. Record the number of food-related messages, what types of foods are advertised, and other observations.
4. How can you integrate knowledge about adolescent nutrition into your potential role as a school nurse at a high school?

---

flossing are adequate, that fluoride is taken if the water supply is not fluoridated, that dental care is obtained to provide for examination of teeth and alignment, and that loose teeth are identified before surgery or sports participation.

Adolescence

Most adolescents need well over 2000 calories daily to support the growth spurt, and some adolescent boys require 3000 or more calories daily. When teenagers are active in a variety of sports, these requirements increase further. The pregnant or breastfeeding adolescent has even more challenging nutrient requirements, and maternity resources should be consulted to plan diets for these periods. Supplementary vitamins and minerals will be needed to enhance the pregnancy outcome. Because adolescents prepare much of their own food and often eat with friends, they need to be taught about good nutrition. Developing a diet that includes a large number of calories, meets vitamin and mineral requirements, and is acceptable to the teen may be a challenge. An adolescent who is hospitalized and does not like the hospital lunch sometimes has a soft drink and chips when a friend comes to visit; however, the teen may be receptive to offers of juice and pizza, a more nutritious meal. Small improvements should be viewed positively as they may lead to further changes.

Fast food represents a significant intake for many adolescents. It is commonly high in fat, calories, and sodium while being low in essential nutrients such as calcium, folic acid, riboflavin, vitamins A and C, and fiber. Many schools are redesigning cafeterias and food programs to entice more teens to eat at school rather than nearby fast-food restaurants. Adding fruits and salads and decreasing access to snack bars can enhance the quality of food intake. School nurses play a vital role in helping to tailor a healthy school nutrition program. Remember that peer group influence is important, so group sessions in which adolescents eat lunch together can provide a forum for influencing food habits. (See Evidence-Based Practice: Adolescent Food Habits.) What other methods can you think of to encourage positive nutritional habits among teens?

■ NUTRITIONAL ASSESSMENT

What is the best indication that the child's nutrition is adequate? Which data collection methods provide the most accurate information about a child's dietary intake? The nurse plays an important role in assessing the diets of children and in seeking additional evaluation from dietitians and nutritionists in complex situations.

Physical and Behavioral Measurement

Growth Measurement

A common method used to evaluate the adequacy of diet is measurement of growth. **Anthropometric measurement** refers to assessment of various parts of the body. Anthropometry of young children commonly includes weight, length, and head circumference. Standing height is substituted for length once the child can stand. Head circumference, also known as occipital-frontal circumference (OFC), is measured until the child is about 5 years. Additional measurements that may be included in special circumstances include chest circumference, mid-upper arm circumference, and skinfold measurement at sites such as triceps, abdomen, and subscapular regions. The *Clinical Skills Manual* presents techniques for accurate measurement of weight, length, height, chest, and head circumference.

Once the measurements are collected, plot the readings on the appropriate standardized growth curves for weight, length to height, head circumference, and body mass index (Figure 14–7 ➤). **Body mass index (BMI)** is a calculation based on the child's weight and height, or length, and is calculated as weight in kilograms/m² of height. This is a useful calculation for determining if the child's height and weight are in proportion. Identify on the plots where the child falls in percentile for each measurement. Children normally fall between the 10th and 90th percentiles. A measurement below the 10th percentile, especially for BMI, may indicate undernutrition, whereas one over the 90th percentile can indicate overnutrition. It is important, however, to look at the differences between measurements. An infant in the 90th percentile for length, weight, and head circumference is proportional and may be a naturally large baby. A child who is consistently in the 10th percentile for all measurements, but is growing steadily and is at a normal development level, may simply be a small child. Much cultural and individual variation exists regarding size. See Appendix A ∞ for standardized growth curves by gender and age for infants, children, and adolescents. Visit the companion website to find out more about the growth curves and a course in accurate assessment techniques.

Plot the child's measurements on the same growth curve with earlier percentiles for the child. When measurements follow the same percentile over time, growth is generally normal for the child and nutrition is likely adequate. However, a sudden or sustained change in percentile may indicate a chronic disorder, emotional difficulty, or a nutritional intake problem. Further assessment of physical status and dietary intake will be needed.

Additional Physical Measurements

Many observations from the physical assessment provide clues to nutritional status. Every body system can be affected by dietary intake, and a combination of certain symptoms may suggest specific nutritional problems. Some of the common clinical manifestations of dietary deficiencies and excesses are outlined on the next page.

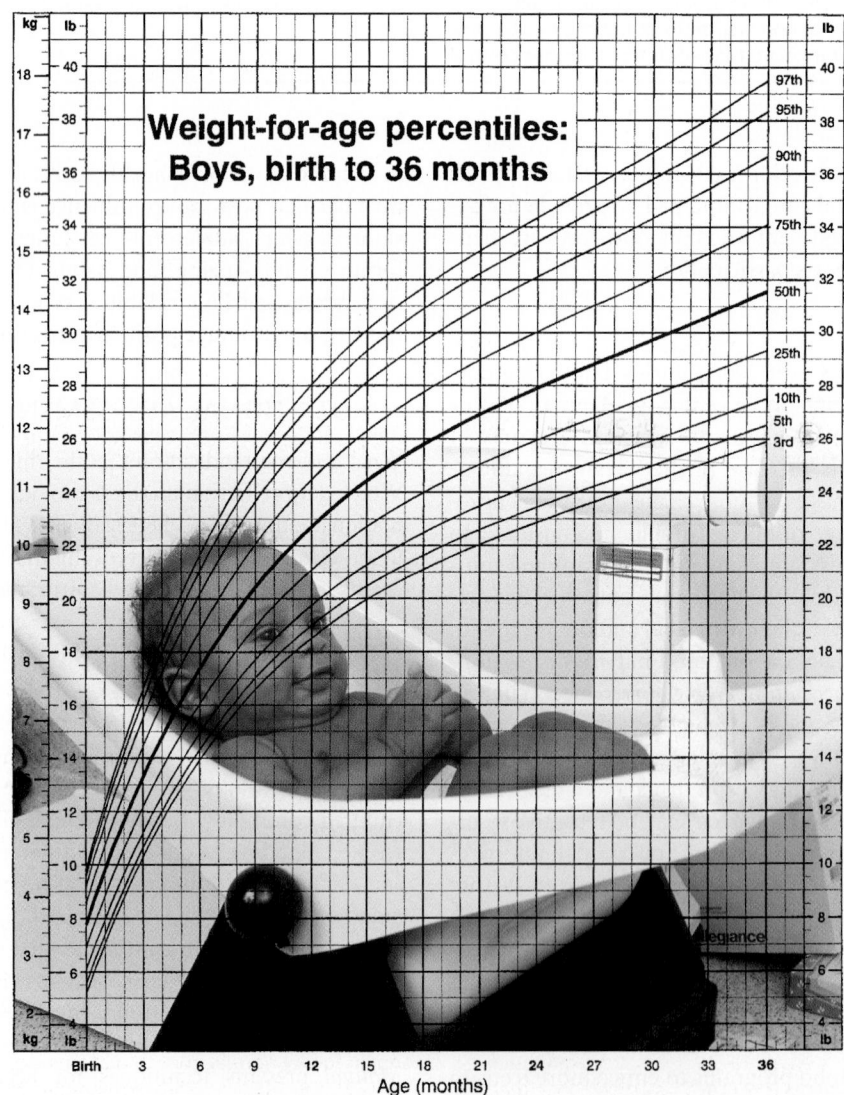

FIGURE 14–7 ➤ The nurse accurately measures the child and then places height and weight on appropriate growth grids for the child's age and gender.

Clinical Manifestations
Dietary Deficiencies/Excesses

Nutrient	Deficiency Manifestation	Excess Manifestation
Vitamin A	Night blindness Skin dryness and scaling	Headache Drowsiness Hepatomegaly Vomiting and diarrhea
Vitamin C	Abnormal hair (coiled shape) Skin abnormalities (dermatitis and lesions) Purpura Bleeding gums Joint tenderness Sudden heart failure	Usually none—excess is excreted in urine
Vitamin D	Rib abnormalities Bowed legs	Drowsiness
B vitamins	Weakness Decreased deep tendon reflexes Dermatitis	Usually none—excess is excreted in urine
Protein	Hepatomegaly Edema Scant, depigmented hair	Kidney failure
Carbohydrate	Emaciation Decreased energy Retarded growth and development	Overweight
Iron	Lethargy Slowed growth and developmental progression Pallor	Vomiting, diarrhea, abdominal pain Pallor Cyanosis Drowsiness Shock

Laboratory measurements can provide useful information when nutritional status is questionable. Some common studies include hematocrit and hemoglobin, serum glucose and fasting insulin, lipids and lipoproteins, and liver and renal function studies. Adding some further measurements such as chest circumference and skinfolds (measurement of fat at certain body sites such as triceps, scapular, and abdominal areas) may also be useful (Lee & Nieman, 2010).

Clinical Tip

If you measure a child and find him or her to be in either very low or very high percentiles, try the following:

1. Measure again to check for accuracy.
2. Examine if length or height, weight, and head circumference are in similar percentiles. Is the child proportional?
3. Observe if the parents are very large or very small.
4. Look at the child's chart to see if the patterns have continued over time or if they represent a sudden change. Changes from one channel to another are of concern. For example, if the child has usually been in the 25th percentile for all measurements, and now suddenly is in the 90th percentile for head circumference or weight, additional assessments must be performed to identify the reason.

Dietary Intake

The mother's dietary intake during pregnancy may provide information about the child's nutritional state, and it can be assessed for pertinent information. Obtain detailed information about the child's dietary intake when there is a potential for nutritional deficiency due to disease, knowledge deficit, or socioeconomic status. After the information is collected, compare the dietary intake with the recommended levels for a child of that age and gender (see Figure 14–1 for Food Guide Pyramid recommendations, and Appendix C ∞ for Dietary Reference Intakes). The 24-hour recall of intake, food frequency

Culture   *Growth Patterns Among Immigrant Children*

The revised growth grids now in use were standardized using a cross-section of the U.S. population and are generally reflective of most children. However, children from some other countries or cultures may fall outside of these curves. For example, new immigrants or adoptees may be in lower percentiles, and "catch up" over several months or years. Children of immigrants from developing countries tend to be larger than their parents. Even when small, children should follow normal growth patterns. For example, a child may remain at the 10th or 25th percentile for height, but continue to slowly grow and not fall to a lower percentile.

questionnaire, and dietary screening history provide a good overview of the infant's or child's intake and eating patterns. A food diary provides information about the child's precise food intake.

24-Hour Recall of Food Intake

The 24-hour diet recall is frequently used to assess adequacy of the diet. People can generally remember their intake in the past day, so results are fairly accurate; it is easy to gather the data and analyze results; only a few minutes are needed. Ask the parent or child to list all foods eaten during the past 24 hours (Figure 14–8 ➤). It is usually helpful to ask for a description of activities in the last day. Then start with the most recent event and move backward, integrating food intake into the daily schedule. For example, you might begin by saying, "You mentioned you got up early to come to the clinic today. What did Sam eat at home before you left? Did he have a snack as you traveled here or after you arrived?" While asking about the foods eaten, inquire specifically about the following:

- All meals and snacks
- Amounts of each food item consumed (have various-size measuring cups, bowls, and plates so accurate amounts can be indicated)
- Types of specific foods used, such as whole milk versus non-fat or 2%, brand names of cereals, specific types of margarine or butter
- Additives used, such as condiments, table salt, spices, milk to mix formula
- Food preparation methods, including adding fats to cook, removal or retention of fats on meats
- Vitamins and supplements, types, and doses
- Whether the intake is representative of the typical diet (in situations such as illness or vacation, intake may be different than usual)

Once the 24-hour recall is obtained, intake analysis is next. First, a quick check can be done to compare servings of various

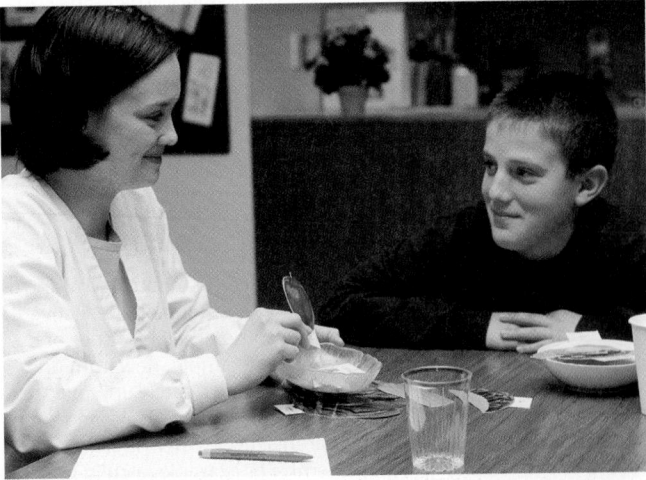

FIGURE 14–8 ➤ The nurse is interviewing a child about foods eaten in the last day. Note the models of food and dishes for accurate assessment of serving sizes.

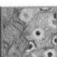

Culture — *Dietary Influences*

Each culture has eating practices that influence dietary intake. It is important to understand the foods commonly eaten by each cultural group and their contribution to the child's total nutrition. Prepare questions for the 24-hour recall that will lead to an accurate profile of intake. Perhaps questions about freshly caught fish or wild game are needed. Home-prepared sausages, cheese, berries, and garden produce may be eaten. Include food preparation techniques for added ingredients. When foods are unfamiliar, ask where they are obtained so that additional information about nutrient intake can be consulted for later nutritional analysis. Geographic location, rural versus urban settings, ethnic and racial identity, and many other factors can all influence food patterns.

food types with MyPyramid, as described earlier. Next, a detailed analysis is done to compute calories, carbohydrate, protein, and fat intake and compare them with recommended amounts. All major vitamins and minerals are also computed and comparisons made to the DRIs. This computation may be done by hand, using a book of nutrients in common foods, or may be done on the computer. Several computer programs are available, and a federal government website provides intake levels and comparisons to the RDAs—try computing your own 24-hour recall or that of a child in your clinical setting using the Healthy Eating Index. See the companion website for more information.

Clinical Tip

Parents seldom control all of the food a child eats. To help parents record an accurate food diary, remind them about all the places a child might be fed or obtain food. Older children often get snacks independently and obtain food from friends. Younger children may be fed in childcare centers.

Food Frequency Questionnaire

Food frequency questionnaires are available that can be easily administered to parents or children. Usually they ask about how often certain types of foods are eaten in a specified period such as a week. Comprehensive questionnaires can evaluate a total diet, or surveys can focus on specific items such as fruit and vegetable intake. A short questionnaire about milk intake or fruit and vegetable intake may be helpful before the start of a teaching project on nutrition to a class of school-age children. Knowing their usual intake of a food item can provide helpful information for the project. See the companion website for an example of a food frequency questionnaire.

Dietary Screening History

Ask the parent about the infant's and child's eating habits using questions in Box 14–2 and Box 14–3. (Questions about adolescents' eating patterns are in Box 14–4.) Responses provide information about the family's and individual youth's eating habits and food beliefs beyond that collected on a 24-hour dietary recall or food frequency questionnaire.

BOX 14–2 Dietary Screening History for Infants

Overview Questions

What was the infant's birth weight?

At what age did the birth weight double and triple?

Was the infant preterm?

Does the infant have any feeding problems such as difficulty sucking and swallowing, spitting up, fatigue, or fussiness?

If Infant Is Breastfed

How long does the baby nurse at each breast?

How many times daily does the infant nurse?

Is the infant growing as recommended?

How many wet diapers does the infant have each day?

Does the baby also take any milk or formula? Amount and frequency? What type?

If Infant Is Formula-Fed

What formula is used? Is it iron fortified?

How is it prepared?

Do you hold or prop the bottle for feedings?

How much formula is taken at each feeding?

How many bottles are taken each day?

Does the baby take a bottle to bed for naps or nighttime? What is in the bottle?

If Infant Is Fed Complementary Foods

At what age did the baby start eating other foods?

Cereal	Finger foods
Fruit/juices	Meats
Vegetables	Other protein sources

Do you use commercial baby food or make your own?

Does the baby eat any table foods?

How often does the baby take solid foods?

How is the baby's appetite?

Do you have any concerns about the baby's feeding habits?

Does the baby take a vitamin supplement? Fluoride?

Have there been any allergic reactions to foods? Which ones?

Does the baby spit up frequently?

Have there been any rashes?

What types of stools does the baby have? Frequency? Consistency?

BOX 14–3 Dietary Screening History for Children

- What foods or beverages does the child dislike?
- What types of food or beverage does the child especially like?
- What is the child's typical eating schedule? Meals and snacks?
- Does the child eat with the family or at separate times?
- Where does the child eat each meal?
- Who prepares the food for the family?
- What method of cooking is used? Baking? Frying? Broiling? Grilling?
- What ethnic foods are commonly eaten?
- Does the family eat in a restaurant frequently? What type?
- What type of food does the child usually order?
- Is the child on a special diet?
- Does the child need to be fed, feed himself or herself, need assistance eating, or need any adaptive devices for eating?
- What is the child's appetite like?
- Does the child take any vitamin supplements (iron, fluoride)?
- Does the child have any allergies? What are the symptoms?
- What types of regular exercise does the child get?
- Are there any concerns about the child's eating habits?

BOX 14–4 Dietary Screening History for Adolescents

- How many times do you eat (meals and snacks) daily? What meals (breakfast, lunch, dinner) do you skip at least three times per week?
- How often do you eat food from fast-food restaurants? Which ones? What are your favorite meals from these restaurants?
- Do you have a special diet? Are there foods you avoid either because of dislike for the food or your own decision, such as vegetarianism?
- Which grains have you eaten in the last few days? Vegetables? Fruits? Milk and dairy products? Meat and meat alternatives? Fats and sweets?
- Are you concerned or satisfied about your weight? Have you tried to lose weight? If so, what methods have you used?
- Do you take vitamin pills? Herbal supplements? Protein powders? Other supplements?
- Do you drink alcohol? How much? Do you use street drugs or other drugs without prescription? If so, which ones?

(Hagan et al., 2008)

Food Diary

Parents are asked to keep a food diary when the child has a nutrition problem or disorder, such as malnutrition, obesity, or type 1 diabetes, that requires dietary management. All meals and snacks, with food preparation methods and quantities eaten over a 1- to 7-day period, are recorded. Eating patterns change significantly for holidays or family gatherings, so ask parents to select typical days for the food diary or to record specific events affecting food intake. Including one weekday and one weekend day may provide the most accurate overview. Food diaries can provide a great deal of helpful information, but take the time and motivation to complete them well (Lee & Nieman, 2010). Be sure instructions are complete and that the form has a place to record amounts, preparation, events occurring, and where food was eaten. The nurse or parent may need to obtain the school lunch menu and talk with the school lunch personnel to add accurate school intake.

The nurse completes the nutritional assessment indicated for a child, and may consult with or refer the family to a dietitian or nutritionist for additional assessment and teaching.

■ COMMON NUTRITIONAL CONCERNS

Childhood Hunger

Although most Americans live in a "land of plenty," significant numbers of children periodically experience hunger. **Food security** is access at all times to enough nourishment for an active, healthy life. In contrast, **food insecurity** indicates an inability to acquire or consume adequate quality or quantity of foods in socially acceptable ways, or the uncertainty that one will be able to do so. About 16% of U.S. children live in households that experience food insecurity at times (USDA, 2009).

A major cause of hunger in children is poverty, and since 17.6% or nearly one in five children is poor, many families may be unable to provide sustainable nutrition at all times (Children's Defense Fund, 2007). Many single-income families have incomes insufficient to provide for family food needs (see Chapter 1 ∞ for a description of Temporary Assistance for Needy Families [TANF]). Families may be ineligible for food assistance programs even though they are unable to purchase enough food for all their members. Children with special nutritional needs are at particular risk because it may be more costly to buy and prepare formula or foods for a child with allergies, diabetes, or an immune disorder.

Children who have insufficient dietary intake are at risk for a wide array of health problems. They may become anemic; experience a high rate of infectious disease due to lowered immune response; have slowed developmental maturation, delayed or stunted physical growth, and learning disorders; and be at greater risk of overweight, cardiovascular disease, and diabetes in adulthood (AAP, Committee on Nutrition, 2009). Subsequently, the national and individual cost of childhood hunger is great.

Nurses evaluate families for food insecurity in a variety of hospital, clinic, school, and home settings. In addition to assessment of the individual child's nutritional status, further questions can determine families with potential problems. Administer a screening tool to identify risk in families (Box 14–5). Many parents go without food themselves in order to feed their children, so food insecurity may not necessarily have directly impacted all children at risk. However, anxiety over providing food can be a very stressful event in families and diet quality deteriorates as insecurity increases. If families have experienced food insecurity or may be likely to at some time, be sure to provide them with access to community agencies and programs that can be of assistance. (See Families Want to Know: Community Resources for Food.) What resources are available in your community to help families with food insecurity?

Overweight and Obesity

After several decades of similar statistics regarding overweight in children, the numbers are now skyrocketing. The current incidence of overweight in the United States is epidemic and is associated with a wide array of health problems, such as the appearance of type 2 diabetes in youth (Institute of Medicine, 2007). See Chapter 30 ∞ for a discussion of diabetes. Additional problems such as stroke, gallbladder disease, arthritis, cardiovascular disease, sleep disturbances, hypertension, dys-

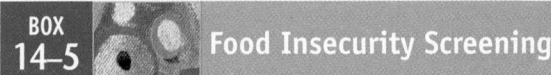

BOX 14–5 — Food Insecurity Screening

1. Does your household ever run out of money to buy food to make a meal?
2. Do you or members of your household ever eat less than you feel you should because there is not enough money for food?
3. Do you or members of your household ever cut the size of meals or skip meals because there is not enough money for food?
4. Do your children ever eat less than you feel they should because there is not enough money for food?
5. Do you ever cut the size of your children's meals or do they skip meals because there is not enough money for food?
6. Do your children ever say they are hungry because there is not enough food in the house?
7. Do you ever rely on a limited number of foods to feed your children because you are running out of money to buy food for a meal?
8. Do any of your children ever go to bed hungry because there is not enough money to buy food?

Scoring: 5–8 yes = hungry; 1–4 yes = risk of hunger

From the Washington State Department of Health.

lipidemia, respiratory problems, certain cancers, interference with physical activity and activities of daily living, social stigma, discrimination, depression, and lower self-esteem have been related to obesity rates. Prevalence of obesity (BMI greater than the 95th percentile) is 18.2% for males and 16% for females from 2 to 19 years (CDC, 2006a). When using the 85th percentile of BMI as a cutoff to indicate overweight, an additional 16% of youth are affected. Thus, 33% of youth are overweight or obese (Institute of Medicine, 2007). Since child/adolescent over-

Families Want to Know
Community Resources for Food

Supplemental Nutrition Assistance Program (SNAP)—Eligibility based on household size and income; refer students and those with low incomes, especially when they have young children; education services often available.

Child Nutrition Programs—School lunch, breakfast, and milk programs; free and lowered cost meals in schools; assist parents to apply.

Special Child Programs—Summer programs, Head Start, childcare centers, and homeless children programs may provide nutritional support in some communities.

Special Supplemental Nutrition Program for Women, Infants, and Children (WIC)—Supplemental foods and nutrition education to pregnant, breastfeeding, and postpartum women and to their young children; assessment of child growth often included.

Nutrition Education and Training Program—Nutrition education for teachers and school food service personnel.

Community Services—May include food banks, field gleaning (collecting produce from farmers' fields that will not be sold due to excess production or small blemishes), and other programs.

Find out what services are available to provide food and nutrition education in your community. Make a list for use in clinical settings with families.

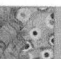
Overweight is more common among some ethnic and socioeconomic groups. Lack of knowledge about foods and physical activity, limited access to fresh produce and safe places to exercise, easy access to increasing numbers of fast foods, and ethnic differences in metabolism may constitute risk factors. Lower income and Hispanic, African American, and Native American ethnic identities are associated with higher incidence of overweight, especially among women. National goals to eliminate health disparities in income and ethnic groups have been set (U.S. Department of Health and Human Services, 2006).

weight and related health problems frequently track into adulthood, the implications for health care are obvious.

Many reasons are cited for the increase in overweight children. The number of calories consumed by children is not generally increasing, but children tend to exercise less, particularly on a daily basis. They infrequently walk or ride bikes, either because of the convenience of driving or due to unsafe neighborhoods. Television viewing is very high among youth; television and other screen activities account for an average of 5.5 hours daily. Even children under 6 years spend an average of 2 hours daily on screen activities, and 26% of those less than 2 years have television sets in their bedrooms (Rideout & Hamel, 2006). Inactive pursuits do not require high caloric energy, leading to an imbalance in intake and demand for calories. Additionally, viewing is often accompanied by ingestion of high-calorie foods, and subjects children to media advertisements for unhealthy foods. Overall obesity prevalence increases with amount of screen time activity (Urrutia-Rojas & Menchaca, 2006).

The percentage of calories from fat consumed in the United States is among the highest in the world. Although no more than 25–35% of calories should come from total dietary fat, and no more than 10% from saturated fat, about 35% of calories consumed by children in the United States are supplied by fat and 12% by saturated fat (Institute of Medicine, 2006). High levels of dietary fat are associated with higher cholesterol levels and decreased activity. The high rate of dietary fat is related to the large amount of fast food consumed. It is also influenced by snacking since snacks are often nutrient poor and calorie dense.

 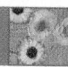
As the rates of obesity increase in youth, new treatments are attempted. Although bariatric surgery has been found to be an effective weight loss strategy for excessive obesity, less is known about its effects in children. Thus far, a few centers have developed criteria for performing bariatric surgery on adolescents. However, obesity itself and bariatric surgery both include risks for adolescents. Bariatric procedures should be preceded by less invasive attempts at treatment, the family must receive comprehensive counseling about risks and benefits, and long-term follow-up is essential (Browne & Inge, 2009; Caniano, 2009). What informed consent is needed in these situations? What ethical dilemmas does this treatment present for health care providers?

Nursing Management

Goals of nursing management are to prevent new cases of overweight, identify children who are overweight, and support youth and families to establish healthy lifestyles that promote weight loss and maintenance of recommended weight (Small, Anderson, & Melnyk, 2007). Perform assessment of height, weight, and BMI. Measure blood pressure and analyze if it is within normal limits. Evaluate amount of screen activities and physical activity levels.

Nurses can assist parents and children in building good nutritional and exercise habits throughout life, thus decreasing the incidence of overweight and its attendant health risks. Advise parents that television viewing should be limited to a maximum of 2 hours daily, and that television and video games should not be placed in children's bedrooms. Daily exercise routines of at least 30–60 minutes can be included in most families. Aim to meet the current recommendation of 60 minutes daily for children with some activity including muscle strengthening and flexibility. Also, teach about the MyPyramid Food Guide and provide guidance for its integration into a healthy life. Healthy snacks include fruits, vegetables, grains, and nuts. "Supersizing" fast foods and eating out often should be avoided.

Risks for poor health often cluster in individuals and families because of both genetic factors and common lifestyles. Be alert for situations in which parents are overweight, or children have elevated blood pressure, exercise infrequently, or are in upper percentiles for weight, BMI, or skinfold. Presence of risk factors necessitates further dietary and risk assessment so that a management plan can be implemented. Nursing care is summarized on the accompanying Nursing Care Plan.

Food Safety

Every year in the United States, about 76 million people contract foodborne illnesses. Some are quite mild, whereas others can be severe. About 300,000 people are hospitalized and 5,000 die from these illnesses (CDC, 2007). Children are at greater risk of severe illness and death from food and water than adults, due to their immature gastrointestinal and immune systems. Children

When girls experience menarche before 11 years of age, they are more frequently overweight. The National Institute of Child Health and Human Development Study of Early Child Care and Youth Development found that higher body mass index (BMI) scores in girls and higher rates of change in BMI from 3 to 6 years of age were associated with early puberty in childhood (Lee, Appugliese, Kaciroti, et al., 2007). Another longitudinal study found that rapid infancy weight gain was associated with increased risk of obesity at 5 and 8 years of age (Dunger, Ahmed, & Ong, 2006). Early weight monitoring, even at the very young ages of infancy, preschool, and early school age, is important. The nurse should also remain alert for signs of breast development in fourth- or fifth-grade students and early menarche (grade 6). Such youth may already be overweight and should be identified for efforts directed at obesity prevention. Such prevention efforts are needed to decrease risks of obesity such as type 2 diabetes.

NURSING CARE PLAN

The Child Who Is Overweight

INTERVENTION	RATIONALE	EXPECTED OUTCOME
1. Imbalanced Nutrition: More than Body Requirements related to excessive intake in comparison to metabolic needs		
NIC Priority Intervention: *Weight reduction assistance:* Facilitating loss of weight and body fat		**NOC Suggested Outcome:** *Weight control:* Personal actions resulting in achievement and maintenance of optimum body weight for health
Goal: Child will demonstrate adequate intake of all nutrients without excessive energy intake.		
■ Perform thorough nutritional assessment of the child.	■ Assessment assists in identification of dietary risks and strengths as well as health conditions related to nutrition.	Child meets dietary requirements while achieving weight and body mass index goal.
■ Share results of the assessment with the child and family by showing weight, height, and body mass index grids.	■ Many families do not consider their child overweight. Concrete information about the child's size in comparison with recommendations assists in establishing the importance of weight management.	
■ Assess access to sufficient nutritious foods for the family at all times.	■ Food insecurity promotes inadequate intake alternating with excess intake of high-caloric foods.	

■ Identify with the child and family two to three target areas to begin weight management. Examples might include:
  ■ Having fast food only once a week.
  ■ Switching to low-fat dairy products.
  ■ Keeping two more fresh fruits and vegetables in the house and two less snack foods.
	■ Changing dietary patterns drastically is difficult and may lead to giving up the attempt at weight management. Partnering with the family to set goals enhances the chance of success.	

■ Integrate nutrition information into each visit. Examples of topics include:
  ■ Dietary requirements for age group.
  ■ Effects of simple sugar and fat intake on weight.
  ■ Beneficial effects of fruits, vegetables, whole grains, and nonfat dairy.
  ■ Reading food labels.
  ■ Healthy choices in fast-food restaurants.
  ■ Calculation of fat content of foods.
	■ Nutrition information is best learned in an ongoing program.	

■ Use growth grids to help the child and family establish a weight reduction or maintenance goal.	■ Goals motivate families to achieve desired health behaviors. The goal for a young child may be weight maintenance so that as the child grows in height, the correct proportion is reached. Weight reduction may be needed for older children or youth who are very obese.	

NURSING CARE PLAN

The Child Who Is Overweight (continued)

INTERVENTION	RATIONALE	EXPECTED OUTCOME
2. Readiness for Enhanced Family Coping related to need to foster health of family member		
NIC Priority Intervention: *Health system guidance:* Facilitating child's use of appropriate nutrition and health services to foster weight control		**NOC Priority Outcome:** *Health promoting behavior:* Actions to promote, sustain, and increase wellness
Goal: Family will assist child to manage stressors and to develop new strategies to support weight control goals.		
▪ Include key family members in some of the counseling sessions with the overweight child.	▪ Key family members are those who purchase food, provide support for the child, and participate in health decisions.	Child expresses satisfaction with family understanding and support of weight management goals.
▪ Encourage the family to eat together at least once daily if possible or to increase the number of meals eaten together each week.	▪ The family is an important support system in weight loss programs. Eating as a family or in a social situation can provide a chance to promote healthy foods; intake is generally lower in fat and calories than when eating alone.	
▪ Seek a resource for the child to be monitored about twice monthly; this may be a health care provider, nutritionist, school nurse, or other person.	▪ This provides an opportunity to monitor the child's progress and offer support, additional information, and problem-solving techniques.	
3. Activity Intolerance related to sedentary lifestyle		
NIC Priority Intervention: *Exercise promotion:* Facilitating regular exercise to maintain and increase endurance and energy use		**NOC Priority Outcome:** *Endurance:* Extent that energy enables the child to sustain activity
Goal: Child will demonstrate activity tolerance by adequate oxygenation, respiratory effort, and ability to speak during brisk walking, biking, or other activity.		
▪ Establish a daily exercise routine beginning with 15–30 minutes of daily walking.	▪ Starting with brief amounts of exercise makes the child feel comfortable and enhances the potential for success.	Child demonstrates ability to engage in moderate activity for 60 minutes with minimal respiratory discomfort.
▪ Gradually increase activity over 1–2 months until 60 minutes of daily exercise is maintained.	▪ A gradual increase as the cardiovascular and respiratory systems adapt is generally comfortable for children; 60 minutes of moderate activity daily is recommended for children.	
▪ Use activities enjoyed by the child and suggest options as necessary; refer the family to community resources such as swimming pools, organized sports, and biking groups.	▪ Activities the child enjoys will be more likely to remain in usual activity patterns; exercising with others in groups increases motivation.	
▪ Have families plan at least one to two activities they can do together each week.	▪ This fosters family relationships and provides the child with support and motivation.	
▪ Limit screen activities to a maximum of 2 hours daily. Have the child keep a log of hours of television, video games, computer, and other similar activities. Tell the child never to snack while doing screen activities.	▪ Increased use of screen activities is related to poor dietary habits, increased sedentary behaviors, and excess weight.	

(continued)

NURSING CARE PLAN

The Child Who Is Overweight (continued)

INTERVENTION	RATIONALE	EXPECTED OUTCOME
■ Ask about use of tobacco in children in fifth grade or higher.	■ Most adults who smoke began the habit in childhood; middle school years are the most common age for smoking initiation.	
■ Inquire about exposure to environmental tobacco smoke at all ages.	■ Smoking by others in the household can be harmful to children.	
■ Perform teaching to discourage tobacco use or offer cessation programs as needed.	■ Smoking decreases respiratory reserves and worsens several cardiovascular disease risks.	

4. Chronic Low Self-Esteem related to weight

NIC Priority Intervention:		NOC Priority Outcome:
Self-esteem enhancement: Assisting the child to increase personal judgment of self-worth		*Quality of life and self-esteem:* Expressed satisfaction with life circumstances and positive judgment of self-worth

Goal: Child expresses positive perception of self-worth and confidence in ability to deal with issues related to weight.

■ Facilitate development of a positive outlook by exposing the child to others who have been successful with weight loss.	■ A positive outlook increases motivation and feelings of self-efficacy.	Child speaks positively about accomplishments in weight control management.
■ Praise the child for weight loss, weight maintenance, increased physical activity, and other achievements. Help the child establish rewards for meeting goals, such as purchase of new clothing.	■ Positive reinforcement enhances judgment of self-worth and pride in accomplishments.	
■ Partner with parents so they understand the value of praise and never label the child by derogatory words such as *fat*.	■ Family members are usually the most intimate support system for the child.	

who are immunocompromised are at even greater risk. The most common pathogens are *Campylobacter*, *Salmonella*, *Shigella*, *Cryptosporidium*, *Listeria*, *Yersinia*, and *Escherichia coli*; infants are at extremely high risk of *Campylobacter*, *Rotavirus*, and *Salmonella* illness (CDC, 2007).

Nursing Alert

Worldwide, over 3 million people die of illness related to unsafe drinking water each year and most of those deaths are among children. The World Health Organization focuses on this important health problem. Children are more prone to illnesses such as diarrhea and dehydration when drinking contaminated water. Caution families with children to be sure water supplies are safe during travel and to use bottled or purified water in areas with potentially unsafe water supplies.

Foodborne illness transmission is associated with food preparation and storage practices, lack of adequate training of retail employees regarding foods and hygiene, and increasing amounts and types of foods being imported from various geographic areas. Some examples of contaminated foods in the last few years include undercooked hamburger meat and cross-contamination of salad bar items from meats, fish, unpasteurized apple cider, milk, raw or undercooked eggs, green onions, raw spinach, prepackaged salad and delicatessen meat, berries, and sprouts. While most infected persons experience acute gastroenteritis (see Chapter 25 ∞), some can develop complications such as hemolytic uremic syndrome (see Chapter 26 ∞) or thrombocytic purpura (see Chapter 23 ∞). A wide array of other symptoms may include neurologic and respiratory problems, fever, jaundice, or arthritis. Health personnel should be alert to symptoms of foodborne illness and integrate teaching regularly so that families can decrease risks. Recommend that families avoid consumption of unpasteurized milk, raw or undercooked oysters, raw or undercooked eggs, raw or undercooked ground beef, and undercooked poultry (CDC, 2007). Find information regarding current outbreaks at the companion website. See Families Want to Know: Foodborne Safety Guidelines.

Food may carry products other than microorganisms that can be harmful. An example is mercury, which may be concentrated in certain types of fish. This metal can cause harm to the developing nervous system of fetuses, infants, and young

Four Key Food Safety Practices:

1. Clean: Wash hands and surfaces often.
2. Separate: Avoid cross-contamination.
3. Cook: Cook to proper temperatures.
4. Chill: Refrigerate promptly.

Data from: Partnership for Food Safety Education, *Safe Food Handling.* Retrieved from http://www.fightbac.org/content/view/6/11/

Culture *Vitamin A Deficiency*

Vitamin A deficiency is common in developing countries. The vitamin is found in liver, dairy products, and fish. Provitamin A sources are yellow and dark green vegetables. The vitamin is fat soluble and stored in the liver. When deficient, children develop night blindness, vision loss, and high rates of infection. Public health efforts have been directed at identifying children with low vitamin A status and providing the vitamin in capsule form or in commonly ingested foods.

children when consumed regularly; infants of mothers consuming high levels of mercury in fish may be born small for gestational age (Ramon, Ballester, Aguinagalde, et al., 2009). The U.S. Food and Drug Administration (FDA) and Environmental Protection Agency (EPA) note that fish are an important part of a healthy diet, but that certain recommendations should be followed to lower the risk of mercury's detrimental effects. The following guidelines are for women who may become pregnant, are pregnant, or are breastfeeding, and for young children:

- Eliminate shark, swordfish, king mackerel, and tilefish from the diet.
- Eat up to 12 ounces (two average meals) a week of a variety of low-mercury fish and shellfish, such as shrimp, canned light tuna, salmon, pollock, and catfish. Albacore or white tuna has more mercury than light tuna, so limit white tuna to one meal per week.
- Check for local advisories about safety of fish caught in your area. In the absence of advice, up to 6 ounces (one meal) per week may be eaten from local waters. Do not eat other fish during that week (U.S. Food and Drug Administration, 2004).

Common Dietary Deficiencies

Although there can be deficits in nearly all nutrients, certain deficiencies are more common in childhood. Either limitations in the food supply or patterns of dietary intake are the cause of most deficiencies. Children with certain disease processes, such as metabolic diseases, may have difficulty absorbing or using nutrients ingested (see Chapter 30 ∞ for a discussion of inborn errors of metabolism). The nutrient deficiencies present in a population are a result of genetic factors, characteristics of the food supply, and intake patterns of particular groups.

Iron

Newborns have a store of iron obtained from their mothers in the uterus, if the maternal nutritional state was satisfactory and the baby is normal gestational age. Breast milk contains little iron, but the iron it does contain has high bioavailability. By 4 to 6 months of age, however, the baby's iron stores begin to decrease. A dietary source of iron must be added by about 6 months of age. Enriched rice cereal is commonly used to meet these initial iron needs. In babies who do not have ade-

quate stores or do not take in enough iron, iron deficiency **anemia** (a reduction in the number of red blood cells) can result (Figure 14–9 ➤). Feeding cow milk during infancy can also cause anemia by irritating the gut and leading to small but consistent loss of blood from the gastrointestinal tract; cow milk should not be fed during the first year of life. When formulas are used, they should be iron fortified to help avoid iron deficiency anemia.

Adolescent females comprise another group commonly deficient in iron related to loss of blood in menses, metabolic need of the growth spurt, and poor dietary balance due to sporadic dieting. Further discussion of the symptoms and treatment of iron deficiency anemia can be found in Chapter 23 ∞. See Table 14–6 for food sources of iron.

Calcium

Calcium is an essential nutrient for bone development during childhood and adolescence. An increased intake of soda pop and fruit juices is related to a decrease in calcium intake, especially among adolescents. During the adolescent growth spurt, almost 40% of the adult bone mass is accumulated (AAP, Committee on Nutrition, 2009). Inadequate intake puts the person at risk for osteoporosis later in life, as there is minimal or no ability to

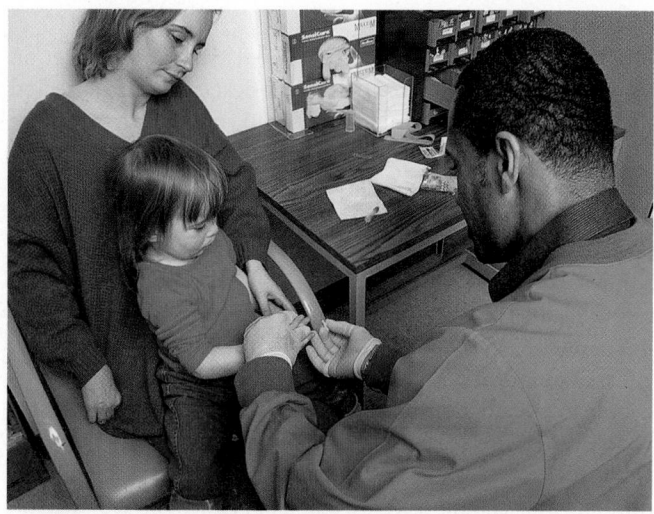

FIGURE 14–9 ➤ Head Start centers participate in screening programs to identify children at risk for anemia. This child sits on the mother's lap while the nurse performs a fingerstick to measure hematocrit. What is the expected hematocrit level in a young child?

TABLE 14–6	Food Sources of Micronutrients		
Iron	Calcium	Vitamin D	Folate
• Meats • Iron-fortified formula • Iron-fortified baby cereal • Enhanced absorption if taken together with vitamin C • Present in breast milk in a small amount, but is very well absorbed	• Milk and milk products • Egg yolks • Grains • Legumes • Nuts • Soybeans	• Milk and formulas fortified with the vitamin • Eggs • Butter • Margarine	• Bread and other products with flour • Yeast • Spinach, avocado, green leafy vegetables • Beans and peas • Liver • Fruits

make up for earlier deficits. Although genetic variables account for some of the influence on adult bone mass, increasing calcium intake has been shown to promote bone formation. While the recommended daily intake for adolescents is 1300 mg, the average intake for adolescent males is 1145 mg and for females is only 700 to 850 mg—only about half of the recommended level (AAP, Committee on Nutrition, 2009; Moore, Bradlee, Di Gao, et al., 2008). See Table 14–6 for common food sources of calcium.

Adolescents at highest risk for impaired bone development include female athletes and others who diet to a magnified degree to maintain slimness. Teens who exercise excessively may manifest the "female athlete triad" of disordered eating and extreme exercise that leads to excessive thinness, amenorrhea, and osteopenia (AAP, Committee on Nutrition, 2009; Hoch, Pajewski, Moraski, et al., 2009; Mendelsohn & Warren, 2010). A high rate of fractures and osteomalacia can result, in addition to an extreme risk of osteoporosis in adulthood. Asking about menstrual patterns, as well as exercise and diet, can be combined with physical measurements of height and weight to obtain pertinent information about the teen athlete. See the discussion of other disordered eating patterns such as anorexia nervosa and bulimia nervosa later in this chapter.

Vitamin D

Vitamin D deficiencies were once believed to be rare; however, an increase in cases of vitamin D–deficient rickets has been observed in recent years. This vitamin is needed to enhance absorption of calcium and ensure bone mineralization. Although the vitamin can be synthesized in the skin upon exposure to sunlight, the amount of sunlight needed for manufacture is variable and determined by the amount of skin exposed, the color of the skin, the latitude, and the time of year. Because of this variability it is now recommended that all infants and children receive a minimum intake of 400 International Units daily. This vitamin is needed to enhance absorption of calcium, so a lack of vitamin D can contribute to calcium deficiency as well. Human milk contains little vitamin D, so breastfed infants should receive 400 International Units of vitamin D daily. Formula-fed infants and older children drinking milk should receive a daily supplement of 400 International Units if consuming less than 1000 mL of formula or milk (1000 mL of formula and of milk contain 400 International Units of vitamin D). Likewise, adolescents who do not consume 400 International Units via diet should receive the amount in a supple-

ment (Wagner, Greer, & Section on Breastfeeding, 2008). See Table 14–6 for common food sources of vitamin D.

Folic Acid

Epidemiologic evidence has linked increasing maternal folic acid (the most common form of folate in the human body) intake with decreased incidence of neural tube defects such as spina bifida in offspring of mothers. Folate levels are low among adolescents, putting them at particular risk of birth defects when they have infants. The FDA approved fortification of cereals and breads with folate to decrease the population risk of related congenital anomalies. All women from 15–45 years should consume 0.4 mg of folic acid daily, and pregnant women should consume 0.6 mg daily. See Table 14–6 for common food sources of folate.

Protein-Energy Malnutrition

While the micronutrient deficiencies previously described are the most common problems in developed countries, macronutrient deficiencies are the most common nutritional problems worldwide. Kwashiorkor indicates protein deficiency, and marasmus is a lack of energy-producing calories; both deficiencies often occur together and are referred to as protein-energy malnutrition (PEM). Protein deficiency manifests with edema, leading to the large abdomens and rounded faces seen in severely malnourished children. Other symptoms include scant, depigmented hair; skin changes; and decreased serum proteins. It can occur following severe diarrhea or other infection in susceptible children. Caloric deficiency results in emaciation, decreased energy levels, and retarded development (see the Clinical Manifestations table on page 345). PEM may occur when a child is weaned in order for the mother to provide breast milk to a new baby. Adoptees and immigrants to developed countries sometimes manifest with at least mild PEM, so careful nutritional assessment is needed to provide adequate nutrition.

Celiac Disease

Celiac disease, or gluten-sensitive enteropathy, is a chronic malabsorption syndrome (van Koppen, Schweizer, Csizmadia, et al., 2009). About 30% of the population has one of the celiac genetic alterations; only about 3% develop the disease (Snyder, Young, Green, et al., 2008). It is more common among members of the same family and in children with Down syndrome and Turner syndrome (National Institute of Diabetes and Digestive and Kidney Disease [NIDDK], 2008).

Celiac disease is an immunologic disorder (Richey, Howdle, Shaw, et al., 2009) characterized by an intolerance for gluten, a protein found in wheat, barley, rye, and oats. Inability to digest glutenin and gliadin (protein fractions) results in the accumulation of the amino acid glutamine, which is toxic to mucosal cells in the intestine. Damage to the villi ultimately impairs the absorptive process in the small intestine.

In the early stages, celiac disease affects fat absorption, resulting in excretion of large quantities of fat in the stools (steatorrhea). Stools are greasy, foul smelling, frothy, and excessive. As changes in the villi continue, the absorption of protein, carbohydrates, calcium, iron, folate, and vitamins A, D, E, K, and B_{12} becomes impaired.

Symptoms usually occur when solid foods containing gluten are introduced to the child's diet (generally between 6 months and 2 years of age), although celiac disease is sometimes first diagnosed in adulthood. The classic features of celiac disease in infancy include chronic diarrhea, growth impairment, and abdominal distention. The child also demonstrates poor appetite, lack of energy, and muscle wasting with hypotonia (Gelfond & Fasano, 2006). Atypical features are present in children diagnosed with delayed-onset celiac disease around 5–7 years of age. Symptoms include nausea, vomiting, recurrent abdominal pain, and bloating. Other symptoms may include delayed growth, iron deficiency, defects in tooth enamel, and abnormal liver function tests (Gelfond & Fasano, 2006).

Diagnosis is confirmed through measurement of fecal fat content, duodenal biopsy, and improvement with removal of gluten products from the diet. Serum screening tests for IgA antiendomysial antibodies (EMA) and IgA antitissue transglutaminase antibodies (tTGA) are used for diagnosis (NIDDK, 2008).

Management of the disease is total exclusion of gluten from the diet. This gluten-free diet is a lifetime treatment. Barley, wheat, and rye are completely eliminated; oats may be tolerated. Symptoms generally improve within a few days to weeks.

The intestinal villi return to normal in about 6 months. Growth should improve steadily, and height and weight should reach normal range within 1 year. Vitamin supplementation may be needed for a period of time if the child has become malnourished.

Nursing Management

Nursing care focuses on supporting the parents in maintaining a gluten-free diet for the child. Thoroughly explain the disease process to the parents. Emphasize the necessity of following a gluten-free diet. Help parents to understand that celiac disease requires lifelong dietary modifications that should not be discontinued when the child is symptom-free. Discontinuation of the diet places the child at risk for growth retardation and the development of gastrointestinal (GI) cancers in adulthood. All children with celiac disease should be seen by a dietitian several times during childhood. Nutritional assessment and continued teaching to maintain a gluten-free diet take place at these visits. Substitutions and recipes using potato, rice, soy, quinoa, buckwheat, or bean flours and foods are provided. Dietary manage-ment is made difficult by hidden gluten in many prepared foods, such as chocolate candy, prepared meats, ice cream, soups, condiments, and food starch.

An infant or toddler's diet is easily monitored at home. When the child enters school, however, ensuring adherence to dietary restrictions becomes more difficult. In addition to easily identified gluten-based foods, such as bread, cake, doughnuts, cookies, and crackers, the child must also avoid processed foods that contain gluten as filler. School-age children and adolescents are often tempted to eat these foods, especially when among peers. Emphasize the need for compliance while meeting the child's developmental needs.

The child's special dietary needs can place a financial burden on the family. Parents need to purchase prepared rice or corn flour products or make their own bread and bakery products. Advise parents that getting a dietary prescription enables them to deduct the cost of these ingredients and commercially prepared products as a medical expense.

Because the entire family must adapt to the diet, parents and siblings need support and management skills. For information and support, refer parents and children to several organizations, including the American Celiac Society, the Celiac Sprue Association/United States of America, and the Gluten Intolerance Group.

Expected outcomes of nursing care include the following:

- The child receives adequate nutrition to support growth and development needs.
- Growth and developmental milestones appropriate for age are achieved.
- The family demonstrates understanding of dietary restrictions and appropriate meal planning.

Feeding and Eating Disorders

Deficiencies in food intake related to available nutrients and safety of the food supply were discussed in the previous section. In addition to these issues of availability, nutrient intake is affected by psychological issues of individuals as well. Disorders of food intake span the entire developmental spectrum, and can affect pregnant women, young children, and adolescents. Some of the most common disorders of feeding and eating are discussed in the following text.

Colic

Colic is a feeding disorder characterized by paroxysmal abdominal pain and severe crying. The crying generally lasts at least 3 hours and occurs at least 3 days per week. Crying episodes peak around 6 weeks of age and generally resolve by 3–4 months of age (Hyman, Milla, Benninga, et al., 2006).

The etiology of colic is unknown. Proposed causes include feeding too rapidly and swallowing large amounts of air.

Characteristically the infant cries loudly and continuously, often for several hours. The infant's face may become flushed. The abdomen is distended and tense. Often the infant draws up the legs and clenches the hands. Episodes occur at the same time each day, usually in the late afternoon or early evening. Crying may stop only when the child is completely exhausted or after passage of flatus or stool.

The symptoms initially may resemble intestinal obstruction or peritoneal infection. These conditions must be ruled out along with sensitivity to formula. Treatment is supportive; no general medical consensus exists on effective treatments or interventions for colic. Some health care providers recommend medications such as simethicone (Mylicon) drops. Some recommend changing formula to a soy formula or an elemental formula such as Pregestimil.

Nursing care requires a thorough history of the infant's diet and daily schedule and the events surrounding episodes of colicky behavior. Assessment of the infant's feeding patterns and diet includes type, frequency, and amount of feeding (if breastfeeding, maternal diet history), and frequency of burping. Inquire about episodes of colic for onset, duration, and characteristics of cry. Ask the parents what measures are used to relieve crying and their effectiveness.

When possible, observe the feeding method. Parents of infants with colic are often tired and frustrated. They require frequent reassurance that they are not to blame for the infant's condition. Suggest ways of alleviating some of the infant's symptoms and discomfort. An important consideration is the significant impact of colic on families. Colic can place extreme stress and fatigue on the family. Active support and counseling for the mother and other family members is essential to reduce the risk of abuse to the infant (Moore, 2009). See Families Want to Know: Suggestions for Alleviating Colic.

Pica

Pica is an eating disorder characterized by ingestion of nonfood items or food items consumed in abnormal quantities or forms. Examples of ingested items include starch, peeling paint, paper, soil components, flour, and coffee grounds. Clinical manifestations include zinc and iron deficiencies as well as symptoms of lead or other heavy metal poisoning (see Chapter 17 ∞) if these substances are contained in peeling paint or other ingested material. Pica most commonly manifests in pregnancy when women have abnormal cravings for nonfood products, and this can seriously impair the developing fetus. Some children also manifest ingestion of abnormal amounts of nonfood items and fail to take in adequate nutrients from food. Treatment for children involves removing them from the substances, ensuring an adequate and nutritious diet, and treating any dietary deficiencies noted.

Rumination

Rumination is a rare and serious form of chronic regurgitation of recently ingested food into the mouth, followed by rechewing and reswallowing or expulsion of the material (Hyman et al., 2006). Chewing movements and mouthing of fingers often precede or accompany regurgitation. Close observation may reveal the infant or child actively initiating gagging with the tongue and fingers.

Rumination is associated with poor maternal–infant bonding and depressive symptoms in children and adolescents (Rood, Roelofs, Bogels, et al., 2009). This behavior is seen in infants deprived of tactile, visual, or auditory stimuli for long periods. The infant substitutes repetitive self-stimulation for the lack of appropriate external stimulation. Rumination can be life threatening because it can lead to weight loss, growth failure, malnutrition,

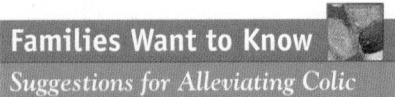

Families Want to Know
Suggestions for Alleviating Colic

Provide Rhythmic Movement

Use front-carrying sling carriers.

Place the baby in an infant swing (battery-operated swing provides continuous motion).

Take the infant for a car ride.

Take the infant for a ride in a stroller.

Alternate Positions

Swaddle the infant in a soft, stretchy blanket with knees flexed up against the abdomen or with legs straight.

Place the infant prone on the parent's arm, supporting the body with one hand under the abdomen and cradling the head in the crook of the other arm.

Reduce Environmental Stimuli

Respond to crying.

Provide quiet, soothing music.

Prevent sudden loud noises.

Avoid smoking.

Provide Various Tactile Stimuli

Offer a pacifier.

Provide a warm bath.

Massage the abdomen.

Alter Intake

Feed smaller amounts and burp frequently.

Use a bottle with a collapsible bag to prevent sucking air.

Breastfeeding mothers: Eliminate milk products and spicy or gas-producing foods.

Hold upright for 30 minutes after feeding.

and electrolyte imbalance. During childhood and adolescence, rumination has been associated in some studies with depression.

Diagnostic evaluation focuses on ruling out an organic cause and determining the degree and type of nutritional deficiencies. The child should be observed ruminating to help confirm the diagnosis. Treatment involves correcting the nutritional deficits and developing normal feeding patterns. An interdisciplinary approach with medical and nursing staff and social services is often needed to help parents meet the child's nutritional and psychologic needs (Hyman et al., 2006).

Nursing care focuses on establishing a warm, caring relationship with the child and the parents. Making eye contact with the infant, providing food regularly, and stimulating the infant through all the senses are ways to break the pattern of rumination. Children and adolescents should receive depression screening and can be referred for psychological care (see Chapter 28 ∞).

Parents need to be included in the infant's or child's care. Discuss proper nutrition and demonstrate feeding techniques and interactions that promote development. Determine the parents' support needs and make a referral to social service agencies as appropriate.

Feeding Disorder of Infancy and Early Childhood (Failure to Thrive)

Feeding disorder of infancy and early childhood, or failure to thrive (FTT), describes a syndrome in which infants or young children fail to eat enough food to be adequately nourished. This disorder accounts for 5–10% of pediatric hospitalizations in children under 1 year of age, and many more children are managed in community settings (Stanton, Jenson, Behrman, et al., 2007).

Etiology and Pathophysiology The cause of FTT can be organic, as in congenital acquired immunodeficiency syndrome (AIDS) (see Chapter 22 ∞), inborn errors of metabolism (see Chapter 3 ∞), esophageal reflux, and neurologic disease (see Chapters 25 and 27 ∞). However, most cases of FTT have no organic cause. FTT resulting from nonorganic causes is called feeding disorder of infancy or early childhood.

Infants and children whose parents or caretakers experience poverty, depression, substance abuse, mental retardation, or psychosis are at risk for this disorder. Parents may be socially and emotionally isolated, or may lack knowledge of infant nutritional and nurturing needs. A multifactorial and reciprocal interaction pattern may exist whereby the parent does not offer enough food or is not responsive to the infant's hunger cues, and the infant is irritable, is not soothed, and does not give clear cues about hunger. Preterm and small-for-gestational-age babies more commonly have eating disorders.

Clinical Manifestations The characteristics of this feeding disorder are persistent failure to eat adequately with no weight gain or with weight loss in a child under 6 years of age, which is not associated with other medical conditions or mental disorders, and is not caused by lack of or unavailability of food. Weight is generally less than the 5th percentile, and weight-for-length is less than 80% of ideal weight (Olsen, 2006; AAP, 2009). Infants with feeding disorders refuse food, may have erratic sleep patterns, are irritable and difficult to soothe, fall well under expected growth patterns, and are often developmentally delayed (Figure 14–10 ➤).

COLLABORATIVE CARE

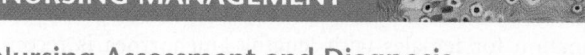

A thorough history and physical examination are needed to rule out any chronic physical illness. The infant or child may be hospitalized so that health care providers can establish a routine for feeding and sleeping. The goals of treatment are to provide adequate caloric and nutritional intake, promote normal growth and development, and assist parents in developing feeding routines and responding to the infant's cues of physical and psychological hunger.

NURSING MANAGEMENT

Nursing Assessment and Diagnosis

Nursing assessment of the child by the nurse is essential for establishing the best intervention plan. Accurate measurement of weight, height, BMI, and percentiles each time any child is seen for health care provides an important record of growth patterns over time. This helps in identification of the child with an eating disorder. The child's activity level, developmental milestones, and interaction patterns provide important information. When feeding the child, the nurse observes how the child indicates hunger or satiety, the ability of the child to be soothed,

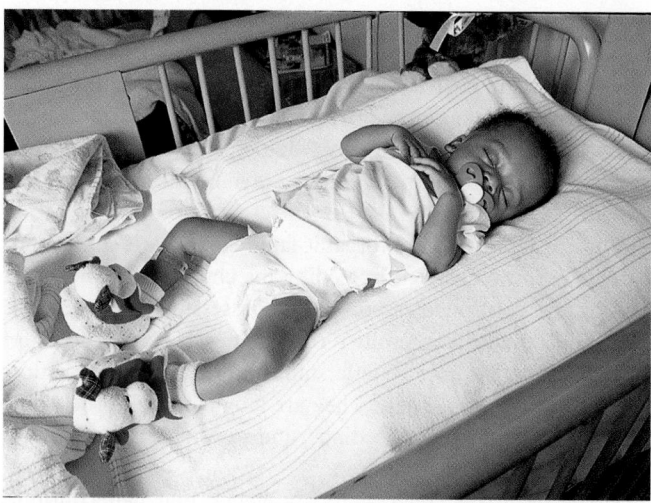

FIGURE 14–10 ➤ Infants with failure to thrive may not look severely malnourished, but they fall well below the expected weight and height norms for their age. This infant, who appears to be about 4 months old, is actually 8 months old. He has been hospitalized for examination of his failure to thrive and treatment of the eating disorder.

and general interaction patterns such as eye contact, touch, and cuddliness.

Parents are questioned about stresses in their lives; these may prevent appropriate interaction with the child. Asking about the pregnancy and delivery can elicit information about early disturbances in the child–parent relationship. Are there other children in the family, and have eating problems occurred with them? Observe the child and parent behaviors while they feed the child; cues given by each person and interactional modes such as rocking, singing, talking, eye contact, and body postures are important.

Following are nursing diagnoses pertinent for the young child with an eating disorder:

- Imbalanced Nutrition: Less than Body Requirements related to inability to ingest proper amounts of food
- Delayed Growth and Development related to inadequate food intake
- Risk for Impaired Parenting related to lack of knowledge about the child's nutritional needs
- Fatigue related to malnutrition

Planning and Implementation

Nursing care centers on performing a thorough history and physical assessment, observing parent–child interactions during feeding times, and providing necessary teaching to enable parents to

Culture — *Growth Measurement*

Each child should maintain a height and weight growth pattern similar to the population standard. Asian American children may normally be below the 5th percentile on growth charts and not have an eating disorder. Suspect an eating disorder when the infant or child falls one standard deviation below his or her own curve and either fails to gain weight or loses weight over several months.

respond appropriately to their child's needs. The child is often hospitalized initially and evaluated for potential organic causes while staff members feed the child. Accurate weights, nutritional assessments, and developmental evaluation should be done to see if the child grows more normally. Additional diagnostic tests may be carried out at this time to rule out organic causes of the poor growth.

Once a diagnosis of nonorganic failure to thrive is confirmed, parents become involved in feeding the child. Observations of feeding and continued careful physical assessments are needed. The child's intake is carefully recorded at each meal or feeding. Parents are taught how to understand and respond to the child's cues of hunger and satiety. They are taught to hold, rock, and touch the infant during feedings, and to establish eye contact with infants and older children.

Upon discharge, referral to an agency that can continue monitoring the home situation is needed. This provides an opportunity to observe feeding during a home visit and evaluate stresses and behavior patterns among family members. Frequent growth measurement and development must be ensured so the child is adequately nourished. Parents may need referral to community resources to help them manage stressful situations in their lives and to enhance their parenting skills.

Evaluation

Expected outcomes of nursing care include the following:

- Adequate growth and normal development of the infant is achieved.
- An improved parent–child relationship is established.

Anorexia Nervosa

Anorexia nervosa is a potentially life-threatening type of disordered eating that occurs primarily in teenage girls and young women. An estimated 5% of young women and 1% of young men in the United States are affected by anorexia nervosa or a related eating disorder (American Dietetic Association, 2006). The typical patient is White and from a middle- to upper-middle-class family. Age at onset varies, and incidence peaks at 12 to 13 years and again at 17 to 18 years.

Etiology and Pathophysiology   Many causes are believed to contribute to the onset of anorexia. Cultural overemphasis on thinness may contribute to the overconcern with dieting, body image, and fear of becoming fat experienced by many adolescents. The media in developed countries portray an image of extreme thinness as positive. Chemical changes have been found in the brain and blood of patients with anorexia, leading to theories about a biological cause. Often a significant life stress, loss, or change precedes the onset of anorexia. Stress hormones are commonly elevated in patients with anorexia, and immune system function may be disturbed (Gluck, 2006).

Many experts view family issues as contributory to anorexia. Intrafamilial conflicts and dysfunctional family patterns may occur when parents are overcontrolling and perfectionistic. The adolescent's eating behaviors may be an attempt to exercise independence and resolve internal psychologic conflicts.

The adolescent often engages in lengthy and vigorous exercise (up to 4 hours daily) to prevent weight gain. Laxatives or diuretics may be used to induce weight loss. As the disorder progresses, the adolescent perceives the ever-thinner body as becoming more beautiful. Youth may share weight loss techniques with friends who are anorectic and search out Internet sites that support anorexia. The body responds to the abnormal eating behaviors as if starvation were occurring. Leukopenia, electrolyte imbalance, and hypoglycemia develop as a result of protein-energy malnutrition. Once the body mass decreases below a critical level, menstruation ceases.

Clinical Manifestations   Adolescents with anorexia are characterized by extreme weight loss accompanied by a preoccupation with weight and food, excessive compulsive exercising, peculiar patterns of eating and handling food, and distorted body image. They may prepare elaborate meals for others but eat only low-calorie foods. Characteristically, the fear of becoming fat does not decrease with continued weight loss. Accompanying signs and symptoms of depression, crying spells, feelings of isolation and loneliness, and suicidal thoughts and feelings are common. The disorder is often associated with mental illness such as obsessive-compulsive disorder, anxiety disorders (see Chapter 28 ∞), and history of abuse (American Dietetic Association, 2006).

Physical findings include cold intolerance, dizziness, constipation, abdominal discomfort, bloating, irregular menses, and malnutrition (Figure 14–11➤). Hypothalamic suppression can lead to disturbances of gynecologic function, osteoporosis, decreased bone density, and fractures. Lanugo (fine, downy body hair) may be present. Fluid and electrolyte imbalances, especially potassium imbalances, are common. The child or adolescent is usually energetic despite significant weight loss. Extreme weight loss often leads to cardiac arrhythmias (bradycardia).

COLLABORATIVE CARE

Collaborative care focuses on early diagnosis of the disorder and referral for treatment, with follow-up to ensure continued interventions when needed.

Diagnostic Tests

Diagnosis is based on a comprehensive history, physical examination revealing characteristic clinical manifestations, and the *DSM-IV* criteria included in Box 14–6. Diagnostic tests commonly include hematocrit and hemoglobin, serum electrolytes, and serum vitamins and vitamin-precursors. Bone density examination for females with lengthy amenorrhea is recommended (American Psychiatric Association, 2006).

Clinical Therapy

The goal of treatment is to address the physiologic problems associated with malnutrition, as well as the behavioral and cognitive components of the disorder. The first phase of therapy involves management and stabilization of the abnormal serum electrolytes. Once that is accomplished, weight management is the major concern. A firm focus is placed on reaching a targeted weight with a gradual weight gain of 0.1 to 0.2 kg/day (0.25 to

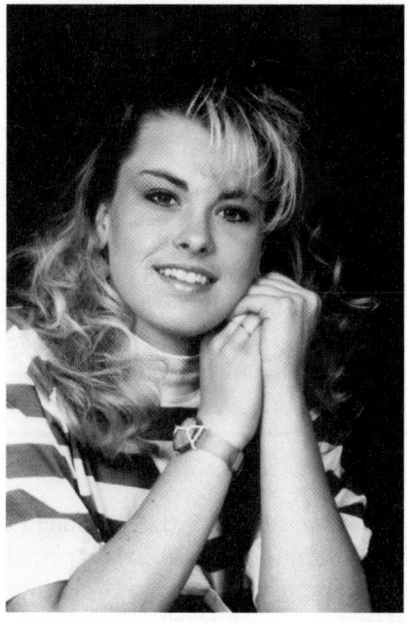
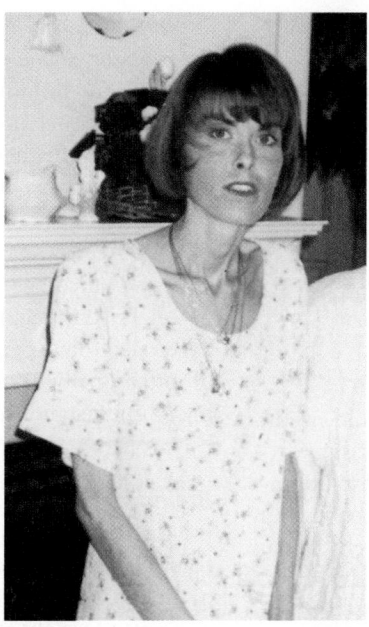

FIGURE 14–11 ➤ This young woman struggled with anorexia and bulimia from the age of 12 years. Her parents were not aware that she had the disorder until she was 15 years of age. In spite of treatment, her condition worsened and she died in her twenties. These photos show her during her teenage years and then shortly before she died.

0.5 lb/day). Weight gain of 2–3 lb/week during hospitalization, or 0.5–1 lb/week during outpatient treatment is expected (American Psychiatric Association, 2006). Enteral feedings or total parenteral nutrition (TPN) may be necessary to replace lost fluid, protein, and nutrients, although the adolescent often perceives these feedings as a punitive measure.

Individual treatment and family therapy are used to address dysfunctional family patterns and assist the family to accept and deal with the adolescent as an independent and less than perfect individual. Family involvement is crucial to effect a lasting change in the adolescent and is most successful with young teens. Nurses, psychologists, family therapists, and dietitians commonly partner to plan and implement therapy.

Long-term outpatient treatment, in either an individual or a group setting, is frequently necessary. Counseling that applies cognitive behavioral therapy may be continued for 2 to 3 years to ensure that weight gain and self-image are maintained. Antidepressant drugs such as imipramine (Tofranil) or desipramine (Norpramin) may be prescribed for co-existing conditions such as depression, anxiety, or obsessive-compulsive disorders. However, they are not generally useful in primary treatment of the disorder (Berkman, Bulik, Brownley, et al., 2006).

Indications for hospitalization include loss of 25–30% of body weight or being at 85% or less of healthy weight, fluid and electrolyte imbalances, cardiac arrhythmias, hypotension, or the need to provide a more intense period of therapy if outpatient treatment fails to produce improvement. Behavior modification techniques are used extensively in combination with counseling and other methods in care of the hospitalized adolescent with anorexia.

NURSING MANAGEMENT

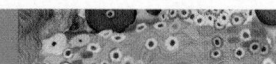

Nursing Assessment and Diagnosis

Obtain a thorough individual and family history. Ask about usual eating patterns, daily caloric intake, exercise patterns, and menstrual history. Ask about medication use; include prescription, nonprescription, and herbal products. Is there a family history of eating disorders? Assess for signs of malnutrition. Obtain height and weight measurements and compare with norms for the general population. Because the patient with anorexia often wears layers of clothes when being weighed, strive to obtain an accurate measurement.

Nursing diagnoses for the adolescent with anorexia nervosa include the following:

• Imbalanced Nutrition: Less than Body Requirements related to inadequate food intake
• Risk for Deficient Fluid Volume related to inadequate fluid intake or fluid volume loss from overuse of laxatives and diuretics

---

BOX 14–6 *DSM-IV* Criteria for Anorexia Nervosa

A. Refusal to maintain body weight at or above a minimally normal weight for age and height (e.g., weight loss leading to maintenance of body weight less than 85% of that expected; or failure to make expected weight gain during period of growth, leading to body weight less than 85% of that expected).

B. Intense fear of gaining weight or becoming fat, even though underweight.

C. Disturbance in the way in which one's weight or shape is experienced, undue influence of body weight or shape on self-evaluation, or denial of the seriousness of the current body weight.

D. In postmenarcheal females, amenorrhea, i.e., the absence of at least three consecutive menstrual cycles. (A woman is considered to have amenorrhea if her periods occur only following hormone, e.g., estrogen, administration.)

Note: Reprinted with permission from the Diagnostic and Statistical Manual of Mental Disorders, *Fourth Edition, Text Revision. Copyright 2000. American Psychiatric Association.*

- Risk for Imbalanced Body Temperature related to excessive weight loss and absence of subcutaneous fat
- Constipation related to inadequate food intake and overuse of laxatives
- Disturbed Body Image related to distorted perception of body size and shape
- Chronic Low Self-Esteem related to dysfunctional family dynamics
- Compromised Family Coping related to parental tendency to be overcontrolling and perfectionistic

Planning and Implementation

Nursing care centers on meeting nutritional and fluid needs, preventing complications, administering medications, supporting psychologic interventions, and providing referral to appropriate resources. Specific treatment measures vary depending on physical complications, length and degree of illness, emotional symptoms accompanying the disorder, and family dynamics. Resistance to treatment is common, and nurses who care for adolescents with anorexia must deal with their own feelings of frustration and anger.

Provide Psychological Support

Care for the adolescent with anorexia necessarily includes psychological support as an important component. The nurse will refer the family to a specialist who can counsel and recommend further treatment. Families should be involved in support groups with the youth with anorexia, and should also receive information about the condition and the youth's plan of care. The adolescent is often treated in individual counseling, and encouragement to participate is needed. Interventions that improve self-concept and lead to a realistic body image are needed. They may include encouragement for participation in sports, praise for participation in the treatment plan, and immediate referral for relapses as treatment progresses.

Meet Nutritional and Fluid Needs

Monitor nutritional and fluid intake, encourage consumption of food, and observe eating behaviors at mealtime. Elimination patterns may be altered as a result of increased intake during hospitalization. Monitor for possible problems, including abdominal distention, constipation, or diarrhea. Daily monitoring of serum electrolytes is necessary.

If TPN is administered, watch for complications such as circulatory overload, hyperglycemia, or hypoglycemia. Use strict aseptic technique when changing tubing or dressings. See the *Clinical Skills Manual.*

Administer Medications

Monitor vital signs if the adolescent is receiving antidepressants. Watch for signs of hypertension and tachycardia. Administering medications after meals helps to prevent gastric irritation. Be alert for substance abuse. Individuals with anorexia often use products such as excess laxatives or ephedra (also known as ma huang) to induce weight loss. Changes in the central nervous system, vital signs, and other findings may indicate over-the-counter or herbal drug use.

Provide Referral to Appropriate Resources

Refer parents and other family members to the American Anorexia and Bulimia Association, National Anorectic Aid Society, and National Association of Anorexia Nervosa & Associated Disorders for further information about the disorder and a list of support groups in their area.

Evaluation

Expected outcomes for nursing care include recommended level of weight gain, maintenance of adequate fluid volume and balanced electrolytes, enhanced positive sense of self-esteem, intake of nutritionally balanced diet, and use of psychologic counseling to understand the disorder.

Bulimia Nervosa

Bulimia nervosa is a disorder characterized by **binge eating** (a compulsion to consume large quantities of food in a short period of time). Usually the episodes of bingeing are followed by various methods of weight control (purging), such as self-induced vomiting, large doses of laxatives or diuretics, or a combination of methods. Bulimia affects 1% of the general population, but 5% or more of young women (Hoek, 2006). Like anorexia, it affects mainly adolescent girls and young women who are White and in the higher socioeconomic classes (Hoek, 2006). The disorder usually begins in middle to late adolescence, frequently emerging during college.

Etiology and Pathophysiology Causes of bulimia nervosa are similar to those of anorexia nervosa: sensitivity to social pressure for thinness, body image difficulties, and longstanding dysfunctional family patterns. Families may be chaotic and distant from the adolescent, rather than overinvolved as with the patient with anorexia. Many individuals with bulimia experience depression. It is not clear whether the depression is a cause or a result of the bulimic individual's inability to control the bingeing and purging cycles. An adolescent with bulimia often binges after any stressful event.

Bingeing usually occurs in secret for several hours until the individual is stopped by abdominal discomfort, by another person, or by vomiting. At first the episodes of binge eating are pleasurable. Immediately following the binge episode, however, feelings of guilt, shame, anger, depression, and fear of loss of control and weight gain arise. As these feelings intensify, the adolescent with bulimia becomes increasingly anxious. This usually initiates the purge behaviors.

Purging eliminates the discomfort from bloating and also prevents weight gain. This relieves the feelings of depression and guilt, but only temporarily. Adolescents with bulimia commonly practice the binge–purge cycle many times a day, losing their ability to respond to normal cues of hunger and satiety.

Clinical Manifestations Bulimia is often a "silent" disorder since it is easily concealed from health care providers. Only about 6% of those with bulimia are believed to receive treatment (Hoek, 2006). Adolescents with bulimia are preoccupied with body shape, size, and weight. They may appear overweight or thin and usually report a wide range of average body weight over the years. Physical findings depend on the degree of purging, starvation, dehydration, and electrolyte disturbance. Erosion of tooth enamel, increased dental caries, and gum recession, which result from vomiting of gastric acids, are common findings. The back of a hand can have calluses from inducing vomiting. Abdominal distention is often seen. Esophageal tears and esophagitis may also occur.

COLLABORATIVE CARE
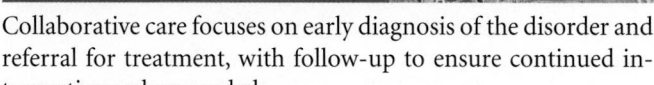

Collaborative care focuses on early diagnosis of the disorder and referral for treatment, with follow-up to ensure continued interventions when needed.

Diagnostic Tests

A comprehensive history is necessary because most adolescents with bulimia appear normal in weight or only slightly underweight. Diagnostic tests include hematocrit, hemoglobin, and serum electrolytes; they may identify signs of altered electrolyte and hematologic status. Lowered potassium levels are related to repetitive vomiting since gastric contents have a high potassium level (American Psychiatric Association, 2006). The diagnosis is confirmed by the presence of specific *DSM-IV* criteria (Box 14–7).

Clinical Therapy

Treatment includes management of physiologic problems, and cognitive-behavior therapy. Medications, such as fluoxetine 60 mg/day for adolescents, may be used (Berkman et al., 2006). Management involves a variety of health care providers such as physicians, nurses, and therapists. Behavior modification focuses on modifying the dysfunctional eating patterns and restoring normal patterns. Until the episodes of bingeing and purging are un-

der control, feelings of discouragement and hopelessness prevail. Thus, the focus early in treatment is on initiating an immediate behavioral change. Once initial interventions have been successful, group therapy sessions work well for persons with anorexia or bulimia. Specific treatment measures may include the following:

- Educating the adolescent about good nutrition (including food choice and caloric content)
- Encouraging the adolescent to keep a log or food journal and assisting the adolescent to make connections between emotional states and stress and the impulse to binge or purge
- Setting up a daily dietary routine of three meals and three snacks a day (using the same foods for each meal and snack every day to change misconceptions about the weight-gaining potential of certain foods and to decrease anxiety about what food must be eaten at the next meal)

Once these initial measures have been taken, the underlying psychosocial issues are explored. The goals of therapy are to provide the adolescent with bulimia adaptive coping skills that improve self-esteem.

Most adolescents with bulimia do not require hospitalization. Serious abnormalities in fluid and electrolyte levels caused by uncontrollable cycles of bingeing and vomiting, accompanied by depression or suicidal activity, indicate the need for hospitalization. The prognosis is good with long-term therapy.

NURSING MANAGEMENT
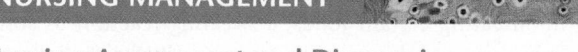

Nursing Assessment and Diagnosis

Obtain a thorough individual and family history, including daily dietary intake and weight fluctuations. Inquire about problems such as abdominal pain or distention, which may indicate an abnormal eating or elimination pattern. Assess the oral mucosa for signs of damage to tooth enamel caused by purging; examine hands for evidence of vomiting-induced calluses.

Following are nursing diagnoses that may be appropriate for the adolescent with bulimia nervosa:

- Imbalanced Nutrition: Less than or More than Body Requirements related to disordered eating patterns
- Risk for Deficient Fluid Volume related to fluid volume loss
- Impaired Oral Mucous Membrane related to chemical effects of vomited gastric acids
- Deficient Knowledge (Adolescent) related to health risks of excessive use of laxatives and diuretics
- Anxiety related to discomfort with weight and eating patterns
- Chronic Low Self-Esteem related to dysfunctional family dynamics
- Ineffective Individual Coping related to life stressors

Planning and Implementation

Nursing care includes monitoring nutritional intake and elimination patterns, preventing complications, and providing appropriate referrals.

> **BOX 14–7** **DSM-IV Criteria for Bulimia Nervosa**
>
> **A.** Recurrent episodes of binge eating. An episode of binge eating is characterized by both of the following:
> 1. Eating, in a discrete period of time (e.g., within any 2-hour period), an amount of food that is definitely larger than most people would eat during a similar period of time and under similar circumstances
> 2. A sense of lack of control over eating during the episode (e.g., a feeling that one cannot stop eating or control what or how much one is eating)
> **B.** Recurrent inappropriate compensatory behavior in order to prevent weight gain, such as self-induced vomiting; misuse of laxatives, diuretics, enemas, or other medications; fasting; or excessive exercise.
> **C.** The binge eating and inappropriate compensatory behaviors both occur, on average, at least twice a week for 3 months.
> **D.** Self-evaluation is unduly influenced by body weight and shape.
> **E.** The disturbance does not occur exclusively during episodes of anorexia nervosa.
>
> *Note: Reprinted with permission from the* Diagnostic and Statistical Manual of Mental Disorders, *Fourth Edition, Text Revision. Copyright 2000. American Psychiatric Association.*

During hospitalization, the patient should keep a food diary. Be alert to the adolescent who hides, gives away, or discards food from the tray or who exits to use the bathroom after meals. The adolescent should be monitored for at least 30 minutes after meals by remaining in a central area in the company of the nurse or other responsible individuals. Withdrawal from laxatives and diuretics is managed with careful observation for alterations in fluid and electrolyte status. Cardiac monitoring may be necessary if potassium levels are seriously altered. Esophageal tearing or esophagitis is treated to promote mucosal healing. Medications such as antidepressants may be administered. Encourage continuation of group and other therapy sessions.

Bulimic adolescents and their families can be referred to organizations such as those previously listed in the section on anorexia for assistance and information about the disorder.

Evaluation

Expected outcomes of nursing care for the adolescent with bulimia include healthy mucous membranes and skin, adequate intake of fluids and food, balanced food intake, maintenance of normal weight, adequate support and healthy psychological balance, and absence of bingeing and purging.

Food Reactions

Food reaction encompasses any adverse reaction to foods or substances ingested in foods. The most common food reaction is **food intolerance**, an abnormal physiologic response to a food that is not IgE mediated. Examples include indigestion or flatulence upon eating certain foods, a sweating reaction to some spices, rhinitis, and hives with urticaria (Burks & Ballmer-Weber, 2006). Milk and grain products are common causes of food intolerance. Chemical additives, antibiotics, preservatives, contaminants in the food, and food colorings also can cause food sensitivity reactions.

The most serious type of food reaction is **food allergy**, an IgE-mediated reaction that is potentially systemic and characteristically rapid in onset. It may be manifested as swelling of the lips, mouth, uvula, or glottis; generalized urticaria; and, in severe reaction, anaphylaxis. Food allergies are the most common cause of anaphylaxis and are most prevalent in children with a family history of allergic reactions to various substances and foods **(atopy)**. The foods that most commonly cause a reaction are fish, shellfish, peanuts, tree nuts, eggs, soy, wheat, corn, strawberries, and cow milk products. Approximately 6% of all children have some type of food allergy, and 1% of children have an allergy to peanuts (Chehade, 2007). A majority of the 150 deaths from food allergies that occur annually in the United States are due to peanut allergy (Palmer & Burks, 2006). Children who have both food allergy and asthma are most at risk of death from anaphylaxis due to a food allergy. See Clinical Manifestations: Food Allergy in the table below. See Chapter 22 ∞ for further information about IgE-mediated reactions and allergy.

Individuals with food allergy need to be aware of "hidden" substances in prepared foods. For example, the child who is allergic to nuts will experience a reaction to a food if nut extracts are used in its preparation.

Nursing Alert

Certain foods can cause either allergy or intolerance, so accurate diagnosis is needed. An example is cow milk, which can cause an allergy with IgE-mediated systemic reaction, or an intolerance from gastrointestinal response to milk proteins (diarrhea, vomiting, abdominal pain) as a result of lack of the enzyme lactase in the gastrointestinal tract.

Culture — *Lactose Intolerance*

Some ethnic groups have a high incidence of lactose intolerance, an inability to digest lactose, due to low amounts of the enzyme lactase in the gut. Although most members of the group have adequate amounts of lactase in childhood to drink milk products, by adulthood 70–100% of some groups are lactose intolerant. African Americans, Native Americans, and Asian Americans often have lactase deficiency that may begin to emerge during childhood (American Academy of Pediatrics, 2009). Abdominal pain, flatulence, and diarrhea occur with ingestion of milk or milk products. When intolerance to milk products develops, suggest alternative sources of calcium and other nutrients found in milk. Some people who have mild indigestion are able to eat yogurt with no problem. Lactase enzyme tablets can be ingested with milk products or sprinkled on those foods to aid digestion. Careful dietary planning may be needed to ensure adequate intake of calcium and vitamin D.

Clinical Manifestations
Food Allergy

System	Manifestations
Skin and mucous membranes	Urticaria of lips, mouth, throat Hives Reddened cheeks Exacerbated eczema/atopic dermatitis Itching of palms and soles of feet
Circulatory	Hypotension Tachycardia Irregular heartbeat
Respiratory	Sneezing Coughing Congestion Difficulty breathing Wheezing Laryngeal edema Recurrent ear infections
Gastrointestinal	Nausea, vomiting, flatulence, diarrhea, abdominal pain
Neurologic	Fatigue Depression, headache Dizziness, syncope Hyperactivity Sleep disturbance Seizures Loss of consciousness, coma, death

Adapted from: Asthma and Allergy Foundation. (2007). Food allergies; Food Allergy and Anaphylaxis Network. (2006). Common food allergens.

Delayed hypersensitivity reactions are attributed to digestive products of food and require a thorough diet history over several days to identify the offending food. These reactions are more difficult to diagnose, because the reaction can occur up to 24 hours after ingestion of the food. There may also be biphasic reactions that occur 1 to 30 hours after an initial anaphylaxis. Such reactions can be severe and life threatening.

Clinical Judgment

Every child with a food allergy who ingests the known allergen should be promptly treated with epinephrine and transported to an emergency facility for further management and monitoring. Delayed hypersensitivity and biphasic reactions can lead to a life-threatening reaction hours after the ingestion.

Diagnostic tests to identify suspected food allergies include measurement of serum IgE levels, scratch tests, and the **radioallergosorbent test (RAST)**, in which radioimmunoassay is used to measure IgE antibodies to specific allergens (see Chapter 22 ∞). A diet diary helps to track the date, types of foods eaten, and reactions, if any. Foods should be eaten singly for several days to determine whether they cause a reaction.

Treatment consists of eliminating the offending foods from the child's diet. Collaborative care involving the child, parents, school, and health care providers is needed to ensure that the child does not get exposed to the offending allergen, and that all children with food reactions can avoid contact with foods to which they are allergic or intolerant.

NURSING MANAGEMENT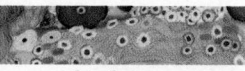

Prevention is the first step. Instruct parents of infants to introduce new foods at a rate of not more than one new food every 3 to 5 days. If a sensitivity is noted, the causative food can be easily identified. Discuss any changes in diet or preparation of formula. Reassure parents that the child's symptoms will disappear when the offending foods are removed from the diet.

Be alert for skin, respiratory, and other characteristic manifestations of sensitivity or allergy. Refer such cases to an allergist immediately for diagnosis. Nursing care of a child with food allergy recognizes that the responsibility for preventing ingestion of an allergenic food for a particular child is shared by the child (when old enough to participate), the family, and the school or other setting (Table 14–7). Children with food allergies should

TABLE 14–7 Food Allergies—Shared Responsibility

Family Responsibility	Child Responsibility	School Responsibility
• Notify and work with the school to develop a Food Allergy Action Plan for the child in all school locations and activities. • Provide written medical documentation, instructions, and prescribed medications; update, label, and replace as needed (e.g., EpiPen). • Provide a current photo of the child for the Food Allergy Action Plan. • Provide emergency contact information. • Educate the child to the level possible, depending on age and cognition, about safe and unsafe foods, avoiding exposure to unsafe foods, symptoms of allergic reactions, how to tell adults about the problem, and how to read food labels. • Institute review of policies/procedures and the Food Allergy Action Plan with the school staff, physician, and child (if old enough) after any reaction.	• Do not trade food with other children. • Do not eat anything known to contain the allergen or when ingredients are unknown. • Notify an adult immediately if an allergen may have been ingested. • Know the location of emergency medication (e.g., EpiPen).	• Inform all personnel and follow federal, state, and district laws relevant to allergies and sharing medical information. • Review health records of all students. • Identify a core team to work with the parents and child to establish a Food Allergy Action Plan (may include school nurse, principal, school food service and nutrition manager/director, counselor). • Include the student who has a food allergy in school activities. • Implement treatment upon possible ingestion of allergen; do not wait for a reaction. • Teach all staff interacting with the child the recognition of food allergy, actions to take in an emergency, and elimination measures of the allergen from meals, educational tools, arts and crafts, incentives, and so forth. • Practice the Food Allergy Action Plan and evaluate results. • Work with the school nurse to allow for safe and accessible storage of emergency medicines; arrange instruction for personnel in administration of medication to ensure proper training regardless of time or location. • Students should be allowed to carry their own epinephrine if age appropriate after approval from the physician/clinic, parent, and school nurse, as allowed by state or local regulations. • Include field trips, transportation on school bus, and sports outings in the Food Allergy Action Plan; enforce a no-eating policy on buses. • Ensure emergency communication from all buses, school events, and field trips. • Be alert for, take seriously, and manage threats or harassment against a student with an allergy. • Institute a review of the plan after any reaction.

Adapted from: School Guidelines for Managing Students with Food Allergies. *Used with permission, 2010. The Food Allergy and Anaphylaxis Network.*

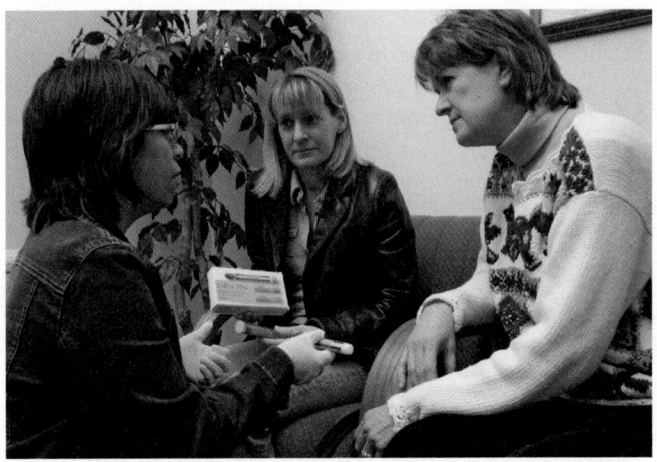

FIGURE 14–12 ➤ The school nurse is providing instruction for a mother and teacher about the use of the EpiPen, which may be needed for treatment of a child with food allergy. They have both received prior instruction and practice but need to review techniques and the child's food allergy plan before a field trip.

wear an alert tag and carry an emergency medication such as EpiPen. Nurses in schools and offices must instruct families, school teachers, and others about the child's allergy and what to do in case of accidental ingestion of the food product. Ensure that a food allergy plan is in place in the school and within each additional setting where the child spends time (Figure 14–12 ➤).

Recognize that food allergies can be life threatening and plan carefully with the family, childcare facilities, schools, and other community contacts to ensure avoidance of the offending food and emergency treatment, if needed. Help the family identify and eliminate the offending foods. Explain to parents all tests, use of a food diary, and care of the child should a reaction occur. The child and school will need an emergency plan for the child in case of accidental ingestion. Emphasize the importance of reading food labels for hidden foods that can trigger an allergic reaction. Refer the family to the Food Allergy Network.

■ NUTRITIONAL SUPPORT

Providing adequate nutrition for all children can be a challenge for families. Nutritional needs change as children grow and develop, family patterns must be integrated into the child's intake, and many social influences intervene to influence dietary patterns. Some children require even more careful management to ensure that they receive necessary nutrients, either due to increased needs or the difficulty in ingesting adequate foods. Several of the particular challenges are discussed in the following text.

Sports Nutrition and Ergogenic Agents
Regular physical activity should be encouraged for all children, with at least 60 minutes of activity recommended daily. However, during vigorous or prolonged exercise, or during hot weather, there may be special nutritional needs of child and adolescent athletes. A well-balanced diet, reflective of the recommended foods, is needed. A wide variety of fresh fruits and vegetables, grains, and complex carbohydrates usually provides for adequate caloric intake. When the child is hungry, extra calories should come from the food groups listed here, rather than

from increased intake of fat. When the child or teen is very active, sports bars or drinks can provide the additional needed calories in a nutritionally balanced manner. As always, the height, weight, and BMI percentiles are the best assurance that the individual is growing adequately over time. Adequate energy to perform the sport and to be attentive and productive at school and for other activities should also be considered (Molinero & Marquez, 2009; Rodriguez, DiMarco, Langley, et al., 2009).

Water should be increased during activity both to minimize the chance of dehydration and to maximize performance. About 1 hour before vigorous exercise, the child should drink one or two glasses (8 to 16 ounces) of water, and should repeat the same amount of fluid just before the exercise begins. Young children may not feel thirsty, and should be encouraged to drink 6 to 12 ounces of fluid every 15 to 20 minutes during exercise (AAP, Committee on Nutrition, 2009). Water is usually the best replacement. During extended exercise, sports drinks may be a good alternative for some of the fluid intake. Additional water is needed after activity. Weight loss of 1 pound indicates a loss of about 0.5 quart of fluid. Be sure the child takes in fluid to replace all losses.

Another type of food product is a **probiotic**, a live microorganism that improves the balance of gut microflora, thereby providing a health benefit. Common probiotics include *Lactobacillus* and *Bifidobacterium,* which are commonly found in the human gastrointestinal tract, are enhanced by eating yogurt with live cultures, and may be helpful in treating diarrhea or atopic dermatitis (Schuerman & Vezeau, 2007; Bowman & Russell, 2006). Inquire about the family's treatment for conditions such as diarrhea. Daily intake of pasteurized yogurt with live cultures can safely be encouraged for children.

Some common nutrients that may be deficient in all teens, but even more often in the athlete, are calcium and iron. The increased blood volume common in the well-conditioned person necessitates greater intake. Calcium foods such as milk products and dark green vegetables, and iron foods such as adequate meats and grains, can guard against deficiencies. Many adolescents believe that they need extra protein during athletic seasons; however, most Americans ingest adequate protein to meet even the increased needs of sports, although the vegetarian child or adolescent may need assistance to plan a diet with adequate protein.

Many teens ingest a wide variety of dietary supplements, believing that they act as **ergogenic aids**, or products that enhance physical performance by influencing energy, alertness, or body composition. Most of the claims of these products are unproven, and their safety has not usually been investigated, especially in the young. Effects on youth whose bodies are still developing are particularly unknown and the risks are high for permanent interference with some normal growth patterns. Offer guidance and help the family, teen, and school personnel to investigate claims before choosing to use a product. Be sure that if youth choose to use supplements, they know recommended doses, desired effects, and potential side effects of supplements. Be aware that some sports coaches may encourage either small size and/or dieting, or use of dietary supplements to increase weight and muscle. Consider that children and adolescents in activities such as ballet, wrestling, track or running, and horse racing may also have health risks associated with inconsistent or poor intake.

Approximately 4% of U.S. high school students (4.8% of males and 3.2% of females) report taking illegal anabolic steroids; up to 6.5% in some communities report use. Interestingly, their use is higher among 9th and 10th graders than 11th and 12th graders (CDC, 2006b). In addition to being illegal, these products can have a wide array of side effects. They may stop growth of long bones, lead to endocrine imbalance, and cause increased tendon rupture. Steroidal hormones are used by some athletes. They cause masculinization of females, disruption of glu-

Pathophysiology Illustrated
Conditions That Influence Nutritional Needs

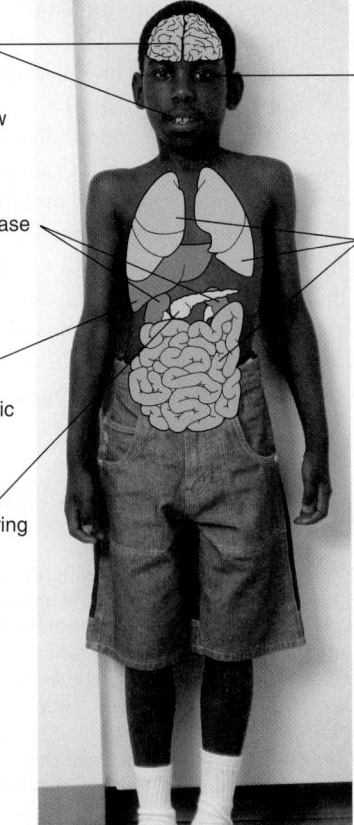

Cerebral palsy or other brain damage can influence the child's ability to chew and swallow food.

Child with renal disease may have trouble regulating fluids and proteins in the body.

Liver disease alters the child's ability to break down metabolic waste products.

Child with diabetes needs close monitoring and regulation of dietary intake.

Lack of sufficient vitamin A intake causes blindness or impaired vision in many children in developing countries.

Cystic fibrosis influences the child's ability to absorb nutrients.

FIGURE 14–13 ➤ While a child's nutritional status influences health, it is important to consider conditions that may affect nutrition in your assessment.

cose balance and insulin sensitivity, premature cardiovascular mortality, and dyslipidemia (Basaria, 2010; Hoffman, Kraemer, Bhasin, et al., 2009).

Some common amino acid nutritional supplements include creatine, carnitine, and glutamine. Although side effects to these substances are minimal, their possible enhancement of performance is temporary and outcomes of long-term use are unknown. Increasing overall intake to meet needs during high activity is a better alternative. Creatine has been studied more than most supplements; it is made by the body and is present in many protein sources. Supplemental creatine increases the creatine level in muscle and may help to increase performance in short bursts of activity, while not affecting endurance sports. The increase in muscle mass that can occur is largely due to water, and the effect will be lost when the supplement is discontinued (Williams, 2006).

Minerals such as chromium, iron, and calcium are used by some youths. Additionally, others use megadoses of sports supplements and combine a number of drugs, greatly increasing the risk of side effects. The nurse can ask careful and sensitive questions, such as "Many athletes take supplements to aid in performance in sports. What supplements do you take or are you considering?" Information can then be provided to enhance the youth's understanding of nutrition and sports performance. Generally, intake of a balanced diet with adequate carbohydrate, protein, and fat will meet the needs of most athletes and lead to maximal sports performance. School nurses can work with physical education teachers and coaches to plan appropriate programs for youth to prevent use of ergogenic agents.

Health-Related Conditions
Many health-related conditions influence the child's nutritional state. Conversely, the child's nutritional state can influence the state of health (Van Riper, Wallace, & American Dietetic Association, 2010). The Pathophysiology Illustrated figure shows some common conditions that influence nutritional needs (Figure 14–13 ➤). These conditions are discussed in various chapters throughout the text. When you read about them, discuss with classmates how you will adjust normal nutritional assessment and teaching due to the presence of a health care concern. Which conditions influence absorption of nutrients? Which cause changes in nutritional intake requirements? Some children benefit from special dietary aids, such as eating utensils and cups that are easy to grasp. Therapists can evaluate and make recommendations about devices that can assist the child at meals.

▲ Health Promotion

Consider a child with developmental disabilities who has difficulty chewing food and feeding self. What nursing care is needed to ensure adequate nutritional intake for the child? What suggestions will you make to the parent and to the child's school?

One example of a child with special nutritional needs is the child with cerebral palsy who may lack the muscular ability to chew and swallow normal foods. Special utensils may be required so the child can grasp them readily. Soft foods or tube feedings may be required to prevent choking on more solid food. Time must be provided within the school day for the child to ingest nutrients. Goals related to self-feeding may be part of the individualized education and health plans. School nurses play a vital role in educating school personnel about the child's nutritional needs. Partnership and collaboration among the office nurse, school nurse, child, family, and school personnel must occur so that the child is consistently offered nutritious intake in a manner that is conducive to ability to ingest (Figure 14–14 ➤).

Vegetarianism

Some families choose to eat vegetarian diets and can be helped and encouraged in their endeavors. Several variations of intake occur. **Vegetarians** eat no poultry, meat, or fish. **Lacto-ovovegetarians** eat eggs and dairy products, while **lacto-vegetarians** eat dairy products. In contrast, **vegans** are strict vegetarians and eat no animal products. When people say they are vegetarian, it is best to ask specific questions about what they will and will not eat.

The vegetarian can be very healthy, but may need some additional help to ensure nutritional adequacy. Some common vegan deficiencies are vitamin D, calcium, vitamin B_{12}, zinc, iron, fiber, calories, protein, and fat.

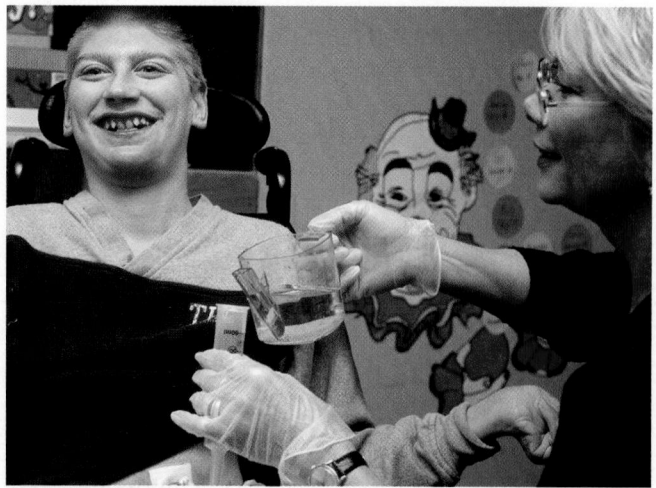

FIGURE 14–14 ➤ This young boy with cerebral palsy has recently returned to school after surgery on his back. He is limited in his ability to chew and swallow and is receiving tube feedings to supplement the limited diet he can ingest by mouth. The school nurse has instructed the teacher (shown here) in safe administration of tube feedings. What information was in her teaching plan for the school personnel?

When a pregnant teen follows a vegetarian diet, additional help will be needed to encourage adequate nutrition (Johnston & Sabate, 2006). A 24-hour or 2-day diet record will help identify nutritional needs. Consider additional pregnancy needs for energy, protein, omega 3 fatty acids, iron, vitamin D, and calcium; note that vitamin B_{12} is recommended as a supplement. Use the Vegetarian MyPyramid available through the American Dietetic Association.

Completing a 24-hour diet recall for the pregnant or lactating woman, and for vegetarian children, with analysis for RDAs can be helpful. Be sure to routinely assess growth and other nutritional measures as well. Provide ideas of various foods to meet nutritional needs and perform other general nutritional teaching. When a vegetarian child is hospitalized, plan with the nutrition department and the child's family to meet intake needs.

Enteral Therapy

Enteral therapy is a form of nutritional support provided by oral or tube feedings when a child cannot take in enough food orally to sustain health. Since it is the closest form of nutritional support to the natural method of eating, it has the least untoward effects and greatest rate of success. Some of the children who use enteral therapy are those with cerebral palsy or other neurological conditions that lead to weakness of the throat and mouth, children with neoplasm or immune dysfunction, and those in acute states of recovery from accidents or illnesses. A tube can be inserted into the nasal opening and placed through the esophagus into the stomach; however, a tube that is surgically placed into the stomach through an abdominal opening is preferred for long-term use. As long as the child can absorb and use nutrients, enteral therapy can be successful in providing calories and essential nutrients. Commercially prepared formulas are available, and specially formulated solutions can be adapted for children with specific dietary needs. Nursing care includes care of the tube and entry site to prevent infection and skin breakdown. See Chapter 25 ∞ and the *Clinical Skills Manual* for suggestions on management of nursing care during tube feedings.

Total parenteral nutrition (TPN) is frequently used in the treatment of children who cannot ingest adequate amounts of foods. In many cases, TPN provides nutrients that offer the child nourishment, leading to an improvement in their condition and, therefore, an improved state of health. However, TPN is expensive and complicated to administer, and it can have adverse side effects. Is this treatment the best option for all children with inadequate nutrition? How are decisions made about when to institute this type of nutritional support? If someone is unconscious or dying, is this method of nutrition started? These ethical issues are often difficult and have no easy answers. Nurses usually administer TPN in the home and hospital and may feel stressed if families, the patient, and other health professionals do not agree on its use. Guidelines are available to help health care professionals make decisions about treatments, and nurses should seek the guidance of ethics professionals in their agencies when needed.

Total Parenteral Nutrition

Parenteral therapy (nutrition introduced outside of the intestinal tract, usually by the intravenous route) has made it possible to provide intravenous nutritional support for individuals who cannot eat or are unable to absorb nutrients from the intestinal tract in a normal manner and are at risk of severe malnutrition. Examples of children who benefit from this method of nutrition are those with congenital malformation of the gastrointestinal tract, brain injury, or severe burns, and those who require support after bone marrow transplant, sepsis, or other critical conditions. A catheter is inserted so that a sterile nutrition solution is infused directly into the bloodstream. A central venous catheter is inserted to promote safe infusion. Fluids usually contain glucose; electrolytes such as sodium, potassium, calcium, magnesium, phosphate, and chloride; vitamins; and proteins. Lipid emulsions are another type of TPN used in some children. Meticulous care is needed, whether in the hospital or at home, to ensure safe TPN infusion and treatment. The nurse performs initial assessment and ongoing evaluation and monitoring of treatment, verifies the solution type and rate of administration, ensures that solution storage recommendations are followed, and administers the solutions in the hospital or other settings. See the protocols for TPN management in the *Clinical Skills Manual.*

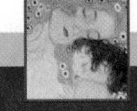

Chapter Highlights

- Adequate nutritional intake is necessary for the normal growth and development of children.
- Children with medical or psychosocial conditions require additional nutritional support.
- Dietary intake patterns vary throughout childhood as the child grows, is able to metabolize different types of food, and gains greater gross and fine motor control.
- Nutritional assessment is an essential part of nursing care and may involve approaches such as growth measurement and intake records.
- Common nutritional concerns in childhood include hunger, overweight, foodborne illness, celiac disease, and dietary deficiencies.
- The child with feeding disorder of infancy and childhood requires comprehensive assessment and ongoing management to foster parent–child interaction and adequate nutritional intake.
- The most common eating disorders of adolescents are anorexia nervosa and bulimia nervosa.
- A combination of behavioral management, counseling, and medication is often used in treatment programs for eating disorders.
- Food allergy represents a life-threatening condition for children, whereas food intolerance can lead to uncomfortable but non-life-threatening symptoms.
- Children engaging in sports and those who eat vegetarian diets may need guidance to meet nutritional needs.
- Alternative feeding methods such as enteral and parenteral feedings are required by some children.

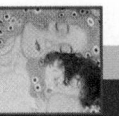

Clinical Reasoning in Action

Recall the family introduced in the chapter opener. Yvonne is a 9-month-old infant who is active and healthy. Her mother, Colleen, has brought her to the Women, Infants, and Children (WIC) Nutrition Program clinic, and they are accompanied by Margarita, the grandmother. Colleen feels unprepared to make decisions about what Yvonne should be eating at this age. Yvonne breastfeeds twice daily since Colleen works, but Colleen wonders if she should continue. The nurse praises Colleen for continuing with these two feedings daily since that ensures the benefits of breastfeeding such as immune protection against some illnesses, and it fosters mother–infant bonding. She reassures Colleen that it is beneficial for her to pump her breasts and suggests that the pumped milk be refrigerated and fed to Yvonne by bottle in the middle of the following day.

1. What fine motor skills would you expect to see in Yvonne at this age that will enable her to perform more self-feeding skills?

2. During the visit, the nurse takes a blood sample for hematocrit. What is the expected level at this age? What factors put infants in the second half of their first year of life at risk for iron deficiency anemia? What teaching can you do to promote intake of iron? Yvonne has a bottle of regular milk in the middle of the day. How could this contribute to anemia? What is recommended for her intake at this age? How can you best support Colleen to encourage her continued breastfeeding of Yvonne?

3. Margarita prepares most of Yvonne's meals during the day and speaks Spanish. How will you prepare teaching for this grandmother so that she can benefit from the teaching that the clinic has designed for parents of infants? How can you make that teaching culturally sensitive?

4. As Colleen looks forward to the next few months, what information will she need to provide nutritious intake for Yvonne? What are expected food patterns at 1 year and 18 months of age?

See Pearson Nursing Student Resources for possible responses.

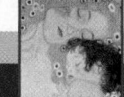

References

Allen, K. N., Taylor, J. S., & Kuiper, R. A. (2007). Effectiveness of nutrition education on fast food choices in adolescents. *Journal of School Nursing, 23,* 337–341.

American Academy of Pediatrics (AAP), Committee on Nutrition. (2009). *Pediatric nutrition handbook* (6th ed.). Elk Grove Village, IL: American Academy of Pediatrics.

American Academy of Pediatrics (AAP), Section on Breastfeeding. (2005). Breastfeeding and the use of human milk. *Pediatrics, 115,* 496–506.

American Dental Association. (n.d.). *ADA statement on early childhood caries.* Retrieved from http://www.ada.org/prof/resources/positions/statements/caries.asp

American Diabetes Association. (2008). Nutrition recommendations and interventions for diabetes. *Diabetes Care, 31,* S61–S78.

American Dietetic Association. (2006). *Nutrition intervention in the treatment of anorexia nervosa, bulimia nervosa, and eating disorders not otherwise specified (EDNOS).* Retrieved from http://www.eatright.org/cps/rde/xchg/ada/hs.xls/advocacy_adapo701_ENU_HTML.htm

American Psychiatric Association. (2006). *Treatment of patients with eating disorders* (3rd ed.). *American Journal of Psychiatry 163* (7 suppl.), 4–54.

Asthma and Allergy Foundation. (2007). *Food allergies.* Retrieved from http://www.aafa.org/display.cfm?id=9&sub=20&cont=286

Basaria, S. (2010). Androgen abuse in athletes: Detection and consequences. *Journal of Clinical Endocrinology and Metabolism, 95*(4), 1533–1543.

Berkman, N. D., Bulik, C. M., Brownley, K. A., Loh, K. N., Sedway, J. A., Rooks, A., & Gartlehnen, G. (2006). *Management of eating disorders* (AHRQ Pub. No. 06.E010). Rockville, MD: Agency for Healthcare Research and Quality.

Blackburn, B. G., Mazurek, J. M., Hlavsa, M., Park, J., Tillapaw, M., & Pariish, M. (2006). Cryptosporisiosis associate with ozonated apple cider. Emerging Infectious Disease. Retrieved from http://www.cdc.gov.ncidod/EID/vol12no04/05-0796.htm

Bowman, B. A., & Russell, R. M. (2006). *Present knowledge in nutrition* (9th ed.). Washington, DC: International Life Sciences Institute.

Browne, A. F., & Inge, T. (2009). How young for bariatric surgery in children? *Seminars in Pediatric Surgery, 18*(3), 176–185.

Burks, W., & Ballmer-Weber, B. K. (2006). Food allergy. *Molecular Nutrition and Food Research, 50,* 595–603.

Caniano, D. A. (2009). Ethical issues in pediatric bariatric surgery. *Seminars in Pediatric Surgery, 18*(3), 186–192.

Centers for Disease Control and Prevention (CDC). (2006a). QuickStats: Prevalence of overweight among persons aged 2–19 years, by sex— National Health and Nutrition Examination Survey (NHANES), United States, 1999–2000 through 2003–2004. *Morbidity and Mortality Weekly Report, 55,* 1229.

Centers for Disease Control and Prevention (CDC). (2006b). Youth Risk Behavior Surveillance— United States, 2005. *Morbidity and Mortality Weekly Report, 55*(SS-5), 1–108.

Centers for Disease Control and Prevention (CDC). (2007). Preliminary FoodNet data on the incidence of infection with pathogens transmitted commonly through food—10 states, 2006. *Morbidity and Mortality Weekly Report, 56,* 336–339.

Centers for Disease Control and Prevention (CDC). (2009). *Breastfeeding.* Retrieved from http://www.cdc.gov/breastfeeding/

Children's Defense Fund. (2007). *The state of America's children.* Washington, DC: Author.

Chehade, M. (2007). IgE and non-IgE-mediated food allergy: treatment in 2007. *Current Opinion in Allergy and Clinical Immunology 7*(3), 264–268.

Dunger, D. B., Ahmed, M. L., & Ong, K. K. (2006). Early and late weight gain and the timing of puberty. *Molecular and Cellular Endocrinology, 254–255,* 140–145.

Food Allergy and Anaphylaxis Network. (2009). *School guidelines for managing students with food allergies.* Retrieved from http://www.foodallergy.org/page/food-allergy-anaphylaxis-network-guidelines

Food Allergy and Anaphylaxis Network. (2006). *Common food allergens.* Retrieved from http://www.foodallergy.org/page/common-food-allergens-index

Gelfond, D., & Fasano, A. (2006). Celiac disease in the pediatric population. *Pediatric Annals, 35*(4), 275–279.

Gluck, M. E. (2006). Stress response and binge eating disorder. *Appetite, 46,* 26–30.

Hagan, J. F., Shaw, J. S., & Duncan, P. M. (2008). *Bright futures: Guidelines for health supervision of infants, children, and adolescents* (3rd ed.). Elk Grove Village, IL: American Academy of Pediatrics.

Hoch, A. Z., Pajewski, N. M., Moraski, L., Carrera, G. F., Wilson, C. R., Hoffmann, R. G., et al. (2009). Prevalence of the female athlete triad in high school athletes and sedentary students. *Clinical Journal of Sport Medicine, 19*(5), 421–428.

Hoek, J. W. (2006). Incidence, prevalence and mortality of anorexia nervosa and other eating disorders. *Current Opinion in Psychiatry, 19,* 389–394.

Hoffman, J. R., Kraemer, W. J., Bhasin, S., Storer, T., Ratamess, N. A., Haff, G. G., et al. (2009). Position stand on androgen and human growth hormone use. *Journal of Strength and Conditioning Research, 23*(5 suppl.), S1–S59.

Hyman, P. E., Milla, P. J., Benninga, M. A., Davidson, G. P., Fleisher, D. F., & Taminiau, J. (2006). Childhood functional gastrointestinal disorders: Neonate/toddler. *Gastroenterology, 130*(5), 1519–1526.

Institute of Medicine. (2006). *Dietary Reference Intakes.* Washington, DC: National Academies Press.

Institute of Medicine. (2007). *Progress in preventing childhood obesity.* Washington, DC: National Academies Press.

Jain, S., Bidol, S. A., Austin, J. L., Berl, E., Elson, F., Lemaile-Williams, M., et al. (2009). Multistate outbreak of Salmonella Typhimurium and Saintpaul infections associated with unpasteurized orange juice—United States, 2005. *Clinical Infectious Diseases, 48*(8), 1065–1071.

Johnston, P. K., & Sabate, J. (2006). Nutritional implications of vegetarian diets. In M. E. Shils, M. Shike, A. C. Ross, B. Caballero, & R. J. Cousins (Eds.), *Modern nutrition in health and disease* (10th ed., pp. 1638–1654). Philadelphia: Lippincott Williams & Wilkins.

Larson, N. I., Neumark-Sztainer, D., & Story, M. (2009). Weight control behaviors and dietary intake among adolescents and young adults: Longitudinal findings from Project EAT. *Journal of the American Dietetic Association, 109*(11), 1869–1877.

Lee, J. M., Appugliese, D., Kaciroti, M., Corwyn, R. F., Bradley, R. H., & Lumeng, J. C. (2007). Weight status in young girls and the onset of puberty. *Pediatrics, 119,* e624–630.

Lee, R. D., & Nieman, D. C. (2010). *Nutrition assessment* (5th ed.). Boston: McGraw-Hill.

Mendelsohn, F. A., & Warren, M. P. (2010). Anorexia, bulimia, and the female athlete triad: Evaluation and management. *Endocrinology and Metabolism Clinics of North America, 39*(1), 155–167.

Molinero, O., & Marquez, S. (2009). Use of nutritional supplements in sports: Risks, knowledge, and behavioural-related factors. *Nutrition in Hospitals, 24*(2), 128–134.

Moore, D. J. (2009). Inflaming the debate on infant colic. *Journal of Pediatrics, 155*(6), 772–773.

Moore, L. L., Bradlee, M. L., Di Gao, A. S., & Singer, M. R. (2008). Effects of average childhood dairy intake on adolescent bone health. *Journal of Pediatrics, 153*(5), 667–673. doi:10.1016/j/jpeds.208.05.016

National Institute of Diabetes and Digestive and Kidney Disease (NIDDK). (2008). *Celiac disease.* Retrieved from http://digestive.niddk.nih.gov/ddiseases/pubs/celiac/#diagnoses

O'Connor, T. M., Yang, S. J., & Nicklas, T. A. (2006). Beverage intake among preschool children and its effect on weight status. *Pediatrics, 118*, e1010–e1018.

Olsen, E. M. (2006). Failure to thrive: Still a problem of definition. *Clinical Pediatrics, 45*, 1–6.

Palmer, K., & Burks, W. (2006). Current developments in peanut allergy. *Current Opinion in Allergy and Clinical Immunology, 6*, 202–206.

Ramon, R., Ballester, F., Aguinagalde, X., Amurrio, A., Vioque, J., Lacasana, M., et al. (2009). Fish consumption during pregnancy, prenatal mercury exposure, and anthropometric measures at birth in a prospective mother-infant cohort study in Spain. *American Journal of Clinical Nutrition, 90*(4), 1047–1055.

Richey, R., Howdle, P., Shaw, E., & Stokes, T. (2009). Recognition and assessment of coeliac disease in children and adults: Summary of NICE guidelines. *British Medical Journal, 338*, b1684. doi: 110.1136/bmj.b1684

Rideout, V., & Hamel, E. (2006). *The media family: Electronic media in the lives of infants, toddlers, preschoolers and their parents.* Menlo Park, CA: Henry J. Kaiser Family Foundation.

Rodriguez, N. R., DiMarco, N. M., Langley, S., American Dietetic Association, Dietitians of Canada, & American College of Sports Medicine. (2009). Position of the American Dietetic Association, Dietitians of Canada, and the American College of Sports Medicine: Nutrition and athletic performance. *Journal of the American Dietetic Association, 109*(3), 509–527.

Rood, L., Roelofs, J., Bogels, S. M., Nolen-Hoeksema, S., & Schouten, E. (2009). The influence of emotion-focused rumination and distraction on depressive symptoms in non-clinical youth: A meta-analytic review. *Clinical Psychology Review, 29*(7), 607–616.

Schuerman, G., & Vezeau, T. (2007). All bugs aren't bad: Probiotics in the treatment of pediatric atopic dermatitis. *American Journal for Nurse Practitioners, 11*(4), 28–36.

Small, L., Anderson, D., & Melnyk, B. M. (2007). Prevention and early treatment of overweight and obesity in young children: A critical review and appraisal of the evidence. *Pediatric Nursing, 33*, 127, 149–161.

Snyder, C. L., Young, D. O., Green, P. H. R., & Taylor, A. K. (2008). Celiac disease. In R. A. Pagon, T. C. Bird, C. R. Dolan, & K. Stephens (Eds.), *GeneReviews* [Internet]. Seattle: University of Washington.

Stanton, B. F., Jenson, H. B., Behrman, R. E., Kliegman, R. M., & Jenson, H. B. (2007). *Nelson textbook of pediatrics* (18th ed.). Philadelphia: Saunders.

Urrutia-Rojas, X., & Menchaca, J. (2006). Prevalence of risk for type 2 diabetes in school children. *Journal of School Health 76*, 189–194.

U.S. Department of Agriculture (USDA). (2009). *Food insecurity in households with children.* Retrieved from http://www.ers.usda.gov/publications/eib56

U.S. Department of Health and Human Services. (2006). *Healthy People 2010: Midcourse Review.* Retrieved from http://www.health.gov/healthypeople/document.html

U.S. Department of Health and Human Services. (2010). *Healthy People 2020: The road ahead.* Retrieved from http://www.healthypeople.gov/hp2020/

U.S. Department of Health and Human Services & U.S. Department of Agriculture. (2005). *Dietary guidelines for Americans.* Washington, DC: Retrieved from http://www.healthierus.gov/dietaryguidelines/

U.S. Food and Drug Administration. (2004). *Backgrounder for the 2004 FDA/EPA consumer advisory: What you need to know about mercury in fish and shellfish.* Washington, DC: U.S. Department of Health and Human Services. Retrieved from http://www.fda.gov/oc/opacom/hottopics/mercury/backgrounder.html

Van Koppen, E. J., Schweizer, J. J., Csizmadia, C., Krom, Y., Hylkema, H. B., van Geel, A. M., et al. (2009). Long-term health and quality-of-life consequences of mass screening for childhood celiac disease: A 10-year follow-up study. *Pediatrics, 123*, e582–e588.

Van Riper, C. L., Wallace, L. S., & American Dietetic Association. (2010). Position of the American Dietetic Association: Providing nutrition services for people with developmental disabilities and special health care needs. *Journal of the American Dietetic Association, 110*(2), 296–307.

Wagner, C. L., Greer, F. R., & Section on Breastfeeding and Committee on Nutrition. (2008). Prevention of rickets and vitamin D deficiency in infants, children, and adolescents. *Pediatrics, 122*, 1142–1152.

Watt, R. G., McGlone, P., Russell, J. J., Tull, K. I., & Dowler, E. (2006). The process of establishing, implementing and maintaining a social support infant feeding programme. *Public Health Nutrition, 9*, 714–721.

Williams, M. H. (2006). Sports nutrition. In M. E. Shils, M. Shike, A. C. Ross, B. Caballero, & R. J. Cousins (Eds.), *Modern nutrition in health and disease* (10th ed., pp. 1723–1740). Philadelphia: Lippincott Williams & Wilkins.

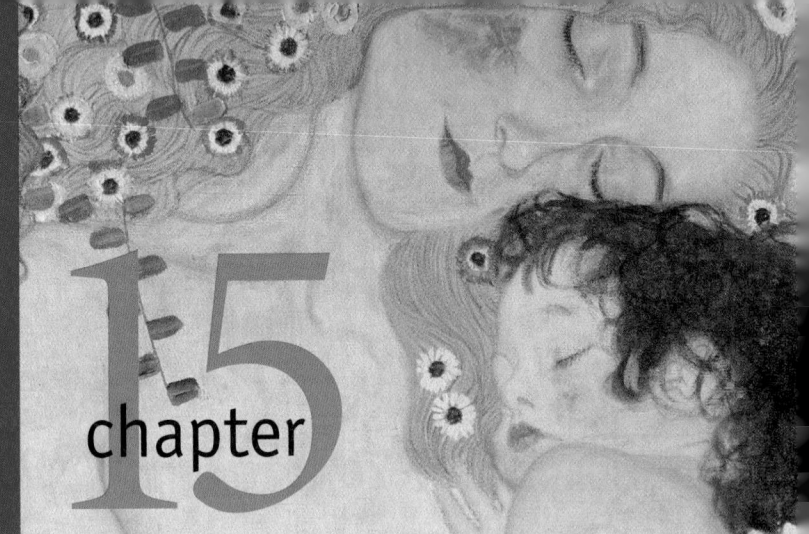

Pain Assessment and Management

chapter 15

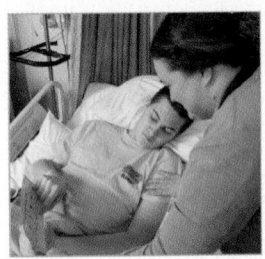

Lucas, 14 years old, is being prepared to undergo orthopedic surgery to stabilize a slipped capital femoral epiphysis. During his preoperative teaching, the nurse shows Lucas how to use a pain scale, explaining what each of the faces means. The nurse tells Lucas that he will be asked to point to the face that matches how much he hurts several times after his operation. Lucas is asked about the most pain he has ever felt, and what caused that pain. The nurse will use this information to help Lucas identify the amount of pain he has during future pain assessments. Lucas is encouraged to tell the nurse or his parents when he has pain after the operation so that he can be given medication to relieve the pain.

The nurse also discusses the importance of assessing and treating pain with Lucas's parents, as Lucas will go home the same day of surgery. The nurse lets them know that controlling Lucas's pain will make it easier for him to move around and promote healing. Why is it important to manage a child's pain? In addition to using the pain scale, what information will the nurse use to assess Lucas's postoperative pain? How is pain treated in children?

Learning Outcomes

After reading this chapter, you will be able to do the following:

1. Summarize the physiologic and behavioral consequences of pain in children.
2. Analyze the behaviors of an infant or a child to assess for pain.
3. Assess a child's readiness to use a self-report pain scale.
4. Calculate an opioid dose and describe the methods used to administer opioids to children.
5. Examine the role of nonpharmacologic (complementary) interventions in effective pain management.
6. Plan the nursing care for an infant or child in acute pain that integrates pharmacologic interventions and developmentally appropriate nonpharmacologic (complementary) therapies.
7. Distinguish between the clinical therapies used for acute and chronic pain.
8. Plan the nursing care for a child to be given sedation and analgesia for a medical procedure.

Every child has his or her own perception of pain. A neurologic response to tissue injury, **pain** is an unpleasant sensory and emotional experience associated with actual or potential tissue damage (Pappagallo & Werner, 2008). Effective pain management is every child's right.

■ PAIN

Pain may be either acute or chronic. **Acute pain** is sudden and of short duration; it may be associated with a single event, such as surgery or injury that can be linked to the pain discomfort. The inflammatory response following the initial tissue injury helps sustain the pain response. See Figure 15–1 ➤ for the pathophysiology of the pain response. The pain often decreases and ends as healing occurs.

Chronic pain is persistent, lasting longer than 3 months; it is often associated with a prolonged disease process such as juvenile rheumatoid arthritis or cancer. Chronic pain may be nociceptive or **neuropathic pain**, initiated or caused by a primary lesion or dysfunction of the nervous system. It does not arouse the sympathetic nervous system in the same way as acute pain. Ongoing stimulation of nociceptors can sensitize the peripheral and central nervous systems leading to neuroanatomical, neurochemical, and neurophysiological changes.

Misconceptions About Pain in Children

Health care professionals once believed that children feel less pain than adults. Undertreatment of pain was based on these attitudes about pain, the difficulty and complexity of pain assessment in children, and inadequate research. Research has shown that past beliefs about children's perception of pain were incorrect. Even the smallest infants do feel pain. For a review of past myths and the contrasting reality, see Table 15–1.

Growth & Development *Newborn and Infant Pain*

Pain impulses in newborns and infants are transmitted along the nonmyelinated C fibers, and the pain signal is less precise. Pain conduction may be slower in neonates, but the distance the pain stimuli must travel is much shorter than in adults. Because the descending neurotransmitters are less developed, newborns are less able to reduce the pain impulses. Premature and newborn infants may be even more sensitive to pain than older children.

Developmental Aspects of Pain Perception, Memory, and Response

A number of factors influence the pain perceived by the child, including maturation of the nervous system, the child's developmental stage, and previous pain experiences (Table 15–2).

Pathophysiology Illustrated
Pain Perception

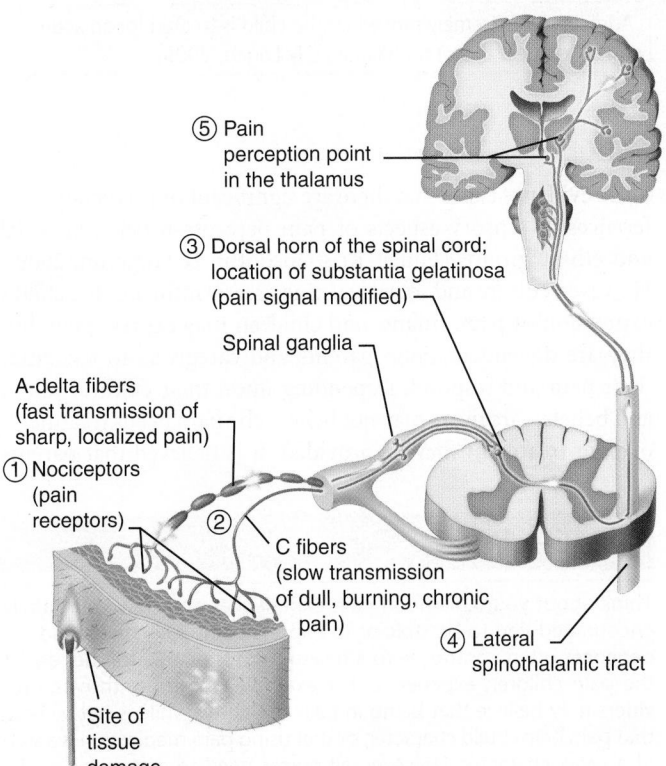

FIGURE 15–1 ➤

1. **Nociceptors** (free nerve endings at the site of tissue damage) transmit information via specialized nerve fibers to the spinal cord.
2. Unmyelinated C fibers slowly transmit dull, burning, diffuse pain as well as chronic pain. Large, myelinated A-delta fibers quickly transmit sharp, well-localized pain. Nociceptors are stimulated by mechanical, thermal, and chemical injury. Biochemical mediators (bradykinin, prostaglandin, leukotrienes, serotonin, histamine, catecholamines, and substance P) are produced in response to tissue damage. These substances help move the pain impulse from the nerve endings to the spinal cord.
3. After the sensory information reaches the substantia gelatinosa in the dorsal horn of the spinal cord, the pain signal may be modified depending on the presence of other stimuli, from either the brain or the periphery.
4. The pain signal is then transmitted through the lateral spinothalamic tract, to the thalamus of the brain where perception occurs.
5. Once the sensation reaches the brain, interpretation of pain occurs, and emotional responses may increase or decrease the intensity of the pain perceived. Due to a two-way control of nociceptive transmission within the spinal tracts, pain perception can be inhibited or changed when a competing nonpain impulse is sent along the same nerve pathways, a simple explanation of the gate control theory of pain. Stimulation of the larger A-beta fibers by ice or massage causes the substantia gelatinosa in the dorsal horn of the spinal cord to "close the gate" and decrease the transmission of pain impulses to the brain. The brain cortex also has control of nociceptive transmission and can inhibit some pain stimuli (Huether, 2010, p. 486). Endogenous opioids, such as endorphins, produced by the brain in response to painful stimuli, help inhibit pain impulses in the spinal cord, brain, and the periphery (Huether, 2010, p. 488).

Figure labels:
- ⑤ Pain perception point in the thalamus
- ③ Dorsal horn of the spinal cord; location of substantia gelatinosa (pain signal modified)
- Spinal ganglia
- A-delta fibers (fast transmission of sharp, localized pain)
- ① Nociceptors (pain receptors)
- ②
- C fibers (slow transmission of dull, burning, chronic pain)
- ④ Lateral spinothalamic tract
- Site of tissue damage

TABLE 15–1 Misconceptions about Pain in Infants and Children	
Myth	Reality
Neonates and infants are incapable of feeling pain. Children do not feel pain with the same intensity as adults because a child's nervous system is immature.	The anatomic and functional structures for pain processing are present early in fetal life. Term infants have the same level of sensitivity to pain as older infants and children.
Infants are incapable of expressing pain.	Infants express pain with both behavioral and physiologic cues that can be assessed.
Infants and children have no memory of pain.	Infants and children do remember pain experiences. Males circumcised as neonates cry significantly longer and have greater pain intensity when getting immunized at age 4 to 6 months (Walden & Carrier, 2009).
Parents exaggerate or aggravate their child's pain.	Parents know their child and are able to identify when the child is in pain.
Children are not in pain if they can be distracted or they are sleeping.	Children use distraction to cope with pain, but they soon become exhausted when coping with pain and fall asleep.
Repeated experience with pain teaches the child to be more tolerant of pain and cope with it better.	Children who have more experience with pain respond more vigorously to pain. Experience with pain teaches how severe the pain can become.
Children tolerate discomfort well. They become accustomed to pain after having it for a while.	Children do not tolerate pain any better than adults, and may have less tolerance after prior painful experiences. They do not become accustomed to pain or cope with it better than adults.
Children recover more quickly than adults from painful experiences such as surgery.	Children heal quickly from surgery, but they have the same amount of pain from surgery as an adult.
Children tell you if they are in pain. They do not need medication unless they appear to be in pain.	Children may be too young to express pain or afraid to tell anyone other than a parent about the pain. The child fears the treatment for pain may be worse than the pain itself.
Children without obvious physical reasons for pain are not likely to have pain.	The cause of pain cannot always be determined. The feeling of pain is subjective and should be accepted by nurses.
Children run the risk of becoming addicted to pain medication when used for pain management.	Addiction is extremely rare when the child is treated for an acute condition (less than 1%) (Plaisance & Logan, 2006).

Newborns and infants develop a memory of pain (Hall & Anand, 2005; Walden & Carrier, 2009). Preschool-age children demonstrate pain memory by making efforts to delay a painful procedure.

Children's responses to acute or chronic pain are also influenced by factors such as their memory of pain, their ability to control what will happen, their use of a pain coping mechanism, and emotions like fear or anxiety (Walco, 2008). Depending on their developmental stage, children use different coping strategies, such as escape, postponement or avoidance, diversion, and imagery, to deal with pain.

Children may not complain of pain for several reasons:

- Young children are unable to give a detailed description of their pain because of their limited vocabulary and pain experiences.
- Some children believe they need to be brave or do not want to worry their parents.
- Preschoolers and adolescents may assume the nurse knows they have pain.
- Some children are afraid that it will hurt more to have the pain treated.

Cultural Influences on Pain

Little evidence exists that there are significant or predictable differences in sensory aspects of pain perception between racial and ethnic groups (Finley, Kristjánsdóttir, & Forgeron, 2009). However, culture and social learning greatly influence the child's expression of pain. Infants and children may express pain, but they are dependent upon parents and caregivers to recognize their pain and respond. Depending upon their cultural values and beliefs, caregivers may not believe the pain needs treatment, or pain treatment may be provided. It is believed that parents

Culture   *Examine Your Experience*

Think about your childhood pain experiences and how your family encouraged you to be stoic or to express pain. Such childhood experiences often contribute to a health professional's attitudes about the pain children experience. For example, some health care providers may believe that being in pain for a little while is not so bad, that pain helps build character, or that using pain medication is a sign of a weak character. However, all nurses need to acknowledge the child's right to pain management, and it is the standard of care.

TABLE 15–2	The Child's Understanding of Pain, Behavioral Responses, and Verbal Descriptions by Developmental Stage		
Age Group	Understanding of Pain	Behavioral Response	Verbal Description
Infant			
Less than 6 months	No understanding of pain; is responsive to parental anxiety	Generalized body movements, chin quivering, facial grimacing, poor feeding	Cries
6–12 months	Has a pain memory; is responsive to parental anxiety	Reflex withdrawal to stimulus, facial grimacing, disturbed sleep, irritability, restlessness	Cries
Toddler			
1–3 years	Does not understand what causes pain and why he or she might be experiencing it	Localized withdrawal, resistance of entire body, aggressive behavior, disturbed sleep	Cries and screams, cannot describe intensity or type of pain Uses common words for pain such as *owie* and *boo-boo*
Preschooler			
3–6 years (preoperational)	Pain is a *hurt* Does not relate pain to illness; may relate pain to an injury Often believes pain is punishment Unable to understand why a painful procedure will help him or her feel better or why an injection takes the pain away	Active physical resistance, directed aggressive behavior, strikes out physically and verbally when hurt, low frustration level	Has the language skills to express pain on a sensory level Can identify location and intensity of pain, may deny pain, may believe his or her pain is obvious to others
School-Age Child			
7–9 years (concrete operations)	Understands simple relationships between pain and disease Understands the need for painful procedures to monitor or treat disease May associate pain with feeling bad or angry May recognize psychologic pain related to grief and hurt feelings	Passive resistance, clenches fists, holds body rigidly still, suffers emotional withdrawal, engages in plea bargaining	Can specify location and intensity of pain and describes physical characteristics of pain in relation to body parts
10–12 years (transitional)	Better understanding of the relationship between an event and pain Has a more complex awareness of physical and psychologic pain, such as moral dilemmas and mental pain	May pretend comfort to project bravery, may regress with stress and anxiety	Able to describe intensity and location with more characteristics, able to describe psychologic pain
Adolescent			
13–18 years (formal operations)	Has a capacity for sophisticated and complex understanding of the causes of physical and mental pain Recognizes that pain has both qualitative and quantitative characteristics Can relate to the pain experienced by others	Wants to behave in a socially acceptable manner (like an adult), shows a controlled behavioral response May immerse self in an activity as a pain distraction May not complain about pain if given cues by nurses or other health care providers who believe it should be tolerated	More sophisticated descriptions as experience is gained; may think nurses are in tune with his or her thoughts, so it is unnecessary to tell the nurse about the pain

begin socializing infants regarding behavioral responses to pain as young as 2 to 4 months of age (Finley et al., 2009).

While some cultural groups (for example, people of Italian and Jewish descent) are reported to use verbal and nonverbal methods to express pain freely, others (such as Anglo-Saxon–Germanic, Irish, Amish, and Appalachian) may encourage a more stoic response with a diminished expression of pain (Purnell, 2009). Be careful to avoid stereotyping. Not all members of a cultural group will demonstrate the same pain response.

Physiologic Consequences of Pain

Unrelieved pain is stressful and has many undesirable physiologic consequences (Table 15–3). For example, the child with acute postoperative pain takes shallow breaths and suppresses coughing to avoid more pain. These self-protective actions increase the potential for respiratory complications. Unrelieved pain may also delay the return of normal gastric and bowel functions and lead to occult gastrointestinal bleeding. Anorexia associated with pain may delay the healing process. The long-term effects of pain on the child's physical or psychologic condition are unknown.

Preverbal children may show conflicting signs of pain (restlessness, agitation or withdrawal, hyperalert or vigilant, grimacing, crying, or anger), making pain assessment and management more challenging.

Children often suffer additional emotional distress and fear that the discomfort will worsen. Depression and aggressive behavior are frequently overlooked as indicators of pain.

■ PAIN ASSESSMENT

The goal of pain assessment is to provide accurate information about the location and intensity of pain and its effects on the child's functioning.

Pain History

Parents can provide a great deal of information about the child's response to pain, such as the following:

- How the child typically expresses pain. Children and parents use similar terms to describe pain, such as a *hurt, owie, boo-boo, stinging, sore, cutting, burning, itching, hot,* and *tight.* Knowing the preferred words makes communication with the child easier. The parent can often inform the nurse about behaviors that will help to identify the child's pain.

Growth & Development · *Pain Words*

Children slowly acquire words for pain over the first 6 years of life. The pain words used spontaneously by children in one study were as follows: *ouch* as early as 17 months, *hurt* and *ow* by 18 months of age, *boo-boo* by 21 months, *ache* by 36 months, *sore* by 45 months, and *pain* by 72 months (Stanford, Chambers, & Craig, 2005). Other pain words include *owie, stinging, sore, cutting, burning, itching, hot,* and *tight.*

- The child's previous experiences with painful situations and reactions.
- How the child copes with and manages pain. The child with several past pain experiences may not exhibit the same types of stressful behaviors as the child with few pain experiences.
- What works best to reduce the child's pain.
- The parent's and child's preferences for analgesic use and other pain interventions.

Ask older children to give a history of painful procedures, but recognize that they may modify their pain descriptions depending on the type of questions asked and what they expect will happen as a result of their response. Examples of questions to ask include the following:

- What kinds of things made you hurt in the past? What made it feel better?

TABLE 15–3 · Physiologic Consequences of Unrelieved Pain in Children

Responses to Pain	Potential Physiologic Consequences
Respiratory Changes	
Rapid shallow breathing Inadequate lung expansion Inadequate cough	Alkalosis Decreased oxygen saturation, atelectasis Retention of secretions
Neurologic Changes	
Increased sympathetic nervous system activity and release of catecholamines	Tachycardia, elevated blood pressure, change in sleep patterns
Metabolic Changes	
Increased metabolic rate with increased perspiration	Increased fluid and electrolyte losses Increased blood glucose and cortisol levels
Immune System Changes	
Depression of immune response	Increased risk of infection
Gastrointestinal Changes	
Increased intestinal secretions and smooth muscle sphincter tone	Impaired gastrointestinal functioning, ileus, stress ulcer
Altered Pain Response	
Increased pain sensitivity	Hyperalgesia, decreased pain threshold, exaggerated memory of painful experiences

Data from: Mitchell, A., & Boss, B. J. (2002). Adverse effects of pain on the nervous systems of newborns and young children: A review of the literature. Journal of Neuroscience Nursing, 34(5), 228–236; Walden, M. (2007). Pain in the newborn and infant. In C. Kenner & J. W. Lott, Comprehensive neonatal nursing: An interdisciplinary approach (4th ed., pp. 360–371). Philadelphia: Elsevier Saunders; Forshee, B. A., Clayton, M. F., & McCance, K. L. (2010). Stress and disease. In K. L. McCance, S. E. Huether, V. L. Brasher, & N. S. Rote (Eds.), Pathophysiology: The biologic basis for disease in adults and children (6th ed., pp. 336–359). St. Louis, MO: Mosby Elsevier.

- Do you tell others about your pain? What do you want them to do for the pain?
- What do you not want done when you are hurting? What would you like the nurse to do for the hurt?
- Where is the hurt, and what does it feel like? What could be causing the hurting?

Pain Assessment Scales

Pain assessment tools for children have been developed and tested primarily to evaluate procedural or postsurgical pain. Many pain tools have been tested for **validity** (the extent to which an instrument or scale measures what it is supposed to measure) and **reliability** (the extent to which the same score is obtained when an instrument or scale is used either by different persons or by the same person at different times). Some of the more commonly used pain assessment tools for different age groups with good validity and reliability are presented on the following pages.

Pain Behavior Scales for Nonverbal Children

Physical and behavioral indicators are used to quantify pain in nonverbal children and rely on the nurse's observation of the child. Pain behavior scales involve assessing behaviors that have been identified as indicators of pain. For example, the Neonatal Infant Pain Scale (NIPS) and the FLACC Behavioral Pain Assessment Scale rely on the nurse's observation of the child's behavior.

Clinical Tip

When assessing pain using a behavioral pain scale, first consider if the child is expected to have pain because of surgery, injury, or health condition. Then, if the score on a behavioral pain scale is low, consider if the tool being used is appropriate to assess the child's pain (e.g., can all elements of the scale be assessed). If the answer is no, one strategy is to have the parent identify behaviors indicating that the child is in pain. If pain is suspected, provide analgesia and evaluate the child's response by observing changes in behavior (Pasero & McCaffery, 2005).

Neonatal Infant Pain Scale   The NIPS is designed to measure procedural pain in preterm and full-term neonates up to 6 weeks after birth. The neonate's facial expression, cry quality, breathing patterns, arm and leg position, and state of arousal are observed. This tool has high interrater reliability and validity. See Table 15–4.

FLACC Behavioral Pain Assessment Scale   The FLACC is designed to measure acute pain in infants and young children following surgery, and it can be used until the child is able to self-report pain with another pain scale. FLACC is an acronym for the five categories that are assessed: face, legs, activity, cry, and consolability. The tool has validity and reliability for evaluation of postoperative pain (Manworren & Hynan, 2003; Willis, Merkel, Voepel-Lewis, et al., 2003). See Table 15–5.

Children with Cognitive Impairments   For nonverbal children with cognitive impairments, parents may be coached to de-

TABLE 15–4 Neonatal Infant Pain Scale (NIPS)

Characteristic	Scoring Criteria Descriptors
Facial Expression	
0 = Relaxed muscles 1 = Grimace	• Restful face with neutral expression • Tight facial muscles; furrowed brow, chin, and jaw (Note: At low gestational ages, infants may have minimal facial expression.)
Cry	
0 = No cry 1 = Whimper 2 = Vigorous cry	• Quiet, not crying • Mild moaning, intermittent cry • Loud screaming, rising, shrill, and continuous (Note: Silent cry may be scored if infant is intubated, as indicated by obvious mouth and/or facial movements.)
Breathing Patterns	
0 = Relaxed 1 = Change in breathing	• Relaxed, usual breathing pattern maintained • Change in drawing breath; irregular, faster than usual, gagging, or holding breath
Arm Movements	
0 = Relaxed/restrained (with soft restraints) 1 = Flexed/extended	• Relaxed, no muscle rigidity, occasional random movements of arms • Tense, straight arms; rigid; or rapid extension and/or flexion
Leg Movements	
0 = Relaxed/restrained (with soft restraints) 1 = Flexed/extended	• Relaxed, no muscle rigidity, occasional random movements of legs • Tense, straight legs; rigid; or rapid extension and/or flexion
State of Arousal	
0 = Sleeping/awake 1 = Fussy	• Quiet, peaceful, sleeping; or alert and settled • Alert and restless or thrashing; fussy

Note: From Lawrence, J., Alcock, D., McGrath, D. P., et al. (1993). The development of a tool to assess neonatal pain. Neonatal Network, 12(6), 61; Taylor, B. J., Robbins, J. M., Gold, J. I., Logsdon, T. R., Bird, T. M., & Anand, K. J. S. (2006). Assessing postoperative pain in neonates: A multicenter observational study. Pediatrics, 118(4), e992–e1000.

velop the Individualized Numeric Rating Scale (INRS). Categories of the FLACC Behavioral Pain Assessment Scale can be used to describe pain behaviors on a Visual Analog Scale. Parents can be asked to recall a time when their child had a painful experience, and then to think about the unique behaviors the child demonstrated using the face, legs, activity, cry, and consolability characteristics that reflected the child's pain, creating an individualized FLACC tool. The parents can write the pain behaviors on the line that corresponds to their interpretation of the child's pain intensity ranging from 0 (no pain) to 10 (worst possible pain). This tool has been evaluated for validity and reliability in the postoperative setting. Findings suggest parents can

TABLE 15–5 FLACC Behavioral Pain Assessment Scale

Categories	Scoring		
	0	1	2
Face	No particular expression or smile	Occasional grimace or frown; withdrawn, disinterested	Frequent to constant frown, clenched jaw, quivering chin
Legs	Normal position or relaxed	Uneasy, restless, tense	Kicking or legs drawn up
Activity	Lying quietly, normal position, moves easily	Squirming, shifting back and forth, tense	Arched, rigid, or jerking
Cry	No cry (awake or asleep)	Moans or whimpers, occasional complaint	Crying steadily, screams or sobs; frequent complaints
Consolability	Content, relaxed	Reassured by occasional touching, hugging, or being talked to; distractible	Difficult to console or comfort

How to Use the FLACC

In patients who are awake: Observe for 1 to 5 minutes or longer. Observe legs and body uncovered. Reposition patient or observe activity. Assess body for tenseness and tone. Initiate consoling interventions if needed.

In patients who are asleep: Observe for 5 minutes or longer. Observe body and legs uncovered. If possible, reposition the patient. Touch the body and assess for tenseness and tone.

Whenever feasible, behavioral measurement of pain should be used in conjunction with self-report. When self-report is not possible, interpretation of pain behaviors and decisions regarding treatment of pain require careful consideration of the context in which the pain behaviors are observed.

Interpreting the Behavioral Score

Each category is scored on the 0–2 scale, which results in a total score of 0–10.

0 = Relaxed and comfortable	**4–6** = Moderate pain
1–3 = Mild discomfort	**7–10** = Severe discomfort or pain or both

Merkel, S. I., Voepel-Lewis, T., Shayevitz, J. R., & Malviya, S. (1997). The FLACC: A behavioral scale for scoring post-operative pain in young children. Pediatric Nursing, *23(3), 293–297; Voepel-Lewis, T., Malviya, S., & Tait, A. (2005). Validity of parent ratings as proxy measures of pain in children with cognitive impairment.* Pain Management Nursing, *l6(4), 168–174.*

give reasonable estimates of their child's pain, and their scores were highly correlated with nurses' scores, although the parents' scores were slightly higher than the nurses' ratings (Voepel-Lewis et al., 2005). See the companion website for a model Individualized Numeric Rating Scale.

Pain Location Young children (3 years and older) can localize pain if given an outline of the front and back of the body. The child can mark where the pain is located or color the areas of pain with crayons. Ask the child to use one color for the area that hurts the most, and another color for less painful areas. See the companion website for body outlines to use for pain assessment.

Self-Report Pain Scales
Other scales depend on the child's self-report of pain intensity. To use pain scales the child must be developmentally ready and

Growth & Development   *Exhibiting Stress*

School-age children and adolescents may not exhibit distress in direct proportion to their pain intensity. Thus, behavioral measures (e.g., facial expression, limited movement) may not match the child's self-report of pain intensity. Children in these age groups can accurately report pain intensity with a pain assessment tool, and the reported pain score should be viewed as valid.

be able to understand the concept of a little or a lot of pain well enough to tell the nurse. Children 2 to 3 years of age are usually able to understand the concept of "more or less." These children cannot be given more than three choices on a pain scale (none, some, a lot) when assessing pain. When the child can understand rank order, such as placing several blocks of different sizes in a row from biggest to smallest, the child is developmentally ready for a numeric scale (Young, 2005).

Oucher Scale The Oucher Scale is a self-report pain scale with versions for Caucasians, African Americans, and Hispanics. It has validity and reliability for children between 3 and 12 years of age (Anthony & Schanberg, 2007). Each version presents a series of six photographs of a child expressing increased intensity of pain in combination with a vertical Visual Analog Scale. See Figure 15–2 ➤. The young child selects a face that best fits his or her level of pain; the older child can select a number between 0 and 10. The nurse should *not* compare the photos with the child's facial expression to determine pain level.

FACES Pain Rating Scale The FACES Pain Rating Scale has a series of six cartoon-like faces with expressions from smiling to tearful that can be used by children starting at 3 years of age. The Wong Baker Faces Scale has been validated in children with acute pain, aged 3 to 6 years, and reliability is adequate (Bailey, Bergeron, Gravel, et al., 2007). See Figure 15–3 ➤. The nurse ex-

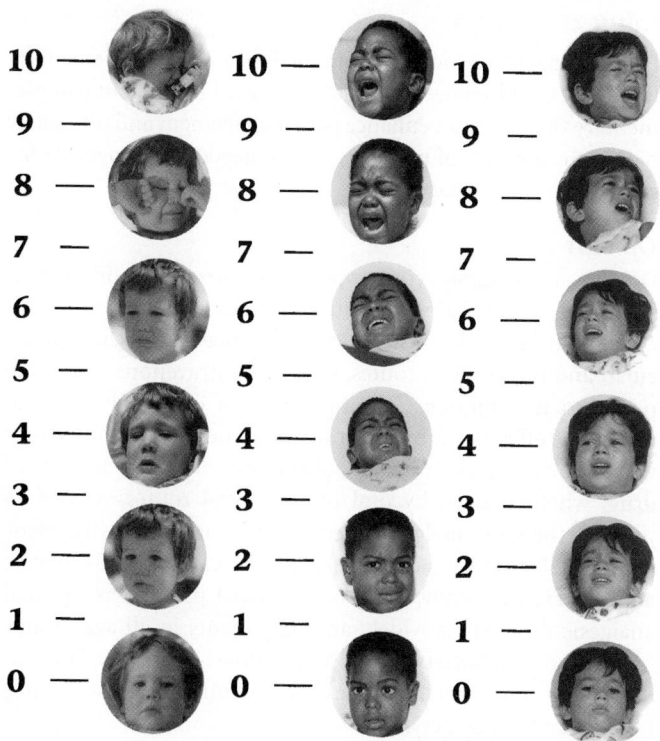

FIGURE 15–2 ➤ Use the Oucher Scale that is the best match for the child's ethnicity. After determining that the child has an understanding of number concepts, teach the child to use the scale. Point to each photo and explain that the bottom picture is "no hurt," the second picture is a "little hurt," the third picture is "a little more hurt," the fourth picture is "even more hurt," the fifth picture is "a lot of hurt," and the sixth picture is the "biggest or most hurt you could ever have." The numbers beside the photos can be used to score the amount of pain the child reports. The Caucasian version of the Oucher was developed and copyrighted by Judith E. Beyer, RN, PhD, 1983. The African American version of the Oucher was developed and copyrighted by Mary J. Denyes, RN, PhD, and Antonio M. Villarruel, RN, PhD, 1990. The Hispanic version of the Oucher was developed and copyrighted by Antonio M. Villarruel, RN, PhD, 1990.

plains the meaning of each face and asks the child to select the face that is the closest match to the pain felt. The nurse should *not* compare the faces with the child's facial expression to determine pain level.

School-age children and adolescents have better number concepts and language skills, so additional tools can be used to assess their pain intensity. The nurse should ask the child to describe the pain and give its location. Providing some words such as *sharp, dull, aching, pounding, cold, hot, burning, throbbing, stinging, tingling,* or *cutting* can help the child describe his or her pain.

Numeric Pain Scale   The Numeric Pain Scale or Visual Analog Scale is a single 10-cm horizontal or vertical line that has descriptors of pain at each end (no pain, worst possible pain). Marks and numbers are placed at each centimeter on the line.

Poker Chip Tool   The Poker Chip Tool uses four checkers or poker chips to quantify pain. The child is asked to pick the number of chips that best matches the pain felt, with one chip being a little pain and four being the most pain he or she could have.

Word-Graphic Rating Scale   The Word-Graphic Rating Scale uses words rather than numbers to describe increasing pain intensity across a 10-cm horizontal line. The child marks the line that is closest to the level of pain felt. A millimeter ruler can be used to quantify the pain and record the pain score. See Figure 15–4 ➤.

Adolescent Pediatric Pain Tool   The Adolescent Pediatric Pain Tool includes a human figure drawing, a 10-cm Word-Graphic Rating Scale, and a list of words to describe pain. Adolescents indicate painful locations on the human figure outline, use the Word-Graphic Rating Scale as described, and use the word choices to characterize the pain felt. See the companion website for the human figure outline and word choices.

■ ACUTE PAIN

Children experience acute pain related to a variety of illnesses and injuries, surgery, and invasive procedures. Just as with adults, children must have their pain assessed and managed.

Clinical Manifestations

Children have both physiologic and behavioral indicators of pain.

Physiologic Indicators

Acute pain stimulates the adrenergic nervous system and results in physiologic changes, including tachycardia, tachypnea, hypertension, pupil dilation, pallor, increased perspiration, and increased secretion of catecholamines and adrenocorticoid hormones. Changes in these signs demonstrate a complex stress response. These signs are not specific to pain, so they cannot be used as the only method for monitoring pain.

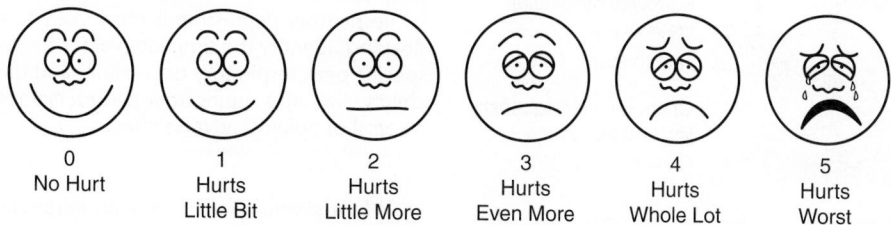

0	1	2	3	4	5
No Hurt	Hurts Little Bit	Hurts Little More	Hurts Even More	Hurts Whole Lot	Hurts Worst

FIGURE 15–3 ➤ The FACES Pain Rating Scale is valid and reliable in helping children to report their level of pain. Make sure the child has an understanding of number concepts, and then teach the child to use the scale. Point to each face and use the words under the picture to describe the amount of pain the child feels. Then ask the child to select the face that comes closest to the amount of pain felt.

Reprinted from Pediatric Nursing, *1988, Volume 14, Number 1, pp. 9–17. Reprinted with permission of the publisher, Jannetti Publications, Inc. Easy Holly Avenue, Box 56, Pitman, NJ 08071-0056; (856) 256-2300; FAX (856) 589-7463; Web site: www.pediatricnursing.net; for a sample copy of the journal, please contact the publisher.*

No Pain	Little Pain	Moderate Pain	Large Pain	Worst Possible Pain

FIGURE 15–4 ➤ The Word-Graphic Rating Scale has words rather than numbers under the line. It may be used by itself or with the Adolescent Pediatric Pain Tool. Teach the child to use the tool by pointing to the side of the line that is no pain. Then run your finger along the line and tell the child that this location is the worst possible pain. If the child has some pain, ask the child to make a mark along the line that is the best match for the amount of pain felt. Use a millimeter ruler to measure from the "no pain" end of the line to the marked location to identify the pain score. Make sure the line is the same length each time pain is assessed so comparisons can be made.

Reprinted from Pediatric Nursing, 1997, Volume 23, Number 1, p. 34. Reprinted with permission of the publisher, Jannetti Publications, Inc. Easy Holly Avenue, Box 56, Pitman, NJ 08071-0056; (856) 256-2300; FAX (856) 589-7463; Web site: www.pediatricnursing.net; for a sample copy of the journal, please contact the publisher.

Behavioral Indicators

Newborns and infants demonstrate knitted brows, squinted eyes with cheeks raised, eyes closed, crying, jerky or flailing movements, and stiff posture in response to pain (Stevens, McGrath, Yamada, et al., 2006). See Figure 15–5 ➤. Children in acute pain may be distressed and anxious, especially if they have experienced pain previously. Behaviors that could indicate pain or anxiety in infants and toddlers include restlessness or agitation, hyperalertness or vigilance, sleep disturbances, and irritability. Children and adolescents may demonstrate the following additional behaviors:

- Short attention span (child is difficult to distract)
- Facial grimacing, biting, or pursing lips
- Posturing (guarding a painful joint by avoiding movement), remaining immobile, or protecting the painful area
- Drawing up knees, flexing limbs, massaging affected area
- Lethargy, remaining quiet, or withdrawal
- Sleep disturbances

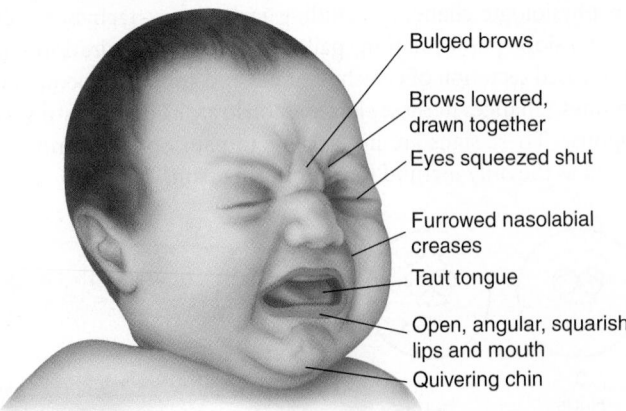

Bulged brows

Brows lowered, drawn together

Eyes squeezed shut

Furrowed nasolabial creases

Taut tongue

Open, angular, squarish lips and mouth

Quivering chin

FIGURE 15–5 ➤ Neonatal characteristic facial responses to pain include bulged brow, eyes squeezed shut, furrowed nasolabial creases, open lips, pursed lips, stretched mouth, taut tongue, and a quivering chin.

Note: Redrawn from Carlson, K. L., Clement, B. A., & Nash, P. (1996). Neonatal pain: From concept to research questions and the role of the advanced practice nurse. Journal of Perinatal Neonatal Nursing, 10(1), 64–71.

Clinical Therapy

Pain management includes both analgesia and complementary therapies. Children need adequate pain medication, but complementary therapies can enhance pain management and ultimately reduce the amount of pain medication needed. See page 381 for complementary therapies.

Opioids

Opioids are analgesics commonly given for severe pain, such as after surgery or for a severe injury. Opioids (e.g., morphine and codeine) may be administered by oral, subcutaneous, intramuscular, and intravenous routes. Oral and intravenous routes are preferred for children. Administration of opioids by an oral route is as effective as by intramuscular and intravenous routes when the drug is given in an **equianalgesic dose** (the amount of drug, whether given by oral or parenteral routes, needed to produce the same analgesic effect) (see the accompanying Medications table on the next page). In some cases opioids may be administered topically, such as a fentanyl patch. The optimal analgesic dose varies widely among patients in all age groups (American Pain Society, 2008). Meperidine is rarely used in children because its metabolite has the potential to cause seizures (American Pain Society, 2008).

Common side effects include sedation, nausea, vomiting, constipation, and itching. A significant potential complication of opioids is respiratory depression. When the child's condition is unstable, as in trauma or critical illness, the dosage of opioids must be carefully calculated to match the child's cardiorespiratory status. Frequent assessments and cardiorespiratory monitoring or pulse oximetry are important safety guidelines when the infant or child has a condition that puts him or her at risk for respiratory depression. Addiction is a rare complication in children treated for painful conditions.

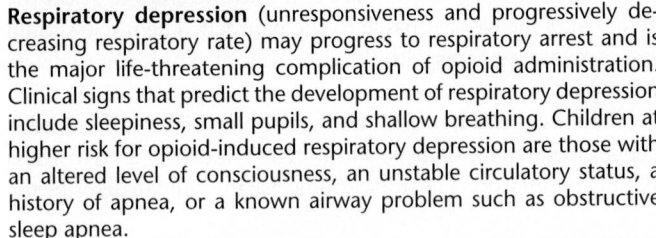

Nursing Alert

Respiratory depression (unresponsiveness and progressively decreasing respiratory rate) may progress to respiratory arrest and is the major life-threatening complication of opioid administration. Clinical signs that predict the development of respiratory depression include sleepiness, small pupils, and shallow breathing. Children at higher risk for opioid-induced respiratory depression are those with an altered level of consciousness, an unstable circulatory status, a history of apnea, or a known airway problem such as obstructive sleep apnea.

Respiratory depression is most likely to occur when the child is sleeping. Identify the time interval for the expected period of drug-specific peak respiratory depression, and then carefully monitor the child's vital signs during that period. Naloxone is the drug used for reversal of opioids' adverse effects.

When given opioids over an extended period, children develop *physical dependence*, the physiologic adaptation to an analgesic or sedative drug at the peripheral and central neurons. These children may experience **withdrawal**, the physical signs and symptoms that occur when a sedative or pain drug is stopped suddenly. **Tolerance** is an adaptation to an opioid

Morphine Animation

Medications Used to Treat

Opioid Analgesics and Recommended Doses for Children and Adolescents*

Drug	Approximate Equianalgesic Oral Dose	Approximate Equianalgesic Parenteral Dose	Recommended Starting Dose (Adults Greater than 50 kg)		Recommended Starting Dose (Children[a] & Adults Less than 50 kg)	
			Oral	Parenteral	Oral	Parenteral
Morphine	30 mg	10 mg	15–30 mg every 3–4 hr	10 mg every 3–4 hr	0.3 mg/kg every 3–4 hr	50–100 mcg/kg every 3–4 hr
Codeine	120 mg	75 mg IV or subcutaneous	30–60 mg every 3–4 hr	60 mg every 2 hr	0.5–1 mg every 3–4 hr[b]	NR
Hydromorphone (Dilaudid)	7.5 mg	1.5 mg	5–10 mg every 3–4 hr	1.5 mg every 3–4 hr	0.1–0.2 mg/kg every 4 hr	10–20 mcg/kg every 3–4 hr
Levorphanol (Levo-Dromoran)	4 mg (acute); 1 mg (chronic)	2 mg (acute); 1 mg (chronic)	2–4 mg every 6–8 hr	2 mg every 6–8 hr	0.04 mg/kg every 6–8 hr	0.02 mg/kg every 6–8 hr
Methadone (Dolophine, others)	10 mg (acute); 2–4 mg (chronic)	5 mg (acute); 2–4 mg (chronic)	5–10 mg every 8 hr	10 mg every 8 hr	0.1–0.2 mg/kg every 12–36 hr	0.1–0.2 mg/kg every 12–36 hr
Oxycodone (Roxicodone)	20 mg	NA	5 mg every 3–4 hr	NA	0.1–0.2 mg/kg every 4 hr[a]	NA
Fentanyl	NA	0.1 mg	5 mcg/kg lozenge	50–100 mcg every 1–2 hr	5–15 mcg/kg Oralet[c]	0.5–1 mcg/kg every 1–2 hr

Data from: American Pain Society. (2008). Principles of analgesic use in the treatment of acute pain and cancer pain (6th ed., pp. 19–21). Glenview, IL; Kraemer, F. W., & Rose, J. B. (2009). Pharmacologic management of acute pediatric pain. Anesthesia Clinics, 27, 241–268.

NR = Not recommended; NA = Not available

*For all parenteral opioids, start with the low dose and titrate to effective pain control.

[a]Infants under 6 months of age should receive a lower per kilogram dose.

[b]Caution: Doses of aspirin and acetaminophen in combination with opioid/NSAID preparation must also be adjusted to the patient's body weight.

[c]The Oralet is not widely used because of nausea and vomiting side effects.

dosage that results in a shorter duration of drug effectiveness over time, and an increasing dose is needed to produce the same level of pain relief. For example, a child might develop physical dependence or tolerance after being in an intensive care setting long term with pain management for life-threatening injuries, multiple surgeries, and invasive procedures. See Table 15–6 for signs and symptoms of withdrawal. Children should be slowly weaned off opioids over 2 to 4 weeks to prevent withdrawal symptoms. One method is to reduce the daily dose by 10–20% over several days. Clonidine is an adjunct medication that may reduce some symptoms of opioid withdrawal.

Acetaminophen and Nonsteroidal Anti-Inflammatory Drugs

Nonsteroidal anti-inflammatory drugs (NSAIDs) such as ibuprofen, primarily given orally, are medications with analgesic properties effective for the relief of mild to moderate pain and chronic pain. Acetaminophen is a nonnarcotic analgesic that is used like an NSAID. It works by raising the pain threshold and is equal to aspirin in analgesic properties. The accompanying Medications table presents recommended dosages of these drugs. They are most commonly used for bone, inflammatory, and connective tissue conditions. An NSAID may be prescribed

TABLE 15–6 Signs and Symptoms of Opioid or Sedative Withdrawal

System	Signs and Symptoms
Central nervous system	Irritability, increased wakefulness, tremulousness, hyperactive deep tendon reflexes, clonus, inability to concentrate, frequent yawning, sneezing, delirium, hypertonicity, visual or auditory hallucinations
Gastrointestinal system	Nausea, vomiting, diarrhea, abdominal cramps, salivation, uncoordinated suck and swallow
Sympathetic nervous system	Tachycardia, tachypnea, increased blood pressure, nasal stuffiness, chills alternating with hot flashes, diaphoresis, fever

Data from: American Pain Society. (2008). Principles of analgesic use in the treatment of acute pain and cancer pain (6th ed.). Glenview, IL: Author; American Pain Society (2005). Guideline for the management of cancer pain in adults and children. Glenview, IL: Author.

Medications Used to Treat
Acetaminophen, NSAIDs, and Recommended Doses for Children and Adolescents

Peak Action Time	Usual Adult Dose	Usual Pediatric Dose	Comments
Non-Opioid Analgesic			
Acetaminophen 0.5–2 hr	500–1000 mg every 4–6 hr	10–15 mg/kg every 4–6 hr	Lacks the peripheral anti-inflammatory activity of other NSAIDs; rectal suppository available
NSAIDs			
Aspirin 1–2 hr	500–1000 mg every 4–6 hr	10–15 mg/kg every 4–6 hr	Do not use in children under 19 years with possible viral illness due to link with Reye syndrome; may cause gastric upset and bleeding; rectal suppository available
Choline magnesium trisalicylate (Trilisate) 2 hr	1000–1500 mg every 12 hr	25 mg/kg every 12 hr	Does not increase bleeding time like other NSAIDs; also available as oral liquid
Ibuprofen (Motrin, others) 0.5 hr	200–400 mg every 4–6 hr	5–10 mg/kg every 6 hr	Available as oral suspension
Naproxen (Naprosyn) 2–4 hr	500 mg initially, then 275 mg every 6–8 hr	5–10 mg/kg every 12 hr	Available as oral liquid
Ketorolac (Toradol) 0.75–1 hr	30–60 mg IV loading dose, then 15–30 mg every 6 hr	1 mg/kg IV loading dose up to 60 mg, then 0.5 mg/kg up to 30 mg IV every 6 hr	IV or IM use only in children less than 50 kg; should not be used for children with bleeding disorder or at risk for bleeding complications; do not use longer than 5 days (Brislin & Rose, 2005)

Adapted from: American Pain Society. (2008). Principles of analgesic use in the treatment of acute pain and cancer pain (6th ed., pp. 6–10). Glenview, IL; Greco, C., & Berde, C. (2005). Pain management for the hospitalized pediatric patient. Pediatric Clinics of North America, 52(4), 995–1027.

in combination with an opioid to increase its effectiveness and to reduce the amount of opioids needed.

Drug Administration

Pain from surgery, major trauma, or cancer is present for predictable periods because of the effects of tissue damage. Pain relief should be provided around the clock. Every effort should be made to give the child analgesics without causing more pain. The preferred routes of administration are intravenous, local nerve block, and oral.

Continuous infusion analgesia is recommended for children with continuous or persistent severe pain because constant drug levels eliminate peaks and valleys in pain control. Analgesics may also be given intravenously on a scheduled basis (e.g., every 3 to 4 hours). Delays in giving analgesics increase the chances of **breakthrough pain** (pain that emerges as the pain medication wears off, resulting in the loss of pain control) and the subsequent anticipation of pain. Giving analgesics on an as-needed (PRN) basis for acute pain also results in the loss of pain control. More medications are often needed to restore pain control than would have been required for continuous infusion analgesia.

Patient-Controlled Analgesia Patient-controlled analgesia **(PCA)** is a method of administering an intravenous analgesic, such as morphine, using a computerized pump programmed by the health care professional and controlled by the child. (See the *Clinical Skills Manual.*) After initial pain control has been achieved with a continuous IV infusion (basal dose) by the nurse, the child presses a button to receive a smaller analgesic dose (bolus dose) for episodic pain relief (Figure 15–6 ➤). This method of pain management is especially useful for pain control in the first 48 hours after surgery when oral pain management is not possible. Safety features to prevent overdoses include the ability to set the maximum number of infusions per hour and the maximum amount of drug received in a given time period. Additional pain medication may be ordered as needed to sup-

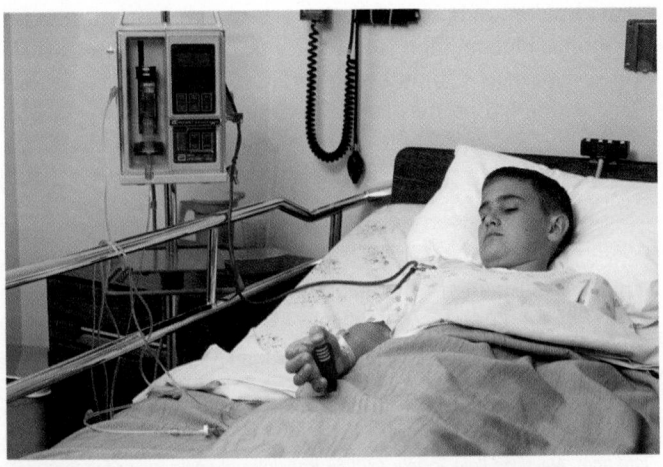

FIGURE 15–6 ➤ By using patient-controlled analgesia, the older child is able to regulate the intake of an intravenous analgesic such as morphine.

plement the continuous and patient-administered infusion when pain control is not maintained.

Children selected for PCA should be able to push the injection button and understand that pushing the button will give them a small amount of additional medication to relieve pain. Children and adolescents benefit from PCA by receiving continuous pain control and having the ability to control their comfort level with no trauma from injections. Once children can take oral analgesics, PCA is discontinued.

PCA is prescribed mostly for children 7 years and older, but may be offered to children as young as 5 years. The child is less likely to administer an overdose as the effect of the medication causes sedation. In rare cases, a parent or nurse is given responsibility for pushing the injection button for a child with disabilities (parent-controlled or **nurse-controlled analgesia**). To reduce the potential for an adverse event, the parent or nurse must follow special guidelines for making pain assessments when responsible for pushing the PCA button (Kraemer & Rose, 2009). See Families Want to Know: Patient-Controlled Analgesia (PCA).

Regional Pain Management Continuous epidural analgesia provides selective analgesia and has become more common for managing severe postoperative pain. The epidural catheter is inserted during general anesthesia into either the lumbar or the caudal space, and advanced up to the space close to the dermatomes to be blocked (Kraemer & Rose, 2009) (Figure 15–7 ➤).

Local nerve blocks, such as a femoral block for anesthesia and analgesia of a leg, are used more frequently for pain control after surgery. A single dose or a continuous infusion of the analgesia with a pump may be used (Kraemer & Rose, 2009). Pain control is achieved without systemic side effects from the medication. Tingling felt in the fingers or toes of the affected extremity is the first sign that the nerve block's effect is ending.

Families Want to Know
Patient-Controlled Analgesia (PCA)

- What is PCA? Analgesia means pain relief: you get to control the amount of medicine you receive by using the machine.

- The machine gives the medicine by passing it through the tube that is connected to your intravenous line. When you push the button, the machine pumps pain medicine into the intravenous line to make you feel better.

- The machine limits the amount of medicine you can get to what the doctor orders. You can get any amount up to the maximum by repeatedly pushing the button. The push button will not let you make a mistake if you drop it or roll on it.

- Whenever you feel pain, hurt, or discomfort, push the button to get more medicine. You should be the only one to push the button.

- No needles for pain shots are needed as long as the intravenous line is in place.

- The PCA may not relieve all of your pain, but it should make you feel comfortable. Let the nurse know if you think your PCA is not working.

- The PCA will be used until you can take pills or drink liquid pain medicine.

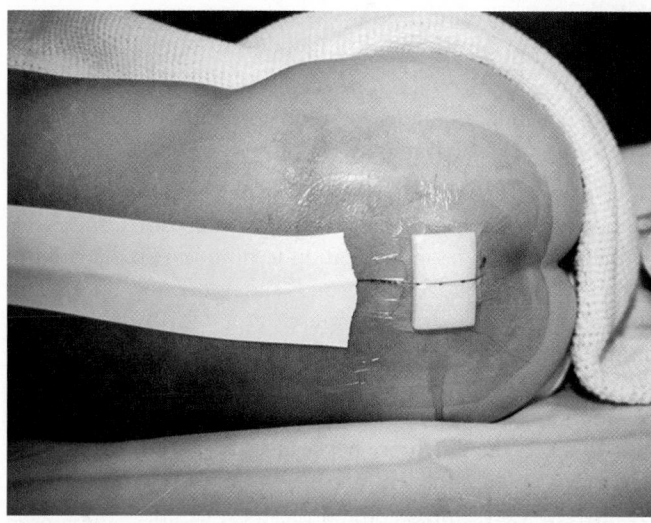

FIGURE 15–7 ➤ An epidural pain block is one example of a regional anesthesia used for postoperative pain management. Once the epidural catheter is placed, it is securely taped and wrapped. Small doses of pain medication may be continuously infused by a pump.
Courtesy of Shriners Hospital for Children, Spokane, WA.

Nonpharmacologic Methods of Pain Management

Complementary therapies are nonpharmacologic methods used for pain management that can enhance the effect of analgesics. If the child has a low pain level, one or more of these methods may provide adequate pain relief without an analgesic.

Cutaneous Stimulation Gently rub the painful area, massage the skin gently, and hold or rock the child. Touching competes with the pain stimuli that are transmitted from the peripheral nerves to the spinal cord and brain and may reduce the pain felt by the child. Swaddling is a method to promote comfort in neonates.

Sucrose Solution Concentrated sucrose solutions (2 mL of 24% solution) may be used as a pain relief measure in preterm and term newborns up to 1 month of age. Sucrose is thought to activate the endogenous opioid system through taste (Taddio, Shah, Hancock, et al., 2008). Give the solution 2 minutes before the procedure, and the analgesic effect of sucrose lasts approximately 3 to 5 minutes. Allow the infant to suck on a pacifier, feed, or breastfeed during the procedure to reduce distress and enhance the effectiveness of the sucrose solution.

Distraction **Distraction** involves engaging a child in a wide variety of pleasant activities that help focus attention on something other than pain and anxiety. Distraction activities may include listening to music, singing a song, blowing bubbles, playing a game, watching television or a video, and playing a computer game. Teach parents how to be distraction coaches and suggest developmentally appropriate activities for the child. Children in severe pain cannot be distracted, but do not assume the pain is gone if a child can be distracted.

Guided Imagery Imagery is a cognitive behavioral process that encourages the child to relax (often with progressive muscle relaxation techniques) and focus on vivid mental images as if they were real. For example, help the child to visualize and explore a favorite place, do a fun activity, remember a funny

Pain Management Kit Video

story, or be a superhero. Ask the child to think about all the sights, sounds, smells, tastes, and feelings that will help enhance the image and experience. Imagery has been used successfully by school-age children and adolescents to reduce pain associated with surgery (Huth, Daraiseh, Henson, et al., 2009).

Relaxation Techniques Relaxation techniques are used to reduce muscle tension that may aggravate pain. Progressive muscle relaxation is one relaxation technique. Ask the child to tense a muscle group for 10 seconds and notice how it feels, and then ask the child to relax the muscle group for 10 seconds and compare the feelings. Teach children to tense and relax different muscle groups, starting with the hands and feet, and then moving to more central muscles. With practice, the child should be able to detect the difference between tense and relaxed muscles and then to reduce the tension.

Breathing Techniques Rhythmic deep breaths can be used with distraction or muscle relaxation during a painful procedure, or as a mechanism to reduce stress. Encourage the child or adolescent to take a deep breath, hold it for 5 seconds, and blow out through the mouth, as if to push the tension out or the needle away. Another breathing technique is patterned, shallow breathing. The child is encouraged to take shallow breaths in through the nose and blow out through the mouth while thinking of a particular image, such as a train with short breaths being the "toot, toot" of the engine.

Hypnosis Hypnosis is an altered state of awareness facilitating heightened concentration, decreased awareness of external stimuli, increased relaxation, and increased suggestibility. In most cases a therapist uses images and the language of the child to induce relaxation and give posthypnotic suggestions for the relief of anxiety, tension, and pain. Hypnosis has been successful in assisting children to control acute postoperative pain, procedural pain and stress, and acute pain associated with conditions such as migraine headaches, hemophilia, and sickle cell anemia. Children can be taught self-hypnosis to give them a sense of mastery and control over pain and distress (Richardson, Smith, McCall, et al., 2006).

Application of Heat and Cold Heat application promotes dilation of blood vessels and increased blood flow enabling pain neurotransmitters and metabolites to be removed from the area (Lane & Latham, 2009). Heat also promotes muscle relaxation, breaking the pain-spasm-pain cycle. To reduce edema, do not apply heat in the first 24 hours after an injury.

The application of cold is believed to slow the speed at which pain fibers transmit pain impulses, reducing the number of pain signals that reach the brain. Cold also controls pain during the acute stage by decreasing bleeding, edema, inflammation, and muscle spasm (Lane & Latham, 2009). Take care to prevent thermal injury. Discontinue cold applications immediately if the skin alternately blanches and reddens afterward.

Electroanalgesia Also known as transcutaneous electrical nerve stimulation (TENS), **electroanalgesia** delivers small amounts of electrical stimulation to the skin by electrodes. This electronic stimulation is stronger than the pain impulses and is thought to interfere with the transmission of pain impulses

from the peripheral nerves to the spinal cord and brain. TENS may be used for both acute and chronic pain management. The only known side effect is skin irritation at the electrode site.

Acupuncture Traditional Chinese treatment for pain relief, acupuncture has been gaining greater acceptance in Western medicine. Acupuncture is based on the theory that energy, or chi, flows along channels through the body (meridians) that are connected by acupuncture points. Pain occurs with obstruction of the energy flow, and inserting needles at the appropriate acupuncture points restores the energy flow (Kundu & Berman, 2007). Placement of acupuncture needles at specific pain points releases endogenous opioid peptides (Wu, Sapru, Stewart, et al., 2009). Limited research has been conducted about the effectiveness of acupuncture use in children.

NURSING MANAGEMENT

Nursing Assessment and Diagnosis

Nurses have an ethical obligation to relieve a child's suffering not only because of the consequences of unrelieved pain but also because appropriate pain management may have benefits such as earlier mobilization, shortened hospital stays, and reduced costs. To provide effective nursing management of children in pain, anticipate the presence of pain and recognize the child's right to pain control.

When assessing pain in children, keep the following questions in mind:

- What is happening in tissues that might cause pain? Assume that children who have had surgery, injury, a vaso-occlusive episode, or illness are experiencing pain, since these events also cause pain in adults. Are there multiple injury sites?
- What external factors could be causing pain? For example, is the cast too tight or is the child poorly positioned in bed?
- Are there any indicators of pain, either physiologic or behavioral?
- How is the child responding emotionally?
- How does the child or parent rate the pain?

Physiologic symptoms such as nausea, fatigue, dyspnea, bladder and bowel distention, and fever may influence the intensity of pain felt by a child. The child's behavior or responses to pain stimuli may be affected by fear, anxiety, separation from parents, anger, culture, age, or a previous pain experience.

When caring for an infant or child, determine which pain assessment tool is the most appropriate for the circumstance and developmental stage. When using a self-report pain scale, use

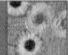
Law & Ethics *Pain Standards*

In 2001, the Joint Commission introduced standards for the assessment and management of pain in patients. All patients have the right to assessment and management of pain, and patient education should include managing pain (Joint Commission, 2008).

the same scale each time you assess for pain or for the evaluation of pain management so you can compare assessment results.

Remember that surgery and trauma can result in multiple sites of pain (incision or laceration, cut or bruised muscles, interrupted blood supply, nasogastric tube placement, insertion sites of intravenous lines). When using pain scales in the assessment of a verbal child, attempt to identify all sites of pain. Then evaluate the intensity of pain at each site.

Examples of nursing diagnoses for children in pain include the following:

- Acute Pain related to injury and femur fracture
- Anxiety related to anticipation of pain from an invasive procedure
- Nausea related to opioids
- Impaired Physical Mobility related to pain

See the Nursing Care Plan for the child with postoperative pain for more nursing diagnoses.

Planning and Implementation

Nursing management involves the following actions to increase and maintain patient comfort: pain medication; complementary therapies; monitoring, evaluating, and documenting the effectiveness of pain control measures to provide optimal comfort; and patient education. See Evidence-Based Practice: Giving Children Adequate Pain Medication.

Pharmacologic Intervention

Give analgesics as ordered by the physician, ensuring that the dose is appropriate for the child's weight. When administering an opioid by intravenous infusion, PCA, or nurse-controlled analgesia, monitor the flow rate and the site for infiltration. For children at risk of respiratory depression, follow facility guidelines for monitoring vital signs and use of a pulse oximeter or cardiorespiratory monitor with an audible alarm set to specified facility parameters. An end tidal CO_2 monitor may be used for a child who is intubated. Vital signs (heart rate and blood pressure) may not change in response to effective analgesia when infection, trauma, or other stressors keep them elevated. Make sure analgesic antagonists such as naloxone are available should complications develop.

Clinical Tip

Naloxone may be used to treat respiratory depression caused by an opioid drug at a dose and slow infusion rate that does not reverse the narcotic's pain control effects. A continuous infusion or repeated doses may be needed for severe overdoses. Dosages are available for children of all ages, including neonates.

NURSING CARE PLAN

The Child with Postoperative Pain

INTERVENTION	RATIONALE	EXPECTED OUTCOME
1. Nursing Diagnosis: Severe Abdominal Pain related to surgery and injury		
NIC Priority Intervention: *Pain management:* Alleviation of pain or a reduction in pain to a level of comfort that is acceptable to the patient		**NOC Suggested Outcome:** *Comfort level:* Feelings of physical and psychologic ease
Goal: The child has pain relief.		
■ Have the child select a pain scale and rate the amount of pain perceived before and 30–60 minutes after analgesia is given to ensure pain relief.	■ The child's pain rating is the best indicator of pain. Maintenance of pain control requires less analgesia than treating each acute pain episode.	The child reports pain relief (to a level acceptable to the child on a pain scale) after administration of analgesia.
■ Assess pain control each hour to ensure that the child's pain control is maintained.	■ Frequent monitoring identifies inadequate pain control before it becomes significant.	
■ Reposition the child every 2 hr to maintain good body alignment.	■ New positions decrease muscle cramping and skin pressure.	
2. Nursing Diagnosis: Disturbed Sleep Pattern related to inadequate pain control		
NIC Priority Intervention: *Sleep enhancement:* Facilitation of regular sleep/awake cycles		**NOC Suggested Outcome:** *Sleep:* Extent and pattern of sleep for mental and physical rejuvenation
Goal: The child will experience fewer disruptions of sleep by pain.		
■ Give analgesia by continuous infusion or every 3–4 hr around the clock.	■ Pain breakthrough occurs even during sleep and disturbs its healing effects.	The child sleeps for the age-appropriate number of hours per day, undisturbed by pain.

(continued)

NURSING CARE PLAN

The Child with Postoperative Pain (continued)

INTERVENTION	RATIONALE	EXPECTED OUTCOME
3. Nursing Diagnosis: Ineffective Individual Therapeutic Regimen Management related to self-management of pain control and use of nondrug pain-control measures		
NIC Priority Intervention: *Self-modification assistance:* Reinforcement of self-directed change initiated by the patient to achieve personally important goals		**NOC Suggested Outcome:** *Treatment behavior pain control:* Personal actions to palliate or eliminate pain
Goal: The child and family will effectively use patient-controlled analgesia (PCA) and complementary therapy pain control measures.		
■ Teach the child how the PCA works and when to push the button.	■ The child must know that pain can be relieved by pushing the PCA button and how the button works.	The child's pain rating stays low.
■ Teach the family and the child how to use age-appropriate complementary therapy pain control measures.	■ Complementary therapies enhance the effect of analgesia and reduce the amount of pain medication needed.	The child and family independently use complementary therapies for pain control.
4. Nursing Diagnosis: Risk for Ineffective Breathing Pattern related to opioid overdose		
NIC Priority Intervention: *Respiratory monitoring:* Collection and analysis of patient data to ensure airway patency and adequate gas exchange		**NOC Suggested Outcome:** *Vital signs status:* Temperature, pulse, respirations, and blood pressure within expected range for the individual
Goal: The child will maintain adequate ventilations.		
■ Verify that the correct dose of opioid is prescribed for the child's weight.	■ Respiratory depression is a significant complication of opioids when too much is given.	There is no episode of respiratory depression associated with the opioid.
■ Monitor vital signs and depth of inspirations before the opioid is administered and at time of peak drug action. Withhold opioid if vital signs fall within parameters established by the physician or by policy.	■ A respiratory depression episode must not progress to respiratory arrest. All opioids act on the brainstem center, which decreases responsiveness to CO_2 tension.	
■ Calculate agonist dose prescribed to be sure it will reverse respiratory depression, but not counteract the effect of analgesia.	■ Valuable time will be saved if an antagonist is needed for an episode of respiratory depression.	
5. Nursing Diagnosis: Constipation related to opioid administration and decreased motility of gastrointestinal tract		
NIC Priority Intervention: *Constipation management:* Prevention and alleviation of constipation		**NOC Suggested Outcome:** *Bowel elimination:* Ability of gastrointestinal tract to form and evacuate stool effectively
Goal: The child will have minimal constipation.		
■ Assess bowel sounds and abdominal distention, and then palpate the abdomen.	■ Signs of constipation must be anticipated and identified.	The child has bowel movements at least every 2 days while on opioid pain control.
■ Request a physician order for a stimulating laxative and stool softener.	■ Opioids increase the transit time of feces and interfere with bile enzymes needed for evacuation.	
■ Provide fluids of choice to increase fluid intake when IV fluids are decreased.	■ Extra fluids will counteract the opioid action of increasing the absorption of water from the large intestine.	
■ Inform the family and child that constipation is a side effect of pain medication.	■ Parents can become partners in managing fluid intake and monitoring bowel movements.	

Problem

A 1-day survey of pain prevalence in a Canadian children's hospital revealed that 77% of 248 interviewed children had pain during admission. Moderate to severe pain was reported by 27% of the children at the time of the survey, and another 64% reported moderate to severe pain in the prior 24 hours. Although analgesics were administered to 58% of the children, only 25% of children got doses of analgesia throughout the day (Taylor, Boyer, & Campbell, 2008). Why does inadequate management of children with acute pain continue to occur?

Evidence

Potential issues associated with undertreating pain in children are the knowledge, beliefs, and values of nurses, and barriers within the hospital that undermine pain management. A survey of pediatric nurse knowledge and attitudes regarding pain management revealed that nurses participating in professional nursing organizations or nursing committees scored higher on pain management competency than nurses who did not participate. Other factors related to a higher score on the knowledge and attitudes regarding pain were nursing education, professional activity, and years of clinical experience (Rieman & Gordon, 2007). Findings of a national study in which three vignettes were used to assess 334 pediatric nurse responses to children's pain did not reveal any personal or professional characteristics of nurses (years of clinical experience, continuing education about pain, education level, and age) related to pain management (Griffin, Polit, & Byrne, 2008). A study conducted in six children's hospitals in Canada revealed that all had policies about pain assessment, but only four had guidelines for pain management (Johnston, Gagnon, Rennick, et al., 2007).

Implications

Research provides variable information regarding the role that nurse characteristics play in pediatric pain management. Institutional barriers may be a bigger factor in increasing pediatric pain management. For example, the lack of pain management guidelines in two Canadian pediatric hospitals is likely a significant institutional barrier to pain management (Taylor et al., 2008). Institutional barriers and infrastructure supports for pain management must be identified so that all nurses know it is an expectation to manage each child's pain.

Critical Thinking Application

In the clinical setting, identify the infrastructure supports to promote pain management of children, such as pain assessment tools, pain flow sheets, pain management policies and guidelines, educational opportunities, and resources for complementary therapies. Identify additional supports that would help you as an inexperienced nurse to gain competence in pediatric pain management.

Check for the presence of other side effects of analgesics, such as sedation, nausea, vomiting, itching, urinary retention, and constipation. If side effects occur, either an alternative opioid is prescribed or the side effects are managed with other medications when long-term analgesia is needed.

Oral NSAIDs are generally ordered for less severe pain or chronic pain. These medications may mask fever. Be alert to the potential complication of gastrointestinal hemorrhage in critically ill children who have increased gastric acids as a physiologic stress response to pain.

Assess the child for pain 15 to 30 minutes following intravenous pain medication and 1 hour after oral pain medication to determine if adequate pain control was achieved. Evaluate the child's level of pain frequently to identify any increase in pain intensity. Use information collected from the child and parent, as well as from an appropriate pain scale. Dramatic reductions in pain should occur, but not all pain may disappear. Use a flow sheet to document pain assessments, medication administration, and results of pain control measures to guide ongoing nursing actions.

Many children sleep after receiving an analgesic. This sleep is not a side effect of the medication or a sign of an overdose, but the result of pain relief. Pain interrupts sleep, and once pain is relieved, the child can sleep comfortably. However, sleep does not always indicate pain control. A child in pain may fall asleep in exhaustion. Look for signs of disturbed sleep such as excess movement or moaning that may indicate pain.

When a regional nerve block is used, the analgesic effect does not recede for several hours after the catheter is removed. Assess the extremity for color, temperature, and capillary refill, and ensure proper positioning to prevent nerve damage. Be careful when ambulating a child with a regional nerve block in an extremity. Protect the extremity from injury because the child has reduced feeling in the limb. Monitor the child for tingling of fingers or toes, an indication that the analgesic effect is receding. Begin oral analgesia to maintain pain control.

Become an advocate for the child when the dose or type of analgesic ordered is inadequate. When the child with severe pain has been taking opioids for several days, an increasing amount of the opioid may be needed to produce or maintain the same level of pain relief. The duration of effective analgesia becomes shorter than expected, and breakthrough pain occurs. Review the child's record to verify that the opioid was given at the appropriate dose and frequency before asking the physician to modify the child's pain medication.

Clinical Tip

Pain is one of the presenting symptoms of many common health problems (e.g., otitis media, pharyngitis, and urinary tract infection). Often the only medication prescribed is an antibiotic to clear the infection. This may leave the child in pain for 48 to 72 hours until the antibiotic brings the infection under control. Give parents recommendations for pain control and comfort measures during this period.

■ Make sure parents have acetaminophen or ibuprofen in an appropriate formulation (drops, elixir, or tablets) for the child's age, and that the medication's expiration date has not passed.

■ Inform the parents about the correct amount of pain medication to use and how frequently it can be given. Ensure that parents have the appropriate medication measuring device.

■ Suggest complementary therapies appropriate for the child's age to help manage the child's pain.

Parents provide security and help reduce the child's anxiety associated with pain and hospitalization. Children often feel more secure telling their parents about their pain and anxiety. When parents are actively participating in the child's care during hospitalization, teach them how complementary therapies can be used to enhance the child's pain management. Help the parents select the age-appropriate complementary therapy for the child:

■ Infants: holding, cuddling, sucking a pacifier, massage
■ Toddlers: massage, stories, bubbles, touch, holding and rocking, music (Figure 15–8 ➤)
■ Preschoolers: engaging in play, stories, music, imagining being a superhero, watching television or a video
■ School-age children: rhythmic breathing, muscle relaxation, guided imagery, talking about pleasant experiences, playing games, listening to radio, watching television or a video
■ Adolescents: rhythmic breathing, muscle relaxation, guided imagery, having visitors, playing games, watching television, listening to CD player or iPod

Nonpharmacologic Intervention

Complementary therapies are nonpharmacologic methods of pain control that can be used with or without analgesics. One or more of these methods may provide adequate relief of low levels of pain. When used with analgesics, nonpharmacologic techniques often increase the effectiveness of the analgesic or reduce the dosage required (see page 381). See Families Want to Know: Helping a Child Cope with Pain to help parents participate in complementary therapies for their child.

Increase Comfort During Painful Procedures

Help the child cope with a painful procedure by telling the child what sensations to expect and what will happen during the procedure. This reduces stress more effectively than just providing information about the procedure. See Chapter 11 ∞ for methods of preparing children of different developmental ages for procedures.

Make every effort to increase the child's comfort during painful procedures, including the use of complementary therapies. Topical anesthetics can be used to reduce the pain associated with an immunization, other injection, intravenous insertion, or venipuncture, or the first needle stick of another procedure. Keep in mind the amount of time needed for the medication to become effective when planning care. Some mechanisms for administration of topical anesthetics include the following:

• Vapocoolant sprays can be used for injections. They are generally effective almost immediately.
• EMLA (eutectic mixture of local anesthetics) cream, an emulsion of 2.5% lidocaine and 2.5% prilocaine, is effective if applied 1 to 2 hours before a needle stick procedure on intact skin in children or 5 to 10 minutes on genital mucosa for neonatal circumcision (Bell, 2009). See Figure 15–9 ➤.

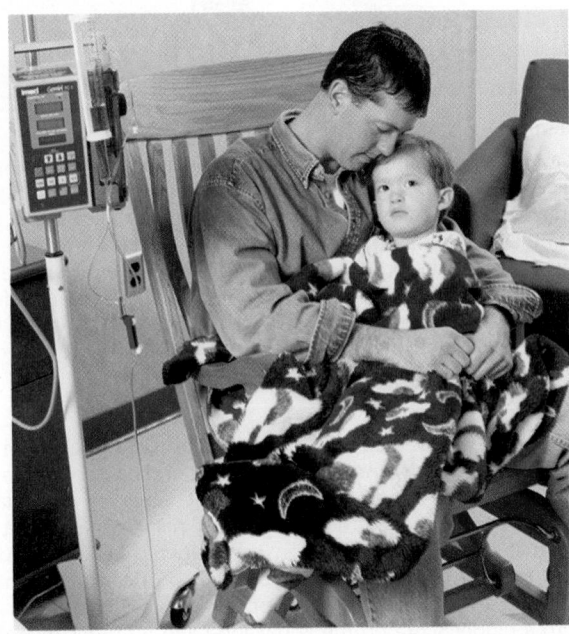

FIGURE 15–8 ➤ The presence of the parent is an important part of pain management. Children often feel more secure telling their parents about their pain and anxiety.

• L-M-X4, 4%, liposomal lidocaine (formerly called ELA-MAX), is effective if applied 30 minutes before needle stick. It is available over the counter.
• **Iontophoresis** involves a patch containing 10% lidocaine hydrochloride and 0.1% epinephrine that is placed over the site of the planned needle stick. A small machine generates electric current to transport anesthetic into the skin in about 10 minutes. However, adverse effects include tingling, itching, and burning (Bell, 2009).
• The Synera anesthetic patch, approved for children 3 years and older, contains a eutectic mixture of lidocaine 70 mg and tetracaine 70 mg. It can be applied for 20 to 30 minutes prior to a venipuncture and intravenous cannulation.

Assemble a pain management kit to promote distraction, imagery, and relaxation in children. Items that might be included are magic wands, pinwheels, bubble liquid, a slinky spring toy, a foam ball, party noisemakers, and pop-up books. It may also be helpful to include items for therapeutic play such as syringes with needles removed, adhesive bandages, alcohol swabs, and other supplies from a medical kit. The pain management kit may

Research ● *Lidocaine Powder*

A study involving 579 children, aged 3 to 18 years, investigated the effectiveness of a lidocaine powder (0.5 mg) provided in a needleless delivery system for venipuncture and intravenous cannulation. Children receiving the lidocaine powder versus placebo reported significantly reduced pain with the procedure. Analgesia occurred within 1 to 3 minutes, and the needleless delivery system did not interfere with the ability to accomplish the venipuncture or intravenous cannulation (Zempsky, Bean-Lijewski, Kauffman, et al., 2008).

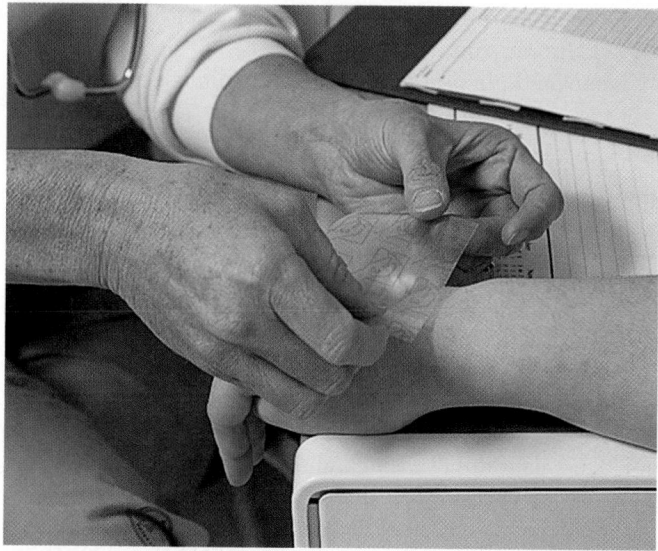

FIGURE 15–9 ➤ When painful procedures are planned, use EMLA or L-M-X4 cream to anesthetize the skin where the painful stick will be made. Apply a thick layer of cream over intact skin and then cover with a transparent adhesive dressing, sealing all the sides. EMLA anesthetizes the dermal surface in about 60 minutes, L-M-X4 in 30 minutes.

be especially helpful for distracting children who are being prepared for surgery or for painful procedures.

Clinical Judgment

What complementary therapies might work best in a preschool-age child having an intravenous start? What about a school-age child?

Discharge Planning and Home Care Teaching

Children are frequently discharged from the hospital with oral analgesics following surgery, injury, or treatment of acute medical conditions. Parents have the responsibility to provide adequate pain control for their child after day surgery. The child usually leaves the surgical center pain-free, and the parents may not anticipate pain. Take the time to discuss the importance of pain management and its benefits in promoting the child's healing. Make sure parents know that a sudden increase in pain intensity may indicate the development of a complication requiring medical attention when efforts to manage the child's pain have been made.

Research — *Post T&A Pain Management*

A study evaluated parent pain management of 261 children aged 2 to 12 years cared for at home following routine tonsillectomy and adenoidectomy (T&A). Parents reported that 86% of children on the first day home and 67% on the third day home had significant pain. Parents were instructed to assess pain with the Bieri Faces Scale and to give pain medication every 4 to 6 hours when the child had pain at a level of 3 or higher. Many children did not receive adequate pain management: 24% of children the first day home and 41% on the third day home received only 0 to 1 doses of analgesia (Fortier, MacLaren, Martin, et al., 2009).

Provide guidance to help parents assess their child's pain, and for school-age children and adolescents to assess their own pain. Teach parents and children about the dosage, frequency of administration, and side effects of the analgesic ordered. Ensure that parents using acetaminophen for short-term pain management identify and temporarily avoid the use of any other medications containing acetaminophen to prevent an overdose. Review nonpharmacologic methods of pain control with parents and children. Encourage children and parents to use the techniques that work best for them.

Evaluation

Expected outcomes of nursing care include:

- The child's pain level is assessed frequently and pain management is effective in improving the child's comfort.
- The child successfully uses a PCA pump to control acute pain.
- Age-appropriate nonpharmacologic methods of pain management enhance the comfort provided by medications.

■ CHRONIC PAIN

Some children have medical conditions that cause chronic pain and episodic acute pain, such as rheumatoid arthritis, cancer, headaches, sickle cell anemia, recurrent abdominal pain, and HIV infection. Children and adolescents with chronic and recurrent pain have functional limitations related to school, social activities and relationships, physical activity, and family responsibilities (Palermo, 2009).

Etiology and Pathophysiology

Chronic pain may be nociceptic or neuropathic, which is caused by abnormal functioning of the nervous system. The sympathetic nervous system is not aroused in the same way it is with acute pain. Chronic pain of long duration that is persistent or continuous permits physiologic adaptation so normal heart rate, respiratory rate, and blood pressure levels are often seen (Huether, 2010).

Clinical Manifestations

Physical and psychologic signs and symptoms should be viewed together. The child may perceive pain but not appear to be in pain. Behavioral indicators of chronic pain may include inactivity, posturing, depression, and difficulty concentrating and sleeping. Chronic pain may be associated with vague and nonspecific symptoms without an easily identifiable cause.

Clinical Therapy

No tools have been developed to assess chronic pain for any pediatric age group. It may be valuable to use multiple tools to assess pain, including a body outline where all pain sites can be marked, a self-report pain scale, and a list of words that describe pain characteristics. Keeping a pain diary including pain characteristics may also be helpful for assessment of recurrent pain.

Children with chronic pain need an individualized pain treatment plan with a primary focus on improved function and comfort. Analgesic medications are prescribed, including NSAIDs, acetaminophen, and opioids, often in combination. Transdermal fentanyl patches may be used for some children with more severe chronic pain needing long-term pain management. Complete pain relief may not be possible, and the child may need additional pain medication for acute flare-ups of the condition. Tricyclic antidepressants may be prescribed for their analgesic properties and because depression may be a co-existing condition. Gabapentin, an antiseizure medication, has efficacy in treating neuropathic pain (Hollan, 2007). Exercise and physical therapy are important to help promote improved function. Complementary therapies are also used.

NURSING MANAGEMENT
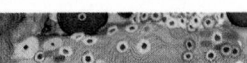

Assessment and evaluation of chronic pain in children should include the following aspects (American Pain Society, 2006):

- Approach pain as the present problem and obtain the history of pain onset, its development over time, intensity, duration, location, what makes it worse or relieves it, and its impact on daily life (sleeping, appetite, school, and social interactions).
- Identify the amount of distress the child and family experience with pain, including anxiety, depression, and hopelessness.
- Determine what the family and child believe causes the pain and their response to it.
- Identify past pain problems in the family and the current methods of treatment.
- Observe the child's appearance, posture, gait, and emotional and cognitive state.
- Assess muscle spasms, trigger points, and areas sensitive to light touch. Perform a complete neurologic examination.

Encourage older children with recurrent episodes of pain to keep a diary to describe the characteristics, timing, activities, and potential pain triggers, and their response to pain treatment measures (Figure 15–10 ➤). A pain assessment scale should be used to rate the pain intensity before and after medications and other pain control measures are used. This record can help improve pain management.

Examples of nursing diagnoses for children with chronic pain include:

- Chronic Pain related to arthritic joint inflammation and degeneration

- Sleep Pattern Disturbed related to ineffective management of chronic pain
- Impaired Physical Mobility related to ineffective management of chronic pain

Children with chronic conditions (e.g., arthritis, sickle cell disease, hemophilia, cancer, recurrent headaches) often need long-term pain management. Strategies for chronic pain management include the following:

- Explain and validate pain and its causes.
- Discuss treatment goals with the child and family and jointly develop a care plan that integrates pharmacologic and nonpharmacologic (complementary) methods.
- Develop a care plan for painful episodes associated with acute flare-ups of their condition.
- Provide effective preventive pain management for procedural pain, as many of these children have numerous medical procedures. If the child's chronic pain is managed with opioids, special consideration is needed to manage the child's procedural pain.

Parents should be actively engaged in pain control for their child. Teach parents the importance of pain control and how to use a variety of complementary therapies with their child to supplement the pain medications administered. Refer children with long-term pain to a pediatric pain program, where they can be evaluated for customized strategies to manage pain.

■ SEDATION AND PAIN MANAGEMENT FOR MEDICAL PROCEDURES

Children undergo a wide variety of painful diagnostic and treatment procedures in the hospital and in outpatient settings. Procedures such as chest tube insertion, arterial puncture, lumbar puncture, bone marrow aspiration, fracture reduction, laceration repair, insertion of a central or peripheral intravenous line, and burn debridement cause significant pain in children. The anticipation of these procedures causes anxiety and emotional distress that can lead to greater intensity of pain.

Clinical Therapy

Sedation is a medically controlled state of depressed consciousness (light to deep) used for painful diagnostic and therapeutic procedures. Children often need light sedation for minimally painful procedures. Children undergoing painful procedures

Date	Time	Pain Intensity	Pain Medication Taken	How Much	Other Pain Relief Methods	Amount of Pain 1 Hour Later

FIGURE 15–10 ➤ A pain diary is an important tool to help record the painful episodes a child experiences with a chronic condition such as rheumatoid arthritis or the recurrent painful episodes that occur with sickle cell anemia. Have the child select a pain scale to be used to record pain intensity.

Clinical Manifestations
Minimal, Moderate, and Deep Sedation

Assessment Factors	Light Sedation	Moderate Sedation	Deep Sedation
Airway	Maintains airway independently and continuously	Maintains airway independently and continuously	Impaired ability to maintain the airway, may need assisted ventilation
Cough and gag reflexes	Reflexes intact	Reflexes intact	Partial or complete loss of reflexes
Level of consciousness	Responds normally to verbal stimuli, but cognitive function is impaired	Easily aroused with verbal or gentle tactile stimulation	Not easily aroused, responds to repeated or painful stimuli

Reprinted from Clinical Pediatric Emergency Medicine, 8, *Mandt, M. J., & Roback, M. G. Assessment and monitoring of pediatric procedural sedation, 223–231. Copyright © 2007, with permission from Elsevier.*

such as burn debridement, laceration repair, bone marrow aspiration, and fracture reduction should be premedicated with analgesia and sedation. Benzodiazepines such as diazepam (Valium) and midazolam (Versed), and pentobarbital are commonly used for sedation. Ketamine, propofol (Diprivan), and etomidate may also be used for sedation (Koh & Palermo, 2007; Buck, 2008). Analgesia must be given in association with sedation because the sedated child can still feel pain but not communicate its presence.

When sedatives are given in lower doses, **light sedation** (formerly called conscious sedation) occurs during which the child maintains protective reflexes and a patent airway, and appropriately responds to verbal stimuli. **Deep sedation** is a controlled state of depressed consciousness or unconsciousness in which the protective reflexes are lost. See the Clinical Manifestations feature above for characteristics of different levels of sedation.

Guidelines should exist in every health care facility where pediatric sedation is performed to ensure safe health care practices. These guidelines often require that the health professionals responsible for monitoring the child have specific qualifications,

Nursing Alert

Whenever sedation is given, be sure to have the resources available to monitor the child's vital signs and to provide advanced life support if the child should progress to deep sedation. If case complications occur, the following equipment should be immediately available: suction apparatus, a bag-valve mask for assisted ventilation, supplemental oxygen, airway equipment, and drugs needed for life support. Antagonists to sedative medication should be premeasured and ready to administer in case of oversedation.

such as Pediatric Advanced Life Support training. With the combined effects of analgesia and sedatives, the child must be carefully monitored for respiratory depression and signs of deep sedation. Antagonist agents (naloxone for opioids and flumazenil for benzodiazepines) must be readily available when the effects of sedation and respiratory depression need to be reversed (Mandt & Roback, 2007).

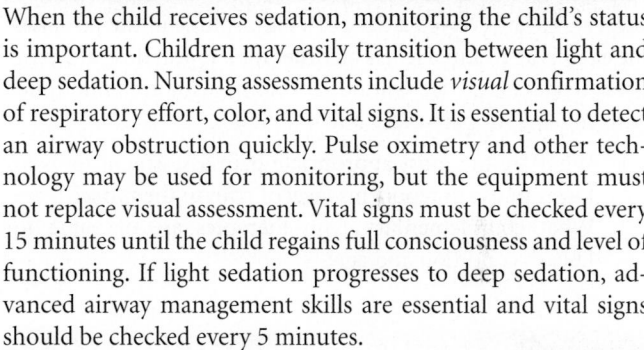

NURSING MANAGEMENT

When the child receives sedation, monitoring the child's status is important. Children may easily transition between light and deep sedation. Nursing assessments include *visual* confirmation of respiratory effort, color, and vital signs. It is essential to detect an airway obstruction quickly. Pulse oximetry and other technology may be used for monitoring, but the equipment must not replace visual assessment. Vital signs must be checked every 15 minutes until the child regains full consciousness and level of functioning. If light sedation progresses to deep sedation, advanced airway management skills are essential and vital signs should be checked every 5 minutes.

Criteria for discharge after sedation include the following:

- The child has satisfactory and stable cardiovascular function and airway patency.
- The child arouses easily and has intact protective reflexes.
- The child is adequately hydrated.
- The infant is able to hold the head up and sit up unassisted if old enough to do so, or the child can stand and walk without assistance.

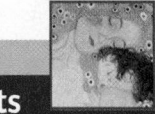

Chapter Highlights

- Pain is an unpleasant sensation that is either acute or chronic, perceived in response to tissue damage. Neuropathic pain is one form of chronic pain.
- Unrelieved pain is stressful for newborns, infants, and children, causing many undesirable physiologic consequences on body systems.

- A child's responses to and understanding of pain depend on age, stage of development, culture, and prior painful experiences.
- Pain assessment should include physical, behavioral, and emotional factors to obtain the most accurate information about the location and intensity of the child's pain and how the child responds to it.

- Pain assessment should include the use of a valid and reliable pain assessment tool that is appropriate for the child's age and condition.
- Every infant, child, and adolescent has the right to adequate pain control.
- Pharmacologic interventions for pain control include opioids, nonsteroidal anti-inflammatory drugs (NSAIDs), and acetaminophen.
- Analgesia for continuous or severe pain should be given around the clock to maintain pain control.
- Complementary therapies for pain management include the following: parental presence, distraction, cutaneous stimulation, sucrose solution, electroanalgesia, guided imagery, breathing techniques, progressive muscle relaxation techniques, hypnosis, application of heat and cold, biofeedback, and acupuncture.

- Epidural and regional nerve blocks are pain control methods used more frequently for postsurgical pain management because they have fewer side effects than systemic medications.
- Parents need education and preparation to provide pain control for children who are discharged home following surgery and injuries.
- Children with recurrent and chronic painful conditions need to have an individualized pain management plan that includes analgesics and complementary therapies.
- Sedation is used to reduce the child's anxiety associated with nonpainful or painful procedures. Analgesia is given with sedation when the procedure will cause pain or discomfort to the child.

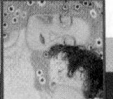

Clinical Reasoning in Action

Recall Lucas, the 14-year-old at the beginning of the chapter who is to have orthopedic surgery for a slipped capital femoral epiphysis (see Chapter 29 ∞). He will go home the same day of surgery. Lucas received a dose of IV morphine in the postanesthesia unit at 10 a.m. He has an order for a repeat dose at 2 p.m., prior to discharge. He will be sent home with acetaminophen with codeine for pain every 3 to 4 hours.

1. What are the most appropriate pain assessment tools for Lucas to use to report his level of pain to the nurse?
2. What complementary pain therapies are of value for Lucas's condition and age?

3. Lucas weighs 52 kg. What is the appropriate dose of morphine for Lucas and the calculated volume (concentration of 2 mg per mL) to be administered?
4. Describe the important nursing assessments for Lucas following morphine administration.
5. Develop a teaching plan for Lucas's home pain management and expected medication side effects.

See Pearson Nursing Student Resources for possible responses.

Pearson Nursing Student Resources

Find additional review materials at
nursing.pearsonhighered.com
Prepare for success with NCLEX®-style practice questions, interactive assignments and activities, web links, animations and videos, and more!

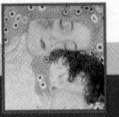

References

American Pain Society. (2005). *Guidelines for the management of cancer pain in adults and children.* Glenview, IL: Author.

American Pain Society. (2006). *Pediatric chronic pain: A position statement from the American Pain Society.* Retrieved from http://www.ampainsoc.org/advocacy/pediatric.htm

American Pain Society. (2008). *Principles of analgesic use in the treatment of acute pain and cancer pain* (6th ed.). Glenview, IL: Author.

Anthony, K. K., & Schanberg, L. E. (2007). Assessment and management of pain syndromes and arthritis pain in children and adolescents. *Rheumatic Disease Clinics of North America, 33,* 625–660.

Bailey, B., Bergeron, S., Gravel, J., & Daoust, R. (2007). Comparison of four pain scales in children with acute abdominal pain in a pediatric emergency department. *Annals of Emergency Medicine, 50*(4), 379–383.

Bell, E. (2009). Update on topical anesthetics. *Infectious Diseases in Children, 22*(7), 12.

Brislin, R. P., & Rose, J. B. (2005). Pediatric acute pain management. *Anesthesiology Clinics of North America, 23,* 789–814.

Buck, M. L. (2008). Use of etomidate for pediatric procedural pain. *Pediatric Pharmacotherapy, 14*(9). Retrieved from http://medscape.com/viewarticle/585288

Finley, G. A., Kristjánsdóttir, Ó., & Forgeron, P. A. (2009). Cultural influences on the assessment of children's pain. *Pain Research & Management,* 14(1), 33–37.

Forshee, B. A., Clayton, M. F., & McCance, K. L. (2010). Stress and disease. In K. L. McCance, S. E. Huether, V. L. Brasher, & N. S. Rote (Eds.), *Pathophysiology: The biologic basis for disease in adults and children* (6th ed., pp. 336–359). St. Louis, MO: Mosby Elsevier.

Fortier, M. A., MacLaren, J. E., Martin, S. R., Perret-Karimi, D., & Kain, Z. N. (2009). Pediatric pain after ambulatory surgery: Where's the pain management? *Pediatrics,* 124(4), e588–e595.

Greco, C., & Berde, C. (2005). Pain management for the hospitalized pediatric patient. *Pediatric Clinics of North America,* 52(4), 995–1027.

Griffin, R. A., Polit, D. F., & Byrne, M. W. (2008). Nurse characteristics and inferences about children's pain. *Pediatric Nursing,* 34(4), 297–305.

Hall, R. W., & Anand, K. J. S. (2005). Short- and long-term impact of neonatal pain and stress: More than an ouchie. *NeoReviews,* 6(2), e69–e74.

Hollan, M. (2007). A practical way to manage chronic pain. *Clinical Advisor,* 10(1), 51–59.

Huether, S. E. (2010). Pain, temperature regulation, sleep, and sensory function. In K. L. McCance, S. E. Huether, V. L. Brashers, & N. S. Rote (Eds.), *Pathophysiology: The biologic basis for disease in adults and children* (6th ed., pp. 481–524). St. Louis, MO: Mosby Elsevier.

Huth, M. M., Daraiseh, N. M., Henson, M. A., & McLeod, S. M. (2009). Evaluation of the Magic Island: Relaxation for kids compact disc. *Pediatric Nursing,* 35(5), 290–295.

Johnston, C. C., Gagnon, A., Rennick, J., Rosmus, C., Patenaude, H., Ellis, J., . . . Byron, J. (2007). One-on-one coaching to improve pain assessment and management practices of pediatric nurses. *Journal of Pediatric Nursing,* 22(6), 467–478.

Joint Commission. (2008). *Health care issues.* Retrieved from http://www.jointcommission.org/NewsRoom/health_care_issues.htm#9

Koh, J. L., & Palermo, T. (2007). Conscious sedation: Reality or myth? *Pediatrics in Review,* 28(7), 243–248.

Kraemer, F. W., & Rose, J. B. (2009). Pharmacologic management of acute pediatric pain. *Anesthesiology Clinics,* 27, 241–268.

Kundu, A., & Berman, B. (2007). Acupuncture for pediatric pain and symptom management. *Pediatric Clinics of North America,* 54(6), 885–889.

Lane, E., & Latham, T. (2009). Managing pain using heat and cold therapy. *Paediatric Nursing,* 21(6), 14–18.

Lawrence, J., Alcock, D., McGrath, P., Kay, J., MacMurray, S. B., & Dulberg, C. (1993). The development of a tool to assess neonatal pain. *Neonatal Network,* 12(6), 61.

Mandt, M. J., & Roback, M. G. (2007). Assessment and monitoring of pediatric procedural sedation. *Clinical Pediatric Emergency Medicine,* 8, 223–231.

Manworren, R. C. B., & Hynan, L. S. (2003). Clinical validation of FLACC: Preverbal patient pain scale. *Pediatric Nursing,* 29(2), 140–146.

Merkel, S. I., Voepel-Lewis, T., Shayevitz, J. R., & Malviya, S. (1997). The FLACC: A behavioral scale for scoring post-operative pain in young children. *Pediatric Nursing,* 23(3), 293–297.

Mitchell, A., & Boss, B. J. (2002). Adverse effects of pain on the central nervous systems of newborns and young children: A review of the literature. *Journal of Neuroscience Nursing,* 34(5), 228–236.

Palermo, T. M. (2009). Assessment of chronic pain in children: Current status and emerging topics. *Pain Research & Management,* 14(1), 21–26.

Pappagallo, M., & Werner, M. (2008). *Chronic pain: A primer for physicians.* Chicago: Remedica.

Pasero, C., & McCaffery, M. (2005). No self-report means no pain-intensity rating. *American Journal of Nursing,* 105(10), 50–53.

Plaisance, L., & Logan, C. (2006). Nursing students' knowledge and attitudes regarding pain. *Pain Management Nursing,* 7(4), 167–175.

Purnell, L. D. (2009). *Guide to culturally competent care* (2nd ed.). Philadelphia: F. A. Davis.

Richardson, J., Smith, J. E., McCall, G., & Pilkington, K. (2006). Hypnosis for procedure-related pain and distress in pediatric cancer patients: A systematic review of effectiveness and methodology related to hypnosis interventions. *Journal of Pain and Symptom Management,* 31(1), 70–84.

Rieman, M. T., & Gordon, M. (2007). Pain management competency evidenced by a survey of pediatric nurses' knowledge and attitudes. *Pediatric Nursing,* 33(4), 307–312.

Stanford, E. A., Chambers, C. T., & Craig, K. D. (2005). A normative analysis of the development of a pain-related vocabulary in children. *Pain,* 114(1–2), 278–284.

Stevens, B., McGrath, P., Yamada, J., Gibbins, S., Beyene, J., et al. (2006). Identification of pain indicators for infants at risk for neurological impairment: A Delphi consensus study. *BMC Pediatrics,* 6(1). Retrieved from http://www.biomedcentral.com/1471-2431/6/1

Taddio, A., Shah, V., Hancock, R., Smith, R. W., Stephens, D., Atenafu, E., . . . Katz, J. (2008). Effectiveness of sucrose analgesia in newborns undergoing painful medical procedures. *Canadian Medical Association Journal,* 179(1), 37–43.

Taylor, B. J., Robbins, J. M., Gold, J. I., Logsdon, T. R., Bird, T. M., & Anand, K. J. S. (2006). Assessing postoperative pain in neonates: A multi-center observational study. *Pediatrics,* 118(4), e992–e1000.

Taylor, E. M., Boyer, K., & Campbell, F. A. (2008). Pain in hospitalized children: A prospective cross-sectional survey of pain prevalence, intensity, assessment, and management in a Canadian pediatric teaching hospital. *Pain Research & Management,* 13(1), 25–32.

Voepel-Lewis, T., Malviya, S., & Tait, A. R. (2005). Validity of parent ratings as proxy measures of pain in children with cognitive impairment. *Pain Management Nursing,* 6(4), 168–174.

Walco, G. A. (2008). Needle pain in children: Contextual factors. *Pediatrics,* 122(Suppl. 3), S125–S129.

Walden, M. (2007). Pain in the newborn and infant. In C. Kenner & J. W. Lott, *Comprehensive neonatal nursing: An interdisciplinary approach* (4th ed., pp. 360–371). Philadelphia: Elsevier Saunders.

Walden, M., & Carrier, C. (2009). The ten commandments of pain assessment and management in preterm neonates. *Critical Care Clinics of North America,* 21, 235–252.

Willis, M. H. W., Merkel, S. I., Voepel-Lewis, T., & Malviya, S. (2003). FLACC behavioral pain assessment scale: A comparison with the child's self-report. *Pediatric Nursing,* 29(3), 195–198.

Wu, S., Sapru, A., Stewart, M. A., Milet, M., Hudes, M., Livermore, L., & Flori, H. (2009). Using acupuncture for acute pain in hospitalized children. *Pediatric Critical Care Medicine,* 10(3), 291–296.

Young, K. D. (2005). Pediatric procedural pain. *Annals of Emergency Medicine,* 45(2), 160–171.

Zempsky, W. T., Bean-Lijewski, J., Kauffman, R. E., Koh, J. L., Malviya, S. V., Rose, J. B., & Gennevois, D. J. (2008). Needle-free powder lidocaine delivery system provides rapid effective analgesia for venipuncture or cannulation pain in children: Randomized, double-blind comparison of venipuncture and venous cannulation pain after fast-onset needle-free powder lidocaine or placebo treatment trial. *Pediatrics,* 121(5), 979–987.

Immunizations and Communicable Diseases

chapter 16

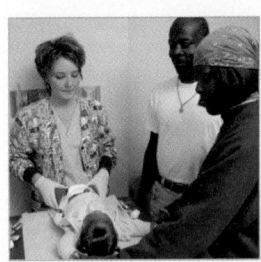

Four-month-old Kendra has been brought by her parents to the community health center for a checkup and immunizations. Kendra is healthy and growing at an appropriate rate. She has not yet had any illnesses. Her parents have enjoyed watching her grow and gain new developmental skills over the past 4 months. During Kendra's health visit, the pediatric nurse practitioner talks with her parents about her food intake and describes how well she is growing.

Kendra's mother reveals that she has heard information about the safety of vaccines on television and asks for more information. She also wants to know why so many shots are given at a time. The nurse practitioner discusses vaccine safety with Kendra's parents and talks about the importance of each of the vaccines Kendra is to receive. She then obtains consent to administer each of the vaccines.

What factors determine the timing of vaccines for administration to infants and children? Why are infants and children at higher risk for infectious diseases? What methods should parents use to reduce the number of infectious diseases in their children? What are signs of a serious infection in an infant and in a child?

Learning Outcomes

After reading this chapter, you will be able to do the following:

1. Explain why children are more vulnerable than adults to communicable diseases.
2. Describe the process of infection and modes of transmission.
3. Summarize the role vaccines play in reduction and elimination of communicable diseases.
4. Prepare a nursing care plan for children of all ages needing immunizations.
5. Differentiate between common communicable diseases.
6. Describe the medical and nursing management of common communicable diseases.

■ COMMUNICABLE DISEASE AS A HEALTH PROBLEM

A **communicable disease** is an illness that is **directly transmitted**, acquired from a person or vector (ticks, mosquitoes, or other animal) by contact with body fluids, or **indirectly transmitted** by contact with contaminated objects. An **infectious disease** is any communicable disease caused by microorganisms that are commonly transmitted from one person to another or from an animal to a person. For a communicable disease to occur, three factors need to be present (Figure 16–1 ➤):

- An infectious agent, or pathogen
- An effective means of transmission or spread of the infectious agent
- A susceptible host

Communicable diseases are a major cause of morbidity in infants and children, and in some cases can cause death. Children can develop complications or secondary infections that require health care intervention and may be an economic burden to families.

Special Vulnerability of Infants and Children

Infants in particular are susceptible to communicable diseases because the immune system is not fully mature at birth and protection through immunization is incomplete. With **passive immunity**, antibodies are produced in another human or animal host. For example, a mother passes **antibodies** (proteins capable of responding to specific infections) to the fetus during the third trimester by the placenta and to the newborn through breast milk. Preterm infants are at greater risk because they receive fewer maternal antibodies prior to birth and their immune system is even less mature (Hall, Noble, & Smith, 2009). Passive immunity decreases in the newborn in the months after birth. Immunodefi-

ciency and poor health may also increase a child's risk of contracting an infectious disease.

The poor hygiene behaviors of young children promote the transmission of infectious diseases in environments with children in close contact. The fecal-oral and respiratory routes are the most common sources of transmission in children. Young children may not wash their hands after toileting unless closely supervised. They then put their fingers in the mouth or rub the nose and eyes. Diapers may leak stool, allowing exposure to fecal organisms. In some cases, the child is contagious before disease symptoms occur (e.g., varicella and parvovirus B-19). See the table beginning on page 410 for more information about these and other communicable diseases.

Infants and children develop **active immunity** with antibody development for specific infections through immunization or exposure to the natural disease through contacts with other children and adults (Figure 16–2 ➤). Subsequent exposure to the same type of organism often results in resistance or in a less severe infection. (See "Focus on the Immune System" in Chapter 22 ∞.)

Public Health and Communicable Diseases

Common preventable communicable diseases are a significant public health problem. Reducing the number of preventable childhood illnesses is a major national goal in *Healthy People 2020*, and nurses are important partners in this effort. Specific objectives are targeted at the reduction or elimination of infectious diseases (U.S. Department of Health and Human Services, 2010):

- Reduce or eliminate cases of vaccine-preventable diseases.
- Reduce hepatitis A, hepatitis B, meningococcal disease, early onset invasive Streptococcal B disease, and invasive pneumococcal disease.

Public health authorities conduct **disease surveillance**, monitoring patterns of disease occurrence from the reported cases of communicable diseases in the United States. National disease surveillance efforts have increased in response to concerns of bioterrorism and a **pandemic**, the emergence and worldwide spread of an infection (e.g., H1N1 influenza) that causes significantly increased morbidity and mortality.

Infection Control

Preventing the spread of infectious diseases is a process that involves several strategies that must be well coordinated. Proper hand hygiene is one

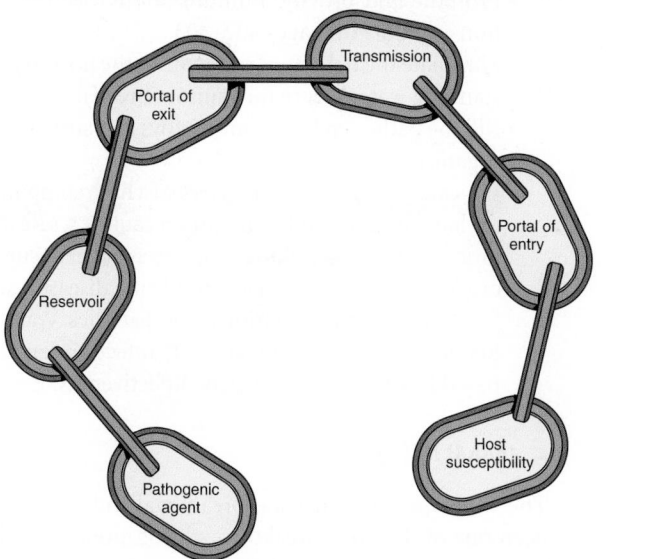

Pathophysiology Illustrated
The Chain of Infection

FIGURE 16–1 ➤ An effective chain of infection transmission requires a suitable habitat or reservoir for the pathogen. To prevent or control the spread of infection, one of the links in the chain must be broken, such as eliminating one or more of the habitats or reservoirs (e.g., insecticide spraying to kill mosquitoes that carry malaria). Isolating an infected individual interferes with disease transmission, and killing the pathogen eliminates the causal agent.

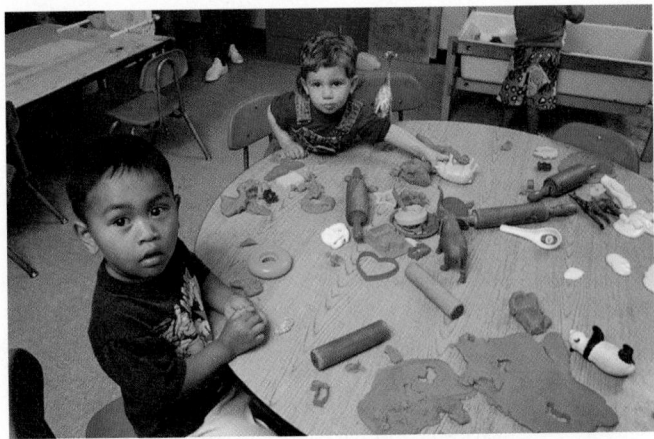

FIGURE 16–2 ➤ Infectious diseases are easily transmitted in settings such as childcare centers where multiple children handle common objects and then put fingers in their mouths.

Culture   *Beliefs About Disease Causation*

In some cultures, infectious diseases are seen as punishment or the result of curses or evil spirits. For example, Native Americans traditionally view illnesses as the result of disharmony or displeasing the spirits. They may not believe in the germ theory of disease causation.

of the most important strategies for everyone. Nurses have a significant role in this process and are responsible for implementing several infection control strategies:

• Use standard and transmission-based precautions.
• Wash hands with soap and water when visibly dirty or contaminated by blood or other body fluids, and after using the toilet (see Figure 16–3 ➤) (World Health Organization, 2009).

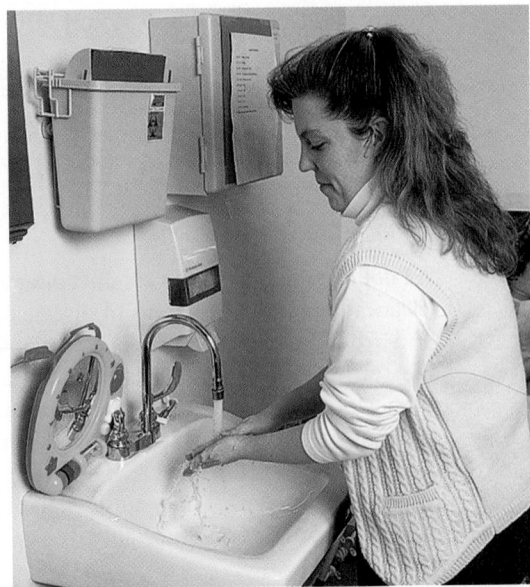

FIGURE 16–3 ➤ Proper handwashing with soap and water for 1 to 2 minutes is one of the most effective measures for preventing disease transmission. Alcohol-based hand sanitizers, which take less than 30 seconds to use, are a good alternative to handwashing.

Families Want to Know
Reducing the Transmission of Infection

The following practices can help families reduce the spread of infection among family members:

■ Use disposable tissues and discard immediately after use.
■ Wash hands thoroughly with soap and water or hand sanitizer after all contact with the child's diaper, runny nose, and mucous membranes.
■ Teach children to cough or sneeze into their elbow rather than their hands.
■ Teach children to wash their hands with soap and water after toileting and before eating.
■ Do not allow children to share dishes and utensils.
■ Wash hands before preparing food, and again several times during food preparation. Follow guidelines for safe food preparation and storage. Wash dishes and cutting boards in warm soapy water or use the sanitizing cycle on the dishwasher.
■ Wipe counters and surfaces that are used for diaper changes or that the child touches with a disinfectant such as bleach solution, Lysol, or isopropyl alcohol. Make sure the diaper-changing area is not near food preparation areas.
■ Dispose of diapers in closed containers.

• Use an alcohol-based hand sanitizer to clean the hands in all other routine clinical situations. Wash hands with soap and water if an alcohol-based hand rub is not available (World Health Organization, 2009).
• Separate or quarantine ill children from well children. Frequently assess children in waiting rooms of clinics and physician's offices to identify children who should be isolated. Separate hospitalized children with infections from children with a high risk for infection, such as those with compromised immune systems.
• Promote and provide immunizations. See the immunization schedule on pages 402–403.
• Eliminate the habitat or reservoir of the host (e.g., eliminate standing water where mosquitoes breed).
• Kill the pathogen (e.g., sanitize toys and surfaces exposed to organisms).
• Educate parents and caregivers of children about the need for hand hygiene and standard precautions, safe food preparation and storage, taking action to avoid exposure to certain organisms (e.g., ticks that cause Lyme disease), and the importance of immunizations. See Families Want to Know: Reducing the Transmission of Infection and Evidence-Based Practice: Hand Hygiene Effectiveness.

■ IMMUNIZATION

The development and widespread availability of vaccines has been one of the great breakthroughs of modern medicine. The average infant born in 2010 will receive immunizations for 14 diseases by the age of 6 years. See the vaccine schedule on pages 402–403. Vaccines have also been developed for older children, adolescents, and adults to protect against pertussis, meningococcus, human papillomavirus, and herpes zoster. Vaccines greatly improve the health of children and reduce the par-

Evidence-Based Practice

Hand Hygiene Effectiveness

Problem

Several studies have investigated the effectiveness of hand hygiene education, handwashing with soap and water, and alcohol-based hand sanitizer in preventing respiratory infections and gastrointestinal infections. What is the most effective hand hygiene method to reduce infections in community settings?

Evidence

A meta-analysis analyzed the effects of different hand hygiene methods to determine which had the greatest effectiveness in community settings, including schools and childcare centers. The most effective intervention was found to be hand hygiene education with the use of non-antibacterial soap. The use of antibacterial soap had little added benefit. Alcohol-based hand sanitizers and hand hygiene education were not strongly associated with reduced rates of respiratory or gastrointestinal illness (Aiello, Coulborn, Perez, et al., 2008). A study investigated the effectiveness of a 4-week learner-centered handwashing program on the frequency of handwashing in 406 second-grade students in seven schools. Children learned about causes of illness and hand hygiene behavior. Techniques were used to enable children to visualize the reduction of organisms after handwashing. Parents were surveyed and 64% reported an increased frequency of handwashing, 50% reported an increase in duration of handwashing, and 79% reported they did not need to remind children to wash their hands before meals. An increase in student handwashing was noted by 94% of teachers (Tousman, Arnold, Helland, et al., 2007).

Implications

Many educational programs teaching hand hygiene to children involve only one session, and this is likely inadequate to change the behavior of young children. Children who see the relationship between handwashing and the difference in organisms on their hands appear to be more likely to have a more long-lasting behavior change.

Critical Thinking Application

When implementing a handwashing program with young children, identify methods to help children visualize the effectiveness of handwashing.

ent's burden of caring for ill children. For example, the rate of pneumonia hospitalizations in children less than age 2 years decreased by 35% after the introduction of the pneumococcal conjugate vaccine in 2000 (Grijalva, Griffin, Nuorti, et al., 2009).

Before the 1950s when infant and childhood immunization programs were initiated, the annual impact of infectious and communicable diseases in the United States was staggering. Thousands of children died or developed permanent disabilities after being infected with diseases such as polio, rubella, measles, diphtheria, pertussis, and *Haemophilus influenzae* type b (Children's Hospital of Philadelphia, 2008).

Etiology and Pathophysiology

Immunization introduces an **antigen** (a foreign substance that triggers an immune system response) into the body. The person produces antibodies and develops active immunity without becoming sick with the disease. Some children need antibodies faster than the body can develop them with a vaccine, such as an unimmunized toddler being treated with chemotherapy who is exposed to chickenpox. Passive immunity is needed to prevent the disease from occurring or to reduce its severity. Varicella immune globulin is given by injection to reduce the child's risk for developing chickenpox. Passive immunity does not confer lasting immunity, so the varicella vaccine is later administered to start the process of antibody development (active immunity).

Types of vaccines against childhood illnesses used in the United States include the following:

- **Killed virus vaccine.** A vaccine that contains a microorganism that has been killed but is still capable of inducing the human body to produce antibodies. Example: inactivated poliovirus vaccine.
- **Toxoid.** A toxin that has been treated (by heat or chemical) to weaken its toxic effects but retain its antigenicity. Example: tetanus toxoid.
- **Live virus vaccine.** A vaccine that contains a microorganism in live but attenuated, or weakened, form. Examples: measles and varicella vaccines.
- Recombinant forms. An organism that has been genetically altered for use in vaccines. Examples: hepatitis B and **acellular vaccine** (a vaccine that uses proteins, such as from pertussis, rather than the whole bacterial cell to stimulate the process of active immunity).
- Conjugated forms. An altered organism joined with another substance to increase the immune response. Example: The *Haemophilus influenzae* type b (Hib) vaccine is conjugated with a protein-carrier like tetanus toxoid, but no immunity to tetanus occurs when it is the protein-carrier.

Today's vaccines are often produced synthetically by means of recombinant DNA technology or genetic engineering to improve vaccine safety and effectiveness, and to reduce side effects.

Clinical Tip

Thimerosal, a bacteriostatic agent that contains ethyl mercury, was previously used to prevent contamination of vaccines in multidose vials. Because of the possible association between mercury poisoning and nerve and brain damage, vaccine manufacturers have removed thimerosal from all vaccines given to children except the influenza vaccine (American Academy of Pediatrics [AAP], 2009, p. 13).

Clinical Manifestations

Children receiving vaccines can have a variety of responses as the body responds to the injected antigen stimulating the immune response. Vaccine recipients commonly have a local reaction that includes erythema, swelling, pain, and induration at the site of the injection. Systemic reactions such as fever, fussiness or irritability, malaise, and anorexia may occur. Other systemic reactions (e.g., rash or arthralgia) are associated with some vaccines.

Allergic reactions to vaccines, such as a wheal or urticaria, occasionally occur within minutes to hours after an injection. A severe local allergic reaction is manifested by warmth, erythema, edema, petechiae, or ulceration occurring 2 to 8 hours after vaccination. A non-life-threatening systemic allergic reaction, such as generalized urticaria or transient petechiae, may occur within minutes. Anaphylaxis is a life-threatening reaction that is manifested by hypotension, generalized urticaria, and angioedema, and it usually occurs within minutes. Laryngeal edema has occurred in rare cases with nearly every vaccine. The reactions to specific vaccines can be found on the Medications table listing common pediatric immunizations on pages 396–400.

Nursing Alert

Be prepared for potential vaccine anaphylaxis. Keep epinephrine 1:1000 and resuscitation equipment immediately available. The dose for epinephrine (aqueous 1:1000) is 0.01 mL/kg per dose up to 0.5 mL intramuscularly. The dose can be repeated every 10–20 minutes for up to a total of three doses. Airway management, supplemental oxygen, and other emergency interventions should be initiated (AAP, 2009, p. 66).

COLLABORATIVE CARE

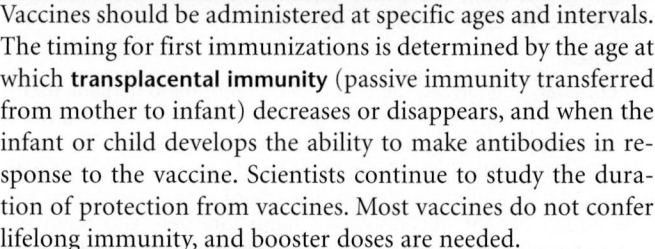

Vaccines should be administered at specific ages and intervals. The timing for first immunizations is determined by the age at which **transplacental immunity** (passive immunity transferred from mother to infant) decreases or disappears, and when the infant or child develops the ability to make antibodies in response to the vaccine. Scientists continue to study the duration of protection from vaccines. Most vaccines do not confer lifelong immunity, and booster doses are needed.

Immunization Schedule

The recommended schedule for immunization is updated at least annually to reflect new vaccines and the need for repeat immunization. The Advisory Committee on Immunization

(Text continues on page 401.)

Medications Used for
Pediatric Immunizations

Immunization Type	Side Effects	Contraindications	Nursing Implications
Diphtheria and Pertussis Vaccines and Tetanus Toxoid (DTaP, Tdap) *Type:* Inactivated. *Route:* Intramuscular. *Dosage:* 0.5 mL. *Age(s) given:* DTaP at 2, 4, 6, 15–18 months; 4–6 years (five doses); 11–12 years (Tdap). Do not restart the series, no matter when the prior dose(s) were given. For a prior serious reaction to the pertussis component of the DTaP vaccine, use DT (children less than 7 years) or Td (children 7 years and older) vaccines. May give at same time as all other vaccines, in a separate site. *Storage:* Refrigerate, do not freeze. Daptacel stopper vial contains latex. Pediarix stopper vial is latex-free.	*Common:* Redness, pain, swelling, nodule at injection site; fever to 38.3°C (101°F); drowsiness, irritability, fussiness; anorexia within 2 days of injection. Increase in frequency and magnitude of local reactions with fourth and fifth doses (e.g., entire limb swelling). *Serious:* Allergic reaction, anaphylaxis; shock or collapse (an episode with sudden loss of muscle tone, pallor, fever, and unresponsiveness), fever above 40.5°C (104.8°F); febrile seizure; persistent inconsolable crying.	Immediate anaphylactic reaction. Encephalopathy within 7 days. Progressive neurologic disorder. Gelatin allergy (do not use Tripedia). *Precautions for DTaP or Tdap administration:* If the child had the following reactions within 48 hours of the previous dose: ■ Fever of 40.5°C (105°F) or higher ■ Inconsolable crying for 3 hours or longer ■ Pale or limp episode or collapse ■ Guillain-Barré syndrome less than 6 weeks after previous dose ■ Seizure within 3 days of dose Delay administration until moderate to severe febrile illnesses have resolved. Postpone Tdap to adolescents with a progressive neurologic disorder or encephalopathy or uncontrolled epilepsy until the condition is stabilized.	Use same brand for all doses if possible. Ask about previous reactions to immunization. In children with a seizure history, give acetaminophen when the vaccine is administered and then every 4 hours for 24 hours. Solution will be cloudy after shaking. Do not use if any clumps are present. Since different product preparations (e.g., single and combination vaccines) may be used for all, one, or some doses, read package inserts carefully. When required, simultaneous administration of tetanus immune globulin or diphtheria antitoxin should be given in separate sites. Inform parents that an increased reaction to the fourth and fifth doses may occur. A tetanus booster may be given for a contaminated wound or burn if 5 or more years have passed since the last dose.

Medications Used for
Pediatric Immunizations *(continued)*

Immunization Type	Side Effects	Contraindications	Nursing Implications
Haemophilus Influenzae Type B Vaccine (Hib) *Type:* Inactivated. *Route:* Intramuscular. *Dosage:* 0.5 mL. *Age(s) given:* 2, 4, 6 months (PRP-T based vaccine) *or* 2, 4 months (PRP-OMP based vaccine) *and* 12–15 months (any Hib vaccine). Do not restart the series, no matter when the prior dose(s) were given. May give at same time as all other vaccines in a separate site. *Storage:* Refrigerate, do not freeze.	*Common:* Pain, redness, or swelling at site. *Serious:* Anaphylaxis (extremely rare); fever.	Prior anaphylactic reaction to this vaccine. *Precautions:* Moderate or severe acute illness with or without fever.	Prior to administration, ask if the child is immunosuppressed. Some children benefit from additional doses (AAP, 2009, p. 320). Solution is clear and colorless. Since different product preparations (e.g., single and combination vaccines) affect the immunization schedule, read package inserts carefully. Follow directions for reconstituting, refrigerating, and discarding unused reconstituted vaccine.
Hepatitis A Vaccine (HepA) *Type:* Inactivated. *Route:* Intramuscular. *Dosage:* 0.5 mL (1 mL over 18 years). *Age(s) given:* 12–23 months; 2–18 years, first dose followed by second dose 6–12 months later. Do not restart the series, no matter when the prior dose was given. May give at same time as all other vaccines in a separate site. *Storage:* Refrigerate, do not freeze.	*Common:* Pain, tenderness, induration at injection site.	Known hypersensitivity to any vaccine component. Prior hypersensitivity or anaphylactic reaction to the vaccine.	Shake well, slightly opaque white suspension. No reconstitution is needed. Can be given for postexposure prophylaxis against hepatitis A in persons not previously immunized. Vaccine brands can be interchanged. Vaqta vials have a latex stopper.
Hepatitis B Vaccine (HepB) *Type:* Inactivated. *Route:* Intramuscular. *Dosage:* 0.5 mL (1 mL at 20 years). *Age(s) given:* Birth, 1–2 months, 6–18 months (three doses). A three-dose series can be started at any age. Do not restart the series, no matter when the prior dose(s) were given. May give at same time as all other vaccines in a separate site. *Storage:* Refrigerate, do not freeze. Newborn dose should be a single vaccine preparation.	*Common:* Pain or redness at injection site; fever. *Serious:* Anaphylaxis is uncommon.	Prior anaphylaxis. Serious hypersensitivity reaction to past dose, perhaps due to a yeast hypersensitivity.	If mother has HBsAg+ or unknown status, give vaccine to infant within 12 hours of birth along with hepatitis B immune globulin in another site. Shake vaccine before withdrawing. Solution will appear cloudy. Various formulations (pediatric, adult, dialysis) and combination vaccines are available. Read package insert carefully and follow directions for the product used. Infants of HBsAG+ mothers should have anti-HBs levels checked at the well-child visit after completion of the HepB series (AAP, 2009, p. 345).

(continued)

Medications Used for
Pediatric Immunizations (continued)

Immunization Type	Side Effects	Contraindications	Nursing Implications
Human Papillomavirus Vaccine (Quadravalent) (HPV) *Type:* Recombinant. *Route:* Intramuscular. *Dosage:* 0.5 mL. *Age(s) given:* Girls 11–12 years, second dose 2 months later, third dose 6 months after first dose. May be administered with hepatitis B vaccine in separate site. *Storage:* Refrigerate, do not freeze.	*Common:* Pain, swelling, erythema at the injection site, pruritus, and fever. *Less common:* Syncope (vasovagal reaction) may occur in some females within 10 minutes of injection (Centers for Disease Control and Prevention [CDC], 2008b). *Potential serious reactions:* Headache, gastroenteritis, bronchospasm, asthma, arthritis.	Hypersensitivity to any vaccine substances (e.g., yeast). Not recommended for pregnant women. Defer vaccine in individuals with moderate or severe illness.	Solution is a white cloudy liquid; shake well before use. Protect vaccine from light to protect its potency. Observe the patient for 15 minutes after injection. May be given to girls at age 9 years and to women less than age 26 years. Vaccine should be administered before onset of sexual activity. Educate about the vaccine's potential to prevent cervical cancer and some human papillomavirus (HPV) infections. Some families may refuse the vaccine for girls and young adolescents due to concerns it may promote sexual promiscuity (Thomas, 2008).
Influenza Vaccine *Type:* Inactivated (TIV), live attenuated (LAIV). *Route:* TIV—intramuscular (all ages), LAIV—intranasal (2 years and older). *Dosage:* 0.25 mL at 6–35 months, 0.5 mL at 3 years and older. *Age(s) given:* Annually, beginning at 6 months. Children receiving TIV or LAIV for the first time should receive a second dose 4 weeks later. May give at same time as all other vaccines in a separate site. *TIV storage:* Refrigerate. Do not use if it has been frozen. *LAIV storage:* Keep frozen.	*Common after TIV:* May have soreness or swelling at injection site, fever, and aches. Mild systemic symptoms such as nausea, lethargy, headache, muscle aches, and chills may occur. Life-threatening allergic reactions are rare. *Common after intranasal vaccine:* Runny nose or nasal congestion, fever, headache or muscle aches, abdominal pain, and occasional vomiting. No life-threatening problems were detected during clinical trials.	Contraindicated in children with history of anaphylactic reaction to egg or chicken protein, hypersensitivity to thimerosal. LAIV is contraindicated in children under 5 years with recurrent wheezing; close contacts with a severely immunosuppressed person. Breastfeeding is not a contraindication for infants to receive the vaccine. Postpone vaccine when child has acute febrile illness until symptoms abate, but may be given with minor illness, with or without fever.	Thawed intranasal vaccine is pale yellow, clear to slightly cloudy. Administered annually in autumn at the time recommended by the CDC. Intranasal dose is split (0.25 mL) with a dose divider clip. Administer in each nostril while child is sitting in an upright position. Insert the tip of the sprayer inside the nose and depress the plunger to spray. Must be reimmunized each year (one dose) as immunity wanes. TIV should be used for any child living in a household with a severely immuno-compromised person.

Medications Used for
Pediatric Immunizations (continued)

Immunization Type	Side Effects	Contraindications	Nursing Implications
Measles, Mumps, Rubella Vaccines (MMR) *Type:* Live attenuated. *Route:* Subcutaneous. *Dosage:* 0.5 mL. *Age(s) given:* 12–15 months; 4–6 years (two doses). May give at same time as all other vaccines in a separate site. *Storage:* Refrigerate. Do not freeze. When reconstituted, keep refrigerated and away from light; discard if unused within 8 hours. Diluent is stored at room temperature or in refrigerator. MMR may be combined with the varicella vaccine (MMRV).	*Common:* Elevated temperature 6–12 days after immunization, lasts 1–2 days; transient noncontagious rash. *Serious:* Febrile seizure; rare incidences of encephalopathy or encephalitis, allergic reaction or anaphylaxis, and thrombocytopenic purpura.	Prior anaphylactic reaction to vaccine. Hypersensitivity to neomycin or gelatin. Immunodeficiency disorder. MMR vaccine is postponed 3–11 months after administration of immune globulin or blood products (time determined by the product), and for 1 month after child receives high doses of oral corticosteroids for 14 days or more (AAP, 2009, pp. 453–454). Pregnancy or possibility of pregnancy within 4 weeks. History of thrombocytopenic purpura. Children with tuberculosis should have therapy initiated prior to MMR.	Reconstituted vaccine is a clear, yellow solution. Prior to immunization, ask if child has allergy to neomycin or gelatin. Inquire about immunosuppression. Children with HIV infection should receive the MMR. Instruct adolescent girls of childbearing age to avoid pregnancy for 3 months after immunization. If giving a tuberculin test, give at same time as MMR or 4–6 weeks later. If MMR and Varivax are not given on the same day, space them 28 or more days apart. Ensure that adolescents going to college have received a second MMR dose.
Meningococcal Vaccine (MCV4 or MPSV4) *Type:* Inactivated. *Route:* MCV4—intramuscular; MPSV4—subcutaneous. *Dosage:* 0.5 mL. *Age(s) given:* 11–18 years. May be given at same time as other vaccines. *Storage:* Refrigerate, do not freeze. MCV4 is the preferred meningococcal vaccine.	*Common:* Pain at injection site, irritability, headache, and fatigue. *Severe:* Guillain-Barré syndrome (GBS).	Hypersensitivity to any component of vaccine, including diphtheria toxoid. MCV4 should not be used in adolescents with a history of GBS; MPSV4 may be used. Pregnant women should receive vaccine if at increased risk of meningococcal disease.	Protect vaccine from light. May be given to children 2 years or older who are immunosuppressed by disease or medication. MCV4 or MPSV4 is recommended for control of meningococcal outbreaks caused by serogroups A, C, W-135, and Y. Vial stopper contains latex.
Pneumococcal Vaccine (PCV or PPSV) *Type:* PCV, conjugated; PPSV, inactive. *Route:* Intramuscular. *Dosage:* 0.5 mL. *Age(s) given:* PCV at 2, 4, 6, 12–15 months. Do not restart the series, no matter when the prior dose(s) were given. Either vaccine may be given at the same time as other vaccines. *Storage:* Refrigerate, do not freeze.	*Common:* Soreness, swelling, redness at injection site; mild to moderate fever. *Severe:* Allergic reaction or anaphylaxis.	Hypersensitivity to diphtheria toxoid.	Clear, colorless, or slightly opalescent liquid. May be given to children up to 9 years. Use PPSV for children 2 years and older at high risk for acquiring pneumococcal infection. PCV should be administered first, followed by PPSV after at least 8 weeks.

(continued)

Medications Used for
Pediatric Immunizations (continued)

Immunization Type	Side Effects	Contraindications	Nursing Implications
Poliovirus Vaccine (IPV) *Type:* Inactivated. *Route:* Subcutaneous or intramuscular; follow manufacturer's guidance for vaccine used. *Dosage:* 0.5 mL. *Age(s) given:* 2, 4, 12–18 months; 4–6 years (four doses). May give at same time as all other vaccines in a separate site. *Storage:* Refrigerate, do not freeze. IPV is a single vaccine or produced in combination with DTaP, Hib, or HepB.	*Common:* Swelling and tenderness, irritability, fatigue. *Serious:* Allergic reaction or anaphylaxis.	Hypersensitivity or anaphylactic response to vaccine components: neomycin, streptomycin, polymyxin B. Pregnancy.	Ask if the child has an allergy to the antibiotic contained in the specific IPV product used. Clear, colorless suspension. Do not use if it contains particulate matter, becomes cloudy, or changes color. All doses must be separated by at least 4 weeks. Do not restart the series, no matter when the prior dose(s) were given.
Rotavirus Vaccine (RV) *Type:* Live. *Route:* Oral. *Dosage:* 2 mL. *Age(s) given:* 2, 4, and 6 months (three doses). Do not start the series if the infant is 15 weeks of age or older. May give at same time as all other vaccines. Use the same manufacturer for all vaccine doses. *Storage:* Refrigerate, do not freeze.	*Common:* Vomiting, diarrhea, irritability. *Potential serious adverse reactions:* Seizures, bronchiolitis, gastroenteritis, pneumonia, fever, urinary tract infection.	Severe hypersensitivity to vaccine components. Severe allergic reaction or anaphylaxis after receiving a dose of vaccine. Postpone vaccine if child has moderate or severe illness.	Pale yellow clear liquid in single dose tube for direct oral administration. Protect vaccine from light. Squeeze the liquid into the infant's mouth toward the inner cheek until the dosing tube is empty. If the infant regurgitates a small amount, do not repeat dose. Discard the empty tube and cap into an approved biological waste container. Complete all doses of vaccine by 8 months of age.
Varicella Virus Vaccine (Var) *Type:* Live attenuated. *Route:* Subcutaneous. *Dosage:* 0.5 mL. *Age(s) given:* 12–15 months; and 4–6 years (two doses). 13 years or older (two doses 4–8 weeks apart). *Storage:* Keep frozen. Use within 30 minutes of reconstitution. Varicella is a single vaccine or combined with MMR.	*Common:* Pain or redness at injection site; fever. Less commonly a rash of 2–5 lesions lasting 2–3 days may appear during first month after the injection. *Severe:* Allergic reaction or anaphylaxis; thrombocytopenia; febrile seizure; central nervous system (CNS) manifestations.	Prior anaphylactic reaction to vaccine. Hypersensitivity to neomycin or gelatin. Immunodeficiency disorder. Active untreated tuberculosis. Var vaccine is postponed 3–11 months after administration of immune globulin or blood products (time determined by the product), and for 1 month after child receives high doses of oral corticosteroids for 14 days or more (AAP, 2009, pp. 453–454). Pregnancy or possibility of pregnancy within 4 weeks.	Ask if the child is immunodeficient or on immunosuppression treatment or has an allergy to neomycin or gelatin. Determine if a family member is immunocompromised. Clear, colorless to pale yellow liquid when reconstituted. Instruct adolescent girls of childbearing age to avoid pregnancy for 3 months after immunization. Antiviral agents should not be used 1 day before vaccine or for 21 days after vaccine. If not given simultaneously with MMR, separate vaccines by at least 28 days.

Data from: American Academy of Pediatrics. (2009). Red book: Report of the committee on infectious disease (28th ed.). Elk Grove Village, IL: Author.

Practices (ACIP) of the Centers for Disease Control and Prevention (CDC), the American Academy of Pediatrics (AAP), and the American Academy of Family Practitioners (AAFP) collaborate to provide a uniform vaccination schedule. See Figures 16–4 and 16–5 ➤ for the recommended schedule of immunizations in the United States. See the companion website for the most current recommended vaccine schedule and for the alternative catch-up immunization schedule. Immunization recommendations vary for children who have recently received immune globulin or immunosuppressive agents. Schedules and recommendations also vary for children who begin immunizations later in childhood or need catch-up doses.

Nursing Alert

Immune globulin inhibits the response to live virus vaccines such as measles, mumps, rubella, and varicella. Ask about recent administration of immune globulin or immunosuppression therapy. Refer to the most current guidelines to identify the appropriate interval (3 to 11 months) between administration of immune globulin or completion of immunosuppression therapy and live virus vaccine administration.

Similarly, if immune globulin must be given within 14 days after administration of a live virus vaccine, the vaccine should be administered again after the period specified in the most current guidelines, unless serologic testing determines that the child developed adequate serum antibodies (AAP, 2009, p. 37).

Immunization of Immigrants

Children less than 10 years of age who are internationally adopted may or may not have written proof of immunizations prior to entry into the United States. Adoptive parents are required to indicate their intent to fully immunize the child when proof is not available (AAP, 2009, p. 177). Often vaccines are administered according to the catch-up schedule when no immunization record exists or there is doubt about the potency of vaccines given. Some vaccines may not have been available in the child's country of origin. Antibody titers may be collected to determine if adequate protection exists for certain diseases, particularly when vaccines are given in a series, for example, DTaP (AAP, 2009, p. 183).

Vaccine Adverse Events

Serious reactions to vaccines occur in rare instances, such as anaphylaxis, encephalopathy, bacterial neuritis, chronic arthritis, thrombocytopenic purpura, and death. Each of these reactions is a reportable event. The National Vaccine Injury Compensation Program was established to support families when significant reactions to a specific vaccine occur. See Table 16–1 on page 404.

Law & Ethics *National Childhood Vaccine Injury Act*

When a link between receipt of a vaccine and a serious adverse effect is found, the National Childhood Vaccine Injury Act of 1986 compensates the family. The Vaccine Adverse Event Reporting System (VAERS) tracks serious vaccine reactions. Follow-up of the patient's condition occurs at 60 days and 1 year after the adverse event. Guidelines for reporting to the VAERS are detailed in Table 16–1 on page 404.

Increasing the Immunization Rate

The effort to increase the numbers of children protected from vaccine-preventable diseases and to monitor immunization status is a national public health initiative. *Healthy People 2020* states important goals for reduction of vaccine-preventable diseases (U.S. Department of Health and Human Services, 2010):

- Achieve and maintain effective vaccination coverage levels for universally recommended vaccines among young children.
- Increase the proportion of children aged 19 to 35 months who receive the recommended vaccines.
- Maintain vaccination coverage levels for children in kindergarten.
- Increase routine vaccination coverage levels for adolescents with vaccines recommended by the Advisory Committee on Immunization Practices.

Many missed opportunities to immunize children have been identified. Children (and siblings present) should have their immunization status assessed during all health care visits, during hospitalizations, and in schools. Efforts to increase immunization levels among children are also supported by health care payers that require contracted health care providers to comply with the pediatric immunization standards. Patient records are audited to ensure compliance.

The reported level of full immunization for children between 19 and 35 months of age in 2007 was 77.4%. Full immunization was defined as four doses of DTP/DT/DTaP; three doses of the IPV, Hib, and HepB vaccines; and one dose of MMR and varicella vaccines. National coverage of four doses of PCV was 75.3% (CDC, 2008a). Immunization rates for adolescents were 87.6% for at least three doses of HepB, 75.7% for one dose of varicella, 32.4% for MCV4, 72.3% for Td or Tdap, and 25.1% for HPV in females (CDC, 2008c).

Challenges in Achieving Optimal Immunization Rates

Lower immunization rates of children are often associated with economic factors, limited access to health care, lack of health care services at hours convenient for working parents, inadequate education regarding the importance of immunization, and religious prohibitions. The federal Vaccines for Children program provides free vaccines for qualified children and adolescents less than 19 years of age and has resolved some of the economic factors associated with vaccine coverage.

An increasing number of parents are choosing not to immunize their children for philosophical reasons and personal beliefs.

Law & Ethics *Vaccines for Children Program*

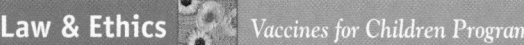

The estimated cost of fully immunizing a child through the adolescent years in 2007 was $1,170 for all approved vaccines (Lee, Santoli, Hannan, et al., 2007). The Vaccines for Children (VFC) program was established in 1994 through the amendment of the Social Security Act by Section 1928. This program makes immunizations available to children who are uninsured, Medicaid recipients, and American Indians/Alaska Natives. The Centers for Disease Control and Prevention buys vaccines at a discount and distributes them by way of public health agencies to private physicians and public health clinics registered as VFC providers (CDC, 2009).

Recommended Immunization Schedule for Persons Aged 0 Through 6 Years—United States • 2010

For those who fall behind or start late, see the catch-up schedule

Vaccine ▼ Age ►	Birth	1 month	2 months	4 months	6 months	12 months	15 months	18 months	19–23 months	2–3 years	4–6 years
Hepatitis B[1]	HepB	HepB			HepB						
Rotavirus[2]			RV	RV	RV[2]						
Diphtheria, Tetanus, Pertussis[3]			DTaP	DTaP	DTaP	see footnote[3]	DTaP				DTaP
Haemophilus influenzae type b[4]			Hib	Hib	Hib[4]	Hib					
Pneumococcal[5]			PCV	PCV	PCV	PCV				PPSV	
Inactivated Poliovirus[6]			IPV	IPV	IPV						IPV
Influenza[7]					Influenza (Yearly)						
Measles, Mumps, Rubella[8]						MMR		see footnote[8]			MMR
Varicella[9]						Varicella		see footnote[9]			Varicella
Hepatitis A[10]						HepA (2 doses)				HepA Series	
Meningococcal[11]										MCV	

Range of recommended ages for all children except certain high-risk groups

Range of recommended ages for certain high-risk groups

This schedule includes recommendations in effect as of December 15, 2009. Any dose not administered at the recommended age should be administered at a subsequent visit, when indicated and feasible. The use of a combination vaccine generally is preferred over separate injections of its equivalent component vaccines. Considerations should include provider assessment, patient preference, and the potential for adverse events. Providers should consult the relevant Advisory Committee on Immunization Practices statement for detailed recommendations: **http://www.cdc.gov/vaccines/pubs/acip-list.htm**. Clinically significant adverse events that follow immunization should be reported to the Vaccine Adverse Event Reporting System (VAERS) at **http://www.vaers.hhs.gov** or by telephone, **800-822-7967**.

1. **Hepatitis B vaccine (HepB).** (Minimum age: birth)
   At birth:
   • Administer monovalent HepB to all newborns before hospital discharge.
   • If mother is hepatitis B surface antigen (HBsAg)-positive, administer HepB and 0.5 mL of hepatitis B immune globulin (HBIG) within 12 hours of birth.
   • If mother's HBsAg status is unknown, administer HepB within 12 hours of birth. Determine mother's HBsAg status as soon as possible and, if HBsAg-positive, administer HBIG (no later than age 1 week).
   After the birth dose:
   • The HepB series should be completed with either monovalent HepB or a combination vaccine containing HepB. The second dose should be administered at age 1 or 2 months. Monovalent HepB vaccine should be used for doses administered before age 6 weeks. The final dose should be administered no earlier than age 24 weeks.
   • Infants born to HBsAg-positive mothers should be tested for HBsAg and antibody to HBsAg 1 to 2 months after completion of at least 3 doses of the HepB series, at age 9 through 18 months (generally at the next well-child visit).
   • Administration of 4 doses of HepB to infants is permissible when a combination vaccine containing HepB is administered after the birth dose. The fourth dose should be administered no earlier than age 24 weeks.

2. **Rotavirus vaccine (RV).** (Minimum age: 6 weeks)
   • Administer the first dose at age 6 through 14 weeks (maximum age: 14 weeks 6 days). Vaccination should not be initiated for infants aged 15 weeks 0 days or older.
   • The maximum age for the final dose in the series is 8 months 0 days
   • If Rotarix is administered at ages 2 and 4 months, a dose at 6 months is not indicated.

3. **Diphtheria and tetanus toxoids and acellular pertussis vaccine (DTaP).** (Minimum age: 6 weeks)
   • The fourth dose may be administered as early as age 12 months, provided at least 6 months have elapsed since the third dose.
   • Administer the final dose in the series at age 4 through 6 years.

4. ***Haemophilus influenzae* type b conjugate vaccine (Hib).** (Minimum age: 6 weeks)
   • If PRP-OMP (PedvaxHIB or Comvax [HepB-Hib]) is administered at ages 2 and 4 months, a dose at age 6 months is not indicated.
   • TriHiBit (DTaP/Hib) and Hiberix (PRP-T) should not be used for doses at ages 2, 4, or 6 months for the primary series but can be used as the final dose in children aged 12 months through 4 years.

5. **Pneumococcal vaccine.** (Minimum age: 6 weeks for pneumococcal conjugate vaccine [PCV]; 2 years for pneumococcal polysaccharide vaccine [PPSV])
   • PCV is recommended for all children aged younger than 5 years. Administer 1 dose of PCV to all healthy children aged 24 through 59 months who are not completely vaccinated for their age.
   • Administer PPSV 2 or more months after last dose of PCV to children aged 2 years or older with certain underlying medical conditions, including a cochlear implant. See *MMWR* 1997;46(No. RR-8).

6. **Inactivated poliovirus vaccine (IPV)** (Minimum age: 6 weeks)
   • The final dose in the series should be administered on or after the fourth birthday and at least 6 months following the previous dose.
   • If 4 doses are administered prior to age 4 years a fifth dose should be administered at age 4 through 6 years. See *MMWR* 2009;58(30):829–30.

7. **Influenza vaccine (seasonal).** (Minimum age: 6 months for trivalent inactivated influenza vaccine [TIV]; 2 years for live, attenuated influenza vaccine [LAIV])
   • Administer annually to children aged 6 months through 18 years.
   • For healthy children aged 2 through 6 years (i.e., those who do not have underlying medical conditions that predispose them to influenza complications), either LAIV or TIV may be used, except LAIV should not be given to children aged 2 through 4 years who have had wheezing in the past 12 months.
   • Children receiving TIV should receive 0.25 mL if aged 6 through 35 months or 0.5 mL if aged 3 years or older.
   • Administer 2 doses (separated by at least 4 weeks) to children aged younger than 9 years who are receiving influenza vaccine for the first time or who were vaccinated for the first time during the previous influenza season but only received 1 dose.
   • For recommendations for use of influenza A (H1N1) 2009 monovalent vaccine see *MMWR* 2009;58(No. RR-10).

8. **Measles, mumps, and rubella vaccine (MMR).** (Minimum age: 12 months)
   • Administer the second dose routinely at age 4 through 6 years. However, the second dose may be administered before age 4, provided at least 28 days have elapsed since the first dose.

9. **Varicella vaccine.** (Minimum age: 12 months)
   • Administer the second dose routinely at age 4 through 6 years. However, the second dose may be administered before age 4, provided at least 3 months have elapsed since the first dose.
   • For children aged 12 months through 12 years the minimum interval between doses is 3 months. However, if the second dose was administered at least 28 days after the first dose, it can be accepted as valid.

10. **Hepatitis A vaccine (HepA).** (Minimum age: 12 months)
    • Administer to all children aged 1 year (i.e., aged 12 through 23 months). Administer 2 doses at least 6 months apart.
    • Children not fully vaccinated by age 2 years can be vaccinated at subsequent visits
    • HepA also is recommended for older children who live in areas where vaccination programs target older children, who are at increased risk for infection, or for whom immunity against hepatitis A is desired.

11. **Meningococcal vaccine.** (Minimum age: 2 years for meningococcal conjugate vaccine [MCV4] and for meningococcal polysaccharide vaccine [MPSV4])
    • Administer MCV4 to children aged 2 through 10 years with persistent complement component deficiency, anatomic or functional asplenia, and certain other conditions placing tham at high risk.
    • Administer MCV4 to children previously vaccinated with MCV4 or MPSV4 after 3 years if first dose administered at age 2 through 6 years. See *MMWR* 2009;58:1042–3.

FIGURE 16–4 ► Recommended Childhood Immunization Schedule for Persons Aged 0 to 6 Years—United States, 2010.

Recommended Immunization Schedule for Persons Aged 7 Through 18 Years—United States • 2010
For those who fall behind or start late, see the schedule below and the catch-up schedule

Vaccine ▼ Age ►	7–10 years	11–12 years	13–18 years
Tetanus, Diphtheria, Pertussis[1]		Tdap	Tdap
Human Papillomavirus[2]	see footnote 2	HPV (3 doses)	HPV series
Meningococcal[3]	MCV	MCV	MCV
Influenza[4]	Influenza (Yearly)		
Pneumococcal[5]	PPSV		
Hepatitis A[6]	HepA Series		
Hepatitis B[7]	Hep B Series		
Inactivated Poliovirus[8]	IPV Series		
Measles, Mumps, Rubella[9]	MMR Series		
Varicella[10]	Varicella Series		

Range of recommended ages for all children except certain high-risk groups

Range of recommended ages for catch-up immunization

Range of recommended ages for certain high-risk groups

This schedule includes recommendations in effect as of December 15, 2009. Any dose not administered at the recommended age should be administered at a subsequent visit, when indicated and feasible. The use of a combination vaccine generally is preferred over separate injections of its equivalent component vaccines. Considerations should include provider assessment, patient preference, and the potential for adverse events. Providers should consult the relevant Advisory Committee on Immunization Practices statement for detailed recommendations: http://www.cdc.gov/vaccines/pubs/acip-list.htm. Clinically significant adverse events that follow immunization should be reported to the Vaccine Adverse Event Reporting System (VAERS) at http://www.vaers.hhs.gov or by telephone, 800-822-7967.

1. **Tetanus and diphtheria toxoids and acellular pertussis vaccine (Tdap).** (Minimum age: 10 years for Boostrix and 11 years for Adacel)
   - Administer at age 11 or 12 years for those who have completed the recommended childhood DTP/DTaP vaccination series and have not received a tetanus and diphtheria toxoid (Td) booster dose.
   - Persons aged 13 through 18 years who have not received Tdap should receive a dose.
   - A 5-year interval from the last Td dose is encouraged when Tdap is used as a booster dose; however, a shorter interval may be used if pertussis immunity is needed.
2. **Human papillomavirus vaccine (HPV).** (Minimum age: 9 years)
   - Two HPV vaccines are licensed: a quadrivalent vaccine (HPV4) for the prevention of cervical, vaginal and vulvar cancers (in females) and genital warts (in females and males), and a bivalent vaccine (HPV2) for the prevention of cervical cancers in females.
   - HPV vaccines are most effective for both males and females when given before exposure to HPV through sexual contact.
   - HPV4 or HPV2 is recommended for the prevention of cervical precancers and cancers in females.
   - HPV4 is recommended for the prevention of cervical, vaginal and vulvar precancers and cancers and genital warts in females.
   - Administer the first dose to females at age 11 or 12 years.
   - Administer the second dose 1 to 2 months after the first dose and the third dose 6 months after the first dose (at least 24 weeks after the first dose).
   - Administer the series to females at age 13 through 18 years if not previously vaccinated.
   - HPV4 may be administered in a 3-dose series to males aged 9 through 18 years to reduce their likelihood of acquiring genital warts.
3. **Meningococcal conjugate vaccine (MCV4).**
   - Administer at age 11 or 12 years, or at age 13 through 18 years if not previously vaccinated.
   - Administer to previously unvaccinated college freshmen living in a dormitory.
   - Administer MCV4 to children aged 2 through 10 years with persistent complement component deficiency, anatomic or functional asplenia, or certain other conditions placing them at high risk.
   - Administer to children previously vaccinated with MCV4 or MPSV4 who remain at increased risk after 3 years (if first dose administered at age 2 through 6 years) or after 5 years (if first dose administered at age 7 years or older). Persons whose only risk factor is living in on-campus housing are not recommended to receive an additional dose. See MMWR 2009;58:1042–3.

4. **Influenza vaccine (seasonal).**
   - Administer annually to children aged 6 months through 18 years.
   - For healthy nonpregnant persons aged 7 through 18 years (i.e., those who do not have underlying medical conditions that predispose them to influenza complications), either LAIV or TIV may be used.
   - Administer 2 doses (separated by at least 4 weeks) to children aged younger than 9 years who are receiving influenza vaccine for the first time or who were vaccinated for the first time during the previous influenza season but only received 1 dose.
   - For recommendations for use of influenza A (H1N1) 2009 monovalent vaccine. See MMWR 2009;58(No. RR-10).
5. **Pneumococcal polysaccharide vaccine (PPSV).**
   - Administer to children with certain underlying medical conditions, including a cochlear implant. A single revaccination should be administered after 5 years to children with functional or anatomic asplenia or an immunocompromising condition. See MMWR 1997;46(No. RR-8).
6. **Hepatitis A vaccine (HepA).**
   - Administer 2 doses at least 6 months apart.
   - HepA is recommended for children aged older than 23 months who live in areas where vaccination programs target older children, who are at increased risk for infection, or for whom immunity against hepatitis A is desired.
7. **Hepatitis B vaccine (HepB).**
   - Administer the 3-dose series to those not previously vaccinated.
   - A 2-dose series (separated by at least 4 months) of adult formulation Recombivax HB is licensed for children aged 11 through 15 years.
8. **Inactivated poliovirus vaccine (IPV).**
   - The final dose in the series should be administered on or after the fourth birthday and at least 6 months following the previous dose.
   - If both OPV and IPV were administered as part of a series, a total of 4 doses should be administered, regardless of the child's current age.
9. **Measles, mumps, and rubella vaccine (MMR).**
   - If not previously vaccinated, administer 2 doses or the second dose for those who have received only 1 dose, with at least 28 days between doses.
10. **Varicella vaccine.**
   - For persons aged 7 through 18 years without evidence of immunity (see MMWR 2007;56[No. RR-4]), administer 2 doses if not previously vaccinated or the second dose if only 1 dose has been administered.
   - For persons aged 7 through 12 years, the minimum interval between doses is 3 months. However, if the second dose was administered at least 28 days after the first dose, it can be accepted as valid.
   - For persons aged 13 years and older, the minimum interval between doses is 28 days.

The Recommended Immunization Schedules for Persons Aged 0 through 18 Years are approved by the Advisory Committee on Immunization Practices (http://www.cdc.gov/vaccines/recs/acip), the American Academy of Pediatrics (http://www.aap.org), and the American Academy of Family Physicians (http://www.aafp.org).
Department of Health and Human Services • Centers for Disease Control and Prevention

CS207330-A

FIGURE 16–5 ► Recommended Childhood Immunization Schedule for Persons Aged 7 to 18 Years—United States, 2010.

TABLE 16–1	National Vaccine Injury Compensation Program—Vaccine Injury Table, November 10, 2008	
Vaccine	**Adverse Event**	**Time Interval**
I. Tetanus toxoid-containing vaccines (e.g., DTaP, Tdap, DTP-Hib, DT, Td, TT)	A. Anaphylaxis or anaphylactic shock B. Brachial neuritis C. Any acute complication or sequela (including death) of above events	0–4 hours 2–28 days Not applicable
II. Pertussis antigen-containing vaccines (e.g., DTaP, Tdap, DTP, P, DTP-Hib)	A. Anaphylaxis or anaphylactic shock B. Encephalopathy (or encephalitis) C. Any acute complication or sequela (including death) of above events	0–4 hours 0–72 hours Not applicable
III. Measles, mumps, and rubella virus-containing vaccines in any combination (e.g., MMR, MR, M, R)	A. Anaphylaxis or anaphylactic shock B. Encephalopathy (or encephalitis) C. Any acute complication or sequela (including death) of above events	0–4 hours 5–15 days Not applicable
IV. Rubella virus-containing vaccines (e.g., MMR, MR, R)	A. Chronic arthritis B. Any acute complication or sequela (including death) of above event	7–42 days Not applicable
V. Measles virus-containing vaccines (e.g., MMR, MR, M)	A. Thrombocytopenic purpura B. Vaccine-strain measles viral infection in an immunodeficient recipient C. Any acute complication or sequela (including death) of above events	7–30 days 0–6 months Not applicable

VI. Polio live virus-containing vaccines (OPV)	A. Paralytic polio
	  —in a non-immunodeficient recipient
	  —in an immunodeficient recipient
	  —in a vaccine-associated community case
	B. Vaccine-strain polio viral infection
	  —in a non-immunodeficient recipient
	  —in an immunodeficient recipient
	  —in a vaccine-associated community case
	C. Any acute complication or sequela (including death) of above events
		
		0–30 days
		0–6 months
		Not applicable
		
		0–30 days
		0–6 months
		Not applicable
		Not applicable

VII. Polio inactivated virus-containing vaccines (e.g., IPV)	A. Anaphylaxis or anaphylactic shock B. Any acute complication or sequela (including death) of above event	0–4 hours Not applicable
VIII. Hepatitis B antigen-containing vaccines	A. Anaphylaxis or anaphylactic shock B. Any acute complication or sequela (including death) of above event	0–4 hours Not applicable
IX. *Haemophilus influenzae* type b polysaccharide conjugate vaccines	A. No condition specified for compensation	Not applicable
X. Varicella vaccine	A. No condition specified for compensation	Not applicable
XI. Rotavirus vaccine	A. No condition specified for compensation	Not applicable
XII. Pneumococcal conjugate vaccines	A. No condition specified for compensation	Not applicable
XIII. Any new vaccine recommended by the Centers for Disease Control and Prevention for routine administration to children, after publication by Secretary, HHS of a notice of coverage[a, b]	A. No condition specified for compensation	Not applicable

From: U.S. Department of Health and Human Services, Health Resources and Services Administration. (2008). National Vaccine Injury Compensation Program. Washington, DC: Author. Retrieved from http://www.hrsa.gov/vaccinecompensation/table.htm

[a] As of **December 1, 2004**, hepatitis A vaccines have been added to the Vaccine Injury Table (table) under this category.
As of **July 1, 2005**, trivalent influenza vaccines have been added to the table under this category. Trivalent influenza vaccines are given annually during the flu season either by needle and syringe or in a nasal spray. All influenza vaccines routinely administered in the United States are trivalent vaccines covered under this category.
[b] As of **February 1, 2007**, meningococcal (conjugate and polysaccharide) and human papillomavirus (HPV) vaccines have been added to the table under this category.

Some of their reasons include the following (Omer, Salmon, Orenstein, et al., 2009): their children are not very susceptible to the communicable diseases, the severity of the diseases is low, and the vaccines have low safety and effectiveness. Vaccine refusal not only increases the child's risk of contracting the disease, it places the entire community at higher risk, particularly infants and children too young to be fully immunized. Geographic clusters of pertussis vaccine refusal have resulted in pertussis outbreaks in those communities (Omer, Enger, Moulton, et al., 2008).

Other common misconceptions about vaccines and communicable diseases that may influence parent decision making are provided in Table 16–2 along with factual information.

All health care providers should be consistent in their message about the value of vaccines and provide parents with an opportunity to have their questions answered prior to giving consent for immunization. It is important to understand that parents want to protect their child from diseases or from the potential harm of the vaccines. A trusting relationship between the health care provider and the parents is an important factor in obtaining consent for immunizations (Benin, Wisler-Scher, Colson, et al., 2006).

NURSING MANAGEMENT

Nursing Assessment and Diagnosis

Nurses are responsible for reviewing a child's health record to determine whether the child needs vaccinations. Identify any potential contraindications to vaccines by asking the following:

- Have there been previous reactions to any immunizations?
- Are there allergies to any vaccine components (e.g., eggs, neomycin, gelatin, or yeast)?
- Does the child have a serious medical condition (e.g., seizures, cancer, HIV infection, immune diseases, asthma, or heart disease)?
- Has the child received any blood products or immune globulin in the past year?
- Has the child received any vaccines in the last 4 weeks?
- If the patient is female, is there a possibility of pregnancy?

Clinical Tip

A screening questionnaire is available from the Immunization Action Coalition to decide if it is safe to give a child or adolescent a vaccine on the day of the health care visit. Information is also provided for health professionals to use in interpretation of responses to questions by parents.

Contraindications may include an acute illness with high fever, hypersensitivity reaction to specific vaccine components, anaphylactic reaction to vaccine, immune globulin therapy in the last 3 to 11 months, cancer treatment, and pregnancy. See the Medications table for specific vaccine contraindications on pages 396–400.

Immunization Action Coalition Website

Health Promotion

Nurses are responsible for reviewing a child's immunization record and determining whether the child needs any vaccines. Use the most current immunization schedule for comparison with the child's record as new vaccines may be approved when the schedule is updated each year. If the child lacks appropriate immunizations for age, determine the best combination of vaccines to give at this visit to better protect the child.

TABLE 16–2 Common Misconceptions About Vaccines

Common Misconceptions	Correct Vaccine Information
Vaccine-preventable diseases have been eliminated.	The incidence of vaccine-preventable diseases is low in the United States, but not completely eliminated. Travelers may reintroduce the disease from a country or a community where the disease still exists. Recent outbreaks of measles, mumps, and pertussis have been linked to groups of children not immunized because of religious and personal beliefs (Nield & Kamat, 2006; Omer, Enger, Moulton, et al., 2008).
Immunization weakens the immune system. Multiple vaccines overload the immune system and cause harmful effects.	Studies have revealed that a child's immune system is capable of responding to large numbers of distinct viruses and bacteria. In addition, this response to vaccines does not place the child at higher risk of getting an infection. The child who becomes infected by a vaccine-preventable disease is at higher risk for secondary infections like pneumonia (Children's Hospital of Philadelphia, 2008).
It would be better to let the child get the disease than get immunized.	Many parents do not understand the dangers inherent in some of these diseases, such as suffering, permanent disability, and even death. Unimmunized children are at a greater risk of getting the disease and of spreading it to pregnant women and to infants and children with serious medical conditions. Risks of getting the disease need to be considered along with the low risks associated with immunizations.
Vaccines do not work; children still get the disease.	No vaccine is 100% effective, and immunity does wane over time, leading to the need for a second immunization.
Vaccines may cause serious conditions, such as autism.	Numerous studies have confirmed the lack of association between the measles vaccine and autism, as well as thimerosal in vaccines and autism (Hornig, Briese, Buie, et al., 2008; Schechter & Grether, 2008).

The accompanying Nursing Care Plan explores two potential nursing diagnoses that may apply to the child needing immunizations. Additional nursing diagnoses may include the following:

- Risk for Impaired Skin Integrity related to vaccine response
- Ineffective Health Maintenance related to cultural beliefs regarding routine immunization
- Risk for Injury related to severe vaccine reaction

Planning and Implementation

Nursing management focuses on being a strong advocate for immunization, protecting the potency of vaccines, educating parents about immunizations and possible side effects, addressing fears about possible reactions, obtaining consent, and reporting adverse reactions.

Improving Immunization Rates

Many missed opportunities to immunize children have been identified. To avoid missed opportunities in administering immunizations, be sure to evaluate the child's immunization record in all health care settings: on acute care units in the hospital, in the emergency department, in health clinics, and in school. A designated nurse vaccine manager is one way to promote an effective immunization program. This nurse can take responsibility for educating staff and developing protocols for immunization, tracking inventory, and ensuring safe storage of vaccines. Some guidelines to reduce the number of missed opportunities for full immunization of children include the following (Joyce, 2007):

- Use combination vaccines to reduce the number of injections.
- Educate staff to review a child's record (and those of accompanying siblings) at each visit and flag the record to remind the health care provider about the child's need for immunizations.
- Send out reminders to parents when it is time for the child's next immunization(s).
- Schedule the appointment for the child's next immunization before the family leaves the health center.
- Immunizations can be given when the child has a minor illness with or without a low-grade fever, with antibiotic treatment, or when the child has been exposed to an infectious disease.
- Give several vaccines at the same visit. Two injections can be given in different sites on the same extremity.

Protect Vaccine Potency

Take special care to ensure vaccine potency. Store vaccines properly in a refrigerator with separate doors for refrigerator and freezer sections. Set the refrigerator at 35°F to 46°F (2°C to 8°C) and the freezer at 5°F (−15°C) or lower as stated in vaccine package inserts. Keep jugs of water in the refrigerator and trays of ice in the freezer to help maintain a consistent temperature. Check the temperature of each unit twice daily and record the temperatures on a log. Review the temperature log weekly, and keep the logs on file for 3 years or use an automatic temperature measurement system (Veraas, 2006). Store the vaccines in the mid-

dle of the units; place the older vaccines in the front. Make sure the facility has an emergency plan for safe storage of vaccines in case of a power outage or natural disaster.

Check the expiration of vaccines prior to use. When reconstituting vaccines, it is important to use the solution provided and follow the manufacturer's directions. Write the date and time on the bottle if it is a multidose vial. Some reconstituted vaccines (varicella and MMR) have a short shelf life and are available only in single-dose vials. See vaccine-specific information in the Medications table on pages 396–400.

Family Education and Informed Consent

Federal legislation requires consent to be obtained before administering a vaccine. In most health care settings, the nurse is responsible for informing the parents or the child's legal guardian, supplying the most current Vaccine Information Statement (VIS) for each vaccine to be administered as required by the National Vaccine Injury Act, and obtaining written consent before the vaccine is administered. The VIS provides concise information about the vaccine, risks and benefits of the vaccine, its recommended schedule, what to do if adverse effects occur, and a description of the National Vaccine Injury Compensation Program.

Explain the risks and benefits of each immunization, as well as common local reactions, using the information in the VIS. In order for parents to provide informed consent, the nurse needs to be able to answer questions to their satisfaction. If the parent chooses not to accept a particular vaccine, document the informed refusal. If there is a disease outbreak, the nonimmunized child must be kept out of childcare and school. Local, city, or state courts decide how to settle any conflicts.

The nurse is required to record the (1) month, day, and year of administration; (2) vaccine given; (3) manufacturer; (4) lot number and expiration date of the immunization given; (5) site and route of administration; and (6) name, title, and address of the person who administers the vaccine. Obtain written consent to give the needed vaccines on the health care facility's standardized form from the parent or guardian. Provide parents with a record of the child's immunizations, and record the vaccines given in the health care agency's official records.

Clinical Judgment

What information should be included in an informed refusal documentation?

Culture — *Vaccine Information Statement (VIS)*

Consider literacy and reading level when giving a VIS to parents. Although written at a sixth-grade level, they may be difficult for some parents to read. It is acceptable to read the VIS to parents, but make sure the parent understands the information. Although they have been translated into 30 languages, use translators to provide verbal explanations and answer questions when necessary. Supplement the VIS with other teaching materials such as videotapes when possible.

NURSING CARE PLAN

The Child Needing Immunizations

INTERVENTION	RATIONALE	EXPECTED OUTCOME
1. Nursing Diagnosis: Risk for Infection related to incomplete immunization series		
NIC Priority Intervention: *Immunization vaccination management:* *Administration:* Monitoring immunization status, facilitating access to immunizations, and provision of immunizations to prevent communicable disease		**NOC Suggested Outcome:** *Immune status:* Adequacy of natural and acquired appropriately targeted resistance to internal and external antigens
Goal: The child will be adequately protected from vaccine-preventable illnesses.		
■ Review the child's immunization record for needed vaccines at each health care visit.	■ Children who have missed needed vaccines can be identified.	The child is adequately protected from vaccine-preventable illnesses.
■ Identify all due vaccines that can be provided simultaneously.	■ Multiple vaccines given at the same visit more adequately protect the child.	
■ Identify potential contraindications to needed vaccines. Review past reactions to vaccines.	■ This reduces the risk for the child and other caretakers to have adverse reactions to vaccines.	
2. Nursing Diagnosis: Effective Therapeutic Regimen Management		
NIC Priority Intervention: *Decision-making support:* Providing information and support for a patient who is making a decision regarding health care		**NOC Suggested Outcome:** *Knowledge: Treatment regimen:* Extent of understanding conveyed about a specific treatment regimen
Goal: Parents will sign consent for vaccines to be given.		
■ Educate the parents and adolescents about the need for specific vaccines and the risk if not given. Obtain signed consent before giving vaccines.	■ Informed consent is required for all treatments.	The parents complete the consent form, which is placed in the child's file.
Goal: Parents and adolescents will state the side effects of vaccines given.		
■ Review past reactions to vaccines and describe common potential reactions and why they occur.	■ Parents should expect common reactions and know they indicate the child's body is building protection to the illness.	Parents report all serious side effects to the health care provider.
■ Describe serious side effects that should be reported to the health care provider.	■ Parents need to be prepared for potential serious side effects so they can obtain care if needed.	
Goal: Parents will manage common side effects of vaccines.		
■ Teach parents general comfort measures for common side effects, for example: • *Cool pack to immunization site(s)* • *Acetaminophen or ibuprofen for fever and discomfort* • *Rocking and holding the infant* • *Gentle movement of affected extremity*	■ Parents will know how to make the child more comfortable during the 24–48 hours after the vaccine is given.	The child is given comfort measures after vaccine administration.

Prior to giving vaccines, provide guidelines for managing expected mild reactions at home. Make sure parents have the correct dosage information for the acetaminophen or ibuprofen formulation that is in the home. See Families Want to Know: Care of the Child After Immunizations.

Reducing Pain and Anxiety

Make an effort to reduce the pain and stress of immunizations, especially since infants and children must return for more injections. Give the injections as efficiently as possible and provide support to the parent and child through the procedure

After your child receives an immunization, observe for any reactions that might occur.

■ Local pain, redness, and swelling are common at the injection site. Use ice on the site for periods of 5 to 10 minutes to help reduce swelling and pain. Acetaminophen or ibuprofen may be given to reduce a fever and pain. The symptoms disappear in a day or two.

■ The child may have a fever, joint pain, muscle aches, or fatigue within hours to days after the vaccine is given. Give acetaminophen or ibuprofen for pain.

■ A few hives around the injection site may indicate a mild allergic reaction to the vaccine.

■ A severe allergic reaction is indicated by a flushed face; swelling of the face, mouth, or throat; wheezing or other difficulty breathing; or shock (confusion, lack of movement or response, or unconsciousness). If these symptoms occur, call 911 or your emergency number so your child can be taken to the emergency department for treatment. Have the child lie down on his or her back and raise the legs to promote blood return to the vital organs until the ambulance arrives.

(Figure 16–6 ➤). Reducing pain will also lessen the anxiety associated with future visits for health care. Some techniques that may reduce pain and anxiety associated with injections include the following:

• Coach the parent to hold and talk with the child during the injections. Let the parent know it is okay to be anxious, but to try to stay calm for the child. Encourage the parent to use an age-appropriate distraction technique. See Chapter 15 ∞.

• Give infants up to 4 months of age 24% sucrose water to suck (use a prepared solution, e.g., Sweet-Ease, or mix 1 packet of sugar in 10 mL of tap water) immediately before the injection. Sucrose water has been demonstrated to reduce pain in newborns. (See Chapter 15 ∞.) Then allow the infant to suck on a pacifier or breastfeed during the injections.

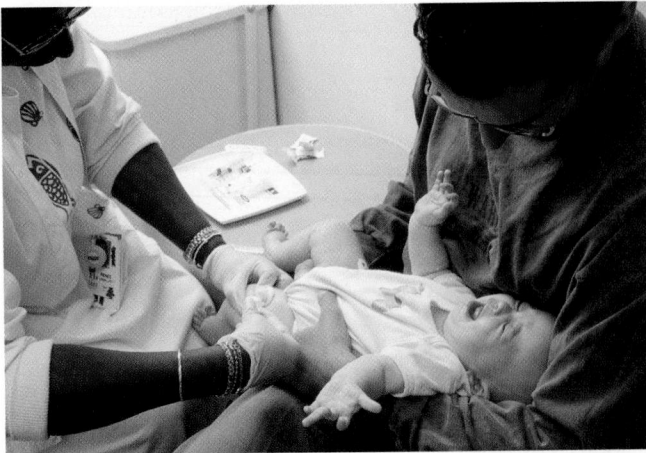

FIGURE 16–6 ➤ Give immunizations quickly and efficiently. Do not prolong the wait and let fear grow. The child will be anxious, especially if more than one injection must be given.

• Apply pressure at the site for 10 seconds before the injection.

• Provide information about obtaining L-M-X4 prior to the next visit. Instruct parents how to apply L-M-X4 to the site(s) prior to the child's appointment.

• Use vapocoolant spray on the skin immediately before the injection, or spray it on a cotton ball and hold it against the skin for a couple of minutes.

• Give two injections simultaneously in different extremities using two different providers.

• Use age-appropriate distraction techniques.

• Encourage the parent to comfort the child after the injection.

Select the correct needle length for intramuscular injections for infants so that medication does not get into the subcutaneous tissue. When the medication reaches the muscle mass, local reactions to immunizations are reduced. A 5/8-inch needle can be used in newborns, including preterm, for injections in the anterolateral thigh. Between 2 and 12 months of age, use a 1-inch needle for the anterior thigh. For toddlers and children, use a 1- to 1 1/4-inch needle for the anterolateral thigh site and a 5/8-inch needle for the deltoid (AAP, 2009, p. 19).

Evaluation

Expected nursing outcomes include the following:

• Parents are fully informed and give consent for immunizations.

• All age-appropriate immunizations are provided for the child at each health visit, or catch-up immunizations are provided as needed.

• Parents are prepared to manage mild reactions to immunizations at home.

• Parents are able to identify and report serious reactions to immunizations.

■ COMMUNICABLE DISEASES IN INFANTS AND CHILDREN

Communicable diseases cause acute illnesses. These diseases are caused by bacterial, viral, protozoan, or fungal organisms. As noted earlier, infants and children develop communicable disease infections more frequently than adults. Active immunity to microorganisms does not occur until there is natural exposure or immunization that leads to the development of antibodies. Therefore, infants and children are more susceptible to the large number of infectious organisms to which they have no resistance.

Epidemiology and Pathophysiology

Microorganisms (bacterial, viral, fungal, and protozoan) use the human body to reproduce. Many microorganisms are pathogens that cause infectious and communicable diseases. They enter the body through direct contact with mucous membranes and injured skin, inhalation, and ingestion. Biting insects or animals (vectors) also inject organisms into the skin and blood.

The microorganisms spread through the lymph and blood to other tissues and organs where they multiply. The initial response of the body to invasion by microorganisms is an inflammatory response. See Chapter 22 ∞ for more information about the inflammatory and immune response.

When antibodies have developed to a specific microorganism to which the child is exposed, they protect the child by:

- Activating the inflammatory response
- Neutralizing bacterial toxins and preventing them from binding with the tissues
- Preventing the initial attachment and entrance of viruses into the cells
- Producing a substance (opsonin) that makes the bacterial outer capsule susceptible to **phagocytosis** (the engulfment and destruction of microorganisms, dead cells, and foreign particles)

Bacteria enter the body and cause inflammation. Endotoxins increase capillary permeability and trigger fever. Antimicrobials may prevent the growth of or destroy microorganisms that have not developed antibiotic resistance.

Pathophysiology Illustrated
Fever

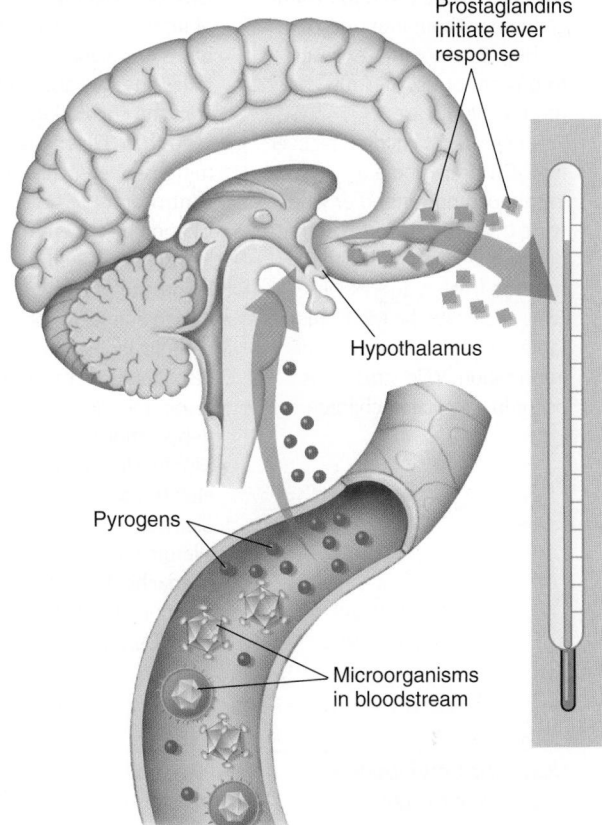

FIGURE 16–7 ➤ The hypothalamus functions as the body's thermostat, directing the body to conserve or dissipate heat. When microorganisms invade the body, endogenous pyrogens are released into the bloodstream. These substances travel to the hypothalamus, where they trigger the production and release of prostaglandins, which initiate the fever response. Blood is diverted from the extremities to more central vessels. This helps increase the core body temperature by decreasing heat loss. Shivering increases both metabolic action and heat production. The hypothalamus then maintains the temperature at the new set-point.

Viruses are parasitic organisms that invade the cells and take them over for their own survival and reproduction. As they reproduce cell to cell, eventually the body's immune response to the virus overwhelms it and the infection is cured. In some cases the virus reproduces at such a slow rate that the infected person is asymptomatic and becomes a carrier of the virus. Secondary bacterial infection can occur in virus-damaged cells. See Chapter 22 ∞ for more information about the immune response and viral infections such as HIV.

Fever

Fever is an increased body temperature of 38°C (100.4°F) taken by the rectal or tympanic route or 37.8°C (100°F) by the oral route. With an infection, **endogenous pyrogens** (interleukins, interferons, and tumor necrosis factor) are released by macrophages in response to an invasive infectious organism. These pyrogens travel through the circulatory system to the hypothalamus, the control center for the regulation of body temperature, and trigger the production of prostaglandin E_2. Prostaglandin E_2 raises the body's thermoregulatory set-point, thus causing the fever to occur (Zomorrodi & Attia, 2008). See Figure 16–7 ➤.

A rise in the hypothalamus's set-point leads to a cold response with shivering and chills, vasoconstriction, and decreased peripheral perfusion. Heat loss from the body is reduced and the body temperature rises to the new temperature set-point. Vasodilation occurs and the skin flushes, becoming warm to the touch. An elevated temperature increases the child's metabolic, heart, and respiratory rates. Each degree of temperature elevation increases the child's oxygen consumption by 13% (Zomorrodi & Attia, 2008).

Infectious and communicable diseases differ in their epidemiology, transmission, and incubation period. Many infectious diseases are communicable between humans, but many are vaccine-preventable. The epidemiology, clinical manifestations, treatment, prevention, and nursing care of selected communicable diseases of childhood are detailed in Table 16–3. Some infectious diseases are transmitted by insects or animals (**zoonosis**) and are not communicable from person to person. See Table 16–4.

See Chapter 19 ∞ for information about conjunctivitis; Chapter 20 for information on tuberculosis; Chapter 22 for information on HIV infection; Chapter 25 for information about hepatitis A, B, and C; Chapter 26 for information on sexually transmitted infections; and Chapter 31 for information about impetigo, methicillin-resistant *Staphylococcus aureus*, scabies, and lice.

Infectious and Communicable Diseases Websites

TABLE 16–3 Selected Infectious and Communicable Diseases in Children

Disease	Clinical Manifestations	Clinical Therapy	Nursing Management
Chickenpox (Varicella)*§ *Causal agent:* Varicella-zoster, human herpesvirus 3. *Epidemiology:* Humans are the source of infection. Peak occurrence is in the late fall, winter, and spring. Maternal antibodies disappear 2–3 months after birth. *Transmission:* Direct contact of the virus to the mucous membranes or conjunctiva primarily through airborne spread of secretions and occasionally with lesion contact. *Incubation period:* 14–21 days. *Period of communicability:* Most contagious 1–2 days before the rash to shortly after onset of rash. Contagious state continues until all lesions are crusted over. This period may be prolonged after passive immunization or in immunodeficient children. 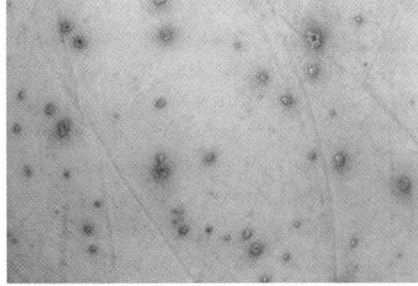 Skin lesions of chickenpox. *Source: Pearson Education.*	Acute onset of mild fever, malaise, anorexia, headache, mild abdominal pain, and irritability occurs before and with eruption. Macular rash for a few hours that progresses to pruritic vesicular lesions for 1–5 days, and then to crusts. Up to 250–500 lesions of all stages may be present at any one time. Crusts may remain for 1–3 weeks. The lesions begin on the trunk, scalp, and face, and then spread to the rest of the body. Ulcerative lesions may be seen in the mucous membranes. Mouth lesions may lead to decreased fluid intake and dehydration. *Complications:* Complications are rare but can include secondary infection (cellulitis, local abscesses, sepsis, meningitis, encephalitis, pneumonia), thrombocytopenia, and Reye syndrome. Chickenpox can be fatal in newborns of infected mothers and immunocompromised children. Children undergoing chemotherapy, steroid treatment, or transplant therapy should be carefully monitored after exposure to the disease.	Fluid from vesicle or scab can be tested using polymerase chain reaction for diagnosis. Medical management is supportive. IV acyclovir is used within 24 hours of rash onset for immunocompromised patients. Oral acyclovir is used for children at high risk of moderate to severe disease (e.g., treated with chronic salicylate therapy or aerosol corticosteroids, or with chronic skin or pulmonary condition) (AAP, 2009). Varicella-zoster immune globulin or immune globulin IV is given within 96 hours of exposure to newborns of infected mothers and to exposed immunocompromised, unimmunized children. The vaccine may be given to healthy children without immunity within 72 hours after exposure to prevent or significantly modify the disease. *Prognosis:* Most children recover fully. Children who are immunocompromised or who were treated with corticosteroids during the incubation period must be treated aggressively. *Prevention:* See the Medications table on page 400 for vaccine information. Wild virus cases occur in vaccinated children.	• Use airborne and contact precautions during contagious period. • Upon hospital admission inquire about varicella immunization or recent exposure. Isolate all exposed children to protect newborns and immunocompromised patients. Ensure that nurses have documented immunity. • Isolate the child at home from all susceptible individuals, especially medically fragile and immunocompromised children or adults, and women early in pregnancy. Notify the school or childcare facility of the child's illness. • Give acetaminophen or ibuprofen to control fever. • Give oral antihistamines for relief of itching. Oatmeal and Aveeno baths or Caladryl lotion applied to lesions may also provide relief. • Trim the child's fingernails and keep them clean. Use soft cotton mittens when itching cannot be controlled. • Change bed linens frequently. • Reassure the child that the lesions will go away. • Observe for signs of complications (e.g., drowsiness, disorientation, meningeal signs, respiratory distress, and dehydration). • Monitor for acyclovir side effects: nausea, vomiting, diarrhea, abdominal pain, allergic skin reactions, or headache. Monitor renal function, if the child has renal insufficiency.
Diphtheria*§ *Causal agent: Corynebacterium diphtheriae.* *Epidemiology:* Occurs mostly in colder months in unimmunized or inadequately immunized persons.	The characteristic lesion is an adherent grayish pharyngeal membrane that in severe cases may extend into the trachea or cause airway obstruction. Attempts to remove the membrane result in bleeding.	Diagnostic tests include a culture from the nose or throat, or from a cutaneous lesion. Medical management includes administration of IV equine antitoxin (for respiratory diphtheria) after the child is	• Place on strict isolation and use transmission-based precautions. • Monitor carefully for increasing respiratory distress and cardiac or neurologic complications.

TABLE 16–3 Selected Infectious and Communicable Diseases in Children *(continued)*

Disease	Clinical Manifestations	Clinical Therapy	Nursing Management
Diphtheria (continued) Cutaneous and wound diphtheria occurs more often in the tropics. The disease is endemic in parts of Africa, Latin America, Asia, the Middle East, and states of the former Soviet Union. *Transmission:* Contact with respiratory droplets, nasal or eye discharge, or skin lesion; or less commonly by contact with contaminated items or unpasteurized milk. *Incubation period:* 2–7 days or longer. *Period of communicability:* Usually 2–4 weeks or until 4 days after antibiotics are started.	A sore throat and enlarged, tender cervical lymph nodes are present. The child may have a swollen neck. *Complications:* Produces an endotoxin that causes myocarditis and peripheral neuropathies that may be confused with Guillain-Barré syndrome.	tested for sensitivity. Dose is based upon duration of symptoms. Antibiotic therapy for 14 days with IV or IM penicillin G, changing to oral erythromycin when the child can swallow. *Prognosis:* Mortality of 5–10% with respiratory diphtheria, even with treatment (Heymann, 2008). *Prevention:* See the Medications table on page 396 for vaccine information. Booster doses are needed every 10 years after primary series. The disease does not confer immunity. This is a reportable disease.	• Have emergency airway equipment available. Provide humidified oxygen as necessary. • Administer antitoxin and antibiotics as prescribed. • Use oral suction gently as necessary. • Allow children to use mouthwash if desired. Gargling is not permitted because it can irritate the pharyngeal surfaces. • Encourage liquids as tolerated. Intravenous fluids may be necessary. • Provide emotional support to the family. • Initiate the search for patient contacts to give antibiotics and immunization boosters.
Enteroviruses *Causal agent:* Group A and B coxsackieviruses, human enteroviruses. *Epidemiology:* Occurs worldwide, most commonly in summer and early fall. More common in settings with poor hygiene and overcrowding. Immunity to specific virus probably occurs after infection, but duration is unknown. *Transmission:* Fecal-oral and respiratory routes. *Incubation period:* 3–6 days. *Period of communicability:* Viral shedding may occur for weeks or months after infection onset.	Each of the viruses causes different manifestations. *Herpangina*—sudden fever onset, sore throat, and small, discrete grayish papulovesicular, ulcerative, pharyngeal lesions that gradually increase in size. *Hand, foot, and mouth disease*—diffuse lesions may occur on the mouth buccal surfaces and tongue; papulovesicular lesions on the hands and feet; last for 7–10 days. Irritability, fever, anorexia, dysphagia, malaise, and a sore throat. *Complications:* Children with immune deficiencies may have more severe manifestations.	Diagnostic tests include a polymerase chain reaction or culture of stool, throat, or other primary site. Medical care is supportive. Immune globulin IV is used in children with severe immunodeficiency disorders (AAP, 2009). *Prognosis:* Recovery is generally good with supportive care. *Prevention:* Avoid contact with infected persons early in the disease.	• Use standard precautions if the child is hospitalized. • Use good hand hygiene. • Apply topical lotions and give systemic medications as ordered to lessen the pain and relieve the irritation. • Offer cool drinks and soft, bland foods (no citrus, salty, or spicy foods). Swallowing may be painful. • Offer warm saline mouth rinses. • Observe for dehydration. • Give nonaspirin antipyretics for fever. • Keep the child out of school or childcare while febrile.
Erythema Infectiosum (Fifth Disease) *Causal agent:* Human parvovirus B-19. *Epidemiology:* Occurs worldwide, most often in winter and spring. The disease also occurs in epidemics every 3–7 years (Heymann, 2008). The incidence is highest in children between the ages of 5 and 14 years. *Transmission:* Respiratory secretions and blood. *Incubation period:* 4–21 days.	The infection begins as a mild illness (fever, headache, malaise, and body aches) followed by the rash in 7–10 days. A fiery-red rash often appears on the cheeks giving a "slapped face" appearance. Circumoral pallor is seen. A lace-like symmetric, erythematous, maculopapular rash appears on the trunk and spreads to the extremities, sparing the palms and soles. It may be mildly pruritic. The rash fades over 1–3 weeks but can reappear if exposed to sunlight or a hot bath.	Diagnosis is made by physical signs, or a positive serum immunoglobulin (Ig) M parvovirus B-19 antibody. Medical treatment is supportive and recovery is usually spontaneous. The child with aplastic crisis may need a blood transfusion. Immunodeficient patients who develop a chronic infection may be treated with IV immune globulin therapy (AAP, 2009). *Prognosis:* Fetal infection may occur, resulting in fetal hydrops or spontaneous abortion.	• Use standard and droplet precautions if children are hospitalized. • Nonaspirin antipyretics may be given to control fever. • Use soothing oatmeal or Aveeno baths if the rash is pruritic. Antipruritics may also help to relieve itching. • Encourage rest and offer frequent fluids. • Keep children out of direct sunlight if possible or cover skin with protective, light, loose clothing.

(continued)

TABLE 16–3 **Selected Infectious and Communicable Diseases in Children** *(continued)*

Disease	Clinical Manifestations	Clinical Therapy	Nursing Management
Erythema Infectiosum (Fifth Disease) (continued) *Period of communicability:* Most infectious before the rash appears. Characteristic lace-like rash of erythema infectiosum (fifth disease). *Courtesy of Maura Connor, Nursing EIC/Pearson Education.*	*Complications:* Children with hemolytic conditions may have transient aplastic crisis. Polyarthropathy is rare in children.	*Prevention:* Avoid contact with infected persons.	• The immune-competent child can return to school or daycare once the rash has appeared (AAP, 2009). • Explain the stages of rash development to parents.
Haemophilus Influenzae, Type B§ *Causal agent:* Several serotypes of *H. influenzae.* *Epidemiology:* Occurs most often in the spring and summer. Most commonly affected are unimmunized or inadequately immunized infants and young children. Neonates may acquire the organism by aspirating amniotic fluid or contact with vaginal secretions. *Transmission:* Direct contact with respiratory secretions or inhalation of droplets. The organism frequently colonizes asymptomatically in the respiratory tract. *Incubation period:* Unknown. *Period of communicability:* 3 days from onset of symptoms.	Begins with an upper respiratory infection. The organism then directly invades the bloodstream and causes severe invasive illnesses, such as meningitis, epiglottitis, pneumonia, septic arthritis, and cellulitis. It may cause sepsis in infants. Sinusitis, otitis media, bronchitis, and pericarditis are other potential infections. Clinical manifestations vary by disease. The vaccine has decreased invasive illnesses 99% (AAP, 2009). *Complications:* Left untreated, severe sequelae and death, especially in young infants from conditions such as meningitis, epiglottitis, sinusitis, pneumonitis, and cellulitis.	Diagnosis by culture of blood, cerebrospinal fluid, or middle ear aspirate. Treatment for invasive disease is IV antibiotics for 10 days. Dexamethasone may be given to reduce neurologic sequelae of meningitis. Rifampin may be given to unprotected household contacts, if another child 4 years or younger has not completed immunizations. Exposed children should receive a dose of vaccine (AAP, 2009). *Prognosis:* Recovery is good with rapid diagnosis and treatment. Delayed treatment may result in disability. *Prevention:* See the Medications table on page 397 for vaccine information.	• Use droplet precautions until 24 hours after the initiation of antibiotics. • Identify potential contacts and identify their immunization status. Determine the need for vaccine dose or rifampin. Inform parents to seek health care rapidly if the exposed child becomes ill. • Administer antipyretics to help the child feel more comfortable. • Perform nursing care measures specific to the illness. • Inform family members that rifampin turns urine and other body fluids orange, and it will cause stains.
Influenza§ *Causal agent:* Orthomyxoviruses, types A, B, and C. *Epidemiology:* Prevalent in the United States from October to March, but the virus is active in other parts of the world year-round. Community outbreaks can last 4–8 weeks or longer. Incidence of infection is often greater in young children who have fewer prior influenza infections and antibodies. H1N1 (swine flu) is a new virus spreading person to person worldwide.	Abrupt onset of fever (38–40°C), chills, dry cough, runny nose, sore throat, malaise, aches, headache, and anorexia. Children may have nausea and vomiting, diarrhea, and abdominal pain. Recovery usually occurs in 3–5 days. *Complications:* Otitis media, invasive secondary infections, myositis, febrile seizures, encephalitis, or severe encephalopathy may occur. Pneumonia, croup, bronchiolitis, and wheezing may occur in infants.	Diagnostic tests include viral culture or rapid antigen testing from throat or nasopharynx; direct fluorescent antibody or indirect immunofluorescent antibody staining. Treatment is supportive. Antiviral therapy for children includes: 1 year and older—oseltamivir, and amantadine; 7 years and older—zanamivir; and 13 years and older—rimantadine (AAP, 2009). Benefit of antiviral therapy is greatest if started within 48 hours, and discontinued 1–2 days after symptoms resolve.	• Use droplet and contact precautions for hospitalized children. • For home care, encourage good hand hygiene and reduce exposure of other family members to the infected child. • Provide fluids to keep nasal secretions moist and to prevent dehydration. • Provide nonaspirin antipyretic for fever management and mild pain. • If antiviral medications are given, be alert for nausea and vomiting. Zanamivir can exacerbate asthma.

TABLE 16-3 Selected Infectious and Communicable Diseases in Children *(continued)*

Disease	Clinical Manifestations	Clinical Therapy	Nursing Management
Influenza (continued) *Transmission:* Spreads by aerosolized particles and direct contact with respiratory secretions or contaminated surfaces. *Incubation period:* 1–4 days, average 2 days. *Period of communicability:* Greatest in first 3–5 days of illness. Virus shedding for up to 7 days in children.	Children under 2 years have the highest complication rate (Heymann, 2008).	*Prevention:* See the Medications table on page 398 for vaccine information.	• Children should be kept home until 24 hours after fever is gone. • Provide rest and quiet diversional activities. • Teach parents to be alert to signs of influenza complications. • Become familiar with community pandemic influenza plans. See the companion website.
Measles (Rubeola)§ *Causal agent: Morbillivirus,* a member of the paramyxovirus group. *Epidemiology:* No longer endemic in the United States. Cases primarily occur due to importation of the virus from other countries and transmission to susceptible individuals (AAP, 2009). In 2008, 91% of cases occurred in unimmunized persons or those of unknown status (CDC, 2008d). Passive maternal immunity lasts until the infant is age 6–9 months (Heymann, 2008). Measles is an endemic disease in developing countries. Global measles control is a World Health Organization goal. *Transmission:* Direct contact with respiratory droplets and airborne spread. *Incubation period:* About 8–12 days. *Period of communicability:* Begins 3–5 days before the rash until 4 days after the rash appears.	Children are quite ill in the 3- to 5-day prodromal phase, with symptoms including fever, conjunctivitis, coryza, cough, anorexia, and Koplik spots (small, irregular, bluish white spots on a red background) on the buccal mucosa. The characteristic red, blotchy maculopapular rash that becomes confluent usually appears 4–7 days after onset of prodromal phase. The rash begins on the face and then becomes generalized. Desquamation occurs in some cases. Symptoms gradually subside after an additional 4–7 days. *Complications:* Diarrhea, otitis media, pneumonia, bronchitis, laryngotracheobronchitis, encephalitis, and death. Complications and death more commonly occur in children who are severely malnourished or immunocompromised. The younger the child, the greater the risk for complications. Measles facial rash, third day of rash. *Courtesy of Centers for Disease Control and Prevention, Atlanta, GA.*	Diagnosis can be made by a serologic test for immunoglobulin (Ig) M measles antibody. Treatment is supportive. No antiviral therapy is available. Vitamin A may be given to malnourished children. Antibiotics are used for secondary bacterial infections. Immune globulin, administered up to 6 days after exposure, may be helpful in preventing or reducing disease severity for infants less than age 1 year, immunocompromised children, and pregnant women. *Prognosis:* Death from respiratory or neurologic complications occurs in 1–3 of every 1,000 cases in the United States (AAP, 2009). *Prevention:* See the Medications table on page 399 for vaccine information. Prevent exposure by susceptible individuals. This is a reportable disease.	• Use airborne precautions when the child is hospitalized. • Use a cool-mist vaporizer to help clear airway passages. • Suction nose and oral cavity very gently as necessary. • Give nonaspirin antipyretics for fever and antipruritics for itching. • Antitussives may be ordered to control coughing. • Teach parents to observe for complications and to seek care as needed. • Keep lights dim, and cover windows if the child has photophobia. • Maintain bed rest and provide diversional activities. Elevate the head of the bed. Keep the room cool with good air circulation. Use light, nonirritating blankets. • Keep skin clean and dry. Avoid the use of soaps. • Offer small amounts of cool liquids frequently to maintain hydration. Blended, pureed, and mashed foods may be most easily tolerated.

(continued)

| TABLE 16–3 | Selected Infectious and Communicable Diseases in Children *(continued)* |

Disease	Clinical Manifestations	Clinical Therapy	Nursing Management
Meningococcus§ *Causal agent: Neisseria meningitidis,* a gram-negative diplococcus. *Epidemiology:* Most often in winter or early spring. Serogroups B, C, Y, or W-135 cause most infections in the United States. Highest rates occur in children under 2 years and among adolescents 15–18 years. Persons living in poverty or crowded conditions are at higher risk. Outbreaks have occurred in childcare centers, college dormitories, and military recruit camps. *Transmission:* Spread by inhalation of respiratory droplets from human carriers. *Incubation period:* 2–10 days. *Period of communicability:* Until 24 hours after antibiotic started to which the organism is sensitive. 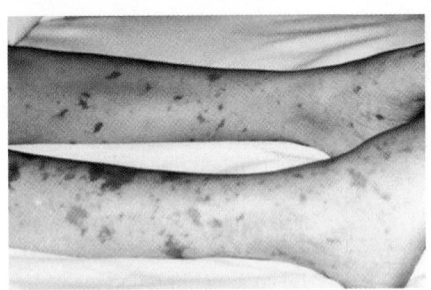 Purpura with meningococcemia. *Used with permission of the American Academy of Pediatrics.*	Children may develop meningitis or meningococcemia, or the two conditions may occur together. Begins with an abrupt onset of fever, chills, malaise, muscle aches, vomiting, and **prostration** (extreme exhaustion). Meningitis neurologic signs include decreased mental status, seizures, or coma. In meningococcemia a maculopapular rash becomes petechial and may progress to purpura and sepsis. Septic shock with leg pain, cold extremities, and pallor may develop (Mola, Nield, & Weisse, 2009). *Complications:* Septic shock; disseminated intravascular coagulation and loss of digits or limbs due to gangrenous necrosis; hearing loss, neurologic disabilities (increased intracranial pressure, cranial nerve palsies, obstructive hydrocephalus), and scarring.	Diagnostic tests include cultures of the blood and cerebrospinal fluid culture, and a Gram stain of petechial skin scrapings. *Treatment:* IV penicillin G (or cefotaxime, ceftriaxone, and ampicillin; chloramphenicol if the child has a penicillin allergy) for 5–7 days. Care is aggressive in the intensive care unit to maintain the airway, assist ventilation, and manage shock with IV fluids and vasopressors. *Prognosis:* Approximately 10% of children die (AAP, 2009). *Prevention:* See page 399 for vaccine information. Close contacts are given rifampin, ceftriaxone, ciprofloxacin, or azithromycin. The vaccine may also be used to prevent secondary cases if the primary case is caused by a serotype covered in the vaccine (AAP, 2009). This is a reportable disease.	• Use standard and droplet precautions until the effective antibiotic has been administered for 24 hours. • Be alert for development of shock and respiratory compromise as the disease progresses rapidly. Have emergency equipment available. • Avoid overloading the child with fluids when giving IV and blood products. Monitor for signs of increased intracranial pressure. (See Chapter 27 ∞.) • Help the family mobilize its support system, and keep the family informed of the child's status as the disease progresses. • Identify close contacts who should receive prophylaxis. Educate them about expected side effects (e.g., orange urine with rifampin). • Teach close contacts about signs of the illness and to seek health care promptly if they occur. • Help coordinate rehabilitation for the child.
Mononucleosis *Causal agent:* Epstein-Barr virus (EBV), gammaherpesvirus. *Epidemiology:* Occurs worldwide in no seasonal pattern. Infection commonly occurs early in life, and spread among family members is common. *Transmission:* Direct contact with saliva or through blood transfusions. EBV can survive in saliva for several hours outside the body. *Incubation period:* Estimated to be 30–50 days.	In very young children, mononucleosis may be mild and have no distinguishing clinical signs. In other children, the disease is characterized by fever, painful sore throat (exudative pharyngotonsillitis), and posterior cervical lymphadenopathy. Hepatosplenomegaly and elevated liver function tests may occur. The syndrome typically lasts 2–3 weeks, but fatigue may continue in some children for weeks longer. *Complications:* Rare side effects include central nervous system symptoms such as encephalitis, aseptic meningitis, cranial nerve palsies, and Guillain-Barré syndrome. Hematologic	Diagnosis is confirmed by a positive heterophil antibody titer and greater than 10% atypical lymphocytes. Serum EBV antibody tests require acute and convalescent specimens to diagnose the disease (AAP, 2009). Treatment is supportive. Corticosteroids may be used to control severe pharyngeal swelling and impending airway obstruction, massive splenomegaly, myocarditis, or hemolytic anemia. Ampicillin and amoxicillin are avoided because they may cause a nonallergic rash (AAP, 2009). *Prognosis:* Rarely fatal. After recovery, the virus remains latent in the lymphoid system	• Use standard precautions if the child is hospitalized. • Give antipyretics and analgesics for fever and sore throat. Offer warm salt water for gargling. Offer soft foods and encourage fluids. • Maintain bed rest during acute phase. • Reassure adolescents who may be worried about keeping up with school work that they can return to school when the fever is gone and swallowing is normal. • Teens should avoid kissing until the fever has been gone several days. • Contact sports should be avoided until the liver and spleen are normal size, usually in about 4 weeks.

TABLE 16–3	Selected Infectious and Communicable Diseases in Children	*(continued)*	
Disease	Clinical Manifestations	Clinical Therapy	Nursing Management
Mononucleosis (continued) *Period of communicability:* Indeterminate, individuals may be asymptomatic carriers for a year or longer (Heymann, 2008).	complications such as splenic rupture, thrombocytopenia, or hemolytic anemia can also occur. Lymphomas or death can occur. EBV causes complex syndromes in immunocompromised patients, such as those with transplants.	and may reactivate in immunodeficient persons. *Prevention:* No known prevention.	• If splenomegaly is present, alcohol should be avoided for 3 months after liver function test results return to normal.
Mumps (Parotitis)§ *Causal agent: Rubulavirus* in the Paramyxoviridae family. *Epidemiology:* Occurs worldwide in unvaccinated children, most often in winter and spring. Infection and vaccination induce lifelong immunity. *Transmission:* Inhalation of or contact with respiratory droplets. *Incubation period:* 12–25 days. *Period of communicability:* 7 days before parotid swelling until 9 days after swelling occurs. This child has mumps with diffuse lymphedema of the neck. *Courtesy of Centers for Disease Control and Prevention, Atlanta, GA.*	Acute onset of malaise, fever, and swelling of one or more salivary glands (parotid, sublingual, or submaxillary). Other signs may include an earache, headache, pain with chewing, and decreased appetite and activity. Mumps may also be asymptomatic in some children. *Complications:* Aseptic meningitis, sensorineural hearing loss, orchitis (inflammation of the epididymis, pain on testicular palpation, and scrotal swelling) may occur in 20–30% of postpubertal males; sterility is relatively rare (Heymann, 2008).	Diagnostic tests include a viral culture (throat, urine, or cerebrospinal fluid) or serologic test for mumps-specific IgM antibodies. Therapy is supportive, focused on symptom relief. *Prognosis:* Mumps is usually self-limiting. *Prevention:* See the Medications table on page 399 for vaccine information. This is a reportable disease. In 2006, a mumps outbreak occurred (more than 6,000 cases) among college students, many of whom had received two doses of the vaccine (CDC, 2006).	• Use standard and droplet precautions for hospitalized children. • Children cared for at home are generally uncomfortable, but rarely very ill. • Avoid exposure to immunocompromised or susceptible individuals. • Give nonaspirin analgesics and antipyretics to control fever and pain. • Encourage fluids. Offer soft foods as swallowing and chewing may be painful. Avoid foods and beverages that increase salivary flow and cause pain (e.g., citrus, spices, and candies). • Talking may be painful. Provide a bell or attention-getting device. • Educate parents about when to seek health care for signs of complications. • Keep children out of school until 5 days after onset of parotid swelling (CDC, 2008e).
Pertussis (Whooping Cough)§ *Causal agent: Bordetella pertussis.* *Epidemiology:* Occurs worldwide. Most common in children under 6 months of age; however, in 2004, adolescents had a higher incidence rate than younger children (Edwards & Johnson, 2007). Epidemic cycles occur every 3–4 years. Pertussis may occur in all persons who have waning immunity, and they can spread the disease to unimmunized infants. Neither pertussis infection nor vaccine immunity is long lasting (AAP, 2009).	The disease begins with nasal congestion, a runny nose, and a cough (catarrhal stage) lasting 1–2 weeks. Fever is minimal. Coughing spasms (paroxysmal stage) develop. A forceful inspiration through a narrowed glottis causes stridor or "whooping." Infants less than age 6 months may have gagging, gasping, or apnea rather than whooping. Sucking may trigger coughing. Coughing may be accompanied by cyanosis, vomiting, and profuse mucous drainage. Paroxysmal coughing may last 1–6 weeks or more. Adolescents	Diagnostic tests include culture from the nasopharynx or polymerase chain reaction (PCR) testing. Treatment includes supportive care and macrolide antibiotics (erythromycin, azithromycin, and clarithromycin). Symptoms may be reduced if initiated in catarrhal stage. If started later they may only reduce communicability. *Prognosis:* The disease is most severe in infants under age 6 months, and most deaths occur in this age group. *Prevention:* See the Medications table on page 396 for vaccine	• When hospitalized, use droplet precautions until 5 days after starting antibiotics. • Continuously assess respirations and oxygen saturation with a cardiac monitor and pulse oximeter. • Remain with the child during coughing spells, when hypoxic and apneic episodes are most likely. Give oxygen if ordered. Have emergency equipment available. • Provide humidification. Gentle suctioning may be necessary. • Encourage frequent rest periods. • Provide small frequent feedings of desired foods.

(continued)

TABLE 16–3	Selected Infectious and Communicable Diseases in Children *(continued)*		
Disease	Clinical Manifestations	Clinical Therapy	Nursing Management
Pertussis (Whooping Cough) (continued) *Transmission:* Inhalation or direct contact with respiratory droplets. *Incubation period:* 7–10 days. *Period of communicability:* Most communicable for first 2 weeks, before the paroxysmal stage, or until 5 days after antibiotic therapy is initiated.	often have upper respiratory symptoms with persistent coughing spasms lasting 3–9 weeks (Edwards & Johnson, 2007). *Complications:* Pneumonia, atelectasis, encephalopathy, seizures, and death.	information. Vaccine protection wanes after 5–10 years. Close contacts should be treated with macrolide antibiotics for prophylaxis, and the vaccine should be given to unimmunized or inadequately immunized adults and children. This is a reportable disease.	• Encourage the child to take fluids. The child may need IV hydration if oral intake is not tolerated. • Provide emotional support to parents. • Teach parents to watch for signs of respiratory distress and dehydration if the child is managed at home.
Pneumococcal Infection*§ *Causative agent:* Streptococcus pneumoniae, many serotypes. *Epidemiology:* The organism is found in the nasopharynx of healthy people. Outbreaks occur in the winter and spring. In temperate climates, 8 of 90 serotypes account for most of the invasive pediatric disease. *Transmission:* Person-to-person spread of respiratory droplets. *Incubation period:* Unknown, may be 1–3 days. *Period of communicability:* Unknown. Probably within 24 hours after beginning effective antibiotic therapy.	The signs and symptoms are related to the focal area of infection. The organism may cause otitis media, sinusitis, pharyngitis, laryngotracheo-bronchitis, pneumonia, meningitis, and bacteremia. See Chapter 19 ∞ for signs of otitis media, Chapter 20 ∞ for signs of laryngotracheobron-chitis and pneumonia, and Chapter 27 ∞ for signs of meningitis. In bacteremia, there is unexplained fever and no localized infection site. Individuals with immunodeficiency (e.g., asplenia, malignancy, sickle cell disease, and nephritic syndrome) are at higher risk for invasive disease. *Complications:* Meningitis, bacteremia, pneumonia, septic arthritis, osteomyelitis, endocarditis, and brain abscess.	Diagnostic tests include bacterial culture from the site of infection. Medical management includes symptomatic care for the specific focus of infection. Antibiotic selection is based upon culture sensitivity. Many pneumococcal strains are resistant to penicillin, cefotaxime, ceftriaxone, and others. Dexamethasone may be an adjunctive therapy for meningitis. *Prevention:* See the Medications table on page 399 for vaccine information. The rate of invasive disease has decreased 99% for serotypes included in the vaccines (AAP, 2009).	• If the child is hospitalized, maintain standard precautions. • Provide nonaspirin antipyretics for fever control and comfort. • Encourage fluids, and monitor intake and output. • Monitor vital signs and level of consciousness to identify signs of worsening condition. • Many children with mild disease will be treated at home. Educate parents about signs indicating a need to seek urgent medical care, proper medication administration, and comfort measures.
Poliomyelitis§ *Causal agent:* Poliovirus is an enterovirus with three serotypes. *Epidemiology:* Global eradication efforts have eliminated polio in all but four countries (Afghanistan, India, Nigeria, and Pakistan), and nearly all cases occur in children less than 5 years (Heymann, 2008). Imported polio is a threat to inadequately immunized children. *Transmission:* Primarily by the fecal-oral route, but also the respiratory route. *Incubation period:* Usually 7–10 days.	More than 90% of infections are asymptomatic. The child may have a nonspecific minor illness with a low-grade fever and sore throat. This minor illness may be followed by aseptic meningitis and paresthesias. Asymmetric flaccid paralysis may occur acutely in up to 2% of cases. Site of paralysis depends on location of injury to the brainstem or spinal cord. Residual paralysis may occur in more than half of those affected (AAP, 2009). *Complications:* Permanent motor paralysis, respiratory arrest, myocardial failure, aseptic meningitis, and post-polio syndrome.	Diagnosis is made by cell culture from stool or throat swabs. Treatment is supportive. No chemotherapeutic agents that directly kill the poliovirus are available. *Prognosis:* If paralysis of the respiratory or swallowing muscles occur, it is life threatening. Motor paralysis may result in long-term disability. *Prevention:* See the Medications table on page 400 for vaccine information. The vaccine induces lifelong immunity. This is a reportable disease.	• Use standard and contact precautions for hospitalized children. • Observe the child for respiratory paralysis (ineffective cough, talking with frequent pauses, shallow and rapid respiratory rate). Keep emergency equipment at the bedside to assist ventilations as needed until mechanical ventilation is set up. • Use moist hot packs to help relieve discomfort. • Encourage fluids. • Keep the child on bed rest and position the child to promote body alignment. • Perform range-of-motion exercises to prevent contractures. Help coordinate rehabilitation services.

TABLE 16–3 Selected Infectious and Communicable Diseases in Children *(continued)*

Disease	Clinical Manifestations	Clinical Therapy	Nursing Management
Poliomyelitis (continued) *Period of communicability:* Highest before and right after clinical symptoms. Virus is excreted in the feces for 3–6 weeks.			• Provide emotional support to the child and family. Keep them informed about the illness.
Roseola (Exanthem Subitum, Sixth Disease) *Causal agent:* Human herpesvirus type 6 (HHV-6). *Epidemiology:* Occurs worldwide, primarily in children 6–24 months of age (after maternal antibodies decline). No seasonal pattern. *Transmission:* Contact with saliva and respiratory secretions. *Incubation period:* 9–10 days. *Period of communicability:* Asymptomatic lifelong viral shedding (AAP, 2009, p. 378).	Sudden-onset fever greater than 39.5°C (103°F) for 3–7 days, during which the child does not appear toxic (normal appetite and behavior) and has no rash or disease-specific signs. An erythematous maculopapular rash appears after the fever resolves, and lasts hours to days. The child's appetite is normal. *Complications:* Febrile seizures in 10–15% of cases (AAP, 2009, p. 378).	Diagnostic testing may include polymerase chain reaction for HHV-6 DNA in blood or cerebrospinal fluid. Medical management is supportive as roseola is self-limiting. *Prognosis:* Roseola is benign in most cases. Nearly all children over 4 years of age have a positive antibody titer to HHV-6 (AAP, 2009, p. 379).	• Children are rarely hospitalized, but use standard precautions if they are. • Give nonaspirin antipyretics to control fever. • Observe closely for any seizure activity, especially during the febrile periods. • Encourage fluids to maintain hydration. • Reassure parents that the rash will disappear in a few days.
Rotavirus *Causal agent:* RNA viruses of the Reoviridae family. Groups A, B, and C infect humans. *Epidemiology:* Occurs more often in cool periods of the year. Most common cause of severe diarrhea in children under 5 years. *Transmission:* Fecal-oral route, possible respiratory route. *Incubation period:* 24 to 72 hours. *Period of communicability:* Virus found in stool for up to 30 days in immunocompromised children (Heymann, 2008).	Acute onset of low-grade fever and vomiting followed by watery diarrhea 1–2 days later. Up to 10–20 diarrheal stools a day. Symptoms last 3–8 days. *Complications:* Dehydration and electrolyte disturbances. Immunocompromised children may develop persistent infection and diarrhea (AAP, 2009, p. 576). Death in rare circumstances.	Diagnosis by enzyme immunoassay or latex agglutination assay to detect group A rotavirus antigen. Treatment involves adequate fluid and electrolyte replacement with oral rehydration solution. Antimotility drugs should not be used (Heymann, 2008). If severely dehydrated, IV fluid resuscitation is performed. No antiviral therapy is available. *Prevention:* See the Medications table on page 400 for vaccine information.	• Use standard and contact precautions if the child is hospitalized. • Encourage parents to use good hand hygiene with soap and water or alcohol-based hand sanitizers. • Clean and disinfect contaminated surfaces. • Assess hydration status frequently. • Breastfeeding is continued during oral rehydration therapy, but wait up to 24 hours before giving formula. • Older children can begin complex carbohydrates and lean meats, yogurt, fruits, and vegetables after 24 hours of oral rehydration therapy.
Rubella (German Measles)* *Causal agent:* A *Rubivirus* in the Togaviridae family. *Epidemiology:* Occurs worldwide and is most prevalent in the winter and spring. No longer endemic in the United States (AAP, 2009, p. 580). Most cases in the United States occur among foreign-born children and adults from countries that have poor vaccine coverage. *Transmission:* Inhalation or direct contact with nasopharyngeal secretions. *Incubation period:* 14–23 days.	May be asymptomatic. Usually a mild disease. An erythematous maculopapular rash appears first on the face and becomes generalized within 24 hours. Other signs include a low-grade fever and lymphadenopathy (posterior auricular and suboccipital, or generalized for 5–8 days), conjunctivitis, or Forchheimer spots (discrete erythematous lesions on the soft palate). Adults may have a low-grade fever, headache, malaise, coryza, and conjunctivitis 1–5 days before the rash.	Diagnostic tests include enzyme immunoassays and a latex agglutination test, cell culture from a nasal swab, and detection of rubella-specific IgM or IgG antibodies. Treatment is supportive as the disease is self-limiting. *Prognosis:* Disease is usually mild and benign. Maternal infection during the first trimester of pregnancy may result in fetal death, congenital defects (ophthalmic, cardiac, auditory, or neurologic), or congenital rubella syndrome.	• Maintain standard and droplet precautions for contagious children. • Maintain contact precautions for infants with congenital rubella syndrome until 1 year of age unless nasopharyngeal and urine cultures are repeatedly negative after 3 months of age (AAP, 2009, p. 581). • Isolate children treated at home from pregnant women. • Give nonaspirin analgesics and antipyretics for any pain and fever. • Encourage fluids and preferred foods.

(continued)

TABLE 16–3	Selected Infectious and Communicable Diseases in Children	(continued)	
Disease	Clinical Manifestations	Clinical Therapy	Nursing Management
Rubella (German Measles) (continued) *Period of communicability:* A few days before to 7 days after the rash onset. Infants with congenital rubella may shed the virus for months after birth.	Congenital rubella syndrome signs: growth retardation, radiolucent bone disease, hepatosplenomegaly, thrombocytopenia, and purpuric skin lesions (giving a "blueberry muffin" appearance). *Complications:* Polyarthralgia and polyarthritis may occur in adolescents.	*Prevention:* See the Medications table on page 399 for vaccine information. 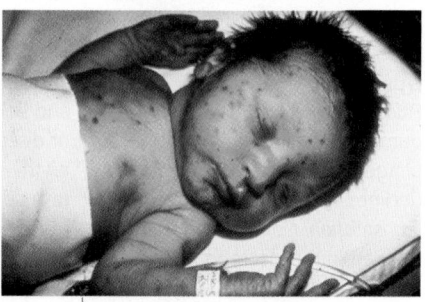 Congenital rubella syndrome. *Courtesy of Centers for Disease Control and Prevention, Atlanta, GA.*	• Provide quiet activities. • Exclude children from childcare or school for 7 days after onset of rash. Notify school and childcare facilities of the child's illness.
Streptococcus A *Causal agent:* Group A streptococci (GAS), numerous serotypes. *Epidemiology:* Pharyngeal infections tend to occur more in late fall, winter, and spring when closer person-to-person contact occurs. Pyodermal infections tend to occur in warmer seasons because of the association with minor skin trauma and insect bites. *Transmission:* Contact with respiratory secretions for pharyngitis or direct contact with skin lesions. *Incubation period:* Pharyngeal: usually 2–5 days; Pyodermal: usually 7–10 days. *Period of communicability:* Highest during acute infection. Noncontagious within 24 hours of starting appropriate antibiotics.	*Pharyngeal:* Abrupt onset with sore throat, dysphagia, tender cervical nodes, malaise, high fever, headache, abdominal pain, anorexia, and vomiting. Pharynx is beefy red with exudate and palatal petechiae may be seen. *GAS respiratory tract infection:* Children under 3 years may develop serous rhinitis, moderate fever, irritability, and anorexia rather than pharyngitis. *Scarlet fever:* A characteristic erythematous, confluent, sandpaper rash most often occurs with pharyngitis. The rash blanches with pressure and concentrates in skin folds. As the rash fades in 3–4 days, the toe tips and finger tips begin to peel. The classic strawberry tongue is seen on day 4–5. *Pyodermal:* Lesions (impetigo) are honey-colored crusts at the site of open lesions. *Complications:* Acute otitis media, sinusitis, peritonsillar or retropharyngeal abscess, cervical lymphadenitis, acute rheumatic fever, acute glomerulonephritis, or toxic shock syndrome.	Diagnosis can be made by a rapid strep antigen test or culture of secretions from the posterior pharynx and tonsils. Cultures of skin lesions are not indicated (AAP, 2009, p. 619). Prompt antibiotic treatment with penicillin V for 10 days is the drug of choice for pharyngitis. Oral cephalosporin or a macrolide or azalide antibiotic is used if the child is allergic to penicillin. Uncomplicated nonbullous impetigo is treated with mupirocin or retapamulin ointment. Invasive strains causing necrotizing fasciitis or myositis need IV antibiotics and surgical intervention (exploration and debridement of dead tissue). *Prognosis:* Recovery is usually good with antibiotic therapy. Up to 15% of healthy children become chronic carriers (AAP, 2009, p. 620). *Prevention:* None.	• Use standard and droplet precautions for pharyngeal infections and contact precautions for skin infections if the child is hospitalized. • Promote bed rest during the febrile stage. • Give nonaspirin antipyretics to control fever. Teach parents signs of a worsening condition. • For pharyngeal infections, offer warm salt water for gargling, and nonacidic beverages. Encourage cool, clear liquids and a soft diet. Swallowing may be difficult. • Emphasize the importance of giving the antibiotics for 10 full days. • Encourage family members with sore throats to have throat cultures taken. • For impetigo, teach the parents to wash the skin, remove crusts, and apply antibiotic ointment. 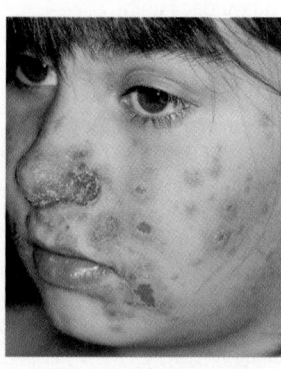 Impetigo. *Courtesy of Jason L. Smith, MD.*

TABLE 16–3 Selected Infectious and Communicable Diseases in Children *(continued)*

Disease	Clinical Manifestations	Clinical Therapy	Nursing Management
Tetanus*§ *Causal agent: Clostridium tetani,* an anaerobic bacillus. *Epidemiology:* The bacillus is common and exists as a spore in soil, dust, and animal excretions. The organism produces an endotoxin that affects the central nervous system. *Transmission:* The organism is transmitted to humans through puncture wounds, burns, or broken skin. Newborns in developing countries are infected when the mother is unimmunized and an unsterile tool is used to cut the umbilical cord, or if the ritual dressing placed on the cord is unknowingly contaminated with tetanus spores, (Heymann, 2008). *Incubation period:* 3 days–3 weeks (average 10 days). *Period of communicability:* No direct person-to-person transmission.	Acute onset of stiffness of the neck and jaw, with painful facial and neck muscle spasms, and difficulty chewing and swallowing. Noise or sudden movement may stimulate spasms. Facial muscle spasms may produce a grinning expression (risus sardonicus). Abdominal rigidity may cause **opisthotonos** (rigid hyperextension of the entire body). Respiratory muscles can be affected and cause airway obstruction and suffocation. Newborns have difficulty with sucking, progressing to an inability to suck, irritability, and nuchal rigidity. *Complications:* Laryngospasm, respiratory distress, and death.	Diagnosis is clinical. Medical management includes giving tetanus immune globulin (intramuscular) or immune globulin (intravenous) to unimmunized persons as soon as possible. Tetanus toxoid is given at the same time in a separate site. The wound is cleaned and debrided. Intensive care is provided with cardiorespiratory monitoring, assisted ventilation, IV metronidazole or penicillin G, nutrition, and supportive care. *Prognosis:* Neonatal mortality is high, especially when intensive care is unavailable. *Prevention:* See the Medications table on page 396 for vaccine information. Tetanus boosters should be updated every 10 years or, if a potentially contaminated wound occurs, in 5 years. Proper surgical debridement of wounds decreases the chance of tetanus.	• Use standard precautions, as the child with tetanus is hospitalized. • Prevent disease by checking immunization records and administering needed vaccines. • Assist with wound debridement. • Monitor the child's condition. Handle as little as possible. Reduce stimulation by placing the child in a quiet, darkened room. • Offer skin and respiratory care. The child may need an endotracheal tube, suctioning, and supplemental oxygen for airway support. • Provide feedings via total parenteral nutrition or feeding tube. • Maintain hydration with IV fluids and electrolytes. • Try to reduce the child's anxiety, as mental status may be unaffected. • Prepare the family for a possible poor prognosis.

* Indicates that a vaccine or antitoxin is available for use in high-risk or as-needed situations.

§ Indicates that the disease has a safe and effective vaccine.

TABLE 16–4 Selected Infectious Diseases Transmitted by Insect or Animal Hosts (Zoonosis)

Disease	Clinical Manifestations	Clinical Therapy	Nursing Management
Lyme Disease *Causal agent: Borrelia burgdorferi,* a spirochete. *Epidemiology:* Occurs in 47 states and the District of Columbia. Most cases occur in the Northeastern, Mid-Atlantic, and North Central states (AAP, 2009, p. 431). Exposure occurs in any outdoor setting where ticks are endemic. The highest incidence is between April and October in children between 5 and 9 years of age in the United States (AAP, 2009, p. 433). *Transmission:* The tick transmits the infected spirochete after feeding for 36 hours. Lyme disease is the most common vector-borne illness in North America.	*Early localized disease (ELD):* Erythema migrans, a painless expanding single annular red rash that may develop central clearing; 5–15 cm in diameter. The rash may look like a bruise in dark-skinned patients. May have fever, body aches, headache, and malaise. *Early disseminated disease (EDD):* in 3–10 weeks after tick bite, multiple smaller erythema migrans lesions, fever, headache, neck pain, malaise, conjunctivitis, enlarged lymph nodes, and cranial nerve palsies may develop. Carditis and meningitis can occur. *Late disseminated disease (LDD):* in 2–12 months Lyme arthritis develops, commonly in the	Diagnosis of ELD is by presence of erythema migrans. An enzyme-linked immunosorbent assay (ELISA) plus the Western blot test may be used in early or late disseminated disease (Kest & Pineda, 2008). Treatment is with oral amoxicillin, cefuroxime, or doxycycline for 14–21 days (ELD), 21–28 days (EDD), and 28 days (LDD). Intravenous antibiotics may be given for up to 28 days for persistent arthritis, carditis, meningitis, or encephalitis. *Prognosis:* Lyme disease may result in significant morbidity. There is no acquired immunity so reinfection may occur.	• Use standard precautions if the child is hospitalized. • Educate parents about the importance of giving the complete course of antibiotics. • Tell parents to have the child avoid sun exposure when taking doxycycline. • Nonaspirin analgesics and antipyretics may provide relief of mild fevers, headaches, and muscle and joint aches. • Children with Lyme disease may tire easily. Promote rest and avoid vigorous activities that may be difficult. • Educate parents and children about the disease and early recognition of the symptoms. • Teach parents to safely remove ticks: grasp the tick gently but

(continued)

TABLE 16–4	Selected Infectious Diseases Transmitted by Insect or Animal Hosts (Zoonosis) *(continued)*		
Disease	Clinical Manifestations	Clinical Therapy	Nursing Management
Lyme Disease *(continued)* *Incubation period:* 1–55 days after an infected tick bite. A rash in 48 hours is an allergic reaction or infection, not Lyme disease. *Period of communicability:* The infection is not contagious from person to person. The appearance of the erythema migrans rash may vary in early Lyme disease. *Courtesy of Pfizer Central Research (1998). Groton, CT.*	knee, with pain, swelling, and effusion. The child may develop encephalitis, polyneuritis, and memory problems. *Complications:* Left untreated, Lyme disease progresses to late disseminated disease with carditis, encephalitis, or meningitis (Kest & Pineda, 2008).	*Prevention:* Avoid areas that are heavily tick infested, and wear protective clothing. Check for ticks (especially hidden in hair) after every outing. Check pets because they may carry home ticks that may transfer to the child. Remove ticks as soon as possible. No vaccine is currently available.	firmly with a fine-point tweezers where the mouthparts are attached. Pull gently until it releases. Clean the area with soap and water (AAP, 2009, p. 191). • If the child is bitten by a tick, tell parents to mark the date on the calendar and monitor the child's health for the rash and flu-like symptoms and to seek medical attention if symptoms develop.
Malaria *Causal agent: Plasmodium*, four species (*P. falciparum, P. vivax, P. ovale, P. malariae*). *Epidemiology:* Occurs in tropics and subtropics in Africa, Americas, Asia, and Oceania. Children have the highest mortality. The disease is acquired during travel to an endemic area. *P. falciparum* causes the most serious disease. *Transmission:* The bite of an infected female *Anopheles* mosquito introduces the parasite to the person. The parasite infects the hepatic cells and reproduces. When the hepatic cell ruptures, parasites are released and infect the red blood cells. Transmission can occur by blood transfusion or transplacentally. *Incubation period:* Varies by type, 7 days up to 1 year. *Period of communicability:* Communicable by blood product transfusion, or the transplantation of organs from an infected person.	Malaria may begin as an illness with high fever, chills, sweating, and headache. Fever and symptoms may reoccur in a cyclic pattern every second or third day. Other signs include nausea, vomiting, diarrhea, cough, tachypnea, arthralgia, and body aches. Hepatosplenomegaly and jaundice may occur. Relapses may occur. *Complications:* The clinical syndrome may develop into an emergency condition (e.g., encephalopathy, renal failure, respiratory failure, severe anemia, vascular collapse, and shock). May cause fetal death if occurs during pregnancy.	Diagnostic tests include blood smears for parasites, or polymerase chain reaction assay. Laboratory tests often reveal anemia and thrombocytopenia. The child is hospitalized for fluid replacement, anemia management, and antipyretics. The blood is regularly monitored for parasite density. Antimalarial medication is selected based on drug resistance by malaria species and include: chloroquine, quinine sulfate and tetracycline, clindamycin, doxycycline, mefloquine, and atovaquone-proguanil. Medications may be given orally or by IV. Hypoglycemia may result from quinine treatment. ICU care is needed in severe disease. Children may need blood transfusions for severe anemia. *Prevention:* While traveling in endemic areas, use DEET insect repellent, screened rooms, DEET-treated mosquito netting, and light-colored clothing that covers the body. There is no vaccine.	• Use standard precautions for the hospitalized patient. • Maintain fluid intake. Monitor intake and output. • Monitor the hematocrit and hemoglobin levels as well as the blood glucose level. • Observe for signs of increasing illness severity such as confusion, seizures, and shock. Be prepared to provide emergency support with an airway and oxygen supplementation until the child can be transferred to the ICU. • Administer antipyretics to control the fever and promote comfort. • Provide information and emotional support to parents. • Educate families traveling to endemic areas about antimalarial chemoprophylaxis and potential side effects of nausea and vomiting. Emphasize the need to take the medication correctly. • Inform parents of other strategies to prevent exposure to mosquitoes.
Rabies (Hydrophobia)* *Causal agent: Lyssavirus* in the Rhabdoviridae family, two types (urban, in dogs; wild, in wildlife). *Epidemiology:* Occurs worldwide. Dogs and cats are usually	May be symptom-free during the incubation period. Illness may begin with headache, fever, malaise, apprehension, and paresthesia at the site.	Diagnosis is confirmed by fluorescent antibody staining of the dead animal's brain tissue, or detection of the virus in the patient's saliva or cerebrospinal fluid.	• Alert local animal control to find and quarantine any animal suspected of having rabies. • Provide emotional support to the family while reinforcing the

TABLE 16–4	Selected Infectious Diseases Transmitted by Insect or Animal Hosts (Zoonosis) *(continued)*		
Disease	Clinical Manifestations	Clinical Therapy	Nursing Management
Rabies (Hydrophobia) (continued) vaccinated. Rabies can occur in many wild animals, particularly bats, foxes, skunks, and raccoons. *Transmission:* Infected saliva from the bite of a rabid animal introduces the virus, which travels along the nerves to the brain. Human-to-human transmission is rare (e.g., by transplantation). *Incubation period:* Highly variable, but usually 3–8 weeks. *Period of communicability:* 3–7 days before onset of symptoms and throughout disease course.	Classic signs of acute neurologic involvement include excitability, hydrophobia (spasms of muscles used for swallowing), delirium, and convulsions. Paralysis of the extremities and respiratory muscles occurs in some cases. The patient progresses to coma and respiratory failure. *Complications:* Usually results in death.	Treatment involves thoroughly washing bites with soap and water and irrigating with a virucidal agent such as povidone-iodine. Avoid suturing the wound (Heymann, 2008). Give human rabies immune globulin (HRIG) and human diploid cell rabies vaccine (HDCV) as soon as possible to persons bitten by animals that may be rabid. Half of the HRIG is infiltrated around the wound and half is given IM. HDCV is repeated on days 3, 7, 14, and 28 after the bite (five doses), but may be stopped if the animal is found free of rabies. If rabies symptoms develop, supportive care is provided. *Prognosis:* Usually results in death. *Prevention:* Immunize all domestic animals against rabies.	urgency for the vaccine and the need for a series of injections. • Educate parents about vaccine side effects—irritation at the injection site, itching, headache, muscle aches, nausea, and dizziness. • Participate in local education about rabies and safe interactions with dogs. See Chapter 31 ∞. • Teach children to avoid contact with all unknown animals, dead or alive. • If the child acquires rabies, he or she will be hospitalized. Institute contact and droplet precautions. • Make the child as comfortable as possible and provide emotional support to the family.
Rocky Mountain Spotted Fever (Tickborne Typhus Fever, Sao Paulo Typhus) *Causal agent: Rickettsia rickettsii.* *Epidemiology:* Occurs throughout the United States, but the highest incidence is in the Southeast, South Atlantic, and South Central states. Occurs between April and September. Infection induces immunity. *Transmission:* Transmitted by bites of dog and wood ticks, which need to be attached for 4–6 hours and feed on blood to transmit the organism. *Incubation period:* 2–14 days (mean 7 days) after the tick bite. *Period of communicability:* No person-to-person transmission.	Early symptoms are nonspecific with fever, malaise, headache, muscle aches, anorexia, nausea, vomiting, and diarrhea. An erythematous maculopapular rash occurs 3–5 days later that becomes petechial. The rash begins on the wrist and ankles and spreads to the palms and soles before becoming widely disseminated. The rash may be difficult to see in children with dark skin. Mental status changes, seizures, photophobia, transient deafness, and other focal neurologic problems may occur (Rim & Eppes, 2007). *Complications:* Death if untreated, disseminated intravascular coagulation (DIC), renal failure, pulmonary edema, and gangrene of the digits, ears, and scrotum (Rim & Eppes, 2007).	Diagnosed clinically. The indirect immunofluorescent antibody test is most accurate 7–10 days after symptom onset (Rim & Eppes, 2007). Treatment of choice is doxycycline regardless of patient age for 7–10 days. Hospitalization is often necessary for patients with severe disease. *Prognosis:* Children less than age 4 years have a mortality rate of 3–4% (Rim & Eppes, 2007). More severe disease may result in hearing loss, peripheral neuropathy, hemiparesis, gangrene, and bowel and bladder incontinence (Rim & Eppes, 2007). *Prevention:* Avoid areas that are heavily tick infested, and wear protective clothing. Check children for ticks and, if found, remove promptly.	• Use standard precautions when the child is hospitalized. • When the child is hospitalized, have hemodynamic monitoring equipment and emergency supplies readily available. • Administer antibiotics as prescribed. • Observe for purpura development and any abnormal bleeding. • Make the child as comfortable as possible. • Provide quiet diversion activities. • Provide emotional support, and keep parents informed about the child's condition. • Educate parents about prevention and appropriate technique for tick removal.

Rash of Rocky Mountain spotted fever.
Courtesy of Pfizer Central Research.
(1998). Groton, CT.

Clinical Manifestations

The child with a communicable disease has several symptoms. Fever is the most common sign. Other common signs and symptoms may include fatigue, weakness, reduced responsiveness, poor appetite, poor concentration, nausea and vomiting, diarrhea, headache, skin rash, and body aches. See the Clinical Manifestations table below for signs and symptoms of infection in infants and children by the system involved.

COLLABORATIVE CARE

Diagnostic Tests

Diagnostic tests include cultures from sites where the infection may potentially be located, such as the skin, pharynx, blood, urine, feces, and cerebrospinal fluid. See the *Clinical Skills Manual* for guidelines related to collection of specimens. Blood may be obtained for condition-specific immunoglobulin antibodies. In some cases, radiographs or special imaging may be used to identify localized infection in an organ such as the lungs.

Clinical Therapy

A fever can be a beneficial physiologic response, helping to slow the growth of organisms that thrive at lower body temperatures. A fever decreases the serum levels of zinc, iron, and copper needed by bacteria for reproduction. It helps to mobilize the immune response by increasing neutrophil production and enhancing phagocytosis (Huether, 2010). Fever is not inherently harmful until it reaches 41°C (105.9°F). For this reason, medical management may include postponing treatment of low-grade fevers under 38.9°C (102°F) in otherwise healthy children to promote the body's natural defenses against an infection.

Fevers are often treated, especially in children with pulmonary or cardiac disorders who may be unable to tolerate the higher metabolic rate and oxygen need. Fevers may also be treated if associated with discomfort. Acetaminophen and ibuprofen are the preferred antipyretics for children. Aspirin is no longer recommended for children because of its association with Reye syndrome. Antipyretics reduce fever by inhibiting prostaglandin synthesis, which results in lowering of the body's temperature set-point.

Administration of antibiotics may also be used for infectious diseases. Antibiotics have been responsible for decreases in morbidity and mortality from infections among children. However,

strains of bacteria have developed resistance to many antibiotics. Children with chronic illnesses such as cystic fibrosis, sickle cell disease, and acquired immunodeficiency syndrome (AIDS) are particularly susceptible to infection by drug-resistant pathogens. Many specialty organizations and medical centers are developing best practice guidelines for the use of antibiotics in treating common infections, such as acute otitis media.

Antiviral medications, such as acyclovir, may be ordered for certain types of viral infections, such as varicella (chickenpox), herpes simplex virus type 1 and 2, influenza, and others. If the child is immunocompromised, the antiviral medication needs to be provided very early in the infectious period to minimize the potentially life-threatening consequences of the infection.

Some infectious or communicable diseases must be reported to the state health department for disease surveillance and to determine the effectiveness of certain preventive measures such as vaccines. Cases can be reported on state-designated websites.

NURSING MANAGEMENT

Nursing Assessment and Diagnosis

Assess the child's hydration status and fluid intake, vital signs, and comfort level, and observe for seizures and for a **toxic appearance** (lethargy, poor perfusion, hypoventilation or hyperventilation, and cyanosis). The child with a fever may be irritable and restless, sleep fitfully, and have nonspecific muscular pain. Identify those children who may be at higher risk for a serious illness in association with a fever, in particular:

- Infants and children having a toxic appearance
- Neonates less than 28 days of age with a temperature over 38°C (100.4°F)

Clinical Manifestations
Infection in Infants and Children by Age Group

System	Infants	Children
Central nervous system	Irritability	Irritability or combativeness
	Decreased responsiveness	Stiff neck
	Lethargy	Back pain
	Bulging anterior fontanel	Decreased responsiveness
	High-pitched cry	Photophobia
	Muscle weakness	Brudzinski sign
	Additional Signs in Newborns:	Kernig sign
	Seizures	Malaise
	Subtle changes in muscle tone or hypotonia	

Clinical Manifestations

Infection in Infants and Children by Age Group (continued)

System	Infants	Children
Cardiovascular	Tachycardia Decreased perfusion Weak peripheral pulses Pallor or mottled skin Flushed, dry skin Delayed capillary refill time *Additional Signs in Newborns:* Cyanosis Hypotension Bradycardia	Tachycardia Decreased perfusion Weak peripheral pulses Pallor or flushed, dry skin Delayed capillary refill time
Respiratory	Tachypnea Increased work of breathing with retractions, nasal flaring Crackles Cough Stridor Decreased oxygen saturation Irregular breathing *Additional Signs in Newborns:* Apnea (new onset or increased episodes) Increased or new-onset oxygen requirement Grunting	Tachypnea Dyspnea Retractions Nasal flaring Crackles Cough Stridor Decreased oxygen saturation
Gastrointestinal	Vomiting Diarrhea Abdominal distention Poor feeding *Additional Signs in Newborns:* Abdominal wall discoloration Paralytic ileus Bloody stool Jaundice or hepatosplenomegaly	Nausea and vomiting Diarrhea Abdominal discomfort Abdominal distention Poor appetite
Renal	White blood cells (WBCs) and bacteria in urine *Additional Signs in Newborns:* Decreased urine output Hematuria, proteinuria	WBCs and bacteria in urine
Hematopoietic (see Appendix D ∞ for expected laboratory values by age)	Neutropenia Increased immature WBCs (bands) in bacterial infections Lymphocytosis in viral infections *Additional Signs in Newborns:* Band cells fraction greater than 0.2 Thrombocytopenia	Leukocytosis Increased immature WBCs (bands) in bacterial infections Lymphocytosis in viral infections
Metabolic	Hyperthermia or hypothermia Hypoglycemia or hyperglycemia	Hyperthermia Chills Hypothermia in septic shock
Other	Rash Dry mucous membranes Poor skin turgor Sunken anterior fontanel Petechiae and/or purpura	Rash Petechiae and/or purpura Dry mucous membranes Poor skin turgor

- Children less than 4 years of age with a temperature over 41°C (105.8°F)
- Children with conditions such as a ventriculoperitoneal shunt, congenital heart disease, asplenia, or sickle cell disease

Observe the child for other signs of infection, such as a rash, nausea and vomiting, or diarrhea, as well as generalized symptoms of a poor appetite, body aches, and malaise.

Examples of nursing diagnoses that may be appropriate for children with infectious and communicable diseases include:

- Hyperthermia related to infectious disease process
- Impaired Skin Integrity related to hyperthermia and self-mutilation of skin lesions
- Impaired Oral Mucous Membrane related to infectious disease process
- Deficient Fluid Volume related to repeated episodes of vomiting and diarrhea
- Ineffective Therapeutic Regimen Management (Family) related to complexity of care required by the child

Planning and Implementation

Most children with communicable diseases are cared for at home; however, children with infections may be evaluated in all health care settings. Nursing care includes assisting with the collection of cultures, treating infection, administering antibiotics on schedule, promoting the child's comfort, and educating parents. The nurse also monitors the child's response to therapy, staying alert for signs that the infection is worsening. Ensure that children have pain management for painful diagnostic procedures such as a lumbar puncture.

Prevent Disease Transmission

In the health care setting, isolate children with suspicious rashes, gastrointestinal infections, and respiratory infections from other children. All items with which the infected child comes into contact are considered contaminated (e.g., linens, toys, medical equipment). The fecal-oral and respiratory routes are the most common sources of infections in children. Use standard precautions and good hand hygiene. Wipe down hard surfaces in the examining room with an antiseptic solution before another child uses the room. If possible, wipe down toys in the waiting room daily with a nontoxic antiseptic solution. Dispose of linens in appropriately marked linen bags. Ensure that all health care professionals are fully immunized or that unimmunized or pregnant health care professionals are not exposed to children with certain infections (e.g., pertussis, rubella, or varicella). See page 394 for information to teach families about reducing the transmission of infection.

Children are often admitted to the hospital for treatment of severe infections. In addition, countless numbers of **nosocomial** (hospital-acquired) **infections** occur each year. Follow your facility's standard precautions and transmission-based precautions to reduce the spread of infectious diseases to staff and other patients. Bring any questions and concerns to your hospital's infection control nurse.

Managing Fevers

Nursing care for treatment of fever includes administering antipyretics, removing unnecessary clothing, and careful continued

Research *Fever*

The practice of alternating acetaminophen and ibuprofen in the care of children with fever has been the subject of two recent studies. These medications have different durations of action (4–6 hours for acetaminophen and 6–8 hours for ibuprofen) and many different preparations. Both studies reported that the children who received an alternating medication regimen achieved a lower temperature than with a single antipyretic. However, each study used a different interval and dosing strategy for the medications. One study only examined a single dose of ibuprofen followed by a single dose of acetaminophen 4 hours later among hospitalized children (Nabulsi, Tamim, Mahfoud, et al., 2006). The other study had parents alternating ibuprofen and acetaminophen every 4 hours in the home over 3 days (Sarrell, Wielunsky, & Cohen, 2006). A risk for overdosing the child exists if the administration schedule and dose are not strictly followed. The potentially synergistic effects of the two medications on the kidneys can cause renal tubular toxicity when used repeatedly for an illness (Miller, 2007). An important patient safety initiative to reduce the risk for overdosing is to encourage parents to use only one antipyretic with the correct dose and administration interval for fever management.

monitoring of temperature progression. Identify clear fluids the child prefers to drink, and encourage the intake of extra fluids.

Care in the Community

Teach parents to care for their child at home, including how and when to give antipyretics, over-the-counter medications, and antibiotics, if ordered; what foods and beverages are appropriate; and how to care for rashes and other topical symptoms. Provide guidelines about the types of fluids to encourage. Identify the antipyretic available in the home and provide the parents with guidelines for the correct dose.

Clinical Tip

Acetaminophen and ibuprofen preparations commonly available in the home are infant drops, liquid syrup, chewable tablets, and adult-strength tablets or capsules. Concentration in liquids and dosage in tablets vary by the type of preparation. The recommended dose of acetaminophen is 10–15 mg/kg/dose and of ibuprofen is 4–10 mg/kg/dose.

Acetaminophen	*Ibuprofen*
Infant drops—80 mg/0.8 mL using dropper in package	Infant drops—50 mg/1.25 mL, using package dropper
Children's liquid—160 mg/5 mL	Children's liquid—100 mg/5 mL
Chewable tablets—80 mg or 160 mg	Chewable and junior tablets—50 mg and 100 mg
Adult tablets or caplets—325 mg and 650 mg	Adult tablets or caplets—200 mg

Parents often fear a fever, believing it is a disease rather than a symptom of an illness. Provide information and reassurance. Help them to recognize signs of the child's worsening condition in association with the child's specific disease. See Families Want to Know: Evaluating and Treating Fever in Children.

Teach parents the importance of proper use of antibiotics when ordered. These guidelines will help reduce the development of antibiotic-resistant bacteria:

Families Want to Know

Evaluating and Treating Fever in Children

About Fevers

■ A fever is not a disease; it is the body's response to an infection. It means the child's body is using natural defenses to fight an infection.

■ If the child has a fever and does not look sick, it may be better to let the child use the body's natural defenses to fight off the virus or bacteria causing the fever, but follow guidelines about when to contact the child's health care provider.

Care for a Fever

■ Use a thermometer to check the child's temperature every 4–6 hours.

■ Use either acetaminophen or ibuprofen to lower a fever (do not use aspirin). Use the correct dose and preparation for the child's weight (drops are more concentrated than syrup). Do not alternate the medications.

■ Remove all but a light layer of the child's clothing.

■ Monitor the child's behavior and response to fever medication. The fever medication will reduce the child's temperature. The temperature may rise again 4 hours after giving acetaminophen or 6 hours after ibuprofen. Check the temperature and give another dose of fever medicine. Do not give more than the number of doses per day recommended on the bottle. The temperature may not return to normal until the child is recovering from the illness.

■ If sponging the child, give fever medication first, and then use tepid water to sponge the child (do not use alcohol). Cool water may increase shivering and discomfort.

Call Your Health Care Provider Immediately if Any of the Following Occur:

■ The infant is under 2 months old and has a fever over 38.0°C (100.4°F).

■ The child has a fever over 40.1°C (104.2°F) and any of the following symptoms are present:

• The child is crying inconsolably or whimpering. The child cries when moved or otherwise touched by the parent or other family members.

• The child is difficult to awaken.

• The child's neck is stiff.

• There are purple spots present on the skin.

• Breathing is difficult and no better after the nose is cleared.

• The child is drooling saliva and is unable to swallow anything.

• The child has a convulsion or seizure.

• The child acts or looks very sick.

Call Your Health Care Provider Within 24 Hours If:

■ The child is 2–4 months old (unless fever occurs within 48 hours of a DTaP shot and the infant has no other serious symptoms).

■ The fever is higher than 40.1°C (104.2°F) (especially if the child is under 3 years old).

■ The child complains of burning or pain with urination.

■ The fever has been present for more than 24 hours without an obvious cause or location of infection.

■ The fever went away for more than 24 hours and then returned.

• Give all the antibiotic dosages as prescribed for the full number of days ordered. Spread the doses around the clock to keep blood levels constant, as much as possible. This will help ensure that the bacteria causing the infection are erad-

icated, rather than having some bacteria left alive to mutate and resist the antibiotic in the future.

• Make sure parents know to give the antibiotic with food or without food to promote optimal absorption.

• Discard the antibiotic when all the doses have been given. Antibiotics have an expiration date and lose potency after that date.

• Do not share the antibiotic with any other family member. There will not be enough antibiotic to fully treat the infection in two people.

Educate parents about methods to reduce disease transmission in the home such as good hand hygiene. Encourage parents to limit the exposure of elderly family members, infants, and visitors to the ill child. Make sure that the ill child's dishes and utensils are washed in hot soapy water or sanitized in a dishwasher. Place dressings with drainage in a plastic bag for disposal to prevent contact by other family members.

Encourage children to rest. Provide quiet diversional activities such as board games, DVDs, and music. Promote fluid intake and provide foods that the child prefers and do not cause discomfort. Reduce itching of rashes with lukewarm baths with Aveeno or oatmeal and topical lotions. Keep hands clean and nails trimmed. Cover hands with clean socks or mittens if scratching cannot be controlled.

Evaluation

Expected outcomes of nursing care include the following:

• Opportunities for spread of infection are minimized between patients and family members.

• The child's fever is effectively managed with antipyretics.

• The full treatment with antibiotics, if ordered, is completed.

■ SEPSIS AND SEPTIC SHOCK

Sepsis is a systemic inflammatory response to infection, such as bacteria invading the bloodstream. Infants in the perinatal period and first year of life are at a high risk for developing sepsis, especially those with low birth weight and those who have several invasive procedures performed. Older infants and children who develop sepsis often have a chronic condition, burns, invasive catheters, compromised immune system, and long-term antibiotics (Hazinski, Mondozzi, & Baker, 2010).

Epidemiology and Pathophysiology

Common microorganisms associated with sepsis include group B streptococcus, *Escherichia coli, Haemophilus influenzae,* and staphylococcus. Newborns have inadequately developed inflammatory and immune system responses, so the microorganisms can rapidly invade, spread, and multiply (see Chapter 22 ∞). Mediators along with procoagulation factors initiate inflammation and coagulation, and inhibit fibrinolysis. White blood cells multiply throughout the body and macrophages produce cytokines, which dilate the blood vessels and increase permeability. Fibrin deposits impede blood flow. Congestion occurs in some tissue beds, reducing the delivery of oxygen and nutrients to the cells, and bacteria may be trapped and multiply unchecked. Interstitial edema and hypovolemia may be followed by multiple organ dysfunction and failure (Moloney-Harmon, 2005). Severe sepsis that progresses to septic shock is a significant health problem with an estimated in-hospital mortality rate of up to 10% (Czaja, Zimmerman, & Nathans, 2009).

Clinical Manifestations

Symptoms of sepsis in newborns are often nonspecific, such as feeding problems; subtle changes in color, tone, and activity; abdominal distention; and vomiting or diarrhea. Newborns often have hypothermia rather than a fever. Nonspecific respiratory distress or apnea may be noted, especially if group B streptococcus is the causative organism. See the Clinical Manifestations table on page 422 for signs of infection in newborns by body system. Early signs of sepsis in children include fever or hypothermia, tachycardia, and tachypnea.

As septic shock begins the child may initially have a fever, tachycardia, tachypnea, warm extremities, bounding pulses, brisk capillary refill, and normal urine output. Responsiveness may be altered. As septic shock progresses, hypotension, prolonged capillary refill time, mottled cool extremities, weak pulses, progressive mental status changes, and decreasing urine output are seen. Fever or hypothermia may be seen. Shock may progress to cardiac arrest if interventions are unsuccessful.

COLLABORATIVE CARE

The site of infection may not be apparent, so cultures of the blood, urine, cerebrospinal fluid, and skin lesions are obtained. Radiographs of the lungs and other potential sites may reveal signs of infection. Blood is obtained for a complete blood count and white blood cell differential. A high white cell count with low neutrophil and high band (immature white blood cell) counts indicate the presence of an infection. C-reactive protein may be elevated.

Clinical therapy focuses on preserving vital organ function with oxygen, aggressive IV fluid resuscitation, and vasopressor medications to manage vasodilation and improve renal perfusion. Laboratory tests (glucose, electrolytes, acid-base balance) are monitored to identify any significant changes needing management. Antibiotics are initiated immediately and changed if necessary to target the specific microorganism causing the infection, once the culture and sensitivities are known. Enteral or parenteral nutritional support may be initiated early.

NURSING MANAGEMENT

Nursing care of the infant or child with sepsis occurs in the neonatal intensive care unit (NICU) or pediatric intensive care unit (PICU). Assess and monitor the vital signs and temperature of infants and children with sepsis. Monitor perfusion, intake and output, and weight. Note any petechiae or purpura that could indicate the development of disseminated intravascular coagulation. Check for perfusion using capillary refill time and temperature of the extremities. Observe for signs that the condition is worsening or resolving.

Attach a cardiorespiratory monitor to detect episodes of apnea in the neonate or bradycardia in the older infant and child. Ensure that the child's airway is maintained and oxygen and ventilatory support are provided as prescribed.

Administer antibiotics and other medications as prescribed. Monitor for side effects of antibiotics, especially when they may cause renal or other organ system damage. Carefully manage the IV fluids to ensure that the infant or child receives the volume needed to maintain perfusion.

See Chapter 13 ∞ for guidelines to support parents when their child has a life-threatening condition. Encourage the parents to participate in the newborn's care as much as possible.

Maintain a high level of suspicion for the development of sepsis in high-risk newborns. Monitor the newborn's condition for signs and symptoms of infection and sepsis, especially high-risk newborns that have invasive procedures performed or are treated with various types of technology. Adhere to hand hygiene guidelines and use aseptic technique for all procedures to reduce the risk for sepsis.

Expected outcomes of nursing care include early recognition of an infant with sepsis, medications administered as prescribed, and effective monitoring to detect changes in the child's condition that require intensive care.

■ EMERGING INFECTION CONTROL THREATS

Public health officials are continuously monitoring the incidence and patterns of infections (disease surveillance) to identify emerging infections, such as *pandemic flu*, a worldwide influenza epidemic. See Table 16–3 for influenza information. Also being monitored are signs of disease related to potential weapons of terrorists such as anthrax, smallpox, plague, botulism, hemorrhagic fever, or tularemia. See Clinical Manifestations: Potential Biological Terrorism Agents. Early recognition of all emerging infections is important so that public health measures to reduce disease transmission and to prepare the mass casualty response are initiated (see Chapter 10 ∞ for further information).

Nursing Management

Nurses have responsibility for maintaining a high level of suspicion when numerous individuals with similar signs and symptoms are present in school or seek care in any health care facility. Initiating infection control measures such as airborne and contact precautions may help reduce the transmission of infection. Instituting isolation before a definitive diagnosis is made is an appropriate nursing action when the level of suspicion is high. Assess children and provide supportive nursing care for the identified infection. Nurses should regularly review guidelines posted by the Centers for Disease Control and Prevention for the management of specific health threats. See the companion website for weblinks to bioterrorism and emerging infections.

Bioterrorism and Emerging Infection Control Threat Websites

Clinical Manifestations
Potential Biological Terrorism Agents

Organisms	Clinical Manifestations	Clinical Therapy
Anthrax *Causal agent: Bacillus anthracis* Cutaneous anthrax. *Courtesy of Centers for Disease Control and Prevention, Atlanta, GA.*	▪ *Cutaneous*—papule that progresses to a vesicle and then to a skin ulcer with a depressed black scab area in the center. Not painful. Child may have fever, malaise, headache, and regional lymphadenopathy. ▪ *Gastrointestinal*—nausea, loss of appetite, bloody diarrhea, hematemesis, fever, stomach pain, and severe abdominal pain followed by fever and septicemia. ▪ *Inhalation*—brief respiratory prodrome with a sore throat, mild fever, malaise, and muscle aches followed by development of dyspnea, cough, chest pain, shortness of breath, and systemic symptoms. Shock, pleural effusion, and meningitis may develop and death may occur without treatment.	▪ IV ciprofloxacin or doxycycline for patients over 12 years. For children under 12 years, IV ciprofloxacin plus clindamycin. ▪ For postexposure prophylaxis: vaccine approved for those over age 18 years (three doses at 0, 2, and 4 weeks) or oral ciprofloxacin or doxycycline for 60 days (Moran, Talan, & Abrahamian, 2008).
Botulism *Causal agent: Clostridium botulinum*	▪ Begins with cranial nerve palsies, often beginning with ptosis, diplopia, blurred vision, and sluggishly reactive pupils. Progressive descending paralysis with speech and swallowing, loss of gag reflex and then symmetric descending flaccid paralysis. Confusion may be present. ▪ May be preceded by abdominal cramps, nausea, vomiting, or diarrhea.	▪ Slow IV infusion of equine antitoxin diluted in normal saline may halt progression of symptoms, but paralysis will not be reversed. ▪ Epinephrine and diphenhydramine for serum sickness or urticaria.
Hemorrhagic Fever *Causal agent: Ebola or Marburg virus*	▪ Abrupt onset of fever, myalgia, headache, nausea, vomiting, abdominal pain, photophobia, diarrhea, chest pain, cough, and pharyngitis. ▪ Maculopapular rash prominent on trunk soon after fever; petechiae, ecchymosis, subconjunctival hemorrhages; shock and circulatory collapse in short period.	▪ Fluid resuscitation to manage hypotension and shock, then maintain fluid and electrolyte balance. ▪ Blood, platelets, and plasma administration for severe hemorrhage. ▪ Ribavirin, but the U.S. Food and Drug Administration has not approved it for this purpose.
Pneumonic Plague *Causal agent: Yersinia pestis*	▪ Severe respiratory illness with high fever, chills, headache, cough, and breathing difficulty. Rapidly developing pneumonia, bloody or watery sputum. May lead to respiratory failure and shock. ▪ May have gastrointestinal symptoms, such as nausea, vomiting, diarrhea, and abdominal pain.	▪ Gentamicin IV or streptomycin IM. Alternate antibiotics include IV doxycycline, ciprofloxacin, or chloramphenicol. ▪ Prophylaxis with doxycycline or quinolone for 6 days.
Smallpox *Causal agent: Variola major virus* Smallpox. *Courtesy of Centers for Disease Control and Prevention, Atlanta, GA.*	▪ Prodrome 2–4 days before rash: abrupt onset with fever (38.3°C [101°F] or higher), malaise, headache, muscle pain, nausea and vomiting, and backache. ▪ Rash begins as red spots in the mouth and on the tongue that develop sores and break open. Then a few macules appear on the forehead, face, and extremities, spreading to become a generalized rash. Macules progress to papules, to tense vesicles, to tense deep pustules with an umbilicated appearance, all in the same stage of development. The temperature usually falls and the patient feels better. The pustules form scabs by the end of the second week, and the scabs fall off after 3–4 weeks.	▪ Supportive care. ▪ Antibiotics for secondary infection. ▪ Vaccine can be effective if given within first few days after exposure.

(continued)

Clinical Manifestations

Potential Biological Terrorism Agents (continued)

Organisms	Clinical Manifestations	Clinical Therapy
Tularemia *Causal agent: Francisella tularensis*	■ Fever, fatigue, chills, headache, malaise, and body aches. ■ Cough, substernal pain, dyspnea, and chest pain. ■ May develop hemorrhagic inflammation of airways that progresses to bronchopneumonia, pleuritis, and hilar lymphadenopathy. ■ May also have pharyngitis, bronchiolitis, and pneumonia with systemic symptoms.	■ Supportive care. ■ Gentamicin IV or streptomycin IM. ■ Alternate antibiotics include IV doxycycline, ciprofloxacin, or chloramphenicol. ■ Prophylaxis with doxycycline or ciprofloxacin.

Data from: Markenson, D. (2005). The treatment of children exposed to pathogens linked to bioterrorism. Infectious Disease Clinics of North America, 19, 731–745; Moran, G. J., Talan, D. A., & Abrahamian, F. M. (2008). Biologic terrorism. Infectious Disease Clinics of North America, 22, 145–187; Centers for Disease Control and Prevention. (2009). Bioterrorism case definitions. Retrieved from http://emergency.cdc.gov/bioterrorism/casedef.asp

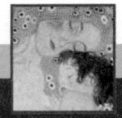

Chapter Highlights

■ Reducing the number of preventable childhood illnesses is a major national public health goal.

■ A communicable disease is an illness caused by microorganisms that are commonly communicated from one host (animal or human) to another.

■ Newborns and infants are especially vulnerable to infectious diseases because their immune systems are immature, their passively acquired maternal antibodies provide limited protection, and disease protection through immunization is not yet complete.

■ For a child to acquire a communicable disease, the following need to be present: an infectious agent or pathogen, an effective means of transmission, and a susceptible host.

■ Infection control measures caregivers can take include the following: performing good hand hygiene with soap and water or alcohol-based gels, disinfecting hard surfaces touched by the child or the child's body fluids, disinfecting toys, and making sure all children are fully immunized.

■ The average infant born in 2009 will receive immunizations for 14 childhood diseases by 6 years of age.

■ The Vaccines for Children program provides free immunizations for low-income children to ensure that finances are not a barrier to full immunization of those children.

■ When parents resist immunizations for religious or philosophical reasons, the nurse should provide them with accurate information and help them understand that their child may be at a significant risk for an infection with potential serious consequences if not immunized.

■ The potency of vaccines must be protected with storage in the refrigerator or freezer at the appropriate temperature.

■ The National Vaccine Injury Acts of 1986 and 1993 provide compensation if a link between immunization and a serious adverse effect is found. The Vaccine Adverse Event Reporting System has been established to track serious vaccine reactions.

■ Immunization information is updated frequently. It is the nurse's responsibility to regularly obtain current information about vaccines, the immunization schedule, and important information to share with parents and adolescents.

■ Infectious and communicable diseases are caused by bacterial, viral, protozoan, or fungal organisms.

■ Fever is often a sign of infectious disease in children. When pathogens invade the body, endogenous pyrogens travel to the hypothalamus, where they trigger the production and release of prostaglandins, which initiate the fever response.

■ The child with a toxic or septic appearance has the following signs: lethargy, poor perfusion, tachypnea or bradypnea, and pallor or cyanosis.

■ The appropriate use and administration of antibiotics to help reduce the development of antibiotic-resistant bacteria includes the following: Give antibiotic dosages as prescribed for the full number of days ordered, do not share with other family members who might be ill, and discard when all doses have been given.

■ Sepsis is a systemic response to infection that has a high mortality rate.

■ The public health system is conducting disease surveillance to detect the emergence of rare infections, an epidemic, or the presence of infectious disease potentially caused by terrorists.

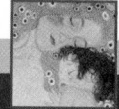

Clinical Reasoning in Action

Recall 4-month-old Kendra and her parents from the opening scenario, who came to the health center for Kendra's immunizations and health assessment. Kendra's growth and development are occurring as anticipated. Kendra has previously received the following vaccines: two doses of HepB, and one dose each of DTaP, IPV, Hib, RV, and PCV.

1. Which vaccines should Kendra receive today? When should she return for the next needed vaccines?
2. What are the nurse's responsibilities before giving Kendra her needed vaccines?
3. What are some potential methods to reduce the pain associated with immunizations?
4. What preparation should the health center have in case Kendra has a serious allergic reaction to a given vaccine?
5. What patient education should be given to Kendra's parents about the expected reactions to the given vaccines?

See Pearson Nursing Student Resources for possible responses.

Pearson Nursing Student Resources

Find additional review materials at **nursing.pearsonhighered.com**

Prepare for success with NCLEX®-style practice questions, interactive assignments and activities, web links, animations and videos, and more!

References

Aiello, A. E., Coulborn, R. M., Perez, V., & Larson, E. L. (2008). Effect of hand hygiene on infectious disease risk in the community health setting: A meta-analysis. *American Journal of Public Health, 98*(8), 1372–1381.

American Academy of Pediatrics (AAP), Committee on Infectious Disease. (2009). *Red book: 2009 Report of the Committee on Infectious Disease* (28th ed.). Elk Grove Village, IL: Author.

Benin, A. L., Wisler-Scher, D. J., Colson, E., Shapiro, E. D., & Holmboe, E. S. (2006). Qualitative analysis of mothers' decision-making about vaccines for infants: The importance of trust. *Pediatrics, 117*(5), 1532–1541.

Centers for Disease Control and Prevention (CDC). (2006). Brief report: Updated mumps activity—United States, January 1–October 7, 2006. *Morbidity and Mortality Weekly Report, 55*(42), 1152–1153.

Centers for Disease Control and Prevention (CDC). (2008a). National, state, and local area vaccination coverage among children aged 19–35 months—United States, 2007. *Morbidity and Mortality Weekly Report, 57*(35), 961–966.

Centers for Disease Control and Prevention (CDC). (2008b). Syncope after vaccination—United States, January 2005–July 2007. *Morbidity and Mortality Weekly Report, 57*(17), 457–460.

Centers for Disease Control and Prevention (CDC). (2008c). Vaccination coverage among adolescents aged 13–17 years—United States, 2007. *Morbidity and Mortality Weekly Report, 57*(40), 1100–1103.

Centers for Disease Control and Prevention (CDC). (2008d). Update: Measles—United States, January–July 2008. *Morbidity and Mortality Weekly Report, 57*(33), 893–896.

Centers for Disease Control and Prevention (CDC). (2008e). Updated recommendations for isolation of persons with mumps. *Morbidity and Mortality Weekly Report, 57*(40), 1103–1105.

Centers for Disease Control and Prevention (CDC). (2009). *Vaccines for children program.* Retrieved from http://www.cdc.gov/vaccines/programs/vfc/default.htm

Children's Hospital of Philadelphia. (2008). *Vaccine education center.* Retrieved from http://www.chop.edu/service/vaccine-education-center/

Czaja, A. S., Zimmerman, J. J., & Nathans, A. B. (2009). Readmission and late mortality after pediatric severe sepsis. *Pediatrics, 123*(3), 849–857.

Edwards, K. M., & Johnson, D. R. (2007). Rising to the challenge of pertussis persistence. *Clinical Advisor, 10*(6), 58–77.

Grijalva, C. G., Griffin, M. R., Nuorti, J. P., & Walter, N. D. (2009). Pneumonia hospitalizations among young children before and after introduction of pneumococcal conjugate vaccine—United States, 1997–2006. *Morbidity and Mortality Weekly Report, 58*(01), 1–4.

Hall, M., Noble, A., & Smith, S. (2009). *A foundation for neonatal care: A multi-disciplinary guide.* New York: Radcliff Publishing.

Hazinski, M. F., Mondozzi, M. A., & Baker, R. A. U. (2010). Shock, multiple organ dysfunction syndrome and burns in children. In K. L. McCance, S. E. Huether, V. L. Brashers, & N. S. Rote, *Pathophysiology: The biologic basis for disease in adults and children* (6th ed., pp. 1727–1754). St. Louis, MO: Elsevier Mosby.

Heymann, D. L. (Ed.). (2008). *Control of communicable diseases manual* (19th ed.). Washington, DC: American Public Health Association Press.

Hornig, M., Briese, T., Buie, T., Bauman, M. L., Lauwers, G., Siemetzki, U., et al. (2008). Lack of association between measles virus vaccine and autism with enteropathy: A case-control study. *PLoS One, 3*(9), e3140–3147.

Huether, S. E. (2010). Pain, temperature regulation, sleep, and sensory function. In K. L. McCance, S. E. Huether, V. L. Brashers, & N. S. Rote, *Pathophysiology: The biologic basis for disease in adults and children* (6th ed., pp. 481–524). St. Louis, MO: Elsevier Mosby.

Immunization Action Coalition. (2009). *Screening questionnaire for child and teen immunization.* Retrieved from http://www.immunize.org/catg .d/p4060.pdf

Joyce, C. (2007). Steps to success: Getting children vaccinated on time. *Pediatric Nursing, 33*(6), 491–496.

Kest, H. E., & Pineda, C. (2008). Lyme disease: Prevention, diagnosis, and management. *Contemporary Pediatrics, 25*(6), 56–64.

Lee, G. M., Santoli, J. M., Hannan, C., Messonnier, M. L., Sabin, J. E., Rusinak, D., et al. (2007). Gaps in vaccine financing for underinsured children in the United States. *Journal of the American Medical Association, 298*(6), 638–643.

Markenson, D. (2005). The treatment of children exposed to pathogens linked to bioterrorism. *Infectious Diseases of North America, 19,* 731–745.

Miller, A. A. (2007). Alternating acetaminophen with ibuprofen for fever: Is this a problem? *Pediatric Annals, 36*(7), 384–388.

Mola, S. J., Nield, L. S., & Weisse, M. E. (2009). Meningococcal disease: Suspect it, treat it, prevent it. *Consultant for Pediatricians, 8*(4), 116–120.

Moloney-Harmon, P. A. (2005). Pediatric sepsis: The infection unto death. *Critical Care Nursing Clinics of North America, 17,* 417–429.

Moran, G. J., Talan, D. A., & Abrahamian, F. M. (2008). Biologic terrorism. *Infectious Disease Clinics of North America, 22,* 145–187.

Nabulsi, M. M., Tamim, H., Mahfoud, Z., Itani, M., Sabra, R., et al. (2006). Alternating ibuprofen and acetaminophen in the treatment of febrile children: A pilot study. *BMC Medicine, 4*(4). Retrieved from http://www.biomedcentral.com/ 1741-7015/4/4

Nield, L. S., & Kamat, D. M. (2006). Vaccine refusal: When parents just say "no." *Consultant for Pediatrics, 5*(10), S5–S8.

Omer, S. B., Enger, K. S., Moulton, L. H., Halsey, N. A., Stokley, S., & Salmon, D. A. (2008). Geographic clustering of nonmedical exemptions to school immunization requirements and associations with geographic clustering of pertussis. *American Journal of Epidemiology, 168,* 1389–1396.

Omer, S. B., Salmon, D. A., Orenstein, W. A., deHart, M. P., & Halsey, N. (2009). Vaccine refusal, mandatory immunizations, and the risks of vaccine-preventable diseases. *New England Journal of Medicine, 360*(19), 1981–1988.

Rim, J. Y., & Eppes, S. (2007). Tick-borne diseases. *Pediatric Annals, 36*(7), 390–403.

Sarrell, E. M., Wielunsky, E., & Cohen, H. A. (2006). Antipyretic treatment in young children with fever: Acetaminophen, ibuprofen, or both alternating in a randomized, double-blind study. *Archives of Pediatric and Adolescent Medicine, 160*(2), 197–202.

Schechter, R., & Grether, J. K. (2008). California data do not support a link between thimerosal in vaccines and autism. *Archives of General Psychiatry, 65,* 19–24.

Thomas, T. L. (2008). The new human papillomavirus (HPV) vaccine: Pros and cons for pediatric and adolescent health. *Pediatric Nursing, 34*(5), 429–431.

Tousman, S., Arnold, D., Helland, W., Roth, R., Heshelman, N., Castaneda, O., et al. (2007). Evaluation of a hand washing program for 2nd-graders. *Journal of School Nursing, 23*(6), 342–348.

U.S. Department of Health and Human Services, Health Resources and Services Administration. (2008). *National Vaccine Injury Compensation Program.* Washington, DC: Author. Retrieved from http://www.hrsa.gov/vaccinecompensation/ table.htm

U.S. Department of Health and Human Services, Office of Disease Prevention and Health Promotion. (2010). *Healthy People.* Washington, DC: Author. Retrieved from http://www.healthypeople .gov/Default.htm

Veraas, K. (2006). Nursing and other medical staff issues in vaccine administration. *Pediatric Annals, 35*(7), 519–521.

World Health Organization. (2009). *World Health Organization guidelines on hand hygiene in health care* (p. 151). Geneva, Switzerland: Author. Retrieved from http://whqlibdoc.who.int/ publications/2009/9789241597906_eng.pdf

Zomorrodi, A., & Attia, M. W. (2008). Fever: Parental concerns. *Clinical Pediatric Emergency Medicine, 9,* 238–243.

Assessment and Management of Social and Environmental Influences

chapter 17

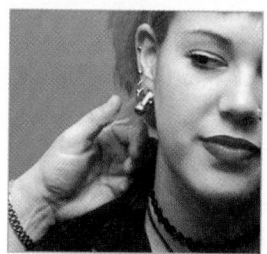

Amy is 15 years old and attends an alternative high school. She recently had an ear piercing that has become painful. She visits the school nurse to get advice. Upon examination, the nurse notices the area around the piercing is inflamed and mildly edematous. The nurse learns that Amy's ear was pierced by a friend, using a needle that had been "sterilized" by passing it through a match flame. Amy has had a slight fever, but otherwise feels fine.

Because her state requires adolescents under 18 years of age to have a parent's signature for body piercings and tattoos, Amy asked a friend to pierce her ears. Her friend has done many ear piercings on others, so Amy thought it was safe. She admits that her parents are not pleased with her body art, but they permit her to do it as long as she stays in high school. She previously had run away and spent several weeks living on the streets.

What health care and social needs does Amy have? How can you support both her and her parents? What signs of resilience does Amy show? This chapter examines the complex social contexts in which children live, learn, and grow, and explores the role of nurses in supporting them to reach their potentials. The challenges of providing comprehensive health care for all children and adolescents, no matter their lifestyles, are discussed.

Key Terms

branding / 448
bullying / 450
chelation / 463
child sexual abuse / 456
cyberbullying / 451
culture shock / 438
cutting / 448
emotional abuse / 456
emotional neglect / 456
hazing / 451
homosexuality / 448
incest / 457
LGBQ / 448
LGBT / 448
physical abuse / 456
physical neglect / 456
toxicants / 462
toxins / 462
violence / 449

Learning Outcomes

After reading this chapter, you will be able to do the following:

1. Identify major social and environmental factors that influence the health of children and adolescents.
2. List external influences that can affect child and adolescent health.
3. Apply the ecologic model and resilience theory to assessment of the social and environmental factors in children's lives.
4. Examine the effects of substance use, physical activity, and other lifestyle patterns on health.
5. Evaluate the environment for hazards to children, such as exposure to substances and potential for poisoning.
6. Develop the nursing role in prevention and treatment of child abuse and neglect, and other forms of violence.
7. Plan nursing interventions for children related to social and environmental situations.

Many of the major causes of mortality and morbidity in children are closely linked with social influences in the child's world. The social contexts for young children growing up today are different from those of even a decade ago. Examining the social contexts in which children live and grow can provide insights into the behavior and health of children and adults, and present opportunities for nursing interventions. All nurses must examine the social influences and apply the knowledge gained to plan health care that will benefit youth as they grow into adulthood.

Children and adolescents are also influenced by their environments. The physical setting, exposure to chemical agents, and other environmental factors are increasingly identified as instrumental in determining health. Nurses assess the environment for its risk and protective factors, and then use this information to plan nursing care appropriate to enhance the health status of children and adolescents.

What are the challenges of today's society that children must often face at a very young age? How can nurses help children to face these challenges and to emerge as healthy and contributing members of society? What roles do nurses play in identifying and applying the protective factors and in minimizing the risk factors of youth? This chapter will help you to examine and apply these social and environmental concepts in a variety of nursing settings.

Examine again the major causes of death for children from 1 year of age through adolescence that are presented in Chapter 1 ∞ (see Figures 1–6A and 1–6B). Did you notice that most morbidity is related to preventable causes linked to present-day lifestyles? Car crashes, fires, drownings, and homicides are a few examples of common causes of death in children.

Now examine the major reasons for hospitalization (see Figure 1–7 ∞). By the time children are 5 years of age, injuries rank as the second cause, and by 10 years, mental disorders and injuries are among the major causes of hospitalization. By the teen years, pregnancy and mental disorders are the most common admitting diagnoses to hospitals. These conditions are related, at least in part, to the environmental settings in which we live. These settings and their influences must be examined to understand how to best intervene with children.

THEORETICAL CONCEPTS

In this chapter, two main theories are used to provide a framework in which to examine societal influences on children: the ecologic model and the theory of resilience. Both of these theoretical approaches were discussed in Chapter 4 ∞, and should be reviewed now (see Figure 4–4 and Tables 4–4 and 4–6).

The *ecologic theory* views the child and the environment as interacting forces, with children influencing systems around them, even while they are influenced by these systems (Bronfenbrenner, 2005). Systems providing daily contact are microsystems, but other systems influencing the child such as parental work and political or cultural environments are also important. Understanding these systems, or the forces in which children function, can provide information that guides care providers. For example, if the parents' employment agencies do not provide health care insurance, their children may not obtain necessary health care such as immunizations, treatment for diseases, and growth monitoring.

Resilience theory examines risk and protective factors in the child's environment because they influence the child's adaptation to stressful events and can often be modified to lead to more productive and healthy outcomes. Families may have protective factors that provide strength and assistance in dealing with crises, and risk factors that promote or contribute to health care challenges. Risk and protective factors can be identified in children, in their families, and in their communities. The combination and interplay of these factors contribute to health status and determine adaptation to a crisis. If a young child is hospitalized for treatment of an acute infectious illness, protective factors might include the ability of one parent to stay with the child at all times, the ability of a grandmother to care for siblings at home, and the child's ability to adapt to new situations and communicate readily with staff members. On the other hand, risk factors might include lack of comprehensive health insurance to pay for the hospitalization, lack of an identified health care "home" (consistent care provider) for the child, and incomplete immunizations. The concepts of resiliency theory can be applied to Amy's family as described in the opening scenario. She experienced disruption in family stability. The risk and protective factors interacted with her personality in ways that resulted in her desire to appear as an independent person, establishing her identity through body art, and finally, a desire to return to school.

Theoretical frameworks are useful when examining social and environmental influences on children because they guide us to assess for certain factors that can be altered. They suggest data to collect and pertinent nursing interventions. They also help foster partnerships with other care providers who use these and similar theories to plan social, psychological, and environmental care for children and their families. Nursing strategies can target risk factors, such as encouraging family behaviors to ensure gun safety by teaching the benefits of gun locks and locked gun cabinets in homes with firearms. In addition, protective factors can be emphasized, such as suggesting regular exercise to help maintain normal weight and cardiovascular function.

Research *Add Health Study*

The National Longitudinal Study of Adolescent Health (called Add Health) was conducted with over 100,000 adolescents and found that parent–family connectedness, school connectedness, a belief in a higher being, and academic success were predictive of youth having the lowest health risks. Interviews are presently being carried out with the participants who are now young adults; the resulting longitudinal data will show what characteristics and influences persist into adult life (Add Health Study, 2007). Nurses can assist adolescents and their families in establishing a sense of attachment to each other. Encourage families to include adolescents in activities, attend their sports and other school events, have meals together regularly, and attend faith-based activities or other community events as a family.

The National Longitudinal Study of Adolescent Health Website

SOCIAL INFLUENCES ON CHILD HEALTH

Poverty

An important risk factor that influences children's health is poverty. Conversely, basic financial stability is a protective factor that contributes to the general health and well-being of children. An estimated 18% of children are poor (Federal Interagency Forum on Child and Family Statistics, 2009). That means they are in a family earning less than $18,310 annually for a family of three persons or less than $22,050 for a family of four. Young children, or those under 5 years of age, are most likely to be poor (Inglehart, 2007; Federal Interagency Forum on Child and Family Statistics, 2009).

Children who are poor are more likely to have unmet health needs, to have difficulty in school, to become teen parents, and to experience multiple health problems, including stunted growth and lead poisoning. Inadequate and unsafe housing, food insecurity, and poor dietary quality are more common (Federal Interagency Forum on Child and Family Statistics, 2009). See Table 17–1 for a list of common health problems among children who are poor and some suggested nursing actions.

Poverty leads to homelessness for some children. Children comprise 25% of the homeless population, and families represent 39%. Families with children are the fastest growing group of homeless people. Each year, from 0.9 to 1.6 million children

TABLE 17–1	Common Health Problems and Nursing Management of Children Who Experience Poverty or Homelessness
Common Health Problems	Nursing Management
Lack of immunizations	Check immunization records. Provide immunizations at schools and in homeless shelters.
Common infectious diseases	Facilitate free clinics in shelters, schools, and community settings. Teach hygiene measures. Provide resources for disease management. Arrange for medications when needed. Provide information about resources for bathing and hygiene.
Sleep deficits	Inform parents about respite facilities. Arrange for children to have quiet sleep time in school if possible.
Vision and hearing deficits	Perform screening for deficits. Provide resources for eyeglasses, hearing aids, and care for ear infections (e.g., service organizations such as Lions Clubs).
Nutritional deficits	Perform height and weight checks and nutritional assessment. Evaluate the family for food security (see Chapter 14 ∞). Be sure the child is registered for school breakfast and lunch programs if available. Ensure that children are linked to summer food programs at the end of an academic year. Link to the Women, Infants, and Children (WIC) Nutrition Program. Inform about resources for meals and field gleaning in the community.
Dental care problems	Teach oral hygiene. Provide toothbrushes and toothpaste. Provide bottled water for use if the child lives in a car or on the street. Perform oral assessment. Refer to dental programs for people with low incomes.
Injuries	Teach basic safety precautions. Visit the living situation if possible to assess for safety hazards. Teach "street safe" skills. Provide helmets, car seats, or other gear needed.
Adolescent pregnancy and sexually transmitted diseases	Provide sexuality teaching. Inform about access to family planning services. Assess for child abuse and prostitution.
Mental illness	Assess for depression. Evaluate for suicide potential. Provide links to services. Plan programs to foster self-esteem. Arrange for a Big Brother or Big Sister. Refer to extracurricular activities in the school and community. Arrange for a school bus stop away from a shelter so other students do not stigmatize the homeless child.

experience homelessness (National Center on Family Homelessness, 2009). The reasons for homelessness are also common risks for a number of the other challenges to health discussed in this chapter, including poor finances, abuse or other violence, and mental instability.

Children who experience homelessness frequently have multiple physical and mental health problems, and lack health insurance to provide care for these problems. Some of the common problems faced by homeless children and families include trauma, substance use, respiratory and skin infections, tuberculosis and HIV, and nutritional disorders. Children may have developmental delays, learning problems, or growth disruptions (National Center on Family Homelessness, 2009). Teens who have been homeless are more likely to engage in other risky behavior, such as unprotected sex with multiple partners and substance use. They are more likely to need emergency care, to be depressed or have other mental illness, and to become pregnant than other teens (Kidd & Davidson, 2006).

Health problems related to homelessness and other family characteristics continue even after finding a place to live. Once families leave homeless shelters, children may become separated from their mothers due to lack of access to resources and inability of parents to provide adequate homes for the children. Complex ongoing care is needed. This may begin in a homeless shelter, but should continue while the family obtains a place to live, accesses other community services, enrolls the children in school, and attains financial and mental stability. Nurses in all of these settings work with families who are homeless and are instrumental in establishing services where the homeless are located, such as in schools, community clinics, and shelters.

Nursing management for families with children that are poor or homeless focuses on identifying poverty, carefully assessing health risks, ensuring that children are referred to school systems, and linking the family to resources that can assist with stability and health. There is often no way to identify a poor child from appearance, and children may hide their status when in school or at a health care facility. Addresses given may not be accurate, or the address of a shelter might be used. Children living at shelters or in cars and on the street may not take the school bus but prefer to walk to avoid stigma. Be alert for children who have multiple health problems and repeated infectious diseases. They are often hungry, and have varying degrees of personal hygiene depending on access to laundry and bathing facilities. See Evidence-Based Practice: Homelessness from the Viewpoint of Mothers and Children.

Stress

The adverse effect of stress on adults is well documented, and the impact of stress on children has been recognized. Stress can be acute, such as when a child has an argument with a friend, a test in school, or a family crisis. Stress can also become chronic when the family frequently does not have enough food, when fighting or abuse are frequent, or when the child is overscheduled and feels under constant pressure to perform (Sparrow, 2007). Children manifest stress in a variety of ways, including regressive behavior, interrupted sleep, hyperactive behavior, gastrointestinal symptoms, crying, and withdrawal from normal events. Common stressful events for children include moving to a new home or school, marital difficulties in the family, abuse, parental deployment in the military, and being expected to achieve at an extremely high level in school or sports (Figure 17–1 ➤). The busy pace of today's lifestyles and the media's impact in encouraging early development of children may put undue stress upon some children and preteens (Elkind, 2007). Adolescents may be stressed by fulfilling many roles, such as student, part-time worker, and active family member. They may also be in school all day, have a sport or music practice for 2 to 3 hours after school, and then have a job for several additional hours. Lack of adequate sleep can add further to stress, in addition to putting the teen at risk for car crashes and poor school performance. For families living in poverty, commonly reported stressors are related to food provision, shelter, transportation, medical care, and personal-time needs.

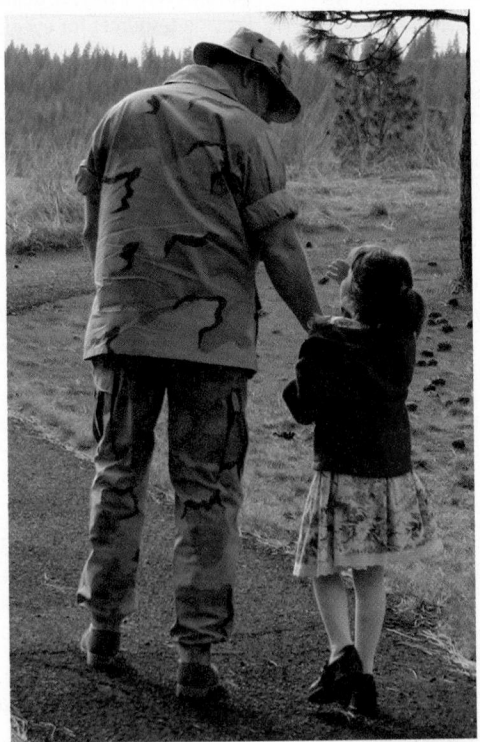

FIGURE 17–1 ➤ The special relationship between a father about to be deployed in the military and his young daughter is clear. This father has two other children and is spending time with each of them, as well as with the family together, before leaving. The cycle of leaving and returning home can be stressful for families. What are the needs of military families?

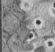

Culture *Poverty*

Ethnic disparities are striking in poverty rates. In married families, 5% of White children, 20% of Hispanic children, and 13% of Black children live in poverty. In female-headed families, 33% of White, 50% of Hispanic, and 50% of Black children live in poverty. However, nearly 80% of children who are poor have at least one parent working full time. Additionally, poverty rates are higher in suburban and rural areas than in central cities (Federal Interagency Forum on Child and Family Statistics, 2009).

Evidence-Based Practice

Homelessness from the Viewpoint of Mothers and Children

Problem

Children are the age group showing the fastest growth in homelessness. Due to their youth, children are vulnerable to developmental delays, mental health problems, and effects of violence. Mothers are the main support for young children, but when they are homeless they may not be able to provide the care children need for health, growth, and development. Most nurses have not been homeless and do not understand the experience of homelessness for children.

Evidence

A qualitative study of 28 homeless women with young children used interviews to learn about the experience of homelessness. Violence was a frequent experience in their lives. The women described stress, but felt respite in the shelter. Poor mental health and a lack of resources were major stresses, both of which directly influenced the mothering ability of the women (Tischler, Rademeyer, & Vostanis, 2007).

Another qualitative research study was conducted by nurses, using interviews with 10 youth, to learn about their experiences of homelessness. The interviews were carried out at a community agency serving the youth. As they described their encounters with health care services, several themes emerged. They felt marginalized and labeled as troublemakers or psychotics. There was a lack of both health care information and adequate time to address their concerns and questions. The teens felt like they had little control over their health care, and felt a lack of coordination throughout care received. Some youth, however, reported that they felt listened to, not judged, and were valued in some health care settings (Darbyshire, Muir-Cochrane, Fereday, et al., 2006). An earlier study by four nurses further describes the homeless experience from the perspective of children. They interviewed 14 children with an average age of 10 years who were located in shelters in a metropolitan area (DeForge, Zehnder, Minick, et al., 2001). The children had been in the shelters from 2 weeks to 6 months, and most had experienced prior periods living in shelters, in hotels, or with relatives. The researchers identified five themes common to the children:

- "I'm not homeless." The children viewed homelessness as having no resources and having to live outside. They felt that they had resources and felt they might be ridiculed if people thought they were homeless.
- "I like living in a shelter sometimes." While the children had mixed feelings about living in shelters, most were glad to have food, a place to sleep, and a feeling of safety. They described friends in the shelter and were glad to have those relationships.
- "Living in a shelter is hard." The children complained about rules and rigid schedules in the shelters. They missed freedom of movement, play space, and privacy.
- "Stop the violence." All children described living in violent neighborhoods and the wish that violence would stop. Fighting back was perceived as important to protecting oneself.
- "I need approval." Children frequently described how important it was to be noticed and praised by teachers and other adults.

Implications

Although these studies were small, there were important findings for nurses. Mothers of young children experience stresses that interfere with their ability to parent young children. The youth had multiple health care and social needs. Positive experiences were noted when care providers took time to discuss the youth's health and explain care. Trust was promoted when a sense of self-worth was enhanced. Clear information was appreciated, and coordinated care resulted in more positive and comprehensive health care.

Critical Thinking Application

Find at least two agencies that provide health care for persons who are homeless in your community. What are some of the common health problems treated? How are youth engaged in school and other community activities? What teaching is provided? Are mothers of young children offered parenting classes and stress reduction interventions? What links are available to other community resources? What is the nursing role in the community agencies you located?

Stress is related to physiological changes in the body and therefore can be related to increased physical and psychological conditions (Balodis, Wynne-Edwards, & Olmstead, 2010). The negative long-term effects of stress on body organs and systems, coupled with the developmental process, suggest that children under stress are at risk for physical and psychological illness and injury.

Nurses help children to manage stress by assessing what is stressful for each child and then encouraging coping strategies. Healthy lifestyles including quality nutrition, exercise, and adequate sleep can be emphasized with all children. Integrate these topics into each health promotion/health maintenance visit, using guidelines found in Chapters 7, 8, and 9 ∞. Parents can be encouraged to provide youth with activities that foster self-esteem and to avoid unrealistic expectations about performance in sports and other activities. Resources to assist with food acquisition, shelter, transportation, and medical care should be provided for families needing assistance. Adolescents may benefit from various approaches for stress management such as massage, rest, physical activity, and yoga.

Assess the family role adaptation needed in military families and provide resources to assist with coping. Connect parents with resources for childcare, mental health services, and arrangements that need to be made to prepare for the absence. Due to frequent moves, the family may not be strongly connected to resources in the community. During deployment the remaining parent may return to the home of origin; some family support may then be present. Help families explain to children why and where the parents are going, and how they will keep in touch during the absence. Children need to know who they will stay with, whether they will attend the same school, and how food and other needs will be provided. Parents, both those being deployed and those remaining at home, benefit from family, mental health, and financial support (Chartrand & Siegel, 2007; Rentz, Marshall, Loomis, et al., 2007).

Families

The families into which children are born provide a profound influence. Children are supported in different ways and acquire different worldviews depending on such factors as whether one or both parents work, how many siblings are present, and whether an extended family is nearby. Note should be made of variations in family structure such as adolescent parent, single parent, gay or lesbian parents, grandparents caring for grand-children, and stepparents. Societal changes have affected family life and the needs of children immensely. Working parents often raise children with little time for quality relationships and without the financial resources needed for optimum development (Annie E. Casey Foundation, 2007). All of these factors influence the physical and mental health of children and can determine their needs for nursing intervention.

Nurses can complete family diagrams during home visits and in other settings to evaluate the people who are important in a child's life (see the ecomap in Chapter 2 ∞ for an example). Both the risk factors of the family (e.g., recent separation, parental stress, and limited health care coverage) and the strengths manifested (e.g., loving relationships, influential grandparents or other extended family members, and general good health) should be identified and used in planning care. See Chapter 2 ∞ for a thorough discussion of family factors as they relate to family-centered care, and strategies for assessment and intervention with families.

School and Childcare

Once a child is 5 or 6 years of age, several hours daily are spent in a school setting. Physical skills are developed through participation in education and sports. Psychosocial stages are met as the child interacts with children and adults and achieves social interaction patterns and pride in accomplishments. The presentation of concepts that challenge thought processes enhances cognitive development.

Although the primary role of schools is educational, they also perform several health-related functions. School health screening programs identify children with such health problems as hearing loss, visual impairment, and scoliosis. Nurses provide assessment, teaching, and clinical management related to some health problems. Consider the case of Amy in the opening scenario. She went to the school nurse when her body piercing was potentially infected; the nurse examined the site, made suggestions for cleaning, and taught Amy the symptoms she needed to be aware of that could indicate a serious infection. Some schools have clinics that examine and provide even more complete health care for children. Many schools teach good nutrition, healthful living, safe sexual practices, and other health-related subjects. A school nurse may be present, at least part time, to plan these classes or to work with teachers. Nurses assist school districts in providing plans for emergency health care when needed. With the increase in mainstreaming, school staff now have the responsibility for administering medications, maintaining urinary catheters, and providing respiratory care and other treatments to ensure the child's proper growth and development. See Chapter 10 ∞ for a further discussion of school nurse activities.

Some children spend part or nearly all of their days in childcare settings (Figure 17–2 ➤). Over 60% of children less than 6 years of age receive some type of childcare regularly. About 19% of these children are in childcare up to 9 hours each week, 38% for 10–19 hours each week, 36% for 30–45 hours each week, and 10% for over 45 hours each week. The closeness of the parent–child re-

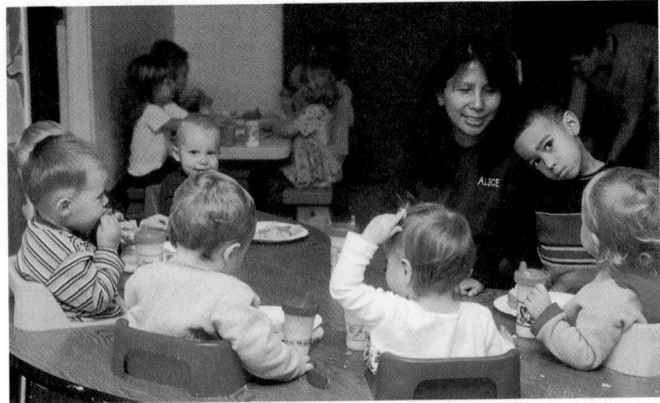

FIGURE 17–2 ➤ Most children will spend time in childcare settings. It is important to explore options and find the best fit for the child's needs.

lationship, the quality of care, and the length of the childcare day are important in determining childcare effects on children. The mother's sensitivity to her child is the best indicator of child behavior regardless of childcare arrangements (Federal Interagency Forum on Child and Family Statistics, 2007; National Institute of Child Health and Human Development, 2007).

Nursing management involves helping parents to explore types of childcare options available and to evaluate programs in their communities (Table 17–2). Care options for young school-age children, either before or after school, can also be shared with parents. Early intervention programs with at-risk children, such as the Zero to Three Project and Head Start, have been influential in contributing to children's health and welfare and should be recommended when available. Nurses frequently manage the health programs in early intervention, providing for screening and health evaluations and establishing early intervention education plans. Nurses assist families in evaluating childcare centers and share information about accreditation (see Families Want to Know: Evaluation of Child Care). The National Association for the Education of Young Children (2007) has established childcare criteria.

Community

The community in which a child lives may support the child's development or, conversely, expose the child to hazards. Social programs such as Head Start preschools, sports activities, after-school programs, and child abuse treatment centers offer valuable services that improve the experience of growing children. However, an economically depressed community with scant services and a high homicide rate is unsupportive and hazardous for growing children.

The physical environment is supportive when the child is provided with sidewalks on which to walk to school, open spaces in which to learn and play, and clean air to breathe. Children who must walk to school on unsafe roads, have access to contaminated drinking supplies, or live near polluting manufacturing companies or in crowded housing or old structures are at risk for injuries and health problems such as lead poisoning (see discussions later in this chapter about lead poisoning and exposure to other environmental contaminants).

TABLE 17–2	**Types of Child Care**		
Type of Care	Description	Advantages	Disadvantages
In home	Caretaker comes to home of the child	Child can remain at home Little exposure to infectious diseases No need for alternative care when child is ill	Limited contact with other children to encourage development Limited ability to rapidly locate alternate care when provider is ill Most costly
Family childcare	Parent brings child to home of a caretaker	Limited number of children Some exposure to other children and encouragement of development Family-type atmosphere	Little governmental regulation or examination
Center care a. Private, nonprofit (e.g., church, YMCA) b. Public (e.g., Head Start) c. Private proprietary	Parent brings child to a center where many children receive care	A learning curriculum plan is in place Contact with other children can enhance development	Exposure to multiple children increases infectious disease risk

Nurses should be aware of the types of neighborhoods in the community. Learn about local resources and hazards. Assessment of every child involves information about the community and the health care that the family needs help to obtain. See Chapter 10 ∞ for techniques that supply comprehensive community assessment. Refer children when appropriate for lead poisoning and safe programs after school, and teach them about injury prevention specific to their communities.

Culture

The child's cultural group may influence the use of traditional and contemporary health care practices. If the parents or children are recent immigrants, they may still be learning the English language and finding out about health care resources. Even in families that have been in the United States for some time, a combination of approaches to health care is common.

Families Want to Know
Evaluation of Child Care

The nurse can help parents to evaluate childcare options and make decisions about placement for their children. Parents should always be welcomed to visit an agency or home childcare—this is essential so they can see the routines in action. Following are suggested questions for them to ask.

Administration

Is the facility licensed?

Who are the administrators? What is their training and experience?

How many staff are employed? What is their training? What is their longevity?

Is there a parent board? What part do they play in administering the center?

Physical Environment, Health, and Safety

What is the neighborhood like? Is transportation to the center convenient?

What is the condition of lighting, heat, cooling, ventilation system, play spaces (inside and out), and the building's general condition?

Is playground equipment safe?

Is there a soft material such as bark, sand, or rubber tiles under climbing equipment?

Is there always supervision for the children?

Are there emergency medical forms and signed forms for field trips?

Who may pick up children? How are they signed in and out?

What is the immunization policy and how are records examined and maintained?

Are criminal background checks of staff done for potential child abuse and other problems?

What is the policy for children with infectious diseases and other illnesses?

How are foods prepared? Are staff licensed in food handling?

What is the state of general cleanliness?

Who changes diapers? Are recommendations for standard precautions to prevent pathogen transfer followed?

What arrangements and routines are made for naps and quiet times?

Developmental Approaches

Is the curriculum appropriate for different age groups?

Are there materials and plans for gross motor, fine motor, language, and social development?

How much time do children spend in structured time? Free time?

How is discipline handled?

Do the children appear occupied and happy?

What reading materials are available?

What type and quantity of field trips are planned?

Is there diversity among the children's backgrounds and experiences?

Adapted from the National Association for the Education of Young Children, 2007.

Children of immigrants may feel stress as they combine their family's traditional culture with the new culture in which the family now lives. They may also have responsibility to interpret for the family, since they frequently speak two languages and understand the practices of the new culture.

Recent immigrants may experience **culture shock**, a state of crisis related to the difference in values and lifestyle between the two cultures they have experienced. This can lead to stress-related symptoms, and create a need for health care intervention. Children whose parents immigrated from another country may feel different from peers and develop conflict with their parents, particularly during adolescence.

All cultural groups have rules regarding patterns of social interaction. Schedules of language acquisition are determined by the number of languages spoken and the amount of speech in the home. The particular social roles assumed by men and women in the culture affect school activities and ultimately career choices. Attitudes toward touching and other methods of encouraging developmental skills vary among cultures.

Nurses must become aware of common characteristics of the cultural groups they are serving in order to establish culturally competent nursing care. Arrange for interpreters when needed. Recognize that traditional and Western health care are often both accepted and used; remain nonjudgmental about traditional healing practices. Provide ethnic foods in health care facilities. Evaluate youth in immigrant families for conflict between family and societal expectations. See Chapter 2 ∞ for further discussion of culture.

▧ LIFESTYLE ACTIVITIES AND THEIR INFLUENCE ON CHILD HEALTH

Many patterns of daily life play a part in determining the length and quality of one's life. The child's use of tobacco products and controlled substances influences both physical and mental health. Patterns of exercise and use of protective gear help to avoid early disabilities. Media use can influence aggressive behaviors, compete with the need for physical activity, or be a positive force in teaching children new concepts. Body art that can introduce pathogens is an example of a lifestyle pattern that influences mental and physical health, as well as body image.

Substance Use

Substance use and abuse occurs in children and adolescents of all socioeconomic levels and is a growing health problem. About 45% of teens claim to have consumed alcohol in the last 30 days, 20% have used marijuana, and 20% have used cigarettes (Centers for Disease Control and Prevention, 2008a). The use of any substance such as tobacco, alcohol, or illicit drugs can pose a serious psychological and physical risk to children and adolescents. Tobacco use and management for the condition is discussed in the following text, followed by sections on alcohol use and drug use, and a management section to address those substances.

Tobacco Use

Tobacco use is the most preventable cause of adult death in the United States. It leads to 438,000 deaths annually, and will be responsible for the premature death of 5 million of today's youth as they reach adult years (U.S. Department of Health and Human Services, 2006). Major health problems linked to tobacco use include cardiovascular disease, cancer, chronic lung disease, increased prevalence of car crashes, low birth weight in babies whose mothers smoke, and other maternal health problems. Even passive smoking or environmental tobacco smoke (ETS) is linked to increased heart disease, increased blood pressure, respiratory problems, and decreased youth academic performance (Reardon, 2007; Collins, Wileyto, Murphy, et al., 2007). Cigarette use is most common; however, chewing tobacco, snuff, cigars, and bidis may also be used. These all pose significant health hazards.

Nursing Alert

Forms of tobacco other than traditional cigarettes may be popular among certain groups or in specific parts of the country. *Smokeless tobacco* in forms of chew, snuff, or dip has been used by 7.9% of youth. This type of tobacco is even used by students in school without staff being aware of the behavior. *Bidis* are small, brown, hand-rolled cigarettes that are popular among some youth. *Cigars* have been used by 13.6% of youth (Centers for Disease Control and Prevention, 2008a). Try to learn what types of tobacco are most common in the local community and plan to integrate history questions during health exams to learn about cigarette and other tobacco use. Never assume a youth is not using tobacco. Ask every youth questions about it, without parents in the room.

Many nurses view tobacco use as an adult issue, but each day 3,000 children and adolescents try their first cigarette, and the major age span for experimenting with tobacco is 9 to 14 years. Early initiation of smoking is an extremely risky behavior because nicotine is very addictive for youth, and 80% of current adult smokers began smoking before 18 years of age (Centers for Disease Control and Prevention, 2006a). Although sale of tobacco products to children and advertisements aimed at this age group are forbidden by federal law, many youth obtain and use tobacco. About 30% of high school students and 13% of middle school students in the United States smoked within the last 30 days (Centers for Disease Control and Prevention, 2006c), and others report use of chewing

Research ▥ *The Youth Risk Behavior Surveillance System*

The Youth Risk Behavior Surveillance System is conducted every other year on large representative numbers of youth by the Centers for Disease Control and Prevention. In 2007, 38 states and 14,103 students were included in reported results (Centers for Disease Control and Prevention, 2008a). The categories of priority health-risk behaviors investigated in each survey are:

- Behaviors contributing to unintentional and intentional injury
- Tobacco use
- Alcohol and other drug use
- Sexual behaviors contributing to unintended pregnancy and sexually transmitted diseases
- Physical inactivity
- Overweight and weight control

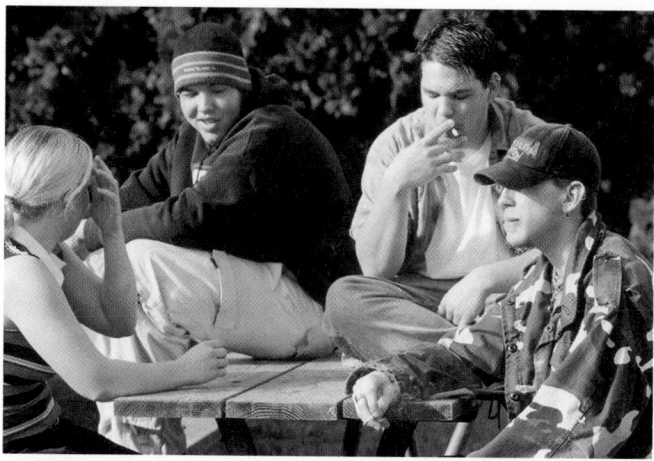

FIGURE 17–3 ➤ Almost 70% of children have tried smoking by their high school years. Early intervention should begin with assessment for and discussions about smoking hazards starting at 9–10 years of age.

Culture 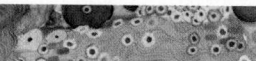 *Smoking Rates Among Youth*

Among youth in the United States, White youth are significantly more likely to smoke than either Hispanic or Black peers. About 23% of White students reported smoking in the previous month, while 17% of Hispanic and 12% of Black students reported smoking. American Indian and Alaska Natives also have high smoking rates, whereas Asian Americans have low rates (Centers for Disease Control and Prevention, 2006a, 2008a).

tobacco and cigars. Approximately 7.8% of females and 14.8% of males from 13 to 15 years report current use of tobacco other than cigarettes (Centers for Disease Control and Prevention, 2006b).

Certain characteristics contribute to the likelihood of tobacco use. They include increasing age, male gender, ethnic group, ease of obtaining tobacco products, and smoking among family members. Low socioeconomic group membership, access to tobacco products, low price of products, advertising, influence of peers, and lack of parental involvement in their children's lives are also associated with tobacco use (Victoir, Eertmans, Van den Broucke, et al., 2006) (Figure 17–3 ➤).

Several programs have been developed to encourage youth to avoid tobacco use. In addition, smoking cessation programs are available to assist youth who are already regular smokers. These programs are successful in achieving the goals of cessation or decrease in tobacco use. Gender differences may exist for youth who are beginning or seeking to quit smoking. For example, girls may be more worried about the smell and effect of tobacco on clothing and appearance, while boys more commonly express concern about smoking's effect on sports or activities (Amos & Bostock, 2006). Use of incentives, and counselor-based, individually tailored telephone interventions have been effective (Liu, Peterson, Kealey, et al., 2007; Backinger, Michaels, Jefferson, et al., 2007). Once a teen is identified as a smoker, using a biological marker such as urine cotinine (a by-product of tobacco) levels can help to identify the frequency of smoking. This information can be used to make suggestions to the teen about the potential outcomes of the behavior and the cessation program that is most likely to be helpful.

NURSING MANAGEMENT

Nursing Assessment and Diagnosis

Nurses are in a unique position to inquire about the incidence of smoking and other tobacco use among youth. Questions should be inserted into all well-child visits, beginning at about 9 to 10 years of age. Inquire about whether family members (es-

pecially parents and siblings) smoke or chew, and ask if some of the child's friends have tried smoking. Assess for associated risk behaviors such as alcohol and drug use, sexual activity, and suicidal thoughts. Determine the child's knowledge and beliefs about the benefits and risks of tobacco use. As the child gets older, more direct and detailed questions are necessary. A nonjudgmental approach will be best to obtain a truthful response. School nurses can make observations about numbers of teens smoking and general attitudes about tobacco use. When children come to hospitals and other health facilities for care, use of tobacco should be part of the general admission questions. Remember to include smokeless tobacco use in questioning.

The following nursing diagnoses may apply to youth who smoke or show potential for this behavior:

- Activity Intolerance related to lowered oxygen supply
- Impaired Gas Exchange related to ventilation-perfusion imbalance
- Chronic Low Self-Esteem related to negative self-appraisal
- Deficient Knowledge regarding dangers of tobacco use related to developmental focus on the present
- Imbalanced Nutrition, Less than Body Requirements related to effects of chemical dependence

Planning and Implementation

The roles of nurses in preventing and intervening in youth smoking are to *inform* youth, *identify* smokers, and *implement* programs for prevention and cessation (Table 17–3). Nurses should provide developmentally appropriate information about the hazards of tobacco use in all settings where youth are present. Posters, flyers, and speakers are particularly useful. Include information about short-term problems such as increased rates of upper respiratory infections and worsening of asthma, as well as long-term effects such as addiction, lung cancer, oral cancer, car crashes, emphysema, and other health problems. Addicted teens who share their stories of difficult withdrawal from tobacco, and adults who have had cancer of the lungs or larynx, may be effective speakers. Find out where teens obtain tobacco products in the community and where they engage in use of the products to target these places. Offer information on available prevention and cessation programs to youth and families in clinics, outpatient surgery centers, community activities, and hospitals. Use opportunities such as adolescent pregnancy and presence of illness to reinforce the hazardous effects of tobacco on the individual and on those nearby. Adolescent mothers should understand the risks for small-for-gestational-age babies when they smoke in pregnancy, and the increased risk of sudden

TABLE 17–3	Nursing Role in Youth Smoking Prevention

Inform

- Hang posters, provide brochures, and facilitate presentations about smoking risks in all settings where youth are present.
- Target smokers with special information about the effects of nicotine on their bodies.

Identify

- Ask questions about smoking and other tobacco use at every health encounter beginning at about 9–10 years of age.
- For users, ask about the amount and type of tobacco.
- Learn where youth obtain tobacco, and be proactive in stopping sales.

Implement

- Encourage young tobacco users to quit.
- Facilitate referral to cessation programs.
- Arrange positive rewards for youth who are successful in cessation.

infant death syndrome (SIDS) when infants are exposed to secondhand smoke (see Chapter 20 ∞ for a detailed discussion of SIDS). Speak to young athletes about the effects of tobacco on athletic performance. Show children the ways in which this product can interfere with their meeting of life goals. Role-play how to say no when tobacco is offered. Establish programs that increase the sense of self-esteem without tobacco use. Be sure to include parents in the programs so that they see and acknowledge their role in setting an example about tobacco use, and in providing guidelines for the child. Information about the influence of environmental tobacco smoke (ETS or secondhand smoke) should also be provided.

Adopt a nonjudgmental attitude when asking questions about smoking so that those who are using tobacco can be identified. Ask questions without parents present and assure the children that the information will not be shared. Encourage youth to cut back and to quit use of tobacco products. Offer them assistance in these efforts. Encourage positive coping techniques for youth who are engaged in cessation. Such techniques include keeping busy, avoiding smoking situations, using oral stimulation such as a toothpick or gum, exercising, relaxing, and using nicotine replacement approaches (Jannone & O'Connell, 2007).

Work with the schools and school districts to help establish preventive and cessation programs. There should be clear guidelines about school policies regarding smoking on school grounds. Keeping occasional youth smokers from becoming regular users should be a goal to avoid nicotine addiction. Find out what positive incentives can be offered to youth who are successful in quitting smoking. Contract with them to achieve their goals.

Evaluation

Expected outcomes of nursing interventions regarding tobacco use are lowered rates of regular use, delayed initiation of use, and success of cessation programs. Use the following proposed *Healthy People 2020* (U.S. Department of Health and Human Services, 2010) objectives as guidelines:

- Reduce tobacco use by adolescents.
- Reduce the initiation of tobacco use among children, adolescents, and young adults.
- Increase smoking cessation attempts by adolescent smokers.
- Reduce the illegal sales rate to minors through enforcement of laws prohibiting the sale of tobacco products to minors.
- Increase the number of States and the District of Columbia, Territories, and Tribes with sustainable and comprehensive evidence-based control programs.
- Increase tobacco-free environments in schools, including all school facilities, property, vehicles, and school events.
- Increase adolescents' disapproval of smoking.
- Reduce the proportion of adolescents and young adults who are exposed to tobacco advertising and promotion.

Alcohol Use

Each day, 7,000 children take their first drink. An estimated 75% have tried alcohol, which is the drug of choice and convenience for youth. By 12th grade, 83% have had alcoholic drinks. Currently, 45% of high school students admit to drinking within the last month, and 26% admit to having engaged in binge drinking, or having five or more drinks within a 2-hour period. Even young children are affected since 44% of 8th graders and 66% of 10th graders have tried alcohol, while 20% of 8th graders and 35% of 10th graders have had alcohol in the last month. Alcohol use frequently starts at an early age; 25.6% of high school students report that their first drink was before age 13 years (Centers for Disease Control and Prevention, 2006c, 2008a).

Numerous health risks are associated with drinking by minors. Perhaps the most obvious is that of motor vehicle accidents. About 5,000 young people annually die from alcohol-related injuries from car crashes, homicides, and suicides (National Institute on Alcohol Abuse and Alcoholism, 2009). Others experience assault such as alcohol-related date rape. Alcohol affects the developing brain, decreasing intellectual capacity and increasing the chance for future alcohol use. Additionally, early drinking significantly increases the chance that someone will become an alcoholic later in life (Surgeon General, 2007; Hingson, Heeren, & Winter, 2006). Endocrine problems, liver abnormalities, and decreased bone density can also occur. The neurologic effects of alcohol on the brain are magnified in the young. Children are much more likely to try alcohol and to become alcoholic when a family member is alcoholic; this is a significant risk as one in five children grow up in a home with an alcoholic adult (National Institute on Alcohol Abuse and Alcoholism, 2009).

Culture	 *Alcohol Use*

There are ethnic differences among youth alcohol consumption. Current use by Blacks is 69%, with 47% of Whites and 48% of Hispanics currently using alcohol. Asian groups traditionally have low alcohol use and Native Americans have high use (Centers for Disease Control and Prevention, 2008a). Nurses can use this information to target groups most at risk of alcohol ingestion, even at these young ages.

Many factors influence the child and adolescent who drink alcohol. Patterns in the family, media advertisements, and social environments in high school and college that honor or expect drinking all contribute to the problem. Access is easy for most youth as older siblings or classmates obtain drinks. It is a "rite of passage" for many at teen birthday parties or college events. Alcohol is the most common and accepted drug in today's society and, as such, youth are exposed and often experience its effects without understanding or considering the implications of its use. A risk factor for initiation of alcohol use is a transition time, such as change from middle to high school, or a major family stress, such as parental separation or divorce (Loveland-Cherry, 2006).

Drug Use

In addition to alcohol, a variety of other drugs are used by youth. Substance use occurs in children and adolescents of all socioeconomic levels and is a growing health problem. Almost 40% of students have used marijuana and 20% have used it in the last month. About 7% have used cocaine, with over 3% having used it in the last month. Inhalant use of glue, paints, or other substances is more common, with 12% reporting use and 4% having used in the last month. Approximately 6% report methamphetamine use, and 2.4% report use of heroin (Centers for Disease Control and Prevention, 2006c). Synthetic drugs such as phencyclidine (PCP) (commonly referred to as "designer" drugs) mimic other narcotics, stimulants, and hallucinogens and are also dangerous. See the companion website for a table of common contemporary drugs and street names.

Over-the-counter (OTC) medications are legal, but frequently abused. Easily obtainable at grocery stores and drugstores, these drugs include antihistamines, atropine, bromides, caffeine, ephedrine, pseudoephedrine, phenylpropanolamine, and amphetamine-like substitutes. Volatile inhalants such as glues are dangerous substances of abuse, and their use is high among school-age children and adolescents. Each incident of "huffing" or inhaling a substance runs the risk of a serious health problem and death, the latter referred to as sudden sniffing death. Children who "huff" while taking amphetamines such as Ritalin for treatment of attention deficit disorder run an elevated risk of a potentially fatal interaction. See Table 17–4 for common inhalant agents. Anabolic steroids are the drugs of abuse most commonly used by athletes; about 4% of students report use of illegal steroids. Use is more common in males (4.8%) than females (3.2%) and lifetime use ranges from 2–6.5% (Centers for Disease Control and Prevention, 2006c).

 Health Promotion

Energy Drinks

Youth may be aware of the caffeine content of herbal products or drinks and choose to use them in excess. Guarana is made from cocoa beans and contains caffeine and other drugs such as theophylline. It is available in supplements and is used in some energy drinks. Yerba mate is formulated from a tree and also contains caffeine, theophylline, and other substances. Some noncaffeinated stimulants include panax (Asian ginseng) and ephedra (ma huang). Question the family, child, and adolescent at each health care visit about consumption of energy drinks and herbal products.

TABLE 17–4	Common Inhalant Agents
Agent	Inhalant
Aerosols	• Cooking spray • Whipped cream • Spray paint • Cosmetic sprays
Adhesives	• Model glues • Rubber cements
Solvents	• Nail polish remover • Paint thinner or cleaner • Lighter fluid • Degreaser
Other	• Gasoline • Helium

Etiology and Pathophysiology In most cases, substance abuse represents a maladaptive coping response to the stressors of childhood and adolescence. Individual, peer, family, and community risk factors all contribute to increased incidence of use (Surgeon General, 2007). A child may begin using alcohol or drugs to deal with stress because family members or peers do so. Children in families with a history of substance abuse are at higher risk of abusing drugs and alcohol. Other risk factors include rebelliousness, aggressiveness, low self-esteem, dysfunctional parental relationships, lack of adequate support systems, academic underachievement, poor judgment, and poor impulse control. Adolescents and young adults use "club drugs" to achieve greater satisfaction during nights of dancing, drinking, and attending clubs. Use of these drugs with alcohol can lead to deadly consequences.

Initial experimentation with alcohol or drugs may be unpleasant. With continued use, however, the adolescent learns to "achieve the high," an illusion of power and well-being. The adolescent wants the high more frequently and actively seeks alcohol or drugs. Tolerance to the substance occurs with continued use, and ever-increasing amounts are required to achieve a pleasurable high. Physical and psychologic dependence ensues as the body's tissues require the substance to function properly. Withdrawal symptoms occur when the child or adolescent is deprived of the substance.

Clinical Manifestations Substance abuse in children and adolescents is commonly overlooked and underdiagnosed by health care providers due in part to the wide range of clinical presentations. These vary according to the type of drug abused, the amount, the frequency, the time of last use, and the severity of drug dependence. See the Clinical Manifestations table on the next page for manifestations of abuse and potential for dependence for several types of drugs.

Common physical manifestations include alterations in vital signs, weight loss, chronic fatigue, chronic cough, respiratory congestion, red eyes, and general apathy and malaise. Lesions in and around the nose and mouth are common. The mental status examination (refer to Chapter 5 ∞) may reveal alterations in level of consciousness, impaired attention and concentration,

Clinical Manifestations
Commonly Abused Drugs

Drug	Potential for Dependence	Clinical Manifestations
Depressants Alcohol, barbiturates (amobarbital, pentobarbital, secobarbital)	*Physical and psychologic:* High; varies somewhat among drugs	*Physical:* Decreased muscle tone and coordination tremors *Psychologic:* Impaired speech, memory, and judgment; confusion; decreased attention span; emotional lability
Stimulants Amphetamines (e.g., Benzedrine), caffeine, cocaine, MDMA	*Physical:* Low to moderate *Psychologic:* High; withdrawal from amphetamines and cocaine can lead to severe depression	*Physical:* Dilated pupils, increased pulse and blood pressure, flushing, nausea, loss of appetite, tremors, vascular heart disease (with MDMA) *Psychologic:* Euphoria; increased alertness, agitation, or irritability; hallucinations; insomnia
Opiates Codeine, heroin, meperidine (Demerol), methadone, morphine, opium, oxycodone (Percodan, OxyContin)	*Physical and psychologic:* High; varies somewhat among drugs; withdrawal effects are uncomfortable but rarely life threatening	*Physical:* Analgesia, depressed respirations and muscle tone (may lead to coma or death), nausea, constricted pupils *Psychologic:* Changes in mood (usually euphoria), drowsiness, impaired attention or memory, sense of tranquility
Hallucinogens Lysergic acid diethylamide (LSD), mescaline, phencyclidine (PCP)	*Physical:* None *Psychologic:* Unknown	*Physical:* Lack of coordination, dilated pupils, hypertension, elevated temperature; severe PCP intoxication can result in seizures, respiratory depression, coma, and death *Psychologic:* Visual illusions and hallucinations, altered perceptions of time and space, emotional lability, psychosis
Volatile inhalants Glues, typing correction fluid, acrylic paints, spot removers, lighter fluid, gasoline, butane	*Physical and psychologic:* Varies with drug used	*Physical:* Impaired coordination, liver damage (in some cases) *Psychologic:* Impaired judgment, delirium
Marijuana	*Physical:* Low *Psychologic:* Usually low; occasionally moderate to high	*Physical:* Tachycardia, reddened conjunctiva, dry mouth, increased appetite *Psychologic:* Initial anxiety followed by euphoria; giddiness; impaired attention, judgment, and memory

impaired thought processes, delusions, and hallucinations. Low self-esteem, feelings of guilt or worthlessness, and suicidal or homicidal thoughts are also common. Paraphernalia reported by parents, such as rags, pipes, and canisters, may indicate use, and chemical odors around the clothing and person should be indicative of possible drug use.

Poor school performance and changes in mood, sleep habits, appetite, dress, and social relationships are nonspecific characteristics of the substance-abusing child. These are often the symptoms first noted by family and friends, and should be the subject of questions at each health promotion visit.

COLLABORATIVE CARE

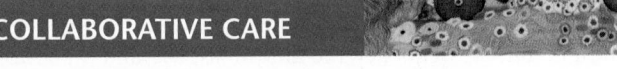

Diagnostic Tests

Multiple psychiatric diagnostic criteria exist for each drug class. Children and adolescents who have other psychosocial disorders commonly use and abuse drugs or alcohol. Therefore, assessment and treatment plans should focus not only on the substance use, but also on the issues underlying the problem. Diagnosis includes assessment of both the family and the substance-abusing child or adolescent. Blood levels of substances and metabolites are sometimes measured.

Clinical Therapy

The primary goal of treatment is to teach the child and other family members to develop and sustain positive coping patterns, and to support them during this process. Most treatment programs offer inpatient and outpatient services, as well as aftercare programs. These programs usually consist of peer support focusing on the development of healthy family relationships, positive coping skills, and a lifestyle free of drugs or alcohol. Family involvement is strongly encouraged. Hospitalization is required if the physical dependence is significant and withdrawal places the child at risk for complications such as seizures, depression, or suicidal behavior.

Clinical Tip

SBI

Screening and Brief Intervention (SBI), presented by the American Public Health Association (2008), is a system of questions to identify alcohol use. It includes a brief discussion with a care provider. Nurses often choose to administer the screening tool in clinical settings. Several tools are available; those with 4–10 items are best for screening. Two that are specific to adolescents are CAGE (Cut down, Annoyed, Guilty, Eye-opener) and CRAFFT (Car, Relax, Alone, Friends, Forget, Trouble). Descriptions and further information can be found at several websites.

Screening Tools Websites

NURSING MANAGEMENT

Nursing Assessment and Diagnosis

Mental health assessment of all older children and adolescents requires screening for alcohol and other substances. Maintaining a confidential approach will increase the ability to obtain truthful information about use of substances (National Institute on Alcohol Abuse and Alcoholism, 2009). Nurses may encounter the substance-abusing child or adolescent in the emergency department or outpatient clinic, in the school and other community settings, or during hospitalization for an injury or other acute problem. Nursing assessment for all children includes taking a thorough history from the parents and child, observing the child's behavior, administering an alcohol screening tool, and performing a physical examination. Maintaining a confidential approach will increase the ability to obtain truthful information about use of substances (National Institute on Alcohol Abuse and Alcoholism, 2009).

Clinical Tip

Alcohol Withdrawal Symptoms

Adolescents who have some or all of the following symptoms may be experiencing alcohol withdrawal: anxiety, headache, tremors, nausea and vomiting, malaise or weakness, insomnia, depressed mood or irritability, and hallucinations. A recurring pattern of these symptoms may indicate youth who have access to alcohol periodically, and then repeatedly experience withdrawal when it is no longer available.

When substance use is known, the history should include the age at which drug use began, the pattern of use, the length of time the drug has been used, the amount of drug used, and the psychologic state while on drugs. A history of parental drug use and noninvolvement in parenting puts the child at higher risk for substance abuse, reflecting the combined effects of genetic and environmental influences. Environmental factors such as access to the substance, use with other teens or adults, and resources for treatment are important to consider. Find out what types of addictions are most common in your community so that assessments can be designed to the risks that are highest for youth in those settings (Figure 17–4 ➤).

Physiological Assessment

Look for physical signs and symptoms of substance abuse, including bloodshot eyes, dilated pupils, skin and mucous membrane lesions, slurred speech, and weight loss. The adolescent may appear sleepy or restless, or may show signs of clumsiness or inconsistent behavior. Consider all types of substance abuse, including model glue, gasoline, club drugs, herbals, and other sources. Assess for current intoxication effects as well as signs of withdrawal.

Psychologic Assessment

Changes in social habits may indicate substance abuse. Parents may report a drop in the school-age child's or adolescent's grades or decreased interest in school activities. The adolescent does not introduce new friends to parents, and has less contact with parents, teachers, and other adults who were previously important. Conversely, the youth may appear more energetic, always appear "on a high," have weight loss, and appear to be high achieving. Note the child's current drug use, potential for violence, and motivation to make changes. Assess the degree of family support available.

Family Assessment

In families with substance-using adults, children may experience neglect and abuse, as well as exposure to drugs. When

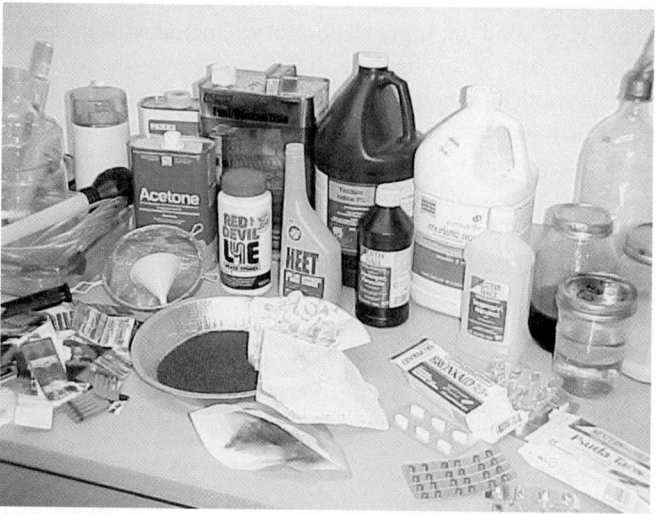

A

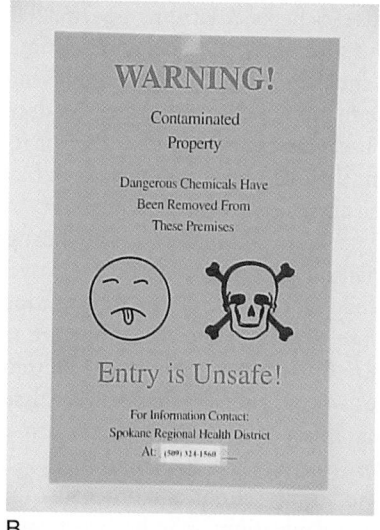

B

FIGURE 17–4 ➤ A, Methamphetamine is a popular drug because it can be manufactured with items that are available to the lay public such as those shown in the picture on the left. Manufacture of the substance in homes has become a concern of health departments and communities at large. Children can be harmed by the chemicals produced, and may experience neglect and abuse when parents are producing. They may suffer even after the home is found and adults are apprehended as they must be placed in foster homes. B, Homes used for methamphetamine production must be decontaminated before they can be safely used.
Photos courtesy of Spokane Regional Health District.

family members are substance users, young children may experience periods when adults cannot provide supervision and cannot encourage healthy activities. The children may be exposed to potentially unsafe or violent episodes. When parents are manufacturing products such as methamphetamine, young children are exposed to toxic chemicals and run the risk of suffering burns and other sequelae from home laboratory production and explosions. Be alert for unusual injuries, signs of inconsistent parenting, and delays in or disturbed growth and development. Be prepared to refer parents for care. Follow protocols for child abuse prevention (see the section on abuse and neglect later in this chapter).

Following are possible nursing diagnoses for children and adolescents who abuse drugs or alcohol:

- Impaired Social Interaction related to altered thought processes
- Chronic Low Self-Esteem related to dysfunctional family and social relationships
- Risk for Injury related to altered perceptions and sensorium
- Risk for Violence: Self-Directed or Other-Directed related to physiologic dependence on drugs, alcohol, and other substances

Planning and Implementation

Care of children and adolescents who abuse drugs, alcohol, and other substances is challenging and often frustrating. Long-term mental health counseling may be necessary to resolve underlying issues and foster lifestyle and behavioral changes.

Prevention is the most desirable intervention. The nurse can teach children and their families about substance abuse (see Families Want to Know: Identifying the Youth Who Is Abusing Substances). Alert parents that prescription drugs from a family medicine cabinet are frequent sources of teen substance use; they should be kept locked and should be safely discarded when no longer in use (Schepis & Krishnan-Sarin, 2009). Education for youth about substances should begin in primary school and continue with intensification during the middle and high school years. Stress reduction resources can help to decrease the need for substance use. Nurses also can play a major role in community education. Various prevention programs have been developed by federal and private organizations.

The child who has begun to use and abuse drugs needs an intensive intervention program. Referral to a psychiatric health specialist is needed for diagnosis and intervention. Group programs and those that integrate the family are most effective. Find out what resources are present in your community to treat youth who are using alcohol or other drugs. Nurses are active in treatment programs as well as sustaining treatment effects and avoiding relapse during visits to community agencies once the youth returns to family, school, and other surroundings. Referral to support organizations may be beneficial for the child, parents, and other family members. Self-help groups, which are available in most communities, include Alcoholics Anonymous, Narcotics Anonymous, Al-Anon, Nar-Anon, and Ala-Teen. Parents may receive support from a group such as Parents Anonymous.

Families Want to Know
Identifying the Youth Who Is Abusing Substances

Families are often confused about the behavior of adolescents and unsure whether it represents normal development or abuse of substances. Some characteristics of normal development that help to differentiate these occurrences follow. When concerned about possible substance use, the parent can provide a forum to discuss the concerns with the child or talk with school nurses or counselors.

- Many youth are periodically distant with parents at times, but remain involved with peers in school sports and other activities. Withdrawal from all activities and friends may indicate substance abuse.
- Adolescents often complain about school, but when teachers report that the student meets expectations and is consistently performing in the classroom, this is normal behavior.
- Teens may be weepy on occasion when having a difficult time with friends or not performing as desired. Continued, consistent weepiness is more likely to indicate depression or substance abuse.
- Teens like to stay up late and are frequently tired in the morning, while abusing teens may "nod off" frequently during the day.
- Many adolescents like to achieve a disheveled look in clothing, but the teen who frequently neglects basic hygiene or does not seem to have the energy to wash and dress may be depressed or abusing substances.
- All teens get some infections, but abusing teens may have reddened eyes, oral sores, and constant respiratory discomfort from "snorting" substances.

The nurse should be aware of the current substance abuse patterns in specific communities. At the present time, methamphetamine (meth) use is increasing in many areas and represents a severe threat to youth because of its extremely addictive capacity and resistance to treatment. An increasing awareness of meth's dangers has led to legislation that pseudoephedrine can only be sold as a "behind-the-counter" controlled substance since it is used in home laboratories manufacturing meth (Gettig, Grady, & Nowosadzka, 2006).

The youth's protective factors against substance abuse can be identified and used in planning appropriate interventions. For example, a child with goals related to a future career can be helped to see the way in which substance use will interfere with goal attainment. Identifying a strong role model through a program like Big Brothers or Big Sisters can assist children who lack that strength in their families.

Evaluation

Expected outcomes of nursing intervention regarding substance abuse include the following:

- The child abstains from alcohol and street drugs.
- The teen successfully participates in substance abuse programs.
- Developmentally normal social interactions are observed in the child.
- School performance at level of potential is achieved.
- The child is safe from injury.

■ PHYSICAL INACTIVITY/SEDENTARY BEHAVIOR

In the past few decades, children have become increasingly physically inactive. This decrease is a reflection of lifestyles in which car travel is valued, computers and televisions are part of daily life, neighborhoods are sometimes unsafe places for play activities, and schools do not routinely require daily physical education classes (Figure 17–5 ➤).

Children and adolescents spend about 20 to 30 hours per week on screen activities, and some spend significantly more. About 37% of high school students watch television over 3 hours each day and about 21% use computer or video games over 3 hours each day (Centers for Disease Control and Prevention, 2006a). The effects of screen activities are multiple: (1) physical inactivity while viewing, (2) lack of active cognition, and (3) tendency to eat high-fat snacks and excessive calories while viewing. Even at very young ages, children are immersed in various types of media.

Physical inactivity leads to many health concerns. A primary outcome is overweight or obesity (see Chapter 14 ∞). Other outcomes can be an increased rate of type 2 diabetes (see Chapter 30 ∞), increased exposure to television/computer game violence and sexual activity at early ages (see violence discussion later in this chapter), and early progression of cardiovascular disease (see Chapter 21 ∞).

Conversely, patterns of physical activity established in childhood can increase exercise behaviors in adulthood and contribute to lower rates of low back pain, overweight, osteoporosis, heart disease, diabetes, colon cancer, and high blood pressure, and a more positive self-image.

Although many children demonstrate low levels of physical activity, a profound decrease in vigorous activity is common in grades 9 through 12. Boys more commonly participate in team sports than girls. Although about 54% of students attend physical education (PE) classes at least once a week, only 33% have daily PE classes (Centers for Disease Control and Prevention, 2006c).

Health professionals can integrate assessment of physical activity into all health care contacts and make recommendations to children and families that will help to increase opportunities for physical activity. Nurses assess height, weight, and body mass index to look for signs of overweight (see Chapter 14 ∞). Ask what a typical day is like and include specific questions about television, computers, and video games. Children should be asked how they like to spend free time. Community and school activities should be encouraged and rewarded. Examples include fun runs, walks of benefit causes, aerobics classes, team sports, roadside cleanups, and fairs and carnivals. Help parents and children learn what they can do for physical fitness. Work with school physical education personnel to plan activities both in and out of PE class that promote lifelong exercise routines. Work toward the goal of 60 minutes of daily moderate-intensity physical activity for all children (U.S. Department of Health and Human Services, 2008). Help children to gradually increase physical activity and decrease sedentary time during regular health promotion visits. See Families Want to Know: Physical Activity Guidelines for Youth.

■ INJURY AND PROTECTIVE EQUIPMENT

In the discussion of causes of childhood and adolescent morbidities and mortalities in Chapter 1 ∞, unintentional injuries are listed as a common problem. In fact, 71% of all deaths from age 10 years onward result from four causes—motor vehicle crashes, other unintentional injury, homicide, and suicide. Chapters 7 through 9 ∞ discuss the frequent injuries seen in children at different developmental ages, and safety precautions to avoid injuries from car crashes, falls, poisonings, and other developmentally related injuries. Many common injuries are preventable by using protective gear and following safety guidelines (Figure 17–6 ➤).

Over 10% of youth rarely or never wear car safety belts in automobiles; 37% of those who ride motorcycles do not wear helmets (Centers for Disease Control and Prevention, 2006a). The

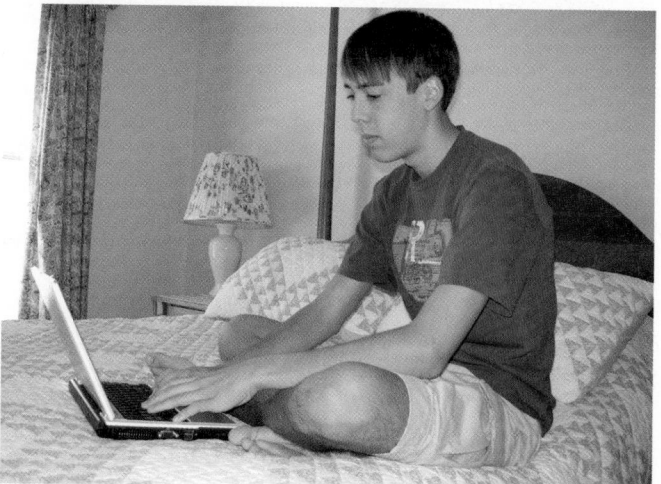
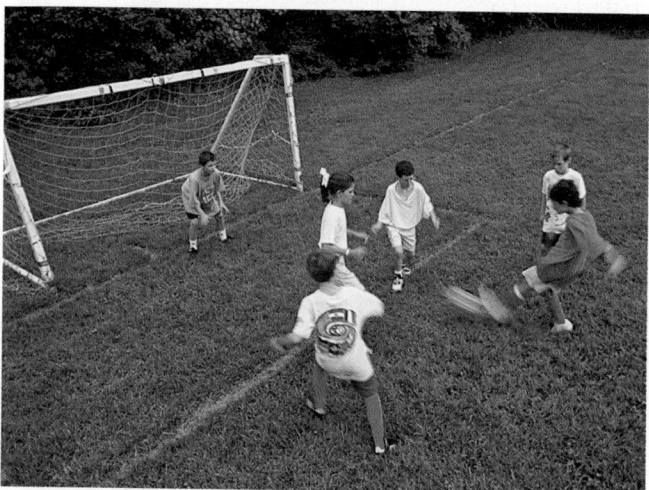

FIGURE 17–5 ➤ Physical inactivity is a growing problem among children, and can contribute to poor health. It is important to balance sedentary activities, such as playing computer games, with physical and social activities. Sports are an excellent way for children to develop their psychosocial, cognitive, and motor skills.
Soccer photo courtesy of Creative Communications, Wake Forest University School of Medicine.

The increasing role of media in children's daily schedules has been known for some time. However, little data have examined the issue in very young children. The Kaiser Family Foundation examined the role of electronic media in the lives of infants, toddlers, and preschoolers and found startling results. A nationally representative survey of 1,065 parents of children from 6 months to 6 years found the following:

- One in four children under 2 years of age has a television in his or her bedroom; 36% of children under 6 years have a television in their bedrooms, while 27% have a VCR or DVD player, 10% have a video game player, and 7% have a computer.
- Those children who have a television in their bedrooms spend significantly less time reading or playing outside than other children.
- Approximately 65% of young children live in a household where the television is on at least half of the time; 36% are in homes where the television is nearly always on.
- Young children spend the same amount of time with electronic media as they spend outdoors (about 2 hours each). About two thirds of young children spend 2 or more hours watching television daily.
- In contrast, these children spend only 39 minutes daily reading or being read to.
- Most young children use computers regularly.

- Much new media is targeted at this very young audience.
- Parents have generally positive views of media, with 72% saying computers mostly help child learning, and about half saying that television and videos are very important to the intellectual learning of children (KidsHealth, 2009; Anderson, Economos, & Must, 2008).

These findings are critical for nurses to consider. Physical inactivity and sedentary behavior are linked to obesity, type 2 diabetes, and other chronic disease risk. Children's ready access to media in the home and other settings directly interferes with recommended levels of physical activity. In all settings with parents of young children, ask about exposure to media. Encourage parents to turn off the television in the house except for select and limited viewing times, avoid media use in the child's bedroom, limit exposure to media, and have the child engaged in physical activity for a greater part of the day than in quiet pursuits. Encourage reading and being read to for young children; parents can schedule reading time to at least equal media viewing. Carefully perform developmental testing on children when exposure to media is high (see Chapter 6 ∞).

What other teaching can you identify to address this issue with parents of young children? How can parents integrate media concerns into the evaluation of childcare settings? What might the effects be on child growth and development with excessive use of media?

---

importance of safe automobile and motorcycle behaviors must be emphasized again in adolescence, with the recognition that risks increase if driving is combined with the use of alcohol and controlled substances. Adolescents sometimes engage in practices that put them at particular risk, and nurses should be alert for activities in their communities. Examples include "extreme" sports and car surfing (standing on the trunk, hood, or roof of a

moving vehicle) or street racing (racing cars down a street at extremely high speed).

About 44 million U.S. children ride bicycles, a beneficial physical activity. However, only 15% are protected by helmet use, even though bicycles are the most common activity connected with injury (Centers for Disease Control and Prevention, 2006a). Helmets could prevent up to 88% of serious brain injuries from bicycle crashes (National Safe Kids, 2007). Strategies to make helmet use more attractive to children and adolescents are needed. Nurses can play a major role in programs to educate

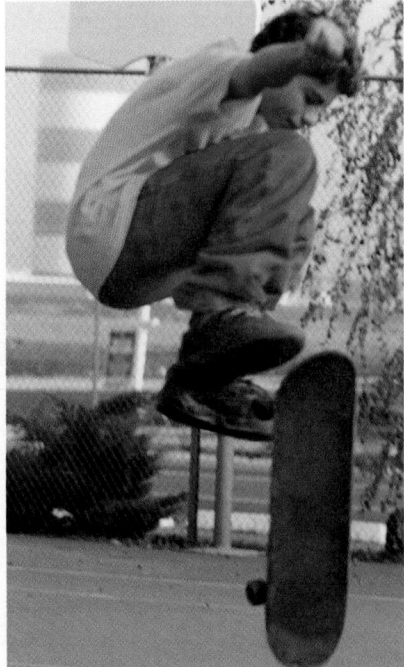

FIGURE 17–6 ➤ What protective gear should children use for skateboarding? How would you convince them to use the protection?

- Engage in moderate to vigorous physical activity (bike riding, walking, baseball, in-line skating, soccer, running, ice hockey) for 60 minutes daily (on at least 3 days/week this should be vigorous activity) (U.S. Department of Health and Human Services, 2008).
- Engage in muscle-strengthening activity at least 3 times weekly.
- Engage in bone-strengthening activity at least 3 times weekly.
- Encourage schools to offer physical education to all students, and have students sign up when this is an elective.
- Encourage walking and bike riding to friends' homes and stores when safe.
- Plan physical activities together as a family.
- Get a pet and plan to walk the pet daily.
- Limit television and other similar sedentary activities to no more than 2 hours daily.
- On days home, allow the child to watch television for up to 1 hour, and then insist that 1 hour of reading, 1 hour of physical activity, and 1 hour of socializing with others take place before returning to more television.

A growing number of children engage in "extreme" sports, those that carry a high degree of risk and have not traditionally been common. Some examples are mountain biking, three wheeling, ski racing, snowboarding through trees and on courses with pikes and other challenges, ice climbing, rock climbing, and wakeboarding. Although the nurse is probably unable to dissuade youth from engaging in these activities, safety measures should be emphasized. Find out what protective gear the youth wears and what is recommended. Keep at hand examples of stories of youth who have been saved by use of such gear. Encourage the youth to engage in sports activities only when others are present and to have a plan for emergencies, including a working cell phone, leaving information with an adult about plans and expected return, and planning for harsh weather with items such as emergency blankets, gear, and food. Encourage the youth to talk with parents and other adults about the risks and responsibilities of these activities.

Culture 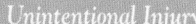 *Unintentional Injury*

Striking ethnic disparity rates exist in unintentional injury among children. These differences are due mainly to living in impoverished communities rather than any innate biological variations. While the unintentional injury rate in children under 14 years of age declined 39% from 1987 to 2000, the smallest reductions were among American Indian/Alaska Natives (20% decline) and African American children (36% decline). Higher reductions were seen in Asian/Pacific Islanders (52% decline) and White children (39% decline). African Americans and Native Americans have rates of injury 1.5 times those of White children (National Safe Kids, 2007). What are the major causes of unintentional injury in your community and state? What ethnic and age groups are at greatest risk? How can you integrate teaching in your practice that is specific to the findings in your community?

and reward children for helmet use, and can assist families to find helmets at a price they can afford. Education should take place in offices and clinics, in school settings, and throughout the community. Nurses can support legislation for helmet use, evaluate proper fits of helmets, and work for incentives and low-cost helmets (Rezendes, 2006). Other physical activities that require special protective gear are listed in Box 17–1.

Nurses can identify youth behaviors in communities and work with schools and other community groups to establish ed-

BOX 17–1 Sports and Activities Requiring Safety Gear

- Rollerblading
- Skateboarding
- Roller hockey
- Ice hockey
- Football
- Soccer
- Baseball
- Scooters
- Skiing or snowboarding

ucational programs. Efforts should also include adequate conditioning for sports, proper treatment of injuries, prevention of overuse injuries, and assessment of risky activities.

■ BODY ART

Body art in the form of painting, tattooing, and piercing has been donned by humans throughout history. However, there has recently been a resurgence of interest in this decorative art by teens. Many adolescents have multiple body piercings and tattoos and may perform these decorations on themselves or friends.

Approximately 51% of adolescents and young adults have piercings, and 22% have tattoos (Mayers & Chiffriller, 2008). In some states, teens must be 18 years of age or have parental permission to obtain body art, but students often report that it is easy to have an adult present who signs and claims to be a parent. Only in some states are tattoo and body piercing businesses required to be licensed and comply with certain regulations. Remember that Amy, who is described in the opening scenario, had her piercing done by a friend. Amy demonstrates some common characteristics of teens who choose to use body art. It may be seen as a way to establish individualism and independence, and helps some teens to feel part of a peer group. Multiple tattoos and piercings are common, as is the case with Amy (Figure 17–7 ➤).

Body art is a common source of infections with skin pathogens, as well as hepatitis B and C. Body piercing and sharing of hardware can be a method of transmission of hepatitis C (Centers for Disease Control and Prevention, 2008b), a disease that may not even become manifested until years later (see Chapter 25 ∞ for a discussion of hepatitis). It can be a source of HIV if proper techniques are not followed. Piercings in parts of the body such as the mouth or navel are most prone to bacterial infection and continued redness and irritation. Serious

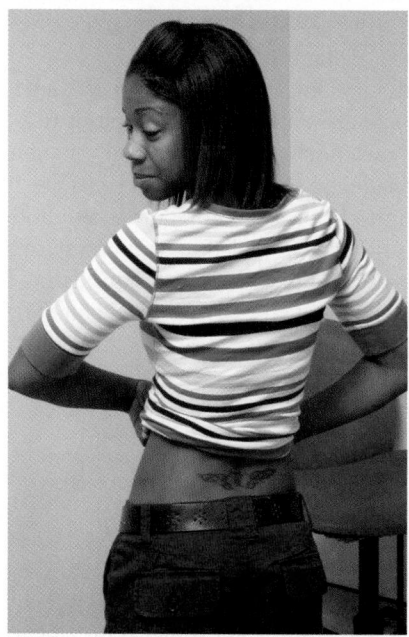

FIGURE 17–7 ➤ Talk openly with adolescents about their health and teach them to avoid health risks connected with tattoos and piercings.

systemic infections such as endocarditis have occurred after some piercings (Leman & Plattner, 2007; Armstrong, DeBoer, & Cetta, 2008). The pierced site may not appear infected, but transfer of organisms causes serious infection and heart damage. Common infective agents include *Neisseria, Staphylococcus, Pseudomonas,* and *Streptococcus* (Larzo & Poe, 2006). When noting signs of systemic infection such as fever, weakness, malaise, and arthralgia (see Chapter 21 ∞ for a full discussion of endocarditis), gather history about body piercings and refer for immediate care to the primary health care provider. Pierced tongues can lead to chipped teeth or even be the cause of choking if jewelry is dislodged from the site.

Prior to getting a tattoo, the teen should consider the relationship of the tattoo to future lifestyle changes. Advise teens to avoid tattooing the name of a person or musical group since relationships change and tastes in music evolve. Be sure they know the meaning of phrases, foreign words, or Asian symbols. Advise them to consider the visibility of the tattoo and its effect on future employment. Tattoos on the face, neck, or other readily visible places may be a detriment during employment interviews. Tattoos should always be considered permanent. Methods for removal may be costly, painful, and unsuccessful.

Another form of body art that is regarded as disfigurement is **branding** or scarification. In this process, the skin is burned to result in a scar. Usually a desired sign, symbol, or word is inscribed. Results are usually not precise and do not adhere to expected designs. This procedure is done on the self or friend, using common household metal implements heated in fires or stoves. Others cut themselves in the form of a desired design, a process called **cutting**. This type of self-harm or self-injury is performed with razor blades, knives, scissors, broken glass, needles, or sharp pencils (Aguirre & Smith, 2007). These self-mutilation practices can result in infection, often do not yield the desired result, and may indicate other mental health problems. Youth who use cutting or other self-mutilation should be referred for further assessment by mental health care providers or counselors (Williams & Bydalek, 2007).

Since teens may choose to obtain body art even if parents object and if there are state laws to prohibit or make it difficult, nursing care must focus on providing information to the teen, assessing sites, identifying infections, and referring if needed (see Families Want to Know: Care for Tattoos and Body Piercings). Care is almost always provided in community settings such as clinics or schools. Ask teens if they are considering body art, because they often do not seek advice before obtaining the art, and may therefore not get adequate teaching. Ask about piercings before all medical procedures since metal needs to be removed for surgery, magnetic resonance imaging, and some other tests.

■ SEXUAL ORIENTATION

Adolescence is a time of identifying emerging sexuality. Most teens establish relationships with members of the opposite sex and learn how to interact in ways that are guided by their peer group, family, and culture. For some youth, the transition into adult sexuality is more challenging, as they feel emotional and sexual attraction to people of the same sex (**homosexuality**). The

Families Want to Know
Care for Tattoos and Body Piercings

Before the Procedure

■ Visit several studios to make comparisons of technique, quality, and cleanliness.

■ Ask to watch a tattoo or piercing done on someone else.

■ Determine the sterilization and hygiene practices of the artist.

■ Ask if the artist is licensed and trained.

■ Look at pictures of completed art and talk with former clients.

■ Insist that new, sterile equipment be opened in front of the person to be decorated.

■ Consider if this permanent body decoration is desired for a lifetime.

■ Consider what the tattoo or piercing will look like in several years.

■ Consider the possible side effects such as infection, future dislike for the art, or allergy to dyes or metals.

■ Be sure that the hepatitis B vaccination is completed before the procedure.

■ Be aware that no immunization is available to protect against hepatitis C and HIV.

Care After the Procedure

■ Touch the area only after careful handwashing.

■ Keep the area elevated and use ice for the first 2 days to minimize swelling.

■ Avoid contact with another person's body fluids until well healed.

■ Turn the piercing jewelry gently several times daily using washed hands.

■ Use antibacterial mouthwash, cleaner, or ointment as recommended.

■ Avoid pressure and rubbing on the site (such as belts on navel piercings).

■ Watch carefully for signs of infection and report them to a health care provider:
  • Increased redness
  • Swelling
  • Pain
  • Hot feeling
  • Discharge

■ Ask the artist how long healing will take. It varies from 2 months in the mouth to 6–8 months in the navel.

■ Metal is dangerous during some medical procedures such as magnetic resonance imaging (MRI) or during surgery. Be sure to tell doctors and nurses about the piercings when hospitalized or receiving medical care, especially if they are not readily visible.

■ If you decide to remove a piece of jewelry soon after placement, then the skin may heal with only a slight scar.

term *gay* is often used for homosexual males and *lesbian* for homosexual females. Other youth are *bisexual,* or attracted to both males and females, and some are *transgendered,* an imprecise term for individuals who cross gender lines. The initials **LGBT** are sometimes used to refer to these minority sexuality choices, and the acronym **LGBQ** is sometimes used for lesbian, gay, bisexual, or questioning. About 3% of high school youth report same-sex activity (Remafedi, 2006).

Sexual attractions and practices that are different from the mainstream are not deviant, but may be viewed as part of a continuum of sexual expression. Although genetic, biologic, and other factors have all been investigated for their influence on sexual preference, no definitive influences have been clearly identified (Santrock, 2008).

LGBT/Q youth are at risk for a variety of problems related to emotional and physical health. These include rejection by family members and peers, verbal harassment, sexual abuse and physical assault, a high rate of suicide, depression, substance abuse, a high rate of homelessness, and sexual risks of HIV and other sexually transmitted diseases. Their health risks need to be identified and appropriate care provided in welcoming and nonjudgmental health care facilities (Meckler, Elliot, Kanouse, et al., 2006).

Nurses can provide health care for youth who are LGBT in a variety of settings. Terminology in assessment should be gender-free. Ask the youth, "Do you have one or more sexual partners?" rather than "Do you have a boyfriend?" When youth identify as LGBT, usual care of all kinds should be provided, including preventive care such as immunizations, sports assessments, and injury prevention teaching. Be alert that the youth may have additional health challenges. Ask about peer and parental support; refer to support groups if needed. Provide resources when the teen is homeless, depressed, or suicidal (see Chapter 28 ∞). Perform testing for sexually transmitted diseases if sexual contact is occurring and teach preventive measures. Foster a positive sense of self-esteem through encouraging activities such as sports, music, and friendships with peers.

Health Promotion

LGBT/Q youth report more depression, drug use, and bullying than other youth; a positive school climate mitigates these risks (Birkett, Espelage, & Koenig, 2009). School nurses can lead efforts to display signs in schools that are inclusive of all sexual preferences. How else can school nurses create a positive school climate that will reduce homophobia and welcome all students to the school and health care offered?

■ VIOLENCE AND ITS EFFECTS ON CHILDREN

Violence is a threatened or actual use of physical force that leads to potential or actual physical or emotional trauma. In the past several years, adults and children alike have been shocked by the violent episodes in homes, schools, and communities. There are many types of violence to which children may be exposed on a regular basis. Children can be the recipients of violence during child abuse and homicides, and they themselves can perform acts of violence on others. They may be touched by violence when parents are killed in gang conflicts, in terrorist attacks, or in wars. The effects of violence are far-reaching and ongoing; they permeate the victim's entire lifetime. This section explores certain types of violence affecting children.

Schools and Communities

At a time when firearm deaths are decreasing overall, unintentional deaths and suicides have increased among children. Many of these deaths are committed with firearms found in the home; about 10% of deaths in children are due to firearm injury (Baxley & Miller, 2006). Approximately 40% of households with chil-

dren have guns, and in 25% of those homes the firearms are stored loaded or are not secured under lock. Additionally, it is common for parents to report that children do not know firearm locations when the children are actually able to state the locations and have handled the guns (Baxley & Miller, 2006).

Nursing Alert

When a group of children is attacked or killed in a school shooting, this tragic occurrence gains media attention. However, this tragedy is really part of daily life in many separate settings across the country. About 8 children are killed by a firearm every day in the United States, or about 56 children per week. An additional 200–300 children experience nonfatal firearm injuries (Children's Defense Fund, 2008). Nurses must intervene in this national tragedy. Become familiar with firearm injury statistics in your community. Teach children, youth, and parents about the dangers of firearms. Urge safe storage. Help schools establish programs to ensure safety for students.

Homicide among children has gained attention in past years due to several notable shootings at schools and universities. Although homicide is an extreme example, other types of violence exist. Children report being threatened verbally and with guns or knives at home, in schools, and in neighborhoods. They may be beaten up, bullied, or harassed. An estimated 3 million children are exposed to acts of domestic violence by adults in their homes (Kolar & Davey, 2007). They may be subjected to dangerous situations in their neighborhoods or during times of homelessness. Date rape or other violence during dating is reported by up to 9% of teens, while 7.5% have been forced to have sexual intercourse (Centers for Disease Control and Prevention, 2006c). Several of these types of violence are specifically addressed in the following sections.

Family risk factors have been identified as more commonly seen in situations when violence has been committed against children. In addition, children who commit violence more commonly have ready access to firearms, are exposed to violence in the home or community, engage in violent media viewing, and have poor self-esteem or depression.

Realizing the impact of violence on and by children, several federal health care initiatives have begun to assist in lowering violence. Some programs have been helpful, and incidents of homicides and most other violence have begun to decrease. Programs that are most successful include individual children, parents, schools, and communities. School health professionals are instrumental in identification of signs of violence (Table 17–5). Provide resources for families and children to decrease violence.

War and Terrorism

Internationally, 40 million children experience violence each year. Decreasing violence against children has become a focus of both the World Health Organization and the United Nations (World Health Organization, 2007). Common forms of violence worldwide are war and terrorism. War affects children in several ways: parents leave home to fight in wars, children may be forced to take on adult roles in families when members leave, children

TABLE 17–5 Assessment Questions to Identify Violence Risk and Protective Factors

Microsystem

- Have you been hurt by your parents or anyone else at home?
- When was the last time you were teased or bullied at school? What did you do?
- Have you ever brought a gun, knife, or other weapon to school?
- Do you have access to guns and knives at home? At friends' houses?
- What stresses are there in your family now?
- Tell me about school—what do you like and dislike?

Mesosystem

- Do your parents attend school meetings? Talk with your teachers?
- Do you participate in any church, synagogue, or mosque services?
- Do you participate in any community activities?

Exosystem

- What stresses do your parents have at work, in their families, or with their health or finances?
- Do you feel like your school helps to keep you safe?
- Are there plans for handling violent episodes at your school if they were to occur?
- Do you feel safe in your neighborhood?
- Where would you go or who would you call if you felt unsafe or were hurt and no one was at home?

become orphans when parents are killed, and some children are trained and forced to fight in battles, carry messages, or otherwise engage in combat themselves (UNICEF, 2009). Depression and mental health problems are common among youth who have experienced war (Bolton, Bass, Betancourt, et al., 2007). Children who live through wars or have a parent or sibling die in war can be permanently affected by these events.

Nursing Alert

Risk factors common in families with child victims of violence include:

- History of mental illness, domestic violence, incarceration, or substance abuse in the home
- Family stresses
- Inadequate childcare or supervision
- Inadequate family social support
- Use of corporal punishment and other inappropriate discipline methods for the child
- Child abuse
- Access to firearms
- Gang membership in family or neighborhood
- High exposure to media violence
- Child hyperactivity and other developmental behavioral disorders

Adapted from: American Academy of Pediatrics, Committee on Injury, Violence and Poison Prevention. (2009). Policy statement: Role of the pediatrician in violence prevention. Pediatrics, 124, 393–402.

Another type of violence is terrorism. The events in the United States of September 11, 2001, and other examples in many countries take a large toll on the mental health of children

and adolescents. The response of children to terrorism is not well studied. Disasters such as the World Trade Center attack can lead to sleep and eating problems, fears of entering tall buildings, regression in school performance and other behaviors, and posttraumatic stress disorder (see Chapter 28 ∞). Most children and adolescents experience profound sadness, cling to adults who provide security, and have a variety of somatic complaints.

Understanding the response of children and adolescents to war and terrorist events can assist health care providers in providing interventions to assist children and families. Some key factors include the following:

- Dose and exposure have a strong impact on the child's response. Repeated events or more intense experiences, such as being personally involved in a shooting episode, create the greatest psychological trauma. Consider that constant exposure by repeated viewing of war and terrorism in the media magnifies the trauma for viewers.
- Children individualize their experiences related to their developmental levels. Younger children are very affected by physical separation from parents whereas older children may worry more about repeat events and their future. Much more research is needed to examine the long-term effects of trauma on various age groups.
- In addition to development, the child's prior experiences with stress may contribute both risk and protective factors to new traumatic situations.
- Interventions to assist children can focus on them, their parents, and others in the community, such as teachers. Interventions should be directed at different phases of violence, such as pre-event preparation (emergency preparation and training) and post-event activity (offering special services and resources).

Several resources have been developed for families and health professionals to help children deal with war and violence. See the companion website for more information.

Bullying

One type of violence that frequently occurs in schools is **bullying**, or aggressive behavior that is intended to cause harm, exists in a relationship with imbalance of power, and occurs repeatedly. Bullies are aggressive and impulsive, and need to dominate others. Bullying behaviors include verbal abuse (taunting, teasing), name calling, threats, spreading rumors, social exclusion, and physical abuse (hitting, shoving, kicking, tripping). About 16% of children in a large national survey had suffered bullying, most commonly in grades 6 through 8, and more frequently among males. Almost 30% of 11- to 15-year-olds have been either victims or perpetrators of bullying. Almost 75% of children from 6 to 13 years report being bullied and 34% report bullying in the past year. Up to 160,000 U.S. children may miss school every day in efforts to avoid bullying (Bauer, Herrenkohl, Lozano, et al., 2006). Although bullying is most commonly reported in schools, it can occur in neighborhoods as children go to and from school, on school buses, in sports teams, and in other settings.

- Indoor air pollution from dust mites, molds, ETS, radon, wood smoke, and other sources.
- Fish that contain high amounts of mercury (e.g., shark, tilefish, and swordfish).
- Plastics containing phthalates and bisphenol A (BPA). Children are exposed from the linings of canned foods (ready-to-feed formulas), baby bottles, and intravenous tubing (Galvez et al., 2009).

NURSING MANAGEMENT

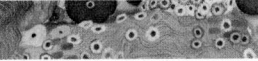

Nurses are instrumental in identifying exposure to environmental toxic agents. Inquire about:

- Parental occupation and whether it involves harmful substances such as dust and chemicals
- Proximity of child's residence to power plants, industrial plants, or toxic waste areas
- Age of home (homes built before 1978 or renovated in the last 6 months are at risk for contamination with chemicals)
- Safety items used in the home to detect radon, carbon monoxide, and smoke
- Child or family member with hobby requiring use of toxic materials (e.g., pesticides with gardening, lead solder for stained glass work, or glue with model building)
- Child's consumption of nonfood products

Assist parents to reduce their child's exposure to environmental toxins. Children should have their hands washed before all meals and snacks, and they should be discouraged from putting nonfood objects into their mouths. If parents work with toxic materials, they should be encouraged to shower and change clothing before leaving work and to wash work clothes separately (Meadows-Oliver, 2006). See the companion website for other prevention ideas.

When delayed development or behavioral problems are evident, consider the possibility of environmental exposure and refer for blood testing and further evaluation. Test blood levels for contaminants such as lead (see next section). Hair, urine, and other testing may be possible as well. Identification of the toxic exposure and its removal from the environment are critical. **Chelation**, administration of a drug that competes with blood and tissue proteins to bind with a substance (e.g., mercury or lead) and increase excretion of that substance in the urine, may be possible. Perform periodic growth and developmental measurements on the child and ensure return for further blood tests and other monitoring.

Lead Poisoning

Lead poisoning has been successfully prevented in the majority of the United States, with a substantial decline in lead levels since the mid-1970s. The average blood lead level (BLL) for children is now 1.9 mcg/dL, down from 15 mcg/dL in 1976. The removal of lead from gasoline and paint in the 1970s reduced lead exposure for children. About 1.6% of children between ages 1 and 5 years have BLLs above the recommended upper level of 10 mcg/dL. There is no known safe level of lead exposure, as even children with BLLs below 10 mcg/dL have been reported to have a de-

> ### Culture | *Lead Sources*
>
> Potential sources of lead include ayurvedic medicine; Chinese and Middle Eastern herbal products for teething, colic, and gastrointestinal distress; and eye cosmetics (kohl, surma) imported from Asia, the Middle East, Africa, and Mexico (Warniment, Tsang, & Galazka, 2010). See the companion website for a more complete list of products containing lead.

crease in intelligence quotient (IQ) (Advisory Committee on Childhood Lead Poisoning, 2007). Children are exposed to lead when they ingest contaminated food, water, and soil or inhale contaminated dust. Children are at greater risk for elevated BLLs because they absorb and retain more lead in proportion to their weight than adults.

> ### Clinical Tip
>
> Paint chips and dust from deteriorating surfaces of homes built before 1978 (before lead paint was banned) is the most common source of exposure for preschool children. External lead paint chips and airborne lead from leaded gasoline have contaminated the soil. Other potential sources of lead include parental occupations and hobbies that involve lead exposure (e.g., plumbing, battery manufacturing, furniture refinishing, stained glass work, pottery glazing); food prepared in improperly fired pottery; drinking water from lead pipes, lead-lined tanks, or teapots soldered with lead; imported toys; and antique toys, cribs, or furniture (Woolf, Goldman, & Bellinger, 2007).

Once in the body, lead accumulates in the blood, soft tissues (kidney, bone marrow, liver, and brain), bones, and teeth. Lead that is absorbed by the bones and teeth is released slowly; thus, exposure to even small doses, over time, can result in dangerously high levels of lead in the body. Lead interferes with normal cell function, primarily of the nervous system, blood cells, and kidneys.

Clinical manifestations depend on the blood level. Few symptoms are noted in children with a blood level lower than 10 mcg/dL, even though impaired mental function can occur at those levels. Anorexia, abdominal pain, vomiting, and constipation may be experienced by children with a blood level higher than 20 mcg/dL. Hyperactivity is noted in children with a history of lead poisoning or with current blood levels of 20–29 mcg/dL or higher (Markowitz, 2007). Neurologic effects of lead poisoning include decreased IQ scores, cognitive deficits, antisocial behavior, and poor education outcomes (Woolf et al., 2007). Severe lead poisoning leading to encephalopathy, coma, and death can occur at BLLs greater than 70 mcg/dL in children and is now rare.

Screening for elevated BLLs is now recommended for all children enrolled in Medicaid and others identified at high risk (based on a state or local risk assessment). Children should be screened at 12 and 24 months, or between 3 and 6 years if no previous screening has been performed. In some higher risk communities, screening is performed at younger ages or more frequently (Advisory Committee on Childhood Lead Poisoning, 2007).

A BLL below 10 mcg/dL is considered acceptable. Obtain an environmental history for children with BLLs between 10 and

19 mcg/dL to identify removable sources of lead. Follow-up testing is required. Children with BLLs between 20 and 69 mcg/dL require a full medical evaluation, including a detailed environmental and behavioral history, physical examination, and tests for anemia and iron deficiency. Interventions to remove sources of lead from the child's environment are necessary. Neurologic and developmental monitoring is initiated. Chelation therapy is administered for children with BLLs greater than 44 mcg/dL. Four potential medications are used for chelation therapy: calcium disodium ethylenediamine tetraacetate (CaNa$_2$ EDTA), dimercaprol (BAL), meso-2,3-dimercaptosuccinic (DMSA), or d-penicillamine. When the BLL is between 45 and 69 mcg/dL, DMSA is prescribed 5 days at a high dose or 14 days at a lower dose. Alternatively the child must be hospitalized and CaNa$_2$ EDTA is prescribed for 5 days, followed by a rest period and a second chelation treatment. When the BLL is greater than 70 mcg/dL and symptoms of lead poisoning are present, the child is hospitalized and CaNa$_2$ EDTA is administered. In some cases BAL and CaNa$_2$ EDTA are both prescribed (Woolf et al., 2007). Lead hazards in the home must be reduced before the child is discharged. Long-term follow-up of children receiving chelation therapy is essential.

NURSING MANAGEMENT
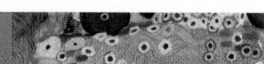

Nursing care centers on screening, education, and follow-up. Nurses often work with public health officials to plan screening for children at high risk of lead exposure. Ask parents about the child's development, eating habits, and potential risk for lead exposure. Educate parents about sources of lead in the environment and techniques to reduce exposure such as the following housekeeping interventions:

- Damp mopping (floors, window sills, baseboards, and wooden furniture)
- Washing the child's hands and face before meals and naptime
- Washing toys and pacifiers frequently
- Removing shoes before entering the house

Teach parents the importance of managing the child's diet. Children who have dietary deficiencies in iron, calcium, vitamin C, or zinc are more susceptible to injury from lead ingestion (Woolf et al., 2007). The child should eat meals at regular intervals, as lead is absorbed more readily on an empty stomach.

Be sure that parents understand the importance of BLL follow-up testing. Referral to a lead prevention program and social services may also be appropriate.

Expected outcomes of nursing care for the child with lead or other environmental contaminants include the following: the child exhibits normal growth, motor, and cognitive development; adequate nutritional intake is ensured for the child; toxins are removed from the child's environment; and the family describes measures to establish a safe environment for the child.

Poisoning

Nearly 2.5 million poisonings occur annually in the United States, and 90% occur in the individual's residence. About 64% (1.6 million) of all poisoning exposures occur in children and adolescents less than age 20 years, with 51% of all poisoning exposures occurring in children under 6 years. However, only 8.2% of poisonings in children and adolescents less than age 20 years were fatal (Bronstein, Spyker, Cantilena, et al., 2008).

Etiology and Pathophysiology

Young children are at risk for ingestion of foreign substances because of their characteristic behaviors, which involve exploration of the environment. Infants and toddlers commonly place objects in their mouths. Although most poisons are ingested, other routes of contamination include dermal, inhalation, and ocular.

The five most common classifications of poisons ingested by children less than 6 years are cosmetics and personal care products, household cleaning products, analgesics, miscellaneous foreign bodies and toys, and topical preparations (Bronstein et al., 2008). Other poisons include plants (e.g., Boston ivy, poinsettia, philodendron, lily-of-the-valley, daffodil bulbs, azalea, and rhododendron), cough and cold preparations, other medications, pesticides, and rodent killers. Some household products are nontoxic and cause little harm; however, products that contain caustic agents or toxic chemicals can cause irreversible damage or death. The Poison Prevention Packaging Act of 1970 mandated child protective devices on the container of all potentially toxic substances, resulting in a reduction in poison exposures among young children. Pharmaceutical agents are the most frequent cause of death in children less than age 20 years (Bronstein et al., 2008).

Nursing Alert

Parents who suspect that their child has ingested a poison should immediately call the Poison Control Center (PCC) at 1-800-222-1222. This number can be accessed from anywhere in the United States and Puerto Rico, and the caller is connected to the closest poison control center.

The PCC will advise parents about treatment to begin at home, and if the child needs treatment in the emergency department. If the child has vomited, the vomitus should be brought to the emergency department. With older children, the possibility of intentional ingestion needs to be considered.

Clinical Manifestations

The manifestations of poisoning depend on the toxin, such as altered mental status, respiratory or cardiac symptoms, seizures, vital sign changes, and gastrointestinal symptoms. Symptoms may be mild initially, but toxicity may be delayed as the toxins are absorbed or have a delayed mechanism of action. See Clinical Manifestations: Commonly Ingested Toxic Agents.

COLLABORATIVE CARE
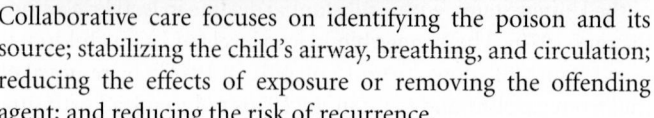

Collaborative care focuses on identifying the poison and its source; stabilizing the child's airway, breathing, and circulation; reducing the effects of exposure or removing the offending agent; and reducing the risk of recurrence.

Diagnostic Tests

A history of medications (including over-the-counter) and household toxins that the child could have accessed should be

Clinical Manifestations
Commonly Ingested Toxic Agents

Type	Sources	Clinical Manifestations	Emergency Care Clinical Therapy
Corrosives (strong acids and alkaline products that cause chemical burns of mucosal surfaces)	Batteries Household cleaners Clinitest tablets Denture cleaners Bleach Toilet bowl cleaners	Vomiting Drooling, difficulty swallowing Burns and pain in the mouth, throat, or stomach Edema of lips, tongue, and pharynx (may cause respiratory obstruction) Agitation	Do not induce vomiting! Dilute toxin with water to prevent further damage.
Hydrocarbons (organic compounds that contain carbon and hydrogen; most are distillates of petroleum)	Gasoline Kerosene Furniture polish Lighter fluid Paint thinners	Gagging and coughing Nausea, vomiting Altered mental status Respiratory symptoms associated with aspiration (tachypnea, cyanosis, retractions)	Do not induce vomiting. Use gastric lavage only for highly toxic hydrocarbons. Provide supportive respiratory care.
Acetaminophen	Many over-the-counter products	Nausea, vomiting, anorexia Sweating Pallor Right upper quadrant pain and tenderness with liver involvement Coagulation and bilirubin abnormalities	Admininister the antidote N-acetylcysteine. Activated charcoal may be used.
Salicylate	Products containing aspirin	Nausea, vomiting Dehydration Diaphoresis Rapid respirations High temperature Bleeding tendencies Agitation, restlessness, confusion Coma	Administer activated charcoal. Correct electrolyte abnormalities. Administer intravenous sodium bicarbonate and fluids.
Iron	Prenatal vitamins or iron supplements	Vomiting, diarrhea Abdominal pain Hematemesis and bloody stools in severe ingestions Drowsiness Hypovolemic shock	Activated charcoal may be used. Administer intravenous fluids and sodium bicarbonate. Deferoxamine chelation therapy may be used.

Data from: Rodgers, G. C., Condurache, T., Reed, M. D., Bestic, M., & Gal, P. (2007). Poisonings. In R. M. Kliegman, R. E. Behrman, H. B. Jenson, & B. F. Stanton, Nelson textbook of pediatrics (18th ed., pp. 339–357). Philadelphia: Elsevier Saunders.

obtained, especially acetaminophen, salicylates, opioids, hydrocarbons, caustic agents, and antidepressants. Obtain information about where and when the child was found, how long unsupervised, history of depression or suicide, allergies, and any other medical problems. Various diagnostic tests are used based on the suspected poison, such as the following: serum glucose, electrocardiogram, serum electrolytes, arterial blood gas, urinalysis, and blood toxicology screens.

Clinical Therapy
In the emergency department the child is evaluated for any life-threatening condition and carefully monitored for changes as some toxins take time to produce symptoms. The goal of treatment is to prevent further absorption of the poison and to reverse or eliminate its effects. The Poison Control Center is consulted to obtain guidance for treatment. An antidote is prescribed if one is available. While no longer routine therapy, children may be treated with gastric lavage or activated charcoal (if within one hour of ingestion). Cathartics or whole bowel irrigation with polyethylene glycol may be used for heavy metals or for long-acting or sustained-release medications (McGregor, Parkar, & Rao, 2009). Vomiting is rarely induced because too much of the poison may be absorbed before the agent causing vomiting is effective.

Nursing Alert

Antidotes and agonists are available for some ingestions, including the following (McGregor et al., 2009):

- Acetaminophen—N-acetylcysteine
- Calcium channel blockers—calcium chloride, glucagon
- Digoxin—digoxin immune Fab
- Opioids—Naloxone
- Organophosphates—atropine
- Warfarin or rodent killers—vitamin K

Children with severe poisoning are admitted to the intensive care unit to carefully monitor the child and provide supportive care for the toxin effects (e.g., arrhythmias, depressed respirations, seizures, hypotension, and electrolyte abnormalities) (Hanhan, 2008). Potential complications of poisoning depend on the toxin and can include respiratory or cardiac arrest, liver failure, renal failure, seizures, and esophageal or tracheal burns.

NURSING MANAGEMENT

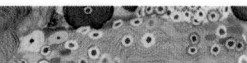

Nursing care focuses on initial emergent care and stabilization of the child with poisoning, and prevention of repeated poisoning.

Nursing Assessment and Diagnosis

Obtain the history about the child's suspected ingestion substance, time, amount, and symptoms. Initial assessment focuses on airway, breathing, circulation, and mental status. Perform a complete physical assessment observing for signs of poisoning such as drooling, diaphoresis, wheezing, respiratory distress, stridor, abnormally large or small pupil size, burns on the lips or mouth, and unusual breath odor. Assess any emesis for the presence of medication or other ingested substances. Determine the child's height and weight.

Nursing diagnoses for the child with ingestion of a toxic substance may include:

- Impaired Gas Exchange related to effects of toxic substance
- Risk for Aspiration related to depressed neurological status and vomiting
- Acute Confusion related to effects of toxic substance
- Risk for Decreased Cardiac Output related to effects of toxic substance
- Risk for Injury related to repeated occurrence of poisoning
- Interrupted Family Processes related to poisoning of a family member

Planning and Implementation

Emergency care focuses on airway and hemodynamic stability, removal of toxic agents, and support of the family. The child is attached to pulse oximetry and a cardiorespiratory monitor. An intravenous line is often started for the administration of an antidote. When activated charcoal is prescribed, it may be in a ready-to-drink solution in an opaque container or it may need to be mixed with sorbitol or apple juice to encourage consumption. Cover the cup and provide a straw so the child does not see the black liquid and to prevent spillage.

Provide support to the parents who may have feelings of anger, guilt, or fear regarding the poisoning event. Wait until the child is out of immediate danger before questioning parents in detail about the incident.

Family Education

Discuss with parents the need to supervise infants and young children at all times. Ask parents how medicines and cleaning agents are stored and whether the house contains any plants. Teach parents proper methods of childproofing the home. The

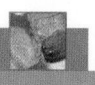

Families Want to Know
Avoiding Childhood Poisoning

Families with children require instructions for avoiding childhood poisoning. Teach family members these interventions to help avoid childhood poisonings:

- Place household cleaners, medications, vitamins, and other potentially poisonous substances out of the reach of children or in locked cabinets.
- Use warning stickers such as Mr. Yuk on all containers.
- Buy products with child-resistant caps.
- Store products in their original containers. Never place household cleansers or other toxic products in food and beverage containers.
- Use caution when visiting other settings that are not childproofed (e.g., grandparents' homes). Remember that visitors may have pills in their purses or pockets that are easily reached by children.

poison control center phone number should be programmed in or beside every phone in the home. Suggest measures for preventing recurrence of poisoning. See Families Want to Know: Avoiding Childhood Poisoning.

Ask parents if syrup of ipecac is stored in the home. Ipecac is no longer standard home treatment of poisons. Instruct the family to return the ipecac to the pharmacy for disposal.

Evaluation

Expected outcomes for nursing care of the child with poisoning include:

- The child maintains effective gas exchange and respiratory pattern.
- The child is free from wheezing, coughing, pneumonia, or other signs indicating aspiration.
- The child's heart rate and blood pressure remain stable and appropriate for age.
- Neurological status is appropriate for age.
- The family and child (if older) verbalize understanding of preventive measures and demonstrate measures to improve home environment safety.

Ingestion of Foreign Objects

Nearly 96,000 cases of ingestion of foreign objects occur annually among children under age 6 years (Bronstein et al., 2008). Coins are the most common objects ingested (Uyemura, 2005). Pins, parts of toys, batteries, and bones from foods are some other commonly ingested objects. The ingestion may be witnessed or the child may report swallowing an object. Small, round, smooth objects often cause no distress unless aspirated. (See Chapter 20 ∞ for care of aspirated foreign bodies.)

Many foreign body ingestions are asymptomatic; however, some objects ingested can cause symptoms. If the foreign body is lodged in the esophagus, the child may present with substernal pain, drooling, and dysphagia. Some children develop wheezing or coughing. Ingestion of a sharp object may result in a perforation. Erosion of the mucosa and strictures may develop at the site of a retained foreign body, such as a button battery.

Bowel obstruction may occur in some cases, causing abdominal distention and pain.

Clinical Judgment

If a foreign body is aspirated rather than ingested, what respiratory symptoms would potentially be present?

Many ingested foreign bodies in children are radio-opaque, so radiographs of the neck, chest, esophagus, and abdomen may be useful in verifying an ingestion and identifying the location of the object.

Most foreign bodies pass spontaneously through the gastrointestinal system and are eliminated through stool. A lodged esophageal foreign body may be removed by endoscopy or advanced into the stomach to reduce complications. Endoscopic examination and retrieval of the ingested foreign body is often urgently performed for sharp objects, magnets, and button batteries.

NURSING MANAGEMENT

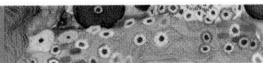

Nursing care centers on supporting the child, collaborating in the identification and removal of the foreign body, and teaching the child and family measures to reduce reoccurrence. Assess the child's airway, breathing, and circulatory status. Assess the child for any symptoms of the ingestion, such as drooling, wheezing, substernal pain, dysphagia, and coughing. Obtain a history about the event, what was ingested, and any symptoms from the family if the ingestion was witnessed.

Explain the needed radiologic studies to the child and family and what information may be discovered. If an endoscopic examination or retrieval is necessary, prepare the child and family for the procedure.

When the foreign object is in the stomach and expected to pass through the intestines without complications, teach the family and child how to monitor the stools for the object. Provide and suggest the use of tongue blades to examine stools for the foreign body. If the object has not passed within the expected time frame (generally 48 hours), encourage the family to return for a radiologic examination to assess the object's progress through the gastrointestinal tract.

Encourage the family to establish a safe home environment for the child and prevent a future ingestion. Advise them to keep all small items out of the child's reach and to ensure the child is monitored at all times.

Expected outcomes for nursing care include removal of the foreign body, reduced risk of a future ingestion, and family description of measures to promote a safe environment for the child.

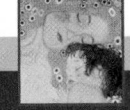

Chapter Highlights

- Many of the major morbidities and mortalities of childhood and adolescence are related to social and environmental factors.
- The theory of ecologic development provides a framework to assess the interactions of children with factors in their environments.
- The theory of resilience examines risk and protective factors of children in order to formulate interventions to assist the child dealing with health problems related to social conditions.
- Poverty is a pervasive and important risk factor that influences many health outcomes.
- Some families that are poor experience homelessness and are at risk for a number of health problems.
- Stressful experiences, family structure, and the community all influence the health of children.
- Tobacco use is high among youth, and the most common time for initiation of tobacco use is the middle school years.
- Tobacco prevention and cessation programs are needed throughout the school years.
- Substance abuse by alcohol and drugs occurs in childhood and adolescence and compounds many health risks.
- A major contributor to overweight and other health problems is the lack of physical activity among children.
- Protective equipment can reduce the number and severity of injuries during risky physical activities.

- Teens need information about body art safety procedures if they choose this method of self-expression.
- Violence can be directed at children, and children can be the perpetrators of violence.
- All families should be regularly assessed for violence, and prevention strategies should be applied when needed.
- Child abuse can take the form of physical abuse or neglect, emotional abuse or neglect, or sexual abuse.
- The nurse plans interventions for an array of abusive situations such as abandoned babies, hazing, domestic violence, and Munchausen syndrome by proxy.
- Environmental contaminants affect the health of children from the prenatal period through childhood; exposure occurs by ingestion, absorption through the skin, and inhalation.
- The most common source of lead exposure for preschool children is paint chips and dust from deteriorating surfaces of homes built before 1978.
- Young children are at risk for poisoning from the ingestion of foreign substances because of their characteristic behaviors—exploring the environment and placing objects in their mouths.
- Most ingested foreign bodies pass spontaneously through the gastrointestinal system and are eliminated in the stool.

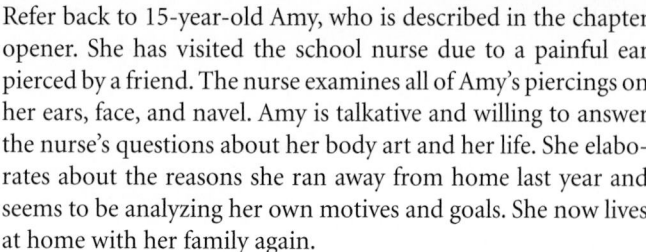

Clinical Reasoning in Action

Refer back to 15-year-old Amy, who is described in the chapter opener. She has visited the school nurse due to a painful ear pierced by a friend. The nurse examines all of Amy's piercings on her ears, face, and navel. Amy is talkative and willing to answer the nurse's questions about her body art and her life. She elaborates about the reasons she ran away from home last year and seems to be analyzing her own motives and goals. She now lives at home with her family again.

1. What is Amy's developmental stage according to Erikson? How can the adults in her life encourage her healthy psychosocial development?

2. Amy has clearly demonstrated many risk and protective factors for physical and psychosocial health. What factors place her at risk of disease or developing unhealthy lifestyles? What factors are protective of her health?

3. List at least three nursing diagnoses based on Amy's risk and protective factors. What interventions will increase her protective factors?

4. Exposure to home piercings and to body art presents several health risks. What are they? What immunization should Amy have to prevent her from acquiring a disease transmitted by blood?

See Pearson Nursing Student Resources for possible responses.

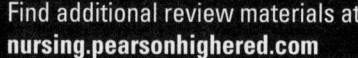

Pearson Nursing Student Resources

Find additional review materials at
nursing.pearsonhighered.com
Prepare for success with NCLEX®-style practice questions, interactive assignments and activities, web links, animations and videos, and more!

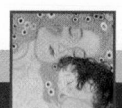

References

Add Health Study. (2007). *Add Health. The National Longitudinal Study of Adolescent Health.* Retrieved from http://www.cpc.unc.edu/addhealth

Advisory Committee on Childhood Lead Poisoning. (2007). Interpreting and managing blood lead levels <10 μg/dL in children and reducing childhood exposures to lead. *Morbidity and Mortality Weekly Report, 56*(RR08), 1–14, 16.

Aguirre, B., & Smith, B. D. (2007). Handling young patients who cut themselves. *Clinical Advisor,* August, 64–69.

American Academy of Pediatrics, Committee on Injury, Violence, and Poison Prevention. (2009). Policy statement—Role of the pediatrician in youth violence prevention. *Pediatrics.* doi: 10.1542/peds.2009-0943

American Public Health Association. (2008). *Alcohol screening and brief interventions: A guide for public health practitioners.* Washington, DC: National Highway Traffic Safety Administration, U.S. Department of Transportation.

Amos, A., & Bostock, Y. (2006). Young people, smoking and gender—a qualitative exploration. *Health Education Research.* doi:10.1093/her/cy075

Anderson, M. E., & Bogdan, G. M. (2007). Environments, indoor air quality, and children. *Pediatric Clinics of North America, 54,* 295–307.

Anderson, S. E., Economos, C. D., & Must, A. (2008). Active play and screen time in US children ages 4 to 11 years in relation to sociodemographic and weight status characteristics: A nationally representative cross-sectional analysis. *BMC Public Health, 8,* 366.

Annie E. Casey Foundation. (2007). *Kids Count 2007.* Retrieved from http://datacenter.kidscount .org/databook/

Armstrong, M. L., DeBoer, S., & Cetta, F. (2008). Infective endocarditis after body art: A review of the literature and concerns. *Journal of Adolescent Health, 43*(3), 217–225.

Backinger, C. L., Michaels, C. M., Jefferson, A. M., Fagan, P., Hurd, A. L., & Grana, R. (2007). Factors associated with recruitment and retention of youth into smoking cessation intervention studies: A review of the literature. *Health Education Research, 19.* doi: 10.1093/her/cym053

Balodis, I. M., Wynne-Edwards, K. E., & Olmstead, M. C. (2010). The other side of the curve: Examining the relationship between pre-stressor physiological responses and stress reactivity. *Psychoneuroendocrinology, 35*(9), 1363–1373.

Bauer, N. S., Herrenkohl, T. I., Lozano, P. L., Rivara, F. P., Hill, K. G., & Hawkins, J. D. (2006). Childhood bullying involvement and exposure to intimate partner violence. *Pediatrics, 118,* 235–242.

Baxley, F., & Miller, M. (2006). Parental misperceptions about children and firearms. *Archives of Pediatrics and Adolescent Medicine, 160,* 542–547.

Birkett, M., Espelage, D. L., & Koenig, B. (2009). LGB and questioning students in schools: The moderating effects of homophobic bullying and school climate on negative outcomes. *Journal of Youth and Adolescence, 38*(7), 989–1000.

Bolton, P., Bass, J., Betancourt, T., Speelman, L., Onyango, G., Clougherty, K., et al. (2007). Interventions for depression symptoms among adolescent survivors of war and displacement in northern Uganda: A randomized control trial. *Journal of the American Medical Association, 298,* 519–527.

Brodowski, M. L., Nolan, C. M., Gaudiosi, J. A., Yuan, Y. Y., Zikratova, L., Oritz, M. J., et al. (2008). Nonfatal maltreatment of infants—United States, October 2005–September 2006. *Morbidity and Mortality Weekly Report, 57,* 336–339.

Bronfenbrenner, U. (2005). *Making human beings human: Bioecologic perspectives.* Thousand Oaks, CA: Sage Publications.

Bronstein, A. C., Spyker, D. A., Cantilena, L. R., Green, J., Rumack, B. H., & Heard, S. E. (2008). 2007 annual report of the American Association of Poison Control Centers' National Poisoning Data System. *Clinical Toxicology, 46,* 927–1057.

Buka, I., Koranteng, S., & Vargas, A. R. O. (2007). Trends in childhood cancer incidence: Review of environmental linkages. *Pediatric Clinics of North America, 54,* 177–203.

Casanueva, C., Martin, S. L., & Runyan, D. K. (2009). Repeated reports for child maltreatment among intimate partner violence victims: Finding from the National Survey of Child and Adolescent Well-Being. *Child Abuse and Neglect, 33*(2), 84–93.

Casanueva, C. E., & Martin, S. L. (2007). Intimate partner violence during pregnancy and mothers' child abuse potential. *Journal of Interpersonal Violence, 22*(5), 603–622.

Centers for Disease Control and Prevention. (2006a). Cigarette use among high school students—United States, 1991–2005. *Morbidity and Mortality Weekly Report, 55,* 724–726.

Centers for Disease Control and Prevention. (2006b). Use of cigarettes and other tobacco products among students aged 13–15 years—worldwide, 1999–2005. *Morbidity and Mortality Weekly Report, 55,* 553–556.

Centers for Disease Control and Prevention. (2006c). Youth risk behavior surveillance—United States, 2005. *Morbidity and Mortality Weekly Report, 55*(SS05), 1–108.

Centers for Disease Control and Prevention. (2008a). Youth risk behavior surveillance—United States, 2007. *Morbidity and Mortality Weekly Report, 57*(SS-4), 1–36.

Centers for Disease Control and Prevention. (2008b). *Body art: Tattoos and piercings.* Retrieved from http://www.cdc.gov

Chartrand, M. M., & Siegel, B. (2007). At war in Iraq and Afghanistan: Children in US military families. *Ambulatory Pediatrics, 7,* 1–2.

Childhelp. (2009). *National child abuse statistics.* Scottsdale, AZ: Author.

Children's Defense Fund. (2008). *Data. Each day in America.* Retrieved from http://www.childrensdefense.org/site/pageServer?pagename=research_national_data_each_day

Collins, B. N., Wileyto, E. P., Murphy, J. F., & Munafo, M. R. (2007). Adolescent environmental tobacco smoke exposure predicts academic achievement test failure. *Journal of Adolescent Health, 41,* 363–370.

Cyr, A. M. (2007). What is Munchausen syndrome by proxy? *Nursing, 37,* 30.

Darbyshire, P., Muir-Cochrane, E., Fereday, J., Jureidini, J., & Drummond, A. (2006). Engagement with health and social care services: Perceptions of homeless young people with mental health problems. *Health and Social Care in the Community, 14,* 553–562.

DeForge, V., Zehnder, S., Minick, P., & Carmon, M. (2001). Children's perspectives of homelessness. *Pediatric Nursing, 27,* 377–383.

Elkind, D. (2007). *The hurried child: 25th anniversary edition.* Cambridge, MA: Da Capo Lifelong Publishing.

Federal Interagency Forum on Child and Family Statistics. (2009). *America's children: Key national indicators of well-being 2009.* Washington, DC: U.S. Government Printing Office.

Fekkes, M., Pijpers, F. I., & Verloove-Vanhorick, S. P. (2006). Effects of antibullying school program on bullying and health complaints. *Archives of Pediatric and Adolescent Medicine, 160,* 638–644.

Feldman, J. M. (2008). Caring for incarcerated youth. *Current Opinion in Pediatrics, 20*(4), 398–402.

Ford, M. D. (2008). Acute poisoning. In L. Goldman & D. Ausiello, *Cecil medicine* (23rd ed., p. 768). Philadelphia: Saunders Elsevier.

Galvez, M. P., Graber, N. M., Sheffield, P. E., Forman, J. A., & Balk, S. J. (2009). Hot topics in pediatric environmental health. *Contemporary Pediatrics, 26*(7), 34–47.

Gettig, J. P., Grady, S. E., & Nowosadzka, I. (2006). Methamphetamine: Putting the brakes on speed. *Journal of School Nursing, 22*(2), 66–73.

Hanhan, U. A. (2008). The poisoned child in the pediatric intensive care unit. *Pediatric Clinics of North America, 55,* 669–686.

Health Resources and Services Administration (HRSA). (2009). *The national bullying prevention campaign.* Washington, DC: Author.

Hingson, R. W., Heeren, T., & Winter, M. R. (2006). Age at drinking onset and alcohol dependence. *Archives of Pediatric and Adolescent Medicine, 160,* 739–746.

Inglehart, J. K. (2007). Insuring all children—the new political imperative. *New England Journal of Medicine, 357,* 70–76.

Jannone, L., & O'Connell, K. A. (2007). Coping strategies used by adolescents during smoking cessation. *Journal of School Nursing, 23,* 177–184.

Johnson, C. F. (2006). Sexual abuse in children. *Pediatrics in Review, 27,* 17–26.

Kellogg, N. D., & Committee on Child Abuse and Neglect. (2007). Evaluation of suspected child physical abuse. *Pediatrics, 119,* 1232–1241.

Kidd, S. A., & Davidson, L. (2006). Youth homelessness: A call for partnerships between research and policy. *Canadian Journal of Public Health, 97,* 445–447.

KidsHealth. (2009). *How TV affects your child.* Retrieved from http://kidshealthoorg.parent/positive/family/tv_affects_child.html

Kliegman, R. M., Behrman, R. E., Jenson, H. B., & Stanton, B. F. (Eds.). (2007). *Nelson textbook of pediatrics* (18th ed.). Philadelphia: Saunders Elsevier.

Klomek, A. B., Marrocco, F., Kleinman, J., Schonfeld, I. S., & Gould, M. S. (2008). Peer victimization, depression and suicidality in adolescents. *Suicide and Life Threatening Behavior, 38*(2), 166–180.

Kolar, K. R., & Davey, D. (2007). Silent victims: Children exposed to family violence. *Journal of School Nursing, 23,* 86–91.

Larzo, M. R., & Poe, S. G. (2006). Adverse consequences of tattoos and body piercings. *Pediatric Annals, 35,* 187–192.

Leman, S. K., & Plattner, M. (2007). When beautification of the body turns ugly. *Clinical Advisor,* February, 27–33.

Liu, J., Peterson, A. V., Kealey, K. A., Mann, S. L., Bricker, J. B., & Marek, P. M. (2007). Addressing challenges in adolescent smoking cessation: Design and baseline characteristics of the HS group-randomized trial. *Preventive Medicine, 45,* 215–225.

Loveland-Cherry, C. J. (2006). Alcohol, children and adolescents. In J. J. Fitzpatrick (Ed.), *Alcohol use, misuse, abuse, and dependence* (pp. 135–177). New York: Springer Publishing.

Markowitz, M. (2007). Lead poisoning. In R. M. Kliegman, R. E. Behrman, H. B. Jenson, & B. F. Stanton, *Nelson textbook of pediatrics* (18th ed., pp. 2913–2918). Philadelphia: Saunders Elsevier.

Mayers, L. B., & Chiffriller, S. H. (2008). Body art (body piercing and tattooing) among undergraduate university students: "Then and now." *Journal of Adolescent Health, 42*(2), 201–203.

McColgan, M. D., & Giardino, A. P. (2005). Internet poses multiple risks to children and adolescents. *Pediatric Annals, 34,* 405–414.

McGregor, T., Parkar, M., & Rao, S. (2009). Evaluation and management of common childhood poisonings. *American Family Physician, 79*(5), 397–403.

Meadows-Oliver, M. (2006). Environmental toxins. *Journal of Pediatric Health Care, 20*(5), 350–352.

Meckler, G. D., Elliot, M. N., Kanouse, D. E., Beals, K., & Schuster, M. A. (2006). Nondisclosure of sexual orientation to a physician among a sample of gay, lesbian and bisexual youth. *Archives of Pediatrics and Adolescent Medicine, 160,* 1248–1254.

National Association for the Education of Young Children. (2007). *Introduction to the NAEYC early childhood program standards and accreditation criteria; Program standards.* Retrieved from http://www.naeyc.org/academy/IntroNewCriteria.asp

National Center on Family Homelessness. (2009). *America's youngest outcasts.* Newton, MA: Author.

National Institute of Child Health and Human Development. (2007). *Add Health Study.* Retrieved from http://www.nichd.nih.gov/health/topics/add_health_study.cfm?renderforprint=1

National Institute of Child Health and Human Development. (2009). *The National Children's Study.* Retrieved from http://www.nationalchildrensstudy.gov

National Institute on Alcohol Abuse and Alcoholism (NIAAA). (2009). *Underage drinking research initiative.* Retrieved from http://www.niaaa.nih.gov/

National Institutes of Health. (2009). *Munchausen syndrome by proxy.* Retrieved from http://www.nlm.nih.gov/medlineplus/ency/article/001555.htm

National Safe Kids. (2007). *Injury facts.* Retrieved from http://www.safekids.org/

Reardon, J. Z. (2007). Environmental tobacco smoke: Respiratory and other health effects. *Clinical Chest Medicine, 28,* 559–573.

Remafedi, G. (2006). Adolescent homosexuality. *Archives of Pediatrics and Adolescent Medicine, 160,* 1303–1304.

Rentz, E. D., Marshall, S. W., Loomis, D., Casteel, C., Martin, S. L., & Gibbs, D. A. (2007). Effect of deployment on the occurrence of child maltreatment in military and nonmilitary families. *American Journal of Epidemiology, 165,* 1199–1206.

Rezendes, J. L. (2006). Bicycle helmets: Overcoming barriers to use and increasing effectiveness. *Journal of Pediatric Nursing, 21,* 35–44.

Rodgers, G. C., Condurache, T., Reed, M. D., Bestic, M., & Gal, P. (2007). Poisonings. In R. M. Kliegman, R. E. Behrman, H. B. Jenson, & B. F. Stanton, *Nelson textbook of pediatrics* (18th ed., pp. 339–357). Philadelphia: Elsevier Saunders.

Santrock, J. W. (2008). *Adolescence* (12th ed.). Boston: McGraw-Hill.

Schepis, T., & Krishnan-Sarin, S. (2009). Characterizing adolescent prescription misusers: A population-based study. *Journal of the American Academy of Child and Adolescent Psychiatry, 48,* 828–836.

Sparrow, J. D. (2007). Understanding stress in children. *Pediatric Annals, 36,* 187–195.

Srabstein, J. (2008). Deaths linked to bullying and hazing. *International Journal of Adolescent Medicine and Health, 20*(2), 235–239.

Stein, J. A., Dukes, R. L., & Warren, J. I. (2007). Adolescent male bullies, victims and bully-victims: A comparison of psychosocial and behavioral characteristics. *Journal of Pediatric Psychology, 32,* 273–282.

Surgeon General. (2007). *The surgeon general's call to action to prevent and reduce underage drinking.* Washington, DC: U.S. Department of Health and Human Services.

Tischler, V., Rademeyer, A., & Vostanis, P. (2007). Mothers experiencing homelessness: Mental health, support and social care needs. *Health and Social Care in the Community, 15,* 246–253.

UNICEF. (2009). *Promoting synergy between child protection and social protection.* Retrieved from http://www.unicef.org/wcaro/wcaro_UNICEF_ODI_5_Child_Protection.pdf

U.S. Department of Health and Human Services. (2006). *Healthy People 2010: Midcourse Review.* Washington, DC: Author.

U.S. Department of Health and Human Services. (2008). *2008 physical activity guidelines for Americans.* Retrieved from http://www.health.gov/paguidelines/

U.S. Department of Health and Human Services. (2010). *Healthy People 2020.* Retrieved from http://www.healthypeople.gov

Uyemura, M. E. (2005). Foreign body ingestion in children. *American Family Physician, 72*(2), 287–291.

Victoir, A., Eertmans, A., Van den Broucke, S., & Van den Bergh, O. (2006). Smoking status moderates the contribution of social-cognitive and environmental determinants to adolescents' smoking intentions. *Health Education Research, 21,* 674–687.

Warniment, C., Tsang, K., & Galazka, S. S. (2010). Lead poisoning in children. *American Family Physician, 81*(6), 751–757.

Willard, N. E. (2007). *Cyberbullying and Cyberthreats: Responding to the challenge of online social aggression, threats, and distress* (2nd ed.). Champaign, IL: Research Press.

Williams, K. A., & Bydalek, K. A. (2007). Adolescent self-mutilation: Diagnosis and treatment. *Journal of Psychosocial Nursing and Mental Health Services, 45*(12), 19–23.

Woolf, A. D., Goldman, R., & Bellinger, D. C. (2007). Update on the clinical management of childhood lead poisoning. *Pediatric Clinics of North America, 54,* 271–294.

World Health Organization (WHO). (2007). *United Nations Surgeon General's study on violence in children.* Retrieved from http://www.violencestudy.org/r25

Clinical Manifestations
Extracellular Fluid Volume Deficit

Clinical Manifestations	Etiology
Weight loss Sunken fontanel (infant)	Decreased fluid volume
Postural blood pressure drop (older children) Dizziness	Inadequate circulating blood volume to offset the force of gravity when in upright position
Increased small-vein filling time Delayed capillary refill time Flat neck veins when supine (older children)	Decreased intravascular volume
Dizziness, syncope	Inadequate circulation to the brain
Oliguria	Inadequate circulation to the kidneys
Thready, rapid pulse	Cardiac reflex response to decreased intravascular volume
Decreased skin turgor	Decreased interstitial fluid volume

pulse, poor skin turgor, dry mucous membranes, seizure activity, and markedly decreased or absent urinary output.

COLLABORATIVE CARE

Diagnostic Tests

The diagnosis of dehydration is best accomplished by clinical observations (see Table 18–3). A major observation that provides clues about the degree of dehydration is percent of weight loss. The serum electrolyte panel may be helpful in severe and continuing dehydration that is complicated by electrolyte imbalance or acidosis. The tests include serum electrolytes, creatinine, and glucose. Elevated blood urea nitrogen (greater than 17 mg/dL) and low serum bicarbonate (less than 16–17 mEq/L) are also useful to identify moderate and severe dehydration (Madati & Bachur, 2008). The results can be used to target the fluid type and amount to best meet the imbalances identified. Urine specific gravity may provide useful information.

Clinical Judgment

Urine specific gravity (concentration of urine) usually increases in older children who are dehydrated. However, the child under 2 years of age is unable to concentrate urine effectively. Do you think a rising specific gravity is usually seen in the child under 2 years who is dehydrated? Why or why not?

Clinical Manifestations
Exertional Heat Illness

Condition	Clinical Manifestations	Etiology
Heat cramps	Acute, painful muscle cramps Thirst Fatigue	Dehydration Electrolyte imbalance Neuromuscular fatigue
Heat syncope	Tunnel vision Pale, sweaty skin Decreased pulse Dizziness, faintness	Peripheral vasodilation Orthostatic hypotension Reduced cardiac output Cerebral ischemia
Heat exhaustion	Sweating, pallor Dehydration Muscle cramps Nausea, anorexia, diarrhea Decreased urinary output Fatigue, fainting, dizziness	Elevated core body temperature Sodium loss
Heat stroke	Tachycardia Hypotension Sweating Hyperventilation Altered mental status, seizures, coma Vomiting, diarrhea Death can occur from severe acidosis, hyperkalemia, renal failure, and disseminated intravascular coagulation	Elevated core temperature (over 104°F or 40°C) Temperature regulation overwhelmed by heat production or absence of adequate heat loss Organ system failure from overheating
Exertional hyponatremia	Disorientation, headache, lethargy Swollen extremities Vomiting Pulmonary or cerebral edema Death can occur from sodium imbalance	Serum sodium less than 130 mmol/L Exercise over 4 hours with water or other low-solute fluids for replenishment

(Adapted from Howe & Boden, 2007.)

Clinical Therapy

Medical management depends on accurate identification of the degree of dehydration. The treatment of extracellular fluid volume deficit is administration of fluid containing sodium. This may be accomplished by oral rehydration therapy or intravenous fluids.

Oral rehydration therapy has been used for a number of years in developing countries without an accessible supply of intravenous fluids. More recently, the benefits of using this therapy early to prevent severe dehydration and to treat mild and moderate dehydration in children in developed countries has been recognized. The therapy is successful in treating the dehydration caused by many gastrointestinal illnesses and prevents hospitalization for many infants and young children. It is the treatment of choice for children with diarrhea who have mild to moderate dehydration (Hartling, Bellemare, Wiebe, et al., 2006; Fontaine, Garner, & Bhan, 2007). Commercially available solutions contain water, carbohydrate (glucose), sodium, potassium, chloride, and lactate. Examples include Pedialyte, Infalyte, Ricelyte, Resol, Nutrilyte, Hydralyte, and Lytren. A World Health Organization/UNICEF solution with high sodium and chloride is used for cholera treatment in developing countries. Some clinicians allow lactose-free milk, breast milk, or half-strength milk to be given in addition to oral rehydration therapy solution.

When the child is severely dehydrated, intravenous fluid will be given, often accompanied with oral rehydration. The intravenous fluid is often Ringer's lactate followed by or accompanied with dilute saline, such as one half or one quarter normal saline (Holliday, Ray, & Friedman, 2007). The fluid combination replenishes the extracellular fluid volume and adds solutes to return the body fluid to normal. The child may be hospitalized or treated with intravenous fluids in a short-stay unit until the dehydration is controlled. Once hydration is completed, the child may resume an age-appropriate diet.

NURSING MANAGEMENT

Nursing Assessment and Diagnosis

Weigh the child daily with the same scale and without clothing. Compare to past weights and calculate weight loss. Carefully measure intake and output, urine specific gravity, level of consciousness, pulse rate and quality, skin turgor, mucous membrane moisture, quality and rate of respirations, and blood pressure (Figure 18–8 ➤). Compare the blood pressure when the child is supine with the pressure when the child is sitting with legs hanging down or standing. If the child is dehydrated, the sitting or standing blood pressure will be lower than the supine blood pressure, because blood accumulates in the dependent legs. The nurse will obtain samples of urine and blood as needed for dehydration evaluation. Evaluate the alertness of the child and any signs of lethargy or weakness.

The nursing diagnosis of Deficient Fluid Volume applies to all children who have an extracellular fluid volume deficit. Other diagnoses depend on the severity of the condition and the age of the child. Several nursing diagnoses that might be appropriate for the mildly to severely dehydrated child are included in the accompa-

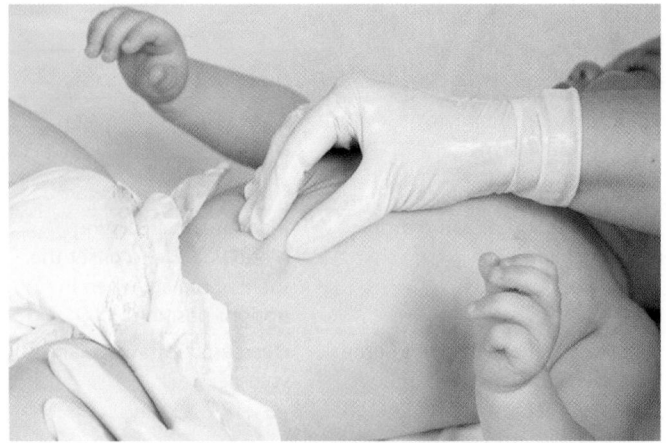

A

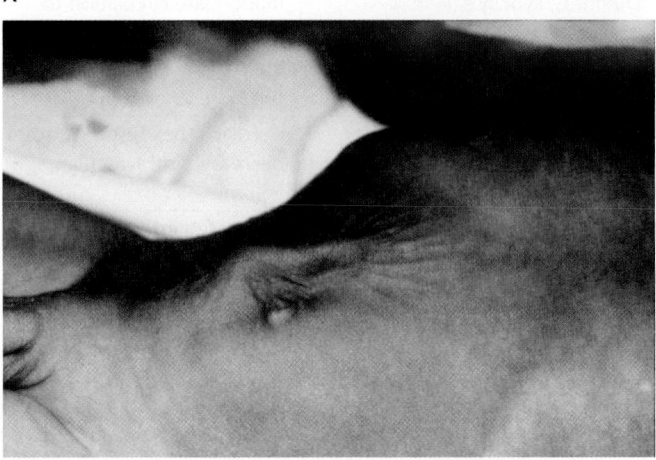

B

FIGURE 18–8 ➤ Assessing skin turgor takes skill and practice. A, In moderate dehydration the skin may have a doughy texture and appearance. B, In severe dehydration, "tenting" of the skin is observed. Diminished turgor is most easily assessed in infants or children with little subcutaneous fat; it is more difficult to assess in those with larger amounts of fat. The chest, abdomen, and upper thighs are locations to measure turgor.

nying Nursing Care Plans. Additional care of the child with dehydration from gastroenteritis can be found in Chapter 25 ∞. Specific examples of nursing diagnoses include the following:

- Fluid Volume (Deficient) related to fluid volume loss or failure of regulatory mechanisms

Clinical Tip

To calculate the percentage of weight loss:

- Subtract the child's present weight from the original weight to find the loss.
- Divide the loss by the child's original weight.

EXAMPLE: In the opening scenario, Vernon weighed 12 kg (26 lb) at the clinic last week. However, when he is weighed today, the scale reads only 11 kg (24 1/2 lb). In this case, subtracting 11 kg from 12 kg yields 1 kg of weight loss. Dividing 1 kg by his original weight of 12 kg reveals that he has lost approximately 8% of his body weight, which indicates moderate dehydration.

- Risk for Ineffective Peripheral Tissue Perfusion related to hypovolemia
- Risk for Injury related to postural hypotension

Planning and Implementation

Nursing care of the dehydrated child focuses on providing oral rehydration fluids, teaching parents oral rehydration methods, and, if necessary, administering intravenous fluids to restore fluid balance.

Clinical Tip

To obtain urine from an infant for testing specific gravity, place two cotton balls in the diaper. When they are wet, push them into a 10-mL syringe and squeeze out the urine with the plunger.

Prevent Dehydration

Nursing care can often prevent dehydration. Carefully monitor temperature probes in radiant warmers and incubators for newborns to prevent overheating and resulting dehydration. Teach parents to use proper clothing for infants to prevent overheating. Nurses can educate parents, youth, school personnel, and coaches about the dangers of heat-related illness. Prevention is key, so that children can exercise safely. Prior to a new exercise regimen, perform assessment for risk factors and refer the child for a physical examination; certain medical conditions such as cystic fibrosis, diabetes, obesity, cardiac conditions, or mental retardation put the child at high risk. Prior history of heat-related illness or recent change from a cooler to hotter environment increases risk. Long exercise periods increase the stress upon the body. The major nursing interventions are partnering with families and athletic coaches to prevent problems and to recognize and treat them promptly. See Families Want to Know: Preventing Heat-Related Illness. Recognize that heat syndromes can result in death, so prevention, prompt recognition, and treatment are essential.

NURSING CARE PLAN

The Child with Mild or Moderate Dehydration

INTERVENTION	RATIONALE	EXPECTED OUTCOME
1. Nursing Diagnosis: Ineffective Management of Therapeutic Regimen related to family knowledge deficit of diarrhea and vomiting		
NIC Priority Intervention: *Family involvement:* Facilitate family participation in care of the child.		NOC Suggested Outcome: *Participation:* Healthcare decisions: Personal involvement in selecting healthcare options
Goal: Parents describe appropriate home management of fluid replacement for vomiting and diarrhea.		
■ Explain how to replace body fluid with an oral rehydration solution. Encourage parents to keep the solution at home and begin use with the first sign of diarrhea.	■ Use of an oral rehydration solution can enable successful treatment of vomiting and diarrhea at home.	Parents choose appropriate fluids for rehydration and are successfully able to treat the child's diarrhea and vomiting at home. The child is adequately hydrated.
■ Teach parents to continue the child's normal diet in addition to providing replacement fluids for diarrhea.	■ Diet plus fluid supplementation leads to faster recovery.	
■ Provide verbal and written instructions to parents at each well-child visit.	■ Parents are provided with a reference for later use.	
2. Nursing Diagnosis: Knowledge Deficit (Parent) related to causes of dehydration		
NIC Priority Intervention: *Teaching:* Teach causes of dehydration.		NOC Suggested Outcome: *Knowledge:* Extent of understanding conveyed about treatment regimen
Goal: Parents will state common causes of childhood dehydration.		
■ Teach parents childhood conditions that commonly lead to dehydration.	■ If parents recognize situations that can lead to dehydration, they will be more alert to its appearance.	Parents recognize conditions of risk for dehydration in children.
3. Nursing Diagnosis: Risk for Fluid Volume, Deficit, related to worsening of child's condition		
NIC Priority Intervention: *Fluid management:* Promote fluid balance.		NOC Suggested Outcome: *Fluid balance:* Balance of water in extra- and intracellular compartments of body
Goal: Parents will seek health care for the child's worsening condition.		
■ Teach parents to seek care when the child's vomiting or diarrhea worsens, or the child's mental alertness changes.	■ Severe dehydration may occur if milder forms are not successfully treated.	Parents seek prompt attention for the child's worsening condition, preventing the development of severe dehydration.

NURSING CARE PLAN

The Child with Severe Dehydration

INTERVENTION	RATIONALE	EXPECTED OUTCOME
1. Nursing Diagnosis: Fluid Volume, Deficient related to excess losses and inadequate intake		
NIC Priority Intervention: *Fluid management:* Promote fluid balance.		**NOC Suggested Outcome:** *Fluid balance:* Balance of water in extra- and intracellular components of the body
Goal: The child returns to normal hydration status and does not develop hypovolemic shock.		
■ Monitor weight daily. Assess intake and output every shift. Assess heart rate, postural blood pressure, skin turgor, small-vein filling time, capillary refill time, fontanel (infant), and urine specific gravity every 4 hours or more frequently as indicated.	■ Frequent assessment of hydration status facilitates rapid intervention and evaluation of the effectiveness of fluid replacement.	The child has signs of normal hydration.
■ Administer intravenous fluids as ordered. Monitor for crackles in dependent portions of the lungs.	■ Replace fluid lost from the body. Excessive replacement of sodium-containing fluids could cause extracellular fluid volume excess.	
2. Nursing Diagnosis: Risk for Injury related to decreased level of consciousness		
NIC Priority Intervention: *Fall prevention:* Institute special precautions.		**NOC Suggested Outcome:** *Fall prevention:* Minimize risk factors that precipitate falls.
Goal: The child does not experience injury.		
■ Raise the side rails of the bed. Ensure that a small child does not become tangled in bedcovers. Keep the call light in reach of the child (if old enough) or parent.	■ Safety measures protect the child.	The child does not fall or suffer other injury.
■ Monitor level of consciousness every 2–4 hours or more often as indicated.	■ Frequent assessment provides evidence of the need for safety interventions and of the effectiveness of therapy.	
■ Monitor serum sodium concentration daily or more often.	■ Elevated serum sodium concentration causes brain cell shrinkage and decreased level of consciousness.	
■ Have the child sit before rising from bed and assist to stand slowly.	■ Slow adjustment to upright posture reduces light-headedness from decreased blood volume.	
3. Nursing Diagnosis: Activity Intolerance related to bed rest/immobility		
NIC Priority Intervention: *Activity therapy:* Plan activities to meet child's developmental needs.		**NOC Suggested Outcome:** *Energy conservation:* Manage energy to sustain activity.
Goal: The child will engage in normal activity for age.		
■ Plan activities appropriate for the age of the child that can be done in bed.	■ Activities will provide distraction and promote recovery.	The child engages in normal developmental activities and receives adequate rest.
■ Group nursing interventions to provide time for the child to rest.	■ The child will require more rest than usual.	
■ Provide assistance during meals and other activities as needed.	■ Prevention of overexertion will conserve body fluid and promote healing.	

Families Want to Know
Preventing Heat-Related Illness

Teach parents, coaches, and youth the following preventive techniques:

■ Precede exercise programs with a physical examination designed to identify risks.

■ Reduce intensity of activity when the temperature or humidity is high.

■ Allow a 10- to 14-day period of acclimation to higher temperatures before reaching usual exercise levels.

■ Ensure hydration before activity begins.

■ During activity, stop for fluids every 15–20 minutes. Children up to 90 pounds should drink 150 mL (5 ounces), and those over 90 pounds should drink 250 mL (9 ounces). A combination of water and sports drink is best.

■ Recognize low urine volume or dark color as a sign of dehydration.

■ Wear light-colored, lightweight clothing. Never use rubber clothing designed to promote weight loss through sweating.

■ Maintain adequate sleep and nutritional status.

(Adapted from Howe & Boden, 2007.)

Provide Oral Rehydration Fluids

In mild or moderate dehydration, oral rehydration fluid is the first intervention (Canavan & Arant, 2009). It is given in frequent small amounts; for example, 1 to 3 teaspoons of fluid every 10 to 15 minutes is a useful guideline for starting oral rehydration. For the first 2 to 4 hours of treatment, 50 mL of fluid for each kilogram of the child's weight should be the target intake. Instruct parents to continue to administer 1 teaspoon every 2 to 3 minutes even if the child vomits, as small amounts of the fluid may still be absorbed. Children are often treated in special sections of emergency departments or outpatient clinics for several hours to begin hydration. Oral or nasogastric tube feedings of oral rehydration are administered while monitoring occurs.

Teach Parents Oral Rehydration Methods

Parents should assess the alertness of the child and ability to take oral fluids. If the child is lethargic or unable to drink normally, the child needs medical care. Instruct parents about the types of fluids and amounts to be given at home. See Families Want to Know: Oral Rehydration Therapy Guidelines. Begin teaching parents of all newborns and reinforce teaching at each well-child visit. Advise parents to continue the child's normal diet in addition to providing the rehydration solution. Cereals, starches, soups, fruits, and vegetables are allowed. Tell parents to avoid simple sugars,

Nursing Alert

Sugar facilitates the absorption of sodium in oral rehydration fluids. Teach parents not to give diet beverages for oral rehydration, because they contain no sugar and will not be effectively absorbed. However, if an oral rehydration solution is too concentrated, it can worsen the diarrhea. Juice and cola are highly concentrated and should be diluted to half strength when given to a child who has diarrhea. Encourage parents to keep an oral rehydration solution in liquid or powder form on hand at all times and to use these solutions rather than juice or soda when the child first develops diarrhea.

Research  *Treatment of Dehydration*

Dehydration is common in children. Oral rehydration therapy is recommended for effective treatment of mild and moderate dehydration, and is successful for the majority of children. However, the condition is commonly treated by intravenous infusion even when oral therapy is likely to be effective. Practitioners should follow guidelines for dehydration treatment. Families prefer to treat their children at home when possible, thus avoiding costly, traumatic care. Careful instructions to parents about administration of fluids and considerations to return for care if the condition persists or worsens ensure proper care for the child if oral rehydration is not successful (Diggins, 2008).

which can worsen diarrhea because of osmotic effects, including soft drinks (if used, they should be diluted with equal parts of water), undiluted juice, Jell-O, and sweetened cereal.

Repeated vomiting of large volumes of fluid or a worsening of the child's condition can indicate the need for intravenous therapy. Teach parents when to seek further medical care. If the child's condition worsens or does not improve after 4 hours of oral rehydration therapy, parents should contact a health care professional.

Monitor Intravenous Fluid Administration

The hospitalized child usually requires administration of intravenous fluids after careful assessment of type of fluid and electrolyte imbalance. The nurse is usually responsible for starting

Families Want to Know
Oral Rehydration Therapy Guidelines

Calculate the specific amounts required for individual children based on the following guidelines, and instruct parents in terminology they understand. A simple way to instruct parents is that infants should get 1 oz hourly, toddlers should get 2 oz hourly, and older children should get 3 oz hourly. Provide measuring devices with proper amounts marked.

■ Children with diarrhea and no dehydration should be continued on age-appropriate diets.

■ For minimal dehydration, if the child weighs less than 10 kg, give 60–120 mL oral rehydration solution (ORS) for each diarrheal stool or vomiting episode; if over 10 kg in weight, give 120–240 mL ORS for each diarrheal stool or vomiting episode. Meanwhile, continue breastfeeding or resume age-appropriate diet after initial hydration.

■ Start slowly, administering 3–5 mL in a small cup or spoon every few minutes. Increase amounts gradually if no vomiting occurs.

■ Recommend or provide samples of ORS. Suggest ready-to-feed or powdered forms for use by parents.

■ For moderate dehydration, give 50–100 mL/kg ORS in 3–4 hours in addition to replacing fluids lost as previously described.

■ For severe dehydration, the child is hospitalized and treated with intravenous fluids. When hydrated adequately or concurrently with intravenous rehydration, begin oral rehydration therapy with 100 mL/kg of fluid in 4 hours and stool replacement as previously described.

■ When rehydration is complete, resume the normal diet.

Note: Adapted from: Managing acute gastroenteritis among children: Oral rehydration, maintenance, and nutritional therapy. (2004). *Pediatrics, 114,* 507; Canavan, A., & Arant, B. S. (2009). Diagnosis and management of dehydration in children. *American Family Physician, 80*(7), 692–696.

BOX 18–1   Calculation of Intravenous Fluid Needs

1. First, calculate the maintenance fluid needs of the child, according to the following guideline:

Usual Weight	Maintenance Amount
Up to 10 kg	100 mL/kg/24 hr
11–20 kg	1000 mL + (50 mL/kg for weight above 10 kg)/24 hr
Greater than 20 kg	1500 mL + (20 mL/kg for weight above 20 kg)/24 hr

Example: Vernon's weight is 12 kg. He needs 1000 mL + (50 × 2), or 1100 mL/24 hr for maintenance fluid.

2. Next, calculate replacement fluid for that lost:

Example: Vernon has lost 1 kg (8%) of his body weight. Multiplying the percentage of body weight × 10 yields the mL/kg/24 hr required:

$$8 \times 10 = 80 \text{ mL/kg/24 hr}$$
$$80 \text{ mL/kg} \times 2 \text{ kg} = 960 \text{ mL}$$

Thus, Vernon's replacement fluid needs are 960 mL/24 hr.

It is also helpful to know that 1 liter of fluid weighs about 1 kilogram. The amount of fluid deficit can be roughly estimated using this formula. In Vernon's case, since he has lost 1 kg of weight, his replacement fluid need is roughly equivalent to 1 L (1000 mL). This is very close to the 960 mL calculated in the previous formula.

3. Finally, calculate continued losses and add to the total maintenance and replacement needs.

---

the intravenous line and administering the prescribed fluids. Be sure that the amount of fluid administered corresponds with the diagnosed dehydration state of the child (Box 18–1). Verify that the type of fluid administered is that which is prescribed. Usually, about half of the 24-hour total maintenance and replacement needs will be given in the first 6 to 8 hours, with a slower rate infused for the remainder of the 24 hours. During the first 1 to 3 hours, the infusion rate may be highest to rapidly expand the vascular space. Rapid infusion of 20 to 30 mL/kg over 1 to 2 hours is sometimes used in outpatient settings, followed by oral fluids. When oral fluids are maintained, the decision for discharge can be made and hospitalization avoided (see Evidence-Based Practice: Home Care for Conditions Causing Dehydration).

Clinical Tip

A normal saline solution is a salt solution that has the same percentage of salt as the human body. This is a 0.9% solution of sodium chloride. The term *normal* indicates that there is the same weight, in grams, of sodium and chloride in the solution. There are 154 mEq/L of sodium and 154 mEq/L of chloride in normal saline. Normal saline or Ringer's lactate (Ringer's lactate contains carbohydrate and additional electrolytes) may be used for early rehydration. Often more dilute sodium solutions follow such as 1/2 normal saline or 1/4 normal saline. If the child is not taking in oral fluids or food, dilute saline solutions with glucose may be prescribed.

Maintain the intravenous line carefully so fluid infusion can be kept on schedule (refer to the *Clinical Skills Manual*). Use a pump to prevent inadvertent, rapid infusion, which can lead to fluid overload and electrolyte imbalance. Play with the toddler and preschool child frequently and use diversionary methods, as necessary, to distract the child from the intravenous line. Monitor the child carefully and implement safety precautions as necessary. Even when an intravenous infusion is used, the child is started on oral rehydration simultaneously. As more oral fluids are tolerated, the intravenous infusion is decreased.

Maintain Safety

The child who is dehydrated is often dizzy and lethargic. Keep side rails up and supervise and assist the child when getting up. Have parents stay at the bedside while the child is being treated in ambulatory units and urge them to maintain safety precautions as they take the child home.

Discharge Planning and Home Care Teaching

Prevention of dehydration is the best approach when possible. Encourage breastfeeding because it is associated with a decreased incidence of gastroenteritis. During health promotion and health maintenance visits, encourage all parents to keep oral rehydration fluids at home in case they are needed. Address the need for increasing fluids in hot weather and when the child is

---

Evidence-Based Practice
Home Care for Conditions Causing Dehydration

Problem

Rotavirus gastroenteritis (RGE) is a common and potentially serious cause of childhood vomiting and diarrhea, and can lead to dehydration among young children.

Evidence

It is estimated that RGE causes 3.5 million cases of diarrhea, 50,000 hospitalizations, and 20 deaths annually in the United States. RGE can generally be successfully treated at home but parents must be aware of assessment and treatment guidelines (Koslap-Petraco, 2006).

Implications

RGE carries a major risk of dehydration in children. Although it may begin as a mild illness, it can quickly progress to severe diarrhea and vomiting. Most children are cared for at home with RGE, but parents often call in to health care facilities. It is important to ask parents about duration and symptoms of severity. Teach them proper administration of oral rehydration therapy, as well as symptoms that require immediate emergency care.

Critical Thinking Application

What questions can you ask on the phone that will help to establish the degree of dehydration of a child at home? What symptoms require immediate medical care? A vaccine for rotavirus is now available for young children; plan the information you need to provide to all parents about this preventive measure (see Chapter 16 ∞ for further details).

exercising. Reinforce safety teaching to decrease incidence of burns, an important cause of dehydration. Teach the signs and symptoms of gastroenteritis and instruct the parent to seek care for the child who has persistent vomiting or diarrhea, or who has decreased urinary output or altered mental status.

Prior to discharge from the hospital or outpatient facility after treatment for dehydration, parents need instructions about types of fluids and amounts to encourage. Teach the signs of dehydration (see Table 18–3) so that if the child does not take in adequate fluids, parents can seek help immediately. Instruct them to begin the child's normal diet once hydration is complete, as determined by adequate urinary output and normal behaviors. Review methods of minimizing the child's chance of acquiring gastrointestinal infections (e.g., avoiding contact with other children who are infected; using careful handwashing and dishwashing procedures when a child in the home is affected).

Nurses should be alert for children in the community who have other health conditions that predispose them to fluid and electrolyte imbalance. Examples include those with cancer, AIDS, cystic fibrosis, and renal disease. When these children are seen for health promotion and health maintenance visits, or because of a health complication, they should be evaluated for fluid and electrolyte imbalance.

Evaluation

Expected outcomes of nursing care for the child with dehydration include the following:

- Water and electrolytes are balanced in intracellular and extracellular compartments.
- Urinary output is within normal limits.
- Adequate fluid intake meets maintenance needs.
- Vital signs are within normal limits.

Extracellular Fluid Volume Excess

Extracellular fluid volume excess occurs when there is too much fluid in the extracellular compartment (vascular and interstitial). This imbalance may also be called saline excess or extracellular volume overload. If this disorder occurs by itself (without saline disturbance), the serum sodium concentration is normal. There is simply too much extracellular fluid, even though it has a normal concentration.

Infants and children who develop an extracellular fluid volume excess have a condition that causes them to retain **saline** (sodium and water) or they have been given an overload of sodium-containing isotonic intravenous fluid (Figure 18–9 ➤). What conditions cause retention of saline? The hormone aldosterone is secreted by the adrenal cortex. One of its normal functions is to cause the kidneys to retain saline in the body (Figure 18–10 ➤). Saline excess can be caused by any condition that results in excessive aldosterone secretion, such as adrenal tumors that secrete aldosterone, congestive heart failure, liver cirrhosis, and chronic renal failure (Figure 18–11 ➤). Most glucocorticoid medications (such as prednisone) have a mild saline-retaining effect when taken long term. Intravenous fluid volume regulation is important, especially in young children. Either inaccurate calculation of needed fluid or inadvertent infusion of excess fluids can cause overload.

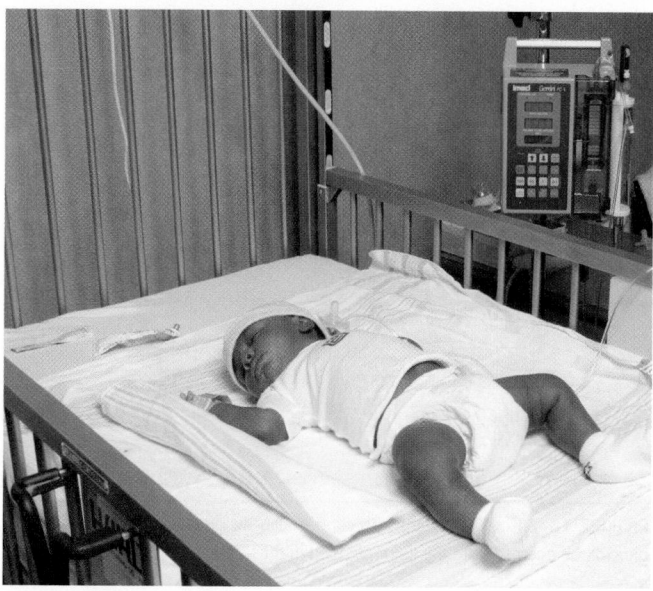

FIGURE 18–9 ➤ If isotonic fluid containing sodium is given too rapidly or in too great an amount, an extracellular fluid volume excess will develop. It is important to monitor fluid intake, excretion, and retention in infants and children.

Because fluid has weight, extracellular fluid volume excess is characterized by weight gain. An overload of fluid in the blood vessels and interstitial spaces can cause clinical manifestations such as bounding pulse, distended neck veins in children (not usually evident in infants), hepatomegaly, dyspnea, orthopnea, and lung crackles. Edema is the sign of overload of the interstitial fluid compartment. In an infant, edema is often generalized. Edema in children with extracellular fluid volume excess occurs in the dependent parts of the body, that is, in the parts closest to the ground. Thus, edema is evident in sacral areas in a child supine in bed. Edema that develops from other causes is described in the next section of this chapter.

Diagnosis of extracellular fluid volume excess is determined by clinical evaluation of weight gain and other manifestations. Serum electrolyte laboratory tests aid in diagnosis, and studies of liver or renal function may provide information about the cause of the condition.

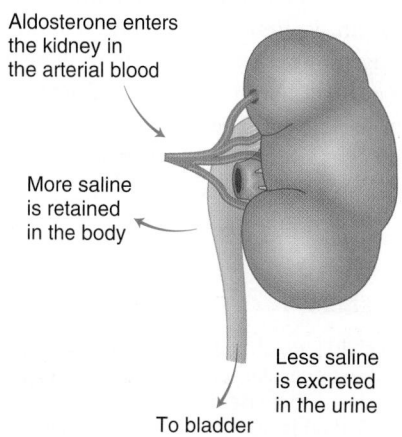

Aldosterone enters the kidney in the arterial blood

More saline is retained in the body

Less saline is excreted in the urine

To bladder

FIGURE 18–10 ➤ Aldosterone has a saline-retaining effect. Increased aldosterone secretion can be caused by adrenal tumors or congestive heart failure.

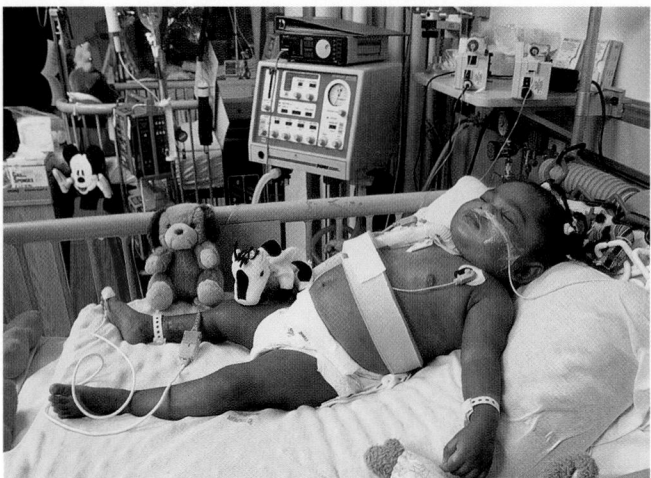

FIGURE 18–11 ➤ This infant with congenital heart disease has signs of generalized edema. Note the fluid retention in the face and abdomen.

Clinical therapy for extracellular fluid volume excess focuses on treating the underlying cause of the disorder in order to reduce the extracellular fluid volume excess. For example, a child who has congestive heart failure is given medications to strengthen the heart's ability to contract (see Chapter 21 ∞). Diuretics may be given to remove fluid from the body, thus reducing the extracellular fluid volume directly.

NURSING MANAGEMENT

Rapid weight gain is the most sensitive index of extracellular fluid volume excess. Therefore, daily weighing is an important nursing assessment. Measure the child's intake and output and weigh the diapers of infants. When treatment is successful, output is greater than intake. Assess the character of the pulse and observe for neck vein distention when the child is sitting (usually visible only in older children). Monitor for signs of pulmonary edema (an indication of severe imbalance) by listening to lung sounds in the dependent lung fields (crackles) and assessing for respiratory distress (rapid respiratory rate, use of accessory muscles of respiration). Observe for edema.

The potential for a child to develop a fluid overload is present whenever an isotonic intravenous solution containing sodium is being administered. Examples of these types of solutions include normal saline (0.9% NaCl), Ringer's solution, and lactated Ringer's solution. Therefore, monitor the infusion rate frequently and carefully and use a pump when possible to aid in accurate administration (Figure 18–12 ➤).

Clinical Tip

You can tell if a child's weight gain is due to normal growth or to the development of extracellular fluid volume excess by looking at the speed with which the increase develops. Sudden weight gain (e.g., 0.5 kg [1 lb] in 1 day) is due to the accumulation of fluid. Gain of 0.5 kg overnight is due to retention of about 500 mL of saline.

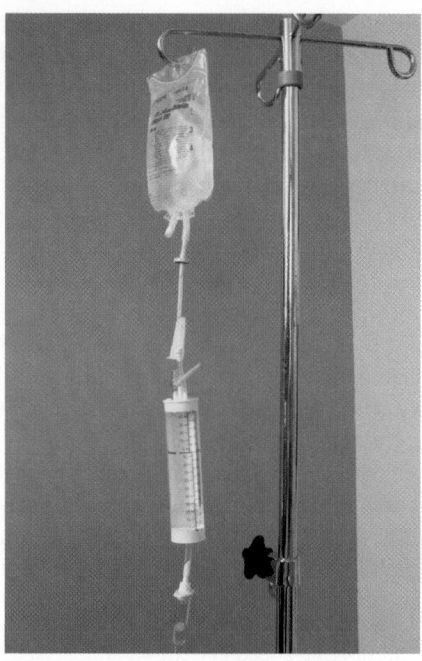

FIGURE 18–12 ➤ The use of a volume control device with an intravenous saline infusion is important to prevent a sudden extracellular fluid volume overload.

If an excess of fluid has already developed, administer the medical therapy as prescribed and monitor for any complications of the therapy. For example, many diuretics increase potassium excretion in the urine, an increase that may lead to an abnormally low plasma potassium concentration unless potassium intake is increased. (Refer to the discussion of hypokalemia later in this chapter.) It is also important to monitor for the development of extracellular fluid volume deficit as a result of diuretic therapy.

If edema is present, provide careful skin care and protection for edematous areas. Teach parents how to provide skin care and perform position changes at home. See the following section for additional interventions related to edema.

If a child has a long-term condition such as chronic renal failure that predisposes him or her to extracellular fluid volume ex-

Nursing Alert

Occasionally intravenous fluid is infused too rapidly, endangering the fluid and electrolyte status of a young child. The nurse can take the following measures to minimize this risk:

■ Use small bags of fluid, so if the fluid were to infuse quickly, the amount infused would be limited.

■ Always use infusion pumps when available so that the rate is programmed and monitored.

■ Check and double-check the machine after setting to be sure it was properly programmed.

■ Have another nurse check your calculation of rates and total fluid to be infused until you are certain of your skill in this area.

■ Finally, remember that even mechanical pumps can have faulty performance, so check the intravenous line, bag, and rate frequently.

cess, a dietary sodium restriction may be prescribed (see Chapter 26 ∞ for further details). Teach parents how to manage sodium restriction. Plan low-sodium meals that fit the family's cultural practices. If the child is old enough to participate, incorporate games into the teaching. If a scale is available, teach parents to take and record an accurate daily weight.

Clinical Tip

An infant's urine output is important in monitoring both dehydration and edema. Weigh the diaper before and after use. A 1-g weight increase in the diaper equals approximately 1 mL of urine volume. Change the diaper frequently to minimize loss from evaporation.

Expected outcomes include electrolyte balance, maintenance of intact skin, and dietary intake as prescribed.

Interstitial Fluid Volume Excess (Edema)

Edema is an abnormal increase in the volume of the interstitial fluid. It may be caused by an extracellular fluid volume excess or it may be due to other causes.

The causes of edema are best understood in the context of normal capillary dynamics. Fluid moves between the vascular and interstitial compartment by the process of filtration. Filtration is the net result of forces that tend to move fluid in opposing directions. The strongest forces will determine the direction of fluid movement.

At the capillary level, two forces (blood hydrostatic pressure and interstitial osmotic pressure) tend to move fluid from the capillaries into the interstitial fluid, while two other forces (blood colloid osmotic pressure and interstitial fluid hydrostatic pressure) tend to move fluid in the opposite direction (from the interstitial fluid into the capillaries). The net result of these forces usually moves fluid from the capillaries into the interstitial compartment at the arterial end of the capillaries and fluid from the interstitial compartment back into the capillaries at the venous end of the capillaries. This process brings oxygen and nutrients to the cells and removes carbon dioxide and other waste products.

Edema occurs if the balance of these four forces is altered so that excess fluid either enters or leaves the interstitial compartment (Figure 18–13 ➤). This may occur through (1) increased blood hydrostatic pressure, (2) decreased blood colloid osmotic pressure, (3) increased interstitial fluid osmotic pressure, or (4) blocked lymphatic drainage. Various clinical conditions are associated with these altered forces (Table 18–4), as described here:

1. *Increased blood hydrostatic pressure.* When extracellular fluid volume excess occurs, the increased fluid volume in the vascular compartment congests the veins. The pressure against the sides of the capillary is increased and more fluid then enters the interstitial compartment.
2. *Decreased blood colloid osmotic pressure.* Much of the osmotic pressure that pulls fluid into the capillaries is due to

TABLE 18–4	Clinical Conditions That Cause Edema
Cause	Clinical Condition
Edema due to increased blood hydrostatic pressure	Increased capillary blood flow • Inflammation • Local infection Venous congestion • Extracellular fluid volume excess • Right heart failure • Venous thrombosis • External pressure on vein • Muscle paralysis
Edema due to decreased blood osmotic pressure	Increased albumin excretion • Nephrotic syndrome (albumin leaks into urine) • Protein-losing enteropathies (excess albumin in feces) Decreased albumin synthesis • Kwashiorkor (low-protein, high-carbohydrate starvation diet provides too few amino acids for liver to make albumin) • Liver cirrhosis (diseased liver unable to make enough albumin)
Edema due to increased interstitial fluid osmotic pressure	Increased capillary permeability • Inflammation • Toxins • Hypersensitivity reactions • Burns
Edema due to blocked lymphatic drainage	Diseases • Tumors • Goiter • Parasites that obstruct lymph nodes • Surgery that removes lymph nodes

the presence of albumin and other plasma proteins made by the liver. The part of the blood osmotic pressure that is due to plasma proteins is often called **oncotic pressure** or blood colloid osmotic pressure. Any condition that decreases plasma proteins will decrease blood colloid osmotic pressure and cause edema. For example, if a clinical condition causes large amounts of albumin to leak into the urine, the liver will not be able to make albumin fast enough to replace it. As a result, the plasma protein level will fall, decreasing the blood osmotic pressure. Without this pulling force to return fluid to the capillaries, edema will occur. This is the cause of the edema that occurs in children who have nephrotic syndrome (see Chapter 26 ∞). Another cause in children is prolonged surgical procedures with significant blood loss. Intravenous fluids and blood may be infused during surgery to replace these losses, but plasma proteins are lost and not fully restored by infusion, causing edema in the postoperative period.

Pathophysiology Illustrated
Capillary Dynamics and Edema

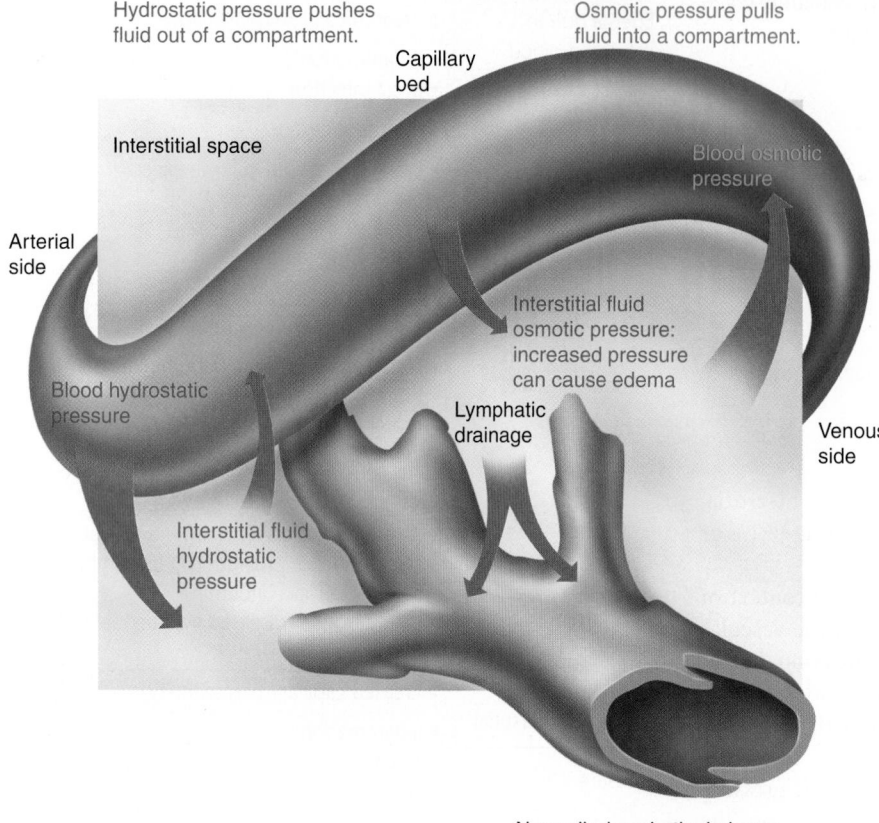

Hydrostatic pressure pushes fluid out of a compartment.

Osmotic pressure pulls fluid into a compartment.

Capillary bed

Interstitial space

Blood osmotic pressure

Arterial side

Interstitial fluid osmotic pressure: increased pressure can cause edema

Blood hydrostatic pressure

Lymphatic drainage

Venous side

Interstitial fluid hydrostatic pressure

Normally, lymphatic drainage removes small proteins and excess interstitial fluid. Blocked lymphatic drainage can cause edema.

FIGURE 18–13 ➤ With normal capillary dynamics, fluid moves out of the compartment by the force of hydrostatic pressure in the blood vessel and is pulled out by interstitial osmotic pressure. Fluid is forced into the compartment by interstitial hydrostatic pressure and pulled in by compartment osmotic pressure. Abnormal capillary dynamics cause edema.

3. *Increased interstitial fluid osmotic pressure.* Ordinarily, only a few small proteins enter the interstitial fluid, and the interstitial fluid osmotic pressure is small. If the capillary becomes abnormally permeable to proteins, however, the influx of large amounts of proteins into the interstitial fluid causes a dramatic increase in interstitial fluid osmotic pressure. This increased pulling force keeps an abnormal amount of fluid in the interstitial compartment. This mechanism plays an important part in the edema caused by a bee sting or a sprained ankle. It occurs to a greater extent in burns, leading to swelling at the same time that there is a great loss of fluid volume through the burned skin (see Chapter 31 ∞).

4. *Blocked lymphatic drainage.* The lymph vessels normally drain small proteins and excess fluid from the interstitial compartment and return them to the blood vessels. If this process is blocked, fluid accumulates in the interstitial compartment. This may occur when a tumor blocks lymphatic drainage.

Edema causes swelling, which may be localized or generalized. The swelling of tissue may cause pain and restrict motion. Edema that is due to extracellular fluid volume excess or right-sided heart failure usually occurs in the dependent portion of the body. In a child who is walking, dependent edema is observed in the ankles; in a child who is supine in bed, it is seen in

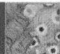 **Culture** *Sodium Use*

Adapt teaching about low-sodium diets to the cultural practices of a family by asking them what types of food they usually eat. Help them to choose low-sodium foods from their diets and to avoid high-sodium foods. This approach is more effective than giving the same list of restricted foods to each family.

For example, some Asians may use monosodium glutamate to flavor foods and can be encouraged to add this at the table for family members who can have extra sodium rather than during cooking. Many Hispanic groups use large amounts of cheese that can provide significant sodium. Encourage them to look for low-sodium cheese and substitute cottage cheese for other types since it is lower in sodium. Low-sodium milk is available and a good option for young children. Canned foods tend to have high sodium, so teach all families to use fresh or frozen produce rather than canned when possible. Teach families how to read and interpret food labels to identify salt (sodium) content.

the sacral area. The skin over an edematous area often appears thin and shiny.

The main focus of clinical therapy for edema is to treat the underlying condition that caused the edema. Such conditions are discussed throughout this book. The edema from inflammation of an injury is initially treated with cold to reduce capillary blood flow and thus reduce blood hydrostatic pressure.

NURSING MANAGEMENT

A child or parent may make comments that alert the nurse to the development of edema. Shoes may become tight by the end of the day (dependent edema); the waistband of pants or a skirt may be "outgrown" suddenly (generalized edema or ascites, which is accumulation of fluid in the peritoneal cavity); the eyes may be puffy (periorbital edema); a ring may be too tight; fingers may "feel like sausages." In many cases visual inspection is sufficient to recognize edema. Observe for the presence of **pitting edema**, a "pit" or concave indentation that remains after an edematous area is pressed downward by the examiner's fingers. To detect changes in the amount of swelling, measure around the edematous part (Figure 18–14 ➤). If the edema is caused by extracellular fluid volume excess, daily measurements of weight and intake and output are a necessary part of the daily assessment. Nursing assessment should also focus on the integrity of the skin, presence of pain, restricted motion, and alterations in the child's body image.

Elevation of an area of localized edema helps to reduce the swelling. The skin over an edematous area needs extra care because it is fragile (Figure 18–15 ➤). Carefully position an infant or child who is on bed rest and turn frequently to prevent pressure sores (see Chapter 31 ∞ for further information on pressure sores). Turning must be performed carefully to avoid skin abrasion by rubbing against the sheets. Pat the skin dry after cleansing rather than rubbing it. Trim the child's fingernails smooth to prevent scratching. Teach parents skin care for the child at home. Teach older children to inspect their skin carefully to identify areas needing special care.

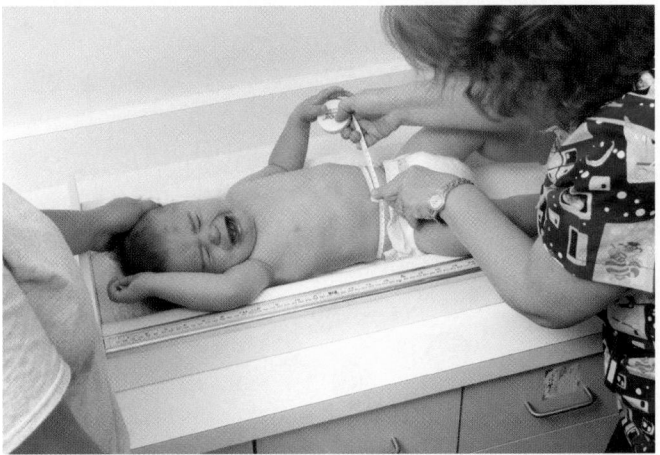

FIGURE 18–14 ➤ Finding the same location each day for measuring circumference to assess edema can be accomplished by use of a reference point. An indelible marker may be used to mark the measurement location on the skin, if this is acceptable to the child and parents.

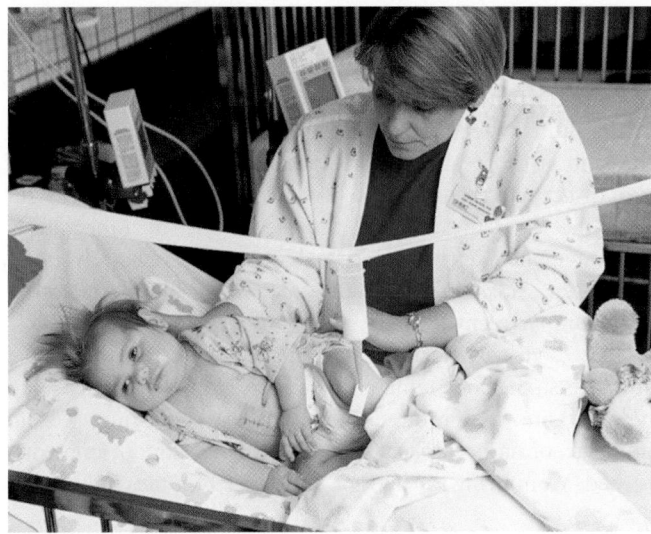

FIGURE 18–15 ➤ Edematous tissue is easily damaged. It must be kept clean, dry, and free of pressure.

If restricted mobility is a problem, specific plans to help the child manage activities are needed. For example, if an edematous finger restricts the motion of a hand, food can be cut into bite-size portions before the meal is served, so that the child can still eat independently.

Discomfort from edema may require creative interventions by the nurse. If the child has a fluid restriction, access to fluids needs to be planned to provide satiety. Distraction with toys or activities appropriate to the child's developmental level can be useful. Interventions to treat the underlying problem can also reduce the edema and its accompanying discomfort. Interventions for edema should be added to the nursing management of the underlying condition that causes the edema. Administration of the prescribed medical therapy and observation for the complications of therapy are nursing responsibilities.

Nursing Alert

Nursing interventions for a child who has a fluid restriction (modify according to the child's developmental level):

- Give cold rather than lukewarm fluids.
- Use an insulated glass that looks bigger than it is.
- Be sure that extra fluids are removed from meal trays before the child sees them.
- Have the child swish fluids around in the mouth before swallowing to relieve thirst.
- Provide frequent oral care.
- Suggest eating meals dry and drinking between meals.
- Provide a chart so an older child can keep intake records.

Discuss with school-age children and adolescents feelings of embarrassment about the edematous appearance. They need to understand the reason for edema and be able to explain it to peers. Arrange for the child to meet other children with similar concerns.

Desired outcomes of care include maintenance of intact skin, normal respiratory sounds and effort, and normal weight patterns.

■ ELECTROLYTE IMBALANCES

All body fluids contain electrolytes, although the concentration of those electrolytes varies, depending on the type and location of the fluid. When a serum electrolyte value is reported from the laboratory, it provides information about the concentration of that electrolyte in the blood. It may not necessarily reflect the concentration of the electrolyte in other body compartments. Refer to Table 18–1 to see which electrolytes are of highest and lowest concentration in the blood and other fluid compartments.

Electrolytes are normally gained and lost in relatively equal amounts so the body remains in balance. However, when a child has an abnormal route of loss, such as vomiting, wound drainage, or nasogastric suction, electrolyte balance can be disturbed. Monitoring for signs of imbalance becomes important.

Sodium Imbalances

The serum sodium concentration reflects the **osmolality** of body fluids, that is, their degree of concentration or dilution. It refers to the number of moles of the substance per kilogram of water in the solution. Serum sodium concentration reflects the proportion of water and sodium in the extracellular compartment. When the osmolality of body fluids becomes abnormal, the cells shrink or swell. These cell size changes are due to *osmosis*, the movement of water across a semipermeable membrane into an area of higher particle concentration. Sodium levels are maintained at high extracellular and low intracellular levels by the sodium-potassium pump, which moves these electrolytes against their expected concentration gradients (Figure 18–16 ➤).

Sodium plays several important roles in the body and is an important **cation** (positively charged particle). It is important in blood pressure regulation and maintenance of fluid volume.

Hypernatremia

Hypernatremia is a condition of increased osmolality of the blood. The body fluids are too concentrated, containing excess sodium relative to water. A serum sodium level above 146 mmol/L in children is diagnostic of hypernatremia (Custer & Rau, 2009).

Hypernatremia results from conditions that cause the body to lose relatively more water than sodium or to gain relatively more sodium than water (Table 18–5). Examples include children who do not have access to adequate water or are developmentally delayed and do not perceive thirst. Special circumstances in which a high solute intake may occur without adequate water include an infant formula that is too concentrated or one that is prepared with salt instead of sugar. A breastfed baby not receiving adequate breast milk who has normal water loss may develop hypernatremic dehydration. This is a particular risk at 2 to 3 days of age, when babies generally have diuresis, if the baby does not feed well, or if the mother does not yet produce an adequate amount of breast milk (Shroff, Hignett, Pierce, et al., 2007).

An infant or child who has hypernatremia is generally thirsty. The urine output is diminished unless the hypernatremia is caused by diabetes insipidus. A decreased level of consciousness manifested by confusion, lethargy, or coma results from shrinking of the brain cells. Seizures can occur when hypernatremia occurs rapidly or is severe. Symptoms in the neonate include decreased activity and alertness, loss of 10% or more of birth weight, and seizures. Severe hypernatremia can be fatal.

The major laboratory test that is diagnostic of sodium imbalance is serum sodium. Normal level for newborns is 131 to 144 mmol/L and for children is 132 to 141 mmol/L. See Table 18–6 for a list of normal serum electrolyte values. Specific gravity of urine is concentrated in hypernatremia. Antidiuretic hormone (ADH) levels and 24-hour urinary output are helpful in diagnosing diabetes insipidus as the cause (see Chapter 26 ∞).

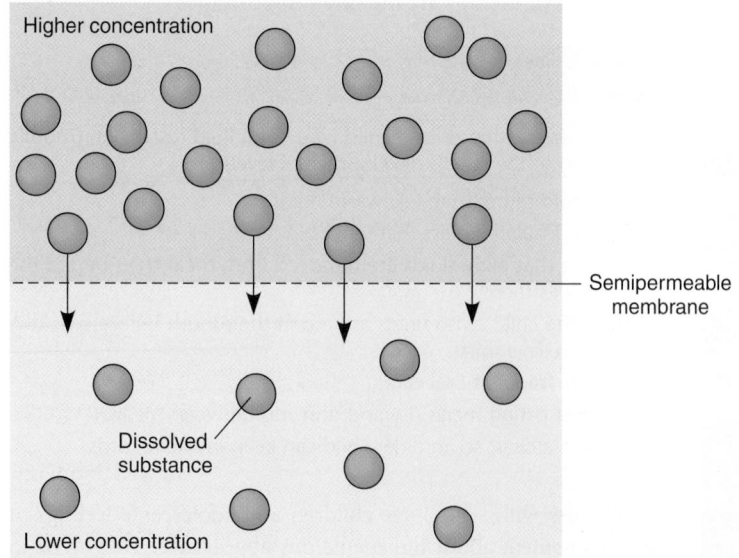

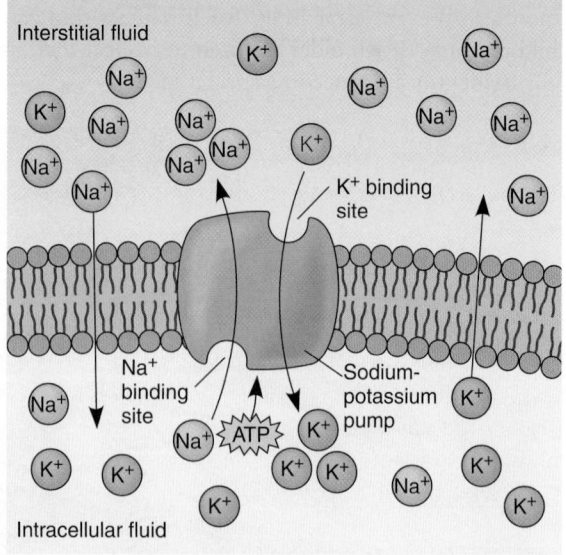

FIGURE 18–16 ➤ A, Water balance is maintained by the simple passage of molecules from greater to lesser concentration across cell membranes. B, Sodium levels are maintained by an active transport system, the sodium-potassium pump, which moves these electrolytes across cell membranes in spite of their concentrations. At times, a pathophysiologic condition causes the pump to not function as quickly and efficiently as needed to maintain balance.

TABLE 18–5	Causes of Hypernatremia	
Loss of Relatively More Water than Sodium	Gain of Relatively More Sodium than Water
Diabetes insipidus (not enough antidiuretic hormone)	Inability to communicate thirst
Diarrhea or vomiting without fluid replacement	Limited or no access to water
Excessive sweating without fluid replacement	High solute intake without adequate water (e.g., tube feedings)
High solute intake without adequate water (causes kidneys to excrete water)	Intravenous hypertonic saline

TABLE 18–6	Normal Serum Values for Electrolytes in Infants and Children	
	Newborn	Infant and Child
Sodium	131–144 mmol/L	132–141 mmol/L
Potassium	Premature 4.5–7.2 mmol/L Term 3.2–5.7 mmol/L	3.3–4.7 mmol/L
Calcium (total)	Premature 1.7–2.3 mmol/L Term 2.10–2.64 mmol/L (8.4–10.6 mg/dL)	2.12–2.64 mmol/L (8.5–10.6 mg/dL)
Magnesium	0.65–1.02 mmol/L (1.6–2.5 mg/dL)	0.7–1.1 mmol/L (1.6–2.7 mg/dL)

Note: Laboratories may have slightly different levels of normal depending on assays performed. Always consult the normal values for your particular laboratory.

Clinical Tip

Normal specific gravity of urine:

Infants to 2 years: 1.001–1.015

Children 2 years: 1.010–1.030

Note: Specific gravity compares the density of urine with the density of water (density of water is 1.000). The infant's kidney is less able to concentrate urine, so urine is more dilute. And remember that the child under 2 years is less able to concentrate urine even when dehydrated, so specific gravity may not indicate the true severity of the infant's fluid and electrolyte imbalance.

Hypernatremia is treated by intravenous administration of **hypotonic fluid**, or fluid that is more dilute than normal body fluid. This therapy dilutes the body fluids back to normal concentration. If a child is dehydrated, **isotonic fluids** (those with the osmolality of body fluids) may be ordered first to replenish the volume, followed by hypotonic fluid to correct the osmolality. The underlying cause of the disorder is also treated.

NURSING MANAGEMENT

Teaching can prevent many cases of hypernatremia. Be sure the breastfeeding mother has instruction and resources about lactation before discharge after delivery. If discharged soon after birth, be sure the infant has an appointment to have weight and alertness checked within the first few days, and instruct the parents about normal output of four to six wet diapers daily. By about 10 days, infants should have regained the birth weight. Assess the infant's alertness and general neurological status.

When an infant is sick or developing slowly, parents sometimes want to feed the infant more concentrated formula to build the child's strength. Parents and caregivers of bottle-fed babies should be taught never to give undiluted formula concentrate or evaporated milk due to the high sodium content.

Clinical Tip

Careful teaching about how to mix powdered formula so that it is not too concentrated can help prevent hypernatremia. Pictures are an important teaching tool if the parents are not able to read labels or instructions.

Children with delayed development are at risk for hypernatremia since they may not be able to recognize thirst or obtain fluids when dehydrated. Teach parents about the child's fluid requirements and ensure that nursing staff offers adequate fluids when the child is hospitalized.

Parents should be cautioned to keep salt out of reach, because eating handfuls of salt has caused hypernatremia. Teach parents to offer extra fluids during hot weather. See Families Want to Know: Preventing Heat-Related Illness on page 483. Teach oral rehydration therapy for use at home during mild vomiting and diarrhea (see page 483).

When a child is hospitalized for hypernatremia, monitor serum sodium level and measure intake and output and urine specific gravity. Specific gravity changes toward normal levels as therapy progresses. Frequently assess responsiveness to monitor the effect of hypernatremia on brain cells. As the concentration of body fluids returns to normal, the child will become more alert and responsive. Watch for rebound hyponatremia while monitoring the fluid replacement. Implement safety interventions such as raised bed rails for protection. Ensure adequate rest and introduce developmentally appropriate activities when the child is alert.

Water deprivation is a form of child neglect or abuse. In neglect, the parents simply do not provide adequate water for the child. A form of child abuse that sometimes includes water deprivation is Munchausen syndrome by proxy (see Chapter 17 ∞). A small child who is hospitalized with hypernatremia that does not have a detectable cause may be subject to water deprivation. Assess the child's general condition, developmental tasks, the family dynamics, and the parent's understanding of formula preparation and the child's fluid intake needs.

Nurses can prevent hypernatremia in hospitalized infants and children by administering water between tube feedings, keeping water available, and offering it frequently. Offering frequent small amounts and using Popsicles and other creative interventions can increase children's intake.

Desired outcomes of treatment for hypernatremia include balance of electrolytes and fluid in the intracellular and extracellular compartments, as well as alert level of consciousness.

Hyponatremia

In hyponatremia, the osmolality of the blood is decreased. The body fluids are too dilute and contain excess water relative to sodium. Hyponatremia is the most common sodium imbalance in children (Kliegman, Behrman, Jenson, et al., 2007). A serum sodium level below 132 mmol/L in children (131 mmol/L in newborns) is diagnostic of hyponatremia.

Etiology and Pathophysiology Hyponatremia results from conditions that cause gain of relatively more water than sodium or loss of relatively more sodium than water (Table 18–7). Oral intake of water causes hyponatremia in unusual conditions such as forced fluid intake. More commonly, parents feed an infant only water or dilute formula to save money instead of regular-strength formula or breast milk. Excessive swallowing of swimming pool water by an infant can have the same effect. Infants are vulnerable to the type of hyponatremia caused by water intoxication, because they have a poorly developed thirst mechanism and may continue to drink, and then are unable to excrete excess water quickly due to immature kidney function. Hospitalized children who are treated with hypotonic saline rather than isotonic solutions can also acquire hyponatremia. Young children are at particular risk because they commonly respond to surgery with increased levels of antidiuretic hormone (ADH) for 3 to 5 days postsurgery, causing decreased excretion of urine; use of hypotonic solutions during this period can cause hyponatremia. Additionally, they have a high brain-to-skull mass and are therefore at high risk of developing the neurologic complications of hyponatremia. Exercise-associated hyponatremia can occur when persons in prolonged physical activity such as marathon running consume hypotonic fluids in the form of water or sports drinks above the levels lost in respiratory, gastrointestinal, skin, and urinary routes (Howe & Boden, 2007).

Clinical Manifestations The child who has hyponatremia has a decreased level of consciousness, which results from edema of brain cells. Manifestations include anorexia, nausea, vomiting, confusion, headache, respiratory distress, muscle weakness, decreased deep tendon reflexes, agitation, lethargy, or confusion. The condition can progress to respiratory arrest, dilated pupils, decorticate posturing, and coma. If hyponatremia arises rapidly or is extreme, seizures may occur. It is a frequent cause of seizures in infants under 6 months of age. Severe hyponatremia can be fatal.

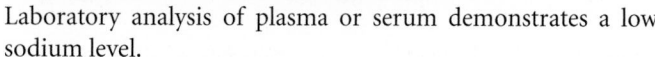

COLLABORATIVE CARE

Laboratory analysis of plasma or serum demonstrates a low sodium level.

Hyponatremia should be prevented in hospitalized children receiving intravenous solutions (particularly postoperatively) by administering isotonic rather than hypotonic solutions. In cases of improper formula preparation or fluid intake, hyponatremia is treated by feeding proper formula or restricting the intake of water. This therapy allows the kidneys to correct the imbalance by excreting excess water from the body. Intravenous **hypertonic fluid** (more concentrated than body fluid) may be administered for severe cases. Use of this concentrated saline is a way to rapidly increase body fluid concentration, but it must be monitored carefully because it can easily cause rebound hypernatremia. For exercise-associated hyponatremia, intravenous access is established at the first aid site, hypertonic saline is administered, and oxygen is delivered (Hew-Butler, Ayus, Kipps, et al., 2008). In cases of diabetes insipidus, treatment for the condition is needed (see Chapter 30 ∞).

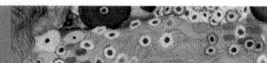

NURSING MANAGEMENT

Nursing Assessment and Diagnosis

Hyponatremia should be prevented in hospitalized children receiving intravenous solutions (particularly postoperatively) by administering isotonic rather than hypotonic solutions. Monitor serum sodium level and measure intake and output. If an infant with hyponatremia has normal ADH levels, and other causes have been ruled out, careful questioning about proper preparation of formula and feeding practices is needed. A toddler or school-age child may be subjected to forced fluid intake as a form of child abuse. Sensitive interviewing and a caring manner on the part of the nurse can help identify such problems in a family.

Because hyponatremia is characterized by a decreased level of consciousness, frequent assessment of responsiveness will be necessary to monitor the response to therapy. The child will become more alert and responsive as the concentration of body fluids returns to normal. Carefully monitor hospitalized children and those exercising for signs of hyponatremia.

The highest priority nursing diagnosis for hyponatremia addresses the Risk for Injury related to the child's decreased level of consciousness and cerebral edema. The following nursing diagnoses might also apply:

- Self-Care Deficit related to weakness and fatigue
- Altered Health Maintenance related to parental information misinterpretation about infant formula
- Ineffective Breast-Feeding related to inadequate sucking by infant or inadequate milk production

TABLE 18–7	Causes of Hyponatremia
Gain of Relatively More Water than Sodium	Loss of Relatively More Sodium than Water
Excessive intravenous D5W (5% dextrose in water) rather than isotonic fluids for hospitalized children Excessive tap water enemas Irrigation of body cavities with distilled water Excessive antidiuretic hormone Forced excessive oral intake of tap water Excessive intake of water during exercise Congestive heart failure	Diarrhea or vomiting with replacement by tap water only instead of fluid containing sodium Excessive sweating such as in cystic fibrosis Diuretics, especially thiazides

Planning and Implementation

Nurses can prevent hyponatremia in hospitalized children by using normal saline instead of distilled water for irrigations and by avoiding tap water enemas. Verify intravenous types and amounts and question use of hypotonic fluids in a child with no intake of sodium. Teach parents to replace body fluids lost through diarrhea or vomiting with oral electrolyte solutions (see the discussion of oral rehydration therapy earlier in this chapter). Teach the person with prolonged exercise to slowly increase exercise times, rehydrate according to thirst, and ensure intake of sodium-containing fluids. The child with diseases such as cystic fibrosis or who is taking thiazide diuretics needs intake above that recommended for usual maintenance needs.

Evaluation

Expected outcomes of nursing care for hyponatremia include the following:

- The child remains safe from injury.
- Balance of fluid and electrolytes is maintained.
- Proper intake of formula, breast milk, and other fluids is established.

Potassium Imbalances

Potassium is an essential **anion** (negatively charged particle) that performs many necessary functions in the body. It is present in high levels in intracellular fluids and is active in enzyme performance in cells. It is needed for contractility of heart and skeletal muscle. Potassium intake in healthy children comes from potassium-rich foods such as fruits and vegetables. Potassium is absorbed easily from the intestine.

A potassium imbalance arises when the serum potassium concentration rises or falls outside the normal range. Potassium imbalances are caused by alterations in potassium intake, distribution, or excretion; or by loss of potassium through an abnormal route such as burns, emesis, or renal failure.

Most of the potassium ions in the body are found inside the cells. The sodium-potassium pump in cell membranes moves potassium ions into cells to maintain the high intracellular potassium concentration (see Figure 18–13). In addition, potassium ions can be shifted into or out of cells by various physiologic factors (Figure 18–17 ➤). Potassium is excreted from the body through urine, feces, and sweat. The hormone aldosterone increases potassium excretion in the urine.

Hyperkalemia

Hyperkalemia, an excess of potassium in the blood, is reflected by a level above 5.5 mmol/L in children or above 5.7 mmol/L in newborns.

Etiology and Pathophysiology   Hyperkalemia is caused by conditions that involve increased potassium intake, shift of potassium from cells into the extracellular fluid, and decreased potassium excretion. Renal insufficiency is a primary cause of hyperkalemia (Custer & Rau, 2009). Increased potassium intake is usually due to intravenous potassium overload. Excessive or

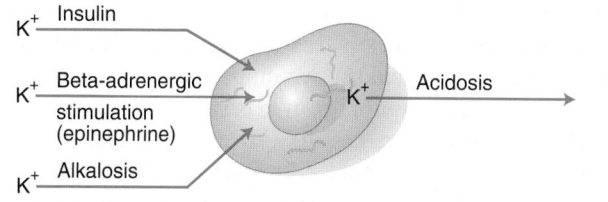

FIGURE 18–17 ➤ Factors that shift potassium ions into or out of cells.

too rapid intravenous administration of potassium-containing solutions can occur if the potassium requirement is overestimated or if the intravenous infusion runs in too quickly.

Blood transfusion is another source of potassium intake that may cause hyperkalemia. Potassium ions leak out of red blood cells that are stored in a blood bank. The longer the blood is stored, the more potassium leaks out of cells and accumulates in the fluid portion of the transfusion. Hyperkalemia from administration of stored blood arises when multiple units are transfused, as when infants receive exchange transfusions or children receive multiple blood transfusions after a serious injury or in surgery.

Shift of potassium from cells into the extracellular fluid occurs when there is massive cell death, as with a crush injury, in sickle cell anemia (hemolytic crisis), or when chemotherapy for a malignancy is rapidly effective. In these situations, the dead cells release their high-potassium contents into the extracellular fluid. Potassium ions also shift out of cells in metabolic acidosis caused by diarrhea and in diabetes mellitus when insulin levels are low.

Decreased potassium excretion occurs with acute or chronic oliguria during renal failure, severe hypovolemia, and conditions that decrease the secretion of aldosterone by the adrenal cortex (lead poisoning, Addison disease, hypoaldosteronism). Several medications can cause hyperkalemia (see the companion website).

Clinical Manifestations   All clinical manifestations of hyperkalemia are related to muscle dysfunction because potassium plays a vital role in muscle activity. Hyperactivity of gastrointestinal smooth muscle causes intestinal colic, cramping, and diarrhea in some children. The skeletal muscles become weak, beginning typically with leg weakness and then ascending up the body. Weakness can progress to flaccid paralysis. The child is often lethargic. Dysfunction of cardiac muscle causes cardiac arrhythmias such as tachycardia and may result in heart failure and cardiac arrest. Abnormalities in the electrocardiogram include a prolonged QRS complex, a peak in T waves, and prolonged PR intervals. Renal signs include oliguria and anuria (Custer & Rau, 2009).

COLLABORATIVE CARE

The major diagnostic tool is the serum laboratory test for potassium. In addition, observations of symptoms and abnormal electrocardiograph are indicative of hyperkalemia. Hyperkalemia is treated by management of the underlying condition that caused the imbalance. For mild cases, intake of potassium is restricted, and loop or thiazide diuretics may be administered. If the serum potassium concentration is very high or is causing

Drugs That May Cause Electrolyte Disturbances Table

dangerous cardiac arrhythmias, treatment to decrease the serum potassium level may be ordered. These treatments may remove potassium from the body or drive it from the extracellular fluid into the cells. Potassium is removed from the body by peritoneal dialysis or hemodialysis, and with a cation exchange resin (Kayexalate) or 70% sorbitol, both of which can be administered orally or rectally. Medical treatments that drive potassium ions into cells are intravenous sodium bicarbonate, intravenous insulin, glucose, and calcium gluconate.

Clinical Tip

If an infant's hyperkalemia was diagnosed using blood obtained from a heel stick, intracellular fluid may have contaminated the sample. A venous sample should be obtained. Additionally, it is possible for a blood sample to be damaged and show increased potassium when tested. If there is an absence of symptoms in the child, obtain a repeat sample for analysis to verify results.

NURSING MANAGEMENT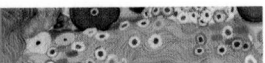

Nursing Assessment and Diagnosis

Monitor serum potassium levels. Ongoing assessment of muscle strength is important, because the muscle weakness may progress to flaccid paralysis. (This paralysis is reversible on correction of the potassium imbalance.) Diarrhea or colic can occur in infants and children. An older child may complain of intestinal cramping. Monitor the pulse rate carefully. Monitor urinary output, particularly in children with renal disease.

Nursing diagnoses for a child who has hyperkalemia depend on the severity of the clinical manifestations. The cause of the imbalance may also lead to useful diagnoses that guide teaching for the child and the parents regarding safety measures and accurate medication administration. The following nursing diagnoses may apply:

- Activity Intolerance related to decreased cardiac output secondary to cardiac arrhythmias
- Risk for Injury related to muscle weakness
- Self-Care Deficit: Hygiene and Dressing related to neuromuscular impairment
- Anxiety related to change in health status
- Ineffective Health Maintenance related to parental lack of exposure to potassium intake in chronic renal failure
- Ineffective Management of Therapeutic Regimen related to complexity of therapy

Planning and Implementation

Nursing care includes measures to prevent hyperkalemia from developing in hospitalized children. If hyperkalemia does develop, care shifts to administering intravenous solutions, monitoring cardiopulmonary status continuously, ensuring safety, promoting adequate nutrition, and preparing the child and family for discharge. For the child in the community, potassium levels are monitored when the child is taking a drug that can cause hyperkalemia, such as those used for cancer treatment. Any child who is receiving an intravenous infusion that contains potassium is at risk for hyperkalemia. Check that urine output is normal (1–2 mL/kg/hr) before administering intravenous potassium solutions. Double-check the potassium order and intravenous dosage with another nurse. Observe the child closely and perform cardiorespiratory monitoring.

Upon diagnosis of hyperkalemia, an electrocardiogram is performed and a cardiac monitor is applied. Monitor for any changes in cardiac status and for cardiac arrhythmias. Report abnormal rate and character of pulse as well as shortness of breath.

Be sure blood or packed red blood cells are fresh, especially for the child receiving multiple transfusions and for all neonates. Be certain that the cardiac monitor is applied and functioning during infusion of these products to watch for arrhythmias.

Once a child is diagnosed as hyperkalemic, ensure that any infusions with added potassium are stopped. Several infusions may need to be managed, including glucose, sodium bicarbonate, and calcium gluconate. Maintain the infusion at the ordered rate and monitor the child's condition frequently.

Since the child is weak, side rails should be raised. Position the child carefully. Assist the child with activities requiring leg muscle strength, such as going to the bathroom, climbing into bed, or pushing up in bed. Encourage quiet activities appropriate for developmental level with frequent rest periods. Document and report any change in muscle weakness.

Adequate caloric intake is necessary to prevent tissue breakdown and the resultant potassium release from cells. Offer the child nourishing snacks if his or her appetite is decreased. Restrict potassium-rich foods.

If the child is discharged to return home with chronic renal failure or another condition that decreases aldosterone secretion, parents and the child need to be taught to restrict foods that are high in potassium (see Table 18–8). Most oral rehydration solutions, including Pedialyte, contain potassium and should not be used to provide fluid for the child. Instruct the family not to use salt substitutes, which commonly contain potassium. Parents should check with the care provider and pharmacist before giving even over-the-counter products to the child, as some of these medications contain potassium. Management of renal failure at home with frequent visits for dialysis and other treatments can be challenging. Refer to Chapter 26 ∞ for further suggestions to help parents handle this condition.

Evaluation

Expected outcomes of nursing care for hyperkalemia include the following:

- The child returns to a state of fluid and electrolyte balance.
- Safety is maintained.

Growth & Development 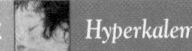 *Hyperkalemia*

The nursing diagnoses for children with hyperkalemia will prompt a nurse to provide safety measures appropriate to the child's developmental level and to assist the child with activities that muscle weakness makes difficult. It is important to provide play and diversional activities that take into account both the child's degree of muscle strength and the appropriate developmental level.

TABLE 18–8	**Food Sources of Electrolytes**
Electrolyte	Food Sources
Potassium-Rich Foods	Apricots Bananas Cantaloupe Cherries Dates Figs Molasses Orange juice Peaches Potatoes Prunes Raisins Strawberries Tomato juice
Calcium-Rich Foods	Cheese Chicken Egg yolks Figs Grains (cream of wheat, farina, bran muffins) Legumes Milk Nuts Pudding Sardines (canned) Yogurt
Magnesium-Rich Foods	Almonds Dark-green vegetables Egg yolk Peanut butter Soy Whole-grain cereal

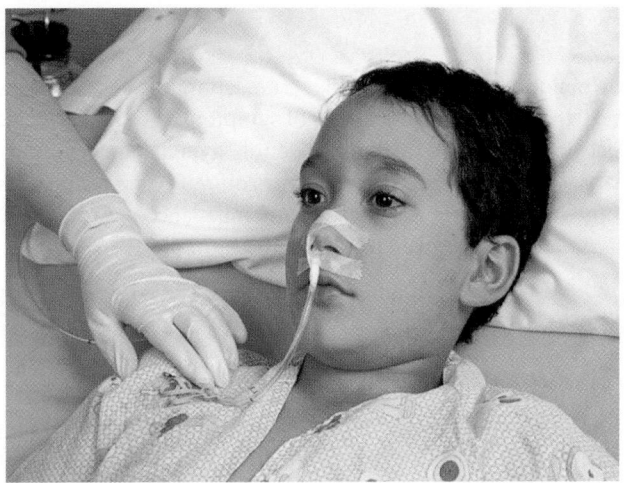

FIGURE 18–18 ➤ Because this child has a nasogastric tube in place that requires suctioning, it is important to monitor his potassium levels. A variety of conditions can lead to hypercalcemia and hypocalcemia.

- The child receives adequate nutritional intake to provide essential potassium.
- Normal cardiac rate and rhythm is maintained.

Hypokalemia

Hypokalemia occurs when the serum potassium concentration is too low. Total body potassium may be decreased, normal, or even increased when the serum level is low, depending on the cause of the imbalance. Serum potassium levels below 3.3 mmol/L in children (3.2 mmol/L for newborns) are diagnostic of hypokalemia.

Etiology and Pathophysiology   Hypokalemia is caused by conditions that involve increased potassium excretion, decreased potassium intake, shift of potassium from the extracellular fluid into cells, and loss of potassium by an abnormal route.

Increased potassium excretion through the gastrointestinal tract is the major cause of hypokalemia in children. Loss of potassium occurs through vomiting and diarrhea (gastroenteritis). In the chapter-opening vignette, Vernon had increased potassium excretion through diarrhea. Self-induced vomiting in bulimia is another example of this cause. Nasogastric suctioning (Figure 18–18 ➤) and intestinal decompression can cause potassium loss.

Causes of increased urinary potassium excretion are osmotic diuresis (glucose present in urine), hypomagnesemia, hypercalcemia, increased aldosterone (hyperaldosteronism, congestive heart failure, nephrotic syndrome, cirrhosis), and increased cortisol (Cushing disease and syndrome) (Custer & Rau, 2009). Eating large amounts of black licorice made from the root of *Glycyrrhiza glabra* increases renal retention of sodium and excretion of potassium.

Decreased potassium intake will lead to hypokalemia slowly, or more rapidly if combined with increased excretion or loss of potassium. Hospitalized children may be placed on NPO status and receive prolonged intravenous therapy without potassium. Adolescents concerned about weight loss or those with anorexia nervosa may embark on diets low in potassium and may take medications that induce diuresis or diarrhea.

Shift of potassium from the extracellular fluid into cells occurs in alkalosis and hypothermia (unintentional or induced for surgery). Hyperalimentation often causes hypersecretion of insulin, which also shifts potassium into cells. Hypokalemia can also be caused by several medications.

Clinical Manifestations   Since the ratio of intracellular to extracellular potassium determines the responsiveness of muscle cells to neural stimuli, it is not surprising that the clinical manifestations of hypokalemia involve muscle dysfunction. Gastrointestinal smooth muscle activity is slowed, leading to diminished bowel tones, abdominal distention, constipation, or paralytic ileus. Skeletal muscles are weak and unresponsive to stimuli, deep tendon reflexes are diminished, and weakness may progress to flaccid paralysis. The respiratory muscles may be impaired. Cardiac arrhythmias can occur, particularly a prolonged QT interval, depressed ST segment, and flat or inverted T waves. Polyuria, polydipsia, and decreased urine specific gravity result from changes in the kidney caused by hypokalemia (Custer & Rau, 2009).

COLLABORATIVE CARE

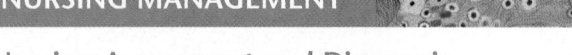

The major diagnostic tool is the serum laboratory test for potassium. In addition, observations of symptoms and an abnormal electrocardiograph are indicative of hypokalemia. Medical management of hypokalemia focuses on replacement of potassium while treating the cause of the imbalance. Potassium replacement may be given intravenously or orally.

NURSING MANAGEMENT

Nursing Assessment and Diagnosis

Monitor serum potassium levels. Observe for muscle weakness, which is frequently detected first in the legs. Parents may report that muscle weakness restricts the child's activities and impairs interactions with peers. Skeletal muscle strength can be difficult to assess if the child is lethargic, as shown with Vernon at the beginning of the chapter.

Muscle weakness may affect the respiratory muscles. Assess the child frequently to determine the need for assisted ventilation. Cardiac monitoring is important for continued assessment of hypokalemia-associated arrhythmias.

Assess for diminished bowel sounds. Ask the parents if the child has recently been awakening to use the toilet at night or has begun bed-wetting after previously being dry at night. These may be symptoms of polyuria associated with chronic hypokalemia.

The most important nursing diagnoses in the child with severe hypokalemia relate to cardiac arrhythmias and respiratory muscle weakness. The following nursing diagnoses may apply:

- Risk for Activity Intolerance related to decreased cardiac output secondary to cardiac dysrhythmias
- Risk for Injury related to muscle weakness
- Constipation related to decreased motility
- Ineffective Health Maintenance related to management of potassium supplements or high-potassium diet
- Imbalanced Nutrition: Less than Body Requirements related to lack of basic nutritional knowledge regarding safe weight-loss diet

Planning and Implementation

Nursing care of the child with hypokalemia focuses on ensuring adequate potassium intake, monitoring cardiopulmonary status, promoting normal bowel function, ensuring safety, providing dietary counseling, and preparing the child and family for discharge.

A child with hypokalemia who is able to eat should be given a high-potassium diet. Teach parents (and the child if old enough) which foods are high in potassium and how to incorporate them into the daily diet (see Table 18–8). Teach parents how to give potassium supplements, if prescribed. Liquid or powdered potassium supplements can be mixed with juice or sherbet to improve the bitter taste. The parent should call the mixture "medicine" so that the child does not learn to dislike all juices. Teach the parents signs of both hypokalemia and hyperkalemia and whom to call to report these

symptoms. The signs must be reported promptly so medications can be adjusted.

Children who have no oral intake for a period of time should receive intravenous fluids that contain potassium. Calculate the dosage to ensure accuracy, and be sure that the infusion runs on schedule. Sometimes the child will complain of burning along the vein when potassium is infused. The infusion may need to be slowed temporarily to relieve pain and maintain the intravenous line. Remain vigilant to maintain patency of the vein to avoid infiltration, which can cause phlebitis and pain. A central line is a better choice than a peripheral line in order to decrease side effects of administration. Consult the hospital formulary for dilution and administration guidelines; it must be administered slowly to avoid arrhythmias and cardiac arrest. Ensure adequate fluid output for the child's age to avoid hyperkalemia from potassium infusion.

Check serum potassium for high or low potassium levels. Analyze other electrolytes and acid-base balance. Monitor urine output. A child with oliguria can develop hyperkalemia when receiving supplements.

Hypokalemia potentiates digitalis toxicity. A child with hypokalemia who is receiving digitalis needs careful surveillance for digitalis toxicity, which is manifested as anorexia, nausea, vomiting, and bradycardia. Observe for these effects. Take the pulse rate and rhythm regularly. Monitor respirations and ease of breathing to watch for decreased respiratory muscle activity.

Ensure adequate fluids and fiber in the diet. Monitor and record the number of stools and report inadequate stools. Keep side rails up. Assist the child as needed to move into and out of bed. Reposition the child frequently to preserve the skin integrity of limbs that are not moved regularly. Perform passive range of motion if the child is not moving. Use supportive pillows to position the child properly.

The adolescent who is trying to lose weight and not consuming a nutritious diet needs dietary teaching. More intensive treatment will be needed for teens who are anorexic or bulimic (see Chapter 14 ∞ for interventions in these cases).

Evaluation

Expected outcomes of nursing care during hypokalemia include the following:

- Normal rate and rhythm of heart and respiratory system is maintained.
- Regular bowel movements are established.
- The child is free from injury.
- The child and family have adequate knowledge regarding food sources of potassium.

Calcium Imbalances

A normal serum calcium concentration is important for many physiologic functions, including muscle and nerve function, secretion of hormones, bone formation and strength, and clotting of the blood. Calcium is the most abundant mineral in the body, and about 99% of it is located in the bones (American Academy of Pediatrics, 2009). There are three forms of calcium in plasma—calcium bound to protein, calcium bound to small organic ions (e.g., citrate), and free ionized calcium (Ca^{++}), the only physiologically active form. A discussion of dietary calcium intake and its importance for bone formation can be found in Chapter 14 ∞.

Calcium imbalances are caused by alterations in calcium intake, absorption, distribution, or excretion. Calcium absorption requires vitamin D for maximum efficiency and is greatest in the duodenum. Calcium distribution involves calcium entry into and exit from bones and the distribution of different forms of calcium in the plasma. Excretion of calcium occurs in urine, feces, and sweat.

Parathyroid hormone is the major regulator of the plasma calcium concentration. It increases this concentration by increasing calcium absorption, increasing calcium withdrawal from bones, and decreasing calcium excretion in the urine. The plasma calcium concentration has an important influence on cell membrane permeability and influences the threshold potential of excitable cells. For this reason, calcium imbalances alter neuromuscular irritability.

Hypercalcemia

Hypercalcemia refers to a plasma excess of total calcium (above 2.6 mmol/L in children or newborns). Because so much calcium is stored in the bones, however, the serum levels of calcium may not reflect body stores.

Etiology and Pathophysiology Hypercalcemia is caused by conditions that involve increased calcium intake or absorption, shift of calcium from bones into the extracellular fluid, and decreased calcium excretion. Hypercalcemia due to increased calcium intake or absorption may occur if an infant is fed large amounts of chicken liver (source of vitamin A) or given megadoses of vitamin D or vitamin A, or if a child or adolescent consumes large amounts of calcium-rich foods concurrently with antacids (milk-alkali syndrome). Infants with very low birth weight can develop hypercalcemia if they have inadequate phosphorus intake, as bone phosphorus and calcium will be resorbed. Hypercalcemia may also occur when children receiving total parenteral nutrition are given doses of calcium that are too high.

Most cases of hypercalcemia in children are due to a shift of calcium from bones into the extracellular fluid. The excessive amounts of parathyroid hormone produced in hyperparathyroidism cause calcium withdrawal from bones. Prolonged immobilization also causes withdrawal of calcium from bones. Often, the excess calcium ions are excreted in the urine. However, if calcium is withdrawn from bones faster than the kidneys can excrete it, hypercalcemia results. Hypercalcemia also occurs with many types of malignancies such as leukemias. The malignant cells produce substances that circulate in the blood to the bones and cause bone resorption. The calcium from the bones then enters the extracellular fluid, causing hypercalcemia. Bone tumors and chemotherapy destroy bone directly, leading to the release of calcium. Familial hypercalcemia and infantile hypercalcemia are rare congenital disorders. Thiazide diuretics (e.g., thiazide and hydrochlorothiazide) decrease calcium excretion in the urine and may contribute to development of hypercalcemia.

Clinical Manifestations Hypercalcemia may have nonspecific symptoms, making diagnosis difficult. Many of the signs and symptoms of hypercalcemia are manifestations of decreased neuromuscular excitability. Constipation, anorexia, nausea, and vomiting can occur. Fatigue and skeletal muscle weakness predominate. Confusion, lethargy, and decreased attention span are common, and polyuria develops. Severe hypercalcemia may cause cardiac arrhythmias and arrest. Neonates with hypercalcemia have flaccid muscles and exhibit failure to thrive. Hypercalcemia increases sodium and potassium excretion by the kidneys and can lead to polyuria and polydipsia.

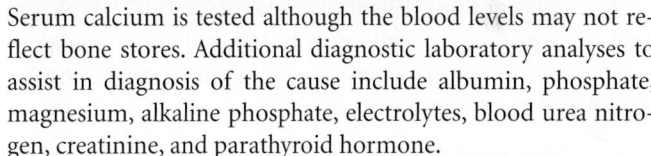

COLLABORATIVE CARE

Serum calcium is tested although the blood levels may not reflect bone stores. Additional diagnostic laboratory analyses to assist in diagnosis of the cause include albumin, phosphate, magnesium, alkaline phosphate, electrolytes, blood urea nitrogen, creatinine, and parathyroid hormone.

Hypercalcemia is treated by increasing fluids and administering the diuretic furosemide (Lasix) to increase excretion of calcium in the urine. Treatment to decrease intestinal absorption of calcium involves effective use of glucocorticoids. Bone resorption can be decreased by administration of glucocorticoids and calcitonin. Phosphate is sometimes given to treat hypercalcemia, but it may cause dangerous precipitation of calcium phosphate salts in body tissues. Dialysis may be used, if necessary. Treatment of the underlying cause for the disorder is needed as well.

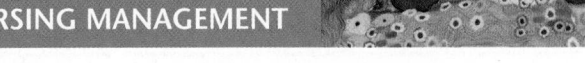

NURSING MANAGEMENT

Nursing Assessment and Diagnosis

Nursing assessment of a child with hypercalcemia includes monitoring serum calcium levels, level of consciousness, gastrointestinal function, urine volume, specific gravity, cardiac rhythm, and pH. With chronic hypercalcemia, assessment of activity tolerance and developmental level becomes important.

Many nursing diagnoses are appropriate for children who have hypercalcemia. Diagnoses that address cardiac and neuromuscular manifestation are especially important. The following nursing diagnoses may apply:

- Risk for Activity Intolerance related to decreased cardiac output secondary to cardiac arrhythmia
- Risk for Injury related to decreased level of response
- Risk for Imbalanced Nutrition: Less than Body Requirements related to anorexia and nausea
- Risk for Impaired Urinary Elimination related to renal calculi

Planning and Intervention

Carefully calculate calcium in total parenteral nutrition and other solutions, administer these solutions with caution, and use cardiac monitoring to prevent hypercalcemia in hospitalized children.

Interventions to increase fluid intake are important for children with hypercalcemia or those who are immobilized. A generous fluid intake, appropriate to the child's age, is necessary to keep the urine dilute and to help reduce constipation (a common symptom of hypercalcemia). An acidic urine helps to keep calcium from forming stones. Because urinary tract infections may cause the urine to be alkaline, nursing interventions to prevent urinary tract infection are necessary. Thiazide diuretics, which decrease calcium excretion, should not be given to the child with hypercalcemia. Provide a high-fiber diet to help reduce constipation.

Increasing mobility through assisted weight bearing helps to decrease the withdrawal of calcium from bones that is caused by immobility. If the hypercalcemia is caused by withdrawal of calcium from bones, the child is at risk for fractures with minor trauma and must be handled with special care. See Chapter 29 ∞ for further discussion of care following fractures and prolonged casting.

Teach parents to avoid giving calcium-rich foods and calcium antacids (e.g., Tums) to children with hypercalcemia. Vitamin D supplements should be avoided as they increase calcium absorption from the gastrointestinal tract.

Clinical Tip

To decrease calcium intake in hypercalcemia, restrict intake of milk, ice cream, and other dairy products. Nondairy fruit-based desserts are acceptable alternatives.

Evaluation

Expected outcomes of nursing care include the following:

- The cardiac pump effectively maintains perfusion.
- The child is free from injury.
- Normal bowel excretion is maintained.
- Adequate nutritional status is maintained.

Hypocalcemia

Hypocalcemia is a serum deficit of calcium (below 2.1 mmol/L in children or newborns). Recall that serum calcium levels may not reflect body stores of this mineral, as most of the body's calcium is stored in bone.

Etiology and Pathophysiology   Hypocalcemia is caused by conditions that involve decreased calcium intake or absorption, shift of calcium to a physiologically unavailable form, increased calcium excretion, and loss of calcium by an abnormal route.

Decreased calcium intake or absorption causes hypocalcemia in children with chronic generalized malnutrition, or with a diet that is low in vitamin D and calcium. Female adolescents trying to lose weight or maintain a low weight often decrease foods that contain calcium and may develop chronic hypocalcemia. In these cases, premature bone loss and inadequate bone formation occur. (See Chapter 14 ∞ for further discussion of calcium in-

take during adolescence.) This deficit cannot be made up later in life, thus increasing the risk of osteoporosis (Heaney, 2006).

Even with a normal calcium intake, hypocalcemia occurs if the mineral is not absorbed. If a child does not have enough vitamin D, calcium is not absorbed efficiently from the duodenum. Sunlight speeds formation of vitamin D in the skin. Children who are institutionalized without access to sunlight (e.g., severely developmentally delayed children), those with very dark skin, or children kept well covered when outside may become hypocalcemic because of the lack of vitamin D (see Chapter 14 ∞). Uremic syndrome is another cause of vitamin D deficiency. It interferes with the kidney's ability to activate vitamin D. High phosphate intake can cause hypocalcemia. Chronic diarrhea and steatorrhea (fatty stools) also reduce calcium absorption from the gastrointestinal tract.

About 40% of calcium is bound to proteins and not available for interactions, 10% is bound to small organic ions such as citrate, and 50% is ionized and physiologically active (American Academy of Pediatrics, 2009). The shift of calcium into a physiologically unavailable form occurs when calcium shifts into bone or when free ionized calcium in plasma binds to proteins or small organic ions in the plasma. Excessive calcium shifts into bones in various types of hypoparathyroidism, including DiGeorge syndrome (congenital absence of the parathyroid glands). Hypomagnesemia impairs parathyroid hormone function and may cause hypocalcemia. Some types of neonatal hypocalcemia are associated with delayed parathyroid hormone function or hypomagnesemia. Calcium shifts rapidly into bone when rickets is treated. A high plasma phosphate concentration causes plasma calcium to decrease. Alkalosis causes more calcium to bind to plasma proteins. The ionized hypocalcemia persists until the alkalosis resolves or the citrate is metabolized by the liver. Citrate in transfused blood products may bind with calcium so it is inactive. Children who receive liver transplants are hypocalcemic for several days because of impaired citrate metabolism.

Increased calcium excretion occurs in steatorrhea, when calcium secreted into the gastrointestinal fluid binds to the fecal fat in addition to the dietary calcium that is bound in the feces. A similar situation occurs in acute pancreatitis.

Loss of calcium by an abnormal route may contribute to hypocalcemia as calcium is lost from the body through burn or wound drainage or sequestered in acute pancreatitis. Many different medications can cause hypocalcemia.

Clinical Manifestations   The signs and symptoms of hypocalcemia are manifestations of increased muscular excitability (tetany). In children they include twitching and cramping, tingling around the mouth or in the fingers, carpal spasm, and pedal spasm. Laryngospasm, seizures, and cardiac arrhythmias are the more severe manifestations of hypocalcemia and may be fatal. Hypocalcemia may cause congestive heart failure, especially in neonates.

Growth & Development *Hypocalcemia*

Hypocalcemia in infants is more frequently manifested as tremors, muscle twitches, and brief tonic-clonic seizures.

Although these symptoms are diagnostic of acute calcium deficiency, a more common state in children and adolescents is chronic low intake of calcium. This may be manifested by spontaneous fractures in infants and in adolescents who exercise excessively.

COLLABORATIVE CARE

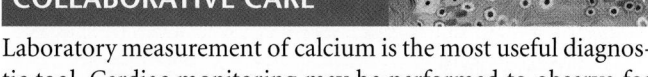

Laboratory measurement of calcium is the most useful diagnostic tool. Cardiac monitoring may be performed to observe for cardiac arrhythmias.

Hypocalcemia is treated by oral or intravenous administration of calcium. The original cause of the imbalance is also treated. If the hypocalcemia is due to hypomagnesemia, the magnesium must be replenished before the calcium replacement can be successful. When the cause is chronic low dietary intake, counseling is needed about high-calcium foods, and perhaps the necessity for vitamin D intake or supplements.

NURSING MANAGEMENT

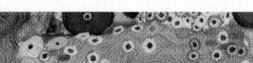

Nursing Assessment and Diagnosis

Carefully assess growth in the young female who is trying to diet. When an adolescent female is very thin, be sure to ask about excessive sports and other activities, and about regularity of menstrual periods. If periods are irregular or not occurring, collect additional dietary information to help determine whether the girl is lacking in intake of calcium, calories, and other nutrients. These assessments are needed even if serum calcium values are normal. Look for signs of inadequate nutrition such as fat and muscle wasting, dry hair, and cold hands and feet.

In those who have acute hypocalcemia, assess for muscle cramps, stiffness, and clumsiness; grimacing caused by spasms of facial muscles and twitching of arm muscles; and laryngospasm. Increased neuromuscular excitability may be detected by testing for Trousseau sign or Chvostek sign. Many healthy newborns have a positive Chvostek sign; however, this assessment should be reserved for children over several months of age.

The effects of increased neuromuscular excitability in the child with hypocalcemia are the basis for the following nursing diagnoses:

- Risk for Injury related to potential for fractures
- Risk for Ineffective Breathing Pattern related to laryngospasm
- Risk for Activity Intolerance related to decreased cardiac output secondary to cardiac arrhythmias
- Imbalanced Nutrition: Less than Body Requirements related to lack of basic nutritional knowledge of sources and recommended amounts of calcium intake

Planning and Implementation

To correct calcium deficiency in the hospitalized child, give oral or intravenous calcium as ordered. Monitor for complications of calcium supplementation. A 10% calcium gluconate solution should be readily available for emergency use in severe hypocal-

Clinical Tip

To test for Trousseau sign, apply a blood pressure cuff to the arm and leave inflated for 3 minutes. If a carpal spasm occurs, the Trousseau sign is positive. To test for Chvostek sign, tap the skin lightly just in front of the ear (over the facial nerve). If the corner of the mouth draws up because of muscle contraction, the Chvostek sign is positive. These findings may be indicative of hypocalcemia or hypomagnesemia.

cemia. Calcium is never given intramuscularly because it causes tissue necrosis. See Medications Used to Treat Acute Hypocalcemia below.

Take measures to ensure safety for the child who is hospitalized with hypocalcemia. Seizure precautions may be necessary. Explain the cause of muscle cramps to parents and older children.

Counsel the family about dairy products and nondairy foods rich in calcium (see Table 18–8). For the adolescent female whose weight and menstrual patterns show irregularities, total calories and calcium intake should be increased. Teaching may also be needed about proper calcium intake and its importance both to athletic performance and to prevention of osteoporosis. Encourage three glasses of nonfat milk per day. Teach ways to use milk in the diet. For example, sprinkle nonfat dry milk on cereal and other foods. If the child is lactose intolerant, emphasize nondairy sources of calcium and advise parents to purchase special milk treated with lactase. As this milk is more costly, inadequate family finances may be an impediment to its use. If a child has a health condition leading to chronic diarrhea, encourage increased intake of calcium-rich foods. Calcium supplements in the form of calcium carbonate tablets may be used.

Evaluation

Expected outcomes of nursing care for hypocalcemia include the following:

- Ingestion of recommended dietary allowances for calcium is maintained.
- The child displays calcium balance.
- The child is free from injury.

Magnesium Imbalances

Magnesium is necessary for enzyme function in cells, acetylcholine release, glycolysis, stimulation of ATPases, and bone formation. Magnesium is a component of chlorophyll; thus, magnesium intake is aided by eating dark green leafy vegetables. Nuts and grains are also good sources of this mineral. Magnesium is absorbed primarily from the terminal ileum. It is distributed among the extracellular fluid (small amounts), the cells (larger amounts), and the bones (largest amounts). Magnesium excretion occurs in urine, feces, and sweat.

Magnesium imbalances are caused by alterations in magnesium intake, distribution, or excretion; by loss through an abnormal route; or by a combination of these factors. The plasma magnesium concentration influences the release of acetylcholine

Medications Used to Treat
Acute Hypocalcemia

Medication/Action	Nursing Implications
10% Calcium Gluconate IV Calcium is a normal body electrolyte and may need to be infused in infants or young children with health problems leading to low calcium. It is also used during exchange transfusion in neonates since citrate in the blood transfusion can bind body calcium. In the form of CaCl, calcium may be used during resuscitation. Calcium regulates excitability of muscles and nerves, and therefore affects cardiac function (inotropic effect); is necessary for blood clotting; plays a role in storage and release of neurotransmitters, in renal function, and in maintaining cell membranes; and is an antidote to excessive magnesium infusion.	Verify dose carefully with the prescriber and another nurse. Monitor heart rate and rhythm—hypotension and bradycardia can occur. Use extreme caution if given to a child with cardiac or renal disease. Maintain IV carefully to avoid extravasation; do **not** administer by peripheral infusion, scalp vein, IM, or SC. It precipitates when given in infusion with bicarbonate.

at neuromuscular junctions. Thus, magnesium imbalances are characterized by alterations in neuromuscular irritability.

Nursing Alert

Oral Calcium

Calcium tablets and powders are available for relief of acid indigestion and to increase calcium intake when it is deficient. Popular products contain calcium carbonate (i.e., Tums), calcium acetate, calcium citrate, tricalcium phosphate, calcium lactate, calcium gluconate, and calcium polycarbophil. Since so many forms exist, be sure that chewable tablets are chewed, sustained-release tablets are swallowed whole, and powders are mixed and administered as recommended. The most common side effect is constipation; other side effects are hypercalcemia and renal calculi.

Intravenous Calcium

Intravenous calcium is administered to treat severe hypocalcemia such as in tetany due to parathyroid disease, in cardiac resuscitation, during exchange transfusions in newborns, and to relieve muscle cramps caused by insect bites. Intravenous calcium has several serious potential side effects, so nursing care centers on maintaining an intact intravenous line, continuous cardiorespiratory monitoring, and monitoring calcium and phosphate levels.

Hypermagnesemia

Hypermagnesemia occurs when the plasma magnesium concentration is too high (above 2.7 mg/dL [1.1 mmol/L]). Keep in mind that the serum levels measured in the laboratory may not reflect body magnesium stores, because most of the magnesium in the body is located in the bones and inside the cells.

Hypermagnesemia is caused by conditions that involve increased magnesium intake and decreased magnesium excretion. Impaired renal function leading to decreased magnesium excretion is the most common cause of hypermagnesemia in children. In both oliguric renal failure and adrenal insufficiency, magnesium ions that cannot be excreted in the urine accumulate in the extracellular fluid.

Less frequently, increased magnesium intake may cause hypermagnesemia. Magnesium sulfate ($MgSO_4$) given to treat eclampsia in the mother before delivery causes hypermagnesemia in the newborn. Abnormally high amounts may also be taken in magnesium-containing enemas, laxatives, antacids, and intravenous fluids. Epsom salt is a readily available product and is a nearly pure magnesium sulfate preparation; its use as an enema has caused death in children. Aspiration of seawater, as in near-drowning, is an uncommon but potentially serious source of excessive magnesium intake. Children with Addison disease can have abnormally high magnesium levels.

Clinical manifestations of hypermagnesemia include decreased muscle irritability, hypotension, bradycardia, drowsiness, lethargy, and weak or absent deep tendon reflexes. In severe hypermagnesemia, flaccid muscle paralysis, fatal respiratory depression, cardiac arrhythmias, and cardiac arrest occur.

Hypermagnesemia is managed primarily by increasing the urinary excretion of magnesium. This is usually accomplished by increasing fluid intake (except in oliguric renal failure) and by the administration of diuretics. Dialysis may sometimes be necessary. See Nursing Management in conjunction with management of hypomagnesemia to follow.

Hypomagnesemia

Hypomagnesemia refers to a plasma magnesium concentration that is too low (below 1.5–1.7 mg/dL [0.62–0.70 mmol/L]). Remember that the serum levels of magnesium may not reflect body stores, as most of the magnesium in the body is found in cells and bones.

Hypomagnesemia is caused by conditions that involve decreased magnesium intake or absorption, shift of magnesium to a physiologically unavailable form, increased magnesium excretion, and loss of magnesium by an abnormal route. Hypocalcemia often accompanies and contributes to hypomagnesemia.

Neonates whose mothers are diabetic sometimes develop hypomagnesemia in the newborn period. Decreased magnesium intake or absorption can occur if a child who is not eating has prolonged intravenous therapy without magnesium. Chronic malnutrition is another cause of decreased magnesium intake. Magnesium absorption is decreased in chronic diarrhea, short bowel syndrome, malabsorption syndromes, and steatorrhea.

A shift of magnesium to a physiologically unavailable form may occur after transfusion of many units of citrated blood products, because magnesium bound to the citrate is not physiologically active. Such transfusions cause prolonged hypomagnesemia in liver transplant patients who have impaired citrate metabolism. Magnesium shifts rapidly into bones that have been deprived of adequate stores.

Increased magnesium excretion in the urine occurs with diuretic therapy, the diuretic phase of acute renal failure, diabetic ketoacidosis, and hyperaldosteronism. Chronic alcoholism, occasionally seen in adolescents, increases urinary magnesium excretion. Magnesium contained in gastrointestinal secretions is bound to fat and excreted in the stool.

Loss of magnesium by an abnormal route occurs with prolonged nasogastric suction and through sequestration of magnesium in acute pancreatitis. Several medications may cause hypomagnesemia.

Hypomagnesemia is characterized by increased neuromuscular excitability (tetany). The clinical manifestations are hyperactive reflexes, skeletal muscle cramps, twitching, tremors, and cardiac arrhythmias. Seizures can occur with severe hypomagnesemia. Hypomagnesemia is associated with high mortality for children in the pediatric intensive care unit.

Magnesium serum levels are measured, along with serum calcium and potassium, since these electrolyte disturbances often occur together. Hypomagnesemia is managed by administering magnesium and treating the underlying cause of the imbalance.

NURSING MANAGEMENT

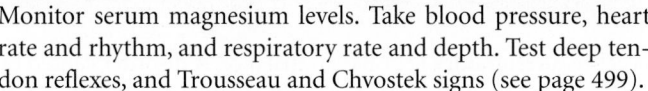

Monitor serum magnesium levels. Take blood pressure, heart rate and rhythm, and respiratory rate and depth. Test deep tendon reflexes, and Trousseau and Chvostek signs (see page 499).

Teach the parents of a child with chronic renal failure and potential for hypermagnesemia not to give milk of magnesia or any antacids that contain magnesium; teach how to read labels to recognize magnesium as an ingredient.

Nursing Alert

Oral Magnesium

Magnesium tablets, capsules, solution, and suspension are available for relief of acid indigestion and to stimulate peristalsis. Popular products contain magnesium citrate, magnesium hydroxide, magnesium oxide, and magnesium salicylate. When used as a cathartic, administer the recommended amount of water to ensure bowel evacuation. The most common side effect is abdominal cramping accompanied by diarrhea; other side effects are dehydration, respiratory depression, and electrolyte imbalance.

Intravenous Magnesium

Intravenous magnesium is administered in the form of magnesium sulfate to treat severe hypomagnesemia, refractory hypocalcemia, and intractable seizures. Intravenous magnesium has side effects of hypermagnesemia, respiratory depression, hypotension, and central nervous system depression. This form of therapy requires close monitoring of body systems and electrolyte status.

Teach parents of a child with hypomagnesemia or continuing risk factors such as chronic diarrhea to include foods containing magnesium in the diet (see Table 18–8). When intramuscular or intravenous magnesium is ordered for hypomagnesemia, administer carefully as directed and monitor vital signs. Electrocardiogram and renal studies may precede drug administration. Have resuscitative drugs and equipment readily available during drug administration. Before administering magnesium supplements, verify that the child's urine output is adequate. Monitor deep tendon reflexes if intravenous magnesium is given, and observe for complications of magnesium supplementation.

Expected outcomes for nursing care include restoration and maintenance of electrolyte balance, normal neuromuscular tone, safety, and regular heart rate and rhythm.

■ CLINICAL ASSESSMENT OF FLUID AND ELECTROLYTE IMBALANCE

How can you assess children appropriately for fluid and electrolyte imbalance without thinking through the clinical manifestations of every possible disorder one after the other? First, perform a rapid risk factor assessment on each child to see which factors are present (Tables 18–9 and 18–10). Remember that most imbalances influence other factors so it is common to find more than one type of fluid and electrolyte problem. Examining several body systems such as cardiovascular, respiratory, and neurologic will be necessary to get a comprehensive picture of the child.

A risk factor assessment may be performed mentally during routine tasks. Look for factors that alter the intake, retention, and loss of isotonic fluid and water. This information is used to evaluate which fluid imbalance is most likely to occur in a particular child. Next, look for factors that alter electrolyte intake and absorption, distribution between plasma and other electrolyte pools, excretion, and abnormal routes of electrolyte loss. This information is used to evaluate which electrolyte imbalances are most likely to occur in the child. A review of pathophysiology is important to understand the role of the other electrolytes and substances, such as phosphorus, in the body. Apply growth and development to realize what types of problems might be most common in various age groups. For example, the newborn is more likely to be dehydrated due to lack of adequate

TABLE 18–9	Risk Factor Assessment for Fluid Imbalances	
Isotonic Fluid (Extracellular Fluid Volume Imbalances)	Water
Source of increased intake?	Source of increased intake?
Aldosterone secretion increased or decreased?	Antidiuretic hormone secretion increased or decreased?
Source of loss from the body?	Source of unusual loss from the body?

TABLE 18-10 Risk Factor Assessment for Electrolyte Imbalances

Electrolyte Intake and Absorption	Electrolyte Shifts	Electrolyte Excretion	Electrolyte Loss by Abnormal Route
• Increased? • Decreased?	• From electrolyte pool to plasma? • From plasma to electrolyte pool?	• Increased? • Decreased?	• Vomiting? • Diarrhea? • Nasogastric suction? • Wound? • Burn? • Excessive sweating?

TABLE 18-11 Summary of Clinical Assessment of Fluid Imbalances

Assessment Category	Specific Assessments	Changes with Fluid Imbalances
Rapid changes in weight	Daily weights	Weight gain—extracellular volume excess Weight loss—extracellular volume deficit; clinical dehydration
Vascular volume	Small-vein filling time Capillary refill time Character of pulse Postural blood pressure measurements Lung sounds in dependent portions Central venous pressure Tenseness of fontanel (infants) Neck vein filling (older children)	Increased—extracellular volume deficit; clinical dehydration Increased—extracellular volume deficit; clinical dehydration Bounding—extracellular volume excess Thready—extracellular volume deficit; clinical dehydration Postural drop—extracellular volume deficit; clinical dehydration Crackles—extracellular volume excess Increased—extracellular volume excess Decreased—extracellular volume deficit; clinical dehydration Bulging—extracellular volume excess Sunken—extracellular volume deficit; clinical dehydration Full when upright—extracellular volume excess Flat when supine—extracellular volume deficit; clinical dehydration
Interstitial volume	Skin turgor Presence or absence of edema	Skin tents—extracellular volume deficit; clinical dehydration Edema—extracellular volume excess
Cerebral function	Level of consciousness	Decreased—clinical dehydration

intake, whereas the toddler more commonly has fluid loss from nausea and vomiting.

After evaluating possible imbalances for the child, perform a clinical assessment. Assessment of fluid imbalances is performed by assessing weight changes, vascular volume, interstitial volume, and cerebral function (Table 18–11). Assessment of electrolyte imbalances is performed by assessing serum electrolyte levels, skeletal muscle strength, neuromuscular excitability, gastrointestinal tract function, and cardiac rhythm. Next, check for other manifestations that are specific to a particular high-risk imbalance (e.g., polyuria in hypokalemia). Evaluate any serum laboratory values available. This method of risk factor assessment followed by clinical assessment provides a rapid yet thorough approach to assessment for fluid and electrolyte imbalances.

See the companion website for a table that summarizes clinical assessment of electrolyte imbalances.

■ ACID-BASE IMBALANCES

There are four acid-base imbalances. Two are the result of processes that cause too much acid in the body and are referred to as acidosis. The other two imbalances are the result of processes that cause too little acid in the body and are called alkalosis. An acid-base disorder caused by too much or too little carbonic acid

is called a respiratory acid-base imbalance. A disorder caused by too much or too little metabolic acid is called a metabolic acid-base imbalance. The types of acid-base imbalance are:

- Respiratory acidosis: Relatively too much carbonic acid
- Metabolic acidosis: Relatively too much metabolic acid
- Respiratory alkalosis: Relatively too little carbonic acid
- Metabolic alkalosis: Relatively too little metabolic acid

See Table 18–12 for normal blood pH and blood gas levels.

Arterial blood gas measurements (ABGs) provide a laboratory evaluation of a child's current acid-base status. In addition to the four components of acid-base balance listed in Table 18–12, oxygenation saturation, or the percentage of hemoglobin saturated with arterial blood, is normally 95–100%. Box 18–2 provides a method that can help to interpret the pH, Po_2, Pco_2, and bicarbonate concentrations, which are the most important acid-base measures. End-tidal CO_2 can provide a continuous noninvasive measurement. (Remember that Pco_2 reflects carbonic acid status, and bicarbonate concentration reflects the metabolic acid status.)

Respiratory Acidosis

Respiratory acidosis is caused by the accumulation of carbon dioxide in the blood. Since carbon dioxide and water can be

TABLE 18-12 Normal Blood pH and Gases			
	Infants	Children	Adolescents
Arterial blood pH	7.18–7.50	7.27–7.49	7.35–7.41
Arterial blood Po_2	60–70 mmHg (8.0–9.3 pKa)	80–108 mmHg (10.7–14.4 pKa)	80–100 mmHg (10.7–13.3 pKa)
Arterial blood Pco_2	27–41 mmHg (3.6–5.5 pKa)	32–48 mmHg (4.3–6.4 pKa)	32–48 mmHg (4.3–6.4 pKa)
Arterial blood HCO_3^- (bicarbonate)	19–24 mmol/L	18–25 mmol/L	20–29 mmol/L

combined into carbonic acid, respiratory acidosis is sometimes called carbonic acid excess. The condition can be acute or chronic. It is controlled by the lungs.

Etiology and Pathophysiology

Any factor that interferes with the ability of the lungs to excrete carbon dioxide can cause respiratory acidosis. These factors may interfere with the gaseous exchange within the lungs, may impair the neuromuscular pump that moves air in and out of the lungs, or may depress the respiratory rate (Figure 18–19 ➤).

BOX 18–2	How to Interpret Arterial Blood Gas Measurements

Ask the following questions to analyze blood gas results:

1. **What is the pH?** If the pH is normal, the child has no imbalance or has compensated for an imbalance. If the pH is below normal, the child has acidosis. If the pH is above normal, the child has alkalosis.

2. **What are the Po_2 and oxygenation saturation?** Lowered levels of both demonstrate hypoxemia. Administering oxygen may help to reverse the hypoxemia and prevent further acid-base imbalance.

3. **What is the Pco_2?** If the Pco_2 is normal, the child does not have an acid-base imbalance. If the Pco_2 is above normal, the child has respiratory acidosis. This may be the primary disorder or may be a compensatory response to metabolic alkalosis. Looking at the bicarbonate concentration helps you decide. If the Pco_2 is below normal, the child has respiratory alkalosis. Again, this can be the primary disorder or may be a compensatory response to metabolic acidosis.

4. **What is the bicarbonate concentration?** If the bicarbonate concentration is within normal range, the child does not have a metabolic acid-base imbalance. If the bicarbonate is above normal, the child has metabolic alkalosis. This can be a primary disorder or can be compensatory in respiratory acidosis. When bicarbonate is below normal, the child has metabolic acidosis, either as a direct disorder or as a compensatory response to respiratory alkalosis.

5. **What do the results together tell you?** If the pH is abnormal and either the Pco_2 or bicarbonate concentration is normal, there is an uncompensated acid-base disorder. If all three values are abnormal, the child has a partially compensated disorder and the pH will provide the definitive answer. If Pco_2, pH, and bicarbonate are all decreased, then partially compensated metabolic acidosis is most likely. If pH is normal and Pco_2 and bicarbonate are abnormal, there is a fully compensated acid-base disorder.

6. **What are the child's history and clinical signs?** Does your interpretation fit with what you know about the child's medical condition and with assessments you are making? This last step helps you to integrate laboratory data with the clinical picture to strengthen your nursing care of the child with an acid-base imbalance.

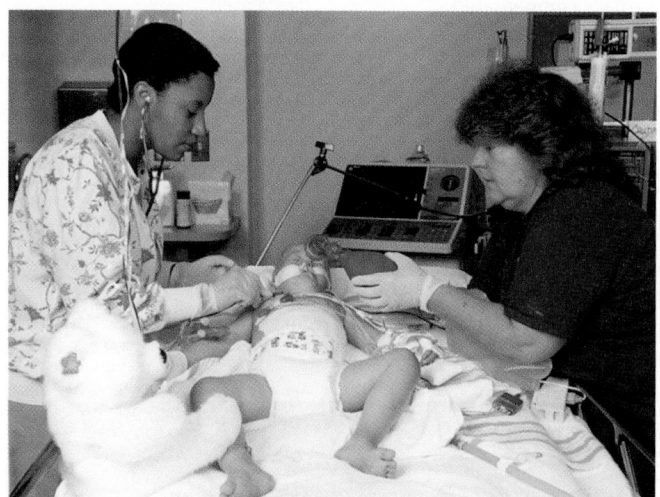

FIGURE 18–19 ➤ This child may develop respiratory acidosis or respiratory alkalosis. If the tidal volume is set too low during mechanical ventilation, carbon dioxide (carbonic acid) will accumulate in the body (respiratory acidosis) because it is not being excreted by the lungs. If the tidal volume is set too high, carbon dioxide will be depleted in the body (respiratory alkalosis) because it is being excreted in great quantities.

As the Pco_2 begins to increase, the pH of the blood begins to decrease. Compensatory mechanisms begin to act in the form of nonbicarbonate buffers, additional hydrogen ion excretion by the kidneys, and decreased bicarbonate excretion by the kidneys. These compensatory mechanisms take several days to become active so the child manifests a changing clinical situation, depending on the underlying cause and the amount of compensation occurring (Table 18–13).

Clinical Manifestations

Acidosis in the brain cells causes central nervous system depression, manifested by confusion, lethargy, headache, increased intracranial pressure, and even coma. Acute respiratory acidosis can lead to tachycardia and cardiac arrhythmias. The child's arterial blood gases always show an increased Pco_2, the laboratory sign of increased carbonic acid. Serum pH can be decreased or normal. See Box 18–2.

COLLABORATIVE CARE

Laboratory tests involve arterial blood gases, as described previously. Treatment of respiratory acidosis requires correction of the underlying cause (see the companion website for a table of causes). For example, treatment may include bronchodilators for bronchospasm, mechanical ventilation for neuromuscular defects, decreasing sedative use, or surgery for kyphoscoliosis.

TABLE 18–13 Laboratory Values in Acid-Base Imbalance

Imbalance	P_{CO_2}	pH	HCO_3^-
Respiratory Acidosis			
Uncompensated	Increased	Decreased	Normal
Partially compensated	Increased	Decreased but moving toward normal	Increasing
Fully compensated	Increased	Normal	Increased
Respiratory Alkalosis			
Uncompensated	Decreased	Increased	Normal
Partially compensated	Decreased	Increased but moving toward normal	Decreasing
Fully compensated	Decreased	Normal	Decreased
Metabolic Acidosis			
Uncompensated	Normal	Decreased	Decreased
Partially compensated	Decreasing	Decreased but moving toward normal	Decreased
Fully compensated	Decreased	Normal	Decreased
Metabolic Alkalosis			
Acute condition; uncompensated	Normal	Increased	Increased
Partially compensated	Increasing	Increased but moving toward normal	Increased
Fully compensated	Full compensation limited by the need for oxygen	Full compensation limited by the need for oxygen	Full compensation limited by the need for oxygen

NURSING MANAGEMENT

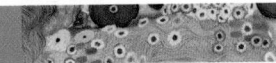

Nursing Assessment and Diagnosis

Nursing assessment plays a pivotal role in decisions about interventions for respiratory acidosis, especially in chronic conditions such as cystic fibrosis and kyphoscoliosis. Assess respiratory rate, rhythm, and depth carefully. Take the apical pulse and be alert for tachycardia or arrhythmia. A cardiac monitor may be used. Obtain serial arterial blood gas measurements in acute conditions to evaluate changing status. Assess the level of consciousness and energy. Observe for chronic fatigue, headache, or decreased level of consciousness.

Several nursing diagnoses may apply to the child with respiratory acidosis. The most important of these addresses the child's risk for injury. Other nursing diagnoses depend on the specific clinical manifestation and the particular cause of the acidosis. Examples include:

- Risk for Injury related to decreased level of consciousness
- Activity Intolerance related to decreased cardiac output secondary to cardiac dysrhythmias
- Ineffective Breathing Pattern (Hypoventilation) related to neuromuscular impairment
- Acute Pain (Headache) related to cerebral vasodilation
- Ineffective Family Management of Therapeutic Regimen related to complexity of bronchodilator therapy

Planning and Implementation

Care in the Community

Teach children at risk for respiratory acidosis and their parents preventive measures to use at home. For the child with a chronic condition such as cystic fibrosis, muscular dystrophy, or kyphoscoliosis, demonstrate deep breathing and encourage its use several times each day. Teach the family signs of infection—including fever, increased respiratory secretions, and discomfort with breathing—so the problems can be treated promptly to prevent further respiratory involvement. Position the child to facilitate chest expansion (Figure 18–20 ➤). Teach parents about proper administration of any necessary medications. For example, the child with cystic fibrosis may receive antibiotics to prevent respiratory infections. Teach parents and older children about home ventilator use (Figure 18–21 ➤).

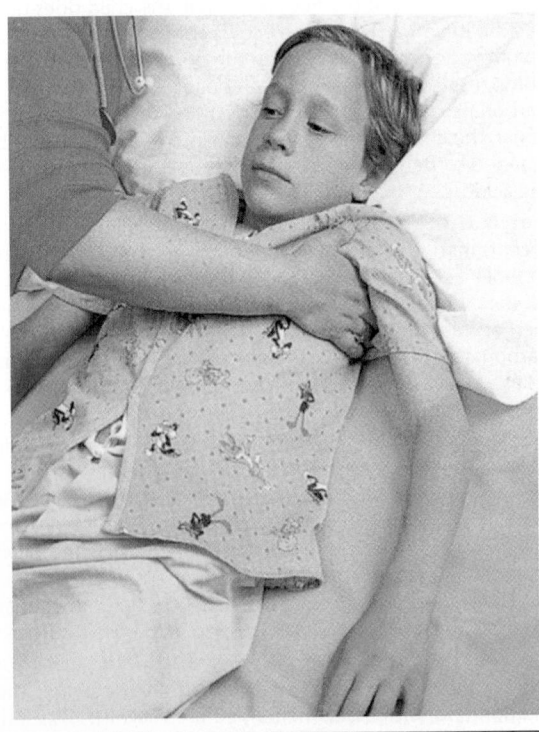

FIGURE 18–20 ➤ Positioning to facilitate chest expansion. If the child is positioned to avoid chest compression or slumping to the side, this will help correct respiratory acidosis.

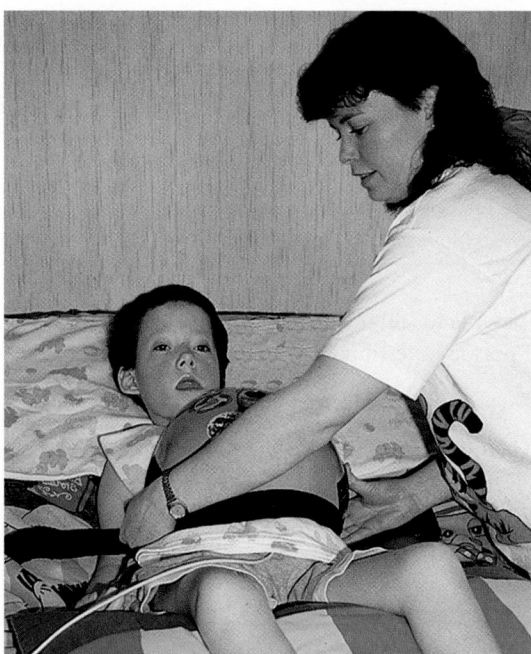

FIGURE 18–21 ➤ This child, who has muscular dystrophy, uses a "turtle" ventilator at home to assist with breathing. His parents required instructions from the nurse on use of the ventilator. The family has a generator to provide electricity for the ventilator during power outages.

Hospital-Based Care

For the hospitalized child, the focus is on ensuring safety. Keep side rails raised, and turn and position the child frequently. Evaluate mental status and document and report any changes in alertness. When laboratory values of blood pH and Pco_2 are available, evaluate them promptly and report any changes or abnormalities. Administer medications as ordered. Carefully watch the doses of sedatives to avoid further respiratory depression. Provide suctioning and encourage deep breathing.

Evaluation

Expected outcomes of nursing care for the child with respiratory acidosis include the following:

• Safety is maintained for the child.
• Adequate rate and rhythm of respirations are manifested.
• Disorders that have contributed to the imbalance are corrected.

Respiratory Alkalosis

Respiratory alkalosis occurs when the blood contains too little carbon dioxide. It is sometimes called carbonic acid deficit.

Excess carbon dioxide loss is caused by hyperventilation, in which more air than normal is moved into and out of the lungs. Common causes of hyperventilation are listed in Box 18–3. Some of the most common causes in young children are hypoxia such as that from severe asthma, salicylate poisoning, and sepsis.

In many cases, respiratory alkalosis only lasts for several hours. Renal compensation does not occur, as these compensatory mechanisms take several days to begin action. An example

BOX 18–3 Causes of Hyperventilation

■ Hypoxemia
■ Anxiety
■ Pain
■ Encephalitis
■ Septicemia caused by gram-negative bacteria
■ Mechanical overventilation
■ Fever
■ Salicylate poisoning
■ Meningitis

is the hyperventilation that occurs with acute anxiety. If the condition persists, however, the kidneys will begin to retain more acid and excrete more bicarbonate. Hydrogen ions will be released from body buffers to decrease plasma bicarbonate. While the imbalance continues, cellular function is thus protected by returning pH to normal levels.

Arterial blood gas measurements show a decreased Pco_2 in respiratory alkalosis. Blood pH is generally elevated. The lack of carbon dioxide causes neuromuscular irritability and paresthesias in the extremities and around the mouth. Muscle cramping and carpal or pedal spasms can occur. The child may be dizzy or confused.

Diagnosis is made by complete arterial blood gas measurements and thorough physical assessment. Clinical therapy focuses on correcting the condition that caused the hyperventilation so that the body's compensatory mechanisms can return carbon dioxide levels to normal. Oxygen therapy may be helpful in cases of hypoxia, salicylates are removed from the body when poisoning is the cause (see Chapter 17 ∞ for further information on poisoning), drugs that have interfered with breathing are changed, sepsis is treated with effective medication, and anxiolytic medications may be used to treat anxiety.

NURSING MANAGEMENT

Nursing Assessment and Diagnosis

Assess the child's level of consciousness and ask if the child feels light-headed or has tingling sensations or numbness in the fingers, in the toes, or around the mouth. Assess the rate and depth of respirations. Monitor the hospitalized child's Po_2 with serial arterial blood gas measurements to evaluate changes in status. A careful assessment is needed regarding the

Nursing Alert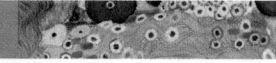

The Po_2 must be checked before any therapy for respiratory alkalosis is started, because it is dangerous to stop hyperventilation if oxygenation is poor. When Po_2 is low, the child's hyperventilation may be a protective mechanism to increase blood oxygenation. Other measures such as oxygen therapy or mechanical ventilation may need to start first, followed by treatment for the cause of respiratory alkalosis.

cause of hyperventilation. Did an occurrence cause anxiety for the child? Is pain present (see Chapter 15 ∞)? Has the child received salicylates in any form? Is the child mechanically ventilated? Is there a central nervous system infection such as meningitis?

Planning and Implementation

Nursing care for the child with respiratory alkalosis centers on teaching stress management techniques, maintaining pain control, promoting respiratory function, ensuring safety, maintaining fluid status, and providing health supervision and home care.

When anxiety is the cause of respiratory alkalosis, instruct the child to breathe slowly, in rhythm with your own breathing. Teach stress control techniques such as relaxation and imagery for situations that cause anxiety (Table 18–14).

Use medications, imagery, distraction, positioning, massage, and other techniques to decrease pain and maintain pain management. Chapter 15 ∞ describes these and other measures to assist with pain control. Have the child cough, or suction as needed. Be certain that mechanical ventilation systems are working properly. Oxygen saturation is usually monitored continuously; observe and record results. Provide a safe environment for the child who has a decreased level of consciousness. Be sure the child is supervised when sitting or standing up. Keep bed rails raised.

Renal compensation to manage ongoing respiratory alkalosis requires adequate urinary output. Regulate fluid intake to ensure urine output unless fluids are restricted due to medical condition.

Teach parents to keep aspirin and other salicylate products out of reach of children, preferably in a locked medicine box. In-

TABLE 18–14	Techniques for Reducing Anxiety in Children
Infant	• Calming touch • Quiet voice • Swaddling • Holding quietly
Toddler and Preschooler	• Stuffed toy to hug • Singing familiar quiet nursery songs • Acknowledging the child's feelings • Holding calmly
Young School-Age Child	• Talking quietly about a happy event • Telling a familiar story • Reading a familiar book together • Explaining that the symptoms will improve • Use of simple guided imagery • Supportive listening
Older School-Age Child and Adolescent	• Explaining the reason for symptoms and when they will improve • Use of guided imagery • Familiar music on tape or radio • Asking what the child does when anxious or "scared" • Teaching coping strategies

struct parents to call the Poison Control Center immediately in case of poison ingestion.

Evaluation

Expected outcomes of nursing care for the child with respiratory alkalosis include the following:

- Normal respiratory rate and rhythm are manifested.
- Safety is maintained for the child.
- Fluid status is appropriately regulated.

Metabolic Acidosis

Metabolic acidosis is a condition in which there is an excess of any acid other than carbonic acid. For this reason, it is sometimes called noncarbonic acid excess.

Etiology and Pathophysiology

Metabolic acidosis is caused by an imbalance in production and excretion of acid or by excess loss of bicarbonate. Excess accumulation occurs by one of two mechanisms. First, a child can eat or drink acids or substances that are converted to acid in the body. Examples include aspirin, boric acid, and antifreeze. Second, cells can make abnormally high amounts of acid that cannot be excreted. This is the case in ketoacidosis of untreated diabetes mellitus, in untreated growth hormone deficiency, in children with bladder construction that uses part of the bowel, or in the starvation that can occur in anorexia or bulimia. A disorder of excretion occurs in conditions such as oliguric renal failure (Figure 18–22 ➤).

Bicarbonate can be lost from the body through the urine or through excessive loss of intestinal fluid. Diarrhea, fistulas, and ileal drainage are all possible sources. Carbonic anhydrase inhibitors can cause loss of excess bicarbonate in the urine.

When the pH of the blood decreases below normal, the chemoreceptors in the brain and arteries are stimulated and respiratory compensation begins. The child's rate and depth of breathing increase and carbonic acid is removed from the body. The blood pH shifts to a more normal range even though the cause is not corrected. The underlying condition and the degree of compensation will alter the clinical laboratory values observed.

Clinical Manifestations

Laboratory values show decreased blood pH and decreased HCO_3^- and Pco_2. An attempt at respiratory compensation causes one of the most important signs of metabolic acidosis, increased rate and depth of respirations (hyperventilation) or **Kussmaul respirations.** Severe acidosis can cause decreased pe-

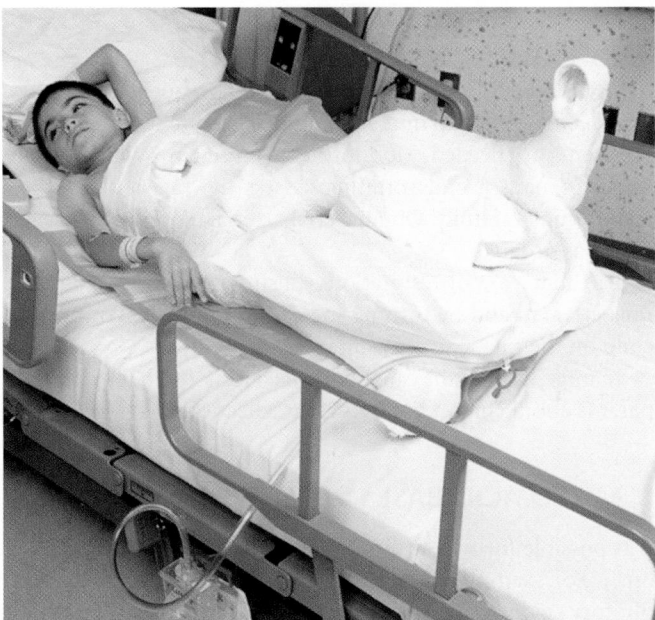

FIGURE 18–22 ➤ With any postoperative or immobilized child, it is important to monitor urine output to detect oliguria. If the kidneys do not produce very much urine, the metabolic acids accumulate in the body and cause metabolic acidosis. Inadequate fluid intake in the postoperative or immobilized child can lead to oliguria and, potentially, metabolic acidosis. Note this child's urine collection device.

ripheral vascular resistance and resultant cardiac arrhythmias, hypotension, pulmonary edema, and tissue hypoxia. Confusion or drowsiness may result, as well as headache or abdominal pain.

COLLABORATIVE CARE

Laboratory tests include blood pH and arterial blood gases. Treatment of metabolic acidosis depends on identification and treatment of the underlying cause (see the companion website for a table of causes). For example, renal failure is treated with medications of dialysis, an intestinal fistula is repaired, and hyperalimentation formula is regulated to decrease acidosis. In severe metabolic acidosis, intravenous sodium bicarbonate may be used to increase the pH and to prevent cardiac arrhythmias. This treatment is difficult to manage, because renal excretion can cause excess retention of bicarbonate; therefore, intravenous sodium bicarbonate is used only in severe situations, such as prolonged cardiac arrest.

NURSING MANAGEMENT

Nursing Assessment and Diagnosis

Teach methods to prevent poisoning at each health promotion visit. For the child being treated for acidosis, assess the rate and depth of respirations. Evaluate the child's level of consciousness frequently. Be alert for signs or complaints of headache and abdominal pain. Serial arterial blood gas measurements will usually be obtained to evaluate changes in status.

The following nursing diagnoses can apply to the child with metabolic acidosis:

- Risk for Injury related to confusion/drowsiness or decreased responsiveness
- Risk for Decreased Cardiac Output related to cardiac dysrhythmias
- Ineffective Tissue Perfusion (Cerebral) related to tissue hypoxia
- Ineffective Family Management of Therapeutic Regimen related to complexity of management of diabetes mellitus

Planning and Implementation

Ensure safety, taking into account the child's level of consciousness and alertness. Turn the child and change his or her position to prevent pressure on the skin. Limit the child's activities to decrease cardiac workload.

Position the child to facilitate chest expansion. Provide oral care during rapid respirations because the mouth may become dry. Monitor intravenous solutions and laboratory values indicating acid-base balance. Report changes promptly.

Once the child is stabilized, provide teaching to compensate for knowledge deficits. This teaching for home prevention should take place at each health promotion visit for all children. Teach parents of young children to keep medications and acids locked in a secure place and out of reach to prevent poisoning (Figure 18–23 ➤). This includes medicines with aspirin as well as substances commonly kept in the garage for car maintenance. Teach about home management of diabetes and about early identification and treatment to avoid diabetic ketoacidosis. Expected outcomes of nursing care relate to prevention of acidosis and restoration of normal body balance during disease processes.

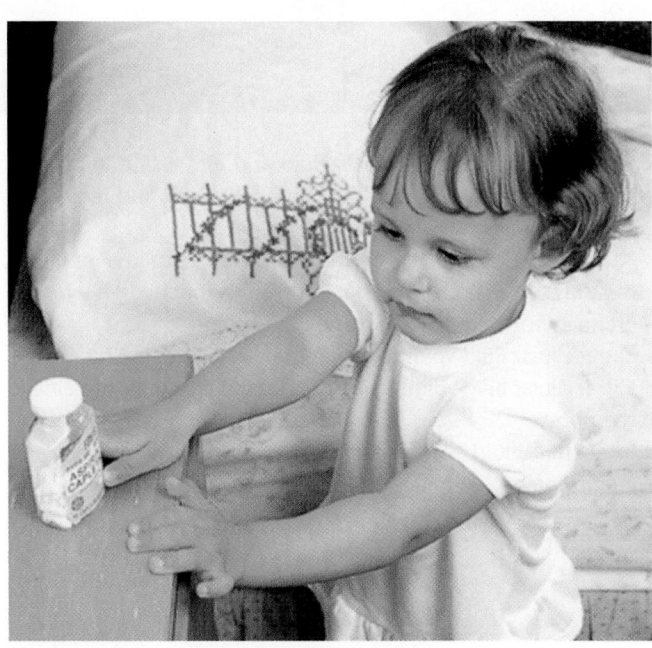

FIGURE 18–23 ➤ Teaching parents to use safety latches on cabinets to keep aspirin away from small children can prevent one cause of metabolic acidosis.

Metabolic Alkalosis

Metabolic alkalosis occurs when there are too few metabolic acids. It is sometimes called noncarbonic acid deficit.

A gain in bicarbonate or a loss of metabolic acid can cause metabolic alkalosis. Bicarbonate is gained through excessive intake of bicarbonate antacids or baking soda or through metabolism of bicarbonate precursors such as the citrate contained in blood transfusions. Increased renal absorption of bicarbonate can occur in profound hypokalemia, primary hyperaldosteronism, or extreme deficit in extracellular fluid volume. Acid can be lost through severe vomiting, such as that seen in infants with pyloric stenosis and in continued removal of gastric contents through suction.

Blood pH, bicarbonate, and Pco_2 are usually elevated in metabolic alkalosis. Hypokalemia often occurs simultaneously (refer to discussion of hypokalemia earlier in this chapter). Respiratory rate and depth usually decrease. Increased neuromuscular irritability, cramping, paresthesia, tetany, seizures, and excitation can occur. Finally, this state can progress to weakness, confusion, lethargy, and coma.

When the chemoreceptors in the brain and arteries detect the rising pH of metabolic alkalosis and respirations decrease, carbonic acid is retained in the body. This carbonic acid can neutralize the bicarbonate and return pH toward normal.

Laboratory tests include blood pH and arterial blood gases. Clinical therapy is directed at treating the underlying cause of the condition (see the companion website for a table of causes). Increasing the extracellular fluid volume with intravenous normal saline is used to facilitate renal excretion of bicarbonate. Medications such as acetazolamide increase renal excretion of bicarbonate as well.

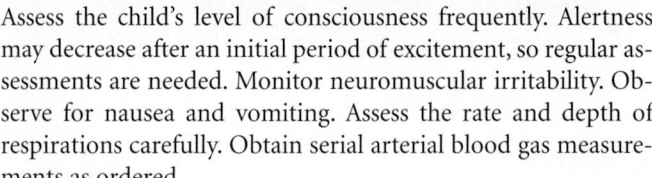

NURSING MANAGEMENT

Assess the child's level of consciousness frequently. Alertness may decrease after an initial period of excitement, so regular assessments are needed. Monitor neuromuscular irritability. Observe for nausea and vomiting. Assess the rate and depth of respirations carefully. Obtain serial arterial blood gas measurements as ordered.

Facilitate ease of respirations. Ensure safety by keeping bed rails elevated and by turning the child frequently. Position the child on the side to avoid aspiration of vomitus.

If antacids were the cause of the alkalosis, teach the child and parents about correct use of these medications.

■ MIXED ACID-BASE IMBALANCES

It is possible for two acid-base imbalances to occur simultaneously. For example, a child with cystic fibrosis can develop respiratory acidosis from lung problems and concurrent metabolic alkalosis from vomiting during an illness. Treatment with diuretics may cause concurrent metabolic alkalosis resulting from extracellular volume depletion and hypokalemia in a child with congestive heart failure and chronic respiratory acidosis. In these cases, all underlying causes must be identified and treated. Care of children with mixed acid-base imbalances is often complicated, requiring hospitalization and careful management. Upon discharge, the nurse can teach parents about signs of imbalance that need to be reported and treated to prevent further complications. Evaluation of care is based on outcomes of adequate respiratory ventilation and metabolic balance.

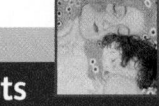

Chapter Highlights

- Young children are at risk for fluid and electrolyte imbalance due to differences in body fluid compartments and regulation systems.
- Nurses institute health promotion and health maintenance measures to maintain normal body fluids for children who exercise in hot weather and those undergoing surgery.
- Extracellular fluid volume deficit manifests as dehydration.
- Extracellular fluid volume excess is due to an excess of saline in the body.
- Interstitial fluid volume excess manifests as edema and weight gain.

- Nurses carefully manage fluid status of young children and teach parents prevention and treatment of fluid imbalances caused by gastroenteritis and other disease states.
- The most common electrolyte imbalances are hypernatremia and hypokalemia, and thus involve sodium and potassium.
- Normal acid-base balance is necessary for proper function of cells in the body.
- The lungs, kidneys, and liver play a role in maintaining acid-base balance.
- Acid-base imbalance can involve alkalosis or acidosis; either can have a respiratory or metabolic origin.

Clinical Reasoning in Action

Consider the scenario involving Vernon at the beginning of this chapter. He is an 18-month-old who has had vomiting and diarrhea for several days. The assessment of body weight loss, skin turgor, and level of activity suggests moderate dehydration. Vernon refuses attempts at feeding him orally, his pulse becomes rapid, and his blood pressure decreases. Voiding is decreased and capillary refill is slow. Vernon is admitted to the short-stay unit and an intravenous infusion is started.

1. Based on his age, what oral fluids might be best to offer to Vernon? What questions will you ask his mother about his normal fluid intake at home?

2. What additional assessment will you perform on Vernon to gather further information about his state of dehydration?

3. Since Vernon has had vomiting and diarrhea, he is probably deficient in an electrolyte present in high quantities in these body fluids. What electrolyte, in addition to sodium, is likely deficient?

4. A major nursing role is to plan care for Vernon while he is in the unit to rehydrate him. Calculate his replacement and maintenance fluid needs. Formulate a plan of care to include the amounts of oral rehydration therapy he should be offered over the next several hours. Use evidence-based findings to provide the rationale for your planned interventions.

See Pearson Nursing Student Resources for possible responses.

Pearson Nursing Student Resources

Find additional review materials at
nursing.pearsonhighered.com
Prepare for success with NCLEX®-style practice questions, interactive assignments and activities, web links, animations and videos, and more!

References

American Academy of Pediatrics. (2009). *Pediatric nutrition handbook* (5th ed.). Elk Grove Village, IL: Author.

Armstrong, L. E., Casa, D. J., Millard-Stafford, M., Moran, D. S., Pyne, S. W., & Roberts, W. O. (2007). Exertional heat illness during training and competition. *Medicine & Science in Sports & Exercise, 39*, 556–572.

Bindler, R., & Howry, L. (2005). *Pediatric drug guide.* Upper Saddle River, NJ: Prentice Hall.

Canavan, A., & Arant, B. S. (2009). Diagnosis and management of dehydration in children. *American Family Physician, 80*(7), 692–696.

Custer, J. W., & Rau, R. E. (2009). *The Harriet Lane handbook* (18th ed.). Philadelphia: Elsevier Mosby.

Diggins, K. C. (2008). Treatment of mild to moderate dehydration in children with oral rehydration therapy. *Journal of the American Academy of Nurse Practitioners, 20*, 402–406.

Fontaine, O., Garner, P., & Bhan, M. K. (2007). Oral rehydration therapy: The simple solution for saving lives. *British Medical Journal, 334*, 2–3.

Hartling, L., Bellemare, S., Wiebe, N., Russell, K., Klassen, T. P., & Craig, W. (2006). Oral versus intravenous rehydration for treating dehydration due to gastroenteritis in children. *Cochrane Database Systematic Reviews*, CD004390.

Heaney, R. P. (2006). Low calcium intake among African Americans: Effects on bones and body weight. *Journal of Nutrition, 136*, 1095–1098.

Hew-Butler, T., Ayus, J. C., Kipps, C., Maughan, R. J., Mettler, S., Meeuwiswse, W. H., et al. (2008). Statement of the second international exercise-associated hyponatremia consensus development conference, New Zealand, 2007. *Clinical Journal of Sport Medicine, 18*, 111–121.

Holliday, M. A., Ray, P. E., & Friedman, A. L. (2007). Fluid therapy for children: Facts, fashions, and questions. *Archives of Disease in Childhood, 92*, 546–550.

Howe, A. S., & Boden, B. P. (2007). Heat-related illness in athletes. *American Journal of Sports Medicine, 35*(8), 1384–1395.

Kliegman, R. M., Behrman, R. E., Jenson, H. B., & Stanton, B. F. (2007). *Nelson textbook of pediatrics* (18th ed.). Philadelphia: Saunders Elsevier.

Koslap-Petraco, M. B. (2006). Homecare issues in rotavirus gastroenteritis. *Journal of the American Academy of Nurse Practitioners, 18*, 422–428.

Madati, P. J., & Bachur, R. (2008). Development of an emergency department triage tool to predict acidosis among children with gastroenteritis. *Pediatric Emergency Care, 24*(12), 822–830.

Mayo Clinic. (2007). *Dehydration and youth sports: Curb the risk.* Retrieved from http://www.mayoclinic.com/health/dehydration/SM00037

Shroff, R., Hignett, R., Pierce, C., Marks, S., & van't Hoff, W. (2007). Life-threatening hypernatraemic dehydration in breastfed babies. *Archives of Disease in Childhood, 91*, 1025–1026.

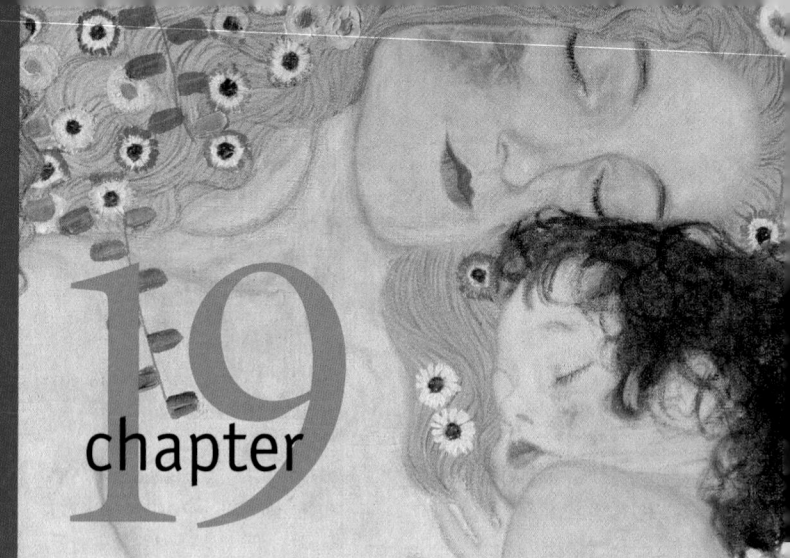

Alterations in Eye, Ear, Nose, and Throat Function

chapter 19

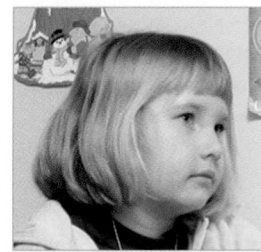

Kate is 5 years old and has had decreased hearing ability from birth. Once Kate's hearing loss was diagnosed, her family explored options to assist her with communication. Kate's parents learned sign language and began using it as she learned language. When Kate was 2 years of age, they decided to have a cochlear implant placed in her inner ear. Kate was slowly introduced to sounds over time and adjusted to her new sense of hearing. She started to make sounds in response to sounds in the environment, and a speech therapist assisted in helping the family introduce her to speech.

Kate communicates verbally now. Each week she visits a speech therapist who helps her learn how to listen for sounds, solve problems, and respond verbally. Both Kate's mother and father attend the therapy sessions so they can learn how to best communicate with Kate at home. The nurse in the office plays an integral part in fostering Kate's development. Ongoing developmental assessments and teaching to enhance Kate's environment so that she learns social and communication skills have been important nursing interventions. In addition, safety teaching and immunizations have been addressed by the nurse in the pediatric health care home.

As Kate begins kindergarten, how can the school nurse collaborate with the office nurse and then work with Kate's family to plan for establishment of an individualized education plan to enhance Kate's learning? What evidence-based practice will the nurse apply to assist the family to prepare for the transition to school and Kate's acquisition of new skills?

Learning Outcomes

After reading this chapter, you will be able to do the following:

1. Identify anatomy, physiology, and pediatric differences in the eye, ear, nose, and throat of children and adolescents.
2. Describe abnormalities of the eye, ear, nose, throat, and mouth in children.
3. Plan for screening programs and identification of children with vision and hearing abnormalities.
4. Integrate evidence-based research to create a nursing care plan for children with vision or hearing impairments.
5. Use the latest recommendations when implementing care and teaching for children with abnormalities of the eye, ear, nose, throat, and mouth.
6. Integrate preventive and treatment principles when implementing care for children related to the eye, ear, nose, and throat.

FOCUS ON

Eyes, Ears, Nose, and Throat

ANATOMY AND PHYSIOLOGY

Sight, hearing, taste, and smell depend on proper functioning of receptor organs and interpretation by the brain. Thus, certain cranial nerves are also an integral part of the anatomy and physiology of the eye, ear, nose, throat, and mouth. Children are prone to both inborn and acquired sensory alterations, as well as a wide array of infections and injuries that can affect the eye, ear, nose, throat, mouth, and upper respiratory system. Since these body parts are connected anatomically, conditions in one necessarily affect the others. Other conditions of the respiratory system, including obstructive sleep apnea, are discussed in Chapter 20 ∞.

Eye

The eye is a complex structure composed of the eyeball and its supporting structures. The *sclera,* or white part of the eye, is the outermost layer. It is transparent in the anterior eye to form the *cornea,* which allows light to enter. The *iris,* or colored part of the

eye, is muscular, allowing it to change the size of the *pupil* and regulate the light that enters the eye. The *lens* is located behind the pupil and focuses light onto the retina. The *anterior chamber,* or the space between the cornea and iris, is filled with a fluid called *aqueous humor.* The *posterior chamber* is located behind the lens and is filled with *vitreous humor.* The innermost, posterior section of the eye is the *retina,* which has an inner layer that receives light impulses and an outer neural layer that transports visual images to the brain by the optic nerve (cranial nerve II). The *rods* in the retina perceive vision in dim light and allow for peripheral vision; the *cones* perceive vision in bright light and are responsible for color discernment. See Figure 19–1 ➤ for normal structures of the child's eye.

As Children Grow

The Eye

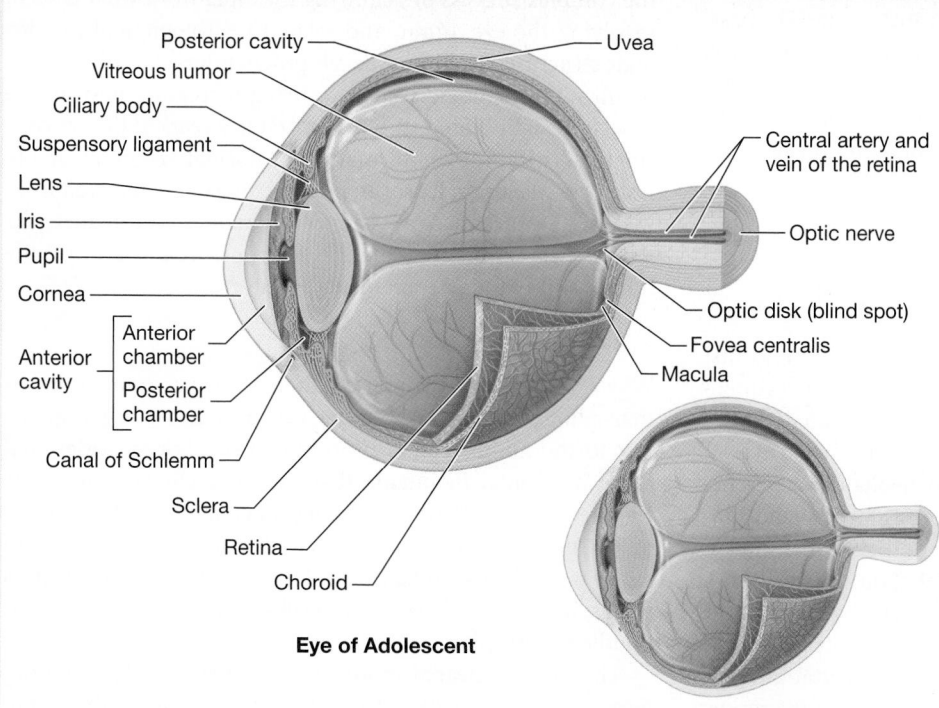

Posterior cavity
Vitreous humor
Ciliary body
Suspensory ligament
Lens
Iris
Pupil
Cornea
Anterior cavity — Anterior chamber / Posterior chamber
Canal of Schlemm
Sclera
Retina
Choroid

Uvea
Central artery and vein of the retina
Optic nerve
Optic disk (blind spot)
Fovea centralis
Macula

Eye of Adolescent

Eye of Young Child

FIGURE 19–1 ➤ The eye is well developed at birth, but there are some variations in the visual acuity of the infant and young child. What influence would the young child's visual acuity have on the types of toys and books that should be made available?

The eye has several supporting structures that assist in the sensation of vision. *Eyebrows, eyelids,* and *eyelashes* protect the eye and add touch sensation. The *conjunctiva* lines the cornea and the inside of the eyelids, lubricating the eye and keeping it viable. The lacrimal apparatus and ducts bathe the eye and produce tears. A series of six muscles allow the eye to move to all planes and maintain the shape of the eyeball. They are innervated by the oculomotor, trochlear, and abducens nerves (cranial nerves III, IV, and V).

Ear

The ear is responsible for the sensory ability of hearing and it establishes the sense of equilibrium. The *external ear* contains the *auricle,* which is visible outside the body; the *external canal;* and the *tympanic membrane.* These structures collect sound waves and direct them to the middle and inner ear. The *middle ear* lies behind the tympanic membrane and contains three bones necessary for sound vibrations: the *incus, malleus,* and *stapes.* Another part of the middle ear, the *eustachian tube,* connects to the nasopharynx and equalizes ear pressure. The *inner ear* contains the bony labyrinth, which in turn houses the *vestibule, semicircular canals,* and the *cochlea.* The vestibule and semicircular canals are responsible for the sense of equilibrium. The cochlea contains the *organ of Corti,* which contains sensory hair cells that are innervated by the acoustic nerve (cranial nerve VIII).

Nose, Throat, and Mouth

The structures of the nose, throat, and mouth are important to all humans. Mucous membranes bathe these body parts and have a high rate of growth. They help to maintain hygiene and protect the body from infectious agents. Salivary apparatus and taste buds are essential parts of the mouth and tongue. The nasal passages contain external nostrils, the sinuses, and the pharynx (or throat). The olfactory, facial, glossopharyngeal, and vagus nerves (cranial nerves I, VII, IX, and X) are responsible for the sense of smell, taste, coordinated swallowing, and the gag reflex, respectively.

PEDIATRIC DIFFERENCES

Eye

How are the eyes of children different from those of adults? Chapter 5 ∞ provides a detailed discussion of the assessment of the eyes and **visual acuity,** the ability to discriminate letters or other objects. The eyes of neonates differ from the eyes of adults in several ways. Visual acuity in neonates ranges between 20/100 and 20/400. The lens is more spherical and cannot accommodate to both near and far objects, which means that the neonate sees best at a distance of about 20 cm (8 in.). Because the optic nerve is not yet completely myelinated, the ability to distinguish color and other details is decreased. If the infant is preterm, especially less than 32 weeks' gestation, retinal vascularization, particularly in the periphery of the retina, may be incomplete. Pupillary reflex reaction is detected by

about 28 to 30 weeks' gestation and so may be sluggish in preterm infants. The rectus muscles that control binocular vision may be somewhat uncoordinated at birth. The eyes should be aligned and movement coordinated by the age of 3 months. Transient **nystagmus** (involuntary rapid eye movement) and **esotropia** (momentary turning inward of eyes) are common in neonates, but decrease in incidence during the first few months of life. Conjunctival and retinal hemorrhages may be observed in the newborn as a result of the trauma of birth; they usually improve gradually and have no lasting effects. The red reflex is examined in children because it is a key method for identifying the presence of retinoblastoma (see Chapter 5 ∞ for the method to evaluate the red reflex and Chapter 24 ∞ for a description of retinoblastoma).

The cornea of the infant and young child occupies a larger portion of the orbit than in the adult; the eyeball is about 3/4 of its adult size. Because the eyeball is relatively unprotected laterally, it is more easily injured. The sclera of the neonate is thin and translucent with a bluish tinge, and the iris is blue or gray. Eye color changes during the first 6 months of life. Infants produce tears to nourish and oxygenate the outer layers of the cornea. However, parents do not see tears when a young infant cries because the infant's lacrimal system drains them efficiently into the nasal cavity.

As infants grow, their eyes mature and their vision improves. The eyeball grows until the third year, when growth slows, until normal adult size is reached by 14 years. By the age of 2 or 3 years, most children have a visual acuity of 20/50, and by the age of 6 or 7 years, it is 20/20. See Figure 19–1 for a summary of pediatric differences of the eye. Visual acuity is measured using standardized letter or picture charts (see Chapter 5 ∞ and the *Clinical Skills Manual*). **Vision** refers to the complex process of acquiring meaning from what is seen, involving the eye, brain, and related neurologic and physiologic structures. Cognitive development interacts with a child's maturing physiologic system to bring increasing meaning to objects in sight (Table 19–1). The first few years of life are considered critical for the formation of normal vision. As acuity improves, the brain learns to interpret messages received from the eyes. Disturbances in vision, even in one eye, can affect the retinal nerve function, muscle function in the eye, or the brain's ability to interpret visual input.

Ear

Why do infants and young children have more ear problems than adults? The eustachian tube, which connects the nasopharynx to the middle ear, is proportionately shorter, wider, and more horizontal in infants than in older children or adults (Figure 19–2 ➤). During sucking, yawning, and other movements, the tube opens for milliseconds, allowing free passage of air between the nasopharynx and the middle ear. These factors predispose young children to development of otitis media or middle ear infection.

The fetus can hear at about 20 weeks' gestation. The auditory nerve function is mature at about 5 months of age in the infant. Before 34 weeks' gestation, the external ear is soft with little car-

TABLE 19-1 Visually Related Developmental Milestones

Age	Milestone
Term neonate	Demonstrates alertness to light and visual stimulus presented 8–12 in. (20–30 cm) from eyes
1 month	Follows an object 60 degrees horizontally and 30 degrees vertically; blinks at an approaching object
2 months	Follows a person or moving object for 180 degrees from 6 ft (2 m) away; smiles in response to a face; raises head 30 degrees from prone
3 months	Tracks an object through 180 degrees; regards own hand; begins visual-motor coordination
4–5 months	Social smile; reaches for a cube 12 in. (30 cm) away; notices a raisin 12 in. (30 cm) away; stares at own hand
7–8 months	Reaches and grasps an object, picks up a raisin by raking, transfers objects from hand to hand
8–9 months	Pokes at holes in a peg board; well-developed pincer grasp; crawls; uncovers toy after seeing it hidden
12–14 months	Stacks blocks; places a peg in a round hole; stands and walks

Data from: Rudolph, C. D., Rudolph, A. M., Hostetter, M. K., Lister, G. E., & Siegel, M. J. (Eds.). Rudolph's pediatrics (21st ed.). New York: McGraw-Hill; Frigelman, S. (2007). The first year. In R. M. Kliegman, R. E. Behrman, H. B. Jenson, & B. F. Stanton, Nelson textbook of pediatrics (18th ed.). Philadelphia: Saunders.

tilage apparent. The external ear canal is small at birth, although the internal ear and middle ear are relatively large. As a result, the tympanic membrane is close to the surface and can be easily injured.

Nose, Throat, and Mouth

Up to the age of 6 months, infants are primarily nasal breathers. Edema and nasal discharge may interfere with adequate air intake and feeding. Mucosal swelling and exudate may block the small nasal passages of young children. The immature immune system of young children (see Chapter 22 ∞ for further description) and the frequent exposure to other children with illnesses causes a high rate of upper respiratory infections in this population.

The palatine tonsils, which are visible on oral examination, are located on each side of the oropharynx. The method for examining a child's throat is discussed in Chapter 5 ∞. Although tonsils vary in size considerably during childhood, they are normally large, especially in school-age children. The nasopharyngeal tonsils (adenoids) lie in the posterior wall of the nasopharynx, just above the oropharynx. In children, the adenoids may become enlarged, harboring bacteria and interfering with breathing.

The mouth is an important organ for the infant because strong muscles are needed for sucking and thereby receiving nutrients. Sucking is an important developmental skill that promotes the muscles needed for later speech development. Taste sensation is present before birth, as evidenced by increased swallowing of amniotic fluid that has been sweetened.

As Children Grow
Eustachian Tube

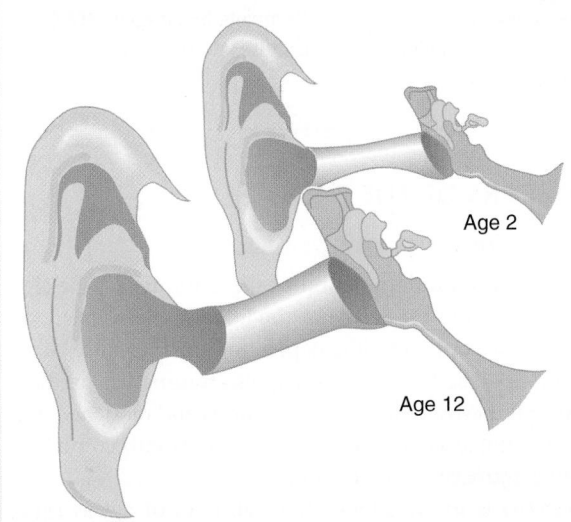

Position of eustachian tube is at less of an angle (more horizontal) in the young child, resulting in decreased drainage.

Age 2

End of eustachian tube in nasal pharynx opens during sucking.

Age 12

Eustachian tube equalizes air pressure between the middle ear and the outside environment and allows for drainage of secretions from middle ear mucosa.

FIGURE 19–2 ➤ Of the three anatomical differences in the eustachian tube between adults and small children (shorter, wider, more horizontal), which do you think could cause more problems for the child and why? Answer: More horizontal. Small children who are bottle-fed in a supine position have a greater probability of developing otitis media because the eustachian tube opens when the child sucks and the horizontal angle provides easy access to the middle ear. In older children, the increased angle helps keep foreign substances and infectious agents away from the middle ear.

Taste sensations increase during childhood. By about 6 months of age the first tooth emerges, and by about 2 years the full set of 20 primary teeth is present. Tooth loss of the primary set begins about 5–6 years, and gradually the secondary teeth (32 total) erupt during childhood. See Chapter 5 ∞ for a further description of teeth eruption.

A variety of diagnostic and laboratory tests are used to evaluate the eye, ear, nose, and throat. See Appendices C and D and Chapter 5 ∞ for details about audiologic screening, newborn hearing screening, tympanogram, complete blood count (CBC), and culture/sensitivity test. See the Assessment Guidelines for the Child with an Alteration of the Eye, Ear, Nose, or Throat.

Assessment Guidelines for the Child with an Alteration of the Eye, Ear, Nose, or Throat

Assessment Focus	Assessment Guidelines
Eyes	■ Describe eye structures and symmetry. ■ Describe visual acuity using the screening test appropriate for age. ■ Measure extraocular movements to all quadrants. Evaluate corneal light reflex, cover-uncover test, and visual fields. ■ Using the ophthalmoscope, elicit and evaluate the red reflex bilaterally. ■ Observe for and report abnormalities such as eye drainage, cloudiness of lens, or abnormal movement.
Ears	■ Describe placement and symmetry of the external ear. ■ Describe auditory acuity using the screening test appropriate for age. ■ Using the otoscope, evaluate the ear canal and tympanic membrane. ■ Ask about pain and discomfort from the ear; observe for drainage.
Nose	■ Describe the nose for symmetry and placement. Are the nares bilaterally patent? Are there lesions or drainage? ■ Can the child identify several smells? ■ Are signs of sinus infection present, such as facial edema or pain, headache, and tenderness upon palpation over the sinus areas?
Mouth and throat	■ Are the oral mucous membranes intact? Is there an odor? ■ How many primary/secondary/loose teeth are present? Are there visible caries? Are there broken or chipped teeth present? ■ Evaluate the soft and hard palate for intactness. ■ Describe the throat and size/appearance of the tonsils. ■ Palpate cervical lymph nodes, noting size and tenderness.

How are conditions of the eye, ear, nose, and throat related? Which conditions have the potential to affect a child's growth, development, and behavior? In what settings do children with eye, ear, nose, and throat conditions receive care?

Because the eye, ear, nose, and throat are connected, a malformation, infection, or other condition in one of these structures may affect them all. Intact sensory structures support the attainment of developmental milestones; thus alterations, especially to the eye and ear, may delay a child's development. (See Chapter 4 ∞ for expected developmental milestones at each age.) In the chapter-opening scenario, Kate's condition was diagnosed when she was very young, and she received a cochlear implant and speech therapy to enhance her development. A variety of diagnostic and laboratory procedures and tests are used to identify abnormalities (Table 19–2). Most children with eye, ear, nose, and throat disorders are treated at home or in the community rather than in the hospital. Infections of the eye, ear, and upper respiratory system are common abnormalities, and most pediatric nurses will need to be experts in assessment and interventions for these conditions.

See Appendices D and E ∞ and descriptions in this chapter for information about these diagnostic procedures and tests.

TABLE 19–2	Diagnostic and Laboratory Procedures/Tests for the Eye, Ear, Nose, and Throat

Diagnostic Procedures	Laboratory Tests
Audiologic screening Newborn hearing screening Tympanogram Vision screening	Complete blood count (CBC) Culture and sensitivity

■ DISORDERS OF THE EYE

Infectious Conjunctivitis

Conjunctivitis is an inflammation of the conjunctiva, the clear membrane that lines the inside of the lid and sclera. There are several types of conjunctivitis, depending on the cause of inflammation. Bacteria, viruses, allergies, trauma, or irritants cause the conjunctiva to become edematous and reddened with a yellow or white discharge (Figure 19–3 ➤). Parents commonly refer to all conjunctivitis as "pink eye."

Conjunctivitis in an infant under 30 days of age is called *ophthalmia neonatorum*. These infections are usually acquired

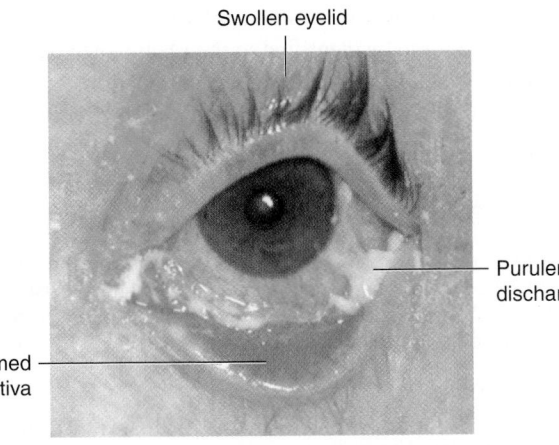

Swollen eyelid

Purulent discharge

Inflamed conjunctiva

FIGURE 19–3 ➤ Acute conjunctivitis. The major difference between bacterial and viral conjunctivitis is that bacterial conjunctivitis has a purulent discharge that may result in crusting whereas the discharge from viral conjunctivitis is serous (watery). Allergic conjunctivitis produces watery to thick drainage and is characterized by itching.
Used with permission from Newell, F. W. (1996). Ophthalmology: Principles and concepts (8th ed.). St. Louis, MO: Mosby Year-Book.

from the mother during vaginal delivery as a result of contact with infected vaginal discharge containing bacterial organisms such as *Chlamydia trachomatis* and *Neisseria gonorrhoeae*. Antibiotics are instilled into the eyes of newborns soon after birth as a prophylactic measure.

In infants who have frequent tearing and mattering (eyelid discharge that has formed a crust) on awakening, a plugged lacrimal duct may mimic conjunctivitis. Treatment involves massaging the tear duct every 4 hours when the infant is awake. Lacrimal ducts that remain plugged after the age of 1 year may have to be opened surgically.

Bacterial conjunctivitis is common in children of any age. It is characterized by edema of the eyelid, reddened conjunctiva, and enlarged preauricular lymph glands. Mucopurulent discharge causes mattering and makes the eyes difficult to open upon awakening. Older children with conjunctivitis complain of itching or burning, mild photophobia, and a feeling of scratching under the lids.

Common infectious organisms include *Staphylococcus aureus*, *Haemophilus influenzae*, *Streptococcus pneumoniae*, *Moraxella catarrhalis*, and *Escherichia coli* (Mah, 2006). Most cases are caused by hand-to-eye contact. The disease can rapidly spread when groups of youth spend time together, such as among young children and adolescents in schools and childcare centers, and among college students in dormitories or on sports teams. The infection can be bilateral but is more commonly unilateral.

Other infections in newborns and children can be caused by viruses. Viral conjunctivitis is commonly bilateral. Adenovirus is a common cause and spreads from respiratory adenovirus infection in a hand-to-eye manner. Signs and symptoms are similar to those of bacterial conjunctivitis, although sometimes milder in severity and slower in onset.

Herpes simplex virus (HSV) can also cause infection, either by transfer from an infected mother to a neonate during birth or

By federal law, all infants born in the United States are given prophylactic eye treatment soon after delivery to help prevent ophthalmia neonatorum. The nurse is responsible for administering this eye ointment. Penicillin, tetracycline, erythromycin, or povidone-iodine ointments are most commonly used.

Sometimes an infant can develop chemical conjunctivitis due to the prophylactic eye ointment. A chemical reaction should be considered as a possible cause when conjunctivitis develops within 24–48 hours after instillation of the medication.

by contact with an infected person at any age. Ophthalmic herpes infection is often accompanied by characteristic vesicular lesions on the skin of the face. A culture of the lesion is performed for diagnosis and any accompanying conjunctivitis is assumed to be caused by HSV. An infection caused by HSV requires prompt and vigorous treatment to prevent eye injury or blindness, which can occur in children with recurrent herpesvirus infections as a result of antibody reaction to the viral antigen. Herpesvirus infections commonly recur, so periodic treatment and sometime prophylaxis may be needed.

Allergic conjunctivitis is a common cause of eye discomfort (Bielory, 2010). When conjunctivitis is caused by an allergy, the child complains of intense itching. Examination reveals reddened eyes with watery discharge and the conjunctivae have a "cobblestone" appearance. The eyes may also appear edematous.

COLLABORATIVE CARE

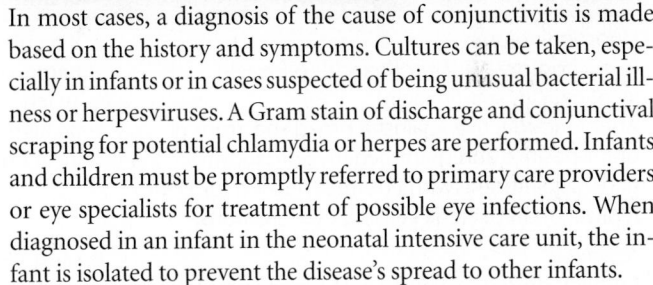

In most cases, a diagnosis of the cause of conjunctivitis is made based on the history and symptoms. Cultures can be taken, especially in infants or in cases suspected of being unusual bacterial illness or herpesviruses. A Gram stain of discharge and conjunctival scraping for potential chlamydia or herpes are performed. Infants and children must be promptly referred to primary care providers or eye specialists for treatment of possible eye infections. When diagnosed in an infant in the neonatal intensive care unit, the infant is isolated to prevent the disease's spread to other infants.

Antibiotic eye medication is prescribed in droplet or ointment form if a bacterial infection is suspected. Treatment may be started after a laboratory sample is obtained but before the results are known. Fluoroquinolones are now frequently used to treat bacterial conjunctivitis; drops or ointment can be used (Lichtenstein, Dorfman, Kennedy, et al., 2006; Wagner & Aquino, 2008). When gonococcal conjunctivitis occurs in newborns, ceftriaxone is recommended; the disease is resistant to penicillin. Chlamydial infections are treated with oral erythromycin or tetracycline. Careful total evaluation of the newborn with conjunctivitis is also performed to watch for other signs of infection. Instructions for instilling eye medications are given in the *Clinical Skills Manual*.

Viral conjunctivitis may be treated with comfort measures such as cleaning drainage away with a warm clean cloth, avoiding bright lights, and avoiding reading. Ophthalmic antibiotics are sometimes given to prevent bacterial invasion due to frequent rubbing of the eyes. Herpes simplex virus infections of the eye are treated promptly by an ophthalmologist, neonatologist, or others who are trained in this serious disease. Topical drugs are used, and often are combined with a systemic antiviral agent such as acyclovir. Neonatal herpes simplex virus is treated vigorously with parenteral acyclovir for 14 days (or longer if central nervous system involvement is found upon lumbar puncture), and with topical ophthalmic medication (trifluridine, iododeoxyuridine, or vidarabine). Recurrent lesions may necessitate suppressive or prophylactic treatment with oral acyclovir (American Academy of Pediatrics, 2009).

If an allergen is diagnosed as the cause of conjunctivitis, systemic or topical antihistamines may be prescribed. Topical steroids and vasoconstrictors may also be used (Bielory, 2010). Decongestants can be combined with systemic antihistamines for short-term therapy. Mast-cell stabilizers may be used to decrease the activation of mast cells that accompanies allergic reactions; their use is safe in children 3 years of age and older. See Medications Used to Treat Conjunctivitis for types of medications used to treat eye conditions.

NURSING MANAGEMENT

Nurses routinely instill prophylactic antibiotics into the eyes of newborns after birth. A careful examination should occur so that any cases of ophthalmia neonatorum are referred promptly to an ophthalmologist. Women infected with gonococcus or chlamydia should be identified so their babies can receive attention and medication at birth to prevent infection. Babies born at home should have ocular examinations soon after birth.

Clinical Tip

During assessment, place a gloved index finger on the child's nose next to the inner corner of the eye and apply gentle pressure for several seconds. If mucopurulent drainage is discharged from the eye, bacterial conjunctivitis may be present.

Nurses also perform assessments of the eyes of infants and children in many settings and refer for care those with identified redness, edema, and discharge. Because bacterial infectious conjunctivitis is extremely contagious, tell parents that children should not return to childcare or school until they have been using an antibiotic for 24 hours. Teach parents the importance of careful hand hygiene and the avoidance of shared towels. Tell parents that children should not rub their eyes; mittens may help prevent infants from doing so. Toddlers may be distracted by activities that keep their hands busy. Teach parents the proper techniques for instilling eye medications (see Families Want to Know: Instilling Eye Medications). For children with allergies, alert parents to signs of infection so that if the child develops

Medications Used to Treat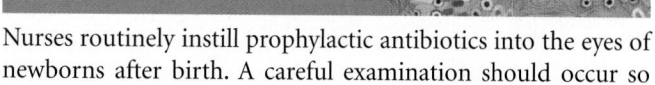
Conjunctivitis

Medication and Action/Indication	Nursing Implications
Fluoroquinolones (e.g., norfloxacin, ciprofloxacin, ofloxacin, levofloxacin, sparfloxacin) Antibiotic effective against a broad spectrum of gram-positive and gram-negative organisms; generally interfere with enzymes needed for DNA replication in bacteria causing eye infections.	■ If a culture and sensitivity test is ordered, perform the test before beginning the antibiotic. ■ Teach parents correct administration of drops or ointment. ■ Be alert for signs of reactivity to medication that might be manifested as local burning, crusting, itching, and edema.
Acyclovir Antiviral drug effective against herpes simplex virus (HSV).	■ Most viral conjunctivitis infections are not treated; good hygiene practices are followed and the infection clears without treatment by medication. However, herpes simplex virus infections must be treated because they can harm vision. Acyclovir is administered intravenously to neonates and some children with HSV; ongoing suppressive oral therapy is used for recurred infections. ■ Teach the family to recognize characteristic herpes skin lesions and report them and all eye redness immediately. Ensure that family members and other care providers understand the possible chronic nature of HSV and engage in careful hygiene to prevent spread when infections are active. ■ Prepare and administer the IV form as ordered, over at least 1 hour. Shake oral suspension when that form is used for children.
Mast-cell stabilizers (e.g., cromolyn, nedocromil, olopatadine) Inhibit release of histamine from mast cells, thereby decreasing allergic response. Used to treat itching and other symptoms of allergic conjunctivitis.	■ Teach the family the correct instillation of medication. Encourage other methods to decrease itching such as cool compresses several times daily to the eyes. ■ Avoid rubbing eyes, which can introduce bacteria or virus to the already inflamed eyes. If medication does not provide relief or additional eye symptoms appear, consult again with the health care provider.

Families Want to Know

Instilling Eye Medications

It can be challenging to safely instill eye medication into the eyes of young children. Give parents the following suggestions:

■ Wash hands well.

■ Be sure the medicine is warmed at least to room temperature.

■ Remove any drainage from the eye with a clean or sterile moist, warm cloth or gauze.

■ Wash hands again.

■ Place the child on the back with eyes closed.

■ Gently pull the lower lid down to form a small pocket.

■ Apply a thin string (for ointment) or drops of the medicine.

■ Allow the eyelid to return to its normal position.

■ Have the child keep the eye closed for several seconds.

■ Help prevent spread of the infection by keeping the child's hands clean.

■ Enhance comfort by keeping the head elevated to decrease swelling and by avoiding exposure to bright light.

---

conjunctivitis, prompt treatment will be obtained. The pruritus of allergic conjunctivitis may be relieved by laying clean washcloths with very cold water over the eyes for several minutes two to three times daily. Avoid use of contact lenses during periods of allergic conjunctivitis since they can further exacerbate the condition.

Periorbital Cellulitis

Periorbital cellulitis is an infection of the eyelid and surrounding tissues that is usually caused by bacteria and is an uncommon complication of sinusitis. The average age for occurrence is 7.5 years (Yang, Quah, Seah, et al., 2009). Children present with edematous, tender, and red or purple eyelids; restricted, painful movement of the area around the eye; and fever. Periorbital cellulitis should be treated promptly to prevent spread of the infection to the posterior orbit, which could lead to serious outcomes such as brain abscess or decreased vision. Orbital cellulitis is a serious outcome that can lead to bacterial meningitis (Nageswaran, Woods, Benjamin, et al., 2006). Clinical therapy includes hospitalization for intravenous administration of antibiotics, drainage of infection in some cases, and the application of hot packs. Children usually respond favorably within 48 to 72 hours.

Nursing management of periorbital cellulitis begins with identification of potential cases and prompt referral for treatment. When the child is hospitalized, the nurse administers antibiotics, provides supportive care, monitors vital signs, and teaches the family about the infection. Desired outcomes are rapid resolution of the infection and return to normal daily activities with no impairment in eye function.

Visual Disorders

Vision, the complex process of acquiring meaning from what is seen, depends on many factors. The eyes must move quickly and in a coordinated manner (see Chapter 5 ∞ for discussion of eye movement assessment). They must function together for clear, single vision to occur. If this ability, called **binocularity**, is not present (perhaps due to strabismus or amblyopia), the child may have double vision and the brain cannot make sense of the images it receives. Normally, perceptions of objects seen are integrated with other senses through eye-hand coordination, and with the brain through visual imagery and discrimination of objects seen. Although visual acuity is essential, the child's movements, mental processes, and other senses all interact to give meaning to objects that are viewed.

About 5–10% of young children have some type of vision impairment, with amblyopia present in 1–4% and refractive errors in 5–7%. If uncorrected, early visual impairment interferes with learning, developmental progression, and school performance; it may even lead to further deterioration of vision and to total blindness (American Academy of Pediatrics, 2007, 2009; Doshi & Rodriguez, 2007; U.S. Preventive Services Task Force, 2005).

Etiology and Pathophysiology

Several common visual disorders involve errors of refraction (Figure 19–4 ➤). As light enters the eye, it is bent or refracted to fall on the retina. Variations in the shape of the eyeball are often genetic in nature and can cause light rays to fall in another area of the eye, where they cannot be interpreted. Common refractive errors include:

- **Hyperopia (farsightedness).** Light rays focus posterior to the retina, resulting in an inability to focus on nearby objects. All children have some degree of hyperopia until 9 to 10 years of age. However, their eyes can accommodate sufficiently to enable them to see near objects clearly. Blurring of vision occurs only in children with excessive hyperopia, or a difference in accommodation between the two eyes. Amblyopia, or a weakening of the poorer eye, can occur in these children if treatment is not obtained.
- **Myopia (nearsightedness).** Light rays focus anterior to the retina, resulting in an inability to see far-off objects. Although children of any age can manifest myopia, it most commonly develops at about 8 years of age. The child may complain of headaches and often squints to improve distance vision.
- **Astigmatism.** Light rays are refracted differently depending on their place of entry to the eye. The curvature of the cornea or lens is not uniformly spherical, causing blurred images. The child with astigmatism often holds pages very close to the face to obtain the best visual image.

Other common visual disorders in children are characterized by abnormal musculature that causes asymmetric eye movement and by other anatomic abnormalities. They include:

- Strabismus
- Amblyopia
- Cataracts
- Glaucoma
- Retinoblastoma

Strabismus, amblyopia, cataracts, and glaucoma are described in Clinical Manifestations: Visual Disorders on pages 519–520. Retinoblastoma is discussed in Chapter 24 ∞.

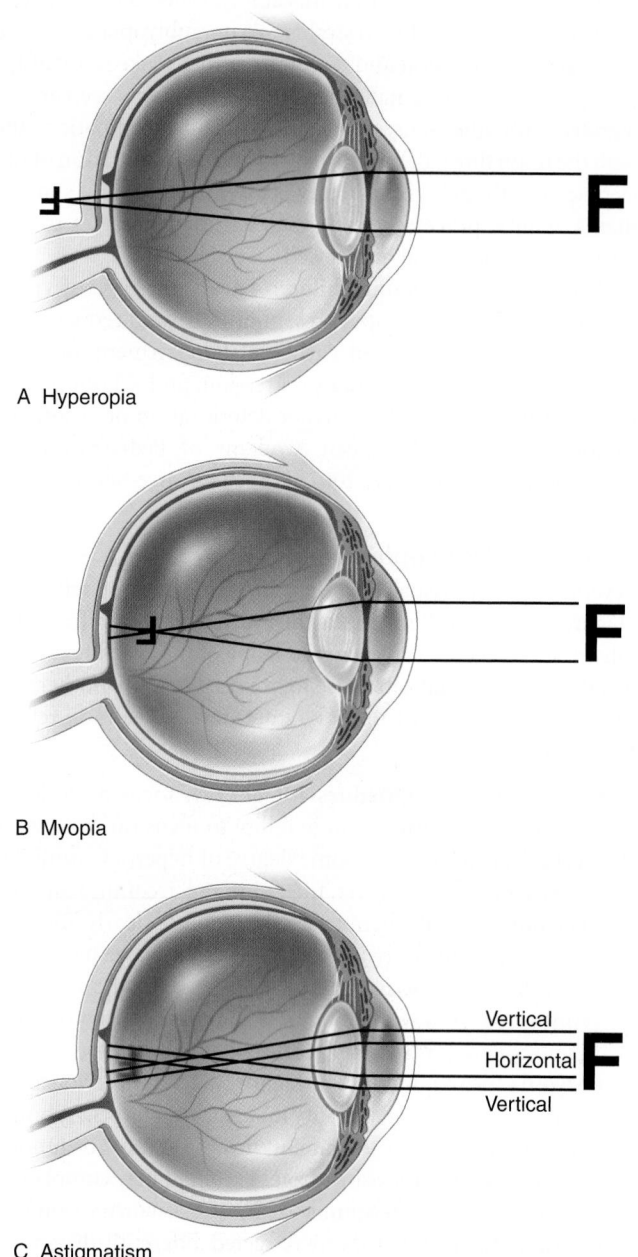

A Hyperopia

B Myopia

C Astigmatism

Vertical
Horizontal
Vertical

FIGURE 19–4 ➤ A, In hyperopia, light rays focus behind the retina, making it difficult to focus on objects at close range. B, In myopia, light rays focus in front of the retina, making it difficult to focus on objects that are far away. C, In astigmatism, light rays do not uniformly focus on the eye due to abnormal curvature of the cornea or lens.

Clinical Manifestations

Children with eye abnormalities may demonstrate a variety of behaviors. An infant who notices objects only on one side or consistently holds the head more to one side may have a decrease in vision in the other eye. Cataracts may be visualized as the lens appears cloudy. Muscular problems may be evident when the eyes do not move symmetrically or one eye deviates inward or outward. Some children squint, cover one eye, hold toys or books close to the face, or have watering eyes. See the Clinical Manifestations table on the following pages for further signs of specific disorders.

COLLABORATIVE CARE

Visual disturbances must be diagnosed and treated promptly to prevent impairment or loss of visual acuity. Most children undergo a simple test for visual acuity during health care visits as soon as they can cooperate with the examiner. Once in school, children's visual acuity is screened every 2 to 3 years during the elementary years. A child who does not pass vision screening is referred to an eye specialist for more detailed examination of near and far vision, eye structure and movement, and color discrimination. During health promotion visits, infants and young children should be examined by using the cover–uncover test, and the red reflex should be examined with an ophthalmoscope. See Chapter 5 ∞ for thorough descriptions of these tests.

Compensatory lenses are prescribed for many visual disorders, particularly refractive disorders. See the section on visual impairment later in this chapter for more details. A significant difference in visual acuity between the eyes is often a result of amblyopia or strabismus, and further treatment by patching or surgery may be needed. The visual acuity of a child with compensatory lenses should be reevaluated every 1 to 2 years. More frequent visits to an eye specialist are needed when a child is being treated for amblyopia or strabismus (Braverman, 2007).

Cataracts are generally treated surgically with removal of the lens, placement of a lens transplant, or use of corrective contact lenses. Glaucoma frequently requires surgery in children to provide outflow for fluid and a resultant decrease in intraocular pressure. Ophthalmic cancers are treated with surgery and chemotherapy.

NURSING MANAGEMENT

The nurse plays an important role in identifying eye disorders in children. Ask questions that will help to identify the child with a decrease in visual acuity (Table 19–3). Perform careful eye examinations of newborns and children. Observe for symmetry of placement and movement, ability to follow objects with each eye, and any abnormalities in appearance. The corneal light reflex, cover–uncover test, and visual acuity testing are essential tests for every child. See Chapter 5 ∞ for a description of eye examination, and the *Clinical Skills Manual* for visual acuity tests. Vision screening should be conducted at birth and at all well-child visits.

Clinical Judgment

Eye assessments of young children must be performed while they engage with their parent or look at you when you speak. How will you interact with a 2-year-old in a health care visit to gather information about symmetry of eye movement and the ability to see small objects?

Nurses in schools also plan and carry out regular visual acuity screening on children. Generally certain grades (such as kindergarten, 2, 4, 6, and 8) are screened annually along with any children new to a district. The nurse performs and records the screening results, and informs the school and families of any

Clinical Manifestations
Visual Disorders

Etiology	Clinical Manifestations	Clinical Therapy
Strabismus Can be congenital or acquired. Seen in 4% of all children; 30–50% of children with strabismus develop amblyopia. Most common types: Esotropia: inward deviation of eyes ("crossed eyes"). Exotropia: outward deviation of eyes ("wall-eyes"). 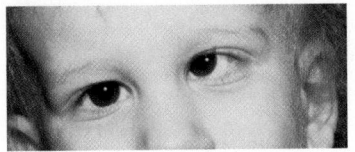 Strabismus. *Reprinted from* Paediatrics, *2e, Thomas & Harvey, p. 130, 1997, by permission of the publisher Churchill Livingstone.*	Eyes appear misaligned to observer. May occur only when child is tired. Symptoms include squinting and frowning when reading, closing one eye to see, having trouble picking up objects, dizziness, and headache. Corneal light reflex and cover–uncover tests confirm diagnosis. Child may have no other abnormalities but certain conditions such as cerebral palsy, hydrocephalus, Down syndrome, and seizure disorder are more commonly accompanied by strabismus.	Occlusion therapy (patching the fixating or good eye for 1–2 hours daily to force use of the weak eye). Compensatory lenses. Surgery of the rectus muscles to correct muscle imbalance. Eye drops to cause blurring of the good eye. Prisms. Vision therapy (eye exercise). If treatment is begun before 24 months of age, amblyopia (reduced vision in one or both eyes) may be prevented.
Amblyopia ("lazy eye") Reduced vision in one or both eyes; affects 4% of children. Amblyopia can result from anything that causes visual deprivation to one eye. The most common causes are untreated strabismus, with the child "tuning out" the image in the deviating eye, congenital cataract, or uncorrected refractive errors causing visual differences between eyes.	Symptoms are the same as for strabismus. Vision testing can be used to diagnose condition.	Compensatory lenses. Occlusion therapy for 2–6 hours daily through patching. Occasionally vision therapy (eye exercises) is used in an attempt to improve the weaker eye. Atropine 1% 1 gtt/day in unaffected eye. Treatment is discontinued when visual acuity no longer improves; 20/20 acuity rarely attained. Treatment is most successful if received by 5–6 years of age.
Cataracts Occurs when all or part of the lens of the eye becomes opaque, which prevents refraction of light rays onto the retina. Seen in 2/10,000 newborns. 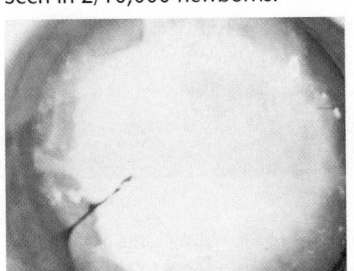 Congenital cataract. *Used with permission from Vaughan, D., Asbury, T., & Riordan-Eva, P. (1992).* General ophthalmology *(13th ed., p. 172). New York: McGraw-Hill Companies.*	Can affect one or both eyes and may be congenital or acquired. Clouding of lens indicates presence of cataract; however, cataracts are not always visible to the naked eye. Symptoms include distorted red reflex, symptoms of vision loss (see *strabismus*), and white pupil. May be present alone but sometimes associated with conditions such as fetal alcohol syndrome, Down syndrome, and Turner syndrome.	Must be diagnosed at a young age for successful treatment; many cases are missed. Specific treatment depends on whether one or both eyes are affected, extent of clouding, and presence of other ocular abnormalities. Surgical removal of lens and corrective lenses; contact lenses frequently used; results of surgery are good; surgery before the age of 2 months is associated with the best results; visual acuity in 55% of children is 20/40 or better. Lens implant may be used. Eye protectors and restraints are used postoperatively to prevent injury; antibiotic or steroid drops may be used for several weeks; treatment for amblyopia may be necessary.

(continued)

Clinical Manifestations
Visual Disorders (continued)

Etiology	Clinical Manifestations	Clinical Therapy
Glaucoma Increased intraocular pressure damages the eye and impairs visual function; the ciliary body of the eye produces aqueous fluid that flows between the iris and lens into the anterior chamber; if enough fluid accumulates, blindness results; affects 1 in 100,000 newborns. May be congenital (occurring in first 3 years of life) or juvenile (occurring from 3–30 years) and affect one or both eyes. Primary glaucoma (50% of cases) is an isolated anomaly of drainage; secondary glaucoma (50% of cases) is associated with other ocular or systemic abnormalities. 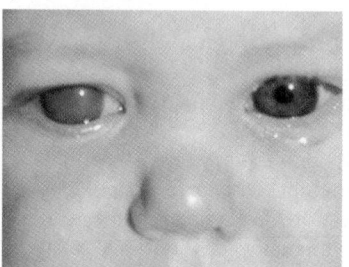 Congenital glaucoma. *Used with permission from Vaughan, D., Asbury, T., & Riordan-Eva, P. (1992). General ophthalmology (13th ed., p. 172). New York: McGraw-Hill Companies.*	Symptoms of congenital glaucoma include tearing, blinking, corneal clouding, eyelid spasms, progressive enlargement of the eye, and photophobia (extreme sensitivity to light). Symptoms of juvenile glaucoma include constant bumping into objects in the child's periphery (painless visual field loss); seeing halos around objects. Diagnosis is made using a tonometer, which measures intraocular pressure.	Surgery to reduce intraocular pressure is the treatment of choice, since medications used to combat glaucoma in adults are not as effective in children. Compensatory lenses are used following surgery. Treatment is not always successful, especially if the child has congenital glaucoma, so parents' feelings regarding care of a child with a visual impairment should be explored.

Data from: Donahue, S. P. (2007). Pediatric strabismus. New England Journal of Medicine, 356, 1040–1047; Nield, L. S., Mangano, L. M., & Kamat, D. (2008, January). Strabismus: A close-up look. Consultant for Pediatricians, 17–25; Doshi, N. R., & Rodriguez, L. F. (2007). Amblyopia. American Family Physician, 75, 361–368; Kliegman, R. M., Behrman, R. E., Jenson, H. B., et al. (2007). Nelson textbook of pediatrics (18th ed., Part XXVIII, Disorders of the Eye, pp. 2569–2615). Philadelphia: Saunders.

TABLE 19–3   Assessment Questions for Identifying Visual Disturbances in Children

Infant	Young Child	School-Age Child
Does your baby follow an object from one side to the other? What is your baby's reaction when you are directly in front and close? Does the baby seem to notice an object to the right and left sides? Do your baby's eyes ever appear to move asymmetrically? What is your baby learning to do right now?	Does your child follow you with his or her eyes as you come into a room? Are other objects followed with ease? Do both eyes work together or does one seem to wander off? At what age did your baby sit, stand, and walk? Does your child have any difficulty picking up objects?	Does your child like to look at pictures and read? Does your child hold toys or books close, or sit very close to the television? Does your child squint or rub the eyes? Is he or she performing at grade level in all subjects? Has your child demonstrated any learning difficulties? Does he or she use a computer, watch television, or play computer games? Does your child play sports and games at the same level of ability as peers?

children with abnormal results who are referred to an eye specialist for care. An important part of the screening process is following up on referrals to be certain that children receive the diagnostic care they need.

Nursing Alert

Some youth use decorative contact lenses, and some even "trade" their lenses with other youth. Contact lenses should only be prescribed and fitted by a qualified eye professional. There have been reports of bacterial conjunctivitis, corneal damage, and allergic reactions to cosmetic lenses. The U.S. Food and Drug Administration (FDA) has noted the dangers of improperly obtained lenses.

When prescriptive lenses are used, the nurse instructs the parent and child on correct wear practices and care. If the child needs surgery, postoperative follow-up is needed, including pain control, observing for signs of infection (ophthalmic or systemic), and administering needed eye medications. Sterile technique is used postoperatively to provide eye care. Promptly report deviations from normal such as increased pain, redness, discharge, or edema of the eye; increased temperature or pulse, which may indicate infection; increased sensitivity to light; or other abnormalities. Children are usually discharged home with instructions to minimize vigorous activities for a certain period of time. Perform postoperative and discharge teaching and emphasize the importance of follow-up visits.

Color Blindness

Color blindness is an X-linked recessive disorder found in 10% of males and rarely in females; it is more common in White than Black males. The most common form affects the ability to distinguish between the colors red and green; blue–yellow discrimination and other colors can also be involved (Subramanian, 2007). Preschool boys are tested for color blindness in some clinics to identify those with the disorder. The Ishihara color blindness test is often used and consists of numbers embedded in a background that are difficult for a person with color blindness to see. Color blindness is not treatable, and management focuses on issues of safety (e.g., problems in distinguishing red–green traffic signals) and techniques to improve discrimination of colors in the affected color groups.

Retinopathy of Prematurity

Retinopathy of prematurity (ROP) occurs when immature blood vessels in the retina constrict and become necrotic. This condition, which may occur in infants of low birth weight or of short gestation, can heal completely or lead to mild myopia or retinal detachment and blindness.

Etiology and Pathophysiology

Retinopathy of prematurity results from injury to the developing capillaries of the retina. Oxygen therapy is associated with the development of ROP (Figure 19–5 ➤), but other factors such as respiratory distress, mechanical ventilation, apnea, bradycardia, cerebral palsy, heart disease, multiple blood transfusions, infection, hypoxia, hypercarbia, acidosis, shock, and sepsis have

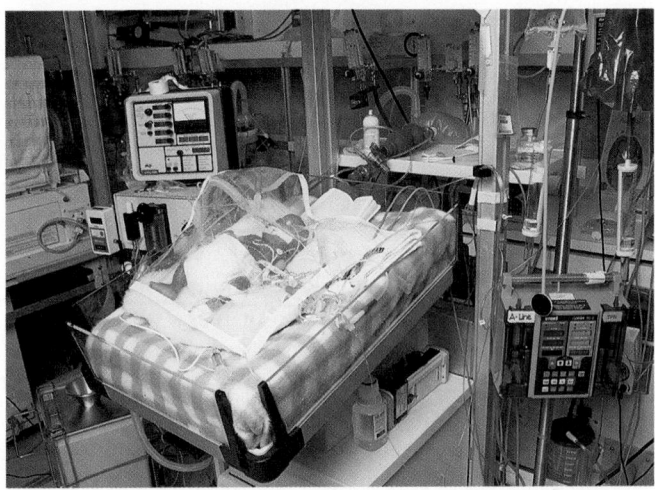

FIGURE 19–5 ➤ This premature infant in the neonatal intensive care unit is receiving artificial ventilation—a risk factor for retinopathy of prematurity. The infant will need careful management of oxygen exposure and periodic eye examinations.

also been linked with the disorder. It is most common in male infants born before 28 weeks' gestation and weighing under 1600 g (3 lb, 8 oz) at birth. A genetic link may be present as White infants are more commonly affected than those of African heritage, and Alaska Natives have a high rate of the disorder. In developed countries, ROP is the second most common cause of blindness, occurring in 12.5% of infants born from 23–26 weeks' gestation (Tasman, Patz, McNamara, et al., 2006; Yang, Donovan, & Wagge, 2006).

The retina is normally vascularized by about 8 months' gestation. For the premature infant, however, this process must continue after birth. The environmental and other conditions listed in the preceding paragraph appear to affect its course. Arteriole constriction, followed by vascular proliferation of abnormal vessels, occurs. In most cases, the abnormal vessels gradually regress and normal vascularization takes place. Sometimes, however, the abnormal vascularization continues into the vitreous cavity, causing abnormalities of the retina, optic disc, and macula. It is not known why the disease progresses in some cases, but progression is directly linked to lower birth weight, greater prematurity, and duration (not necessarily concentration) of oxygen therapy.

Although the developing capillaries are lost, in up to 90% of cases some degree of revascularization occurs later (Tasman et al., 2006). The degree of visual loss, varying from slight to total, is determined by the degree of revascularization that occurs.

Clinical Manifestations

Retinopathy of prematurity is characterized by progressive changes in the retinal blood vessels and, in severe disease, by retinal detachment. Premature and low-birth-weight infants at risk for the disease are given frequent ocular examinations to ensure early detection of these changes. For infants who do not receive ophthalmologic examinations, the resulting visual impairment may be detected only later in infancy when the child progresses slowly in meeting developmental milestones, fails to reach for objects, and does not follow objects or faces with the eyes. When visual impairment is present, the child usually manifests myopia. Total loss of vision can occur in the child who suffers a retinal detachment.

COLLABORATIVE CARE

Diagnostic Tests

Diagnosis is made by ophthalmologic examination. A classification system that includes zone (area of retina with abnormal vasculature), stage (severity of disease), and plus disease (vascular dilation and tortuosity in the posterior pole near the optic nerve) is used to describe the location, extent, and severity of the disease (Alme, Mulhern, Hejkal, et al., 2008; International Committee for the Classification of Retinopathy of Prematurity, 2005; Tasman et al., 2006). See Table 19–4. All infants at risk, namely those born before 32 weeks' gestation and under 1500 g (3 lb, 7 oz) at birth, or those born after 32 weeks' gestation with birth weight from 1500 to 2000 g (3 lb, 7 oz to 4 lb, 3 oz), are assessed frequently with binocular ophthalmoscopy by an ophthalmologist who is experienced with the condition. The disease is not manifested before 4 to 6 weeks after birth, so it is important that the infant receive regular eye examinations until the risk is discounted. Eye examinations continue every 1 to 3 weeks, with the frequency determined by the location of disease, progress of disease, and the infant's degree of immature vascularization. Involvement of blood vessels in the periphery of the retina rarely leads to visual impairment. With involvement in other areas of the retina, risk of visual problems is more common (Alme et al., 2008).

Clinical Therapy

Treatment of infants with severe retinopathy of prematurity often involves laser therapy to stop progression of the disease process. Other surgical procedures such as a scleral buckle procedure and vitrectomy have been used in retinal detachments. Prompt treatment of accompanying problems such as strabismus, amblyopia, and myopia can promote maximal development.

NURSING MANAGEMENT

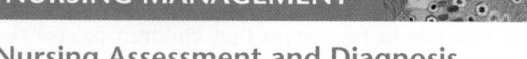

Nursing Assessment and Diagnosis

Assessment of the infant at risk for retinopathy of prematurity begins at birth by identification of infants who may require oxygen therapy, assisted ventilation, or both. Evaluate risk factors such as prematurity and low birth weight. Assess the infant's breathing efforts and report changes and abnormalities. Be certain the ventilation equipment is properly set to deliver the correct ventilatory pressure and amount of oxygen. (See the *Clinical Skills Manual.*) Ventilatory equipment is meticulously monitored. The nurse weans the infant from oxygen as indicated by an oxygen saturation reading in concordance with standing orders in the neonatal intensive care unit. Note the cumulative risks in a particular case (longer exposure to oxygen increases risk) and ensure referral to an ophthalmologist for evaluation and monitoring.

The accompanying Nursing Care Plan outlines several nursing diagnoses for a child with a visual impairment secondary to retinopathy of prematurity. Following are other nursing diagnoses that may be appropriate for an infant with the potential to develop ROP or a child with resulting visual impairment:

- Altered Visual Sensory Perception related to abnormal transmission of impulses
- Potential Impaired Gas Exchange related to ventilation-perfusion imbalance
- Delayed Growth and Development related to effects of visual impairment
- Altered Family Processes related to a child with a visual impairment

Planning and Implementation

The nurse plays an important role in preventing retinopathy of prematurity. Encourage early and regular prenatal care to prevent unnecessary premature births. Administer oxygen only to newborns who need it, and in the amount specified by the

TABLE 19–4	**Diagnosis of Retinopathy of Prematurity**		
Zone (Area of Retina Involved with Abnormal Vasculature)	Stage (Severity of ROP Wherever It Is Present)	Plus Disease (Vascular Dilation and Tortuosity Noted in Posterior Pole in Area Near Optic Nerve)	Threshold (Measure of Severity of Disease; Used to Judge When Treatment Is Needed)
Zone I (most posterior and near optic nerve head)	Stage 1 (line divides vascular and avascular retina)	Presence	Threshold I (stage 3 ROP in Zone I or II and five continuous or eight cumulative "clock hour" areas with plus disease; treatment is required)
Zone II (outside or area anterior to Zone I)	Stage 2 (line of demarcation is elevated)	Absence	
Zone III (only present on temporal side of eye; nasal quadrants are adequately vascularized)	Stage 3 (new vascularization is present in the demarcation area)		

Data from: Alme, A. M., Mulhern, M. L., Hejkal, T. W., Meza, J. L., Qiu, F., Ingvoldstad, D. D., & Margalit, E. (2008). Outcomes of retinopathy of prematurity patients following adoption of revised indications for treatment. BMC Ophthalmology, 13(8), 23.

NURSING CARE PLAN

The Child with a Visual Impairment Secondary to Retinopathy of Prematurity

INTERVENTION	RATIONALE	EXPECTED OUTCOME
1. Nursing Diagnosis: Disturbed Visual Sensory Perception related to altered reception, transmission, and integration resulting from retinopathy of prematurity		
NIC Priority Intervention: *Visual deficit enhancement:* Assistance in accepting and learning alternate methods for living with diminished vision		**NOC Suggested Outcome:** *Developmental progression:* Compensate for sensory deficits by maximizing use of impaired senses.
Goal: The child will receive adequate sensory input.		
■ Provide kinesthetic, tactile, and auditory stimulation during play and in daily care (e.g., talking and playing). Provide music while bathing an infant using bells and other noises on each side of the infant. Verbally describe to a child all actions being carried out by an adult.	■ Because visual sensory input is not present, the child needs input from all other senses to compensate and provide adequate sensory stimulation.	The child demonstrates minimal signs of sensory deprivation.
2. Nursing Diagnosis: Risk for Injury related to impaired vision		
NIC Priority Intervention: *Fall prevention:* Instituting special precautions with patients at risk for injury		**NOC Suggested Outcome:** *Risk control:* Actions to eliminate or reduce modifiable health threats
Goal: The child will be protected from safety hazards that can lead to injury.		
■ Evaluate the environment for potential safety hazards based on age of child and degree of impairment. Be particularly alert to objects that give visual cues to their dangers (e.g., stairs, stoves, fireplaces, candles). Eliminate safety hazards and protect the child from exposure. Take the child on a tour of new rooms (e.g., schools, hotel room, hospital room).	■ The child may be at risk for injury related to both developmental stage and inability to visualize hazards.	The child will experience no injuries.
3. Nursing Diagnosis: Risk for Altered Growth and Development related to impaired vision		
NIC Priority Intervention: *Developmental enhancement:* Facilitating or teaching parents and caregivers to facilitate optional growth and development of children		**NOC Suggested Outcome:** *Child growth and development:* Milestones of developmental progression
Goal: The child has experiences necessary to foster normal growth and development.		
■ Help parents plan early, regular social activities with other children.	■ The child with a visual impairment benefits developmentally from contact with other children.	The child demonstrates normal growth and development milestones.
■ Provide opportunities for and encourage self-feeding activities.	■ To obtain adequate nutrients, the child needs to feel comfortable feeding self.	
■ Provide an environment rich in sensory input.	■ Sensory input is needed for normal development to occur.	
■ Assess growth and development during regular examinations to identify the child's strengths and needs.	■ Regular examinations aid in early identification of growth problems or developmental delays, so that appropriate interventions can be planned.	

(continued)

NURSING CARE PLAN

The Child with a Visual Impairment Secondary to Retinopathy of Prematurity (continued)

INTERVENTION	RATIONALE	EXPECTED OUTCOME
4. Nursing Diagnosis: Risk for Compromised Family Coping related to child's prolonged disability from sensory impairment		
NIC Priority Intervention: *Family mobilization:* Utilization of family strengths to influence child's health positively		**NOC Suggested Outcome:** *Positive coping:* Extent to which family can mobilize resources to deal with the child's needs
Goal: The family identifies methods for coping with their child's visual impairment.		
■ Provide explanation of visual impairment as appropriate.	■ The parents may feel guilt about the child's visual impairment, which can be allayed by knowledge of the cause.	The family successfully copes with the experience of having a child with a visual impairment.
■ Refer parents to organizations, early intervention programs, and other parents of children with visual impairments.	■ The parents will receive needed information and support from others.	
■ Assist parents to plan for meeting developmental, educational, and safety needs of their child. Offer resources for changing the home environment to assist the child.	■ The child may require an enhanced environment in order to foster developmental progress.	

physician to maintain prescribed oxygen saturation. Ensure that the proper ventilatory settings are used. Be alert for infants with multiple risk factors and refer them, when appropriate, for ophthalmologic examination. Parents of infants at risk for ROP require information about the disorder, as well as support, as the long-term effects on the child's vision are often identified only after subsequent examinations as the child grows. Families may be frustrated that a prognosis cannot be made at the time of the first eye examination. Explanations and consistent updates on the infant's condition can be reassuring. Reinforce to parents the importance of follow-up eye examinations. Teach methods of stimulating development for the child with a visual impairment (refer to the next section).

Evaluation

Expected outcomes of nursing care for the child with retinopathy of prematurity include the following:

- Visual impairment will be identified early in the child's life and an intervention program will be established.
- The child will achieve normal developmental milestones. The child's visual condition will be effectively managed by the family.

Visual Impairment

Visual impairment accounts for 11% of chronic medical conditions in children. Overall, 2.5% of children have visual impairment or blindness; the rate rises to 3.3% for children from 6 to 17 years of age. Low vision, or the inability to correct vision to a normal level, is present in 1.2 to 1.3 children per 1,000, or 13.5 million children in the United States. Amblyopia is the most common cause of low vision in children, affecting 2–3% of children (Center for Health and Health Care in Schools, 2007).

Many conditions discussed earlier in this chapter lead to temporary or permanent visual impairment. Infants who are premature; whose mothers were infected prenatally with rubella, toxoplasmosis, or other viruses; or who have certain congenital and hereditary conditions have a high risk of visual problems (Table 19–5). Fetal alcohol syndrome (FAS) is a major cause of visual disturbance (Green, 2007). See Chapter 28 ∞ for a further description of FAS.

The signs of visual impairment depend on the cause and degree of the problem and the age of the child (Table 19–6). The child's eyes may appear crossed or watery, and the lids may be crusty. Verbal children may complain of itching; dizziness; headache; or blurred, double, or poor vision.

COLLABORATIVE CARE

The American Optometric Association and American Public Health Association recommend comprehensive vision examination starting at 6 months of age. The American Academy of Ophthalmology and American Academy of Pediatrics recommend screening by 3 years of age (Center for Health and Health Care in Schools, 2007). The U.S. Preventive Services Task Force (USPSTF) recommends screening to detect amblyopia, strabismus, and defects in visual acuity in children younger than 5 years (American Academy of Pediatrics, 2007; U.S. Preventive Services Task Force, 2005). All young children should have vision examinations in order to identify vision problems early in life.

Clinical therapy depends on the child's condition and may include surgery, medication, and supportive aids. In the case of a disorder that results in permanent visual impairment, an interdisciplinary team of specialists works with the child and

TABLE 19–5	Common Causes of Visual Impairment in Children
Cause	Visual Impairment

Congenital or Hereditary	• Cataracts
	• Glaucoma
	• Tay-Sachs disease
	• Marfan syndrome
	• Down syndrome
	• Fetal alcohol syndrome
	• Prenatal infections (maternal infection)
	  • Rubella
	  • Toxoplasmosis
	  • Herpes simplex
	• Retinoblastoma

Acquired	• Injury to eye or head
	• Infections
	  • Rubella
	  • Measles
	  • Chickenpox
	• Brain tumor
	• Retinopathy of prematurity
	• Cerebral palsy

TABLE 19–6	Signs of Visual Impairment
Age Group	Manifestation
Infants	• May be unable to follow lights or objects • Do not make eye contact • Have a dull, vacant stare • Do not imitate facial expressions
Toddlers and Older Children	• May rub, shut, or cover eyes • Tilt or thrust head forward • Blink frequently • Hold objects close • Bump into objects • Squint

family. As members of this team, nurses collaborate with families and with other health care professionals to plan appropriate interventions.

NURSING MANAGEMENT

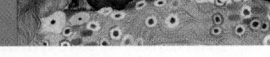

Nursing Assessment and Diagnosis

Prevention of low vision, early identification of the condition, and interventions to enhance development of children with low vision provide the focus for nursing care. (See Evidence-Based Practice: Nursing Role in Vision Screening and Follow-Up.) Vision screening facilitates early detection and treatment of conditions that can lead to vision loss. Visual testing can be done at any age, including immediately after birth. Developmental milestones that require vision, such as following bright lights, reaching for objects, or looking at pictures in a book, can be used to assess vision. For children over the age of

3 years, visual acuity is most frequently measured by means of an age-appropriate acuity test (see Chapter 5 ∞ and the *Clinical Skills Manual*). The photoscreener is a device that can be used to take a photo of the child's eyes. It is useful for infants, toddlers, and preschoolers. The photo can be used to diagnose refraction errors, eye opacities, and misalignment (Donahue, Lorenz, & Johnson, 2008). Visual fields and the ability to discriminate colors are tested at school age, when children can cooperate.

Children who are visually impaired may lag in development of cognitive and other skills. Sighted children use four senses—sight, touch, hearing, and taste—to obtain the information necessary to connect a word, such as *cup*, with the object it represents. In contrast, children with visual impairments rely on only three senses—touch, hearing, and taste. They learn concepts through differences in sounds, textures, and shapes. Many visual disorders are linked with conditions that influence development. Thus, a child with cerebral palsy or fetal alcohol syndrome should be assessed frequently to identify a visual disorder, as well as to evaluate normal developmental milestones.

Nursing diagnoses for the child with impaired vision may include the following:

- Disturbed Sensory Alteration (Visual) related to altered sensory perception
- Risk for Injury related to poor vision
- Risk for Delayed Growth and Development related to visual impairment
- Risk for Ineffective Family Coping related to demands of a child with a sensory impairment

Planning and Implementation

Promote safety in sports and other activities to prevent visual impairment when possible. Encourage protective eyewear in sports such as hockey, handball, and football. Work with school personnel to establish guidelines for protective eyewear for chemistry or other science or industrial education courses that may present a risk to eyes. Keep laser pointers away from children since they can cause retinal damage, especially when stared at for 10 seconds. Young children do not blink as often as adults or older children and so are at greater risk of retinal damage from lasers.

Clinical Tip

Strategies for nurses working with children who are visually impaired:

- Call the child's name and speak before touching the child.
- Tell the child when you are leaving the room.
- Describe what each procedure will feel like (e.g., blood pressure cuff, otoscope).
- Let the child touch the equipment to establish familiarity.
- Describe what foods are present and their locations on the food tray.

Nursing care focuses on encouraging the child's use of all senses, promoting socialization, helping parents to meet the child's developmental and educational needs, and providing

Evidence-Based Practice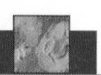
Nursing Role in Vision Screening and Follow-Up

Problem

Screening for visual ability is important to identify children with impairments. The American Academy of Pediatrics recommends that children be screened at every well-child visit, beginning in the newborn period, to include vision history, vision assessment, external inspection of the eyes and lids, eye movement assessment, pupil examination, and elicitation of the red reflex. Once the child can cooperate, usually by about 3 years, a vision test such as HOTV or tumbling E, along with ophthalmoscopic examination, should be added to the examination (American Academy of Pediatrics, 2007; U.S. Preventive Services Task Force, 2005). Nurses often conduct vision examinations, evaluate results, and provide follow-up care. They participate in well-child health visits and often perform assessments of vision in schools. What evidence is available to assist nurses in this important role?

Evidence

A study of 1,677 children in preschool, kindergarten, and first grade applied the HOTV acuity test and two types of photoscreening devices. (See the *Clinical Skills Manual* for a further description of these types of screening.) Photoscreening was found to be significantly more effective in identifying children with visual impairment, and was faster to perform (Leman, Clausen, Bates, et al., 2006).

Once visual impairment is identified, an essential nursing role is to refer for appropriate care and to follow up to determine if that care is received. A study attempted to determine the contributing factors to lack of follow-up care after a failed vision screening. An interview was conducted with 66 families who had a child referred for

eye examination after school screening. The researchers found that 85% of the families had low incomes. The barriers to eye care they identified included financial reasons, logistical problems (no ability to get to appointments), social or family issues (large family with adults all working or recent change in residence), and perceptual barriers (did not believe results or perceive the importance of the referral) (Kimel, 2006).

Implications

Nurses play a vital role in ensuring that children receive early, periodic, and regular visual and eye screening. Evidence that suggests the most accurate methods should be closely examined. Photoscreening machines represent an important new addition to the tools that nurses can use. While identification of problems is important, the nursing roles of referral for care, identifying barriers to care, and ensuring that follow-up care has been received are also integral to vision care.

Critical Thinking Application

What vision screening methods are available in the offices, clinics, and schools in your community? How could you perform vision screening in the hospital setting if a child did not demonstrate expected visual ability for age? Design a follow-up program for a school that screens all children in kindergarten and first grade for visual acuity. What questions will you ask parents during a well-child visit for a 2-year-old to determine if vision is normal? How will you combine your knowledge of developmental milestones with screening for vision?

emotional support to parents. These interventions are known as vision rehabilitation, a major *Healthy People 2020* goal (U.S. Department of Health and Human Services, 2010). Refer the parents to an early intervention program upon diagnosis. Be sure that a regular series of developmental screenings is performed either in the early intervention program or during health care visits (see Chapter 6 ∞). Developmental screening should be done about every 2 months during infancy, and every 6 months from 1 to 5 years. As the child grows, assess for physical activity, since children with visual impairments are less likely than sighted children to achieve physical activity milestones. Suggest exercise that is safe and continues to challenge physical development. Dancing, balance and coordination activities, as well as running, can all be encouraged. Nearly all care will occur in community and home settings. Instruct parents on care of glasses or lenses.

Clinical Tip

Clean the child's glasses daily with warm water and a clean, soft dry cloth. Follow the prescriber's directions for care of contact lenses. General guidelines include:

■ Allow the child to wear the lenses for the recommended time only.
■ Store each lens in the right or left container as labeled.
■ Wash hands carefully before contact with the child's eyes or lenses.
■ Use a cleaning solution on the lens after its removal.
■ Rinse the lens with the recommended rinsing solution.
■ Keep the lenses in the case with the disinfecting solution.
■ Note on medical charts that the child wears lenses.

Encourage Use of All Senses

Children who are partially sighted or blind use other senses to a great extent. Encouraging the use of the eyes as much as possible is important even if a child has poor vision. See Families Want to Know: Enhancing Development of the Child with a Visual Impairment.

Promote Socialization

The child's interactions and socializations should be as normal as possible (similar to those of sighted children of the same age and development).

● Stroke, rock, and hug infants and children who are visually impaired. Sing and talk to them. These infants do not make eye contact and have rather blank expressions.
● Teach parents to read body language and vocalization as expressions of emotion. Facial expressions give a great deal of information, but infants and children with poor vision do not have the ability to learn by visual imitation. Show parents how to use tactile means to teach appropriate facial ex-

Growth & Development *Visual Impairment*

Infants with visual impairment use kinesthesia, touch, and language to socialize. They will appreciate and use touch more than other children and will respond to verbal explanations when others use nonverbal communication. Vision affects both fine and gross motor skills, so skills such as hand-to-mouth coordination and walking may be delayed in children who are visually impaired.

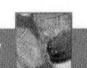

- Encourage a toddler or preschooler who is visually impaired to look at pictures in well-lit settings. Have a school-age child read large-print books. Computers designed for children with visual impairments are also available. The Optacon (a device that raises print so it can be felt by the child) and View Scan (which magnifies print) are instruments that improve the ability to read.
- Expose the infant and child to everyday sounds.
- Encourage the infant to use the sense of touch to explore people and objects. Have the parents purchase toys with sound and texture in mind. Directional concepts can be taught using games. Responding to the infant's and child's vocalizations encourages the use of speech.
- Teach specific techniques for toileting, dressing, bathing, eating, and safety.
- When the child becomes mobile, furniture and other objects in the environment should be kept in the same positions so the child can safely move around independently. Extra care must be taken to prevent injuries when a child does not see.
- Emphasize the child's abilities. Adolescents can use seeing-eye dogs or a white cane to function independently.
- Encourage the child to function independently within normal developmental parameters.
- If in the hospital or another strange environment, orient the child to the placement of objects and do not rearrange them.
- Teach those around the child to:
  - Announce their presence to the child when approaching.
  - When walking with a child who is blind, walk slightly ahead of the child so he or she can sense your movements.
  - Let the child hold the seeing person's arm rather than the reverse.
  - Identify the contents of meals and encourage the child to feed self.

pressions. For example, a touch on the arm can be soft and stroking to indicate a smile, but firmer to indicate dismay or a frown.

- Explain to parents that discipline and rewards for children with poor vision should be the same as those for other children in the family. The child should be given age-appropriate tasks.
- Encourage contact with peers as the child grows older. Teach the child to look directly at persons who are talking to him or her. Play, sports, and other activities can be modified to give the child the same social experiences as a sighted child.
- Foster physical activity for children with visual impairments by encouraging involvement in early intervention programs; recommending programs that increase cardiovascular strength, endurance, upper body strength, and flexibility; and facilitating participation in and reward for sports and athletics.

Care in the Community

Public laws require that each state provide educational and related services for children with disabilities (see Chapter 10 ∞). Parents and professionals should develop an individualized ed-

ucation plan (as discussed in Chapter 10) that maximizes the child's learning ability. If possible, the child with a vision problem should attend childcare and preschool with children who have normal visual acuity. While some developmental skills such as feeding and dressing may develop slower than in sighted children, plans for encouraging development tailored to the child's needs can assist in learning skills. Provide parents with information about educational options before their child reaches school age. Education should take place in a setting that allows the child to have contact with other children and to participate in social activities. Familiarize the child with each new environment and allow time for adjustment. The child may be mainstreamed with a tutor, be partially mainstreamed in a resource room, attend special classes, or be tutored at home. If the child is to attend public school, suggest to parents that they contact the school well before enrollment to ensure that school personnel understand the child's disability.

Make sure that items such as large-print books, Braille materials, and audio or computer equipment are available. Ensure that frequent eye examinations are performed and assist with proper use and care of prescribed glasses or contact lenses, as necessary.

Provide Emotional Support

Family members often need help to understand the child's abilities and disabilities. Support them as they learn about the child's visual problems, tell friends and family, and then adjust to support the child.

- Encourage habilitation as soon as realistically possible. Make the adjustment easier by providing information about the child's specific type of visual impairment, available community services, and groups or associations for children with similar vision conditions. Suggest resources to families of children with visual disorders.
- Be supportive and listen to the family's concerns regarding the child's visual deficit.
- Ensure that parents meet their own physical and emotional needs so they are better able to care for and provide support to their child.

Nursing Alert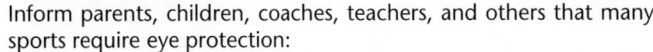

Inform parents, children, coaches, teachers, and others that many sports require eye protection:
- Badminton
- Baseball
- Basketball
- Bicycling
- Fencing (requires face mask)
- Handball
- Hockey (field, ice, roller, street)
- Lacrosse
- Racquetball
- Soccer
- Squash
- Swimming (requires swim goggles)

Evaluation

Expected outcomes of nursing care for the child with a visual impairment include the following:

- The child will remain safe from injury.
- The child will achieve growth and developmental milestones to maximum potential.
- An individualized education plan will be established and followed for the child.
- The family members will express effective stress management.

Injuries of the Eye

In the United States, eye injuries are common in children from 9 to 11 years of age, particularly in males. Boys from 11 to 15 years have four times more eye injuries than girls. About 42,000 sports injuries occur annually, with about half of these in children. Sports, darts, fireworks, air-powered BB guns, blunt and sharp objects, chemical and thermal burns, physical irritants, and abuse may cause eye trauma (Kliegman, Behrman, Jenson, et al., 2007). Recreational activities such as sports and projectile toys are common causes. Older children may be injured by chemicals in school science laboratories.

Some injuries can be treated at home, but many necessitate a trip to the emergency department or require hospitalization. Personnel take a careful history of the injury, perform assessment of the eye, and measure visual acuity. See Clinical Manifestations: Emergency Treatment of Eye Injuries.

Nursing Alert

Be sure to check the immunization status of the child with an eye injury. If the child has not had a tetanus booster within 5 years, this immunization should be given.

Nursing Management

Prevention of injury is an important nursing intervention. Nurses should also be informed about emergency treatment of eye injuries, inform parents and school personnel of care, and manage transfer to medical facilities when eye injury occurs. See the Clinical Manifestations table on the next page for emergency care.

▲ Health Promotion

Nurses should perform teaching at each health promotion examination about ways to avoid eye injuries in children. Protective eyewear should be used by participants in all sports with a risk of eye injury, with extreme caution in those with diminished vision or only one functional eye. Plan strategies to teach children about prevention of eye injuries. What questions will you ask to identify risk factors? What teaching is needed for school-age children? For adolescents?

■ DISORDERS OF THE EAR

Otitis Media

Otitis media, or inflammation of the middle ear, is sometimes accompanied by infection. This condition is one of the most common childhood illnesses. About 70% of infants have at least one case of acute otitis media during the first year of life, and 93% have been diagnosed with the problem by age 7 years. Peak incidence is in the first 2 years of life, particularly from 6–20 months of age (Bernius & Perlin, 2006). Otitis media occurs more frequently among boys and in children who attend childcare centers, in those with allergies, in children exposed to tobacco smoke, and in those who use pacifiers several hours daily. It is most common during the winter months. Children with conditions such as cleft lip and palate or Down syndrome more often experience otitis media. Breastfeeding appears to be protective against otitis media.

Etiology and Pathophysiology

The specific cause of otitis media is unknown, but it appears to be related to eustachian tube dysfunction. Often an upper respiratory infection precedes the development of otitis media. This infection causes the mucous membranes of the eustachian tube to become edematous. As a result, air that normally flows to the middle ear is blocked, and the air in the middle ear is reabsorbed into the bloodstream. Fluid is pulled from the mucosal lining into the former air space, providing a medium for the rapid growth of pathogens. The tympanic membrane and fluid behind it become infected. The most common causative organisms are *Streptococcus pneumoniae, Haemophilus influenzae,* and *Moraxella catarrhalis* (Pichichero, Casey, Hoberman, et al., 2008).

Conditions such as enlarged adenoids or edema from allergic rhinitis can also obstruct the eustachian tube and lead to otitis media. Pacifier use raises the soft palate and thus alters dynamics in the eustachian tube, providing for entry of microorganisms from the nasopharynx (Neto, Hemb, & Silva, 2006). Ethnicity appears to play a role in the incidence of otitis media. Recurrent otitis media has an increased frequency in children of parents who smoke. Children with multiple siblings and those who attend childcare centers have increased rates of recurrent acute otitis media (Daly, Hoffman, Kvaerner, et al., 2009).

Clinical Manifestations

Otitis media is the general term for inflammation of the middle ear. *Acute otitis media* (AOM) is diagnosed when the child has acute onset of ear pain, marked redness of the tympanic membrane upon otoscopy, and middle ear effusion (Figure 19–6 ➤). Recurrent acute otitis media indicates repeated bouts of AOM, such as three in 6 months, or four in 12 months. *Otitis media with effusion* (OME) is evidence of fluid in the middle ear without inflammation (Figure 19–7 ➤). OME sometimes becomes chronic in nature (continuing more than 3 months) and is more commonly associated with hearing loss.

Infants and young children have characteristic behaviors that indicate otitis media may be present. Pulling at the ear is a sign of ear pain. Diarrhea, vomiting, and fever are typical of otitis media. Irritability and "acting out" may be signs of a related hearing impairment. The child with otitis media often has night awakenings with crying due to increased ear pressure when prone or supine. See Clinical Manifestations: Acute Otitis Media and Otitis Media with Effusion for further details.

Otitis Media Video

Clinical Manifestations

Emergency Treatment of Eye Injuries

Condition and Etiology	Clinical Manifestations	Clinical Therapy
Subconjunctival hemorrhage (caused by coughing, mild trauma, or increased physical activity)	Reddened area in conjunctiva	Usually heals spontaneously; the child should see an ophthalmologist if most of the sclera is covered or if the condition does not clear up in 1–2 weeks.
Periorbital ecchymosis	"Black eye" or bruising of the skin around the eye	Apply ice to the eye area (both eyes) for 5–15 minutes every hour for the first 1–2 days after injury (even if only one eye is affected, both eyes may discolor); then apply warm compresses beginning the second day after injury.
Foreign body on conjunctiva	Intense pain or feeling of something in the eye	Do not let the child rub the eye; remove material on the eye surface by closing the upper lid over the lower lid, irrigating or everting the upper lid, visualizing material, and removing it with a slightly damp handkerchief. Patch the eye and transport the child to the emergency department if the foreign body cannot be removed.
Corneal abrasion	Intense pain and redness	Superficial corneal abrasions are diagnosed by touching a sterile fluorescein strip to the lower conjunctiva; dye remains where corneal epithelial cells are disrupted; most corneal abrasions heal spontaneously although antibiotic ointment may be prescribed and eyes patched in some children.
Burns (alkaline burns readily penetrate cornea and are more serious than acid burns)	Pain or complaints of "blindness" or vision loss	For a child with a chemical burn, irrigate the eye for 15–30 minutes; transport the child to the emergency department, where irrigation should continue (see the *Clinical Skills Manual*); pupils are dilated to reduce pain and prevent adhesions; after irrigation is complete, eyes are patched and antibiotics are prescribed.
Penetrating and perforating injuries	Pain	Obtain medical assistance immediately; never try to remove an object that has penetrated the child's eye; such objects should be removed by an ophthalmologist; prevent the child from rubbing the injured eye; cover both eyes with a shield before transportation to the emergency department.
Eye injuries caused by severe blows to head and eye (blunt trauma can seriously injure all eye structures, including orbit, which can be fractured)	Pain and redness	Transport immediately to the ophthalmologist's office or emergency department for evaluation and treatment. Personnel should be aware that retinal hemorrhage is a common presentation of the type of child abuse called "shaken child syndrome" (see Chapter 17 ∞ for further discussion of child abuse).

Culture  *Otitis Media*

American Indian and Alaska Native (AI/AN) children have a very high rate of otitis media, perhaps due to culturally related bony structures of the ear, nose, and mouth. AI/AN children are seen about 3 times more frequently in outpatient clinics for otitis media than are other U.S. children (Hunter, Davey, Kohtz, et al., 2007). Black children have a higher incidence of the condition than White children (Centers for Disease Control and Prevention, 2008). Be alert for the common incidence in these population groups, plan prevention programs, and ensure prompt care and teaching about treatments for families of children affected. What prevention measures would you emphasize with these families?

COLLABORATIVE CARE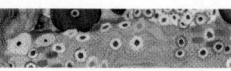

Diagnostic Tests

Diagnosis of otitis media is based on otoscopic examination. Acute otitis media is diagnosed with certainty when there is a history of acute onset, presence of middle ear effusion (bulging or decreased mobility of the tympanic membrane, air and fluid behind the membrane or otorrhea or discharge), and signs and symptoms of inflammation (erythema of tympanic membrane or discomfort that makes sleep and other activities difficult for the child) (American Academy of Pediatrics, Subcommittee on Management of Acute Otitis Media, 2004; Daly et al., 2009). Otoscopic examination includes visualization and pneumatic otoscopy. The trained clinician can perform

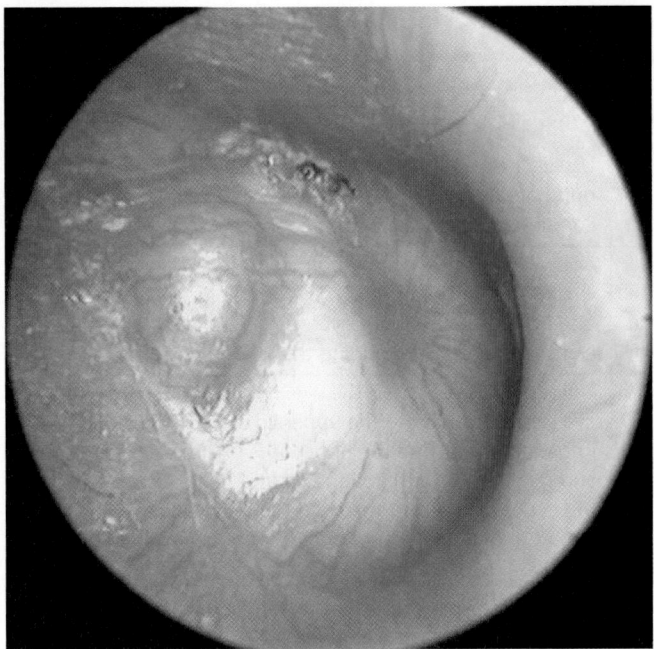

FIGURE 19–6 ➤ Acute otitis media is characterized by abrupt onset, pain, middle ear effusion, and inflammation. Note the injected vessels and altered shape of the cone of light. See Chapter 5 ∞ for a normal tympanic membrane.
Courtesy of Kevin Kavanagh, MD, FACS.

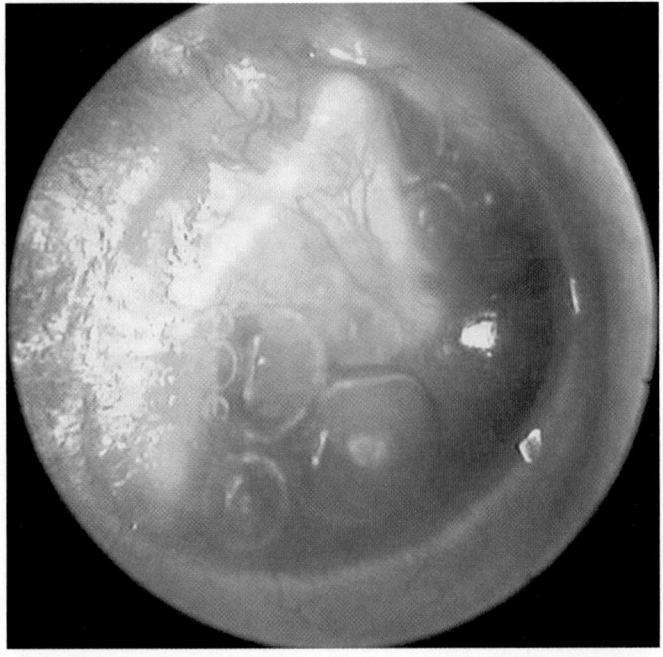

FIGURE 19–7 ➤ Otitis media with effusion is noted on otoscopy by fluid line or air bubbles. Pneumatic otoscopy or tympanometry shows a nonmobile tympanic membrane. Note that the light reflex is not in the expected position due to a change in tympanic membrane shape from air bubbles. Where would you expect to see the cone of light? See Chapter 5 ∞ for a description of normal findings.
Courtesy of Kevin Kavanagh, MD, FACS.

pneumatic otoscopy in which positive air pressure in the external canal is used to measure movement of the tympanic membrane (see Chapter 5 ∞ for a further description of this technique).

Special gradient acoustic reflectometry (SGAR) measures the condition of the middle ear by introducing a sound and mea-

suring the tympanic membrane response (Windmill & Windmill, 2006). A flat tympanogram, indicating absence of normal movement for the tympanic membrane, is also suggestive of otitis media. (The tympanogram is described later in this chapter in the section on hearing impairment.)

Clinical Manifestations
Acute Otitis Media and Otitis Media with Effusion

Etiology	Clinical Manifestations	Clinical Therapy
Acute Otitis Media—bacterial infection in the middle ear from pathogens transferred from the nasopharynx; most common infectious agents are *S. pneumoniae*, *H. influenzae*, *M. catarrhalis*	*Behavioral*—ear pain, pulling at ear, rapid onset, irritability, malaise, poor feeding *Examination*—bulging tympanic membrane; air or fluid bubbles present behind tympanic membrane; immobile or poorly mobile tympanic membrane; red tympanic membrane (or other color change such as white, gray, or yellow with bulging present); reduced visibility of tympanic membrane landmarks with displaced light reflex	Treat ear pain with anesthetic ear drops, herbal pain products instilled into the auditory canal, or systemic acetaminophen or ibuprofen. Verify that the tympanic membrane is intact before instilling ear drops. Observe the child's condition for 48–72 hours and, if not improved, treat with course of antibiotics.
Otitis Media with Effusion—collection of fluid in the middle ear behind the tympanic membrane, which is not infected with bacteria	*Behavioral*—difficulty hearing or responding as expected to sounds *Examination*—signs of acute inflammation are NOT present; tympanic membrane is retracted or neutral; immobile or partly mobile tympanic membrane; yellow or gray tympanic membrane; opaque or thickened tympanic membrane with visibility of landmarks reduced	Symptomatic treatment of pain Careful assessment of hearing acuity over several months Speech assessment if loss of hearing acuity occurs Developmental assessment

Occasionally, the middle ear fluid is cultured so that the causative organism can be identified. If the tympanic membrane is not intact, the culture is easy to obtain; in cases with repeated antibiotic treatment failures, a tympanocentesis may be done to aspirate some fluid from the middle ear through the tympanic membrane.

Since otitis media with effusion may only involve fluid in the middle ear, it is best diagnosed by pneumatic otoscopy and tympanometry. This type of otitis media is most commonly associated with hearing loss, so audiological testing should be performed in the pediatric health care home (medical home) if the effusion persists for 3 months or longer. A referral to an audiologist should be made for children who fail testing in the pediatric office.

Clinical Therapy

Concern has developed about the increasing appearance of drug-resistant microbials as causative agents in otitis media. The American Academy of Pediatrics and the American Academy of Family Physicians joined in 2004 to establish treatment recommendations (American Academy of Pediatrics, Subcommittee on Management of Acute Otitis Media, 2004; Leach & Morris, 2007; Lett, DeMaria, Huot, et al., 2007). Acute otitis media is now treated with antibiotic therapy for 10 days in children under 6 years, and 5–7 days for children 6 years and over. Consistent with current guidelines, acute otitis media treatment is delayed for 48–72 hours after diagnosis in children 6 months to 2 years with nonsevere illness at presentation AND uncertain diagnosis, or in children 2 years and older without severe symptoms OR with uncertain diagnosis.

When prescribed, the choice of antibiotic depends on the probable organism, ease of administration, cost, previous effectiveness, and any history of allergies. First-line therapy is amoxicillin; amoxicillin with clavulanate or cefuroxime are second-line drugs. If an intramuscular drug is preferred, cefdinir, cefpodoxime, or cefuroxime can be prescribed. See Medications Used to Treat Acute Otitis Media for more details about common medications used.

When antibiotic therapy is not prescribed initially, the child can be given ibuprofen or acetaminophen for pain relief and should return for further treatment if symptoms continue. When the tympanic membrane is intact, topical anesthetic ear drops are sometimes prescribed for several days to provide pain relief.

OME is not treated with antibiotics but is evaluated periodically to be sure there is not an additional AOM requiring treatment. Children with OME generally improve within 3 months. Since this type of otitis is more commonly associated with hearing loss and cochlear damage, follow-up with audiology is essential. If hearing is abnormal, speech testing should be performed (Otitis Media with Effusion, 2004).

Neither decongestants nor antihistamines have been shown to be effective in the treatment of otitis media with or without effusion. Steroids also do not appear to have any long-term beneficial effect. If infection recurs despite antibiotic treatment for acute otitis media or if OME continues 4 months or more with

Complementary Therapy
Naturopathic Extract for Ear Pain in Otitis Media

Because many children with otitis media experience ear pain that can disrupt their sleep, as well as that of family members, anesthetic ear drops have been used for their analgesic effect on the tympanic membrane. Naturopathic Herbal Extract Ear Drops (a naturopathic herbal extract of *Allium sativum, Verbascum thapsus, Calendula flores, Hypericum perforatum,* lavender, and vitamin E) with a local anesthetic of amethocaine and phenazone is preferred by some families. However, a collective analysis of several studies concluded that there is as yet insufficient evidence to describe whether naturopathic treatment is effective for treatment of ear pain in children (Foxlee, Johansson, Wejfalk, et al., 2006).

Medications Used to Treat
Acute Otitis Media

Medication and Action/Indication	Nursing Management
Amoxicillin Broad-spectrum antibiotic that inhibits mucoprotein synthesis in cell wall of bacteria; used to treat some gram-positive and gram-negative infections.	■ Assess for previous allergy to drug, penicillins, and cephalosporins. ■ Take as instructed for entire period prescribed. ■ If oral suspension is given, refrigerate and shake well before administration. ■ Teach parents how to administer drug to the child. ■ Have family report side effects such as rash and diarrhea.
Amoxicillin and clavulanate potassium Action and use are similar to amoxicillin. However, clavulanate is a β-lactamase inhibitor that enhances the effect of amoxicillin.	See *amoxicillin.*
Cefuroxime A second-generation cephalosporin that binds to one or more of the penicillin-binding proteins in cell walls of bacteria; useful in treatment of most gram-negative and some gram-positive infections.	■ Assess for previous allergy to drug, penicillins, and cephalosporins. ■ Take as instructed for entire period prescribed. ■ If oral suspension is given, refrigerate and shake well before administration. ■ Teach parents how to administer drug to the child. ■ Have family report side effects such as rash and diarrhea.

persistent hearing loss present, **myringotomy** (surgical incision of the tympanic membrane) may be performed and **tympanostomy tubes** (pressure-equalizing tubes) may be inserted to drain fluid from the middle ear.

NURSING MANAGEMENT

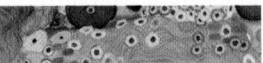

Nursing Assessment and Diagnosis

Assess the tympanic membrane for color, transparency, mobility, presence of landmarks, and light reflex. Ask the parents if the child has had a fever, fussiness, or pulling at the ears. Observe for signs of impaired hearing, including the child's ability to hear whispered or soft sounds.

Inquire about what the family has done at home to treat the ear infection and its associate pain. Some home remedies, such as rocking and singing to the child, are safe. Some other practices may be harmful.

Several nursing diagnoses that may apply to the child with otitis media are included in the accompanying Nursing Care Plan. Additional nursing diagnoses may include the following:

- Risk for Imbalanced Body Temperature: Hyperthermia related to infectious process
- Fatigue (Child and Parent) related to sleep deprivation
- Disturbed Sensory Perception (Auditory) related to chronic ear infections and altered hearing reception

Planning and Implementation

Preventive measures should be emphasized. Exposure to second-hand smoke in the home increases the incidence of otitis media in children; therefore, parents who smoke should be encouraged to avoid smoking near the child or in the home. Wood-burning stoves should also be avoided when possible. If young children are in childcare with fewer than 10 children, incidence decreases. Breastfeeding provides some protection from the disease. Placing babies to sleep with a pacifier may increase incidence and should be avoided in the infant with prior infections. Encourage immunizations for *Haemophilus influenzae* and *Pneumococcal pneumoniae* to prevent otitis media caused by these infective agents.

Most children with otitis media are not hospitalized; therefore, nursing management centers on care of the child in the home. The accompanying Nursing Care Plan summarizes nursing care for the child with otitis media. Review for parents the purpose of a waiting period before prescriptions for antibiotics. When antibiotics are prescribed, review administration techniques, side effects, and the need for a repeat appointment when the medication is completed. Encourage parents to bring the child back for care if the condition worsens or has not improved in the recommended time.

Likewise, parents of children with OME need explanations about why there is a waiting period of about 3 months with no medications or other medical care. Explain that antibiotics, steroids, and antihistamines/decongestants have not been effective and that most children improve in 3 months. Assure parents that if the effusion continues beyond that time, the child will be tested for hearing acuity and, if indicated, for speech development.

Families Want to Know

Care of the Child with Tympanostomy Tubes

After Surgery

- Encourage the child to drink generous amounts of fluids.
- Reestablish a regular diet as tolerated.
- Give pain medication (acetaminophen) as ordered for discomfort and at bedtime. Observe and report excess drowsiness or lethargy.
- Place drops in the child's ears, if instructed.
- Restrict the child to quiet activities. Report any drainage.

Following Postoperative Period

- Follow the physician's instructions regarding swimming and water (some caution against swimming and other activities that might get water in ears; others do not).
- Ear plugs can be used to prevent water from getting into the ears.
- Be alert for tubes becoming dislodged and falling out, and alert the physician when this happens (they usually fall out within 1 year).
- Report purulent discharge from the ear, which may indicate a new ear infection. Contact the care provider.

The chronic nature of otitis media in some children can create many problems for the family. The child's waking at night with ear pain results in lack of sleep and parental fatigue. Parents often become frustrated and disillusioned because of the inability of the health care system to cure the child and may fear a permanent hearing impairment. Reassure parents that as the child grows older, the recurrent infections eventually cease. Provide pain relief techniques such as teaching correct administration of ear drops, oral administration of acetaminophen, and positioning the baby with the head slightly elevated, which often decreases pressure and pain. Provide hearing and language examinations at regular intervals, inform parents of results, and refer to an audiology specialist if hearing problems are identified. For the child with hearing loss due to otitis media with effusion, a home environment that fosters cognitive skills can overcome the effects of lowered hearing during the time of infection. Nurses should focus interventions on helping parents to read and talk with children frequently who have otitis media with effusion.

The child who is having tympanostomy tubes inserted is generally treated in a day surgery setting. Parents and the child will need preparation about what to expect and instructions for safe care upon discharge. (See Families Want to Know: Care of the Child with Tympanostomy Tubes.)

Evaluation

Expected outcomes of nursing care for the child with otitis media include:

- The child returns to normal sleep and feeding patterns.
- The child maintains normal hearing and speech development.
- Effective pain and temperature management are achieved for the child.
- The parents indicate adequate understanding of the treatment regimen.

NURSING CARE PLAN

The Child with Otitis Media

INTERVENTION	RATIONALE	EXPECTED OUTCOME
1. Nursing Diagnosis: Acute Pain related to inflammation and pressure on tympanic membrane		
NIC Priority Intervention: *Pain management:* Alleviation or reduction in pain to a level of comfort acceptable to patient and family		**NOC Suggested Outcome:** *Pain level:* Amount of reported or demonstrated pain
Goal: The child or parent will indicate absence of pain.		
■ Give an analgesic such as acetaminophen. Use analgesic ear drops.	■ Analgesics alter perception or response to pain.	The verbal child states that pain is relieved. The nonverbal child has improved disposition and comfort.
■ Have the child sit up, raise head on pillows, or lie on unaffected ear.	■ Elevation decreases pressure from fluid.	
■ Apply a heating pad or a hot water bottle filled with warm water.	■ Heat increases blood supply and reduces discomfort.	
■ Have the child chew gum or blow on a balloon to relieve pressure in the ear.	■ Attempts to open the eustachian tube may help aerate the middle ear.	
2. Nursing Diagnosis: Infection related to presence of pathogens		
NIC Priority Intervention: *Infection control:* Minimizing the acquisition and transmission of infectious agents		**NOC Suggested Outcome:** *Risk control:* Actions to eliminate or reduce health threats
Goal: The child will be free of infection.		
■ Encourage breastfeeding of infants.	■ Breastfeeding affords natural immunity to infectious agents.	The child's temperature is normal, symptoms have disappeared, and the tympanic membrane shows no signs of infection.
■ Instruct the parents to administer analgesics and antibiotics exactly as directed and to complete the prescribed course of antibiotic.	■ Taking antibiotics as prescribed minimizes the chance for overgrowth of pathogens. Analgesics provide pain relief.	
■ Telephone the parents 2–3 days after initial examination.	■ If symptoms have not improved in 48–72 hours, treatment should be evaluated.	
■ Examine the ear 3–4 days after completion of the antibiotic treatment.	■ A check-up determines if treatment is effective.	
3. Nursing Diagnosis: Risk for Delayed Growth and Development related to hearing loss		
NIC Priority Intervention: *Developmental enhancement:* Facilitating optimal growth and development of the child		**NOC Suggested Outcome:** *Growth and development:* Milestones of developmental progression
Goal: The child will have normal hearing.		
■ Access hearing ability frequently.	■ Monitoring detects hearing loss early.	The child's general health and hearing improve, and incidence of the condition decreases.
Goal: The child will have normal motor and language development.		
■ Assess motor and language development at each health care visit.	■ Early detection of developmental delays can lead to appropriate intervention.	The child has language and motor development within norms for age group.

Otitis Externa

Otitis externa is an inflammation of the skin and surrounding soft tissue of the ear canal. It is sometimes called "swimmer's ear" because it is common in children who swim frequently, especially during hot and muggy weather. The ear canal can also be injured by use of cotton-tipped applicators, foreign objects, or sprays used near the face. If the tympanic membrane is not intact because of tympanostomy tubes or breakage of the membrane, there may be drainage visible in the canal; this drainage may irritate the canal and lead to otitis externa. Any irritation of the canal can become infected with bacteria, virus, or fungi; sometimes it represents an allergic reaction. The child usually complains of pain and itching, and may have intense pain when the examiner presses on the tragus, or skin tab in front of the ear. Sometimes the ear appears swollen, and redness or drainage of the canal may be seen upon otoscopic examination.

Treatment of otitis externa requires removing the dried and flaking epithelium and cerumen. Burow's solution or normal saline is used to irrigate and clean the canal if the tympanic membrane is intact. Steroid ear drops are used to decrease inflammation, and antibiotic drops are also used if a bacterial infection is suspected. If the child has tympanostomy tubes or a perforated tympanic membrane, a non-ototoxic ear antibiotic such as quinolone antibiotic ear drops is used (Rosenfeld, Brown, Cannon, et al., 2006). Ibuprofen or acetaminophen is commonly used for pain control. The child should be seen by the health care provider if the condition has not improved by 48 to 72 hours. The child should not return to swimming for about 5 days. The ear canal should then be kept dry by using ear plugs or a swim cap for swimming and gently blow-drying the canal after bathing. Cotton-tipped applicators or other objects should not be placed in the ear canal so that the skin in the canal can heal. If hair sprays or other solutions are irritating, they should not be used by the child or adolescent.

Nurses should be aware of the signs of otitis externa such as a painful ear, drainage, and irritated canal. Verify that the tympanic membrane is intact during otoscopic examination. Teach families to avoid the irritants identified such as cotton-tipped applicators, sprays, and frequent swimming. Demonstrate proper instillation of drops (see the *Clinical Skills Manual*) and give instructions for use of acetaminophen for pain relief in the acute period.

Hearing Impairment

Approximately 1 million children (3 of every 1,000 births) in the United States have some form of hearing impairment (Joint Committee on Infant Hearing, 2007). Hearing impairment is expressed in terms of **decibels** (dB), which are units of loudness, and rated according to severity (Table 19–7). Children who have only a mild hearing loss (35 to 40 dB) may miss 50% of everyday conversation and are considered at high risk for difficulty in school. Children with a hearing loss of more than 90 dB are considered legally deaf. Between 2 and 6 children per 1,000 have a hearing loss.

Etiology and Pathophysiology

About 50% of hearing loss is genetically caused, generally in a recessive inheritance pattern with GJB2 gene abnormalities

TABLE 19–7	Severity of Hearing Loss	
Type of Loss	Decibel Level (dB)	Hearing Ability
Slight/mild	26–40	Some speech sounds are difficult to perceive, particularly unvoiced consonant sounds.
Moderate	41–60	Most normal conversational speech sounds are missed.
Severe	61–80	Speech sounds cannot be heard at a normal conversational level.
Profound	81–90	No speech sounds can be heard.
Deaf	Greater than 90	No sound at all can be heard.

Data from: American Speech-Language-Hearing Association. (2008). Type, degree, and configuration of hearing loss. Retrieved from http://www.asha.org/public/hearing/disorders/types.htm

(Yaeger, McCallum, Lewis, et al., 2006). Another 25% is due to environmental causes around the time of birth (Weichbold, Nekahm-Heis, & Wizl-Mueller, 2006); the remainder is due to unknown causes. Although many infants with hearing loss have no known risk factors, identified risks include:

- A family history of congenital hearing loss
- Positive titer for TORCH infections (toxoplasmosis, rubella, cytomegalovirus, syphilis, herpes)
- Craniofacial abnormalities
- Very low birth weight (less than 1500 g)
- Neonatal intensive care unit for over 5 days, or need for extracorporeal membrane oxygenation (ECMO), assisted ventilation, administration of ototoxic medications (e.g., gentamicin, tobramycin) or loop diuretics (e.g., furosemide), or hyperbilirubinemia that requires exchange transfusion
- Chemotherapy, particularly with aminoglycoside medications over 5 days
- Low Apgar score at 1 or 5 minutes
- Bacterial or viral meningitis
- Head trauma, especially basal skull/temporal bone fractures requiring hospitalization
- Presence of syndromes associated with hearing loss (Down syndrome, Pierre Robin syndrome, Arnold-Chiari malformation)

(Joint Committee on Infant Hearing, 2007)

Common causes of conductive hearing loss include impacted cerumen, the most frequent reason for conductive loss; otitis externa ("swimmer's ear"); trauma; or a foreign body. Conductive loss also occurs if the tympanic membrane does not fully vibrate, as in otitis media. In these cases, loss may be restored after the infection clears. Chronic and untreated ear infections may lead to ear structural changes and permanent hearing impairment. The loss of acuity may be gradual or rapid and results in diminished hearing in all ranges.

Conditions leading to sensorineural hearing loss may be congenital (maternal rubella), genetic (Tay-Sachs disease), or acquired (such as from ototoxic drugs, bacterial meningitis, or loud noise). In sensorineural hearing loss, high-frequency sounds are most affected. Such hearing loss may be preceded by **tinnitus** or ringing in the ears. Teenagers who use earphones at high volumes or attend many rock concerts are at risk for hearing loss. Other noise hazards include firecrackers, guns, and power and farm equipment.

Clinical Manifestations

Hearing is both an innate and a learned behavior. Infants and children who have hearing impairment exhibit a range of behaviors, depending on the child's age and the severity of the deficit (Table 19–8). Infants who hear normally respond to sound in both obvious and subtle ways that do not occur in those with hearing impairment. As children with hearing impairments mature, language skills are affected. Hearing loss is often manifested as a cognitive deficit, a behavioral problem, or both.

Hearing disorders can be classified according to the location of the deficit. **Conductive hearing loss** occurs when conditions

TABLE 19–8	Behaviors Suggestive of Hearing Impairment
Age	Behavior
Infant	Has a diminished or absent startle reflex to loud sound Does not awaken when environment is very noisy Awakens only to touch Does not turn head to sound at 3–4 months Does not localize sound at 6–10 months Babbles little or not at all
Toddler and preschooler	Speaks unintelligibly, in a monotone, or not at all Communicates needs through gestures Is unable to follow directions Appears developmentally delayed, especially in social interactions Appears emotionally immature, yells inappropriately Does not respond to doorbell or telephone Appears more interested in objects than people and prefers to play alone Focuses on facial expressions rather than verbal communications
School-age child and adolescent	Asks to have statements repeated Answers questions inappropriately, except when able to view speaker's face Daydreams and is inattentive Performs poorly at school or is truant Has speech abnormalities or speaks in a monotone Sits close to or turns television or radio up loudly Prefers to play alone

Adapted from: Council on Children with Disabilities, 2006; Dunlap, 2008.

Children and adolescents may have hearing impairments due to noise exposure from loud music, often in ranges not screened during school auditory testing (Zhao, Manchaian, French, et al., 2010). Preventing these hearing losses is possible, so nurses should identify and find sources of noise in the child's environment. They may include stereos, airplanes, firearms, power tools, machinery, and toys. Encourage use of ear plugs during hazardous activities (Quintanilla-Dieck, Artunduaga, & Eavey, 2009). Be aware of the potential harm from iPods or other music since it is in very close contact with the ear and the sound is usually loud and directed into the ear canal with no dissipation into surrounding air. Additionally, the current practice of using headphones for extended parts of the day increases the risk of injury.

in the external auditory canal or tympanic membrane prevent sound from reaching the middle ear. **Sensorineural hearing loss** occurs when the hair cells in the cochlea or along the vestibulo-cochlear (acoustic) nerve (cranial nerve VIII) are damaged. This leads to permanent hearing loss. A **mixed hearing loss** indicates a hearing loss having a combination of conductive and sensorineural causes.

COLLABORATIVE CARE

Diagnostic Tests

Early identification of hearing loss is a key element in successful treatment. Detection of hearing loss in infants is important to ensure optimal development. Universal screening of all infants is recommended before 1 month of age, with diagnostic audiologic evaluation before 3 months, and beginning of early intervention programs by 6 months of age for those with hearing impairment (Windmill & Windmill, 2006). Many state laws now mandate screening of newborns. Observations of response to noise in all newborns should be accompanied by more sophisticated testing such as auditory brainstem response or transient evoked otoacoustic emissions, especially in those at high risk of deficits (Figure 19–8 ➤). See Table 19–9 for a description of the common tests used for newborn hearing.

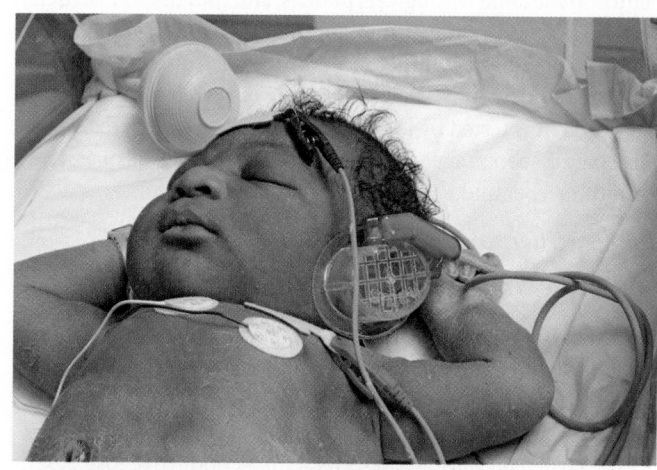

FIGURE 19–8 ➤ Newborn hearing screening is an effective tool in diagnosing some cases of hearing impairment very early in life.

TABLE 19–9	Screening Tests for Newborn Hearing
Test	Mechanism of Action
Otoacoustive Emission (OAE) (either Transient-Evoked [TEOAE] or Distortion-Product [DPOAE])	A measure of low-intensity sounds from the cochlear hair cells in response to clicks from a probe placed in the ear canal Sensitive in frequency range above 1500 Hz May show false negative for loss below 1000–1500 Hz Detects inner ear hearing loss by evaluating cochlear and hair cell function Does not detect neural damage to eighth cranial nerve Can be sensitive to outer ear canal obstruction or middle ear effusion, leading to false positive result
Auditory brainstem response (ABR)	Electrical response to auditory stimuli from three surface scalp electrodes Reflects activity of cochlea, cranial nerve VIII, and auditory brainstem pathways Detects hearing loss from 1000–8000 Hz May show false negative results for losses in the 500–2000 Hz levels Will give a positive result if there is damage to cranial nerve VIII or brainstem pathways even if cochlear loss is not present

An otoscopic examination with a tympanogram can be performed on an older infant to determine conductive hearing loss. The **tympanogram** is a test that provides a graph of the middle ear's ability to transmit sound. An airtight probe is inserted into the external ear canal and a tone is emitted. The pressure is measured by the probe and plotted on a graph. A flat tympanogram suggests conductive hearing loss (Figures 19–9A and B➤). **Audiography** can be used with cooperative children over 3 years of age. Sounds of various frequencies and intensities are presented to the child through earphones, and the child is instructed to raise a hand upon hearing the sound. Although audiography cannot detect hearing loss caused by middle ear effusion, it can indicate sensorineural loss. The hearing of preschool and school-age children is tested by asking them to repeat whispered words. Hearing of school-age children and adolescents is also assessed with the Weber and Rinne tests (see Chapter 5 ∞).

Clinical Therapy

If a hearing loss is uncorrectable, a multidisciplinary team composed of the pediatrician, audiologist, otolaryngologist, speech-language pathologist, nurse, teacher, and social worker should assist the child and family with adaptation to the disability. If the deficit is due to recurrent ear infections, tympanostomy tube insertion may improve hearing.

A hearing aid may be prescribed for a conductive loss. A sensorineural loss is more difficult to treat, but bone conduction hearing aids have been used in some children. Some families choose to have a child treated with a cochlear implant. A cochlear

Growth & Development *Hearing Loss*

Infants and young children respond automatically with a blink or the startle reflex to unexpected or loud noises. As they mature, they localize the sound source, then understand speech, and then communicate verbally. When these responses are missing, the child may be hard of hearing. Children with hearing loss can easily fall behind their peers in language milestones since they cannot hear and speak in the same manner as other children. Without interventions to enable them to learn language, they can also fall behind in reading, literacy skills, related cognitive processes, and social-emotional development (Joint Committee on Infant Hearing, 2007). Carefully evaluate hearing and all developmental milestones during each regularly scheduled health care visit. Refer infants and children with abnormalities for further evaluation. When hearing loss is identified as a cause of delayed development, interventions guided by health care professionals with expertise in hearing loss are needed.

implant is a small electronic device that helps to provide sound for those who are deaf or profoundly hard of hearing (National Institutes of Health, 2007). It consists of:

- A microphone to pick up sound that is located outside of the body; it is worn as a headpiece behind the ear.
- A speech processor that organizes sound from the microphone; it is worn behind the ear or on a belt.
- A transmitter that transfers the sound into electrical impulses; it is part of the headpiece behind the ear.
- Electrodes that send the signals to the brain; this receiver is implanted in the skin behind the ear with a wire leading to the cochlear fluid in the middle ear.

Kate, the child introduced in the opening scenario, had a cochlear implant inserted at about 2 years of age (Figure 19–10 ➤). Children with cochlear implants need ongoing speech therapy to teach them the meaning of the new sounds they hear after the implant. There is an elevated risk of bacterial meningitis following implant, so immunization against pneumococcal disease and ongoing monitoring for this potential complication are needed (U.S. Food and Drug Administration, 2008).

For children with uncorrectable hearing loss, several approaches are used to enhance communication (Table 19–10). Children with hearing impairment may receive speech therapy and instructions in lip-reading, signing, cuing, and finger-spelling.

NURSING MANAGEMENT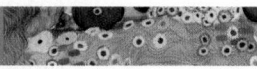

Nursing Assessment and Diagnosis

Nurses conduct newborn hearing tests soon after birth and make observations of the infant's responses to sound. As the child grows, hearing should be assessed at every well-child visit. The best judges of hearing are parents; ask them if they have concerns about their child's hearing. Be alert for parents who believe that their children do not have normal hearing since they are often the first to diagnose a hearing impairment. Recall Kate in the opening scenario; her father designed an experiment by clanging pans behind her when he suspected she did not hear. An infant's reaction to rattles, bells, or hand clapping 30 cm

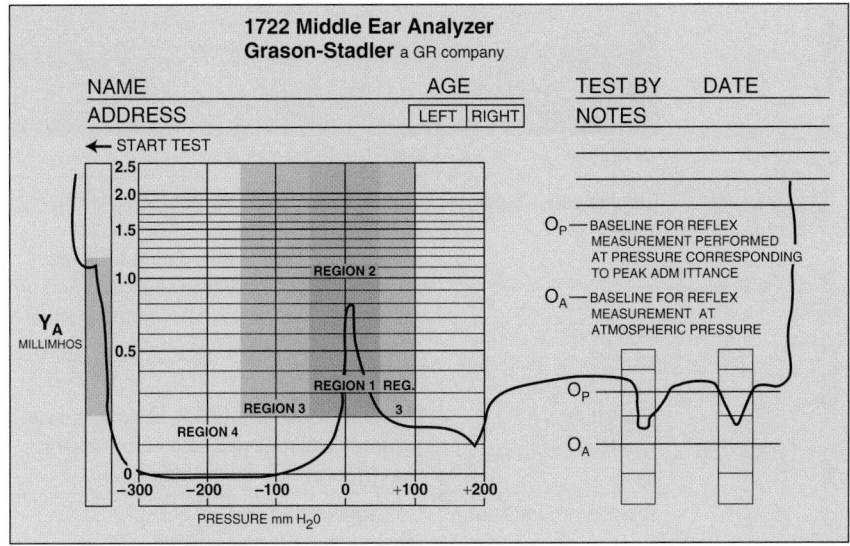

A

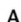

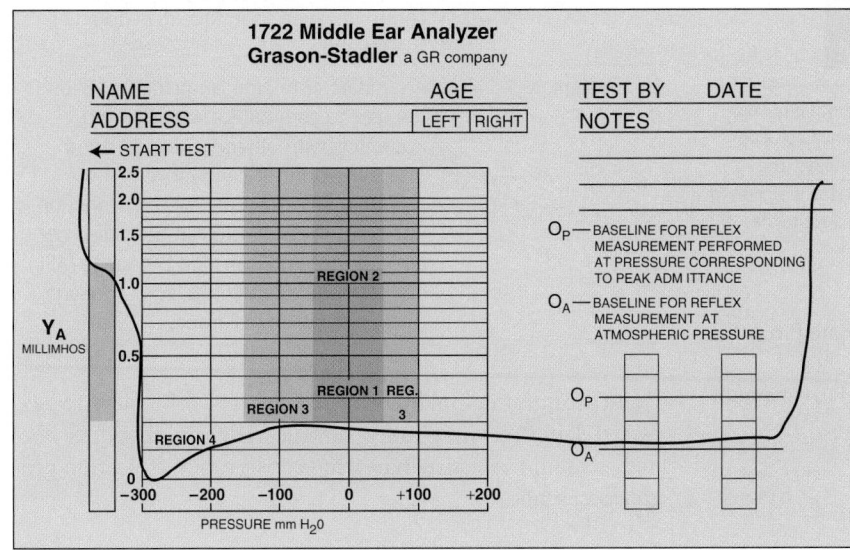

B

FIGURE 19–9 ➤ A, This tympanogram demonstrates normal hearing as evidenced by the curve showing the tympanic membrane's movement when a sound wave is emitted into the ear canal. Mobility is between 0.2 mL and 1.0 mL, the normal range. B, In contrast, note the flat pattern in the second tympanogram, which shows very restricted mobility of the tympanic membrane in response to sound.

(12 in.) from the ear is an important observation. Language milestones should be evaluated when the older infant and child are examined. Language development is a major area of focus in children who are deaf. Infants who are deaf begin to babble at about 5 to 6 months of age, the same age as hearing infants. However, this babbling ceases several months later in the child with a hearing impairment.

School nurses use audiometers to evaluate hearing during screening programs in schools and refer children who do not pass the screening test. See the *Clinical Skills Manual* for techniques in performing hearing screening. Nurses in offices often use tympanometers to evaluate ear function.

Following are common nursing diagnoses for the child with impaired hearing:

- Disturbed Sensory Perception related to abnormal sound transmission
- Risk for Impaired Verbal Communication related to hearing loss

Law & Ethics — *Deafness and Cochlear Implants*

Many people who are deaf consider deafness similar to an ethnic group or a group with other common traits and experiences. They believe that they are fully functional, communicate, and socialize with others satisfactorily, and they do not view deafness as a defect. They believe that it is an affront to their culture to consider that someone should try to change from being deaf to hearing. Others note that only a select few can obtain cochlear implants due to their cost and the fact that health insurance may not cover the surgery, instrumentation, or speech therapy. Some are opposed to use of cochlear implants for children because of the surgical risk involved and the fact that children are not old enough to make their own decision about choosing the surgery. However, the earlier the child has the surgery and hears sounds, the more likely speech is to develop. Read about the controversy in resources such as M. Hyde & D. Power. (2006). *Cochlear implants in children: Ethics and choices.* Washington, DC: Gallaudet University Press. Imagine the difficulty parents have as they try to make the choice about treatment for the child who is hearing impaired. How can nurses support the family as they consider alternatives and then once the treatment decision is made?

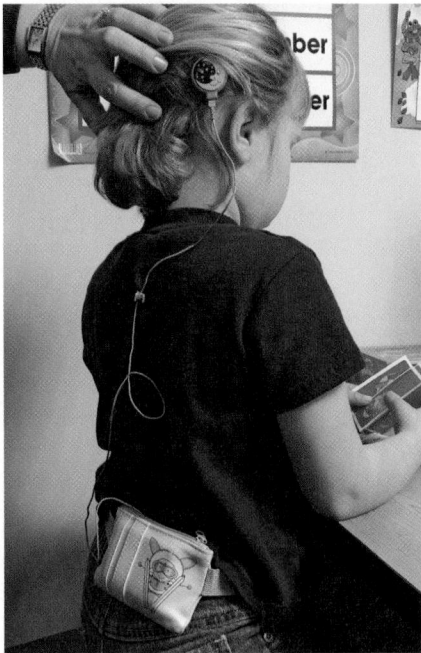

FIGURE 19–10 ➤ The child with a cochlear implant wears a speech processor, like the one present in this child's waist pack, as well as a microphone to pick up sounds and a transmitter that transfers the sound into electrical impulses. The microphone and transmitter are seen behind the ear. Electrodes that send signals to the brain are implanted in the skin behind the ear with a wire that leads to the middle ear.

- Risk for Delayed Growth and Development related to communication impairment
- Readiness for Enhanced Family Coping related to caring for a child with a hearing impairment

Planning and Implementation

Prevention and Early Identification

Nurses can encourage prevention of hearing loss from exposure to loud noises such as from power and farm equipment and music. Music should be turned down and ear protection should be worn for other activities. Early identification of hearing loss in infants and children is facilitated by newborn screening, developmental assessment, and childhood screening programs. Infants should be tested for hearing loss by 3 months of age; in cases of loss, intervention should begin before 6 months of age

Nursing Alert

Both parents and children should be instructed never to put any object in the child's ear. Some parents believe that the ear canal should be cleaned with a cotton-tipped swab. If the cleaning is too vigorous or the child moves unexpectedly, a ruptured tympanic membrane could result.

If an alkaline button battery (like those found in many toys or watches) is inserted in a child's ear, it can rapidly destroy tissue, causing perforation of the tympanic membrane, destruction of the ossicles, and local tissue ulceration. Removal should be performed with the child under sedation or general anesthesia.

TABLE 19–10	Communication Techniques for Children Who Are Hearing Impaired
Technique	**Description**
Cued speech	Supplement to lip-reading; eight hand shapes represent groups of consonant sounds, and four positions about the face represent groups of vowel sounds; based on the sounds the letters make, not the letters themselves; the child can "see-hear" every spoken syllable a hearing person hears.
Oral approach	Uses only spoken language for face-to-face communication; avoids use of formal signs; uses hearing aids and residual hearing.
Total communication	Uses speech and sign, finger-spelling, lip-reading, and residual hearing simultaneously; the child selects a communication technique depending on the situation.
Sign language	A separate or foreign language that allows the user to communicate quickly and accurately with others who understand signs. The signs or hand movements represent words or concepts. When a sign is not available, the word can be spelled out using signs. American Sign Language (ASL) is most often used; British Sign Language (BSL) is common in Europe.

(Joint Committee on Infant Hearing, 2007). Be alert for expected language milestones during early childhood. School nurses should be active in hearing conservation education programs in school.

Care in the Community

Most of the care for children with hearing impairments takes place in the community. The nurse integrates special care into the health promotion and health maintenance visit of children with hearing impairments. Nursing care of the child with a hearing impairment focuses on facilitating the child's ability to receive spoken language and to send information, on helping parents to meet the child's schooling needs, and on providing emotional support to parents. Refer the parents to an early intervention program as soon as the diagnosis of hearing impairment is made, in order to foster the child's development. If a cochlear implant is planned, the child needs surgical care and follow-up to monitor results and integrate sound gradually into the child's life. Parents often need help to decide on the best method for hearing and language enhancement for the child. You may need to interpret information, refer to the Internet and other resources, and help parents connect with other parents who have chosen various approaches for their own children.

Children with cochlear implants need regular speech therapy after surgery. Refer parents to appropriate resources. Due to the increased rate of bacterial meningitis in cochlear recipients, particularly that caused by pneumococcus, immunization status is important. The child should be up to date for pneumococcal recommendations by 2–3 weeks before implant surgery. Following surgery, recommendations of the Centers for Disease Control and Prevention and cochlear implant manufacturer should be followed. Parents should be taught the signs and symptoms of meningitis (see Chapter 27 ∞) so that they can seek prompt care, if needed.

Facilitate Ability to Receive Spoken Language

Be aware of how the child compensates for hearing loss and use these strategies in communication:

- If hearing loss is mild or temporary or if the child reads lips, first obtain the child's visual attention by lightly touching the child or saying his or her name.
- Position your face 1 to 2 m (3 to 6 ft) from the child's face and make sure that the child's eyes are focused on your face and lips. Make sure the room is well lit, with no backlighting. Speak at a normal rate and tone, and use facial expressions that show caring or concern. If the child does not understand, rephrase the information in shorter, simpler sentences. Use specific, concrete explanations, and give the child time to comprehend. Watch for subtle signs of misinterpretations and give consistent and immediate feedback.
- Be familiar with the different types of hearing aids. Hearing aids, which are microphones that amplify all sounds, can be worn in or behind the ear, in the frame of glasses, or on the body with a wire attached to the ear. When talking to a child with a hearing aid, speak slowly and be positioned 15 to 45 cm (6 to 18 in.) from the microphone using a normal conversational tone. Talk to the child even if the child is not looking at you. Make sure the batteries are fresh for the best reception. All sound is amplified, so reduce background noise as much as possible (see Families Want to Know: Care of the Hearing Aid).
- Acoustic feedback, an audible whistling sound that cannot always be heard by the child, is a common problem with hearing aids. To eliminate this sound, readjust the hearing aid to ensure that it is inserted properly and that no hair or ear wax is caught between the ear mold and canal. Turning down the volume may also help.
- A remote microphone system is another type of device designed to improve hearing. This is often used in the classroom situation because it eliminates background noise. The speaker wears a transmitter that picks up the voice and transmits it to a receiver worn by the child.

Facilitate Ability to Send Information

Maintain the child's hearing aid in proper condition. Many children with impaired hearing communicate using speech, which is enhanced through speech therapy. In addition, they are taught to sign, finger-spell, or use cued speech (Figure 19–11 ➤). Articulation may be difficult, and understanding what the child is trying to say may be frustrating for both the nurse and the child. Taking time to listen carefully is important.

Measures to promote speech and communication development as well as safety are implemented. Ask the parents to ex-

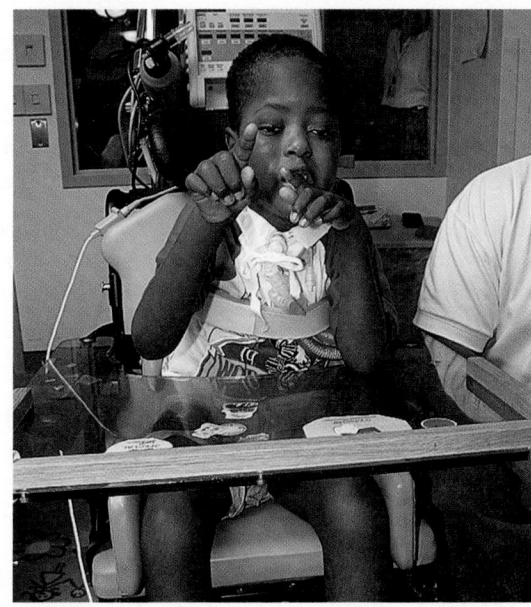

FIGURE 19–11 ➤ This child with a hearing impairment and tracheostomy is communicating by means of American Sign Language.

plain the child's communication techniques and to help interpret words. Have younger children point to pictures. Use assisted technologies such as a computer or picture board, as well as drawings or gestures, if necessary. This technique is especially helpful for communicating feelings of pain and hunger during hospitalization. If the child signs or finger-spells, be sure you understand the signs for important functions. Give older children a paper and pencil to write requests. People other than parents should be able to understand what the child is trying to communicate. Have an interpreter available if the child uses American Sign Language. Learn some common signs to communicate simple words or phrases. Orient the child carefully to new settings such as the hospital room or a new school.

Families Want to Know
Care of the Hearing Aid

Families need to know how to maintain the child's hearing aid in proper condition to ensure its function. They can be taught when the child receives the first hearing aid, with at least annual updates to check on knowledge and questions. Items to include in teaching are as follows:

- The three types of hearing aids are those that fit totally in the ear canal, those that fit in the external ear canal, and those that fit behind the ear.
- The hearing aid should be cleaned each day with a damp cloth.
- Change the batteries as needed, usually about once a week. Remove the battery when not in use.
- Place the hearing aid in the ear with the volume off, and then slowly turn the volume up to half volume. Adjust as needed.
- Be sure the hearing aid fit is checked yearly, as the child's growth may necessitate a new fitting.

Help Parents to Meet the Child's Educational Needs

Public laws apply to the education of children who are hearing impaired (see Chapter 1 ∞). After diagnosis, the parents and professionals together agree on an individualized education plan (see discussion in Chapter 10 ∞). Childcare and preschool are recommended for children with hearing problems.

- Provide parents with information about adjustments that may have to be made for the child with a hearing impairment who attends public school. By sitting at the front of the classroom, the child can hear and see more clearly. The teacher should always face the child when speaking, and background noise should be reduced.
- Tell parents that children who are hearing impaired have the same intelligence quotient (IQ) distribution as children without hearing impairment. However, communication and learning can be difficult, and extra support is needed.
- Children with hearing impairment should reach their intellectual potential, although development in certain areas may take place more slowly than it does in children with no hearing impairment.

Provide Emotional Support

By recognizing the effects of the diagnosis on the family, the nurse can help family members deal with their reactions to the child's hearing loss. Help the parents understand the child's disability and its effect on speech and language development. Supporting healthy coping is an important intervention to help the parents carry on with their lives. Tell the family about the community services available for medical, nursing, psychologic, and financial assistance.

Evaluation

Expected outcomes of nursing care for a child with hearing impairment include:

- The child will demonstrate successful establishment of a communication method or assistive listening device (U.S. Department of Health and Human Services, 2010).
- The child will manifest growth and developmental milestones to maximum potential.
- An effective individualized education plan will be established and implemented for the child.
- The family will demonstrate positive methods of coping with stress.

Injuries of the Ear

Ear injuries of many types commonly occur in children. Lacerations, infections, and hematomas may occur in the external ear structures, especially the pinna. Children may place foreign objects in the ear, and insects may enter the ear canal.

Rupture of the tympanic membrane may result from head injuries, blows to the ear, or insertion of objects into the ear canal. Serous drainage from the ear can indicate a basilar skull fracture. Be alert for ruptured tympanic membranes in combination with conjunctival and retinal hemorrhage, and other signs of shaken child syndrome (see Chapters 6 and 26 ∞ for further explanation of this syndrome).

See Table 19–11 for information on the emergency treatment of ear injuries. Any injury resulting in earache, decreased hearing, persistent bleeding, or other discharge should be seen by a physician.

TABLE 19–11 Emergency Treatment of Ear Injuries

Injury	Treatment
Pinna	
Minor cuts or abrasions	Wash thoroughly with soap and water and rinse well; leave exposed to air if possible or apply an adhesive bandage; monitor for infection.
Hematomas	Needle aspiration should be performed and a pressure dressing applied; undrained hematomas may become fibrotic; "cauliflower ear" deformity may develop.
Cellulitis or abscesses	Apply moist heat intermittently; make sure that the prescribed antibiotic is taken; minor surgery may be performed for an abscess.
Deep lacerations	Apply pressure to stop bleeding; transport to the physician's office or emergency department for suturing.
Ear Canal	
Foreign bodies	Have the child lie on the back and turn the head over the edge of the bed, with affected side down; wiggle the earlobe and have the child shake the head; the foreign object may fall out as a result of gravity; if the object remains in the ear, call a physician; do not try to remove a foreign body with tweezers because this may push the object further into the ear.
Insects	Shine flashlights into the ear to try to attract the insect; instilling a few drops of mineral oil, olive oil, or alcohol kills the insect, and irrigating the ear canal gently may remove it (see the *Clinical Skills Manual*).
Tympanic Membrane	
Ruptures	Call a physician if a child has persistent ear pain after a blow, blast injury, or insertion of a foreign object; cover the external ear loosely with a piece of sterile cotton or gauze; if the tympanic membrane has been ruptured, systemic antibiotics are prescribed.

■ DISORDERS OF THE NOSE AND THROAT

Epistaxis

Epistaxis, or nosebleed, is common in school-age children, especially boys. Kiesselbach plexus, an area of plentiful veins located in the anterior nares, is a usual source of bleeding, commonly caused by irritation from nose picking, foreign bodies, or low humidity. Other causes include forceful coughing, allergies, or infections resulting in congestion of the nasal mucosa. Posterior nosebleeds have a variety of causes, some of which may indicate systemic disease (e.g., bleeding disorder) or injury.

Children with nosebleeds are sometimes brought to the emergency department by a parent who has been unable to stop the flow of blood within a few minutes. Both parent and child may be frightened. Ask the parent briefly about any history of nosebleeds and other contributing factors, including medications. Take the child's pulse and blood pressure to assess for excessive blood loss. Carefully examine the nasal mucosa by asking the child to blow any clots out gently, if possible. Suctioning may be necessary.

Observing the flow may help determine if the blood is coming from an anterior or a posterior location. A nosebleed confined to one side of the nose is almost always anterior, but posterior bleeding can flow on one or both sides. If blood cannot be seen, the child may be swallowing it, resulting in nausea. Suspect posterior bleeding in children who have sustained blunt trauma to the head.

The child with anterior bleeding should sit upright quietly. The head should be tilted forward to prevent blood from trickling down the throat, which can lead to vomiting. The nares should be squeezed just below the nasal bone and held for 10 to 15 minutes while the child breathes through the mouth. If the bleeding does not stop, a cotton ball or swab soaked with Neo-Synephrine, epinephrine, thrombin, or lidocaine may be inserted into the affected nostril by the primary care provider to promote topical vasoconstriction or anesthesia. Once the bleeding has stopped, the nostril may have to be cauterized with silver nitrate or electrocautery. If the bleeding cannot be stopped, absorbable packing may be used.

Posterior bleeding must also be stopped by packing, and the child must be monitored carefully. Arterial ligation is occasionally needed. History of repeated or severe nosebleeds should be referred to an otolaryngologist.

Nursing Management

Assess the child's hematocrit or hemoglobin if significant bleeding has occurred. Children with frequent epistaxis should have a complete history taken and physical examination performed to rule out systemic disease.

After the nosebleed has stopped, the child is more vulnerable to recurrent bleeding and should avoid bending over, stooping, strenuous exercise, hot drinks, and hot baths or showers for the next 3 to 4 days. Sleeping with the head elevated on two or three pillows and humidifying the air with a vaporizer may also prevent a recurrence. Provide parents with suggestions for prevention and home management of epistaxis. See Families Want to Know: Prevention and Home Management of Epistaxis.

Families Want to Know
Prevention and Home Management of Epistaxis

Prevention
- Humidify the child's room, especially during the winter.
- Discourage the child from picking or rubbing the nose or inserting foreign objects into the nose.
- Instruct the child to blow the nose gently and release sneezes through the mouth.

Home Management
- Keep the child calm.
- Sit the child upright with head tilted slightly forward so blood does not run down the nasopharynx.
- Press a roll of cotton under the upper lip to compress the labial artery.
- Apply steady pressure to both nostrils just below the nasal bone with the thumb and forefinger for 15–20 minutes, timed by a clock or watch.
- Apply an ice pack or cold compress to the bridge of the nose or the back of the neck.
- Call the health care provider if the bleeding does not stop after the above treatments.
- Avoid vigorous exercise and aspirin or other noncoagulant drugs during the first few days after an epistaxis episode.

Note: Adapted from Health Care Guide, 2008.

Nasopharyngitis

Nasopharyngitis, also known as upper respiratory infection (URI) or the "common cold," causes inflammation and infection of the nose and throat and is probably the most common illness of infancy and childhood. More than 200 viruses and numerous bacteria can cause this condition. The most common viruses include rhinovirus and coronavirus, and the most frequently occurring bacterium is group A streptococcus. See Chapter 20 ∞ for a discussion of respiratory syncytial virus (RSV), a common cause of both upper and lower respiratory illness. URI organisms incubate in 1 to 3 days, and the infection is communicable several hours before symptoms develop and for 1 to 2 days after they begin. Symptoms may last 4 to 10 days or longer. The pathogens spread when the infected person touches the hand of an uninfected person, who then touches his or her mouth or nose, resulting in self-inoculation with infected droplets.

A red nasal mucosa with clear nasal discharge and an infected throat with enlarged tonsils may be apparent in children with nasopharyngitis. Vesicles may be present on the soft palate and in the pharynx. Accompanying symptoms may vary, depending on the child's age (Table 19–12).

Between episodes of nasopharyngitis, the child should be asymptomatic. If a child continues to have upper respiratory infections, the presence of an underlying condition such as allergy, asthma, or polyps should be ruled out.

Nursing Management

For infants who cannot breathe through the mouth, normal saline nose drops can be administered every 3 to 4 hours, especially

TABLE 19–12 Symptoms of Nasopharyngitis		
Infants Younger than 3 Months of Age	Infants 3 Months of Age or Older	Older Children
• Lethargy • Irritability • Feeding poorly • Fever (may be absent)	• Fever • Vomiting • Diarrhea • Sneezing • Anorexia • Irritability • Restlessness	• Dry, irritated nose and throat • Chills, fever • Generalized muscle aches • Headache • Malaise • Anorexia • Thin nasal discharge, which may later become thick and purulent • Possible sneezing

Families Want to Know

Teaching About Over-the-Counter Cough and Cold Medications

Parents may try to treat children who have upper respiratory infections with the same medications they are accustomed to taking for a cold. Prepare them during a health promotion visit and help them plan for how to handle medications for the child. Guidelines are as follows:

- Do NOT use cough and cold products in children under 2 years unless given specific directions to do so by a health care provider.
- Read the label to be sure the medication is recommended for the child's age and condition. Give only the dose recommended for the child's age and weight. Do NOT use products packaged for adults.
- Be sure you know how to measure the medication. Tablespoon and teaspoon are NOT the same, and using household spoons may lead to incorrect dosing. Use the measuring device that is provided with liquid medications for greatest accuracy.
- Consult the pharmacist, nurse, or doctor if you have questions, if the medication is not recommended for the age of your child, if the child's condition does not improve, or if other symptoms appear.
- Use the child-resistant cap after each opening of the bottle. Store the medication out of reach of all children, preferably in a locked location.
- If you use home remedies or other herbal products to treat colds, be sure to check on their safety for a child with your health care provider first.
- Inspect containers and do not buy those that may have tears, imperfections, or tampering.
- Review all of the information in the "Drug Facts" box on the package label. If you do not understand instructions on the package, contact a health care provider before using it.
- If the child becomes more ill or does not improve, stop the medicine and contact the health care provider.

Adapted from: Goldman, R. D. (2009). Cough and cold medications are risky for children. *Journal of Pediatrics, 155*(3), 451–452; U.S. Food and Drug Administration. (2007). *Public Health Advisory—Nonprescription cough and cold medicine use in children.* Retrieved from http://www.fda.gov/cder/drug/advisory/cough_cold.htm

before feeding. (See the *Clinical Skills Manual.*) For infants over 9 months of age, nasal stuffiness can be treated with normal saline nose drops. Children over 6 years of age can use nasal sprays.

Decongestant nose drops should not be used for more than 4 or 5 days, or more often than recommended, since effectiveness will decrease and incidence of side effects increases. Antihistamines may be helpful for children with allergic rhinitis or profuse nasal drainage. Long-acting nasal sprays and medications with several ingredients are not recommended.

Room humidification may help prevent drying of nasal secretions. Antipyretics such as acetaminophen reduce fever and make the child more comfortable. Aspirin is not recommended because of its association with Reye syndrome (refer to Chapter 27 ∞).

Children should avoid strenuous physical activity and engage in quiet play such as reading, listening to music or stories, or watching television or videotapes. Children should not be forced to eat, but the intake of favorite fluids to liquefy secretions should be encouraged. Parents should be told that no medicine or vaccine can prevent the common cold, but eliminating contact with infected persons can reduce the spread of infection. (See Families Want to Know: Teaching About Over-the-Counter Cough and Cold Medications.) Proper hand hygiene and disposal of tissues help to decrease the spread of the infection. Clean counters, toys, door knobs, and other surfaces daily and discourage sharing of food, dishes, and utensils.

Sinusitis

Sinusitis is an inflammation of one or more of the paranasal sinuses. These sinuses, which have respiratory epithelium and are continuous with the respiratory tract, include the maxillary, ethmoid, frontal, and sphenoid sinuses. The sinuses commonly become infected following a viral upper respiratory infection; of the 6–8 respiratory infections children get annually, 5–10% of them are followed by sinusitis (Demetroulakos, 2007; DeMuri & Wald, 2010). In most cases, the child's history reveals a URI for several days, followed by improvement in symptoms, but an increase in purulent nasal drainage. There is accompanying facial pain, headache, and fever (Bernius & Perlin, 2006). Chronic sinusitis may occur in children, more commonly in children with

allergies, asthma, or cystic fibrosis; see Chapter 20 ∞ for assessment of these conditions.

Signs and symptoms of sinusitis in children are sometimes nonspecific. A history of recent upper respiratory infection is common, persistent cough from postnasal drip can occur, and nasal discharge or swelling can be apparent. Malodorous breath, fever, mouth breathing, hyponasal speech, and cervical lymphadenopathy may be present (Bernius & Perlin, 2006). Young children may be anorexic or have difficulty feeding while older children may complain of headache.

A diagnosis of sinusitis is usually based on history and physical examination findings. Percussion and illumination of sinuses are not generally useful in children. Computed tomography (CT), magnetic resonance imaging (MRI), and radiographs may be performed but they can be costly, require sedation of young children, and may be inconclusive. For the child with repeated sinusitis or who appears toxic, aspiration of sinus aspirate may be performed for culture by an otolaryngologist.

Collaborative Care

The goals of collaborative care are relief from pain and promotion of ulcer healing. Most mouth ulcers and other oral lesions are diagnosed by history and appearance. Culture of exudate may be helpful in identifying an infective cause. Biopsy may be performed if the cause is not clear or a mouth cancer is possible. Occasionally laboratory blood analysis is done and may show leukocytosis in infectious cases and Stevens-Johnson syndrome.

Most mouth ulcers are treated symptomatically. Since the oral mucosa is fast growing, the cells can rapidly heal. Keeping the mouth clean and administering systemic or topical analgesics can assist with comfort. Foods should be mild and nonirritating. Acyclovir may be administered for treatment of herpes infections. Antibiotics are needed for bacterial infection of oral lesions. Stevens-Johnson syndrome necessitates removing the drug that causes the reaction, and treating the child with oral antihistamines and supportive therapy.

Nursing Management

Nurses assess the oral cavity of all children beginning in the neonatal period. Structural abnormalities are promptly referred for further diagnostic work. Mouth ulcers are examined for size, location, drainage, and pain. For those at risk, such as children on chemotherapy, regular careful examination of the oral mucosa is an important part of care. Some of the appropriate nursing diagnoses for children with oral ulcers include:

- Acute Pain related to injury of oral cavity
- Impaired Oral Mucous Membrane related to chemotherapy or infection
- Imbalanced Nutrition: Less than Body Requirements related to inability to ingest adequate foods

Nurses play an important role in the treatment of oral ulcers. Ensure that children have good oral care, including brushing teeth with a soft bristle brush or by use of mouth sponges. Rinse the mouth after all meals and snacks. Teach the family correct administration of oral medications and topical preparations designed to treat infection or provide comfort. When oral mucosa ulcers are predicted, such as with chemotherapy or in AIDS, begin oral protocols before lesions occur to decrease their appearance and severity (Shetty, 2006). Encourage a diet of mild foods, and avoid spicy, sweet, sour, and acidic items; cold foods may be soothing. Monitor hydration status to ensure adequate fluid intake. Teach parents correct administration of analgesic treatment. Use standard precautions to protect the child from infections and prevent their flora from being transferred to other children or family members. Encourage parents to keep children with herpes gingivostomatitis out of contact with other children if active lesions or drooling are present.

Desired outcomes of nursing care for children with oral problems include a decrease in reported oral pain or disruptive effects on dietary intake, structural intactness and normal function of oral mucosal membranes, and ingestion of adequate amounts of fluids and nutrients.

Mouth and Dental Emergencies

Children may experience trauma to the mouth and teeth during falls, sporting activities, and motor vehicle crashes. A predominance of cases occurs in the toddler years as children become more mobile (Bernius & Perlin, 2006). Nurses inform parents of proper treatment for injuries and may provide emergency treatment in schools and other community settings. Injury prevention is encouraged through use of protective gear during sports. See Chapter 24 ∞ for a discussion of oral care during treatment for cancer, and Chapter 17 ∞ for a discussion of protective sporting gear and of body piercing, which may include the oral cavity.

Because the mouth has a profuse blood supply, bleeding may be extensive for even minor injuries. It is best to use clean cloths to absorb the blood and prevent choking on it, and get the child to an emergency facility to have the lesion carefully examined.

Dental injuries may involve fracture of a tooth, luxation (partial extrusion), or avulsion (complete removal). The periodontal ligament holds the tooth in the socket, but its attachment is torn during a tooth avulsion. The child should be transported immediately to an emergency facility. If otherwise stable, an emergency dental visit is the best choice. When avulsion has occurred, fast care improves the chance that a permanent tooth can be reimplanted and kept alive. When reimplanted within 30 minutes, the tooth's chances of survival are best (American Association of Endodontics, 2010). Nurses can perform care or teach parents what to do in case of dental emergency. See Families Want to Know: Care of a Tooth Avulsion. Refer to dental resources as needed. See Chapters 7, 8, and 9 ∞ for specific dental health promotion and health maintenance strategies at each age during childhood and adolescence.

Families Want to Know
Care of a Tooth Avulsion

When a tooth is removed during an injury, prompt treatment may influence the chance that it can be reimplanted. If the child's condition is stable, try to reimplant the tooth and then transfer the child to an emergency dental facility.

- Handle the tooth only by the crown (its top) rather than the root in order to avoid further damage.
- Gently rinse the tooth with a stream of water or sterile saline.
- Insert the tooth into the socket if possible.
- Have the child provide gentle pressure by biting a piece of gauze or a moistened tea bag.

If the child is unstable or has other injuries, enlist emergency medical transportation (call 911). In this case, the tooth is transported with the child to the health care facility. During that time it must be kept moist.

- If a dental aid kit is available, it may contain an emergency transport liquid. If these are not available, alternatives include cold milk, saliva, saline, or water with a pinch of salt.

Note: Adapted from American Association of Endodontists. (2010). *Saving a knocked-out tooth.* Retrieved from http://www.aae.org/patients/patientinfo/references/avulsed.htm

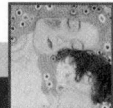

Chapter Highlights

- Health conditions affecting the eyes and ears are common in childhood, partially due to anatomical differences in structure.
- Disorders of the eye and ear can lead to developmental and communication delays.
- Conjunctivitis can occur throughout childhood, and can be caused by bacteria, viruses, and allergy.
- Conjunctivitis in the newborn, ophthalmia neonatorum, can be acquired during birth from the mother, and can pose a serious health threat.
- Children manifest a wide array of visual disorders such as hyperopia, myopia, and astigmatism.
- Conditions that can seriously affect vision are strabismus, amblyopia, cataracts, and glaucoma.
- Retinopathy of prematurity is an iatrogenically caused visual disorder.
- Nurses commonly screen vision of children in schools and health facilities to identify those with visual impairment.
- Interventions for the child with visual impairment center on providing input through other senses to maximize the child's development.

- Otitis media is the most common childhood health condition and has increased in incidence in the past decade.
- Overgrowth of resistant organisms has made treatment of otitis media difficult.
- Treatment of otitis media may begin with up to 3 days of monitoring, followed by antibiotic therapy if the child's condition worsens.
- Newborns should be screened for response to sounds; those at high risk of hearing impairment should be carefully monitored in early childhood.
- Hearing loss may be conductive, sensorineural, or mixed.
- Nursing plan interventions maximize development and communication in the child with a hearing impairment.
- Common disorders of the nose and throat in children include epistaxis, nasopharyngitis, pharyngitis, and tonsillitis.
- Common disorders of the mouth in children are structural abnormalities and oral ulcers.
- Nurses are influential in providing care in dental emergencies and referring families for adequate dental care.

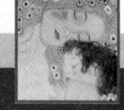

Clinical Reasoning in Action

Recall Kate, who was described in the opening scenario. She was deaf and had a cochlear implant at 2 years of age. She is now 5 years of age. She hears sounds, is working to integrate sounds with meaning, and attends speech therapy each week. Kate is fortunate that she has two parents who are able to attend speech therapy with her and reinforce learning at home. They are concerned about finding the best kindergarten for her to attend next year.

1. Describe the normal speech patterns of a 5-year-old. How are Kate's patterns likely to differ?
2. Refer back to the Denver II Developmental Screening Test described in Chapter 7 ∞. Are there any items for the 5-year-old that might be difficult for Kate? If so, which ones?
3. Which immunization is especially important for Kate to receive in order to prevent a risk of meningitis with her cochlear implant? How will you counsel parents about this and help them find a resource for immunizations?
4. Provide a list of questions that Kate's parents can ask as they visit and evaluate kindergartens. What characteristics will be especially important for them to consider?

See Pearson Nursing Student Resources for possible responses.

References

Alme, A. M., Mulhern, M. L., Hejkal, T. W., Meza, J. L., Qiu, F., Ingvoldstad, D. D., & Margalit, E. (2008). Outcome of retinopathy of prematurity following adoption of revised indications for therapy. *BMC Ophthalmology, 8,* 23.

American Academy of Pediatrics. (2007). Recommendations for preventive pediatric health care. *Pediatrics, 120,* 1376.

American Academy of Pediatrics. (2009). Clinical report—Hearing assessment in infants and children: Recommendations beyond neonatal screening. *Pediatrics, 124,* 1252–1263.

American Academy of Pediatrics, Committee on Infectious Diseases. (2009). *Red book* (28th ed.). Elk Grove Village, IL: Author.

American Academy of Pediatrics, Subcommittee on Management of Acute Otitis Media. (2004). Diagnosis and management of acute otitis media. *Pediatrics, 113,* 1451–1465.

American Association of Endodontists. (2010). Traumatic dental injury. Retrieved from http://www.aae.org/patients/patientinfo/faqs/traumaticdentalinjuries.htm

Bernius, M., & Perlin, D. (2006). Pediatric ear, nose, and throat emergencies. *Pediatric Clinics of North America, 53,* 195–214.

Bielory, L. (2010). Allergic conjunctivitis and the impact of allergic rhinitis. *Current Allergy and Asthma Reports, 10*(2), 122–134.

Bindler, R. M., & Howry, L. B. (2005). *Pediatric drug guide.* Upper Saddle River, NJ: Prentice Hall-Health.

Bonsignori, F., Chiappini, E., & De Martino, M. (2010). The infections of the upper respiratory tract in children. *International Journal of Immunopathology and Pharmacology, 23* (1 suppl.), 16–19.

Braverman, R. (2007). Diagnosis and treatment of refractive errors in the pediatric population. *Current Opinion in Ophthalmology, 18,* 379–383.

Center for Health and Health Care in Schools. (2007). *Childhood vision: Public challenges and opportunities.* Retrieved from http://www.healthinschools.org

Centers for Disease Control and Prevention. (2008). *Streptococcus pneumoniae disease.* Retrieved from http://www.cdc.gov/ncidod/dbmd/diseaseinfo/streppneum_t.htm

Council on Children with Disabilities. (2006). Identifying infants and young children with developmental disorders in the medical home: An algorithm for developmental surveillance and screening. *Pediatrics, 118*(1), 405–420.

Daly, K. A., Hoffman, H. J., Kvaerner, K. J., Kvestad, E., Casselbrant, M. L., Homol, P., & Rovers, M. M. (2009). Epidemiology, natural history and risk factors: Panel report from the 9th International Research Conference on Otitis Media. *International Journal of Pediatric Otolaryngology, 74*(3), 231–240.

Demetroulakos, J. L. (2007). Sinusitis. *MedlinePlus.* Retrieved from http://nih.gov

DeMuri, G. P., & Wald, E. R. (2010). Acute sinusitis: Clinical manifestations and treatment approaches. *Pediatric Annals, 39*(1), 34–40.

Donahue, S. P. (2007). Pediatric strabismus. *New England Journal of Medicine, 356,* 1040–1047.

Donahue, S. P., Lorenz, S., & Johnson, T. (2008). Photo screening around the world: Lions Clubs International Foundation experience. *Seminars in Ophthalmology, 23*(5), 294–297.

Doshi, N. R., & Rodriguez, L. F. (2007). Amblyopia. *American Family Physician, 75,* 361–368.

Dudas, R. (2006). Retropharyngeal abscess. *Pediatrics in Review, 27,* 45–46.

Dunlap, L. L. (2008). *An introduction to early childhood special education.* Upper Saddle River, NJ: Pearson Allyn & Bacon.

Foxlee, R., Johansson, A., Wejfalk, J., Dawkins, J., Dooley, L., & Del Mar, C. (2006). Topical analgesia for acute otitis media. *Cochrane Database Systematic Review, 19,* CD005657.

Galito, N. J. (2008). Peritonsillar abscess. *American Family Physician, 77,* 199–202, 209.

Goldman, R. D. (2009). Cough and cold medications are risky for children. *Journal of Pediatrics, 155*(3), 451–452.

Green, J. H. (2007). Fetal alcohol spectrum disorders: Understanding the effects of prenatal alcohol exposure and supporting students. *Journal of School Health, 77*(3), 103–106.

Health Care Guide. (2008). *Epistaxis.* Retrieved from http://www.health-care-guide.org/epistaxis.htm

Hunter, L. L., Davey, C. S., Kohtz, A., & Daly, K. A. (2007). Hearing screening and middle ear measure in American Indian infants and toddlers. *International Journal of Pediatric Otorhinolaryngology, 71,* 1429–1438.

Hyde, M., & Power, D. (2006). *Cochlear implants in children: Ethics and Choices.* Washington, DC: Gallaudet University Press.

International Committee for the Classification of Retinopathy of Prematurity. (2005). The international classification of retinopathy of prematurity revisited. *Archives of Ophthalmology, 123,* 991–999.

Joint Committee on Infant Hearing. (2007). Year 2007 position statement: Principles and guidelines for early hearing detection and intervention programs. *Pediatrics, 120,* 898–921.

Kimel, L. S. (2006). Lack of follow-up exams after failed school vision screenings: An investigation of contributing factors. *Journal of School Nursing, 22,* 156–162.

Kliegman, R. M., Behrman, R. E., Jenson, H. B., & Stanton, B. F. (2007). *Nelson textbook of pediatrics* (18th ed.). Philadelphia: Saunders.

Leach, A. J., & Morris, P. S. (2007). Antibiotics for the prevention of acute and chronic suppurative otitis media in children. *Cochrane Reviews, 2,* 697–760.

Leman, R., Clausen, M. M., Bates, J., Stark, L., Arnold, K. K., & Arnold, R. W. (2006). A comparison of patched HOTV visual acuity and photoscreening. *Journal of School Nursing, 22,* 237–243.

Lett, S. M., DeMaria, A., Huot, J., Wesson, J., Karumuri, S., Truong, L., et al. (2007). Emergence of antimicrobial-resistant serotype 19A *Streptococcus pneumoniae*—Massachusetts, 2001–2006. *Morbidity and Mortality Weekly Report 56*(41), 1077–1080.

Lichtenstein, S. J., Dorfman, M., Kennedy, R., & Stroman, D. (2006). Controlling contagious bacterial conjunctivitis. *Journal of Pediatric Ophthalmology & Strabismus, 43,* 19–26.

Lim, J., & McKean, M. C. (2009). Adenotonsillectomy for obstructive sleep apnoea in children. *Cochrane Database Systematic Review, 15*(2), CD003136.

Mah, F. (2006). Bacterial conjunctivitis. *Pediatric Clinics of North America, 53*(Suppl. 1), 7–10.

Marseglia, G. L., Poddighe, D., Caimmi, D., Marseglia, A., Caimmi, S., Ciprandi, G., et al. (2009). Role of adenoids and adenoiditis in children with allergy and otitis media. *Current Allergy and Asthma Reports, 9*(6), 460–464.

Martin, J. M. (2010). Pharyngitis and streptococcal throat infections. *Pediatric Annals, 39*(1), 22–27.

Nageswaran, S., Woods, C. R., Benjamin, D. K., & Shetty, L. (2006). Orbital cellulitis in children. *Pediatric Infectious Disease Journal, 25,* 695–699.

National Institutes of Health. (2007). *Cochlear implants.* Washington, DC: Author.

Neto, J. F., Hemb, L., & Silva, D. B. (2006). Systematic literature review of modifiable risk factors for recurrent acute otitis media in childhood. *Journal of Pediatrics (Rio J), 82,* 87–96.

Nield, L. S., Mangano, L. M., & Kamat, D. (2008). Strabismus: A close-up look. *Consultant for Pediatricians,* January, 17–25.

O'Connor, A. R., Wilson, C. M., & Fielder, A. R. (2007). Ophthalmological problems associated with preterm birth. *Eye, 21,* 1254–1260.

Otitis Media with Effusion. (2004). Clinical practice guideline. *Pediatrics, 113,* 1412–1429.

Page, N. C., Bauer, E. M., & Lieu, J. E. C. (2008). Clinical features and treatment of retropharyngeal abscess in children. *Otolaryngology—Head and Neck Surgery, 138,* 300–306.

Pichichero, M. E., Casey, J. R., Hoberman, A., & Schwartz, G. (2008). Pathogens causing recurrent and difficult-to-treat acute otitis media, 2003–2006. *Clinical Pediatrics, 47*(9), 901–906.

Quintanilla-Dieck, M. L., Artunduaga, M. A., & Eavey, R. D. (2009). Intentional exposure to loud music: The second MTV.com survey reveals an opportunity to educate. *Journal of Pediatrics, 155*(4), 550–555.

Rosenfeld, R. M., Brown, L., Cannon, C. R., Dolor, R. J., Ganiats, T. G., Hannley, M., et al., & American Academy of Otolaryngology—Head and Neck Surgery Foundation. (2006). Clinical practice guideline: Acute otitis externa. *Otolaryngology—Head and Neck Surgery, 134*(4 Suppl.), S4–23.

Shetty, K. (2006). Oral lesions commonly associated with pediatric HIV infection—presentation, management, and review of the literature. *General Dentistry, 54,* 284–287

Subramanian, M. (2007). *Color blindness.* Retrieved from http://medlineplus.gov

Tasman, W., Patz, A., McNamara, J. A., Kaiser, R. S., Trese, M. T., & Smith, B. T. (2006). Retinopathy of prematurity: The life of a lifetime disease. *American Journal of Ophthalmology, 141,* 167–174.

U.S. Department of Health and Human Services. (2010). *Healthy People 2020.* Retrieved from http://www.healthypeople.gov

U.S. Food and Drug Administration. (2007). *Public health advisory. Nonprescription cough and cold medicine use in children.* Retrieved from http://www.fda.gov;Drugs/DrugSafety/PublicHealthAdvisories/UCM051282

U.S. Food and Drug Administration. (2008). Cochlear implants and bacterial meningitis. *ORL Head and Neck Nursing, 26*(1), 24.

U.S. Preventive Services Task Force. (2005). Screening for visual impairment in children younger than five years: Recommendation statement. *American Family Physician, 71,* 333–336.

Wagner, R. S., & Aquino, M. (2008). Pediatric ocular inflammation. *Immunology and Allergy Clinics of North America, 28*(1), 169–188.

Weichbold, V., Nekahm-Heis, D., & Welzl-Mueller, K. (2006). Universal newborn hearing screening and postnatal hearing loss. *Pediatrics, 117,* 3631–3636.

Weichbold, V., & Zorowka, P. (2007). Can a hearing education campaign for adolescents change their music listening behavior? *International Journal of Audiology, 46,* 128–133.

Windmill, S., & Windmill, I. M. (2006). The status of diagnostic testing following referral from universal newborn hearing screening. *Journal of the American Academy of Audiology, 17,* 367–378.

Yaeger, D., McCallum, J., Lewis, K., Soslow, L., Shah, U., Potsic, W., . . . Krantz, I. D. (2006). Outcomes of clinical examination and genetic testing of 500 individuals with hearing loss evaluated through a genetics of hearing loss clinic. *American Journal of Medical Genetics, 140,* 827–836.

Yang, M., Quah, B. L., Seah, L. L., & Looi, A. (2009). Orbital cellulitis in children—medical treatment versus surgical management. *Orbit, 28*(2–3), 124–136.

Yang, M. B., Donovan, E. F., & Wagge, J. R. (2006). Race, gender, and clinical risk index for babies (CRIB) score as predictors of severe retinopathy of prematurity. *Journal of American Association for Pediatric Ophthalmology and Strabismus, 10,* 253–261.

Zhao, F., Manchaian, V. K., French, D., & Price, S. M. (2010). Music exposure and hearing disorders: An overview. *International Journal of Audiology, 49*(1), 54–64.

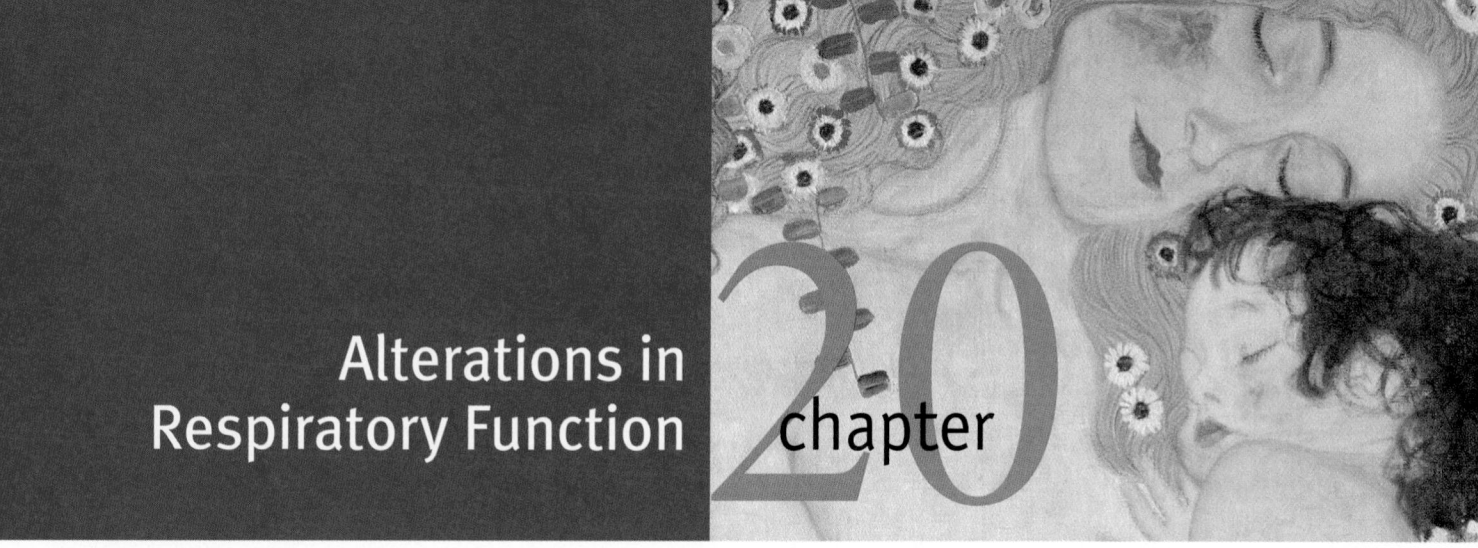

Alterations in Respiratory Function

chapter 20

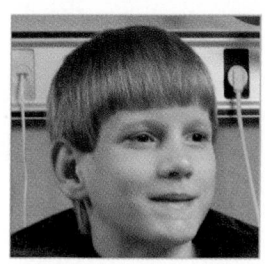

Shaun, a 13-year-old with cystic fibrosis, lives with his mother and a sister who does not have cystic fibrosis. He is in the seventh grade and enjoys riding his bicycle. He usually spends a few days in the university medical center each year for intensive therapy sessions to clear his lungs.

It takes a lot of time each day to manage cystic fibrosis. All of Shaun's care must be scheduled around school and recreation. In most cases, the treatments cut into his recreational time. Shaun has learned to manage many aspects of his care, relieving his mother of some tasks. Shaun sets up his nebulizer and correctly measures the amount of DNase to use. After the nebulizer treatment, he uses an oscillating vest for airway clearance for about 20 minutes. Coughing up the sputum during and after the treatment is very tiring.

Shaun needs extra calories to grow and to meet metabolic demands. His mother works hard to prepare and provide the extra calories he needs throughout the day, and he takes pancreatic enzymes to help him digest food. Because Shaun sometimes has difficulty getting enough calories to support adolescent growth, he has a gastrostomy tube for nighttime feedings.

Why are children with cystic fibrosis at higher risk for respiratory infections? What are signs of a respiratory infection and respiratory distress in infants and children? What nursing care should be provided to a child with a respiratory condition?

Learning Outcomes

After reading this chapter, you will be able to do the following:

1. Describe unique characteristics of the pediatric respiratory system anatomy and physiology.
2. Contrast the respiratory conditions and injuries that can cause respiratory distress in infants and children.
3. Distinguish between mild, moderate, and severe respiratory distress in a child, and plan the appropriate nursing care for each level of respiratory distress severity.
4. Assess the child's respiratory status and analyze the need for oxygen supplementation.
5. Differentiate between the signs and symptoms of a child with an upper airway and a lower airway respiratory condition.
6. Create a nursing care plan for a child with a common acute respiratory condition.
7. Plan the nursing care for the child with a chronic respiratory condition.
8. Demonstrate the nursing assessment for a child with an acute lung injury.

FOCUS ON

The Respiratory System

ANATOMY AND PHYSIOLOGY

The respiratory system is composed of both the upper and lower airways. The upper airway, containing the nasopharynx and oropharynx, serves as the pathway for gases exchanged during **ventilation**, the movement of oxygen into the lungs and carbon dioxide out of the lungs. The larynx divides the upper and lower airways. See Figure 20–1 ➤. The lower airways (trachea, bronchi, and bronchioles) serve as the pathway of gases to the alveoli in the lungs. The left lung is divided into two lobes, and the right lung is divided into three lobes. Alveolar sacs surrounded by capillaries are located at the end of the airways and are the site of gas exchange, where oxygen diffuses across the alveolocapillary membrane. Surfactant secreted by alveolar cells coats the inner surface of the alveolus to allow expansion during inspiration. The lung tissue surrounding the airways keeps them from collapsing as the oxygen moves in and carbon dioxide moves out during ventilation. The lungs are positioned in the thoracic cavity, where the ribs and muscles protect the lungs from injury.

The intercostal muscles work with the diaphragm to perform the work of breathing. The diaphragm is a muscle that separates the abdominal and thoracic cavity contents. When the diaphragm contracts, it creates negative pressure that increases the thoracic volume and pulls air into the lungs. The lungs and chest wall have the ability to expand during inspiration (**compliance**) and then to recoil or return to the resting state with expiration. The work of breathing is tied to the muscular effort required for ventilation, which can be increased in cases of disorders that increase the stiffness of the lungs or obstruct the airways.

The respiratory center in the brain controls respiration, sending impulses to the respiratory muscles to contract and relax. Breathing is usually involuntary as the nervous system automatically adjusts the ventilatory rate and volume to maintain normal gas exchange (Brashers, 2010b). Chemoreceptors monitor the pH, $PaCO_2$, and PaO_2 in the arterial blood and send signals to the respiratory center to increase ventilation in cases of

As Children Grow

Airway Development

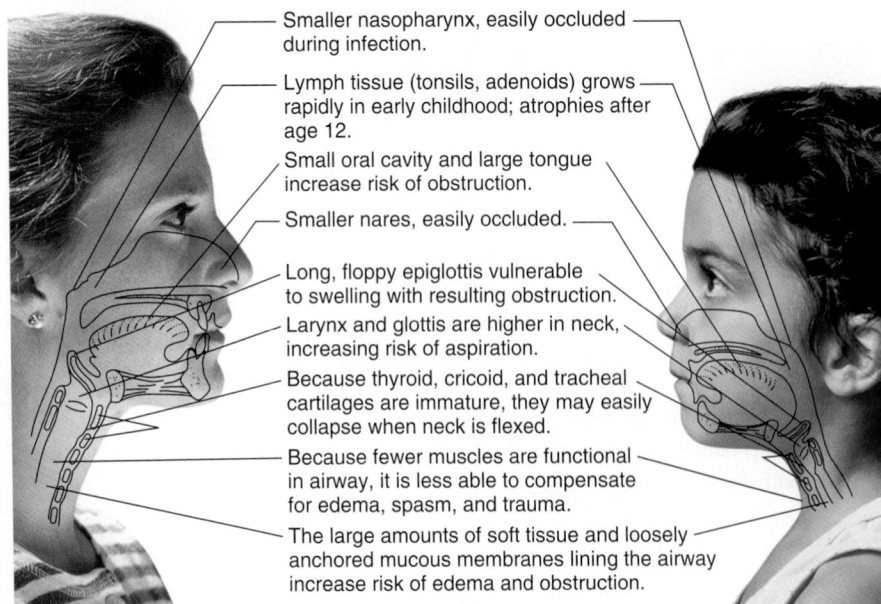

Smaller nasopharynx, easily occluded during infection.

Lymph tissue (tonsils, adenoids) grows rapidly in early childhood; atrophies after age 12.

Small oral cavity and large tongue increase risk of obstruction.

Smaller nares, easily occluded.

Long, floppy epiglottis vulnerable to swelling with resulting obstruction.

Larynx and glottis are higher in neck, increasing risk of aspiration.

Because thyroid, cricoid, and tracheal cartilages are immature, they may easily collapse when neck is flexed.

Because fewer muscles are functional in airway, it is less able to compensate for edema, spasm, and trauma.

The large amounts of soft tissue and loosely anchored mucous membranes lining the airway increase risk of edema and obstruction.

FIGURE 20–1 ➤ It is easy to see that a child's airway is smaller and less developed than an adult's airway, but why is this important? An upper respiratory tract infection, allergic reaction, positioning of the head and neck during sleep, and the small objects children play with can have serious consequences in the child.

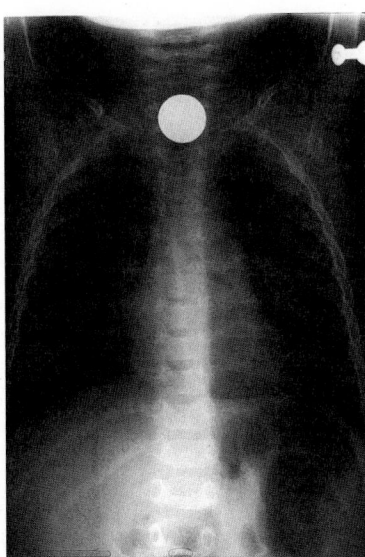

FIGURE 20–5 ➤ An aspirated foreign body (coin) is clearly visible in the child's trachea on this chest radiograph.
Courtesy of Rockwood Clinic, Spokane, WA.

changes in breath sounds, from noisy to decreasing to absent, on the affected side. This can indicate that the object is moving and blocking a mainstem bronchus. Attach the child to a cardiorespiratory monitor and pulse oximeter to assess the child for subtle signs of increasing hypoxia. See the *Clinical Skills Manual.* Be concerned if the pulse oximetry reading (SpO_2) drops to less than 95%.

Clinical Tip

The accuracy of pulse oximetry readings (SpO_2) may be affected by placing the sensor probe over nailbeds with dark nail polish or when the sensor is in bright light or sunshine. Some pulse oximeters may be less accurate if the sensor is on a moving extremity. Make sure the heart rate detected by the pulse oximeter matches the child's heart rate by direct assessment for accuracy. An inaccurate reading may also occur if peripheral blood flow is decreased due to vasoconstriction, arrhythmias, or shock (Valdez-Lowe, Ghareeb, & Artinian, 2009).

Psychosocial Assessment

The unexpected and acute nature of the event creates anxiety for the parents. The child will be fearful because of difficulty breathing. Assess their coping ability and level of stress.

Developmental Assessment

As the child's condition stabilizes, observe how well the child's abilities match the parents' understanding of age-appropriate behaviors. See Chapters 7 and 8 ∞.

Common nursing diagnoses for a child with an AFB include:

- Ineffective Airway Clearance related to obstruction by foreign body
- Impaired Spontaneous Ventilations related to respiratory muscle fatigue
- Anxiety (Child) related to difficulty breathing, unfamiliar surroundings and procedures
- Risk for Injury related to small objects in environment

Planning and Implementation

When the airway is totally obstructed, administer chest thrusts and back blows to an infant or abdominal thrusts to a child in an effort to remove the AFB. (See the *Clinical Skills Manual.*) When the child has a partial obstruction, remain with the child and have resuscitation equipment at the bedside. Permit the child to stay in a position of comfort. Avoid performing procedures that increase the child's anxiety as sudden movements and increased respiratory efforts may cause the obstruction to move and completely obstruct the airway.

After the AFB is removed, the child is stabilized and observed for a few hours in a short-stay unit to ensure that there are no respiratory complications.

Discharge Planning and Home Care Teaching

Discharge planning centers on anticipatory guidance about childproofing the home (see Chapters 7 and 8 ∞). Encourage the parents to learn cardiopulmonary resuscitation (CPR), back blows, chest thrusts, and abdominal thrusts.

Evaluation

Expected outcomes of nursing care include:

- The child ventilates spontaneously after removal of the foreign body.
- Parents complete a safety check of the home to prevent future aspiration incidents.

Respiratory Failure

Respiratory failure occurs when the body can no longer maintain effective gas exchange, and often results from a serious acute or chronic respiratory or neuromuscular condition. Acute lung injury can result from sepsis, pneumonia, meconium aspiration, aspiration of stomach contents, smoke inhalation, and drowning. Many of these conditions are discussed later in the chapter. See Chapter 27 ∞ for information about drowning. The acute lung injury causes an inflammatory-immune response and alveolar-capillary membrane damage.

The physiologic process that ends in respiratory failure begins with hypoventilation of the alveoli. Hypoventilation occurs when the body's need for oxygen exceeds actual oxygen intake, the airway is partially occluded, lung injury has occurred, or the exchange of oxygen and carbon dioxide in the alveoli is disrupted. This disruption may occur for the following reasons:

- A malfunction of respiratory center stimulation occurs (the alveoli do not receive the message to diffuse, e.g., due to an opioid overdose).
- The muscles of ventilation are fatigued and do not work effectively (e.g., a severe asthma exacerbation).
- The relationship between ventilation and blood flow to the alveoli is impaired (see the companion website for more information).

Gas Exchange Animation

Poor ventilation of the alveoli results in **hypoxemia** (lower-than-normal blood oxygen level) and **hypercapnia** (an excess of carbon dioxide in the blood). See Appendix D ∞ for expected laboratory values by age. When the blood levels of oxygen and carbon dioxide reach abnormal levels, **hypoxia** (lower-than-normal oxygen in the tissues) occurs and respiratory failure begins.

Signs of impending respiratory failure include irritability, lethargy, mottled color or cyanosis, and increased respiratory effort such as dyspnea, tachypnea, nasal flaring, and intercostal retractions. **Grunting** (a moaning or crying-like sound that is produced by forceful expiration against closed vocal cords in an effort to prevent alveolar collapse) helps maintain lung volume and alveolar pressures. It is a sign of severe distress in the newborn and may signal the onset of respiratory failure (Cifuentes & Carlo, 2007). *Hypoxemia that persists when supplemental oxygen is given is a sign of respiratory failure.* See the Clinical Manifestations table on this page.

Nursing Alert

When the child in respiratory distress has had increased respiratory effort over a prolonged period, a decreasing respiratory rate is a critical sign of impending respiratory arrest. The ventilatory muscles are so fatigued that the child will soon stop breathing.

Pulse oximetry and arterial blood gases are used to assess respiratory failure. See Appendix D ∞ for expected laboratory values. Refer to Chapter 18 ∞ for interpretation of acidosis and alkalosis that must be considered simultaneously.

Medical management is focused on treating the cause of respiratory failure and reversing the severe hypoxemia with oxygen, mechanical ventilation, and continuous positive airway pressure (CPAP). See Figure 20–6 ➤. These children are admitted to the intensive care unit (ICU) for monitoring and ventilatory support.

As the level of responsiveness decreases, the tongue may obstruct the airway. Endotracheal (ET) intubation is a short-

Clinical Manifestations
Respiratory Failure and Imminent Respiratory Arrest

Physiologic Cause	Clinical Manifestations
Initial Respiratory Failure The child is trying to compensate for oxygen deficit and airway blockage. Oxygen supply is inadequate; behavior and vital signs reflect compensation and beginning hypoxia.	Restlessness Tachypnea Tachycardia Diaphoresis
Early Decompensation The child uses accessory muscles to assist oxygen intake; hypoxia persists and breathing efforts now waste more oxygen than is obtained.	Nasal flaring Retractions Grunting Wheezing Anxiety and irritability Mood changes Headache Hypertension Confusion
Severe Hypoxia and Imminent Respiratory Arrest The oxygen deficit is overwhelming and beyond spontaneous recovery. Cerebral oxygenation is dramatically affected; central nervous system changes are ominous.	Dyspnea Bradycardia Cyanosis Stupor and coma

term, emergency measure to stabilize the airway. The ET tube must be protected and stabilized to prevent its displacement. End-tidal CO_2 monitoring to measure carbon dioxide expiration is helpful to ensure that the tube is positioned in the trachea. (See the *Clinical Skills Manual.*) A tracheostomy is the creation of a surgical opening into the trachea through the anterior neck at the cricoid cartilage when longer term airway

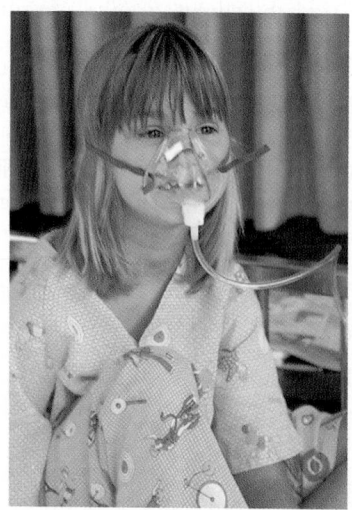 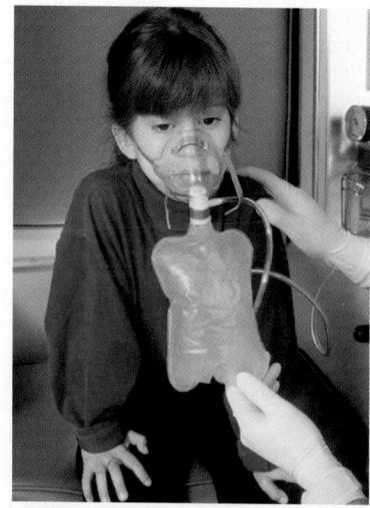 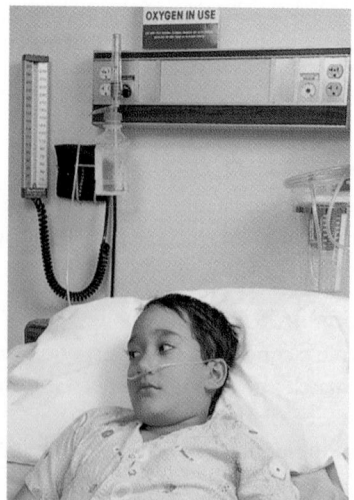

FIGURE 20–6 ➤ Various oxygen delivery devices are used to give supplemental oxygen to children. Oxygen delivery devices are selected to match the concentration of oxygen needed by the child. In respiratory failure, a higher concentration of oxygen is needed to reverse the hypoxemia. Which oxygen delivery device should be used? Are there any contraindications to oxygen use in a child who is hypoxic?

management is needed. The child may be sedated to optimize ventilation. CPAP is used to improve oxygenation and lung compliance. Death results if respiratory failure cannot be successfully managed.

Nursing Management

Early recognition of impending respiratory failure is an important nursing function for a child with any signs of respiratory compromise. Signs and symptoms can progress rapidly, and detection of subtle early signs is essential so that intervention can begin and prevent progression to cardiopulmonary arrest. When the child has a chronic respiratory condition, development of respiratory failure may be gradual. Be particularly alert to behavior changes in addition to respiratory signs. Serial blood gases may be needed to monitor the child.

Nursing Alert

As the child tires from the prolonged effort of breathing, the respiratory rate may begin to decrease. This is an ominous sign and may progress to respiratory arrest without intervention.

Excessive crying and anxiety deplete metabolic reserves and increase oxygen demand. Comfort the child and avoid invasive procedures that will increase distress. Place a child who has respiratory distress in an upright position (by elevating the head of the bed).

Assess respiratory quality and rate, followed by apical pulse rate and temperature. Monitor oxygen saturation with pulse oximetry. Administer oxygen as ordered and keep respiratory emergency equipment at the child's bedside. Monitor the child for changes in vital signs, respiratory status, and level of responsiveness. Be prepared to assist ventilations if respiratory status deteriorates. (See the *Clinical Skills Manual.*)

Because endotracheal and tracheostomy tubes prevent vocal cord vibration, intubated children cannot cry or talk. Infants and young children often express initial frustration when they realize they cannot communicate verbally. When the child is alert, give suggestions for ways to make noise and gain attention, such as striking the mattress. A communication board can be used with older children. Suction airway secretions as needed and provide tracheostomy care. (See the *Clinical Skills Manual.*)

Many children are discharged from the hospital and cared for at home for an extended period with a tracheostomy tube in place. It is essential to teach parents how to maintain the airway, clean the tracheostomy site, and change the tube. A home health care nurse can provide follow-up care and support for the child and family.

■ APNEA

Periodic breathing, an irregular rhythm with pauses of *up to* 20 seconds between breaths, occurs commonly in newborns. This breathing pattern is not apnea. **Apnea** is the cessation of respiration lasting longer than 20 seconds, or any pause in respiration associated with cyanosis, marked pallor, hypotonia, or bradycardia. Apnea may be the first major sign of respiratory dysfunction in the neonate.

Complementary Therapy
Vanilla

The introduction of a pleasant odor (vanillin) into the incubator of a preterm infant with apnea of prematurity was associated with decreased episodes of apnea greater than 20 seconds without bradycardia. The 14 infants exposed to the pleasant odor had been unresponsive to traditional treatment for apnea of prematurity with caffeine or doxapram. No side effects to the therapy were noted (Marlier, Gaugler, & Messer, 2005).

Apnea of Prematurity

Apnea of prematurity is defined as apnea in an infant younger than 37 weeks' gestation and is often associated with immature respiratory control. Although the cause is unknown, it may occur when the infant's baseline CO_2 (the physiologic stimulus for breathing) decreases below the apnea threshold (Al-Saif, Alvard, Manfreda, et al., 2008). Apneic episodes often occur during periods of active sleep. Infants are treated with methylxanthines (usually caffeine). Episodes usually disappear when the newborn's respiratory system matures, usually by 37 weeks' gestational age (Silvestri, 2009).

Apparent Life-Threatening Event (ALTE)

An ALTE is defined as an episode of apnea accompanied by a color change (e.g., cyanosis or pallor), limp muscle tone, choking, or gagging. The majority of these events involve a significant cardiovascular event. The episodes often occur in infants at a median age of 2 months, but less than 12 months (Silvestri, 2008). These episodes may occur during sleep, wakefulness, or feeding. Some children have repeated episodes. Do not confuse ALTE with sudden infant death syndrome (SIDS); see page 561.

A cause is identified in more than 50% of infants who experience ALTE. The most common causes include prematurity, gastroesophageal reflux, sepsis, lower respiratory tract infections, seizures or other neurologic problems, child abuse, and Munchausen syndrome by proxy (Silvestri, 2008). In some cases, no cause is identified. The ALTE episode frightens the parent, who often fears the infant has died. Vigorous stimulation or resuscitation is required to stop the episode.

Clinical therapy is focused on identifying the cause of ALTE and then providing effective treatment. The infant is usually admitted to the hospital for evaluation and cardiorespiratory monitoring. Blood, urine, and cerebrospinal fluid are collected to rule out hematology, electrolyte, infectious, metabolic, and toxicology conditions. Studies for gastroesophageal reflux may be performed. An electroencephalogram may be performed to investigate seizures as a cause. An electrocardiogram and other cardiac testing may be performed to identify any cardiac defects or arrhythmias. Radiographic imaging of the chest and brain may be performed. The diagnostic testing selected will be initially focused on the most likely cause identified by history and physical examination. No minimum set of diagnostic tests have been identified to evaluate individual children (Silvestri, 2008). An infant may be sent home with an apnea monitor and event recorder for 4 to 6 weeks when the infant is at risk for additional events and no cause has been identified (Silvestri, 2009).

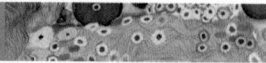

Nursing Alert

Home apnea monitors do not detect obstructive apnea or hypoxemia. The monitor interprets the struggle to breathe as respiratory activity. By the time the monitor detects bradycardia and the absence of breathing, the infant may have profound hypoxemia and be challenging to resuscitate (Halbower, 2008).

NURSING MANAGEMENT

Nursing care includes collecting a detailed history of the event, observing and monitoring cardiorespiratory status, providing supportive care to the infant and family, participating in the diagnostic process, and anticipating the need for emergency resuscitation.

Obtain a Detailed History

Obtain information about the characteristics and duration of the event and the intervention used by the parent to end it. Identify whether the infant was awake or asleep when the episode occurred.

Monitor Cardiorespiratory Status

Cardiorespiratory monitoring records heart rate and respiratory rate while the infant is awake and asleep. Pulse oximetry provides a noninvasive continuous evaluation of the infant's oxygenation. A pulse oximetry reading (SpO_2) less than 95% indicates hypoxemia. Because the infant who has had ALTE may be at risk for cardiopulmonary arrest, keep emergency resuscitation equipment and drugs readily accessible at all times.

Provide Emotional Support

Establishing rapport and open communication with the parents will help them develop a sense of trust. Parents are naturally fearful and anxious about the infant's prognosis. Explanations of tests and treatment help to decrease their anxiety and increase their understanding of the situation.

During hospitalization the infant should be held and cuddled to provide a sense of security and well-being. Encouraging parents' participation in the infant's care helps to meet these needs. Often parents are hesitant to touch the infant because they are afraid of disconnecting the monitoring cable. Wrapping the cable inside the infant's blanket helps secure the wires, increasing parents' feelings of confidence in handling the infant.

Support the mother to continue breastfeeding and maintain a supply of breast milk by pumping, if necessary. Ensure that the mother gets adequate fluids and nutrition.

Discharge Planning and Home Care Teaching

Identify and address home care needs well in advance of discharge. Teach parents how to use and operate a home apnea monitor recorder if one is prescribed. See Families Want to Know: Using a Home Apnea Monitor. Parents also need to learn what to do when the infant has an apneic episode, and how to perform CPR and choking-management techniques.

Obstructive Sleep Apnea

Obstructive sleep apnea syndrome (OSAS) is defined as recurrent episodes of partial and complete upper airway obstruction that disrupts normal sleep and interferes with adequate respiration (Perez & Davidson Ward, 2008). This results in breathing difficulty and snoring when the child sleeps. OSAS occurs more commonly between 2 and 8 years of age when tonsils and adenoids are at their largest in contrast to the airway's size. Conditions that increase the risk for OSAS include obesity, craniofacial abnormalities, Down syndrome, sickle cell disease, and cerebral palsy.

Epidemiology and Pathophysiology

The upper airway contains about 30 muscles that permit the pharynx to collapse, enabling the child to talk and swallow, but also maintain airway patency. When the child is awake, muscle tone is maintained and the airway remains patent even when ob-

Families Want to Know
Using a Home Apnea Monitor

Emergency Preparation

■ Have an emergency plan and complete an emergency information form about the infant's health problem.

■ Post important phone numbers (e.g., rescue squad, physician, equipment company, power company, neighbor, parents' work numbers) and CPR guidelines in several places in the home; add extra phone handsets or carry a cell phone.

■ Learn CPR, back blows, and chest thrusts for airway obstruction.

■ Keep the apnea monitor battery fully charged.

Safety Precautions

■ Place the monitor on a firm surface, away from water and other appliances (television, microwave oven).

■ Ensure that alarms are audible from all locations.

■ Ensure that the monitor is turned on.

■ Thread cable and wires through the lower end of the infant's clothes.

Routine Care

■ Understand reasons for the apnea monitor and frequency of use. Review the manual for troubleshooting.

■ Learn how to attach and detach infant chest leads and belt. Care for the skin by moving patches correctly, and use no oils or lotions on the chest. Evaluate skin for irritation or sores under the electrodes; move electrode if skin is irritated.

Responding to an Alarm

■ First observe the infant to determine if the alarm is for a real event or a loose lead.

■ Stimulate the infant if bradycardia is present, respiration is absent, or the infant is lethargic. Start by gently touching and proceed to vigorous touch if needed.

■ If no response, proceed with CPR.

Loose Lead

■ Check the electrode patch. Is it loose? Dirty? Belt loose?

■ Check wires from the electrode or monitor cable.

■ Check power supply. Is battery low? Power failure? Monitor malfunctioning?

structions such as enlarged adenoids and tonsils, craniofacial anomalies, or obesity are present. During sleep, the airway muscles relax, the pharynx becomes obstructed, and airway resistance is increased. Obstruction then results in apnea episodes that lead to hypoventilation, hypoxia, hypercapnia, and an elevated blood pressure. Without treatment, complications develop that can include growth failure, systemic and pulmonary hypertension, and metabolic disorders such as insulin resistance and dyslipidemia (Perez & Davidson Ward, 2008).

Clinical Manifestations

Children with OSAS snore loudly, especially in the supine position. Signs of labored breathing during sleep may include retractions and paradoxical breathing. After pauses in snoring or lack of airflow, the child may be noted to snort, gasp, choke, move, or arouse to take a breath. Sleep is restless and the child may sleep in unusual positions to hyperextend the neck and airway. The child may mouth breathe when awake. Daytime sleepiness and other symptoms of sleep deprivation (poor attention, increased activity, aggression, acting-out behavior, poor school performance) may be noted.

COLLABORATIVE CARE

Diagnosis is made by **polysomnography**, a sleep study that simultaneously records the brain activity, eye movement, apnea episodes, oxygen desaturation, and sleep disturbances. Adenoidectomy and tonsillectomy is the most common treatment for OSAS, and resolution of the condition occurs in the majority of children. Children with obesity have a greater risk for persistent OSAS after surgery (Hoban & Chervin, 2007). Continuous positive airway pressure (CPAP) or bilevel positive airway pressure (BPAP) is used for children with surgical contraindications or those with persistent OSAS after adenotonsillectomy. Intranasal corticosteroids and a leukotriene modifier may be prescribed for persistent OSAS.

NURSING MANAGEMENT

In the community setting, all children should be screened for snoring as part of their routine health care. Assess the child for signs of nasal obstruction, mouth breathing, and enlarged tonsils. Determine if the child has symptoms of sleep deprivation or if a condition is present that places the child at high risk for OSAS. When snoring is present, encourage the parents to keep a sleep diary. Coordinate referral for a more extensive evaluation and polysomnogram, and explain the purpose of the test. Discuss how to prepare the child for the strange setting and wires that will be attached during the sleep study. Most pediatric centers will allow the parent to stay with the child during the study.

Following adenoidectomy and tonsillectomy, the hospital nurse monitors the child for bleeding and respiratory distress. Continuous pulse oximetry is used to detect oxygen desaturation. These children are at increased risk for respiratory distress after surgery due to complications of obstructive sleep apnea.

They should be carefully monitored postoperatively. Pain is often managed by nonopioid analgesics (acetaminophen) and complementary therapies to avoid the risk for respiratory distress. See Chapter 19 ∞ for care of the child having an adenoidectomy and tonsillectomy. The child with obesity should be referred to a weight management program.

Sleep center nurses provide education and support to families of children who need to use CPAP or BPAP to treat the OSAS. The nurse helps identify the best-fitting mask or nasal prong system. Parents may need guidance about helping children to sleep wearing the mask until they become accustomed to it.

Sudden Infant Death Syndrome

Sudden infant death syndrome (SIDS) is defined as the sudden death during sleep of an infant under 1 year of age that remains unexplained after a thorough investigation, including an autopsy, a review of the circumstances of death, and the clinical history. It was the third leading cause of death in infants less than 12 months of age in 2006 (Heron, Hoyert, Murphy, et al., 2009). Most SIDS deaths occur in infants between 2 and 4 months of age. It is currently unpredictable and in some cases unpreventable.

The interaction of multiple factors may lead to SIDS or infant asphyxia (Kinney & Thach, 2009; Fleming & Blair, 2007):

- An underlying vulnerability of the infant (e.g., a genetic cardiac dysrhythmia, such as long QT syndrome, or a defect in neural networks that control respiration, sleep, and arousal).
- A critical developmental period (such as before cardiorespiratory system maturation).
- An additional stressor (e.g., rebreathing exhaled air, being overheated, or a respiratory infection).
- Homicide may be associated with up to 5% of SIDS deaths.

See Box 20–1 for infant and maternal factors that place infants at risk for SIDS. Protective factors may be completed immunizations for age and use of a pacifier when the infant is put down to sleep (Adams, Good, & Defranco, 2009).

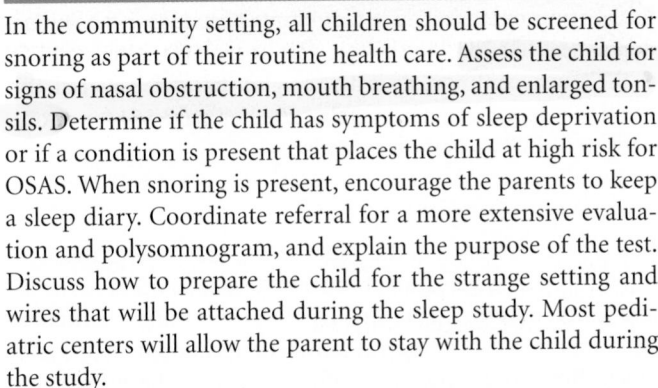

BOX 20–1 Risk Factors for Sudden Infant Death Syndrome (SIDS)

Infant Risk Factors

- Native American and Black infants at higher risk (may be a genetic factor); Whites and Asians at lower risk
- Males at higher risk (may be genetic factor)
- Preterm or low birth weight
- Maternal smoking, alcohol intake, or substance use
- Socioeconomic disadvantages (e.g., single parenthood, younger mother, fewer years of education, unemployment)

Environmental Risk Factors

- Prone or side-lying sleep position
- Bed sharing
- Soft bedding or the use of pillows, quilts, or soft toys with bedding

Data from: Fleming, P., & Blair, P. S. (2007). Sudden infant death syndrome. Sleep Medicine Clinics, 2, *463–476; Kinney, H. C., & Thach, B. T. (2009). The sudden infant death syndrome.* New England Journal of Medicine, 361(8), *795–805.*

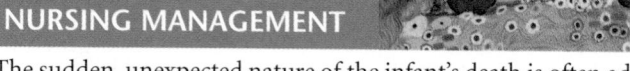

A recent population-based case-control study in 11 California counties explored how the use of a fan or open window affected the risk for SIDS. It was thought that fan use could reduce the infant's risk of re-breathing exhaled carbon monoxide trapped by the bedding near the airway. Fan use during last sleep was associated with a 72% reduction in the rate of SIDS among the study population. The effect was greater when the infant was in a warmer environment, shared a bed, and was not using a pacifier (Coleman-Phox, Odouli, & De-Kun, 2008).

The first symptom is a cardiac arrest. Clinical findings include evidence of a struggle or change in position during sleep and the presence of frothy, blood-tinged secretions from the mouth and nares. Typically parents find the infant dead in the crib in the morning or after a nap and report having heard no cries or disturbances during the night.

NURSING MANAGEMENT

The sudden, unexpected nature of the infant's death is often addressed in the emergency department. The nurse's role is to be empathetic and provide support to the family during one of its greatest crises. Special support is needed during the communication of bad news and the shock of the infant's death. See the companion website and Chapter 13 ∞ for guidelines to support the bereaved family.

Clinical Tip

Guidelines for the support of families experiencing SIDS should include baptism services, religious support, grief counseling, assistance with funeral arrangements, counseling on cessation of breast-feeding if appropriate, and sibling reactions.

Reassure the parents that they are not responsible for the infant's death, and help them contact other family members and mobilize support. Older children may need reassurance that SIDS will not happen to them. Siblings may also believe that bad thoughts or wishes about their baby brother or sister caused the death. Support groups can help parents, siblings, and other family members express these fears and work through their feelings about the infant's death. The First Candle organization can help families locate a support group in their area; see the companion website for SIDS resources.

Prevention of SIDS

Nurses play an important role in SIDS prevention. Educate the parents of all newborns and infants about the recommended infant sleep position—on the back. The Back to Sleep Campaign initiated in 1992, encouraging the placement of infants in supine position for sleeping, has led to a 50% reduction in the number of SIDS deaths. In 2008, 15% of all infants were estimated to sleep in prone position; however, the rate of prone or side-lying position for sleep is much higher among African American infants (38%) (Carrier, 2009). Ask parents to make sure the supine position is used when the infant is cared for by another family member or childcare provider. Parents should

also use a firm mattress and avoid the use of loose bedding, toys, and pillows. Bed sharing with the parent or other individual during sleep should be discouraged. Use a sleeper rather than a blanket to keep the infant warm while sleeping, and to keep covers off the face. Educate pregnant women about the dangers of exposing the fetus to tobacco smoke. Referral to a smoking cessation program should be encouraged.

Clinical Tip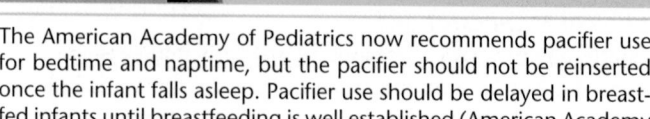

The American Academy of Pediatrics now recommends pacifier use for bedtime and naptime, but the pacifier should not be reinserted once the infant falls asleep. Pacifier use should be delayed in breast-fed infants until breastfeeding is well established (American Academy of Pediatrics, Task Force on Sudden Infant Death Syndrome, 2005).

Infants should have supervised tummy time when awake to promote motor development and to reduce infant skull flattening. See Chapter 27 ∞ for issues related to infant skull flattening (positional plagiocephaly) from the supine sleeping position.

■ CROUP SYNDROMES

Croup is a term applied to a broad classification of upper airway illnesses that result from inflammation and swelling of the epiglottis and larynx. The swelling usually extends into the trachea and bronchi. The subglottic area is the only region of the airway that has a complete cartilaginous ring that prevents the airway's outward expansion when edematous, so 1 mm of swelling can reduce the normal airway size by more than 50% (Sobol & Zapata, 2008). See Figure 20–3. Viral croup syndromes include spasmodic laryngitis and laryngotracheobronchitis (LTB). Bacterial croup syndromes include bacterial tracheitis and epiglottitis (Figure 20–7 ➤). The term *croup* is most often used to refer to LTB.

LTB and bacterial tracheitis affect a large number of children across all age groups in both sexes. Epiglottitis, previously a common serious respiratory illness, is rare in the United States due to the *Haemophilus influenzae* type b immunization. The initial symptoms of all three conditions include inspiratory stridor, a "seal-like" barking cough, and hoarseness. Although LTB is the most common disorder, epiglottitis and bacterial tracheitis are more serious. See Table 20–2 on page 564 for a comparison of LTB and croup syndromes.

Laryngotracheobronchitis

LTB is a viral invasion of the upper airway that extends throughout the larynx, trachea, and bronchi. Most cases occur in the fall and winter months. Acute viral LTB is most common in children 6 months to 3 years of age but can occur in children up to 8 years of age. Boys are affected more often than girls. The episode may last 3 to 7 days.

Etiology and Pathophysiology

Airway tissues respond to the invading virus with inflammation and edema. The laryngeal inflammation causes the airway di-

Pathophysiology Illustrated

Airway Changes with Croup

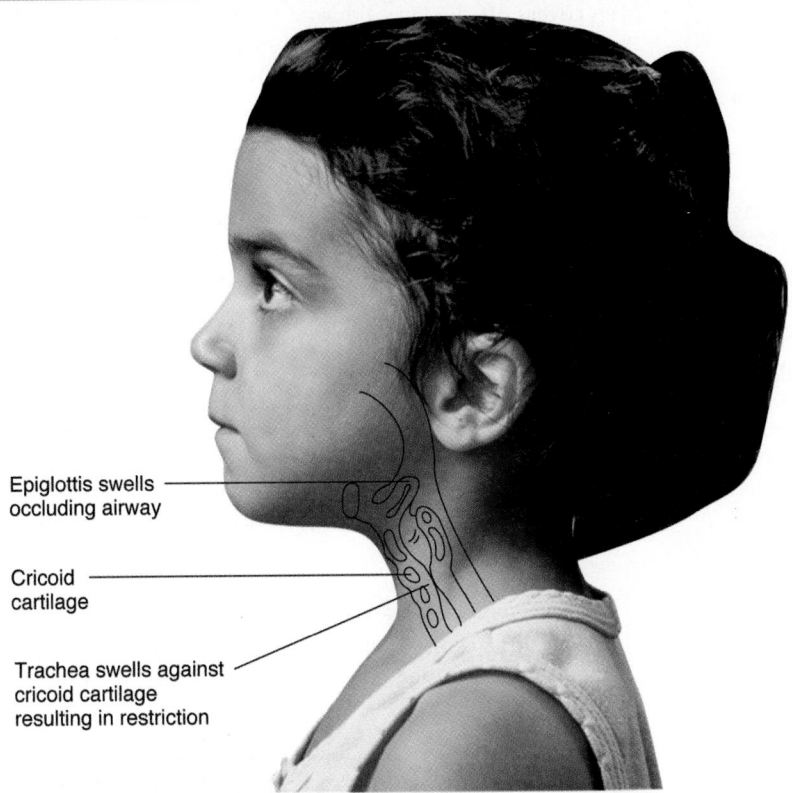

Epiglottis swells
occluding airway

Cricoid
cartilage

Trachea swells against
cricoid cartilage
resulting in restriction

FIGURE 20–7 ➤ There are two important changes in the upper airway in croup: The epiglottis swells, thereby occluding the airway, and the trachea swells against the cricoid cartilage, causing restriction and narrowing the airway.

ameter to narrow in the subglottic area, the airway's narrowest part. Copious, tenacious secretions further increase the child's respiratory distress. Even small amounts of mucus or edema can quickly obstruct the airway. Both the large and small airways can be affected. Table 20–2 compares LTB and other croup syndromes.

Clinical Manifestations

Most children brought to the emergency department with LTB have been ill for a couple of days with upper respiratory symptoms. These symptoms progress to a cough and hoarseness. Fever may or may not be present. The presence of expiratory stridor, severe tachypnea, retractions, and a low SpO_2 are associated with a more severe airway inflammation and swelling. Changes in mental status may indicate hypoxemia and potential respiratory failure.

COLLABORATIVE CARE

Diagnostic Testing

Diagnosis is often made by clinical signs. Pulse oximetry is used to detect hypoxemia. If the diagnosis of LTB is in question, anteroposterior (AP) and lateral radiographs of the upper airway may be taken; these may show symmetric subglottic narrowing called a "steeple sign." A stridor assessment score is often used to provide an objective and quantifiable measure of respiratory difficulty that can be compared with future scores (Table 20–3).

Throat cultures and visual inspection of the inner mouth and throat are contraindicated in children with LTB and epiglottitis. These procedures can cause laryngospasms (spasmodic vibrations that close the larynx) as a result of the child's anxiety or of probing this reactive and already compromised area. A complete airway obstruction may result.

Clinical Therapy

Management consists of maintaining and improving respiratory effort with medications and supplemental oxygen when the SpO_2 level is less than 92%. See Medications Used to Treat Symptomatic Laryngotracheobronchitis on page 565. Children who respond well to medications are often sent home from the emergency department after an observation period. Children with moderate to severe symptoms after nebulizer medications are admitted for further observation and treatment. Airway obstruction is a potential complication of LTB. The child may require intubation and transfer to the ICU to maintain airway patency if obstruction is imminent. Most children, however, respond positively to the medications and oxygen therapy and are discharged within 48 to 72 hours.

NURSING MANAGEMENT

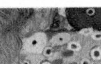

Nursing Assessment and Diagnosis

The initial and ongoing physical assessment of the child with LTB focuses on adequacy of respiratory functioning. Attach a cardiorespiratory monitor and pulse oximeter. Use a stridor assessment scale every 2–4 hours, or more frequently if distress increases. See Table 20–3.

Place the child in an area where continuous visual monitoring is possible to identify changes in airway patency. Pay particular attention to the child's respiratory effort, breath sounds, preferred position, and responsiveness. Note any change in behavior such as agitation or irritability. Physical exhaustion can diminish the intensity of retractions and stridor. As the child uses the remaining energy reserve to maintain ventilation, breath sounds may actually diminish. Noisy breathing (audible airway congestion, coarse breath sounds) in this situation verifies adequate energy stores. Responsiveness decreases as hypoxemia increases.

The following nursing diagnoses might be appropriate for the child with acute LTB:

- Ineffective Breathing Pattern related to tracheobronchial obstruction, decreased energy, and fatigue

TABLE 20–2 Overview of Viral and Bacterial Croup Syndromes

Characteristics	Viral Syndromes		Bacterial Syndromes	
	Acute Spasmodic Laryngitis (Spasmodic Croup)	Laryngotracheobronchitis (LTB)	Bacterial Tracheitis	Epiglottitis (Supraglottitis)
Severity	Least serious	Serious; progresses if untreated	Guarded; requires close observation	Most life threatening (medical emergency)[a]
Age affected	3 months–3 years	3 months–8 years	1 month–13 years[a]	2 years–8 years
Onset	Abrupt onset; symptoms peak at night, rapidly resolves over 24–48 hours, recurs[a]	Gradual onset; starts as URI, progresses to symptoms of respiratory distress; symptoms worse at night	Progressive from URI (1–2 days)	Progresses rapidly (hours)[a]; may progress to complete airway obstruction
Clinical manifestations	Afebrile; mild respiratory distress; barking-seal cough	*Early:* mild fever (less than 40°C [102.2°F]); barking-seal, brassy, croupy cough; hoarse voice; rhinorrhea; sore throat; stridor (inspiratory); apprehension; restless or irritable May progress to retractions; increasing stridor; cyanosis	High fever (higher than 39°C [102.2°F]); URI appears as viral croupy cough; croup initially; stridor (tracheal); purulent secretions; often prefers to lie flat	High fever (higher than 39°C [102.2°F]); URI; intense sore throat; dysphagia[a]; drooling[a]; increased pulse and respiratory rate; prefers upright position (tripod position with chin thrust)[a]; cherry red epiglottis
Etiology	Unknown; suspect viral with allergic/emotional influences	Parainfluenza, types 1 and 2, respiratory syncytial virus, influenza, *Mycoplasma pneumoniae*; may develop a bacterial superinfection	*Staphylococcus, Moraxella catarrhalis,* and non-typeable *Haemophilus influenzae*; may follow viral LTB	*Haemophilus influenzae,* streptococcus and staphylococcus

[a]Classic parameter or key point (distinguishes condition).

- Risk for Deficient Fluid Volume related to inadequate fluid intake prior to admission
- Fear (Child) related to dyspnea, unfamiliar surroundings, procedures, and separation from support system

Planning and Implementation

Maintain Airway Patency

Allow the child to assume a comfortable position with the head elevated, or sitting upright if desired. A means of communica-

TABLE 20–3 Clinical Scoring System for Assessing Children with Stridor

Signs	Criteria for Scoring					
	0	1	2	3	4	5
Stridor	None	Only with agitation or excitement	Mild at rest, heard with stethoscope	At rest, heard without stethoscope		
Retractions	None	Mild	Moderate	Severe		
Air entry	Normal	Decreased	Severely decreased			
Cyanosis	None				With agitation	At rest
Level of consciousness	Normal					Altered mental status

Scoring: To quantify the severity of stridor, add the individual scores for each of the sign categories. A score between 0 and 18 is possible. Mild respiratory distress is less than 3, moderate respiratory distress is a score of 3–6, and severe respiratory distress is a score greater than 6.

Note: From Sobol, S. E., & Zapata, S. (2008). Epiglottitis and croup. Otolaryngology Clinics of North America, 41, 551–566.

Medications Used to Treat
Symptomatic Laryngotracheobronchitis

Medication, Route, and Action	Nursing Management
Beta-agonists and beta-adrenergics (e.g., albuterol, racemic epinephrine) Aerosolized through face mask. Rapid-acting bronchodilator, decreases bronchial and tracheal secretions and mucosal edema.	■ May cause tachycardia (160–200 beats/min) and hypertension; dizziness, headache, and nausea; may necessitate stopping medication. ■ Provides temporary relief in about 30 minutes, lasting about 2 hours, until the corticosteroid begins to work; reduces need for an artificial airway.
Corticosteroids (e.g., dexamethasone) IM, PO, nebulized budesonide Anti-inflammatory, used to decrease edema. Has a long half-life of 36–54 hours.	■ May cause cardiovascular symptoms (hypertension); observe closely for individual response. ■ Stridor resolves faster, children less frequently need emergency airways.

tion (sign language or simple word cues) must be established so the older child can alert nursing staff to respiratory difficulty. Cool mist may be used for some children. Supplemental oxygen with humidity may be needed for hypoxemia. Be immediately available to attend to the child's respiratory needs, and keep resuscitation equipment at the bedside.

Meet Fluid and Nutritional Needs
The respiratory distress may have interfered with the child's ability and desire to drink fluids and therefore compromised the child's fluid status. Recognizing fluid deficit and monitoring the child's hydration and nutritional status are essential tasks. Fluids help thin secretions and provide calories for energy and metabolism.

Children with LTB usually prefer cool, noncarbonated, nonacidic drinks such as oral rehydration fluids. The parents can be encouraged to give the child oral fluids. An intravenous infusion may be necessary to rehydrate the child, maintain fluid balance, or provide emergency access. Observe the child closely for difficulty in swallowing, which may be an early sign of epiglottitis or bacterial tracheitis.

Discharge Planning and Home Care Teaching
During the child's observation period, take every opportunity to assess the parents' knowledge of symptoms of LTB and discuss actions to take if symptoms recur. For example, instruct parents to call the child's physician if:

• Mild symptoms do not improve after 1 hour of exposure to cool night air or air conditioning.
• The child's breathing is rapid and labored.

Research ▓ *Mist Therapy*

High humidity has been a mainstay of treatment for croup and LTB. However, a study comparing the use of high- and low-humidity mist therapy in 140 children with moderately severe croup revealed that mist therapy is not beneficial. No differences in croup scores were found within 1 hour of mist therapy (Scolnik, Coates, Stephens, et al., 2006).

• The child does not drink adequate fluids and the urine output is reduced.

Evaluation
Expected outcomes of nursing care include:

• The child responds to medications with decreased respiratory distress.
• The child has adequate fluid intake for age.

Epiglottitis
Epiglottitis is an inflammation of the epiglottis (supraglottis), the long narrow structure that closes off the glottis during swallowing. (See Table 20–2 for a comparison of epiglottitis and other croup syndromes.)

Epiglottitis is caused by bacterial invasion of the soft tissue of the larynx by *Streptococcus* and *Staphylococcus*, and by *Haemophilus influenzae* type b (Hib) in unimmunized children. The resulting inflammation and edema in the epiglottis and surrounding tissues lead to airway obstruction. It is considered a life-threatening condition. The Hib vaccination has resulted in a decreased incidence of epiglottitis by 99% in children less than 5 years (Sobol & Zapata, 2008).

Characteristically, a previously healthy child suddenly becomes very ill with a sore throat and a high fever (greater than 39°C [102.2°F]). The condition rapidly progresses to **dysphagia** (difficulty in swallowing). The intense throat pain keeps the child from swallowing, resulting in drooling. Talking is painful and the patient may speak with a muffled voice (dysphonia). As the larynx becomes obstructed, inspiratory stridor and respiratory distress develop. To open the airway and improve air intake, the child sits up and leans forward with the jaw thrust forward in the classic "sniffing" or tripod posture and refuses to lie down (Figure 20–8 ➤). The child's anxiety increases as it becomes more difficult to breathe.

Diagnosis is often based on physical signs and a lateral neck radiograph, which reveals a narrowed airway and an enlarged, rounded epiglottis, seen as a mass at the base of the tongue. Laryngospasm and airway obstruction can occur as a result of the severe irritation and hypersensitivity of the airway muscles.

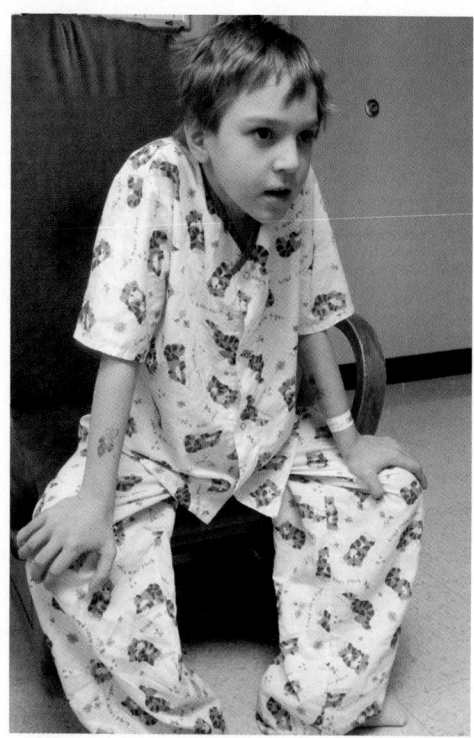

FIGURE 20–8 ➤ Children with severe respiratory distress and a narrowed airway often sit in a tripod position with arms on the legs leaning forward. The head and neck are extended with the jaw thrust forward to help keep the airway open. This position may also be seen in a child with a severe asthma flare.

For this reason, *visual inspection of the mouth and throat is contraindicated in children with suspected epiglottitis.*

Immediate clinical therapy usually involves insertion of an endotracheal tube (often in the operating room) to maintain the airway, and the epiglottis is cultured. The child is admitted to the pediatric intensive care unit (PICU). If the child develops an airway obstruction, assisted ventilation is performed until the endotracheal tube can be inserted. Antibiotics effective for gram-positive organisms and *H. influenzae* are given until culture sensitivities are available. Racemic epinephrine and corticosteroids are not effective. If *H. influenzae* is the causative organism, rifampin prophylaxis should be given to any child contact under age 48 months with incomplete Hib immunization (American Academy of Pediatrics [AAP], 2009, p. 315). Antipyretics (acetaminophen, ibuprofen) may be useful in managing fever and sore throat pain.

Nursing Management

Nursing management consists of airway management, drug therapy, hydration, and emotional and psychosocial support of the child and parents.

> **Nursing Alert**
>
> Observe the child continuously for inability to swallow, absence of voice sounds, increasing degree of respiratory distress, and acute onset of drooling (an ominous sign of supraglottic obstruction). If any of these signs occur, get medical assistance immediately. The quieter the child, the greater the cause for concern.

Until the child is intubated, allow the child to assume a position of comfort, often sitting. Observe the child's respiratory and airway status continuously. Note any change in level of consciousness. Anxiety-provoking procedures, such as obtaining cultures or starting an IV line, are postponed until the airway is stabilized. Crying stimulates the airway, increases oxygen consumption, and can precipitate laryngospasm. Supplemental humidified oxygen may be used initially to reverse hypoxemia.

The child is usually managed in the ICU until the endotracheal tube is removed, usually after 1 to 2 days. (See the *Clinical Skills Manual.*) Administer antibiotics to treat bacterial infection and antiviral medications for viral cause. Most children show rapid improvement once oxygen, antibiotics, and fluid therapy are started. Because the child was febrile with a sore throat before admission, fluid intake may have been compromised.

The life-threatening condition causes stress for the parents. The loss of voice, unfamiliar hospital environment, and strange equipment can be frightening to a child. Reassure the parents that the child's voice loss is temporary and explain the need for the various pieces of equipment.

Home care may involve completing the course of antibiotics. Parents need instructions on proper administration and potential problems of drug therapy.

Bacterial Tracheitis

Bacterial tracheitis is a secondary infection of the upper trachea after viral laryngotracheitis that is most often caused by *Staphylococcus aureus*, *group A streptococcus*, *Moraxella catarrhalis*, or *Haemophilus influenzae*. The child may begin with signs similar to croup, followed by the rapid onset of high fever, cough, respiratory distress, and a toxic or seriously ill appearance. Drooling is rarely present, and the child may prefer to lie flat (Shah & Sharieff, 2007). Purulent secretions can obstruct the airway and become life threatening. Table 20–2 compares bacterial tracheitis and other croup syndromes.

Because of the similarity of symptoms, bacterial tracheitis is often misdiagnosed initially as LTB. Instead of improving with therapy, however, the child's condition becomes worse. Blood cultures are often negative. Diagnosis is often made by endoscopic visualization of the upper trachea. The subglottis is edematous with ulceration and thick mucopurulent exudate that should be cultured. Intravenous antibiotics are given initially and changed to oral as the child's condition improves over the 10- to 14-day course. Most children need an endotracheal tube to secure the airway for 3 to 11 days and ventilatory support.

Nursing Management

The child with bacterial tracheitis is frequently cared for in the PICU after endotracheal intubation. Suctioning of the thick tracheal secretions that pool high in the upper airway helps maintain a patent airway. (See the *Clinical Skills Manual.*) Provide humidified air or oxygen. Antibiotics are administered as ordered. The earlier section on epiglottitis discusses other nursing care interventions that may also be appropriate for the child with bacterial tracheitis.

■ LOWER AIRWAY DISORDERS

The lower airway, or bronchial tree, lies below the trachea and includes the bronchi, bronchioles, and alveoli. Lower airway disorders occur because a structural or functional problem interferes with the lungs' ability to complete the respiratory cycle. Lower airway disorders include bronchitis, bronchiolitis, bronchopulmonary dysplasia, pneumonia, and tuberculosis.

Bronchitis

Acute bronchitis, inflammation of the trachea and bronchi, rarely occurs in childhood as an isolated problem. The bronchi can be affected simultaneously with adjacent respiratory structures during a respiratory illness. Bronchitis occurs most often in the winter months.

The classic symptom of bronchitis is a coarse, hacking cough, which increases in severity at night. The cough may or may not be productive. The child may swallow sputum and vomit as a result. The chest and ribs may be sore because of the deep and frequent coughing. Over several days, breath sounds may become coarse with fine crackles, and some scattered high-pitched wheezing may be heard. Treatment is palliative unless a secondary bacterial infection develops and requires antibiotic therapy.

Nursing Management

Nursing management includes supporting respiratory function through rest, humidification, hydration, and symptomatic treatment. Refer to the sections on asthma and pneumonia for detailed information on treatment measures.

Home care should emphasize the self-limiting nature of the disorder. Advise parents who smoke that quitting or refraining from smoking in the child's presence may benefit the child.

Bronchiolitis and Respiratory Syncytial Virus

Bronchiolitis is a lower respiratory tract illness that occurs when an infecting agent (virus or bacterium) causes inflammation and obstruction of the small airways, the bronchioles. Bronchiolitis is a leading cause of hospital admission among infants under age 12 months, but it causes fewer than 500 deaths annually (Zorc & Phelan, 2008). Children with bronchiolitis have an increased incidence of reactive airway disease and asthma later in childhood (Willis, 2007).

Etiology and Pathophysiology

Bronchiolitis is associated with the *respiratory syncytial virus* (RSV) in 70% of bronchiolitis cases and the metapneumovirus in 5–15% of cases (Zorc & Phelan, 2008). Other organisms causing bronchiolitis include influenza, adenovirus, rhinovirus, and parainfluenza. RSV occurs in annual epidemics during the winter and early spring. It is transmitted through direct contact with contaminated secretions or surfaces. Nearly all children have been infected with RSV by 2 years of age, and reinfection is common as infection does not confer immunity (AAP, 2009, pp. 560–561). Infants at risk for severe infection with RSV are those who are preterm, have cyanotic or complicated congenital heart disease, have chronic lung disease of prematurity, or have immunodeficiency disease or immunosuppression.

Viruses, acting as parasites, are able to invade the mucosal cells that line the small bronchi and bronchioles. The invaded cells die when the virus bursts from inside the cell to invade adjacent cells. The membranes of the infected cells fuse with adjacent cells, creating large masses of cells or *syncytia*. The resulting cell debris clogs and obstructs the bronchioles and irritates the airway. In response, the airway lining swells and produces excessive mucus. Despite this protective effort by the bronchioles, the actual effect is partial airway obstruction and bronchospasms.

The cycle is repeated throughout both lungs as the airway cells are invaded by the virus. The partially obstructed airways allow air in, but the mucus and airway swelling block expulsion of the air. This creates the wheezing and crackles in the airways. Air trapped below the obstruction also interferes with normal gas exchange, leading to hypoxemia. The infant with severe RSV infection is at risk for apnea and respiratory failure as hypoxemia and hypercarbia develop.

Clinical Manifestations

Some children have mild symptoms such as rhinitis, cough, low-grade fever, wheezing, tachypnea, poor feeding, vomiting, and diarrhea. Dehydration may be present if the child has been sick for several days. Parents report that the infant or child is acting more ill—appearing sicker, less playful, and less interested in eating. Infants, especially, may refuse to feed or may spit up what they eat along with thick, clear mucus.

The infant or child with a more severe infection has tachypnea greater than 70 breaths per minute, grunting, increased wheezing, retractions, nasal flaring, irritability, lethargy, poor fluid intake, and a distended abdomen from overexpanded lungs. As hypoxia develops, the infant becomes cyanotic and has decreasing mental status. As the airflow continues to decrease, breath sounds diminish. Thus the noisier the lungs, the better, as this indicates that the child is still able to move air in and out of the lungs. While RSV bronchiolitis resolves in 5 to 7 days, increased airway resistance and airway hypersensitivity may persist for weeks or even months.

COLLABORATIVE CARE

Diagnostic Testing

The history and physical examination provide the data needed to diagnose bronchiolitis. Chest radiographs show hyperinflation, patchy atelectasis, and other signs of inflammation. Enzyme-linked immunosorbent assay (ELISA) or immunofluorescent assay performed on a posterior nasopharyngeal specimen are laboratory tests used to identify the virus causing bronchiolitis (see the *Clinical Skills Manual*).

Clinical Therapy

Treatment is supportive as no effective therapy for RSV exists. Children who test positive for RSV are isolated or roomed together to minimize the spread of the virus to other hospitalized children. Humidified oxygen is provided to maintain the SpO_2 at readings greater than 90% (Willis, 2007). Other supportive care includes hydration with oral or IV fluids and nasal suctioning. Chest physiotherapy may have no benefit (AAP Subcommittee on the Diagnosis and Management of Bronchiolitis, 2006). The use of CPAP for children with severe bronchiolitis is being evaluated (Seiden & Scarfone, 2009). The child with apnea or respiratory failure will be cared for in the critical care unit, usually intubated and ventilated when too fatigued to breathe effectively (see the *Clinical Skills Manual*).

Supportive care is provided. Few medications are prescribed for RSV and bronchiolitis. Antipyretics may be used. A short trial of inhaled albuterol may be used to see if wheezing improves. The use of dexamethasone and antibiotics is not recommended. Ribavirin, an antiviral drug specifically available for RSV treatment, is reserved for cases of severe disease such as infants with potential life-threatening infection (AAP, 2009, p. 562).

Prevention of RSV is a focus for children at high risk for severe bronchiolitis, including the following groups of children during RSV season (AAP, 2009, pp. 564–568):

- Children under age 24 months with chronic lung disease of prematurity who have needed medical therapy within 6 months of the start of RSV season
- Children under age 24 months with significant congenital heart disease, such as congestive heart failure, pulmonary hypertension, and cyanotic heart disease
- Infants born at 28 weeks' gestation or less, during their first 12 months of life
- Infants born at 29 to 32 weeks' gestation, up to 6 months of age
- Infants born at 32 to 35 weeks' gestation, with two or more of the following risk factors: childcare attendance, has a sibling less than age 5 years, born less than 3 months before onset of RSV season, congenital abnormalities of the airway, or severe neuromuscular disease

Prophylaxis with an intramuscular injection of palivizumab (Synagis) at a dose of 15 mg/kg every 30 days is given for 5 months beginning in October or November, at the onset of RSV season. Palivizumab is expensive, but less costly than hospitalization for an infant with RSV. Palivizumab does not interfere with administration of normal recommended childhood vaccines (AAP, 2009, p. 568).

NURSING MANAGEMENT

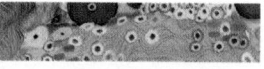

Nursing Assessment and Diagnosis

The nursing assessment focuses on airway and respiratory function because the infant may tire with the extra work of breathing and the development of respiratory failure.

Physiologic Assessment

Assess airway and respiratory function carefully. Good observation skills are important to ensure timely interventions for worsening respiratory symptoms and prevention of respiratory distress (see Assessment Guidelines on page 554 and Clinical Manifestations: Respiratory Failure and Imminent Respiratory Arrest on page 558). An oxygen saturation level below 90% is the best indicator of the disease's severity.

Psychosocial Assessment

Observe children and their parents for signs of fear and anxiety. The unfamiliar hospital environment and procedures can increase stress and have an impact on respiratory status. Parents' questions, as well as their nonverbal cues, help direct nursing interventions during admission and throughout hospitalization.

The accompanying Nursing Care Plan: The Child with Bronchiolitis lists common nursing diagnoses for the child with bronchiolitis. Others that might also be appropriate include:

- Ineffective Airway Clearance related to increased airway secretions in bronchioles
- Activity Intolerance related to imbalance between oxygen supply and demand
- Interrupted Family Processes related to sudden acute illness of the infant

Clinical Judgment

What assessment should be initiated if you notice that an infant who has had tachypnea for several hours begins breathing slower than the expected rate for age?

Planning and Implementation

Nursing management focuses on maintaining respiratory function, supporting overall physiologic function and hydration, reducing the child's and family's anxiety, and preparing the family for home care. An important nursing action is to educate parents of infants at high risk for RSV to obtain the monthly injections of palivizumab and to promptly seek care if respiratory symptoms develop. Encourage good hand hygiene.

Maintain Respiratory Function

Close monitoring is essential to evaluate the child's improvement or to spot early signs of deterioration. Supplemental oxygen with humidity may be provided via nasal cannula, mask, hood, or tent. When the child resists or is frightened by the oxygen apparatus, engage the parent to soothe the child and promote acceptance of the therapy. Patent nares are important to promote oxygen intake. A bulb syringe and saline nose drops can be used to quickly clear the nasal passages. Elevate the head of the bed to ease the work of breathing and drain mucus from the upper airways.

Support Physiologic Function

Grouping nursing tasks promotes rest and decreases stress. Medications may be administered to control temperature and promote comfort as needed. Infants may have feeding difficulty and are at risk for aspiration. Smaller volumes and frequent

NURSING CARE PLAN

The Child with Bronchiolitis

INTERVENTION	RATIONALE	EXPECTED OUTCOME
1. Nursing Diagnosis: Ineffective Breathing Pattern related to increased work of breathing		
NIC Priority Intervention: *Respiratory Monitoring:* Collection and analysis of patient data to ensure airway patency and adequate gas exchange		**NOC Suggested Outcome:** *Vital Signs Status:* Temperature, pulse, respiration, and blood pressure within expected range for the child's age
Goal: The child will return to respiratory baseline and will not experience respiratory failure.		
▪ Assess respiratory status (Table 20–1) when the child is calm and not crying at least every 2–4 hours, or more often as indicated for an increasing or decreasing respiratory rate and episodes of apnea.	▪ Changes in breathing pattern occur quickly when the child's energy reserves are depleted. Baseline and subsequent assessments help detect changes in the respiratory rate and quality of respiratory effort.	The child returns to respiratory baseline within 48–72 hours.
▪ Attach a cardiorespiratory monitor and pulse oximeter with alarms set. Record and report changes promptly to the physician.	▪ The alarm can alert the nurse to any sudden respiratory changes and lead to more rapid interventions.	
Goal: The child's oxygenation status will return to baseline.		
▪ Administer humidified oxygen via mask, nasal cannula, hood, or tent.	▪ Humidified oxygen loosens secretions, helps maintain oxygenation status, and eases respiratory distress.	The child's respiratory effort eases. The SpO_2 level remains at 95% or higher during treatment.
▪ Assess and compare the child's SpO_2 level when on room air and on supplemental oxygen.	▪ Comparison of SpO_2 levels provides information to assess condition improvement.	
▪ Note the child's response to ordered medications.	▪ Medications act systemically to improve oxygenation and decrease inflammation.	The child tolerates therapeutic measures with no adverse effects.
▪ Position the head of the bed up or place the child in a position of comfort on the parent's lap, if crying or struggling in the crib or bed.	▪ Position facilitates improved aeration and promotes decreased anxiety (especially in toddlers) and energy expenditure.	The child rests quietly in a position of comfort.
▪ Assess tolerance to feeding and activities.	▪ This provides an assessment of condition improvement.	
2. Nursing Diagnosis: Risk for Deficient Fluid Volume related to inability to meet body requirements and increased metabolic demand		
NIC Priority Intervention: *Fluid Management:* Promotion of fluid balance and prevention of complications resulting from abnormal or undesired fluid levels		**NOC Suggested Outcome:** *Hydration:* Amount of water in intracellular and extracellular compartments of body
Goal: The child's immediate fluid deficit is corrected.		
▪ Evaluate the need for intravenous fluids. Maintain IV, if ordered.	▪ Previous fluid loss may require immediate replacement.	The child's hydration status improves during the acute phase of illness as demonstrated by appropriate urine output and moist mucous membranes.
Goal: The child will be adequately hydrated, be able to tolerate oral fluids, and progress to a normal diet.		
▪ Calculate maintenance fluid requirements and give oral fluids, IV fluids, or both.	▪ Assessment of fluid requirements enables the nurse to maintain hydration while transitioning the child to oral fluids.	The child takes adequate oral fluids to maintain hydration.
▪ Offer clear fluids and incorporate parents in care. Offer fluid choice when tolerated.	▪ Choice of fluid offered by a parent gains the child's cooperation.	The child accepts a beverage of choice from the parent or nursing staff.

(continued)

NURSING CARE PLAN

The Child with Bronchiolitis (continued)

INTERVENTION	RATIONALE	EXPECTED OUTCOME
■ Maintain strict intake and output monitoring and evaluate specific gravity at least every 8 hours.	■ Monitoring provides objective evidence of fluid loss and ongoing hydration status.	
■ Perform daily weight measurement on the same scale at the same time of day.	■ This provides further evidence of improvement of hydration status.	The child's weight stabilizes after 24–48 hours; skin turgor is supple.
■ Assess mucous membranes and presence of tears. Evaluate skin turgor.	■ Moist mucous membranes and tears are signs of adequate hydration.	The child shows evidence of improved hydration.

3. Nursing Diagnosis: Anxiety (Child and Parent) related to acute illness, hospitalization, uncertain course of illness and treatment, and home care needs

NIC Priority Intervention: *Anxiety Reduction:* Minimizing apprehension, dread, foreboding, or uneasiness related to an unidentified source of anticipated danger		NOC Suggested Outcome: *Anxiety Control:* Ability to eliminate or reduce feelings of apprehension and tension from an unidentifiable source

Goal: The child and parents will demonstrate behaviors that indicate less anxiety.

■ Encourage parents to express fears and ask questions; provide direct answers and discuss care, procedures, and condition changes.	■ Parents have the opportunity to vent feelings and receive timely, relevant information. This helps reduce parents' anxiety and increase trust in nursing staff.	Parents and child show less anxiety as symptoms improve and as they feel more secure in the hospital environment. *Parents* freely ask questions and participate in the child's care. The *child* cries less and allows staff to hold or touch him or her.
■ Incorporate parents in the child's care. Encourage parents to bring familiar objects from home. Ask about the home routines for feeding and sleeping, and incorporate them in the care plan.	■ Familiar people, routines, and objects decrease the child's anxiety and increase parents' sense of control over an unexpected, uncertain situation.	

Goal: Parents will verbalize knowledge of bronchiolitis symptoms and use of home care methods before the child's discharge from the hospital.

■ Explain symptoms, treatment, and home care of bronchiolitis.	■ Anticipating the potential for recurrence assists the family to be prepared for a potential recurrence of respiratory symptoms after discharge.	Parents accurately describe respiratory symptoms and initial home care actions.
■ Provide written instructions for follow-up care arrangements, as needed.	■ Written and verbal instructions reinforce knowledge. Parents may not "hear" and remember details if only given verbally.	
■ Make sure parents can read the instructions; provide them in the family's primary language.	■ Many families have reading difficulty and may read a language other than English.	

feedings will help conserve energy in infants who are formula- or breastfed. When the risk of aspiration is high, nasogastric tube feedings may be used to provide nutrition. An IV infusion may be ordered to rehydrate and maintain fluid balance until the child is capable of taking sufficient oral fluids.

Reduce Anxiety

The parents may be frightened and stressed by the child's continued respiratory difficulty and the equipment at the bedside. Provide parents with thorough explanations and daily updates, and encourage their participation in the infant's care. Reassure them that holding or touching the infant will not dislodge wires or tubing, and that their presence will calm the infant.

If the infant has been ill for a few days before admission, the parents are likely to be tired. Acknowledging parents' physical and emotional needs creates a spirit of caring and enhances communication between staff and family. Encourage the parents to take turns at the child's bedside and to take breaks for meals and rest.

Discharge Planning and Home Care Teaching

Children are discharged once they show sufficient stability in maintaining adequate oxygenation (as evidenced by easing of respiratory effort, decreased mucus production, and absence of coughing). In most children, symptoms decrease within 24 to 72 hours; however, resolution of all symptoms may take weeks. Coughing may continue for a few weeks after discharge.

Families Want to Know
Discharge Teaching for Bronchiolitis

General care instructions:

■ Use a bulb syringe to keep the infant's nose clear.

■ Give fluids to help keep secretions thin, and provide small frequent feedings.

■ Encourage active toddlers to rest and take naps during recovery.

Advise parents to call the physician if:

■ Breathing is rapid or difficult.

■ Respiratory symptoms interfere with sleep or eating.

■ Symptoms persist in a child who is less than 1 year old, has heart or lung disease, or was premature and had lung disease after birth.

■ The child acts sicker—appears tired, less playful, and less interested in food (parents just "feel" the child is not improving).

Teach the parents proper administration of medications. Acetaminophen may be prescribed for persistent low-grade fevers and general discomfort. Advise parents that RSV infection can recur; therefore, they need to know how to recognize symptoms and when to call the physician. See Families Want to Know: Discharge Teaching for Bronchiolitis.

Evaluation

In addition to the expected outcomes of nursing care provided in the Nursing Care Plan, the infant at high risk receives all doses of palivizumab.

Pneumonia

Pneumonia is an inflammation or infection of the bronchioles and alveolar spaces of the lungs, occurring most often in infants and young children. The incidence of community-acquired pneumonia in the United States is 36 to 40 cases per 1,000 children under age 5 years, and 11 to 16 cases per 1,000 children 5 to 14 years of age (Woods, 2008).

Pneumonia may be viral, mycoplasmal, or bacterial in origin. In children under age 5 years, pneumonia is most often caused by viruses such as RSV; influenza A and B; parainfluenza virus 1, 2, and 3; adenovirus; and human metapneumovirus. While bacterial pneumonia is more common in children over 5 years, it occurs in all age groups. Common bacterial organisms include *Streptococcus pneumoniae, Chlamydophila pneumoniae,* and *Staphylococcus aureus.* Group B *Streptococcus,* enteric gram-negative bacilli, and *Chlamydia trachomatis* are found in infants 3 months of age or less. Children with cystic fibrosis or immunosuppression are susceptible to other bacterial, parasitic, or fungal infections. Children often have a viral illness preceding bacterial pneumonia.

Bacterial and viral invaders act differently within the lungs:

• Bacterial invaders circulate through the bloodstream to the lungs, where they damage cells. Cellular debris and mucus cause airway obstruction. Bacteria tend to be distributed evenly throughout one or more lobes of a single lung, termed *lobar pneumonia.*

• Viruses frequently enter from the upper respiratory tract, infiltrating the alveoli nearest the bronchi of one or both lungs. The virus invades the cells, replicating and bursting out forcefully, killing the cells and sending out cell debris. Adjacent areas are invaded, resulting in a scattered, patchy pattern referred to as bronchopneumonia.

• Aspiration of food, emesis, gastric reflux, or hydrocarbons causes a chemical injury and an inflammatory response, setting the stage for bacterial invasion.

Regardless of the causative agent, symptoms commonly include fever, cough, and tachypnea. Rhonchi, crackles, wheezes, dyspnea, nasal flaring, restlessness, chest pain, and malaise may also be seen. Decreased breath sounds may be noted if lung consolidation is present. The child also may have poor oral intake, nausea, vomiting, and abdominal pain.

Diagnosis is made by chest radiograph, which shows an abnormal density of tissue, such as a lobar consolidation or patchy consolidation associated with bronchopneumonia. Children over age 8 years may be able to produce enough sputum for culture. A nasopharyngeal aspirate can be tested with polymerase chain reaction or immunofluorescence tests to identify respiratory viruses. Clinical management for all types of pneumonia includes symptomatic therapy (pain and fever control) and supportive care through airway management, fluids, and rest. Mycoplasma and other bacterial pneumonias are treated with organism-sensitive antibiotics; viral pneumonias usually improve without antibiotics. Some children with significant pneumonia are hospitalized for careful monitoring and to receive oxygen and IV fluids to maintain hydration. Complications such as an empyema (a collection of pus in the pleural space) or a pleural effusion are treated by drainage with a thoracostomy tube. (See the *Clinical Skills Manual.*)

Nursing Management

Most children with pneumonia are cared for at home. When a child is hospitalized, assess the child, paying particular attention to respiratory rate, heart rate, and temperature, and observe color for pallor or cyanosis. Attach a pulse oximeter to monitor the SpO_2 level. Assess hydration status. Assess for the presence of pain with coughing.

In addition to ongoing respiratory assessment and supportive therapies (chest physiotherapy, supplemental oxygen, and hydration), the child may need relief from pain when coughing and deep breathing. Teach the child and parent how to splint the chest by hugging a small pillow, teddy bear, or doll to make coughing less painful. Pain medication (acetaminophen or ibuprofen) can provide the added benefits of temperature control and may aid in sleep.

The goal of nursing care is to restore optimal respiratory function. Medications, especially antibiotics, must be taken at prescribed intervals and for the full course. Teach parents the proper administration of drugs and any side effects. Follow-up may include a chest radiograph to see if the lungs are clear. Symptoms of pneumonia usually disappear long before the lungs are completely healed. Most children recover uneventfully, but some children continue to have worsening reactive airway problems or abnormal pulmonary function test results.

Full immunization of infants is one preventive measure against pneumonia. The pneumococcal conjugate vaccine (PCV7) administered during infancy has significantly reduced the incidence of invasive pneumococcal illness, including pneumonia (Poehling, Talbot, Griffin, et al., 2006). A 23-valent pneumococcal vaccine (PPV23) is recommended for children over 2 years of age who are immunosuppressed or have chronic diseases (see Chapter 16 ∞).

Tuberculosis

Tuberculosis (TB) is caused by an organism of *Mycobacterium tuberculosis* complex, which is transmitted through the air in infectious particles called droplet nuclei. In 2005, 863 children under age 15 years in the United States acquired TB. Nearly 25% of these children were foreign born, and 75% were Hispanic or non-Hispanic Black (Starke, 2007). TB is a significant health problem in developing countries.

Epidemiology and Pathophysiology

Children usually acquire a TB infection from infected adults who cough, sneeze, speak, or sing, and send out tiny droplets containing the bacillus. When inhaled, the bacillus is small enough to travel directly to the alveoli and cause infection. When the organism reaches the alveoli, macrophages surround and wall off the bacillus where it multiplies. When the organisms number 1,000 to 10,000 after 2 to 10 weeks, a cellular immune response to TB can be elicited with the TB skin test. In persons with intact cell-mediated immunity, activated T cells and macrophages form granulomas that limit bacillus multiplication. Small numbers of viable bacilli may remain in the granuloma, and these individuals have latent tuberculosis infection (LTBI), a positive tuberculin skin test, and no clinical or radiographic signs of disease. However, they are not infectious and cannot transmit the disease.

Active TB can develop as the bacilli grow, divide within the macrophage, and break free of the macrophage. Infants and adolescents have the greatest risk of transitioning from LTBI to active TB. Factors increasing that risk include immunosuppressive therapy, HIV co-infection, malnutrition, vitamin D deficiency, chronic medical conditions, TB infection in the past 2 years, and viral infections such as measles (Newton, Brent, Anderson, et al., 2008; AAP, 2009, p. 662). The greatest risk for LTBI transition to active TB occurs within 2 to 12 months after initial infection (Ranganathan & Sonnappa, 2009). Children under age 10 years with active TB are rarely contagious, because they have small pulmonary lesions, they have an unproductive cough, and few or no bacilli are expelled (AAP, 2009, p. 682).

Extrapulmonary TB occurs in 10–20% of children (Peredo-Pinto & Jacobs, 2008). Tuberculosis meningitis can occur 3 to 6 months after primary infection and is one of the most severe forms of childhood TB (Newton et al., 2008). If a tubercle extends into a blood vessel, TB can also spread to the liver, spleen, kidney, or bone marrow.

Clinical Manifestations

Infants, children, and adolescents with latent TB infection will have no symptoms. Clinical manifestations of active TB in in-

fants include a persistent cough, weight loss or failure to gain weight, and low-grade fever. Wheezing and decreased breath sounds may be present. Children with active TB may have fatigue, cough, anorexia, weight loss or growth delay, night sweats, chills, a low-grade fever, and enlarged lymph nodes. Hemoptysis is a late sign of advanced pulmonary TB. When TB spreads outside the pulmonary system, additional signs are specific to the system invaded:

- Superficial lymphadenitis: firm, nontender, matted lymph nodes
- Meninges: high fever, vomiting, lethargy, headache, seizures, nuchal rigidity, and irritability; also hepatosplenomegaly and generalized lymphadenopathy
- Osteoarticular: inflammation, pain, swelling, fever, and limited range of motion of the affected bone or joint

COLLABORATIVE CARE

Diagnostic Testing

Screening to identify a child's risk for LTBI should occur during the first health visit, then every 6 months until age 2 years, and then annually. Administer an intradermal tuberculin skin test (PPD) if one or more of these risk factors are present (AAP, 2009, p. 685):

- The child was born in any country or region except the United States, Canada, Australia, New Zealand, or Western Europe.
- The child traveled outside the United States and had contact with the resident population for more than a week in any country or region except those listed above.
- The child has a family member or contact with TB.
- A family member had a positive tuberculin skin test.

A positive test indicates that the child has been exposed to and infected with TB, and antibodies have been produced against the bacillus. A PPD cannot distinguish between LTBI and active TB.

An interferon-gamma release assay, QuantiFERON-TB Gold (QFT-G), may be beneficial to support PPD findings. It is most useful when a child vaccinated with bacille Calmette-Guérin (BCG) has a borderline positive response to a PPD, when a repeat PPD may cause a boost response, or when the child cannot return in 48 to 72 hours for a PPD reading (Ranganathan & Sonnappa, 2009). Like the PPD, the QFT-G cannot distinguish between latent and active TB. Other diagnostic tests include acid-fast stains of blood, sputum cultures, gastric aspirate in children unable to produce sputum, and a chest radiograph.

Clinical Therapy

Active and latent TB are treated with antitubercular drugs, including isoniazid, rifampin, pyrazinamide, and ethambutol. Therapy for active TB usually involves a daily 6-month regimen consisting of isoniazid, rifampin, pyrazinamide, and ethambutol for the first 2 months, followed by treatment with isoniazid and rifampin for the remaining 4 months. LTBI is treated with a single daily dose of isoniazid for 9 months (or rifampin for 6 months if TB is drug resistant to isoniazid). Therapeutic agents are modified if a drug-resistant strain of TB is causing the infection. To ensure treatment adherence for both active TB and LTBI, direct-observed drug therapy administered by a nurse or other health care provider three times a week for the duration of treatment is recommended (Ranganathan & Sonnappa, 2009).

Cases of active TB are reported to the public health department so that disease contacts can be found. A child diagnosed with TB is considered a sentinel case, and the adult contact with active TB must be identified.

NURSING MANAGEMENT

Nursing Assessment and Diagnosis

Nurses have an important role in identifying children with one or more risk factors for TB infection, such as foreign-born children and children with potential exposure. Children at risk should have a PPD applied and read within 48 to 72 hours using the guidelines for interpretation in Box 20–2.

Children who are hospitalized with active TB have their respiratory status assessed as well as energy level, nutritional intake, and weight. Children who have no cough and negative sputum acid-fast bacillus smears do not need to be isolated (AAP, 2009, p. 698). If the patient is contagious, airborne isolation is needed.

The following nursing diagnoses may be appropriate for the child with TB:

- Effective Therapeutic Regimen Management related to directly observed medication administration
- Risk for Infection (Active TB) related to exposure to infected contact
- Imbalanced Nutrition: Less than Body Requirements related to anorexia and infection

Planning and Implementation

Nursing care centers on administering medications and providing supportive care. Teach parents about the disease process, medications, possible side effects, and the importance of adhering to medication therapy for the prescribed 6 to 12 months.

Clinical Tip

Children with active tuberculosis should receive "directly observed drug therapy" administered by a nurse or another health care provider to ensure the drug is being taken. Direct observation should occur two or three times a week for the duration of treatment. If any concern about medication adherence exists, even children with LTBI should receive directly observed drug therapy twice a week.

Encourage proper nutrition and rest to promote normal growth and development. The child can return to school or childcare when effective therapy has been instituted, adherence to therapy has been documented, and clinical symptoms have diminished substantially (AAP, 2009, p. 699). Most children with TB can lead essentially normal lives. See the discussion of pneumonia on page 571 and of meningitis in Chapter 27 ∞ for other nursing care measures.

Tuberculosis is a reportable disease. Public health nurses need to investigate the child's contacts to identify the primary case of TB and other potentially infected family members.

Evaluation

Expected outcomes of nursing care include:

- The child with latent TB infection completes therapy and does not develop active TB.
- The child's contacts are evaluated for TB and those infected are treated.

BOX 20-2 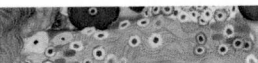 Interpreting Tuberculin Skin Test Results in Infants, Children, and Adolescents*

Induration greater than 5 mm

- Children in close contact with known or suspected contagious cases of tuberculosis disease
- Children suspected to have tuberculosis disease: with findings on chest radiograph consistent with active or previously active tuberculosis or clinical evidence of potential tuberculosis disease (i.e., meningitis)
- Children receiving immunosuppressive doses of corticosteroids or having immunosuppressive conditions, including HIV infection

Induration greater than 10 mm

- Children at increased risk of disseminated disease: younger than 4 years of age; with other medical conditions, including Hodgkin disease, lymphoma, diabetes mellitus, chronic renal failure, or malnutrition
- Children with likelihood of increased exposure to tuberculosis disease: born in high-prevalence regions of the world; frequently exposed to adults who are HIV infected, homeless, users of illicit drugs, residents of nursing homes, incarcerated or institutionalized, or migrant farm workers; or travel to high-prevalence regions of the world

Induration greater than 15 mm

- Children 4 years of age or older without any risk factors

These definitions apply regardless of previous bacille Calmette-Guérin (BCG) immunization.
From: American Academy of Pediatrics. (2009). Red book: 2009 Report of the Committee on Infectious Diseases (28th ed., p. 681). Elk Grove Village, IL: Author.

CHRONIC LUNG DISEASES

Asthma

Asthma is a common chronic disorder of the airways that is complex and characterized by variable and recurring symptoms, airflow obstruction, bronchial hyperresponsiveness, and an underlying inflammation (National Asthma Education and Prevention Program [NAEPP], 2007, p. 12). In the United States, approximately 9% (6.7 million) of children aged 0 to 17 years have asthma and approximately 4.1 million (5.6%) children report at least one asthma episode in the past 12 months (Hill & Wood, 2009; Moorman, Rudd, Johnson, et al., 2007). Asthma accounts for 3% of all hospitalizations among children and 2.8% of all pediatric emergency department visits. The asthma mortality rate is 2.5 per million children (Hill & Wood, 2009). Most children experience their first asthma symptoms before the age of 5 years.

Etiology and Pathophysiology

Asthma is a chronic inflammatory disease of the lungs in children who are genetically susceptible. It is caused by multiple interacting factors including exposure to tobacco smoke, indoor air contaminants (e.g., pet dander, cockroach feces), outdoor air pollutants, recurrent respiratory viral infections, and allergic disease (e.g., atopic eczema, food allergies). Protective factors include a large family size, later birth order, childcare attendance, dog in the family, and living on a farm. Protective factors increase exposure to infections early in life, enabling the child's immune system to develop along a nonallergic pathway (NAEPP, 2007, p. 23).

Inflammation causes the normal protective mechanisms of the lungs (mucous formation, mucosal swelling, and airway muscle contraction) to overreact in response to a stimulus. Airway responsiveness is enhanced through inflammatory mechanisms. A **trigger**, an inflammatory or noninflammatory stimulus that initiates an asthma episode, increases the frequency and severity of smooth muscle contraction (bronchospasm). Triggers include exercise, infectious agents, allergens, fragrances, food additives, pollutants, weather changes, and emotions.

The trigger may activate IgE and sensitized mast cells, leading to the release of inflammatory mediators (e.g., histamines, prostaglandins, and leukotrienes). The inflammatory mediators release pro-inflammatory cytokines causing chronic airway inflammation that may be associated with **airway remodeling** (permanent airway damage that involves thickening of the subbasement membrane, subepithelial fibrosis, airway smooth muscle hypertrophy and hyperplasia, blood vessel proliferation and dilation, and mucous gland hyperplasia and hypersecretion) (Brashers, 2010a). Decreased lung function results.

Airway narrowing results from bronchial constriction, airway swelling, and production of copious amounts of mucus. Mucus clogs small airways, trapping air below the plugs (Figure 20–9 ➤). Decreased perfusion of the alveolar capillaries results from hypoxic vasoconstriction and increased pressure due to hyperinflation of the alveoli.

Pathophysiology Illustrated
Asthma

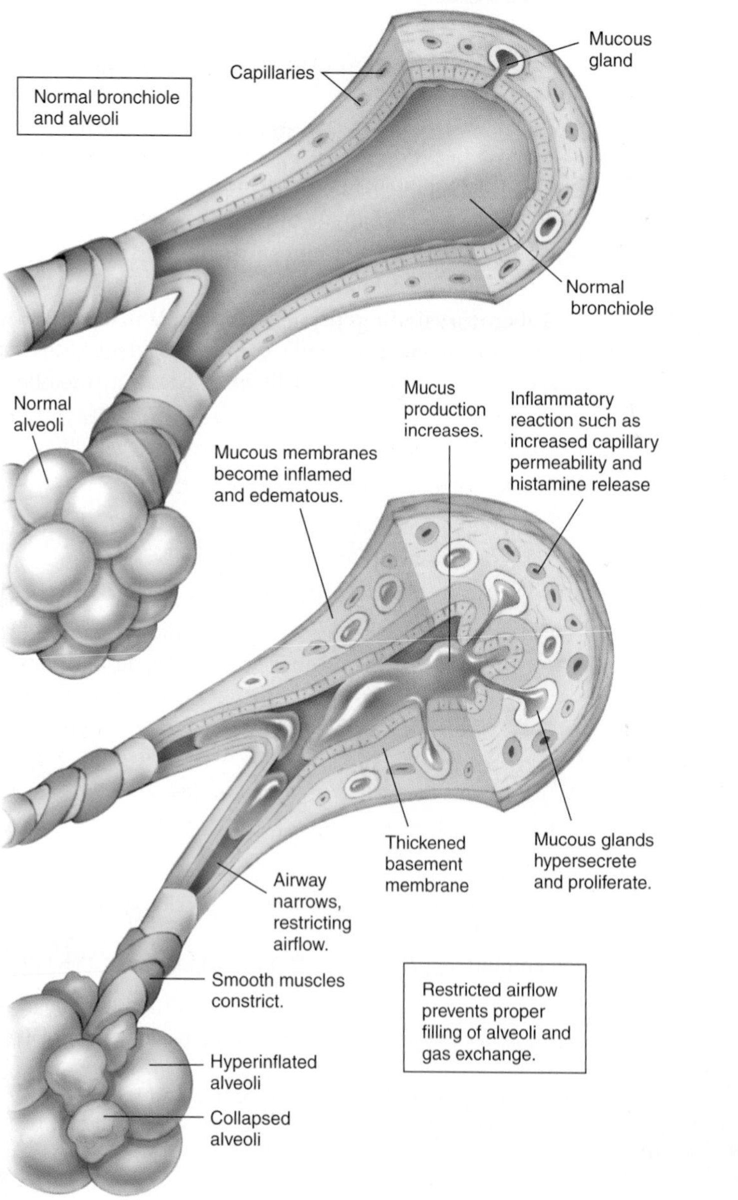

Normal bronchiole and alveoli

Capillaries

Mucous gland

Normal bronchiole

Normal alveoli

Mucous membranes become inflamed and edematous.

Mucus production increases.

Inflammatory reaction such as increased capillary permeability and histamine release

Thickened basement membrane

Mucous glands hypersecrete and proliferate.

Airway narrows, restricting airflow.

Smooth muscles constrict.

Restricted airflow prevents proper filling of alveoli and gas exchange.

Hyperinflated alveoli

Collapsed alveoli

FIGURE 20–9 ➤ Some asthma triggers are exercise, infection, and allergies. The figure shows how asthma obstructs airflow through constriction and narrowing of the airway, along with increased production of mucus.

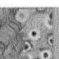

Culture · *Asthma Prevalence*

Asthma prevalence rates vary by cultural group, and even among Hispanic children of different origins. Non-Hispanic Black children have an asthma prevalence rate of 15.8%, and 7.45% had an asthma episode in the past year. Non-Hispanic White children have an asthma prevalence of 12.7%, and 5.8% had an asthma episode in the past year. Hispanic children have an asthma prevalence rate of 12.4%, and 5.1% had an asthma episode in the past 12 months. Of Hispanic children, Puerto Ricans have the highest prevalence rate (26%) and 11.8% had asthma episodes in the past year. Cuban and Dominican children have prevalence rates similar to non-Hispanic Black children, and Mexican children have the lowest prevalence rates of all groups (Lara, Akinbami, Flores, et al., 2006). This type of information may help researchers identify potential genetic and environmental factors associated with asthma in these cultural groups.

Clinical Manifestations

The sudden appearance of breathing difficulty (cough, wheeze, or shortness of breath) is often referred to as an asthma episode or flare. The infant or child who has had episodes of frequent coughing or frequent respiratory infections should be evaluated for asthma. Frequent coughing, especially at night, is the warning signal that the child's airway is very sensitive to stimuli, and it may be a sign in "silent" asthma.

During an acute episode, respirations are rapid and labored, and the child often appears tired from the ongoing effort to breathe. Nasal flaring and intercostal retractions may be visible. The child exhibits a productive cough and expiratory wheezing, use of accessory muscles, decreased air movement, and respiratory fatigue. The child may complain of chest tightness. Anxiety occurs with respiratory distress, and it intensifies the child's physical responses.

In cases of severe obstruction, wheezing may not be heard because of the lack of airflow. Head bobbing may be seen in young children if the accessory muscles (sternocleidomastoids) are used to breathe. Hypoxia and the cumulative effect of medications may cause behaviors ranging from wide-eyed agitation to lethargic irritability. In children who have repeated acute episodes, a barrel chest and the use of respiratory accessory muscles are common findings.

The symptoms of exercise-induced bronchospasm are cough, wheeze, chest pain or tightness, shortness of breath, and fatigue. Symptoms peak 5 to 10 minutes after completing the exercise session, and subside within 30 to 60 minutes (Cuff & Loud, 2008).

Life-Threatening Asthma Exacerbation In some cases unrelenting, severe respiratory distress and bronchospasm persists despite pharmacologic and supportive interventions. These children are in acute respiratory distress. Clinical manifestations include the use of accessory muscles, restlessness and anxiety, altered mental status, inability to say more than a word or two without gasping for a breath, diaphoresis, and cyanosis. Signs of impending respiratory failure include an inability to speak, inability to lie down, altered mental status, intercostal retraction, and worsening fatigue (Camargo, Rachelefsky, & Schatz, 2009).

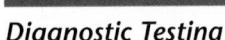

COLLABORATIVE CARE

Diagnostic Testing

Diagnosis is made by a review of the history, physical examination, and spirometry or pulmonary function testing that shows evidence of episodic airflow obstruction (that is at least partially reversible) and airway hyperresponsiveness. Children are generally able to cooperate with spirometry testing at age 5 to 6 years. Spirometry readings are most commonly measured as forced expiratory volume in 1 second (FEV_1) and expressed as a percentage of predicted FEV_1 for the child's height, age, gender, and race. A chest radiograph may help determine if a foreign body could account for symptoms. Skin testing may be used to identify allergens that could be asthma triggers.

Clinical Tip

When spirometry testing is performed, coach the child to give the best effort each time. Encourage the child to seal the lips tightly around the mouthpiece. Then, instruct the child to breathe out as hard as possible, and then to breathe in deeply.

Laboratory findings for the child who needs admission to an intensive care unit may include hypoxemia (may be masked by supplemental oxygen), a $PaCO_2$ of 42 mmHg or greater, respiratory acidosis, and sometimes metabolic acidosis (Gott & Froh, 2010). A peak expiratory flow meter (PEFM) reading of less than 30–50% of the predicted level indicates severe airway obstruction.

Clinical Therapy

Asthma may go into remission or increase in severity over time. Asthma severity is categorized by the child's amount of impairment and risk (or the number of episodes needing oral system corticosteroid therapy). See Tables 20–4 and 20–5 for the classification of asthma severity in children of different age groups. This asthma severity classification guides the recommended therapy protocol. Although current asthma treatment is effective in controlling symptoms, reducing airflow limitations, and preventing exacerbations, the underlying severity of asthma is not prevented (NAEPP, 2007, p. 28).

Clinical therapy includes medications, hydration, education, and support of the parents and child. Pharmacologic treatment is matched to the severity of asthma for daily control and for management of acute episodes. See Medications Used to Treat Asthma. The goal is to maintain asthma control long term, using the least amount of medication and reducing the risk for adverse effects.

A stepwise approach to medication therapy is recommended that matches the child's asthma severity, adding and changing specific medications if the severity progresses or diminishes while maintaining control (NAEPP, 2007, p. 284). The child's response to therapy after 2 to 6 weeks guides the need to further step up the medications to better control symptoms. See

TABLE 20–4 **Classification of Asthma Severity in Children Birth to 4 Years of Age**

Components of Severity		Classification of Asthma Severity (0 to 4 years of age)			
		Intermittent	Persistent		
			Mild	Moderate	Severe
Impairment	Symptoms	2 or fewer days a week	Greater than 2 days a week, but not daily	Daily	Throughout the day
	Nighttime awakenings	0	1 to 2 times a month	3 to 4 times a month	Greater than 1 time a week
	SABA* use for symptom control (not prevention of exercise-induced bronchospasm)	2 or fewer days a week	Greater than 2 times a week, but not daily	Daily	Several times a day
	Interference with normal activity	None	Minor limitation	Some limitation	Extremely limited
Risk	Exacerbations requiring oral systemic corticosteroids	0 to 1 time a year	← 2 or more times a year →		
		← Consider severity and interval since last exacerbation. → Frequency and severity may fluctuate over time for patients in any severity category.			
Recommended step for initiating therapy (see Figure 20–10)		Step 1	Step 2	Step 3 and consider short course of oral systemic corticosteroids	
		In 2 to 6 weeks, depending on severity, evaluate level of asthma control that is achieved. If no clear benefit is observed in 4 to 6 weeks, consider adjusting therapy or alternative diagnoses.			

*SABA = short-acting beta₂-agonist.

From: National Asthma Education and Prevention Program. (2007). Expert panel report 3: Guidelines for the diagnosis and management of asthma (p. 307). Bethesda, MD: National Heart Lung and Blood Institute, National Institutes of Health. Retrieved from http://www.nhlbi.nih.gov/guidelines/asthma/

Figure 20–10 ➤ on page 580 and the companion website for the nationally recommended stepwise approach by age group. Recommendations for children with persistent asthma include the use of daily inhaled corticosteroids and additional long-term control medications as severity increases. Children with intermittent asthma may only need short-acting beta₂-agonists. If asthma control is difficult to achieve, refer the child to an asthma specialist. Treatment also involves reducing exposure to or the impact of triggers causing asthma episodes.

Clinical Tip

Signs of well-controlled asthma in children under age 12 years include symptoms 2 or fewer days a week; no more than one nighttime awakening a month; no interference with normal activity, school, or exercise; use of a short-acting beta₂-agonist for symptom control 2 or fewer days a week; greater than 80% of predicted peak flow (in children 5 years and older); and no more than 1 asthma episode a year requiring oral corticosteroids (NAEPP, 2007, pp. 309, 310, 345).

Most children with acute exacerbations respond to aggressive management in the emergency department. Children who do not respond or who are already being managed at home on corticosteroids have a greater chance of being admitted.

Severe Asthma Exacerbations Some children with a severe (potentially life threatening) asthma exacerbation need aggressive and immediate intervention in the intensive care unit.

Complementary Therapy
Asthma

Massage, osteopathic manipulative treatment, and hypnosis have all been demonstrated in small studies to be beneficial complementary therapies for the treatment of asthma. When asthma episodes are emotionally triggered, mind-body techniques that include training in breathing exercises, behavioral techniques to manage asthma, and relaxation techniques help reduce the duration of asthma episodes (Bukutu, Le, & Vohra, 2008).

These children may progress to respiratory failure and die. The child is placed on a cardiorespiratory monitor and pulse oximetry. Continuous nebulized albuterol, inhaled ipratropium, intravenous corticosteroids, magnesium, and aminophylline may be implemented (Mannix & Bachur, 2007). Electrolytes are carefully monitored. If the child's condition progresses to respiratory failure, noninvasive positive pressure ventilation or intubation may be performed. See nursing management of respiratory failure on page 559 for more information.

Exercise-Induced Asthma Children with exercise-induced asthma have a history of coughing, breathlessness, chest pain, or wheezing that occurs during and after exercise. A spirometry or peak expiratory flow rate (PEFR) indicating a 15% decrease with exertion is diagnostic. Treatment is a short-acting beta₂-agonist 5 to 60 minutes before exercise or long-acting beta₂-agonist 30 to 60 minutes before exercise (Banasiak, 2007).

TABLE 20–5	Classification of Asthma Severity in Children 5 Years to Adulthood			
Components of Severity		Classification of Asthma Severity (5 to 11 years of age and 12 years to adulthood)		
		Intermittent	Persistent	
			Mild / Moderate / Severe	

Components of Severity		Intermittent	Mild	Moderate	Severe
Impairment	Symptoms	2 or fewer days a week	Greater than 2 days a week, but not daily	Daily	Throughout the day
	Nighttime awakenings	2 times or less per month	3 to 4 times a month	Greater than 1 time a week, but not nightly	Often 7 times a week
	SABA for symptom control (not prevention of exercise-induced bronchospasm)	2 or fewer days a week	Greater than 2 times a week, but not daily	Daily	Several times a day
	Interference with normal activity	None	Minor limitation	Some limitation	Extremely limited
	Lung function (5 to 11 years)	• Normal FEV_1 between exacerbations • FEV_1 greater than 80% predicted • FEV_1/FVC greater than 85%	• FEV_1 greater than 80% predicted • FEV_1/FVC greater than 80%	• FEV_1 equals 60–80% predicted • FEV_1/FVC equals 70–80%	• FEV_1 less than 60% predicted • FEV_1/FVC less than 75%
Normal FEV_1/FVC: 8–19 years 85%	Lung function (12 years to adulthood)	• Normal FEV_1 between exacerbations • FEV_1 greater than 80% predicted • FEV_1/FVC normal	• FEV_1 greater than 80% predicted • FEV_1/FVC normal	• FEV_1 equals 60–80% predicted • FEV_1/FVC reduced 5%	• FEV_1 less than 60% predicted • FEV_1/FVC reduced more than 5%
Risk	Exacerbations requiring oral systemic corticosteroids	0 to 1 time a year	← 2 or more times a year →		
		← Consider severity and interval since last exacerbation. → Frequency and severity may fluctuate over time for patients in any severity category.			
Recommended step for initiating therapy (5 to 11 years) (see the companion website for the stepwise approach to management)		Step 1	Step 2	Step 3, medium dose ICS option	Step 3, medium dose ICS option, or step 4
				Consider short course of oral system corticosteroids	
Recommended step for initiating therapy (12 years to adulthood) (see the companion website for the stepwise approach to management)		Step 1	Step 2	Step 3	Step 4 or 5
				Consider short course of oral system corticosteroids	

Evaluate level of asthma control achieved in 2–6 weeks and adjust therapy accordingly.

* FEV_1 = forced expiratory volume in 1 second; FVC = forced vital capacity; SABA = short-acting beta$_2$-agonist; ICS = inhaled corticosteroids.

Adapted from: National Asthma Education and Prevention Program. (2007). Expert panel report 3: Guidelines for the diagnosis and management of asthma (pp. 308 and 344). Bethesda, MD: National Heart Lung and Blood Institute, National Institutes of Health. Retrieved from http://www.nhlbi.nih.gov/guidelines/asthma/

Medications Used to Treat
Asthma

Quick Relief Medication, Route, and Action	Nursing Management
Short-acting beta$_2$-agonists (SABA) Albuterol, levalbuterol, pirbuterol *Metered dose inhaler (MDI) or nebulizer* Relaxes smooth muscle in airway leading to rapid bronchodilation (within 5 to 10 minutes) and mucus clearing. Drug of choice for acute therapy.	■ Use before inhaled steroid, wait 1–2 minutes between puffs, wait 15 minutes to give inhaled steroid. Child should hold breath 10 seconds after inspiring. Then rinse mouth and avoid swallowing medication. Use a spacer. ■ Differences in potency exist, but all products are comparable on a per-puff basis. ■ Some dose-related side effects include tachycardia, nervousness, nausea and vomiting, and headaches. ■ Regular use more than 2 days a week for symptom control indicates a loss of control and need for additional therapy.

Acute Intervention Medication, Route, and Action	Nursing Management
Corticosteroids Methylprednisolone, prednisone, prednisolone *Oral* Diminishes airway inflammation and obstruction, enhances bronchodilating effect of beta$_2$-agonists. Used for short courses to establish control when initiating therapy or during periods of deterioration.	■ Short-term therapy should continue until child achieves 80% peak expiratory flow personal best or symptoms resolve. ■ Give with food to reduce gastric irritation. ■ Give oral dose in early morning to mimic normal peak corticosteroid blood level. ■ Assess for potential adverse effects of long-term therapy, such as decreased growth, unstable blood sugar, and immunosuppression.
Anticholinergic Ipratropium *Metered dose inhaler or nebulizer* Inhibits bronchoconstriction and decreases mucus production.	■ Not for primary emergency treatment because of delayed onset. ■ Rinse mouth afterward to get rid of bitter taste. ■ Side effects include increased wheezing, cough, nervousness, dry mouth, tachycardia, dizziness, headache, and palpitations. ■ Prevent medication contact with eyes.

Daily Control Medications, Route, and Action	Nursing Management
Long-acting beta$_2$-agonists (LABA) Salmeterol, formoterol *Dry powder inhaler (DPI)* Relaxes smooth muscle in airway, used for nocturnal symptoms and prevention of exercise-induced bronchospasm.	■ Should not be used for acute asthma flare. Should only be used in combination with inhaled corticosteroids. ■ Take pre-exercise dose 30 to 60 minutes before activity. Do not use additional dose before exercise if already using twice daily doses which should be 12 hours apart. ■ Caution against overdosage as side effects such as tachycardia, tremor, irritability, and insomnia will last 8 to 12 hours. ■ Report failure to respond to usual dose as this may indicate need for stepped-up therapy.
Inhaled corticosteroids (ICS) Beclomethasone, budesonide, flunisolide, fluticasone, mometasone, triamcinolone *Metered dose inhaler or nebulizer* Anti-inflammatory, controls seasonal, allergic, and exercise-induced asthma; effectively reduces mucosal edema in airways; effective for control of asthma, but ICS does not prevent development of chronic asthma (Guilbert, Morgan, Zeiger, et al., 2006).	■ Administer with spacer or holding chamber. ■ Rinse mouth and gargle following treatment to remove drug from oropharyx to reduce chance of cough, thrush, and dysphonia. ■ Separate parts and clean inhaler daily. ■ Monitor growth; however, recommended doses do not have long-term or irreversible effects on vertical growth (Fong & Levin, 2007). ■ Prevent eye exposure through proper MDI, nebulizer, or DPI administration. ■ Monitor for headache, gastrointestinal upset, dizziness, and infection. ■ Use exactly as prescribed.

Medications Used to Treat
Asthma (continued)

Daily Control Medication, Route, and Action	Nursing Management
Methylxanthines Theophylline *Oral* Relaxes muscle bundles that constrict airways; dilates airway; provides continuous airway relaxation; sustained release for prevention of nocturnal symptoms.	▪ Tablet should not be crushed or chewed. ▪ Used for long-term control; works best when a therapeutic serum level (10–20 mcg/L) is maintained; give at the same time each day. ▪ Requires serum level checks and dose adjustment. ▪ Limit caffeine intake. ▪ Side effects include tachycardia, dysrhythmias, restlessness, tremors, seizures, insomnia, hypotension, severe headaches, vomiting, and diarrhea.
Mast-cell inhibitors Cromolyn sodium, nedocromil *Metered dose inhaler or nebulizer* Anti-inflammatory, inhibits early- and late-phase asthma response to allergens and exercise-induced bronchospasm; may be used for unavoidable allergen exposure.	▪ Not used at time of symptom development or acute exacerbation. ▪ Must be used up to 4 times a day to be effective. ▪ Therapeutic response seen in 2 weeks, maximum benefit may not be seen for 4 to 6 weeks. ▪ Adverse reactions include wheezing, bronchospasm, throat irritation, nasal congestion, and anaphylaxis. Immediately report these symptoms to a physician.
Leukotriene receptor antagonist (LTRA) Montelukast, zafirlukast *Oral* Reduces inflammation cascade responsible for airway inflammation; improves lung function and diminishes symptoms and need for quick relief medications.	▪ Available in granules for infants and chewable tablets for young children. ▪ Administer montelukast in the evening for maximum effectiveness; may be given with food or without. ▪ Make sure child chews montelukast chewable tablet rather than swallowing whole; granules may be mixed in applesauce or ice cream, do not mix in liquid. ▪ Administer zafirlukast 1 hour before or 2 hours after a meal. ▪ Report fever, acute asthma episodes, flu-like symptoms, severe headaches, or lethargy. ▪ Take as prescribed; do not withdraw abruptly.
Immunotherapy Omalizumab A therapeutic antibody that targets IgE, blocking it from causing reactions leading to asthma symptoms.	▪ Approved for children 12 years and older with moderate or severe persistent asthma. ▪ Injections required every 2 to 4 weeks based on serum IgE levels.
Other Hyposensitization (allergy shots), subcutaneous Series of injections with gradual dose increase that can increase the child's tolerance of unavoidable allergens (e.g., mold, pollen).	▪ May be of value for child with persistent asthma having allergies that can be addressed by immune therapy.

Data from: Banasiak, N. C. (2007). Childhood asthma: Part two: Management update. Journal of Pediatric Health Care, 21(3), 184–191; Bindler, R., & Howry, L. (2005). Pediatric drug guide with nursing implications. Upper Saddle River, NJ: Pearson Prentice Hall; Fong, E. W., & Levin, R. H. (2007). Inhaled corticosteroids for asthma. Pediatrics in Review, 28(6), e30–e35; National Asthma Education and Prevention Program. (2007). Expert panel report 3: Guidelines for the diagnosis and management of asthma (pp. 311–318). Bethesda, MD: National Heart Lung and Blood Institute. Retrieved from http://www.nhlbi.nih.gov/guidelines/asthma/

NURSING MANAGEMENT

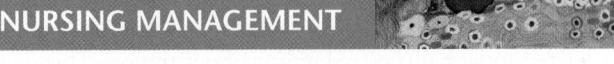

Nursing Assessment and Diagnosis

The nurse usually encounters the child and family in the emergency department or nursing unit. In these settings, acute care has become necessary because the child's level of respiratory compromise cannot be managed at home.

Physiologic Assessment

Identify the child's current respiratory status first by assessing the ABCs—airway, breathing, and circulation—to make sure the child's condition is not life threatening. If the child is moving air or talking, assess the quality of breathing. Assess the respiratory rate. Inspect the chest for retractions to assess the severity of respiratory distress. Auscultate the lungs for the quality of breath sounds and for the presence or absence of wheezing. Observe the child's color and assess the heart rate. Note whether a cough or stridor is present.

Attach a pulse oximeter to monitor the SpO$_2$. Assess PEFR, skin turgor, intake and output, and urine specific gravity. Because asthma can be a symptom of another illness, perform a head-to-toe assessment to identify other associated problems. See the Assessment Guidelines on page 554.

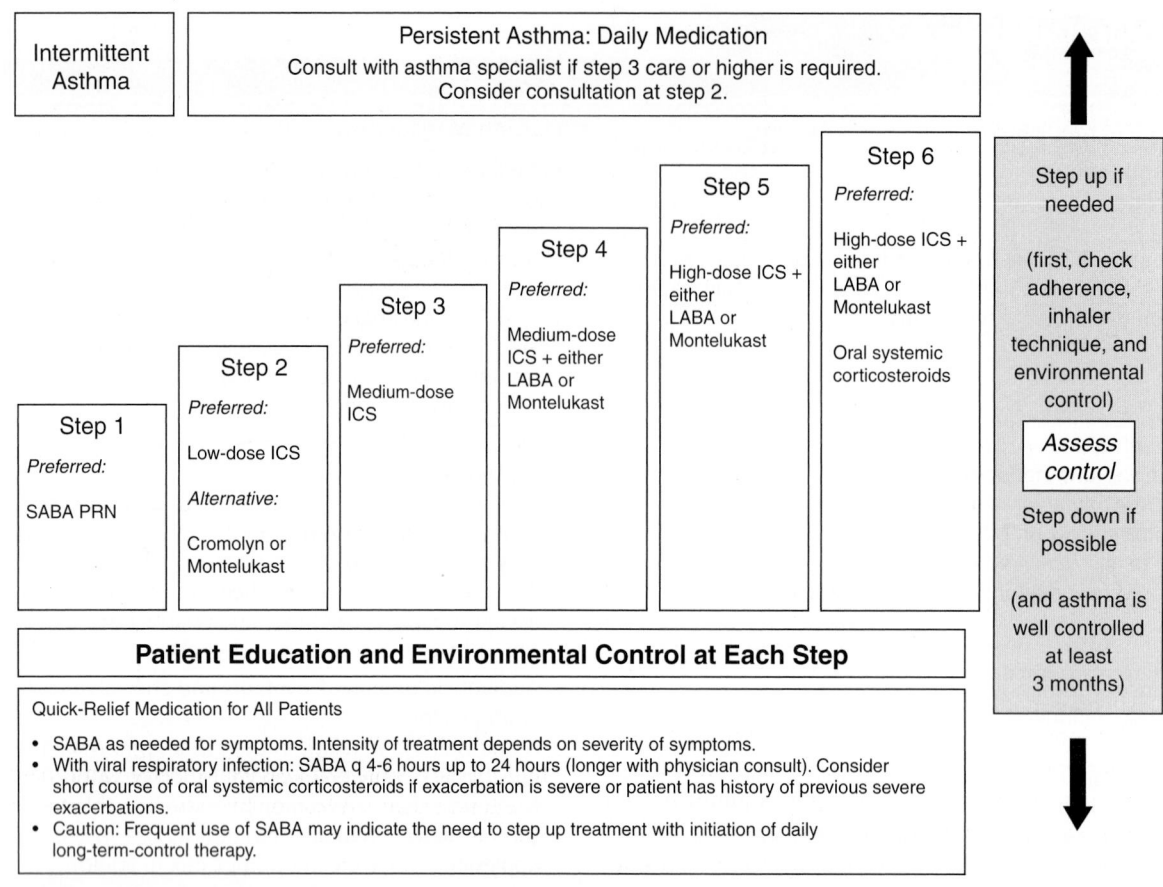

Intermittent Asthma

Persistent Asthma: Daily Medication
Consult with asthma specialist if step 3 care or higher is required.
Consider consultation at step 2.

Step 1
Preferred:
SABA PRN

Step 2
Preferred:
Low-dose ICS
Alternative:
Cromolyn or Montelukast

Step 3
Preferred:
Medium-dose ICS

Step 4
Preferred:
Medium-dose ICS + either LABA or Montelukast

Step 5
Preferred:
High-dose ICS + either LABA or Montelukast

Step 6
Preferred:
High-dose ICS + either LABA or Montelukast
Oral systemic corticosteroids

Step up if needed
(first, check adherence, inhaler technique, and environmental control)
Assess control
Step down if possible
(and asthma is well controlled at least 3 months)

Patient Education and Environmental Control at Each Step

Quick-Relief Medication for All Patients

- SABA as needed for symptoms. Intensity of treatment depends on severity of symptoms.
- With viral respiratory infection: SABA q 4-6 hours up to 24 hours (longer with physician consult). Consider short course of oral systemic corticosteroids if exacerbation is severe or patient has history of previous severe exacerbations.
- Caution: Frequent use of SABA may indicate the need to step up treatment with initiation of daily long-term-control therapy.

Key: **Alphabetical order is used when more than one treatment option is listed within either preferred or alternative therapy.** ICS, inhaled corticosteroid; LABA, inhaled long-acting beta$_2$-agonist; SABA, inhaled short-acting beta$_2$-agonist

FIGURE 20–10 ➤ Stepwise approach for managing asthma in children 0 to 4 years of age. See the companion website for the stepwise approach for managing asthma in children 5 to 11 years and children 12 years and older.
Source: From National Asthma Education and Prevention Program. (2007). Guidelines for the diagnosis and management of asthma (p. 305). Bethesda, MD: National Institutes of Health, National Heart Lung and Blood Institute.

Assess Asthma Management

Key questions to consider asking parents and older children or adolescents include the following (NAEPP, 2007, p. 332):

- Which medicines is the child currently taking? How often?
- How is the medication administered?
- How many times a week is a medication dose missed?
- Have you had problems related to giving the medicine (cost, time, lack of perceived need)?
- What concerns you about the prescribed asthma medication?
- What other treatments for asthma are you using (e.g., complementary therapies)?

Psychosocial Assessment

Assess the child's anxiety or fear related to the asthma episode or hospitalization. How are parents responding to the latest episode? Are they anxious, concerned, or frustrated? Do they potentially have concerns about finances, missing work, or other family members at home? Assess whether the child thinks this episode could have been avoided if medications had been used.

Examples of nursing diagnoses for the child experiencing an acute asthma episode include the following:

- Ineffective Airway Clearance related to airway compromise, copious mucous secretions, and coughing
- Impaired Gas Exchange related to airway obstruction
- Risk for Deficient Fluid Volume related to inability to drink adequate fluids when in respiratory distress
- Anxiety/Fear (Child and Parents) related to difficulty breathing
- Ineffective Management of Therapeutic Regimen (Family) related to lack of understanding about the need for daily management of a chronic disease

Planning and Implementation

Pharmacologic and supportive therapies are used to reverse the airway obstruction and promote respiratory function. Nursing interventions center on maintaining airway patency, meeting fluid needs, promoting rest and stress reduction for the child and parents, supporting the family's participation in care, and educating the family to more effectively manage the child's disease.

Maintain Airway Patency

If the child is exhibiting breathing difficulty, give supplemental oxygen by nasal cannula or face mask. Humidified oxygen should be used to prevent drying and thickening of mucous secretions. Place the child in a sitting (semi-Fowler) or upright position to promote and ease respiratory effort. Evaluate the effectiveness of positioning and oxygen administration by pulse oximeter and by observing for improved respiratory status.

Clinical Judgment

If the mental status of a child with an asthma episode changes to less responsive, what could be the cause and what nursing actions should be initiated?

The respiratory distress and need for supplemental oxygen can be stressful for parents and the child (Figure 20–11 ➤). Encouraging the parents' presence can be reassuring for the child. Keep the parents informed of procedures and results, and get their input when developing the treatment plan.

Most medications are given by inhalation (Figure 20–12 ➤). This route of administration enables the pulmonary blood vessels to rapidly absorb the medication while minimizing the systemic effects. (See the *Clinical Skills Manual.*) The inhaled droplets provide the added benefit of moisture. Continuous inhalation treatments by nebulizer may be used for some children with severe exacerbations. See Growth and Development: Medication Administration for considerations in administering

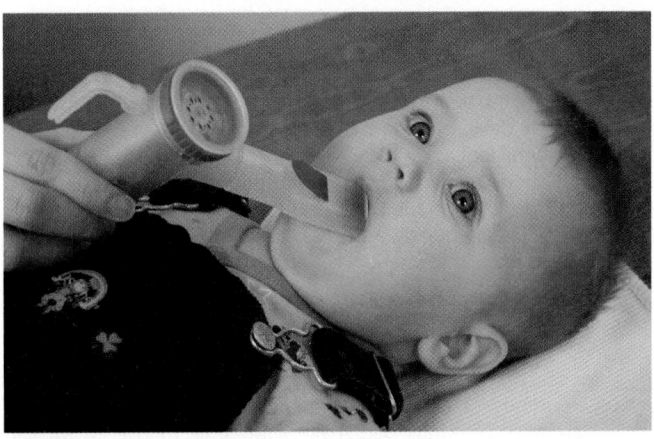

FIGURE 20–12 ➤ Medications given by aerosol therapy are effective because they reach the bloodstream rapidly, and nebulizers require no breathing and medication administration coordination.

medications with inhalation devices. Monitor the child for medication side effects. The frequency of vital sign assessment is determined by the severity of symptoms.

Meet Fluid Needs

Fluid therapy is often necessary to restore and maintain adequate fluid balance. Adequate hydration is essential to thin and break up trapped mucous plugs in the narrowed airways. If an adequate oral intake is not possible because of the child's compromised respiratory status, an intravenous infusion may be needed. Additional medications and glucose may also be provided through the IV. Monitor the child's intake, output, and specific gravity to avoid overhydration and to prevent pulmonary edema in severe asthma attacks.

As respiratory difficulty diminishes, slowly offer oral fluids. The child's fluid preferences should be determined and choices given where possible. Involve parents to help gain the child's cooperation in taking oral fluids.

Clinical Tip

Iced beverages precipitate bronchospasms in some children with asthma. It is safest to offer the child room-temperature or slightly cooled fluids without ice.

Promote Rest and Stress Reduction

The child with an acute asthmatic episode is usually very tired when admitted to the nursing unit. Labored breathing and low oxygen status have left the child exhausted. Put the child in a quiet, private room if possible, but accessible for frequent monitoring, to promote relaxation and rest. Group nursing tasks to avoid repeatedly disturbing the child.

Support Family Participation

The parents may stay with the child, but they may be exhausted after hours of their child's respiratory distress. Give parents the option of assisting with the child's treatments, rather than

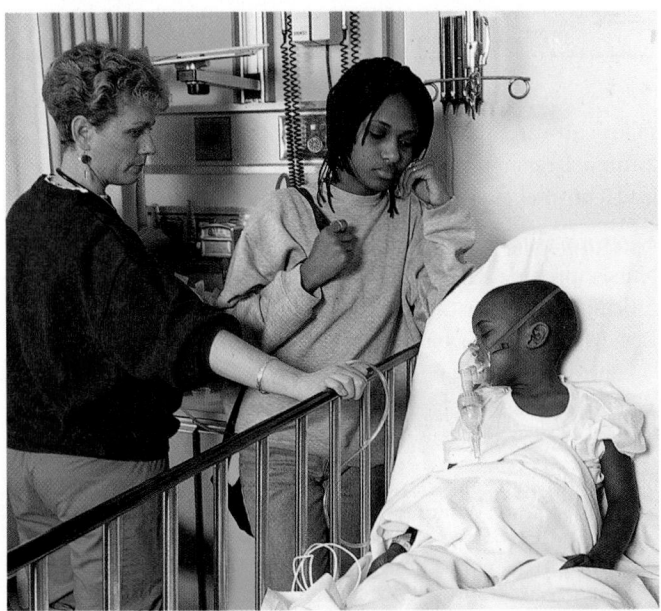

FIGURE 20–11 ➤ Acute exacerbations of asthma may require management in the emergency department. The child is placed in a semi-sitting position to facilitate respiratory effort. Providing support to both the child and parent is an important part of nursing care during these acute episodes. This mother is exhausted after a sleepless night of caring for her son.

Growth & Development *Medication Administration*

Metered-dose inhalers (MDIs), nebulizers, and dry powder inhalers (DPIs) are the devices used for inhalation therapy. These devices are relatively inefficient and have special challenges for infants and young children. Many devices require cooperation, coordination, and appropriate technique that is taught and reinforced frequently. Clean all devices regularly and wash the child's face when a face mask is used for administration.

■ Children over 5 years usually have the ability to use an MDI, co-ordinating medication release and inspiration; however, they may prefer to use a holding chamber or spacer with a valve. With proper technique, 10–15% of the dose may reach the lower airways (Virchow, 2005). Spacers can double the amount of drug delivered to the lungs and make it possible to use an MDI in younger children (Bell, 2006). Spacers have a mouthpiece or mask attachment. Use a spacer with a mask sized to fit the face of an infant or young child. Teach the parents that the mask must conform to the face to prevent an air leak. It may be difficult to maintain a seal when the child is uncooperative. Crying leads to prolonged exhalation and short inspiration, reducing lung deposition. Try to improve cooperation for medication delivery with play and distraction. Wash the plastic spacer with household detergent and permit it to air-dry. This reduces the electrostatic charge and frees more of the drug for delivery (Meadows-Oliver & Banasiak, 2005).

■ Steps in using an MDI include: shake the canister and put the spacer on if used, breathe out, actuate the MDI (release a puff), put the mouthpiece between the lips and teeth (or the mask over the face), inhale deeply over 4 to 5 seconds (with a mask, the child should take 4 to 6 breaths), remove the mouthpiece, and hold the breath 10 seconds. Clean the MDI regularly with water to ensure that the sprayer does not get clogged. Teach the child

to use an MDI without a spacer, by breathing slowly through a straw.

■ Some inhalers have a whistle. In some it warns that the inhaled breath is too fast or too shallow, but in other devices it indicates that an adequate breath has been taken. Be sure to inform the child and family about what the whistle on the child's inhaler indicates.

■ Dry powder inhalers are activated when the patient takes a breath, so puffs do not need to be coordinated with inhalation. No spacer is required and no propellant is used. Children must be able to take rapid, deep, and sustained breaths to effectively use the device (Fong & Levin, 2007). Drug delivery to the lower airway varies from 15–30% dependent upon the type of inhaler. Children less than 6 years of age who are wheezing may not be able to inspire at a rate fast enough to obtain the optimal amount of medication.

■ Essential steps for using a DPI include: remove the lid, load the dose (puncturing the blister or capsule), blow out away from the device, put the mouthpiece between the lips and teeth, and breathe in deeply and forcefully.

■ Nebulizers change liquid medication into aerosol particles. No co-ordination of breathing is required, making them easier for young children to use. Nebulizers are not more efficient than MDIs with a spacer, but they may lead to better outcomes because the child only needs to breathe normally. The nebulizer mouthpiece should be in the mouth, and breathing through the mouth is important for drug delivery. A face mask can be used for children who cannot coordinate mouth breathing. Nebulizers take 8 to 10 minutes for the treatment, and it may be difficult for infants and young children to cooperate for that duration.

Data from: Brand, P. L. P. (2005). Key issues in inhalation therapy in children. Current Medical Research and Opinion, 21(Suppl. 4), S27–S32; Dolovich, M. B., Ahrens, T. C., Hess, D. R., et al. (2005). Device selection and outcomes of aerosol therapy: Evidence-based guidelines. Chest, 127, 335–371; Everard, M. L. (2006). Aerosol delivery to children. Pediatric Annals, 35(9), 630–636; Meadows-Oliver, M., & Banasiak, N. C. (2005). Asthma medication delivery devices. Journal of Pediatric Health Care, 19(2), 121–123; Virchow, J. C. (2005). What plays a role in the choice of inhaler device for asthma therapy? Current Medical Research and Opinion, 21(Suppl. 4), S19–S25.

expecting them to assist. Their role should be to comfort the child. Provide frequent updates about the child's condition and encourage the parents to take breaks as needed.

The length of hospitalization depends on the child's response to therapy. Any underlying or accompanying health problem, such as pre-existing lung disease or pneumonia, can complicate and extend the child's hospital stay. Frequently communicate with the family of the hospitalized child about the child's condition.

Discharge Planning and Home Care Teaching

Parents need a thorough understanding of asthma—how to prevent attacks, maintain the child's health, and avoid unnecessary hospitalization. When possible, educate parents when they are rested, and also refer the child to a health care provider for more extensive education. Make sure the child receives an appointment with an allergist or asthma specialist if moderate to severe persistent asthma exists. Support of parents and the child should focus on helping them to understand and cope with the diagnosis and the need for daily management to promote near-normal respiratory function while the child continues to grow and develop normally. Ensure that the child and family receive an appointment for

follow-up care and education about the daily management of asthma. Reassure the family that most children with asthma can lead a normal life with some modifications.

Nursing Care in the Community

Nurses provide care to children with asthma in pediatricians' offices, specialty asthma clinics, schools, and summer camps. Review the family's daily plan for monitoring the child's respi-

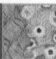

Culture *Asthma Health Beliefs*

Black and Latino children are less likely to use asthma controller medication than Whites. A recent telephone and mail interview study conducted in English and Spanish with 668 parents of children with persistent asthma revealed some interesting differences. Parents of Black and Latino children had lower expectations for their child's functioning with asthma (e.g., a greater number of symptomatic days was expected) than White parents. Black and Latino parents were also more concerned than White parents about medication effects of prescribed daily controller medications, which may lead to less regular use. This study suggests that different health beliefs may be a factor in asthma management (Wu, Smith, Bokhour, et al., 2008).

ratory status. See Families Want to Know: Using a Peak Expiratory Flow Meter. Encourage the school-age child or parent of younger children to use a symptom diary for 2 weeks prior to a health visit to record all daytime and nighttime symptoms and peak expiratory flow measurements. Assess the parent's ability to identify the timing and appropriate medication and care needed to manage worsening symptoms. The goal is to bring asthma episodes under control with stepped-up care before emergency care is needed. See the companion website for a symptom diary and asthma action plan. See the Nursing Care Plan for the child with asthma in the community setting.

Health Maintenance Provide routine health promotion and maintenance care, including immunizations; however, live virus vaccines may need to be postponed if the child has used oral corticosteroids recently. Assess the child's growth pattern if the child is treated with inhaled corticosteroids (ICS) and courses of oral corticosteroids as these medications may affect overall growth.

Assess the amount of activity and exercise the child gets, as well as any symptoms experienced such as chest tightening, wheezing, or shortness of breath. Exercise-induced asthma typically occurs 5 to 10 minutes after stopping the activity and resolves in another 20 to 30 minutes. Children who have symptoms with usual play activities should get a step up in medication management (NAEPP, 2007, p. 297). First determine that the child gets some exercise. Then identify how frequently the child has exercise-induced asthma symptoms, and compare that to the classification of asthma severity in Tables 20–4 or 20–5. For example, if the child has daily exercise-induced asthma symptoms, that is classified as *moderate persistent* asthma. Make sure the daily control and quick relief medication asthma action plan is used by the child.

▲ Health Promotion

Exercise has benefits for children with asthma. Children with asthma may need to learn correct breathing techniques for swimming before learning strokes, and they may need to modify the breathing-stroke ratio. The benefits of swimming were found by one program to increase the child's involvement in other sport and nonsport activities, reduce absences from school, and reduce hospitalizations. Children felt less disadvantaged because of asthma (Wardell, Huang, & Isbister, 2006). Improved cardiovascular fitness and self-esteem were added benefits.

Child and Family Education Once the stress of the acute episode has passed, take advantage of opportunities to provide more extensive education at each health visit. See Families Want to Know: Home Care for the Child with Asthma for a guide to topics that should be discussed in asthma education.

Engage the child in learning about asthma and beginning the steps toward self-management as appropriate. An activity or coloring book may be a good teaching tool. Encourage the child to ask questions about his or her asthma. Provide printed educational materials and referral to a local support group to help parents gain additional knowledge and confidence that will enable them to help their child lead a normal life. Many hospitals have family resource centers that can assist the parents to find helpful

Families Want to Know
Using a Peak Expiratory Flow Meter

Use of a peak expiratory flow meter (PEFM) can help assess the severity of asthma. This device measures the child's ability to push air forcefully out of the lungs. Changes in the PEFM signal worsening lung function and the beginning of an asthma episode. To use a PEFM:

■ Set the device at zero or the base level.

■ Stand up and take as deep a breath as possible.

■ Put the mouthpiece of the meter in the mouth and firmly close the lips around it. Do not cough or let your tongue block the mouthpiece. Blow out as hard and fast as possible over 1 to 2 seconds.

■ Write down the reading.

■ Repeat the process two times and record the highest of three numbers on the chart.

■ Measure and record the best PEFM reading twice a day for 2 to 3 weeks to determine the child's personal best reading. (The child should be optimally treated with medications during the day so the best reading is obtained.)

■ The physician will use the child's personal best average readings to individualize the color zones to guide treatment in the child's asthma action plan.

Zone	PEFM Rate (Best and Predicted for Age)	Action Needed
Green	80–100%	Good asthma control. No asthma symptoms. Take usual medications.
Yellow	50–80%	Caution! Asthma is worsening. Follow guidelines for additional medications in the asthma action plan. Call the health care provider if the child stays in this zone after receiving the additional medications.
Red	Less than 50%	Danger! Severe asthma episode. Use quick relief medications. Call the health care provider or go to the emergency department if PEFM rate does not return to the yellow or green zone.

Adapted from: American Academy of Allergy, Asthma, and Immunology (AAAAI). (2009). *Peak flow meter.* Retrieved from http://www.aaaai.org/

Research ▒▒ *Child's Need for Information*

One study of 63 children (mean age 9 years) with the onset of asthma investigated their needs for psychosocial support and satisfaction with care received. Half of the children reported a need for more information about asthma from their health professionals, especially about handling future asthma episodes. Many children wanted to talk with other children their age with asthma about handling asthma at school. Several of these children were worried about having another asthma episode and being sick with their asthma (McNelis, Musick, Austin, et al., 2007).

Asthma Resources

NURSING CARE PLAN

The Child with Asthma in the Community Setting

INTERVENTION	RATIONALE	EXPECTED OUTCOME
1. Readiness for Enhanced Family Coping related to increased control of asthma with daily medication		
NIC Priority Intervention: *Family Support:* Promotion of family interests and goals		**NOC Suggested Outcome:** *Family Normalization:* Ability of family to maintain routines and management strategies that contribute to optimal functioning when a family member has a chronic illness or disability
Goal: The child and parents will work in partnership with the nurse to improve the child's asthma management.		
■ Listen to the family's concerns about asthma management and respond with information to correct any misconceptions.	■ The parents' concerns may differ from the nurse's. If the parents' concerns are not addressed, the parents may not adhere to recommended care.	The parents express greater confidence in averting and managing their child's asthma flares.
■ Emphasize the importance of daily controller medications to keep asthma under control.	■ Daily medications control the inflammation that triggers asthma flares.	The number of asthma flares requiring medical intervention is reduced.
■ Teach the child and parents to use a peak expiratory flow meter (PEFM), identifying the child's personal best and the range indicating asthma symptom onset.	■ The PEFM helps quantify changes in respiratory status before symptoms are detected.	
■ Teach the family skills (assessment, use of equipment, and giving medications) for managing the child's asthma, and when to seek medical advice or emergency treatment.	■ Proper use of equipment and appropriate medication dosage will help avert and alleviate asthma symptoms. Parents need guidelines for judging the severity of asthma flares.	Parents appropriately call to ask questions about initiating home management or going to the emergency department for an asthma flare.
■ Teach the child and family to monitor the child's response to medications with the PEFM.	■ Monitoring the response gives the family information to determine when home care is inadequate and medical intervention is needed.	
■ Provide telephone consultation to the parents during management of the first few asthma flares.	■ Support and reinforcement of learning during an asthma flare will increase the parents' confidence in managing future flares.	
2. Ineffective Health Maintenance related to lack of school asthma action plan		
NIC Priority Intervention: *Health System Guidance:* Facilitating a patient's location and use of appropriate health services		**NOC Suggested Outcome:** *Health Promoting Behavior:* Actions to sustain or promote optimal wellness, recovery, and rehabilitation
Goal: The child's asthma symptoms will be managed promptly in the school setting.		
■ Provide the family with educational materials to share with the school nurse, teacher, and administrators.	■ School personnel need the latest information about effective asthma management in school settings.	An IHP is developed and an asthma action plan is used to treat the child's asthma flares. The number of school absences for asthma flares that occur during school hours is decreased.
■ Encourage the family to develop an individualized health plan (IHP) with school personnel. Include an asthma action plan for management of an asthma flare.	■ An asthma action plan provides guidance to school personnel for the initial treatment of an asthma flare.	
■ Make sure that the IHP and asthma action plan are available for school sports and for field trips.	■ Participation, even with modification or premedication, prior to activities promotes self-esteem and peer relationships.	

NURSING CARE PLAN

The Child with Asthma in the Community Setting (continued)

INTERVENTION	RATIONALE	EXPECTED OUTCOME
■ Help the family to obtain extra equipment and medications that can be provided to the school.	■ Schools will provide care, but the families must provide all equipment and medications.	
■ Ensure that an additional person other than the school nurse is educated to provide needed medications for an asthma flare.	■ School nurses often travel between several schools. A school administrator or secretary may serve as the backup care provider.	

information on the Internet. See the companion website for educational resources.

Teach the child and family about the importance of the daily control medication program, and collaborate with the physician to develop a written asthma action plan for the child and family. The plan should include the daily control medications, quick relief medications for an asthma flare, and when symptoms require care by a health professional. School-age children should be encouraged to assume more responsibility for care, including avoidance of known triggers, early symptom recognition, relaxation breathing, and the proper use of inhaled medication. Help the child learn the early signs of an asthma episode (coughing, breathlessness) so that treatment can be obtained before signs become more serious. Determine if the family uses any complementary and alternative therapies for asthma management. See Evidence-Based Practice: Improving Asthma Management.

Assess family support systems and family response to the chronic illness. Establish a partnership with the child and family that supports their ability to manage daily control medication regimens. Reasons middle school-age children give for nonadherence include the following: treatment is time consuming and annoying, they forget to carry medication with them, and medications taste bad (Ayala, Miller, Zagami, et al., 2006). Suggest that the child use a fanny pack to carry the inhaler and rinse the mouth with water or flavored mouthwash after the inhaler treatment.

Families Want to Know
Home Care for the Child with Asthma

Identify current knowledge about the condition and its impact on the child:

■ Review the parents' and older child's understanding of asthma pathophysiology and its effect on the child. Ask:

- What causes asthma? What happens in the lungs during an asthma flare?
- What are the early warning signs of an asthma flare in the child?
- What are the child's symptoms and how does he or she respond to them? Does the child wake up at night? Does the child cough a lot? When?
- Is the child involved in any exercise activity? If no, why not? Do asthma symptoms occur?
- Does asthma interfere with social activities or activities with friends?

■ Ask about the child's personal asthma triggers. (Suggest that the parents and child keep a log of symptoms that occur during the day and night, and where symptoms occur to help identify triggers, e.g., home, school, outdoors, with exercise.)

Set up a schedule for parents to learn asthma management:

■ Make sure the parents understand that asthma is a chronic condition that needs daily management and environmental control to reduce or prevent asthma flares.

■ Work with the physician to develop an asthma action plan for daily management, quick relief, and when to call the physician or to seek emergency care.

■ Assess the child's PEFM technique, and correct technique as needed. Discuss how to interpret and use the PEFM results for asthma control. Keep a record of PEFM readings for 2 weeks prior to each health visit.

Review parents' understanding of medication therapy:

■ Provide information about medications: name, type of drug, dose, method of administration, expected effect, and possible side effects. Make sure families understand that control medications help prevent asthma flares, and the child will not feel them working as with quick relief medications. Address the parents' fears about maintaining their child on "steroid" medication, and make sure they understand this is different from the anabolic steroids abused by athletes.

■ Assess the child's technique for the use of an MDI or DPI and correct as needed.

■ When parents use a nebulizer for an infant or young child, suggest diversions that might help the child cooperate during the 8- to 10-minute treatment.

Address associated issues:

■ What are the financial considerations of medication cost and lifestyle changes?

■ What arrangements have been made for the child's use of medications at childcare or school?

■ Does the child with persistent asthma have a medical identification bracelet or tag?

■ Would a self-help group or camp experience be helpful for the child?

Problem

Many children with asthma have less-than-optimal medication management to control symptoms. What are some effective strategies to improve asthma management among children?

Evidence

A recent meta-analysis of studies evaluating asthma education interventions revealed that pediatric asthma education reduces the mean number of hospitalizations and emergency department visits, but not the mean number of urgent physician visits (Coffman, Cabana, Halpin, et al., 2008). The use of nonprofessional community health workers in reducing rehospitalization of 191 low-income African American children (aged 2 to 8 years) with asthma in an urban city was studied. Half of the children received the community health worker intervention and half received their usual asthma education and treatment. Community health workers coached parents in asthma management behaviors (e.g., use of controller medications, use of asthma reliever medications at the time of first symptoms, use of an asthma action plan, the effects of tobacco smoke, and cockroach environmental control). The asthma coach intervention significantly reduced hospitalizations

more than the usual treatment for this population (Fisher, Strunk, Highstein, et al., 2009). A study of 290 children in 36 schools, half receiving school-supervised asthma controller medication and half receiving parent-supervised medication, evaluated the impact on asthma control over a 15-month period. Findings revealed that the school-supervised asthma therapy improved asthma control among this group of predominantly low-income Black children (Gerald, McClure, Mangan, et al., 2009).

Implications

While education should be provided to all families and children with asthma, interventions to improve asthma management should be developed to support what is successful for the culture and social characteristics of the family.

Critical Thinking Application

Think about the cultural and social characteristics of the children in your practice setting. Identify a strategy that would potentially improve asthma management. What resources are needed to implement that strategy? What role would you have in helping to implement that strategy?

Environmental Control Environmental control is an important part of asthma management. If pets and plants are important to the family, make sure they are not allowed in the child's bedroom. An effort should be made to control the dust mites that live in the carpets, mattresses, upholstered furniture, bedcovers, soft toys, and clothes, especially in the child's bedroom. The child's mattress and pillow should be encased in plastic covers. Cockroach eradication should be initiated. Educate parents about the dangers of passive tobacco smoke, and of smoke from woodstoves and fireplaces. See Families Want to Know: Removing Common Allergens from the Home on page 670 and the companion website for information about asthma-friendly childcare.

School Management Encourage parents to work with school personnel to develop an individualized health plan for management of the child's asthma flares during school, including medication for exercise-induced asthma. Make sure the child has a supply of medications at school or childcare as well as at home.

Exercise is beneficial and should be included in the individualized health plan. Make sure teachers of young children can help recognize signs of an asthma flare and reduce a child's anxiety about going to the nurse for quick relief medications. Many schools are attempting to become "asthma friendly" by improving the environment to reduce asthma triggers, providing awareness programs for students and staff, and coordinating with families to better manage asthma and reduce absenteeism (Centers for Disease Control and Prevention, 2006).

 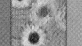

All 50 states have passed legislation that entitles a child to carry and self-administer asthma medications at school (Allergy and Asthma Network, 2010). See the companion website for links to specific state laws.

Evaluation

Expected outcomes of nursing care include the following:

- The child recognizes early asthma symptoms and promptly uses quick relief medications, hydration, and relaxation breathing before severe respiratory distress occurs.
- The child learns to avoid asthma triggers.
- The child and family implement a daily treatment plan for asthma and reduce the number of asthma episodes the child has.
- The child with a serious asthma episode responds to oxygen, fluids, and medication therapy, avoiding hospital admission.

Bronchopulmonary Dysplasia

Bronchopulmonary dysplasia (BPD), also called chronic lung disease, is the need for supplemental oxygen for at least 28 days after premature birth. Its severity is determined by the respiratory support required at term. BPD is a major cause of mortality and long-term morbidity in infants, and respiratory function abnormalities persist into adolescence (Doyle, Faber, Callanan, et al., 2006).

Etiology and Pathophysiology

BPD usually occurs in infants born at a gestational age of 30 weeks or less with a very low birth weight, less than 1250 g (Walsh, Szefler, Davis, et al., 2006). Provision of oxygen and positive pressure ventilation at birth in which tidal volume and inspiratory pressure are not monitored is thought to damage the developing alveolar sacs in the immature lungs. Fewer and larger alveoli with less functional surface area result, and reduced capillary growth in the alveolar region leads to ventilation-perfusion mismatch. Pulmonary hypertension, interstitial fibrosis, and smooth muscle hypertrophy may also develop (Gott & Froh, 2010). Pneumonia, sepsis, meconium aspiration syndrome, di-

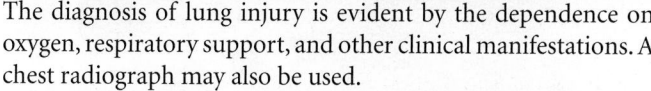

A study involving 150 premature infants with BPD (chronic lung disease) evaluated developmental outcomes at 12 months of adjusted age. Infants were assigned to receive follow-up care by a medical center–based multidisciplinary team (social worker, neonatologist, and nurse specialist) or by a community-based nurse specialist who made frequent telephone calls to the parents. The community-based telephone model was designed to provide social and emotional support to the families, referrals to needed services, developmental surveillance, and care coordination, just as the medical center model did. Both models of follow-up care were provided in collaboration with the infant's primary care physician. Outcomes revealed that infants in the community-based and medical center model of care had no significant differences in development. The community-based model may be a safe model of coordinated care when a family lives far from a medical center (O'Shea, Nageswaran, Hiatt, et al., 2007).

aphragmatic hernia, and lung hypoplasia are causes of BPD in term or near-term newborns (Baraldi & Filippone, 2007). The use of surfactant replacement therapy and antenatal steroids have reduced the risk for respiratory distress syndrome and resulting BPD in more mature preterm newborns (Askin & Diehl-Jones, 2009).

Severity of BPD in infants born at a gestational age of less than 32 weeks is categorized by the need for 21% oxygen for at least 28 days plus these characteristics (Askin & Diehl-Jones, 2009):

- **Mild**—breathing room air at 36 weeks' postmenstrual age or at discharge
- **Moderate**—need less than 30% supplemental oxygen at 36 weeks' postmenstrual age or at discharge
- **Severe**—need greater than or equal to 30% supplemental oxygen at 36 weeks' postmenstrual age and/or positive pressure ventilation or nasal CPAP at 36 weeks' postmenstrual age or at discharge

Clinical Manifestations

The infant with BPD has persistent signs of increased respiratory effort, including tachypnea, irritability, nasal flaring, grunting, and retractions. The infant may have wheezing, crackles, and pulmonary edema. Feeding can create increased oxygen demands the infant cannot meet, fatigue, and poor intake, leading to failure to thrive. The infant has intermittent bronchospasms, mucous plugging, and air trapping that may cause episodes of sudden respiratory deterioration. The air trapping persists and in time causes the chest to assume a barrel shape. Cyanosis may be seen in severe cases.

COLLABORATIVE CARE

The diagnosis of lung injury is evident by the dependence on oxygen, respiratory support, and other clinical manifestations. A chest radiograph may also be used.

Children with BPD may have frequent respiratory illnesses, feeding difficulties, growth failure, and rehospitalizations. Medical management involves symptomatic treatment that supports respiratory function and good nutrition, which helps to accelerate lung maturity. Supplemental oxygen with humidity is used. A tracheostomy may be needed for long-term airway management to prevent narrowing of the trachea. Infants with severe BPD are carefully weaned off assisted ventilation. Some children need gastrostomy or nasogastric tube feeding to get adequate calories.

Chest physiotherapy and medications (diuretics, bronchodilators, anti-inflammatories, and methylxanthines) are used (see Medications Used to Treat Bronchopulmonary Dysplasia). Corticosteroids are not recommended for routine use in premature infants, and their use is controversial in surviving infants (Baraldi & Filippone, 2007). Antibiotics are used to aggressively treat infections. Palivizumab is given monthly to prevent RSV infection (see page 568). With improvement and adequate weight gain, the child is weaned off oxygen, diuretics, and bronchodilators. Some infants die due to respiratory failure and infection.

NURSING MANAGEMENT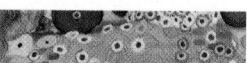

Nursing management focuses on assessing and managing the infant's acute episodes, educating the family to provide home care and adequate nutrition, and promoting growth and development.

Nursing Assessment and Diagnosis

Infants with BPD are often managed in the home. At each health visit, assess the child's respiratory status, any signs of infection, as well as growth and development. Many of these infants have poor weight gain because the work of breathing requires extra calories. Assess how well the family is managing care for the child in the home and any stressors that might exist.

> ▲ **Health Promotion**
>
> Assess the infant's length, weight, and head circumference and plot measurements on a growth chart corrected for gestational age at each health care visit. Identify whether the infant is continuing to grow within an established percentile, indicating that adequate calories are being ingested to support growth.

Infants with BPD may become acutely ill at any time and require hospitalization. Assess airway and respiratory function, vital signs, color, and behavior changes to identify signs of worsening respiratory symptoms, even when oxygen is provided. During hospitalization for acute infections, a cardiorespiratory monitor and pulse oximeter are used. Observe for airway obstruction when the infant has a tracheostomy, and suction as needed. See the *Clinical Skills Manual*.

Nursing diagnoses that may be appropriate include:

- Impaired Gas Exchange related to ventilation-perfusion imbalance
- Caregiver Role Strain related to 24-hour responsibility for infant with BPD
- Imbalanced Nutrition: Less than Body Requirements related to high metabolic needs and fatigue associated with feeding
- Risk for Delayed Development related to chronic condition and limited opportunities to practice motor skills

Planning and Implementation

Organize care for the hospitalized child who will have increased respiratory effort to reduce unnecessary physical stimulation. Position the infant to facilitate breathing.

Medications Used to Treat
Bronchopulmonary Dysplasia

Medication and Action	Nursing Management
Bronchodilators (beta$_2$-adrenergics, anticholinergics, theophylline, albuterol nebulizer) Decreases airway resistance; increases expiratory flow in small airways; stimulates mucous clearance.	▪ Monitor vital signs and for signs of toxicity. ▪ Administer medications at same time each day. ▪ Encourage fluid intake.
Anti-inflammatories (cromolyn sodium) Decreases inhibition of inflammatory mediators from mast cells.	▪ Ensure parents use proper technique for inhaler and spacer. ▪ Clean inhaler daily, rinsing and drying parts.
Diuretics (furosemide, chlorothiazide, spironolactone) Removes excess fluid from lungs; decreases pulmonary resistance and increases pulmonary compliance; may cause electrolyte imbalances.	▪ Follow guidelines for allowable fluid intake. ▪ Monitor serum potassium and sodium levels. ▪ Teach families about sodium- and potassium-rich foods to eat or avoid, depending upon diuretic prescribed.
Potassium chloride Prevents electrolyte imbalances associated with diuretics.	▪ Monitor serum potassium level. ▪ Teach families about potassium-rich foods to avoid or use in moderation.
Methylxanthines (caffeine, theophylline) Increases respiratory drive, decreases apnea, and relaxes muscle bundles that constrict airways.	▪ Monitor vital signs and respiratory status. ▪ Monitor for adverse effects such as irritability, tremor, tachycardia, nausea, and vomiting.

Administer medications as prescribed. Provide fluids and nutrition to meet energy needs. Fluid management is essential as excess fluids can lead to pulmonary edema. Support the mother who desires to breastfeed. A high-calorie formula (24 to 30 calories/oz) may be given to promote weight gain. Some children need nasogastric or gastrostomy tube feedings to ensure adequate calories for growth.

Once home, infants may need ventilation therapy (e.g., CPAP), supplemental oxygen, tracheostomy care, multiple medications, fluid restrictions, and high-calorie feedings (Figure 20–13 ➤). Make referrals for needed oxygen, respiratory supplies, and an early intervention program. Some families need home health nursing assistance, especially during the initial transition period. Ensure that parents have needed medications and scheduled follow-up care at the time of discharge. Teach parents to provide the complex care needed by the infant and to identify the signs of respiratory compromise indicating a need for rapid intervention. Suggest ways to promote the infant's normal development, such as reaching for or moving toward toys and objects of interest.

Evaluation

Expected outcomes of nursing care may include:

- The infant receives adequate calories to sustain growth.
- The family identifies acute illness episodes rapidly and seeks appropriate care.
- The infant's acute respiratory episodes are effectively managed.

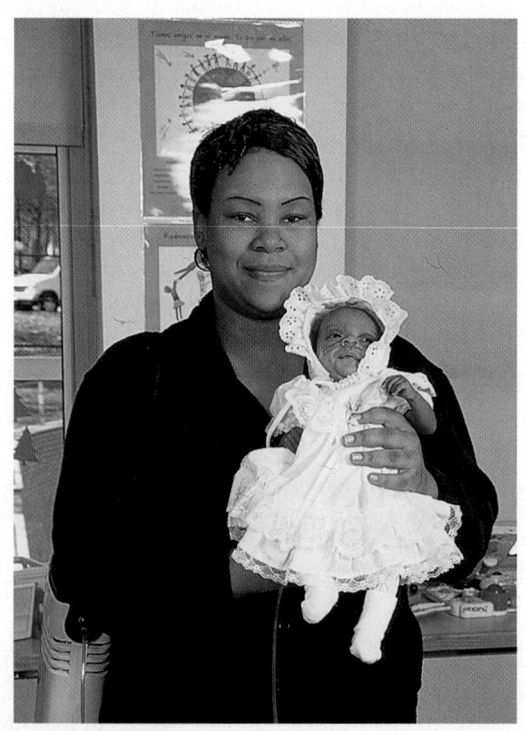

FIGURE 20–13 ➤ Many children with BPD are cared for at home, with the support of a home care program to monitor the family's ability to provide airway management, oxygen, and ventilator support. This premature infant girl, who is now 4 months old but weighs only about 5 pounds, requires respiratory support, which is provided by a portable oxygen tank.

Cystic Fibrosis

Cystic fibrosis (CF) is a common inherited autosomal recessive disorder of the exocrine glands that results in physiologic alterations in the respiratory, gastrointestinal, integumentary, and reproductive systems. The incidence of CF varies by race— 1:3,200 in Whites, 1:7,000 in Hispanics, 1:15,000 in Blacks, and 1:31,000 in Asian Americans (Strausbaugh & Davis, 2007; Kaye & Committee on Genetics, 2006). Gender is not a factor in disease incidence. Approximately 30,000 children and adults have CF in the United States, and approximately 45% are older than 18 years. The median life span for individuals with cystic fibrosis is 37 years (Cystic Fibrosis Foundation, 2009a).

Etiology and Pathophysiology

More than 1,500 mutations of the CF transmembrane conductance regulator (CFTR) gene on chromosome 7 can cause cystic fibrosis (Strausbaugh & Davis, 2007). An estimated 4–5% of all Whites in North America are carriers of the defective CFTR gene (Montgomery & Howenstine, 2009).

Chloride-ion transport across the exocrine and epithelial cells is impaired due to the defective CFTR protein. Decreased chloride secretion and increased sodium absorption results, causing the body to produce unusually thick, sticky mucus that clogs the lungs, leading to infections, and obstructs the pancreatic secretion of natural enzymes that enable the body to digest and absorb food (Strausbaugh & Davis, 2007; Cystic Fibrosis Foundation, 2009a).

In infants with CF, the usual viral illnesses from which healthy children normally recover often progress to bacterial pneumonias. Children develop a classic cough because the respiratory cilia in the lungs cannot clear the thick mucus. Air becomes trapped in the small airways, leading to hyperinflation, atelectasis, and secondary respiratory infections. Bacteria and fungi colonize in the airways over time. Lung inflammation persists, damaging the lungs even after antibiotic therapy. Chronic infection and inflammation lead to bronchiectasis (a persistent abnormal dilation of the bronchi). Pneumothorax and hemothorax may occur in older children. The rate of progression is variable among affected children. End-stage lung disease is the cause of death in 80% of patients with CF (Liou, Woo, & Cahill, 2006).

Failure of the obstructed pancreatic ducts to secrete the natural enzymes needed to digest fats and proteins results in poor digestion, and nutritional deficits may cause failure to thrive. The pancreas may stop producing sufficient insulin in some older children, leading to the development of cystic fibrosis–related diabetes mellitus.

Failure to secrete enough chloride and fluid into intestines may cause a meconium ileus (a small bowel obstruction in newborns), affecting 14% of newborns with cystic fibrosis (Hazle, 2010). Older children may have intermittent and recurrent episodes of partial small bowel obstruction. Chronic inflammation may lead to the development of Crohn disease. Some children develop liver disease (Strausbaugh & Davis, 2007). Nearly all males with CF are sterile because of blocked or absent vas deferens. Females have difficulty conceiving, and if they become pregnant, their pulmonary and nutritional health may be affected.

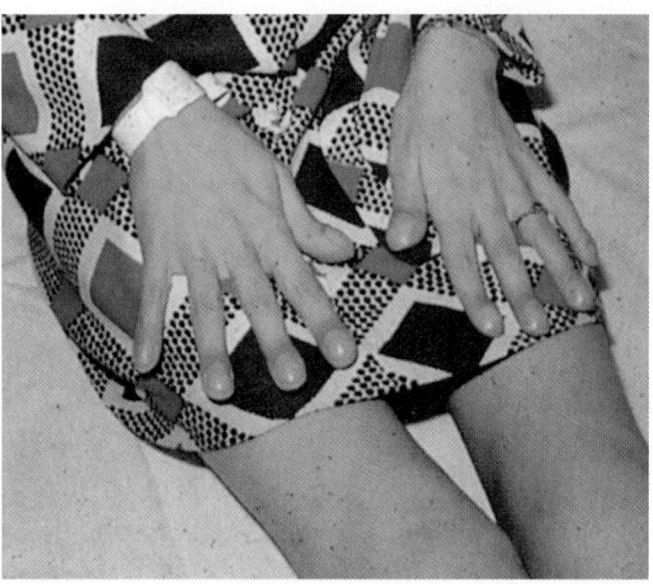

FIGURE 20–14 ➤ Digital clubbing.

Thickened biliary secretions may lead to gallbladder disease and liver dysfunction.

Clinical Manifestations

One of the first signs of CF noticed by the parents is a salty taste to the skin. A meconium ileus may occur in affected newborns. Stools of the child with cystic fibrosis characteristically are frothy (bulky and large quantity), smell foul, contain fat (are greasy), and float. Constipation is common and intestinal obstruction may occur in older children. Rectal prolapse may occur in a small number of children.

Respiratory signs and symptoms include a chronic moist, productive cough and frequent respiratory infections. The child often has wheezing, tachypnea, decreased breath sounds, and fine crackles on auscultation. Clubbing and a barrel chest develop over time (Figure 20–14 ➤). Chronic sinus infections and nasal polyps are found in many children with CF.

Most children have difficulty maintaining and gaining weight despite a voracious appetite because of malabsorption and an increased metabolic rate associated with frequent infections. Infants and children may have a delayed bone age, short stature, and delayed onset of puberty.

COLLABORATIVE CARE

Diagnostic Testing

Cystic fibrosis is usually diagnosed in infancy or early childhood with one of four major presentations: newborn meconium ileus, malabsorption or failure to thrive, chronic recurrent respiratory infections, or intussusception (see Chapter 25 ∞).

Newborn screening can be performed on dried blood samples to detect immunoreactive trypsinogen (IRT) concentrations, which are high in newborns with CF. If the reading is high, a chromosome mutation analysis can be performed on the dried blood spot, or a second IRT test can be performed in 2 to

3 weeks. If the level is still high, an extensive chromosome analysis can be performed to identify less common mutations causing CF (Kaye & Committee on Genetics, 2006). Newborn screening for CF is performed in 48 states and the District of Columbia (Cystic Fibrosis Foundation, 2009b). Genetic testing is also available to identify carriers of CF gene mutations.

A sweat chloride test by pilocarpine iontophoresis is used to confirm the diagnosis when the IRT or newborn screening tests are positive (Kaye & Committee on Genetics, 2006). A sweat chloride concentration of 50 to 60 mEq/L is suspicious. A sweat chloride concentration greater than 60 mEq/L is diagnostic with other signs (meconium ileus, high IRT level, or positive family history). The test is often repeated to confirm the diagnosis (Figure 20–15 ➤).

A spirometer is used on children older than 6 years to monitor pulmonary function. Sputum cultures are obtained to identify infectious organisms and antibiotic sensitivities.

Clinical Therapy

Clinical therapy focuses on maintaining respiratory function, managing infection, promoting optimal nutrition and exercise, and preventing gastrointestinal blockage (Table 20–6). Newly diagnosed children without symptomatic lung disease are aggressively treated to slow the development of chronic respiratory infections and reduction in pulmonary function, and to improve nutrition and support growth. Treatment is focused on controlling inflammation and infection, and on reducing mucus accumulation with an airway clearance technique appropriate for the child's age and development.

Frequent prolonged courses of antibiotics for infections are often prescribed to improve pulmonary function, exercise tolerance, and quality of life. Inhaled tobramycin is given to children with chronic *Pseudomonas aeruginosa* infection to suppress bacterial growth; it is given in alternating months (Montgomery & Howenstine, 2009). Children who have evidence of *Pseudomonas aeruginosa* or *Burkholderia cepacia* infections have a poorer outcome. Medications are used to reduce sputum viscos-

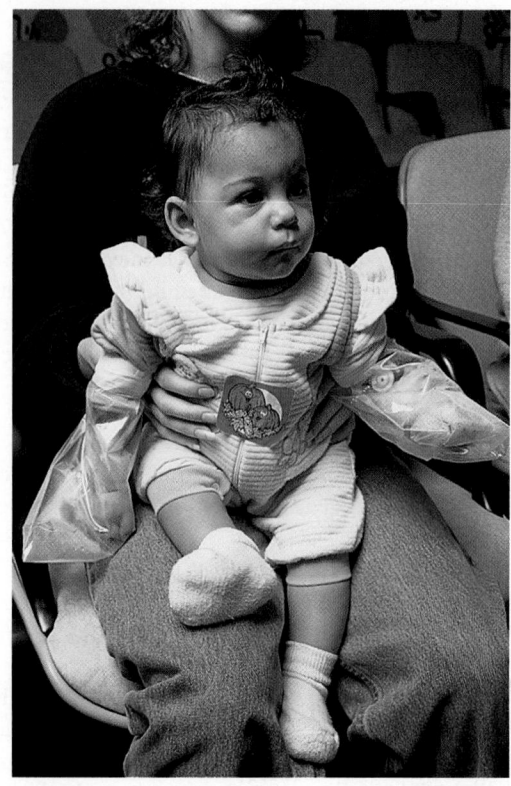

FIGURE 20–15 ➤ This 6-month-old girl is being evaluated for cystic fibrosis using the sweat test.

ity and to dilate the airways. Anti-inflammatory treatment is sometimes prescribed. Vitamins and pancreatic enzymes are also provided to improve the child's nutritional status. See Medications Used to Treat Cystic Fibrosis.

Lung transplantation is occasionally performed, and approximately 60% of cases survive for the first 5 years (Hazle, 2010). Unfortunately, little improvement in survival and long-term outcomes has occurred over the past 20 years (Visner & Gold-

TABLE 20–6	**Clinical Therapy for Cystic Fibrosis**
Clinical Therapy	Rationale
Respiratory Therapy	
Exercise and physical fitness	Promote maintenance of lung function.
Airway clearance techniques—chest physiotherapy twice a day by percussion or vibration, oscillating chest vests, other expiratory techniques (see page 592)	In association with coughing and breathing techniques, airway clearance techniques help move secretions to the bronchi from smaller airways.
Immunizations	Prevent viral and some bacterial infections.
Gastrointestinal Tract Therapy	
Acid suppression preparation	Gastroesophageal reflux worsens lung function; enteric coating of enzyme supplements is affected by high acid content in duodenum.
Hyperosmolar enemas, isotonic fluid lavage of the intestines (oral or nasogastric tube)	Enema relieves meconium ileus in most infants; fluid lavage reduces distal intestinal obstruction.
Nutritional Needs	
Well-balanced diet with 110–200% of Recommended Dietary Allowance (RDA) for calories (Stallings, Stark, Robinson, et al., 2008)	Promotes weight gain and stature growth that is associated with increased lung capacity and survival.

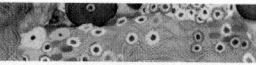

Medications Used to Treat
Cystic Fibrosis

Medications and Actions	Nursing Management
Bronchodilators (aerosol) Increases expiratory flow in small airways; stimulates mucous clearance.	Use before airway clearance techniques. Have the child hold the breath 10 seconds after inspiring. Avoid swallowing the medication, and rinse the mouth.
Dornase alfa (aerosol) Loosens, liquefies, and thins pulmonary secretions.	Keep refrigerated until placed in nebulizer. Monitor for improvement in dyspnea and sputum clearance.
Hypertonic saline (7%) (aerosol) Hydrates the airway mucus and stimulates coughing (Montgomery & Howenstine, 2009).	Use following the bronchodilator.
Ibuprofen (oral) Slows the rate of pulmonary function decline (Flume, O'Sullivan, Robinson, et al., 2007).	Educate child and parents to monitor for signs of gastrointestinal bleeding. Ensure that the child does not take aspirin or other NSAIDs unless approved by physician.
Antibiotics (oral, IV, and inhalation) Used to treat and suppress infections; selected based upon culture sensitivities.	Higher doses than normal and prolonged courses may be needed because of rapid clearance. Teach the child and family to develop a schedule to give the correct dose at appropriate intervals.
Pancreatic enzyme supplements (Cotazym-S, Pancrease, Viokase) Assists in digestion of nutrients, decreasing fat and bulk in the intestines.	Give prior to food ingestion. Ensure that enzymes are taken with meals and snacks.
Vitamins A, D, E, and K (oral)	Ensure that vitamins are prescribed in non-fat-soluble form to promote absorption. Give twice a day.

farb, 2007). Immunosuppressive medications can cause significant problems in individuals infected with *Pseudomonas aeruginosa* or *Burkholderia cepacia*.

NURSING MANAGEMENT

Care of the child with previously diagnosed CF is the focus of the following discussion.

Nursing Assessment and Diagnosis

Physiologic Assessment

Physical assessment of the child focuses on adequacy of respiratory function. Inquire about the frequency and character of the child's cough and sputum characteristics. Compare this information with the child's baseline. Changes in the cough may be more important than its presence or absence related to the development of a new infection. Auscultate the chest for breath sounds, crackles, and wheezes. Note any cyanosis or clubbing of the extremities. Obtain oxygen saturation and spirometry readings if changes in respiratory status are suspected.

Evaluate the child's growth, plotting the weight and height on a growth curve. Determine whether the child is maintaining an appropriate growth pattern. Children with significantly lower percentiles for height and weight should be considered malnourished. Inquire about the child's appetite and dietary intake. Ask how nutritional supplements, pancreatic enzymes, and vitamins are used. Observe the adolescent for the appearance of secondary sex characteristics, which are often delayed due to nutritional status.

Assess the child's stooling pattern. Identify whether the child has problems with abdominal pain or bloating, and whether these problems can be related to eating, stooling, or other activities. Palpate the abdomen for liver size, fecal masses, and evidence of pain.

Psychosocial Assessment

The emotional stress of this chronic disease may not be readily apparent on admission, particularly if the child's symptoms are mild and not imminently life threatening. Ongoing observation of the child's and parents' behavior helps direct nursing interventions throughout hospitalization. Parents may feel guilt as carriers of the disease. Siblings may also show signs of difficulty in dealing with the illness, particularly if not affected by the disease. Siblings with CF may be affected if the child is showing signs of significant deterioration, being forced to acknowledge their own future course with the disease.

Ask parents how the child's illness has affected day-to-day functioning, whether there have been any potential conflicts with family activities, and how they have adapted to the child's plan of care. Investigate the need of and options for respite. The nurse should ask what parents have told the child and siblings about the disease. What kinds of questions have the child and siblings asked about CF, and how have parents answered them? Has the child ever asked about his or her life expectancy? If not, what would parents say if asked?

Common nursing diagnoses for the child with cystic fibrosis include the following:

- Ineffective Airway Clearance related to thick mucus in lungs
- Risk for Infection related to the presence of mucous secretions and airway obstruction
- Imbalanced Nutrition: Less than Body Requirements related to the need for increased calories to meet metabolic needs
- Parental Role Conflict related to interruptions in family life due to the home care regimen and child's frequent exacerbations

Planning and Implementation

Nursing management involves supporting the child and family when the diagnosis is made, during subsequent hospitalizations, and during visits to specialty and primary health care providers. The nurse's role begins with implementing specific medical therapies and providing nursing care to meet the child's physiologic and psychosocial needs. Airway clearance techniques, medications, and nutrition must be coordinated to promote optimal body function. Psychosocial support and reinforcement of the child's daily care needs are important in preparation for home care.

Children with cystic fibrosis require periodic hospitalization when a severe infection occurs or for a pulmonary and nutritional assessment. The child is usually placed in a single room to reduce the spread of infectious organisms with standard precautions. Children with CF are not co-roomed to reduce the risk for cross-infection with *Pseudomonas aeruginosa* and *Burkholderia cepacia*.

Respect the parents' experiences as the child's primary care provider and include them in the child's routine care as much as possible. However, parents may view the hospital stay as a break from the rigorous daily pulmonary routine at home and need support in taking advantage of some "down" time. While the family is often proficient at providing physical care to the child, the nurse should take the opportunity to review basic and new information about respiratory care, medications, and nutrition. This is especially important as the child matures and begins to assume some responsibility for self-care.

Promote Airway Clearance

Chest physiotherapy is often performed on children under 2 years one to three times per day before meals to clear secretions from the lungs, as coughing may stimulate vomiting (see the *Clinical Skills Manual*). Aerosol treatments with a bronchodilator, as well as DNase and hypertonic saline to help thin respiratory secretions, may precede airway clearance techniques. Respiratory therapists and nurses often collaborate in teaching parents and other family members the skills for these necessary treatments. Older children may use an oscillating vest or forced expiratory airway clearance techniques (Figure 20–16 ➤). Exercise and aerobic conditioning is recommended for children with CF as it promotes airway clearance (Hazle, 2010).

Administer Medications and Meet Nutritional Needs

Antibiotics for acute exacerbation are provided by oral, inhalation, and intravenous routes. Because children with CF have an increased clearance of most antibiotics, they need higher doses and long treatment courses. Serum antibiotic drug levels may be ordered to ensure therapeutic dosing. In some cases, a portacath or central line may be placed for home IV therapy to enable an earlier discharge.

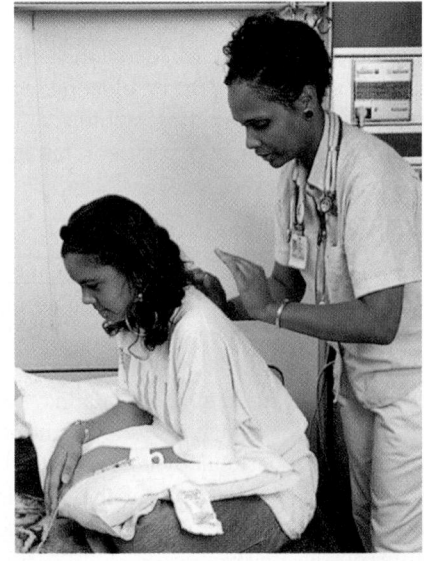
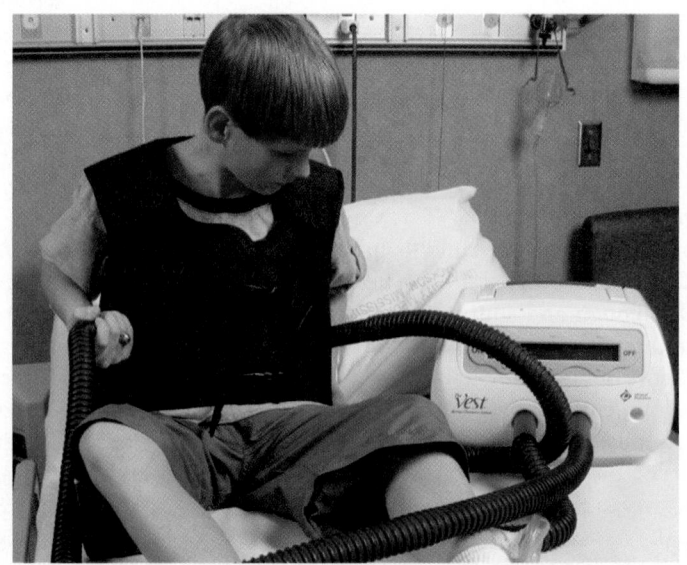

FIGURE 20–16 ➤ A, Postural drainage can be achieved by clapping with a cupped hand on the chest wall over the segment to be drained to create vibrations that are transmitted to the bronchi to dislodge secretions. B, Oscillating vibration vest that this child can independently set up to perform chest physiotherapy.

Digestive problems can be eased with pancreatic enzymes and dietary modification. Pancreatic enzyme supplements come in powder sprinkles and capsule form. They are taken orally with all meals and large snacks. The amount needed is individualized, based on the child's nutritional needs and digestive response to these supplements. Families need to learn which foods if any to avoid that contribute to a child's gastrointestinal problems. The goal is to achieve near-normal, well-formed stools and adequate weight gain.

Because of the child's high metabolic rate, some children need nutritional supplements or supplemental nasogastric or gastrostomy feedings to gain and maintain weight. The diet should be well balanced, with an emphasis on high caloric value. Fats and salt are both necessary in the diet.

Provide Psychosocial Support

Help the parents and child learn what they must do to maintain health after discharge. Emotional support is essential because the diagnosis of this disorder creates anxiety and fear in both the parents and the child. They need assistance with emotional and psychosocial issues relating to discipline, body image (stooling and odor), frequent rehospitalization, the potential fatal nature of the illness, the child's feeling of being different from friends, and overall financial, social, and family concerns. Because the disorder is inherited, families may have more than one child with cystic fibrosis. Refer families to genetic counseling and support groups; see the companion website for resources.

Discharge Planning and Home Care Teaching

The financial burden of medications, supplies, and medical follow-up may not be recognized immediately by a family overwhelmed by the diagnosis. Initially, parents need assistance in obtaining necessary equipment. If the family requires financial assistance, they should be referred to the appropriate social services. Home care of the child with cystic fibrosis is expensive and can be draining on the family's finances.

Nursing Care in the Community

Nurses may encounter the child with CF in specialty clinics, health centers, and schools. Assess the child as described on page 554. Observe the child's physical appearance, noting overall body proportions and any changes characteristic of CF. Respiratory function tests are usually performed every 6 months during CF visits. Assess hearing acuity on a regular basis, especially if the antibiotic tobramycin is used.

A psychosocial assessment is especially important when the child is going through major developmental stages. School-age children and adolescents are often embarrassed at being viewed as different from peers, such as small and thin for age, or eating large quantities of food. Ask how the child or adolescent feels about the need for a special diet, medications, and the daily routine of respiratory management.

Review the child's use of bronchodilators and airway clearance techniques. If additional short-term therapies are prescribed to help improve pulmonary status, educate the child and family about the techniques to use and help them identify the best time to fit the additional treatment into the daily schedule. Chest physiotherapy or other airway clearance techniques prescribed three

or four times a day is a significant impact on the family time. Alternative bronchial hygiene therapy techniques such as an oscillating vest may be more easily accepted by the family, especially since the parent does not have to physically perform the percussion and vibration. A regular vigorous exercise regimen is also beneficial in improving lung function, respiratory muscle strength, endurance, and airway clearance.

Children with CF need a balanced diet enhanced with calorie-dense snacks and supplements to support growth. Parents often have difficulty encouraging the child with CF to eat the extra calories needed for optimal nutrition, setting the stage for a potential mealtime battleground. Parents need guidance about managing negative mealtime behaviors, in addition to guidelines for preparing nutritional calorie-dense foods. Increase calorie intake by offering high-calorie snacks between meals and before bed. Extra intervention, such as a gastrostomy tube for nighttime feedings, may be needed when the child's weight is 85–90% of ideal weight for height. Children with adequate nutrition have a longer life expectancy.

Clinical Tip

Use of cream or half and half added to soups, casseroles, and puddings; cream cheese spread on breads, muffins, and crackers; sour cream added to casseroles; and powdered milk added to regular milk, meatloaf, and custards are all ways to increase the calories in food eaten. Ensure Plus, Boost, or Carnation Instant Breakfast can be added to ice cream and fruit to make a milk shake (Pitts, Flack, & Goodfellow, 2008).

Children with CF lose more than normal amounts of salt in their sweat. This loss can become intensified during hot weather, strenuous exercise, and fever. During periods of exercise and increased sweating, the child should be encouraged to drink more fluids and increase salt intake. Parents should allow the child to add extra salt to food and should permit some salty snacks (pretzels with salt, pickles, carbonated soda). Teach parents to recognize early symptoms of salt depletion, including fatigue, weakness, abdominal pain, and vomiting, and to contact the child's health care provider if these symptoms occur.

Adolescents with CF need special assistance in coping with their disorder, especially since the median survival is now more than 37 years. Help them identify normal adolescent changes versus those related to CF. Adolescents must learn how to cope

Research ○ *Self-Care Indicators*

A study of 123 adolescents with CF investigated predictors of universal health self-care (e.g., eating a nutritious diet) and of CF-related self-care (e.g., airway clearance techniques, taking medications). Satisfaction with family was a predictor of universal self-care and CF-related self-care. A greater sense of life being meaningful and manageable, plus ego strength, attention to health, health knowledge, and decision-making capability were predictive of universal self-care. Adolescents who engaged in higher levels of universal self-care were more likely to engage in CF-related self-care (Baker & Denyes, 2008).

with the difference they know exists between themselves and peers. Provide information about potential infertility along with guidelines for safe sexual practices to reduce the risk for sexually transmitted infections. Females with CF may be able to conceive and should be offered contraception.

The child's gradual assumption of responsibility for daily disease management is necessary. Adherence with the daily disease management may be a problem during adolescence. Individualized planning to achieve adolescents' daily care regimen while enabling them to interact with peers and participate in school activities may be most helpful. Link adolescents to services to assist with planning appropriate educational and occupational goals for their future. Palliative care planning should be initiated as the disease progresses to respiratory failure.

Evaluation

Expected outcomes of nursing care include:

- The child and family become proficient in daily pulmonary care and reduce the incidence of respiratory infections.
- The child and family develop a schedule and routine for daily pulmonary care that fits into family and school activities.
- The child consumes adequate calories and pancreatic enzymes to support growth and to stay within desirable weight ranges.

■ INJURIES OF THE RESPIRATORY SYSTEM

Airway compromise after an unintentional injury can cause death if not managed quickly and effectively. Children are vulnerable to changes in respiratory function after injury. The child's airway may become obstructed because of its small size. The airway may be obstructed by the tongue; small amounts of blood, mucus, or foreign debris; as well as swelling in the respiratory tract or adjacent neck tissue. If the child's neck is flexed or hyperextended, the soft laryngeal cartilage may also compress and obstruct the airway.

Smoke Inhalation Injury

Exposure of the child's face and airway to fire or thermal conditions causes dramatic responses in a child's respiratory tract. Smoke and heat inhalation injury increases the child's risk for airway obstruction, carbon monoxide poisoning, acute respiratory distress syndrome, and late complications such as pneumonia and pulmonary embolism (Antoon & Donovan, 2007). The child's higher respiratory rate also increases the exposure to noxious chemicals.

The severity of the smoke inhalation injury is influenced by the type of material burned. The injury is more severe if the child is found in a closed space. The composition of materials determines how easily they ignite, how fast they burn, and how much heat they release. Smoke, a product of the burning process that is composed of gases and particles, is generated in varying volumes and density. The type and concentration of toxic gases, which are usually invisible, affect the severity of pulmonary damage. The duration of exposure to the smoke produced and any toxic gases contribute significantly to the child's prognosis.

Exposure to extreme heat, common in house fires, leads to surface injury and upper airway damage. The upper airway normally removes heat from inhaled gases, sparing the lower airway from thermal damage. Airway edema develops rapidly over a few hours and places the small child at risk for airway obstruction and potentially for acute respiratory distress syndrome.

Carbon monoxide (CO) is a clear, colorless, odorless gas present in all fire conditions as the fire consumes oxygen. The CO molecule binds more firmly to hemoglobin than does oxygen. As a result, CO replaces oxygen in the blood cells and hypoxia rapidly results. The brain receives inadequate oxygen, resulting in confusion. This accounts for the inability of fire victims to escape as confusion progresses to loss of consciousness.

Damage to the lower airway most often results from chemicals or toxic gas inhalation. Smoke particles are carried deep into the lungs. These particles combine with lung moisture to produce acid chemicals that burn the lung tissue, causing loss of cilia, loss of surfactant, and edema. Tissue destruction, pulmonary edema, and disruption of gas exchange produce the initial insult to the lungs and potential airway obstruction. Days later, the damaged tissue sloughs off, obstructing the airways. The lungs become a breeding ground for microorganisms, leading to pneumonia. Healing leaves scars in the damaged alveoli, which can greatly reduce future lung function.

Clinical manifestations of inhalation injury include burns of the face and neck, singed nasal hairs, soot around the mouth or nose, and hoarseness with stridor or voice change, even when the child initially has no respiratory distress. Edema develops rapidly over a few hours and may lead to airway obstruction with signs such as tachypnea, stridor, coughing, and wheezing. Respiratory distress develops and can lead to respiratory failure. If carbon monoxide poisoning is present the child will be confused or unconscious, and have cardiac arrhythmias.

Nursing Management

Most children who survive smoke inhalation injury are admitted for close observation, airway management, and ventilatory support, if indicated. Initial treatment is 100% humidified oxygen administered through a nonrebreather mask (see the *Clinical Skills Manual*). Carefully assess the child for respiratory function, and assess for behavior changes that can indicate increasing hypoxia. Provide oxygen as ordered. Position the child to promote respiratory function. If respiratory distress develops, aggressive airway management with an endotracheal tube, mechanical ventilation, and monitoring are usually provided in an intensive care unit. Care is provided as described for the child with respiratory failure.

Blunt Chest Trauma

Blunt chest trauma in children often occurs with other system injuries. Blunt chest trauma in infants and toddlers is most often due to motor vehicle crashes and abuse. Bicycles, scooters, skateboards, and skates are more commonly associated with blunt chest trauma in school-age children. Injuries from high-energy motor vehicle crashes and hitting the steering wheel are more common causes of blunt chest trauma in adolescents (Pitetti & Walker, 2005). Chest injuries may not be obvious and can be extremely difficult to evaluate.

Most children who die after sustaining severe blunt chest trauma were hypoxic because of poor airway and ventilatory control. A child's elastic, pliable chest wall and thin abdominal muscles provide minimal protection to underlying organs. This elasticity of the ribs often prevents rib fractures, but the energy from blunt trauma is transferred from an external force to the internal organs, often causing a pulmonary contusion or pneumothorax. A rib fracture in children under 12 years old indicates trauma of significant force.

Pulmonary Contusion

A pulmonary contusion is defined as bruising damage to the tissues of the lung that often occurs without bony injury to the thorax. This causes bleeding from the capillaries of the alveoli, which may lead to capillary rupture in the air sacs. Pulmonary edema develops in the lower airways as blood and fluid from damaged tissues accumulate. The lower airway becomes obstructed, leading to poor perfusion of the alveoli, poor compliance, hypoxemia, and hypoventilation (Pitetti & Walker, 2005).

Initially the child may appear asymptomatic. Respiratory distress, along with fever, wheezing, hemoptysis, and crackles, often develops over several hours. Careful observation is required during the first 12 hours after the injury to detect decreased perfusion related to ventilatory impairment.

The child with severe injury will need mechanical ventilation with low airway pressures, fluid restriction, supplemental oxygen, pain control, and incentive spirometry. It is important to avoid prolonged immobilization. Pneumonia is a potential complication that can progress to respiratory failure (Pitetti & Walker, 2005).

Nursing Management

Nursing care centers on providing necessary physiologic support, such as oxygen therapy, positioning, positive pressure ventilation, fluid management, and comfort measures.

Observe for hemoptysis (fresh blood in the emesis), dyspnea, decreased breath sounds, wheezes, crackles, and a transient temperature elevation. Inspect the thorax for symmetric chest wall movement and equal presence of breath sounds in both lungs. The child may initially appear well but requires careful and thorough monitoring to detect signs of deterioration. The child's level of consciousness is an excellent indicator of respiratory function. Agitation and lethargy can signal increasing hypoxia.

Nursing Alert

When monitoring the status of a child who has a pulmonary contusion, do not rely on the child's color as an indicator of adequate oxygenation. Cyanosis in children is often a late indicator of respiratory distress.

Children with significant injuries are cared for in the ICU with ventilator support. Intake and output should be carefully monitored to reduce the severity of pulmonary edema. Incentive spirometry should be performed while assisting the child to reduce discomfort associated with coughing (see the *Clinical Skills Manual*).

Support the parents who are anxious about the potential life-threatening nature of the child's injury. See Chapter 13 ∞ for suggested support for families and siblings.

Pneumothorax

A **pneumothorax** occurs when air enters the pleural space because of tears in the tracheobronchial tree, the esophagus, or the chest wall. If blood collects in the pleural space, it is called a *hemothorax*. If blood and air collect, it is called a *pneumohemothorax*.

A pneumothorax may be open, closed, or tension. An open pneumothorax, sometimes referred to as a sucking chest wound, results from any penetrating injury that exposes the pleural space to atmospheric pressure, thereby collapsing the lung. A sucking sound may be heard as the air moves through the opening on the chest wall.

A closed pneumothorax is sometimes caused by blunt chest trauma with no evidence of rib fracture. The chest may be compressed against a closed glottis (such as may occur with breath holding), causing a sudden increase in pressure within the thoracic cavity. The pressure increase is transferred to the alveoli, causing them to burst. A single burst alveolus may be able to seal itself off, but the lung collapses when many alveoli burst. Breath sounds are decreased or absent on the injured side, and the child is in respiratory distress. A chest radiograph often reveals air in the chest. Treatment usually involves a thoracostomy and insertion of a chest tube. A closed drainage system is attached to help remove the air and reinflate the lung by reestablishing negative pressure.

A tension pneumothorax is a life-threatening emergency that results when the air leaks into the chest during inspiration but cannot escape during expiration (Figure 20–17 ➤). Internal pressure continues to build, compressing the chest contents and collapsing the lung. Venous return to the heart is impaired as the trachea, heart, vena cava, and esophagus are compressed toward the unaffected lung when the mediastinum shifts, leading to decreased cardiac output. Signs of tension pneumothorax include increasing respiratory distress, decreased breath sounds, and paradoxical breathing.

Nursing Management

Nursing management focuses on airway management and maintaining lung inflation. The child arrives on the nursing unit with a chest tube and drainage system in place. Continued close observation for respiratory distress is essential. Carefully monitor vital signs and respiratory function. When the chest tube is removed, the site is covered with an occlusive dressing and the child's respiratory status is monitored for signs of respiratory distress. If a hemothorax occurs, monitor blood draining into the chest tube drainage system and the child's physiologic status for hypovolemic shock. See Chapter 21 ∞ for management of the child in hypovolemic shock.

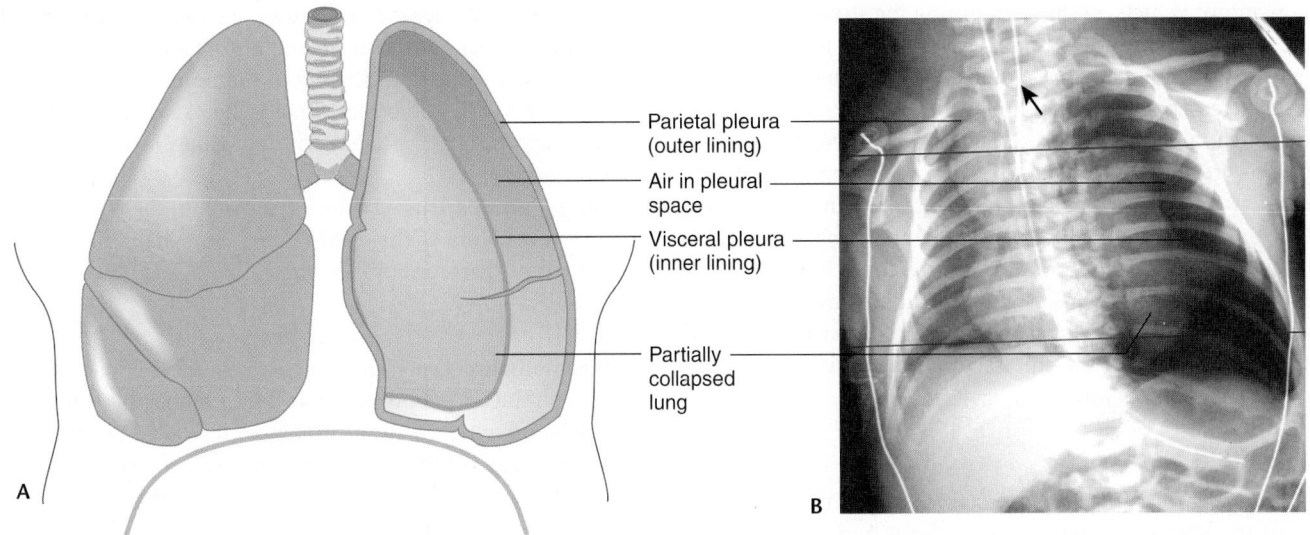

FIGURE 20–17 ➤ A, A pneumothorax is air in the pleural space that causes a lung to collapse. Whether the air results from an open injury or from bursting of alveoli due to a blunt injury, it is important to focus on airway management and maintain lung inflation. B, Tension pneumothorax. Note the collapsed lung on the patient's left side and the deviation of the child's heart and trachea to the right side of the chest.
Note: B, Courtesy of Dorothy I. Bulas, M.D., Professor of Radiology and Pediatrics, Children's National Medical Center, Washington, DC.

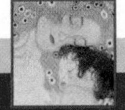

Chapter Highlights

- Respiratory conditions are a leading cause of hospitalization for all children between 1 and 19 years of age.
- The child's airway is shorter and narrower than an adult's, increasing the risk for obstruction. The lungs have no muscles; the diaphragm and intercostal muscles power ventilation.
- Foreign body aspiration is a major health problem for infants and toddlers, often related to their increasing mobility and tendency to put small objects such as food and toy parts in the mouth.
- Signs of impending respiratory failure in infants and children include worsening respiratory distress, irritability, lethargy, mottled color or cyanosis, diaphoresis, and increased respiratory effort such as dyspnea, tachypnea, nasal flaring, grunting, and retractions.
- An apparent life-threatening event (ALTE) is an episode of apnea accompanied by a color change (e.g., cyanosis or pallor), limp muscle tone, choking, or gagging in an infant less than 12 months of age.
- Obstructive sleep apnea syndrome (OSAS) in children is commonly caused by enlarged tonsils and adenoids. Children snore loudly and have labored breathing during sleep.
- Sudden infant death syndrome (SIDS) is a leading cause of death in infants. Onset of the fatal episode occurs during sleep and remains unexplained after a thorough investigation, including an autopsy, a review of the circumstances of death, and the clinical history.
- Laryngotracheobronchitis (LTB) is a viral croup syndrome with signs of an upper respiratory illness, hoarseness, tachypnea, in-

spiratory stridor, and a seal-like barking cough. Fever may or may not be present.
- Epiglottitis is a potentially life-threatening airway obstruction caused by bacterial invasion of the laryngeal soft tissue causing inflammation and edema of the epiglottis and surrounding tissues. Classic signs include dysphonia, dysphagia, drooling, and distressed respiratory effort.
- Respiratory syncytial virus (RSV) is the most common cause of bronchiolitis, a lower respiratory tract infection that causes inflammation and obstruction of the bronchioles.
- Symptoms of pneumonia in infants and children include elevated temperature, rales, crackles, wheezes, cough, dyspnea, tachypnea, restlessness, and decreased breath sounds if consolidation occurs.
- Children under 2 years are at increased risk for developing active tuberculosis, including tubercular meningitis and disseminated TB.
- An asthma flare or episode results from inflammation and a stimulus causing excessive mucous formation, mucosal swelling, and airway muscle contraction, leading to airway obstruction.
- Chronic lung disease or bronchopulmonary dysplasia (BPD) usually develops in neonates with a birth weight of 1000 g or less. Treatment with oxygen and positive pressure ventilation causes inflammation and damages the bronchioles, resulting in fibrosis, edema of the bronchioles, and smooth muscle hypertrophy.
- In cystic fibrosis, defective chloride-ion transport across the exocrine and epithelial cell walls results in an abnormal accu-

mulation of viscous, dehydrated mucus that affects the respiratory, gastrointestinal, and reproductive systems.

■ Signs of smoke inhalation injury in children include burns of the face and neck, singed nasal hairs, soot around the mouth or nose, and hoarseness with stridor or voice change.

■ A pneumothorax may become life threatening when air leaking into the chest cavity during inspiration cannot escape during expiration, increasing compression. Venous blood return to the heart is impaired as the mediastinum shifts toward the unaffected lung.

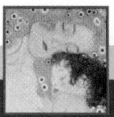

Clinical Reasoning in Action

Recall Shaun, the 13-year-old from the opening scenario. He is in the hospital for infection management and aggressive respiratory therapy. Because he has cystic fibrosis and infectious organisms in his lungs, he is in a single room. He is not permitted to interact with the other children on his unit. Shaun uses a mask when he leaves his room and the nursing unit. He is not feeling ill and welcomes company and distractions. His mother and sister are only able to visit after work. This is an optimal time to continue teaching Shaun to manage his condition.

1. What is Shaun's developmental stage, and what information and self-care skills should be included in a teaching plan for Shaun to correspond to that stage?

2. What information should be reviewed with Shaun about his condition and the treatments needed to keep it from progressing?

3. What signs should Shaun learn to recognize that might indicate a new infection?

4. What approaches might be taken to help Shaun schedule his treatments around school and recreational activities that might increase adherence to the schedule?

See Pearson Nursing Student Resources for possible responses.

Pearson Nursing Student Resources

Find additional review materials at
nursing.pearsonhighered.com
Prepare for success with NCLEX®-style practice questions, interactive assignments and activities, web links, animations and videos, and more!

References

Adams, S. M., Good, M. W., & Defranco, G. M. (2009). Sudden infant death syndrome. *American Family Physician, 79*(10), 870–874.

Allergy and Asthma Network. (2010). *Medications at school.* Retrieved from http://www.aanma.org/advocacy/meds-at-school/

Al-Saif, S., Alvard, R., Manfreda, J., Kwatkowski, K., Cates, D., Qurashi, M., & Rigatto, H. (2008). A randomized controlled trial of theophylline versus CO_2 inhalation for treating apnea of prematurity. *Journal of Pediatrics, 153*(4), 513–518.

American Academy of Allergy, Asthma, and Immunology (AAAAI). (2009). *Peak flow meter.* Retrieved from http://www.aaaai.org/

American Academy of Pediatrics (AAP). (2009). *Red book: 2009 Report of the Committee on Infectious Diseases* (28th ed.). Elk Grove Village, IL: Author.

American Academy of Pediatrics (AAP) Subcommittee on Diagnosis and Management of Bron-

chiolitis. (2006). Diagnosis and management of bronchiolitis. *Pediatrics, 118*(4), 1774–1793.

American Academy of Pediatrics (AAP), Task Force on Sudden Infant Death Syndrome. (2005). The changing concept of sudden infant death syndrome: Diagnostic coding shifts, controversies regarding the sleeping environment, and new variables to consider in reducing risk. *Pediatrics, 116*(5), 1245–1255.

Antoon, A. Y., & Donovan, M. K. (2007). Burn injuries. In R. M. Kliegman, R. E. Behrman, H. B. Jenson, & B. F. Stanton, *Nelson textbook of pediatrics* (18th ed., pp. 450–458). Philadelphia: Elsevier Saunders.

Arnold, L. D. (2006). Ingested and aspirated foreign bodies: Making sure what went in comes out. *Contemporary Pediatrics, 23*(11), 32–44.

Askin, D. F., & Diehl-Jones, W. (2009). Pathogenesis and prevention of chronic lung disease in the

neonate. *Critical Care Nursing Clinics of North America, 21,* 11–25.

Ayala, G. X., Miller, D., Zagami, E., Riddle, C., Willis, S., & King, D. (2006). Asthma in middle schools: What students have to say about their asthma. *Journal of School Health, 76*(6), 208–214.

Baker, L. K., & Denyes, M. J. (2008). Predictors of self-care in adolescents with cystic fibrosis: A test of Orem's theories of self-care and self-care deficit. *Journal of Pediatric Nursing, 23*(1), 37–48.

Banasiak, N. C. (2007). Childhood asthma: Part two: Management update. *Journal of Pediatric Health Care, 21*(3), 184–191.

Baraldi, E., & Filippone, M. (2007). Chronic lung diseases after premature birth. *New England Journal of Medicine, 357*(19), 1946–1955.

Bell, E. (2006). Pulmonary pharmacotherapy options changing for cystic fibrosis patients. *Infectious Diseases in Children, 19*(10), 12–13.

Brand, P. L. P. (2005). Key issues in inhalation therapy in children. *Current Medical Research and Opinion, 21*(Suppl. 4), S27–S32.

Brashers, V. L. (2010a). Alterations in pulmonary function. In K. L. McCance, S. E. Huether, V. L. Brashers, & N. R. Rote, *Pathophysiology: The biologic basis for disease in adults and children* (6th ed., pp. 1266–1304). St. Louis, MO: Mosby Elsevier.

Brashers, V. L. (2010b). Structure and function of the pulmonary system. In K. L. McCance, S. E. Huether, V. L. Brashers, & N. R. Rote, *Pathophysiology: The biologic basis for disease in adults and children* (6th ed., pp. 1242–1265). St. Louis, MO: Elsevier.

Bukutu, C., Le, C., & Vohra, S. (2008). Asthma: A review of complementary and alternative therapies. *Pediatrics in Review, 29*(8), e44–e49.

Camargo, C. A., Rachelefsky, G., & Schatz, M. (2009). Managing asthma exacerbations in the emergency department: Summary of the National Asthma Education and Prevention Program Expert Panel Report 3: Guidelines for the management of asthma exacerbations. *Journal of Allergy and Clinical Immunology, 124,* S5–14.

Carrier, C. T. (2009). Back to sleep: A culture change to improve practice. *Newborn & Infant Nursing Reviews, 9*(3), 163–168.

Centers for Disease Control and Prevention, Division of Adolescent and School Health. (2006). *Resources for addressing asthma in schools.* Retrieved from http://www.cdc.gov/HealthyYouth/asthma/pdf/pubs-links.pdf

Cifuentes, J., & Carlo, W. A. (2007). Respiratory system. In C. Kenner & J. W. Lott, *Comprehensive neonatal care: An interdisciplinary approach* (4th ed., pp. 1–17). St. Louis, MO: Elsevier Saunders.

Coffman, J. M., Cabana, M. D., Halpin, H. A., & Yelin, E. H. (2008). Effects of asthma education on children's use of acute care services: A meta-analysis. *Pediatrics, 121*(3), 575–586.

Coleman-Phox, K., Odouli, R., & De-Jun, L. (2008). Use of a fan during sleep and risk of sudden infant death syndrome. *Archives of Pediatrics and Adolescent Medicine, 162*(10), 963–968.

Cuff, S., & Loud, K. (2008). Exercise-induced bronchospasm. *Contemporary Pediatrics, 25*(9), 88–95.

Cystic Fibrosis Foundation. (2009a). *About cystic fibrosis: What you need to know.* Retrieved from http://www.cff.org/AboutCF/

Cystic Fibrosis Foundation. (2009b). *Newborn screening for cystic fibrosis.* Retrieved from http://www.cff.org/GetInvolved/Advocate/NewbornScreening/

Dolovich, M. B., Ahrens, R. C., Hess, D. R., Anderson, P., Dhand, R., Rau, J. L., et al. (2005). Device selection and outcomes of aerosol therapy: Evidence-based guidelines. *Chest, 127,* 335–371.

Doyle, L. W., Faber, B., Callanan, C., Freezer, N., Ford, G. W., & Davis, N. M. (2006). Bronchopulmonary dysplasia in very low birth weight subjects and lung function in late adolescence. *Pediatrics, 118*(1), 108–113.

Everard, M. L. (2006). Aerosol delivery to children. *Pediatric Annals, 35*(9), 630–636.

Fisher, E. B., Strunk, R. C., Highstein, G. R., Kelley-Sykes, R., Tarr, K. L., Trinkaus, K., & Musick, J. (2009). A randomized controlled evaluation of the effect of community health workers on hospitalization for asthma. *Archives of Pediatrics and Adolescent Medicine, 163*(3), 225–232.

Fleming, P., & Blair, P. S. (2007). Sudden infant death syndrome. *Sleep Medicine Clinics, 2,* 463–476.

Flume, P. A., O'Sullivan, B. P., Robinson, K. A., Goss, C. H., Mogayzel, P. J., et al. (2007). Cystic fibrosis pulmonary guidelines: Chronic medications for maintenance of lung health. *American Journal of Respiratory and Critical Care Medicine, 176,* 957–969.

Fong, E. W., & Levin, R. H. (2007). Inhaled corticosteroids for asthma. *Pediatrics in Review, 28*(6), e30–e35

Gerald, L. B., McClure, L. A., Mangan, J. M., Harrington, K. F., Gibson, L., Erwin, S., et al. (2009). Increasing adherence to inhaled steroid therapy among schoolchildren: Randomized, controlled trial of school-based supervised asthma therapy. *Pediatrics, 123*(2), 466–474.

Gibson, W. A. (2007). Choking: Strategies for evaluation and management. *Consultant for Pediatricians, 6*(12), 640–644.

Gott, K., & Froh, D. L. (2010). Alterations in pulmonary function in children. In K. L. McCance, S. E. Huether, V. L. Brashers, & N. R. Rote (Eds.), *Pathophysiology: The biologic basis for disease in adults and children* (6th ed., pp. 1310–1343). St. Louis, MO: Mosby Elsevier.

Guilbert, T. W., Morgan, W. J., Zeiger, R. S., Mauger, D. T., Boehmer, S. J., Szefler, S. J., et al. (2006). Long-term inhaled corticosteroids in preschool children at high risk for asthma. *New England Journal of Medicine, 354*(19), 1985–1997.

Halbower, A. C. (2008). Pediatric home apnea monitors: Coding, billing, and updated prescribing information for practice management. *Chest, 134*(2), 425–429.

Hazle, L. A. (2010). Cystic fibrosis. In P. J. Allen, J. A. Vessey, & N. A. Shapiro, *Primary care of the child with a chronic condition* (5th ed., pp. 405–426). St. Louis, MO: Mosby Elsevier.

Heron, M., Hoyert, D. L., Murphy, S. L., Xu, J., Kochanek, K. D., & Tejada-Vera, B. (2009). Deaths: Final data for 2006. *National Vital Statistics Reports, 57*(14), 1–135.

Hill, V. L., & Wood, P. R. (2009). Asthma epidemiology, pathophysiology, and initial evaluation. *Pediatrics in Review, 30*(9), 331–335.

Hoban, T. F., & Chervin, R. D. (2007). Sleep-related breathing disorders of childhood: Description and clinical picture, diagnosis, and treatment approaches. *Sleep Medicine Clinics, 2,* 445–462.

Kaye, C. I., & Committee on Genetics, American Academy of Pediatrics. (2006). Newborn screening fact sheets. *Pediatrics, 118*(3), e934–e963.

Kinney, H. C., & Thach, B. T. (2009). The sudden infant death syndrome. *New England Journal of Medicine, 361*(8), 795–805.

Lara, M., Akinbami, L., Flores, G., & Morgenstern, H. (2006). Heterogeneity of childhood asthma among Hispanic children: Puerto Rican children bear a disproportionate burden. *Pediatrics, 117*(1), 43–53.

Liou, T. G., Woo, M. S., & Cahill, B. C. (2006). Lung transplantation for cystic fibrosis. *Current Opinion in Pulmonary Medicine, 12*(6), 459–463.

Mannix, R., & Bachur, R. (2007). Status asthmaticus in children. *Current Opinion in Pediatrics, 19,* 281–287.

Marlier, L., Gaugler, C., & Messer, J. (2005). Olfactory stimulation prevents apnea in premature newborns. *Pediatrics, 115*(1), 83–88.

McNelis, A. M., Musick, B., Austin, J. K., Larson, P., & Dunn, D. W. (2007). Psychosocial care needs of children with recent-onset asthma. *Journal for Specialists in Pediatric Nursing, 12*(1), 3–12.

Meadows-Oliver, M., & Banasiak, N. C. (2005). Asthma medication delivery devices. *Journal of Pediatric Health Care, 19*(2), 121–123.

Montgomery, G. S., & Howenstine, M. (2009). Cystic fibrosis. *Pediatrics in Review, 30*(8), 302–309.

Moorman, J. E., Rudd, R. A., Johnson, C. A., King, M., Minor, P., Bailey, C., et al. (2007). National surveillance for asthma—United States, 1980–2004. *Morbidity and Mortality Weekly Report, 56*(SS-8), 1–60.

National Asthma Education and Prevention Program (NAEPP). (2007). *Expert panel report 3: Guidelines for the diagnosis and management of asthma.* Bethesda, MD: National Institutes of Health, National Heart Lung and Blood Institute. Retrieved from http://www.nhlbi.nih.gov/guidelines/asthma/

National Center for Health Statistics. (2009). *National Hospital Discharge Survey.* Unpublished data.

Newton, S. M., Brent, A. J., Anderson, S., Whittaker, E., & Kampmann, B. (2008). Paediatric tuberculosis. *Lancet Infectious Diseases, 8*(8), 498–510.

O'Shea, T. M., Nageswaran, S., Hiatt, D. C., Legault, C., Moore, M. L., Naughton, M., & Goldstein, D. J. (2007). Follow-up care for infants with chronic lung disease: A randomized comparison of community- and center-based models. *Pediatrics, 119*(4), e947–e957.

Peredo-Pinto, H., & Jacobs, N. M. (2008). A 17-month infant with a calf lesion and generalized hypotonia. *Pediatric Annals, 37*(2), 96–98.

Perez, I. A., & Davidson Ward, S. L. (2008). The snoring child. *Pediatric Annals, 37*(7), 465–470.

Pitetti, R. D., & Walker, S. (2005). Life-threatening chest injuries in children. *Clinical Pediatric Emergency Medicine, 6,* 16–22.

Pitts, J., Flack, J., & Goodfellow, J. (2008). Improving nutrition in the cystic fibrosis patient. *Journal of Pediatric Health Care, 22*(2), 137–140.

Poehling, K. A., Talbot, T. R., Griffin, M. R., Craig, A. S., Whitney, C. G., Zell, E., et al. (2006). Invasive pneumococcal disease among infants before and after introduction of pneumococcal conjugate vaccine. *Journal of the American Medical Association, 295*(14), 1668–1674.

Ranganathan, S. C., & Sonnappa, S. (2009). Pneumonia and other respiratory infections. *Pediatric Clinics of North America, 56,* 135–156.

Scolnik, D., Coates, A. L., Stephens, D., DaSilva, Z., Lavine, E., & Schuh, S. (2006). Controlled delivery of high vs low humidity vs mist therapy for croup in emergency departments: A randomized controlled trial. *Journal of the American Medical Association, 295,* 1274–1280.

Seiden, J. A., & Scarfone, R. J. (2009). Bronchiolitis: An evidence-based approach to management. *Clinical Pediatric Emergency Medicine, 10,* 75–81.

Shah, S., & Sharieff, G. Q. (2007). Pediatric respiratory infections. *Emergency Medicine Clinics of North America, 25,* 961–979.

Silvestri, J. M. (2008). Apparent life-threatening events in the young infant and neonate. *Clinical Pediatric Emergency Medicine, 9,* 184–190.

Silvestri, J. M. (2009). Indications for home apnea monitoring (or not). *Clinical Perinatology, 26,* 87–99.

Sobol, S. E., & Zapata, S. (2008). Epiglottitis and croup. *Otolaryngology Clinics of North America, 41,* 551–566.

Stallings, V. A., Stark, L. J., Robinson, K. A., Feranchak, A. P., Quinton, H., & Clinical Practice Guidelines on Growth and Nutrition Subcommittee: Ad Hoc Working Group. (2008). Evidence-based practice recommendations for nutrition-related management of children and adults with cystic fibrosis and pancreatic insufficiency: Re-

sults of a systemic review. *Journal of the American Dietetic Association, 108*(5), 832–839.

Starke, J. R. (2007). New concepts in childhood tuberculosis. *Current Opinion in Pediatrics, 19*(3), 306–313.

Strausbaugh, S. D., & Davis, P. B. (2007). Cystic fibrosis: A review of epidemiology and pathobiology. *Clinics of Chest Medicine, 28,* 279–288.

Valdez-Lowe, C., Ghareeb, S. A., & Artinian, N. T. (2009). Pulse oximetry in adults. *American Journal of Nursing, 109*(6), 52–57.

Virchow, J. C. (2005). What plays a role in the choice of inhaler device for asthma therapy? *Current Medical Research and Opinion, 21*(Suppl. 4), S19–S25.

Visner, G. A., & Goldfarb, S. B. (2007). Posttransplant monitoring of pediatric lung transplant recipients. *Current Opinion in Pediatrics, 19*(3), 321–326.

Walsh, M. C., Szefler, S., Davis, J., Allen, M., Van Marter, L., Abman, S., et al. (2006). Summary proceedings from the bronchopulmonary dysplasia group. *Pediatrics, 117*(3), S52–S56.

Wardell, C., Huang, S., & Isbister, C. (2006). When children with asthma go swimming, the benefits can be many and long-lasting. *Contemporary Pediatrics, 23*(10), 89–96.

Willis, K. C. (2007). Bronchiolitis: Advanced practice focus in the emergency department. *Journal of Emergency Nursing, 33*(4), 346–351.

Woods, C. R. (2008). Acute bacterial pneumonia in childhood in the current era. *Pediatric Annals, 37*(10), 694–702.

Wu, A. C., Smith, L., Bokhour, B., Hohman, K. H., & Lieu, T. A. (2008). Racial/ethnic variation in parent perceptions of asthma. *Ambulatory Pediatrics, 8*(2), 89–97.

Zorc, J. J., & Phelan, K. J. (2008). An update on the AAP's bronchiolitis guidelines and the latest evidence on assessment and treatment. *Contemporary Pediatrics, 25*(2), 55–62.

Alterations in Cardiovascular Function

chapter 21

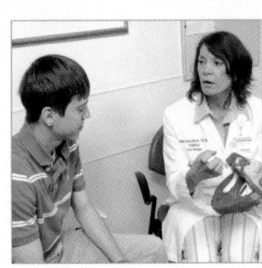

Tim Howard, who is 16 years old, had surgical repair for tetralogy of Fallot as an infant. Other than the usual childhood illnesses, Tim grew and developed as expected during childhood. His parents made sure he had regular health promotion care, and they tried to follow the pediatrician's advice to treat him as a normal child.

A year ago, Tim felt dizzy and tired more quickly with exercise and activity. After a comprehensive cardiac evaluation, Tim was found to have an episodic slow ventricular heart rate. A pacemaker was determined to be his best treatment option. Tim's exercise limitations include no strenuous activities, competitive sports, or biking, which had been a favorite activity. He is now seen every 6 months in the pediatric cardiac clinic to monitor for further changes in his condition.

Tim is trying to adjust to his new limitations. He has average grades in school, but he does not know if his heart condition will limit his career options. He has a lot of friends, but wonders if he will keep them with his activity limitations. His parents have always made the decisions about his visits and treatment. What information does Tim need as he prepares for his future? What are some school and community activities that might allow Tim to maintain his friendships? What kinds of careers should Tim consider?

Learning Outcomes

After reading this chapter, you will be able to do the following:

1. Describe the anatomy and physiology of the cardiovascular system, focusing on the flow of blood and action of the heart valves.
2. Contrast the pathophysiology associated with congenital heart defects with increased pulmonary circulation, decreased pulmonary circulation, and obstructed systemic blood flow.
3. Create a nursing care plan for the infant with a congenital heart defect cared for at home prior to corrective surgery.
4. Plan the nursing care for the child undergoing open heart surgery.
5. Recognize the signs of congestive heart failure in an infant and child.
6. Plan the nursing care for a child with congestive heart failure.
7. Differentiate between the heart diseases acquired during childhood and congenital heart defects.
8. Distinguish between the pathophysiology of hypovolemic shock, distributive shock, and cardiogenic shock.

FOCUS ON

The Cardiovascular System

ANATOMY AND PHYSIOLOGY OVERVIEW

The heart is divided into four chambers: two atria and two ventricles. Atrioventricular valves (tricuspid and mitral) separate the atria from the ventricles. They open and close to control the flow of blood to the ventricles. The semilunar valves (pulmonary and aortic) open when the ventricles pump blood and close to prevent the backflow of blood to the ventricles. The great arteries (aorta and pulmonary artery) carry blood away from the heart to either the body or the lungs. Pulmonary veins and the superior and inferior venae cavae return blood to the heart. See Figure 21–1 ➤ for the anatomy of the heart.

The heart is the pump that circulates the blood through the systemic and pulmonary systems. Blood flows to the lungs for oxygen and carbon dioxide exchange. The oxygenated blood returns to the heart for distribution to the systemic circulation, organs, and tissues. See Table 21–1 for **hemodynamics** (passage of blood through the heart and pulmonary system and pressures generated by the blood) of the normal heart. The heart's electrical conduction system controls the rhythmic pumping (Figure 21–2 ➤).

Transition from Fetal to Pulmonary Circulation

Blood flows from the placenta to the fetus through the umbilical vein to the ductus venosus (the fetal vascular channel between the umbilical vein and the inferior vena cava) and into the right atrium of the heart. The foramen ovale, an opening between the atria of the fetal heart, allows blood to flow from the right atrium to the left atrium and then into the left ventricle. Blood is then pumped into the aorta and systemic circulation. Some blood returns from the head and upper extremities to the superior vena cava and right atrium. Some blood travels to the right ventricle where it is pumped into the pulmonary artery. The majority of this blood passes through the ductus arteriosus, the vascular channel between the pulmonary artery and the aorta, and into the systemic circulation. A small amount of the blood from the pulmonary artery goes to the fetal lungs. Blood

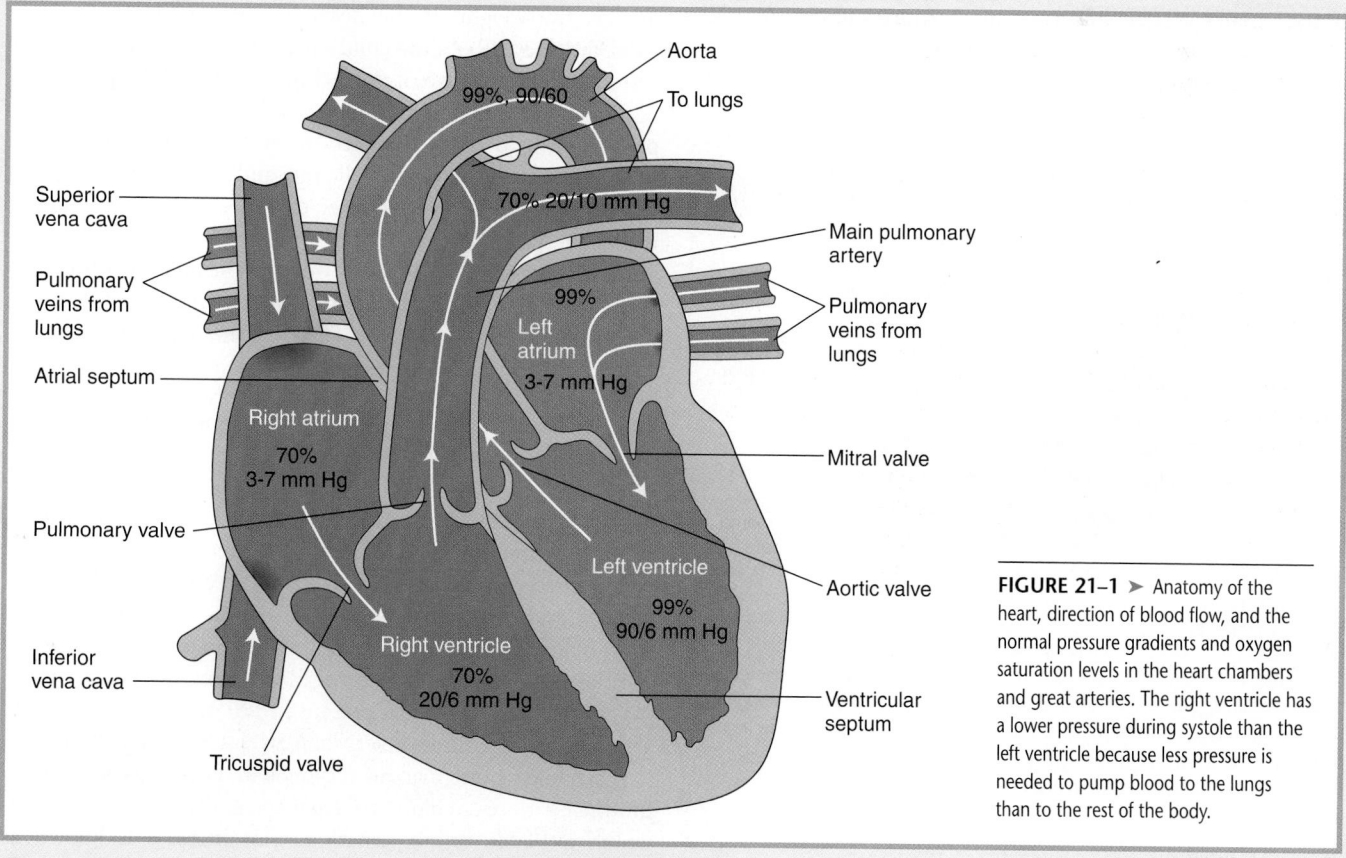

FIGURE 21–1 ➤ Anatomy of the heart, direction of blood flow, and the normal pressure gradients and oxygen saturation levels in the heart chambers and great arteries. The right ventricle has a lower pressure during systole than the left ventricle because less pressure is needed to pump blood to the lungs than to the rest of the body.

TABLE 21–1 Hemodynamics of the Normal Heart

Action	Right Side of Heart	Left Side of Heart
Blood return to heart	Systemic circulation by way of the superior and inferior venae cavae.	Lungs by way of the left and right pulmonary veins.
Diastolic phase	Pulmonary valve closes and tricuspid valve opens. Blood flows from the venae cavae through the right atrium and tricuspid valve into the right ventricle.	Aortic valve closes and mitral valve opens. Blood flows from the pulmonary veins through the left atrium and mitral valve into the left ventricle.
Systolic phase	Tricuspid valve closes and pulmonary valve opens. Blood is pumped into the pulmonary artery and passes into the right and left pulmonary arteries and lungs.	Mitral valve closes and aortic valve opens. Blood is pumped into the aorta where it enters the systemic circulation.

eventually returns to the placenta by way of the umbilical arteries. After the umbilical cord has been cut, the newborn must quickly adapt to receiving oxygen from the lungs.

The transition from fetal to pulmonary circulation occurs within a few hours of birth (Figure 21–3 ➤). The first breath expands the lungs, and blood that previously flowed through the ductus arteriosus to the aorta begins flowing to the lungs. Pulmonary blood flow increases and pulmonary vascular resistance decreases. Pressure in the left atrium increases as increased blood flow is returned from the lungs through the pulmonary veins.

Systemic vascular resistance (the force or resistance of the blood in the body's blood vessels that helps return blood to the heart) increases and right atrial pressure falls after the umbilical cord is cut. Increased pressure in the left atrium stimulates closure of the foramen ovale unless there is excess pressure on the right side of the heart. The ductus arteriosus, responding to higher oxygen saturation, normally constricts and closes within 10 to 15 hours after birth. Permanent closure occurs by 10 to 21 days after birth, unless oxygen saturation remains low. Fetal tissues are accustomed to low oxygen saturation. This may explain why newborns with heart conditions with decreased pulmonary blood flow (cyanotic defects) appear relatively comfortable even when their arterial partial pressure of oxygen (PaO_2) is very low.

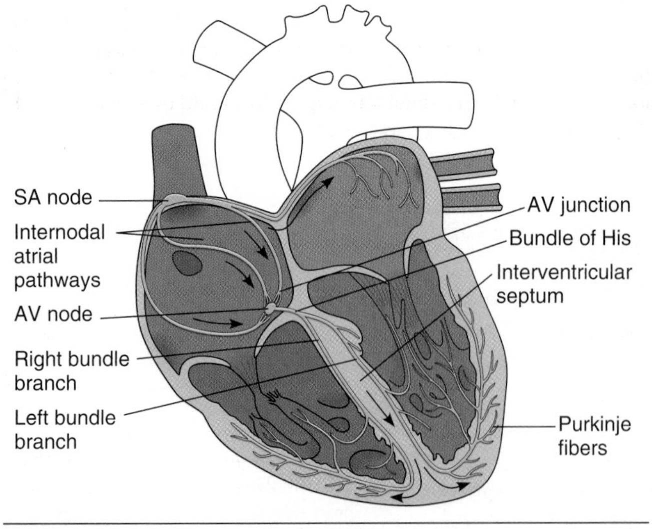

Pediatric Differences

Cardiac Functioning

Infants have a greater risk of heart failure than older children because the immature heart is more sensitive to volume or pressure overload. During infancy the heart's muscle fibers are less developed and less organized, resulting in limited functional capacity. Less **compliance** (amount of distention or expansion the ventricles can achieve to increase stroke volume) of the heart muscle means that the **stroke volume** (amount of blood ejected with each contraction) cannot increase substantially. The heart muscle fibers develop during early childhood, and by 9 years of age, the weight of the heart has increased by six times (McDaniel, 2010). As the child's heart grows and develops, the systolic blood pressure rises, reaching adult levels by puberty.

The infant maintains a high heart rate and high **cardiac output** (volume of blood ejected from the left ventricle each minute) to meet high metabolic rate and oxygen requirements. Infants and children with a fever, exercise, stress, or respiratory distress respond with tachycardia rather than increased stroke volume to increase their cardiac output. The infant has little cardiac output reserve capacity until oxygen requirements begin to decrease at about 2 months of age (McDaniel, 2010).

Oxygenation

Oxygen bound to hemoglobin is transported to the tissues by the systemic circulation. Hematocrit and hemoglobin concentrations appropriate for the child's age are necessary for adequate oxygen transport (see Chapter 20 ∞). The arterial **oxygen saturation** is the amount of oxygen that can potentially be delivered to the tissues. **Desaturated blood** results when oxygenated and unoxygenated blood mix because of a congenital heart defect. Cyanosis, which indicates **hypoxemia** (lower-than-normal amounts of oxygen in the blood), results when 5 g of deoxygenated hemoglobin is present in 100 mL of blood or from arterial oxygen saturation less than 80% (Callahan, 2008).

The child's bone marrow responds to chronic hypoxemia by producing more red blood cells to increase the amount of hemoglobin available for oxygenation. This increase is known as

SA node
Internodal atrial pathways
AV node
Right bundle branch
Left bundle branch
AV junction
Bundle of His
Interventricular septum
Purkinje fibers

FIGURE 21–2 ➤ Electrical conduction system of the heart. Depolarization normally follows a sequence that begins in the sinoatrial (SA) node and travels through the atrial muscle to the atrioventricular (AV) junction, and then through the AV node to the ventricular muscles. The pathway in the ventricles begins in the bundle of His and divides into the right and left bundle branches. The pathway terminates in the Purkinje system so that the impulse spreads across the myocardium.

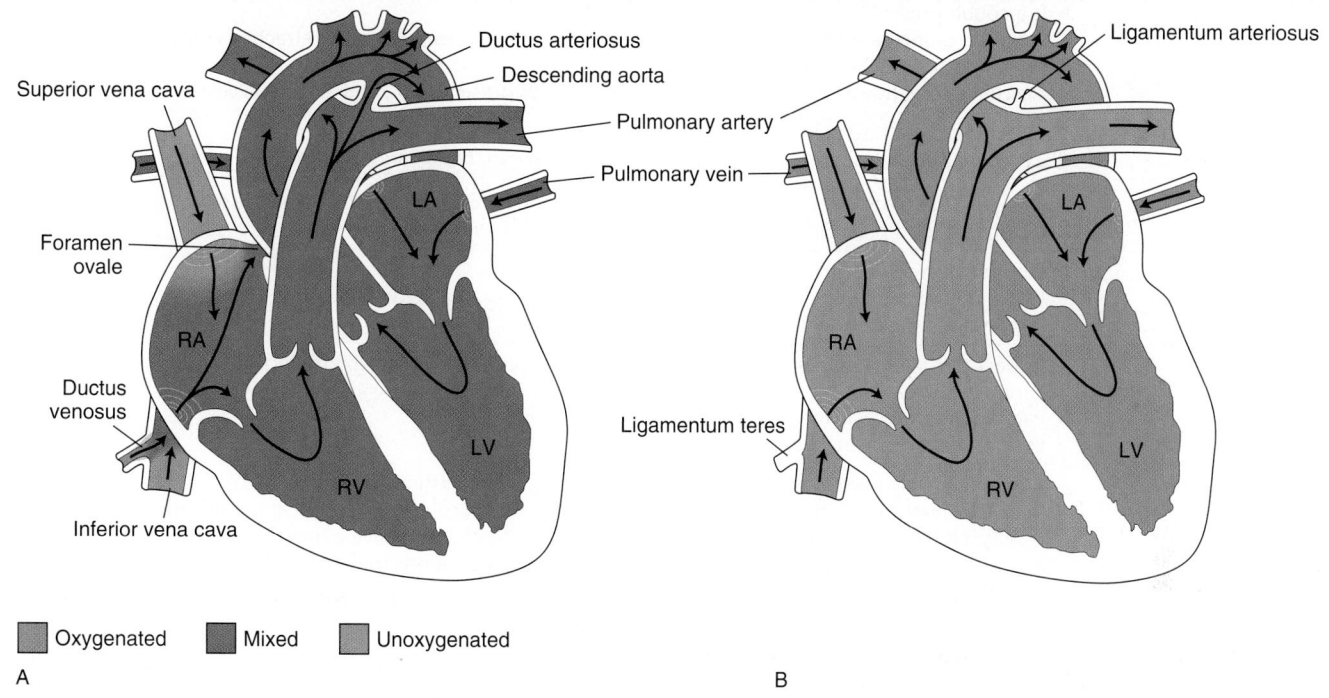

FIGURE 21–3 ➤ The arrows indicate the flow of blood through the heart while the color indicates level of oxygen saturation in the blood. A, Fetal circulation. B, Pulmonary circulation. LA, left atrium; LV, left ventricle; RA, right atrium; RV, right ventricle.

polycythemia. A hematocrit value of 50% or higher is common in children with heart defects with decreased pulmonary blood flow.

Children respond to severe hypoxemia with bradycardia. Cardiac arrest in children generally results from prolonged hypoxemia related to respiratory failure or shock rather than from a primary cardiac insult as in adults. Bradycardia is therefore a significant warning sign of cardiac arrest. Appropriate management of hypoxemia often reverses bradycardia and prevents cardiac arrest.

Nursing Alert

Hemoglobin greater than 20 g/dL and a hematocrit greater than 55–60% are dangerous and put the child at risk for a thromboembolism, especially if dehydration occurs (Schultz & Kreutzer, 2006, p. 53).

Cardiac Assessment

Numerous diagnostic procedures and laboratory tests are used for the diagnosis of cardiac conditions. See Table 21–2.

Performing a nursing assessment of the child with a potential or actual cardiac condition involves a careful review of the signs and symptoms in many body systems and analysis of their relationship to cardiac functioning. Use the Assessment Guidelines on page 604 to perform a comprehensive nursing assessment of the cardiovascular system.

Clinical Tip

A pulse oximeter provides a noninvasive measurement of the arterial oxygen saturation level (SpO$_2$). A reading of 95–98% is normal in children. Newborns usually achieve readings this high within the first 2 hours of life (Schultz & Kreutzer, 2006). A pulse oximetry reading less than 94% in a quiet infant or child should be considered abnormal (Sivarajan, Vetter, & Gleason, 2006, p. 3).

TABLE 21–2 Diagnostic Procedures and Laboratory Tests Used to Evaluate Cardiac Conditions*

Diagnostic Procedures	Laboratory Tests
Cardiac catheterization	Complete blood count
Chest radiograph	Arterial blood gases
Echocardiogram (transthoracic and transesophageal)	Antistreptolysin-O antibody titer
Exercise testing	Erythrocyte sedimentation rate
Ambulatory electrocardiography (Holter monitor)	C-reactive protein
Hyperoxitest	Serum lipid panel
Computed tomography	Serum drug tests (e.g., digoxin)
Magnetic resonance imaging	

*See Appendices D and E ∞ for information about these diagnostic procedures and expected laboratory values.

Assessment Guidelines for the Child with a Cardiac Condition*

Assessment Focus	Assessment Guidelines
Respirations	▪ What is the respiratory rate and depth? ▪ Is a cough present? ▪ Are signs of increased respiratory effort present (e.g., tachypnea, dyspnea, retractions, nasal flaring, or expiratory grunting)? ▪ Auscultate breath sounds. Are any adventitious sounds present (e.g., wheezes, crackles)?
Pulses	▪ Assess the pulse rate, rhythm, and quality. ▪ Compare pulse sites for rate and strength (apical, brachial, radial, and femoral).
Blood pressure	▪ Compare the blood pressure to expected value for age, sex, and height percentiles (see Appendix B ∞). ▪ Compare blood pressure values between an upper and lower extremity.
Color	▪ Observe overall color: note pallor, dusky color, or cyanosis. ▪ Compare the color in peripheral and central locations (e.g., nailbeds to mucous membranes). Does crying improve or worsen color?
Chest	▪ Inspect the anterior chest for skeletal abnormalities, bulging, or *heaving* (lifting of the chest wall during contraction). ▪ Palpate the chest wall for pulsations, heaves, or vibrations. ▪ Locate the point of maximum intensity.
Heart auscultation	▪ Auscultate heart sounds and their quality (loud versus weak, distinct versus muffled). ▪ Are extra heart sounds or murmurs present? Describe murmurs by intensity, location, radiation, timing, and quality. NOTE: Not all murmurs indicate pathology; some children have a functional murmur. ▪ Auscultate the heart with the child in sitting and reclining positions to detect differences in heart sounds.
Fluid status	▪ Observe for signs of periorbital, facial, or peripheral edema, or for dehydration. ▪ Observe for abdominal distention. ▪ Palpate the liver to detect hepatomegaly. ▪ Assess capillary refill.
Activity and behavior	▪ Is exercise intolerance present? Does the child tire with feeding? ▪ Note presence of diaphoresis and when it occurs. ▪ Identify changes in activity level or behavior.
General	▪ Assess growth.

See Chapter 5 ∞ for actual techniques of assessment.

Alterations in cardiovascular function may be the result of a congenital defect, acquired infection, or injury. Congenital heart disease is the leading cause of death, excluding prematurity, during the first year of life. It is estimated that about one third of children born with congenital heart disease die as a result of their cardiac disease, and about one third of those deaths occur in the first year of life (Connor, 2006). Rapid advances in the treatment of congenital heart defects allow children to have surgery at younger ages. As a result, the nursing care required to identify and manage responses of infants and children with heart disease has become more challenging.

▪ CONGENITAL HEART DISEASE

Congenital heart disease (CHD) refers to a defect in the heart or great vessels, or persistence of a fetal structure after birth. It is one of the most common birth defects, with an incidence of 6 per 1,000 live births (Zeigler, 2008). More than 35 types of heart defects have been documented. Of infant deaths due to congenital malformations, CHD causes 46% of them. However, approximately 96% of newborns with congenital heart disease who survive their first year will still be alive at age 16 years (Sadowski, 2009).

Etiology and Pathophysiology

Most congenital heart defects develop during the first 8 weeks of gestation. Many are the result of a combined or interactive effect of genetic and environmental factors, such as (McDaniel, 2010):

- Fetal exposure to drugs (e.g., phenytoin, lithium, valproic acid), alcohol, and secondary tobacco smoke.
- Maternal viral infections such as rubella or coxsackie B5.
- Maternal metabolic disorders such as phenylketonuria, diabetes mellitus, and hypercalcemia.
- Increased maternal age.
- Genetic factors (family recurrence patterns).
- Chromosomal abnormalities (e.g., Turner, Noonan, Marfan, DiGeorge, and trisomy syndromes) that are associated with specific CHDs.

The incidence of congenital heart defects is expected to slowly rise as children with such abnormalities survive and have children of their own.

Congenital heart defects are generally categorized by pathophysiology and hemodynamics. These categories include:

- Increased pulmonary blood flow (see page 607).
- Decreased pulmonary blood flow (see page 613).

Congenital Heart Defects Video

- Obstructed systemic blood flow (see page 620).
- Mixed defects (with combined defects that increase and decrease pulmonary blood flow). These defects have similar clinical characteristics, clinical therapy, and nursing management to those with decreased pulmonary blood flow, and will be discussed in that section (see page 613).

Clinical Manifestations

The presence of a heart murmur is often the first indication of a congenital heart defect. A loud murmur indicates blood is flowing with higher pressure than normal to get through a narrowed valve or vessel, or through a **shunt** (movement of blood between the systemic and pulmonary circulation through an abnormal anatomic opening, such as through the right and left ventricles). Other clinical manifestations and the timing of their appearance vary by the pathophysiology and severity of the defect. See Clinical Manifestations: Heart Defects by Pathophysiology. Newborns may become symptomatic as soon as the umbilical cord is cut or within the first few days of life. Some children may be asymptomatic except for a heart murmur.

Nursing Alert

Exercise-induced dizziness, chest pain, arrhythmias, and **syncope** (brief loss of consciousness due to transient cerebral hypoxia) in older children with congenital heart disease are serious signs indicating a need for medical intervention. Sudden death may also occur.

COLLABORATIVE CARE

Diagnostic Tests

The history and physical examination findings may lead to a suspicion of a CHD. See Table 21–2 for laboratory tests and procedures used to diagnose cardiac defects. A hematocrit and hemoglobin may be used to assess for anemia or polycythemia. Arterial blood gases may be obtained, especially when cyanosis or a complex heart defect is suspected.

Clinical Therapy

One third of infants born with CHDs develop life-threatening symptoms in the first few days of life. Treatment depends on the severity of symptoms and whether the condition is imminently life threatening.

Interventional cardiac catheterization is performed to manage some CHDs. A balloon may be used to create a larger opening in the atrial septum (atrial septostomy), to dilate a narrowed pulmonic or aortic valve, and to expand a coarctation of the aorta. A stent can be inserted to keep the ductus arteriosus patent, or a coil can be used to occlude it. A septal closing device may be used for some atrial and ventricular septal defects.

A **palliative procedure** (a procedure that does not create normal anatomic or hemodynamic results) may be performed in children with a potentially fatal or lethal condition. It may also be performed as an initial procedure, allowing an infant to grow before definitive corrective surgery. Table 21–3 lists the types of interventions during cardiac catheterization and surgical procedures performed on children with CHDs.

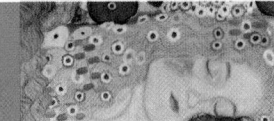

NURSING MANAGEMENT FOR CARDIAC CATHETERIZATION

Cardiac catheterization is often performed on an outpatient basis, but some children will be admitted for observation afterward to monitor for complications or for scheduled surgery. The child is given nothing by mouth (NPO) for several hours, except for medications, and arrives at the catheterization laboratory 1 to 2 hours before the procedure. Before entering the laboratory, the child is asked to void and is given an oral sedative.

Assessment and Diagnosis

Before the procedure, assess the child using the guidelines on page 604. Pay attention to the child's vital signs, hematocrit, hemoglobin, and capillary refill time. Collect baseline data on skin

Clinical Manifestations
Heart Defects by Pathophysiology

Pathophysiology	Clinical Manifestations
Increased pulmonary blood flow (PDA, ASD, VSD, AV canal)	Tachypnea, tachycardia, murmur, congestive heart failure, poor weight gain, diaphoresis, periorbital edema, frequent respiratory infections
Decreased pulmonary blood flow (PS, TOF, pulmonary or tricuspid atresia)	Cyanosis, hypercyanotic episodes, poor weight gain, polycythemia
Obstructed systemic blood flow (COA, AS, HLHS, MS, interrupted aortic arch)	Diminished pulses, poor color, delayed capillary refill time, decreased urine output, congestive heart failure with pulmonary edema
Mixed defects—postnatal survival is dependent upon mixing of systemic and pulmonary blood (TGA, TAPVR, truncus arteriosus, double outlet right ventricle)	Cyanosis, poor weight gain, pulmonary congestion, or congestive heart failure may occur with increased shunting

AS—aortic stenosis, ASD—atrial septal defect, AV—atrioventricular, COA—coarctation of aorta, HLHS—hypoplastic left heart syndrome, MS—mitral stenosis, PDA—patent ductus arteriosus, PS—pulmonic stenosis, TAPVR—total anomalous pulmonary venous return, TOF—tetralogy of Fallot, TGA—transposition of great arteries, VSD—ventricular septal defect.

TABLE 21–3 Clinical Interventions for Congenital Heart Defects

Cardiac Catheterization Interventions and Therapeutic Use	Description
Balloon atrial septostomy—Rashkind, or with transatrial needle puncture and balloon dilation Palliative for TGA	Creation of larger defect (at the foramen ovale) between atria to increase blood mixing; performed during cardiac catheterization.
Balloon dilation procedure Corrective for PS and MS, palliative for AS, COA	A balloon is inserted and inflated to stretch the opening of a narrowed valve or blood vessel. A stent may be inserted to keep the vessel open.
Device closure Corrective for PDA, ASD, small VSDs	Closure of ductus arteriosus by an umbrella or coil device, and closure of a septal defect by a septal occluder.
Surgical Procedures	Purpose
Aorta end-to-end anastomosis Corrective, COA	Resection of the narrowed section of the aorta and connecting the proximal and distal sections.
Blalock-Taussig shunt, modified Palliative, TOF, single-ventricle lesions with pulmonary outflow obstruction	Creation of aortopulmonary conduit (from the brachiocephalic artery to pulmonary artery) to increase pulmonary blood flow.
Brock Corrective, PS	Blind incision of pulmonary valve.
Damus-Kaye-Stansel Corrective for TGA Palliative for complex single-ventricle defects	Pulmonary artery is cut in two with the proximal section attached to the ascending aorta, the distal end sewn over, and a shunt created between the systemic circulation and pulmonary artery to send blood to the lungs.
Fontan Palliative, HLHS, single-ventricle defects	Creation of conduit between inferior vena cava and pulmonary artery to increase pulmonary blood flow—total right heart bypass. This permits the single ventricle to assume the responsibility for the systemic circulation and eject blood into the aorta.
Glenn, Bidirectional Glenn Palliative, HLHS, single-ventricle defects	Superior vena cava connected to right pulmonary artery along with closure of aortopulmonary shunt. Systemic venous blood from the head is sent to the lungs directly without ventricular pumping.
Jatene (arterial switch) Corrective, TGA	Aorta and pulmonary arteries are transected and reattached to opposite stumps; coronary arteries are moved to new aorta area.
Norwood Palliative, aortic hypoplasia, single-ventricle defects (e.g., HLHS)	Atrial septectomy, anastomosis of the main pulmonary artery to the aorta, and an arterial-pulmonary shunt.
Norwood with Sano modification Palliative, HLHS	Creation of a right ventricle to pulmonary artery conduit so that both the direct pulmonary and aorta blood flow originates in the right ventricle.
Patch aortoplasty Corrective, COA	Insertion of a Dacron patch or opened left subclavian vein to expand the lumen of the aorta.
Pulmonary artery banding Palliative, VSD, AV canal, single-ventricle defects	Placement of constricting band around pulmonary artery to reduce pulmonary blood flow and pressure.
Rastelli Corrective, TGA with pulmonic stenosis, TOF, tricuspid atresia, truncus arteriosus, and double outlet right ventricle	Creation of a conduit between the right ventricle to pulmonary artery with closure of the ventricular septal defect. In the case of truncus arteriosus, the pulmonary arteries are removed from the truncus.
Ross Corrective, AS	The diseased aortic valve is replaced with the patient's pulmonic valve (pulmonary autograft), and a homograft (valve from an animal or human donor) replaces the pulmonic valve.
Subclavian flap aortoplasty Corrective, COA	Division of the distal subclavian artery and insertion of a flap into the aorta through the coarcted segment.
Transplant Corrective, HLHS, complex defects, cardiomyopathies	Replacement of diseased heart with donor heart.

AS—aortic stenosis, ASD—atrial septal defect, AV—atrioventricular, COA—coarctation of aorta, HLHS—hypoplastic left heart syndrome, MS—mitral stenosis, PDA—patent ductus arteriosus, PS—pulmonic stenosis, TOF—tetralogy of Fallot, TGA—transposition of great arteries, VSD—ventricular septal defect.

temperature, color, and strength of pedal and popliteal pulses for comparison with postcatheterization assessments.

For several hours after the procedure, monitor the child for potential complications such as arrhythmia, bleeding, hematoma development, thrombus formation, and infection. No bleeding should occur at the catheterization site. Assess vital signs, perfusion of the lower extremities (pulses, temperature, color, capillary refill time, and sensation), and the pressure dressing over the catheterization site every 15 minutes for 1 hour and then every 30 minutes for 1 hour, or as directed by agency guidelines. Check under the buttocks to make sure blood does not ooze out and run under the child. The child's vital signs should remain stable. Seek immediate medical intervention if reduced limb warmth, decreased perfusion in the extremity, or bleeding is noted. Monitor intake and output because the contrast medium may cause diuresis.

The following nursing diagnoses may apply to the child who undergoes cardiac catheterization:

- Fear related to separation from support system in a stressful situation
- Risk for Imbalanced Fluid Volume related to inadequate fluid intake due to NPO status and diuretic effect of contrast medium
- Impaired Tissue Perfusion (Cardiopulmonary) related to mechanical reduction of arterial and venous blood flow

Planning and Implementation

Prepare the child for cardiac catheterization with age-appropriate information. Because the child will be sedated but arousable for the procedure, explain the sensations that might be experienced.

Nursing care during a cardiac catheterization focuses on monitoring the child's vital signs, reassuring the child, and providing emergency care if necessary. After the catheters and guidewires are removed at the end of the procedure, direct pressure must be applied for 15 minutes. A pressure dressing is then placed over the site for 6 hours.

Families Want to Know
Home Care After Cardiac Catheterization

- ■ Check for the following signs of complications several times in the first 24 hours after catheterization, and notify the health care provider immediately if any of these signs are noted:
  - Fever
  - Bleeding or a bruise increasing in size at the catheterization site
  - Foot on side of catheterization site is cooler than other foot
  - Loss of feeling in foot on side of catheterization
  - Signs of dehydration (dry mucous membranes, absence of tears, and concentrated urine) if the child is treated with diuretics
- ■ Encourage fluids to help flush the dye out of the body and to prevent dehydration.
- ■ Allow quiet play such as games, puzzles, and videos for the first 24 hours after the procedure.

The child is kept on bed rest for 4 to 6 hours with an effort to keep the leg straight for several hours. Do not elevate the head of the bed as flexion of the hips is not permitted during this period. Activity is then limited for 24 hours. Provide quiet diversional activities to keep the child occupied.

Encourage the child to drink small amounts of clear liquids initially, and then progress to other fluids and food as the child tolerates them. Provide adequate fluids to maintain hydration by keeping intake and output balanced. If the infant or child is treated with diuretics, a greater potential for dehydration exists.

Discharge Planning and Home Care Teaching

Children are routinely discharged several hours after the cardiac catheterization. Teach the parents to watch the child for signs of complications, and make sure they know when to notify the physician. See Families Want to Know: Home Care After Cardiac Catheterization.

Evaluation

Expected outcomes of nursing care include the following:

- Any potential complications (thrombosis or hemorrhage) following cardiac catheterization are rapidly identified and treated.
- The child maintains fluid balance.

Congenital Heart Defects That Increase Pulmonary Blood Flow

Etiology and Pathophysiology

The most common congenital heart defects allow blood to flow between the left and right side of the heart, such as through an opening in the septum or a connection between the great arteries (patent ductus arteriosus). The higher pressures on the left side of the heart cause blood to be shunted to the right side, increasing the amount of blood pumped to the lungs. The size of the opening or connection and amount of blood passing through it determines how quickly the child develops congestive heart failure (CHF). The increased blood flow to the lungs causes increased pulmonary vascular resistance (constriction of the pulmonary vascular bed) in an effort to reduce the blood flow, as well as pulmonary hypertension (see page 630). Right ventricular hypertrophy (RVH) develops to overcome the increasing pulmonary vascular resistance and deliver the blood to the lungs.

Clinical Manifestations

The infant's heart rate, respiratory rate, and metabolic rate are increased due to the high pulmonary blood flow. Feeding takes energy, and diaphoresis often occurs. The infant may be unable to ingest enough calories to support the metabolic rate and growth, leading to poor weight gain. If CHF develops, signs include dyspnea, tachypnea, intercostal retractions, and periorbital edema (see page 620). Frequent respiratory infections occur as the wet environment in the lungs supports bacterial growth. See Table 21–4 for the pathophysiology, clinical manifestations, and clinical therapy for specific CHDs with increased pulmonary blood flow.

TABLE 21–4	Pathophysiology, Clinical Manifestations, and Clinical Therapy for Heart Defects That Increase Pulmonary Blood Flow

Pathophysiology, Clinical Manifestations, and Clinical Therapy	Anatomy

Patent Ductus Arteriosus (PDA)

A common congenital defect caused by persistent fetal circulation that accounts for 5–10% of all congenital heart defects (Park, 2008). When pulmonary circulation is established and systemic vascular resistance increases at birth, the aorta pressure is higher than in the pulmonary arteries. Blood shunts from the aorta to the pulmonary arteries, increasing circulation to the pulmonary system. It is a common problem of preterm infants as the ductus arteriosus is not as responsive to the increased oxygen after conversion to pulmonary circulation, and it is less likely to close spontaneously (Joshi & Sekhavat, 2006).

Clinical Manifestations

Dyspnea; tachypnea; tachycardia; full, bounding pulses; widened pulse pressure; hypotension may be noted when cardiac output is low.
CHF, intercostal retractions, hepatomegaly, and growth failure when a large PDA exists.
Continuous "machinery" murmur during systole and diastole, and a thrill in the pulmonic area. Full-term infants may have a murmur without other signs.
High risk for frequent respiratory infections and pneumonia.

Diagnostic Procedures

The chest radiograph and ECG show left ventricular hypertrophy.
The PDA can be visualized, and the left-to-right shunt can be measured on echocardiogram.

Clinical Therapy

Ligation of PDA is the treatment of choice, often using video-assisted thoracoscopic surgery. Transcatheter closure by an obstructive device is attempted in some older children.
Intravenous ibuprofen or indomethacin often stimulates closure of the ductus arteriosus in premature infants.
Prognosis: No long-term sequelae occur if treated before pulmonary vascular disease develops. If PDA is not treated, the child's life span is shortened because pulmonary hypertension and pulmonary vascular obstructive disease develop.

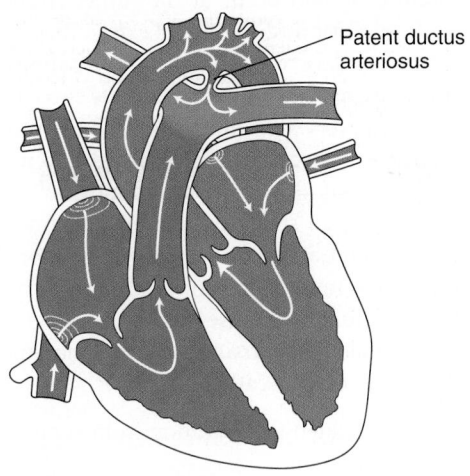

Patent ductus arteriosus

■ Mix of oxygenated and unoxygenated blood

Atrial Septal Defect (ASD)

This opening in the atrial septum permits left-to-right shunting of blood. This defect occurs frequently, either in isolation (5–10% of cases) or as a part of a cardiac defect (in 30–50% of children with a congenital heart defect) (Park, 2008). The opening may be small, as when the foramen ovale fails to close, or large, as when the septum may be completely absent.

Clinical Manifestations

Infants and young children usually have no symptoms. Small and moderate-size ASDs may not be diagnosed until preschool years or later.
CHF, easy tiring, and poor growth occur with a large ASD.
A soft systolic ejection murmur occurs in the pulmonic area with fixed wide splitting of S_2 through all phases of respiration.

Diagnostic Procedures

Echocardiogram identifies a dilated right ventricle due to blood overload and the shunt size.
The chest radiograph and ECG reveal little information unless the ASD is large and has excessive shunting, and right ventricular hypertrophy is present.

Clinical Therapy

Spontaneous closure of some ASDs occurs within the first 4 years of life. No activity limitations are needed.
Surgery to close or patch the ASD is performed when significant increased pulmonary blood flow causes CHF, or when spontaneous closure has not occurred by 4 years of age. Some ASDs may be closed by a transcatheter device (septal occluder) during cardiac catheterization.
Prognosis: Many persons with uncorrected small- and moderate-sized ASDs have lived to middle age without symptoms, but a risk for embolism exists. CHF and pulmonary hypertension may develop in untreated adults. Atrial arrhythmias may also occur in adults.

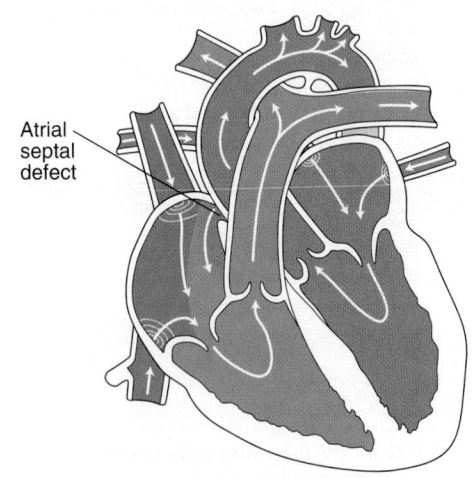

Atrial septal defect

| TABLE 21–4 | Pathophysiology, Clinical Manifestations, and Clinical Therapy for Heart Defects That Increase Pulmonary Blood Flow *(continued)* |

| Pathophysiology, Clinical Manifestations, and Clinical Therapy | Anatomy |

Ventricular Septal Defect (VSD)

An opening in the ventricular septum causes increased pulmonary blood flow. Blood is shunted from the left ventricle directly across the open septum into the pulmonary artery. This most common CHD occurs in isolation in 15–20% of cases, or in combination with other defects (Park, 2008).

Clinical Manifestations

Moderate- and large-sized VSDs may be associated with CHF, an increased number of pulmonary infections, or pulmonary hypertension.

A systolic murmur is auscultated at the third or fourth left intercostal space at the sternal border.

Diagnostic Procedures

A chest radiograph and electrocardiogram (ECG) reveal little when VSDs are small. An enlarged heart and pulmonary vascular markings on chest radiograph may be seen when a large VSD causes shunting. Right and left ventricular hypertrophy may be seen on ECG. Echocardiogram establishes the diagnosis if shunting is present.

Cardiac catheterization may be used in preparation for surgery. Findings reveal increased oxygen in the right ventricle and increased systolic pressure in the right ventricle and pulmonary artery.

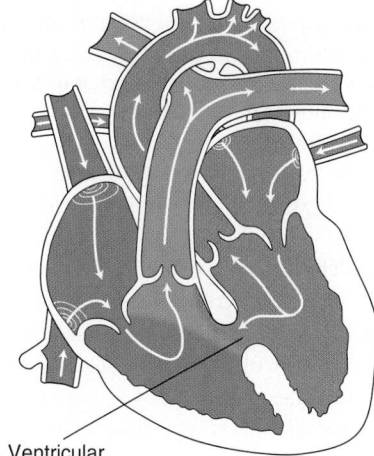

Ventricular
septal defect

Clinical Therapy

Most small VSDs close spontaneously within the first 6 months of life. Treatment is conservative when no signs of CHF or pulmonary hypertension are present.

Surgical patching of VSD during infancy is performed when poor growth is evident.

Device closure of VSD during cardiac catheterization may be attempted for some defects (Gillespie, Schneider, & Rome, 2006).

Prognosis: Highest risk associated with surgical repair is in the first few months of life. Children respond well to surgery and experience substantial catch-up growth. Tachyarrhythmias and right bundle branch block are possible complications.

Atrioventricular Canal (Endocardial Cushion) Defect (AV Canal)

Endocardial cushions are fetal growth centers for mitral and tricuspid valves and the atrioventricular (AV) septum. The most complex AV canal defect has one AV valve and large septal defects between both atria and ventricles. A total or partial AV canal defect occurs in about 2% of congenital heart defect cases (Park, 2008). This defect is associated with Down syndrome.

Clinical Manifestations

Severity of symptoms depends on amount of left-to-right shunting of blood across the septum. May be asymptomatic.

Infants have CHF, tachypnea, tachycardia, poor growth, recurrent respiratory infections, and repeated respiratory failure.

A **holosystolic** (heard the entire phase of systole) murmur is loudest at the left lower sternal border, and the intensity reflects the amount of mitral regurgitation. S_1 is accentuated and S_2 is split.

Diagnostic Procedures

On chest radiograph, cardiomegaly and pulmonary vascular markings are present.

On ECG, atrial enlargement, right ventricular hypertrophy, and an incomplete right bundle branch block are noted.

Echocardiogram reveals dilation of the ventricles, septal defects, and details of valve malformation.

Cardiac catheterization reveals increased oxygen in the right atrium, and increased right ventricle and/or pulmonary artery pressure.

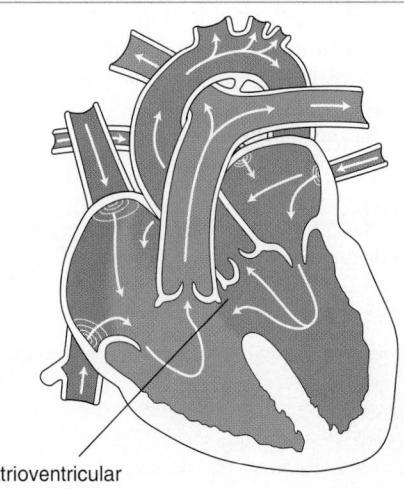

Atrioventricular
canal defect

Clinical Therapy

Surgery is performed during infancy to prevent pulmonary vascular disease. Patches are placed over septal defects, and valve tissue is used to form functioning valves. The mitral valve may be replaced.

Palliative pulmonary artery banding may be used to reduce blood flow to the lungs and CHF so the infant can grow before corrective surgery. CHF is treated (see page 620). Oxygen may be required until surgery, but it may increase pulmonary blood flow and worsen CHF.

Infective endocarditis prophylaxis is required until 6 months after corrective surgery.

Prognosis: Long-term survival following successful surgery is unknown. Arrhythmias and mitral valve insufficiency occur postoperatively. Infants with and without Down syndrome have similar short-term survival rates.

COLLABORATIVE CARE

Diagnostic Tests

See Table 21–4 for tests used to diagnose defects that cause increased pulmonary blood flow. Coagulation studies, platelet counts, and serum electrolytes are often obtained for children in preparation for open heart surgery, in addition to a chest radiograph, complete blood count, and urinalysis.

Clinical Therapy

Surgery to correct or manage defects that cause significant increased pulmonary blood flow is performed early in infancy to prevent irreversible pulmonary hypertension, the major complication of these defects. Unless complications develop before surgery, the child should make a complete recovery without limitations.

Conservative treatment, such as waiting until the child is symptomatic or older, may be selected for some children with these defects. See Figure 21–4 ➤. For example, small ventricular or atrial septal defects may close spontaneously, or repair of an atrial septal defect may be postponed until preschool or early school-age years. Indomethacin may be given to preterm infants with a patent ductus arteriosus when immediate closure of the ductus is needed. Interventional cardiac catheterization may be performed for defects. See Table 21–3.

Postpericardiotomy syndrome occurs as a complication in approximately 25–30% of children when surgery involves an incision through the pericardium, leading to pericardial and pleural inflammation (Park, 2008, p. 377). It is believed to result from an autoimmune response to a damaged myocardium or pericardium, or to blood in the pericardial sac. The syndrome generally develops within a few weeks to a few months after surgery, more often in children over 2 years than in infants. It is characterized by a high fever up to 40°C (104°F) and severe chest pain that worsens with deep inspiration and in supine position. The median duration of the condition is 2 to 3 weeks. Mild cases are treated with bed rest and nonsteroidal anti-inflammatories (NSAIDs). Severe cases may need corticosteroids, emergency pericardiocentesis, or diuretics (Park, 2008).

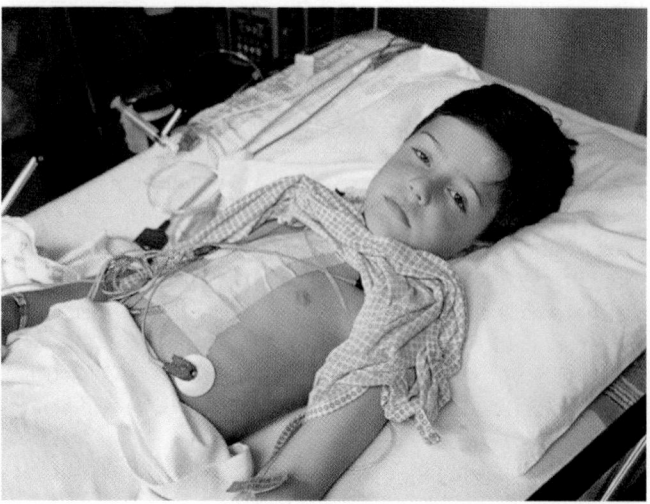

FIGURE 21–4 ➤ A child with atrial septal defect repair. Surgery is performed with this type of defect to prevent pulmonary hypertension.

NURSING MANAGEMENT PRIOR TO SURGERY

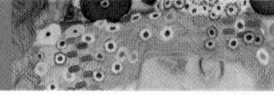

Nursing Assessment and Diagnosis

Physiologic Assessment

Prior to surgery, the infant or child is seen regularly to assess growth and to detect signs of worsening CHF. Many infants with a small defect will have no growth problems. Failure to gain weight is an indication of an increased metabolic rate and inability to consume adequate calories for both metabolic function and growth. Assessment of length and head circumference helps to determine the full impact of the condition on growth.

Psychosocial Assessment

Assess the parents' ability to cope with the infant's diagnosis. Parents may initially be in shock and feel guilty or anxious. Parents need an opportunity to express their feelings and learn to cope with the child's illness. The initial period of diagnosis, hospitalization, and early care of the infant at home are very stressful. Parents need special support if their infant has a life-threatening heart defect.

Examples of nursing diagnoses associated with heart defects having increased pulmonary blood flow and their complications include:

- Excess Fluid Volume related to heart failure and pulmonary vasculature overload
- Ineffective Infant Feeding Pattern related to shortness of breath and fatigue
- Risk for Infection related to pulmonary vascular congestion and chronic illness
- Interrupted Family Processes related to crisis of child's serious illness

Planning and Implementation

When the child has a large defect, CHF may be present. See page 623 for nursing management guidelines.

Family Education

Participate with members of the cardiology team to provide information and educate the family about the child's condition. Information may include the following:

- General information about the CHD, including a description of the heart's anatomy and physiology and the defect
- Information about genetic and environmental influences associated with congenital heart disease
- Overview of the child's prognosis and timing of medical and surgical interventions

Clinical Tip

Resources for parents of a child with a congenital heart defect include:

■ *It's My Heart* by the Children's Heart Foundation
■ *The Parent's Guide to Children's Congenital Heart Defects* by Gerri Freid Kramer and Shari Maurer, Three Rivers Press
■ *The Heart of a Child: What Families Need to Know About Heart Disorders in Children* by C. A. Neill, E. A. Clark, and C. Clark, Johns Hopkins Press

Psychosocial Support

Parents often need support for anxiety about an uncertain surgical outcome. Determine if parents have a support system as they learn about the infant's diagnosis and make difficult decisions about the child's surgery. Some parents may be concerned that consenting to surgery places the child in even more danger of illness or even death. Identify resources for support, such as social services, pastoral services, or a parent of a child with a similar heart defect. See the companion website for resources.

Parents should be offered genetic counseling if planning a future pregnancy.

Home Care

Children are often managed at home until surgery. Parents should encourage feeding to promote growth, but allow the infant to feed no longer than 40 minutes, or as directed by health professionals for infants with complex CHDs or CHF. Breastfeeding is encouraged if growth is adequate, and it is less stressful than bottle-feeding (Cook & Higgins, 2010). Infants should be held at a 45-degree angle to reduce tachypnea. Transpyloric, nasogastric, or gastrostomy tube feedings may also be given at night or 24 hours a day to ensure that adequate calories are ingested. See Figure 21–5 ➤. When tube feedings are used, encourage the infant to take some formula orally to provide positive oral stimulation. See feeding suggestions for the infant with CHF on page 627.

Reduce the infant's exposure to infectious diseases and encourage frequent hand hygiene. Respiratory infections make hypoxemia worse in children with cyanosis. Fever increases the metabolic rates and oxygen demands. Vomiting and diarrhea

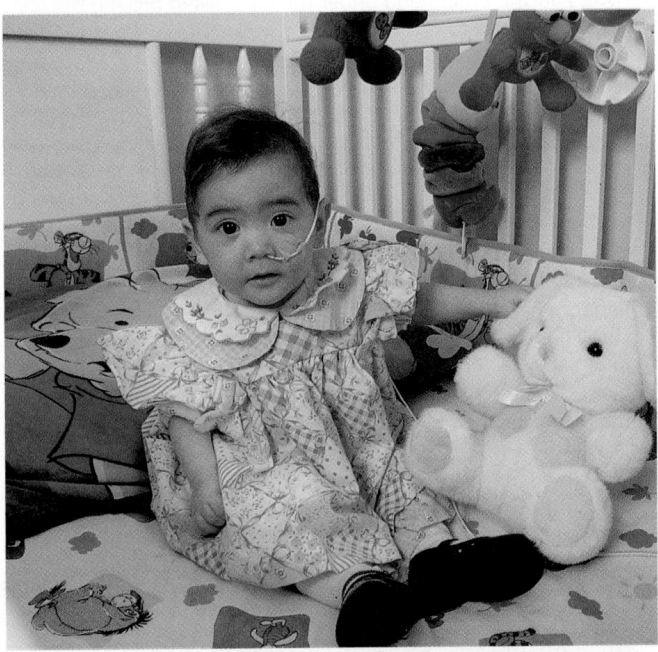

FIGURE 21–5 ➤ Infants with cardiac conditions often require supplemental feedings to provide sufficient nutrients for growth and development. The parents of this infant girl have been taught how to give her nasogastric feedings at home.

may cause an electrolyte disturbance and digoxin toxicity (Cook & Higgins, 2010). The physician should be notified about fever, poor feeding, vomiting, and diarrhea.

Health promotion visits are important. Provide all immunizations according to the recommended schedule. Monthly prophylaxis for respiratory syncytial virus (RSV) with palivizumab should be provided during the peak season. See Chapter 20 ∞.

Preparation for Surgery

When the child is preschool age or older, prepare the child for the settings, equipment, and experiences to expect before and after surgery. Follow guidelines for preoperative treatment described in Chapter 11 ∞. If an infant or toddler is having surgery, provide parents with information about how the child will look, equipment that will be used, and what care will be provided in the immediate postoperative period.

Evaluation

Expected outcomes include the following:

- Nutritional intake is adequate with oral feeding and supplemental tube feeding as necessary.
- The child maintains a growth pattern that follows the established growth curve percentile.
- The child receives all immunizations and RSV prophylaxis to reduce the potential for acute illnesses.

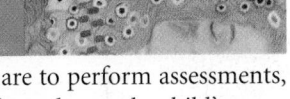

NURSING MANAGEMENT AT THE TIME OF SURGERY

The goals of nursing management are to perform assessments, provide supportive care to the family, and meet the child's nursing care needs before and after surgery.

Nursing Assessment and Diagnosis

At the time of surgery, the child needs a careful history and physical examination to detect any acute illnesses. Assess the child's behavioral patterns, heart function, respiratory function, weight, and fluid status.

In the immediate postoperative period, the child will be cared for in the intensive care unit. When the child returns to the general nursing unit, assessment focuses on signs of surgical complications such as infection, arrhythmias, and impaired tissue perfusion. Pain assessment is also important. Monitor the child's temperature and inspect the surgical incision site. Fever, excessive incisional pain, spreading erythema around the incision, and wound drainage beginning 3 to 4 days postoperatively may be early signs of infection. Assess the chest and lungs for breath sounds, respiratory effort, and signs of distress that may indicate pneumonia or fluid in the pleural space.

Monitor the vital signs, including blood pressure. As the discharge date nears, the child may not be on a cardiac monitor, so auscultate the apical pulse to detect an irregular heart rate or bradycardia, both signs of reduced cardiac output that require immediate intervention. Check pulse oximetry, capillary refill, extremity warmth, pedal pulses, level of consciousness, and urine output to assess impaired tissue perfusion. Reduced urine output is another sign of decreased cardiac output.

Examples of nursing diagnoses following cardiac surgery include the following:

- Ineffective Breathing Pattern related to respiratory muscle fatigue
- Acute Pain related to surgical incision and expansion of chest with coughing and deep breathing exercises
- Risk for Imbalanced Fluid Volume related to impact of surgery on heart's pumping action
- Risk for Infection related to surgery and chronic disease status

Planning and Implementation

Pain Management

Pain management with 24-hour intravenous opioids or ketorolac should be provided for 1 to 2 days postoperatively until the child is taking fluids. Once the child is taking oral fluids and foods, an oral analgesic may be given around the clock. Follow the guidelines for pain management provided in Chapter 15 ∞. Teach parents and caregivers to lift and move the child carefully and avoid stress on the incision to reduce potential pain.

Promote Respiratory Function

Encourage the child to take deep breaths and cough or to perform spirometry exercises regularly to promote full lung expansion. (See the *Clinical Skills Manual*.) Provide tips for splinting the chest (a pillow or stuffed animal) to reduce the pain from coughing and deep breathing. Chest physiotherapy may be performed in children under 3 years of age.

Clinical Judgment

What are some suggestions to encourage deep breathing in children of different ages after cardiac surgery?

Manage Fluids and Nutrition

Encourage the infant or child to begin oral fluids and nutrition when permitted. Although oral fluids are rarely limited for children with CHDs that increase pulmonary volume, intake and output are carefully monitored. Parents may be encouraged to bring in favorite foods for the child when they can be tolerated. Promote bowel elimination following surgery, especially when opioids are used for pain management.

Administer antibiotics as ordered. If intravenous antibiotics are continued after the child's oral intake is normal, the line can be converted to a heparin or saline lock.

Activity

Encourage the child to increase activity gradually with longer periods out of bed every day, but ensure adequate rest periods to promote healing. Provide diversional activities and opportunities for therapeutic play so the child can better manage the stresses associated with pain and frightening procedures.

Discharge Planning and Home Care Teaching

Infants and children may be discharged from the hospital within a few days of surgery. Parents need information spread over several days to prepare for care of the child at home. See Families Want to Know: Care of the Child After Cardiac Surgery.

Prepare parents for potential behavior problems of young children that may result from the stress of hospitalization, such as nightmares, separation anxiety, and overdependence on parents. Encourage parents to reassure children about their security, and to promote play and other means to deal with their feelings. If the child's behavioral symptoms continue for several weeks, a referral for psychological evaluation and care may be needed for posttraumatic stress disorder (see Chapter 28 ∞).

Reassure parents of children with a complete correction of the cardiac defect that there should be no further cardiovascular problems. Provide parents with full information about the child's defect and the surgery performed to share with the child's current and future health care providers. Encourage parents to allow the child to live a normal and active life.

Families Want to Know
Care of the Child After Cardiac Surgery

- Place infants and children in car safety seats for travel home from the hospital. Place a small blanket over the incision to prevent the straps from rubbing.
- Sponge bathe the infant or use a tub bath with a low water level. Avoid soaking the incision until sutures are out, the Steri-Strips are off, or Dermabond has flaked off, and the incision is healed. Cover the incision with a clean shirt or bib to keep it clean and dry. Clean the newly healed incision daily with gentle baby or pH-balanced soap. Do not use oils, creams, lotions, or ointments on the incision.
- Pick up infants and young children by placing one hand under the head and the other hand under the hips. Avoid picking the child up under the arms.
- Allow the child to increase activity gradually as tolerated, starting with quiet play for the first week at home. Report increased fatigue or decreased activity tolerance to the physician. Postpone rough play, bike riding, and strenuous activities for 6 weeks until the sternum and incision have healed completely. Allow the child to return to school in about 3 weeks, but no backpack should be carried for several weeks.
- Encourage a nutritious diet and snacks for the infant or child to promote healing and catch-up growth.
- Report any signs of wound infection, fever, flulike symptoms, chest pain, increased respiratory rate or respiratory distress, appetite change, or irritability to the physician.
- Acetaminophen or ibuprofen can be given for pain control. Use the recommended dose for the child's weight.
- Antibiotic prophylaxis for infective endocarditis should be prescribed for dental and invasive respiratory procedures for 6 months after corrective surgery when a prosthetic heart valve or prosthetic material is used. See the Medications table on page 631. Report any unexplained fever or illness during the first 2 months following surgery because the child is at higher risk for infective endocarditis during that time.
- Live virus vaccines should be postponed after cardiac surgery when blood products have been administered (5 months for packed red blood cells, 6 months for whole blood) (American Academy of Pediatrics, 2009, p. 448).

Evaluation

Examples of expected outcomes of nursing care include the following:

- The child's pain is effectively managed.
- Full lung expansion is maintained with incentive spirometry exercises or chest physiotherapy.
- The child's incision heals without infection.
- Catch-up growth occurs over the next few months to years.

Defects Causing Decreased Pulmonary Blood Flow and Mixed Defects

Information about these CHD categories is combined because the clinical therapy and nursing interventions are similar. Distinguishing features are described by etiology, pathophysiology, and clinical manifestations.

Etiology and Pathophysiology

Defects Causing Decreased Pulmonary Blood Flow Defects that obstruct the pulmonary blood flow result in little or no blood reaching the lungs to get oxygenated. If an atrial or ventricular septal opening exists between the left and right side of the heart, right-sided pressures exceed those on the left, resulting in right-to-left shunting. In this case, cyanosis often results.

The bone marrow is stimulated to produce more red blood cells to increase the hemoglobin available to carry oxygen. Polycythemia may result and place the child at risk for thromboembolism. Over time, platelet survival is reduced and clotting factors are impaired, increasing the infant's risk of bleeding with surgery. Brain abscesses are more common in cases of polycythemia and septal defects; bacteria may cross into the systemic circulation rather than getting filtered out by the lung capillaries (Park, 2008, p. 145).

When infants and children with cyanosis rise in the morning, they may experience an abrupt decrease in systemic resistance and pulmonary blood flow. This physiologic change can trigger a **hypercyanotic** (hypoxic or "tet") **episode** when combined with a sudden increase in cardiac output and venous return associated with crying, feeding, exercise, a warm bath, and straining with defecation. The partial pressure of oxygen (PO_2) is lowered, and the partial pressure of carbon dioxide (PCO_2) rises. Hypoxemia becomes progressively worse as the respiratory center in the brain overreacts, increasing the respiratory effort. The extra respiratory effort further increases the cardiac output and contributes to a life-threatening decline unless rapid intervention is successful.

Mixed Defects Many complex congenital heart defects involve a combination of defects that make the newborn dependent upon mixing pulmonary and systemic circulations for survival during the postnatal period. This mixing of oxygen-saturated and desaturated blood results in a general desaturated systemic blood flow and cyanosis. Pulmonary congestion occurs because of increased pulmonary blood flow and obstruction of systemic flow.

Clinical Manifestations

Defects Causing Decreased Pulmonary Blood Flow Clinical manifestations in infants initially include cyanosis shortly after birth, dyspnea, and a loud murmur. The skin may initially be ruddy or mottled before cyanosis is observed. Cyanosis that does not respond as expected to supplemental oxygen is a classic sign. Signs and symptoms of chronic hypoxemia include fatigue, clubbing of the fingers and toes, exertional dyspnea, and delayed developmental milestones. The infant may need to stop sucking periodically during feedings to breathe, and diaphoresis may be seen with the increased work of feeding. These infants have a higher metabolic rate, and inadequate calories may be consumed, resulting in poor weight gain. See Table 21–5 for the pathophysiology, clinical manifestations, and clinical therapy for these defects.

When the infant or child has severe obstruction to pulmonary blood flow, hypercyanotic episodes can occur suddenly. The knee–chest position or squatting by a toddler reduces the cardiac output by decreasing the venous return from the lower extremities and by increasing the systemic vascular resistance. Hypercyanotic episodes usually appear between 2 months and 2 years of age. Signs include increased rate and depth of respirations, increased heart rate, increased cyanosis or pallor, poor tissue perfusion, diaphoresis, irritability and crying, and seizures and loss of consciousness.

Older children may have additional symptoms such as exercise-induced dizziness and syncope, which are serious signs indicating a need for medical evaluation.

Mixed Defects These complex congenital heart defects cause varying degrees of cyanosis and CHF. See Table 21–6 for the pathophysiology, clinical manifestations, and clinical therapy for these complex mixed defects.

COLLABORATIVE CARE

Diagnostic Tests

See Tables 21–5 and 21–6 for diagnostic tests and clinical therapy for these individual defects.

Clinical Therapy

Early management of these defects is important to prevent secondary damage to the heart, lungs, and brain, including the adverse effects of hypoxemia on the child's cognitive and psychomotor development. Corrective surgery is often performed on the neonate or young infant when possible. A palliative procedure may be performed first to preserve life in children with potentially lethal CHDs or CHDs with complications. With some defects, corrective surgery can be postponed with a palliative procedure, giving the infant an opportunity to grow and improve the success of corrective surgery. See Figure 21–6 ➤ for various palliative shunts (surgically created channels for blood flow) that may be performed.

See Tables 21–5 and 21–6 for clinical therapy for specific congenital heart defects. If closure of the ductus arteriosus causes life-threatening cyanosis in newborns, prostaglandin E_1 (PGE_1) is given to reopen the ductus arteriosus and to improve pulmonary or systemic blood flow. Treatment with PGE_1 provides time to transfer the newborn to a cardiac center for diagnostic evaluation and medical or surgical intervention. Adverse effects include respiratory depression and apnea, so the infant must be closely monitored and sometimes ventilation must be assisted.

TABLE 21–5	Pathophysiology, Clinical Manifestations, and Clinical Therapy for Defects with Decreased Pulmonary Blood Flow

Defect Pathophysiology, Clinical Manifestations, and Clinical Therapy	Anatomy

Pulmonic Stenosis (PS)

Stenosis is narrowing of the valve, valve area, or great artery above the valve. Stenosis obstructs blood flow into the pulmonary artery, which increases **preload** (the volume of blood in the ventricle at the end of diastole that stretches the heart muscle before contraction) and results in right ventricular hypertrophy. Isolated PS accounts for 8–12% of all congenital heart defects, but it also is associated with tetralogy of Fallot (Park, 2008). Stenosis in the subvalvular area may develop as the heart muscle grows.

Clinical Manifestations

Children with mild stenosis may have no symptoms and grow normally. In moderate stenosis, dyspnea and fatigue occur on exertion. Signs of CHF and hepatosplenomegaly are rare but may result from chronic pressure overload. Heart failure and chest pain on exertion occur in severe cases. A loud systolic ejection murmur with a widely split S_2 and thrill may be found in the pulmonic listening area.

Diagnostic Procedures

The chest radiograph may show an enlarged pulmonary artery with normal heart size and normal pulmonary vascularity.
The ECG may show right atrial enlargement and right ventricular hypertrophy.
An echocardiogram provides information about the pressure gradient across the valve and size of valve ring.
Cardiac catheterization findings include increased right ventricular pressure and a normal or slightly lowered pulmonary artery pressure.

Clinical Therapy

Dilation by balloon valvuloplasty, performed during cardiac catheterization, treats simple pulmonic stenosis.
Surgical valvotomy may be used when other defects such as VSD are present.
Surgical resection may be needed for narrowing above the valve area. Pulmonary regurgitation may result, but is not a significant problem.
Prognosis: Pulmonic stenosis does not typically increase in severity. Lifelong infective endocarditis prophylaxis is necessary.

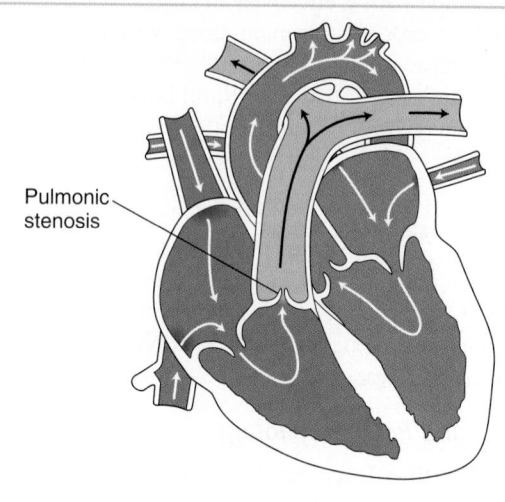

Pulmonic stenosis

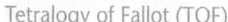 Decreased unoxygenated blood flow

Tetralogy of Fallot (TOF)

Four defects—pulmonic stenosis, right ventricular hypertrophy, ventricular septal defect (VSD), and overriding of aorta—make up the condition. Some children have a fifth defect, an open foramen ovale or atrial septal defect (ASD). About 5–10% of children with CHD have TOF (Park, 2008). Elevated pressures in the right side of the heart cause a right-to-left shunt.

Clinical Manifestations

The infant becomes hypoxic and cyanotic as the ductus arteriosus closes. The degree of pulmonary stenosis determines the severity of symptoms. A systolic murmur in the pulmonic area and a single S_2 is auscultated. A thrill may be palpated in the pulmonic area.
Polycythemia, hypoxic episodes, metabolic acidosis, poor growth, clubbing, and exercise intolerance may develop.
Toddlers with uncorrected defects instinctively squat (assume a knee–chest position) to decrease the return of systemic venous blood to the heart.

Diagnostic Procedures

A chest radiograph shows the boot-shaped heart due to the large right ventricle, decreased pulmonary vascular markings, and a prominent aorta. The ECG shows right ventricular hypertrophy.
The echocardiogram shows the VSD, obstruction of pulmonary outflow, an overriding aorta, and the size of the pulmonary arteries.
Cardiac catheterization provides details about the anatomic defects.
Blood tests reveal an elevated hematocrit and hemoglobin and an increased clotting time.

Clinical Therapy

Management of hypercyanotic episodes is described on page 615. Monitoring the child for metabolic acidosis or prolonged unconsciousness is critical.
Some children need palliative surgery (modified Blalock-Taussig shunt) to allow the infant to grow prior to surgery that corrects the defect. Some infants have surgery to correct the defect as the first surgery.
Prognosis: Not all children are cured by surgery, but most have improved quality of life and improved longevity. Arrhythmias may result from surgery. Ventricular arrhythmias may occur many years after surgery and may cause sudden death (Park, 2008, p. 243).

Pulmonic stenosis

Overriding aorta

Ventricular septal defect

Right ventricular hypertrophy

Decreased unoxygenated blood flow

Mixed oxygenated and unoxygenated blood

TABLE 21–5	Pathophysiology, Clinical Manifestations, and Clinical Therapy for Defects with Decreased Pulmonary Blood Flow *(continued)*

Defect Pathophysiology, Clinical Manifestations, and Clinical Therapy	Anatomy

Pulmonary or Tricuspid Atresia

Pulmonary atresia is the absence of communication between the right ventricle and the pulmonary artery, either at the site of the pulmonary valve or in the main pulmonary artery. In tricuspid atresia (1–3% of CHDs), the tricuspid valve is absent resulting in no communication between the right atrium and ventricle, and the right ventricle is **hypoplastic** (small and nonfunctional) (Park, 2008, p. 254). Blood flows to the left side of the heart through the foramen ovale. The ductus arteriosus provides the only flow of blood to the pulmonary arteries.

Clinical Manifestations

Cyanosis is present at birth.
Tachypnea, CHF, pulmonary edema, hepatomegaly, acidosis, hypoxic episodes, clubbing, polycythemia, and growth delays occur.
A continuous murmur from the PDA is heard in the pulmonic area. A single S_2 is heard in the aortic area, and a harsh systolic murmur may be heard in the tricuspid area.

Diagnostic Procedures

The chest radiograph may reveal a normal size or slightly enlarged heart.
The ECG may reveal right atrial hypertrophy.
The echocardiogram shows a small hypoplastic right ventricular cavity and tricuspid valve, an absent right ventricular outflow tract, a dilated right atrium, and right-to-left shunting across the atrial septum.

Clinical Therapy

Prostaglandin E_1 is given immediately to maintain a patent ductus arteriosus. Digoxin and diuretics are also used.
The Rashkind balloon atrial septostomy is performed to increase the atrial opening size.
A Rastelli or modified Fontan procedure results in improved survival.
Prognosis: Outcome depends upon the size of the pulmonary outflow tract developed by surgery and the fibrosis in the right ventricle. The child with tricuspid atresia has a 5-year survival rate of 80% and a 10-year survival rate of 70% (Park, 2008, p. 262).

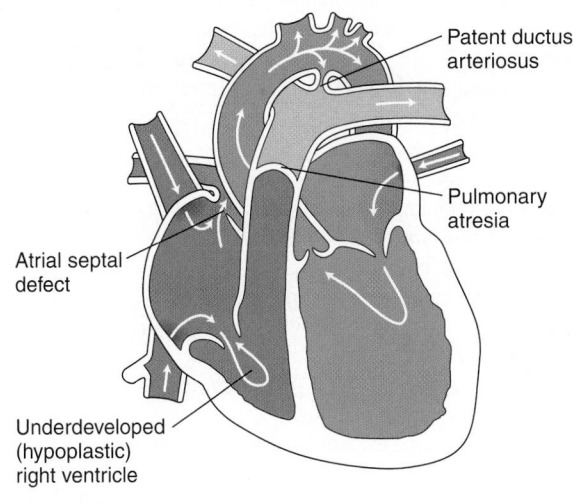

Patent ductus arteriosus
Pulmonary atresia
Atrial septal defect
Underdeveloped (hypoplastic) right ventricle

☐ Decreased unoxygenated blood flow
■ Mixed oxygenated and unoxygenated blood

FIGURE 21–6 ➤ Anatomic location of the modified Blalock-Taussig and Glenn shunts for palliative procedures.

Bidirectional Glenn shunt
Aorta
Subclavian artery
Modified Blalock-Taussig shunt
Right pulmonary artery
Superior vena cava
Main pulmonary artery

CHF is treated aggressively (see page 623). The child's hemoglobin and hematocrit values are monitored for polycythemia or anemia. If the blood viscosity becomes too high, red cell pheresis may be performed. These infants also do not tolerate anemia well as they have less oxygen-carrying hemoglobin. Packed red blood cells may be administered to improve oxygen delivery to the tissues when the child is anemic.

Hypercyanotic Episodes Oral propranolol may be prescribed to prevent hypercyanotic episodes (Park, 2008, p. 239). Hypercyanotic episodes are aggressively treated. To increase the systemic vascular resistance, the infant is immediately placed in knee–chest position. To decrease the pulmonary vascular resistance, the initial treatment involves calming the child, giving supplemental oxygen, administering morphine and propranolol intravenously, and giving intravenous fluids to expand circulatory volume. Postpone all unpleasant procedures. Dopamine or phenylephrine (Neo-Synephrine) is also given. Once a hypercyanotic episode has occurred, immediate palliative or corrective surgery is often scheduled.

Infective Endocarditis Prophylactic antibiotics for infective endocarditis are required for most children with complex cardiac defects prior to surgery and for 6 months after surgery. See Medications Used to Treat: Prophylaxis for Infective Endocarditis on page 631. Children whose surgery involves prosthetic patches

TABLE 21–6 Pathophysiology, Clinical Manifestations, and Clinical Therapy for Mixed Defects

Defect Pathophysiology, Clinical Manifestations, and Clinical Therapy   Anatomy

Transposition of the Great Arteries (TGA)

The pulmonary artery is the outflow tract for the left ventricle, and the aorta is the outflow tract for the right ventricle, creating parallel circulations. The condition is life threatening at birth, and survival initially depends on an open ductus arteriosus and foramen ovale. This condition occurs in about 5–7% of children with CHDs (Park, 2008). An ASD or VSD may also be present with TGA.

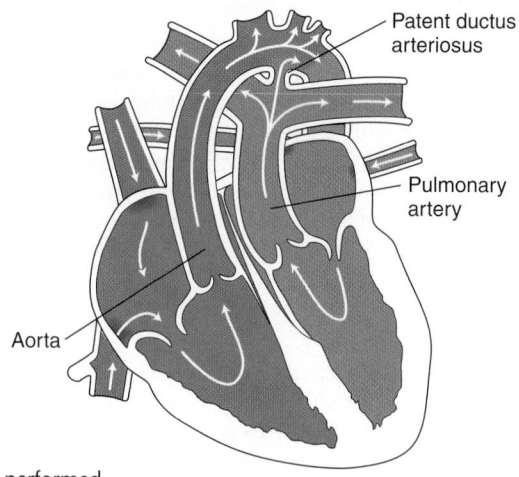

Clinical Manifestations

Cyanosis, apparent soon after birth, progresses to hypoxia and acidosis. Cyanosis does not improve with supplemental oxygen. Cyanosis may be less apparent when a large VSD is present.

CHF may develop immediately or over days or weeks. Tachypnea (60 breaths per minute) is often present without retractions or other signs of dyspnea.

A systolic murmur is present if a VSD is present; no other murmur is generally heard. S_2 is loud.

Infants take a long time to feed and need frequent rest periods because of rapid respiratory rate and fatigue.

Growth failure may be evident as early as 2 weeks of age if corrective surgery is not performed.

Diagnostic Procedures

A chest radiograph may reveal a classic egg-shaped heart on a string (narrow superior mediastinum) with enlarged ventricles and increased pulmonary vascular markings.

The ECG reveals right ventricular hypertrophy.

The echocardiogram often shows the abnormal position of the great arteries rising from the ventricles.

A hyperoxitest (see Appendix E ∞) confirms a congenital heart defect causing cyanosis.

Cardiac catheterization shows increased right ventricular pressure, and the catheter can enter the aorta through the right ventricle.

Blood tests reveal an increased hematocrit and hemoglobin or polycythemia.

Clinical Therapy

Prostaglandin E_1 is ordered to maintain a patent ductus arteriosus until a palliative procedure can be performed. Oxygen is administered for severe hypoxemia.

Balloon atrial septostomy may be performed during cardiac catheterization in newborns as a first stage while surgery is planned within days. The septostomy is corrected surgically.

Corrective surgery (arterial switch) is usually performed between 1 and 3 weeks of age.

Prognosis: Survival without surgery is impossible. Few complications occur with the arterial switch procedure. Arrhythmias are rare and ventricular function is usually normal (Park, 2008, p. 225). Arrhythmias, decreased right ventricular function, pulmonary vascular disease, and sudden death may be long-term complications associated with previously used surgical procedures (e.g., Mustard and Senning) (Park, 2008).

Truncus Arteriosus

A single large vessel empties both ventricles and provides circulation for the pulmonary, systemic, and coronary circulations. A VSD is usually present. This occurs in less than 1% of congenital heart defects (Park, 2008).

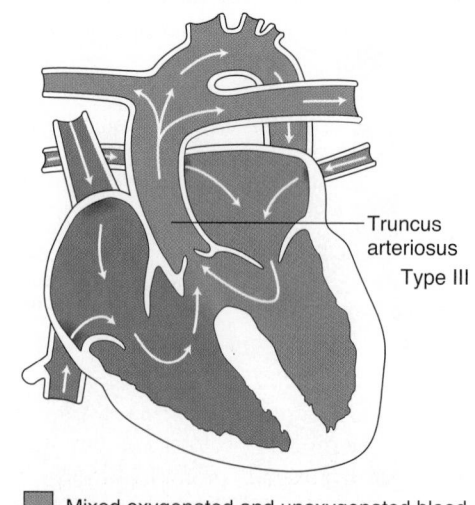

Clinical Manifestations

Cyanosis develops soon after birth; however, this is also a condition of increased pulmonary blood flow. Severe CHF, dyspnea, retractions, fatigue, poor feeding, poor growth, polycythemia, clubbing, increased pulse pressure, bounding peripheral pulses, a widened pulse pressure, frequent respiratory infections, and cardiomegaly occur.

The VSD produces a harsh systolic murmur in the lower sternal border. A systolic click may be heard in the apex and pulmonic area.

Diagnostic Procedures

The chest radiograph shows cardiomegaly, a large aorta, and increased pulmonary vascular markings.

The ECG reveals bilateral ventricular hypertrophy.

The echocardiogram shows a VSD, a large single great artery, and one semilunar valve.

■ Mixed oxygenated and unoxygenated blood

Clinical Therapy

A Rastelli procedure is performed to close the VSD, enable the left ventricle to empty into the truncus, and create a passage to the pulmonary arteries. Repeated surgery is necessary to enlarge the pulmonary artery conduit.

Digoxin and diuretics are given.

Prognosis: Mortality from surgery ranges from 10–30% (Park, 2008, p. 281). The long-term prognosis is unknown. Ventricular arrhythmias may develop. The child should not participate in competitive or strenuous sports.

TABLE 21–6 Pathophysiology, Clinical Manifestations, and Clinical Therapy for Mixed Defects *(continued)*

Defect Pathophysiology, Clinical Manifestations, and Clinical Therapy | Anatomy

Total Anomalous Pulmonary Venous Return

The pulmonary veins empty into the right atrium or veins leading to the right atrium rather than into the left atrium. The foramen ovale must remain patent for mixed blood from the right atrium to pass to the systemic circulation. Any obstruction of the pulmonary veins increases the condition's severity. It occurs in about 1% of children with a congenital heart defect (Park, 2008).

Clinical Manifestations

Mild cyanosis and tachypnea are present. Increased cyanosis may occur with feedings as the filled esophagus compresses the common pulmonary vein. The S_2 has a wide, fixed split when there is no pulmonary vein obstruction. A gallop rhythm is present, but no heart murmur is usually auscultated. Crackles and hepatosplenomegaly are usually present.

Diagnostic Procedures

The chest radiograph may show cardiac enlargement, and the lung fields may reveal pulmonary edema.
The ECG reveals hypertrophy of the right atrium and ventricle.
The echocardiogram shows enlargement of the right atrium and ventricle, with a small left atrium and ventricle, dilated pulmonary arteries, and a patent foramen ovale.

Clinical Therapy

Prostaglandin E_1 may be given to maintain patent ductus arteriosus.
Digoxin and diuretics are given to treat CHF.
Balloon atrial septostomy may be performed to increase blood flow to the left side so surgery can be delayed until the infant is stabilized.
Surgery to connect or baffle the pulmonary veins to the left atrium is performed.
Prognosis: Survival without surgery is not possible. Children may develop pulmonary vein obstruction or atrial arrhythmias.

Anatomy labels: Superior vena cava; Total anomalous pulmonary venous connection; Pulmonary vein; Pulmonary vein; Atrial septal defect

---

or devices and those who have unrepaired cyanotic CHD, including palliative shunts and conduits, need lifelong infective endocarditis prophylaxis (Wilson, Taubert, Gewitz, et al., 2007).

Long-Term Clinical Therapy Children with complex congenital heart defects require long-term care following palliative or corrective heart surgery. Some need multiple stages of surgery, revisions of previous surgeries, valve replacements, or interventional cardiac catheterization to reopen valves or vessels that have become stenotic. An implanted pacemaker may be needed for arrhythmias associated with anomalies of the conduction system or unavoidable surgical incisions in areas of the sinoatrial node or sinoventricular node, such as the Fontan procedure. The Mustard, Senning, and Fontan procedures, as well as tetralogy of Fallot (TOF) repairs, are associated with increased risk of arrhythmias. A pacemaker may be used in older children with life-threatening AV block or ventricular arrhythmias, as described for Tim in the opening scenario (Park, 2008, pp. 451–455).

Although most children with congenital heart disease have normal IQ scores, and children with corrected simple defects can lead normal lives, neurologic insults can occur for many reasons. CHF, prolonged hypoxemia, profound acidosis, and low cardiac output increase the infant's risk for neurologic sequelae. Inadequate nutrition during rapid brain growth in the first year, intraventricular hemorrhage, hypoxic-ischemic injury, or periventricular leukomalacia (focal necrotic lesions in the periventricular white matter) can cause neurologic problems (Zeltser & Tabbutt, 2006, pp. 38–39). Cardiopulmonary bypass and deep hypothermic circulatory arrest used during most surgeries are other potential neurologic insults. See Evidence-Based Practice: Neurodevelopmental Outcomes in Children with Complex Congenital Heart Disease on the next page.

Children with complex CHDs are at risk for visuospatial, visual motor, and speech deficits even when IQ scores fall within normal ranges (Brosig, Mussatto, Kuhn, et al., 2007). Children with hypoplastic left heart syndrome (HLHS) are at higher risk for neurocognitive impairment because of a higher incidence of congenital brain abnormalities, ductal-dependent systemic blood flow, severe acidosis at diagnosis, deep hypothermic cardiac arrest during surgery, and postoperative challenges of maintaining adequate systemic blood flow and cerebral perfusion. It is thought that some infants with complex congenital defects have abnormal brain development (Miller, McQuillen, Hamrick, et al., 2007).

NURSING MANAGEMENT

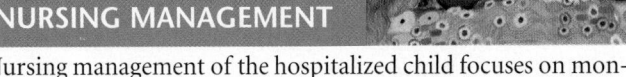

Nursing management of the hospitalized child focuses on monitoring PGE$_1$ therapy for newborns, treating hypercyanotic episodes, supporting families to care for the child at home, and providing postsurgical care.

Nursing Assessment and Diagnosis

Physiologic Assessment Before Surgery

Newborns receiving PGE$_1$ infusion therapy are cared for in an intensive care nursery where their cardiovascular status can be closely monitored until palliative procedures are performed.

Neurodevelopmental Outcomes in Children with Complex Congenital Heart Disease

Problem

In the last two decades, surgery for infants with complex CHDs has been performed at younger ages, reducing the time infants are exposed to prolonged hypoxemia, profound acidosis, and low cardiac output. Children with complex CHDs have more central nervous system abnormalities than the general population (Miller et al., 2007). What information do parents and school officials need to plan for educational supports for children who have had surgery for complex CHDs?

Evidence

A study of 109 school-age children who had surgery as newborns for a complex CHD revealed 53 (49%) were receiving remedial education services and 15% were in special education classes. A significant number had inattention and hyperactivity (Shillingford, Glanzman, Ittenbach, et al., 2008). A group of 94 infants with complex heart defects having open heart surgery were followed and evaluated at school age to assess functional (motor and neurologic) outcomes. Mild fine and gross motor impairments were present, but few were severe. An association was found between increasing surgical circulatory arrest time and fine and gross motor function delays (Majnemer, Limperopoulos, Shevell, et al., 2006). A study of 43 children with simple and complex CHDs and 43 healthy children without CHDs, aged 8 years, was conducted, excluding children with obvious neurodevelopmental problems. Testing revealed that children with CHDs scored within the expected range on the Wechsler Intelligence Test, but significantly lower than healthy controls. Children with CHDs performed significantly lower in domains of sensorimotor functioning, language, attention and executive functioning, and memory (Miatton, De Wolf, Fançois, et al., 2007). A study evaluating the outcome of 26 children, 3.5 to 6 years of age, who had had surgery for TGA and HLHS found that children with HLHS had more problems with visual-motor skills, expressive language, attention, and behavior than the children with TGA (Brosig et al., 2007).

Implications

CHDs and treatment regimens are associated with motor problems in some children or difficulties in coordination and balance, handwriting, language, and attention. Children may need special educational assessment and developmental screening to identify specific neurodevelopmental problems. Children may need an individualized education plan when disabilities affect learning.

Critical Thinking Application

Develop an outline of important information for the parent of a child with a complex CHD to discuss with the child's teacher, school nurse, and school officials when the child enters school.

Common side effects of PGE$_1$ therapy include cutaneous vasodilation, bradycardia, tachycardia, hypotension, seizure activity, fever, and apnea.

Prior to or between stages of surgery, the infant or child is seen regularly to assess growth and monitor for signs of CHF (tachycardia, tachypnea, crackles, frothy secretions, low urine output, and pulmonary edema). The child's poor growth may affect height, weight, and head circumference, so plot serial measurements on the same growth curve to monitor the significance of the growth problems. Monitor physiologic status using the Assessment Guidelines on page 604.

The infant needs careful observation for signs of increased cyanosis in the morning or at other high-risk times. Observe for neurologic signs of thromboembolism due to polycythemia such as headache, dizziness, excessive irritability, and paralysis. Older children with cyanotic defects may have clubbing of the fingers and toes or squat into a knee-chest position (Figure 21–7 ➤).

Assessment Following Surgery

Children are admitted to the intensive care unit following surgery. Children undergoing video-assisted thoracoscopic surgery may go to the postanesthesia unit for discharge the same day. Once the child returns to the general nursing unit, monitor the child's heart functioning. Assess vital signs, pulse oximetry, skin color, and skin perfusion by capillary refill and distal pulses. Monitoring fluid intake and output following surgery is critical. A sudden sustained increase in pulse and respirations and a de-crease in peripheral perfusion may be early signs of hemorrhage. Signs of respiratory distress may indicate the development of a pneumothorax or CHF.

Psychosocial Assessment

Assess the parents' need for information and emotional support. In many cases, the infant's condition is first identified at birth; however, a defect could have been identified prenatally by sonogram. The parents will be grieving the loss of a perfect newborn and be extremely anxious about the infant's condition and prognosis.

Examples of nursing diagnoses that may apply to a child with decreased pulmonary blood flow include:

- Decreased Cardiac Output related to ventricular restriction and an obstructed outflow tract
- Risk for Infection related to unfiltered bacteria in the blood and sites of blood shunting that promote bacterial growth
- Ineffective Family Therapeutic Regimen Management related to complexity of therapeutic regimen: assessment and management of unpredictable hypercyanotic spells
- Activity Intolerance related to cyanosis and dyspnea on exertion
- Delayed Growth and Development related to congenital anomaly and hypoxemia

Planning and Implementation

Home Care of the Child Before Surgery

Infants with tetralogy of Fallot and other serious defects are often managed at home to grow and potentially improve surgical outcome. Parents are usually anxious during the wait for surgery. They may fear that the infant will not survive until surgery or that they

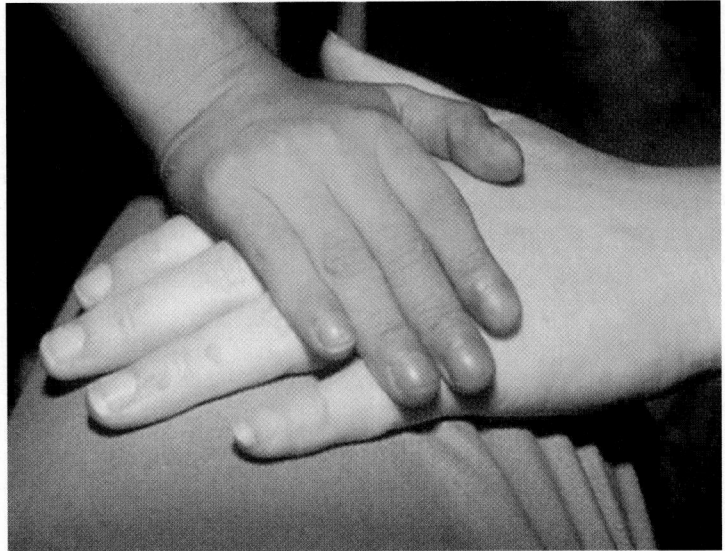
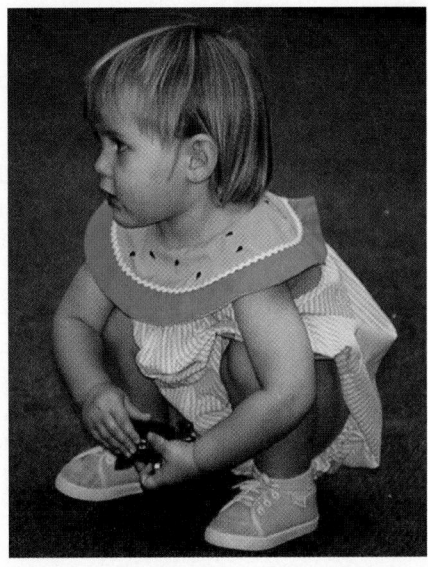

FIGURE 21–7 ➤ A, Clubbing of the fingers in an older child is one manifestation of a heart defect that reduces pulmonary blood flow. B, A young child with an uncorrected or partially corrected defect that reduces pulmonary blood flow may squat (assumes a knee–chest position) to reduce systemic blood flow return to the heart.

will be unable to manage any problems the infant may have. Provide information and teach parents how to care for the infant at home. Arrange for home health care nursing and other community services that may be required. Many of these children require supplemental nutrition and oxygen for emergencies. Because unoxygenated and oxygenated blood mix, supplemental oxygen does not improve the child's usual oxygen saturation (SpO_2) level.

Promoting Development Cyanosis with or without CHF often results in delayed gross motor skills. Make referrals to community-based early intervention programs to help parents learn about realistic developmental goals and to promote the child's development. Encourage parents to treat the infant as normally as possible. Children with mild cyanotic lesions do not need to adjust activity. The child with moderate to severe disease should be able to tolerate crying for a few minutes without difficulty. Comfort the infant when crying is prolonged, because it causes fatigue and further hypoxia.

Caring for a Hypercyanotic Episode Hypercyanotic episodes become life threatening if not treated immediately. The child becomes progressively more hypoxic and limp, loses consciousness, is likely to have a seizure or cerebrovascular accident, and may die. Teach parents to observe for signs of

worsening cyanosis, particularly in the morning, that could signal the beginning of a hypercyanotic episode. Some families use a pulse oximeter daily; they need to know the child's typical SpO_2 and what change may indicate an emergency.

Provide guidelines for the initial care of the hypercyanotic episode. The parents should call for an ambulance and try to calm and reassure the infant. The infant should be placed in knee–chest position with the parent holding the infant facing the chest, placing one arm under the knees, and folding the legs upward toward the infant's chest. Use the other arm to support the infant's back. Alternately, the infant can be placed supine with knees bent up to the chest. If oxygen is available, provide it in a manner that does not further upset the infant. If none is available in the home, it will be administered in the ambulance during transport to the emergency department.

Preventing Serious Illnesses Teach parents to report signs of illness to the physician. Vomiting and diarrhea may lead to dehydration, which is a particular risk in children with polycythemia because the blood can become even more viscous. Fever increases the metabolic rate and causes further stress on the heart. Aggressive management with antipyretic medication and fluid volume replacement is sometimes necessary.

Signs of infective endocarditis (low-grade fever, fatigue, and malaise) occurring within 2 months of surgery or a high-risk procedure should be reported. Parents should be taught about the need to request antibiotic prophylaxis for the child.

Although parents may travel with cyanotic children, they should talk with the physician before taking them to areas of high altitude. Supplemental oxygen when traveling on an airplane may be necessary.

Hospital-Based Care of the Infant and Child

If a hypercyanotic episode occurs in an infant or toddler prior to surgery, immediately place the child in the knee–chest position

---

Clinical Tip

Develop an emergency plan for the infant in anticipation of acute problems such as a hypercyanotic episode or respiratory distress. The parents should learn cardiopulmonary resuscitation. Provide the parents with a card or brief history form with information about the child's condition, medications, necessary emergency care, and the physician's name so emergency care providers have vital information for medical care.

and administer oxygen. Administer morphine as ordered. Immediately notify the physician. Ask for further orders if these procedures are ineffective and the episode continues. Avoid any unpleasant or anxiety-provoking procedures.

Following surgery, the child is initially cared for in the intensive care unit until heart function has stabilized. Once the child returns to the general nursing unit, nursing care is the same as described for the child having surgery for increased pulmonary blood flow. See page 611.

Community-Based Care After Surgery

Adolescents need to be supported as they transition to assuming responsibility for their own care. Practice guidelines now recommend coordinated care of adults with complex CHD through regional centers with expertise in the care of these adults (Warnes, Williams, Bashore, et al., 2008).

 Health Promotion

Adolescents with congenital heart defects need annual preventive care and health education. Provide all recommended immunizations. Provide information about the adolescent's specific defect, prior procedures and surgeries, medications, and any signs or symptoms of the condition that need immediate attention. Be sure to include general health education needed by all adolescents including exercise, weight management, pregnancy prevention, as well as the risks for tobacco, alcohol, other substances of abuse, and unprotected sexual activity.

Evaluation

Examples of expected nursing care outcomes include the following:

- The parents recognize a hypercyanotic episode and initiate appropriate emergency treatment.
- The parents manage fever and medical illnesses to prevent dehydration and thromboembolism.
- The child becomes stable following surgery and has no complications.
- The child attains expected development following surgical repair of the congenital heart defect.

Defects Obstructing Systemic Blood Flow

Etiology and Pathophysiology

An anatomic stenosis (narrowing of a valve, of the area around the valve, or in the great artery above the valve) causes obstruction to blood flow, resulting in a pressure load on the left ventricle and decreased cardiac output. The greater the narrowing, the more obstructed blood flow is to the circulation. Neonates with severe left outflow obstruction or left ventricular dysfunction may develop decreased cardiac output and shock.

Clinical Manifestations

Low cardiac output is responsible for the following clinical manifestations: diminished pulses, poor color, delayed capillary refill time, and decreased urinary output. The blood cannot move past the obstruction, so it backs up into the left

atrium and then the lungs, causing congestive heart failure and pulmonary edema. In children with mild obstruction, the child may have leg cramps, cooler feet than hands, and stronger pulses and higher blood pressure in the upper extremities than the lower extremities. Decreased blood supply to the gastrointestinal tract may lead to necrotizing enterocolitis. See Chapter 25 ∞. See Table 21–7 for the pathophysiology, clinical manifestations, and clinical therapy for the congenital heart defects that obstruct systemic blood flow.

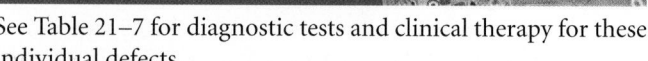 **Clinical Tip**

The blood pressure reading is usually 10 to 15 mmHg higher in the legs than in the arms unless the child has a coarctation of the aorta, a defect that obstructs systemic blood flow.

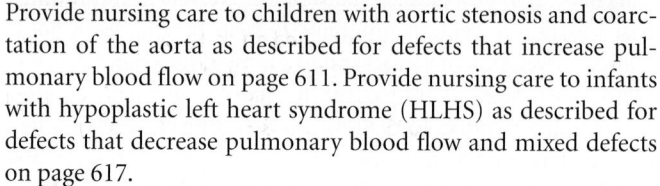 **COLLABORATIVE CARE**

See Table 21–7 for diagnostic tests and clinical therapy for these individual defects.

Neonates with severe systemic outflow obstruction or left ventricular dysfunction may develop decreased cardiac output and shock. PGE_1 and inotrope medications may be required to support the systemic circulation until the obstruction is relieved or ventricular function improves.

NURSING MANAGEMENT

Provide nursing care to children with aortic stenosis and coarctation of the aorta as described for defects that increase pulmonary blood flow on page 611. Provide nursing care to infants with hypoplastic left heart syndrome (HLHS) as described for defects that decrease pulmonary blood flow and mixed defects on page 617.

Parents of children with life-threatening defects such as HLHS must make decisions very quickly about the best treatment for their child. There is no cure, and a decision must be made that is best for their individual situation (Norwood or Sano procedure, heart and lung transplant, or palliative care). Parents are faced with the potential death of the newborn before having an opportunity to grieve the loss of a normal infant. Nurses play an important role in supporting parents through this difficult decision-making period. Ensure that parents are fully informed about each treatment option and the associated mortality, the intense care needed by the surviving infant, potential neurocognitive and neurodevelopmental outcomes, and unknown long-term survival. If parents choose comfort or palliative care, interventions such as PGE_1 are discontinued and the infant is given appropriate pain medication and comfort. Seek the support of clergy, social workers, or other supportive individuals in the family's life to assist them through this period. Reassure parents that they are good parents, no matter what decision they make. See Chapter 13 ∞.

Defect Pathophysiology, Clinical Manifestations, and Clinical Therapy   Anatomy

Aortic Stenosis (AS)

Narrowing of the aortic valve obstructs blood flow to systemic circulation. The valve often has two valve leaflets (bicuspid) rather than three. The pressure gradient across the valve usually increases as the child grows and cardiac output increases. Aortic stenosis accounts for up to 10% of congenital heart defects (Park, 2008).

Clinical Manifestations

Most infants and children are asymptomatic with normal growth and development. Life-threatening aortic stenosis is detected in some newborns. CHF develops in infants with significant stenosis.

The blood pressure is normal, but a narrow pulse pressure may be noted. Peripheral pulses may be weak. The child may complain of chest pain after exercise, but exercise intolerance is uncommon. Syncope and dizziness are serious signs that require intervention.

A systolic heart murmur and thrill occur in the aortic or pulmonic areas with transmission to the neck. An ejection click may be heard. Splitting of the S_2 may be noted with severe aortic stenosis. Interventions may result in aortic insufficiency, causing a high-pitched diastolic decrescendo murmur along the left sternal border near the mitral area.

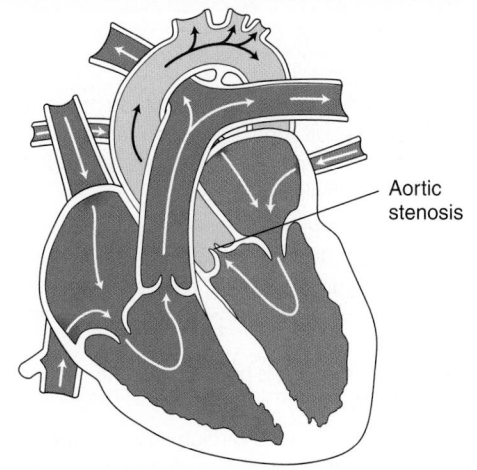

Aortic stenosis

☐ Decreased oxygenated blood flow

Diagnostic Procedures

The chest radiograph is usually normal, but may reveal a slight prominence of the left ventricle and aorta with increased severity.
The ECG is usually normal in mild cases, but may show mild left ventricular hypertrophy and inverted T waves with increased severity.
An echocardiogram reveals the number of the valve cusps, pressure gradient across valve, and size of the aorta.
Exercise testing may be used in asymptomatic children to determine the amount of obstruction present with exercise.

Clinical Therapy

Newborns with life-threatening aortic stenosis need PGE_1 to maintain a patent ductus arteriosus until the aortic valve can be dilated. Treatment involves balloon dilation during cardiac catheterization or surgical valvotomy. Surgical treatment is palliative rather than curative. Aortic valve replacement (Ross procedure) is performed when stenosis is severe or if significant regurgitation results from other interventions.
Prognosis: Chest pain, syncope, and sudden death can occur in children with severe AS. Stenosis may recur following intervention, and may worsen as the valve calcifies. Valve replacement may be necessary once the child reaches adulthood, often requiring lifelong anticoagulant therapy. Lifelong infective endocarditis prophylaxis is required.

Coarctation of the Aorta (COA)

Narrowing or constriction in the descending aorta, often near the ductus arteriosus or left subclavian artery, obstructs the systemic blood outflow. COA occurs in 8–10% of children with congenital heart disease and is common in girls with Turner syndrome (Park, 2008; Schneider & Goldmuntz, 2006).

Clinical Manifestations

Many children are asymptomatic and grow normally. Infants with severe constriction may have cyanosis in the lower extremities, heart failure, and shock as the ductus arteriosus closes. Renal failure and necrotizing enterocolitis may develop. Infants with moderate constriction may have poor feeding, failure to thrive, increased respiratory effort, and CHF.

Blood pressure in legs is lower than in the arms. Brachial and radial pulses are typically bounding, but femoral pulses are weak or absent.
Older children may complain of weakness and pain in the legs after exercise.
S_2 is loud and single on auscultation. A systolic ejection murmur may be heard at the upper right and middle or lower left sternal border. A thrill may be palpated in the suprasternal notch.

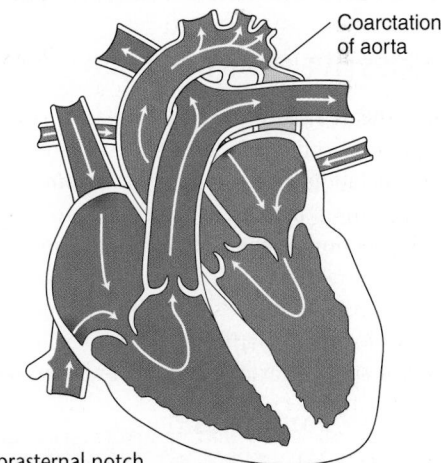

Coarctation of aorta

Diagnostic Procedures

The chest radiograph may reveal cardiomegaly, pulmonary venous congestion, and indentation of the descending aorta. Rib notching is rarely seen before 10 years of age. CT scan and MRI show the site of coarctation.
ECG shows left ventricular hypertrophy; right ventricular hypertrophy may be seen in severe cases.
Echocardiogram shows the size of the aorta, the actual coarctation, and the function of the aortic valve and left ventricle.

Clinical Therapy

In symptomatic newborns, PGE_1 is given to reopen the ductus arteriosus and promote blood flow to the lower extremities. Treatment to prevent CHF may be initiated with **inotropic medications** (a drug that increases myocardial contractility), diuretics, and oxygen (Park, 2008). Surgical resection is often preferred initially rather than balloon dilation to reduce the risk for recoarctation. Balloon dilation may be performed for recoarctation (Park, 2008). Balloon dilation and surgical resection are palliative, as coarctation may recur with either procedure.
Prognosis: Chronic systemic hypertension is more likely to occur in children older than 1 year at the time of repair (Marino, Ostrow, & Cohen, 2006).

(continued)

TABLE 21–7	Pathophysiology, Clinical Manifestations, and Clinical Therapy for Defects That Obstruct the Systemic Blood Flow *(continued)*

Defect Pathophysiology, Clinical Manifestations, and Clinical Therapy	Anatomy

Hypoplastic Left Heart Syndrome (HLHS)

The mitral and aortic valves are absent or stenosed along with an abnormally small left ventricle and small aorta. It accounts for about 1% of congenital heart defects and 9% of defects in critically ill newborns. Up to 29% of infants with this defect have a brain abnormality (Park, 2008).

Clinical Manifestations

With closure of the ductus arteriosus the newborn has progressive cyanosis, tachycardia, tachypnea, dyspnea, retractions, and decreased peripheral pulses. Poor peripheral perfusion, pulmonary edema, and CHF lead to shock, acidosis, and sometimes death.
A single loud heart sound is present, and often no murmur is present.

Diagnostic Procedures

The chest radiograph shows cardiomegaly and increased pulmonary vascularity. The echocardiogram shows the small left ventricle. This condition may be diagnosed prenatally.

Clinical Therapy

Prostaglandin E$_1$ is given to maintain a patent ductus arteriosus.
Supplemental oxygen is avoided.
Three treatment options include the Norwood and Sano procedures, heart transplantation (see page 629), and comfort or palliative care.
The Norwood procedure is performed in the first week of life, followed by the Glenn procedure at about 3 to 8 months of age, and the Fontan procedure between 18 months and 3 years of age (Khairy, Poirer, & Mercier, 2007).
Heart transplantation outcomes are not as good as with the Norwood. Few infant hearts are available for transplantation. Each heart transplant is likely to last 10 to 15 years (Kon, 2005).
Prognosis: Improved surgical management has resulted in increased survival of infants with HLHS, up to 85% for the first two stages of surgery (Cook & Higgins, 2010). The single ventricle causes physical activity limitations and fails over time. A heart transplant may be required during adolescence or adulthood. Many children have significant neurocognitive and neurodevelopmental impairment regardless of surgical intervention (Mahle, Visconti, Freier, et al., 2006). Arrhythmias and thromboemboli are other potential complications (Khairy et al., 2007).

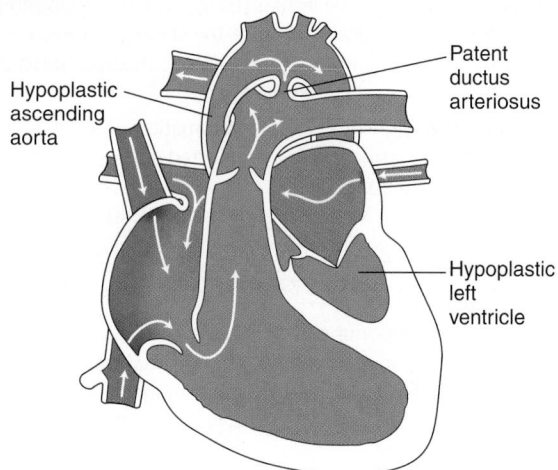

Mixed oxygenated and unoxygenated blood

■ CONGESTIVE HEART FAILURE

Congestive heart failure (CHF) is a disorder of circulation in which cardiac output is inadequate to support the body's circulatory and metabolic needs. It may result from a congenital heart defect that causes increased blood flow to the lungs or obstructed blood flow to the systemic circulation, from problems with heart contractility, or from pathologic conditions that require high cardiac output, such as severe anemia, acidosis, or respiratory disease. In addition, CHF results from acquired heart disease such as cardiomyopathy or Kawasaki disease.

Etiology and Pathophysiology

Blood volume overloads associated with CHDs are the most common cause of CHF in infants. Up to 90% of infants who develop CHF do so within the first 6 to 12 months of life (Connor, 2006). Some defects allow blood to flow from the left side of the heart to the right so that extra blood must be pumped to the pulmonary system rather than through the aorta when the left ventricle contracts. This overloads the pulmonary system, and if prolonged can lead to pulmonary hypertension (see page 630). Obstructive congenital defects (i.e., abnormally small pulmonary vessels) restrict the flow of blood so the heart muscle hypertrophies to work harder and force blood through these structures.

When cardiac output remains insufficient, the body's organs and tissues do not receive adequate oxygen. A sympathetic nervous system response increases the heart rate, heart muscle contractility, and peripheral vascular resistance. The kidneys respond to the lowered circulating volume by activating the renin-angiotensin mechanism to retain salt and water. The heart muscle fibers stretch to accommodate the increased blood volume, and the myocardium hypertrophies to manage the increased ventricular pressure. These responses increase cardiac output to the vital organs. The compensatory mechanisms increase their intensity and further compromise the heart. Progressive systemic edema and pulmonary congestion occur, leading to right- or left-sided heart failure, and eventually bilateral failure.

Complementary Therapy
Dangerous Medication Interactions

Caution parents of children with CHDs treated with anticoagulants, digoxin, or diuretics to avoid using herbal products because of potential interaction with prescribed medications. Ginkgo and ginseng increase the effect of anticoagulants, while St. John's wort interacts with warfarin to decrease the drug level. Ginseng may interact with furosemide and cause drug resistance. St. John's wort interacts with digoxin and decreases the drug level (Holcomb, 2009).

Clinical Manifestations
Congestive Heart Failure

Cause	Clinical Manifestation
Pulmonary venous congestion	Tachypnea, wheezing, crackles, retractions, cough, grunting, nasal flaring, tiring with feeding and play, irritability
Systemic venous congestion	Hepatomegaly, ascites, peripheral edema, fluid retention Jugular venous distention and dependent edema in older children
Impaired cardiac output	Tachycardia, weak pulses, hypotension, capillary refill time greater than 2 seconds, pallor, cool extremities, oliguria
High metabolic rate	Failure to thrive or slow weight gain, diaphoresis

Clinical Manifestations

Initial signs of CHF may be subtle and not immediately recognized. The infant tires easily, especially during feeding. Weight loss or lack of normal weight gain, diaphoresis, irritability, and frequent infections may be evident. Older children may have exercise intolerance, dyspnea, abdominal pain or distention, and peripheral edema.

As the disease progresses, symptoms such as tachypnea, tachycardia, pallor or cyanosis, nasal flaring, grunting, retractions, cough, or crackles may occur. A third heart sound may be auscultated. Generalized fluid volume overload is seen more commonly in toddlers and older children. Periorbital and facial edema and hepatomegaly are signs of fluid volume excess. Jugular vein distention is seen in older children. See Clinical Manifestations: Congestive Heart Failure.

Cardiomegaly, enlargement of the heart by hypertrophy of its walls, occurs as the heart attempts to maintain cardiac output. Cyanosis, weak peripheral pulses, cool extremities, hypotension, and heart murmur are precursors of cardiogenic shock, which can occur if CHF is not adequately treated. (Cardiogenic shock is discussed on page 640.)

COLLABORATIVE CARE

Diagnostic Tests
Diagnosis is based primarily on clinical manifestations such as tachycardia, respiratory distress, and crackles. A chest radiograph study reveals cardiac enlargement and venous congestion or signs of pulmonary edema. Echocardiography may be performed to diagnose specific cardiac defects or dysfunction. An electrocardiogram may show tachycardia, bradycardia, or ventricular hypertrophy. Electrolytes, lactic acid, arterial blood gases, and a complete blood count are obtained.

Clinical Therapy
The goals of medical management are to make the heart work more efficiently and to remove excess fluid. This decreases the heart's work and improves systemic circulation without flooding the pulmonary system. Diuretics, such as furosemide, bumetanide, chlorothiazide, and spironolactone, are given to promote fluid excretion. Inotropic medicines and afterload-reducing agents (angiotensin-converting enzyme inhibitors) are sometimes prescribed to lessen the heart's workload and help it to work more efficiently.

Digoxin is the drug most commonly used to improve the heart's ability to contract and therefore increase its output. Occasionally a higher-than-normal dose is given initially, followed by a lower maintenance dose. This process, called **digitalization**, helps the child achieve therapeutic blood levels more quickly. Beta-blockers, such as propranolol and carvedilol, are being evaluated for safety and effectiveness for children with CHF (Menteer, Hogarty, & Chrisant, 2006). See Medications Used to Treat Congestive Heart Failure.

Nursing Alert

Digoxin and digitoxin are both digitalis preparations, but they are not the same drug. Digoxin is the drug of choice in pediatrics. Digitoxin is 10 times more powerful than digoxin, and is rarely used in children. Read labels carefully and double-check doses to ensure that you give the child the right dose of the right drug.

Surgery or interventional cardiac catheterization to correct a congenital heart defect may become the treatment of choice. Cardiac transplantation may be performed for children with end-stage cardiomyopathy or a complex CHD, such as hypoplastic left heart syndrome.

Other medical therapy is supportive. Airway management, ventilatory support, rest, and fluid and dietary management are also part of the treatment plan. Oxygen may be ordered (Figure 21–8 ➤). Most children improve rapidly after medication is administered.

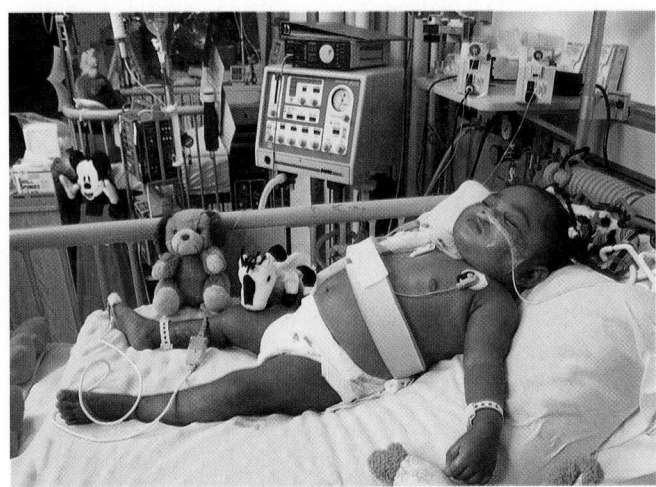

FIGURE 21–8 ➤ This infant is receiving intravenous fluids and oxygen. Her condition is being continuously monitored for congestive heart failure.

Medications Used to Treat
Congestive Heart Failure

Medications and Actions	Nursing Management
Digoxin (Lanoxin) Increases myocardial contractility by improving systemic circulation.	Assess the heart rate for bradycardia for 1 minute prior to giving a dose (see page 625) or for changes in heart rhythm or quality. Monitor the child for digitoxicity. See page 627 for more nursing management.
Furosemide (Lasix) Rapid diuresis; blocks reabsorption of sodium and water in renal tubules; potassium depletion.	Monitor patients during rapid diuresis for vital signs, intake and output, and fluid and electrolyte imbalances.
Thiazides (Diuril) Chlorothiazide (suspension) Hydrochlorothiazide (tablets) Maintenance diuresis, decreases absorption of sodium, water, potassium, chloride, and bicarbonate in renal tubules.	Monitor blood pressure and intake and output rates and patterns. Monitor lab values for hypokalemia. Assess for digitoxicity if hypokalemia is present.
Spironolactone (Aldactone) Maintenance diuresis (potassium-sparing).	Assess for signs of fluid and electrolyte imbalance, and digitoxicity.
ACE (angiotensin-converting enzyme) inhibitor (e.g., captopril, enalapril) Promotes vascular relaxation and reduced peripheral vascular resistance.	Assess for common side effects such as cough, hyperkalemia, and worsening renal function.
Propranolol (Inderal) Increases contractility.	Monitor vital signs and peripheral perfusion. Monitor intake and output ratio and daily weight. Dietary sodium is usually restricted.
Carvedilol (Coreg) Improves left ventricular function, promotes vasodilation of systemic circulation for chronic heart failure and dilated cardiomyopathy.	Monitor for signs of CHF improvement. Monitor for dizziness and hypotension. Monitor digoxin levels as drug may increase plasma digoxin concentration. Monitor liver function periodically.

Data from: Bindler, R. M., Howry, L. B., Wilson, B. A., Shannon, M. T., & Stang, C. L. (2005). Pediatric drug guide. Upper Saddle River, NJ: Prentice Hall; Wilson, B. A., Shannon, M. T., & Shields, K. M. (2009). Nurses' drug guide 2009. Upper Saddle River, NJ: Prentice Hall.

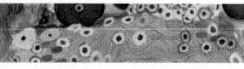

NURSING MANAGEMENT

Nursing Assessment and Diagnosis

As diagnosis of CHF depends primarily on physical symptoms, nursing observations are important. Psychosocial assessment is important in learning how the family is coping with the demands and stresses of the child's condition.

Physiologic Assessment

Assess the child's vital signs, behavioral patterns (e.g., playfulness, irritability), cardiac function, respiratory function, and fluid status using the Assessment Guidelines on page 604. Use the age-specific heart and respiratory rates in Chapter 5 ∞ to identify tachycardia and tachypnea (see pages 138 and 141). Obtain a detailed history of the onset of symptoms from the parents, as CHF often develops slowly.

Clinical Judgment

What changes in vital signs, behavior, and fluid status would indicate that an infant's or child's CHF is progressing in severity?

Measure intake and output carefully. Weigh the infant's diapers before and after changing to measure urine output (1 g = 1 mL urine). Observe for changes in peripheral edema and circulation. Weigh the child daily at the same time. If ascites is present, take serial abdominal measurements to monitor changes. See the *Clinical Skills Manual.* Turn the child frequently, and provide skin care when edema is present.

Psychosocial Assessment

Review the child's previous hospitalizations, and assess the family's knowledge about the child's condition. Families of children with CHF are anxious and fear the potentially serious outcome of the problem and the need to provide ongoing care. Assess the family's anxiety level and coping strategies. Evaluate the family's economic status. Medication is crucial to treatment, and a family's inability to afford or obtain the necessary medications jeopardizes the child's survival. Determine if another family member is available who could assist parents or provide respite care.

Developmental Assessment

Since fatigue limits the activities of the child with CHF, the child does not have the opportunity to practice the skills needed to attain normal developmental milestones. Assess development with a tool such as the Denver II (see Chapter 7 ∞), and ask parents when the child attained expected developmental milestones such as sitting, manipulating objects, standing, or walking. Ask parents about contact and play with other children and a typical day's activity schedule. Parents may limit the child's contact with other children because of frequent infections and exercise intolerance. When CHF is well controlled, the child's energy level increases and developmental skills often improve. In infants and toddlers, assessments every 2 to 3 months are useful to observe development and evaluate disease management.

Several nursing diagnoses that may apply to the child with CHF can be found in the accompanying Nursing Care Plan: The Child Hospitalized with Congestive Heart Failure. The primary nursing diagnosis is Decreased Cardiac Output related to cardiac anomaly.

Planning and Implementation

Nursing care for the child with CHF focuses on administering and monitoring effects of medications, maintaining adequate oxygenation and myocardial function, promoting rest, fostering development, providing adequate nutrition, and providing emotional support to the child and family.

Administer and Monitor Prescribed Medications

Children with CHF usually receive digoxin and furosemide. These medications are potent and must be correctly administered. Observe the child carefully for digoxin toxicity. Early signs include cardiac arrhythmias in children. Early indicators in adults (nausea, vomiting, anorexia, diarrhea, visual disturbance) are rarely the initial signs of toxicity in children. Obtain a serum digoxin level at least 6 hours after the daily dose. Monitor serum digoxin levels closely during antibiotic therapy as altered intestinal flora may precipitate digoxin toxicity.

Nursing Alert

Before giving the digitalizing dose of digoxin, establish baseline vital signs, the quality of peripheral pulses, and clinical symptoms, and also obtain an ECG. Check serum electrolytes, and hepatic and renal function. Assess hydration status, and hydrate if hypovolemic.

Before giving any dose of digoxin, take the apical pulse for 1 minute. Call for a physician's advice *before* administering the digoxin in the following conditions:

■ The heart rate is less than 60 to 100 beats/min, depending upon age, or is higher or lower than the guideline noted in the physician's order.

■ Changes in heart rhythm or quality are noted.

Maintain Oxygenation and Myocardial Function

Oxygen therapy may be ordered. Make sure that tubing is patent, the oxygen flow rate is correct, the oxygen delivery device is working properly, and humidification is provided. Keep the child calm and quiet. Position the child in a semi-Fowler or 45-degree angle position to promote maximum oxygenation.

Promote Rest

Group assessments and interventions together to ensure that the child has some uninterrupted rest each hour. Rocking is restful for infants. Encourage older children to engage in quiet activities such as playing board games or watching television.

Foster Development

Encourage parents to play with the child, using toys to stimulate eye–hand coordination and fine motor movements. Such toys include rattles, blocks, and stuffed animals for infants, and books, paper and pencil, and dolls for older children. Encourage sitting, standing, or walking for short periods with adequate rest afterward to promote the development of large muscles. Singing, talking, and playing music facilitate cognitive and language skills.

Provide Adequate Nutrition

Teach parents about feeding techniques. Encourage the mother who chooses to breastfeed the infant, as the antibodies in breast milk reduce infections and the milk is naturally low in sodium. However, the sucking involved in breastfeeding or bottle-feeding may cause dyspnea that forces the infant to rest frequently during feeding. Infants should be burped frequently to permit rest and prevent vomiting. In addition, they may need small frequent feedings and longer feeding periods. Make sure parents understand that changes in feeding habits (decreased intake, vomiting, sleeping through feedings, increased perspiration with feedings) may indicate deteriorating cardiac status.

Clinical Tip

Positioning the baby in an infant seat at a 45-degree angle decreases venous return to the heart and decreases its metabolic demand. This is a favorable position for feeding and interacting with the infant to promote development (Cook & Higgins, 2010).

The infant needs adequate nutrition to support growth. Some infants need a higher caloric formula (24 to 27 calories per ounce) to obtain adequate nutrition. It is not unusual for infants with heart problems to develop failure to thrive as the result of feeding difficulties (see Chapter 14 ∞). When infants have significant dyspnea with feeding, special feeding techniques are needed such as nutritional supplementation by nasogastric, transpyloric, or gastrostomy tube (see Figure 21–5). (See the *Clinical Skills Manual*.)

Parents are often advised to give the infant a chance to feed orally for a specific period (such as 20 to 30 minutes) that varies according to how much dyspnea the infant has with feeding. The remainder of the formula is then given by nasogastric or gastrostomy tube.

Provide Emotional Support

When a child is hospitalized with CHF, the family is often anxious about his or her condition. Give parents a chance to express their concerns. Explain the child's treatment regimen, and make sure family members understand the child's need for nutrition and rest. Refer parents to the appropriate support groups as talking with parents of children with cardiac conditions may be a source of emotional support.

NURSING CARE PLAN

The Child Hospitalized with Congestive Heart Failure

INTERVENTION	RATIONALE	EXPECTED OUTCOME
1. Nursing Diagnosis: Decreased Cardiac Output related to cardiac anomaly (VSD)		
NIC Priority Intervention: *Hemodynamic regulation:* Optimization of heart rate, preload, afterload, and contractility		**NOC Suggested Outcome:** *Cardiac pump effectiveness:* Extent to which blood is ejected from the left ventricle per minute to support systemic perfusion pressure
Goal: The child's cardiac output will be sufficient to meet the body's metabolic demands.		
▪ Administer digoxin as ordered.	▪ Digoxin increases contractility of the heart and force of contraction.	The child's cardiac output is sufficient as indicated by increased energy, adequate feeding intake, and decreased edema.
▪ Regularly count the apical pulse and listen to heart sounds, especially before each dose of digoxin. Record the apical pulse rate with each dose of digoxin.	▪ Digoxin may cause bradycardia. Pulse and heart sounds provide information about heart functioning.	
▪ Use a cardiac monitor if prescribed.	▪ The monitor notes bradycardia and arrhythmias.	
▪ Monitor serum potassium level and for digitoxicity.	▪ Hypokalemia increases risk of digoxin toxicity.	The child maintains normal serum potassium levels and therapeutic levels of digoxin.
▪ Provide for rest periods each hour.	▪ Rest decreases the need for high cardiac output.	The child rests hourly and has adequate energy to eat and play.
Goal: The child will manifest adequate oxygenation.		
▪ Evaluate respiratory rate and breath sounds. Use pulse oximetry to determine oxygen saturation readings.	▪ This provides information about oxygenation and ease of respiration.	The child maintains a normal SpO_2 level and respiratory rate for age without evidence of adventitious sounds or diaphoresis.
▪ Provide oxygen and humidification if prescribed. Observe for diaphoresis, a sign of increased respiratory effort.	▪ Supplemental oxygen decreases tachypnea, and humidification moistens secretions to keep the airway clear.	
▪ Place the child in a semi-Fowler position.	▪ This position facilitates lung expansion.	
2. Nursing Diagnosis: Excess Fluid Volume related to heart failure		
NIC Priority Intervention: *Fluid management:* Promotion of fluid balance and prevention of complications resulting from abnormal or undesired fluid levels		**NOC Suggested Outcome:** *Fluid balance:* Balance of water in the intracellular and extracellular compartments of the body
Goal: The child's peripheral and central edema will decrease. Intake and output will be balanced once excess fluid is excreted.		
▪ Administer diuretics as ordered.	▪ Diuretics mobilize fluids and facilitate excretion.	The child's intake and output are proportional, and electrolyte levels remain within normal ranges.
▪ Measure intake and output carefully. Weigh diapers to assess output of infants. Weigh daily. Measure abdominal girth daily. Observe for peripheral edema.	▪ Adequate output is a good indicator of renal perfusion. Assessments demonstrate effectiveness of treatment.	
▪ Monitor electrolytes.	▪ Electrolyte imbalance is common when diuretics are given.	
Goal: The child's peripheral and central edema will decrease.		
▪ Change the child's position frequently.	▪ Position changes promote circulation to skin over pressure points.	The child has no skin breakdown after edema resolves.
▪ Inspect skin frequently for redness and skin breakdown over pressure points.	▪ Inspection identifies earliest stages of skin breakdown.	

NURSING CARE PLAN

The Child Hospitalized with Congestive Heart Failure (continued)

INTERVENTION	RATIONALE	EXPECTED OUTCOME
3. Nursing Diagnosis: Imbalanced Nutrition: Less than Body Requirements related to high metabolic needs and rapid tiring while feeding		
NIC Priority Intervention: *Nutrition management:* Assistance with or provision of a balanced dietary intake of food and fluids		**NOC Suggested Outcome:** *Nutrition status:* Extent to which nutrients are available to meet metabolic needs
■ Hold the infant at a 45-degree angle for feeding.	■ This position facilitates breathing while eating.	The infant or child gains recommended weight according to growth grids. All dietary requirements are met, and mealtimes are pleasant.
■ Record intake carefully.	■ Evaluation of intake indicates whether caloric and other nutritional needs are met.	
■ Weigh the child daily.	■ Weight indicates growth (in absence of fluid retention).	
■ Give frequent small meals with rest periods in between.	■ Digesting small meals requires less energy.	
■ Use high-calorie formula or give high-calorie snacks.	■ High-calorie formulas and snacks provide calories efficiently.	
■ Use soothing approaches such as holding infants for feeding and having parents eat with the older child.	■ A restful approach facilitates intake with minimum cardiac work.	
■ Transition to supplemental tube feedings if the infant is not able to gain weight.	■ Tube feedings provide added calories without taxing the infant's energy.	

Discharge Planning and Home Care Teaching

Identify and address home care needs well in advance of discharge. Show parents how to feed the child to maximize nutritional intake. While the child is hospitalized, teach the family about the signs of a worsening condition (e.g., increased feeding difficulty, irritability, lethargy, breathing difficulty, and puffiness around the eyes or extremities). Parents are frequently taught to take the child's pulse and to report any significant change to the physician. An increase in pulse rate can signal CHF, and a decrease can indicate digoxin toxicity. Teach parents to identify signs of dehydration when the child is managed on diuretics. An acute illness could lead to dehydration more quickly when the child takes these medications.

Demonstrate administration of drugs, and then supervise while the parents measure and administer medications. Teach parents about the toxic effects of digoxin and other drugs. Advise them to notify the physician immediately if any of these side effects occur. (See Families Want to Know: Administering Digoxin.)

Arrange for home care nursing visits to reinforce the education provided, to monitor the child's condition, and to assess the family's ability to manage the child's care. Ensure that the family has a phone contact for emergency assistance.

Care in the Community

Parents play a critical role in the care of the child with heart disease by facilitating normal development and limiting the incidence of CHF. See Nursing Care Plan: The Child with Congestive Heart Failure Being Cared for at Home.

Families Want to Know

Administering Digoxin

■ Take the child's pulse prior to giving digoxin. Report to the physician when the pulse rate falls below or rises above guidelines provided.

■ Administer the medication exactly as prescribed at the same time each day. The parents should decide if the medication will be given with food or without food, and be consistent in giving it the same way each day.

■ Do not repeat the digoxin dose if the child vomits unless directed to do so by the physician.

■ Do not give the child over-the-counter medications for colds, coughs, allergies, gastrointestinal upset, or obesity without approval.

■ Do not give the child on digoxin herbal preparations such as ginseng, ma huang, or ephedra. They interact with digoxin and may cause digoxin toxicity or arrhythmias.

■ Keep the medication locked and out of reach of children. In case of accidental ingestion, immediate medical care is needed. Be sure to keep the Poison Control Center number on all phones.

■ Remind the child's health care providers about the potential interaction between digoxin and certain antibiotics (e.g., tetracycline, erythromycin, rifampin, neomycin) so that safe antibiotics can be prescribed when needed (Park, 2008, p. 471).

Evaluation

Expected outcomes of nursing care can be found in the Nursing Care Plans on pages 626–627 and 628–629.

NURSING CARE PLAN

The Child with Congestive Heart Failure Being Cared for at Home

INTERVENTION	RATIONALE	EXPECTED OUTCOME
1. Nursing Diagnosis: Delayed Growth and Development related to effects of physical disability		
NIC Priority Intervention: *Developmental enhancement:* Teaching parents to facilitate optimal gross motor, fine motor, language, cognitive, social, and emotional growth of preschool children		**NOC Suggested Outcome:** *Child development (2 years):* Milestones of physical, cognitive, and psychosocial progression by 2 years of age
Goal: The child will meet developmental milestones for age group.		
■ Perform baseline developmental assessment.	■ Assessment provides comparison for later assessments and a basis for planning specific games, toys, and activities.	The child displays normal language, fine motor, and gross motor activity.
■ Plan for short play periods after rest.	■ Short play periods maintain energy and facilitate play.	
■ Introduce age-appropriate toys and activities such as rattles and blocks for infants and art projects for older children.	■ Play activities facilitate learning and mastery of developmental tasks.	
■ Plan for interactions with healthy children.	■ Social skills are learned through contact with others.	
2. Nursing Diagnosis: Ineffective Therapeutic Regimen Management related to complexity of therapeutic regimen		
NIC Priority Intervention: *Mutual goal setting:* Collaborating with the family to identify and prioritize care goals, and then developing a plan for achieving those goals		**NOC Suggested Outcome:** *Compliance behavior:* Actions taken on the basis of professional advice to promote wellness, recovery, and rehabilitation
Goal: Parents will demonstrate correct administration of medications.		
■ Have parents prepare the medication dosages and administer the digoxin, diuretics, and other medications to the child under the supervision of the home health nurse.	■ Demonstrating techniques used to administer medications provides opportunities to identify dosage errors and to suggest methods to help ensure the child gets all needed medications.	Parents report that the child continues to demonstrate improvement and adequate cardiac output without signs of congestive heart failure.
Goal: Parents will state side effects of medications and symptoms of congestive heart failure.		
■ Describe side effects of medications. Give parents handouts with the telephone number to call to ask questions or report side effects.	■ If side effects are understood, serious complications can be avoided.	
■ Describe subtle onset of CHF and its symptoms (increasing weakness, exhaustion, irritability, difficulty feeding, cough or difficult respirations, edema).	■ Parents can evaluate the child regularly and note subtle changes requiring medical management.	
3. Nursing Diagnosis: Imbalanced Nutrition: Less than Body Requirements related to chronic illness and tiring while feeding		
NIC Priority Intervention: *Weight gain assistance:* Facilitation of body weight gain		**NOC Suggested Outcome:** *Nutritional status: Food and fluid intake:* Amount of food and fluid taken into the body over a 24-hour period
Goal: The infant or child will demonstrate normal weight gain for age.		
■ Teach parents methods to promote food intake related to positioning, size of feedings, and food choices.	■ Positioning, frequency of feedings, size of feedings, and use of high-caloric foods can enhance nutritional intake.	The infant or child shows normal weight gain.
■ Observe feeding during a home visit.	■ Feedback can assist parents in integrating positive feeding techniques.	Parents report and demonstrate successful feedings of child.

NURSING CARE PLAN

The Child with Congestive Heart Failure Being Cared for at Home (continued)

INTERVENTION	RATIONALE	EXPECTED OUTCOME
4. Nursing Diagnosis: Activity Intolerance (Child) related to poor cardiac output		
NIC Priority Intervention: *Energy management:* Regulating energy use to treat or prevent fatigue and optimize function		**NOC Suggested Outcome:** *Energy conservation:* Extent of active management of energy to initiate or sustain activity
Goal: The child will perform all necessary activities of daily living without undue tiring.		
▪ Help parents alternate activities and rest throughout the child's day.	▪ Activities to promote development must be alternated with rest due to decreased cardiac output.	The child performs necessary activities and rests frequently each day.
▪ Have parents limit the child's exposure to persons with contagious disease.	▪ When the child is ill and tired, the immune system can be compromised.	
▪ Help the family plan quiet surroundings to provide for the child's rest.	▪ The home setting may need to be altered to promote rest.	
5. Nursing Diagnosis: Caregiver Role Strain (Parent) related to 24-hour responsibility for child's care		
NIC Priority Intervention: *Caregiver support:* Provision of the necessary information, advocacy, and support to facilitate primary patient care by someone other than a health care professional		**NOC Suggested Outcome:** *Caregiver endurance potential:* Factors that promote family care provider continuance over an extended period of time
Goal: Parents will express the ability to meet their own needs.		
▪ Assess family and community supports. Provide information related to respite care.	▪ Variable family and community supports are available.	Parents report some time away from the child and report renewal in caring for the child.
▪ Encourage parents to seek activities to meet personal needs.	▪ Parents need time for their personal needs to successfully care for the child.	

■ CARDIOMYOPATHY

Cardiomyopathy is a serious disorder of the heart's muscle that affects the ventricular systolic function, diastolic function, or both (Towbin, Lowe, Colan, et al., 2006). The highest incidence of cardiomyopathy in the pediatric population occurs during the first year of life. Males have a higher incidence than females. Almost 40% of children with symptoms of cardiomyopathy die of the condition within 2 years or receive a heart transplant (Cox, Sleeper, Lowe, et al., 2006).

Dilated cardiomyopathy is the most common form, in which the four chambers dilate and systolic contraction is weakened. Myocarditis and neuromuscular disorders, such as muscular dystrophy, are the most common identified causes of this type of cardiomyopathy; however, 66% of cases have no known cause (Towbin et al., 2006). The child usually presents in CHF with tachypnea, wheezing, and poor cardiac output. Arrhythmias may develop that can cause cardiac arrest. Treatment involves diuretics, digoxin, an ACE inhibitor, antiarrhythmics, anticoagulants, and carvedilol or metoprolol. Ultimately a heart transplant may be considered.

In hypertrophic cardiomyopathy, the heart muscle is thickened and one or more chambers are small or normal in size. About 50% of hypertrophic cardiomyopathy cases are genetically transmitted

as an autosomal dominant trait (Park, 2008). Palpitations may occur because of atrial or ventricular arrhythmia. Symptoms include exertional dyspnea, fatigue, dizziness, fainting, and chest pain; sudden unexpected death may occur. Treatment involves beta-blockers, calcium channel blockers, and antiarrhythmics. A heart transplant may be considered. Sudden death may be associated with sports or vigorous exercise (Park, 2008).

NURSING MANAGEMENT

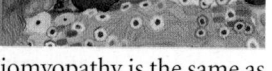

Nursing management for dilated cardiomyopathy is the same as for children with CHF unless or until a heart transplant is performed. Nursing management for hypertrophic cardiomyopathy involves frequent visits to assess the child's condition and to review progress with antiarrhythmic medications.

■ HEART TRANSPLANTATION

Approximately 260 heart transplants are performed in children each year for end-stage cardiomyopathy or complex CHDs with ventricular failure such as hypoplastic left heart syndrome (Sudan, Bacha, John, et al., 2007). Ventricular assist devices and extracorporeal membrane oxygenation (ECMO) use prior to and following transplantation improves the child's recovery from end-organ failure and enhances transplantation outcome (Blume, Naftel, Bastardi, et al., 2006). Up to 75% of children are surviving after 5 to 8 years (Morales, Dreyer, Denfield, et al., 2007).

Rejection is a major cause of mortality and morbidity. The immunosuppression regimen usually includes calcineurin inhibitors (cyclosporin or tacrolimus), azathioprine or mycophenolate mofetil, and corticosteroids. Signs of acute organ rejection in infants and children are often nonspecific. Tachycardia and irregular rhythm are associated with acute rejection. Endomyocardial biopsy is performed during cardiac catheterization, frequently during the first year after transplant to detect rejection and then annually if no rejection occurs.

Statin medications are prescribed to control hyperlipidemia, and hypertension is treated with calcium channel blockers. Hyperlipidemia and blood vessel thickening in the transplanted heart has become the leading cause of death for long-term survivors. Because the transplanted heart does not have the usual nerve connections, the child or adolescent does not usually experience chest pain (Sudan et al., 2007).

NURSING MANAGEMENT

Depending upon the age at time of transplant, the child may not have had all immunizations (see Chapter 16 ∞). Live virus vaccines are contraindicated in children with heart transplants. Help parents arrange for school and childcare center administrators to immediately alert the family if any cases of measles, mumps, rubella, and chickenpox occur. Preventive treatment for the child can be provided as necessary. Good hand hygiene to reduce the spread of infection should be encouraged at home and at school.

After recovery from surgery, children may have near-normal exercise capabilities, normal heart function, and return to school and other activities. Immunosuppressive medications will be continued long term and can cause a variety of side effects such as hair growth, gum hyperplasia, weight gain, moon face, acne, rashes, and osteoporosis. Children and adolescents may need support to develop a positive self-esteem.

Organ rejection is a major concern of families. Educate the parents and child about the need to adhere to the immunosuppression protocol and to keep appointments for procedures to assess rejection status. Adolescents need special attention to promote adherence to the immunosuppression protocol.

■ PULMONARY HYPERTENSION

Pulmonary hypertension is a complication of a cardiac condition that causes a sustained increase in the pulmonary artery pressure, such as a large ventricular septal defect or patent ductus arteriosus with systemic to pulmonary shunting, pulmonary disease (e.g., meconium aspiration syndrome, or acute respiratory distress in a newborn), and congenital diaphragmatic hernia. Excessive pulmonary blood flow over time leads to pulmonary vascular vasoconstriction to decrease the blood flow to the lungs. The smooth muscle in the small pulmonary arteries increases to sustain vasoconstriction if the excess pulmonary blood flow is not controlled. The pulmonary artery pressure must increase to push blood across the vascular bed. Inflamma-

tion, hypertrophy of pulmonary vessels, and fibrosis develop. The increased pressure leads to a right-to-left shunt, and right heart function is impaired. The condition may become irreversible and progressive (Rothstein, Paris, & Quizon, 2009).

Hypoxemia results from pulmonary hypertension and helps maintain the vasoconstriction. Infants display tachypnea, cyanosis, retractions, and fatigue. Tiring with feeding and failure to thrive are seen. As right-sided heart failure occurs, signs of CHF develop. Older children may have dyspnea, chest pain, and syncope on exertion.

Diagnosis should involve a chest radiograph, an ECG, and echocardiogram. Clinical therapy involves cardiac surgery to correct an obstructive lesion or close a defect. Therapy for pulmonary hypertension related to pulmonary conditions involves supplemental oxygen and correcting the pulmonary condition causing pulmonary hypertension. Newborns may be treated with supplemental oxygen, inhaled nitric oxide, or ECMO. A heart transplant may be performed.

NURSING MANAGEMENT

Nursing care focuses on promoting rest for oxygen conservation, monitoring fluid intake and output carefully, and administering medications and oxygen. Airplane travel may be possible with supplemental oxygen. Exercise should be tailored to avoid dyspnea. Give parents needed support and information about their child.

■ ACQUIRED HEART DISEASES

Infective Endocarditis

Infective endocarditis is a potentially life-threatening but uncommon infection in an individual with endocardial cell damage. The endocardium is injured by a high velocity or turbulent blood flow due to a heart defect or an indwelling catheter in the right side of the heart. Infectious organisms in the bloodstream adhere to the injured **endocardium** (the tissue lining of the heart chambers), colonize, and in some cases form a vegetation. The time between bacteremia and development of symptoms is estimated to be 7 to 14 days (Wilson et al., 2007). Infectious endocarditis may be associated with a congenital heart defect, rheumatic heart disease, a central venous catheter or heart surgery, or intravenous drug abuse.

Symptoms can be mild and develop slowly, or they can be severe and develop rapidly. Common symptoms are fever, fatigue, joint and muscle aches, weight loss, headache, and diaphoresis. Other signs may include a heart murmur, hepatosplenomegaly, and congestive heart failure. Children with indwelling catheters may initially have pulmonary signs related to septic pulmonary embolism.

Infective endocarditis is diagnosed primarily by blood culture; however, urine and cerebrospinal fluid also may be cultured. Elevated erythrocyte sedimentation rate, anemia, elevated C-reactive protein level, increased white blood cell count, alterations in the electrocardiogram, and changes in heart sounds and murmurs are indicators of the condition. Transesophageal and transthoracic echocardiography is used to identify vegeta-

Medications Used to Treat
Prophylaxis for Infective Endocarditis

Antibiotic Recommendations	Nursing Management
Amoxicillin for oral use	▪ One large dose is given 30 to 60 minutes before procedures. If the preprocedure dose is not taken, the dose may be taken up to 2 hours postprocedure.
Ampicillin or cefazolin or ceftriaxone IM or IV when unable to take oral medication	▪ Teach parents and the child to keep at least one dose in the home to take before dental visits or for dental emergencies.
Cephalexin or clindamycin or azithromycin or clarithromycin when allergic to penicillin or ampicillin	▪ Have parents inform each health care provider of the child's need for prophylaxis.
Cefazolin or ceftriaxone OR clindamycin IV or IM when allergic to penicillin or ampicillin and unable to take oral medication	▪ Dentists and physicians can write the prescription.

Modified from: Wilson, W., Taubert, K. A., Gewitz, M., Lockhart, P. B., Baddour, L. M., et al. (2007). Prevention of infective endocarditis: Guidelines from the American Heart Association Rheumatic Fever, Endocarditis, and Kawasaki Disease Committee, Council on Cardiovascular Disease in the Young, and the Council on Clinical Cardiology, Council on Cardiovascular Surgery and Anesthesia, and the Quality of Care and Outcomes Research Interdisciplinary Working Group. Circulation, 116, 1736–1754.

tion or infective lesions in the heart, the extent of valve damage, and cardiac function.

Clinical therapy consists of intravenous antibiotics such as penicillin G, ceftriaxone, vancomycin, nafcillin, oxacillin, gentamicin, ciprofloxacin, and cefazolin for 2 to 8 weeks until the infective organism is eradicated. Serum levels of antibiotics are monitored to maintain a therapeutic range. Surgery may be necessary to replace a heart valve or because of risk of embolism. If CHF occurs, bed rest and medications such as digoxin and furosemide are prescribed.

Prevention of infective endocarditis is preferred. Antibiotic prophylaxis is recommended for dental procedures and invasive respiratory procedures for selected individuals at highest risk for adverse outcomes from infective endocarditis (see page 615). A previous episode of infective endocarditis is also a risk factor for reinfection. See Medications Used to Treat: Prophylaxis for Infective Endocarditis.

NURSING MANAGEMENT

Nursing care focuses on assessing the child's respiratory and cardiovascular status, administering medications, and teaching the parents about the child's care. Take the child's vital signs. Assess oxygen saturation and level of consciousness as CHF and embolism may occur. The parents will be anxious about the child's condition, especially if this occurs following surgery for a congenital heart defect or in a critically ill child or newborn. Monitor the parents' coping skills and need for information.

Administer medications as ordered and monitor serum antibiotic levels. Monitor for side effects of antibiotics and for infiltration at the infusion site. Keep invasive procedures to a minimum. Use careful aseptic technique when managing central lines and venous access devices.

The child is often lethargic and on bed rest. Encourage parents to participate in the child's care and plan quiet age-appropriate activities. Home infusion therapy is often ordered so care can continue on an outpatient basis. Instruct parents about care procedures and reinforce the importance of follow-up visits. Home schooling may be needed during the recovery period.

Nursing care also focuses on prevention of endocarditis. Good oral hygiene and regular dental care are important preventive measures. Stress the importance of telling future health care providers, including dentists and surgeons, about the child's infective endocarditis risk so prophylactic antibiotics can be given for invasive dental and respiratory procedures (Wilson et al., 2008).

Rheumatic Fever

Rheumatic fever is an inflammatory disorder of connective tissue that follows an initial infection by some strains of group A beta-hemolytic streptococcal pharyngitis. Although this is a significant health problem in developing countries, the incidence is very low in the United States (Gerber, Baltimore, Eaton, et al., 2009). This disorder causes changes in the heart, joints, brain, and skin tissues.

The hallmark signs of rheumatic fever may occur 1 to 3 weeks after an untreated streptococcal pharyngitis infection. The Jones criteria outline the major signs important for diagnosis (Park, 2008):

- Carditis involving the mitral or aortic valve may be detected by the development of a new murmur. Chest pain may be caused by pericardial inflammation.
- Polyarthritis may be detected in which two or more large joints become inflamed with pain, swelling, tenderness, erythema, and heat. Signs may shift from joint to joint (migratory polyarthritis).
- Subcutaneous nodules may be palpated over bony prominences and along extensor tendons.
- Erythema marginatum, a nonpruritic skin rash with pink macules and blanching in the middle of the lesions, appears on the trunk but not on the face and hands.
- Sydenham chorea (St. Vitus dance), characterized by aimless movements of the extremities plus facial grimacing, occurs if the central nervous system is affected.

Diagnosis of acute rheumatic fever using the Jones criteria is based on the presence of two or more of the major signs noted above and evidence of a recent streptococcal infection, such as a positive throat culture or an elevated or rising antistreptolysin O titer. Rheumatic fever is suspected when one major sign, evidence of a recent streptococcal infection, and one or more minor signs (arthralgia, fever of at least 38.8°C [102°F], elevated erythrocyte sedimentation rate or C-reactive protein, or a prolonged PR interval on electrocardiogram) are present (Park, 2008).

Clinical therapy includes antibiotics (penicillin, sulfadiazine, or erythromycin) to eradicate the streptococcal infection. Aspirin is used for fever, arthritis, and arthralgias. Corticosteroids may be used to reduce the inflammation and for severe carditis causing CHF (Park, 2008). Most children recover fully, but they are at risk for subsequent episodes of rheumatic fever. Children should be monitored carefully by echocardiogram for potential cardiac complications. Long-term antibiotic prophylaxis may be prescribed (intramuscular benzathine penicillin, oral penicillin V, or oral sulfadiazine in persons allergic to penicillin) to reduce the risk for recurrent episodes and rheumatic heart disease.

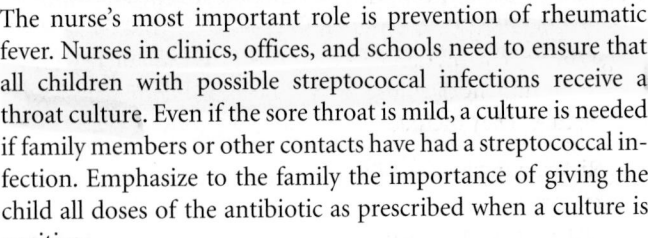

NURSING MANAGEMENT

The nurse's most important role is prevention of rheumatic fever. Nurses in clinics, offices, and schools need to ensure that all children with possible streptococcal infections receive a throat culture. Even if the sore throat is mild, a culture is needed if family members or other contacts have had a streptococcal infection. Emphasize to the family the importance of giving the child all doses of the antibiotic as prescribed when a culture is positive.

In a case of severe rheumatic fever, the child is hospitalized for a period of time. During the acute inflammatory phase, take the child's temperature at least every 4 hours and monitor vital signs. The child is on bed rest while monitoring for the onset of carditis, and for 4 weeks if carditis develops. Auscultate the child's heart and note any unusual sounds. Observe the child for changes in skin, joints, or behavior. Be sure family members have throat cultures done to identify subclinical cases or asymptomatic streptococcal carriers.

Administer antibiotics and aspirin as ordered. The child is usually lethargic and often has joint pain. Aspirin often relieves pain dramatically after a few doses. Position and handle the child's joints carefully. Provide quiet activities, as the child is often confined to bed. Encourage visits or telephone calls from family members and friends. Provide emotional support to the child with *chorea* (purposeless involuntary movements) that can last for 5 to 15 weeks and be disturbing. Encourage the family to participate in the child's hospital care.

During the recovery phase, the child is generally cared for at home. Activities may be limited, especially if heart damage is suspected. Help parents plan quiet activities, such as playing board games, working with computers, or reading, and arrange rest periods after the child returns to school. Reassure the child and parents that the effects of chorea will eventually subside.

Make sure the child and parents understand the importance of taking prescribed prophylactic antibiotics until adulthood to prevent future infection and possible heart damage from recurrent rheumatic fever. Make sure the parents understand that the child's future sore throats may be streptococcal and that a throat culture should be taken even when the child is taking daily antibiotics. The child may need additional different antibiotics for

the infection. Emphasize the importance of follow-up care to prevent new infections and to monitor heart function.

Kawasaki Disease

Kawasaki disease is an acute febrile, systemic vascular inflammatory disorder that is the leading cause of acquired heart disease in children in the United States (Vetter, 2006). Children under 4 years of age account for 80% of cases, and 50% of cases occur in children under 2 years (American Academy of Pediatrics, 2009, p. 414). Although this disorder is most common in children of Asian and Pacific Islander origin, it is seen in all racial and ethnic groups (Park, 2008).

Etiology and Pathophysiology

The etiology of Kawasaki disease is unknown, but it is thought to be caused by an unidentified infectious agent. The disorder appears to result in an exaggerated immune response in a genetically susceptible child (Vetter, 2006). A multisystem inflammatory disease involves the small- and medium-sized arteries, including the coronary arteries. As the coronary arteries heal, they can become stenotic, leading to reduced blood flow and potential infarcts (Milana & Chandran, 2006).

Clinical Manifestations

The three stages of the disease are acute, subacute, and convalescent.

- The acute stage of Kawasaki disease, lasting 1 to 2 weeks, is characterized by irritability, high fever that persists for more than 5 days, hyperemic conjunctivae, red throat, swollen hands and feet, maculopapular or erythema multiforme-like rash on the trunk and perineal area, unilateral enlargement of the cervical lymph nodes, diarrhea, and hepatic dysfunction.
- The subacute stage, lasting 2 to 4 weeks, is characterized by cracking lips and fissures, desquamation of the skin on the tips of the fingers and toes, joint pain, cardiac disease, and thrombocytosis (Figure 21–9 ➤).
- In the convalescent stage, 6 to 8 weeks after disease onset, the child appears normal but lingering signs of inflammation may be present.

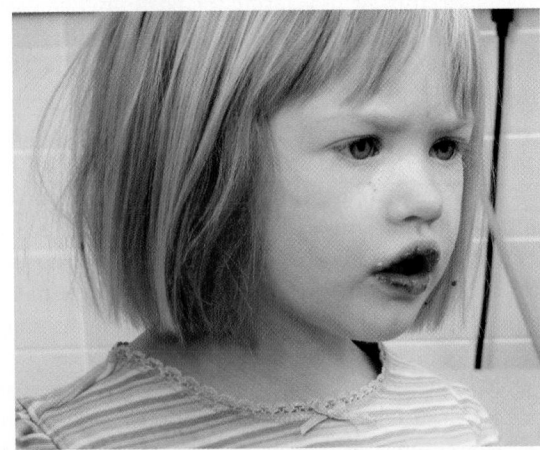

FIGURE 21–9 ➤ This child has returned for one of her frequent follow-up visits to assess her cardiac status after treatment for Kawasaki syndrome. Notice the lips that show inflammation and cracking.

Other clinical signs that may occur during the acute phase include arthralgias, abdominal pain with diarrhea, liver dysfunction, and aseptic meningitis.

COLLABORATIVE CARE

Diagnostic Tests

Kawasaki disease is diagnosed when a high spiking fever over 39°C (102.2°F) for 5 days or longer is present along with four of five principal features not explained by another disease process (see Table 21–8). When fewer than four criteria are present, but echocardiography or angiography reveals coronary artery abnormalities, Kawasaki disease is also diagnosed. Initial and repeat echocardiography is used to identify specific vascular changes in the heart and coronary arteries.

Clinical Therapy

Kawasaki disease is treated with intravenous immunoglobulin (IVIG) at a dose of 2 g/kg given in a single infusion, and aspirin. High doses of aspirin (80 to 100 mg/kg/day in four divided doses) are given while the fever is high. The aspirin dose is decreased to 3 to 5 mg/kg/day or less once the fever has dropped for its antiplatelet activity. High doses of IVIG given before the 10th day of fever reduce the incidence of coronary artery lesions and aneurysms, as well as decrease fever and inflammatory signs (Milana & Chandran, 2006). If the child does not respond well to IVIG, corticosteroids or infliximab, a monoclonal antibody, may be used (Son, Gauvreau, Ma, et al., 2009).

Children are usually hospitalized for 3 or more days, depending upon the presence of cardiac lesions and how long the fever persists. Most children recover fully. Careful monitoring for cardiac disease continues for several weeks or months. Coronary aneurysms may develop in 5% of children treated with intravenous immune globulin (Newburger, Sleeper, McCrindle, et al., 2007). Many smaller coronary aneurysms resolve spontaneously in 1 to 2 years after treatment (Milana & Chandran, 2006). Some children with stenosed coronary arteries may need angioplasty or coronary artery bypass grafts.

NURSING MANAGEMENT

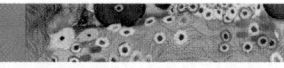

Nursing care focuses on promoting comfort, monitoring for early signs of complications or disease progression, and supporting the family.

Nursing Assessment and Diagnosis

Assessment is important in identifying signs of Kawasaki disease, as the acute phase of this disorder is commonly confused with other diseases. The nurse in the community must be alert to early signs and symptoms.

When the child is hospitalized, take the temperature every 4 hours and before each dose of aspirin. Carefully assess the extremities for edema, redness, and desquamation every 8 hours. Examine the eyes for conjunctivitis and the mucous membranes for inflammation. Monitor the child's dietary and fluid intake and weigh the child daily. Carefully assess heart sounds and rhythm.

Several nursing diagnoses may apply to the child with Kawasaki disease. They include:

- Risk for Imbalanced Body Temperature related to inflammatory process
- Impaired Oral Mucous Membranes related to inflammation and decreased fluid intake
- Impaired Skin Integrity due to edema, diaphoresis, and skin desquamation
- Interrupted Family Processes due to child's acute and potentially life-threatening illness

Planning and Implementation

Administer aspirin and IVIG as ordered. Monitor for side effects of aspirin such as bleeding and gastrointestinal upset. Administer IVIG as a blood product, carefully regulating the infusion rate to run slowly according to the physician's orders, and watching for any reactions to the infusion. The infusion rate should not be over 1 mL/min. If symptoms of reaction occur, stop the infusion immediately (see Chapter 22 ∞).

Promote the child's comfort. Keep the child's skin clean and dry, and lubricate the lips. Use cool compresses to make the feverish child more comfortable. Change the child's clothes and bed linens frequently. Give the child frequent small feedings of soft foods and liquids that are neither too hot nor too cold.

Use passive range of motion exercises to facilitate joint movement. Because the child with Kawasaki disease is often lethargic and irritable, plan rest periods and quiet age-appropriate activities. Encourage the parents to participate in their child's care. This comforts and reassures the child. Give the parents information about the disease and the child's treatment.

Before the child is discharged, teach the parents to administer aspirin as ordered and to watch for side effects. Inform the parents that the aspirin is being used only for this diagnosis. If the child has a subsequent fever, acetaminophen or ibuprofen may be needed. Advise the parents that the child may need to avoid contact sports or other activities that could cause bleed-

TABLE 21–8	Diagnostic Criteria for Kawasaki Disease When Fever Is Present 5 Days or Longer
Body Part Affected	Principal Features
Eyes	Bilateral bulbar conjunctivitis without exudate
Skin	Intense erythema of the buccal and pharyngeal surfaces with dry, swollen, cracked, and fissuring lips and a strawberry tongue Erythema of the palms and soles, edema of the hands and feet, and then desquamation after 2 or more weeks of symptoms Dermatitis of the trunk with an erythematous maculopapular rash
Lymph nodes	Cervical lymphadenopathy, frequently unilateral, with a lymph node over 1.5 cm in diameter found early in the disease

Modified from: Vetter, V. L. (2006). Kawasaki disease. In V. L. Vetter, Pediatric cardiology: The requisites in pediatrics (p. 132). St. Louis, MO: Elsevier Mosby.

ing. Limitation of strenuous activity is recommended for all children with coronary aneurysms or stenoses. Emphasize the need for follow-up care to monitor for cardiac complications.

Nursing Alert

Postpone the immunization of a child with Kawasaki disease with live vaccines (e.g., measles or varicella) for 11 months after IVIG administration as it interferes with the child's immune response to the live virus vaccine. If the child is at high risk of exposure to measles or varicella, immunize the child before this time has passed, then reimmunize the child 11 months after IVIG treatment. Do not postpone immunization with inactivated vaccines (American Academy of Pediatrics, 2009, p. 418).

Evaluation

Examples of expected nursing care outcomes include:

- The child's skin care promotes healing and protects from further damage and infection.
- The parents are educated to monitor the child for complications and to provide ongoing care to the child.

■ CARDIAC ARRHYTHMIAS

Cardiac **arrhythmias** (abnormal rhythms or dysrhythmias) occur frequently in children, but less often than in adults. These include tachyarrhythmias (sinus tachycardia) and bradyarrhythmias (sinus bradycardia) that occur with acute conditions such as hypoxia, acidosis, increased intracranial pressure, hypothermia, and hypoglycemia. Most of these arrhythmias resolve once the condition is treated. Less common arrhythmias are often associated with congenital heart disease, including atrial fibrillation, atrial flutter, ventricular fibrillation, and heart block. Arrhythmias must be recognized because they cause decreased cardiac output and CHF, or an even more serious arrhythmia may develop that could result in sudden death. See the companion website for Clinical Manifestations and rhythm strips of some common arrhythmias.

Bradycardia

Bradycardia is a heart rate less than the lower limit of normal for the child' age, usually a rate less than 80 beats per minute in infants and less than 60 beats per minute in children and adolescents (Doniger & Sharieff, 2006). Some athletes may normally have a heart rate of 60.

For sinus bradycardia due to an acute condition, treatment with oxygen, ventilation, and medications such as epinephrine or atropine are used until the condition resolves. Other chronic bradycardias due to heart block often require a pacemaker.

Supraventricular Tachycardia

Supraventricular tachycardia (SVT), the most common pediatric pathologic arrhythmia, is an abrupt and unpredictable onset of a very rapid heart rate (Schlechte, Boramanand, & Funk, 2008). Neonates and young children may be predisposed to the condition because of a congenital heart defect or Wolff-Parkinson-

White syndrome. Short periods of arrhythmia (several seconds), which may be caused by paroxysmal atrial tachycardia, are rarely dangerous. Cardiac output is affected because diastolic filling cannot occur with such a rapid heart rate. Prolonged episodes of SVT (e.g., 24 to 48 hours) may progress to CHF or cardiogenic shock if untreated (Schlechte et al., 2008).

Clinical manifestations in infants include nonspecific signs such as poor feeding, vomiting, irritability, diaphoresis, and increased sleepiness. The presenting heart rate in infants with SVT may be 220 to 280 beats/min. Older children may have palpitations, chest pain, dizziness, shortness of breath, and decreased exercise tolerance. In older children, a heart rate may be 180 to 240 beats/min. Adolescents report many of the same signs as older children, but they may also have pallor, a feeling of palpitations in the neck, and diaphoresis. Recurrent attacks are common.

Electrocardiography, including a 24- to 48-hour rhythm recording with a Holter monitor after the acute episode, is commonly performed. However, an electrophysiology study performed under sedation may be needed to confirm the diagnosis.

Vagal stimulation such as applying ice or iced saline solution to the face of an infant may reduce the heart rate. An older child can perform the Valsalva maneuver (holding the breath and straining, or blowing forcefully on the thumb) to increase intrathoracic and venous pressures and thus slow the heart rate. Adenosine may be administered intravenously when vagal stimulation does not work. Calcium channel blockers may be administered to children over age 1 year. Synchronized cardioversion may be used for life-threatening episodes unresponsive to medications. Digoxin, a beta-blocker (e.g., atenolol), amiodarone, or propranolol may also be used for chronic management of SVT.

Nursing Alert

When applying ice or iced saline to the face of an infant, take care to avoid pressure on the eyes as retinal damage could occur. Also ensure that the child's airway is unobstructed by the ice packs.

Ablation is the use of radiofrequency energy or liquid nitrous oxide (cryoablation) to destroy a very small section of the myocardium through which an accessory conduction pathway passes that triggers tachycardia. The procedure is performed in a cardiac catheterization laboratory; when successful, medications taken to control SVT can be discontinued.

Long QT Syndrome

Long QT syndrome is a rhythm disturbance of autosomal dominant and autosomal recessive inheritance that puts children at risk for ventricular fibrillation and sudden death. The ventricular tachycardia with a prolonged QT interval impairs cardiac output leading to syncope or seizures. Electrolyte abnormalities (hypokalemia, hypocalcemia, and hypomagnesemia) and medications may also cause the disorder (Doniger & Sharieff, 2006). It is thought to be associated with some cases of sudden infant death syndrome. Males younger than 15 years are at higher risk for sudden death due to the syndrome (Hobbs, Peterson, Moss, et al., 2006).

The arrhythmia may be triggered by demanding physical exercise, extreme emotional stress, or an abrupt loud noise (e.g., doorbell or alarm clock). Arrhythmia may occur without warning and result in sudden death. Presenting signs include syncope, seizure, cardiac arrest, or palpitation during exercise or when experiencing strong emotion.

If the child is resuscitated or evaluated because of early signs, the arrhythmia is commonly detected by electrocardiogram. The disorder is treated by beta-blockers (propranolol) in doses that lessen the chance of drug-induced bradycardia (Park, 2008). A cardiac pacemaker or implantable cardioverter-defibrillator may be used in patients considered at high risk for sudden death. Children with the condition should not engage in competitive sports. In addition, swimming should be supervised.

NURSING MANAGEMENT

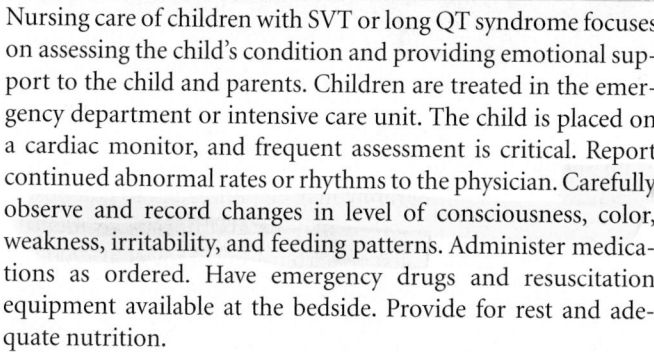

Nursing care of children with SVT or long QT syndrome focuses on assessing the child's condition and providing emotional support to the child and parents. Children are treated in the emergency department or intensive care unit. The child is placed on a cardiac monitor, and frequent assessment is critical. Report continued abnormal rates or rhythms to the physician. Carefully observe and record changes in level of consciousness, color, weakness, irritability, and feeding patterns. Administer medications as ordered. Have emergency drugs and resuscitation equipment available at the bedside. Provide for rest and adequate nutrition.

Episodes of arrhythmia are frightening for both the child and parents. Carefully explain the treatment plan and home care. Teach parents to take the child's apical pulse. Make sure parents are trained in cardiopulmonary resuscitation and know how to seek emergency care. Emphasize that prescribed medications help prevent or reduce the frequency of the episodes. Help the child and family recognize and avoid medications that can trigger another episode. The child with SVT should not use cardiac stimulant drugs such as decongestants. For the child with long QT syndrome, teach the parents and adolescents to remind the primary care provider not to prescribe medications that prolong the QT interval (e.g., antihistamines, antidepressants, and macrolide antibiotics). An updated list of these medications can be found online at the companion website.

■ DYSLIPIDEMIA

Dyslipidemia is a condition in which one or more lipids (total cholesterol, low-density lipoproteins, triglycerides, high-density lipoproteins) have an abnormal level in the blood. It is important to identify children who have a genetic history or lifestyle that makes them more susceptible to future coronary heart disease and to implement preventive health measures to reduce the child's risk of disease and premature death as an adult. Improving lipid and lipoprotein concentrations during childhood and adolescence may help lower the child's risk of adult cardiovascular disease.

Abnormalities in lipid levels may be the result of excessive production, lack of clearance of the lipoprotein particles, a ge-

Research *Cardiovascular Risk Factors*

A study of 94 families revealed that screening and identification of children with cardiovascular risk factors (obesity, blood pressure, dyslipidemia, hyperglycemia, and metabolic syndrome) was highly correlated to their parents' cardiovascular risk factors (Reis, Kip, Marroquin, et al., 2006). Some parents may not be aware of their own risk factors because they have fewer primary care visits than their children. Identifying risk factors in children provides an important education opportunity to encourage parents to seek care for their own cardiovascular risk factors.

netic defect in lipid metabolism, or other defects such as enzyme deficiencies. Some children have primary dyslipidemia due to familial hypercholesterolemia. Obesity is the secondary leading cause of dyslipidemia.

A blood test identifies hyperlipidemia. Recommended and abnormal values for recommended tests are as follows (Daniels, Greer, & Committee on Nutrition, 2008):

- **Total Cholesterol:** Recommended—less than 170 mg/dL, Abnormal—greater than 200 mg/dL
- **Triglyceride:** Recommended—less than 150 mg/dL, Abnormal—greater than 150 mg/dL
- **High density lipoproteins:** Recommended—greater than 35 mg/dL, Abnormal—less than 35 mg/dL
- **Low density lipoproteins:** Recommended—less than 110 mg/dL, Abnormal—greater than 130 mg/dL

All children over 2 years of age with the following risk factors should be screened for dyslipidemia with a fasting lipid profile: a family history of dyslipidemia or premature cardiovascular disease, current dyslipidemia in men of 55 years or less, or women of 65 years or less, unknown family history of dyslipidemia, other risk factors such as overweight or obesity (body mass index greater than 85%), hypertension, cigarette smoking, or diabetes mellitus (Daniels et al., 2008).

The primary management of dyslipidemia in most children includes dietary modifications, exercise, and other changes in lifestyle. The child's diet is carefully analyzed and changes are made to satisfy the dietary guidelines so that saturated fats are less than 7% of total caloric intake, and cholesterol intake is less than 200 mg per day for treatment of elevated LDL levels (Gidding, Dennison, Birch, et al., 2005). A healthy total fat intake is 20–35% of daily calories. If the child is obese, weight loss is encouraged. Intensive dietary and exercise programs have resulted in modest reductions in LDL-C (Belay, Belamarich, & Tom-Revzon, 2007).

If the child continues to have high serum lipid levels, pharmacologic treatment may be initiated for children 8 years and older. Cholestyramine or colestipol (which bind bile acid in the intestine) niacin, and statins may be prescribed. The initial goal is to lower LDL concentration to less than 160 mg/dL. However, target LDL concentration may be as low as 130 mg/dL or even 110 mg/dL when there is a strong family history of cardiovascular disease and other risk factors such as obesity and diabetes mellitus (Daniels et al., 2008).

NURSING MANAGEMENT

Nursing care focuses on identifying children at risk for dyslipidemia, providing education about diet and exercise, and monitoring eating patterns. Identification and management of dyslipidemia takes place in many community settings. Office and clinic nurses identify children who need to have serum lipid measured. Nurses in schools provide education on ways to reduce risk factors. The child's history of exercise patterns, body mass index, and dietary intake provides important information. Obtain information on familial heart disease, hypertension, diabetes, and smoking to determine risk factors. Although a screening for total cholesterol level does not require fasting, the child needs to fast for 12 hours before blood is drawn for a complete lipid evaluation.

Work with nutritionists to provide dietary teaching and monitor family eating patterns. The food plan for the child and entire family should consist primarily of fruit, vegetables, whole grains, low-fat and nonfat dairy products, lean meat and fish, legumes, and nuts. Help parents understand that modeling food choices helps children learn to make better food choices and reduce lipid levels. For children with familial hypercholesterolemia, lifelong dietary control is essential.

Help the child select an enjoyable moderate to intense activity for daily participation, and then obtain 30 minutes of aerobic exercise (e.g., jogging, swimming, biking, in-line skating, soccer) at least 3 to 4 times a week to promote cardiovascular fitness. Discourage smoking by the child or the parents as it increases the risk for cardiovascular disease.

Educate children and adolescents taking statin medications to report any adverse effects to their health care provider, such as myalgia, muscle soreness, weakness, tenderness, or dark-colored urine. Include the entire family in the treatment plan; it is difficult for a single family member to change eating and exercise patterns.

■ HYPERTENSION

Hypertension in children and adolescents is defined as a systolic or diastolic blood pressure reading that is equal to or greater than the 95th percentile for age, sex, and height percentile (see Appendix B ∞ for the blood pressure tables). Normal blood pressure is defined as a systolic or diastolic reading that falls below the 90th percentile for age, sex, and height percentile. Hypertension is now estimated to occur in 5% of the pediatric population, possibly related to the number of obese children (Brady, Siberry, & Solomon, 2008). Increasing rates of hypertension in childhood is a significant concern because it is a major risk factor for heart disease and stroke during adulthood.

Primary hypertension is less common in children than adults. Secondary causes of hypertension may include conditions such as coarctation of the aorta, renal disorders, neoplasms, endocrine disorders, and obstructive sleep disorder (Brady et al., 2008).

Children often have no symptoms of hypertension, and the condition is usually detected during a health examination. Hypertension symptoms include nausea, vomiting, epistaxis, blurry vision, or diplopia.

COLLABORATIVE CARE

The diagnosis of hypertension is based on three or more separate readings a week apart in which the systolic or diastolic reading is greater than or equal to the 95th percentile for gender, age, and height percentile (Feld & Corey, 2007). Blood chemistry (BUN, creatinine, glucose, and electrolytes), complete blood count, fasting lipids, thyroid function tests, urinalysis, urine culture, renal ultrasound, echocardiogram, and a retinal exam should be performed to detect secondary causes of hypertension. Polysomnography may be performed to diagnose a sleep disorder. A drug screen may be appropriate to identify substances that could cause hypertension (Brady et al., 2008).

Nonpharmacologic measures for reduction of blood pressure include weight reduction and increased exercise. Dietary modification involves reduced sodium and saturated fats, three to five fruit servings daily, and an adequate intake of calcium and dietary fiber. Smoking, alcohol, and drugs should be strongly discouraged. Children also need 30 to 60 minutes of physical activity each day.

Medications are used for children with persistent, severe hypertension that is not resolved with nonpharmacologic therapies. Angiotensin-converting enzyme (ACE) inhibitors and calcium channel blockers are most commonly prescribed for children because of their low side effects (Brady et al., 2008).

NURSING MANAGEMENT

All children age 3 years and older should have a blood pressure reading at each health visit. If high blood pressure is identified,

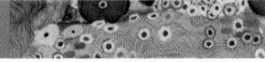

Research *Hypertension*

A study conducted with 48 African American students, aged 14 to 17 years, investigated the risk factors (positive family history, diet, exercise, and blood pressure) for their development of hypertension as adults. Findings revealed many factors placing these adolescents at risk for hypertension: 31 (65%) had a positive family history; the average intake of fruits and vegetables was 2.4 servings a day; 41 (85%) reported exercising less than 3 times a week, and females exercised less often than males; and 14 (29%) were prehypertensive or hypertensive (Covelli, 2007). Behavioral risk factors (e.g., diet and exercise) may potentially be addressed with education about how to eat healthy and the importance of exercise.

Culture *Blood Pressure*

A recent study contrasted the blood pressure of 13- and 14-year-old children in the eighth grade in three states. The sample of 1,740 children had the following racial and ethnic heritage: White (14.3%), Black (22%), Hispanic (50%), Native American (2%), and mixed heritage (11.7%). No significant differences in blood pressure were found to be related to racial or ethnic origin; however, a larger number of children than expected (23.9%) had high blood pressure. High blood pressure was most often attributable to body mass index (BMI) (Jago, Harrell, McMurray, et al., 2006).

Blood Pressure Animation

Transcendental Meditation for Stress Management and Blood Pressure Control

Meditation is a mind-body therapy that may help adolescents with stress management and blood pressure control. It is thought that meditation might work by reducing activity in the sympathetic nervous system and increasing activity in the parasympathetic nervous system, slowing the heart and breathing rates, dilating blood vessels to improve blood control, and increasing digestive juices (National Center for Complementary and Alternative Medicine, 2009). One study of 69 African American adolescents with high normal resting blood pressure compared the impact of a 2-month transcendental meditation program with lifestyle education sessions offered in the school setting. The treatment and control groups had similar numbers of males and females. Meditation was practiced 4 minutes a day (20 minutes a week) with a teacher, and students were asked to practice meditation at home. Control group students had weekly 20-minute sessions on high blood pressure prevention and cardiovascular disease risk factor reduction. They were asked to do 20-minute daily walks. Study results revealed that transcendental meditation shows promise as a potential therapy to help children to maintain their high normal resting blood pressure rather than progress to hypertension (Barnes, Davis, Murzynowski, et al., 2004).

a complete history is taken to identify potential risk factors such as a family history for hypertension, smoking, or a systemic disease. Identify symptoms associated with a potential health condition. Is the child obese? Learn about the child's diet, including the number of daily servings of fruits and dairy products, and salt and caffeine intake. What are the child's daily exercise routines? Review any medications or other potential agents used by the child or adolescent.

Assess the child's blood pressure and consistently use the right arm and an appropriately sized cuff (see the *Clinical Skills Manual*). Compare the leg blood pressure to that in the arm. Compare readings to the expected blood pressure reading for gender, age, and height percentile. Monitor the child's blood pressure every 3 to 6 months.

Teach both the child and the parents how to improve the diet and develop exercise routines. Provide suggestions about substitute seasonings for salt and a list of salty foods to avoid. Increasing intake of low-fat dairy products and fruits can contribute to blood pressure control.

Emphasize the importance of avoiding smoking. Discuss ways to increase activity and reduce time watching television or playing computer games. Provide suggestions for the management of stress and stressful situations. Teaching that involves the entire family is usually the most effective. Instruct the family on correct administration of prescribed medications when used.

■ INJURIES OF THE CARDIOVASCULAR SYSTEM

Shock

Shock is an acute, complex state of circulatory dysfunction resulting in failure to deliver sufficient oxygen and other nutrients to meet cell and tissue demands. It can be caused by a variety of conditions such as hemorrhage, dehydration, sepsis, obstruction of blood flow, and cardiac pump failure.

Hypovolemic Shock

Hypovolemic shock is a clinical state of inadequate tissue and organ perfusion resulting from the movement of blood or plasma out of the intravascular compartment leading to inadequate intravascular volume (Figure 21–10 ➤). The blood or plasma in the vascular space may be decreased because of hemorrhage or fluid movement into the interstitial spaces.

Etiology and Pathophysiology   Major causes of decreased intravascular blood volume include:

- Hemorrhage from significant injury
- Plasma loss from burns, nephrotic syndrome, and sepsis
- Fluid and electrolyte loss associated with dehydration, diabetic ketoacidosis, and diabetes insipidus

Decreased intravascular blood volume results in inadequate delivery of oxygen and nutrients to cells and the accumulation of toxic wastes in the capillaries, leading to a decrease in cardiac output and mean arterial pressure. Cellular hypoxia and acidosis develop simultaneously. The accumulation of toxins and inadequate tissue oxygenation cause cellular damage.

The child's body attempts to compensate by the following measures:

- The renin-angiotensin-aldosterone system is stimulated to retain sodium and water when perfusion of the kidneys is decreased.
- The antidiuretic hormone is secreted when the atria have reduced blood volume leading to water retention.
- The heart rate and myocardial contractility increase to improve cardiac output.
- The respiratory rate increases to improve oxygenation and decrease waste accumulation in the cells.
- The hydrostatic pressure falls, permitting fluid to shift into the vascular space and increasing the circulating blood volume.
- The peripheral vasculature constricts to maintain the systemic vascular resistance and to increase perfusion to the vital organs as long as possible.

The child can compensate until 20–25% of volume loss occurs, and then life-threatening hypotension results.

Clinical Manifestations   Signs of early hypovolemic shock in children are nonspecific but need to be recognized before hypotension occurs. See the Clinical Manifestations table on the next page comparing the signs of early and uncompensated shock. If treatment is not begun, the condition progresses until the child can no longer compensate. Reduced cerebral blood flow ultimately results in a decreased level of consciousness. If shock is not reversed, the condition progresses to cardiopulmonary failure.

Clinical Therapy   No laboratory tests can be used to evaluate the volume deficit rapidly enough to diagnose hypovolemic shock. The child is examined for characteristic signs to confirm

Pathophysiology Illustrated
Hypovolemic Shock

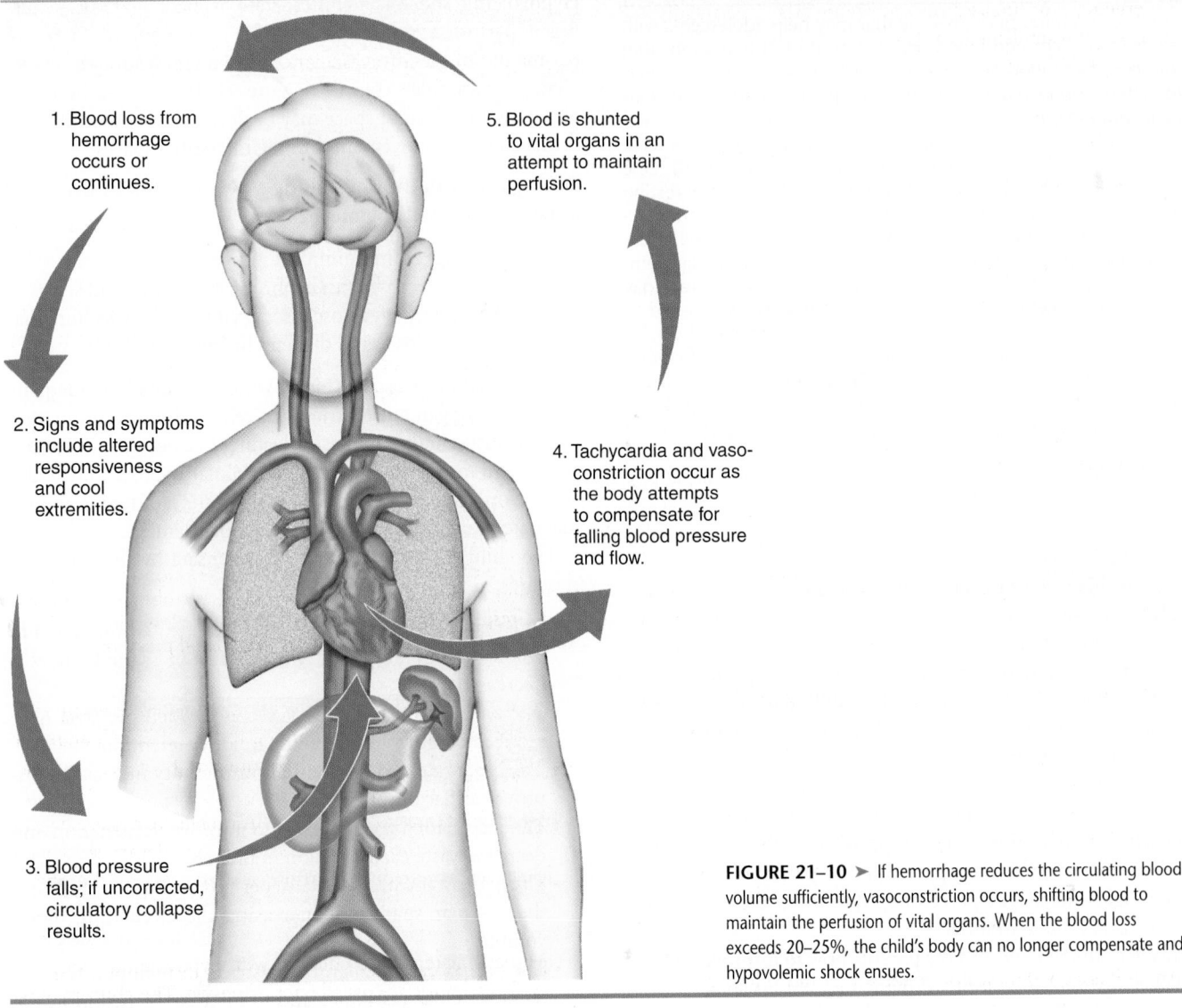

1. Blood loss from hemorrhage occurs or continues.

2. Signs and symptoms include altered responsiveness and cool extremities.

3. Blood pressure falls; if uncorrected, circulatory collapse results.

4. Tachycardia and vaso-constriction occur as the body attempts to compensate for falling blood pressure and flow.

5. Blood is shunted to vital organs in an attempt to maintain perfusion.

FIGURE 21–10 ➤ If hemorrhage reduces the circulating blood volume sufficiently, vasoconstriction occurs, shifting blood to maintain the perfusion of vital organs. When the blood loss exceeds 20–25%, the child's body can no longer compensate and hypovolemic shock ensues.

Clinical Manifestations
Hypovolemic Shock

System	Early Shock	Uncompensated Shock
Cardiac	Mild tachycardia, weak distal pulses, strong central pulses	Moderate tachycardia, thready distal pulses, weak central pulses, decreasing systolic blood pressure
Respiratory	Mild tachypnea	Moderate tachypnea
Neurologic	Normal, restless, less interactive	Restless, agitated, diminished responses
Skin	Mottled appearance; capillary refill time greater than 2 seconds; cool, clammy extremities	Pallor; capillary refill time greater than 3 seconds; cold, dry extremities; sunken eyes
Renal	Decreased urine output, increased specific gravity in older infants and children (newborns cannot concentrate urine)	Oliguria, increased specific gravity

Data from: Dieckmann, R. A. (Ed.). (2006). Pediatric education for prehospital professionals (2nd ed., pp. 83–84). Sudbury, MA: Jones and Bartlett; McKiernan, C. A., & Lieberman, S. A. (2005). Circulatory shock in children: An overview. Pediatrics in Review, 26(12), 451–459; Ralston, M., Hazinski, M. F., Zaritsky, A. L., Schexnayder, S. M., & Kleinman, M. E. (2006). Pediatric advanced life support: Provider manual (p. 100). Dallas, TX: American Heart Association.

the diagnosis. Laboratory tests commonly performed after hypovolemic shock is diagnosed include hematocrit and hemoglobin, arterial blood gases, serum electrolytes, glucose, osmolality, blood urea nitrogen, and urinalysis.

Emergency care focuses on improving tissue perfusion. An open airway is established, oxygen is administered, and ventilation is assisted if necessary. Bleeding is controlled, and an intravenous or intraosseous line is started to provide large volumes of crystalloid fluids.

Ringer's lactate solution is the preferred fluid for initial resuscitation. A fluid volume of 20 mL/kg is administered rapidly over 5 minutes. The same amount of fluid is administered 5 minutes after the first if the child's physiologic condition does not improve. If no improvement is seen after the second fluid bolus, blood or albumin is usually ordered.

Once the child's physiologic condition is stabilized, the cause of the hypovolemic shock becomes the focus of examination and treatment. If no external bleeding is evident, determine whether an injury may be causing internal bleeding. For example, injury to the liver or spleen, highly vascular organs, may cause significant bleeding and cause hypovolemic shock. Prolonged vomiting and diarrhea due to gastroenteritis may cause dehydration and hypovolemic shock.

NURSING MANAGEMENT

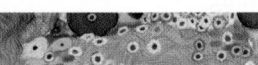

Nursing Assessment and Diagnosis

Ask the parent (or child, if appropriate) about possible injuries or the duration and severity of acute illnesses. If external bleeding is apparent, determine the amount of blood lost. Although children lose the same amount of blood from a laceration as adults, the total volume of blood lost is proportional to their weight.

Frequently assess the child's heart rate, respiratory rate, blood pressure, capillary refill time, level of consciousness with the Glasgow Coma Scale (see Chapter 27 ∞), color, and skin temperature to identify any changes that indicate improvement or deterioration in the child's condition. Monitor urine output and specific gravity hourly, as it is a good indicator of adequate fluid volume.

Assess the parents' response and coping mechanisms to the child's potentially life-threatening injury. Families are unprepared for the abrupt change in the child's condition because of the unpredictability of the injury. See Chapter 13 ∞.

Several nursing diagnoses may apply to the child with hypovolemic shock. They include:

- Decreased Cardiac Output related to hypovolemia
- Deficient Fluid Volume related to active fluid volume loss from vomiting and diarrhea

 Growth & Development *Blood Volume*

The child's total blood volume varies by weight. The child has approximately 80 mL of blood for every kilogram of body weight.

- Newborn: 3 kg × 80 mL = 240 mL (1 cup)
- 5-year-old child: 25 kg × 80 mL = 2000 mL (2 quarts)
- 13-year-old child: 50 kg × 80 mL = 4000 mL (1 gallon)

- Ineffective Tissue Perfusion (Cardiopulmonary, Renal, and Cerebral) related to impaired transport of oxygen across the alveolar and capillary membrane
- Compromised Family Coping related to life-threatening condition of the child

Planning and Implementation

Nurses in the emergency department and intensive care unit participate in resuscitation of the child in hypovolemic shock, often using protocols or guidelines for nursing interventions. Assist with the child's assessment and the establishment of intravenous access. Calculate and prepare the amount of intravenous fluid needed for administration according to the child's weight (20 mL/kg). Ensure rapid administration of warmed fluids by intravenous push or pressure bag. Warmed intravenous fluids are used for resuscitation because hypothermia may interfere with the child's response to treatment. Monitor the child's physiologic response to the fluid bolus within 5 minutes. Prepare a second and third fluid bolus. Keep the child covered or use heat lamps to reduce body heat loss.

Clinical Tip

Signs that a child with hypovolemic shock is responding to fluid resuscitation include slowing of the heart rate, improved color, improved responsiveness, increased warmth of extremities, a faster capillary refill time, and increased systolic blood pressure.

When packed red blood cells are administered, verify that the correct blood has been obtained for the child. Change the intravenous fluid to normal saline solution to prevent clotting during blood administration. (See the *Clinical Skills Manual*.) Assess the child carefully for a transfusion reaction (see Chapter 23 ∞). Monitor the child's physiologic circulatory responses for improvement or deterioration in status. Notify the physician of any deterioration.

Provide support to the child and family during the acute phase of treatment. Parents and children with hypovolemic shock resulting from injury are usually apprehensive. The child may be fearful because of the sudden hospitalization or agitated because of an altered level of consciousness. Determine the causes of the child's anxiety. As the parents often fear for the child's life in cases of severe injury, update them about the child's condition frequently. Explain the care being provided and how it helps the child. Listen to their concerns and correct any misconceptions.

Evaluation

Examples of expected nursing care outcomes include:

- The child receives adequate fluid resuscitation to prevent progression to uncompensated shock.
- The family copes with the stress of the child's injury.

Distributive Shock

Distributive shock is an abnormal distribution of blood volume, usually resulting from a decrease in systemic vascular resistance. The blood accumulates in the extremities because of vasodilation and capillary permeability. Less blood is returned to the heart, so preload (amount of blood in the ventricle at the end of diastole that stretches the heart muscle before contraction) drops and cardiac output falls. Causes of distributive shock include anaphylaxis, sepsis, and spinal cord injury. See Chapter 16 ∞ for information about sepsis.

NURSING MANAGEMENT

The child with distributive shock is cared for in an intensive care unit. Nursing care focuses on detecting and managing subtle changes in the child's condition that improve the child's chances for survival. Parents are supported as described in Chapter 13 ∞.

Obstructive Shock

Obstructive shock occurs when a blockage of the main bloodstream interferes with tissue perfusion (Figure 21–11 ➤). Causes in children include compression of the vena cava, pericardial tamponade, pulmonary embolism, tension pneumothorax, pleural effusion, and congenital heart defects with outflow obstruction (e.g., coarctation of the aorta). Management is focused on treatment of the underlying condition.

NURSING MANAGEMENT

The child is usually cared for in the intensive care unit with nursing care focused on supporting the child's respiratory and cardiovascular functioning. See Chapter 20 ∞, page 595 for care of the child with a tension pneumothorax.

Pathophysiology Illustrated
Mediastinal Shift in Obstructive Shock

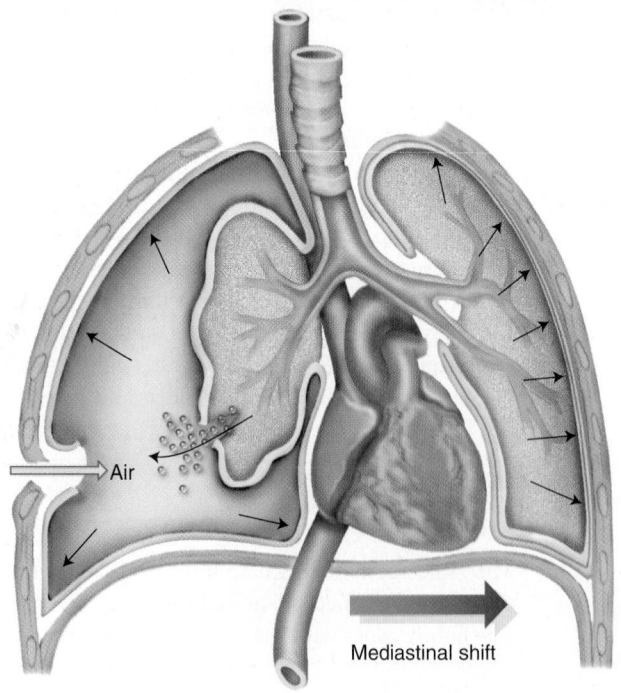

FIGURE 21–11 ➤ Compression of the great arteries can occur when a tension pneumothorax causes a mediastinal shift of the heart and great arteries and obstructs blood flow to and from the heart.

Cardiogenic Shock

Cardiogenic shock is an abnormality of myocardial function in which the heart fails to maintain adequate cardiac output and tissue perfusion (Figure 21–12 ➤). Causes of cardiogenic shock in children may include pump failure, severe obstructive congenital heart disease such as hypoplastic left heart syndrome, cardiomyopathy, arrhythmias, sepsis, poisoning, or myocardial injury (Ralston et al., 2006, p. 76).

Clinically, cardiogenic shock resembles hypovolemic shock with low cardiac output. Tachycardia, tachypnea, decreased oxygen saturation, hypotension, diminished peripheral pulses, and cool, pale extremities are common signs. The child becomes disoriented and restless as the compensatory mechanisms fail. Compensatory responses divert blood to the heart and brain; however, reduced blood flow to the kidneys, liver, and intestines can lead to ischemia and end-organ failure. Increased systemic vascular resistance puts more stress on the failing heart. Each contraction causes more blood to accumulate in the heart and pulmonary vessels, eventually leading to CHF, metabolic acidosis, and circulatory collapse.

The goals of medical treatment are rapid restoration of myocardial function with adequate ventilation, resolution of the initial metabolic insult, correction of arrhythmias, management of fluids, and administration of diuretics and inotropic drugs.

NURSING MANAGEMENT

The child will be cared for in the intensive care unit. Nursing care focuses on monitoring and supporting the respiratory and cardiovascular status, fluid management, and medication administration. See Chapter 13 ∞ for care of the child with a life-threatening condition.

Myocardial Contusion

Myocardial contusion, a rare injury in children, results from a strong, blunt force against the chest wall that injures the heart muscle. Blood flow to areas of the heart muscle is disrupted, or myocardial cells are directly destroyed. This potentially life-threatening condition is often associated with a motor vehicle–related injury. It most often occurs in adolescents who have struck the steering wheel of a motor vehicle during a crash or children who have been struck in the chest with a baseball.

A myocardial contusion should be suspected in cases of injury to the anterior chest. The child

Pathophysiology Illustrated
Cardiogenic Shock

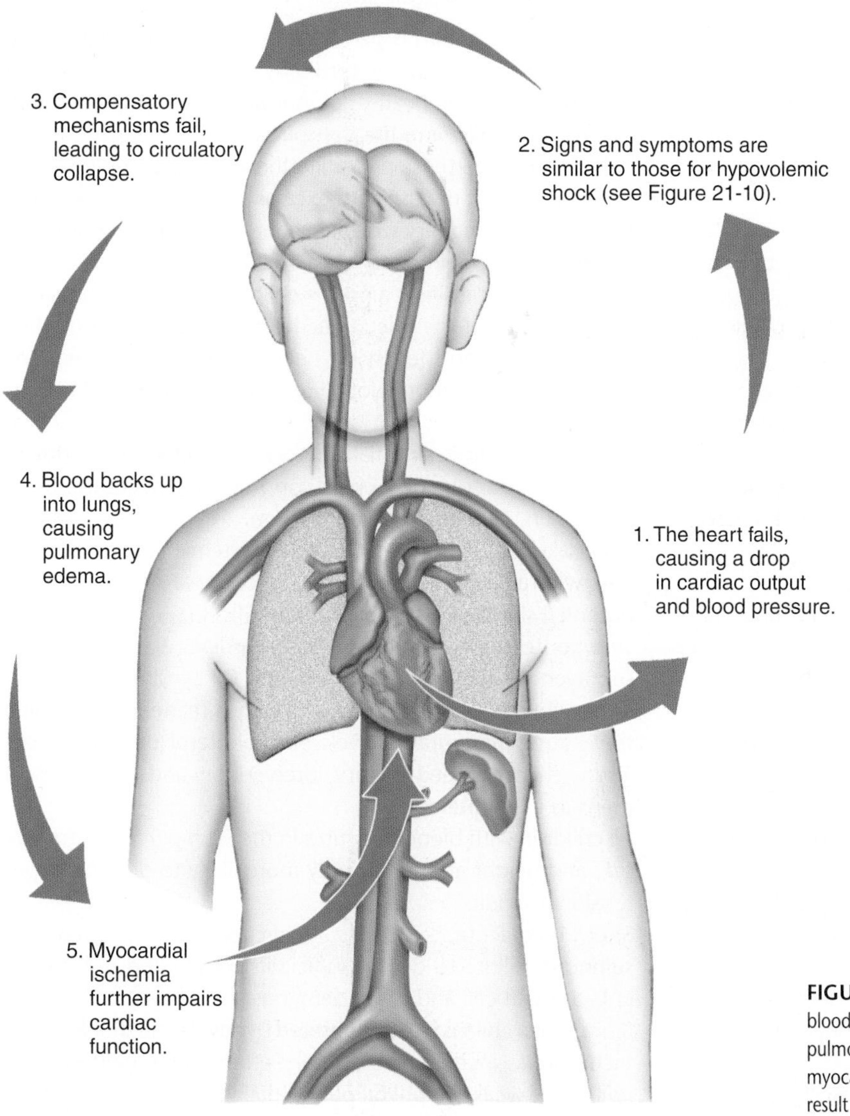

3. Compensatory mechanisms fail, leading to circulatory collapse.

2. Signs and symptoms are similar to those for hypovolemic shock (see Figure 21-10).

4. Blood backs up into lungs, causing pulmonary edema.

1. The heart fails, causing a drop in cardiac output and blood pressure.

5. Myocardial ischemia further impairs cardiac function.

FIGURE 21–12 ➤ When the heart fails, cardiac output and blood pressure decrease. Blood backs up into the lungs, causing pulmonary edema. Inadequate amounts of oxygen reach the myocardium, further impairing the heart's pumping action. The result is cardiogenic shock.

typically has chest discomfort because of fractured ribs or a chest wall contusion. An electrocardiogram reveals arrhythmias or signs of myocardial infarct. A two-dimensional echocardiogram may show an abnormality in heart wall movement. Cardiac troponin I levels and cardiac isoenzyme concentrations may be monitored for elevation. Because of the risk of sudden arrhythmias, the child is admitted to the intensive care unit for cardiac monitoring. Long-term problems could potentially include aneurysm, myocardial rupture, and cardiac tamponade (Roddy, Lange, & Klein, 2005).

NURSING MANAGEMENT
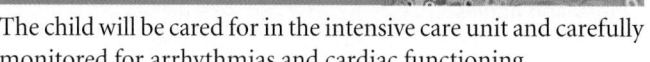

The child will be cared for in the intensive care unit and carefully monitored for arrhythmias and cardiac functioning.

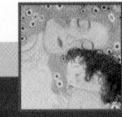

Chapter Highlights

- Infants are at risk of heart failure because they are more sensitive to volume or pressure overload.
- Increasing cardiac output is primarily heart rate dependent in infants and children under 5 years of age. After that age, the muscle fibers in the myocardium are developed enough to stretch and increase ventricular volume.
- Most congenital heart defects develop during the first 8 weeks of pregnancy, often the result of combined or interactive genetic and environmental factors.
- Congenital heart defects are categorized by pathophysiology and hemodynamics:
  - Defects that increase pulmonary blood flow include the following: patent ductus arteriosus, atrial septal defect, ventricular septal defect, and atrioventricular canal.
  - Defects that decrease pulmonary blood flow include the following: pulmonic stenosis, tetralogy of Fallot, pulmonary atresia, and tricuspid atresia.
  - Defects that decrease systemic blood flow include the following: aortic stenosis, coarctation of the aorta, and hypoplastic left heart syndrome.
  - Transposition of the great arteries and truncus arteriosus are examples of mixed defects that require mixing of the pulmonary and systemic circulations for survival during the neonatal period.
- Cardiac catheterization may be used to evaluate the hemodynamics and pressure gradients within the heart or to correct some heart defects.
- Infants with congenital heart defects that increase pulmonary blood flow are at high risk for development of congestive heart failure.
- The child with a congenital heart defect that decreases pulmonary blood flow may have life-threatening hypercyanotic episodes requiring emergency treatment.
- Congenital heart defects that obstruct systemic blood flow cause signs and symptoms associated with low cardiac output: diminished pulses, poor color, prolonged capillary refill time, and decreased urinary output.
- Signs of congestive heart failure may include tachypnea, tachycardia, pallor or cyanosis, nasal flaring, grunting, retractions, cough, crackles, periorbital and facial edema, jugular vein distention, and hepatomegaly.
- Cardiomyopathy during childhood occurs most often in infancy and adolescence.
- Heart transplantation is performed in infants and children for complex heart defects or cardiomyopathy. Rejection and infection are the major causes of mortality and morbidity during the first year following the transplant.
- Pulmonary hypertension is a life-threatening complication of congenital heart disease with excessive pulmonary blood flow. Irreversible pulmonary vascular changes include inflammation, hypertrophy of pulmonary vessels, and fibrosis.
- Infective endocarditis is a risk for children who have some congenital heart defects, rheumatic heart disease, or a central venous catheter, and following heart surgery or interventional cardiac catheterization. Not all cases of infectious endocarditis are preventable.
- Rheumatic fever is an inflammatory connective tissue disease following a streptococcal infection that may affect the heart, joints, skin, or central nervous system.
- Kawasaki disease is an acute febrile, systemic inflammatory illness with an unknown etiology. Coronary artery damage is a potential significant complication.
- Two potentially life-threatening cardiac arrhythmias are supraventricular tachycardia and long QT syndrome.
- Some children have familial or lifestyle-related dyslipidemia that causes undesirable levels of cholesterol or triglycerides. These children need dietary intervention and exercise regimens as initial therapies.
- All children with blood pressures in the 90th percentile for age, sex, and height are significantly more likely to develop hypertension as adults.
- Shock is an acute, complex state of circulatory dysfunction resulting in failure to deliver sufficient oxygen and other nutrients to meet cell and tissue demands.
- Signs that a child is in compensated hypovolemic shock include tachycardia, increased respiratory effort, prolonged capillary refill time, weak peripheral pulses, pallor, and cold extremities.
- Distributive shock is an abnormal distribution of the blood volume that results from a decrease in vascular resistance. It may be caused by anaphylaxis, sepsis, or spinal cord injury.
- Obstructive shock occurs when the main bloodstream is blocked (e.g., compression on the vena cava due to tension pneumothorax, pulmonary embolism, or coarctation of the aorta) and interferes with tissue perfusion.
- Myocardial contusion results from a strong, blunt force against the chest wall that injures the heart muscle.

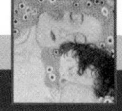

Clinical Reasoning in Action

Recall Tim, 16 years old, in the opening scenario who was born with the tetralogy of Fallot congenital heart defect. Despite successful corrective surgery as an infant, he recently had a pacemaker placed to help manage the episodic slow ventricular heart rate.

Tim is the oldest of two children; his brother is 10 years old. Tim had been able to participate in all usual school and childhood activities except sports until the past year. He has many friends, and he is friendly with several girls. Tim is becoming more aware of how different he is from his peers due to his heart defect and recent pacemaker implantation. His parents had previously made all of his health care decisions, but at the time the pacemaker was needed, Tim became more involved in the patient education and decision-making process. Now Tim is real-

izing that he must become much more involved in his health care, but does not know how to assume that responsibility.

1. What is the potential explanation for the development of an arrhythmia so many years after the original heart surgery?
2. What emotional and behavioral responses should be expected from Tim when learning more about his physical limitations and future health care needs?
3. Develop a teaching plan to educate Tim about his congenital heart condition and self-management to maintain his health status.
4. Develop a transition plan for Tim to begin taking primary responsibility for all aspects of his health care.

See Pearson Nursing Student Resources for possible responses.

Pearson Nursing Student Resources

Find additional review materials at
nursing.pearsonhighered.com
Prepare for success with NCLEX®-style practice questions, interactive assignments and activities, web links, animations and videos, and more!

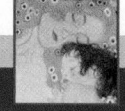

References

American Academy of Pediatrics, Committee on Infectious Disease. (2009). *Red book: Report of the Committee on Infectious Disease* (29th ed., pp. 413–418). Elk Grove Village, IL: Author.

Barnes, V. A., Davis, H. C., Murzynowski, J. B., & Treiber, F. A. (2004). Impact of meditation on resting and ambulatory blood pressure and heart rate in youth. *Psychosomatic Medicine, 66*, 909–914.

Belay, B., Belamarich, P. F., & Tom-Revzon, C. (2007). The use of statins in pediatrics: Knowledge base, limitations, and future directions. *Pediatrics, 119*(2), 370–380.

Bindler, R. M., Howry, L. B., Wilson, B. A., Shannon, M. T., & Stang, C. L. (2005). *Pediatric drug guide.* Upper Saddle River, NJ: Prentice Hall.

Blume, E. D., Naftel, D. C., Bastardi, H. J., Duncan, B. W., Kirklin, J. K., Webber, S. A., et al. (2006). Outcomes of children bridged to heart transplantation with ventricular assist devices: A multi-institutional study. *Circulation, 113*, 2313–2319.

Brady, T., Siberry, G. K., & Solomon, B. (2008). Pediatric hypertension. *Contemporary Pediatrics, 25*(11), 46–56.

Brosig, C. L., Mussatto, K. A., Kuhn, E. M., & Tweddel, J. S. (2007). Neurodevelopmental outcome in preschool survivors of complex congenital

heart disease: Implications for clinical practice. *Journal of Pediatric Health Care, 21*(1), 3–12.

Callahan, J. M. (2008). Pulse oximetry in emergency medicine. *Emergency Medicine Clinics of North America, 26*, 869–879.

Cook, E. H., & Higgins, S. S. (2010). Congenital heart disease. In P. J. Allen, J. A. Vessey, & N. A. Shapiro, *Primary care of the child with a chronic condition* (5th ed., pp. 385–404). St. Louis, MO: Mosby Elsevier.

Covelli, M. M. (2007). Prevalence of behavioral and physiological risk factors of hypertension in African American adolescents. *Pediatric Nursing, 33*(4), 323–332.

Cox, G. F., Sleeper, L. A., Lowe, A. M., Towbin, J. A., Colan, S. D., Orav, E. J., et al. (2006). Factors associated with establishing a causal diagnosis for children with cardiomyopathy. *Pediatrics, 118*(4), 1519–1531.

Daniels, S. R., Greer, F. R., & Committee on Nutrition. (2008). Lipid screening and cardiovascular health in childhood. *Pediatrics, 122*(1), 198–207.

Dieckmann, R. A. (Ed.). (2006). *Pediatric education for prehospital professionals* (2nd ed., pp. 83–84). Sudbury, MA: Jones and Bartlett.

Doniger, S., & Sharieff, G. Q. (2006). Pediatric dysrhythmias. *Pediatric Clinics in North America, 53*, 85–105.

Feld, L. G., & Corey, H. (2007). Hypertension in childhood. *Pediatrics in Review, 28*(8), 283–297.

Gerber, M. A., Baltimore, R. S., Eaton, C. B., Gewitz, M., Rowley, A. H., Shulman, S., & Taubert, K. A. (2009). Prevention of rheumatic fever and diagnosis and treatment of acute streptococcal pharyngitis. *Circulation, 119*, 1541–1551.

Gidding, S., Dennison, B. A., Birch, L. L., Daniels, S. R., Gillman, M. W., Lichtenstein, A. H., et al. (2005). Dietary recommendations for children and adolescents: A guide for practitioners. Consensus statement from the American Heart Association. *Circulation, 112*, 2061–2075.

Gillespie, M. J., Schneider, H. E., & Rome, J. (2006). The use of cardiac catheterization to diagnose and treat heart diseases in pediatric patients. In V. L. Vetter, *Pediatric cardiology: The requisites in pediatrics* (pp. 195–221). St. Louis, MO: Elsevier Mosby.

Hobbs, J. B., Peterson, D. R., Moss, A. J., McNitt, S., Zareba, W., Goldenberg, I., et al. (2006). Risk of aborted cardiac arrest or sudden cardiac death during adolescence in the long-QT syndrome.

Journal of the American Medical Association, *296*(10), 1249–1254.

Holcomb, S. S. (2009). Common herb drug interactions: What you should know. *Nurse Practitioner,* *34*(5), 21–29.

Jago, R., Harrell, J. S., McMurray, R. G., Edelstein, S., El Ghormli, L., & Bassin, S. (2006). Prevalence of abnormal lipid and blood pressure values among ethnically diverse population of eighth-grade adolescents and screening implications. *Pediatrics,* *117*(6), 2065–2073.

Joshi, V. M., & Sekhavat, S. (2006). Acyanotic congenital heart defects. In V. L. Vetter, *Pediatric cardiology: The requisites in pediatrics* (pp. 79–96). St. Louis, MO: Elsevier Mosby.

Khairy, P., Poirer, N., & Mercier, L. (2007). Univentricular heart. *Circulation, 115,* 800–812.

Kon, A. A. (2005). Discussing nonsurgical care with parents of newborns with hypoplastic left heart syndrome. *Newborn and Infant Reviews,* *5*(2), 60–68.

Mahle, W. T., Visconti, K. J., Freier, M. C., Kanne, S. M., Hamilton, W. G., Sharkey, A. M., et al. (2006). Relationship of surgical approach to neurodevelopmental outcomes in hypoplastic left heart syndrome. *Pediatrics,* *117*(1), e90–e97.

Majnemer, A., Limperopoulos, C., Shevell, M., Rosenblatt, B., Rohlicek, C., & Tchervenkov, C. (2006). Long-term neuromotor outcome at school entry of infants with congenital heart defects requiring open-heart surgery. *Journal of Pediatrics,* *148*(1), 72–77.

Marino, B. S., Ostrow, A. M., & Cohen, M. S. (2006). Surgery for congenital heart disease. In V. L. Vetter, *Pediatric cardiology: The requisites in pediatrics* (pp. 277–320). St. Louis, MO: Elsevier Mosby.

McDaniel, N. L. (2010). Alterations of cardiovascular function in children. In K. L. McCance, S. E. Huether, V. L. Brashers, & N. R. Rote, *Pathophysiology: The biologic basis for disease in adults and children* (6th ed., pp. 1209–1241). St. Louis, MO: Mosby Elsevier.

McKiernan, C. A., & Lieberman, S. A. (2005). Circulatory shock in children: An overview. *Pediatrics in Review, 26*(12), 451–459.

Menteer, J., Hogarty, A. N., & Chrisant, M. R. K. (2006). Heart failure in pediatrics. In V. L. Vetter, Pediatric Cardiology: The requisites in pediatrics (pp. 159–169), St. Louis: Mosby Elsevier.

Miatton, M., De Wolf, D., François, K., Thiery, E., & Vingerhoets, G. (2007). Neuropsychological performance in school-aged children with surgically corrected congenital heart disease. *Journal of Pediatrics, 151*(1), 73–78.

Milana, C., & Chandran, L. (2006). What's new in Kawasaki disease? *Contemporary Pediatrics, 23*(7), 40–47.

Miller, S. P., McQuillen, P. S., Hamrick, S., Xu, D., Glidden, D. V., Charlton, N., et al. (2007). Abnormal brain development in newborns with congenital heart disease. *New England Journal of Medicine, 357*(19), 1928–1938.

Morales, D. L. S., Dreyer, W. J., Denfield, S. W., Heinle, J. S., McKenzie, E. D., Graves, D. E., et al. (2007). Over two decades of pediatric heart transplantation: How has survival changed? *Journal of Thoracic and Cardiovascular Surgery, 133*(3), 632–639.

National Center for Complementary and Alternative Medicine (NCCAM). (2009). *Meditation: An introduction.* Retrieved from http://nccam.nih .gov/health/meditation/overview.htm

Newburger, J. W., Sleeper, L. A., McCrindle, B. W., Minich, L., Gersony, W., Vetter, V. L., et al. (2007). Randomized trial of pulsed corticosteroid therapy for primary treatment of Kawasaki disease. *New England Journal of Medicine, 356*(7), 663–675.

Park, M. K. (2008). *Pediatric cardiology for practitioners* (5th ed.). St. Louis, MO: Mosby.

Ralston, M., Hazinski, M. F., Zaritsky, A. L., Schexnayder, S., & Kleinman, M. E. (2006). *Pediatric advanced life support: Provider manual.* Dallas, TX: American Heart Association.

Reis, E. C., Kip, K. E., Marroquin, O. C., Kiesau, M., Hipps, L., & Peters, R. E. (2006). Screening children to identify families at increased risk for cardiovascular disease. *Pediatrics, 118*(6), e1789–e1797.

Roddy, M. G., Lange, P. A., & Klein, B. L. (2005). Cardiac trauma in children. *Clinical Pediatric Emergency Medicine, 6,* 234–243.

Rothstein, R., Paris, Y., & Quizon, A. (2009). Pulmonary hypertension. *Pediatrics in Review, 30*(2), 39–45.

Sadowski, S. L. (2009). Congenital cardiac disease in the newborn infant: Past, present, and future. *Critical Care Nursing Clinics of North America, 21,* 37–48.

Schlechte, E. A., Boramanand, N., & Funk, M. (2008). Supraventricular tachycardia in the pediatric primary care setting: Age-related presentation, diagnosis, and management. *Journal of Pediatric Health Care, 22*(5), 289–299.

Schneider, H. E., & Goldmuntz, E. (2006). The genetics of congenital heart disease. In V. L. Vetter, *Pediatric cardiology: The requisites in pediatrics* (pp. 145–157). St. Louis, MO: Elsevier Mosby.

Schultz, A. H., & Kreutzer, J. (2006). Cyanotic heart disease. In V. L. Vetter, *Pediatric cardiology: The requisites in pediatrics* (pp. 51–78). St. Louis, MO: Elsevier Mosby.

Shillingford, A. J., Glanzman, M. M., Ittenbach, R. F., Clancy, R. R., Gaynor, J. W., & Wernovsky, G. (2008). Inattention, hyperactivity, and school performance in a population of school-aged children with complex congenital heart disease. *Pediatrics, 121*(4), e759–e766.

Sivarajan, V. B., Vetter, V. L., & Gleason, M. M. (2006). Pediatric evaluation of the cardiac patient. In V. L. Vetter, *Pediatric cardiology: The requisites in pediatrics* (pp. 1–30). St. Louis, MO: Elsevier Mosby.

Son, M. B. F., Gauvreau, K., Ma, L., Baker, A., Sundel, R. P., Fulton, D. R., & Newburger, J. W. (2009). Treatment of Kawasaki disease: Analysis of 27 US pediatric hospitals from 2001 to 2006. *Pediatrics, 124*(1), 1–8.

Sudan, D., Bacha, E. A., John, E., & Bartholomew, A. (2007). Childhood organ transplantation. *Pediatrics in Review, 28*(12), 439–453.

Towbin, J. A., Lowe, A. M., Colan, S. D., Sleeper, L. A., Orav, E. J., Clunie, S., et al. (2006). Incidence, causes, and outcomes of dilated cardiomyopathy in children. *Journal of the American Medical Association, 296*(15), 1867–1876.

Vetter, V. L. (2006). Kawasaki disease. In V. L. Vetter, *Pediatric cardiology: The requisites in pediatrics* (pp. 131–144). St. Louis, MO: Elsevier Mosby.

Warnes, C. A., Williams, R. G., Bashore, T. M., Child, J. S., Connolly, H. M., Dearani, J. A., et al. (2008). ACC/ACH guidelines for the care of adults with congenital heart disease: A report of the American College of Cardiology and the American Heart Association task force on practice guidelines. *Circulation, 118,* e714–e833.

Wilson, B. A., Shannon, M. T., & Shields, K. M. (2009). *Nurses' drug guide 2009.* Upper Saddle River, NJ: Prentice Hall Health.

Wilson, W., Taubert, K. A., Gewitz, M., Lockhart, P. B., Baddour, L. M., Levison, M., et al. (2007). Prevention of infective endocarditis: Guidelines from the American Heart Association Rheumatic Fever, Endocarditis, and Kawasaki Disease Committee, Council on Cardiovascular Disease in the Young, and the Council on Clinical Cardiology, Council on Cardiovascular Surgery and Anesthesia, and the Quality of Care and Outcomes Research Interdisciplinary Working Group. *Circulation, 116,* 1736–1754.

Zeigler, V. L. (2008). Congenital heart disease and genetics. *Critical Care Nursing Clinics of North America, 20,* 159–169.

Zeltser, I., & Tabbutt, S. (2006). Critical heart disease in the newborn. In V. L. Vetter, *Pediatric cardiology: The requisites in pediatrics* (pp. 31–50). St. Louis, MO: Elsevier Mosby.

Alterations in Immune Function

chapter 22

Raymond, a 2-year-old child, has had recurrent infections since he was born. In the last 3 months, he has had bronchitis twice, otitis media three times, and several colds. Raymond has had fever, vomiting, and diarrhea for several days, and does not appear to be improving. His mother brings him to an ambulatory clinic for evaluation.

After a thorough history is taken, blood tests are performed to assess Raymond's immune function. On the basis of an evaluation of Raymond's clinical symptoms and the results of the laboratory tests, he sees a specialist and is diagnosed with acquired immunodeficiency syndrome (AIDS). Raymond is admitted to a special unit of the hospital for children with human immunodeficiency virus (HIV)/AIDS so that his treatment can begin. Like many of the other children, Raymond is often irritable and difficult to console. Because he vomits frequently, the nurses pay particular attention to Raymond's nutritional problems, giving him frequent small feedings.

Raymond is diagnosed as having failure to thrive, a common sequela of AIDS. Broad-spectrum antibiotics are given, and he is assessed frequently for the development of new infections. Drugs for treatment of HIV are initiated. A multidisciplinary team of nurses, physicians, nutritionists, and social services professionals are involved in planning Raymond's care. In addition to medications, what are important components of the treatment plan for Raymond? What are the nursing priorities for his care?

Learning Outcomes

After reading this chapter, you will be able to do the following:

1. Describe the structure and function of the immune system.
2. Apply knowledge of the immune system to the care of children with immunological disorders.
3. Explain the differences between primary and secondary immunodeficiency.
4. Summarize infection control measures to prevent the spread of infection to children with an immunodeficiency.
5. Develop a nursing care plan in partnership with the family for a child with human immunodeficiency virus (HIV).
6. Contrast the differences between immune deficiency diseases and autoimmune diseases.
7. Plan nursing care for the child with an autoimmune condition such as systemic lupus erythematosus or juvenile idiopathic arthritis.
8. Describe exposure prevention measures for the child with latex allergy.
9. Apply nursing interventions and prevention measures for the child experiencing other hypersensitivity reactions.

FOCUS ON

The Immune System

ANATOMY AND PHYSIOLOGY

The function of the immune system is to recognize any foreign substances within the body—in simple terms, to distinguish "nonself" from "self"—and to eliminate foreign substances as efficiently as possible. When the body recognizes the presence of a substance that it cannot identify as part of itself, the body protects itself through the immune response. Normally, the immune system responds to an invasion of foreign substances, or antigens, in numerous ways. It produces **antibodies**, or proteins that work against **antigens**, the foreign substances that trigger the immune response. There are many types of antibodies, which are described later in this section. The immune system also produces other types of cells, such as T lymphocytes and natural killer (NK) cells.

Immunity is either natural or acquired. **Natural immunity** comprises the defenses present at birth, such as intact skin, body pH, natural antibodies from the mother, and inflammatory and phagocytic properties. **Acquired immunity** consists of humoral (antibody-mediated) and cell-mediated immunity and is not fully developed until a child is about 6 years of age.

Humoral immunity is responsible for destroying bacterial antigens. B lymphocytes, produced in the bone marrow, gut, and other lymphoid tissue, are the central factor in humoral immunity, and develop into plasma cells that produce antibodies. Antibodies are a type of protein called **immunoglobulins**, of which there are five types: IgM, IgG, IgA, IgD, and IgE (Table 22–1). IgM, IgG, and IgA act to control a number of body infections, whereas IgE is useful in combating parasitic infections and is part of the allergic response. The role of IgD is unknown (Diamond & Grimaldi, 2009).

Antibodies are found in serum, body fluids, and certain tissues. When a child is first exposed to an antigen, the B-lymphocyte system begins to produce antibodies that react specifically to that antigen (Figure 22–1 ➤). It takes approximately 3 days for this process, known as a **primary immune response**, to occur. Subsequent encounters with the antigen trigger memory cells, resulting in a **secondary immune response** within 24 hours.

Cellular immunity or *cell-mediated immunity* uses T lymphocytes, produced mainly in the thymus, to provide cellular immunity and protect against most viruses, fungi, slowly developing bacterial infections such as tuberculosis, and tumors. In addition, they control the timing of the response in delayed hypersensitivity reactions, such as the purified protein derivative (PPD) test, and they are responsible for the rejection of foreign grafts, such as transplants. Specialized types of T lymphocytes include killer T cells, suppressor T cells, and helper T cells. Suppressor T cells inhibit B lymphocytes from differentiating into plasma cells. Helper T cells aid in the proliferation and immunologic function of other cells. T lymphocytes have proteins on their surfaces that attract and trap receptors; they can be used to measure the immune activity of these cells. For example, some of the common proteins are CD2, CD3, CD4, CD5, CD7, and CD8. Natural killer (NK) cells (also known as non-B/non-T lymphocytes) originate in the bone marrow and thymus and migrate to the blood and spleen. They play a role in control of viral infection, tumors, and autoimmune diseases.

Complement is a component of blood serum consisting of 11 protein compounds. It is an inactive enzyme that activates in response to antigen-antibody functions, resulting in a generalized inflammatory reaction that kills foreign cells. It also plays a role in causing some autoimmune diseases.

Immune cells also secrete proteins called **cytokines** that carry messages for immune system function. Lymphocytes, monocytes, and macrophages all secrete cytokines that have a variety of effects on the target cells. Effects may include stimulation of growth through proliferation of cells, differentiation of cellular actions, production of inflammation, sensitization to pain, and other actions. Interleukins, a type of cytokine, were first identified in white blood cells but now are known to be present in many cells. Many types of interleukins have been identified and some are known to influence the function of the immune system.

PEDIATRIC DIFFERENCES

Immune system development is a complex and multifactorial process. Early in-utero experiences, environmental exposures after birth, and other factors influence this important feedback system. It protects children from harmful diseases but also leads to conditions such as asthma (Chapter 20 ∞), food allergy (Chapter 14 ∞), or skin atopy (Chapter 31 ∞).

TABLE 22–1	Classes of Immunoglobulins
IgM	Present in intravascular spaces
IgG	Present in all body fluids
IgA	Present in secretions of gastrointestinal, respiratory, and genitourinary tracts
IgD	Present in blood, lymph, and surfaces of B cells
IgE	Present in internal and external body fluids

Primary and Secondary Immune Response Video

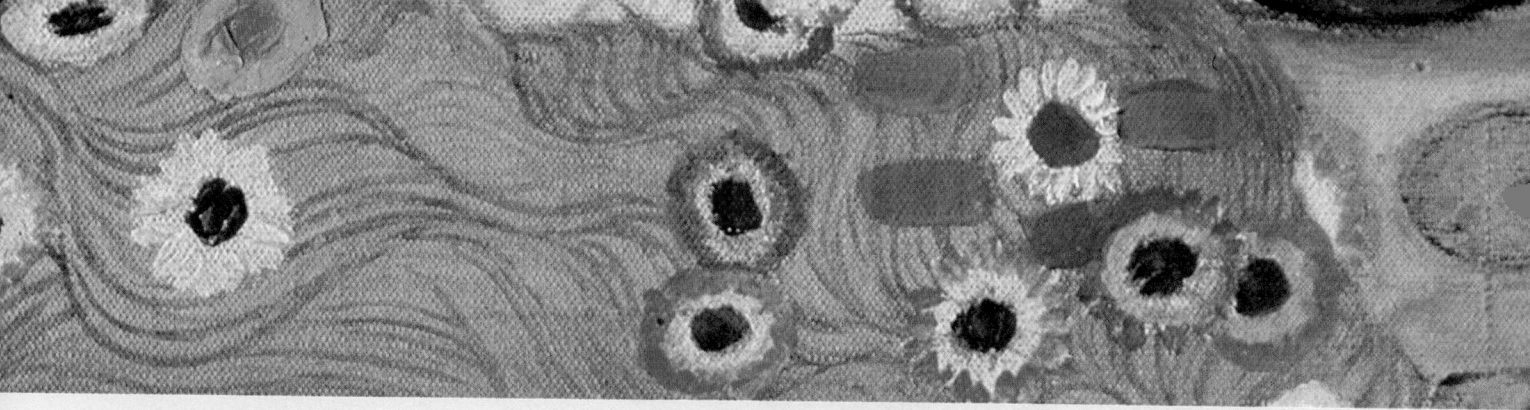

Pathophysiology Illustrated

Primary Immune Response

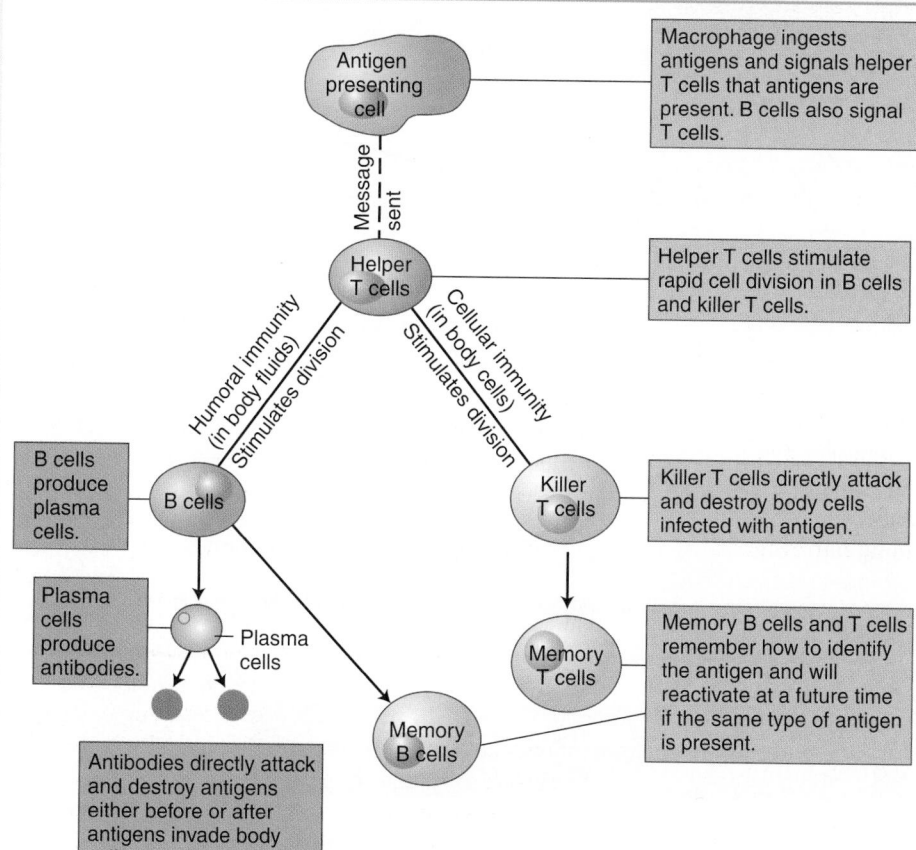

Antigen presenting cell

Macrophage ingests antigens and signals helper T cells that antigens are present. B cells also signal T cells.

Message sent

Helper T cells

Helper T cells stimulate rapid cell division in B cells and killer T cells.

Humoral immunity (in body fluids)
Stimulates division

Cellular immunity (in body cells)
Stimulates division

B cells produce plasma cells.

B cells

Killer T cells

Killer T cells directly attack and destroy body cells infected with antigen.

Plasma cells produce antibodies.

Plasma cells

Memory T cells

Memory B cells and T cells remember how to identify the antigen and will reactivate at a future time if the same type of antigen is present.

Memory B cells

Antibodies directly attack and destroy antigens either before or after antigens invade body cells.

FIGURE 22–1 ➤ The primary immune response encompasses a cascade of events that involve humoral and cellular immunity.

Infants and children have differing amounts of some immunoglobulins. IgG is the only immunoglobulin that crosses the placenta; as a result, a newborn's levels are similar to those of the mother (Buckley, 2007). This maternal IgG disappears by 6 to 8 months of age. The infant's IgG then increases gradually until mature levels are reached at 7 to 8 years. IgM levels are low at birth, rise markedly at 1 week of age, and continue to increase until adult levels are reached at about 1 year. IgA and IgE are not present at birth. Manufacture of these immunoglobulins begins by 2 weeks of age; however, normal values are not achieved until 6 to 7 years. It is thus easy to see why children under 6 years of age become ill so often—they do not have a full complement of immunoglobulins.

In contrast, cell-mediated immunity achieves full function early in life. Early in fetal life, the thymus begins producing T cells. By birth, many of these cells are present. The thymus is large at birth, grows during childhood, reaches peak size just before puberty, and then decreases in size (Buckley, 2007). Other lymphoid tissues, such as the spleen and tonsils, are also comparatively large in young children. Because of the well-developed cellular immunity, any blood infused into newborns is generally irradiated to prevent **graft-versus-host disease**

Growth & Development *Newborns and Immunity*

Newborns are most prone to development of infection, particularly when born premature, since they have lower levels of their own immune protections, as well as less IgG obtained from the mother. Feeding of human milk is protective against newborn infections (Heird, 2007).

(a series of immunologic reactions in response to transplanted cells) from transfused lymphocytes (Figure 22–2 ➤).

Newborns have somewhat lower numbers of NK cells than older children and adults, decreasing their ability to respond to certain antigens. The levels of some complement proteins are lower in newborns than in older children and adults, thus delaying and hampering response to certain infections. Levels of monocytes and macrophages are low (Marodi, 2006).

Examples of diagnostic and laboratory tests used to evaluate immune system function are provided in Table 22–2. Use the Assessment Guidelines below to perform a nursing assessment of the immune system.

As Children Grow

Immunoglobulins Throughout Childhood

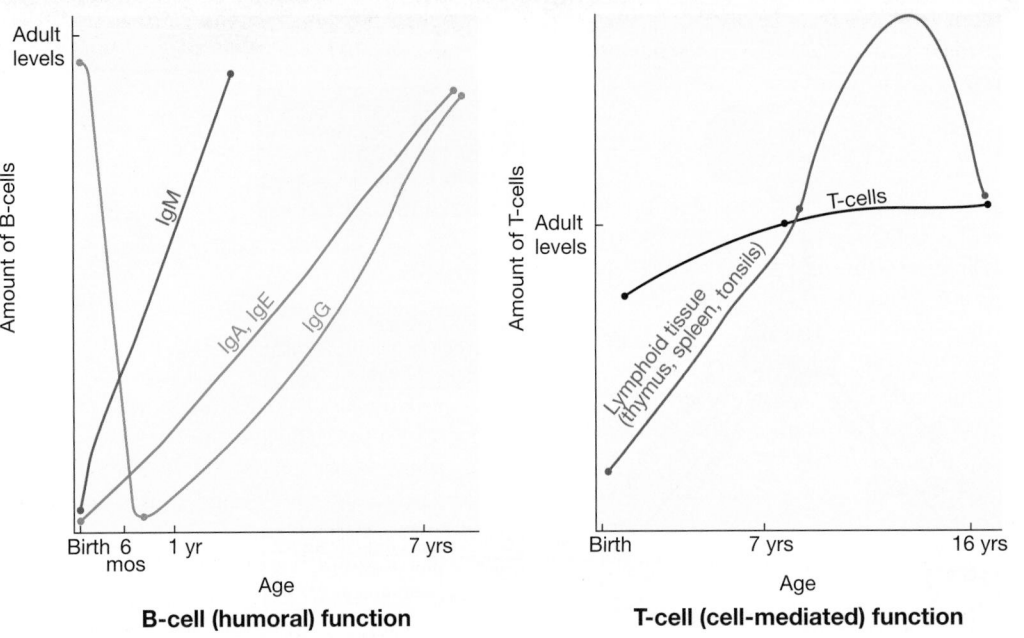

FIGURE 22–2 ➤ Different types of immunoglobulins mature at variable times throughout childhood. Children have high levels of some types of immunoglobulins, while others may be low at certain periods during development.

TABLE 22–2 **Diagnostic Tests and Laboratory Procedures for the Immune System***	
Diagnostic Test	Laboratory Test
HIV tests—see Table 22–5	Complete blood count
Radioallergosorbent test (RAST)—see page 670	Complement
Skin reactions (intradermal skin testing)—see Figure 22–7	Immunoglobulins

*See Appendices D and E ∞ for information about these diagnostic procedures and tests.

Assessment Guidelines for the Child with an Immune System Alteration

Assessment Focus	Assessment Guidelines
Family history	▪ Does a family member have a history of allergy? ▪ Does the mother or other family member have a history of HIV or other immune system disorder? ▪ Has the child been treated prophylactically for HIV due to the mother's positive status?
Growth and development	▪ Is growth regular? Is the child meeting developmental milestones? What is the child's food intake and appetite?
Skin and mucous membranes	▪ Is the skin intact? Are there lesions of the mucous membranes? ▪ Do lesions heal quickly without additional infection?
Evidence of disease	▪ Does the child have a history of recurring or unusual infections?

What are the signs and symptoms of immunologic disorders in children? Many times they are nonspecific. Raymond's admitting signs and symptoms, described in the opening scenario, are characteristic of several different immunodeficiency disorders. The immune system is one of the few body systems that regulates, either directly or indirectly, all other body functions. Thus, a problem with the immune system can have multisystem consequences and may be life threatening. Allergic reactions to food or frequent episodes of otitis media may indicate a disorder of immune function. Immune conditions can be mild to severe and can be life threatening. Congenital abnormalities sometimes signal a defect in cellular immunity. In this chapter, some of the common disorders of immune function will be examined, with a discussion of nursing care for children and their families.

IMMUNODEFICIENCY DISORDERS

Immunodeficiency, a state of decreased responsiveness of the immune system, can occur to varying degrees in response to any number of events. Children with congenital immunodeficiency, or **primary immune deficiency**, are born with a failure of humoral antibody formation (B-cell disorder), a deficient cellular immune system (T-cell disorder), or a combination of both defects. In congenital disorders, the immune deficiency is not caused by another condition. However, immunodeficiency may also be acquired, as in human immunodeficiency virus (HIV) infection. Acquired immunodeficiency is also called **secondary immune deficiency**.

B-Cell and T-Cell Disorders

In B-cell disorders, immunoglobulins may be present in inadequate numbers or nearly absent. X-linked hypogammaglobulinemia, selective IgA deficiency, and common variable immunodeficiency are examples of such disorders (Michaels & Green, 2007). Because newborns are protected from infection by maternal antibodies in the first months after birth, symptoms of B-cell disorders usually become apparent after 3 months of age. Infants with these disorders have frequent recurrent bacterial infections and failure to thrive. With treatment, consisting of in-

travenous immunoglobulins and antibiotics, most children survive into adulthood. Prognosis depends on the degree of antibody deficiency.

T-cell disorders are characterized by inadequate numbers of T lymphocytes or absence of T-cell functions. Isolated T-cell disorders are rare, usually accompanied by a B-cell disorder, and may be associated with congenital abnormalities (as in DiGeorge syndrome) or of unknown cause. Table 22–3 compares laboratory values for selected congenital immunodeficiency disorders.

DiGeorge syndrome, a T-cell disorder caused by chromosome deletion at 22q11.2, is usually diagnosed soon after birth. In the general population the estimated incidence is 1 per 2,000–4,000 (Bawle, 2008). The syndrome is characterized by absence (complete DiGeorge) or hypoplasia (partial DiGeorge) of parathyroid or thymus glands, hypocalcemia with tetany within 24–48 hours after birth, cardiac defects, low-set ears, hypertelorism (widely set eyes), and viral and bacterial infections in the neonatal period (Buckley, 2007, 2008). Generally a mild to moderate decrease in T-lymphocyte counts is found (McLean-Tooke, Spickett, & Gennery, 2007). Prophylactic antibiotics are used to prevent bacterial infections. Children with partial DiGeorge are treated with calcium and vitamin D supplements. Those with complete DiGeorge need thymus transplantation in order to survive (Buckley, 2008).

Immunodeficiency with hyper-IgM is a T-cell disorder that primarily affects males and causes decreased T-cell function, variable abnormal levels of immunoglobulins, and high titers of some antibodies. It is usually X-linked but is autosomal in some cases. Recurrent bacterial infections including pneumonia, upper respiratory tract infections, and otitis media occur in children with this disorder (Lewis, Nadeau, & Cohen, 2009). Treatment with intravenous immune globulin (IVIG) therapy is helpful although later malignancies and liver disease can occur (Nagaraj, Egwim, & Adler, 2007).

Severe Combined Immunodeficiency Disease

Severe combined immunodeficiency disease (SCID) is a congenital condition characterized by absence of both humoral and

TABLE 22–3 Laboratory Findings for Selected Congenital Immunodeficiency Disorders

Disorders	Laboratory Findings
B cell	
X-linked hypogammaglobulinemia	Reduced IgA, IgM, IgE, IgG (less than 100 mg/dL), absence of B cells in peripheral blood, normal T cells
Selective IgA deficiency	IgA less than 10 mg/dL
Common variable immunodeficiency	IgA, IgM reduced; IgG less than 250 mg/dL
T cell	
DiGeorge syndrome	Lymphopenia; absent T-cell functions, decreased T cells, normal B cells
Immunodeficiency with hyper-IgM	Reduced IgG, IgA; elevated IgM; mutations in T-cell surface proteins
Combined	
Severe combined immunodeficiency syndrome (SCID)	Complete absence of T- and B-cell and NK immunity
Wiskott-Aldrich syndrome	Thrombocytopenia, low platelet volume, nonfunctional B cells, normal IgG, decreased IgM, increased IgA, increased IgE; inability to respond to polysaccharide antigens

cellular immunity that is manifested by lack of appropriately functioning T cells and B cells (Joshi & Davies, 2009; Yee, DeRavin, Elliott, et al., 2008). SCID occurs in X-linked recessive and autosomal recessive forms. In some cases, SCID may be the result of chromosomal abnormalities. The disorder is much more common in males than females and is estimated to occur in 1 per 50,000 live births (Lewis et al., 2009). Without appropriate treatment, children born with SCID usually do not survive more than 1 year (Joshi & Davies, 2009; Kobrynski, 2006).

Etiology and Pathophysiology

Severe combined immunodeficiency disease is caused by genetic mutations that lead to impaired lymphoid development in children with low T and NK cells. The B lymphocytes may appear normal in number but their function is compromised due to the severe T-cell deficiency (Bonilla & Geha, 2006; Buckley, 2007).

Clinical Manifestations

Symptoms of SCID develop early in life. The infant often demonstrates a susceptibility to infection, presenting during the first few months of life with persistent respiratory infections and diarrhea (Buckley, 2007). Recurrent oral candidiasis, failure to thrive, and skin infections are also frequently seen in children. Additionally, failure to completely recover from infection, frequent reinfection, and infection with viruses such as cytomegalovirus and the bacterium *Pneumocystis carinii* (*jiroveci*) are common to the child with SCID (Buckley, 2007; Kobrynski, 2006). Children are also highly susceptible to serious infections such as meningitis, skin or organ infection, osteomyelitis, or sepsis.

COLLABORATIVE CARE

A marked reduction in lymphocyte counts is indicative of SCID. Patients with SCID generally have very few T cells and NK cells (Joshi & Davies, 2009). The B-lymphocyte count may be decreased, elevated, or normal, although these cells do not function normally. Immunoglobulin levels are significantly reduced (Joshi & Davies, 2009; Kobrynski, 2006). Refer to Table 22–3 on page 649 for laboratory findings in SCID. Diagnosis is usually made only after extensive laboratory testing. In addition to a complete blood count, erythrocyte sedimentation rate, and B- and T-cell lymphocyte counts, other studies including IgA, IgG, and IgM antibody titers; neutrophil count; and titer levels of immunizations received and neutrophil count may be performed (Table 22–4). A chest radiograph is conducted to assess thymus size.

The standard therapy for severe combined immunodeficiency disease is the administration of IVIG, which is administered to provide protection until humoral immunity is established. Hematopoietic stem cell transplantation offers the best hope for children with SCID (see Chapter 23 ∞). T-cell function is restored with the transplantation, and new cells appear 3 to 4 months after infusion of the donor stem cells. Prognosis for the child is poor without aggressive therapy and transplant.

With the identification of the genetic defect for SCID in recent years, gene therapy has been successfully attempted to treat a small number of children. Due to the subsequent development of leukemia in some of these patients, this form of treatment is under review (Bonilla & Geha, 2006; Puck & Malech, 2006).

Prevention and prompt treatment of infection are essential. Antibiotic therapy is targeted at infectious agents. Antibiotic prophylaxis and specific immunization recommendations for immunodeficiency are needed. Children with T-cell deficiencies should receive cytomegalovirus-negative irradiated blood products due to the risk of infection and graft-versus-host disease from lymphocytes in donor blood (Kobrynski, 2006).

NURSING MANAGEMENT

Nursing Assessment and Diagnosis

Obtain a thorough history of infections, including age of onset, type of causal organism, frequency, and severity. Assess family history, and find out if the child has had any unusual reactions to vaccines, medications, or foods. Measure the child's height and weight accurately to identify failure to thrive. Assess the child's nutritional intake and fluid and electrolyte balance. Assess for evidence of infections involving the skin, subcutaneous tissues, respiratory system, and mucous membranes. Palpate the abdomen for hepatomegaly and the lymph nodes for lymphadenopathy. Perform a developmental assessment and assess for delays in achievement of developmental milestones. Assess family support systems and coping mechanisms when a child is diagnosed with the disorder.

TABLE 22–4 Cells Evaluated in Laboratory Studies for Immune Conditions	
Test, Type of Cell, and Action	Implication of Increased or Decreased Levels
White blood cell (WBC) count	
Neutrophil Phagocytic cell that defends against bacteria	Increased in bacterial infection, inflammatory processes, and some malignancies
Eosinophil Associated with antigen–antibody reaction	Increased in allergic reaction Decreased in children receiving corticosteroids
Lymphocytes (T, B, non-B/non-T [NK]) Major components of immune system	Increased in many infections Decreased in children with immune deficiency
Immunoglobulins	
(IgM, IgG, IgA, IgD, IgE) Many roles in a number of immunologic reactions	Increased in presence of infection or allergic response; decreased in children with immune deficiency

The primary nursing diagnosis for a child with SCID is Risk for Infection related to immunodeficiency. Other nursing diagnoses may include the following:

- Imbalanced Nutrition: Less than Body Requirements related to chronic illness
- Risk for Impaired Skin Integrity related to immunologic deficit
- Risk for Caregiver Role Strain related to a child with a chronic, life-threatening illness
- Risk for Delayed Growth and Development related to chronic illness

Planning and Implementation

Nursing care of the child who is immunodeficient focuses on preventing infection. However, even with the use of environmental controls, such as keeping children inside special units to maintain a sterile environment, these children are prone to **opportunistic infections** (those caused by organisms that are usually nonpathogenic but can cause infections in persons who lack normal immunity).

Prevent Systemic Infection

Frequent and thorough hand hygiene is important. Standard precautions are always used, with transmission-based precautions when indicated. Implement sterile aseptic technique when caring for all sites where needles, catheters, central lines, endotracheal tubes, pressure-monitoring lines, and peripheral intravenous lines enter the child's body. Food and other items entering the hospital room may need special treatment. The child should be placed in a private room, and contact with infectious individuals should be avoided. Inform parents that live vaccines are avoided for the child because of the risk of infection. See Chapter 16 ∞ and the Centers for Disease Control and Prevention (CDC) website for information about immunization recommendations in the immunocompromised child.

Promote Skin Integrity

The skin is the only intact defense for many children who are immunodeficient. Provide thorough and frequent skin care, and observe all possible pressure areas closely for signs of breakdown or infection. Reposition the child frequently and encourage range of motion exercises.

Promote Nutritional Balance

Encourage adequate fluid and nutritional intake. Provide foods that the child prefers and those with high nutritional value. Offer small frequent feedings of high-calorie, protein-rich foods. Monitor development and weigh the child daily. Refer to a dietitian as needed to plan with parents the best individualized diet for the child.

Manage Medication Therapy

Many of the medications used in the long-term treatment of children with SCID have numerous side effects. Monitor closely for side effects of antibiotics, such as overgrowth of resistant organisms (e.g., thrush infections in the mouth, *Clostridium difficile* infections of the gastrointestinal tract) and administer IVIG safely. See Medications Used to Treat Immune Disorders.

Provide Emotional Support and Referral

SCID is a life-threatening and devastating disease. Even with aggressive therapy, the prognosis is poor. Evaluate the family's knowledge about the disease and provide education on infection control measures and signs of infection. Encourage the parents to assist in and manage care for their child (see Families Want to Know: Reducing Risk of Infection). The parents may feel guilt because of the genetic nature of the disease and the difficulties of treatment. Listen closely to their concerns and encourage them to discuss their fears. Refer them to an appropriate support group or counselor if needed. Encourage genetic counseling if the parents plan to have more children. Evaluate the family's ability to care for the child at home. Provide opportunities for the child to have contact with other children when it is safe to do

Medications Used to Treat
Immune Disorders

Medication/Action and Indication	Side Effects	Nursing Management
Immune Globulin Intravenous immune globulin (IVIG) is prepared from pools of multiple samples of human plasma and contains globulin (primarily IgG). It is used after exposure to diseases such as hepatitis B, and in idiopathic thrombocytopenic purpura, Kawasaki disease, AIDS, and other disorders. Specific types of immune globulin are effective against specific diseases. For example, HBIG is effective to prevent infection after exposure to hepatitis B.	Local inflammatory reaction, malaise, fever, nausea, vomiting, and arthralgia; hypersensitivity reaction with fever, chills, and anaphylactic shock; infusion reaction with nausea, flushing, chills, headache, difficulty breathing, and pain in back or abdomen.	▪ Have emergency drugs and equipment readily available to treat a hypersensitivity reaction or infusion reaction. ▪ The child may be treated with an antipyretic or antihistamine before the infusion. Follow manufacturer directions for reconstitution, dilution, and intravenous infusion rates. Do not mix with other medications for infusion. ▪ Monitor vital signs throughout infusion. Stop infusion immediately and notify the physician when any signs of hypersensitivity occur. ▪ Activate the emergency system as needed. ▪ Have the family instruct health care providers about IVIG therapy because immunization recommendations will be altered.

Data from: Bindler, R. M., & Howry, L. B. (2005). Pediatric drug guide with nursing implications. *Upper Saddle River, NJ: Prentice Hall.*

Families Want to Know
Reducing Risk of Infection

■ Wash all bottles, nipples, and pacifiers with hot water and soap, or in the dishwasher.

■ Do not allow the child to share utensils, cups, bottles, or pacifiers.

■ Use safe food preparation practices such as peeling fruit and vegetables and using different surfaces and utensils for preparing meats and other foods.

■ Change diapers frequently. Cleanse skin with mild soap and dry thoroughly.

■ Perform hand hygiene before handling the child, after changing diapers, and before feeding the child.

■ Maintain clean pets and keep the pet's environment clean.

■ Avoid exposing the child to others with illnesses, such as respiratory and skin infections.

so. Suggest activities that will foster development. Offer financial resource information and other referrals as needed.

The family of a child who undergoes hematopoietic stem cell transplantation requires additional support and referrals. The transplantation procedure involves surgery for both the ill child and the donor, often another child in the family (refer to the discussion in Chapter 23 ∞). After the transplant, the ill child will be hospitalized for several months until T-lymphocyte levels are sufficient to provide resistance to infection. During this period, parents may need to rely on social services to help manage the family situation, particularly if the child is hospitalized at a medical center far from the family's home. Assess the family's situation and make appropriate referrals to social services and to support groups. Introduce parents to other families with a child undergoing transplantation.

Evaluation

Expected outcomes of nursing care include the following:

• The child will be free from infection.
• The child will demonstrate adequate nutritional status as determined by normal growth patterns.
• Intact skin will be maintained.
• The family will demonstrate adaptive coping to the demands of a chronic illness.
• The child will demonstrate developmental progress consistent with expectations.

Wiskott-Aldrich Syndrome

A combined congenital immunodeficiency syndrome, Wiskott-Aldrich syndrome (WAS) is an X-linked disorder that causes mutation in the WAS gene and changes in WAS protein. The gene resides on Xp11.22 (Kobrynski, 2006). The incidence is 4 in 1 million live male births (Dibbern & Routes, 2009). The IgG and IgA levels are normal, IgM levels are decreased, and IgE levels may be increased (Kobrynski, 2006).

The diagnosis is made in the early neonatal period on the basis of the thrombocytopenia, which leads to bleeding as evidenced by petechiae, hematuria, bloody diarrhea, and hematemesis. Wiskott-Aldrich syndrome is characterized by eczema and recurrent infections in infancy and childhood such

as otitis media, bacterial pneumonia, and skin infections (Ochs & Thrasher, 2006).

Treatment includes antibiotic prophylaxis, platelet transfusions, and intravenous gamma globulin. Hypersplenism is a complication of WAS that may necessitate a splenectomy; however, this is done sparingly because of the risk of life-threatening infection following the procedure. The treatment of choice and the only cure for WAS is hematopoietic stem cell transplantation (HSCT). Following HSCT, the child is at risk for both rejection and graft-versus-host disease (see page 670) (Kobrynski, 2006; Ochs & Thrasher, 2006).

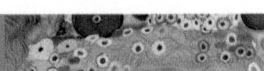
NURSING MANAGEMENT

Nursing care is similar to that for the child with SCID. Refer the parents for genetic counseling to help them understand the transmission of the disease and the probability of having another child with the same disorder. Arrange for psychologic support for those parents who may be overwhelmed with guilt from learning that the illness is inherited.

Help the parents and family cope with the knowledge that the child has a chronic and potentially fatal illness. Referral to family counseling may be appropriate. Provide support during the process of transplantation. Expected outcomes are a return to normal immunologic function or successful coping with a life-threatening illness.

Human Immunodeficiency Virus and Acquired Immune Deficiency Syndrome

Acquired immune deficiency syndrome (AIDS) is caused by the human immunodeficiency virus (HIV-1 primarily; HIV-2 less commonly) (American Academy of Pediatrics [AAP], 2009). As HIV destroys the body's ability to fight infection, opportunistic infections that would normally not affect healthy people destroy the immune system. AIDS, the advanced stages of HIV infection, may result if treatment is not initiated.

Most cases of HIV in children are the result of perinatal transmission. The CDC estimates that 100–200 infants are born with HIV infection each year in the United States compared with the peak incidence of 1,650 in 1991 (CDC, 2007). This improvement is primarily due to more effective identification and treatment of mothers who are infected with HIV and infants exposed to HIV. The leading cause of newly acquired HIV infection in teens is unprotected sexual intercourse, while intravenous substance abuse is responsible for most other cases. In some cases, both of these factors are involved.

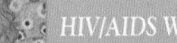
Culture *HIV/AIDS Worldwide*

While major progress has been made in the United States and several other developed countries to decrease the number of HIV/AIDS cases in children, developing countries have not been able to afford testing or treatment. Subsequently, some have large numbers of children with HIV/AIDS. The countries most acutely affected are in Africa: in Botswana, 57.7% of childhood deaths are due to AIDS; in Zimbabwe, 42.2%; in Swaziland, 40.6%; in Namibia, 36.5%; and in Zambia, 33.6%. In contrast, the world rate of child deaths that are related to AIDS is 4% (Kline, 2006).

The virus affects multiple systems and eventually destroys the ability of the child's immune system to respond to infection. An understanding of the natural history of HIV disease is still evolving, as there are several important differences in the disease progression and clinical manifestations of pediatric and adult HIV infection.

Etiology and Pathophysiology

Children can acquire HIV in a form of **vertical transmission** from their mothers transplacentally or during delivery. Transmission can occur during birth from blood, amniotic fluid, and exposure to genital tract secretions, and after birth through breast milk from mothers infected with HIV. However, risk for perinatal transmission has been significantly reduced since mothers identified as infected receive antiretroviral therapy (ART) during pregnancy, undergo a cesarean section, and are advised not to breastfeed. If the mother is not treated, there is a 25% chance that the newborn will be infected compared with a 2% or less chance if the mother is treated (CDC, 2007). Prenatal testing is essential to further reduce the incidence of HIV infection in children.

HIV selectively targets and destroys T cells, thereby decreasing and eventually eliminating cellular immunity. HIV destroys the CD4 T cells (helper cells) that are crucial to normal function of the immune system. HIV selectively targets T cells, decreasing cellular immunity and affecting humoral immunity as well. Thus, the child is left unprotected against a myriad of bacterial, viral, fungal, and opportunistic infections, which are ultimately fatal. Every organ system can be affected (Figure 22–3 ➤).

Clinical Manifestations

The neonate is asymptomatic at birth. Most children with HIV infection have nonspecific findings, including lymphadenopathy,

hepatosplenomegaly, nephropathy, oral candidiasis, failure to thrive and weight loss, diarrhea, chronic eczema and dermatitis, and fever of unknown origin. The time period for the development of opportunistic infections varies. Specific symptoms usually appear within 2 years in children who acquire HIV infection perinatally and include conjunctivitis (pink eye), ear infections, and tonsillitis. Bacterial and opportunistic infections, such as *Streptococcus*, *Haemophilus influenzae*, *Salmonella*, and *Pneumocystis jiroveci* pneumonia (formerly known as *Pneumocystis carinii*), and malignancies, such as Burkitt lymphoma, frequently occur as the disease progresses. Lymphoid interstitial pneumonitis (LIP) is a common manifestation of pediatric AIDS. Frequently children develop encephalopathy resulting in developmental delay or a deterioration of motor skills and intellectual functioning (Kline, 2006; Plowfield, 2007). Raymond, described at the beginning of this chapter, had several of these findings, such as a history of recurrent, acute infections (bronchitis, otitis media, and upper respiratory infections). See Clinical Manifestations: Human Immunodeficiency Virus in Children.

COLLABORATIVE CARE

Diagnostic Tests

Most children with HIV infection are diagnosed early in life. Serologic tests for detection of the virus are monitored in infants born to mothers infected with HIV. These tests are performed within 48 hours of birth. Infants who initially test negative should be retested at 1 to 2 months. Tests are repeated at 3 and 6 months, and then again between 12 and 18 months. Because an infant born to a mother infected with HIV may have maternal antibodies up to 18 months of age, routine antibody tests are not helpful for diagnosing HIV infection in infants (Alvarez & Rathore, 2007). The preferred tests are the HIV DNA polymerase chain reaction (PCR) or the HIV RNA assay (viral load). Any positive result is confirmed by retesting. In addition, CD4+ percentage or counts should be performed at least every 3 to 4 months to evaluate the child's immune status (U.S. Department of Health and Human Services, 2009a). See Table 22–5.

Law & Ethics — *HIV Screening in Prenatal Care*

The CDC recommends HIV testing for all pregnant women. Pregnant women should be offered repeat HIV screening in the third trimester in areas with elevated HIV rates (CDC, 2007).

Clinical Manifestations
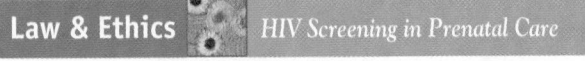
Human Immunodeficiency Virus in Children

Etiology	Clinical Manifestations	Nursing Management
Frequent, chronic, or unusual infections due to poor immune response	Chronic bilateral otitis media Oral candidiasis *Pneumocystis jiroveci* pneumonia (PCP) Skin disorders Fever	Teach families the importance of antimicrobial therapy for treatment of infections and the need for recommended immunizations. Limit exposure to groups of people or to individuals with known infections of any kind.
Poor nutritional intake due to lack of appetite caused by disease and medications	Failure to thrive (eating disorder of childhood) Weight and body mass index below 10th percentile Chronic diarrhea Skin irritation	Monitor growth. Provide supplemental intake such as enteral feedings at night, and total parenteral nutrition (TPN) if needed. Provide meticulous skin care to prevent breakdown.
Immune system overgrowth to compensate for lack of proper immune response	Hepatosplenomegaly and lymphadenopathy	Assess the abdomen frequently. Teach about safe transport to avoid injury to the liver and spleen.

Note: Be alert for the possibility of HIV infection in infants with combinations of listed clinical manifestations, especially in infants known to be at risk.

Pathophysiology Illustrated

Human Immunodeficiency Virus

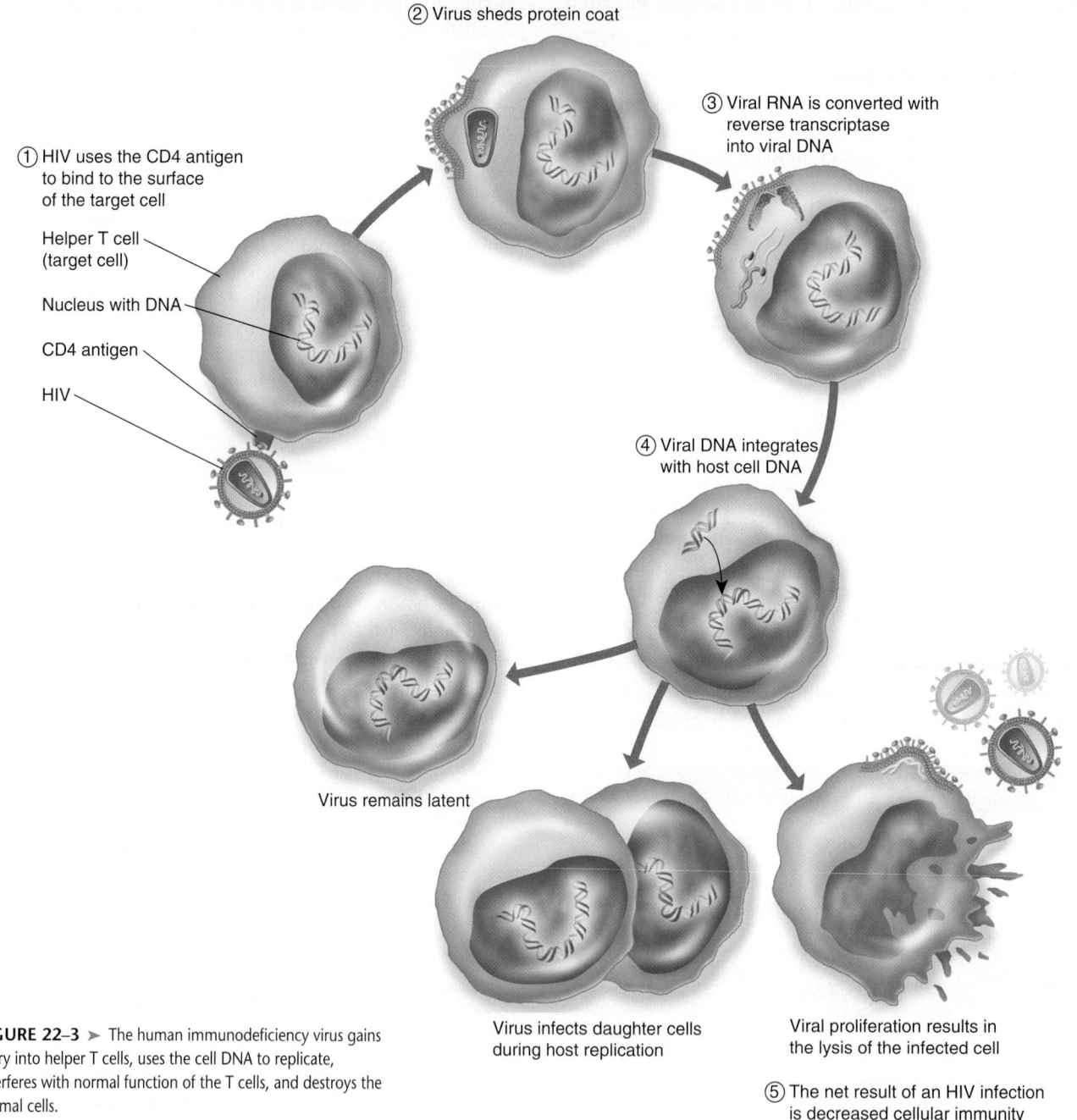

② Virus sheds protein coat

① HIV uses the CD4 antigen
to bind to the surface
of the target cell

Helper T cell
(target cell)

Nucleus with DNA

CD4 antigen

HIV

③ Viral RNA is converted with
reverse transcriptase
into viral DNA

④ Viral DNA integrates
with host cell DNA

Virus remains latent

Virus infects daughter cells
during host replication

Viral proliferation results in
the lysis of the infected cell

⑤ The net result of an HIV infection
is decreased cellular immunity

FIGURE 22–3 ➤ The human immunodeficiency virus gains entry into helper T cells, uses the cell DNA to replicate, interferes with normal function of the T cells, and destroys the normal cells.

An antibody test to see if the maternal HIV antibodies have disappeared should be performed at 12 months of age. If the test is still positive it should be repeated at 15 to 18 months of age (U.S. Department of Health and Human Services, 2009a). If the antibody test is still positive at 18 months of age, the child is considered to be infected with HIV. Antibody tests that are used include enzyme-linked immunosorbent assay (ELISA) or enzyme immunoassay (EIA). These tests are confirmed with the Western blot test or the indirect immunofluorescence assay (IFA) (Alvarez & Rathore, 2007). The CDC considers children less than 13 years of age to be infected if their symptoms meet the CDC criteria for HIV infection. The CDC criteria address two issues: the diagnosis of HIV and the clinical classification of children infected with HIV (AAP, 2009) (Table 22–6).

Clinical Therapy

Medical management begins with prevention of the spread of HIV from mother to newborn. Due to the rapidity of disease progression in perinatally transmitted HIV infection, early identification of infected infants is important to ensure the

Test	Description
CD4+ cell counts and percentages	Used to assess immune status at diagnosis and ongoing.
Enzyme immunoassay (EIA) and enzyme-linked immunosorbent assay (ELISA)	Commonly used test to identify HIV; detects antibodies to the virus. Positive results are verified by the Western blot test.
HIV DNA polymerase chain reaction (PCR)	A test that makes copies of a DNA sequence which can then be analyzed; useful to detect HIV or other conditions with only small amounts of blood. Preferred for detection of HIV infection in infants.
HIV RNA assay (viral load)	A test that makes copies of an RNA sequence which can then be analyzed to evaluate the severity of the infection at diagnosis and the response to treatment. May be used to confirm HIV infection in infants.
Western blot test	The definitive and confirmatory test for HIV. Allows visualization of particular antibodies to each viral protein.
Rapid HIV tests	Tests that use saliva and produce results in 60 minutes or less. Useful for quick screening, but results must be confirmed with serum tests because false positives can occur. See Box 22–1.

TABLE 22–5 Commonly Used HIV Tests

Source: Data from Alvarez, A. M., & Rathore, M. H. (2007). Hot topics in pediatric HIV/AIDS. Pediatric Annals, 36(7), 423–432; Delaney, K. P., Branson, B. M., Uniyal, A., Kerndt, P. R., Keenan, P. A., Jafa, K., et al. (2006). Performance of an oral fluid rapid HIV-1/2 test: Experience from four CDC studies. AIDS, 20, 1655–1660; Plowfield, L. A. (2007). HIV disease in children 25 years later. Pediatric Nursing, 33(3), 273–278.

most effective treatment. Mothers infected with HIV should be identified during pregnancy, and their infants should undergo periodic laboratory testing, as previously described. All infected mothers should receive combination antiretroviral therapy after the first trimester of pregnancy. Monotherapy is no longer recommended in the United States; however, if a mother with HIV infection is in labor and has not been on an antiretroviral regimen, this type of treatment may be used (Cibulka, 2006).

All infants of infected mothers with indeterminate HIV infection status should start prophylaxis against PCP by 4 to 6 weeks of age and continue to 1 year of age unless the diagnosis of HIV infection is excluded. Prompt therapy with anti-infectives is used for bacterial and viral opportunistic infections. The need for prophylaxis after 1 year of age is dependent on the child's degree of immunosuppression (AAP, 2009; Baker, 2007).

TABLE 22–6 Clinical Staging of Pediatric HIV Infection

Diagnosis of HIV infection in children

- HIV infected (two or more positive tests for HIV or clinical signs and symptoms of HIV infection or an AIDS-defining illness)
- Perinatally exposed (born to a mother known to be infected with HIV)
- Seroconverter (born to a mother known to be infected with HIV but has had two negative HIV tests)

When infected, the child with HIV is classified as

- Category N (not symptomatic)
- Category A (mildly symptomatic)
- Category B (moderately symptomatic)
- Category C (severely symptomatic; multiple, recurrent serious bacterial infection)

Adapted from: American Academy of Pediatrics. (2009). Red Book: 2009 Report of the Committee on Infectious Diseases (28th ed., pp. 382–390). Elk Grove Village, IL: Author.

Treatment for the child diagnosed with HIV involves highly active antiretroviral therapy (HAART). Initial medication therapy should include a combination of several antiretroviral (ARV) drugs. At least 3 drugs from a minimum of 2 different categories should be used. Of the 22 AVRs currently being manufactured, 16 have an approved pediatric treatment indication and are available as a pediatric formulation or capsule size (see Medications Used to Treat Human Immunodeficiency Virus in Children) (Marón, Gaur, & Flynn, 2010; U.S. Department of Health and Human Services, 2009a, 2009b). Families should be advised that these drugs neither cure HIV nor prevent transfer from the person infected to others.

Clinical Judgment

The cost of antiretroviral therapy has decreased over the years as more generic drugs have become available. Worldwide, however, only about 24% of individuals who need ART receive it (Alvarez & Rathore, 2007). What can be done to improve access to these drugs for children worldwide?

BOX 22–1 Rapid HIV Tests

Many people who are at risk of HIV infection may not have HIV testing readily available. To reduce barriers to early detection of the virus, rapid HIV tests have been made available. Specimens are obtained from saliva or fingerstick for a blood sample. Oral fluids are obtained by gently swabbing both the upper and lower outer gum of the mouth. Results are available in 1 hour or less and some do not require blood draws. FDA-approved options include OraQuick Rapid HIV-1/2 Antibody Test, Reveal Rapid HIV-1 Antibody Test, Uni-Gold Recombigen HIV Test, and Multispot HIV-1/HIV-2 Rapid Test. Health professionals must be prepared to offer counseling when the test is administered. Traditional laboratory tests are used to confirm positive rapid HIV tests (Delaney et al., 2006; Greenwald, Burstein, Pincus, et al., 2006).

Medications Used to Treat
Human Immunodeficiency Virus in Children

Medication	Action	Nursing Management
Nucleoside/Nucleotide Reverse Transcriptase Inhibitors (NRTIs)		
Abacavir Didanosine Emtricitabine Lamivudine Stavudine Zidovudine (AZT)	Inhibits action of viral reverse transcriptase, an enzyme in the conversion of RNA to DNA	Baseline data include physical assessment and laboratory studies (especially measurement of white and red blood cell counts). Monitor at least monthly for changes. Common side effects include fever, headache, insomnia, myalgia, nausea, vomiting, diarrhea, anorexia, bone marrow suppression with resulting granulocytopenia and anemia, dyspnea, cough, and skin rash. Teach signs and symptoms of infection.
Protease Inhibitors		
Atazanavir Darunavir Fosamprenavir Lopinavir/Ritonavir Nelfinavir Ritonavir Tipranavir	Blocks the function of the enzyme protease needed for viral formation and growth	Baseline data include physical assessment and laboratory studies such as serum electrolytes, CBC, liver function studies, blood glucose, hemoglobin A$_{1c}$, serum amylase, and creatine phosphokinase (CPK). Monitor at least monthly for changes. Side effects include central nervous system changes, cardiovascular changes, life-threatening hematologic changes, respiratory distress, and allergy; monitor for specific side effects of the particular drug administered. Oral forms are taken within 2 hours of a full meal.
Nonnucleoside Reverse Transcriptase Inhibitors (NNRTIs)		
Efavirenz Nevirapine	Binds to viral reverse transcriptase and disrupts the conversion of RNA to DNA	Baseline data include physical assessment and laboratory studies (such as liver and kidney function tests, CBC and differential). Monitor at least monthly for changes. Side effects include fever, headache, nausea, diarrhea, hepatitis, altered liver function, anemia, neutropenia, drowsiness and fatigue, altered mental status, rash, and Stevens-Johnson syndrome. Teach the family to notify the health care provider immediately if a rash appears.
Fusion Inhibitors		
Enfuvirtide	Prevents viral entry	This medication requires subcutaneous injection twice a day. There is a high incidence of local reaction at the injection site, limiting the use of this medication in children.

Source: Data from U.S. Department of Health and Human Services. (2009a). Guidelines for the use of antiretroviral agents in pediatric HIV infection. Retrieved from http://aidsinfo.nih.gov/contentfiles/PediatricGuidelines.pdf; U.S. Department of Health and Human Services. (2009b). Pediatric antiretroviral drug information. Retrieved from http://aidsinfo.nih.gov/contentfiles/PediatricGL_Supl.pdf; Alvarez, A. M., & Rathore, M. H. (2007). Hot topics in pediatric HIV/AIDS. Pediatric Annals, 36(7), 423–432; Marón, G., Gaur, A. H., & Flynn, P. M. (2010). Antiretroviral therapy in HIV-infected infants and children. Pediatric Infectious Disease Journal, 29(4), 360–363.

Children on antiretroviral therapy should be monitored closely for side effects and toxicity related to the medications. A complete blood count and blood chemistry along with a clinical history should be evaluated prior to beginning treatment, 4 to 8 weeks later, and then every 3 to 4 months. In addition, CD4+ cell counts and HIV RNA levels are recommended at the same time intervals to evaluate compliance with the medication regimen and effectiveness of the treatment. A lipid panel is also recommended every 6 to 12 months to monitor for signs of elevated cholesterol and triglyceride levels (U.S. Department of Health and Human Services, 2009a).

The earlier the child develops AIDS, the poorer the prognosis. An estimated 20% of children with HIV infection develop AIDS in the first year of life, and most of them die by 4 years of age. The other 80%, however, may not develop serious disease until school age or adolescence. With rapid advances in the treatment of HIV infection ongoing, the life span of children and adolescents cannot be predicted as these treatments are significantly extending their lives (Plowfield, 2007).

NURSING MANAGEMENT

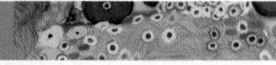

Nursing Assessment and Diagnosis

When the mother is HIV positive, the infant will need to be screened for HIV infection according to CDC guidelines as described in the previous section. Facilitate the screening and explain the necessity to the family.

NURSING CARE PLAN

The Child with Acquired Immunodeficiency Syndrome (continued)

INTERVENTION	RATIONALE	EXPECTED OUTCOME
3. Nursing Diagnosis: Risk for Impaired Skin Integrity related to skin infection, immobility, or diarrhea		
NIC Priority Intervention: *Skin surveillance:* Collection and analysis of patient data to maintain skin integrity		**NOC Suggested Outcome:** *Tissue integrity:* Skin and mucous membranes: Structural intactness and normal physiological function of skin and mucous membranes
Goal: The child will have intact skin.		
■ Observe all pressure areas closely for signs of infection or breakdown.	■ Skin care is important in the immunocompromised child. The skin may be the only intact defense the child has.	The child is free of preventable skin breakdown.
■ Keep skin clean and dry. Provide perineal care to minimize irritation from diarrhea.	■ Skin care prevents breaking or cracking of skin.	
4. Nursing Diagnosis: Deficient Knowledge (Parent) related to home care of child with AIDS		
NIC Priority Intervention: *Teaching, treatment:* Preparing a patient and family to understand and mentally prepare for a treatment		**NOC Suggested Outcome:** *Knowledge, treatment regimen:* Extent of understanding conveyed about treatment of HIV infection
Goal: The parent(s) will demonstrate knowledge about home care including medication regimen, measures to prevent infection, and signs and symptoms to report to health care providers.		
■ Explain the importance of optimizing the child's health status and reducing risk of complications through diet, rest, and meticulous personal hygiene. Be sure that parents and other family members understand how HIV infection is spread and take appropriate precautions.	■ Knowledge about the disorder and preventive measures is necessary to provide safe and effective home care for the child.	The parent describes appropriate home care and preventive measures for a child with AIDS.
■ Be sure that parents understand the need for adherence to the medication regimen and understand how to administer medications.	■ Knowledge of rationale increases compliance.	
■ Inform the family about signs and symptoms of infection that should be reported promptly to the physician or nurse (fever, chills, cough, mild erythema).	■ Early recognition leads to prompt treatment.	

secretions. Bathe the newborn as soon as possible after delivery and wash the eyes and face before administration of prophylactic eye drops or ointment. Avoid invasive procedures in the newborn and encourage the mother to formula-feed the baby rather than breastfeed.

Frequent hand hygiene and limiting exposure of the child to individuals with upper respiratory or other infections are the best interventions to protect the child with HIV from acquiring other infections. Because the risk of serious outcomes for measles disease is great, a live measles-mumps-rubella vaccine is administered at 12 to 15 months unless the child is severely immunocompromised. Vaccination with the live varicella vaccine is considered safe and effective in children with no or mild symptoms of HIV infection. The benefits and risks of the vaccine are weighed, and the child should receive the immunization if appropriate. Tuberculosis is more common in children with AIDS; therefore, annual skin tests that are read by health professionals are recommended (AAP, 2009). See Chapter 16 ∞ for further recommendations about the child who is immunocompromised and immunization recommendations.

Educate sexually active adolescents about the importance of practicing safe sex and the ramifications of high-risk sexual behaviors and intravenous drug use.

Health care workers who come in contact with blood or other body fluids of children infected with HIV are at risk for exposure to the virus. Standard precautions should be used in caring for all children, as HIV status and presence of other infections may not be known (refer to the *Clinical Skills Manual*).

A study of 46 children between the ages of 6 and 18 years who had acquired HIV infection perinatally and had been receiving antiretroviral therapy (ART) for at least 1 year evaluated three adherence measures. Pharmacy refill, caregiver report, and appointment maintenance data were evaluated as they related to viral load suppression. Although individual measures were not predictive of viral response, when all three measures were in agreement, viral suppression could be predicted (Burack, Gaur, Marone, et al., 2010). Since adherence is essential for positive outcomes in these patients, nurses must continue to evaluate methods of promoting adherence to the medication regimen in children and adolescents with HIV infection.

Promote Medication Regimen Adherence

The treatment regimen with the use of antiretroviral therapies for the child with HIV infection may be complex, time consuming, and costly, presenting an overwhelming challenge to the child and the family. Adherence to the prescribed antiretroviral treatment regimen is imperative as nonadherence will likely result in increased morbidity and mortality. Some common reasons for nonadherence include frequent dosing, the child's displeasure with medication (pill size, number of pills or amount of liquid, bad taste), and the caregiver's lack of knowledge related to the disease (Plowfield, 2007).

Strategies for achieving optimal management of the treatment regimen include educating the parent or care provider, as well as the child when old enough to understand, regarding the purpose of the medication, the benefits of adhering to the regimen, and the potential consequences of failure to adhere to the regimen. Behavior modification techniques, using positive rein-

forcement, can be very effective in promoting the child's adherence. Support should be provided to the family, and the medication regimen should be tailored to the family's routine. Praise should be offered to the child and parent for adhering to the regimen. If problems exist in management of the treatment regimen, carefully listen to the family to help determine the cause. Collaborate with the family in establishing goals to help meet the prescribed treatment regimen. Consider the effect of cultural beliefs on medication adherence (see Evidence-Based Practice: Adolescents with HIV Infection and Medication Regimen Adherence). If further intervention is required, other options include direct observational therapy or home visits.

Work with the family of the child with HIV infection to establish a plan for medication administration. Assist them to establish a time schedule that limits the administration of several large amounts of medication at the same time. Stress the importance of disguising the taste of bitter medications to increase the child's willingness to take the medication.

Promote Respiratory Function

Because many children with AIDS develop pneumonia, encourage the child to cough and deep breathe every 2 to 4 hours. In the community, regular physical activity encourages lung aeration. When in the hospital, blowing cotton balls with a straw, blowing bubbles or pinwheels, or other games may engage the interest of a younger child. Reposition infants frequently so all areas of the lungs can aerate. Rest periods to conserve energy and lower the body's demand for oxygen are important.

 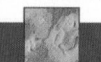
Problem

HIV infection is a significant health problem among adolescents in the United States (Mahat et al., 2008). Adherence to highly active antiretroviral therapy (HAART) has been shown to decrease morbidity and mortality; however, medication adherence in this age group is not adequate (Naar-King, Templin, Wright, et al., 2006). What factors are most frequently associated with medication nonadherence in adolescents with HIV infection?

Evidence

A study of 65 adolescents and young adults ages 16–25 years examined three psychosocial factors that affect adherence to a HAART regimen: self-efficacy, social support, and psychological distress. The study found that rates of adherence were inadequate for effective disease management. Psychological distress and self-efficacy were associated with nonadherence. Social support was not associated with adherence to the medication regimen but was associated with self-efficacy (Naar-King et al., 2006).

Another study examined predictors of adherence to an antiretroviral medication regimen over the previous 3 days. The study examined 2,088 children and adolescents ages 3–18 years enrolled in the Pediatric AIDS Clinical Trials Group (PACTG). While adherence rates were 84% overall, the rate for adolescents ages 15–18 years was the

lowest at 76%, compared with 83–89% for younger children. In addition to age, other factors that were related to nonadherence included stress, repeating a grade in school, and a diagnosis of anxiety or depression (Williams, Storm, Montepiedra, et al., 2006).

Implications

Adherence to the HAART regimen is problematic in the adolescent population. In addition to age, factors associated with nonadherence include lack of self-efficacy, stress, depression, and anxiety. Research indicates that adherence to the HAART regimen significantly improves outcomes. It is essential that adolescents receive comprehensive education related to the importance of adherence to their medication regimen. Discuss strategies with adolescents that will assist them in remembering to take their medication. Referrals for counseling and stress management along with treatment for depression are indicated in some cases.

Critical Thinking Application

What are some barriers that may lead to medication nonadherence in the HIV-positive adolescent? What support does the adolescent need to improve medication adherence? What measures can the nurse take to improve medication adherence in the adolescent?

Promote Adequate Nutritional Intake

Because many children with AIDS have failure to thrive, nutrition is an important part of their care. (See Chapter 14 ∞ for information to include in a detailed nutritional assessment.) A nutritionist should be involved in planning an appropriate diet for the child that provides necessary calories, protein, and other nutrients. Vitamins may be especially lacking in the diets of infected children. Antioxidants (vitamin A, vitamin E, zinc, and selenium) are known to enhance general immune system function and should be consumed at recommended levels. Periodic dietary analysis and teaching are needed. Adequate nutrition is sometimes provided by total parenteral nutrition or tube feedings.

Diarrhea resulting from gastrointestinal infection and lactose intolerance is a common finding in children with HIV infection and complicates other nutritional disturbances. Alternative formulas may be recommended. Although antidiarrheal medications are not generally used in infants, they may be prescribed for older children. Carefully monitor hydration status, skin turgor, and urine output. Provide careful perineal skin care to prevent infection.

The frequency of *Candida* infections leads to blisters, cracking, and discharge involving the oral mucous membranes. To keep the child's lips and mouth moist, mouth care should be performed every 2 to 4 hours with a non-alcohol-based solution such as normal saline.

Provide Emotional Support

The family of the child with HIV infection is under emotional stress; this is compounded if the mother and others in the family are also infected. The infected teen may see progression of disease in the parent and lose hope. Integrate social services and support groups into the care of the child as soon as the diagnosis is made. Spend time talking with the family about their fears and feelings. In many parts of the United States, HIV infection still carries a tremendous stigma, and the family may not be able to discuss their feelings outside the health care environment. Safeguard the family's wishes about the privacy of the diagnosis. Refer to Chapter 12 ∞ for information related to the child with a chronic illness.

Clarify any misconceptions the older child with HIV infection may have about the transmission of the disease. Routes of transmission and the need for safe sexual practices must be clearly discussed with adolescents. Providing support for adolescents is particularly important, as the dependence that this chronic and terminal disease brings can make it difficult to meet the developmental task of independence. Adolescents may benefit from contact with other infected peers.

Law & Ethics — *Confidentiality*

Disclosure of patient information is a breach of confidentiality that may subject a nurse to legal action. Disclosure of confidential information occurs when a patient's condition—for example, a diagnosis of HIV infection—is discussed inappropriately with any third party.

Discharge Planning

The diagnosis of HIV infection is surrounded by strong emotions and fears. Be honest and direct. Education is essential. Explain that there is no evidence that casual contact among family members can spread the infection. For the child who has been hospitalized, home care needs should be identified well in advance of discharge.

Discuss the family's finances as well as health insurance coverage for the child's care. Assess the family's ability to provide nutritious food, required medications, and a supportive environment. Refer to services as needed to ensure provision of quality care for the child after discharge.

Support groups, home health care nursing services, financial assistance, respite care, and psychological counseling are usually needed at some point during the child's illness, and the family should be aware that such services are available. Assist the family with coping mechanisms to deal with feelings of guilt about the child's condition.

Care in the Community

Much of the care of the child with HIV infection takes place in the community. With the continued success of aggressive therapy, the majority of children infected with HIV can be expected to attend school. Additionally, a substantial number of these children will reach adolescence, and some will reach adulthood. Assess the family and community support systems and provide resources and referrals as needed to help them provide adequate care for their child and to assist adolescents as they transition to adulthood (see Chapter 12 ∞). Many children with HIV infection are placed in foster homes, and these families need careful instruction to manage this multifaceted illness.

School guidelines recommend unrestricted school or childcare center attendance for children with HIV infection. In addition, children should be allowed to participate in all activities to the extent that their health and other recommendations for management of infectious diseases permit (AAP, 2009). Contraindications to school attendance include lack of control of body secretions, biting, and open wounds that cannot be covered. CDC guidelines for standard precautions should always be followed in the school, childcare, and home settings. The nurse may also be responsible for providing medicines or other care at school for the child infected with HIV (Plowfield, 2007).

Assist the family to alter the home environment in order to provide standard precautions during care. Make sure the child and family understand that HIV is transmitted through blood, urine, stool, and other body fluids. Educate family members about the importance of hygiene measures. Encourage careful hand hygiene and tell parents to use precautions when handling body fluids. Explain that they should wear gloves when changing diapers; disposing of urine, stool, and emesis; or treating the child's cuts and scrapes. In addition, teach them to wash their hands immediately after contact with blood or other body fluids. Instruct parents to use a bleach solution for disinfection of objects when necessary and to avoid contact with persons with infectious illnesses. Precautions to guard against foodborne illness are particularly important for the child infected with HIV. (See Families Want to Know: Food Safety and HIV.) Parents will also need instruction

Families Want to Know
Food Safety and HIV

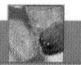

The child with HIV infection is more prone to foodborne disease. Instruct parents to practice the following:

1. Use a separate cutting board for meats, and wash it with hot soapy water after use.
2. Wash all utensils with hot soapy water between any uses.
3. Wash and peel fresh fruits and vegetables.
4. Use a disposable cloth or cloth that is washed after each meal to clean dishes. A sponge can harbor organisms and should not be used.
5. Have well water checked for contaminants regularly if that is the source of drinking water.
6. Do not allow the child to eat raw or undercooked meats, fish, eggs, or cookie dough.
7. Use a bleach solution for cleaning surfaces in the kitchen.

on correct administration and side effects of any medications the child is taking. Giving a child a complicated combination of drugs can be challenging for all families, so use teaching that is tailored to the particular family and perform repeated evaluation of the family's success with medication administration.

Emphasize the importance of promoting the child's development. Perform frequent developmental screenings. Teach the parents how to support the child in achieving developmental milestones. Encourage contact with other children and adults, provide for appropriate toys, teach parents how to encourage the child's communication, and praise the family for what the child has already accomplished. Children who manifest decreasing developmental milestones or other neurologic symptoms should be assessed by the primary care provider for HIV-induced encephalopathy.

Evaluation

Expected outcomes of nursing care include the following:

- Decreased numbers of cases of pediatric HIV due to vertical transmission from known infected mothers will be demonstrated.
- Interventions will be successful in preventing infectious diseases in children with the virus.
- Children will have adequate respiratory function and perfusion.
- Nutritional intake of affected children will support normal growth patterns and prevent malnutrition.
- The family who has a child with HIV will demonstrate adequate coping with the stress of chronic disease.
- The child will be able to attend school and receive other supports in the educational process.

■ AUTOIMMUNE DISORDERS

In an immune system damaged by pathologic changes, an immune response may occur to some of the body's own proteins, resulting in the production of autoantibodies. These pathologic conditions in which the body directs the immune response against itself—identifying "self" as "nonself"—are called autoimmune disorders.

The primary feature of autoimmune disorders is tissue injury caused by a probable immunologic reaction of the host with its own tissues. Structural or functional changes occur as immune cells attack other cells in the body. Autoimmune disorders are grouped into systemic and organ-specific diseases. *Systemic diseases*, which generally involve more than one organ, include systemic lupus erythematosus and juvenile idiopathic arthritis, which are discussed in this chapter. *Organ-specific diseases*, which primarily affect a single organ, include type 1 diabetes and thyroiditis (see Chapter 30 ∞). Idiopathic (or immune) thrombocytic purpura, an immune disease affecting blood platelets and clotting, is discussed in Chapter 23 ∞ .

Systemic Lupus Erythematosus

Systemic lupus erythematosus (SLE) is a chronic inflammatory, autoimmune disease of unknown origin that involves many organ systems (Tucker, 2007). Although it is primarily diagnosed in adulthood, approximately 20% of cases are diagnosed in childhood prior to age 16 (Brunner, Higgins, Wiers, et al., 2009). SLE is more common among Native Americans, African Americans, Hispanics, and Asians than Caucasians; more severe disease is seen in African Americans and Hispanics (Gottlieb & Ilowite, 2006). SLE is seven times more common in females than males (Brunner et al., 2009).

Etiology and Pathophysiology

The exact etiology of SLE is unknown. A genetic component is suspected as the disease is often more prevalent in members of the same family. It is believed that in those genetically disposed, an outside environmental agent causes the body to initiate an abnormal immune system response to its own tissues (Lupus Foundation of America, 2008; Pongmarutani, Alpert, & Miller, 2006). The body produces autoantibodies and combines with antigens to form immune complexes. These antigen-antibody complexes are then deposited in the connective tissue, triggering an inflammatory response. The chronic inflammation then destroys connective tissue. The tissue damage varies according to the organ involvement, though the tissues most likely to be affected are the small blood vessels, glomeruli, joints, spleen, and heart valves. Because many systems can be affected simultaneously, organ damage with subsequent multisystem failure may occur.

Clinical Manifestations

Manifestations of SLE may be acute, with onset of nephritis, arthritis, or vasculitis; or it may be noted as a gradual onset with nonspecific symptoms. Symptoms depend on the organ involved and the amount of tissue damage that has occurred. Initial symptoms include recurrent fever, chills, fatigue, malaise, and weight loss. The most common symptoms are rash, fever, mucositis, and arthritis. A butterfly rash on the face, consisting of a pink or red rash over the bridge of the nose extending to the cheeks, is a characteristic finding (Gottlieb & Ilowite, 2006)

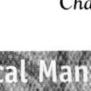

FIGURE 22–4 ➤ This child displays a "butterfly" rash across the cheeks and bridge of the nose. It is often seen in the child with SLE.

Source: From Zitelli, B. J., & Davis, H. W. (Eds.). (2002). Atlas of pediatric physical diagnosis (3rd ed., p. 238). St. Louis, MO: Mosby.

(Figure 22–4 ➤). See Clinical Manifestations: Childhood-Onset Systemic Lupus Erythematosus.

Systemic lupus erythematosus is characterized by periods of remission and exacerbation (flares). Flares are triggered by a variety of causes including sun exposure, an upper respiratory or other infection, and stress. The child or family may be able to identify other triggers to flares, such as particular events, activities, or situations.

COLLABORATIVE CARE

Blood tests reveal anemia, an elevated blood urea nitrogen (BUN), abnormal plasma proteins, abnormal erythrocyte sedimentation rate (ESR), presence of antinuclear antibodies, and a positive lupus erythematosus (LE) cell reaction, which indicates nonspecific inflammation. The Coombs test is positive. Radiologic examinations include chest radiographs and computed tomography (CT) scans, as well as magnetic resonance imaging (MRI) of the affected joints. A 24-hour urine collection and imaging studies, as well as renal biopsies, may be performed to evaluate lupus nephritis. Urinalysis may reveal proteinuria.

The goals of medical management are to create a remission of symptoms and to prevent complications. Corticosteroids, such as prednisone or methylprednisolone, are prescribed to control inflammation. Antimalarial preparations, such as hydroxychloroquine, are used to treat symptoms associated with skin lesions and renal and arthritic problems. Although the exact action of these drugs with regard to SLE is not known, they often permit continued remission with a lowered dose of steroids. Nonsteroidal anti-inflammatory drugs (aspirin, ibuprofen, naproxen) are used to relieve muscle and joint pain. Immunosuppressant drugs, such as cyclophosphamide, azathioprine, mycophenolate mofetil, cyclosporine, and methotrexate, have been used to help control SLE (Gottlieb & Ilowite, 2006; Marinescu & Ilowite, 2007). (See Medications Used to Treat Systemic Lupus Erythematosus.) Diet may

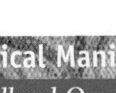

Clinical Manifestations
Childhood-Onset Systemic Lupus Erythematosus

System	Clinical Manifestations
Integumentary	A butterfly rash on the face, consisting of a pink or red rash over the bridge of the nose extending to the cheeks (a characteristic finding) Photosensitivity Alopecia Mouth or nose ulcers
Hematologic	Fatigue Fever Easy bruising Bloody stools Nosebleeds
Musculoskeletal	Joint pain Swollen inflamed joints Myalgias Muscle weakness
Neurological	Headache Peripheral neuropathy Psychosis Seizures Mood disorder Cognitive disorder Stroke
Pulmonary	Chest pain Dyspnea Pulmonary hypertension Pulmonary embolism
Cardiac	Arrhythmias Chest pain Friction rub Raynaud phenomenon (fingers turning white and/or blue in the cold)
Renal	Hematuria Hypertension Proteinuria Edema
Gastrointestinal	Abdominal pain (may rotate to the shoulder)

Source: Adapted from Gottlieb, B. S., & Ilowite, N. T. (2006). Systemic lupus erythematosus in children and adolescents. Pediatrics in Review, 27(9), 323–328; Klein-Gitelman, M. S. (2010). Systemic lupus erythematosus. Retrieved from http://emedicine.medscape.com/article/1008066-overview; Tucker, L. B. (2007). Making the diagnosis of systemic lupus erythematosus in children and adolescents. Lupus, 16, 546–549.

be restricted if the child has excessive weight gain or fluid retention from steroids and renal damage.

The prognosis depends on the severity of the internal organ involvement. Whereas SLE was once considered a fatal disease, the 5-year survival rate for juvenile-onset SLE is 92% and the 10-year survival rate is 85% (Gottlieb & Ilowite, 2006). Kidney failure is managed by hemodialysis or peritoneal dialysis. Renal transplantation has been very successful for treatment of renal failure secondary to lupus nephritis.

▲ Health Promotion

Adolescents are generally very concerned about their appearance. The side effects of corticosteroids, immunosuppressants, and antimalarial drugs used in the treatment of children with SLE are significant and include hair loss, susceptibility to infection, "moon face," retinal damage, and bone loss. These side effects can affect the adolescent's body image and decrease self-esteem. Teens with SLE may need special teaching, guidance, and support. Support groups or Internet chat rooms may be helpful.

Medications Used to Treat
Systemic Lupus Erythematosus

Medication	Action/Indication	Nursing Management
Corticosteroids Prednisone Methylprednisolone	To control inflammation	■ Monitor for side effects including weight gain, mood changes, insomnia, and elevated serum glucose. ■ *Caution:* Corticosteroids may interfere with normal growth and increase susceptibility to infection. ■ Avoid live vaccines in the child on high-dose steroids.
Antimalarial preparations Hydroxychloroquine (Plaquenil)	To treat symptoms associated with skin lesions and renal and arthritic pain	■ Administer with milk or meals to reduce gastric irritation. ■ Teach the family to report the following serious side effects: • Weakness • Visual symptoms • Hearing loss • Bruising • Unusual bleeding • Skin eruptions
Nonsteroidal anti-inflammatories (NSAIDs) Naproxen Ibuprofen	To relieve muscle and joint pain	■ Monitor for side effects including abdominal pain, bleeding, and gastrointestinal complications. ■ Teach the family to monitor for side effects and to avoid administration of additional NSAIDs.
Immunosuppressants Cyclophosphamide Azathioprine Methotrexate Cyclosporine Mycophenolate mofetil	To help control SLE during acute exacerbations	■ Monitor for infection. ■ Implement measures to reduce risk of infection. ■ Monitor for thrombocytopenia. ■ Teach the family that the child should avoid exposure to sunlight and wear sunscreen and sunglasses. ■ Follow vaccine guidelines for children with immunodeficiency.

Source: Data from: Gottlieb, B. S., & Ilowite, N. T. (2006). Systemic lupus erythematosus in children and adolescents. Pediatrics in Review, 27(9), 323–329; Marinescu, L. M., & Ilowite, N. T. (2007). Update on pediatric rheumatology: Growth spurt in the knowledge base. Consultant for Pediatrics, 6(7), 397–404.

NURSING MANAGEMENT
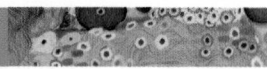

Nursing management focuses on thorough assessments, due to the multitude of systems that can be affected by SLE, and teaching to enhance general health practices.

Nursing Assessment and Diagnosis

Thorough assessments are needed, as symptoms are widespread. Based on the combination of symptoms that are manifested, a unique group of nursing diagnoses is identified.

Physiologic Assessment

Assess the child's nutritional status including baseline weight and history of recent weight loss or weight gain. The skin is assessed for rashes, ulcers, photosensitivity, ecchymosis, petechiae, cyanosis, and hair loss. Respiratory assessment includes breath sounds and respiratory rate and assessing for pleural effusion or pleuritis. Cardiovascular assessment includes vital signs, heart sounds, and symptoms of pericarditis or friction rub. Musculoskeletal assessment includes joint pain, joint deformity, other pain, weakness, and ability to perform activities of daily living. Neurological assessment includes changes in affect or cognitive abilities and seizure activity. Gastrointestinal assessment includes splenomegaly.

Psychosocial Assessment

Because SLE is a chronic disease that affects primarily adolescents, psychosocial assessment is indicated. Assess family interactions, exploring stressful situations such as divorce or trauma. Treatment-related restrictions and changes in appearance can lead to withdrawal, depression, and suicidal tendencies. Perform psychological assessments periodically as the child grows and adapts to the disorder or faces new developmental challenges with a chronic disease. The following nursing diagnoses may apply to the child with SLE:

- Risk for Ineffective Management of Therapeutic Regimen (Family) related to complexity of therapeutic regimen
- Risk for Ineffective Tissue Perfusion (Renal) related to interrupted blood flow in kidneys
- Risk for Impaired Skin Integrity related to immunologic deficit
- Risk for Activity Intolerance related to chronic disease
- Risk for Disturbed Body Image related to side effects of medications and skin alterations
- Risk for Infection related to immunosuppressive medications
- Acute Pain related to joint inflammation and injury

Planning and Implementation

The goals of nursing care are to assist the child to manage and cope with a chronic disease, prevent infection, maintain fluid balance, promote adequate nutrition, promote skin integrity, promote rest and comfort, manage side effects of medication, avoid triggers for disease flares, and provide emotional support.

Prevent Infection
Infections are a leading cause of death for patients with SLE. Instruct the patient and family to inform all health care providers of the disease in order to plan for prophylactic measures. Educate the patient and family on the importance of adhering to the immunization schedule, and to obtain a yearly influenza vaccine to prevent infection. Instruct the family on hand hygiene and infection control measures in the home, and warn adolescents about the dangers of tattooing and body piercing because of the risk of infection.

Maintain Fluid Balance
Because most children with SLE have renal involvement, nursing care includes maintaining accurate intake and output measurements and frequent evaluation of the child's fluid and electrolyte status and weight.

Promote Adequate Nutrition
Currently, there are no specific dietary plans for the child with SLE; however, the diet may be restricted according to renal involvement, weight gain, weight loss, or other complications. The child is at risk for weight gain associated with treatment with steroids and a decreased activity level during exacerbations of this disease. A well-balanced, nutritious diet with calcium and vitamin D supplements to support bone density as well as appropriate fluid intake for age should be encouraged.

Promote Skin Integrity
Presence of ulcers on mucous membranes can cause weakening of the tissues, placing the child at increased risk for infection. Provide instructions on oral care to maintain intact oral mucosa. Encourage the use of good hygiene measures and a mild soap for the skin. Recommend that adolescents limit their use of cosmetics, especially oil-based. Reinforce the importance of avoiding sunlight as much as possible, as well as the use of sun protection factor (SPF) of 30 or higher at all times when in the sun. Encourage the child to wear protective clothing to limit exposure to sunlight. (See Chapter 31 ∞ for a discussion of sun exposure.) Additionally, avoidance of unprotected fluorescent lighting is recommended, since exacerbations of SLE have been reported following this exposure. Educate adolescents that the use of tanning beds will cause the same reaction as sun exposure (Lupus Foundation of America, 2008). Provide instructions on oral care to maintain intact oral mucosa. Provide instructions on care of the head if alopecia occurs.

Promote Rest and Comfort
The child with SLE experiences fatigue and joint pain, leaving little energy reserve during acute episodes of the disease. Encourage frequent rest periods and a nutritious diet to maximize energy stores. A physical therapist can plan a program to encourage mobility and increase muscle strength. Implement measures such as application of heat to painful areas.

Manage Side Effects of Medications
Observe for side effects of medications used for treatment, and teach the child and family about these effects. For example, immunosuppressant drugs can promote infection anywhere in the body; and nonsteroidal anti-inflammatory drugs commonly cause gastric distress and bleeding of the gastrointestinal tract. The antimalarial drug hydroxychloroquine increases the risk of retinopathy and blindness; therefore, routine eye examinations are essential (Gottlieb & Ilowite, 2006). Corticosteroid side effects include cushingoid effects, weight gain, and hypertension. Sulfa drugs should be avoided because they increase photosensitivity.

Provide Emotional Support
Adolescents may have an altered body image as a result of rash, alopecia, arthritic changes in the joints, and chronic disease. Referral to a lupus support group, social services, or counseling may be helpful. The Lupus Foundation of America can provide information to help parents and children adjust to the disease. The family needs ongoing support and information to deal with the complexity of the disease.

Avoidance of Triggers for Disease Flares
Many children and their parents can recognize the signs of an impending flare and the triggers that precede them. Work with the parents and child to implement measures to avoid these triggers. Discuss preventive behaviors such as avoiding sun exposure and avoiding stressors. Adolescents should be warned that alcohol, smoking, and drugs also pose an increased risk due to the potential to stimulate flares. Female adolescents who are sexually active should avoid birth control pills that contain the hormone estrogen since the extra estrogen may exacerbate symptoms. In addition, alternative birth control methods should be discussed with the adolescent.

Evaluation
Successful outcomes of nursing care involve management of this chronic disease. Expected outcomes of nursing care include the following:

- Adequate intake and output levels are maintained, with demonstrated fluid and electrolyte balance.
- Intact skin is maintained.
- No signs of infection are evident.

Complementary Therapy
SLE and Stress

Systemic lupus erythematosus exacerbations have been linked to stress. Stress-reducing techniques such as guided imagery, reading, and quiet games can benefit the child or adolescent and reduce these exacerbations. Since SLE is most common in adolescents, what stress reduction might be possible? Consider a busy teen who plays sports, has many social activities, and excels in school; how can you assist this teen to see the importance of and identify techniques for stress reduction? How can stress reduction be integrated into the daily life of an active teen?

Autoimmune Disorder Resources

• A balance of rest and activity is maintained to promote development.
• The child or adolescent develops a positive body image.

Juvenile Idiopathic Arthritis

Arthritis in children has long been referred to as juvenile rheumatoid arthritis, or JRA, in the United States. In recent years, the International League of Associations for Rheumatology has adopted the term *juvenile idiopathic arthritis* (JIA) to describe arthritis with an unknown cause in children (Nistala, Woo, & Wedderburn, 2009).

Juvenile idiopathic arthritis refers to inflammation involving one or more joints, lasting more than 6 weeks, diagnosed prior to 16 years of age, and without any other known cause (Coren, Ciervo, & Mason, 2008; Nistala et al., 2009). This disease results in decreased mobility, swelling, and pain. The peak age of onset for JIA is between 1 and 3 years of age, with the illness occurring twice as often in females as in males (Nistala et al., 2009). Approximately 18 of every 100,000 children develop JIA each year, and the prevalence is estimated to be up to 150 of every 100,000 children (Bernatsky, Duffy, Malleson, et al., 2007). It is estimated that 40–60% of children with JIA will continue with symptoms into adulthood (Sarma, Misra, & Aggarwal, 2008).

Juvenile idiopathic arthritis affects joints and surrounding tissues in addition to potential effects on other organs such as the heart, lungs, liver, and eyes. During the disease's course, the child may experience pain, impaired mobility, and interference with normal growth and development. Children may enter remission or manifest continued symptoms of a chronic disease. Remission may last for months, years, or a lifetime. Rarely, the disease is unresponsive to treatment or the child may suffer lasting impairment such as bone and joint changes. Children with early onset have a better prognosis for complete recovery.

Etiology and Pathophysiology

The cause of JIA is unknown, but it is thought to have an autoimmune basis. Inflammation begins in the joint and leads to pain and swelling (Figure 22–5 ➤). Scar tissue eventually develops, resulting in limited range of motion. Although terminology varies among the different classifications, according to the most current classification the three major types of JIA are oligoarthritis, polyarthritis, and systemic arthritis (Nistala et al., 2009).

• *Oligoarthritis* involves four or fewer joints. Approximately 60% of children with JIA have oligoarthritis (Sanzo, 2008). Uveitis occurs in approximately 30% of children with oligoarthritis (Nistala et al., 2009).
• *Polyarthritis* involves five or more joints. This type of arthritis affects approximately 30% of the children with JIA. This classification is further identified as rheumatoid factor positive or negative. Uveitis occurs in approximately 10% of children with polyarthritis (Nistala et al., 2009).
• *Systemic arthritis* is characterized by high fever; swollen, painful joints; and rash. Systemic arthritis affects internal organs and joints. Approximately 10% of children with JIA have systemic arthritis (Sanzo, 2008).

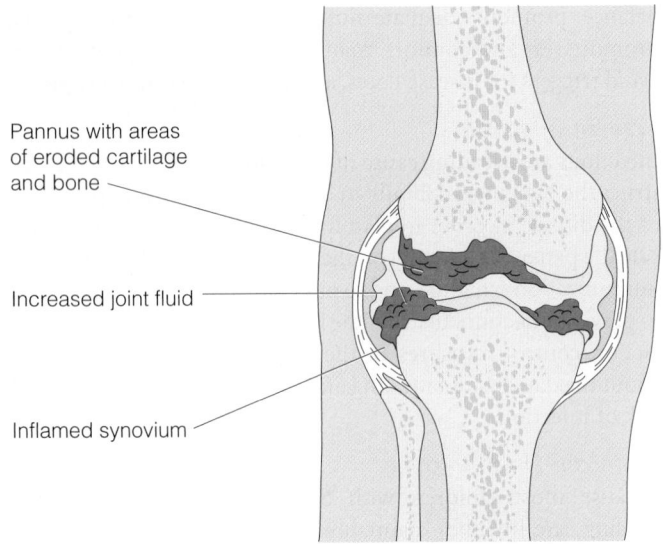

Pannus with areas of eroded cartilage and bone

Increased joint fluid

Inflamed synovium

FIGURE 22–5 ➤ Joint inflammation and destruction in idiopathic arthritis.

Clinical Manifestations

JIA may be restricted to a few joints or be systemic with involvement of multiple joints. Symptoms can include fever, rash, lymphadenopathy, splenomegaly, and hepatomegaly. The child may develop a limp or obviously favor one extremity over the other. A slow rate of growth or uneven growth of extremities may also be noted. Pain, stiffness, loss of motion, and swelling occur in the large joints such as the knees. Older children may develop symmetric involvement of the small joints of the hand. The disease is frequently chronic, extending over several years after an initial manifestation with pain and other symptoms. Remissions and exacerbations are characteristic.

COLLABORATIVE CARE

Diagnosis is made primarily on the basis of the history and assessment findings: in particular, arthritis having an onset before 16 years of age and persisting for at least 6 weeks, with no other identifiable cause (Marinescu & Ilowite, 2007). There are no specific laboratory tests to confirm the diagnosis although there are tests to help support the diagnosis. In some children, test results are positive for rheumatoid factor, human leukocyte antigen (HLA) B27, and antinuclear antibody (ANA). Erythrocyte sedimentation rate (ESR) and C-reactive protein (CRP) tests may be helpful in determining the amount of inflammation (Cassidy & Petty, 2005). Radiographs are generally performed to exclude other causes of pain and inflammation, such as fractures, and for monitoring for joint damage and bone development.

The goals of treatment are to relieve pain, control inflammation, manage systemic complications, preserve joint function and range of motion, and promote normal physical, psychosocial, behavioral, and vocational development (Cassidy & Petty, 2005). Nonsteroidal anti-inflammatory drugs (NSAIDs) such as aspirin, ibuprofen, and naproxen are used to reduce inflammation and pain. Children who do not respond to NSAIDs may be treated with disease-modifying antirheumatic drugs such as sulfasalazine and methotrexate. Corticosteroids such as prednisone and methylprednisolone may be used with children with more severe forms of JIA. Biologic response modifiers such as etanercept have also been used to treat JIA (Cassidy & Petty 2005; Marinescu & Ilowite, 2007; Sanzo, 2008). Physical therapy, occupational therapy, or both are performed to increase strength and mobility of joints while protecting them from injury. The physical therapist or occupational therapist tailors an exercise regimen specifically to the child. Range of motion exercises are essential to maintain joint mobility. Surgery is occasionally performed to relieve pain and maintain or improve joint function in children with joint contractures.

Complications such as chronic uveitis, which results from chronic eye inflammation, may occur in children with JIA. Children less than 6 years of age with oligoarthritis or polyarthritis who have a positive ANA test should have an eye exam every 3–4 months. Children 7 or older or those with a negative ANA test need an exam every 6 months. Because uveitis is rare in children with systemic arthritis, the recommended frequency for eye exams is every 12 months (Marinescu & Ilowite, 2007).

Growth interference for the child with JIA is a potential complication. The specific disorder may result in contractures or effusions of the joints. The administration of corticosteroids can also inhibit growth.

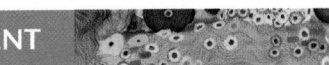

NURSING MANAGEMENT

Nursing Assessment and Diagnosis

A careful history is important, as it is sometimes the primary mode of diagnosis. Assess for joint redness, swelling and deformities, pain, decreased range of motion, morning stiffness, fever, nodules under the skin, growth delays, and enlarged lymph nodes.

The following nursing diagnoses may apply to the child with JIA:

- Activity Intolerance related to chronic pain
- Impaired Physical Mobility related to joint stiffness
- Anxiety (Child and Family) related to stress of chronic illness
- Chronic Pain related to joint inflammation
- Disturbed Body Image related to illness

Planning and Implementation

Nursing care focuses on promoting mobility, encouraging adequate nutrition, and teaching the parents and child about the disease and its management. Most care will occur in the community, including physical therapy, with only occasional hospitalizations at the time of an exacerbation of the disease.

Promote Improved Mobility

The goals of physical therapy are to maintain joint function, strengthen muscles, increase tone, maintain body alignment, and prevent permanent deformities such as contractures. Range of motion exercises, stretching, hydrotherapy, and swimming

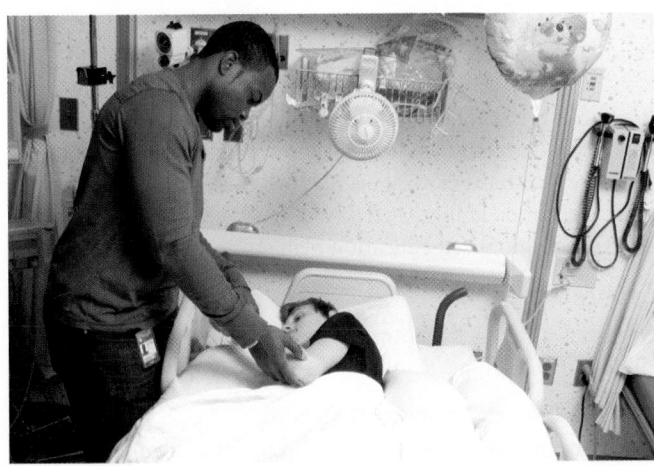

FIGURE 22–6 ➤ Passive range of motion exercises are an important aspect of physical therapy for a child or adolescent who has juvenile idiopathic arthritis.

help to prevent deformities (Figure 22–6 ➤). Encourage the child to perform activities of daily living. Medications may be given to reduce joint swelling and inflammation. In addition, warm compresses to the involved joints are soothing.

Encourage Adequate Nutrition

Promote general health by encouraging a well-balanced diet. Children with decreased mobility may have reduced metabolic needs, and excess weight causes additional muscle strain. Periodically perform diet recalls and nutritional assessments. Plot growth carefully and watch for changes in growth and body mass index (BMI) percentiles. (See Chapter 14 ∞ for additional information regarding nutritional assessment.)

Care in the Community

The child with JIA may never, or rarely, be hospitalized. Most care takes place during visits to health care offices, clinics, and physical therapy. Educate parents about the child's condition and prognosis, and answer their questions about the child's treatment. The child and family may need support to adjust to the diagnosis of a chronic illness. (See Chapter 12 ∞.) Encourage the child to maintain contact with peers and to attend school when possible. Explain to the child and parents that overexertion may lead to exacerbation of the disease. Inform parents about possible complications of JIA, such as altered growth related to early closure of epiphyseal plates, small joint contractures, and synovitis. Teach parents about signs of infection, encourage recommended immunizations, and encourage health promotion activities such as nutritious diet and adequate rest. Parents and children can be referred to the Arthritis Foundation and the American Juvenile Arthritis Foundation for further information and support.

Clinical Judgment

Children with JIA may receive aspirin therapy as part of their treatment regimen, placing them at increased risk for developing Reye syndrome (see Chapter 27 ∞). Which vaccines should the nurse ensure that these children have received in order to decrease their risk?

Collaborate with the family and school officials to meet the child's needs. Accommodations at school may include providing a set of books for the home so the child is not required to carry the books home daily. Additional time may be required for the child to move from class to class. Adaptive computers and tutors during exacerbations may also be helpful. School nurses work with the child, family, and school personnel to establish the child's individualized education plan (IEP).

Evaluation

Expected outcomes of nursing care for the child with JIA include the following:

- The child maintains joint mobility.
- The child expresses comfort and freedom from pain.
- The child develops a positive body image.
- The child is free from infection.
- Parents express adequate understanding, support, and management of the therapeutic regimen.

■ ALLERGIC REACTIONS

For unclear reasons, there continues to be a rise in the number of children diagnosed with conditions related to allergies. Why are some children allergic to cats, for instance, although no one else in the family has allergies? To answer this question, the nurse requires a basic understanding of the mechanisms of allergy.

An **allergy** is an abnormal or altered reaction to an antigen. Antigens responsible for clinical manifestations of allergy are called **allergens**. Allergens can be ingested in food or drugs, injected or absorbed through contact with unbroken skin, or inhaled. Common allergens in children include medications such as penicillin; animal dander; dust mites, mold, and plant pollens; and foods such as nuts, seafood, or egg white. An allergic reaction is an antigen-antibody reaction and can manifest itself as anaphylaxis, atopic disease, serum sickness, or contact dermatitis. Therefore, the symptoms can be mild to severe or life threatening, and they can be localized or systemic. Characteristic findings in children with allergies are summarized in Table 22–7.

TABLE 22–7	Characteristic Findings in Children with Allergies
System	Clinical Manifestations
Respiratory	Asthma, rhinitis (seasonal and perennial), serous otitis media, cough, pneumonia, croup, edema of glottis
Gastrointestinal	Abdominal pain and colic, stomatitis, constipation, diarrhea, bloody stools, geographic tongue, vomiting
Skin	Angioedema, urticaria, atopic eczema, erythema multiforme, purpura, drug and food rashes, contact dermatitis
Nervous	Headache, tension, fatigue, convulsions, Ménière disease, tremor
Eye	Conjunctivitis, cataract, ciliary spasm, iritis
Blood	Thrombocytopenic purpura, hemolytic anemia, leukopenia, agranulocytosis
Musculoskeletal	Arthralgia, myalgia, arthritis, torticollis
Genitourinary	Dysuria, vulvovaginitis, enuresis
Miscellaneous	Anaphylactic shock, serum sickness, autoimmune diseases

The **hypersensitivity response**, an overreaction of the immune system, is responsible for allergic reactions. Hypersensitivity reactions have been classified into four types (Table 22–8). Type I hypersensitivity reactions are immediate reactions that occur within seconds or minutes of exposure to the antigen. The release of chemical substances such as histamine is responsible for the signs and symptoms. The first time a child is exposed to the allergen, there is no reaction. With every exposure thereafter, however, the child who is allergic may have a reaction to the allergen.

Type II sensitivity reactions occur within 15 to 30 minutes after exposure to the antigen. Type III hypersensitivity reactions may be difficult to distinguish from type II reactions. Hypersensitivity reactions generally peak within 6 hours.

TABLE 22–8	Types of Hypersensitivity Reactions		
Type	Etiology	Clinical Manifestations	Examples
Type I Localized or systemic reactions (anaphylaxis)	Antibodies bind to certain cells, causing release of chemical substances that produce an inflammatory reaction.	Hypotension, wheezing, gastrointestinal or uterine spasm, stridor, urticaria	Extrinsic asthma, hay fever
Type II Tissue-specific reactions	Antibodies cause activation of a complement system, which leads to tissue damage.	Variable; may include dyspnea or fever	Transfusion reaction, ABO incompatibility, hemolytic disease of the newborn
Type III Immune-complex reactions	Immune complexes are deposited in tissues, where they activate complement, which results in a generalized inflammatory reaction.	Urticaria, fever, joint pain	Acute glomerulonephritis, serum sickness
Type IV Delayed reactions	Antigens stimulate T cells that release lymphokines, which cause inflammation and tissue damage.	Variable; may include fever, erythema, itching	Contact dermatitis, tuberculin skin test, graft-versus-host disease, allograft rejection

Anaphylaxis is an exaggerated hypersensitivity reaction that may manifest with itching; localized or generalized hives on the hands, feet, or mucosa; soft-tissue swelling; cough; dyspnea; pallor; sweating; and tachycardia. Severe reactions may lead to respiratory distress or death. Nursing roles involve preventing anaphylactic reactions by teaching families how to minimize exposure and by alerting all health care personnel in hospitals and clinics to the child's allergy. In addition, knowledge of emergency procedures is important in all facilities such as schools, homes, and hospitals.

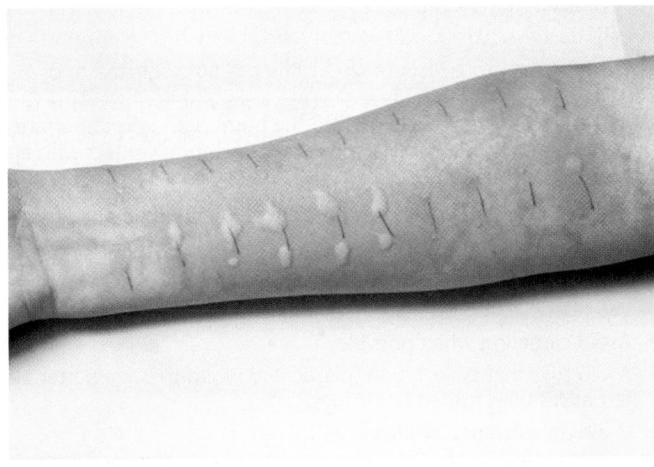

FIGURE 22–7 ➤ Results of intradermal skin testing on the forearm. Injections are given on each side of the markings. Note the positive results marked by induration and erythema in response to certain antigens.
Photo Researchers, Inc.

Type IV reactions are delayed responses that do not appear until several hours after exposure and require 24 to 72 hours to develop fully. A type IV reaction, which is not confined to any specific tissue, is elicited by relatively complex antigens such as those of bacteria and viruses and by simple antigens such as drugs and metals. (See Chapter 31 ∞ for a description of contact dermatitis.)

Assessment of the child with allergy includes a complete physical examination; laboratory, radiograph, and pulmonary function studies; tests of nasal function; and skin testing. Treatment generally involves avoidance of the allergen, such as substitution of a different drug when the child has a drug allergy. Desensitization may sometimes be used, with increasing doses of the allergen administered intradermally in an office where resuscitation is readily available. This treatment is useful for allergy to bees or some pollens. For skin allergies, the allergen is avoided, skin is kept well lubricated, and topical steroids may be used. Oral antihistamines are sometimes used to treat allergy. Emergency medical care may be required to treat anaphylaxis.

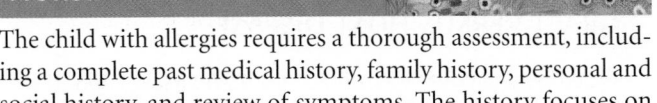

NURSING MANAGEMENT

The child with allergies requires a thorough assessment, including a complete past medical history, family history, personal and social history, and review of symptoms. The history focuses on the following areas:

- What symptoms does the child experience? Encourage the child to describe the difficulty in his or her own words.
- Are the symptoms continuous or intermittent? What are the frequency and duration of episodes?
- When did the child first begin to experience symptoms? Did the child have eczema or a feeding problem in infancy or childhood? Did the infant have frequent episodes of colic or skin problems when new foods were introduced? Was there a change in symptoms at puberty? Are the symptoms becoming worse or spontaneously improving?
- What known agents in the environment cause difficulties?
- Are there seasonal variations in symptoms? At what time of the day or night do symptoms usually occur?

The nurse may be responsible for performing intradermal skin tests for allergies (Figure 22–7 ➤). Nursing care focuses on treating the symptoms, alleviating the anxiety of the child and parents, and identifying the allergens. Teaching the child and family how to minimize or avoid exposure to allergens is im-

portant. Parents of children who have had severe reactions to bee or wasp stings should be taught how to take precautions and how to provide emergency treatment if the child is stung.

Instruct the family on proper use of epinephrine (see Families Want to Know: Using an EpiPen). Families may also need instructions on allergy-proofing the home. Pets, dust, carpets, fabrics, feather pillows and bedding, and cigarette smoke can all cause allergic reactions (see Families Want to Know: Removing Common Allergens from the Home). If families are reluctant to give up pets, frequent baths can reduce dander, which is the usual allergen.

When the child has type I reactions to an environmental substance, avoidance of the allergen is most critical. In addition, care providers, families, and school personnel must be able to treat anaphylaxis if exposure to the allergen occurs. When the child is hospitalized, be sure to label the child's chart and bed, and apply a red armband to alert others to allergies. School nurses keep records about children's allergies and inform school personnel about the allergies and cautions that need to be followed. Nurses must be aware of the resuscitation procedures and equipment in

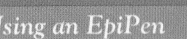

Families Want to Know
Using an EpiPen

If the child has had a severe or systemic reaction in the past, ensure that the parents know how to handle an anaphylactic reaction if the child experiences another reaction.

- Kits with syringes of premeasured epinephrine are available by prescription.
- Ensure that family members understand how to use the kit.
- Encourage the child to wear a medical alert bracelet.
- Instruct the family on proper storage of the kit and to avoid exposing the kit to sun or high temperature.
- Instruct the family to frequently check the expiration date of the epinephrine.
- Emphasize to the family that a kit should be readily available at school, camp, childcare, or other settings, with someone instructed in its use.

Exposure to the known allergens in the home setting is important. Several measures that families can take to minimize contact with allergens are as follows:

- Remove household pets, or keep them out of the child's bedroom.
- Control dust by frequent cleaning.
- Clean with moist cloths and mops to remove dust.
- Use plastic covers on mattresses and pillows.
- Avoid carpeting when possible.
- Avoid toys that collect dust (plastic and wood toys are better alternatives than stuffed fabric toys).
- Use high-efficiency air filters.
- Repair homes to prevent entry of water and subsequent molds.
- Consider dehumidification in moist climates.

all facilities such as hospital units, offices, childcare centers, and schools. See Chapter 14 ∞ for information on serious allergies to food such as peanut allergy, Chapter 20 ∞ for information on airway maintenance and asthma, and the *Clinical Skills Manual* for resuscitation procedures.

Latex Allergy

Latex is a sap from the rubber tree. Latex allergy is caused by an IgE-mediated response that develops after repeated exposure to latex. A reaction to latex products can be manifested as an irritant reaction of the skin; as a type IV delayed hypersensitivity with redness, inflammation, and blisters on the skin; or as a type I hypersensitivity, which is immediate and often has systemic manifestations (itchy eyes, asthma, or anaphylaxis) (De Queiroz, Combet, Berard, et al., 2009; Paskawicz, 2005).

Latex allergy is a common finding among certain occupations, including health care workers, and in specific types of patients. An estimated 5–15% of health care workers and approximately 60% of children with spina bifida are allergic to latex (Asthma and Allergy Foundation of America, 2010). In addition, children who have frequent medical procedures or multiple surgeries involving latex are at increased risk of developing allergy to latex (Asthma and Allergy Foundation of America, 2010; De Queiroz et al., 2009).

Children and adolescents at high risk should receive allergy testing for latex; the radioallergosorbent test (RAST) is most often used. RAST is a common laboratory test used to detect IgE antibodies. It measures circulating IgE antibodies to many allergens and generally correlates well with skin test results. Health

 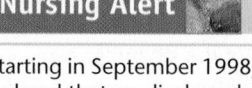
Starting in September 1998, the U.S. Food and Drug Administration ordered that medical products with latex carry a warning label that reads: "Caution: This product contains natural rubber latex, which may cause allergic reactions." Check the products in your health care facility to find this label. What products do you expect to need the label? When children have latex allergy, have the family investigate all medical supplies for the warning label.

care personnel should use alternative products when caring for those persons at risk.

When a positive skin test has occurred or when the person has had a reaction to latex, all latex products must be removed from the individual's environment. Alternative products, such as nonlatex gloves and catheters, must be used when providing health care. These individuals should also wear a medical identification bracelet at all times, and should have an epinephrine kit readily available at home and school. Nurses should be alert for any signs of hypersensitivity when the child is receiving health care, and be prepared with drugs and equipment to treat anaphylaxis. This is especially important in operative settings when acute anaphylaxis is often life threatening. Nurses should emphasize to parents and children that many everyday products contain latex, including latex balloons and pacifiers (Box 22–2).

■ GRAFT-VERSUS-HOST DISEASE

Graft-versus-host disease can occur when organs are transplanted or when bone marrow or stem cells are transfused into a recipient, typically as treatment for leukemia or severe combined immunodeficiency disease. The donated cells attach to the recipient child's bone marrow and begin production. The child's lymphocyte production increases and immune response develops. However, despite prior blood and tissue typing, sometimes the donor cells are incompatible with the recipient cells and the new cells begin to mount an immunologic response in the child who has received the transplant. The incidence of the disease is lower in matched siblings than in matched nonsibling transplants (Velardi & Locatelli, 2007).

Graft-versus-host disease may be either acute or chronic. Acute disease occurs in the first 100 days after transplant. The skin is most commonly affected, and the condition manifests as a pruritic and macular-papular rash that begins on the ears, palms, and soles, progressing to the trunk. Blistering and a burning sensation may occur. Gastrointestinal effects may include nausea, vomiting, anorexia, diarrhea, cramping, and abdominal pain. Impaired liver function is evident from jaundice and abnormal liver function tests (Velardi & Locatelli, 2007). Chronic graft-versus-host disease occurs after the 100 days posttransplant; this reaction is similar to an autoimmune reaction in the recipient's body (Negrin & Blume, 2006).

Careful physical examination and laboratory tests assist in determining presence of the disease and stage of reaction. Early identification is key to beginning therapy and stopping progression of the life-threatening condition. Several drugs are used in treatment, commonly cyclosporine, tacrolimus, and prednisone (Velardi & Locatelli, 2007).

Nursing care focuses on careful physical assessment of all children who have received transplants to assist in early identification of the disease process. All body systems can be involved, especially in chronic disease, so frequent and thorough assessments are needed. Place particular emphasis on skin examina-

tion and report rashes that occur. Monitor gastrointestinal functioning by asking about nausea, vomiting, diarrhea, abdominal pain, bloody stools, and dietary intake. Weigh and measure the child and compare to earlier findings. Auscultate the lungs and be alert for signs of infection. Inquire about pain in joints or other body parts. Perform regular eye examinations and ask about burning or itching of eyes. Perform prescribed blood tests to monitor for liver and bone marrow function.

Nursing care for the child who has had a bone marrow or stem cell transplant is complex. Emphasize the need for regular examinations to identify any signs of disease. Children and their families need information and support about this immune system complication of transplantation of bone marrow or stem cells.

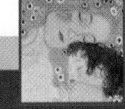

Chapter Highlights

- The infant is born with natural immunity from the mother and develops acquired immunity gradually in the first 6 years of life.
- Acquired immunity is humoral (antibody mediated) and cell mediated.
- B cells, T cells, natural killer (NK) cells, and complement proteins are the major components of a healthy immune system.
- Disorders of the immune system can be due to genetic causes (primary immunodeficiency) or can be acquired (secondary immunodeficiency).
- Severe combined immunodeficiency disease (SCID) is life threatening and requires careful medical and nursing management.
- Human immunodeficiency virus (HIV) can lead to acquired immune deficiency syndrome (AIDS); care focuses on prevention of this viral infection.
- When the child is infected with HIV, support for nutrition, infection control, and developmental stimulation is needed.
- Nurses provide support for families of children with severe immune deficiency with a focus on finances, provision of complex medical care, and emotional support.
- Autoimmune disorders such as eczema, juvenile idiopathic arthritis, and systemic lupus erythematosus occur when the body perceives its own tissue as foreign and mounts a defense against it.

- Systemic lupus erythematosus (SLE), a generalized disorder mainly occurring in females, is a chronic inflammatory, autoimmune disease of unknown origin that involves many organ systems.
- Juvenile idiopathic arthritis is a chronic autoimmune inflammatory disease characterized by joint inflammation resulting in decreased mobility, swelling, and pain that occurs twice as often in females as in males.
- There continues to be a rise in the number of children diagnosed with some types of allergy. A thorough assessment and careful teaching can help the child with allergies to successfully manage reactions.
- Allergy to latex products is commonly seen in children, health care workers, and the general population. Children most at risk for latex allergy include those with spina bifida and those undergoing frequent medical procedures or multiple surgeries involving latex.
- Graft-versus-host disease is a type IV hypersensitivity reaction in which the donor T lymphocytes are stimulated by the recipient's antigen-presenting cells.

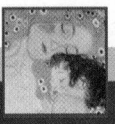

Clinical Reasoning in Action

Recall Raymond, the 2-year-old introduced at the beginning of this chapter, who, after repeated infections, was diagnosed with AIDS. Raymond had no other risk factors for HIV and AIDS, so the health care team recommended that Raymond's mother be tested for the infection. She was subsequently diagnosed with HIV infection whereas Raymond's 5-year-old sister tested negative for

HIV. The family is dealing with the diagnosis for both Raymond and his mother as well as learning to care for Raymond.

1. Raymond is having difficulty eating. After you consider his age of 2 years and the recommended intake at this age, plan a daily menu for him with several small feedings.

2. You have just been assigned to care for Raymond during a day shift. Organize your morning assessment of Raymond. Plan to observe the systems constituting the most frequent sources of infection in children with HIV.

3. What is the most common cause of Raymond's infection with HIV? How might the family react when they learn about perinatal transmission?

4. Dealing with the challenges of HIV in a young child taxes the family's resources. Plan nursing care that involves HAART medication administration and interventions to promote Raymond's development.

See Pearson Nursing Student Resources for possible responses.

Pearson Nursing Student Resources

Find additional review materials at
nursing.pearsonhighered.com

Prepare for success with NCLEX®-style practice questions, interactive assignments and activities, web links, animations and videos, and more!

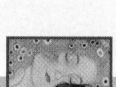

References

Alvarez, A. M., & Rathore, M. H. (2007). Hot topics in pediatric HIV/AIDS. *Pediatric Annals, 36*(7), 423–432.

American Academy of Pediatrics (AAP). (2009). *Red book: Report of the Committee on Infectious Diseases* (28th ed.). Elk Grove Village, IL: Author.

Asthma and Allergy Foundation of America. (2010). *Latex allergy.* Retrieved from http://www.aafa.org/display.cfm?id=9&sub=21&cont=383

Baker, C. J. (2007). *Red book atlas of pediatric infectious diseases.* Elk Grove Village, IL: American Academy of Pediatrics.

Bawle, E. W. (2008). *DiGeorge syndrome.* Retrieved from http://emedicine.medscape.com/article/886526-overview

Bernatsky, S., Duffy, C., Malleson, P., Feldman, D. E., St. Pierre, Y., & Clarke, A. E. (2007). Economic impact of juvenile idiopathic arthritis. *Arthritis & Rheumatism, 57*(1), 44–48.

Bindler, R., & Howry, L. (2005). *Pediatric drugs and nursing implications.* Upper Saddle River, NJ: Prentice Hall Health.

Bonilla, F. A., & Geha, R. S. (2006). Update on primary immunodeficiency diseases. *Journal of Allergy and Clinical Immunology, 117,* S435–S441.

Brunner, H. I., Higgins, G. C., Wiers, K., Lapidus, S. K., Olson, J. C., Onel, K., et al. (2009). Health-related quality of life and its relationship to patient disease course in childhood-onset systemic lupus erythematosus. *Journal of Rheumatology, 36*(7), 1536–1545.

Buckley, R. H. (2007). The T-, B-, and NK-cell systems. In R. M. Kliegman, R. E. Behrman, H. B. Jenson, & B. F. Stanton (Eds.), *Nelson textbook of pediatrics* (18th ed., pp. 873–879). Philadelphia: Saunders Elsevier.

Buckley, R. H. (2008). DiGeorge. In *Merck manual online.* Whitehouse Station, NJ: Merck Research

Laboratories. Retrieved from http://www.merck.com.ch164/ch164h.html?qt=DiGeorge&alt=sh

Burack, G., Gaur, S., Marone, R., & Petrova, A. (2010). Adherence to antiretroviral therapy in pediatric patients with human immunodeficiency virus (HIV-1). *Journal of Pediatric Nursing, 25*(6), 500–504.

Cassidy, J. T., & Petty, R. E. (2005). Chronic arthritis in childhood. In J. T. Cassidy, R. E. Petty, R. M. Laxer, & C. B. Lindsley (Eds.), *Textbook of pediatric rheumatology* (5th ed., pp. 206–260). Philadelphia: Elsevier Saunders.

Centers for Disease Control and Prevention (CDC). (2007). *Mother to child (perinatal) HIV transmission and prevention.* Retrieved from http://www.cdc.gov/hiv/topics/perinatal/resources/factsheets/pdf/perinatal.pdf

Centers for Disease Control and Prevention (CDC). (2009). *HIV/AIDS among African Americans.* Retrieved from http://www.cdc.gov/hiv/topics/aa/resources/factsheets/pdf/aa.pdf

Cibulka, N. J. (2006). Mother-to-child transmission of HIV in the United States. *American Journal of Nursing, 106*(7), 56–63.

Coren, J. S., Ciervo, C. A., & Mason, D. (2008, June). Ten-month-old with joint swelling in left hand and left knee. *Consultant for Pediatricians, 7*(6), 245–247.

Delaney, K. P., Branson, B. M., Uniyal, A., Kerndt, P. R., Keenan, P. A., Jafa, K., et al. (2006). Performance of an oral fluid rapid HIV-1/2 test: Experience from four CDC studies. *AIDS, 20,* 1655–1660.

De Queiroz, M., Combet, S., Berard, J., Pouyau, A., Genest, H., & Mouriqua, P. (2009). Latex allergy in children: Modalities and prevention. *Pediatric Anesthesia, 19,* 313–319.

Diamond, B., & Grimaldi, C. (2009). B cells. In G. S. Firestein, R. C. Budd, E. D. Harris, I. B. McInnes,

S. Ruddy, & J. S. Sergent, *Kelley's textbook of rheumatology* (8th ed., pp. 177–199). Philadelphia: Saunders-Elsevier.

Dibbern, D. A., & Routes, J. M. (2009). *Wiscott-Aldrich syndrome.* Retrieved from http://www.emedicine.com/med/topic1162.htm

Gottlieb, B. S., & Ilowite, N. T. (2006). Systemic lupus erythematosus in children and adolescents. *Pediatrics in Review, 27*(9), 323–328.

Greenwald, J. L., Burstein, G. R., Pincus, J., & Branson, B. (2006). A rapid review of rapid HIV antibody tests. *Current Infectious Disease Reports, 8,* 125–131.

Hahn, E. K. (2009). Incorporating the CDC recommendations for adolescent HIV screening into practice. *Journal for Nurse Practitioners, 5*(4), 265–273.

Heird, W. C. (2007). The feeding of infants and children. In R. M. Kliegman, R. E. Behrman, H. B. Jenson, & B. F. Stanton (Eds.), *Nelson textbook of pediatrics* (18th ed., pp. 214–224). Philadelphia: Saunders Elsevier.

Joshi, S. A., & Davies, S. M. (2009). Hematopoietic stem cell transplantation for immunodeficiencies and genetic diseases. In R. Hoffman, E. J. Benz, S. J. Shattil, B. Furie, L. E. Silberstein, P. McGlave, & H. Heslop (Eds.), *Hematology: Basic principles and practice* (5th ed., pp. 1577–1586). Philadelphia: Churchill Livingstone-Elsevier.

Klein-Gitelman, M. S. (2010). *Systemic lupus erythematosus.* Retrieved from http://emedicine.medscape.com/article/1008066-overview

Kline, M. W. (2006). Perspectives on the pediatric HIV/AIDS pandemic: Catalyzing access of children to care and treatment. *Pediatrics, 117,* 1388–1393.

Kobrynski, L. J. (2006). Combined immune deficiencies in children. *Journal of Infusion Nursing, 29*(4), 213.

Lewis, D. B., Nadeau, K. C., & Cohen, A. C. (2009). Disorders of lymphocyte function. In R. Hoffman, E. J. Benz, S. J. Shattil, B. Furie, L. E. Silberstein, P. McGlave, & H. Heslop (Eds.), *Hematology: Basic principles and practice* (5th ed., pp. 721–745). Philadelphia: Churchill Livingstone-Elsevier.

Lupus Foundation of America. (2008). *About lupus.* Retrieved from http://www.lupus.org/webmodules/webarticlesnet/templates/new_aboutintroduction.aspx?articleid=311&zoneid=9

Mahat, G., Scoloveno, M. A., DeLeon, T., & Frenkel, J. (2008). Preliminary evidence of an adolescent HIV/AIDS peer education program. *Journal of Pediatric Nursing, 23*(5), 358–363.

Marinescu, L. M., & Ilowite, N. T. (2007). Update on pediatric rheumatology: Growth spurt in the knowledge base. *Consultant for Pediatricians, 6*(7), 397–404.

Marodi, L. (2006). Innate cellular immune response in newborns. *Clinical Immunology, 118*, 137–144.

Marón, G., Gaur, A. H., & Flynn, P. M. (2010). Antiretroviral therapy in HIV-infected infants and children. *Pediatric Infectious Disease Journal, 29*(4), 360–363.

McLean-Tooke, A., Spickett, G. P., & Gennery, A. R. (2007). Immunodeficiency and autoimmunity in 22q11.2 deletion syndrome. *Scandinavian Journal of Immunology, 66*, 1–7.

Michaels, M. G., & Green, M. (2007). Infections in immunocompromised persons. In R. M. Kliegman, R. E. Behrman, H. B. Jenson, & B. F. Stanton (Eds.), *Nelson textbook of pediatrics* (18th ed., pp. 1100–1107). Philadelphia: Saunders Elsevier.

Naar-King, S., Templin, T., Wright, K., Frey, M., Parsons, J. T., & Lam, P. (2006). Psychosocial factors and medication adherence in HIV-positive youth. *AIDS Patient Care and STDs, 20*(1), 44–47.

Nagaraj, N., Egwim, C., & Adler, D. G. (2007, April). X-linked hyper-IgM syndrome associated with poorly differentiated neuroendocrine tumor presenting as obstructive jaundice secondary to extensive adenopathy. *Digestive Diseases and Sciences, 52*(9), 2312–2316.

Negrin, R. S., & Blume, K. G. (2006). Principles of hematopoietic cell transplantation. In M. A. Lichtman, E. Beutler, T. J. Kipps, U. Seligsohn, K. Kaushansky, & J. T. Prchal, *Williams hematology* (7th ed.). Retrieved from http://www.accessmedicine.com

Nistala, K., Woo, P., & Wedderburn, L. R. (2009). Juvenile idiopathic arthritis. In G. S. Firestein, R. C. Budd, E. D. Harris, I. B. McInnes, S. Ruddy, & J. S. Sergent, *Kelley's textbook of rheumatology* (8th ed., pp. 1657–1675). Philadelphia: Saunders-Elsevier.

Ochs, H. D., & Thrasher, A. J. (2006). The Wiskott-Aldrich syndrome. *Journal of Allergy and Clinical Immunology, 117*(4), 725–738.

Paskawicz, J. (2005). Latex allergy revisited. *Clinician Reviews, 15*(11), 66–75.

Plowfield, L. A. (2007). HIV disease in children 25 years later. *Pediatric Nursing, 33*(3), 274–278, 273.

Pongmarutani, T., Alpert, P. T., & Miller, S. K. (2006). Pediatric systemic lupus erythematosus: Management issues in primary practice. *Journal of the American Academy of Nurse Practitioners, 18*, 258–267.

Puck, J. M., & Malech, H. L. (2006). Gene therapy for immune disorders: Good news tempered by bad news. *Journal of Allergy and Clinical Immunology, 117*(4), 865–869.

Sanzo, M. (2008). The child with arthritis in the school setting. *Journal of School Nursing, 24*(4), 190–196.

Sarma, P. K., Misra, R., & Aggarwal, A. (2008). Physical disability, articular, and extra-articular damage in patients with juvenile idiopathic arthritis. *Clinical Rheumatology, 27*, 1261–1265.

Spina Bifida Association. (2007). *Latex (natural rubber) in the hospital environment* and *Latex (natural rubber) in the home and community.* Retrieved from http://www.spinabifidaassociation.org/atf/cf/%7BEED435C8-F1A0-4A16-B4D8-A713BBCD9CE4%7D/2007%20Latex%20Lists.pdf

Tucker, L. B. (2007). Making the diagnosis of systemic lupus erythematosus in children and adolescents. *Lupus, 16*, 546–549.

U.S. Department of Health and Human Services. (2009a). *Guidelines for the use of antiretroviral agents in pediatric HIV infection.* Retrieved from http://aidsinfo.nih.gov/contentfiles/PediatricGuidelines.pdf

U.S. Department of Health and Human Services. (2009b). *Pediatric antiretroviral drug information.* Retrieved from http://aidsinfo.nih.gov/contentfiles/PediatricGL_SupI.pdf

Velardi, A., & Locatelli, F. (2007). Graft versus host disease (GVHD) and rejection. In R. M. Kliegman, R. E. Behrman, H. B. Jenson, & B. F. Stanton (Eds.), *Nelson textbook of pediatrics* (18th ed., pp. 930–931). Philadelphia: Saunders Elsevier.

Williams, P. L., Storm, D., Montepiedra, G., Nichols, S., Kammerer, B., Sirois, P. A., et al. (2006). Predictors of adherence to antiretroviral medications in children and adolescents with HIV infections. *Pediatrics, 118*(6), e1745–e1757.

Yee, A., DeRavin, S. S., Elliott, E., Ziegler, J. B., & Contributors to the Australian Paediatric Surveillance Unit. (2008). Severe combined immunodeficiency: A national surveillance study. *Pediatric Allergy and Immunology, 19*, 298–302.

Alterations in Hematologic Function

chapter 23

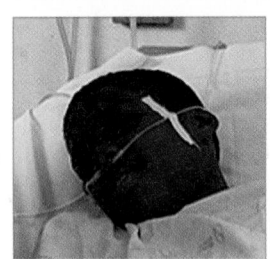

Michael, a 12-year-old boy, is admitted to the hospital with severe abdominal pain. He was diagnosed with sickle cell anemia at 1 year of age and has been in fairly good health. He has, however, been hospitalized on two previous occasions with complications of the disease. Recently, Michael has had several viral illnesses, leading his physician to suspect that his spleen is filled with abnormal cells that are impairing his immune function.

Michael is small for his age and has several bruises on his lower legs. His respirations are rapid and he appears anxious. Michael's parents are knowledgeable about sickle cell anemia, as his uncle also has the disease. They know that Michael is experiencing an episode of sickle cell crisis.

An intravenous infusion is started, and Michael is medicated for pain. The nurse attempts to perform multiple tests and procedures together to allow Michael time to rest in between. Michael is receiving oxygen by nasal cannula to increase his oxygen saturation to normal levels.

What immediate and long-term care does Michael require? What do Michael and his parents need to know about this crisis? How could you help them manage the challenges of this condition? This chapter will assist you in planning care for children like Michael who have disorders of the hematologic system.

Learning Outcomes

After reading this chapter, you will be able to do the following:

1. Describe the function of red blood cells, white blood cells, and platelets. 475-76
2. Summarize the etiology, clinical manifestations, and nursing care for a child with iron deficiency anemia. 476
3. Distinguish pathophysiology and clinical manifestations for chronic disorders of red blood cells.
4. Plan nursing care for the child with a chronic disorder of red blood cells.
5. Distinguish pathophysiology and clinical manifestations for the major bleeding disorders affecting the pediatric population.
6. Prioritize nursing interventions for a child with a major bleeding disorder.
7. Summarize nursing implications for a child receiving hematopoietic stem cell transplantation (HSCT).

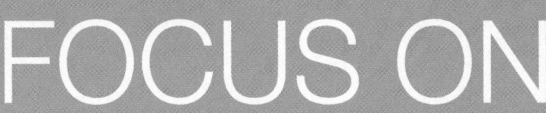

FOCUS ON

The Hematologic System

ANATOMY AND PHYSIOLOGY

Blood has two components: a fluid portion called plasma and a cellular portion known as the formed elements of the blood. Plasma contains proteins, electrolytes, clotting factors, antibodies, and anticoagulants. The cellular elements are red blood cells or RBCs (**erythrocytes**), white blood cells or WBCs (**leukocytes**), and platelets (**thrombocytes**) (Figure 23–1 ➤). Table 23–1 gives normal values for these blood components in children.

Red Blood Cells

Red blood cells, or erythrocytes, are the most abundant of the cellular elements of blood. They are formed through a process called **erythropoiesis**. The primary function of red blood cells is to transport oxygen from the lungs to the tissues. These cells also help to carry carbon dioxide back to the lungs. Hemoglobin, a red pigment composed of protein and iron which is contained in the RBC, is essential to this function. The normal life span of a red blood cell is about 120 days. See Chapter 21 ∞ for a discussion of fetal hemoglobin and its unique characteristics, as well as its effect on hemoglobin levels in the newborn period.

    Polycythemia is an above-average increase in the number of red cells in the blood. Any condition that causes the quantity of oxygen transported to the tissues to decrease ordinarily increases the rate of red blood cell production. When a child becomes anemic secondary to hemorrhage, for instance, the bone marrow immediately begins to produce large quantities of red cells. **Anemia** is a reduction in the number of red blood cells; the various types of anemia will be discussed in this chapter.

White Blood Cells

White blood cells, or leukocytes, are the mobile units of the body's protective system. They are formed in bone marrow and lymph tissue. There are five types of white blood cells, each with a distinct function (Table 23–2). A differential blood count indicates the percentages of the different types of white cells present in the blood and is sometimes useful in identifying the cause of an illness. For example, infections cause an increase in neutrophils, and allergies are related to an increase in eosinophils. The role of lymphocytes is discussed with acquired immunodeficiency syndrome in Chapter 22 ∞. A decrease in the number of white blood cells is called **leukopenia**, and can be caused by immune or bone marrow disorders.

Platelets

Platelets, or thrombocytes, are cell fragments that can form hemostatic plugs to stop bleeding. They are synthesized from components in the red bone marrow and are stored in the spleen. A deficiency of platelets can lead to a bleeding disorder and is termed **thrombocytopenia**.

PEDIATRIC DIFFERENCES

Production of *red blood cells* occurs in the fetus by the second week of gestation, with white blood cell and platelet production beginning at 8 weeks. Most of this early production occurs first in the embryonic yolk sac and then in the liver; however, by 20 to 24 weeks' gestation, liver production decreases as bone marrow production begins to predominate (Chamley, Carson,

TABLE 23–1	Mean Values for Common Hematology Tests in Children Ages 2–12 Years
Test	Mean Value
Red blood cell (RBC)	$3.89–5.03 \times 10^{12}$/L
Hemoglobin (Hb)	10.2–13.4 g/dL
Hematocrit (HCT)	31.7–39.8%
White blood cell (WBC)	$4.86–11.4 \times 10^{9}$/L
Platelets	$150–400 \times 10^{9}$/L

Adapted from: Soldin, S. J., Brugnara, C., & Wong, E. C. (2007). Pediatric reference ranges (6th ed.). Washington, DC: AACC Press; Kliegman, R. M., Behrman, R. E., Jenson, H. B., & Stanton, B. F. (2007). Nelson textbook of pediatrics (18th ed.). Philadelphia: Saunders Elsevier.

TABLE 23–2	White Blood Cells and Their Functions
Cell Type	Function
Neutrophils	Phagocytosis
Eosinophils	Allergic reactions
Basophils	Inflammatory reactions
Monocytes (macrophages)	Phagocytosis, antigen processing
Lymphocytes	Humoral immunity (B cell), cellular immunity (T cell)

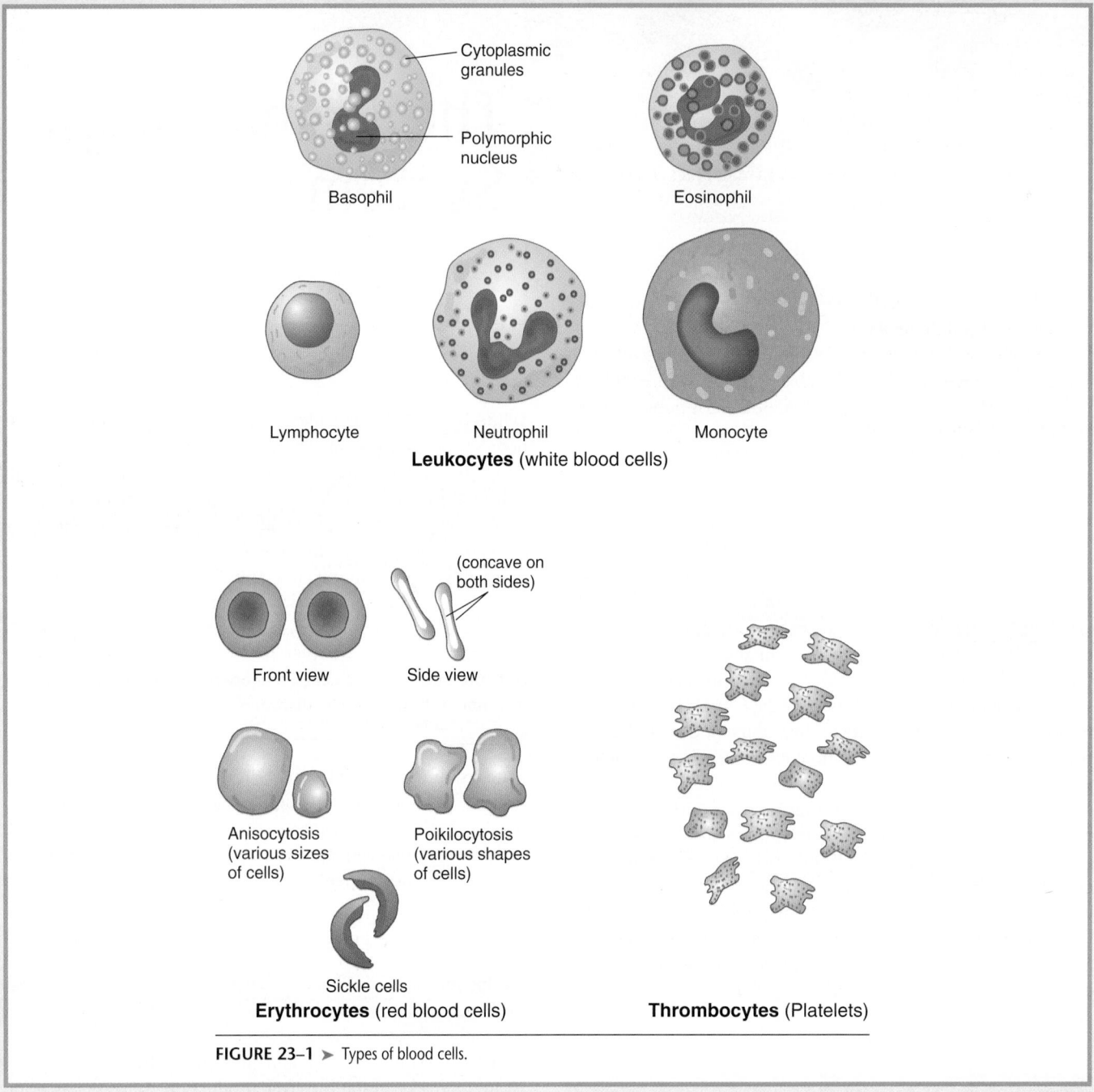

Leukocytes (white blood cells)

Cytoplasmic granules

Polymorphic nucleus

Basophil

Eosinophil

Lymphocyte

Neutrophil

Monocyte

(concave on both sides)

Front view

Side view

Anisocytosis (various sizes of cells)

Poikilocytosis (various shapes of cells)

Sickle cells

Erythrocytes (red blood cells)

Thrombocytes (Platelets)

FIGURE 23–1 ➤ Types of blood cells.

Randall, et al., 2005; Ohls & Christensen, 2007). At birth, **hematopoiesis**, or blood cell production, occurs in the marrow of almost every bone. The flat bones, such as the sternum, ribs, pelvic and shoulder girdles, vertebrae, and hips, retain most of their hematopoietic activity throughout life.

Fetal RBCs contain fetal hemoglobin, which has a high level of affinity for oxygen. The fetus must extract oxygen from the maternal circulation, which has lower oxygen saturation than the atmosphere, so the developing fetus needs this enhanced ability. Fetal hemoglobin is present in decreasing amounts after birth, with normal hemoglobin gradually increasing.

Blood volume of the newborn term infant is approximately 85 mL/kg of body weight (London, Ladewig, Ball, et al., 2011). At birth, the newborn has a naturally occurring elevation in RBCs and hemoglobin due to a high level of erythropoietin, which stimulates red cell production. Additional contributors to these higher RBC levels are the transfusion of blood from the placenta at birth and low extracellular fluid volume from low oral intake after birth. Once the newborn begins breathing air and the oxygen level in the blood increases, the RBC production slows. Levels of RBCs and hemoglobin fall until about 2 to 3 months of age (to about 9–11 g/dL), and then begin increasing. Adult levels are reached during adolescence. Teenage males have red blood cell levels slightly higher than teenage females (see Appendix D ∞).

The *white blood cell* count is highest at birth, although levels vary greatly among infants. By 1 week of age, white blood cell values stabilize. Throughout childhood, there is a very slow decrease in white blood cell count (Boxer, 2007).

Platelet levels in newborns are lower than in older children and adults. Levels of many clotting factors, particularly those requiring vitamin K for activation (factors II, VII, IX, X, and anticoagulant factors—proteins C and S), are also lower in infants. For this reason, all newborns receive a prophylactic injection of vitamin K at birth. Values of platelets and other coagulation products soon reach normal childhood levels (Scott & Montgomery, 2007).

Examples of diagnostic and laboratory tests used to evaluate the hematologic system are provided in Box 23–1; see Appendices D and E ∞ for more detailed descriptions. Use the assessment guidelines on this page to perform a nursing assessment of this system.

The hematologic system is one of the few body systems that regulate, directly or indirectly, all other body functions. Because blood is involved in the function of all tissues and organs, changes in the blood may result in altered functioning of many body organs and structures. A tendency toward easy bruising is a characteristic sign of many bleeding disorders. Other signs include nosebleeds, pallor, frequent infections, and lethargy. This chapter discusses the most common disorders of the blood and blood-forming organs in children. (See Chapter 24 ∞ for a discussion of leukemia.)

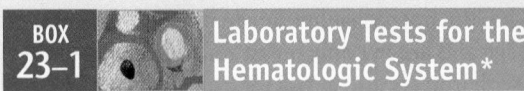

BOX 23–1

Laboratory Tests for the Hematologic System*

- Complete blood count
- Clotting indices (prothrombin time, thrombin time, platelets, reticulocyte count)
- Fetal hemoglobin level
- Hemoglobin electrophoresis
- Iron indices (ferritin, iron, iron-binding capacity)
- Red blood cell indices (mean corpuscular volume [MCV], mean corpuscular hemoglobin [MCH], mean corpuscular hemoglobin concentration [MCHC])
- White blood cell differential

*See Appendix D ∞ for information about these laboratory tests.

Assessment Guidelines for the Child with a Hematologic Condition

Assessment Focus	Assessment Guidelines
Family history	■ Does a family member have sickle cell anemia/trait or other blood disorder? ■ Does a family member have hemophilia or other inherited clotting alteration?
Growth and development	■ Is the child reaching developmental milestones? ■ Plot height and weight on standardized growth charts. ■ Is the child receiving enough calories? Is the child receiving enough iron?
Skin	■ Assess for pallor, flushing, rashes, and ecchymosis. ■ Observe for prolonged bleeding/clotting time. Does the child have a history of easy bruising or frequent nosebleeds?
Joints	■ Observe for edema, pain, inflammation, and range of motion.
Additional assessments	■ Assess pain in various body parts. ■ Identify frequency of infections. ■ Does the child have a history of fatigue and lethargy?

■ ANEMIAS

Anemia is defined as a reduction in the number of red blood cells, the quantity of hemoglobin, and the volume of packed red cells to below-normal levels. This condition can be caused by loss or destruction of existing red blood cells or by an impaired or decreased rate of red cell production. Anemia also can be a clinical manifestation of an underlying disorder, such as lead poisoning or hypersplenism (a syndrome characterized by splenomegaly and blood cell deficiencies). Common childhood anemias are discussed in this section.

Iron Deficiency Anemia

Iron deficiency anemia is the most common type of anemia and the most common nutritional deficiency in children. Iron deficiency anemia can occur secondary to blood loss, malabsorption, or poor nutritional intake. Increased physiologic demands (such as rapid growth periods) for blood production can also lead to this type of anemia.

Etiology and Pathophysiology

The body requires iron for the production of hemoglobin. Insufficient quantities of iron limit hemoglobin production, in turn affecting the production of red blood cells. RBCs are needed to carry oxygen throughout the body, so anemia results in less oxygen reaching cells and tissues. See Chapter 14 ∞ for a discussion of iron deficiency anemia due to deficits in nutritional intake. Increased physiologic demands (such as rapid growth periods) for blood production can also lead to anemia.

Infants who do not consume adequate solid foods after 6 months of age and are fed only breast milk or formula that is not fortified with iron are also at risk for iron deficiency because neonatal iron stores have been depleted by this time and their iron needs are not being met. In addition, if the mother's nutritional status during pregnancy was inadequate, or the infant was born prematurely or as part of a multiple birth, insufficient iron may have been stored in the latter part of pregnancy, placing the infant at higher risk for anemia in the first months of life. Rapidly growing adolescents whose diets are high in fat and low in vitamins and minerals are particularly susceptible to iron deficiency anemia. Female adolescents are at risk for anemia secondary to menstrual blood loss (American Academy of Pediatrics, Committee on Nutrition, 2009), especially those who have **menorrhagia** (heavy menstrual bleeding).

Clinical Manifestations

Clinical manifestations and severity of symptoms are directly related to the amount of iron deficiency or degree of iron deficiency anemia. Pallor, fatigue, and irritability are characteristic findings. Nailbed deformities, growth retardation, developmental delay, tachycardia, and systolic heart murmur can occur with prolonged anemia. *Pica*, or consumption of nonfood items, is also associated with iron deficiency anemia.

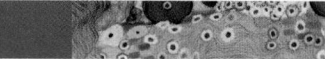
COLLABORATIVE CARE

Diagnostic Tests

Diagnosis is made on the basis of clinical presentation and laboratory studies. The hemoglobin, hematocrit, RBC count, mean corpuscular volume (MCV), and the mean corpuscular hemoglobin (MCH) are evaluated to confirm the diagnosis and help determine the cause of anemia. Serum iron, serum ferritin, and transferrin levels reflect iron storage and assist in a diagnosis of iron deficiency anemia. Microscopic analysis (Figure 23–2 ➤) reveals RBCs are microcytic (small) and hypochromic (pale) (Borgna-Pignatti & Marsella, 2008). A diet history and analysis can provide information about food intake; see Chapter 14 ∞ for guidelines about diet history.

Clinical Therapy

Treatment involves correction of iron deficiency anemia with oral elemental iron preparations for about 4 months. Ferrous sulfate at a dose of 3 to 6 mg/kg/day is a common treatment, followed by evaluation for its effectiveness (Borgna-Pignatti & Marsella, 2008). Oral iron preparations cause side effects such as constipation and gastrointestinal discomfort; therefore, the child may receive iron medications to restore blood levels of

Culture   *Chi*

According to traditional Chinese beliefs, a person who does not feel well is lacking in chi (inner energy) and blood. Those who follow traditional practices may be hesitant to have blood drawn for laboratory studies for fear of causing bodily weakness.

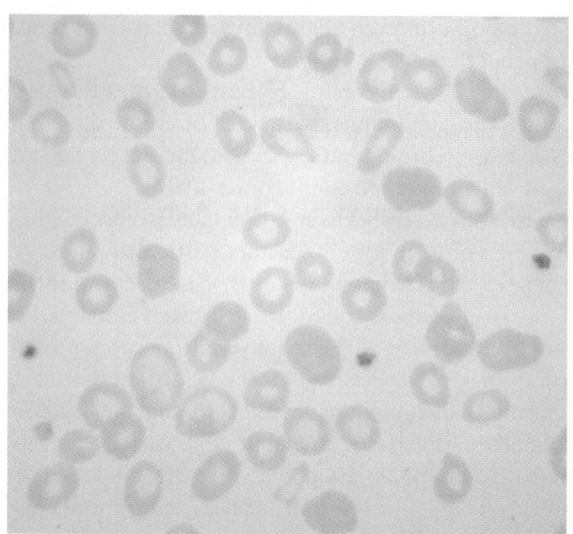

FIGURE 23–2 ➤ In iron deficiency anemia, red blood cells appear hypochromic as a result of decreased hemoglobin synthesis.
Courtesy of Dr. Ed Wong, Laboratory Medicine, Children's National Medical Center, Washington, DC.

iron while the iron content of the diet is increased above the recommended dietary allowances (RDAs). Oral iron medications can then be tapered off once the child's food intake can supply the needed iron; the child is evaluated in about 6 months for recurring anemia.

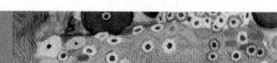
NURSING MANAGEMENT

Nursing Assessment and Diagnosis

Children with iron deficiency anemia are usually identified and treated in the community unless they have another serious illness. Nursing care focuses on screening for the disorder and educating the parents and children about the causes of iron deficiency anemia, dietary management, and the importance of complying with the medication regimen.

Screening for anemia is recommended at 9–12 months of age and at 15–18 months of age for young children. During adolescence, males should be screened at routine physical examinations during peak growth spurts. Females should be screened at all routine physical examinations during adolescence (American Academy of Pediatrics, Committee on Nutrition, 2009). A hematocrit or hemoglobin level is obtained for screening. More detailed tests are performed if the blood test is abnormal. Children at high risk for nutritional deficiencies, such as those in low-income groups and Women, Infants, and Children (WIC) programs, may require tests at earlier ages. Most children in Head Start are screened annually by nurses. In addition, children showing signs of anemia such as low energy and pallor should be screened. Height and weight measurements should be obtained at each health care visit, plotted on growth charts, and compared with percentiles obtained at previous visits. Slow downward trends in percentiles are of concern and require further nutritional analysis. A diet history and analysis provide information related to food intake (see Chapter 14 ∞ for guidelines about diet analysis). Developmental screening tests should be performed to assess for developmental delays (see Chapter 6 ∞).

Nursing diagnoses that may apply to the child with iron deficiency anemia include:

- Imbalanced Nutrition: Less than Body Requirements related to dietary intake of iron
- Activity Intolerance related to decreased oxygen-carrying capacity
- Risk for Delayed Growth and Development related to decreased tissue perfusion
- Readiness for Enhanced Knowledge related to management of iron deficiency anemia

Planning and Implementation

Dietary management is the preferred long-term treatment for iron deficiency anemia. Teach the family and child about foods that are rich in iron. Include teaching about foods with vitamin C as well since this vitamin enhances absorption of iron (Borgna-Pignatti & Marsella, 2008) (Table 23–3). The infant over 6 months of age should have a diet that includes breast milk or iron-fortified formula and baby cereals with iron fortification. Avoid cow milk in the first year of life since it can cause bleeding from the gastrointestinal tract, contributing to anemia. If the older infant or toddler consumes large quantities of milk and refuses to eat solid food, restriction of milk intake may be required. Older infants and toddlers can be provided with finger foods such as thinly sliced meats. Adolescents can be encouraged to eat foods with a high iron content and vitamin C such as a hamburger with a slice of tomato.

Oral iron preparations, usually ferrous sulfate, are given to correct anemia (see Medications Used to Treat Iron Deficiency Anemia below). Instruct the family about side effects such as black, green, or "tarry" stools; constipation; and a foul aftertaste. Emphasize the importance of drinking fluids and eating foods high in dietary fiber to minimize constipation. Store medication safely to avoid accidental poisoning.

TABLE 23–3 Food Sources of Iron and Vitamin C	
Iron-Rich Foods	Vitamin C-Rich Foods
Meats, fish, poultry	Orange juice
Vegetables	Citrus fruits
Dried fruits	Strawberries
Legumes	Tomatoes
Enriched grain products	Broccoli
Whole-grain cereals	Green leafy vegetables
Iron-fortified dry cereals	Potatoes
	Some dry cereals

Evaluation

Expected outcomes of nursing care include the following:

- The child's laboratory results manifest a normal red blood cell level.
- The family verbalizes understanding of the treatment regimen.
- The child consumes the recommended dietary intake.
- The child is free of side effects of oral iron therapy.

Normocytic Anemia

In normocytic anemia, there is an increase in the destruction of red blood cells or decreased production of red blood cells. This type of anemia may be related to chronic hemolytic anemia, pancytopenia, disseminated intravascular coagulation (DIC; see the discussion later in this chapter), G6PD (glucose-6-phosphate dehydrogenase) deficiency, hemolytic-uremic syndrome (see Chapter 26 ∞), some autoimmune diseases, or several other conditions (Coyer, 2005). Normocytic anemia can be caused by an infection such as septic arthritis or meningitis. It may also be found in a child with an inflammatory illness such as juvenile arthritis or chronic liver disease. Clinical manifestations of normocytic anemia are similar to those seen in iron

Medications Used to Treat
Iron Deficiency Anemia

Medication/Action and Indication	Nursing Management
Ferrous Sulfate Corrects anemia caused by iron deficiency. A variety of doses and preparations are available, such as tablets, capsules, syrup, elixir, and drops.	▪ Common side effects include gastrointestinal symptoms such as nausea, anorexia, constipation, abdominal distress, and black stools. ▪ Give on an empty stomach if possible; if gastric distress occurs, give with or immediately after meals. ▪ Monitor bowel movements and suggest increased fluid and fiber. ▪ Monitor development, sleep, and activity/fatigue patterns. ▪ Monitor hemoglobin and reticulocytes to measure effectiveness of therapy. ▪ Mix liquid preparations with water or fruit juice and give through a straw to prevent teeth staining. For infants the preparation may be placed on the back of the tongue. ▪ Instruct families to keep this drug locked and out of reach of children; poisoning is a serious risk.

deficiency anemia, with the possible occurrence of hepatomegaly and splenomegaly.

Treatment of normocytic anemia depends on the underlying cause. When the anemia is associated with inflammation or infection, the underlying condition is treated. For anemia caused by renal failure, recombinant human erythropoietin is administered. When hemorrhage is the underlying cause, the source of the bleeding is identified and treated. In acute emergencies, blood products are infused to replenish some of the losses.

Nursing management of normocytic anemia depends on the cause of the decreased red blood cells. Children with inflammatory or infectious diseases require careful assessment and management of medication and other treatment regimens. Administer blood products and other intravenous fluids as ordered to restore blood volume. Follow-up and home visits are used to assess hematocrit, hemoglobin, and dietary intake. (Refer to the discussion later in this chapter for management of DIC, to Chapter 25 for management of intestinal infections, and to Chapter 26 ∞ for management of hemolytic-uremic syndrome.)

Sickle Cell Disease

Sickle cell disease is a hereditary **hemoglobinopathy** characterized by the partial or complete replacement of normal hemoglobin with abnormal hemoglobin S (Hb S) in red blood cells (Table 23–4). This causes occlusion of small blood vessels, ischemia, and damage to affected organs. Sickle cell trait (carrying one gene for the disease) affects 1 in 12 African Americans and 1 in 16 Hispanic Americans (American Sickle Cell Anemia Association, 2007). Approximately 2 million Americans carry the sickle cell gene (Hb SA). Individuals with sickle cell trait have one sickle cell hemoglobin gene and one normal hemoglobin gene. They are carriers of the disease and generally do not have symptoms, although symptoms have been known to occur when the body is under severe stress (Platt & Eckman, 2006).

Etiology and Pathophysiology

Sickle cell anemia is an autosomal recessive disorder. If both parents have the trait, with each pregnancy the risk of having a child with the disease is 25%. (See Chapter 3 ∞ for a discussion of recessive gene transmission.)

In sickle cell anemia, the hemoglobin in the RBC acquires an elongated crescent or sickle shape (Figure 23–3 ➤). The sickled cells are rigid and obstruct capillary blood flow. Microscopic obstructions lead to engorgement and tissue ischemia. This local tissue hypoxia causes further sickling and ultimately large infarctions. Organ tissues become damaged by infarctions leading to scarring and impaired function. The spleen is the first organ affected by sickling. Approximately 90% of children with Hb SS disease have functional asplenia by 6 years of age (Driscoll, 2007). Children with sickle cell anemia may suffer from splenic sequestration when blood is trapped in the spleen, a life-threatening complication. Many children must undergo splenectomy in early childhood, leading to severely compromised immunity. Infection rate is high due to impaired immunity. Bacterial infections are the leading cause of death in young children with sickle cell disease.

TABLE 23–4 Types of Sickle Cell Disease (SCD)

Disorder	Characteristics
Sickle Cell Anemia (Hb SS)	Most common type of sickle cell disease (65% of SCD cases). RBCs are crescent shaped. Homozygous condition (child has two sickle hemoglobin genes). Child is subject to sickle cell crises. Average life span is 45 years of age.
Sickle C Disease (Hb SC)	Child inherits one Hb S gene and one Hb C gene (25% of SCD cases). RBCs are C shaped. Anemia is generally milder than in Hb SS disease. Painful crises occur about 50% as often as in Hb SS disease. Average life span is 65 years of age.
Sickle Beta + Thalassemia Disease (Hb+ Sβ) and Sickle Beta 0 Thalassemia Disease (Hb0 Sβ)	Combination of sickle cell trait and thalassemia trait. In sickle cell beta + there is a reduced amount of hemoglobin A, and life span is near normal. In sickle cell beta 0 there is no hemoglobin A and the life span is mid-50s.

Data from: Debaun, M. R., & Vichinsky, E. (2007). Hemoglobinopathies. In R. M. Kliegman, R. E. Behrman, H. B. Jenson, & B. F. Stanton (Eds.), Nelson textbook of pediatrics (18th ed., pp. 2025–2038). Philadelphia: Saunders Elsevier; Wang, W. (2007). Central nervous system complications of sickle cell disease in children: An overview. Child Neuropsychology, 13, 103–119; Saunthararajah, Y., & Vichinsky, E. P. (2009). Sickle cell disease: Clinical features and management. In R. Hoffman, E. J. Benz, S. J. Shattil, B. Furie, L. E. Silberstein, P. McGlave, & H. Heslop (Eds.), Hematology: Basic principles and practice (5th ed., pp. 577–601). Philadelphia: Churchill Livingstone-Elsevier; Mehta, S. R., Afenyi-Annan, A., Byrns, P. F., & Lottenberg, R. (2006). Opportunities to improve outcomes in sickle cell disease. American Family Physician, 74(2), 303–310; Driscoll, M. C. (2007). Sickle cell disease. Pediatrics in Review, 28(7), 259–268.

Stroke is a significant risk to children with sickle cell anemia and can lead to developmental delay, cognitive impairment, and other neurologic deficits (Driscoll, 2007; King, Herron, McKinstry, et al., 2006). Other complications of sickle cell disease may include acute chest syndrome with pulmonary hypertension, pulmonary infiltrate, and infection; aplastic crisis or temporary cessation of bone marrow blood cell production; **priapism**, sustained and painful penile erection; and gallstone formation (Inati, Koussa, Taher, et al., 2008).

Sickling may be triggered by fever, hypoxia, emotional stress, or physical stress. Precipitating factors for sickle cell crisis include increased blood viscosity (such as from a low fluid intake or fever) and hypoxia or low oxygen tension. Potential causes of hypoxia or low oxygen tension include high altitudes, poorly pressurized airplanes, hypoventilation, vasoconstriction when cold, or an emotionally stressful event. Any condition that increases the body's need for oxygen or alters the transport of oxygen (such as infection, trauma, or dehydration) may result in sickle cell crisis.

Sickled cells can resume a normal shape when rehydrated and reoxygenated. The membrane of these cells becomes more

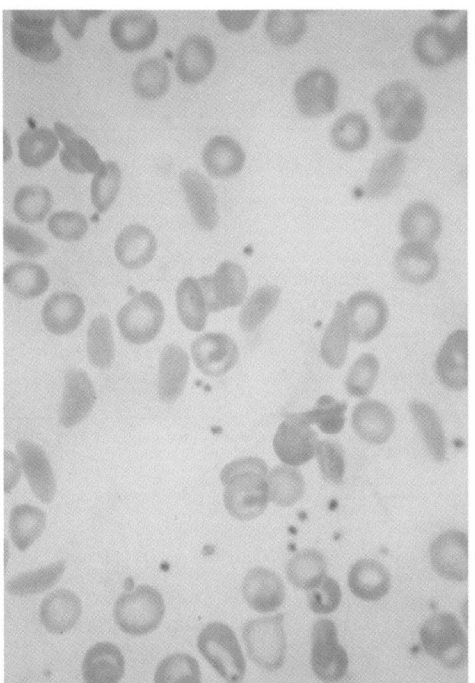

FIGURE 23–3 ➤ Many of these red blood cells show an elongated crescent shape characteristic of sickle cell anemia.
Courtesy of Dr. Ed Wong, Laboratory Medicine, Children's National Medical Center, Washington, DC.

and result in multiple signs and symptoms (Figure 23–5 ➤). Affected children are usually asymptomatic until 4 to 6 months of age because sickling is inhibited by high levels of fetal hemoglobin. Clinical manifestations are directly related to the shortened life span of blood cells (hemolytic anemia) and tissue destruction resulting from **vaso-occlusion** (blockage of a blood vessel). Illness results from recurrent vaso-occlusive events that involve painful crises and chronic organ damage. Sickle cell crises are acute exacerbations of the disease that vary markedly in severity and frequency. Table 23–5 outlines the most common types of crises affecting children with sickle cell disease, and Box 23–2 lists some of the common precipitating factors. Notice that infections, impaired respirations, neurologic symptoms, pain, and skin changes are common manifestations of the disease. Crises in these systems may occur individually or in combination. Michael, the boy described at the beginning of this chapter, is in sickle cell crisis. Both his lungs and spleen are affected by the present crisis.

fragile, however, and cell life is shortened to about 15 days rather than the usual 120 days. In response, bone marrow spaces enlarge to produce more RBCs. Continuous formation and destruction of the child's RBCs contributes to the severe hemolytic anemia that is characteristic of sickle cell anemia (Platt & Eckman, 2006). See Figure 23–4 ➤.

Clinical Manifestations

The manifestations of sickle cell disease occur in nearly all of the organ systems. Pathologic changes occur in most body systems

BOX 23–2	Precipitating Factors Contributing to Sickle Cell Crisis

- Fever
- Dehydration
- Altitude
- Extremes in temperature
- Vomiting
- Emotional distress
- Fatigue
- Alcohol consumption
- Pregnancy
- Elevated hemoglobin levels
- Elevated reticulocyte counts
- Excessive exercise or physical activity
- Acidosis

TABLE 23–5	Types of Sickle Cell Crises
Type of Crisis	**Characteristics and Clinical Manifestations**
Vaso-occlusive Crisis (Pain Crisis)	• Most common type of crisis • Precipitated by dehydration, temperature extremes, infection, localized hypoxemia, and physical or emotional stress • Caused by stasis of blood with clumping of cells in the microcirculation, ischemia, and infarction • Thrombosis and infarction of local tissue may occur if the crisis is not reversed • Cerebral occlusion can result in stroke, manifested by paralysis or other central nervous system complications • Extremely painful; symptoms include fever, tissue engorgement, painful swelling of joints in hands and feet, priapism, and severe abdominal pain
Splenic Sequestration	• Life-threatening crisis; death can occur within hours • Caused by pooling of blood in the spleen • Clinical manifestations include profound anemia, hypovolemia, and shock
Aplastic Crisis	• Diminished production and increased destruction of red blood cells • Triggered by viral infection or depletion of folic acid • Clinical manifestations include profound anemia and pallor

Data from: De, D. (2008). Acute nursing care and management of patients with sickle cell. British Journal of Nursing, 17(13), 818–823; Geller, A. K., & O'Connor, M. K. (2008). The sickle cell crisis: A dilemma in pain relief. Mayo Clinic Proceedings, 83(3), 320–323; Inati, A., Koussa, S., Taher, A., & Perrine, S. (2008). Sickle cell disease: New insights into pathophysiology and treatment. Pediatric Annals, 37(5), 311–321.

Sickle Cell Disease Animation

Pathophysiology Illustrated

Sickle Cell Anemia

Hemoglobin S and Red Blood Cell Sickling

Sickle cell anemia is caused by an inherited autosomal recessive defect in Hb synthesis. Sickle cell hemoglobin (HbS) differs from normal hemoglobin only in the substitution of the amino acid valine for glutamine in both beta chains of the hemoglobin molecule.

When HbS is oxygenated, it has the same globular shape as normal hemoglobin. However, when HbS loses its oxygen, it becomes insoluble in intracellular fluid and crystallizes into rodlike structures. Clusters of rods form polymers (long chains) that bend the erythrocyte into the characteristic crescent shape of the sickle cell.

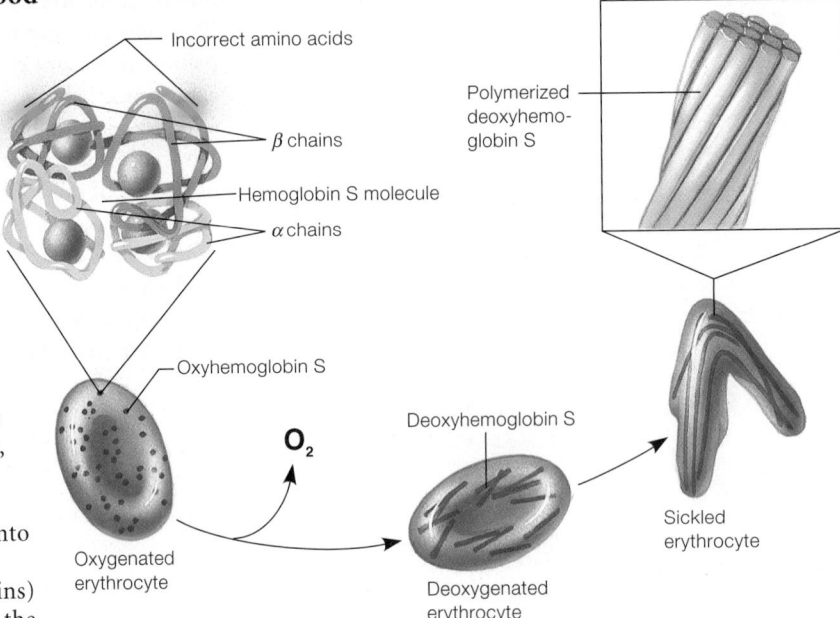

The Sickle Cell Disease Process

Sickle cell disease is characterized by episodes of acute painful crises. Sickling crises are triggered by conditions causing high tissue oxygen demands or that affect cellular pH. As the crisis begins, sickled erythrocytes adhere to capillary walls and to each other, obstructing blood flow and causing cellular hypoxia. The crisis accelerates as tissue hypoxia and acidic metabolic waste products cause further sickling and cell damage.

Sickle cell crises cause microinfarcts in joints and organs, and repeated crises slowly destroy organs and tissues. The spleen and kidneys are especially prone to sickling damage.

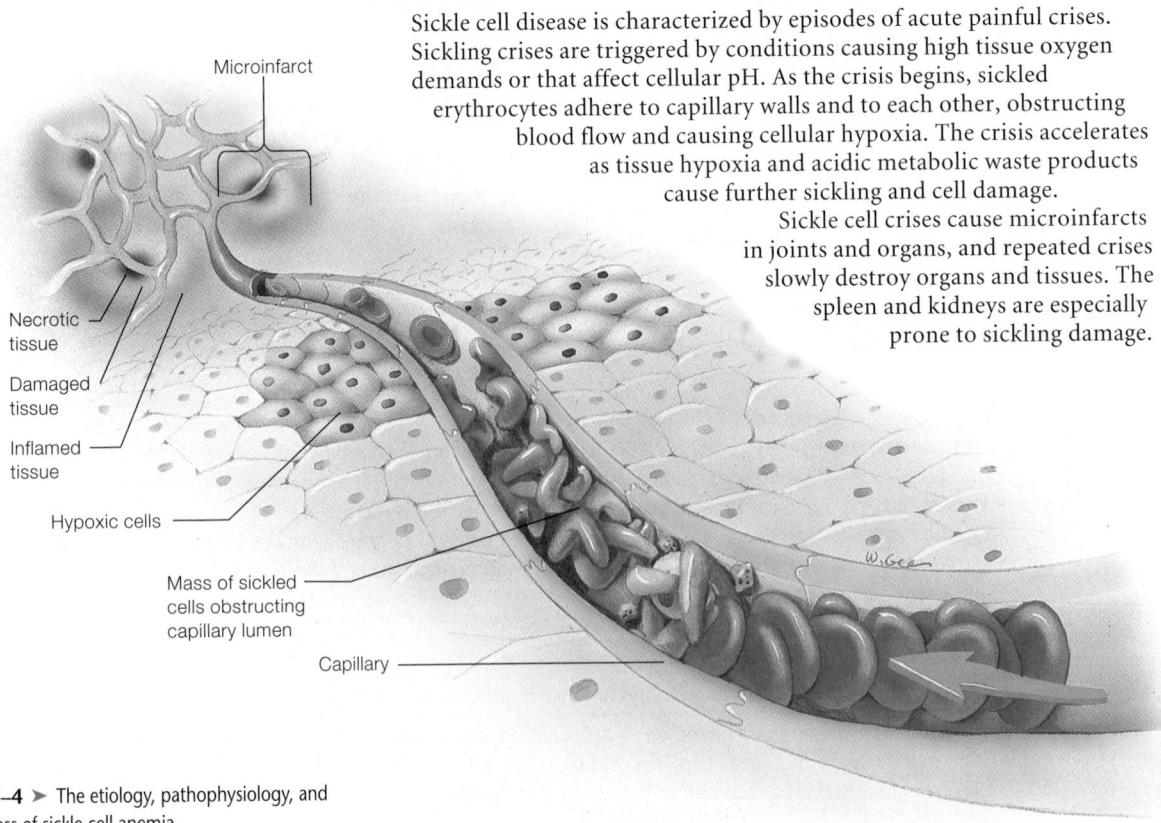

FIGURE 23–4 ➤ The etiology, pathophysiology, and disease process of sickle cell anemia.

Pathophysiology Illustrated

Clinical Manifestations of Sickle Cell Anemia

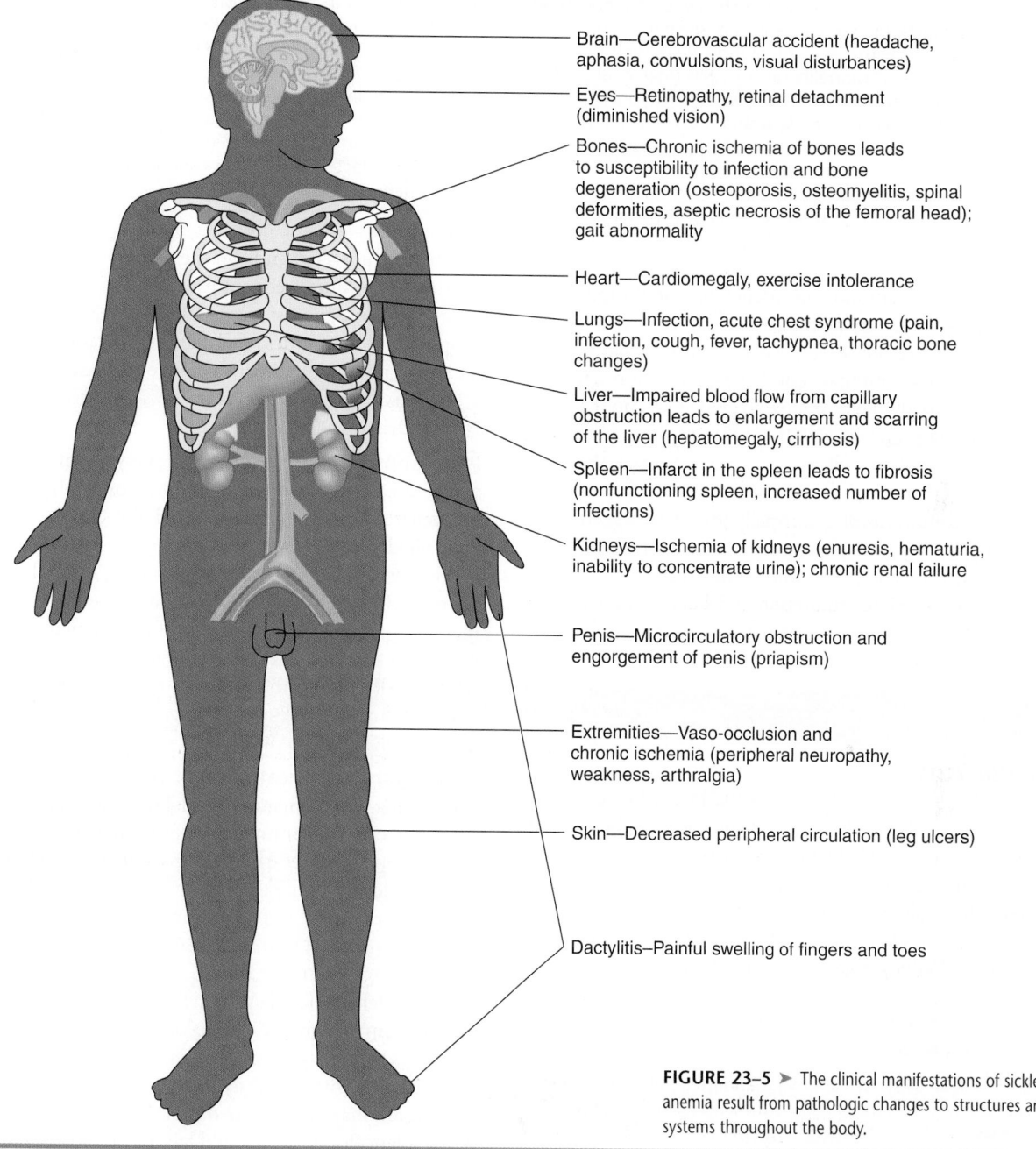

Brain—Cerebrovascular accident (headache, aphasia, convulsions, visual disturbances)

Eyes—Retinopathy, retinal detachment (diminished vision)

Bones—Chronic ischemia of bones leads to susceptibility to infection and bone degeneration (osteoporosis, osteomyelitis, spinal deformities, aseptic necrosis of the femoral head); gait abnormality

Heart—Cardiomegaly, exercise intolerance

Lungs—Infection, acute chest syndrome (pain, infection, cough, fever, tachypnea, thoracic bone changes)

Liver—Impaired blood flow from capillary obstruction leads to enlargement and scarring of the liver (hepatomegaly, cirrhosis)

Spleen—Infarct in the spleen leads to fibrosis (nonfunctioning spleen, increased number of infections)

Kidneys—Ischemia of kidneys (enuresis, hematuria, inability to concentrate urine); chronic renal failure

Penis—Microcirculatory obstruction and engorgement of penis (priapism)

Extremities—Vaso-occlusion and chronic ischemia (peripheral neuropathy, weakness, arthralgia)

Skin—Decreased peripheral circulation (leg ulcers)

Dactylitis–Painful swelling of fingers and toes

FIGURE 23–5 ➤ The clinical manifestations of sickle cell anemia result from pathologic changes to structures and systems throughout the body.

The most common reason for hospitalization of the child with sickle cell anemia is acute painful episodes (Inati et al., 2008). The sickled RBCs cause vaso-occlusion, microinfarction, and ischemia. Pain results from avascular necrosis of the bone marrow, and is typically experienced in the back, abdomen, chest, and joints. Children with sickle cell anemia can also develop acute chest syndrome (ACS), a life-threatening complication of sickle cell disease. ACS is the second most common reason for hospitalization in patients with sickle cell disease (Gladwin & Vinchinsky, 2008). See Box 23–3.

Clinical Judgment

During the initial assessment of a 10-year-old with sickle cell anemia, the nurse notes that the child's breathing is shallow and his respiratory rate is 32 breaths per minute. The child rates the pain in his chest at a 4 on a scale of 1–10, and he has a temperature of 100.5°F. What complication of sickle cell anemia is the nurse most concerned about based on these symptoms? What actions should the nurse initiate?

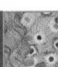

BOX 23–3 Acute Chest Syndrome

Acute chest syndrome describes new pulmonary findings on radiograph. Common causes are rib, bone marrow, or pulmonary infarction; acute infections; pain crises; and surgery. Acute chest syndrome affects approximately 40% of individuals with sickle cell anemia and has an overall mortality rate of 1.8% (Inati et al., 2008). Common symptoms include chest pain, fever, tachypnea, coughing, and wheezing (Hernandez & Patterson, 2009). The child with acute chest syndrome is frequently admitted to pediatric intensive care for close monitoring of oxygen levels and symptoms. Treatment includes analgesics, oxygen, hydration, incentive spirometry, antibiotics, and transfusion for severe anemia or hypoxemia.

Pain intensity and duration vary depending on the individual and the location. Pain may be transient in a localized area, such as the wrist, or it may be severe, generalized pain that lasts for several days or weeks and may require hospitalization. The pain is often severe enough to require opioid analgesics and the use of a patient-controlled analgesic (PCA) pump. Children with sickle cell trait rarely have sickle cell crises. However, because they have some abnormal hemoglobin, they may develop symptoms of the disease under conditions of abnormally low oxygen such as flying in an unpressurized airplane over 7,000 feet or during anesthesia. The most common symptoms experienced by those with sickle cell trait are splenic infarction and hematuria. However, most persons who carry the trait never have symptoms, even with low oxygen concentrations.

COLLABORATIVE CARE

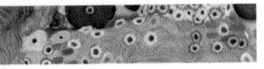

Diagnostic Tests

The initial diagnosis of sickle cell anemia in newborns is often made by testing cord blood using hemoglobin electrophoresis. The sickle-turbidity test (Sickledex) may be used for quick screening purposes in children over 6 months of age, once the fetal hemoglobin levels have fallen. Hemoglobin electrophoresis is performed to verify positive Sickledex test results. Newborn screening of infants for hemoglobinopathies occurs in most states.

Clinical Tip

When a child with sickle cell anemia is admitted with a reticulocyte count that is lower than the child's normal level, this signifies that the marrow may not be responding appropriately. Parvovirus may be suspected (see Chapter 16 ∞) (DeBaun & Vichinsky, 2007). The child should be placed on isolation precautions per hospital policy to prevent spread of the disease (Servey, Reamy, & Hodge, 2007). If parvovirus is ruled out, isolation precautions can be discontinued.

Clinical Therapy

Management focuses on pain control, hydration, oxygenation, prevention of infection, and prevention of associated complications. Treatment of crises involves aggressive hydration, oxygen, pain management, and bed rest to reduce energy expenditure. Neonatal screening, early intervention, prophylactic antibiotics, and parent education have allowed children with sickle cell disease to live into adulthood.

Historically, sickle cell disease has been thought of as only occurring in the African American population. In recent years, the disease has been diagnosed in those of Mediterranean, South American, Arabian, and East Indian descent (Kral, Brown, Connelly, et al., 2006). All newborns should be screened for sickle cell disease as part of the newborn screening panel (March of Dimes, 2008). Although African American families may be familiar with the need for screening, parents of children from other cultures may question this practice. Explain the importance of early diagnosis of sickle cell disease and reinforce the fact that heritage cannot be predicted from appearance or name alone.

The prognosis depends on the severity of the child's disease; children with more frequent exacerbations and hospitalization have poorer prognoses. Neonatal screening, early intervention, prophylactic antibiotics, and parent education have extended life spans in individuals with sickle cell disease. The median survival age is 45 for those with HbSS disease and 65 for those with HbSC (Driscoll, 2007).

Pain Control, Hydration, and Oxygenation   Parenteral analgesics, such as morphine and hydromorphone (Dilaudid), are generally administered around the clock or via patient-controlled analgesia. In addition to parenteral narcotics, the child may receive intravenous ketorolac (Toradol) or oral ibuprofen (Motrin) every 6 hours around the clock as adjunctive therapy. Oral and intravenous fluid replacement also promotes pain relief since dehydration is often a cause of crisis. Fluids reduce the viscosity of the blood, so adequate hydration is essential. Oxygen is usually administered to provide comfort and decrease incidence of pulmonary complications.

Prevention and Treatment of Infection   To prevent life-threatening infection, it is essential that the child with sickle cell disease receive recommended immunizations, including the 7-valent pneumococcal conjugate vaccine, Hib vaccine, and influenza vaccine (Chapter 16 ∞). In addition, children with SCD 2 years of age and older should have the 23-valent pneumococcal vaccine (Yanni, Grosse, Yang, et al., 2009). Children 2 years of age and older should also receive the meningococcal vaccine (Mehta, Afenyi-Annan, Byrns, et al., 2006).

Penicillin prophylaxis is recommended for children from 2 months to 5 years of age to prevent a potentially life-threatening infection with the *Streptococcus pneumoniae* bacteria. The medication may be continued past 5 years of age if the child has had a splenectomy, if the child has a history of severe pneumococcal sepsis, or if the health care provider feels the child is still at high risk for infection caused by *S. pneumoniae* (Saunthararajah & Vichinsky, 2009).

Infection in a child with sickle cell anemia is a serious condition requiring immediate attention. When an infection is suspected, cultures (blood, urine, and throat) are obtained to identify the source of infection and the offending organism. Aggressive antibiotic therapy is implemented immediately.

Transfusion of Red Blood Cells   Blood transfusions improve tissue oxygenation, reduce sickling, and temporarily reduce the percentage of Hb S. Chronic transfusions may be indicated in the child with sickle cell anemia who has had a stroke (Mirre, Brousse,

Research  *Compliance with Deferasirox Therapy*

The use of once-a-day oral deferasirox (DFX) has the potential to simplify treatment of iron overload caused by chronic transfusions. Twenty-one patients ages 7–21 years with sickle cell anemia were enrolled in a prospective study to evaluate adherence to the DFX regimen. Intake of greater than or equal to 80% of the prescribed dose was defined as good adherence. Adherence was evaluated by pill counts, calendars, and questionnaires at regular intervals over a 12-month period. Pill counts indicated continued good adherence in only 43% of the patients because of poor bottle return at follow-up visits. Questionnaire responses indicated 71% compliance over the study period. Overreporting may have occurred through the self-report method, thus true adherence was difficult to evaluate. Reasons for noncompliance included forgetting to take the medication and undesirable side effects associated with the medication. Adherence was better when parents were involved with medication administration and in patients 16 years of age or less (Alvarez et al., 2009).

Berteloot, et al., 2010). However, frequent transfusions may result in an overload of iron in the body. The iron is stored in tissues and organs (**hemosiderosis**) because the body has no way of excreting it. For this reason, an iron-chelating drug such as deferoxamine (Desferal), which binds excess iron so it can be excreted by the kidneys, is administered. An oral chelator, deferasirox (Exjade), has been used in some patients since approval by the U.S. Food and Drug Administration (FDA) in 2005 and has demonstrated similar efficacy to deferoxamine infusion (Alvarez, Rodriguez-Cortes, Robinson, et al., 2009). Deferasirox could potentially simplify treatment and improve compliance by use of once-daily oral administration for patients requiring chelation therapy (Ault & Jones, 2009).

Other Therapies Treatment with hydroxyurea has been helpful in adults, and is being used more frequently in children. This cytotoxic medication improves fetal hemoglobin levels (Brawley, Cornelius, Edwards, et al., 2008). The presence of fetal hemoglobin reduces sickling and subsequently the frequency of painful crises secondary to vaso-occlusion. In the pediatric population, hydroxyurea has been used most in adolescents, but recent studies have shown it to be effective in children as young as 6 months (Anderson, 2006).

Hematopoietic stem cell transplantation (HSCT) is the only known cure for sickle cell anemia and has been used in children younger than 16 years with complications related to the disease. The treatment, however, is limited to children who have a family donor who is genotypically identical. The survival rate for children who have been able to receive an HLA-identical sibling donor stem cell transplant is 93% (Platt & Eckman, 2006). (See the discussion regarding HSCT later in this chapter.)

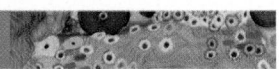

NURSING MANAGEMENT

Nursing Assessment and Diagnosis

The nurse may be involved in sickle cell gene testing to identify carriers and children who have the disease. Once a child is diagnosed with the disease, a comprehensive physical assessment is essential because sickle cell anemia can affect any body system.

Law & Ethics *Genetic Testing and Confidentiality*

Information about genetic testing is confidential and must not be shared with persons other than those tested. In the 1970s, when genetic testing for sickle cell disease and trait first became available, discrimination in jobs and insurance occurred against Blacks who had the trait for sickle cell disease.

Physiologic Assessment

In children who are known to have sickle cell anemia, obtain a detailed history from the parents or child about past crises, precipitating events, medical treatment, and home management. Measure the child's height and weight accurately and compare them with past measurements, since failure to thrive is common. Ask about chronic or acute pain that the child is experiencing. Pain may occur in nearly any body part, but most commonly manifests as headache, extremity pain, or abdominal discomfort. Use a pain scale and identify pain perception in each body part where pain exists (see Chapter 15 ∞). Assess the pain management protocols the family has used and what has been most successful.

The ill child with sickle cell disease should receive a careful multisystem assessment. Fever, neurological changes such as decreased alertness or behavioral changes, and respiratory symptoms are emergency conditions that necessitate prompt treatment. When the child is in crisis, assess pain and note the presence of any signs of inflammation or infection. Carefully monitor the child for signs of shock (see Chapter 21 ∞).

Psychosocial Assessment

The child with sickle cell disease experiences a chronic illness that interferes with activities of daily living. Disturbed self-concept and body image, guilt about disturbing the family routines, depression, and isolation can occur. Carry out an assessment of the child's developmental status with a concentration on friends, family support, and self-concept.

The family of a child with sickle cell disease requires a thorough psychosocial assessment. Ask if other family members have the diagnosis. If the child is newly diagnosed with the disorder, the family will need assistance to deal with the disease's serious, life-threatening nature. Assess parents' understanding of the disease transmission and ask whether genetic counseling has been obtained. Determine whether the family has adequate health care coverage to pay for the child's medical expenses and whether the child qualifies for assistance. Ask older children about their knowledge of the disease, and explore their feelings related to the management of a chronic condition. When siblings or other family members are carriers, counseling is needed periodically so that implications for dating, marriage, and having children can be understood.

Several nursing diagnoses that may apply to the child with sickle cell anemia are presented in the accompanying Nursing Care Plan. Other nursing diagnoses may include the following:

- Risk for Impaired Tissue Perfusion (Cerebral) related to interrupted blood flow
- Caregiver Role Strain related to child's chronic illness

NURSING CARE PLAN

The Child with Sickle Cell Anemia

INTERVENTION	RATIONALE	EXPECTED OUTCOME
1. Nursing Diagnosis: Ineffective Tissue Perfusion related to decreased hemoglobin concentration in blood		
NIC Priority Intervention: *Circulatory care:* Promotion of arterial and venous circulation		**NOC Suggested Outcome:** *Tissue perfusion, peripheral:* Extent to which blood flows through the small vessels of the extremities and maintains tissue function
Goal: The child will show few signs and symptoms of tissue hypoxia.		
■ Instruct the child to avoid physical exertion, emotional stress, low-oxygen environments (e.g., airplanes, high altitudes), and known sources of infection.	■ Decreased activity and exposure reduce the body's need for oxygen.	The child has no shortness of breath and shows no signs of hypoxia.
■ Administer blood transfusions as ordered.	■ Packed cells increase the number of red blood cells available to carry oxygen to tissue cells. Transfusions promote circulation.	
■ Perform several caregiving activities together whenever possible.	■ Grouping activities allows for optimum rest.	
■ Give oxygen as ordered.	■ A high concentration of oxygen in the alveoli increases the diffusion of gas across membranes.	
Goal: Repeated strokes will be avoided.		
■ Administer and teach the family about prophylactic transfusions for the child who has had a stroke.	■ Prophylactic transfusions lower the potential for a future stroke	The child does not suffer a stroke.
2. Nursing Diagnosis: Risk for Deficient Fluid Volume related to inadequate fluid intake and dehydration		
NIC Priority Intervention: *Fluid management:* Promotion of electrolyte balance and prevention of complications resulting from abnormal or undesired fluid levels		**NOC Suggested Outcome:** *Hydration:* Amount of water in the intracellular and extracellular compartments of the body
Goal: The child will maintain or be restored to adequate hydration.		
■ Calculate the child's daily fluid requirements. Monitor the child's usual fluid consumption and make necessary adjustments. Encourage the child to take fluids. Observe for signs of dehydration.	■ Optimizing fluid intake ensures that the child gets needed fluid. Dehydration exacerbates crises.	The child shows signs of adequate hydration.
■ Record intake and output.	■ Early intervention can be effective in minimizing complications from dehydration. The child may need oral or intravenous rehydration therapy.	
3. Nursing Diagnosis: Pain related to chronic physical disability and clustering of sickled cells		
NIC Priority Intervention: *Pain management:* Alleviation of pain or a reduction in pain to a level of comfort acceptable to the patient		**NOC Suggested Outcome:** *Comfort level:* Feelings of physical and psychologic ease
Goal: The child will verbalize that pain is controlled.		

NURSING CARE PLAN

The Child with Sickle Cell Anemia (continued)

INTERVENTION	RATIONALE	EXPECTED OUTCOME
■ Administer analgesics, such as morphine or hydromorphone (Dilaudid), as ordered. Continuous intravenous infusion is used for the duration of a painful crisis.	■ The pain of sickle cell crises is excruciating.	The child is pain-free or pain control is significantly improved.
■ Position carefully.	■ Joints and extremities can be extremely painful.	

4. Nursing Diagnosis: Risk for Infection related to chronic disease and splenic malfunction

NIC Priority Intervention:		NOC Suggested Outcome:
Infectious control: Minimizing the acquisition and transmission of infectious agents		*Risk control:* Actions to eliminate or reduce actual, personal, and modifiable health threats

Goal: The child will not develop infection.

■ Ensure adequate nutrition by providing a high-calorie, high-protein diet.	■ Children with a chronic illness are at greater risk of infection.	The child is free of infection.
■ Make sure that the child's immunizations are up to date and that children less than age 5 years are receiving prophylactic antibiotics.		
■ Report any signs of infection to the physician immediately.		
■ Isolate the child from possible sources of infection. Instruct parents about signs of infection and encourage them to seek prompt health care.	■ Restriction of persons with infection decreases the child's contact with infectious agents. Prompt care for infection reduces the chance of a sickle cell crisis.	

• Risk for Interrupted Family Processes related to having a child with a chronic illness
• Delayed Growth and Development related to effects of physical disability
• Impaired Physical Mobility related to pain
• Deficient Knowledge (Child and Parents) related to lack of exposure to information about sickle cell anemia

Planning and Implementation

The accompanying Nursing Care Plan summarizes nursing care for the child with sickle cell anemia. Nursing management for the child in crisis focuses on increasing tissue perfusion, promoting hydration, controlling pain, preventing infection, ensuring adequate nutrition, preventing complications, and providing emotional support to the child and family. Refer to Michael in the opening scenario and determine how many of the following interventions apply.

Promote Increased Tissue Perfusion

Administer blood transfusions and oxygen as ordered. To prevent hemolysis, the intravenous fluid used before and after a blood transfusion must be saline rather than D₅W. Monitor for transfusion reactions. (See Clinical Manifestations: Blood Trans-

fusion Reactions.) Encourage the child to rest. Work with the child and family to avoid emotional stress. Any activities that increase cellular metabolism also result in tissue hypoxia. Schedule caregiving activities and play during hospitalizations and clinic visits to allow for optimal rest.

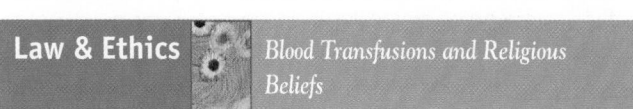

Law & Ethics — *Blood Transfusions and Religious Beliefs*

Jehovah's Witnesses and some other religious groups are opposed to the transfusion of blood products. Ethical issues arise when blood transfusion is the treatment of choice for a childhood disease, since parents may choose not to consent to treatment. The courts generally accept that the child's life is of the greatest importance and temporarily make the child a ward of the court to allow medical personnel to administer the needed blood product. Recent advances in synthetic clotting factor production and research into blood volume expanders that can successfully treat some conditions have decreased the incidence of disagreement between religious and medical interventions. However, nurses may care for children and families when court-ordered therapy is being carried out. Sensitivity to the family's beliefs, a caring approach to the child, and provision of information about care are needed (Woolley, 2006).

Clinical Manifestations
Blood Transfusion Reactions

Type of Reaction and Etiology	Clinical Manifestations	Nursing Management
Allergic reaction related to immune response to protein in the blood	Urticaria, itching, respiratory distress	Stop the transfusion; call the physician; administer antihistamines as ordered. Monitor vital signs; keep the intravenous line open with normal saline; check urine for hematuria.
Hemolytic reaction related to mismatched blood, history of multiple transfusions, or infusion with a solution containing dextrose or other additives	Fever, chills, hematuria, headache, chest pain; can progress to shock	
Febrile or septic related to contamination of blood; may also be caused by idiopathic conditions	Chills, fever, headache, decreased blood pressure, nausea and/or vomiting, leg and back pain	Call the physician. Administer medications as ordered.
Circulatory overload related to infusion of excessive amounts of fluid or too rapid administration	Labored breathing, chest or lower back pain, productive cough with rales heard on auscultation, distended neck veins; central venous pressure may increase	Call the physician. Administer diuretics if ordered.

Nursing Alert

Nurses should consider the following principles when administering blood and blood products:

- Become familiar with the transfusion policies and procedures at your workplace.
- Verify the blood type, patient number, donor number, and Rh factor with another registered nurse (Figure 23–6 ➤).
- Check the blood for sediment, or any nonuniform or unusual characteristics.
- Use a blood-warming coil to bring blood to room temperature as infusion of cold blood may increase sickling.
- Assess the child's history for previous transfusion reactions.
- Blood reactions can occur as soon as the blood transfusion begins. Administer the first 20 mL of blood slowly and observe the child carefully for a reaction.
- Repeatedly assess the child, including vital signs, according to hospital policy.
- Remain with the child during the first 20 minutes of the transfusion to monitor for undesirable reactions.
- If a transfusion reaction occurs, immediately discontinue the transfusion, change the IV to normal saline, and notify the primary health care provider.

Refer to the *Clinical Skills Manual* for further information related to administering blood or blood products.

Growth & Development   *Encouraging Fluid Intake*

To encourage fluid intake in a small child:

- Use a favorite cup or glass.
- Use straws.
- Take advantage of times the child is thirsty, such as on awakening or after play.
- Leave a cup within easy reach of the child.
- Offer frozen juice pops, crushed ice drinks, and flavored ice chips.

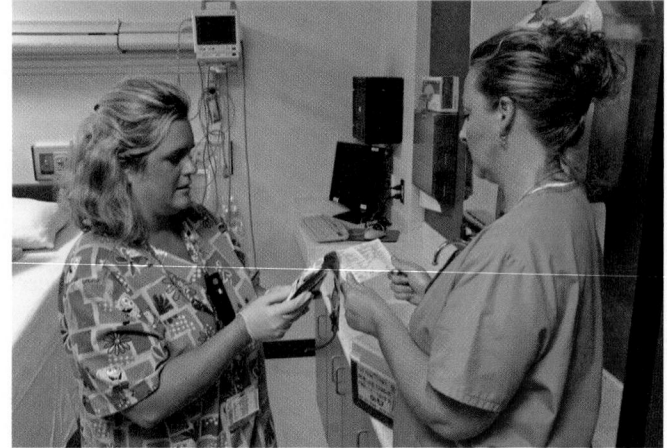

FIGURE 23–6 ➤ Blood must be checked by two nurses prior to administration to verify that the child is receiving the correct blood product.

Promote Hydration

The child with sickle cell anemia is adversely affected by dehydration. Calculate the child's fluid maintenance requirements (minimum daily fluid intake) (see Chapter 18 ∞) and monitor the child's oral fluid intake. Administer intravenous fluids as ordered. Adjust oral intake as necessary to keep the child well hydrated.

Pain Management

Administer prescribed analgesics around the clock during crises. If patient-controlled analgesia is used, be sure that the constant infusions run as ordered and that the parent or child understands the use of bolus infusions, when needed (see Chapter 15 ∞). Help the child assume a comfortable position. Avoid putting stress on painful joints. See Evidence-Based Practice: Sickle Cell Anemia and Pain Management.

Complementary Therapy

Sickle Cell Disease

A survey of parents of 57 children with sickle cell disease identified that 54% used some type of complementary and alternative medicine (CAM) with their children. Spiritual practices (including prayer) and relaxation techniques were identified as the most commonly used techniques in these children who frequently experience pain. CAM use was increased in children with more severe disease (Sibinga, Shindell, Casella, et al., 2006).

Nursing Alert

Neither hot nor cold compresses should be used for pain management in the child who has sickle cell anemia. Ischemic tissue is fragile and has reduced sensation, increasing the risk of burn injury. Cold compresses promote sickling.

Prevent Infection

Infection makes the child more susceptible to a crisis, and the crisis increases susceptibility to infection. Teach the parents how to administer antibiotics for prophylaxis or treatment of infection. Because infections are particularly virulent in these children, tell parents to seek immediate care when the child is ill.

Emphasize the importance of immunizations. See the earlier discussion on page 684 and Chapter 16 ∞ for further information about recommended and supplemental immunizations.

Ensure Adequate Nutrition

Emphasize the importance of adequate nutrition to promote growth. Encourage the child to eat a high-protein, high-calorie diet. Stress the importance of folic acid and vitamin C supplements as prescribed. Perform regular growth measurements and, if slow growth is apparent, perform 24-hour diet recalls and other nutritional assessments.

Prevent Complications of Crises

Observe the child for signs of increasing anemia and shock (e.g., mental status change, pallor, vital sign changes). Maintain ongoing monitoring of the child's neurologic status for evidence of altered cerebral function. Assess for an enlarged spleen by gentle palpation. Administer blood transfusions and observe the child for any adverse reaction. Assess growth and developmental milestones.

Provide Emotional Support

Sickle cell anemia is a chronic disease that is accompanied by life-threatening episodic crises. Family members often need help to deal with their feelings about the diagnosis and its implications.

Evidence-Based Practice

Sickle Cell Anemia and Pain Management

Problem

Severe episodes of vaso-occlusive sickle cell crisis require hospitalization for pain management. Relief of pain is the primary goal for health care providers and is most significant to the child experiencing pain. Research has found that this goal is not always met (Jacob, Miaskowski, Savedra, et al., 2006). Different pain management regimens may be used during each hospitalization, and effective regimens are not well documented. How effective are pain management strategies utilized in children hospitalized with vaso-occlusive crisis?

Evidence

As part of a larger study, nurse researchers evaluated analgesic use in 27 children with sickle cell disease hospitalized with vaso-occlusive crisis. Specifically the study (1) quantified analgesic use using the Medication Quantification Scale and (2) examined the relationship between pain scores, body outline drawings with painful areas identified and word descriptors describing pain quality, and the amount of pain medication the children received. The children ranged in age from 5 to 19 years. Results indicated that the majority of the children received subtherapeutic doses of analgesics. There was a significant correlation between pain characteristics as outlined above and the Medication Quantification Scale (Jacob, Miaskowski, Savedra, et al., 2007).

This same team of authors evaluated the effect of pain on sleep, food intake, and activity levels. Children hospitalized in pain crisis reported disruption in their nighttime sleep, but sleeping more during the day. Food intake was markedly decreased throughout the hospitalization. Activity levels also remained relatively low throughout the hospitalization (Jacob et al., 2006).

Implications

Hospitalized children with pain related to sickle cell disease may not receive therapeutic doses of pain medication, inhibiting the child's ability to achieve adequate pain relief. The inability to achieve pain relief affected the child's ability to sleep and the desire to eat and remain active.

For children using PCA whose pain is unrelieved, consider whether a higher dosage in the basal infusion would help pain control. Also evaluate whether the child is self-administering appropriately. For children receiving intravenous and oral analgesics administered on an as-needed basis by the nurse, collaborate with the health care provider to determine if administering these medications on a scheduled basis increases pain control. In addition, children and families have developed many effective pain relief measures at home that may not be included in hospital care. More information is needed about methods of integrating these techniques into hospital care.

Recommendations include the need to evaluate whether increasing analgesic use to at least the amount prescribed would increase the amount of pain relief and in turn improve the child's sleeping, eating, and exercise patterns. Additional research is needed to determine the effectiveness of different pain regimens including PCA and long-acting oral analgesics and to evaluate the effectiveness of pain management algorithms.

Critical Thinking Application

How will you determine if the child in sickle cell crisis is obtaining adequate pain relief? (Consult Chapter 15 ∞ for ideas.) What personal beliefs of health care providers may influence effective pain management? How can these beliefs be addressed? If the primary health care provider has prescribed a subtherapeutic dosage of pain medication for a child in sickle cell crisis, what action could you take?

Assess their knowledge of signs of infection and of sickle cell crisis and when to seek medical care for the child. Refer the parents for genetic counseling, particularly if they plan to have more children. Encourage adolescents and young adults in the family to receive genetic counseling and testing, as well. Referrals to support groups and contact with others with the disease can be helpful.

Collaborate with family members and provide them with ongoing support to deal with the stress of having a child with a chronic condition. (See Families Want to Know: Home Care Considerations for the Child with Sickle Cell Anemia.) Provide resources, respite care for parents, and information as needed for siblings. Sickle cell disease and some other hematologic disorders of childhood require that parents provide ongoing monitoring and care for their children with these chronic conditions. Refer to Chapter 12 ∞ for a discussion of chronic disorders in children. Refer parents to support groups such as the National Association of Sickle Cell Disease for further information.

Discharge Planning and Home Care Teaching

Home care needs should be identified and addressed well in advance of discharge. Provide parents with information about sickle cell disease and the child's treatment. Even parents of a child previously diagnosed with the disorder and adolescents may benefit from information about the disease process and its management. Explain the basic effect of tissue hypoxia and the effects of sickling on circulation. Assist the family to explore resources in the home and community, and determine if parents will be able to administer medications and fluids and to provide adequate nutrition.

Teach parents to look for signs of dehydration, such as dry mucous membranes, weight loss, and sunken fontanels in infants. Give specific instructions about how many ounces of liquid the child needs to drink each day. Emphasize that increased fluid intake is needed to replace the fluids lost from overheating or exposure to hot weather. Make sure both the child and family understand the triggers and precipitating factors for sickle cell crises. Encourage them to avoid situations that cause

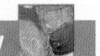

Families Want to Know

Home Care Considerations for the Child with Sickle Cell Anemia

■ Follow recommended schedules for well-child care visits.

■ Be sure the child is up to date with immunizations, including hepatitis B, annual influenza, pneumococcal vaccine, meningococcal vaccines, and a tuberculosis skin test.

■ Special testing, such as heart and eye examinations, may be needed periodically to check for any sequelae of the disease.

■ Special medications, such as antibiotics, may be needed; pain relief medicine and blood transfusions may be administered.

■ Dehydration is dangerous. Be sure the child gets extra fluids in hot weather, when ill, during physical activity, and during travel.

■ As the child develops, provide information about the disease and encourage self-care. Be sure the school personnel understand the child's diagnosis and any care required during school hours.

■ Contact your health care provider if the child has a high fever, a common illness that lasts more than a day, seizures, change in behavior, severe pain, abnormal skin color or breathing pattern, or any other symptoms of concern.

crises. Instruct the child and parents about signs and symptoms of crises that should be reported to their health care provider.

When regular blood transfusions are used, the resulting iron overload is damaging to body organs. Provide the family with instructions about the treatment for iron overload. Tell parents that it is important to inform all treating physicians and dentists of the child's medical condition. The child should also wear medical identification (e.g., a medical identification bracelet). Special precautions are necessary when the child undergoes surgery of any kind, as hypoxia resulting from anesthesia is a major surgical risk.

Family members need ongoing support to deal with the stress of having a child with a chronic condition. Provide resources, respite care for parents, and information as needed for siblings.

Encourage older children with sickle cell anemia to participate in activities with other children between crises but to avoid strenuous physical exertion and contact sports. Play and social interactions that promote learning and development are important.

Care in the Community

The child may receive home care nursing for transfusion therapy or may need to travel frequently for treatment at a medical center. The nurse partners with the child and family to establish a plan of care. An individualized school health plan will need to be established. The nurse can assist the family and school with establishing this plan.

School personnel must be aware of the child's disease, since prompt care is essential if the child exhibits any sign of sickle cell crisis. The nurse can identify key staff members in the school and partner with them to ensure essential management actions are understood by all staff members. Members of the school staff should be instructed in management of emergencies, and contact numbers for parents should be readily available.

Children who have episodes of sickle cell crisis miss school for prolonged and repeated periods. In addition, if they have experienced strokes as a disease complication, they often have learning difficulties and neurological changes. Teachers may have difficulty understanding why children with a blood disease are frequently absent and why they may have trouble with concepts in the classroom that they previously understood. School and other community-based nurses are ideally situated to provide information to teachers about sickle cell disease so that they understand the challenges faced by children with the disease. Assist the family and school to plan an appropriate schedule of activities without overprotecting the child. Children with sickle cell disease

Clinical Tip

Although teachers commonly have some knowledge about sickle cell disease, they are often not fully aware of the neurological sequelae and the importance of the individualized education plan and its frequent evaluation and revision (King, Tang, Ferguson, et al., 2005). Outline the topics that you would address to inform teachers about the effect of sickle cell anemia on a child's ability to learn.

should not engage in activities, such as running and heavy exercise, that may increase oxygen demand, resulting in sickling.

Evaluation

Expected outcomes of nursing care for the child with sickle cell anemia include the following:

- The child reports effective pain management.
- The child demonstrates adequate hydration to prevent cell sickling.
- The child displays no side effects of disease in the respiratory system, central nervous system, and body organs.
- The child has normal immune status and freedom from infection.
- The family and health care personnel promptly recognize and treat complications of the disease.
- The child meets normal growth and developmental milestones.
- The family demonstrates adequate knowledge of the disease and treatment regimens.

Thalassemias

The thalassemias are a group of inherited blood disorders of hemoglobin synthesis characterized by anemia that can be mild to severe. One of the two pairs of polypeptide chains (alpha and beta polypeptides) in the hemoglobin chain is affected. There are three types of beta-thalassemias (β-thalassemias). β-thalassemia major, also known as Cooley anemia, is the most common type. Alpha-thalassemias (α-thalassemias) vary from the trait to the fatal disorder α-thalassemia major, in which all four alpha-forming genes are defective.

The thalassemias occur most often in people who live in the Mediterranean basin and those who live in tropical and subtropical regions of Asia and Africa (Giardina & Forget, 2009). There are an estimated 200,000 people with β-thalassemia in the Mediterranean area alone, not including those in other parts of the world (Yesilipek, 2007). β-thalassemia is an autosomal recessive disorder, so if both parents carry the abnormal gene, with each pregnancy there is a 25% chance of passing the disorder on to the child.

Etiology and Pathophysiology

Beta-thalassemia In β-thalassemia, defective hemoglobin is synthesized as a result of impaired production of the beta chain of hemoglobin A (Hb A). To compensate for decreased Hb A, production of Hb F (fetal hemoglobin) increases. The RBCs are fragile and are easily destroyed, shortening their life span (Figure 23–7 ➤). As hemolysis increases, **hemosiderin** (iron-containing pigment accumulated from hemoglobin as the red blood cells are destroyed) is deposited in the skin, causing a bronze appearance. Chronic anemia leads to hyperplasia of the bone marrow cavity and thinning of the bone marrow cortex as the bone marrow attempts to compensate for the anemia. Pathologic fractures and skeletal deformities may occur as a result of these bone marrow changes. Splenomegaly results from hyperactivity in removing damaged RBCs and from pooling of cells.

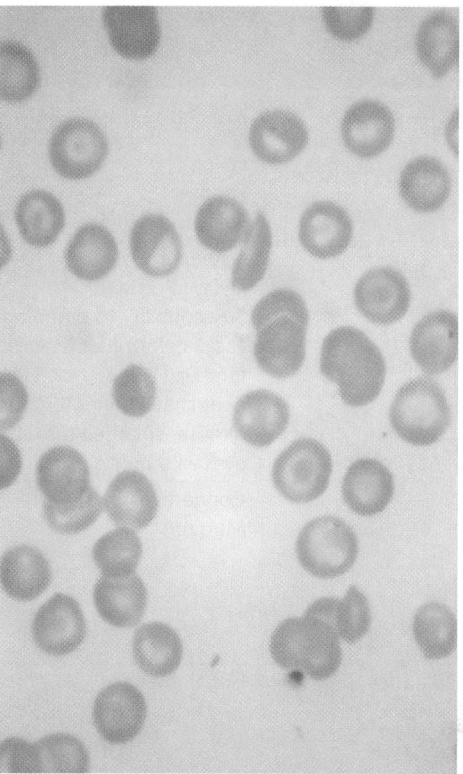

FIGURE 23–7 ➤ Red blood cell appearance in β-thalassemia. What characteristic abnormalities can be seen on this microscopic view?
Courtesy of Dr. Ed Wong, Laboratory Medicine, Children's National Medical Center, Washington, DC.

The three types of β-thalassemia are (Richardson, 2007):

- β-thalassemia minor, or thalassemia trait (produces mild anemia)
- β-thalassemia intermedia (produces moderate anemia, may require transfusions)
- β-thalassemia major (produces anemia requiring transfusion)

Long-term complications related to hemosiderosis include liver failure, endocrine complications such as diabetes and hypothyroidism, and heart failure (Piga, Galanello, Forni, et al., 2006). Skeletal changes include pathologic fractures and skeletal deformities such as an enlarged head and thickened cranial bones. Death is generally the result of cardiac complications related to iron overload (Piga et al., 2006). Other causes of death include liver disease and infection. However, with improved treatment, survival is now possible through the second and third decades of life.

Alpha-thalassemia In α-thalassemia, the defect occurs on the alpha chain of adult hemoglobin. As with beta-thalassemia, the severity of the disorder is dependent on the number of genes that are defective.

The four types of α-thalassemia are (DeBaun & Vichinsky, 2007; Richardson, 2007):

- α-thalassemia silent carrier—defect in a single alpha chain–forming gene
- α-thalassemia trait—defect in two genes
- Hemoglobin H disease—defect in three genes
- α-thalassemia major—defect in all four alpha-forming genes

Clinical Manifestations
β-Thalassemia

Body Organs	Clinical Manifestations	Clinical Therapy
Red blood cells (anemia)	Pallor Fatigue Folic acid deficiency	Administer hypertransfusion program. Administer folic acid and increase dietary consumption of folic acid and vitamin C.
Skeletal changes	Osteoporosis Delayed growth Susceptibility to pathologic fractures Facial deformities: enlarged head, prominent forehead due to frontal and parietal bossing, prominent cheek bones, broadened and depressed bridge of nose, enlarged maxilla with protruding front teeth, eyes with mongolian slant and epicanthal fold	Assess growth and plot on chart—monitor for delays in growth. Teach safety precautions to avoid fractures.
Heart	Congestive heart failure Murmurs	Monitor for signs of congestive heart failure (Chapter 21 ∞). Chest radiograph may be conducted to evaluate heart size. Electrocardiogram (ECG) and echocardiogram may be conducted to assess heart function.
Liver/gallbladder	Hepatomegaly	Magnetic resonance imaging (MRI) or computed tomography (CT) scans may be conducted to evaluate the liver and gallbladder. Liver biopsy may be performed.
Spleen	Splenomegaly	MRI or CT scans may be conducted to evaluate the spleen. Monitor for signs of infection.
Endocrine system	Delayed sexual maturation Symptoms of diabetes (Chapter 30 ∞)	Assess sexual maturation using the Tanner stages.
Skin	Darkening of skin	Assess for skin changes.

Source: Data from DeBaun, M. R., & Vichinsky, E. (2007). Hemoglobinopathies. In R. M. Kliegman, R. E. Behrman, H. B. Jenson, & B. F. Stanton (Eds.), Nelson textbook of pediatrics (18th ed., pp. 2025–2038). Philadelphia: Saunders Elsevier; Piga, A., Galanello, R., Forni, G. L., Cappellini, M. D., Origa, R., Zappu, A., et al. (2006). Randomized phase II trial of deferasirox (Exjade, ICL670), a once-daily, orally-administered iron chelator, in comparison to deferoxamine in thalassemia patients with transfusional iron overload. Haematologica, 91, 873–880; Richardson, M. (2007). Microcytic anemia. Pediatrics in Review, 28(1), 5–14.

Clinical Manifestations

Beta-thalassemia Clinical manifestations of β-thalassemia are caused by the defective synthesis of hemoglobin, structurally impaired red blood cells, and the shortened life span of the RBCs. The infant with β-thalassemia major manifests pallor, failure to thrive, hepatosplenomegaly, and severe anemia that leads to chronic hypoxemia (Richardson, 2007). See Clinical Manifestations: β-Thalassemia. The liver enlarges as a result of hemosiderosis, and the spleen enlarges as a result of extramedullary hematopoiesis and increased hemolysis of red blood cells.

Alpha-thalassemia The child with a one-gene defect (alpha-thalassemia silent carrier) is generally symptom-free. The child with a two-gene defect (alpha-thalassemia trait) may have mild anemia. Manifestations of hemoglobin H disease include anemia and splenomegaly. Alpha-thalassemia major results in hydrops fetalis, intrauterine congestive heart failure, cardiomegaly, hepatomegaly, and death. Bone marrow transplant is the only cure (DeBaun & Vichinsky, 2007; Richardson, 2007).

COLLABORATIVE CARE

The goal of collaborative care is to maintain normal hemoglobin levels and to prevent long-term complications associated with the disorder.

Diagnostic Tests

Diagnosis is made by hemoglobin electrophoresis, which reveals a decreased production of one of the globin chains in hemoglobin and an elevated F and A hemoglobin. A complete blood count (CBC) reveals a decreased hemoglobin, hematocrit, and reticulocyte count (DeBaun & Vichinsky, 2007). Thalassemia can be detected early in infancy. Characteristic erythrocyte cell changes are often recognized in infants by 6 weeks of age. Prenatal testing using chorionic villus sampling (CVS) or amniocentesis can detect or rule out thalassemia in the fetus.

Clinical Therapy

Treatment for thalassemia is supportive. A hypertransfusion program, in which blood transfusions are administered every 2 to 4 weeks, is the conventional therapy used to treat children

β-Thalassemia and Transplantation

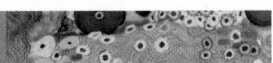

The only cure for β-thalassemia is allogeneic hematopoietic stem cell transplantation (HSCT) (Mathews, George, Deotare, et al., 2007). (See page 701 for a description of different types of HSCT.) The number of people who can receive transplantation is limited to the availability of a compatible donor, usually a sibling. An estimated 70% of affected individuals do not have a compatible donor (Yesilipek, 2007).

with severe disease. Since iron overload is a side effect of this treatment, children may be required to receive an iron-chelating drug such as deferoxamine (Desferal) or Exjade. (See previous discussion beginning on page 684.) A splenectomy may be required for the child with splenomegaly. Hematopoietic stem cell transplantation (HSCT) may be offered as an alternative therapy for children newly diagnosed with the disorder (Box 23–4).

NURSING MANAGEMENT

Nursing care focuses on observing for complications of transfusion therapy, supporting the child and family in dealing with a chronic life-threatening illness, and referring the family for genetic counseling.

Nursing Assessment and Diagnoses

Assess for the classic manifestations, which are pallor, failure to thrive, severe anemia, skin discoloration, and hepatosplenomegaly. Assess for signs of infection including frequent evaluation of temperature. Assess for signs of congestive heart failure, including respiratory distress, fatigue, and edema (Chapter 21 ∞).

Nursing diagnoses for the child with thalassemia may include:

- Risk for Infection related to splenectomy or functional asplenia
- Deficient Knowledge related to disease process and management
- Activity Intolerance related to anemia
- Disturbed Body Image related to discoloration of skin
- Ineffective Tissue Perfusion (all systems) related to anemia

Planning and Implementation

Care for the child receiving blood transfusions as previously discussed. Teach the parents techniques for administration of deferoxamine or regimen for oral deferasirox to prevent iron overload. See discussion on pages 684–685 and 690.

Chronic toxicity may result from high doses of deferoxamine, and resulting complications include hearing loss and renal calcium loss. Blurred vision, decreased visual acuity, and night blindness may occur. Blurred vision should be reported immediately. Periodic ophthalmologic examinations are recommended. Inform the parents and child that deferoxamine discolors urine to a reddish color.

Diet is normal for age and should include folic acid and ascorbic acid (vitamin C). Iron should not be administered and foods rich in iron should be avoided.

If the child has undergone a splenectomy, the risk for infection is increased. Teach the parents and child infection control measures, including proper handwashing and aseptic technique for infusion. Long-term prophylactic antibiotics are generally prescribed.

Provide parents information about thalassemia and its treatment, and encourage them to obtain genetic counseling. Provide emotional support to the child and parents and assist them in coping with a chronic life-threatening illness (see Chapters 12 and 13 ∞).

Encourage parents to take an active role in the child's treatment regimen. Partner with the parents and child to provide opportunities for physical activities, such as swimming, that do not increase the risk of fractures. Collaborate with the family and school to establish individualized health and education plans. Discuss potential body image changes with the child and provide an opportunity for the child to express concerns. The child may require referral for counseling in helping to cope with the body image changes.

Compliance with transfusion therapy often becomes an issue as children reach adolescence. Offering the adolescent a choice regarding treatment options, such as when to undergo transfusion, can help to improve compliance. Adolescents with β-thalassemia and parents of newly diagnosed children can be referred to the Thalassemia Action Group, a national organization for patients, or to the Cooley's Anemia Foundation.

Evaluation

Expected outcomes of nursing care for the child with thalassemia include:

- The child will be free of infection.
- The family will verbalize understanding of treatment regimen and signs of potential complications.
- The child will participate in age-appropriate, safe activities.
- The child will develop a positive body image.
- The child will demonstrate signs of effective tissue perfusion throughout the body.

Hereditary Spherocytosis

Hereditary spherocytosis (HS) is an autosomal dominant hemolytic disorder occurring in 1 in 5,000 births in North America and Northern Europe (Tracy & Rice, 2008). The red blood cell membrane is fragile due to a defect in the protein spectrin. The red blood cell assumes a spherical doughnut shape. The blood cells are sequestered and hemolyzed in the spleen, leading to anemia in the child (Gallagher, 2010; Linker, 2008).

Clinical manifestations generally appear in the neonatal period or during early infancy. Severity of the anemia varies from mild to severe, requiring blood transfusion. Signs and symptoms include jaundice, splenomegaly, and gallstones. A complete blood count reveals anemia, and microscopic examination reveals the abnormally shaped cells (Iolascon, Piscopo, & Boschetto, 2008).

Hyperbilirubinemia in the newborn may require phototherapy or exchange transfusions (Iolascon et al., 2008). Surgical removal of the spleen, generally around the age of 5 years, produces a clinical cure by eliminating hemolysis; however, it does not correct the red blood cell defect. Removal of the spleen increases the risk of infection and sepsis. Nursing care for the child with hereditary spherocytosis is the same as care for the child with anemia.

Aplastic Anemia

Aplastic anemia is a deficiency of the blood cells that results from failure of the bone marrow to produce adequate numbers of circulating blood cells. The condition may be congenital or acquired. Most aplastic anemia is immune-mediated and results from a combination of environmental exposure and an individual's genetically determined response to the causative environmental agent (Young, Calado, & Scheinberg, 2006).

Congenital aplastic anemia (Fanconi anemia) is a rare autosomal recessive syndrome consisting of multiple congenital anomalies. Symptoms can include **purpura** (bleeding into the tissues), **petechiae** (pinpoint lesions), bleeding, fatigue, and pallor. Laboratory findings include **neutropenia** (decreased number of neutrophils) or anemia, and thrombocytopenia (low platelet count) that progresses to **pancytopenia** (decreased number of blood cell components).

Children with congenital aplastic anemia are at risk for developing malignancies such as acute nonlymphocytic leukemia (Freedman, 2007). Acquired aplastic anemia in children is either idiopathic or occurs from a drug reaction. It can develop after exposure to ionizing radiation or insecticides or after ingestion of drugs such as sulfonamides, chloramphenicol, quinacrine, benzene solvents in model airplane glue, or lead. This type of anemia can also be a result of an infectious process such as viral hepatitis or mononucleosis.

Clinical manifestations are related to the degree of bone marrow failure and can include petechiae, purpura, bleeding, pallor, weakness, tachycardia, and fatigue. Diagnosis is made by blood studies, which reveal leukopenia (low white blood cell count) with marked neutropenia, thrombocytopenia, and pancytopenia; and by bone marrow aspiration, which reveals yellow, fatty bone marrow instead of red bone marrow.

After identification of the disorder, the child is removed from any causal agents and the underlying disorder is treated. Therapy involves preventing complications associated with neutropenia, thrombocytopenia, and anemia. Supportive treatment includes transfusions of packed cells, platelets, or both. Immunosuppressive drug therapy is effective for many children because it is believed the child's immune system is reacting against the bone marrow. Immunosuppressive agents include antithymocyte globulin (ATG) and cyclosporine (Young et al., 2006). Antibiotics are administered if infection is confirmed. The treatment of choice is hematopoietic stem cell transplantation from a compatible sibling or family member donor. The family and child require psychosocial support during this life-threatening illness.

NURSING MANAGEMENT

Nursing care is similar to care provided for the child with leukemia (see Chapter 24 ∞). Nursing actions focus on pre-

venting bleeding, administering and monitoring blood transfusions, preventing infection, encouraging mobility as tolerated, educating the parents and child about the disorder, and providing emotional support.

The nurse partners with the child and family to assist the child with activities of daily living and cluster patient care to conserve energy since fatigue, poor tissue oxygenation, and weakness may be experienced. Observe for complications associated with administration of blood products, including transfusion reaction and fluid overload. For the child receiving hematopoietic stem cell transplantation, refer to the section discussing HSCT later in this chapter.

Families require support in dealing with a child who has a life-threatening disease. A collaborative approach with the use of social services, spiritual care, and other support services offers comfort and education to families with these special needs. Expected outcomes of nursing care include maintenance of normal levels of white and red blood cells and platelets to support body functions.

■ BLEEDING DISORDERS

The body depends on a complex mechanism to ensure proper clotting of blood. Platelets and several clotting factors are required. Platelets can be decreased (the condition known as thrombocytopenia) for several reasons:

- Injury of the bone marrow or inability to produce platelets (see aplastic anemia discussion on this page)
- Loss or excessive dilution of blood
- Pooling of blood in the spleen (see discussion of sickle cell disease on page 680)
- A variety of medical conditions such as disseminated intravascular coagulation (see page 698), hemolytic-uremic syndrome (see Chapter 26 ∞), or infection
- Immune response (immune thrombocytopenic purpura; see description beginning on page 699) (Buchanan, 2005)

Clotting factors are most often deficient due to genetic causes; see the discussions of hemophilia and von Willebrand disease that follow.

Hemophilia

Hemophilia refers to a group of hereditary bleeding disorders that result from a deficiency in specific clotting factors. In the United States, about 1 in 5,000 male births result in hemophilia. Hemophilia A, or classic hemophilia, is caused by a deficiency of clotting factor VIII in the blood and accounts for 85% of persons with hemophilia. Hemophilia B, also known as Christmas disease, is caused by a deficiency of factor IX. Of persons with hemophilia, 10–15% have hemophilia B (Ohls & Christensen, 2007). The severity of the disease may range from mild to severe bleeding tendencies. Hemophilia C, a deficiency in factor XI, is an autosomal disease, occurring equally in males and females. The bleeding in factor XI deficiency is generally less severe than in factors VIII and IX deficiencies (Siegel, 2009). The following discussion is focused on hemophilia A and B.

Etiology and Pathophysiology

Genes for clotting factors VIII and IX are located near the terminal long arm of the X chromosome (Scott & Montgomery, 2007). Hemophilia A and B are X-linked recessive traits, which manifest almost exclusively as affected males and carrier females. A daughter who inherits the trait from her father has a 50% chance at each pregnancy of transmitting it to her sons (refer to Chapter 3 ∞ for a description of genetic transmission). However, as many as one third of the children affected by hemophilia do not have a family member with a history of a clotting disorder. In these cases, the disorder is caused by a new mutation (Scott & Montgomery, 2007).

The degree of bleeding is related to the amount of clotting factor, which is dependent upon the phase of coagulation affected and the severity of the injury. Potential complications of hemophilia include internal hemorrhaging, transfusion reactions, shock, and death.

Clinical Manifestations

Hemophilia is manifested in different children by bleeding tendencies that range from mild to moderate or severe. Children with hemophilia often do not manifest symptoms until after 6 months of age as they become more mobile and incur injuries and bleeding from falls or from tooth eruption. Spontaneous bleeding, **hemarthrosis** (bleeding into a joint space), and deep tissue hemorrhage occur. Affected children frequently experience bleeding into the joint spaces of the knees, ankles, and elbows. Bleeding into joint spaces or bursae causes the child to have limited motion because of pain, tenderness, and swelling. Bone changes, contractures, and disabling deformities can result from immobility and from the effects of blood in the joint structures.

Male children may have bleeding after circumcision. Other signs and symptoms include easy bruising (**ecchymosis**), nosebleeds, hematuria, and bleeding after tooth extraction, minor trauma, or minor surgical procedures. Large subcutaneous and intramuscular hemorrhages sometimes occur. Bleeding into the tissues of the neck, mouth, or chest is particularly serious because of the potential for airway obstruction. Retroperitoneal and intracranial bleeding may also occur and can be life threatening.

Females who carry the trait for hemophilia do not usually manifest symptoms of the disease. However, they may have prolonged bleeding during dental work, surgery, or trauma.

COLLABORATIVE CARE

Diagnosis of affected individuals and carriers can be done before birth through chorionic villus sampling or amniocentesis. Genetic testing of family members is increasingly being used to identify carriers. Diagnosis can also be made on the basis of the history, physical examination, and laboratory data. Laboratory tests will show low levels of factor VIII or IX, and prolonged activated partial thromboplastin time (aPTT). Prothrombin time (PT), thrombin time (TT), fibrinogen, and platelet count are normal. See Table 23–6.

TABLE 23–6 Diagnostic Tests for Bleeding Disorders

Test*	Normal Value
Fibrinogen	175–400 mg/dL
Partial thromboplastin time, activated (aPTT)	22–34 seconds
Platelet count	150–400 × 10⁹/L
Prothrombin time (PT)	11–15 seconds
Thrombin time (TT)	14–16 seconds

Data from: Kliegman, R. M., Behrman, R. E., Jenson, H. B., & Stanton, B. F. (2007). Nelson textbook of pediatrics (18th ed.). Philadelphia: Saunders Elsevier; Corbett, J. V. (2008). Laboratory tests and diagnostic procedures with nursing diagnoses (7th ed.). Upper Saddle River, NJ: Pearson Prentice Hall.

*See Appendix E ∞ for information about these tests.

The goal of medical management is to control bleeding by replacing the missing clotting factor. Desmopressin (DDAVP), an analog of vasopressin, stimulates the release of factor VIII stored in the blood vessels, thereby increasing the percentage of available factor by approximately threefold. DDAVP is used in some patients with mild and moderate hemophilia A (Manno & Larson, 2009).

The child with severe hemophilia may be on a prophylactic regimen of factor concentrate therapy several times per week, whereas the child with mild to moderate hemophilia may only receive episodic therapy. Even with prophylaxis, the child with severe hemophilia may have a bleeding episode and need episodic treatment as well (Manco-Johnson, Abshire, Shapiro, et al., 2007; Rodriguez & Hoots, 2008). Prompt and adequate treatment is needed to prevent serious bleeding episodes and their sequelae.

The outlook for children with hemophilia has been greatly improved by the availability of transfusion therapy. In the past, many children with factor VIII deficiency died in the first 5 years of life. Today, children with moderate or mild hemophilia can lead normal lives. See Table 23–7 for types of blood products available for infusion in hemophilia and other disorders. Additional products have recently been approved for treatment of hemophilia (Box 23–5).

BOX 23–5 New Products for Treatment of Hemophilia A

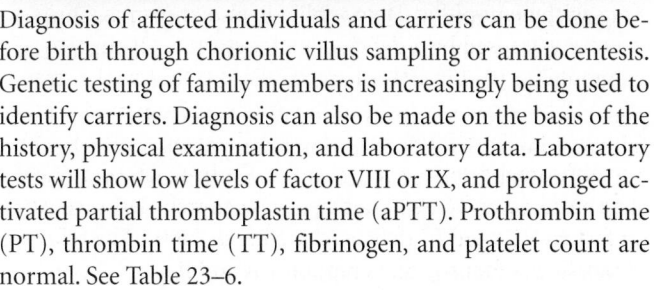

Xyntha, a recombinant antihemophilic factor, is used to prevent and control bleeding episodes in hemophilia A and is produced without the use of additives such as albumin, decreasing the risk for infection after use of this product (Thompson, 2008). Kogenate FS is a version of factor VIII that was first approved in 1993 to control bleeding or prevent bleeding episodes during surgery. Recently it has been approved for use in children with severe hemophilia A to decrease the frequency of bleeding episodes and to reduce joint damage. Clinical trials demonstrated that boys who received daily doses of Kogenate FS had 6 times less joint damage and 8 times less bleeding than those boys who only received the product at the time of a bleeding episode (Foster, 2008).

TABLE 23–7	Type of Blood and Blood Products for Administration to Children with Hematologic Disorders
Type of Blood or Blood Product	Indication for Use
Whole blood	To replace blood volume Generally given in hypovolemic shock
Packed red blood cells	To increase oxygen-carrying capacity in anemia and some leukemias, also given in cases of hypovolemic shock
Fresh frozen plasma	To expand blood volume
Albumin	To expand blood volume in shock and trauma
Factor VIII concentrate	To treat factor VIII deficiency (hemophilia A) and von Willebrand disease
Factor IX concentrate	To treat factor IX deficiency (hemophilia B)

Research *Gene Therapy*

Gene therapy is being explored for treatment of hemophilia. Efforts in animal models such as dogs are under way. These research approaches offer the promise of new treatment options in the future (Warrington & Herzog, 2006).

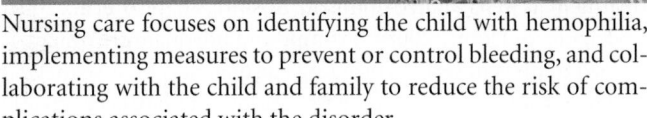

NURSING MANAGEMENT

Nursing care focuses on identifying the child with hemophilia, implementing measures to prevent or control bleeding, and collaborating with the child and family to reduce the risk of complications associated with the disorder.

Nursing Assessment and Diagnosis

Physiologic Assessment

Obtain a complete medical history from the parents or child. In particular, inquire about previous episodes of bleeding and the occurrence of hemophilia or any other bleeding disorders in family members. The history of bleeding will vary depending on the severity of the disease. Observe for prolonged bleeding or oozing of blood. At times, children with mild disorders are diagnosed after incidents such as prolonged nosebleeds or seeping after a venipuncture.

Assess the child for any joint pain, swelling, or permanent deformity, particularly around the knees, elbows, ankles, and shoulders. Assess for pain in any body part. Note the presence of hematuria and mild flank pain. Assess skin for evidence of ecchymoses or petechiae. A neurological assessment is conducted, as the risk for intracranial hemorrhage and bleeding can lead to peripheral neuropathies.

Psychosocial Assessment

It is difficult for families to manage care of the child with hemophilia, especially if the disease is severe. Assess the family's coping mechanisms and support systems. Determine the family's ability to manage procedures and treatment; the factor concentrates and infusion equipment are costly. Inquire if the parents have respite care that enables them to take time for themselves while knowing that the child is cared for safely. Assess older children's understanding of the disease, limitations, and their adaptation to it.

Developmental Assessment

Because the child with hemophilia may have physical activity restrictions, physical skills may be delayed. Perform frequent developmental assessments, being particularly attentive to fine and gross motor skills.

The most important nursing diagnosis for the child with hemophilia is Risk for Injury related to bleeding disorder. Following are other nursing diagnoses that may apply:

- Acute Pain related to bleeding episodes
- Impaired Physical Mobility related to joint stiffness or contractures
- Deficient Knowledge related to lack of exposure to information about hemophilia
- Interrupted Family Processes related to family role shift required to care for a child with a chronic illness
- Delayed Growth and Development related to effects of physical disability

Planning and Implementation

Nursing care focuses on preventing and controlling bleeding episodes, limiting joint involvement and managing pain, and providing emotional support. Both short-term interventions and long-term management are necessary.

Prevent and Control Bleeding Episodes

Bleeding problems are rare in infants with hemophilia. As children learn to walk and develop other motor skills, however, they often fall and suffer cuts and bruises. The risk of injury can be reduced by emphasizing to parents the need for close supervision and a safe environment. Parents should encourage children to play with toys that are safe and age-appropriate. When the child is learning to walk, a helmet is recommended to protect the head from injury during falls. The home environment should be adapted to promote safety, such as by removing rugs that cause tripping and padding furniture with sharp edges.

If dental surgery or tooth extraction is necessary, it is performed in a controlled environment by experienced staff. Use of a dental irrigation device is often recommended if the child has excess bleeding from gums. Advise adolescents to shave only with an electric razor.

Control any superficial bleeding by applying pressure to the area for at least 15 minutes. Immobilize and elevate the affected area, and apply ice packs to promote vasoconstriction. Follow prescriptions for administration of factor replacement. Carefully monitor the child's condition for any side effects when factor replacement therapy is administered. If the child sustains a head, abdominal, or other major injury, immediate medical attention is required.

When the child is hospitalized, use nursing approaches to minimize the chance of bleeding. Ensure that the hospital environment is safe by orienting the child to the room and keeping the floor and room clear of hazards as much as possible.

Limit Joint Involvement and Manage Pain

During bleeding episodes, hemarthrosis is managed by elevating and immobilizing the joint and applying ice packs. Administer analgesics as ordered. Once bleeding has been controlled, range of motion exercises are performed to strengthen muscles and joints and to prevent flexion contractures. Physical therapy may be required. Because excessive weight can place an added stress on joints, encourage the child to maintain an appropriate weight. Oral or intravenous opioids may be required for pain relief.

Clinical Tip

Use the acronym RICE (rest, ice, compression, elevation) to help you remember important measures to control a bleeding episode.

Clinical Tip

Take the following precautions when caring for children with bleeding disorders:

- Avoid taking temperatures rectally or giving suppositories.
- Check blood pressure by cuff as infrequently as possible.
- Avoid intramuscular or subcutaneous injections.
- Use only paper or silk tape for dressings.
- Except for factor replacement therapy, avoid all venipunctures.
- Use a peripheral fingerstick to obtain blood samples.
- Do not give aspirin or aspirin-containing products.
- Check the child's ears with an otoscope very gently (and only when necessary), using rounded or cushioned specula.

Provide Emotional Support

The needs of families with children who have hemophilia are best met through a comprehensive team approach. Refer the parents for genetic counseling as soon as possible after diagnosis. It is important to identify family members who carry the trait, as they may suffer excessive bleeding during surgery.

Encourage the parents to verbalize their feelings. Be understanding and sensitive to their needs. Mothers may feel guilty about having transferred the disease to the child and may benefit from assistance in dealing with these feelings. Refer to counseling as appropriate. Partner with the family to explain the disorder and how it affects both the child and other family members. Refer the parents and child to organizations such as the National Hemophilia Foundation for further information.

Discharge Planning and Home Care Teaching

The child may be hospitalized briefly during the first manifestation of bleeding or diagnosis and management. Most care will subsequently take place in the home. Home care needs should be identified and addressed well in advance of discharge. Advise parents to have the child wear a medical identification tag. Dentists and other health care providers should be aware of the diagnosis.

Explain the cause of bleeding so both the child and parents understand the disease process. Teach the child and family how to identify internal bleeding. Signs and symptoms such as joint pain, abdominal pain, and obvious bleeding are indicators for immediate factor infusion. Make sure the child and parents know what situations could cause bleeding to occur. Teach parents to give acetaminophen instead of aspirin or aspirin-containing products.

Instruct the parents and the child, when appropriate, in the preparation and administration of intravenous factor concentrate. If infusion of the missing factor is scheduled on a regular basis, bleeding episodes can be controlled or avoided. Have the parents demonstrate the procedure and make sure they can properly administer the product. The parents need to be familiar with properties of the factor concentrate to correctly prepare the mixture. As the child advances in age, he or she can assume some of the management responsibilities of care.

The child will need an individualized school health plan (see Chapter 12 ∞). Members of the school staff should be instructed in management of emergencies, and infusion equipment should be readily available. The nurse can identify key staff members in the school and teach them the actions that need to be taken.

Help the family and school to plan an appropriate schedule of activities without overprotecting the child. Children with hemophilia should not engage in contact sports such as football and soccer, which may result in injury and trauma. Instead, sports such as swimming, hiking, and bicycling should be encouraged.

Explain how the parents can coordinate their child's care with a number of health professionals. Provide ongoing case management, assisting the family to take on this task, if able.

Hemophilia is a debilitating disorder for the child, and it can also be financially draining for the family. Frequent outpatient visits, emergency department visits, hospital admissions, and the cost of factor concentrate can exhaust a family's resources. If indicated, referral should be made to appropriate social services (e.g., the state's maternal and child health program for children with special health care needs) and organizations such as the National Hemophilia Foundation. Sharing experiences with other families of children with hemophilia can provide support.

Hemophilia Resources

Growth & Development *The Adolescent with Hemophilia*

Encourage adolescents with hemophilia to participate in leisure activities such as computer games, reading clubs, and crafts. They should use knee pads, elbow pads, and helmets when participating in any physical sports. Swimming and other noncontact sports are good choices for physical activity. Contact sports such as soccer and football should be avoided. Activities important to development can be encouraged when coaches, teachers, and others know how to treat bleeding episodes. Advise adolescents to shave only with an electric razor.

Investigate the availability of summer camps for children and teens with hemophilia and provide this information to families.

Evaluation

Expected outcomes of nursing care include the following:

- The child will be free from injury that could cause bleeding.
- Normal joint mobility will be maintained.
- Pain will be successfully managed to a level of comfort for the child.
- Safe and timely infusions will be provided as needed to treat the disease and prevent complications.
- The child will demonstrate normal growth and developmental progression.
- The child and family will demonstrate adequate knowledge of disease management, including recognition of bleeding and prompt initiation of infusions.
- Family members will verbalize that they have adequate support to provide care for the child with hemophilia and to deal with genetic implications of the disease.

Von Willebrand Disease

Von Willebrand disease is the most common hereditary bleeding disorder (Robertson, Lillicrap, & James, 2008). A variety of subtypes of this disorder are classified based on the amount and functionality of the von Willebrand factor (vWF), a plasma protein and the carrier for clotting factor VIII. The most common form of the disorder is transmitted as an autosomal dominant trait, and can occur in both males and females. The gene for the disease is located on chromosome 12 (Geil, 2009).

Normally, vWF concentration increases in the area of an injury and binds to platelets to facilitate their binding to the damaged vessel wall. With von Willebrand disease, the vWF is not sufficient in quantity or is dysfunctional; therefore, clot forming and bleeding control is impaired.

The characteristic manifestations are prolonged and excessive mucocutaneous bleeding. In children this generally is exhibited through gingival bleeding, epistaxis, bruising, bleeding from the gums, and minor wounds or lacerations. Increased bleeding also occurs during surgery and dental extractions. The disease may not be diagnosed until a surgical or dental procedure leads to bleeding. Affected teenage girls may have menorrhagia (increased menstrual bleeding) (Robertson et al., 2008). Gastrointestinal bleeding can occur. Hemarthrosis is uncommon.

Diagnosis of von Willebrand disease is made after laboratory studies reveal decreased von Willebrand factor levels, von Willebrand factor antigen levels, and factor VIII activity; reduced platelet agglutination; prolonged or normal bleeding time; and prolonged or normal activated partial thromboplastin time (APPT) (Robertson et al., 2008).

Treatment is similar to that for the child with hemophilia and involves infusion of von Willebrand protein concentrate. Desmopressin (DDAVP) is administered to promote release of stored vWF and to prevent bleeding associated with dental or surgical procedures. Locally administered medications such as aminocaproic acid are sometimes used to manage bleeding in the mucous membranes.

NURSING MANAGEMENT

Nursing care is the same as for a child with hemophilia. See page 696. Teach parents about the disorder and instruct them not to give the child any aspirin or other drugs that can cause bleeding or inhibit platelet function. Teach management of bleeding episodes and intravenous infusion techniques, as for hemophilia. The prognosis is good, and children with von Willebrand disease usually have a normal life expectancy. Expected outcomes of nursing care include prompt management of bleeding and prevention of disease complications.

Disseminated Intravascular Coagulation

Disseminated intravascular coagulation (DIC) is a life-threatening, acquired pathologic process in which the clotting system is abnormally activated, resulting in widespread clot formation in the small vessels throughout the body. The most common cause of DIC is sepsis (see Chapter 16 ∞). Infections caused by gram-negative and gram-positive bacteria, fungi, viruses, and protozoa may lead to DIC (LeMone & Burke, 2008).

The disorder results from increased protease activity that is caused by unregulated release of thrombin. Excess thrombin is generated, followed by deposition of fibrin strands in body tissues. These changes slow the circulating blood and cause tissue hypoxia, resulting in eventual tissue necrosis. The circulating fibrin fragments later begin to interfere with platelet aggregation and other aspects of the clotting mechanism, resulting in bleeding or hemorrhage. The disease process commonly interferes with function in the respiratory, cardiovascular, hepatic, renal, neurologic, and gastrointestinal systems (Oren, Cingoz, Duman, et al., 2005).

COLLABORATIVE CARE

The prothrombin time and partial thromboplastin time are prolonged, platelet count and fibrinogen levels are increased, and levels of fibrin-fibrinogen split products are high.

Management is supportive and includes identification and treatment of the underlying disorder; replacement of depleted coagulation factors, fibrinogen, and platelets; and anticoagulant therapy (heparin).

NURSING MANAGEMENT

DIC is a complex disorder that is managed by a critical care team. Nursing care focuses on assessing the bleeding, preventing further injury, and administering prescribed therapies.

Because all body systems can be involved, careful assessment of all systems is needed on a continual basis. Assess extremities for capillary refill, warmth, and pulses. Frequently assess vital signs and level of consciousness. Observe petechiae, ecchymoses, and all body orifices and skin breaks for oozing blood every 1 to 2 hours. Careful monitoring of dependent areas is essential, as blood will pool in these locations. Intravenous sites are particularly prone to oozing and should be assessed every 15 minutes. Examine stool for the presence of blood, and measure blood loss as accurately as possible. Assess intake and output. Monitor urine for presence of blood. Blood urea nitrogen (BUN) and creatinine are monitored to assess renal function.

Institute bleeding control precautions and administer replacement therapy of blood products as prescribed. Monitor vital signs frequently and report any signs of complications. Monitor for signs of hypovolemic shock.

Monitor oxygen saturations and arterial blood gases. The child may require mechanical ventilation. Maintain patency of airway and implement safety measures to preserve endotracheal tube position.

Implement measures to maintain skin integrity, such as gentle repositioning. Implement a nutritional plan of tube feedings or total parenteral nutrition. Identify the family's coping strategies and support system to facilitate their ability to manage this life-threatening crisis. See Chapter 13 ∞.

Expected outcomes of nursing care are management of bleeding and adequate functioning of all body systems, as well as effective family coping.

Immune Thrombocytopenic Purpura

Immune thrombocytopenic purpura (ITP), also known as idiopathic thrombocytopenic purpura, is a disorder characterized by increased destruction of platelets in the spleen, even though platelet production in the bone marrow is normal. Platelets are destroyed as a result of the binding of autoantibodies to platelet antigens. When the rate of platelet destruction exceeds the rate of platelet production, the number of circulating platelets decreases and blood clotting slows.

Etiology and Pathophysiology

ITP is the most common bleeding disorder in children. It occurs annually in 4 children per 100,000 (Belletrutti, Kaiser, Barnard, et al., 2007). The acute condition occurs most frequently in children 1 to 10 years of age, and the chronic condition is most common in children over 9 years (Panepinto & Brousseau, 2005).

The cause of ITP is unknown, but it frequently follows an infectious illness. It is seen as an uncommon complication in 1 in 25,000 children after the measles-mumps-rubella vaccination (Blanchette & Bolton-Maggs, 2008). An antibody that acts against platelets binds to the platelet surface, reacts with membrane glycoproteins, and causes platelet destruction in the liver and spleen (Buchanan, 2005; Panepinto & Brousseau, 2005).

Clinical Manifestations

Symptoms include multiple ecchymoses and petechiae. Mucosal bleeding such as in the mouth or nose is a common presentation. The child has typically been well, has a history of recent infection, and then develops sudden bruising or petechiae (Blanchette & Bolton-Maggs, 2008).

COLLABORATIVE CARE

Diagnosis is made by history and thorough physical and laboratory findings, which reveal a decreased platelet count (less than 20,000 mm³/dL). The child has normal hemoglobin and white blood cell counts. If the presentation is atypical, further labora-

tory testing involves a bone marrow aspiration to rule out other diagnoses (Buchanan, 2005).

If they have minor thrombocytopenia and minimal bleeding, some children with ITP are initially monitored closely rather than treated. Most children improve without treatment within 6 months (Buchanan, 2005). Families need instructions to identify bleeding, especially intracranial, and to seek care immediately. Children must avoid contact sports until platelet counts return to normal. The primary goal of treatment for ITP is to prevent intracranial hemorrhage, which occurs in 0.2–1% of patients with ITP, generally when the platelet count is less than 20,000/mm³ (Beck, Nathan, Parkin, et al., 2005).

The modalities of treatment for ITP vary among health care providers, but may include corticosteroids, intravenous immune globulin (IVIG), and intravenous anti-D immunoglobulin (Blanchette & Bolton-Maggs, 2008; Son, Jeon, Yang, et al., 2008). Platelet administration is not usually indicated unless intracranial hemorrhage occurs. With ITP, platelet administration will control bleeding temporarily, since the administered platelets will be destroyed.

It is estimated that 20–25% of patients with ITP will develop chronic disease (Blanchette & Bolton-Maggs, 2008). Children who fail to respond to treatment for acute ITP and persist with thrombocytopenia for longer than 6 months are diagnosed with chronic ITP (Belletrutti et al., 2007). For children who do not respond to drug therapy over a period of 6 months to 1 year, splenectomy may be the treatment of choice since the platelets are destroyed in the spleen.

NURSING MANAGEMENT

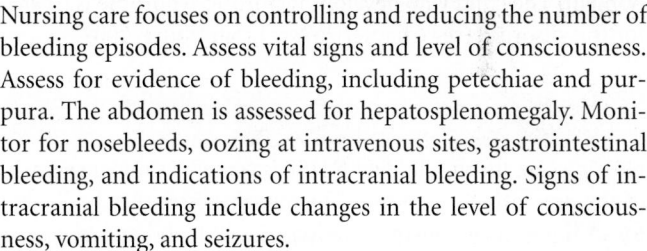

Nursing care focuses on controlling and reducing the number of bleeding episodes. Assess vital signs and level of consciousness. Assess for evidence of bleeding, including petechiae and purpura. The abdomen is assessed for hepatosplenomegaly. Monitor for nosebleeds, oozing at intravenous sites, gastrointestinal bleeding, and indications of intracranial bleeding. Signs of intracranial bleeding include changes in the level of consciousness, vomiting, and seizures.

Measures to prevent bleeding are similar to those for the child with hemophilia. Teach parents to use acetaminophen to manage pain and fever, rather than aspirin or other drugs that influence bleeding time. The child should avoid contact sports and other activities that may increase the risk of injury. Ensure that the family and child are aware of the signs and symptoms indicating bleeding, including signs of intracranial bleeding.

Expected outcomes of nursing care are prevention of bleeding and restoration of normal coagulation patterns with no serious sequelae.

Henoch-Schönlein Purpura

Henoch-Schönlein purpura (HSP) is described as a **vasculitis** (inflammation of the blood vessels) of the small vessels. It is the most common vasculitis in children, affecting approximately 10 children per 100,000 each year. The disease predominates in childhood with a mean age of 6 years. Approximately 90% of children affected are under 10 years of age (Saulsbury, 2007).

HSP is twice as common in males as it is in females (Roberts, Waller, Brinker, et al., 2007).

The cause of HSP is unknown; however, IgA is known to play a role in the development of the illness which generally follows an upper respiratory infection (Barillas-Arias, Adams, & Lehman, 2008; Roberts et al., 2007; Saulsbury, 2007).

The child with HSP typically presents with slightly raised purpuric lesions (palpable purpura), joint pain (arthritis), colicky abdominal pain, gastrointestinal bleeding represented by blood in the stool, and hematuria (Chen, Chang, Chu, et al., 2007; Saulsbury, 2007). HSP is generally a self-limiting disease. The severity of the renal involvement (nephritis) is the primary prognostic factor with 30–50% having long-term problems (Saulsbury, 2007).

COLLABORATIVE CARE

Management of HSP focuses on supportive care directed at the systems involved. The child should also be monitored for rare but serious complications including hemorrhage in any body system (Roberts et al., 2007).

Although the IgA concentration is elevated in approximately 50% of patients with HSP, there is no defining laboratory test that confirms the diagnosis. The symptoms described previously are generally sufficient criteria for the diagnosis; tests may be performed to rule out other illnesses (Roberts et al., 2007; Saulsbury, 2007).

Supportive care for the child with HSP focuses on controlling gastrointestinal symptoms, joint pain, and renal involvement. Corticosteroids have been used successfully in controlling both gastrointestinal and joint pain. They are helpful in managing the severity of the nephritis, but not in preventing its development. The child who develops nephrotic syndrome is treated for this disorder (see Chapter 26 ∞) (Saulsbury, 2007).

NURSING MANAGEMENT

Nursing care for the child with HSP is centered on management of the presenting symptoms. The nurse assesses the child's skin for changes in the purpuric lesions. Careful abdominal assessment is necessary to detect increased abdominal pain and distention that might be associated with gastrointestinal hemorrhage or nephritis. Joint assessment helps monitor progression of the disease. Management of joint pain is an essential aspect of care and promotes comfort and tolerance of symptoms. Stools should be evaluated for occult blood. Evaluation of urinary output is essential in monitoring the child's renal function. Urine should be tested for the presence of blood. The child should have daily weights and careful assessment for the development of edema associated with renal involvement. A full multisystem assessment aids in detection of complications related to hemorrhage in body systems. Any abnormalities should be reported to the physician.

Teaching related to corticosteroid therapy is essential. If the child is being discharged on steroids or is being managed at home (in mild cases), the family must understand the dosage schedule and the side effects of this medication (see Chapter 26 ∞). HSP generally is self-limiting, but the nurse should be diligent not only in monitoring the child for progression of the disease but also in supporting the family during the illness.

Meningococcemia

Meningococcemia is a virulent disease process that develops in some individuals infected with *Neisseria meningitidis* (see Chapter 16 ∞). *N. meningitidis* is a gram-negative bacteria that is transmitted primarily via the respiratory route (Woods, 2007). Onset is sudden. Often, a respiratory infection is followed by fever, myalgias, weakness, headache, diarrhea, and vomiting. The petechial rash characteristic of this disease may develop before other serious symptoms and progresses rapidly (Milonovich, 2007; Woods, 2007). The child's condition may deteriorate rapidly within a few hours. The clotting cascade is initiated resulting in bleeding and thrombosis in the tissues (Milonovich, 2007). The child is critically ill and demonstrates multisystem disease. Frequently the skin is pink and then black as the tissues are damaged from reduced oxygen delivery.

Treatment consists of antibiotics, removal from sources of infection, and multisystem shock management (refer to Chapter 21 ∞ for a description of distributive shock). Prompt administration of antibiotics to the child who manifests fever with purpura can decrease the severity of outcome. Depending on the child's condition, total parenteral nutrition, sedation and pain relief, dialysis, or amputation may be required. Close contacts of the child should receive prophylactic antibiotics.

NURSING MANAGEMENT

Nursing care of the child with meningococcemia is complex, and treatment must begin quickly. The child generally has a lengthy hospitalization in a pediatric intensive care unit followed by years of care that may involve plastic surgery or prosthetic adaptation. Thorough assessments of all body systems are performed. Ongoing assessment of vital signs is essential.

Administer intravenous infusions when ordered to ensure correct and timely administration of antibiotics and other therapies. Measure urinary output to evaluate kidney function. Meticulous skin care is necessary to preserve the integrity of tissues. Take care to prevent further infections. Nutritional support in the form of total parenteral nutrition is common. The family needs support to deal with the changing critical nature of the child's illness and the possibility that death or permanent, severe deformities will result. When the child improves, continuing comprehensive care in the hospital and then in the community is needed to manage complex issues related to growth, development, nutrition, amputations, and prosthetics. Expected outcomes of nursing care include prevention of further infection, maintenance of body systems during the acute phase of illness, and positive adjustment to amputations and deformities resulting from the disease.

■ HEMATOPOIETIC STEM CELL TRANSPLANTATION (HSCT)

Hematopoietic stem cell transplantation is a treatment used for diseases such as severe combined immunodeficiency disease, severe and unresponsive aplastic anemia, and leukemia (refer to Chapters 22 and 24 ∞). Hematopoietic stem cells exist primarily in the bone marrow but also circulate in the peripheral blood. These cells can grow into new body cells and so have become useful to treat immune and hematologic diseases when restoration of normal cells is needed. Stem cells can be obtained from bone marrow, cord blood, or peripheral blood and frozen for later use (Rowley & Donato, 2008).

COLLABORATIVE CARE

Hematopoietic stem cell transplants are either autologous or allogeneic. In **autologous transplantation**, the child's own marrow is taken, treated, stored, and reinfused after the child has received chemotherapy. **Allogeneic transplantation** may be **syngeneic** (from an identical twin), related, or unrelated. In allogeneic transplantation, the donor, often a sibling (related), has a compatible human leukocyte antigen (HLA). Human leukocyte antigens are proteins found on the surface of nearly all nucleated cells within the body, and they are responsible for regulating the immune response. When no relative is found to match the child, a histocompatible donor (unrelated) may be sought from the National Marrow Donor Program or a cord blood bank (Brunstein & Wagner, 2008; Petersdorf & Anasetti, 2008). With the development of this registry, bone marrow transplantation from HLA-matched unrelated donors has become possible for some children.

Clinical Therapy

Pretransplant Phase After a thorough evaluation of the child, including HLA typing, evaluation of organ functions, and laboratory studies, the child receives high doses of chemotherapy and, sometimes, total body irradiation directed at destroying circulating blood cells and the diseased bone marrow in the ill child. Common chemotherapeutic agents used include cyclophosphamide, busulfan, etoposide, melphalan, cytarabine, and thiotepa. The chemotherapy program for destruction of bone marrow ranges from 7 to 10 days (Moore, 2005). During this time, the child is cared for in strict isolation in a special unit that provides a positive pressure environment (Figure 23–8 ➤).

Transplant Phase Following the immunosuppression procedure, the child receives an intravenous transfusion with the donor stem cells. This procedure is similar to administration of a blood product. The healthy stem cells migrate to the bone marrow. Healthy bone marrow, capable of making blood cells, is the anticipated result. If the transplantation is successful, the cells implant in the child's marrow and begin to produce blood cells within approximately 2 to 4 weeks.

Posttransplant Phase Pancytopenia (marked decrease in RBCs, WBCs, and platelets) lasts for several weeks following the transplantation. The major risks during this period are infection, anemia, bleeding, and severe mouth sores. Transfusion of red blood cells and platelets may be required. The child's illness and the side effects related to the chemotherapy may alter nutritional status. Total parenteral nutrition (TPN) may be implemented to meet the child's nutritional needs during this period.

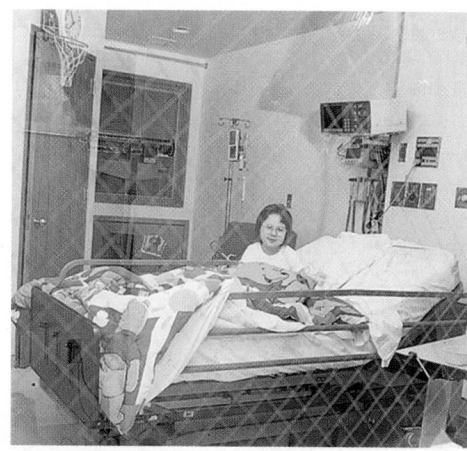

FIGURE 23–8 ➤ The child undergoing bone marrow transplantation is hospitalized in a special sterile unit while receiving chemotherapy before the transfusion. The child remains in the unit for several weeks afterward until the new marrow produces enough cells to maintain health.

Except for children receiving syngeneic transplants, immunosuppressive agents are administered to prevent graft-versus-host disease. Once the bone marrow begins to produce new cells, graft-versus-host disease (rejection) is the major threat. Refer to Chapter 22 ∞ for a discussion of this disease.

NURSING MANAGEMENT
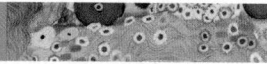

Monitor the child undergoing HSCT by assessing the skin, mucous membranes, gastrointestinal function, respiratory function, cardiac function, and hydration status. Multisystem assessment is needed. Because graft-versus-host disease may occur at any time, even after the child returns home, frequent thorough assessments are necessary after discharge.

> ▲ Health Promotion
>
> For the child who has undergone HSCT, hearing and vision screening is advised at each primary care visit. Hearing loss may occur as a result of ototoxic drug therapy, and corticosteroid use can cause cataracts. Additionally, graft-versus-host disease can result in keratoconjunctivitis, and cytomegalovirus (CMV) can cause retinitis.

Supportive care after the transplantation procedure focuses on preventing infection, controlling bleeding, maintaining adequate nutrition and hydration, monitoring for signs of rejection, and providing psychosocial support. The treatment is lengthy, the child is often critically ill, and parents may have traveled to a medical center many miles from home for the procedure. Ask parents about other family members and how they are managing. Provide information about inexpensive housing available near the medical center, such as in a Ronald McDonald house. Encourage parents to discuss their feelings with other parents of children receiving bone marrow transplantation. Organizations such as the Bone Marrow Transplant Family Support Network can serve as resources for families.

When the child is ready for discharge, be sure the family is prepared to administer medications, recognize signs of graft-versus-host disease, provide adequate nutrition for the child, and perform other necessary care. Arrange for follow-up visits and provide the names of local health care contact persons who can offer support and provide information. The child may need tutors or other educational assistance to promote integration back into the school setting.

The major expected outcome of nursing care is the proper activity of bone marrow in the child with resulting normal levels and function of blood cells. Other outcomes are provision of family support, ongoing care and education for the child, adequate nutrition, and prevention of infection.

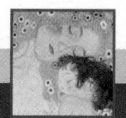

Chapter Highlights

- Erythrocytes (red cells) are a major component of the blood and transport oxygen from the lungs to body tissues.
- Polycythemia is an increase in the number of red blood cells. Anemia is characterized by a decrease in red blood cell number. Leukocytes (white cells) are important in the cell's defenses against disease.
- Thrombocytes (platelets) are necessary for normal clotting of blood.
- The major anemias of childhood include iron deficiency anemia, thalassemia, aplastic anemia, normocytic anemia, and sickle cell anemia.
- Sickle cell anemia is a genetic disease in which an abnormal shape, or sickling, of red blood cells prevents the normal flow of blood.
- Nurses assist families in dealing with chronic diseases such as sickle cell anemia by providing information about the disorder and resources that can provide assistance, monitoring child growth and development, instituting preventive care, and managing exacerbations of the disease.
- Hereditary spherocytosis is an autosomal dominant disorder caused by an abnormality of proteins by an unknown cause. The cells have an unusual characteristic cell structure and become sequestered and hemolyzed in the spleen.
- The thalassemias are a group of genetic diseases of red blood cells, which cause defective synthesis of hemoglobin.
- Aplastic anemia is a deficiency of all blood cells related to poor bone marrow function; it can be congenital or acquired after exposure to certain drugs or harmful environmental toxins.
- Hemophilia is a bleeding disorder transmitted by genes; hemophilia A is most common and results in a decrease in clotting factor VIII.

- The goal of treatment for hemophilia is to control bleeding by preventive care and replacement of the missing factor.
- Major nursing concerns for the child with hemophilia include managing bleeding episodes, controlling pain during bleeds, minimizing physical immobility, supporting the family in learning management of this chronic disease, and explaining genetic implications of the disease.
- Von Willebrand disease is a hereditary bleeding disorder characterized by a deficiency of von Willebrand factor, a plasma protein that is a carrier for clotting factor VIII.
- Disseminated intravascular coagulation is a serious condition in which clotting mechanisms are disturbed, leading to extensive clotting and tissue damage.
- Immune thrombocytopenic purpura causes destruction of platelets and most frequently follows a childhood viral disease.
- Management of immune thrombocytopenic purpura includes corticosteroids and immunoglobulins since the disease is considered to be autoimmune in nature.
- Henoch-Schönlein purpura is a small vessel vasculitis that occurs primarily in the pediatric population.
- Occasionally, infection with organisms such as *Neisseria meningitidis* is followed by a severe systemic disease known as meningococcemia.
- Hematopoietic stem cell transplant (HSCT) is a useful treatment in some diseases of the hematologic system and some cancers; it involves infusion of bone marrow, peripheral stem cells, or neonatal stem cells from a donor into the blood of the recipient where it circulates, implants into the bone marrow, and begins making new blood cells.
- Nursing care before and after HSCT includes infection prevention, careful physical assessment, administration of medications, and support for the family.

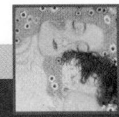

Clinical Reasoning in Action

Recall Michael, the child in the opening scenario who is admitted with sickle cell crisis. Michael is receiving intravenous and oral fluids, oxygen, and opioids via a patient-controlled analgesia (PCA) pump. His hemoglobin on admission was 7.7 g/dL, and hematocrit was 22%. Michael's father has returned to work and he visits in the evenings. Michael's mother remains at the hospital with her son.

1. Considering Michael's age and developmental stage, what communication techniques will the nurse implement when teaching Michael about his disease and treatment?

2. Refer to Chapter 15 ∞ to plan the pain assessment and management techniques that can be used with Michael.

3. What are the expected levels of hemoglobin and hematocrit at Michael's age? Why are his levels abnormal? Describe how sickle cell disease influences blood values.

4. What are the most immediate care needs while Michael is hospitalized? What additional immediate care will he require at home?

See Pearson Nursing Student Resources for possible responses.

Pearson Nursing Student Resources

Find additional review materials at
nursing.pearsonhighered.com
Prepare for success with NCLEX®-style practice questions, interactive assignments and activities, web links, animations and videos, and more!

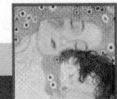

References

Alvarez, O., Rodriguez-Cortes, H., Robinson, N., Lewis, N., Sang, C. D. P., Lopez-Mitnik, G., & Paley, C. (2009). Adherence to deferasirox in children and adolescents with sickle cell disease during 1-year of therapy. *Journal of Pediatric Hematology/Oncology, 31*(10), 739–744.

American Academy of Pediatrics, Committee on Nutrition. (2009). Iron. In *Pediatric nutrition handbook* (6th ed., pp. 403–422). Elk Grove Village, IL: American Academy of Pediatrics.

American Sickle Cell Anemia Association. (2007). *How common is sickle cell anemia?* Retrieved from http://www.ascaa.org/How_Common_Is_Sickle_Cell_Anemia.asp.

Anderson, N. (2006). Hydroxyurea therapy: Improving the lives of patients with sickle cell disease. *Pediatric Nursing, 32*(6), 541–543.

Ault, P., & Jones, K. (2009). Understanding iron overload: Screening, monitoring, and caring for patients with transfusion-dependent anemias. *Clinical Journal of Oncology Nursing, 13*(5), 511–517.

Barillas-Arias, L., Adams, A., & Lehman, T. (2008). Pediatric vasculitic syndromes: Henoch-Schonlein purpura. *Consultant for Pediatricians, 7*(9), 361–367.

Beck, C. E., Nathan, P. C., Parkin, P. C., Blanchette, V. S., & Macarthur, C. (2005). Corticosteroids versus intravenous immune globulin for the treatment of acute immune thrombocytopenic purpura in children: A systematic review and meta-analysis of randomized controlled trials. *Journal of Pediatrics, 147*, 521–527.

Belletrutti, M., Kaiser, A., Barnard, D., Blanchette, V., Chan, A., David, J. M., et al. (2007). Chronic immune thrombocytopenic purpura in children: A survey of the Canadian experience. *Journal of Pediatric Hematology/Oncology, 29*(2), 95–100.

Blanchette, V., & Bolton-Maggs, P. (2008). Childhood immune thrombocytopenic purpura: Diagnosis and management. *Pediatric Clinics of North America, 55*, 393–420.

Borgna-Pignatti, C., & Marsella, M. (2008). Iron deficiency in infancy and childhood. *Pediatric Annals, 37*(5), 329–337.

Boxer, L. A. (2007). Leukopenia. In R. M. Kliegman, R. E. Behrman, H. B. Jenson, & B. F. Stanton (Eds.), *Nelson textbook of pediatrics* (18th ed., pp. 909–915). Philadelphia: Saunders Elsevier.

Brawley, O. W., Cornelius, L. J., Edwards, L. R., Northington, G. V., Green, B. L., Inturrisi, C., et al.

(2008). National Institutes of Health Consensus Development Conference Statement: Hydroxyurea treatment for sickle cell disease. *Annals of Internal Medicine, 148*, 932–938.

Brunstein, C. G., & Wagner, J. E. (2008). Umbilical cord blood transplantation. In R. Hoffman, E. J. Benz, S. J. Shattil, B. Furie, L. E. Silberstein, P. McGlave, & H. Heslop (Eds.), *Hematology: Basic principles and practice* (5th ed., pp. 1643–1664). Philadelphia: Churchill Livingstone-Elsevier.

Buchanan, G. R. (2005). Thrombocytopenia during childhood: What the pediatrician needs to know. *Pediatrics in Review, 26*, 401–409.

Chamley, C., Carson, P., Randall, D., & Sandwell, W. (2005). *Developmental anatomy and physiology of children.* St. Louis, MO: Elsevier.

Chen, M. J., Chang, W. H., Chu, C. H., Wang, T. E., Lin, S. C., & Shih, S. C. (2007). Rapid response of Henoch-Schönlein purpura to corticosteroids: Correlation between skin and gastric mucosal lesions. *Digestive Diseases and Sciences, 52*, 1706–1708.

Corbett, J. V. (2008). *Laboratory tests and diagnostic procedures with nursing diagnoses* (7th ed.). Upper Saddle River, NJ: Pearson Prentice Hall.

Coyer, S. M. (2005). Anemia: Diagnosis and management. *Journal of Pediatric Health Care, 19*(6), 380–385.

De, D. (2008). Acute nursing care and management of patients with sickle cell. *British Journal of Nursing, 17*(13), 818–823.

DeBaun, M. R., & Vichinsky, E. (2007). Hemoglobinopathies. In R. M. Kliegman, R. E. Behrman, H. B. Jenson, & B. F. Stanton (Eds.), *Nelson textbook of pediatrics* (18th ed., pp. 2025–2038). Philadelphia: Saunders Elsevier.

Driscoll, M. C. (2007). Sickle cell disease. *Pediatrics in Review, 28*(7), 259–268.

Foster, M. (2008). FDA approves use of blood product for patients with hemophilia. *Infectious Diseases in Children, 21*(11), 15.

Freedman, M. H. (2007). The pancytopenias. In R. M. Kliegman, R. E. Behrman, H. B. Jenson, & B. F. Stanton (Eds.), *Nelson textbook of pediatrics* (18th ed., pp. 2047–2053). Philadelphia: Saunders Elsevier.

Gallagher, P. G. (2010). The red blood cell membrane and it's disorders: Hereditary spherocytosis, elliptocytosis, and related disorders. In M. A. Lichtman, T. J. Kipps, U. Seligsohn, K. Kaushansky, & J. T. Prchal, *Williams hematology* (8th ed.). Retrieved from http://www.accessmedicine.com

Geil, J. D. (2009). *Von Willebrand disease.* Retrieved from http://emedicine.medscape.com/article/959825-overview

Geller, A. K., & O'Connor, M. K. (2008). The sickle cell crisis: A dilemma in pain relief. *Mayo Clinic Proceedings, 83*(3), 320–323.

Giardina, P. J., & Forget, B. G. (2009). Thalassemia syndromes. In R. Hoffman, E. J. Benz, S. J. Shattil, B. Furie, L. E. Silberstein, P. McGlave, & H. Heslop (Eds.), *Hematology: Basic principles and practice* (5th ed., pp. 535–563). Philadelphia: Churchill Livingstone-Elsevier.

Gladwin, M. T., & Vinchinsky, E. (2008). Pulmonary complications of sickle cell disease. *New England Journal of Medicine, 359*(21), 2254–2265.

Hernandez, S., & Patterson, G. E. (2009, June). What you need to know about acute chest syndrome. *Nursing,* 42–45.

Inati, A., Koussa, S., Taher, A., & Perrine, S. (2008). Sickle cell disease: New insights into pathophysiology and treatment. *Pediatric Annals, 37*(5), 311–321.

Iolascon, A., Piscopo, C., & Boschetto, L. (2008). Red cell membrane disorders in pediatrics. *Pediatric Annals, 37*(5), 295–301.

Jacob, E., Miaskowski, C., Savedra, M., Beyer, J. E., Treadwell, M., & Styles, L. (2006). Changes in sleep, food intake, and activity levels during acute painful episodes in children with sickle cell disease. *Journal of Pediatric Nursing, 21*(1), 23–34.

Jacob, E., Miaskowski, C., Savedra, M., Beyer, J. E., Treadwell, M., & Styles, L. (2007). Quantification of analgesic use in children with sickle cell disease. *Clinical Journal of Pain, 23*(1), 8–14.

King, A., Herron, S., McKinstry, R., Bacak, S., Armstrong, M., White, D., & DeBaun, M. (2006). A multidisciplinary health care team's efforts to improve educational attainment in children with sickle-cell anemia and cerebral infarcts. *Journal of School Health, 76*(1), 33–37.

King, A. A., Tang, S., Ferguson, K. L., & DeBaun, M. R. (2005). An education program to increase teacher knowledge about sickle cell disease. *Journal of School Health, 74,* 11–14.

Kliegman, R. M., Behrman, R. E., Jenson, H. B., & Stanton, B. F. (2007). *Nelson textbook of pediatrics* (18th ed.). Philadelphia: Saunders Elsevier.

Kral, M. C., Brown, R. T., Connelly, M., Cure, J. K., Besenski, N., Jackson, S. M., & Abboud, M. R. (2006). Radiographic predictors of neurocognitive functioning in pediatric sickle cell disease. *Journal of Child Neurology, 21,* 37–44.

LeMone, P., & Burke, K. M. (2008). Nursing care of clients with hematologic disorders. In P. LeMone & K. Burke, *Medical surgical nursing: Critical thinking in client care* (4th ed., pp. 1101–1152). Upper Saddle River, NJ: Prentice Hall.

Linker, C. A. (2008). Hematology. In S. J. McPhee, M. A. Papadakis, & L. M. Tierney, Jr., *Current medical diagnosis and treatment 2008.* McGraw-Hill's Access Medicine.

London, M. L., Ladewig, P. W., Ball, J. W., Bindler, R. C., & Cowen, K. J. (2011). *Maternal & child nursing care* (3rd ed.). Upper Saddle River, NJ: Prentice Hall Health.

Manco-Johnson, M. J., Abshire, T. C., Shapiro, A. D., Riske, B., Hacker, M. R., Kilcoyne, R., et al. (2007). Episodic treatment to prevent joint disease in boys with severe hemophilia. *New England Journal of Medicine, 357*(6), 535–544.

Manno, C. S., & Larson, P. J. (2009). Transfusion therapy for coagulation factor deficiencies. In R. Hoffman, E. J. Benz, S. J. Shattil, B. Furie, L. E. Silberstein, P. McGlave, & H. Heslop (Eds.), *Hematology: Basic principles and practice* (5th ed., pp. 2247–2256). Philadelphia: Churchill Livingstone-Elsevier.

March of Dimes. (2008). *Sickle cell disease.* Retrieved from http://www.marchofdimes.com/professionals/14332_1221.asp

Mathews, V., George, B., Deotare, U., Laksbmi, K. M., Viswabandya, A., Daniel, D., et al. (2007). A new stratification strategy that identifies a subset of class III patients with an adverse prognosis among children with β-thalassemia major undergoing a matched related allogeneic stem cell transplantation. *Biology of Blood and Marrow Transplantation, 12,* 889–894.

Mehta, S. R., Afenyi-Annan, A., Byrns, P. F., & Lottenberg, R. (2006). Opportunities to improve outcomes in sickle cell disease. *American Family Physician, 74*(2), 303–310.

Milonovich, L. M. (2007). Meningococcemia: Epidemiology, pathophysiology, and management. *Journal of Pediatric Health Care, 21*(2), 75–80.

Mirre, E., Brousse, V., Berteloot, L., Lambot-Juhan, K., Verlhac, S., Boulat, C., . . . De Montalembert, M. (2010). Feasibility and efficacy of chronic transfusion for stroke prevention in children with sickle cell disease. *European Journal of Haematology, 84* (3) 259–265.

Moore, T. (2005). *Bone marrow transplantation.* Retrieved from http://www.emedicine.com/ped/topic2909.htm

Ohls, R. K., & Christensen, R. D. (2007). Development of the hematopoietic system. In R. M. Kliegman, R. E. Behrman, H. B. Jenson, & B. F. Stanton (Eds.), *Nelson textbook of pediatrics* (18th ed., pp. 1997–2003). Philadelphia: Saunders Elsevier.

Oren, H., Cingoz, I., Duman, M., Yilmaz, S., & Irken, G. (2005). Disseminated intravascular coagulation in pediatric patients. *Pediatric Hematology and Oncology, 22,* 679–688.

Panepinto, J. A., & Brousseau, D. C. (2005). Acute idiopathic thrombocytopenic purpura of childhood—diagnosis and therapy. *Pediatric Emergency Care, 21,* 691–695.

Petersdorf, E. W., & Anasetti, C. (2008). Unrelated donor hematopoietic cell transplantation. In R. Hoffman, E. J. Benz, S. J. Shattil, B. Furie, L. E. Silberstein, P. McGlave, & H. Heslop (Eds.), *Hematology: Basic principles and practice* (5th ed., pp. 1619–1631). Philadelphia: Churchill Livingstone-Elsevier.

Piga, A., Galanello, R., Forni, G. L., Cappellini, M. D., Origa, R., Zappu, A., . . . Alberti, D. (2006). Randomized phase II trial of deferasirox (Exjade, ICL670), a once-daily, orally-administered iron chelator, in comparison to deferoxamine in thalassemia patients with transfusional iron overload. *Haematologica, 91,* 873–880.

Platt, A. F., & Eckman, J. (2006, February). Relieving the symptoms of sickle cell disease. *Clinical Advisor, 54,* 59–62, 67.

Richardson, M. (2007). Microcytic anemia. *Pediatrics in Review, 28*(1), 5–14.

Roberts, P. F., Waller, T. A., Brinker, T. M., Riffe, I., Sayre, J. W., & Bratton, R. L. (2007). Henoch-Schönlein purpura: A review article. *Southern Medical Journal, 100*(8), 821–824.

Robertson, J., Lillicrap, D., & James, P. D. (2008). von Willebrand disease. *Pediatric Clinics of North America, 55,* 377–392.

Rodriguez, N. I., & Hoots, W. K. (2008). Advances in hemophilia: Experimental aspects and therapy. *Pediatric Clinics of North America, 55,* 357–376.

Rowley, S. D., & Donato, M. L. (2008). Practical aspects of stem cell collection. In R. Hoffman, E. J. Benz, S. J. Shattil, B. Furie, L. E. Silberstein, P. McGlave, & H. Heslop (Eds.), *Hematology: Basic principles and practice* (5th ed., pp. 1695–1712). Philadelphia: Churchill Livingstone-Elsevier.

Saulsbury, F. T. (2007). Clinical update: Henoch-Schönlein purpura. *Lancet, 369,* 976–978.

Saunthararajah, Y., & Vichinsky, E. P. (2009). Sickle cell disease: Clinical features and management. In R. Hoffman, E. J. Benz, S. J. Shattil, B. Furie, L. E. Silberstein, P. McGlave, & H. Heslop (Eds.), *Hematology: Basic principles and practice* (5th ed., pp. 577–601). Philadelphia: Churchill Livingstone-Elsevier.

Scott, J. P., & Montgomery, R. R. (2007). Hemorrhagic and thrombotic diseases. In R. M. Kliegman, R. E. Behrman, H. B. Jenson, & B. F. Stanton (Eds.), *Nelson textbook of pediatrics* (18th ed., pp. 2060–2089). Philadelphia: Elsevier Saunders.

Servey, J. T., Reamy, B. V., & Hodge, J. (2007). Clinical presentations of parvovirus, B19 infection. *American Family Physician, 75*(3), 373–376.

Sibinga, E. M. S., Shindell, D. L., Casella, J. F., Duggan, A. K., & Wilson, M. H. (2006). Pediatric patients with sickle cell disease: Use of complementary and alternative therapies. *Journal of Alternative and Complementary Medicine, 12*(3), 291–298.

Siegel, J. E. (2009). *Factor XI deficiency.* Retrieved from http://emedicine.medscape.com/article/209984-overview

Soldin, S. J., Brugnara, C., & Wong, E. C. (2007). *Pediatric reference ranges* (6th ed.). Washington, DC: AACC Press.

Son, D. W., Jeon, I., Yang, S. W., & Cho, S. H. (2008). A single dose of anti-D immunoglobulin raises platelet count as efficiently as intravenous immunoglobulin in newly diagnosed immune thrombocytopenic purpura in Korean children. *Journal of Pediatric Hematology/Oncology, 30*(8), 598–601.

Thompson, C. A. (2008). Additional antihemophilic factor to be available. *American Journal of Health-System Pharmacy, 65,* 592.

Tracy, E. T., & Rice, H. E. (2008). Partial splenectomy for hereditary spherocytosis. *Pediatric Clinics of North America, 55*(2), 503–519.

Wang, W. (2007). Central nervous system complications of sickle cell disease in children: An overview. *Child Neuropsychology, 13,* 103–119.

Warrington, K. H., & Herzog, R. W. (2006). Treatment of human disease by adeno-associated viral gene transfer. *Human Genetics, 119,* 571–603.

Woods, C. R. (2007). Neisseria meningitidis. In R. M. Kliegman, R. E. Behrman, H. B. Jenson, & B. F. Stanton (Eds.), *Nelson textbook of pediatrics* (18th ed., pp. 1164–1169). Philadelphia: Saunders Elsevier.

Woolley, S. (2006). Children of Jehovah's Witnesses and adolescent Jehovah's Witnesses: What are their rights? *Archives of Disease in Children, 90,* 715–719.

Yanni, E., Grosse, S. D., Yang, Q., & Olney, R. S. (2009). Trends in pediatric sickle cell disease-related mortality in the United States, 1983–2002. *Journal of Pediatrics, 154*(4), 541–545.

Yesilipek, M. A. (2007). Stem cell transplantation in hemoglobinopathies. *Hemoglobin, 31*(2), 251–256.

Young, N. S., Calado, R. T., & Scheinberg, P. (2006). Current concepts in pathophysiology and treatment of aplastic anemia. *Blood, 108*(8), 2509–2519.

The Child with Cancer   chapter 24

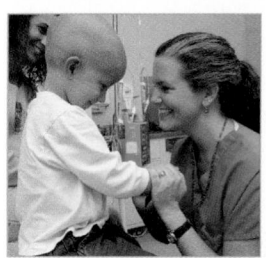

Sam, a 4-year-old, had several bruises on his legs that puzzled his parents since he had not been engaged in any activities that would have caused them. He also appeared to be lethargic compared to his usual energetic self. Suspecting an influenza after he also began to manifest a respiratory infection, Sam's parents brought him to the pediatric office. The physician's assessment showed hepatosplenomegaly, so a complete blood count was obtained. Low amounts of red blood cells and platelets were seen with high levels of white blood cells. The physician suspected leukemia and referred Sam to the oncology center that afternoon. Sam's mother was devastated; she had never suspected this diagnosis.

The next few days were a blur of making phones calls, arranging care for two older children, and then staying with Sam during his lumbar puncture, bone marrow aspiration, several body scans, and placement of a central line. Sam remained in the hospital for induction therapy and then went home. He is now returning for his next series of consolidation therapy treatments at the oncology clinic. The nurse who planned care in the immediate diagnostic period prepared him appropriately for every procedure, and now sees Sam at each visit. Although Sam has remained well, the nurse provided information for his parents about common side effects of chemotherapy drugs and the treatment regimen. She offered information about nutritional intake and answered his mother's questions at each visit. What support will Sam's two older siblings need to understand his condition and feel that they are part of his care? How can the nurse identify the family's resources, such as psychosocial support, and their greatest needs?

Key Terms

apoptosis / 707
benign / 707
biotherapy / 713
cachexia / 711
carcinogens / 709
chemotherapy / 713
complementary therapies / 715
debulk / 713
extravasation / 726
leukocytosis / 737
leukopenia / 737
malignant / 707
metastasis / 707
myelosuppression / 727
neoplasms / 707
neutropenia / 727
oncogene / 710
pancytopenia / 737
phantom pain / 741
polypharmacy / 727
protocol / 713
proto-oncogene / 710
radiation / 713
secondary cancer / 720
staging / 712
thrombocytopenia / 718
tumor suppressor gene / 710

Learning Outcomes

After reading this chapter, you will be able to do the following:

1. Differentiate between characteristics of cancer in adulthood and childhood.
2. Describe the incidence, known etiologies, and common clinical manifestations of childhood cancer.
3. Synthesize information about diagnostic tests and clinical therapy for cancer to plan comprehensive care for children undergoing these procedures.
4. Integrate the pathophysiology of oncologic emergencies into plans for monitoring all children with cancer.
5. Recognize the most common solid tumors in children, describe their treatment, and plan comprehensive nursing care.
6. Plan care for children and adolescents of all ages who have a diagnosis of leukemia.
7. Recognize the most common soft-tissue tumors in children, describe their treatment, and plan comprehensive care.
8. Describe the impact of cancer survival on children and use this information to plan for ongoing physiological and psychosocial care.

Cellular Growth

ANATOMY AND PHYSIOLOGY

Abnormal cellular growth can occur in any area of the body. Why are some growths called cancer and others are not? Changes in cellular growth within the body are called **neoplasms** (meaning new growth). A neoplasm is further classified as benign or malignant. **Benign** means that a growth does not endanger life or health; it tends not to recur after treatment. **Malignant** means that progressive growth of the tumor will, if not checked by treatment, spread to other sites in the body (**metastasis**), resulting in death. The common term for this type of cellular growth is *cancer*.

PEDIATRIC DIFFERENCES

Cancers in children often have different etiology than those in adults. Most adult cancers are epithelial in origin, whereas in children the nonepithelial or embryonal cell types predominate (Twombly, 2007). While many adult cancers are slow-growing and result from exposure to carcinogens over time, most childhood cancers are fast-growing, so that a child who appears healthy becomes ill over a period of days or weeks. Different types of cancers predominate at various ages in childhood, demonstrating the multiple causes and their relationship to age and development (Figure 24–1 ➤). Occasionally, an environmental exposure is linked to the incidence of cancer in children.

Although not common, some neonates have cancer that is diagnosed soon after birth. The types of cancers most common in this age group include brain tumors, neuroblastoma, leukemia, retinoblastoma, and teratomas (arising from primary germ layers). While treatments are usually as effective in neonates as in older children, rapid growth at this age makes side effects of therapy more serious.

A major physiologic difference between adults and children that affects cellular growth involves the immune system, which plays a part in preventing some cancers but functions immaturely in the young child (see the following text for further description of immune immaturity). The rate of cell growth in children can also play a role in the rapidity with which some childhood cancers progress. The continuing presence of fetal cells in small children is related to some cancers. These immature cells decrease and finally disappear as children grow, but can be related to cancers such as neuroblastoma in very young children.

The immune system defends the body against foreign organisms and substances through two responses: nonspecific and specific. In a nonspecific response, the components of the immune system attack a variety of targets. Nonspecific components include phagocytic (cell destroying) cells such as mononuclear leukocytes, polymorphonuclear (PMN) leukocytes, natural killer (NK) cells, and complements (noncellular proteins) that work together to destroy invading cells and substances. During the first month of a child's life, the nonspecific response is immature, so phagocytic cells have little ability to move toward cancer cells and fulfill their function. The nonspecific response is also impaired in premature and small-for-gestational-age (SGA) infants.

In a specific response, T lymphocytes and immunoglobulin (Ig) attack only one type of invader. The specific response capability also is immature in infants. B-cell production of various proteins called immunoglobulins (IgM, IgG, and IgA) is below adult levels, so that the infant is vulnerable to bacterial and viral infections. (For a discussion of immune function, see Chapter 22 ∞.)

In children, many cells are growing quickly; this fast growth can lead to the proliferation of both cancerous and normal cells. Cell division that is out of control may normally trigger a mechanism called **apoptosis**, whereby the cell "realizes" something is wrong and destroys itself. The process of apoptosis or physiologic cell death limits the growth of cancerous cells but may not be well developed in young children.

Examples of diagnostic and laboratory tests used to evaluate cancer are provided in Table 24–1; see Appendices D and E ∞ for further information about these diagnostic procedures and tests common in cancer care.

Use the Assessment Guidelines on page 709 to identify and monitor alterations in cellular growth.

As Children Grow

Types of Cancer by Age Group

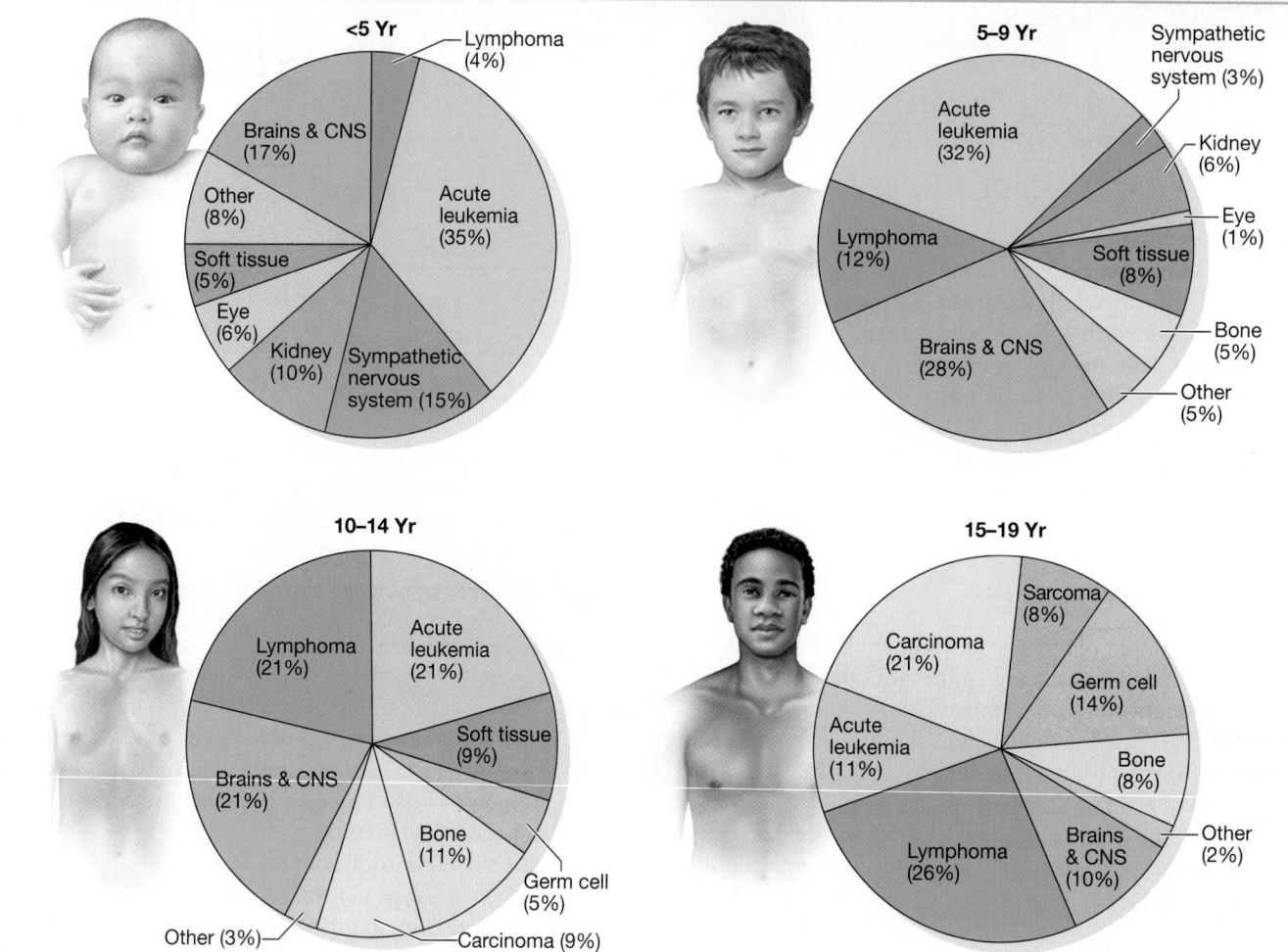

FIGURE 24–1 ➤ Percentage of primary cancers by site of origin for different age groups.

Data from: Kadan-Lottick, N. S. (2007). Epidemiology of childhood and adolescent cancer. In R. M. Kliegman, R. E. Behrman, H. B. Jensen, & B.F. Stanton (Eds.), Nelson textbook of pediatrics (18th ed., p. 2098). Philadelphia: Saunders.

TABLE 24–1 Diagnostic Procedures and Laboratory Tests for Cancer

Diagnostic Procedures	Laboratory Tests
Biopsy	Complete blood count (CBC) with differential
Bone marrow aspiration and biopsy	Red and white blood cell indices
Computed tomography (CT) and computerized axial tomography (CAT)	Serum chemistry panel
Lumbar puncture	Tumor markers
Magnetic resonance imaging (MRI) Positron emission tomography (PET) scan and single-photon emission computed tomography (SPECT)	Urinalysis
Radiograph (X-ray)	
Nuclear medicine scans	
Ultrasound	

Assessment Guidelines for the Child with an Alteration in Cellular Growth

Assessment Focus	Assessment Guidelines
Growth and development parameters	▪ Assess the child's weight and height and plot on growth grids; be alert for weight loss. ▪ Inquire about nutritional intake and any recent changes in appetite. ▪ Perform developmental assessment and be alert for slow progress or regression. ▪ Ask about school performance for children enrolled in school; include this information in every assessment of children who were treated for cancer in the past.
Pain	▪ Pain is abnormal if there is no known acute injury or chronic condition; assess any pain for length, duration, and type. ▪ Does the child exhibit limping, headache, decreased activity level, or other symptoms indicative of pain?
Skin	▪ Is there bruising and other signs of bleeding on the skin? ▪ Is there pallor and other signs of anemia? ▪ Describe skin lesions.
Eyes, ears, nose, and throat (EENT) and sensory	▪ Inspect the symmetry and general condition of the eyes, ears, mouth, throat, head, and neck. ▪ Inspect eye movements, corneal light reflex, and red reflex. ▪ Evaluate hearing and vision and note any recent changes.
Chest, heart, and respiratory system	▪ Inspect the shape of the chest, respiratory rate, and ease of respirations. ▪ Auscultate heart and lungs. ▪ Ask about endurance and activity levels.
Abdomen	▪ Be alert for abdominal masses. Stop palpation immediately if any are noted and inform the physician. ▪ Is there repeated vomiting, anorexia, or weight loss?
Urinary and gastrointestinal systems	▪ Evaluate frequency of urination and feces. ▪ Assess for intake and evidence of vomiting or food intolerance. ▪ Ask about blood or other discoloration in urine or stool. ▪ Be alert for urinary tract infections.
Musculoskeletal system	▪ Observe for expected developmental tasks. ▪ Is there asymmetry of bone or muscle? ▪ Does the child limp or have other abnormalities of gait?

▪ CHILDHOOD CANCER

The care of children who have cancer is a challenging specialty in pediatric nursing. Cancer treatments may last for several years; they have improved the prognosis in many cases, but in some, the prognosis still requires that the family deal with a life-threatening illness (see Chapter 13 ∞). The child is cared for at home with outpatient visits for treatments and occasional hospitalizations when needed. The periods of hospitalization are times of intense physical vulnerability for the child and intense emotional vulnerability for both the child and the family. To monitor the child closely, nurses need a sound knowledge of physiologic and psychologic responses, medical interventions, and nursing care. Effective communication skills are also necessary to support the child and family and promote realistic hope.

During 2006, cancer was diagnosed in the United States in approximately 12,500 children under 20 years of age; 9,500 of these children were 14 years or younger. In children under 15 years of age, cancer is the leading cause of disease-related death, and the fourth leading cause of overall death (Pollack, Stewart, Thompson, et al., 2007). In 2006, about 1,560 U.S. children died of cancer. One third of the deaths were from leukemia (American Cancer Society, 2006). However, mortality rates have declined by about 48% since 1975, and the rates continue to improve. The overall survival rate is 80% for childhood. Survival rates vary for different types of cancer, ranging from 66% for neuroblastoma to 95% for Hodgkin disease (American Cancer Society, 2006; Pollack et al., 2007).

Etiology and Pathophysiology

Alterations in cellular growth occur in response to external and internal stimuli. Neoplasms are caused by one or a combination of three factors: (1) external stimuli that cause genetic mutations, (2) immune system and gene abnormalities, and (3) chromosomal abnormalities.

External Stimuli

External stimuli may affect the child's general health and cause mutations in body cells. **Carcinogens** are chemicals or industrial processes that, when combined with genetic traits and in interaction with one another, result in cancer. Several carcinogens cause cancers that are diagnosed during childhood. Others cause cancers that begin in childhood but are not identified until adulthood. Chemicals suspected of causing childhood cancer include diethylstilbestrol or DES (maternal use of therapeutic estrogen hormones), anabolic androgenic steroids, alkylating chemotherapy agents, and immunosuppressants used for organ transplantation. Radiation exposure has been known to cause cancers such as leukemia and thyroid tumors in children exposed to nuclear fallout from atomic bombs, other nuclear accidents, and other excessive radiation sources.

External stimuli may also lead to secondary cancers in children, or those occurring after treatment for a primary cancer and of a different cellular type than the primary cancer. Secondary cancers can result when the child is treated for a primary cancer with high doses of radiation. Excessive exposure to ultraviolet radiation from the sun predisposes children to development of skin cancer in adolescence and adulthood (see Chapter 31 ∞). See Families Want to Know: Cancer Prevention.

Immune System and Gene Abnormalities

One critical function of a normal immune system is immune surveillance, in which phagocytic cells circulate throughout the body, detecting and destroying abnormal and cancerous cells. Children with congenital immune deficiencies, such as Wiskott-Aldrich syndrome, in which immune surveillance may fail are at high risk for cancer. A form of non-Hodgkin lymphoma develops in some children treated with drugs that suppress the immune system. Children with acquired immunodeficiency syndrome (AIDS) may be at higher risk of certain types of cancer, such as Hodgkin disease, non-Hodgkin lymphoma, leiomyosarcoma, and Kaposi sarcoma (Stanescu, Foarfa, Georgescu, et al., 2007).

Viruses and other substances may act in the body to alter the immune system, thereby allowing cancer to occur (Figure 24–2 ➤). Their action is based on changing certain genes that normally regulate cellular growth and development (called **proto-oncogenes**) to related genes that allow unregulated cell division and cancerous growth (called **oncogenes**). Among cancers thought to be linked to virus action and the change of proto-oncogenes to oncogenes are certain leukemias, rhabdomyosarcoma, Burkitt lymphoma, and some forms of Hodgkin disease.

Pathophysiology Illustrated
Proto-oncogene Alteration

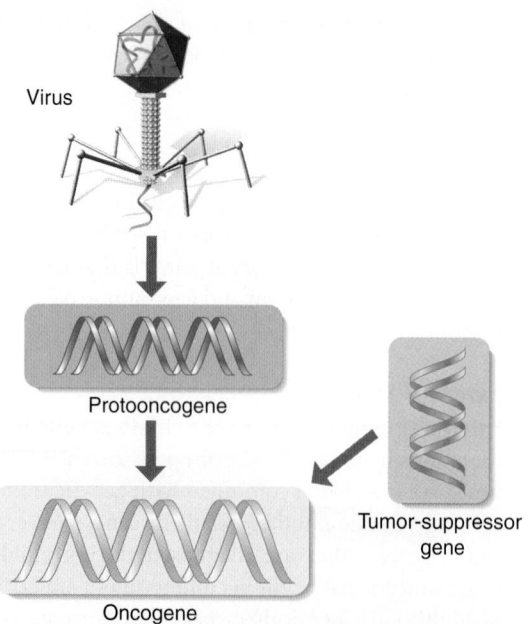

Virus

Protooncogene

Tumor-suppressor gene

Oncogene

FIGURE 24–2 ➤ A proto-oncogene normally regulates cellular growth and development. When altered by a virus or other external cause, it can change to an oncogene, which allows unregulated genetic activity and tumor growth. Tumor-suppressor genes regulate the effects of oncogenes to decrease wildly proliferating cellular growth.

Genetic changes (mutations) can include autosomal dominant, autosomal recessive, and X-linked transfer. Cancers of these types typically occur early in life and are aggressive. There is increasing ability to perform genetic testing for certain familial cancers. Examples of cancers that are sometimes caused by genetic abnormalities within families include retinoblastoma (described later in this chapter); Wilms tumor (described in this chapter); multiple endocrine neoplasia, type 2 (thyroid cancer); and familial adenomatous polyposis (invasive colon cancer). Not all cases of these cancers are familial, but their incidence suggests the need for careful history taking to identify any other cases in the family.

Tumor suppressor genes counteract the effect of oncogenes, keeping cellular growth within normal limits. When tumor suppressor genes are missing, unstemmed cellular growth can occur. These genes are commonly missing in children with retinoblastoma and Wilms tumor.

Chromosomal Abnormalities

Normal chromosomes undergo change as a part of the genetic process. Although most of the changes are not harmful, some changes result in chromosomal abnormalities such as hyperploidy (a greater-than-normal number of chromosomes), deletion, translocation, and breakage.

Some of these chromosomal abnormalities have been linked to an increased incidence of cancer. Children with Down syndrome have a relative risk 20–30 times higher for developing leukemia than nonaffected children. Acute myeloid and lymphoblastic leukemia are more common in children with Down syndrome (Zwaan, Reinhardt, Hitzler, et al., 2010). Children who are missing a band of genetic material on chromosome 13 often have retinoblastoma. Similarly, a Wilms tumor often develops in children missing part of the genetic material from chromosome 11. Regardless of the location and cause of abnormal cellular growth, the pathophysiologic process of cancer is similar. The altered cell begins to multiply as directed by the altered genetic structure of its DNA and the absence or inactivation of tumor suppressor genes. Each new cell transmits the new or altered pattern to the next generation. As the abnormal cells replicate, they form a growing neoplastic mass. Normal cells usually die as the increased metabolic rate of the neoplastic cells depletes available nutrition. The altered DNA in the tumor cells may also cause the abnormal cells to invade adjoining tissue. Through continued growth, the mass invades, disrupting a major vessel or a vital organ.

Families Want to Know
Cancer Prevention

Many parents ask what they can do to decrease the incidence of cancer in children as they grow into adulthood. Five major teaching areas to address are as follows:

1. Have children increase their intake of fruits, vegetables, and whole grains. Aim for five or more servings of fruits and vegetables daily. Most children do not eat enough of these foods, and higher intake throughout life is associated with lower rates of several cancers in adulthood.
2. Protect skin with sunscreen. Early excessive exposure to sun and having one or more sunburns during childhood increase chances of skin cancers developing in adulthood.
3. Discourage smoking among children and be sure children are not exposed to environmental tobacco smoke. This will decrease future chances of developing lung cancer.
4. Have homes tested for radon. Be alert for exposure to any potential hazardous substances in the home or on parents' clothing if they work in industries with chemicals or other harmful substances.
5. When there is a history of cancer in the family, particularly if a type associated with familial incidence such as some breast and ovarian cancers, encourage the family to learn more about the cancer and teach the child or adolescent about recommendations for regular surveillance.

Clinical Manifestations

Each type of childhood cancer signals its presence differently. Because many of the presenting signs and symptoms of cancer are typical of common childhood illnesses, a delay in diagnosis can occur. In some cases, no symptoms are noted until the cancer is advanced. Children commonly present with presence of cancer in a site other than its origin at the time of diagnosis. Some of the common presenting symptoms of cancer follow:

- *Pain* may be the result of a neoplasm either directly or indirectly affecting nerve receptors through obstruction, inflammation, tissue damage, stretching of visceral tissue, or invasion of susceptible tissue. The pain may be in any body part, such as abdominal pain, bone and joint discomfort, or headache.
- ***Cachexia*** is a syndrome characterized by anorexia, weight loss, anemia, asthenia (weakness), and early satiety (feeling of being full).
- *Anemia* may be experienced during times of chronic bleeding or iron deficiency. In chronic illness the body uses iron poorly. Anemia is also present in cancers of the bone marrow when the number of red blood cells (RBCs) is reduced, in part because of the presence of large numbers of other bone marrow products. Treatment of cancer often promotes further anemia.
- *Infection* is usually a result of an altered or immature immune system. In addition, infection occurs when bone marrow cancers inhibit maturation of normal immune system cells. Infection may also occur in children who are treated with corticosteroids. Because their immune response is altered, the normal signs of infection may not appear.

- *Bruising* or ecchymosis can occur if the bone marrow cannot produce enough platelets. Prolonged bleeding also occurs after minor trauma.
- *Neurologic symptoms* may result from impingement on the brain or nervous system. Signs of increased intracranial pressure, decreased or altered consciousness, eye abnormalities, or other neurologic or behavioral changes may be evident.
- *Palpable mass* may be present for certain cancers. This is most commonly abdominal but may be mediastinal, or in the neck or other sites.

A variety of other symptoms can occur depending on the location of the cancer. Subcutaneous nodules may appear if leukocytosis is present. Superior vena cava syndrome (obstruction of the superior vena cava by a mass and leading to increased venous pressure and involvement of the lungs and other mediastinal structures) or respiratory difficulty can occur with mediastinal tumors (such as neuroblastoma) (Cheng, 2009), and enlarged lymph nodes are common with lymphomas.

COLLABORATIVE CARE

Diagnostic Tests

The most common diagnostic tests performed on children with cancer are complete blood count with differential, bone marrow aspiration, bone marrow biopsy, lumbar puncture, radiographic examination, magnetic resonance imaging (MRI), computed tomography (CT), ultrasound, and biopsy of tumors (Figure 24–3 ➤). See Table 24–1 for diagnostic procedures and laboratory tests commonly used in cancer and Table 24–2 for normal values.

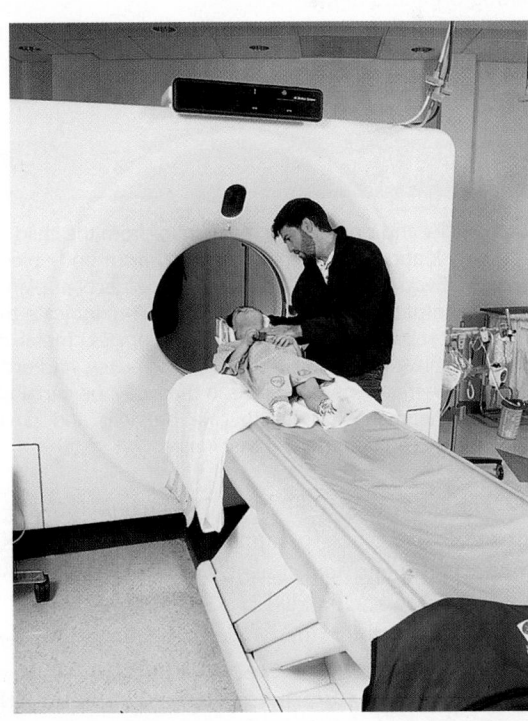

FIGURE 24–3 ➤ Computed tomography (CT) can be a frightening procedure for children. This 2-year-old boy is comforted by his father before the procedure.

TABLE 24–2 Selected Diagnostic Test Results for Childhood Cancer

Test	Purpose	Normal Laboratory Values	Diagnostic Values
Bone marrow aspiration	Examines bone marrow	Less than 5% blast cells (immature)	Greater than 25% blast cells in acute lymphoblastic leukemia, most with hypercellular marrow
Lumbar puncture	Examines cerebrospinal fluid	Cell count (microLiters) Polymorphonuclear leukocytes 0 Monocytes 0–5 RBCs 0–5	Presence of malignant cells indicates central nervous system (CNS) involvement
Complete blood count and differential	Examines cellular components of blood	WBCs less than 10,000/microLiter Platelets 150,000–400,000/microLiter Hemoglobin 12–16 g/dL	WBCs greater than 10,000/microLiter Platelets 20,000–100,000/microLiter Hemoglobin 7–10 g/dL
Absolute neutrophil count (ANC)	Blood component ratio: % of segmental neutrophils plus % of bands (immature neutrophils) times WBC count	ANC greater than 1000	ANC less than 500 indicates risk of infection

Additional studies diagnostic for certain cancers are nuclear medicine scans with radioactive isotopes such as gallium or iodine, bone scan with technetium 99m, or positron emission tomography (PET) and single-photon emission computed tomography (SPECT) that combine nuclear medicine with CT (Yang, Kim, & Inoue, 2006). Specific tests such as pulmonary function tests and echocardiograms may be used to determine if the lungs or heart may be affected by the cancer. Detailed blood analysis is also performed and includes:

- Red blood cells (RBCs), white blood cells (WBCs), and platelets.
- Hemoglobin and hematocrit.
- RBC indices (e.g., mean corpuscular volume [MCV], mean corpuscular hemoglobin concentration [MCHC], and mean corpuscular hemoglobin [MCH]).

Nursing Alert

Remove all jewelry and clothes with metal snaps from the child before an MRI scan. Ask about and remove all metal from body piercings; they may not always be visible. Some metallic objects implanted in the body are compatible with MRI but others contraindicate the use of MRI. Metallic objects include orthodontic braces, metal dental bridgework, cochlear implants, surgical clips or plates, and orthopedic rods. When there are metal objects in the body, be certain to report them to the managing health care provider and radiology technician so they can determine if MRI is safe.

- WBC indices (manual differential) which include the percent of all five types (basophils, eosinophils, monocytes, lymphocytes, neutrophils; neutrophils are further divided into segmented and banded).
- Absolute neutrophil count (ANC), which uses both the segmented (mature) neutrophils and bands (immature neutrophils) as a measure of the body's infection-fighting capability; calculated by adding percentage of segmented neutrophils to percentage of bands, and then multiplying this percentage by the WBC count.

- Serum chemistry, which includes electrolytes, including sodium, potassium, chloride, calcium, magnesium, phosphorus, and carbon dioxide.
- Additional studies that provide important diagnostic clues in some cases; for example, renal function studies such as blood urea nitrogen (BUN) and creatinine; liver studies such as total bilirubin, alanine aminotransferase (ALT), aspirate aminotransferase (AST), and lactic dehydrogenase (LDH); alkaline phosphatase may be elevated; uric acid is commonly elevated in leukemia.
- Certain substances, or markers, that are elevated with some specific tumors; for example, α-fetoprotein may be elevated in liver tumors, vanillylmandelic acid (VMA) and homovanillic acid (HVA) may be elevated in adrenal tumors, and elevated catecholamines are found in neuroblastoma.

Urinalysis is performed, as the presence of abnormal cells such as RBCs (hematuria) may assist in diagnosis of some kidney tumors. Histological or laboratory analysis of tumor cells is often critical in diagnosis. A needle biopsy or endoscopic procedures of some tumors can be performed to obtain tumor cells. If the tumor is removed during surgery, the entire tumor is available for study. The borders are examined to be certain it has been totally removed, and lymph nodes may also be removed to analyze possible spread via the lymph system.

Tests are aimed at identifying the source of the cancer and any metastases to additional sites. This enables the oncology specialist to stage the cancer. **Staging** refers to the process of labeling the type, severity, and spread of cancer cells, which will determine the recommended treatment. Stage number 1 indicates less severe cancer without spread to other parts of the body, while higher numbers indicate both greater severity and spread to other sites.

Clinical Therapy

Clinical therapy for cancer is extremely complex and is managed by a specialist in pediatric oncology. The cancer itself is treated, its effects on the body must be addressed, and the side effects of treatment also require management. All children and adolescents suspected of having cancer should be referred to a pediatric cancer center and have their care coordinated by that center.

Cancer is treated with one or a combination of therapies: surgery, chemotherapy, radiation, biotherapy, and bone marrow or hematopoietic stem cell transplantation. Some families also choose to use complementary therapy, in addition to traditional medical approaches. The treatment plan is determined by the type of cancer, the site of primary tumor, and the degree and sites of metastasis (spread to other sites in the body).

The goal of treatment may be curative, supportive, or provision of end-of-life care. Curative treatment rids the child's body of the cancer. Supportive treatment includes transfusions, pain management, antibiotics, and other interventions to assist the body's defenses and increase the child's comfort. End-of-life treatment is designed to make the child as comfortable as possible when no curative treatment is possible (see Chapter 13 ∞ for a detailed discussion of end-of-life care for children). Whatever combination of treatment is used, families have many questions and need resources for information.

Surgery   Surgery is used to remove or **debulk** (reduce the size of) a solid tumor. An example of a cancer that is commonly treated with surgery is a Wilms tumor. Surgery is also used to determine the stage and type of cancer since the tumor cells can be examined microscopically once removed, and various body organs can be inspected for signs of cancer during the surgery.

Chemotherapy   Chemotherapy is the administration of specific drugs that kill both normal and cancerous cells. The administration of various chemotherapeutic drugs is timed to achieve the greatest cellular destruction. The schedule is determined by the cell's cycle of replication (Figure 24–4 ➤). Several chemotherapeutic drugs are administered simultaneously to maximize their lethal impact on cells at all stages of activity. See Medications Used to Treat Cancer Through Chemotherapy on pages 716–717.

Whereas DNA in a normal cell can repair itself after chemotherapy, the DNA in a neoplastic cell cannot. The particular chemotherapy treatment protocol used is based on research into different types of cancer cells. A **protocol** is a plan of action for chemotherapy that is based on the type of cancer, its stage, and the particular cell type (Figure 24–5 ➤).

Other drugs used in the treatment of children with cancer include colony-stimulating factors, antiemetics, and nutritional supplements. Colony-stimulating factors are hormone-like glycoproteins that enhance blood cell production and counteract the myelosuppressive effects of chemotherapy drugs (see Medications Used to Treat Cancer: Colony-Stimulating Factors on page 718). For example, erythropoietin is produced in the kidney, and a recombinant form (epoetin) is available which can be used to treat anemia of cancer, thereby decreasing the number of transfusions needed. Filgrastim (Neupogen) increases production of neutrophils by the bone marrow. Antiemetics, such as ondansetron (Zofran), are used to treat the nausea and vomiting that are common side effects of therapy. Nutritional supplements can be given to maintain nutritional status. Some children need periodic treatment with antibiotics or antiviral drugs to treat infections that occur as a result of decreased immune response.

Radiation   Radiation therapy involves the use of unstable isotopes that release varying levels of energy to cause breaks in the DNA molecule and thereby destroy cells. Radiation has been used as a treatment method since shortly after its discovery in the early 1900s. It is often used for the local and regional control of cancer, and in combination with surgery and chemotherapy. Long-term side effects of radiation in children include stunted bone growth, learning difficulties, and behavioral changes (American Cancer Society, 2009b).

The area to be irradiated (treatment field) includes the tumor site and sometimes other involved areas, such as lymph glands. The goal is to irradiate the tumor but not irradiate healthy adjacent tissue. The total dose of radiation is divided (or fractionated) and given over several weeks. A common course of radiation treatment might be once daily 4 or 5 days per week for a period of 2 to 7 weeks. Examples of cancers treated with radiation include Hodgkin disease, Wilms tumor, retinoblastoma, rhabdomyosarcoma, and central nervous system (CNS) disease in leukemia.

Nursing Alert

Nurses who care for a child receiving implant radiation or who work in a radiation department must wear a dosimeter film badge at all times. The cumulative radiation exposure is thus measured. The nurse must avoid radiation exposure for a period of time if recommended levels are exceeded.

Biotherapy   Biotherapy is the use of biologic retooling and molecular intervention to produce targeted cancer therapy. Biologic retooling uses parts of the human body that are programmed to destroy cells, and applies them to the cancer cells. An example of this technique includes development of antibodies that are tumor-specific to certain cancers and are produced by the body in response to antigens of cancer cells (Hantel, Lewrick, Schneider, et al., 2010). These antibodies promote apoptosis or death of the cancerous cells. Another example is the group of drugs that stimulate the body's own immune response (Fry & Lankester, 2008). The actions of many of these agents are not completely understood, and some agents have more than one effect. For example, interferon has both antiviral and antiproliferative effects on some malignant cells. Interferon and tumor necrosis factor (TNF) are undergoing clinical trials to study their effectiveness and to develop protocols for their safe use against selected cancers. Cancer vaccines are under development that may work to help the body fight cancers; already available is human papillomavirus vaccine (see Chapter 16 ∞).

Molecular targeting involves interference with metabolic pathways (for example, through enzyme disruption) in the tumor cells. It may therefore disturb the cell's growth and development and thereby depress proliferation. For example, the signaling system in cancer cells that leads to proliferation is triggered by kinases, a specific type of enzyme that leads to transfer of phosphates among molecules. Drug therapy can interfere with the action of specific kinases, leading to cancer cell proliferation arrest (Faivre, Djelloul, & Raymond, 2006). Astrocytoma (discussed later in the section on brain tumors), for example, is a

Pathophysiology Illustrated
Chemotherapy Drug Action

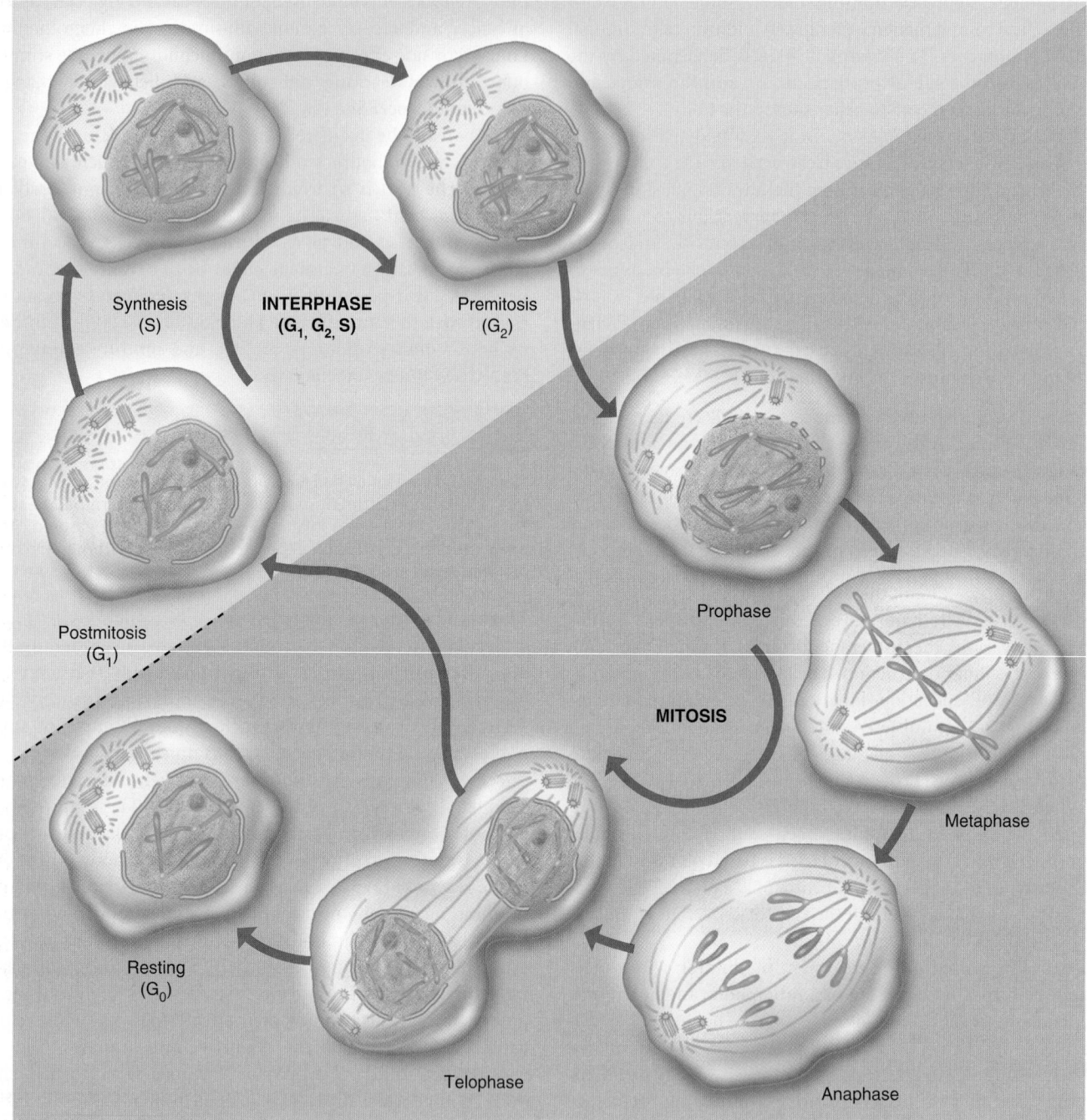

FIGURE 24–4 ➤ Chemotherapy drugs either act at specific parts of the cell cycle or are nonspecific for action (act throughout all cell phases).

cancer in which research on therapy to interfere with metabolic pathways is proving useful (Butowski, Sneed, & Chang, 2006).

An additional type of biological therapy is gene therapy, an attempt to replace a faulty gene with one that is normal. Genetic technology is rapidly growing and shows promise for treatment of cancer and some other childhood diseases in the future. This complex field includes research to identify genes that lead to dis-

ease, recombinant techniques to enable genetic engineering, and studies of enzymes active in DNA and RNA formation. Nurses will need to have increased knowledge of this important work in the future as technologies are used more frequently in cancer treatment (American Nurses Association & International Society of Nurses in Genetics, 2007; National Human Genome Research Institute, 2009).

Protocol = Map or plan of action

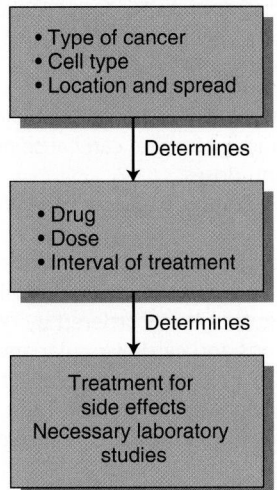

FIGURE 24–5 ➤ Chemotherapy protocol. A protocol is a map or plan of action that directs therapy by identifying the drug and its accompanying treatment.

Bone Marrow and Hematopoietic Stem Cell Transplantation Bone marrow and hematopoietic stem cell transplantation are used to treat leukemia, neuroblastoma, and some noncancerous conditions such as aplastic anemia (National Cancer Institute, 2008). The goal of therapy is to administer a lethal dose of chemotherapy and radiation that will kill the cancer, and then to resupply the body with bone marrow stem cells either from the child's own marrow that was previously removed and stored (autologous transplant) or from a compatible donor (allogeneic transplant). Umbilical cord blood is another source of stem cells used for transplant. Peripheral blood stem cells are increasingly being used for transplant. The donor, whether autologous or allogeneic, can be given growth factors prior to donation to stimulate production of stem cells.

Transplantation has become the treatment of choice for some cancers in the event a relapse occurs while the child is receiving another form of cancer therapy (Handgretinger, Kurtzberg, & Egeler, 2008). First, a histocompatible donor must be located. The child then receives intensive chemotherapy, often followed by total body irradiation. Beginning 7 to 10 days before the transplant, this treatment kills all circulating blood cells and bone marrow contents. Supportive care is needed to treat the effects of nausea, diarrhea, and pain. Following this treatment, the child is intravenously transfused with the transplant stem cells. New blood cells usually form within 2 to 8 weeks. (See Chapter 22 ∞ for a complete description of care for the child undergoing transplantation.)

Complementary Therapies Some families use **complementary therapies** to treat a child's cancer. These approaches accompany conventional care; examples include nutritional supplements, herbal ingestion, touch therapy, and mind-body interventions. Little research has been done on complementary therapies, although about 80% of patients have used at least one such therapeutic approach (Decker, 2008). The National Center for Complementary and Alternative Medicine at the National Institutes of Health leads research and education about these therapies. See Chapter 2 ∞ for further information on complementary care.

Mind-body therapies and touch such as acupuncture and Reiki are the most frequently used approaches. Some people use nutrition and herbal therapies with foods such as carrots, garlic, green tea, cabbage, citrus fruits, ginger root, shark or bovine cartilage, and willow bark, which are thought to be effective in the prevention and treatment of cancer (Decker, 2008). Health care providers should be aware of these practices, inquire in a nonjudgmental manner about what therapies are used, and attempt to learn about specific therapies and practices. Although some herbs and nutritional products such as St. John's wort may decrease serum concentration of chemotherapeutic agents, and others may act as hormones in the body, most are not known to negatively affect contemporary medical treatment. The families should be assisted in seeking information and supported in use of their chosen therapies. Some herbs are useful in the treatment of nausea and vomiting, and others can boost the immune system's function or treat pain.

End-of-Life Care In spite of modern medicine practices and complementary therapies, some children do not survive childhood cancer. In these cases, the focus of health care is to provide comfort through physical care and emotional support for the child and family. Too often, health care providers feel uncomfortable when a child is expected to die and may withdraw from close contact with the child or family, fail to provide adequate comfort measures, and leave the family without access to needed resources. When delay in the recognition of prognosis occurs, children experience greater suffering and less integration of needed care. Some of the symptoms for which children are commonly undertreated include pain, dyspnea, nutrition, elimination, and fatigue. Additionally, care may be required by a wide array of specialists that can lead to fragmentation of care and lack of integrated approaches (Baker, Hinds, Spunt, et al., 2008).

The presence of an end-of-life care team and an integrated plan of care; collaboration between families, the primary care provider, and other practitioners; and focus on the child's developmental level and the needs of the family can enhance the care provided for the child who is dying. An advance directive that outlines the care plans for the child is helpful in preserving the child's quality of life and increases the child's comfort (Baker et al., 2008). See Chapter 13 ∞ for a detailed description of end-of-life care for children with terminal disease.

Special Issues in Childhood Cancer

Oncologic Emergencies Oncologic emergencies may result from the cancer itself or as a side effect of treatment. They can be organized into three groups: metabolic, hematologic, and those involving space-occupying lesions.

Metabolic Emergencies Several types of emergencies can arise from metabolic changes in the body. The first of these metabolic emergencies results from the lysis (dissolving or decomposing) of tumor cells and rapid release of their contents into the blood, a process called *tumor lysis syndrome*. This cell destruction releases high levels of uric acid, potassium, and phosphates into the blood and can lower serum sodium levels, possibly resulting in cardiac arrhythmias and renal failure. This

Medications Used to Treat
Cancer Through Chemotherapy

Medication	Action/Indication	Nursing Management
Cell Cycle Specific Agents Antimetabolites ■ 5-Azacytidine ■ 5-Fluorouracil ■ 6-Mercaptopurine ■ 6-Thioguanine ■ Cytosine arabinoside (cytarabine) ■ Hydroxyurea ■ Methotrexate	The antimetabolites work at the synthesis phase of cell division, interface with function of nucleic acid, and inhibit DNA or RNA synthesis.	■ Most common side effects are nausea and vomiting, myelosuppression, and stomatitis. Specific agents such as methotrexate and cytarabine can cause neurologic toxicity with high doses. ■ Consult drug books and package inserts for a detailed list of side effects. ■ Obtain baseline CBC, liver function, and renal function. ■ Monitor intake and output, and body weight. Ensure hydration and output levels ordered by the oncologist. ■ Monitor vital signs and cardiovascular and respiratory function. ■ Watch for bleeding and signs of infection. ■ Monitor carefully during administration for signs of anaphylaxis.
Vinca alkaloids ■ Etoposide ■ Teniposide ■ Irinotecan ■ Paclitaxel ■ Vinblastine ■ Vincristine	Act during mitosis; bind with cell proteins to inhibit nucleic acid and protein synthesis.	■ Common side effects include nausea and vomiting, abdominal cramping and diarrhea, constipation, paralytic ileus, hair loss, hypotension or hypertension, peripheral neuropathy, and neurological toxicity (latter especially with vinblastine and vincristine). ■ Obtain baseline blood work. ■ Consult specific drug information for the period of maximum myelosuppressive effect. ■ Be alert for bruising, infection, and other signs of myelosuppression. ■ Monitor carefully during administration for signs of anaphylaxis.
Miscellaneous—G_1 phase activity ■ L-asparaginase	Causes depletion of asparagine, needed by cancer cells; makes cell in G_1 phase vulnerable to other agents; interferes with prosynthesis. Used in combination with other agents in leukemia and other cancers.	■ Administered intravenously. ■ Major side effects are severe nausea and vomiting, hypersensitivity (monitor for anaphylaxis), renal failure, myelosuppression, and acid-base imbalance. ■ CBC, serum amylase, glucose, coagulation factors, bone marrow function, and liver function tests are performed before therapy and twice weekly. ■ Monitor intake and output, neurologic status, gastrointestinal symptoms, and abdominal pain.
Miscellaneous—G_2 phase activity ■ Etoposide	Works at G_2 phase; binds cellular proteins to cause metaphase arrest; also acts on S phase of DNA synthesis. Used with other agents, particularly in recurrent disease.	■ Administered orally and intravenously. ■ Common side effects are nausea and vomiting, myelosuppression, hair loss, and diarrhea. Can cause anaphylaxis; hypotension and IV site pain with rapid infusion. ■ Perform baseline CBC, and liver and renal function tests. ■ Check IV site frequently since extravasation can cause necrosis. ■ Monitor vital signs during infusion and stop the drug if hypotension occurs.

Medications Used to Treat
Cancer Through Chemotherapy (continued)

Medication	Action/Indication	Nursing Management
Cell Cycle Nonspecific Agents Alkylating agents ▪ Cyclophosphamide ▪ Carboplatin ▪ Cisplatin ▪ Busulfan ▪ Chlorambucil ▪ Ifosfamide ▪ Thiotepa ▪ Mechlorethamine ▪ Melphalan ▪ Procarbazine ▪ Dacarbazine	Substitute an alkyl group for a hydrogen atom, leading to blockage of DNA replication. Used for treatment of many cancers, either alone or in conjunction with other agents.	▪ Most are administered orally and/or intravenously. Array of side effects, depending on the specific drug. Some common side effects are nausea and vomiting, diarrhea, myelosuppression, hair loss, neuropathies, pulmonary toxicity, hemorrhagic cystitis, and renal damage. Secondary tumors later in life are associated with some agents. ▪ Obtain CBC and full blood work before and during treatment. ▪ Monitor for side effects of the specific agents administered. Ensure generous hydration and monitor intake and output. Teach family the importance of long-term monitoring for secondary tumors.
Antibiotics ▪ Doxorubicin ▪ Mitomycin-C ▪ Dactinomycin ▪ Bleomycin ▪ Daunorubicin ▪ Idarubicin ▪ Mitoxantrone	Interfere with nucleic acid, inhibiting DNA or RNA synthesis. Used in combination with other agents to treat leukemia and other childhood cancers.	▪ Most are administered intravenously. ▪ Common side effects include nausea and vomiting, myelosuppression, oral ulcers, and skin and pulmonary toxicity. Several have cumulative dose toxicity and lifetime maximum dose recommendations, such as cardiac abnormalities (doxorubicin) and skin/pulmonary (bleomycin); total dose the child has received must be monitored. ▪ Obtain baseline CBC and other blood studies and monitor throughout therapy. ▪ Monitor vital signs, lung function, cardiac function, and neurologic status throughout and following therapy. Be alert for signs of myelosuppression and mucosal ulcers.
Nitrosoureas ▪ Carmustine ▪ Lomustine	Cross breakage in DNA strands so that DNA and RNA replication cannot occur. Used in lymphomas and other childhood cancers. Can cross blood-brain barrier.	▪ Administered orally (lomustine) or intravenously (carmustine). The major side effect is myelosuppression. ▪ Others include pulmonary fibrosis, eye infarction, skin changes, hair loss, nausea, and vomiting. ▪ Obtain baseline and periodic CBC and other studies. ▪ Monitor pulmonary function, skin, and signs of infection or bleeding.
Hormones ▪ Prednisone ▪ Prednisolone ▪ Dexamethasone	Analog of hydrocortisone; anti-inflammatory; delayed and depressed immune response. Used in conjunction with other agents for many types of childhood cancer.	▪ Often administered orally. ▪ Numerous side effects include edema, moon face, mood lability, increased appetite, disturbed sleep, immunosuppression, disturbed glucose control, and osteoporosis. ▪ Teach the child and family the effects of the drug. Minimize exposure to persons with infection. Monitor for infections in all systems. ▪ Monitor weight and vital signs. Teach to take drug as directed. Drug may or may not be tapered at the end of therapy.
Topoisomerase I inhibitor ▪ Irinotecan ▪ Mitoxantrone ▪ Topotecan	Inhibit the enzyme topoisomerase I in the cell nucleus, relaxing DNA and preventing its duplication. Used in conjunction with other agents to treat acute lymphocytic leukemia and other childhood cancers.	▪ Administered intravenously; topotecan can be given intrathecally. ▪ Common side effects include nausea and vomiting, diarrhea, fever, dehydration, and myelosuppression. Can alter liver function and cause skin changes. ▪ Obtain baseline and periodic CBC and other studies, including liver function. ▪ Monitor for signs of myelosuppression, gastrointestinal distress, and change in liver function.

Medications Used to Treat
Cancer: Colony-Stimulating Factors

Medication	Action/Indication	Nursing Management
Epoetin alfa (human recombinant erythropoietin)	This glycoprotein stimulates the bone marrow in RBC formation; useful when numbers of RBCs are low due to chemotherapy effects.	■ Give subcutaneously or intravenously. ■ Do not shake and do not use if discolored or if particles are present. Single-dose vials only, so discard any solution that is not used. ■ Obtain blood tests before therapy and periodically after; improvement in hematocrit should be seen in 7–14 days. ■ Monitor blood pressure before and during therapy as hypertension can result. ■ Monitor for change in neurologic response and headache; both seizures and strokes are possible side effects.
Filgrastim (Neupogen) and pegfilgrastim (Neulasta)	This human granulocyte colony-stimulating factor (G-CSF) increases production of neutrophils by the bone marrow.	■ Administered subcutaneously and intravenously; prepare as directed for IV infusion to prevent its absorption by IV tubing. ■ Single-dose vials only, so discard any solution that is not used. ■ Incompatible with many medications; check package insert; do not give within 24 hours before or after chemotherapy drugs or their effect may be decreased. ■ Obtain baseline and twice weekly CBC. ■ Monitor for side effects such as bone pain and heart arrhythmias; report fevers and be alert for other signs of infection when neutrophil count is low.
Oprelvekin (Neumega)	A hematopoietic growth factor, interleukin-11, that increases platelet count; useful in low platelet count due to chemotherapy effects on bone marrow.	■ Administered subcutaneously. ■ Single-dose vials only, so discard any solution that is not used. ■ Obtain baseline CBC and platelet count; monitor platelets throughout treatment. ■ Monitor for side effects such as edema, fever, CNS changes, tachycardia, respiratory problems, and skin rash. ■ Take daily weights and monitor for fluid retention.

syndrome is seen most commonly in children with non-Hodgkin lymphoma and acute lymphocytic leukemia (Bleyer, 2007; Rampello, Fricia, & Malaguarnera, 2006; Zonfrillo, 2009). See the Clinical Manifestations: Tumor Lysis Syndrome table for more details on manifestations and management of tumor lysis syndrome.

A second type of metabolic emergency is septic shock. During periods of immune suppression the child is vulnerable to overwhelming infection, resulting in circulatory failure, hypothermia or hyperthermia, tachypnea, mental changes, inadequate tissue perfusion, and hypotension (da Silva, Koch Nogueira, Russo Zamataro, et al., 2008). Septic shock can be fatal (see Chapter 21 ∞ for a description of septic shock); early and aggressive therapy is needed. Factors contributing to massive infection include inadequate neutrophil production, abnormal granulocytes (not able to be actively phagocytic), erosions through normal barriers such as blood vessels and mucous membranes, and altered bone marrow production caused by chemotherapy and some forms of radiation. Such infections must be vigorously treated with antimicrobial therapy and hydration management.

A third type of metabolic emergency occurs when large amounts of bone are destroyed by treatment and decreased renal tubular excretion, resulting in hypercalcemia (elevated calcium in the serum). Hypercalcemia is most common in children with acute lymphocytic leukemia and rhabdomyosarcoma. Treatment includes hydration, bisphosphonates, glucocorticoids, and adequate intake of phosphate by oral supplement (Spinazze & Schrijvers, 2006).

Some children develop syndrome of inappropriate antidiuretic hormone (SIADH) and have excessive release of ADH. The resulting decreased urinary output leads to water intoxication. See Chapter 30 ∞ for a detailed description of SIADH.

Hematologic Emergencies Hematologic emergencies result from bone marrow suppression or infiltration of brain and respiratory tissue with high numbers of leukemic blast cells (hyperleukocytosis). Bone marrow suppression results in anemia and **thrombocytopenia** (decreased platelets) with resultant hemorrhage. Disseminated intravascular coagulation (DIC) occurs in some children and is a life-threatening complication. (See Chapter 23 ∞ for a thorough description of this condition.) Gastrointestinal and central nervous system bleeding (strokes) are common. Disruption of normal WBC production and resulting hyperleukocytosis can lead to obstruction of small blood vessels throughout the body.

Treatment involves infusion of packed red blood cells for anemia; and platelet transfusion, vitamin K, and fresh frozen plasma for thrombocytopenia and hemorrhage. Hyperleukocy-

Clinical Manifestations
Tumor Lysis Syndrome

Etiology	Clinical Manifestations	Clinical Therapy	Nursing Management
Breakdown of malignant cells releases intracellular components into blood.	Hyperuricemia Hyperkalemia Hyperphosphatemia Hypocalcemia	■ Vigorous hydration with 2–4 times maintenance fluid ■ Correction of electrolyte imbalances ■ Administration of allopurinol or urate oxidase (rasburicase) to reduce conversion of metabolic by-products to uric acid	■ Administration of fluids, beginning before therapy ■ Careful intake and output measures ■ Daily weight ■ Urine specific gravity (should remain less than 1.010) ■ Monitoring for desired and side effects of drug therapy
Electrolyte imbalance causes metabolic acidosis and serious abnormalities.	Cardiac arrhythmias Impaired renal function Tetany, neurological and mental status changes	■ ECG monitoring ■ Medications such as furosemide to facilitate potassium excretion ■ Dialysis may be needed	■ Administration of electrolytes and medications ■ Urine pH (should remain 7.0 to 7.5) ■ Perform Trousseau and Chvostek signs for tetany monitoring and assess neurological function ■ Perform mental status examination ■ Obtain laboratory specimens as needed

tosis is treated by hydration, diuresis, respiratory support, and plasmapheresis, if needed (Rheingold & Lange, 2006).

Space-Occupying Lesions Extensive tumor growth may result in spinal cord compression, increased intracranial pressure, brain herniation, seizures, massive hepatomegaly, and superior vena cava syndrome (obstruction of the superior vena cava by tumor). These emergencies are often caused by neuroblastoma, medulloblastoma, astrocytoma, Hodgkin disease, or lymphoma. After biopsy of the mass, treatment involves radiation therapy, chemotherapy, and corticosteroids.

Psychosocial Needs The diagnosis of cancer is devastating for families. They cannot believe that their vibrant young child or adolescent has a potentially life-threatening disease. Families are in a state of crisis when the diagnosis is made; their first response is typically shock. Despite this, parents must gather resources to support the child, make treatment decisions, and adjust family life to integrate the needs of the child with cancer. Some families need to travel a great distance for the child's treatments, and others may have financial constraints that make health care costs a major concern. For nearly everyone, parental work schedules, as well as arrangements for other children, must be adjusted. Most cancer treatment will last for a minimum of several months up to several years, necessitating nearly constant adaptation. Parents, siblings, and extended families should all be included in plans of care (Brody & Simmons, 2007). See Families Want to Know: Cancer Therapy.

The child reacts to the diagnosis based on age and developmental stage. Infants and toddlers are unaware of the severity of the disease, while preschoolers are beginning to understand the illness. However, they may think they caused their illness, and are confused about why the parent cannot make the illness go away. School-age children can understand a diagnosis of cancer

and benefit from opportunities to talk about the experience. Adolescents find contact with others who have gone through their experience reassuring and supportive. Children and adolescents are commonly anxious about the treatments and disturbed schedules and routines (Kersun & Elia, 2007). Nearly all children are hospitalized after diagnosis, and care should

Families Want to Know
Cancer Therapy

Most parents are not aware of the effects of cancer treatment and how they can help children through this experience. Depending on the stage and type of treatment, there are several ways to help:

■ Children in radiation and chemotherapy are fatigued. Provide extra rest periods with shorter activity periods between them.

■ Have essential items packed in case the child develops a complication and needs to be taken to stay in the hospital for a few days. Several hospital stays of a few days are normal during treatment.

■ When concerned about a symptom in the child, talk to the care provider. Parents are often key in identifying problems early.

■ Parents are usually concerned about central line care, but feel more comfortable after a few days of caring for the line.

■ Children may not feel hungry, so nutritional intake is needed when they are ready to eat.

■ Remember that the child is still at the normal developmental age. Treat children based on their ages, not as if they are older or younger.

■ Try to maintain contact with the child's peer group and family members.

■ Seek information from other parents and resources on cancer care.

■ Remind parents to get time away and relax so that parental energy remains high and they are better able to deal with the child's therapy.

include close proximity to parents, involvement in self-care appropriate for age, positive relationships with staff, and emotional care (Bjork, Nordstrom, & Hallstrom, 2006). Group therapy sessions, computer programs about cancer and treatment, and school reintegration all show potential for assisting youth who are adjusting to cancer.

Cancer Survival   Children with cancer have a variety of common psychologic and physiologic challenges, regardless of their specific types of cancer. They and their families are dealing with a complex illness that influences their lives for years. The impact of this experience extends into all areas of function. Over the past 20 to 30 years, treatment for childhood cancers has been increasingly successful and 80% of children with cancer will have long-term survival (Oeffinger, Nathan, & Kremer, 2008). The success of new modalities and treatment combinations has, however, created special health care needs for many survivors (Figure 24–6 ➤).

Surgery can have many results. Body organs may be removed and manipulated, leading to adhesions, intestinal obstruction, visual impairment, neurologic disruption, and sterility. Removal of the spleen can lead to serious infections. Amputation necessitates the need for prosthetic devices and physical rehabilitation.

Radiation has several long-term effects. It can impair the growth of bones, teeth, and eyes, leading to conditions such as scoliosis, leg length discrepancy, low bone mineral density, cataracts, or poor dental health. Chronic pain can result from skeletal toxicity (Kaste, 2008). Hypothyroidism can be observed in those who have had head and neck radiation (Skinner, Hamish, Wallace, et al., 2006). Cardiotoxicity and pulmonary toxicity can result from mediastinal radiation, and delayed puberty and sterility can result from radiation effects to the cranium and spinal regions. Impaired neurocognitive performance may occur as a long-term effect of treatment, especially with higher doses of radiation. Some studies have found lower behavioral and social competence in treated children, and higher rates of posttraumatic stress syndrome (Rourke, Hobbie, Schwartz, et al., 2007).

Secondary cancers, most commonly solid tumors, occur in some survivors. **Secondary cancers** are also called second malignant neoplasm (SMN). They occur subsequent to the primary cancer and treatment but are of a different histologic type. Cancers of the thyroid, CNS, breast, and skin are examples of described secondary neoplasms. Other chronic conditions, such as congestive heart failure, cognitive dysfunction, and reproductive problems, are more common in cancer survivors who are adults than in the general population (Twombly, 2007).

Chemotherapy can cause a wide variety of effects, both during its administration and for years afterward. See Clinical Manifestations: Common Side Effects of Chemotherapy on page 728. Cardiomyopathy can occur with some drugs, especially the anthracyclines. Temporary or permanent pulmonary toxicity and renal complications can develop. Neurologic effects of some drugs can lead to hearing loss (e.g., cisplatin and ifosfamide), cataracts, and paraplegia (e.g., intrathecal methotrexate for leukemia). Learning disabilities and change in intelligence quotient (IQ) occur in some children. Infertility may also result. Although radiation is responsible for most secondary tumors, some chemotherapy drugs have also been implicated.

The diagnosis and stress of treatment, along with the risk of recurrence, are significant stressors for the child with cancer. Families may find it difficult to obtain full insurance coverage

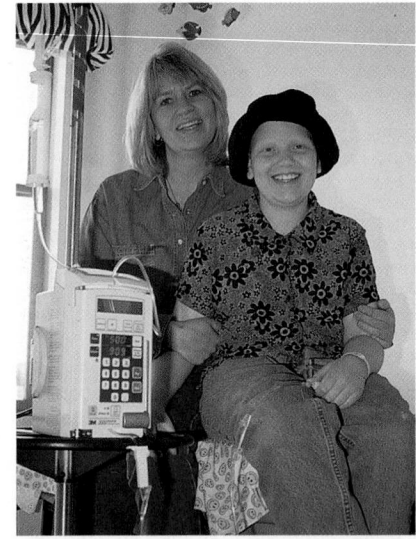

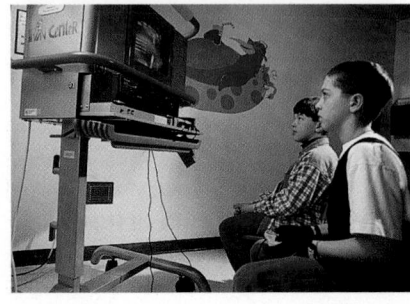

A

B

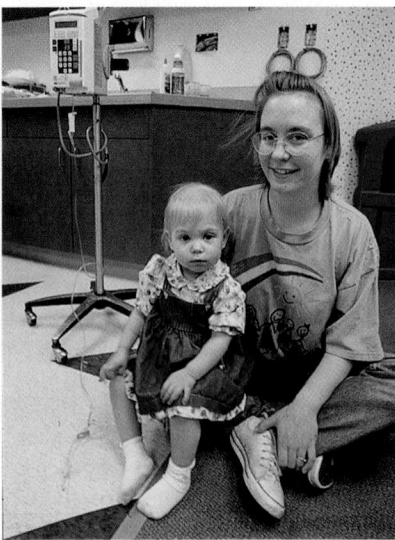

C

FIGURE 24–6 ➤ Survivors of childhood cancer. A, Nicole, 11 years old, is undergoing chemotherapy for Ewing sarcoma. Her mother emphasizes, "It's our faith that has gotten us through this. The hardest part is how busy you are coming to treatments all the time. Nicole's younger brother sometimes feels neglected." B, According to Jesse, who is 10 years old and waiting for a bone marrow transplant, "The thing that has helped me the most [in dealing with acute lymphoblastic leukemia] is all the mail I got from my friends." His mother adds, "We're just really positive and think that everything will turn out all right." C, Cassie, 19 months old, has been diagnosed with neuroblastoma. At this age, it is hard for her to understand what is happening. Her mother has stayed with her each time she has come to the hospital, which has helped Cassie adjust to therapy. Her caregivers are confident that she will respond well to her treatment.

for the child who has had a prior cancer. Employment can be a potential problem for cancer survivors if employers have concerns about the earlier cancer diagnosis. Most people with cancer report fear of recurrence of the disease, which is another stressor. Depression, suicidal thoughts, and concerns about appearance may be more common in survivors of childhood cancer, although this finding is not consistent among all studies (Zebrack, Zevon, Turk, et al., 2007).

Conversely, hopefulness and the sense of having an added purpose in life can be positive outcomes for many cancer survivors. Some meet with others who have recently been diagnosed or work on fund-raising events that support cancer research. The highest risk for long-term psychological distress in adult survivors of childhood cancer occurs in those with poor health status, low income, low education, and unemployment. Thus, encouraging children with cancer to meet educational goals will maximize their chances of psychological adaptation (Zebrack et al., 2007).

A consensus group of experts identified barriers to optimal care for cancer survivors, including:

- Lack of knowledge about survivorship by health care professionals
- Lack of knowledge about risks and care recommendations by the cancer survivor
- Lack of awareness about cancer survivorship by the general public
- Paucity of research on survivorship

Therefore, additional education of health care professionals and the public, as well as research into survivor issues, are recommended (Houldin, Curtiss, & Haylock, 2006).

NURSING MANAGEMENT
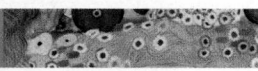

Nursing Assessment and Diagnosis

Children who have cancer have all of the usual health promotion and health maintenance requirements; in addition, they require astute assessments to identify any of the possible outcomes of cancer and its treatment. Nurses who work with children and adolescents will find useful references through the Association of Pediatric Hematology and Oncology Nurses.

History

During health promotion visits, nurses should determine if there is a history of cancer in the family. In particular, if more than one person has had cancer, and if young children in the extended family have been affected, complete a genogram to isolate cases in the family (see Chapter 3 ∞). A history of exposure to known carcinogens is also important. Does a parent work in an industry with chemicals or asbestos that might remain on clothing worn home? Was the child treated with radiation or chemotherapy for a previous cancer? Does the child have an identified condition such as Down syndrome? Does the child have any recognized congenital anomalies? A number of conditions are more commonly associated with certain types of cancer.

Physiologic Assessment

When performing any physiologic assessment on children, the nurse considers the possible signs and symptoms of cancer. These include anemia, frequent infections, bleeding disorders, loss of weight, fatigue, pain, and changes in mental health and neurological status. Assessment of children with the most significant types of childhood cancers is presented in separate sections throughout this chapter.

Once cancer has been diagnosed, a thorough physical assessment of all systems is needed to help identify the presence and extent of cancer (see Chapter 5 ∞), particularly neurologic, respiratory, cardiac, and gastrointestinal systems. Assess hydration status and the tumor site if it is visible. These assessments will be completed regularly at each treatment and monitoring visit. Height and weight should be carefully measured and compared with prior findings for the child. Nutritional intake histories may be pertinent as well. Observe immunization status, developmental milestones, gait and coordination, as well as any changes in mental status. Evaluate pain, fatigue, infections, bruising, shortness of breath, and elimination problems, and perform periodic laboratory studies.

Psychosocial Assessment

Assessment of stress and coping abilities, as well as knowledge of the condition and cognitive level, support systems, developmental level, and body image, provides data that help determine the appropriate nursing interventions for the child with cancer and his or her family.

> ### ▲ Health Promotion
>
> #### Adolescents and Cancer
> Adolescence is a distinct developmental stage that overlaps both childhood and adulthood, characterized by increased independence in decision making and reliance on a peer support group (Linder, 2008). Health promotion visits should continue during cancer treatment, providing a forum for joint discussions with the health care providers, parents, and teens, and individual sessions when the adolescent meets alone with the health care team. During these visits, ask for adolescents' perspectives to best understand the experience of cancer and offer the support they need. Inquire about what has changed in the adolescent's life and what has been challenging to manage. Provide the opportunity to discuss feelings; offer assistance to locate other teens with cancer for further discussion and support. Continue to provide health promotion regarding nutrition, activity, and other important topics (see Chapter 9 ∞).

Stress and Coping The diagnosis of cancer is a major stressor for both the child and his or her family. Although each child's prognosis and each family's coping mechanisms are unique, most families deal with the diagnosis in a manner similar to that of other families who have a child with a life-threatening illness (see Chapter 13 ∞). Assess the family (and child, if old enough) for their understanding and acceptance of the diagnosis. Evaluate if the family has told the child about the diagnosis and whether the family needs assistance in deciding how to do this. Ask what the parents have told siblings; if they need suggestions, help and support them to decide how much and when to share information with the child's siblings.

Assess the level of anxiety during health care visits and scheduled treatments. Evaluate the family's methods of coping, such as the ability to integrate relaxing and meaningful activities into family life, the use of support systems in the extended family and the community, and the ability to alter expectations to take into account the child's health status (Figure 24–7 ➤). Some families demonstrate resilience and the ability to assist the child and all of their members. Other families, however, may be experiencing multiple stresses, making adaptation to the new diagnosis difficult (Kazak, Rourke, Alderfer, et al., 2007). Concurrent stressors increase the family's difficulty in coping with childhood cancer. Evaluate the family for stressors such as illness or death of another family member, occupational changes, financial problems, relocation, and changes in vacation plans. Evaluate the family's knowledge of the U.S. Family and Medical Leave Act benefits, which enable parents to use sick time, vacation, and leave without pay to care for an ill family member while safeguarding employment.

Knowledge People who are anxious tend to narrow their scope of attention and may read unintended messages into the behaviors of health care personnel. Anxiety also limits a person's ability to retain information.

The child's knowledge of cancer and its treatment should be assessed throughout the treatment period. As the child matures cognitively, new evaluations of knowledge are needed. Cancer and its treatment are complex topics, and parents are exposed to information in various forms, including written material, news reports, Internet websites, and other resources. Evaluate their knowledge and information sources, and provide them with opportunities to ask questions. Evaluate the learning styles of the child and family in order to adapt approaches to meet their needs.

Support Systems Cancer treatment generally occurs over a long period of time. The extended family is crucial in providing necessary support to the child, parents, and siblings. Identify key

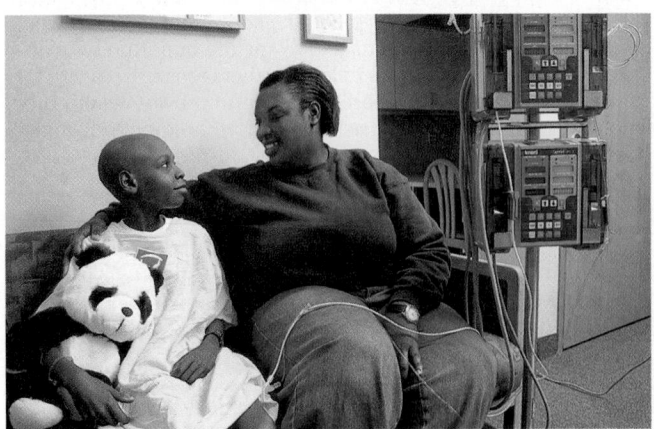

FIGURE 24–7 ➤ The child with cancer depends on parents and family members to provide support. Nurses can assist families to draw upon their strengths to help the child.

Research *The Father's Perspective*

Much of the research concerning family support for the child with cancer focuses on the mother, but the father often alters his role to support the child and facilitate the child's treatment. Fathers often find support from extended family, religious faith, and health care professionals. Those who are able to work fewer hours and participate in the family are most able to cope positively (Bennett Murphy, Flowers, McNamara, et al., 2008; Brody & Simmons, 2007).

persons in the family. They may be the parents, grandparents, or aunts and uncles. Thoroughly assess the coping strategies used by the family to meet the various challenges posed by the child's illness. This information helps to predict the success of interventions, such as home care with intravenous medications, and to decide when referrals for other supportive therapies are needed.

Assess family resources to identify support systems available to help the family during crises and if a child is not expected to live. Extended supports include friends, jobs, insurance coverage, faith-based affiliations, cultural support systems, the health care system, and the school system (Figure 24–8 ➤). Inquire if the insurance carrier provides for a case manager in complex health needs such as cancer. Parents commonly lose contact with close friends following the diagnosis of cancer in a child. This is an additional stressor for the family. Jobs are often a source of support because coworkers may have gone through the same experience. It may also be comforting for parents to return to a job where they can feel a sense of security in tangible accomplish-

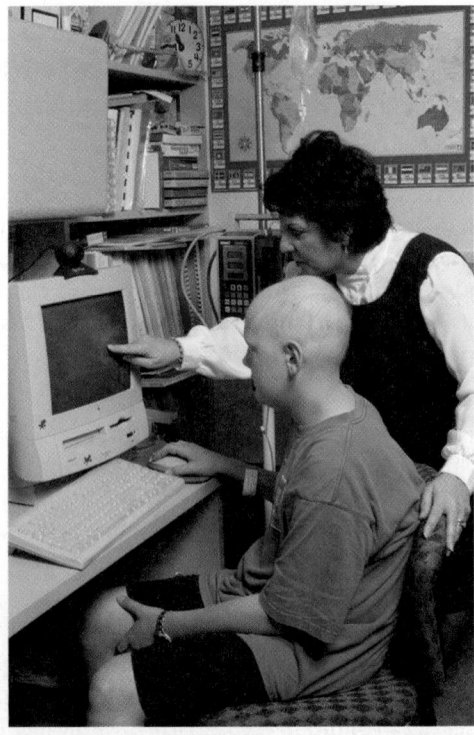

FIGURE 24–8 ➤ This teacher is able to come to the pediatric oncology center to work with students while their chemotherapy is administered. What are the benefits of having her work with students in this setting?

ments. However, jobs can also be a source of stress if employers are unsympathetic to the demands of the child's hospitalization and clinic or office visits.

Faith-based affiliations can be an important source of support. Evaluate whether such affiliations are meaningful for the family and, if so, plan for visits from the appropriate clergy. In some cultures, spiritual leaders are an important part of the family's support. Enable a healer to visit the child and conduct a healing ceremony if that will be supportive to the family and child.

The child's return to school may pose difficulties for the child with cancer, or, alternatively, it may be a source of support to be connected again to peers. The child is encouraged to go to school, even if only for half a day per week, to stay connected to peers. Evaluate the school's ability to accept a medically vulnerable child into the classroom. Nurses who work in the oncology department of the hospital or clinic can ask if the family will give consent to visit the school, meet with the school nurse, and plan together to meet the child's educational needs. Assess whether the other children and teachers have been prepared for the appearance and needs of the child with cancer. Arrangements can be made for tutors to help the child keep up with school work if he or she cannot attend school. An individualized education plan is needed (see a description of the IEP in Chapter 10 ∞). Parents need information about the legal right to this plan since the child is newly ill and they will likely not have been exposed to this in the past.

Developmental Assessment Developmental assessment of children should be performed regularly during treatment for cancer. This assessment should be done at times when the child feels well so that results are accurate. Children under 6 years of age who have cancer should receive regular developmental assessment with a standardized tool such as the Denver II Developmental Screening Test (see Chapter 6 ∞). A home health care nurse, or a nurse in the pediatric health care home (medical home) who sees the child for a general health supervision visit, can perform such testing. Assessment of the child's physical and neurologic development helps in determining the progress made during treatment and provides a baseline for evaluating the long-term effects of treatment. Recommend referral to a neuropsychologist for testing early in treatment and determine if changes in developmental performance are noted. Observe developmental milestones at each contact with the child and refer for further assessment if regression has occurred. Performance in school and social activities with friends also provide important information about expected developmental milestones in older children.

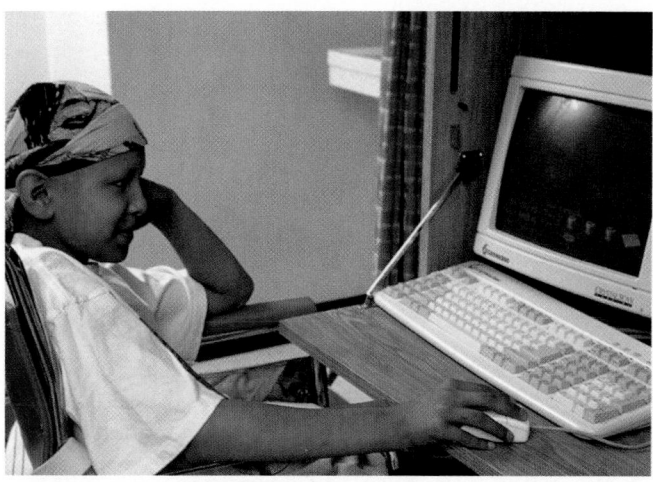

FIGURE 24–9 ➤ One of the most common threats to a child's body image at any age is hair loss induced by chemotherapy. Use of hats can improve self-concept.

Body Image Body image disturbances occur when a child cannot integrate changes and continues to cling to old images despite their inconsistency with reality. Common means for assessing body image are drawings, colored pictures cut out by the child to form a collage, discussion, and observation. Drawing is an especially powerful tool that assists children in handling the stress of the disease and enhances communication with health care providers. See Chapter 11 ∞ for further discussion of these and other assessment techniques that can be used with children.

Hair loss, surgical scars, and cushingoid changes are three common treatment-induced threats to body image. Most children being treated for cancer experience hair loss (Figure 24–9 ➤). Children who have cranial surgery lose hair as part of the surgical preparation. Chemotherapy also frequently results in some degree of hair loss. The speed of hair loss is unique to the child and can be as rapid as overnight or slower, evidenced by hair left on the pillow and in the hairbrush. Assess for hair loss and assist the child to deal with it in the method he or she chooses.

A second challenge to the child's body image is surgery. The scars of cranial and neck surgery are obvious, as are amputation and limb salvaging. Abdominal surgery for lymphoma is more easily concealed but is still a threat to the child's body image.

A third source of altered body image is the cushingoid features such as round and flushed face, prominent cheeks, double chin, and generalized obesity that result from the use of corticosteroids (Figure 24–10 ➤). As the child's weight increases, stretch marks similar to those women experience in pregnancy may occur. These stretch marks often remain after the corticosteroids are decreased.

Growth & Development *Cancer and Age Considerations*

Children of different ages experience differing threats to body image as a result of cancer treatment. A preschool girl may be most upset at hair loss, since she will look like a boy. A school-age child has the most difficult time with changes that interfere with the developmental task of industry. Amputation, which decreases the child's ability to participate in activities such as sports, dancing, and school work, can be a major challenge during the school-age years. Adolescents are often most worried about such changes as hair loss and cushingoid features, which cause them to look different from peers.

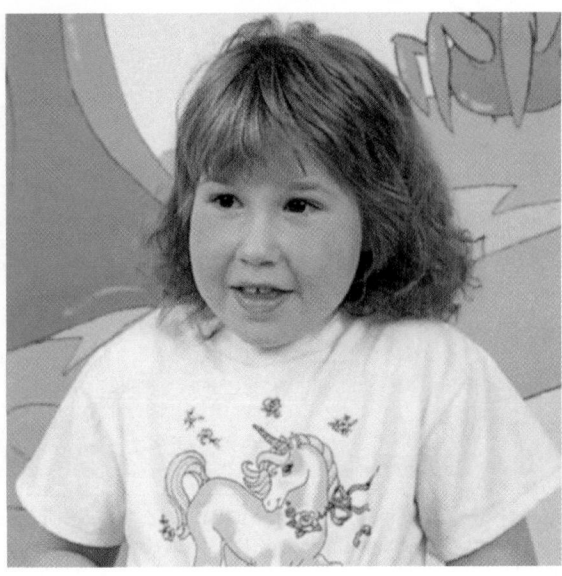

FIGURE 24–10 ➤ The child with cushingoid changes frequently has a rounded face and prominent cheeks.

Assessment for Impact of Cancer Survival Nurses are involved with families when a diagnosis of cancer is made, during the therapy process, and in the years that follow. The family needs support as treatment concludes and the child is integrated back into his or her usual home and community roles. For a child who survives cancer, ongoing care is essential (Hudson & Findlay, 2006; Kurt, Armstrong, Cash, et al., 2008; Oeffinger et al., 2008). Evaluate the child regularly with thorough physical, psychosocial, developmental, and cognitive assessments. Carefully monitor all body systems (e.g., cardiovascular; respiratory; musculoskeletal; eye, ear, nose, and throat; genitourinary). Record height, weight, and general growth patterns. Ask about the child's interactions with peers and performance at school. Children who have received cranial radiation and intrathecal chemotherapy need regular scholastic evaluations. Be alert for signs and symptoms that could indicate a secondary tumor.

> **Clinical Tip**
>
> For many parents, especially those with daughters, the loss of the child's hair can be devastating. Ask the parents and the child what this issue is like for them. Prepare them for the fact that the hair loss can be rapid or slow. Find out how they will plan to cope. Some children want their hair cut very short so its loss will not be as traumatic. Offer resources for wigs, hats, or other ideas. Put them in touch with children who have lost hair and with those who have regrown it.

Assess the need for physical rehabilitation, support related to visual impairment, or treatment for cardiac or musculoskeletal abnormalities. Facilitate periodic evaluations in a health care agency so that serious outcomes of treatment can be identified early. Ask the parents about insurance coverage and other financial difficulties with ongoing care.

The accompanying Nursing Care Plan includes several diagnoses that may be appropriate for the child with cancer who is receiving care in the hospital. Among the many other diagnoses that may be appropriate for a child with cancer are the following:

- Impaired Oral Mucous Membrane related to chemotherapy and radiation therapy
- Impaired Skin Integrity related to altered nutritional state, effects of medication, radiation, and immobilization
- Ineffective Individual Coping related to situational crises of chronic and acute illness
- Disturbed Sleep Pattern related to biochemical agents, anxiety, and unfamiliar surroundings
- Deficient Diversional Activity related to frequent lengthy treatments
- Disturbed Body Image related to chronic illness and treatments
- Deficient Knowledge (Child or Parents) related to lack of exposure to disease or treatments

Planning and Implementation

The nursing care of children newly diagnosed with cancer and their families includes immediate physiologic and psychologic support, along with anticipatory guidance about imminent and future medical interventions. The family should be assisted and supported in making decisions about types of treatment that are appropriate for their child.

Ensure Optimal Nutritional Intake

The high metabolic rate of cancer growth depletes the child's nutritional stores. In addition, the catabolic effect of chemotherapy and radiation on normal cells necessitates additional cellular replacement. The child needs increased nutritional intake at a time when nausea and vomiting are occurring as drug side effects, when taste and smell have been altered, and when decreased activity, fatigue, pain, and general health status result in diminished appetite. This often leads to extreme concern on the part of parents, who may focus excessive attention on the child's intake. See Families Want to Know: Nutrition and the Child with Cancer on page 727.

The goals of nutrition therapy during treatment for cancer are to prevent or reverse any nutritional deficiencies, preserve the child's lean body mass, minimize any side effects that influence nutritional state, allow for the child's growth needs, and improve overall quality of life. Administer antiemetic drugs to lessen nausea from chemotherapy. Offer frequent, small meals. It may be helpful to offer the child's favorite foods at times when nausea and vomiting are decreased. Ask the family what treatments they use to decrease the child's nausea and vomiting. Perform 24-hour dietary recalls to assess the child's intake, and evaluate height and weight regularly. Special nutritional products may be given orally, nasogastric or nasoduodenal tube feedings may be given, or total parenteral nutrition may be necessary. When the child's nutritional status is deteriorating or parenteral nutrition is used, perform weekly studies of serum electrolytes, liver chemistry, glucose, and triglycerides. Partner with both the oncologist and the dietitian to plan interventions appropriate for meeting the needs of individual children.

End-of-life care is provided when a child is not expected to recover. Nutritional support becomes especially important

NURSING CARE PLAN

Hospital Care of the Child with Cancer

INTERVENTION	RATIONALE	EXPECTED OUTCOME
1. Nursing Diagnosis: Chronic Pain related to tissue injury		
NIC Priority Intervention: *Pain management:* Alleviation or reduction in pain to a level of comfort acceptable to patient		**NOC Suggested Outcome:** *Comfort level:* Feelings of physical and psychologic ease
Goal: The child will report reduced pain that is manageable.		
■ Give analgesics as ordered.	■ Adequate medications can reduce pain.	The child experiences pain reduced to the level that allows the child to interact appropriately and gain rest.
■ Teach relaxation techniques, deep breathing, and distraction.	■ Nonpharmacologic methods work with the medication to reduce pain.	
2. Nursing Diagnosis: Imbalanced Nutrition: Less than Body Requirements related to inability to ingest or digest food or absorb nutrients		
NIC Priority Intervention: *Nutrition management:* Assistance with and provision of a balanced dietary intake		**NOC Suggested Outcome:** *Nutritional status:* Extent to which nutrients are available to meet metabolic needs
Goal: The child will maintain adequate nutritional intake. The child will experience reduced side effects of chemotherapy (i.e., nausea and vomiting).		
■ Offer small feedings. Encourage favorite foods. Refer to a dietitian for special meals. Weigh daily.	■ These measures can increase caloric intake. Taste changes and mouth sores alter the desire for food.	The child maintains admission weight.
■ Teach the child distraction and relaxation techniques. Give antiemetics according to orders.	■ Pharmacologic and nonpharmacologic methods are effective in helping to reduce nausea.	The child has minimal or no nausea and vomiting.
3. Nursing Diagnosis: Risk for Constipation related to change in usual foods and eating patterns		
NIC Priority Intervention: *Constipation management:* Prevention and alleviation of constipation		**NOC Suggested Outcome:** *Bowel elimination:* The ability of the gastrointestinal tract to form and evacuate stool effectively
Goal: The child will reestablish normal bowel pattern.		
■ Record all output by size and description. Administer stool softeners. Test stool for guaiac. Report changes in stool to the physician. Encourage adequate fluid intake.	■ Chemotherapy or tumor may create constipation, diarrhea, or blood in stool.	The child has normal bowel pattern.
4. Nursing Diagnosis: Fluid Volume Excess or Deficient related to medications		
NIC Priority Intervention: *Fluid management:* Promotion of fluid balance and prevention of complications resulting from abnormal fluid levels		**NOC Suggested Outcome:** *Fluid balance:* Balance of water in the intracellular and extracellular compartments of the body
Goal: The child will be adequately hydrated.		
■ Record all intake. Monitor intravenous rate and solution as appropriate.	■ Some drugs (e.g., cyclophosphamide) necessitate a high level of fluid intake to prevent complications.	The child demonstrates adequate hydration. Mucous membranes are hydrated.
■ Test specific gravity of urine daily.	■ Renal function may be affected by chemotherapy.	Specific gravity remains within normal range.

(continued)

NURSING CARE PLAN

Hospital Care of the Child with Cancer (continued)

INTERVENTION	RATIONALE	EXPECTED OUTCOME
5. Nursing Diagnosis: Risk for Infection related to immunosuppression, invasive procedures, malnutrition, or pharmaceutical agents		
NIC Priority Intervention: *Infection protection:* Prevention and early detection of infection in patient at risk		**NOC Suggested Outcome:** *Risk control:* Actions to eliminate or reduce health threats
Goal: The child will remain free of infection.		
■ Wash hands often. Maintain in isolation if needed.	■ Handwashing is effective to reduce organisms. Transmission-based precautions may be needed to safeguard the child.	The child remains infection-free.
■ Monitor temperature. Report elevation to the physician.	■ Elevated temperature is a sign of infection.	
■ Administer intravenous antibiotics as ordered. Monitor temperature. Use a cooling mattress as ordered. Report elevations over 38°C (101°F) to the physician.	■ Multiple antibiotics are needed to deal with bacterial and lung infections during neutropenia. Blood cultures may be taken to identify the organism.	The child with an infection is effectively treated.
6. Nursing Diagnosis: Ineffective Individual Coping related to situational crisis		
NIC Priority Intervention: *Coping enhancement:* Assisting a patient to adapt to stressors that interfere with meeting life demands and roles		**NOC Suggested Outcome:** *Coping:* Actions to manage stressors that tax an individual's resources
Goal: The child will demonstrate normal adaptive coping methods.		
■ Encourage drawings and other therapeutic play for expression of feelings. Allow for expression of angry feelings, such as hitting dolls and throwing sponge balls. Discuss how to behave during treatments.	■ Expression of feelings helps identify avoidance coping for further intervention. Play is a normal way for the child to express self and ideas. Misinterpretations can be corrected. Knowledge of appropriate and helpful behaviors supports self-esteem.	The child continues to use usual coping strategies expected for developmental stage.

during this time to improve quality of life, enhance comfort, and support the immune system. Children should be offered foods that they like and which are easy to eat. Soft, nonspicy foods like puddings, eggs, and purées offer high-energy density as well as ease in consumption and digestion. Ensure adequate fluids, and supplement fluids with powdered milk or energy supplements.

Administer Medications

An important intervention of the oncology nurse is administering medications safely. Most chemotherapeutic drugs are prescribed and calculated as dose per meter squared (dose/m²), with m² calculated from the child's height and weight, or as mg/kg. (Refer to the section on administering medications in the *Clinical Skills Manual*.)

Several chemotherapeutic drugs are often used in combinations. These drugs are prepared with special techniques under laminar flow devices to minimize potential toxic effects on health care providers. Gloves and other hazardous drug protocols are used. Care must be taken to avoid **extravasation** of intravenous drugs (leakage into the soft tissue around the infusion site), as this can cause permanent tissue damage.

Clinical Tip

Several precautions must be taken during administration of chemotherapy drugs. Usually the child receiving intravenous medications has a central line or implantable port. The line is maintained carefully; if any drugs are given through a peripheral line, extreme caution and frequent monitoring are used to prevent extravasation, which can seriously injure tissues. Likewise, health care providers must avoid inadvertent contact with these potent drugs. The Occupational Safety and Health Administration (OSHA) publishes an instruction manual entitled *Controlling Occupational Exposure to Hazardous Drugs* that outlines general guidelines, protective equipment, and procedures.

Special techniques such as generous hydration and accompanying medications help to decrease side effects. In addition to chemotherapy drugs, the nurse administers other medications, such as antiemetics to control nausea, vitamin supplements, and antibiotics. Antiemetics such as ondansetron are given prophylactically when a cancer agent is administered that has known emetic effects. Parents are asked about complementary therapy and medications they are obtaining from other sources and us-

OSHA Website

Families Want to Know
Nutrition and the Child with Cancer

Because of the effects of cancer and chemotherapy or other treatment, the child often has a poor appetite. Mucosal sores lead to difficulty chewing and swallowing. Parents can enhance the child's nutritional intake in the following ways:

- Provide frequent small feedings rather than three meals daily.
- Integrate the child's favorite foods into daily menus.
- Have nutritious snacks available for times when the child feels like eating.
- Sprinkle dried milk on top of cereals and other foods.
- Serve smooth, soft foods. Milkshakes with added peanut butter, puddings, and soft casseroles may be well tolerated and preferred. Try a variety of liquid protein-calorie supplements to find those the child likes.
- Avoid making food an area for disagreement. Do not force foods, but make them readily available.
- If the child is vomiting due to therapy, do not encourage food at that time. Food aversions may develop to foods that are vomited.
- Administer antiemetics as ordered during therapy because they can prevent nausea and vomiting.
- Report weight loss and increased fatigue.
- Bring the child in for scheduled health visits so growth, development, and effects of therapy can be monitored.
- Request a temporary feeding tube to ensure adequate nutrition. Feedings at night can often increase intake and promote health. Occasionally a central line is inserted to provide total parenteral nutrition.
- Recognize that supplements and tube feedings will usually be covered by insurance if the provider writes an order for them.

ing at home. All medications must be safely administered, and the child should be monitored for side effects. **Polypharmacy** (the use of several drugs at one time to treat multiple health conditions) can lead to multiple side effects and can challenge the body's ability to metabolize and excrete drugs.

Nursing Alert

A treatment known as *leucovorin rescue* is used in conjunction with high-dose methotrexate chemotherapy. Leucovorin (citrovorum factor) is a form of folic acid that helps to protect normal cells from the destructive action of methotrexate (Warnick & Auger, 2009). It is started within 24 hours of methotrexate administration and is given along with hydration therapy. Usual administration is every 6 hours for 72 hours or until serum methotrexate is at the desired level.

Likewise, mesna is a detoxifying agent used to inhibit hemorrhagic cystitis, a side effect of ifosfamide. It interacts with the toxic metabolites of the drug, thereby decreasing hematuria. Mesna is administered with every dose of ifosfamide (Wilson, Shannon, & Shields, 2009).

Parents and children must become well informed about the drugs to be administered and the side effects that may occur. Telephone numbers, websites, and other resources are needed for provision of information when questions arise. Inform the family about the phases of drug trials if the child is asked to participate, and provide other resource links.

Law & Ethics *Clinical Trials*
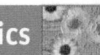

When unapproved investigational drugs are given in a clinical trial, permission for the child to participate must be obtained from parents. They should understand the potential benefits and harm to the child. Children who are cognitively able should actively participate by learning about and providing assent, if that is their wish, orally or in writing (Unguru, Coppes, & Kamani, 2008). This assent can usually be obtained from children by the age of 7–9 years, depending on the child's level of understanding. Conferences that are held with the families, including children, to discuss the disease and potential treatments, identify risks and benefits of treatment, and ensure that the choices are voluntarily made are an important part of oncology practice (Chappuy, Doz, Blanche, et al., 2006; American Cancer Society, 2009a). Even when the family has given consent for a clinical trial, they may have additional questions. Nurses can clarify information and refer the family to the research investigator for further explanations.

Manage Treatment Side Effects

All cancer treatments affect some normal body cells as well as cancer cells, causing a wide variety of side effects. A frequent occurrence is **myelosuppression,** or suppression of blood cell production in the bone marrow. Be alert for signs of a decreased white blood cell count, such as infections. **Neutropenia** is present when the absolute neutrophil count (ANC) is less than 500 cells/mm³ or if between 500 and 1000 cells/mm³ when chemotherapy is being given and falling levels are anticipated. Children with neutropenia and fever are treated with a broad-spectrum antibiotic; granulocyte colony-stimulating factor (G-CSF) may also be given (see the Medications table on page 718). Take the child's temperature, isolate the child from others with infections, and perform serum laboratory studies as ordered. See Clinical Manifestations: Common Side Effects of Chemotherapy.

Protect the child from bruises and be alert for signs of bleeding such as petechiae, nosebleeds, dark colored or bloody stools, and presence of blood in vomit and urine. These are all effects of decreased platelets. When thrombocytopenia occurs, minimize needlesticks and other intrusive procedures. Be ready to deal with nosebleeds and watch for bleeding gums. Report any bleeding episodes to the physician. Be sure parents know that the child should avoid contact sports or other rough activities and that any health care provider, such as a dentist, should be informed of the child's treatment and condition. Infusions to increase platelets are sometimes administered.

Inadequate red blood cell production can result in anemia. Encourage the child to eat iron-rich foods, and administer nutritional supplements as needed. Blood transfusions are sometimes required to treat severe anemia.

Chemotherapy affects all rapidly growing cells in the body, but especially those of the mucous membranes. Provide good oral hygiene with a soft toothbrush, foam wand, or water irrigation device. Report oral breakdown promptly. (See Families Want to Know: Oral Care.) Be alert for blood in vomitus and stool, which can be indicators of bleeding in the gastrointestinal tract.

Ensure Adequate Hydration

Hydration management can be a challenge as the child may not be thirsty but is excreting large numbers of cell fragments and

Clinical Manifestations
Common Side Effects of Chemotherapy

Side Effect	Manifestations	Clinical Therapy
Bone marrow supipression	Evidence of suppression usually appears 7–10 days after administration of chemotherapy. Recovery is usually complete within 3–4 weeks.	Blood transfusions are administered based on laboratory findings of CBC and platelets, as well as the clinical condition of the child. Some institutions use a low dose microbial to decrease the possibility that infectious organisms will colonize the intestine. Septra is used for *Pneumocystis jirovecii* pneumonia prophylaxis; nystatin and oral vancomycin are used for antifungal and antibacterial prophylaxis. Instruct the family and child about the importance of protecting the body from bruising during periods of mild to moderate thrombocytopenia (platelet count less than 5000/mm^3). Nonsteroidal anti-inflammatory agents are avoided in thrombocytopenia. Careful handwashing is essential. Encourage use of masks if family or staff have nasopharyngeal infections.
Nausea and vomiting	Symptoms may occur immediately, a few hours later, or any time during the treatment.	Antiemetics, such as Zofran, Kytril, Reglan, and Benadryl, are used to treat this side effect. Teach relaxation techniques, hypnosis, and systematic desensitization (a hypnotic process that progressively reduces reactions to objects that cause strong emotional or physical responses) to help to decrease the child's symptoms. Encourage mild exercise and change of diet (eating only easily digestible foods) 12 hours before chemotherapy.
Anorexia and weight loss	May occur at any time.	Hyperalimentation is necessary if dietary changes are unsuccessful in halting the child's weight loss. Pay careful attention to changes in taste that affect food preferences. Referral to a dietitian may be helpful to achieve successful modification of the child's diet.
Mouth ulcers	The oral mucositis resulting from chemotherapy usually occurs within 3–4 days and is often a contributing factor in anorexia.	Antifungal agents, such as nystatin or clotrimazole, lessen the possibility of candidal infection. Promote good oral hygiene. Use a soft foam wand or water irrigation to clean teeth; commercial mouthwashes are not recommended because they contain alcohol and increase drying of the oral cavity; specially formulated pharmacological mouthwash may promote comfort.
Constipation	Can occur at any time in treatment but becomes more common as therapy progresses and dietary intake and physical activity decrease.	Stool softeners and laxatives are used to treat this side effect (e.g., MiraLax). Advise parents to increase fluids and fibrous foods in the child's diet.
Pain	Pain can occur at any time and is best understood by subjective explanations of the child.	Acetaminophen, morphine or other narcotics, steroids, nonsteroidal anti-inflammatory drugs, and antidepressants may be used to manage pain; careful monitoring is needed to avoid masking signs of infection with use of acetaminophen for treatment of pain. Careful pain assessment is important. The location of the pain may provide a clue to its cause, for example, metastasis to the skull, infiltration of joints, or damage to soft tissue. Pain associated with chemotherapy may also be related to oral mucositis, myalgia, or tumor embolization; painful polyneuropathy can follow treatment with vincristine or cisplatin. Pharmacologic, nonhypnotic (deep breathing, self-control), and hypnotic methods often prove helpful to children with pain from multiple etiologies.

Since cancer treatment and poor nutritional status can adversely affect the oral status of children, families need help to plan and carry out prophylactic and treatment measures. Children continue to lose teeth, have new teeth erupt, and require nutrients to help in building teeth not yet erupted, even during cancer treatment. Some suggestions are:

- Provide a visit to the dentist early in treatment for assessment, treatment of dental disease, and establishment of a prevention plan.
- Floss and brush teeth twice daily with a soft bristle brush and rinse with water. Use mouthwash as prescribed (normal saline or chlorhexidine are most common).
- Toothpaste can be used unless it causes discomfort.
- Avoid hot, spicy foods and choose mild flavors and soft textures.
- When granulocyte counts fall below 500/mm³ or platelets fall below 40,000/mm³, Toothettes or gauze can be used to clean the teeth. Avoiding brushes will help to prevent bleeding and infection.
- Medications may be used to prevent infection. They may include antibacterial mouthwash, antibacterial lozenges, and suspension to treat mucositis. Continue oral fluoride if it is not present in the drinking water.
- If bleeding, infection, or other oral care needs emerge, consult with the dentist and pediatric oncologist to develop a treatment plan.

Radiation can cause burns to the skin. Examine the skin daily during hospitalization or weekly when making home visits. Leave the marks on the skin that outline the radiation target area. Avoid use of lotions, powders, and soaps on the target skin area. Some children may need to be anesthetized to ensure correct positioning for radiation; postanesthesia care will then be needed.

other substances as a result of treatment. Offer frequent small amounts of fluid. Include frozen ice pops or other fluid-containing foods such as Jell-O. Measure intake and output. To ensure adequate excretion, a number of chemotherapy drugs are given with intravenous fluids. It is important to administer fluids as ordered, monitor intravenous lines carefully, and ensure that the recommended urinary output excretion rate is maintained after drug administration.

Prevent and Treat Infection

Children with cancer have an altered immune system, both from the disease and from the effects of immunosuppressant drugs, and must be kept away from persons with known infections. Teach parents to avoid taking the child to places that attract large gatherings of people, such as department stores, once the child returns home. Emphasize the need to report any exposure to contagious diseases, especially chickenpox. Signs of infection may be masked by some drugs, so be alert for any signs of mild infection. Fever, malaise, and mild respiratory infection must be reported promptly. Follow recommendations for the immunization of children with cancer as published by the Centers for Disease Control and Prevention and the American Academy of Pediatrics. Usually no immunizations are given to the child until 6 months after receiving chemotherapy. Immunity may be lost from some prior immunizations, requiring titer levels and repeat immunization later.

Teach administration of any drugs being used to prevent infection such as pentamidine or sulfa preparations for pneumocystis pneumonia prophylaxis. Management of infections is critical. Children are often hospitalized, and central lines are used for antibiotic administration. Blood cultures and cultures of infected body parts help to establish the causative organisms. Due to lowered immune status, unusual organisms are sometimes identified. Administer medication treatment on time and as ordered. Ensure that standard precautions and transmission-based precautions are followed. Temperature, vital signs, and assessment of all body systems are performed at admission and at least every 4 hours. (See Families Want to Know: Reportable Events for Children Receiving Chemotherapy.)

Manage Pain

The child with cancer may experience pain from the disease itself and from the medical interventions, such as lumbar puncture, bone marrow aspiration, and frequent intravenous infusions and blood draws. Use all possible pain management techniques to keep the child comfortable, as this will assist with comfort and encourage cooperation throughout the long treatment period. (See Chapter 15 ∞ for suggestions on methods of pain management.) Nurses must examine research on effective pain management for children and integrate findings into practice (Figure 24–11 ➤).

Sedation (see Chapter 15 ∞) may be used for some procedures. Administer sedation as ordered for young children who are undergoing lumbar punctures, radiation, and other procedures, and monitor them during and after the procedures. Coordinate painful or intrusive tests so they can be done together while the child is sedated. Topical anesthetics such as EMLA cream may be used to numb the skin before a blood draw or an intravenous start.

Report the following events to your child's oncologist if they occur while the child is receiving chemotherapy:

- Temperature above 38°C (101°F)
- Any bleeding, such as nosebleeds, blood in stool or urine, petechiae, or bruising
- Pain or discomfort with urination or defecation
- Sores in the mouth
- Vomiting or diarrhea
- Persistent pain anywhere, including headache
- Signs of infection, such as cough, fever, runny nose, or tugging at ears
- Signs of infection in central lines, such as redness, drainage, or tenderness
- Exposure to communicable diseases, especially varicella (chickenpox)

Inform dentists and other health care providers that the child is receiving chemotherapy prior to procedures. Prophylactic antibiotics should be given before and after dental care.

Note: Adapted from Bindler, R. M., & Howry, L. B. (2005). *Pediatric drug guide.* Upper Saddle River, NJ: Prentice Hall.

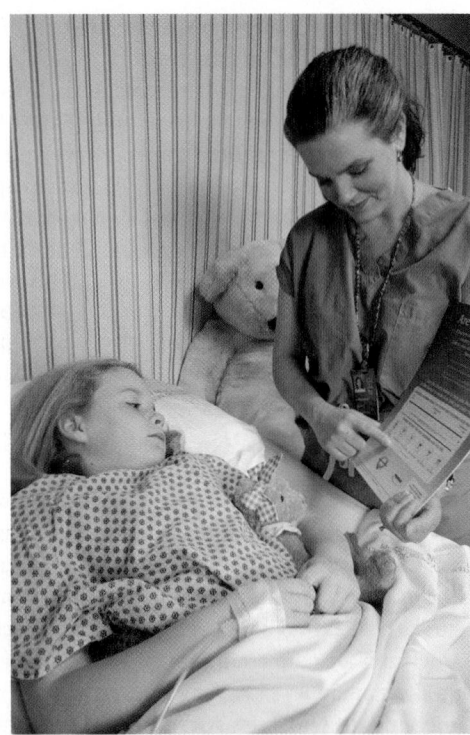

FIGURE 24–11 ➤ The nurse is having the child rate her pain by pointing to the face that most closely matches the way she feels. Note her stuffed animals that provide comfort.

When possible, include the parents in comforting the child during and after painful procedures. Find what techniques work at home to relieve pain and insert them into care of the child in the health facility.

Clinical Tip

EMLA cream, or eutectic mixture of local anesthetics, is a combination of lidocaine 2.5% and prilocaine 2.5% in an emulsion. Apply a thick layer of the cream to intact skin and cover with an occlusive dressing. Leave in place 1 hour for minor procedures and 2 hours for major procedures. Parents can apply at home prior to a scheduled painful procedure. Do not use EMLA on infants who are a gestational age of less than 37 weeks, under 20 kg, or under 12 months and receiving treatment with methemoglobin-inducing agents. For all infants, be certain that parents realize the importance of limiting the area and duration as ordered. Instruct them to keep the cream in a safe place in the home to avoid ingestion by any children. Similarly, LMX4 (lidocaine 4%) can be applied prior to procedures to provide local anesthetic effects.

Other pain prevention measures include fast-acting sprays, intradermal injection of anesthesia with lidocaine, iontophoresis (local anesthetic and electrical current), and sedation. (See the *Clinical Skills Manual* for sedation monitoring.)

Provide Psychosocial Support

A diagnosis of cancer generates many emotions within the family. Initially parents experience shock and anger. They need basic information about the disease and the purpose of the tests that will be performed. Instructions often need to be repeated as parents may not process information the first time it is presented due to their increased stress levels. Assist the parents to

Complementary Therapy
Pain Management

Children have many painful and invasive procedures during cancer treatment. In addition to use of medication, they will be helped by a variety of other pain management techniques. These include:

- The parent's presence during procedures as a support person.
- Use of distraction and relaxation. Either a parent or health care provider can work with the child and integrate techniques, such as singing, counting, telling stories, and blowing bubbles. Children and teens can be taught to visualize positive scenes, use rhythmic breathing, or listen to music.
- Use of hypnosis. This technique has been used successfully to manage both pain and nausea/vomiting during cancer treatment with children from 5–18 years (Richardson, Smith, McCall, et al., 2006).

plan how and when to tell the child the diagnosis. What the child needs to know is based on his or her developmental level and understanding.

After progressing from the initial state of shock about the diagnosis, the family needs to learn more about the disease, including the pathophysiology, treatment, and expected outcome or the prognosis. Clarify the family's understanding of these areas and be ready to answer questions. Provide oral explanations and written material. Parents may talk with friends, purchase books, or search the Internet for information. Find out where they are getting information and provide additional resources when appropriate. Correct misconceptions and misinformation.

The family needs many strategies to deal with the challenge of long-term treatment for cancer. As the child experiences remissions and exacerbations or complications, the family feels alternately hopeful and discouraged. Help the family to identify support systems and intervene as needed to enhance these systems. Facilitate contact with extended family members who might be of help, faith-based or spiritual connections, social service agencies, and other resources such as the Internet and parent support groups. Assist parents who are concerned about job obligations and financial issues. In addition, consider the impact on siblings when a child is being treated for cancer. They may alternately resent and feel guilty for the sibling's illness. They may not understand the treatments or disease. School progress may be slowed and teachers may not be aware of the sibling's stress.

The child undergoing treatment for cancer needs support appropriate to his or her developmental stage and cognitive level. (See Chapters 4 and 11 ∞ for developmental levels and effective support strategies for children of different ages.) Younger children primarily need support during painful procedures and separation from parents. They need to learn about procedures and feel comfortable touching the equipment that is used in their care. Older children also need intervention strategies to assist in working through feelings related to treatments (Figure 24–12 ➤). A major developmental task of adolescence is to attain independence and control, but cancer often interferes with adolescents' ability to achieve this task. Therefore, plan nursing strategies that empower adolescents. Children and adolescents gain strength from participating in usual routines such as school

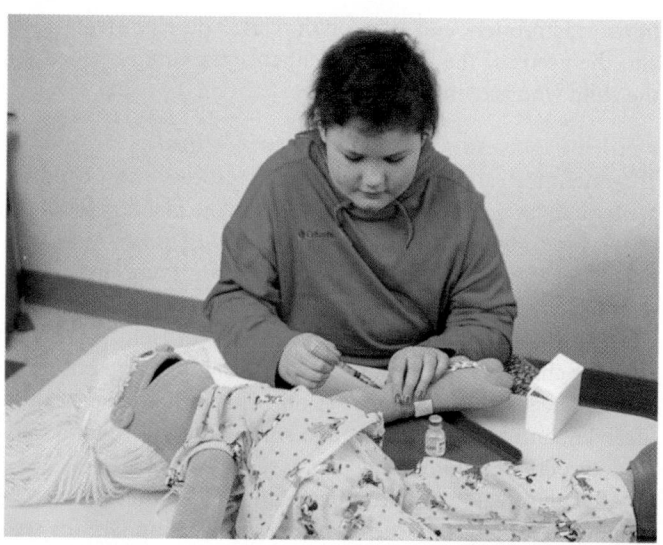

FIGURE 24–12 ➤ A child in a pediatric oncology clinic is giving injections to a doll. This type of play therapy helps the child deal with fear, thus lowering his or her stress level.

as much as possible (Breen, Coombes, & Bradbourne, 2009). (See Evidence-Based Practice: Cancer and Sleep.)

Talk with the child's teachers before he or she returns to school after treatment to explain the child's condition. Arrange for tutors if necessary to assist the child with school work during hospitalization and home care. Explore the option of summer camp for children with cancer. The Make-a-Wish Foundation strives to make dreams come true for children who are ill by sponsoring them for a desired activity or outing. Refer the child to this foundation, if appropriate.

The siblings of a child who has cancer are often stressed by the changes in the family. They may grieve over the ill brother or sister and may feel sad and depressed. They also may experience anger, guilt, or resentment and may have a lack of knowledge about the disease and treatment. Inquire about siblings and ask what they know about the child's condition. Find out who is caring for siblings and whether their teachers have been informed about the family situation. Include siblings in the child's care when possible. Invite them to visit and to participate both during hospitalization and at home care visits. They can be involved in play therapy sessions and recreational activities with the ill child. Ask the parents if the siblings are demonstrating symptoms such as depression, behavioral changes, or decrease in school performance and suggest interventions as appropriate. They may benefit from speaking with a school counselor or can be referred to a support group for siblings of children with cancer. Some cancer summer camps welcome siblings as well as children with cancer.

The family of a child with cancer is faced with a life-threatening illness. Refer to Chapter 13 ∞ for strategies to assist the family in coping with this stress. For some types of cancer, the child may experience a remission with treatment, but then a recurrence of disease later as cancer cells grow again. In this case, the family may become angry or depressed about the relapse. Repeated treatments challenge the family's support systems. Waiting for the outcome of diagnostic tests can be an especially challenging time, so provide information as soon as possible. If the child's illness progresses, refer the family to hospice to assist them in caring for the child who is terminally ill and in working through the grieving process. Explore support groups and information related to cancer in order to share this information with families as well.

Care in the Community

Preparation for home care centers on creating a normal environment while supporting the child's physiologic and psychosocial responses to the cancer and treatments. Education is the

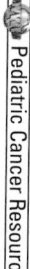

Pediatric Cancer Resources

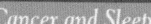

Evidence-Based Practice

Cancer and Sleep

Problem

Inadequate amounts and quality of sleep are common problems among youth. Busy schedules, use of screen technologies, and other causes often lead to poor sleep habits. Daytime sleepiness and other outcomes can result (Sedeh, Dahl, Shahar, et al., 2009). The child or adolescent with cancer is even more likely to have disturbed sleep, due to cancer itself, the treatment protocols, and associated symptoms or worry.

Evidence

A systematic review examined the measurement of sleep in adolescence, by measures such as questionnaires, sleep diaries, and actigraphy (use of a watch-like device that measures movement and accurately shows sleep) (Erickson, 2009). Primary reasons for disturbed sleep in cancer treatment include pain, frequent awakenings or fragmented sleep, and symptoms such as nausea.

A study of nine children with leukemia and their parents found that there were more frequent awakenings than prior to diagnosis, and that the children reported pain symptoms at night. Resultant daytime fatigue also was reported (Gedaly-Duff, Lee, Nail, et al., 2006).

Implications

Cancer interfaces with normal developmental progression in several ways, one of which is sleep. Adolescents as a group are frequently sleep-deprived and experience daytime sleepiness. Adolescents with cancer are even more likely to have sleep problems, exacerbated by the cancer itself and side effects of symptoms or treatment. Sleep patterns should be questioned at each oncology visit, suggestions for sleep hygiene should be provided, and the teen can be referred to the oncology specialist for additional interventions to handle sleep disruptions. Provide instructions about methods for ensuring adequate sleep, such as removing televisions and cell phones from bedrooms, providing rest periods each day, and maintaining routines that enable sleep. (See Chapter 9 ∞ for further information about sleep hygiene.)

Critical Thinking Application

Plan a series of questions to ask an adolescent about the amount of sleep obtained on weekdays and weekends, patterns of sleep, use of screen media during the night, and any changes in sleep that have occurred since cancer was diagnosed. Inquire about daytime sleepiness and fatigue. Plan a list of sleep hygiene measures that assist adolescents in acquiring needed sleep time and quality.

primary focus of discharge planning. Teach the parents how to ensure adequate nutritional intake, to be alert for signs of infection, to protect the child from exposure to communicable diseases during times of neutropenia, to administer medications at home, and to handle vomiting and pain. Assist the parents and child to deal with any obstacles to normal development and functioning. Teach the parents and family about symptoms that need to be treated immediately.

Home management of a vascular access device or central line, such as a Broviac catheter (refer to the *Clinical Skills Manual*), is an initial challenge for parents (Figure 24–13 ➤). Alternatively, an implanted port may be used and allows the child freedom to swim and engage in other activities. Parents will need information about whatever device the child has received. Details about cleaning the site, keeping the line open, and other needed care are demonstrated and reviewed. After teaching the parents, observe them performing the procedure before the child is discharged.

Emphasize the need for the child and family to have usual family activities, including recreational activities. Play distracts the child and is essential in reducing fears. Children, parents, and siblings often benefit from participation in cancer support groups and cancer summer camps. These activities create additional support systems, build the child's self-esteem, and enhance coping skills through role modeling.

Make home visits to evaluate the family's strengths and needs. Refer to support services and websites as appropriate. Be sure that the family has adequate support from a hospice and other end-of-life services when the child's condition is terminal. The presence of a palliative care team; an integrated plan of care; collaboration between families, the primary care provider, and

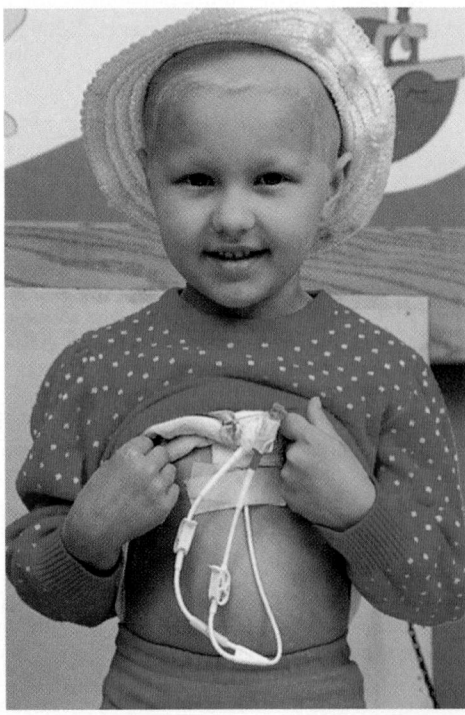

FIGURE 24–13 ➤ A vascular access device allows chemotherapeutic agents to be administered without the need for repeated "sticks" to the child.

other practitioners; and focus on the child's developmental level and the needs of the family can enhance the care provided for the child who is dying.

Health Promotion and Health Maintenance

Treatment for cancer is generally a long process; most children are treated for a period of 2–3 years. Since normal developmental stages progress during this time, health promotion and health maintenance visits should still occur. Some usual care may have to be altered, but many of the same developmental concerns of all children should be addressed. Help parents to view the child as a "normal" child who is ill for a period of time, but still needs to have limits set on behavior, develop healthy lifestyles, and have environmental stimulation to learn to talk, read, or perform motor and cognitive tasks.

After the treatment is complete, the child should be closely monitored for any sequelae of cancer survivorship (see the section earlier in the chapter about issues of survivorship). The possibility of treatment-related physical and psychological side effects necessitates clear instructions to the family, with increasing information provided to the child as cognitive development proceeds. Periodic laboratory and diagnostic tests may be needed, in addition to thorough physical and psychological examinations. Guidelines for health care professionals and survivors have been developed by the Childhood Cancer Survivor Study (Armstrong, 2010; Leigh, 2008; Oeffinger et al., 2008). When the child transfers to the care of a health care professional who serves adults, provide a clear and complete summary of the cancer and treatment so that appropriate follow-up can be maintained.

Evaluation

The following expected outcomes of nursing care for the child with cancer relate to the specific disease, treatments, and responses:

- The child has adequate nutritional intake to promote normal growth.
- Hydration is adequate to support body processes and ensure drug and cancer cell product elimination.
- Side effects of the cancer and therapies are promptly identified and treated.
- Pain is managed to a level of comfort satisfactory to the child and family.
- The family uses resources to provide necessary support during hospitalizations and treatments.
- The child and family demonstrate knowledge of management needed for treatment regimens.
- All family members accept the prognosis in order to support the child.

■ SOLID TUMORS

Brain Tumors

Central nervous system or brain tumors are the most commonly occurring solid tumors in children and the second most common malignancy, after leukemia. Each year in the United States approximately 1,700 children up to 14 years, and about 2,200 youth up to 20 years are diagnosed with tumors of the brain and central nervous system, accounting for one in five childhood cancers (Blaney, Kun, Hunter, et al., 2006; Bleyer, 2007).

Etiology and Pathophysiology

The cause of most brain tumors is unknown; about 5–10% are genetic in origin. Exposure to radiation is a risk factor, such as CNS radiation used for treatment of some other cancers. There is a higher incidence in children with certain other disease such as retinoblastoma, renal tumors, neurofibromatosis, tuberous sclerosis, or endocrine syndromes (Blaney et al., 2006).

Brain tumors in children usually occur below the roof of the cerebellum and involve the cerebellum, midbrain, and brainstem (Figure 24–14 ➤). In contrast, brain tumors in adults are usually located above the areas between the cerebrum and cerebellum.

Clinical Manifestations

Brain tumors can manifest in children through behavioral and nervous system changes; these result from increased intracranial pressure and may occur either rapidly or more slowly and subtly. Some common symptoms include headache (most common manifestation), nausea, vomiting, abnormal gait, dizziness, change in vision or hearing, fatigue, and mental status changes, such as educational or behavioral problems (Wilne, Collier, Kennedy, et al., 2007; Wilne, Ferris, Nathwani, et al., 2006).

Brainstem tumors can present with weight deficits, and may be mistakenly diagnosed as an eating disorder of infancy and childhood (failure to thrive). This may delay proper treatment. See Clinical Manifestations: Brain Tumors.

Clinical Tip

Some children with brain tumors have nonspecific signs. They may have a slight behavior change, perform poorly at school, or show some incoordination. Be alert to such signs and to the parents' statement that they notice a change in the child. Report such findings so appropriate assessments can be made.

Medulloblastomas, brain tumors in the external layer of the cerebellum, account for 10–20% of childhood brain tumors, and commonly occur in children ages 5 to 6 years. They are fast-growing and therefore often present with sudden onset of symptoms such as increased intracranial pressure, manifested by increased head circumference in infants, vomiting, headache, ataxia, and vision changes. *Astrocytomas* arise from glial cells and can be either above or below the area between the cerebrum and cerebellum. They comprise 40–60% of childhood brain tumors, and vary from low-grade cerebellar to low-grade cerebral or high-grade tumors. The presenting symptoms vary depending

Pathophysiology Illustrated
Sites of Brain Tumors in Children

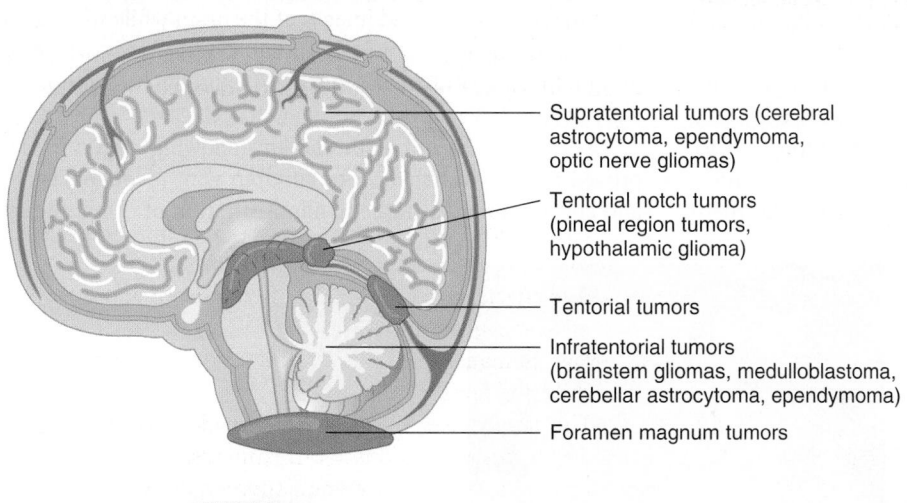

- Supratentorial tumors (cerebral astrocytoma, ependymoma, optic nerve gliomas)
- Tentorial notch tumors (pineal region tumors, hypothalamic glioma)
- Tentorial tumors
- Infratentorial tumors (brainstem gliomas, medulloblastoma, cerebellar astrocytoma, ependymoma)
- Foramen magnum tumors

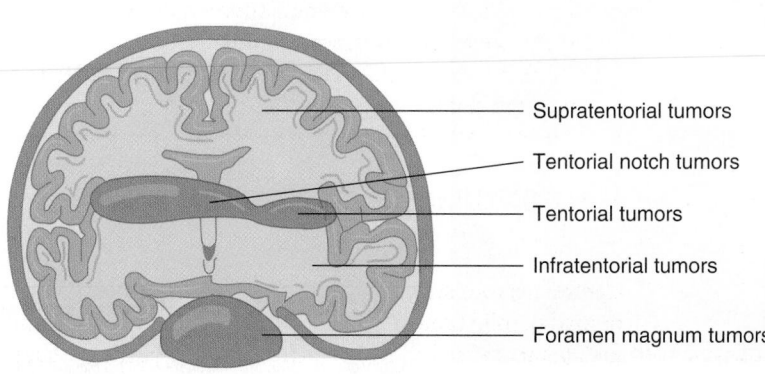

- Supratentorial tumors
- Tentorial notch tumors
- Tentorial tumors
- Infratentorial tumors
- Foramen magnum tumors

FIGURE 24–14 ➤ Approximately 3,000 children and adolescents under the age of 15 years are diagnosed with tumors of the brain and central nervous system each year. The four most common brain tumors in children are medulloblastoma, cerebral astrocytoma, ependymoma, and brainstem glioma.

Clinical Manifestations
Brain Tumors

Tumor	Location	Clinical Manifestations	Clinical Therapy
Medulloblastoma	External layer of cerebellum	Headache, vomiting, ataxia	Surgery; chemotherapy with lomustine, vincristine, prednisone, cisplatin; radiation
Astrocytomas	Glial cells, supratentorial or infratentorial	Seizures, visual disturbances, increased intracranial pressure, vomiting	Surgery; chemotherapy with vincristine, dactinomycin; radiation
Ependymoma	Fourth ventricle, posterior fossa	Hydrocephalus	Surgery, radiation
Brainstem gliomas	Pons	Cranial nerve (VI and VII) tract signs, nystagmus, ataxia, motor symptoms	Surgery, radiation

on the location of the tumor. Endocrine, vision, and behavioral changes are all possible, as well as increased intracranial pressure and seizures. *Ependymomas* commonly occur in the fourth ventricle of the posterior fossa and comprise 5–10% of childhood brain tumors. Impaired growth, hydrocephalus, seizures, and cranial nerve impairments are the most common manifestations. *Gliomas*, which can occur in the brainstem or as supratentorial lesions, account for 15% of brain tumors in children. Brainstem gliomas are located in the pons and typically spread into the surrounding tissue. Cranial nerve impairments, mental status changes, seizures, and motor symptoms occur.

COLLABORATIVE CARE

Diagnostic Tests

The first step in diagnosing brain tumors is a detailed health history and physical examination. Onset of symptoms, severity, and presentation of neurological symptoms are recorded. Brain tumors are then definitively diagnosed by means of computed tomography (CT; Figure 24–15A ➤), magnetic resonance imaging (MRI; Figure 24–15B), positron emission tomography (PET), single-photon emission computed tomography (SPECT), myelography, and angiography. Neurophysiologic tests (electroen-cephalography and brainstem evoked potentials) are used to assess sensory pathway integrity and disease- or drug-related sensory dysfunction. Other tests that may be performed are use of tumor markers such as α-fetoprotein and human chorionic gonadotropin. Analysis of DNA is also useful in some types of cancer when a genetic basis is related to the cancer type. Lumbar puncture is used to identify abnormal cells in the cerebrospinal fluid. Bone marrow aspiration identifies any extracranial primary neoplastic growth, as cancers in other sites can metastasize to the brain.

Clinical Therapy

Treatment depends on the type of brain tumor. Surgery is a common treatment, and may be performed to obtain a biopsy specimen, to debulk (reduce the tumor size by partial removal) or excise the tumor, or to treat any hydrocephalus that may be present. During surgery, radiology images allow the neurosurgeon to see computerized images of the brain while stimulating nerves to determine their functioning. Laser surgery, which has delicate precise control and accuracy, is used when tumors are close to sensitive neural or vascular structures.

Use of radiation and chemotherapy following surgery has improved the survival chances of children with medulloblastoma and ependymoma. Intrathecal administration of chemotherapy

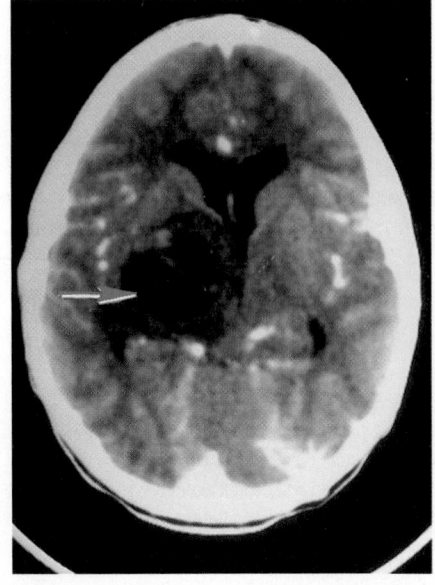

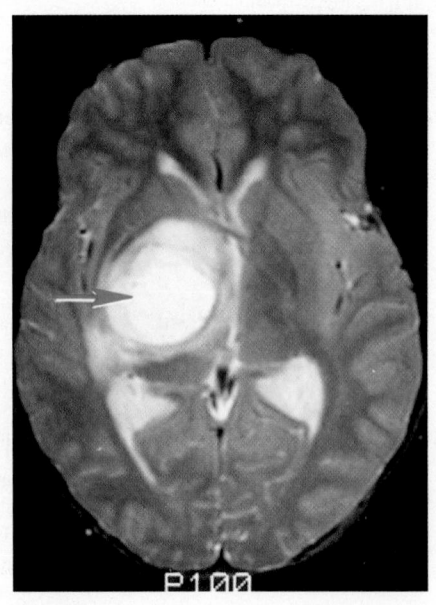

A   **B**

FIGURE 24–15 ➤ Radiologic imaging of a child with a brain tumor. A, CT scan. B, MRI.

Courtesy of Carlos Sivit, MD, Children's National Medical Center, Washington, DC.

is useful in some cases. However, the blood-brain barrier is a factor in the effectiveness of chemotherapy for children with brain tumors. For example, when methotrexate is administered intrathecally (in the spinal canal), only a small amount crosses normal brain capillaries. Bone marrow and stem cell transplantation is an increasingly used treatment option.

Many new approaches are being investigated and some are expected to emerge as viable treatments in the years ahead. New combinations of chemotherapeutic agents, precision-guided delivery of medications and radiation, gene therapy, and cytokine-producing therapy to activate the immune system are examples of emerging treatments (Robertson, 2006).

Complications of treatment for children with brain tumors are significant. They include severe infections (associated with high-dose chemotherapy), seizure activity, sensorimotor defects, hydrocephalus, and growth problems. Care is taken to treat infections early and aggressively. If a cerebrospinal shunt is used, infection or blockage can occur (see Chapter 27 ∞ for further discussion of cerebrospinal shunts in children). Anticonvulsants are commonly given prophylactically following surgery. Endocrine problems, such as growth hormone changes, hypothyroidism, and panhypopituitarism, may occur when the tumor is in the hypothalamic-pituitary area. Treatment may also lead to impaired cognitive function and emotional or behavioral problems in some children. Memory deficits and selective attention deficits are the most common problems.

Diabetes insipidus is a special consideration in children with midline brain tumors, such as those that compress the hypothalamus, pituitary stalk, or posterior pituitary gland. Manifestations of diabetes insipidus include voiding of large amounts of dilute urine with a specific gravity of less than 1.005 to 1.010 (see Chapter 30 ∞).

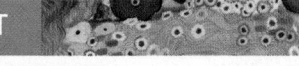

NURSING MANAGEMENT

Nursing Assessment and Diagnosis

The focus of physiologic assessment of the child with a brain tumor is determined by its presentation (Table 24–3). Presenting signs can be categorized as follows:

- Nonspecific signs related to increasing intracranial pressure
- Secondary signs related to displacement of intracranial structures
- Focal signs suggesting direct involvement of the brain and cranial nerves

Thorough neurologic examination before surgery is essential to provide a record of baseline functioning and allow evaluation of the child's changing physiologic status before surgery. Ask if the child has manifested slow changes over time or has had quickly developing symptoms. Measurement of head circumference and assessment of the anterior fontanel are necessary in children under the age of 18 months.

Perform developmental screening on young children using the Denver II or other developmental tests (see Chapter 7 ∞). Ask about the child's social interactions, school performance, and any behavior changes that have occurred.

The following nursing diagnoses can be identified for the child with a brain tumor, depending on the type and location of the tumor:

- Imbalanced Nutrition: Less than Body Requirements related to loss of appetite
- Impaired Physical Mobility related to tumor pressure on coordination centers
- Delayed Growth and Development related to effects of disability
- Impaired Memory related to neurologic disturbance
- Acute Pain related to compression of brain tissue and diagnostic tests

Planning and Implementation

The child with a brain tumor requires multidisciplinary care by a neurologist, neurosurgeon, pediatrician, dietitian, social worker, and other specialists. The nurse can act as a case manager to coordinate the complex care needed by the child and help the family to understand treatment.

For the nursing care of children immediately following surgery, refer to Chapter 11 ∞. In addition, close monitoring of neurologic status is needed postoperatively (see Chapter 27 ∞). Subtle alterations such as visual differences, behavior or alertness variations, and gait changes can herald serious problems from the tumor or pressure in the brain. Many children return from surgery with a ventricular-peritoneal shunt. Be especially alert for signs of increased intracranial pressure and infection. Observe for seizure activity. Administer drugs such as antibiotics and anticonvulsants as ordered.

Signs and symptoms of diabetes insipidus may occur following brain surgery (see Chapter 30 ∞ for a description of diabetes insipidus). Nursing care includes hourly measurement of intake and output, measurement of serum sodium levels every 4 to 6 hours, accurate fluid replacement, and frequent assessment

TABLE 24–3 Physiologic Assessment of Brain Tumors	
Clinical Manifestations	Assessment
Nonspecific signs: headache, morning vomiting, somnolence, irritability	Level of consciousness, pupil response, pupil shape and size
Secondary signs: disturbances of cranial nerves; other signs depend on site of tumor	All cranial nerves
Focal signs: truncal ataxia (midline brain tumors), general nystagmus, head tilting	Motor ability, head positions when watching television or looking at people (double vision, sixth cranial nerve involvement)

of neurologic status. An indwelling urinary catheter is useful for accurate measurement of urinary output.

Discharge Planning and Home Care Teaching

Teach the parents to watch for an increase in voiding of dilute urine. Be sure they can recognize the signs of infection and changes in the child's neurologic status. Once the child is ready for discharge, chemotherapy or radiation may begin; inform parents of the reason for these treatments and their potential side effects. Assist the family in obtaining any special equipment they may need to care for the child at home, such as a wheelchair, bed rails, or dressings. The American Cancer Society is a potential resource for assistance with these needs.

Children with brain tumors, especially those who have received radiation, often have some permanent sequelae. They may have slowed development, incoordination, learning disabilities, or other effects. These sequelae are most common in children who are 3 years of age or younger at the time of radiation therapy. Perform accurate height and weight measurements at each health care visit. Assess developmental milestones. Ask about progress in school and any special services that might be needed. Perform thorough neurologic assessments. Support the family as they learn to deal with unknown or changed expectations for the child's performance.

Evaluation

Expected outcomes of nursing care for the child with a brain tumor depend on the site of the tumor, clinical therapy, and medical outcome. Possible outcomes include the following:

- Nutritional intake will be adequate to support growth and prevent malnutrition.
- A safe environment will be maintained for the child.
- Physical mobility to maximum level allowed by developmental level and alterations of disease will be attained.
- An environment will be provided to meet normal developmental milestones within the child's capability.
- Pain will be successfully managed to reach a comfort level.
- Parents display understanding of the diagnosis and treatment plan.

Neuroblastoma

Neuroblastoma is the solid tumor most commonly occurring outside the cranium of children. It is responsible for 8–10% of childhood cancers and 15% of cancer deaths in children. The average age at onset is 2 years; it is the most common tumor in infants during the first year of life. Nearly all cases are diagnosed before 5 years of age (Ater, 2007; Park, Eggert, & Caron, 2008). Prognosis varies, depending on the staging of the tumor (Table 24–4) and the age of the child, with more favorable outcomes in infants under 1 year of age, and in presenting sites in the pelvis or thorax. Less favorable outcomes are associated with the presence of N-myc oncogene amplification. Survival rates are 98% for stages 1 and 2, but drop to 22% for stage 4 (Kim & Chung, 2006).

Neuroblastoma is commonly a smooth, hard, nontender mass that can occur anywhere along the sympathetic nervous

TABLE 24–4	International Neuroblastoma Staging System
Stage	Description
1	Localized tumor confined to the area of origin; complete gross excision, with or without microscopic residual disease; identifiable ipsilateral and contralateral lymph nodes negative microscopically
2A	Unilateral tumor with incomplete gross excision; identifiable ipsilateral and contralateral lymph nodes negative microscopically
2B	Unilateral tumor with complete or incomplete gross excision; with positive ipsilateral regional lymph nodes; identifiable contralateral lymph nodes negative microscopically
3	Tumor infiltrating across the midline with or without regional lymph node involvement; or unilateral tumor with contralateral regional lymph node involvement; or midline tumor with bilateral regional lymph node involvement
4	Dissemination of tumor to distant lymph nodes, bone, bone marrow, liver, and/or other organs (except as defined in stage 4S)
4S	Localized primary tumor as defined for stage 1 or 2 with dissemination limited to liver, skin, and/or bone marrow in an infant less than 1 year of age; bone marrow involvement should be minimal (less than 10% of cells); if greater it is stage 4 disease

Note: Data from National Cancer Institute. (2007a). Neuroblastoma treatment: Stage information.

system chain. A frequent location is the abdomen, although other sites are the adrenal, thoracic, and cervical areas.

Etiology and Pathophysiology

Neuroblastoma originates in primitive neurocrest cells that form the adrenal medulla, paraganglia, and sympathetic nervous system of the cervical sympathetic chain and the thoracic chain. Approximately 50% of neuroblastomas develop in the adrenal medulla; 30% develop in the cervical, thoracic, or pelvic ganglia; and the remaining are elsewhere along the sympathetic chain (Ater, 2007). Lymph node metastasis is common.

The cause of neuroblastoma is unknown. Theories center on the possible effects of environmental factors such as prenatal drug exposure from the mother and disturbed cellular nerve growth factors. A genetic defect found in many cases of neuroblastoma is a deletion of the short arm of chromosome 1 (1p del); other abnormalities include 11q, 14q, and 17q. Oncogenes are present in neuroblastoma cells in a DNA sequence known as N-myc, located on chromosome 2. High levels of the N-myc oncogene are associated with rapid disease progression and a poorer prognosis (Ater, 2007).

Clinical Manifestations

The location of the mass determines the symptoms. Altered bowel and bladder function occur when the mass is retroperitoneal; characteristic signs are weight loss, abdominal fullness, irritability, fatigue, and fever. Dyspnea or infection may occur when the tumor is mediastinal. Neck and facial edema may result from vena cava syndrome if the tumor is mediastinal and large. Intracranial lesions may be present with periorbital ecchymosis. Malaise, fever, and a limp can occur if there has been metastasis to the bone. Bone marrow disease can manifest as **pancytopenia** (abnormal depression of all cellular blood components) with neutropenia (causing infections) and anemia (causing fatigue). Metastatic spread can result in an array of symptoms affecting multiple organs.

COLLABORATIVE CARE

Diagnostic Tests

The International Neuroblastoma Staging System (INSS) recommends different diagnostic and laboratory evaluations for diagnosis of the primary disease and of metastases (Table 24–5).

Routine blood cell counts are needed, including CBC with differential. The test may reveal anemia and thrombocytopenia. There is no classic WBC response, although thrombocytopenia may occur in association with disseminated intravascular coagulation. **Leukocytosis** (higher than normal leukocyte count) and **leukopenia** (lower than normal leukocyte count) have been observed with bone marrow involvement. Serum electrolytes, liver function studies, LDH, coagulation studies, and urinalysis are performed. Baseline cardiac function is evaluated if doxorubicin will be used in treatment.

Tumor markers include VMA, HVA, dopamine, ferritin, NSE, LDH, and a ganglioside GD2. Vanillylmandelic acid (VMA) and homovanillic acid (HVA) are by-products of adrenal hormones, and their levels are usually elevated in the urine and blood (see Appendix C ∞ for normal values). Urinary catecholamines are increased. Elevations in dopamine, ferritin, NSE (an enzyme in neural tissue), LDH, and GD2 (a sugar and lipid molecule on the surface of neural cells) are seen. All of these laboratory findings are used initially to diagnose the disease and later to follow its progress. A biopsy or surgical removal of the tumor will be followed by analysis of its type and genetic abnormalities. Areas of necrosis and calcification in major organs are readily identifiable with radiologic tests and MRIs. These tests also help in the staging of the disease by identifying metastases.

TABLE 24–5 Diagnostic Tests for Neuroblastoma

Tests for Initial Diagnosis	Tests for Metastases
Tumor tissue diagnosis by light microscopy, or Biopsy of tumor cells plus laboratory evaluation showing increased urine or serum catecholamines (two separate measures each more than 3 standard deviations above the norm for age)	Bone marrow aspirate and biopsy Radiolabeled scanning with metaiodobenzylguanidine (MIBG) Bone scan Skeletal radiograph CT or MRI of abdomen, liver, brain, eye orbits MRI of spine Chest radiograph, with added CT or MRI if radiograph shows lesions

Clinical Therapy

The stage of the tumor (see Table 24–4) determines the treatment protocol. Surgical excision of the mass is performed and may be the only treatment in low-risk stages. With higher risk, surgery is followed by chemotherapy consisting of a combination of drugs. Several courses of chemotherapy may be needed prior to surgery when the mass is large or wrapped around major blood vessels. Chemotherapy may include medications such as cyclophosphamide, ifosfamide, doxorubicin, carboplatin, teniposide, etoposide, and cisplatin.

Radiation is often used, especially in disseminated disease or when tumors are not receptive to chemotherapy. Stem cell transplantation may be performed for advanced disease, sometimes followed by the biological modifier *cis*-retinoic acid and fenretinide (to promote apoptosis). Studies are being conducted involving GD2, natural killer cells, gene therapy to interrupt growth of abnormal cells, antitumor vaccines, monoclonal antibodies with growth factors, and high-dose chemotherapy (Ater, 2007).

NURSING MANAGEMENT

Nursing Assessment and Diagnosis

The presenting site of the tumor, such as the neck or abdomen, is assessed by observation and inspection. Palpation is contraindicated. Carefully document related functioning, such as bowel and bladder function. Take vital signs to watch for elevated temperature and vital sign changes caused by a thoracic mass. Observe gait and coordination. Take weight and height measurements and compare them with earlier percentiles for the child. Specific assessments during treatment will depend on the treatment methods used (refer to the earlier discussions of chemotherapy and radiation treatment). Psychosocial and emotional assessments of the family are needed.

Clinical Judgment

Why is palpation of the tumor contraindicated when the child has a neuroblastoma? How can you notify other health care providers that palpation should not occur?

The following nursing diagnoses may be appropriate for the child with neuroblastoma, depending on the location and extent of the presenting disease:

- Impaired Gas Exchange related to ventilation-perfusion imbalance
- Impaired Physical Mobility related to neuromuscular impairment
- Disturbed Sensory Perception Alteration (Visual) related to loss of vision
- Chronic Pain related to pressure of tumor and injury to tissues
- Anticipatory Grieving (Family) related to potential loss of significant person

Planning and Implementation

Nursing management of the child with neuroblastoma can encompass the three phases of medical treatment: chemotherapy, surgery, and radiation. Specific postsurgical care depends on the size and site of the tumor. Normal postoperative care includes providing fluid support and respiratory care and preventing infection.

Nursing care during the chemotherapy phase includes minimizing side effects, preventing infection, teaching parents about the medications their child is receiving, and monitoring the young child's physical and emotional growth and development. When radiation is part of the treatment, use common nursing measures described earlier in the chapter. Topics for parent and family teaching and discharge planning are presented in Families Want to Know: The Child with Neuroblastoma. Ongoing support and connection to resources to assist in management of the child's treatment at home will be needed. When the prognosis is poor, parents may appreciate referrals to hospice, to other parents who have experienced similar child illnesses, and to other community resources. See Chapter 13 ∞ for additional nursing care for end of life.

Clinical Tip

Many oncology centers provide notebooks with information on chemotherapy and other relevant treatment approaches to families shortly after diagnosis. Information that is pertinent to the child is highlighted during the teaching sessions. Blank pages are included to encourage parents to use the notebook for recording information, tests and results, personal thoughts, and questions.

Evaluation

Expected outcomes of nursing care for the child with neuroblastoma include the following:

- Ventilatory exchange adequate to support daily activities
- Physical mobility to level possible considering developmental age
- Management of sensory/perceptual alterations to provide for safety and sensory input
- Pain management to level of comfort
- Acceptance and integration of diagnosis into lives of family members

Wilms Tumor (Nephroblastoma)

Nephroblastoma is a common intrarenal abdominal tumor of childhood and accounts for 6% of all childhood tumors (Dome, Perlman, Ritchey, et al., 2006). The incidence is approximately 7.6 cases per million children annually. The most common type is Wilms tumor, which occurs most frequently between 41 and 47 months of age, with young ages more commonly associated with bilateral disease (Dome et al., 2006; Jaffe & Huff, 2007; Kim & Chung, 2006).

Etiology and Pathophysiology

Wilms tumor is associated with several congenital anomalies: aniridia (absence of the iris), hemihypertrophy (abnormal growth of half of the body or a body structure), genitourinary anomalies, nevi, and hamartomas (benign, nodule-like growths).

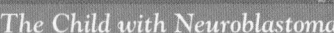

Families Want to Know
The Child with Neuroblastoma

Surgery phase

- Teach the parents to observe for signs of infection at the wound site and to take the child's temperature, if necessary.
- Assist the family to provide pain management including medication administration and various comfort measures.
- Teach the parents the importance of keeping accurate records of urine output and bowel movements and to notify the health care provider if the child does not have a bowel movement at least every 3 days.
- Continue with progression to a regular diet.

Chemotherapy phase

- The child frequently has a central line placed early in the chemotherapy phase. The central line greatly reduces the emotional trauma associated with chemotherapy and blood tests.
- Teach the child how to help the parents with cleaning of the central line.
- Teach the child how to protect the central line.
- Teach the parents how to clean and dress the site of the central line.
- Have the parents practice central line care with a model and then on the child before discharge to increase the parents' confidence.
- Give the parents written and illustrated information about care of a central line.
- Arrange for home care dressing supplies before discharge.
- Give the parents detailed chemotherapy information.
- Teach administration of any medications that the parent will perform via central line or other routes.
- Refer the family to the American Cancer Society for coloring books and other resources for children receiving chemotherapy.

These connections suggest a genetic link; chromosome deletions at 11p13 and 11p15 (locations for WT1 and WT2 genes) have been associated with Wilms tumor. There is a high incidence with Beckwith-Wiedemann syndrome, which is characterized by macroglossia and hypoglycemia. However, most children with Wilms tumor have no other abnormalities. A tumor suppressor gene has been identified that acts to promote normal kidney development. This gene and others may be missing in children with Wilms tumor. Wilms tumor grows very quickly, doubling its size in 11 to 13 days. Such fast growth generally contributes to a large tumor by the time of diagnosis. However, chemotherapy drugs have significantly increased survival rates for children with Wilms tumor, with even stage III and IV groups having a 10-year survival rate, or 75% and 55%, respectively (Kutluk, Varan, Buyukpamukcu, et al., 2006). Tissue type is associated with outcome, with anaplastic tumors having a less favorable prognosis.

Clinical Manifestations

Wilms tumor is usually an asymptomatic, firm, lobulated mass located to one side of the midline in the abdomen. Often a parent discovers the mass during the child's bath. Hypertension caused by increased renin activity related to renal damage is reported in 25% of cases. Hematuria or abdominal pain is sometimes present.

COLLABORATIVE CARE

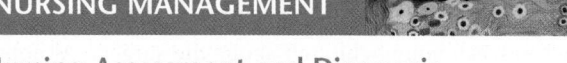

The diagnosis of Wilms tumor is based on an ultrasound study of the abdomen and an intravenous pyelogram. CT scanning or MRI of the lungs, liver, spleen, and brain may be performed to identify any metastasis. This information is used in staging the tumor (Table 24–6). A complete blood count is obtained, as well as BUN and creatinine levels, and liver function tests are performed. Histologic examination is performed for tissue typing once the tumor is removed.

Treatment is multifaceted and increasingly successful. About 90% of early stages and 70% of metastatic cases have long-term survival (Kutluk et al., 2006). Surgery is performed to remove the affected kidney, to examine the opposite kidney, and to look for other sites of metastasis. Chemotherapy or radiation therapy, alone or in combination, is sometimes used before surgery to reduce the size of the tumor. Children with stage III and IV disease often receive vincristine, dactinomycin, and doxorubicin; cyclophosphamide is sometimes added as well. Radiation may also follow surgery, especially in disseminated disease. Children whose tumors are almost completely excised and who have a favorable prognosis do not require irradiation of the tumor bed.

Long-term complications of treatment include liver damage, portal hypertension, and mild cirrhosis, which may occur in children treated for right-sided Wilms tumor. Radiation damage (such as thinning or weakening) of the skeleton, pelvis, and thorax has been reported. Kyphosis and scoliosis may occur from irradiation of vertebral bodies and the pelvis. Glomerular damage to the remaining kidney may also occur. Secondary malignancies in the original radiation field have occurred with orthovoltage radiation, but recent changes in radiation therapy have reduced this risk.

NURSING MANAGEMENT

Nursing Assessment and Diagnosis

Perform a thorough baseline assessment of the child. Do not palpate the abdomen, as this may potentially spread the cancerous cells. Monitor the child's blood pressure carefully because hypertension is a common finding that may require treatment.

Nursing Alert

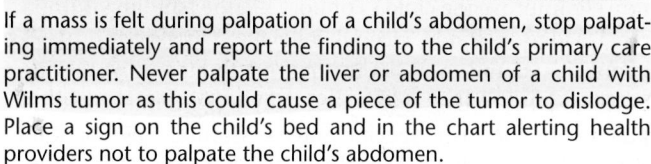

If a mass is felt during palpation of a child's abdomen, stop palpating immediately and report the finding to the child's primary care practitioner. Never palpate the liver or abdomen of a child with Wilms tumor as this could cause a piece of the tumor to dislodge. Place a sign on the child's bed and in the chart alerting health providers not to palpate the child's abdomen.

Nursing diagnoses for a child with Wilms tumor will differ depending on the phase of treatment. Common nursing diagnoses may include the following:

- Risk for Infection related to inadequate defenses
- Impaired Urinary Elimination related to anatomic obstruction
- Ineffective Cardiopulmonary Tissue Perfusion related to hypertension caused by mechanical reduction of blood flow
- Risk for Caregiver Role Strain related to child's illness severity

Planning and Implementation

Nursing management can be divided into two phases: the postrenal surgery phase and the chemotherapy phase. (See

TABLE 24–6	National Wilms Tumor Study Staging System
Stage	Description
I	The tumor is limited to the kidney and completely excised. The surface of the renal capsule is intact. The tumor is not ruptured before or during removal. No residual tumor is apparent beyond the margins of the excision.
II	The tumor extends beyond the kidney but is completely excised. Regional extension of the tumor is present (i.e., penetration through the outer surface of the renal capsule into the perirenal soft tissues). Vessels outside the kidney substance are infiltrated or contain tumor thrombus. Biopsy may have been performed on the tumor, or local spillage of tumor confined to the flank has occurred. No residual tumor is apparent at or beyond the margin of excision.
III	Residual nonhematogenous tumor is confined to the abdomen. Any of the following may occur: Lymph nodes on biopsy are found to be involved in the hilus, the periaortic chains, or beyond. Diffuse peritoneal contamination by the tumor has occurred, such as by spillage of tumor beyond the flank before or during surgery, or by tumor growth that has penetrated through the peritoneal surface. Implants are found on peritoneal surfaces. The tumor extends beyond the surgical margins either microscopically or grossly. The tumor is not completely resectable because of local infiltration into vital structures.
IV	Hematogenous metastasis: deposits are present beyond stage III (e.g., lung, liver, bone, and/or brain).
V	Bilateral renal involvement is present at diagnosis. An attempt should be made to stage each side according to the above criteria on the basis of extent of disease before biopsy.

Note: Data from National Cancer Institute. (2007b). *Wilms tumor and other childhood kidney tumors: Stage information.*

Chapter 11 ∞ for general care of the child after surgery.) Drawings and special teaching dolls with removable kidneys can be used to teach young children about the surgery. Although chemotherapy may occur at two different times, before and after surgery, nursing management considerations remain the same.

Nursing care during the postrenal surgery phase focuses on pain management and close monitoring of fluid levels. A large incision is necessary to remove the kidney, and the resultant postoperative shift of organs and fluid in the abdominal cavity may create discomfort for the child. Frequently reposition the child and use noninvasive and pharmacologic pain interventions to improve the child's comfort. Gentle handling is important. Monitor fluids closely following surgery to prevent hypovolemia and to assess the shift of fluids out of the third space and out of the body. Assess daily weight, intake and output (I&O), and urine specific gravity. Monitor the function of the remaining kidney. Take blood pressure measurements frequently to watch for signs of shock and to assess the functioning of the remaining kidney.

During the chemotherapy phase, monitor the child for side effects of drugs, the potential for infection from the central line site, and the function of the remaining kidney. Advise parents about home care needs, administration of medications, and monitoring for drug side effects and ongoing needs for health monitoring. Ensure that care is well coordinated among all the health care providers.

Evaluation

Desired outcomes for nursing care of the child with nephroblastoma include balanced intake and output, normal vital signs, recovery from surgery, and successful family management of postsurgical care and ongoing treatments.

Bone Tumors

Osteosarcoma

Osteosarcoma is the most common tumor affecting the skeleton of children, with an incidence of 5.6 cases per million children. Its peak incidence is during the rapid growth years, at 13 years for girls and 14 years for boys (Hartford, Wodowski, Rao, et al., 2006). The tumor is usually located at the metaphysis of the distal femur, proximal tibia, or proximal humerus.

Etiology and Pathophysiology   Bone tissue produced by osteosarcoma never matures into compact bone. Although the cause of osteosarcoma is unknown, radiation exposure (either environmental or treatment related) is associated with its development. Survivors of retinoblastoma have a greatly increased incidence of osteosarcoma. An abnormality of gene p53 has been noted in some cases of this cancer, leading to oncogene malformations and possibly to an absence of tumor suppressor genes (Heare, Hensley, & Dell'Orfano, 2009).

Clinical Manifestations   The common initial symptoms of osteosarcoma are pain, swelling, and a limp. The pain can be referred to the hip or back, which can delay diagnosis. Deep bone pain causing night awakenings should be investigated (Arndt, 2007). Pulmonary metastasis occurs in 20% of cases. Other metastatic sites include the kidney, adrenals, brain, and pericardium. When lung metastasis is the only site, lung resection may be successful for treatment. Disseminated metastases and bone lesions have poorer prognoses.

COLLABORATIVE CARE

Diagnosis of osteosarcoma is made through radiographic studies of the affected area, bone scan, CT or MRI scans of involved bone, blood test for serum alkaline phosphatase and lactic dehydrogenase (level may be elevated), and tumor biopsy. Complete blood count, liver studies, and renal studies are performed to investigate possible metastases. Arteriography may be performed if limb-salvage surgery is contemplated. Cardiac assessments are performed to establish baseline function prior to treatment with doxorubicin.

Treatment involves both surgery and chemotherapy. The surgery is either a limb-salvage procedure or limb amputation. In limb-salvage procedures, the tumor is removed and an internal prosthesis is inserted. A limb-salvage procedure is possible if bone growth has taken place and a neurobundle (area where several nerves converge) is not involved in the tumor. If these two criteria are not met, limb amputation is necessary. Physical rehabilitation will be needed after either amputation or limb-salvage procedure. At the time of diagnosis, most children have metastases (even though they may not be identifiable), so chemotherapy is needed. Chemotherapy may be started before surgery, especially in cases where limb-salvage surgery is performed. It is also given postoperatively to treat and prevent metastasis. Aggressive chemotherapy following surgery has improved the survival rate. Drugs commonly used for osteosarcoma include doxorubicin, cisplatin, ifosfamide with MESNA rescue, and methotrexate with leucovorin rescue.

Radiation is generally not effective in treating osteosarcoma, although it may be used with chemotherapy for recurrence at other sites.

Ewing Sarcoma

Ewing sarcoma is a malignant, small, round cell tumor usually involving the diaphyseal (shaft) portion of the long bones. The most common sites are the femur, pelvis, tibia, fibula, ribs, humerus, scapula, and clavicle, but any bone may be involved. Ewing sarcoma occurs in two children per million. It is more common in Whites and Hispanics and less common in Black and Asian children, and it is more common in males. Translocations on chromosomes 11 and 22 have been identified in children with Ewing sarcoma; these are t(11;22)(q24;q12). In addition, these tumors express a proto-oncogene, c-myc (Heare et al., 2009).

The symptoms are similar to those of osteosarcoma and may include pain, swelling, fever, an elevated WBC count, elevated erythrocyte sedimentation rate, and elevated C-reactive protein. Some children present with a fracture of the affected bone. A tumor biopsy is necessary for diagnosis. Diagnostic tests are the same as those for osteosarcoma.

Initial treatment for Ewing sarcoma is chemotherapy to reduce the tumor, followed by surgical removal of the entire bone or intensive high-dose irradiation of the entire bone (Lahl,

Fisher, & Laschinger, 2008). Limb-salvage procedures are now commonly performed rather than amputation. Surgery is preferred because of the possibility of a secondary cancer from radiation. Chemotherapy is always used following initial treatment, as undetectable metastases are nearly always present. Medications used to treat Ewing sarcoma include drugs such as vincristine, doxorubicin, cyclophosphamide, dactinomycin, etoposide, and ifosfamide.

NURSING MANAGEMENT

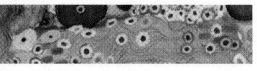

Nursing Assessment and Diagnosis

Carefully evaluate any child or adolescent who has a limp or complains of pain in an extremity. Confirm the onset and whether the symptoms were associated with injury. Refer for further evaluation if the discomfort persists or is not associated with injury.

Physiologic assessment of the child with a bone tumor includes assessment of the site before surgery. Assess the child's pain or discomfort, mobility, and gait. Take careful vital signs, especially noting temperature and respirations. Psychologic assessment of the child and family is needed, especially if amputation is planned. Body image disturbances occur when a limb is lost, particularly with school-age children and adolescents. Assess the child's understanding of the treatment and of care after surgery. Inquire about support systems that are available for assistance to the family.

Observe the wound postoperatively for infection and hemorrhage. Assess circulation above and below the operative site. If edema is found, elevate the limb. If a limb-salvage procedure is performed, the child's extremity will be intact but it will not function as before, because muscle insertion sites and mass have been removed with the tumor during surgery. Detailed charting of the condition of the surgical site and limb function is important.

If the limb has been amputated, assess the child for the following signs indicating a disturbed body image:

- Refusal to look at or touch the altered or missing body part
- Preoccupation with loss or change
- Feelings of shame or embarrassment, either verbalized or demonstrated
- Distorted perception of normal body (easily seen in the child's drawings of the body)
- Fears of rejection or unwanted attention from others
- Overexposure or hiding of the affected body part
- Actual or perceived change in the structure and function of the body or body parts

Psychosocial assessment of the child and family is discussed in more detail earlier in this chapter in the Childhood Cancer section (see pages 721–724).

Appropriate nursing diagnoses for the child with a bone tumor are based on the treatment and needs of each child:

- Risk for Infection related to amputation
- Impaired Skin Integrity related to mechanical forces of prosthesis
- Impaired Physical Mobility related to musculoskeletal impairment
- Impaired Adjustment related to disability and lifestyle change
- Disturbed Body Image related to treatment and injury
- Chronic Pain related to physical injury of tissues

Planning and Implementation

Care of the child after surgery involves general postoperative care (see Chapter 11 ∞). The child who has had an amputation has special needs regarding skin care and rehabilitation. Inspect the tissue at the surgical site, using sterile technique, and turn the child at least every 2 hours. The site needs to heal completely before chemotherapy can begin and a prosthesis can be made. Pain management is a major nursing care need. When amputation has occurred, the adolescent will often experience **phantom pain**. This pain, which feels as if it is in the amputated extremity, is caused by trauma to the nerves in the area of the amputation. Acknowledge the pain as real since the nerve endings are intact and the patient is perceiving real discomfort. Medicate adequately and use additional pain control measures such as repositioning the limb using gentle movement, supporting the limb, and using distraction or deep breathing.

Discuss insurance and other financial arrangements with the parents, as prosthetics can be expensive. Physical rehabilitation will be needed as well. Referral to a Shriners Hospital is an option for some families.

Implement plans to help the child deal with body image disturbance. Plan for a visit from another child who is well adjusted to a prosthesis. Help the child to gradually learn how to care for the stump. Slow progress may be made as the child first looks briefly, then for longer periods, and finally is willing to touch the stump. Show the child how it is possible to continue with sports such as baseball, skiing, or biking with a prosthesis. A discussion group with others can be very useful for adolescents. Plan with the child how to tell friends about the surgery and what issues he or she may face upon return to school. Make plans for elevator access if needed and emergency evacuation procedures. Some children or adolescents may need referral for counseling to assist in dealing with body image disturbance.

The child will receive physical rehabilitation while hospitalized and after discharge. When the child is discharged, explain to the family the importance of bringing the child for outpatient chemotherapy and physical rehabilitation visits. Special arrangements may be needed at the child's school to facilitate a wheelchair, crutches, or ambulation with a new prosthesis. Call or visit the school to evaluate the presence of buttons to open doors, wide doorways to facilitate passage, and any limitations of the building. Contact school personnel to plan for the child's return. The child will need careful management of a schedule that permits both healing of the surgical site with rehabilitation and then the demands of chemotherapy.

Follow-up care is needed to monitor for progress and to be alert for signs of metastases. See the discussion of cancer survivorship earlier in this chapter. Fracture may be a sign of recurrent tumor. All body systems such as the lungs, heart, kidneys, and liver are monitored for signs of recurrence. Consider carefully the drugs the child received and the long-term side effects, such as cardiac change with doxorubicin.

Evaluation

The following expected outcomes of nursing care for the child with a bone tumor focus on the treatments required and adaptation to changes in lifestyle:

- The surgical site heals with no signs of infection.
- The child adapts to changes in mobility status.
- The child manifests successful adjustment to changes required in school settings.
- Healthy, intact skin is maintained at the surgical site.
- The child shows evidence of positive body image.
- Pain is managed to a comfort level.
- The child and family successfully integrate continuing medical therapy into family life.

■ LEUKEMIA

Leukemia is among the most commonly diagnosed pediatric malignancies in children under 14 years of age. A cancer of the blood-forming organs, leukemia is characterized by a proliferation of abnormal white blood cells in the body. Several types of leukemia are differentiated, depending on the blood cells affected. The main types are acute lymphoblastic leukemia (ALL), acute myeloid leukemia (AML), and the rare chronic leukemias of childhood.

The most common type of childhood leukemia is ALL, which accounts for 25% of all childhood cancer and 78% of leukemias in children. Sam, described in the opening scenario, has ALL. The peak age at onset is 2 to 3 years. ALL is more common among Whites and in boys (Figure 24–16 ➤) (American Cancer Society, 2009c). Subtypes of ALL are based on the French-American-British (FAB) system of classification, and the three subtypes are L1, L2, and L3.

Acute myeloid leukemia refers to all leukemias from myeloid cells. About 17% of childhood leukemias are AML. It is most common in children younger than 2 years of age and in adolescents. It is more common in males than females, and in

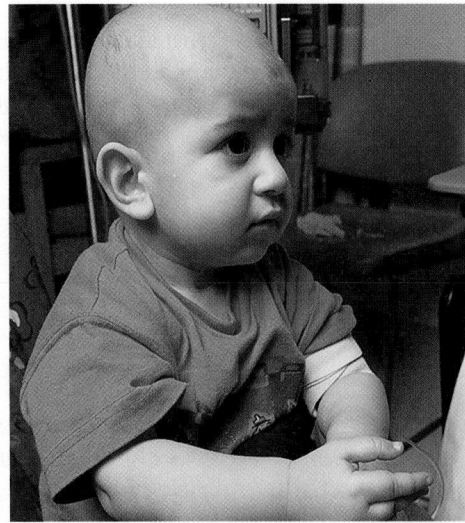

FIGURE 24–16 ➤ Acute lymphoblastic leukemia is the most common type of leukemia in children and the most common cancer affecting children under 5 years of age.

 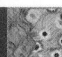
Asians/Pacific Islanders, Hispanics, and Whites than in Blacks (Brown, 2006). There are several subtypes of AML in the FAB classification:

- M0 = AML without maturation
- M1 = AML with poor maturation
- M2 = AML with maturation
- M3 = acute promyelocytic leukemia
- M4 = acute myelomonocytic leukemia
- M5 = acute monocytic leukemia
- M6 = erythroleukemia
- M7 = acute megakaryocytic leukemia

Because chronic leukemias such as chronic myelocytic, chronic myelomonocytic, and chronic lymphocytic leukemia are rare in children, the following discussion will focus on ALL and AML.

Etiology and Pathophysiology

The causes of leukemia are not well understood. Some investigators theorize that exposure to infectious agents can predispose children to leukemia. Genetic factors are also believed to play a role in some types of the disease. For instance, children with chromosomal defects such as Down syndrome, neurofibromatosis type I, Bloom syndrome, and Shwachman syndrome have an increased incidence of ALL, and a variety of genetic abnormalities are present in most children with ALL (Pieters & Carroll, 2008). Children with immune deficiency states, such as ataxia-telangiectasia, congenital hypogammaglobulinemia, and Wiskott-Aldrich syndrome, have an increased risk of ALL. Certain racial and ethnic groups have poorer outcomes from leukemia.

Ionizing radiation when in utero, and chemical agents, such as treatment of an earlier cancer with chemotherapy (alkylating agents and topoisomerase II inhibitors), are thought to play some role in the development of AML. There are several chromosomal and genetic abnormalities associated with AML. For example, trisomy 8 is associated with all subtypes of the disease (Jaff, Chelghoum, Elhamri, et al., 2006).

Leukemia occurs when the stem cells in the bone marrow produce immature WBCs that cannot function normally. These cells proliferate rapidly by cloning instead of through normal mitosis, causing the bone marrow to fill with abnormal WBCs. The abnormal cells then spill out into the circulatory system where they steadily replace the normally functioning WBCs. As this occurs, the protective lymphocytic functions such as cellular and humeral immunity are reduced, leaving the body vulnerable to infections. The malignant WBCs rapidly fill the bone marrow, replacing stem cells that produce erythrocytes (red blood cells) and other blood products such as platelets, thereby decreasing the amount of these products in circulation. The stem cells are replaced by leukemic clones, eventually resulting in anemia. Children with leukemia commonly experience abnormal bleeding because of the reduced platelet amounts.

Clinical Manifestations

Children with ALL and AML usually have fever, pallor, overt signs of bleeding, lethargy, malaise, anorexia, and large joint or bone pain. Petechiae, frank bleeding, and joint pain are cardinal signs of bone marrow failure. Enlargement of the liver and spleen (hepatosplenomegaly) and changes in the lymph nodes (lymphadenopathy) are common. If the leukemia has infiltrated the central nervous system (entered it by means of the circulatory or lymphoid system), the child may exhibit signs such as headache, vomiting, papilledema, and sixth cranial nerve palsy (inability to move the eye laterally). These findings are caused by the leukemic cells massing and putting pressure on nerves. The testicles, spinal cord, and bone marrow are common sites for infiltration. The leukemic cells in the testicle become a mass that causes the testicle to enlarge, often painlessly.

COLLABORATIVE CARE

Diagnostic Tests

Diagnosis is based initially on blood counts and bone marrow aspiration. Blood counts reveal anemia, thrombocytopenia, and neutropenia. Bone marrow aspiration, the definitive test, reveals immature and abnormal lymphoblasts and hypercellular marrow. The percentage of blast cells in marrow is measured; 25% lymphoblasts is definitive for the disease (Brown, 2006). Neutropenia, thrombocytopenia, and anemia are commonly noted. Other abnormal laboratory findings include elevated serum uric acid and elevated calcium, potassium, and phosphorus levels. New laboratory studies such as rapid flow cytometric assay are making the measurement of even very small numbers of leukemic cells possible, so that treatment can be used to improve the prognosis in children with minimal residual disease. Leukemic cells are examined and classified by FAB type, and DNA analysis may provide clues about genetic changes; all of these considerations are used to establish the protocol for treatment. Blood cells of children with ALL are either B cell or T cell; these classifications are also used to establish treatment protocols.

Clinical Therapy

Treatment of ALL involves radiation and chemotherapy. Radiation is used for central nervous system disease, in T-cell leukemia, and for testicular involvement. Chemotherapy is organized into four phases—induction, consolidation, delayed intensification, and maintenance. Maximum cell death occurs during the *induction phase*. The cells that remain after this period are more resistant to treatment. After 3 to 4 weeks, when a remission has occurred, central nervous system prophylaxis begins. Drugs are used in combination with cranial irradiation. During the *consolidation phase*, chemotherapy with L-asparaginase and doxorubicin is administered. *Delayed intensification* uses additional drugs to target the leukemic cells that have survived. Treatment during the *maintenance phase* is aimed at destroying the remaining leukemic cells. Maintenance therapy may continue for 2 to 3 years, causing decreased resistance to infection for this prolonged period of time. Similarly, treatment of AML involves use of a wide variety of drugs during the induction and consolidation phases. AML treatment is often shorter in duration than that for ALL but intensive in dosing.

Combinations of active drugs are used to prevent resistance. Many complications can occur with such high doses and combinations of drugs; therefore, much of the clinical therapy is aimed at managing these effects. In addition, long-term complications such as central nervous system toxicity; damage to the pituitary, liver, kidneys, gastrointestinal tract, heart, lungs, gonads, blood, and immune system; and secondary malignancies can occur.

Some of the drugs commonly used throughout treatment for leukemia include prednisone, vincristine, methotrexate, L-asparaginase, daunorubicin, doxorubicin, coxorubicin, ara-C, cyclophosphamide, 6-mercaptopurine, 6-thioguanine, mitoxantrone, cytarabine, etoposide, and teniposide. Intrathecal methotrexate can be used for central nervous system infiltration by leukemic cells.

The prognosis for children with leukemia is much improved with current therapy. However, several risk factors affect the long-term outcome. The most favorable findings are as follows:

- Age at onset between 2 and 10 years
- Initial hemoglobin level less than 10 g/dL
- Low initial WBC count
- Lack of B- or T-cell antigens
- Absence of extramedullary (outside bone marrow or spinal cord) involvement
- Rapid response to chemotherapy

The most important factor is the initial leukocyte count. A higher leukocyte count (over 50,000/mm³) at diagnosis leads to a more guarded prognosis; even higher risk ALL has a 75–80% survival rate with current treatments (Pui & Evans, 2006). Infants under 12 months of age have lower survival rates. Treatment methods and duration are adjusted for each child, depending on that child's risk factors.

Nursing Alert

Laboratory values in leukemia:

	Usual	Common Values in Leukemia
Leukocytes	Less than 10,000/microLiter	Greater than 10,000/microLiter
Platelets	15,000–400,000/microLiter	20,000–100,000/microLiter
Hemoglobin	12–16 g/dL	7–11 g/dL

Leukemia Video

Approximately 10% of children have a relapse within a year after completing treatment. Treatment for relapse consists of additional chemotherapy drugs. The prognosis is best if the relapse occurs late after the initial diagnosis and after the initial treatment is completed. Bone marrow transplantation is a treatment option for the child who has a relapse with ALL who then achieves a second remission; the transplant is given when the child is in remission. Transplant is also used for children with AML; they do not need to be in remission for the transplant to be performed. Chemotherapy itself can create numerous complications, affecting all body organs. Secondary malignancies sometimes occur later in life. Central nervous system toxicity; damage to organs such as pituitary, liver, kidneys, heart, and lungs; and secondary malignancies sometimes occur (Pieters & Carroll, 2008).

NURSING MANAGEMENT

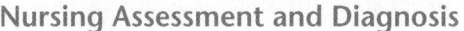

Nursing Assessment and Diagnosis

Thorough physical assessment is important to ensure prompt identification of problems without injuring the child who has deficient coagulation and immune function. Perform assessments every 8 hours or more often depending on the chemotherapy regimen. Observe carefully for bruising and other new sites of bleeding, and for fever or other signs of infection. Once chemotherapy has begun, closely monitor renal functioning through specific gravity, I&O, and daily weight measurement. Monitor dietary intake, nausea, vomiting, and constipation. Observe for mucosal sores in the mouth. A central line is usually in place for intravenous infusion of medications, so careful assessment of the line for proper functioning and for signs of infection is needed. Ask the parents about any behavioral changes. Central nervous system infiltration can affect the child's level of consciousness, causing irritability, vomiting, and lethargy. However, these nonspecific signs can also be induced by chemotherapeutic drugs and antiemetics. Frequent venipunctures, bone marrow aspirations, and lumbar punctures require pain assessment and an evaluation of the level of knowledge and coping skills of the child and family.

Leukemia causes many changes in the body, and confirmation of the disease is difficult for families to face. Among the many nursing diagnoses that might be appropriate for the child with leukemia are the following:

- Imbalanced Nutrition: Less than Body Requirements related to inability to ingest food
- Risk for Infection related to altered immune system functioning
- Risk for Injury related to bleeding
- Activity Intolerance related to generalized weakness
- Chronic Pain related to chemotherapy and disease process
- Disturbed Sleep Pattern related to chemotherapy drugs and disease process
- Anxiety (Child and Parent) related to change in health status

Planning and Implementation

Bone marrow suppression necessitates transmission-based precautions (refer to the *Clinical Skills Manual*). Instruct parents in the prevention of infection and use nursing care measures to prevent infection as well. Perform careful hand hygiene; take temperature frequently; give mouth care with antibacterial mouthwashes; and inspect the skin, mouth, rectal area, and central line site for any signs of infection. Care of mouth ulcers and other side effects of chemotherapy are presented in the Nursing Care Plan: Hospital Care of the Child with Cancer, earlier in this chapter.

Special attention to renal function is needed when the child receives cyclophosphamide. Gross hematuria is a side effect of this drug. Hydration with intravenous fluids to attain a specific gravity of less than 1.010 prevents or reduces the severity of hematuria. It also prepares the kidneys to manage products of tumor cell breakdown. To achieve this desired specific gravity, the child receives intravenous fluids at 1.5 times maintenance volume for at least 6 to 8 hours before and at least 1.5 hours after administration of the drug. Other chemotherapy drugs have different infusion times, and some do not require hydration prior to infusion. Check drug references carefully for recommendations with each drug. Evaluate the infusion site before and frequently during infusion. Although extravasation is not as common with central lines used in cancer treatment as in peripheral lines, it still can occur. Many chemotherapy agents are extremely toxic to tissues. In addition, lysis of the cancer cells can produce toxic side effects (see oncologic emergencies described earlier in the chapter). Careful monitoring of I&O is required to record the intravenous fluids, assess kidney functioning, and monitor excretion of by-products from destroyed tumor cells. Monitor specific gravity every 8 hours, as well as before and during administration of the drug, and when the intravenous fluids are reduced to maintenance volume levels. Daily weight measurements are important to assist in planning adequate hydration during chemotherapy, as well as to measure nutritional status.

Drug side effects may necessitate infusion of platelets or packed red blood cells. See the *Clinical Skills Manual* for techniques to be used in these situations.

Many children are treated in an oncology clinic, staying in the hospital only on the day of intravenous drug administration, and receive oral medications at home. The time at the hospital is used to assess how the family is managing issues such as nutrition, sleep, medication administration, and obtaining psychosocial support. Careful teaching for the family is needed to ensure safe drug administration and identification of issues requiring further care.

Nurses play a key role in the long-term multidisciplinary treatment of children with leukemia. The impact of a diagnosis of leukemia and the long-term nature of treatment can severely stress the coping abilities of both the child and the family. Consider the shock to the family when Sam, described in the chapter opener, was diagnosed with leukemia, a possibility they had never considered. Ongoing psychosocial assessment and emotional support are essential (see the general discussion of psychosocial assessment in the Childhood Cancer section, pages 721–724). Referral to support groups and social services may be beneficial. Assist the family in exploration of alternative therapies such as relaxation, imagery, and nutritional support that may aid the child. Be alert for any interactions that could occur between alternative therapies and the medical regimen. (See Families Want to Know: Chemotherapy for Leukemia.)

Evaluation

Following are expected outcomes for nursing care of the child with leukemia:

- The child is adequately hydrated to allow for elimination of drugs and cell components.
- The child maintains normal urinary output.
- The child remains free from infection.
- Blood values are maintained within normal limits.
- The family successfully adapts to parenting a child with a chronic illness.
- The parents demonstrate adequate knowledge related to the disease process and treatment regimens.

■ SOFT-TISSUE TUMORS

Hodgkin Disease

Hodgkin disease, a disorder of the lymphoid system, usually arises in a single lymph node or an anatomic group of lymph nodes (Figure 24–17 ►). Hodgkin disease is rare before 10 years of age; it accounts for just 5% of cancers in children under 14 years, but 15% of cancer in youth from 15–19 years. The disease has a bimodal peak with higher incidence in the early 20s and after 50 years (Cairo & Bradley, 2007). There is a slightly increased incidence in males, which is more pronounced in the disease when manifested in younger children (Hudson, Onciu, & Donaldson, 2006).

Etiology and Pathophysiology

Hodgkin disease occurs in clusters and has been reported in families. This suggests a possible genetic link as well as an infectious agent or environmental hazard (Cairo & Bradley, 2007).

Clinical Manifestations

The main symptom of Hodgkin disease is nontender, firm lymphadenopathy, usually in the supraclavicular and cervical nodes but occasionally in the mediastinal area. A mediastinal growth can cause respiratory difficulty because of pressure on the trachea or bronchi. A characteristic large cell with multiple nuclei, called the Reed-Sternberg cell, is characteristic of Hodgkin, though the cell is found also in infectious mononucleosis and some other lymphomas. Fever, night sweats, and weight loss occur in one third of children with Hodgkin disease; these symptoms and elevated sedimentation rate are associated with a more aggressive form of the disease. The leukocyte count and erythrocyte sedimentation rate (ESR) may be elevated.

COLLABORATIVE CARE

Diagnosis is based on lymph node biopsy; Reed-Sternberg cells are present. A staging classification is used to determine disease severity (Table 24–7). The basis for staging is data obtained from the history, physical examination, chest radiograph study (for metastasis), chest CT scan, CT or MRI scans of the retroperitoneal nodes, lymphangiogram if there is retroperitoneal involvement, laboratory studies (complete blood count, erythrocyte sedimentation rate, serum copper level, C-reactive protein, liver and renal function tests), and a radionuclide scan with gallium. Bone marrow biopsy, bone scan, or a staging laparotomy may be performed in certain situations when advanced disease is suspected. Minimally invasive surgery can be used to biopsy or remove the spleen for diagnosis, avoiding the potential complications of major surgery (Hudson et al., 2006).

Clinical Tip

An oral contrast medium is often given to children having CT scanning of the abdomen and pelvis. Mixing this contrast medium with fruit juice or punch makes it more palatable. Mix it in a small amount so the child can easily drink it all.

Pathophysiology Illustrated

Hodgkin Disease

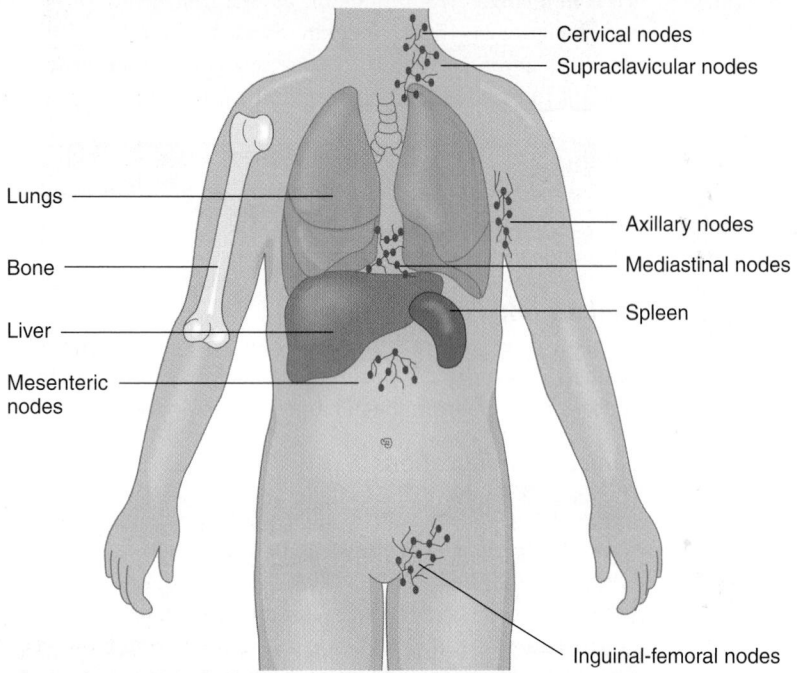

FIGURE 24–17 ➤ Lymph nodes and organs affected in Hodgkin disease in children.

Treatment is commonly performed in outpatient settings unless complications develop that require hospitalization. A four-drug chemotherapy combination has been found to be the most effective drug treatment. Drugs commonly used include doxorubicin, bleomycin, dacarbazine, etoposide, vinblastine, prednisone, cyclophosphamide, procarbazine, methotrexate, and mechlorethamine.

Radiation is commonly added, with low doses for children who are still growing, and larger doses for those who are physically mature or whose disease is more advanced at diagnosis. The 5-year survival rate is approximately 85–90%, depending on the stage of the disease at diagnosis. Autologous or allogeneic stem cell transplantation is a treatment option in children with advanced disease or relapse.

Non-Hodgkin Lymphoma

There are three types of pediatric non-Hodgkin lymphoma: (1) lymphoblastic lymphoma (30–40%), (2) small noncleaved cell (Burkitt) lymphoma (40–50%), and (3) large cell lymphoma (15%) (Mann, Attarbaschi, Steiner, et al., 2006). Lymphomas of all types are the third most common group of malignancies in children, following leukemia and brain tumors. Non-Hodgkin lymphomas are malignant tumors of lymphoreticular (internal framework of the lymph system) origin. The peak incidence for lymphomas occurs between the ages of 7 and 11 years, and they are three times more common in boys than in girls.

Lymphoblastic non-Hodgkin lymphomas are caused by T-cell abnormalities. These abnormal T cells are diffuse, highly malignant, and very aggressive, and do not mature. T-cell lymphomas produced by these cells often occur in children with congenital or acquired immunodeficiency states, chronic immune stimulation, or autoimmune disease. Some lymphomas have B-cell abnormalities, most specifically Burkitt lymphoma; 8q24 chromosomal translocation may be found in these cases, and it is sometimes associated with Epstein-Barr virus infection. Large cell lymphomas are variable in cell type affected and may also manifest chromosomal translocations (Mann et al., 2006).

The incidence of lymphomas shows geographic variability. For example, a high incidence of Burkitt lymphoma is found in equatorial Africa, where it causes 50% of childhood cancer. Incidence in Hispanic children is higher than in Whites, and Blacks have the lowest incidence. Males are affected more than females, and children with immune system compromise are most commonly affected. Epstein-Barr virus has been associated with Burkitt lymphoma (Cairo & Bradley, 2007).

Children with non-Hodgkin lymphoma frequently present with fever and weight loss. The lymph glands are usually enlarged or nodular, with the most frequent sites being the cervical, axillary,

Stage	Description
I	Disease within a single lymph node region
IE	Disease within a single extralymphatic organ or site outside of the lymphatic system (extralymphatic organ)
II	Disease within two or more lymph node regions on the same side of the diaphragm
IIE	Disease within an extralymphatic organ, and of one or more lymph node regions on the same side of the diaphragm
III	Disease of lymph node regions on both sides of the diaphragm; stage III(1) indicates involvement of the upper abdomen above the renal vein while stage III(2) indicates involvement of the pelvic or other lower abdominal nodes
IIIE	Disease of lymph node regions on both sides of the diaphragm with involvement of an extralymphatic organ
IIIS	As in III, plus disease within the spleen
IIIE+S	As in III, plus disease in extralymphatic organs and the spleen
IV	Disseminated disease within one or more lymphatic organs with or without lymph node involvement

TABLE 24–7 Staging System for Hodgkin Disease

Data from National Cancer Institute (2010).

inguinal, and femoral nodes. However, the disease may be diffuse, without nodular glands. The anterior mediastinum is the primary site for T-cell lymphomas. Tumors that occur in this area may compress the airway (causing breathing difficulty) or superior vena cava (leading to swelling of the face, neck, or arms), and can cause pain. Jaw involvement is common in Burkitt lymphoma. An abdominal mass may cause pain, nausea, and vomiting.

The symptoms of lymphoma are often nonspecific, and treatments may already have been tried with antibiotics or other medication if a mass is thought to be an infection. A careful history will help determine the progression and possible location of disease. CBC is performed; additional blood tests include renal and liver function, electrolytes, uric acid, and LDH. Bone marrow aspiration and lumbar puncture are performed. Chest radiograph, bone scan, gallium scan, CT, and MRI can help to isolate affected body organs. Diagnosis is confirmed by tissue biopsy.

A staging system is used to describe the tumor mass and extension to other body areas (Table 24–8). Treatment is tailored to the type of cancer and its stage. Stages I and II may be treated with drugs such as vincristine, cyclophosphamide, prednisone, and methotrexate for several months. Intrathecal medication is added if head and neck cancers are present. Stages III and IV are treated with additional drugs (up to nine total) for longer periods of time (1–2 years). Radiation is uncommonly used and may be helpful to treat a tumor that is impinging on a body part. Surgery is used to biopsy the tumor mass and treat any complications caused by the cancer. Bone marrow transplantation or hematopoietic stem cell transplantation is used for children with recurrent disease.

Rhabdomyosarcoma

Rhabdomyosarcoma is the most common soft-tissue sarcoma diagnosed in children, and is especially common in children under 5 years of age. The 5-year survival rate is 64% (Punyko, Gurney, Baker, et al., 2006). It occurs most often in the muscles around the eyes (extraorbital), in the neck, and less commonly in the abdomen, genitourinary tract, and the extremities. Genitourinary, bladder, and prostate cancers are more common in children under 5 years, while paratesticular and extremity can-

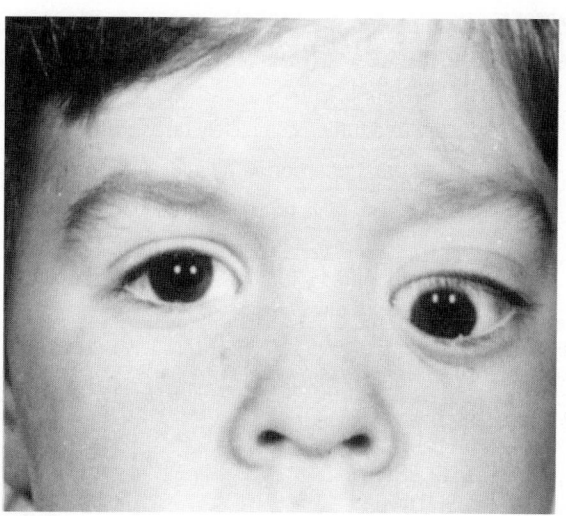

FIGURE 24–18 ➤ Rhabdomyosarcoma is characterized by ptosis and swelling. *The McGraw-Hill Companies.*

cer is more common among adolescents. Rhabdomyosarcoma occurs more often in Whites than in Blacks or Asians. It is uncommon in newborns; if it is present in this age group, abdominal or pelvic sites are the most common locations.

The cause of rhabdomyosarcoma is unknown. However, it is more common in children with neurofibromatosis and Li-Fraumeni syndrome. Mutations in a tumor suppressor gene p53 are sometimes seen. The abnormal cells arise from mesenchyme, which normally grows into muscle, fat, and bone.

Tumors occurring close to the eye produce swelling, ptosis, visual disturbances, and eye movement abnormalities (Figure 24–18 ➤). When the tumor occurs in the genitourinary tract, the result can be obstruction, hematuria, dysuria, vaginal discharge, and a protruding vaginal mass. Rhabdomyosarcoma occurring in the abdomen may be asymptomatic. There is rapid metastasis to the lungs, bones, bone marrow, and distant lymph nodes.

Diagnosis is confirmed by CT, MRI, PET, bone marrow aspiration, and biopsy. CBC, renal and liver studies, and urinalysis are performed. Lumbar puncture may be used in head and neck tumors. A useful biologic marker, desmin, allows differentiation of rhabdomyosarcoma from other round cell tumors. A significant number of children have metastatic disease at the time of diagnosis, so chest and lung CT scans are performed; regional lymph node biopsies also help to establish the extent of disease (Rodeberg & Paidas, 2006).

Treatment includes surgical removal of the tumor when possible. However, if the tumor involves other structures, removal may not be possible. Many children have metastasis at the time of diagnosis, so the primary tumor is removed. Surgery is followed by wide-field radiation and chemotherapy with a combination of drugs. Some commonly used drugs include vincristine, actinomycin, and cyclophosphamide (in combination known as "VAC therapy").

Prognosis depends on the site, staging (Table 24–9), and histologic findings, with about 70% of children now surviving (Rodeberg & Paidas, 2006).

TABLE 24–8	St. Jude Children's Research Hospital Staging Classification for Non-Hodgkin Lymphoma
Stage	Description
I	Single tumor or node area involved; no tumor in the abdomen or mediastinum
II	Single tumor with lymph node involvement; or two node areas or tumor on the same side of the diaphragm; or gastrointestinal tumor in one site
III	Two tumors or node areas on different sides of the diaphragm; or a primary mediastinal, intra-abdominal, or epidural tumor
IV	Any involvement with CNS or bone marrow metastases

Adapted from: Hussong, M. R. (2002). In C. R. Baggott, K. P. Kelly, D. Fochtman, & G. V. Foley, Nursing care of children and adolescents with cancer (3rd ed., p. 539). Philadelphia: Saunders.

Group	Description
	TABLE 24–9 Classification of Rhabdomyosarcoma
I	Localized tumor, completely resected disease
II	Total gross resection with regional microscopic spread
III	Locally extensive tumor with residual microscopic spread
IV	Any size primary tumor with distant metastatic disease present

Note: From Wexler, L. H., Meyer, W. H., & Helman, L. J. (2006). Rhabdomyo-sarcoma and the undifferentiated sarcomas. In P. A. Pizzo & D. G. Poplack (Eds.), Principles and practices of pediatric oncology (5th ed., p. 982). Copyright 2006: Lippincott, Williams & Wilkins.

Retinoblastoma

Retinoblastoma is an intraocular malignancy of the retina. It may be bilateral (20–30%) or unilateral. In 40% of children, the disease is inherited by an autosomal dominant gene. Family history is therefore important to collect, although many cases occur after a recent mutation. The RB1 gene is on chromosome 13q14 (de Andrade, da Hora Barbosa, Vargas, et al., 2006; Herzog, 2007; Hurwitz, Shields, Shields, et al., 2006).

The first sign of retinoblastoma is a white pupil, termed leukokoria or cat's-eye reflex (Figure 24–19 ➤). The red reflex is absent, asymmetrical, or of a differing color in the affected eye. Other symptoms may include a fixed strabismus (a constant deviation of one eye from the other), orbital inflammation, glaucoma, and heterochromia (irises of different colors).

Retinoblastoma is usually diagnosed when the child is between 1 and 2 years of age. A family history should alert health care providers so that regular ophthalmologic examinations can be performed frequently on infants and young children in the family. The appearance of a unilateral tumor demands regular examinations of the healthy eye since bilateral disease can develop. In some children a pineal gland tumor can also de-

velop, causing central nervous system symptoms. The overall tumor-free survival rate is 90%, 5 to 10 years after diagnosis (Kids Data, 2006).

Children at risk for retinoblastoma due to family history can be tested for the RB1 gene. Diagnostic tests include full ocular examination and CT or MRI scans of the eye orbit. All children with a history of retinoblastoma in the family should be examined by an ophthalmologist after birth, at 6 weeks, every 2–3 months until 2 years, every 4 months until 3 years, and then annually (de Andrade et al., 2006) to aid in early diagnosis. Tumors are classified according to a staging system, from a very small localized tumor (group I) to tumors involving more than half the retina and with seeding into the vitreous (group V).

Treatment for retinoblastoma may include removal of the eye (enucleation) when there is permanent retinal damage or failure to respond to other treatment. Other surgical treatments involve cryotherapy or photocoagulation (argon laser therapy). Radiation is nearly always used, either as the sole treatment or before surgery to shrink the tumor. Chemotherapy is occasionally used but is generally ineffective as the drugs often fail to penetrate sufficiently into the eye. Chemotherapy drugs include carboplatin, etoposide, vincristine, and cyclosporine. Multiple therapies are more commonly used in children with bilateral retinoblastoma. Children with retinoblastoma are at increased risk of developing a secondary tumor, including another retinoblastoma or a sarcoma, most commonly osteogenic sarcoma. However, most young children who have been treated for the disease have good health and normal mental abilities several years after treatment. Over 90% of children with small unilateral tumors survive. Increased size and invasion by a tumor decrease success of treatment. The most common sequela of retinoblastoma is a decrease in visual acuity.

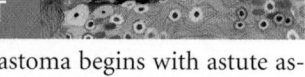

NURSING MANAGEMENT

Nursing management of retinoblastoma begins with astute assessments that may identify the condition, extends through the treatment process in support for the child and family, and includes ongoing care to ensure the child's normal developmental progression.

Nursing Assessment and Diagnosis

Physiologic Assessment

Careful family histories can sometimes identify children at risk who need frequent physical examinations. For example, if a family history of retinoblastoma is present, the child should receive frequent eye examinations. Physiologic assessment of the child with a soft-tissue tumor, such as Hodgkin disease, non-Hodgkin lymphoma, rhabdomyosarcoma, and other lymphomas, focuses on the child's general condition. Accurate height and weight measurements are essential to provide a baseline against which to measure the child's growth during treatment, as well as for calculation of chemotherapeutic drug dosages.

Observe the area of the tumor, such as the face, neck, and abdomen, and describe any changes. Monitor respiratory status if

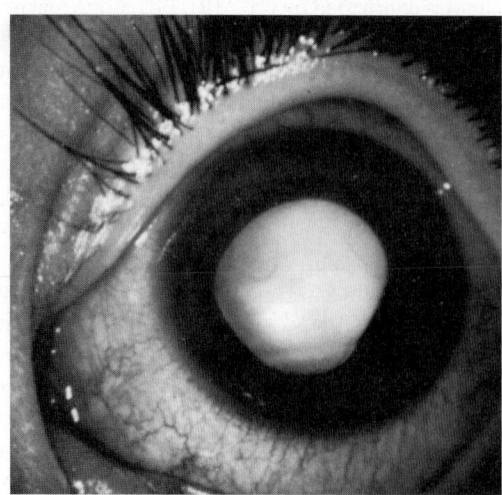

FIGURE 24–19 ➤ Retinoblastoma is characterized by leukokoria, a white reflection in the pupil.

Used with permission from Hathaway, W. E., Hay, W. W., Jr., Groothuis, J. R., & Paisley, J. W. (1993). Current pediatric diagnosis and treatment (11th ed.). New York: McGraw-Hill Companies.

the tumor is on the face or neck. Report any changes in respiratory pattern to the oncology specialist. Avoid palpation of any tumor site or enlarged area, as metastasis can be influenced by injudicious palpation and manipulation of a tumor site. Notify the primary health care provider of a change in any lymph node or any other area of the body.

Gastrointestinal and genitourinary function can be altered by the presence of a tumor and by treatment such as chemotherapy and radiation. Careful monitoring of the child's intake and output measurement is essential. Abdominal tumors may affect defecation, so charting of all bowel movements is important. Explain to the family and child why keeping accurate records is necessary.

Observe wounds closely for lack of healing as a result of chemotherapy or radiation. Examine the mouth and extremities for wounds or ulcers. Nutritional changes caused by treatment will affect the body's ability to support healthy cells and heal wounds.

A thorough eye examination is warranted for any child who has a family history of retinoblastoma or has undergone treatment for a prior tumor. Assess the color and position of the iris, eye movements, cover–uncover test, and other eye tests described in Chapter 5 ∞. Ask whether the child has been evaluated by an ophthalmologist.

Psychosocial Assessment

Assessment of the family's psychosocial status and coping mechanisms is an essential component of nursing care. Refer to the general discussion of psychosocial assessment in the Childhood Cancer section earlier in this chapter. Assessment of body image is needed when the child has a soft-tissue tumor affecting the appearance of the head and neck. Even after treatment is successfully completed, lasting mental health changes may be apparent. Survivors of childhood lymphoma more commonly report depression and somatic distress (symptoms such as pains in the heart or chest, dizziness, weakness) than other individuals (Zebrack et al., 2006). Ask about symptoms of depression such as loneliness, lack of interest, anxiety, and suicidal thoughts. Survivors of rhabdomyosarcoma are less likely to complete high school than their siblings, and they report higher incidences of pain (Punyko et al., 2006).

The location and type of soft-tissue tumor determine the specific nursing diagnoses for a particular child. Common nursing diagnoses may include the following:

- Altered Tissue Perfusion (Peripheral) related to interruption of blood flow
- Ineffective Breathing Pattern related to effect of tumor deformity on neck or chest wall
- Impaired Swallowing related to acquired tumor
- Delayed Growth and Development related to effects of treatment
- Disturbed Sensory Perception (Visual) related to illness

Planning and Implementation

Nursing management of children with soft-tissue tumors varies depending on the specific tumor. (See Families Want to Know: The Child with a Soft-Tissue Tumor.) Children with lymphoma affecting the mediastinum may need respiratory

---

Families Want to Know
The Child with a Soft-Tissue Tumor

- Teach the family about the chemotherapy drugs and their side effects.
- Teach about the care of surgically placed venous access devices.
- Provide written and illustrated information about the chemotherapy protocol(s).
- Provide radiation and surgery education specific to the tumor treatment.
- Refer the family to nutrition resources such as dietitians to improve the child's nutritional status.

---

support. Position the child so that the head is elevated. Administer chemotherapy drugs as ordered, maintaining adequate fluids to facilitate excretion of the resultant breakdown products. Monitor the central line used for chemotherapy administration, and teach parents care of the central line when the child is at home.

For the child with a rhabdomyosarcoma involving the bladder, monitor urinary output carefully. Report hematuria and painful urination. Monitor the changes that occur during therapy. For example, in children with eye tumors, observe for a decrease in ptosis, which may indicate successful treatment. Administer pain medications as needed and use distraction and other techniques to decrease the child's discomfort. Emphasize to parents the need for follow-up CT and MRI scans after completion of treatment.

When the child with retinoblastoma undergoes removal of the eye, the parents and child will need detailed instructions on postsurgical care. Demonstrate to the parents care of the socket and use of a conformer to maintain the eye socket's shape. When healing is complete and the child receives a prosthetic eye, instruct parents about its insertion and care. The child can gradually be taught to take over this care when old enough. Encourage periodic health care visits to monitor for signs of a tumor in the other eye. Interventions to encourage normal developmental milestones are adapted if sensory alteration has resulted.

Attention is directed at the body changes of the cancer and its treatment. Children and adolescents may need suggestions to deal with hair loss, disfigurement, and issues related to living with a serious illness. Referral to other children and teens with similar concerns may be helpful. Parents of all children need help to encourage normal development in the child with cancer.

The child with a soft-tissue tumor often receives chemotherapy or radiation, or sometimes both modalities. Nursing management during chemotherapy and radiation was discussed earlier in this chapter in the general sections on these treatment measures (see page 713) and in the Nursing Care Plan: Hospital Care of the Child with Cancer. Generally, the family will need help to adjust to the diagnosis of a life-threatening disease and to the care of the ill child. Refer to Chapter 11 ∞ for a description of postsurgical care. Consult Chapter 19 ∞ for strategies to assist the child and family if the child has a visual impairment resulting from a retinoblastoma. Topics for parent and family teaching and discharge planning are similar to those previously presented. Referral resources to support the families of children with these types of cancer can be found at the companion website.

Care in the Community

Reinforce with families the importance of long-term follow-up after treatment for a soft-tissue tumor. Increased risk for secondary cancers is possible for two to three decades, and early identification can help with prompt diagnosis (Hudson & Findlay, 2006). Partner with other health care providers to supply instructions to the family as the child transitions from oncology treatment back to the pediatrician so they understand the importance of telling all care providers about the cancer and treatment. Establish oncology clinics to track and examine survivors. As children grow into the teen and young adult years, help them to take over this important task in their care. Some recommended annual examinations include:

- CBC
- Physical examination with special attention to skin, abdomen, and thyroid
- Monitoring for signs of hypo- and hyperthyroidism
- Neurological and developmental examinations; monitoring of school performance
- First mammogram at 25 years in those with chest radiation
- Pap and pelvic exams for teen and young adult women
- Mental status assessment

Evaluation

The following expected outcomes of nursing care for the child with a soft-tissue tumor are examples that illustrate the varied tumor presentations:

- Treatment side effects are successfully managed.
- The surgical site heals with no signs of infection.
- The child successfully adapts to sensory loss.
- The child achieves growth and development to maximum potential.
- The parents and family achieve anticipatory grieving in cases of terminal disease.

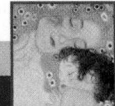

Chapter Highlights

- Cancer is a leading cause of illness and death among children.
- Cancer may be influenced by chromosomal or genetic messages, environmental carcinogens, or infectious processes. Often a combination of factors seems to be present.
- Cancer treatments include surgery, chemotherapy, radiation, biotherapy, and alternative therapies. End-of-life care is needed when disease has relapsed and cure is no longer possible.
- Oncologic emergencies are life-threatening conditions caused by cancer or its treatment.
- Main types of oncologic emergencies are metabolic, hematologic, or space occupying.
- Key signs of childhood cancer are pain, cachexia, anemia, infection, bruising, and neurological symptoms.
- A protocol is a plan of action for chemotherapy that is based on the type of cancer, its stage, and the particular cell type.
- Nursing assessment for children with cancer involves detailed physical data, as well as psychological factors and developmental achievements.
- Common physical nursing interventions for children with cancer involve nutrition, medication administration, hydration, infection prevention, pain management, and measures to decrease side effects of treatment. Families require ongoing psychosocial support, information, and referral to diverse resources when caring for a child with cancer.
- While the number of children who are long-term survivors continues to grow, it is known that some of these children experi-

ence lasting effects such as cognitive or behavioral problems, recurrent or secondary cancers, or discrimination.
- Nursing care after cancer treatment is completed includes monitoring for any long-term physiological or psychosocial sequelae.
- Common brain tumors in children include medulloblastoma, astrocytoma, ependymoma, and gliomas.
- Headache, vomiting, ataxia, seizures, increased intracranial pressure, hydrocephalus, and sensory disturbances are the major clinical manifestations of brain tumors.
- Neuroblastoma is a tumor that is located along the sympathetic nervous system chain.
- Nephroblastoma (Wilms tumor) is an intrarenal tumor; when suspected, the abdomen should not be palpated.
- Common bone tumors in childhood are osteosarcoma and Ewing sarcoma; both are most common among adolescents.
- Leukemia is a common childhood malignancy, with the major types being acute lymphoblastic leukemia (ALL) and acute myeloid leukemia (AML).
- A variety of soft-tissue tumors are seen in children and adolescents; they include Hodgkin disease, non-Hodgkin lymphoma, rhabdomyosarcoma, and retinoblastoma.
- Nurses assist families during a diagnosis for cancer, while therapy is carried out, in adjustment to school and other life tasks, and in providing end-of-life care for children who do not survive.

Clinical Reasoning in Action

Recall 4-year-old Sam, who was described in the opening scenario. He was recently diagnosed with acute lymphocytic leukemia (ALL) and has begun treatment. Both his mother and father are strong supports, and his older siblings, Jeffrey (6 years) and Blake (8 years), are worried about and protective of their younger brother. On a recent clinic visit, Sam's hemoglobin was found to be 6 g/dL.

1. Sam has had several procedures already that are painful and have required sedation. Plan to prepare him for a lumbar puncture for which he will be sedated. Consider his age as you plan how far ahead to tell him, how to explain the room he will be in, and how you will include his parents in the procedure.
2. Lack of all blood cellular components is a side effect of leukemia treatment. Explain why Sam's hemoglobin is low.

What is the expected level? What colony-stimulating factor might be used in his treatment to increase RBCs? What dietary teaching can you do to enhance hemoglobin levels?

3. Infection is a frequent complication of treatment for leukemia. During Sam's clinic visit, what assessments will you make to monitor for infection?
4. Jeffrey and Blake are attending one of Sam's clinic visits when he receives chemotherapy. What questions and activities will you plan for them during the visit? What can you do to increase their knowledge and help them feel like they are part of Sam's care? Could their concern for Sam influence their own school performance? What should their teachers know about the fact that they have a sibling who has leukemia?

See Pearson Nursing Student Resources for possible responses.

Pearson Nursing Student Resources

Find additional review materials at
nursing.pearsonhighered.com
Prepare for success with NCLEX®-style practice questions, interactive assignments and activities, web links, animations and videos, and more!

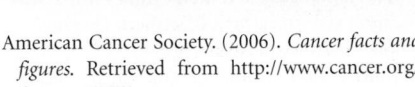

References

American Cancer Society. (2006). *Cancer facts and figures.* Retrieved from http://www.cancer.org/docroot/STT/stt_o.asp

American Cancer Society. (2009a). *Clinical trials: What you need to know.* Retrieved from http://www.cancer.org/docroot/ETO/content/ETO_6_3_clinical_Trials_-_patient_Participation.asp

American Cancer Society. (2009b). *Childhood cancer: Late effects of cancer treatment.* Retrieved from http://www.cancer.org/docrot/cri/content/cri_2_6x_late_effects_of_childhood_cancer.asp

American Cancer Society. (2009c). *What are the key statistics about childhood leukemia?* Retrieved from http://www.cancer/.org/cancer/Leukemiain Children/DetailedGuide/childhood-leukemia-key-statistics

American Nurses Association & International Society of Nurses in Genetics. (2007). *Genetics/genomics nursing: Scope and standards of practice.* Silver Spring, MD: American Nurses Association.

Armstrong, G. T. (2010). Long-term survivors of childhood central nervous system malignancies: The experience of the Childhood Cancer Survivor

Study. *European Journal of Paediatric Neurology, 14*(4), 298–303.

Arndt, C. A. S. (2007). Malignant tumors of bone. In R. M. Kliegman, R. E. Behrman, H. B. Jenson, & B. F. Stanton (Eds.), *Nelson textbook of pediatrics* (18th ed., pp. 2146–2149). Philadelphia: Saunders.

Ater, J. A. (2007). Neuroblastoma. In R. M. Kliegman, R. E. Behrman, H. B. Jenson, & B. F. Stanton (Eds.), *Nelson textbook of pediatrics* (18th ed., pp. 2137–2140). Philadelphia: Saunders.

Baker, J. N., Hinds, P. S., Spunt, S. L., Barfield, R. C., Allen, C., Powell, B. C., et al. (2008). Integration of palliative care practices into the ongoing care of children with cancer: Individualized care planning and coordination. *Pediatric Clinics of North America, 55*(1), 223–250.

Bennett Murphy, L. M., Flowers, S., McNamara, K. A., & Houng-Saleme, T. (2008). Fathers of children with cancer: Involvement, coping and adjustment. *Journal of Pediatric Health Care, 22*(3), 182–190.

Bindler, R. M., & Howry, L. B. (2005). *Pediatric drug guide.* Upper Saddle River, NJ: Prentice Hall.

Bjork, M., Nordstrom, B., & Hallstrom, I. (2006). Needs of young children with cancer during their initial hospitalization: An observational study. *Journal of Pediatric Oncology Nursing, 23*(4), 210–219.

Blaney, S. M., Kun, L. E., Hunter, J., Rorke-Adams, L. B., Lau, C., Strother, D., & Pollack, I. F. (2006). Tumors of the central nervous system. In P. A. Pizzo & D. G. Poplack, *Principles and practice of pediatric oncology* (5th ed., pp. 786–864). Philadelphia: Lippincott Williams & Wilkins.

Bleyer, A. (2007). Principles of diagnosis; Principles of treatment. In R. E. Behrman, R. M. Kliegman, & H. B. Jenson (Eds.), *Nelson textbook of pediatrics* (18th ed., pp. 2108–2116). Philadelphia: Saunders.

Breen, M., Coombes, L., & Bradbourne, C. (2009). Supportive care for children and young people during cancer treatment. *Community Practice, 82*(9), 28–31.

Brody, A. C., & Simmons, L. A. (2007). Family resiliency during childhood cancer: The father's perspective. *Journal of Pediatric Oncology Nursing, 24*(3), 152–165.

Brown, P. (2006). Answers to key questions about childhood leukemias. *Contemporary Pediatrics, 23*(3), 81–84, 87, 90.

Butowski, N. A., Sneed, P. K., & Chang, S. M. (2006). Diagnosis and treatment of recurrent high-grade astrocytoma. *Journal of Clinical Oncology, 10,* 1273–1280.

Cairo, M. S., & Bradley, M. B. (2007). Lymphoma. In R. M. Kliegman, R. E. Behrman, H. B. Jenson, & B. F. Stanton (Eds.), *Nelson textbook of pediatrics* (18th ed., pp. 2123–2127). Philadelphia: Saunders.

Chappuy, H., Doz, F., Blanche, S., Gentet, J. C., Pons, G., & Treluyer, J. M. (2006). Parental consent in paediatric clinical research. *Archives of Disease in Childhood, 91,* 112–116.

Cheng, S. (2009). Superior vena cava syndrome: A contemporary review of a historic disease. *Cardiology Review, 17*(1), 16–23.

Da Silva, E. D., Koch Nogueira, P. C., Russo Zamataro, T. M., de Carvalho, W. B., & Petrilli, A. S. (2008). Risk factors for death in children and adolescents with cancer and sepsis/septic shock. *Journal of Pediatric Hematology and Oncology, 30*(7), 513–518.

De Andrade, A. F., da Hora Barbosa, R., Vargas, F. R., Ferman, S., Eisenberg, A. L., Fernandes, L., & Bonvicino, C. R. (2006). A molecular study of first and second RB1 mutational hits in retinoblastoma patients. *Cancer Genetics and Cytogenetics, 167,* 43–46.

Decker, G. M. (2008). The marriage of conventional cancer treatments and alternative cancer therapies. *Nursing Clinics of North America, 43*(2), 221–242.

Dome, J. S., Perlman, E. J., Ritchey, M. L., Coppes, M. J., Kalapurakal, J., & Grundy, P. E. (2006). Renal tumors. In P. A. Pizzo & D. G. Poplack, *Principles and practice of pediatric oncology* (5th ed., pp. 905–932). Philadelphia: Lippincott Williams & Wilkins.

Erickson, J. M. (2009). Approaches to measure sleep-wake disturbances in adolescents with cancer. *Journal of Pediatric Nursing, 24*(4), 255–269.

Faivre, S., Djelloul, S., & Raymond, E. (2006). New paradigms in anticancer therapy: Targeting multiple signaling pathways with kinase inhibitors. *Seminars in Oncology, 33,* 407–420.

Fry, T. J., & Lankester, A. C. (2008). Cancer immunotherapy: Will expanding knowledge lead to success in pediatric oncology? *Pediatric Clinics of North America, 55*(1), 147–168.

Gedaly-Duff, V., Lee, K. A., Nail, L., Nicholson, H. S., & Johnson, K. P. (2006). Pain, sleep disturbance and fatigue in children with leukemia and their parents: A pilot study. *Oncology Nursing Forum, 33*(3), 641–646.

Handgretinger, R., Kurtzberg, J., & Egeler, R. M. (2008). Indications and donor selections for allogeneic stem cell transplantation in children with hematologic malignancies. *Pediatric Clinics of North America, 55*(1), 71–96.

Hantel, C., Lewrick, F., Schneider, S., Zwermann, O., Perren, A., Reiricke, M., et al. (2010). Anti insulin-like growth factor 1 receptor immoliposomes: A single formulation combining two anticancer treatments with enhanced therapeutic efficiency. *Journal of Clinical Endocrinology and Metabolism, 95*(2), 943–952.

Hartford, C. M., Wodowski, K. S., Rao, B. N., Khoury, J. D., Neel, M. D., & Daw, N. C. (2006). Osteosarcoma among children age 5 years or younger. *Journal of Pediatric Hematology and Oncology, 28,* 43–47.

Hawks, R. (2006). Complementary and alternative medicine research initiative in the children's oncology group and the role of the pediatric oncology nurse. *Journal of Pediatric Oncology Nursing, 23,* 261–264.

Heare, T., Hensley, M. A., & Dell'Orfano, S. (2009). Bone tumors: Osteosarcoma and Ewing's sarcoma. *Current Opinion in Pediatrics, 21,* 365–372.

Herzog, C. E. (2007). Retinoblastoma. In R. M. Kliegman, R. E. Behrman, H. B. Jenson, & B. F. Stanton (Eds.), *Nelson textbook of pediatrics* (18th ed., pp. 2151–2152). Philadelphia: Saunders.

Houldin, A., Curtiss, C. P., & Haylock, P. J. (2006). Executive summary: The state of the science on nursing approaches to managing late and long-term sequelae of cancer and cancer treatment. *American Journal of Nursing, 106*(3), 54–59.

Hudson, M. M., & Findlay, S. (2006). Health-risk behaviors and health promotion in adolescent and young adult cancer survivors. *Cancer, 107*(7 Suppl.), 1695–1701.

Hudson, M. M., Onciu, M., & Donaldson, S. S. (2006). Hodgkin lymphoma. In P. A. Pizzo & D. G. Poplack, *Principles and practice of pediatric oncology* (5th ed., pp. 695–721). Philadelphia: Lippincott Williams & Wilkins.

Hurwitz, R. L., Shields, C. L., Shields, J. A., Chevez-Barrios, P., Hurwitz, J. Y., & Chintagumpala, M. M. (2006). Retinoblastoma. In P. A. Pizzo & D. G. Poplack, *Principles and practice of pediatric oncology* (5th ed., pp. 865–886). Philadelphia: Lippincott Williams & Wilkins.

Hussong, M. R. (2002). Non-Hodgkin lymphoma. In C. R. Baggott, K. P. Kelly, D. Fochtman, & G. V. Foley, *Nursing care of children and adolescents with cancer* (3rd ed., p. 539). Philadelphia: WB Saunders.

Jaff, N., Chelghoum, Y., Elhamri, M., Tigaud, I., Michallet, M., & Thomas, X. (2006). Trisomy 8 as sole anomaly or with other clonal aberrations in acute myeloid leukemia: Impact on clinical presentation and outcome. *Leukemia Research, 31,* 67–73.

Jaffe, N., & Huff, V. (2007). Neoplasms of the kidney. In R. M. Kliegman, R. E. Behrman, H. B. Jenson, & B. F. Stanton (Eds.), *Nelson textbook of pediatrics* (18th ed., pp. 2140–2143). Philadelphia: Saunders.

Kadan-Lottick, N. S. (2007). Epidemiology of childhood and adolescent cancer. In R. M. Kliegman, R. E. Behrman, H. B. Jensen, & B. F. Stanton (Eds.), *Nelson textbook of pediatrics* (18th ed.). Philadelphia: Saunders.

Kaste, S. C. (2008). Skeletal toxicities of treatment in children with cancer. *Pediatric Blood Cancer, 50*(2 Suppl.), 469–473, 486.

Kazak, A. E., Rourke, M. T., Alderfer, M. A., Pai, A., Reilly, A. F., & Meadows, A. T. (2007). Evidence-based assessment, intervention and psychosocial care in pediatric oncology: A blueprint for comprehensive services across treatment. *Journal of Pediatric Psychology, 32,* 1099–1110.

Kersun, L., & Elia, J. (2007). Depressive symptoms and SSRI use in pediatric oncology patients. *Pediatric Blood Cancer, 49,* 881–887.

Kids Data. (2006). *Net five-year cancer survival rates.* Retrieved from http://www.kidsdata.org

Kim, S., & Chung, D. H. (2006). Pediatric solid malignancies: Neuroblastoma and Wilms' tumor. *Surgical Clinics of North America, 86,* 469–487.

Kurt, B. A., Armstrong, G. T., Cash, D. K., Krasin, M. J., Morris, E. B., Spunt, S. L., et al. (2008). Primary care management of the childhood cancer survivor. *Journal of Pediatrics, 152,* 458–466.

Kutluk, T., Varan, A., Buyukpamukcu, N., Atahan, L., Caglar, M., Akyuz, C., & Buyukpamukcu, M. (2006). Improved survival of children with Wilms' tumor. *Journal of Pediatric Hematology and Oncology, 28,* 423–426.

Lahl, M., Fisher, V. L., & Laschinger, K. (2008). Ewing's sarcoma family of tumors: An overview from diagnosis to survivorship. *Clinical Journal of Oncology Nursing, 12*(1), 89–97.

Leigh, S. A. (2008). The changing legacy of cancer: Issues of long-term survivorship. *Nursing Clinics of North America, 43*(2), 243–258.

Linder, L. A. (2008). Developmental diversity in symptom research involving children and adolescents with cancer. *Journal of Pediatric Nursing, 23*(4), 296–307.

Mann, G., Attarbaschi, A., Steiner, M., Simonitsch, I., Strobl, H., Urban, C., et al. (2006). Early and reliable diagnosis of non-Hodgkin lymphoma in childhood and adolescence. *Pediatric Hematology and Oncology, 23,* 167–176.

National Cancer Institute. (2007a). *Neuroblastoma treatment: Stage information.* Retrieved from http://www.cancer.gov/cancertopics/pdq/treatment/neuroblastoma/HealthProfessional/page3

National Cancer Institute. (2007b). *Wilms' tumor and other childhood kidney tumors: Stage information.* Retrieved from http://www.cancer.gov/cancertopics/pdq/treatment/wilms/HealthProfessional/page3

National Cancer Institute. (2008). *Bone marrow transplantation and peripheral blood stem cell transplantation.* Retrieved from http://www.cancer.gov/cancertopics/factsheet/Therapy/bone-marrow-transplant

National Cancer Institute. (2010). *Staging and diagnostic evaluation. Childhood Hodgkin lymphoma treatment.* Retrieved from http://www.cancer.gov/candertopics/pdq/treatment/childhodgkins/HealthProfesionals

National Human Genome Research Institute. (2009). *Essential nursing competencies and curricula guidelines for genetics and genomics.* Retrieved from http://www.genome.gov/17517037

Oeffinger, K. C., Nathan, P. C., & Kremer, L. C. M. (2008). Challenges after curative treatment for childhood cancer and long-term follow up of survivors. *Pediatric Clinics of North America, 55*(1), 251–274.

Park, J. R., Eggert, A., & Caron, H. (2008). Neuroblastoma: Biology, prognosis, and treatment. *Pediatric Clinics of North America, 55*(1), 97–120.

Pieters, R., & Carroll, W. L. (2008). Biology and treatment of acute lymphoblastic leukemia. *Pediatric Clinics of North America, 55*(1), 1–20.

Pollack, L. A., Stewart, L., Thompson, T. D., & Li, J. (2007). Trends in childhood cancer mortality—

United States, 1990–2004. *Morbidity and Mortality Weekly Report, 56,* 1257–1261.

Pui, C. J., & Evans, W. E. (2006). Treatment of acute lymphoblastic leukemia. *New England Journal of Medicine, 354,* 166–178.

Punyko, J. A., Gurney, J. G., Baker, K. S., Hayashi, R. J., Hudson, M. M., Liu, Y., et al. (2006). Physical impairment and social adaptation in adult survivors of childhood and adolescent rhabdomyosarcoma: A report from the Childhood Cancer Survivors Study. *Psycho-Oncology, 16,* 26–37.

Rampello, E., Fricia, T., & Malaguarnera, M. (2006). The management of tumor lysis syndrome. *National Clinical Practice in Oncology, 3*(8), 438–447.

Rheingold, S. R., & Lange, B. J. (2006). In P. A. Pizzo & D. G. Poplack, *Principles and practice of pediatric oncology* (5th ed., pp. 1202–1230). Philadelphia: Lippincott Williams & Wilkins.

Richardson, J., Smith, J. E., McCall, G., & Pilkington, K. (2006). Hypnosis for procedure-related pain and distress in pediatric cancer patients: A systematic review of effectiveness and methodology related to hypnosis interventions. *Journal of Pain and Symptom Management, 31,* 70–84.

Robertson, P. L. (2006). Advances in treatment of pediatric brain tumors. *NeuroRx, 3*(2), 276–291.

Rodeberg, D., & Paidas, C. (2006). Childhood rhabdomyosarcoma. *Seminars in Pediatric Surgery, 15,* 57–62.

Rourke, M. T., Hobbie, W. L., Schwartz, L., & Kazak, A. D. (2007). Posttraumatic stress disorder (PTSD) in young adult survivors of childhood cancer. *Pediatric Blood & Cancer, 49*(2), 177–182.

Rubnitz, J. E., Lensing, S., Razzouk, B. I., Pounds, S., Pui, C. H., & Ribeiro, R. C. (2007). Effect of race on outcome of white and black children with acute myeloid leukemia: The St. Jude experience. *Pediatric Blood & Cancer, 48,* 10–15.

Sedeh, A., Dahl, R. E., Shahar, G., & Rosenblat-Stein, S. (2009). Sleep and the transition to adolescence: A longitudinal study. *Sleep, 32*(12), 1602–1609.

Skinner, R., Hamish, W., Wallace, B., & Levitt, G. A. (2006). Long-term follow-up of people who have survived cancer during childhood. *Lancet, 7,* 489–498.

Spinazze, S., & Schrijvers, D. (2006). Metabolic emergencies. *Critical Reviews in Oncology/Hematology, 58,* 79–89.

Stanescu, L., Foarfa, C., Georgescu, A. C., & Georgescu, I. (2007). Kaposi's sarcoma associated with AIDS. *Romanian Journal of Morphology and Embryology, 48,* 181–187.

Twombly, R. (2007). Childhood cancer survivor study doubles to examine late effects of new treatments. *Journal of the National Cancer Institute, 99,* 1574–1576.

Unguru, Y., Coppes, M. J., & Kamani, N. (2008). Rethinking pediatric assent: From requirement to ideal. *Pediatric Clinics of North America, 55*(1), 211–222.

Warnick, E., & Auger, D. (2009). Management of patients with primary central nervous system lymphoma treated with high-dose methotrexate. *Clinical Journal of Oncology Nursing, 13*(2), 177–180.

Wexler, L. H., & Helman, L. J. (2006). Rhabdomyosarcoma and the undifferentiated sarcomas. In P. A. Pizzo & D. G. Poplack, *Principles and practice of pediatric oncology* (5th ed., pp. 971–1001). Philadelphia: Lippincott Williams & Wilkins.

Wilne, S., Collier, J., Kennedy, C., Koller, K., Grundy, R., & Walker, D. (2007). Presentation of childhood CNS tumours: A systematic review and meta-analysis. *Lancet Oncology, 8,* 685–695.

Wilne, S. H., Ferris, R. C., Nathwani, A., & Kennedy, C. R. (2006). The presenting features of brain tumors: A review of 200 cases. *Archives of Disease in Childhood, 91,* 502–506.

Wilson, B. A., Shannon, M. T., & Shields, K. M. (2009). *Nurse's drug guide.* Upper Saddle River, NJ: Pearson Prentice Hall.

Yang, D. J., Kim, E. E., & Inoue, T. (2006). Targeted molecular imaging in oncology. *Annals of Nuclear Medicine, 20,* 1–11.

Zebrack, B. J., Zevon, M. A., Turk, N., Nagarajan, R., Whitton, J., Robison, L. L., & Zeltzer, L. K. (2007). Psychological distress in long-term survivors of solid tumors diagnosed in childhood: A report from the Childhood Cancer Survivor Study. *Pediatric Blood & Cancer, 49*(1), 47–51.

Zonfrillo, M. R. (2009). Management of pediatric tumor lysis syndrome in the emergency department. *Emergency Medical Clinics of North America, 27*(3), 497–504.

Zwaan, M. C., Reinhardt, D., Hitzler, J., & Vyas, P. (2010). Acute leukemias in children with Down syndrome. *Pediatric Clinics of North America, 55*(1), 53–70.

Alterations in Gastrointestinal Function

25 chapter

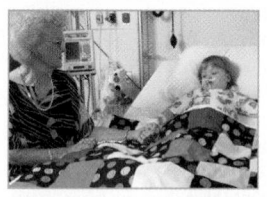

Jenna is a 4-year-old who has just been admitted to the pediatric unit following surgery for a ruptured appendix. She had complained of her stomach hurting last night, but this morning her condition appeared worse and she had a temperature of 102°F. Worried that this was not just a virus, her mother took her to the pediatrician. On the way to the doctor's office, Jenna told her mother that her pain "just went away." While at the pediatrician's office she complained of feeling bad all over. On examination her abdomen was rigid and no bowel sounds were heard. A complete blood count revealed a white blood cell (WBC) count of 22,000 mm³. The pediatrician diagnosed that Jenna had appendicitis and most likely had a ruptured appendix. He referred Jenna to the emergency department for assessment and surgical consultation. A computed tomography (CT) scan confirmed a diagnosis of appendicitis. During surgery the appendix was found to have ruptured.

Jenna had an open appendectomy with wound closure. A dry dressing is in place. Jenna now has a peripherally inserted central catheter (PICC) line for intravenous fluids, pain medication, and intravenous antibiotics. She also has a nasogastric tube to suction and a Foley catheter.

Jenna's parents feel guilty that the appendix was ruptured and wonder if they could have done something to prevent it. This is Jenna's first hospitalization. Jenna's parents are worried that she will have a lot of pain and wonder how she will cope with the hospitalization. What is the priority of nursing care for Jenna in the immediate postoperative period? What should the nurse include when teaching Jenna's parents about the postoperative course?

Key Terms

atresia / 758
bilirubin / 756
cholestasis / 779
chronic vomiting / 767
constipation / 771
cyclic vomiting / 767
deamination / 757
diarrhea / 771
encopresis / 788
gastroschisis / 768
gluconeogenesis / 757
hepatitis / 794
hernia / 773
hyperbilirubinemia / 792
intussusception / 769
omphaloceles / 767
ostomy / 774
peristalsis / 757
projectile vomiting / 764
stoma / 774
strangulation / 774
volvulus / 770

Learning Outcomes

After reading this chapter, you will be able to do the following:

1. Describe the anatomic and physiologic characteristics of the developing gastrointestinal system.
2. Discuss the pathophysiological processes associated with specific gastrointestinal disorders in the pediatric population.
3. Identify signs and symptoms that may indicate a disorder of the gastrointestinal system.
4. Summarize preoperative and postoperative family-centered care for the child born with cleft lip/palate.
5. Contrast nursing management for the child with a gastrointestinal condition having abdominal surgery versus nonoperative management.
6. Summarize etiology, pathophysiology, symptoms, and management for the child with a parasitic or viral infection of the gastrointestinal system.
7. Analyze developmentally appropriate approaches for nursing management of gastrointestinal disorders in the pediatric population.
8. Plan nursing care for the child with an injury to the gastrointestinal system.

FOCUS ON

The Gastrointestinal System

ANATOMY AND PHYSIOLOGY REVIEW

The gastrointestinal (GI) tract includes the esophagus, stomach, pancreas, small intestine, and large intestine (Figure 25–1 ➤). Through the GI tract, a child ingests and absorbs the foods and fluids necessary to sustain life and promote growth. Elimination of waste products is another role of the GI tract. Other organs located in the abdominal region include the gallbladder, liver, and spleen. The abdomen is generally divided into four quadrants for purposes of assessment. (Refer to Figure 5–36 on page 143 for the abdominal organs and structures in each quadrant.)

Esophagus and Stomach

The esophagus is a continuous tube that allows food to pass to the stomach. Food enters the esophagus through the mouth, where it is chewed. Initial enzyme secretion then occurs to begin food digestion. (See Chapter 19 ∞ for more information related to the mouth and pharynx.) The stomach is located in the left upper quadrant (LUQ) of the abdomen. The role of the stomach is to store food and to secrete enzymes and digestive juices that aid in the digestion of the food (Table 25–1). Hydrochloric acid stimulates the stomach's pepsinogens to become pepsins which break down proteins and are active in acidic levels (pH of 3 or less). The stomach propels food that is partially digested into the duodenum (a part of the small intestine).

Pancreas

The pancreas is located behind the stomach and has several functions. The pancreas secretes enzymes, electrolytes, and

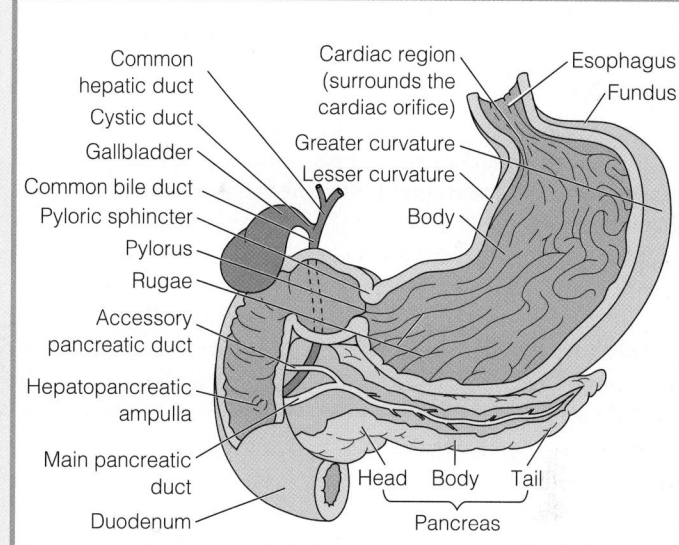

FIGURE 25–1 ➤ The internal anatomic structures of the stomach, including the pancreatic cystic and hepatic ducts, the pancreas, and the gallbladder.

TABLE 25–1	Enzymes Used in Digestion	
Enzyme	Source	Function
Amylase	Secreted by salivary glands	Converts starches to disaccharides
Hydrochloric acid	Secreted by stomach	Stops action of amylase; converts pepsinogen to pepsin that is instrumental in converting proteins to polypeptides
Amylase	Secreted by pancreas	Converts starches to disaccharides
Enterokinase	In small intestine	Converts chymotrypsinogen and trypsinogen to trypsin
Chymotrypsin and trypsin	In small intestine	Converts polypeptides to di- and tripeptides and then to amino acids
Bile salts	From bile and secreted to small intestine	Emulsifies fats
Lipase	From pancreas and small intestine	Converts fats to fatty acids and glycerol

Adapted from: Chamley, C. A., Carson, P., Randall, F., & Sandwell, M. (2005). Developmental anatomy and physiology of children. St. Louis, MO: Elsevier.

bicarbonate that aid in the digestion and absorption of fats, proteins, and carbohydrates (Werlin, 2007). Another key function of the pancreas is to regulate blood glucose metabolism through production of insulin, glucagon, and gastrin.

Liver and Gallbladder

The liver, the largest organ in the abdomen, is located in the right upper quadrant (RUQ). Its primary functions include production of blood clotting factors, fibrinogen and prothrombin; secretion of bile and **bilirubin** (yellow pigment produced from the breakdown of red blood cells); metabolism of fat, protein, and carbohydrates; detoxification of hormones, drugs, and other substances; and storage of vitamins A, D, E, and K and glycogen. The gallbladder is a small organ located behind the liver. The gallbladder stores and concentrates the bile that is produced in the liver. It then releases stored bile as needed into the duodenum. Bile includes a variety of substances such as water, salts, bilirubin, and cholesterol. A major role of bile is to emulsify fats so that fatty acids become soluble and absorbable (Bates & Balistreri, 2007).

Spleen

The spleen is located in the LUQ of the abdomen and is a very vascular organ. The spleen contains about 30% of the circulating platelets and is a site for red blood cell production as well.

Defense against infection is another key role of the spleen. Through phagocytosis, infectious organisms are filtered from the blood (Warkentin & Kelton, 2005).

Small and Large Intestine

The small intestine consists of the duodenum, the jejunum, and the ileum. Each part of the small intestine plays a vital role in the digestion and absorption of carbohydrates, amino acids, fats, and vitamins. About 90% of absorption takes place in the small intestine (Chamley et al., 2005). The intestinal wall is covered with small villi, the brush border, through which absorption occurs. Absorption occurs both through diffusion (commonly monosaccharides, amino acids, fatty acids, and glycerol) and active transport (commonly disaccharides, dipeptides, and tripeptides). A complex system of innervation and secretions maintains a basic pH that facilitates metabolism and absorption. The large intestine includes the cecum, the appendix, the colon (consisting of ascending, transverse, descending, and sigmoid portions), and the rectum, which passes to the exterior through the anus. The primary function of the large intestine is reabsorption of fluid and electrolytes from the GI tract and excretion of wastes (Wyllie, 2007a). Large intestine bacteria synthesize vitamin K and facilitate some vitamin B absorption.

As Children Grow

Stomach Capacity Increases

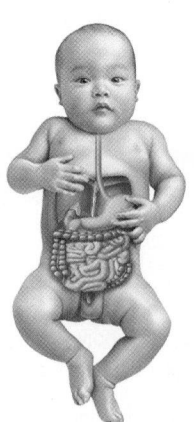

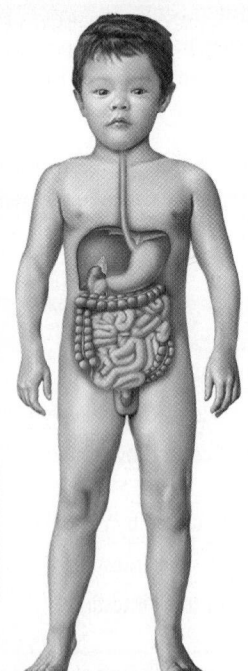

Stomach capacity throughout early childhood	
Age	*Capacity (mL)*
Newborn	10 to 20
1 week	30 to 90
2 to 3 weeks	75 to 100
1 month	90 to 150
3 months	150 to 200
1 year	210 to 360
2 years	500

FIGURE 25–2 ➤ Parents should be reminded that the young infant has a small stomach as compared to the older child or adolescent. Amounts per feeding should be determined accordingly using the guidelines seen here.

From: Chamley, C. A., Carson, P., Randall, D., & Sandwell, M. (2005). Developmental anatomy and physiology of children (p. 193). St. Louis, MO: Elsevier.

PEDIATRIC DIFFERENCES

Although the fetus makes sucking and swallowing movements in utero and ingests amniotic fluid, the GI system is immature at birth. The processes of absorption and excretion do not begin until after birth because the placenta provides nutrients and removes waste. Sucking is a primitive reflex that occurs whenever the lips or cheeks are stroked. The infant does not have voluntary control over swallowing until about 6 weeks of age.

The stomach capacity of the newborn is quite small, and intestinal motility (**peristalsis**) is greater than in older children (Figure 25–2 ➤). These characteristics explain the newborn's need for small, frequent feedings and the increased frequency and liquid consistency of bowel movements. Because of the relaxed cardiac sphincter, infants frequently regurgitate small amounts of feedings.

Digestion takes place in the duodenum. Infants have a deficiency of several enzymes: amylase (which digests carbohydrates), lipase (which enhances fat absorption), and trypsin (which catabolizes protein into polypeptides and some amino acids). Enzymes are usually not present in sufficient quantities to aid digestion until 4 to 6 months of age. Thus, abdominal distention from gas is common.

Liver function is also immature. After the first few weeks of life the liver is able to conjugate bilirubin and excrete bile. The processes of **gluconeogenesis** (formation of glycogen from noncarbohydrates), plasma protein and ketone formation, vitamin storage, and **deamination** (removal of amino group from amino compound) remain immature during the first year of life.

TABLE 25–2	Diagnostic Tests and Laboratory Procedures for the Gastrointestinal System	
Diagnostic Procedures	Laboratory Tests
Abdominal ultrasound	Complete blood count
Barium or contrast enema	Bilirubin
CT of the abdomen	Electrolytes
Endoscopy	Liver enzymes
GI series	Stool for occult blood
Intraesophageal pH probe monitoring	Stool for ova and parasites
Abdominal radiographs	

*See Appendices D and E ∞ for information about these diagnostic procedures and tests.

By the second year of life, digestive processes are fairly complete. Stomach capacity increases to accommodate a three-meals-per-day feeding schedule. At about the same time, myelination of the spinal cord becomes complete and voluntary control over excretory functions can be achieved.

Use the assessment guidelines below to perform a nursing assessment of the gastrointestinal system. A list of diagnostic and laboratory tests used to evaluate gastrointestinal conditions is provided in Table 25–2. See Appendices D and E ∞ for further information about lab values and test and procedures for the gastrointestinal system.

Assessment Guidelines for the Gastrointestinal System

Assessment Focus	Assessment Guidelines
Abdomen—inspection	▪ Observe the shape of the abdomen. ▪ Note any abdominal distention. ▪ Observe the umbilicus for protrusion ▪ Observe for peristaltic waves (visible rhythmic contractions of the intestinal wall smooth muscle).
Abdomen—auscultation	▪ Auscultate for bowel sounds in all four quadrants prior to palpation.
Abdomen—palpation	▪ Palpate the abdomen and note if it is soft or firm. ▪ Palpate the size of the umbilical ring. ▪ Does the child complain of pain or tenderness during palpation? Does the infant cry? ▪ Describe any masses palpated by location, shape, size, and consistency. ▪ Palpate the liver for size and tenderness. ▪ Palpate the spleen for size and tenderness.
Mouth and esophagus	▪ Note the presence of increased oral secretions. ▪ Note the presence of cleft lip or palate.
Nutrition	▪ Note tolerance of feedings, spitting up, emesis, and recurrent respiratory infections. ▪ Observe amount, color, and frequency of emesis. ▪ Note if emesis is associated with feeding and whether it is projectile. ▪ Note amount of intake, frequency of feedings, and growth.
Stool	▪ Observe color, consistency, and size of stool. Note any changes in stool patterns.
Family history	▪ Ask about history of gastrointestinal illness with genetic influences such as celiac disease and inflammatory bowel disease.

▧ STRUCTURAL DEFECTS

Structural defects can involve one or more areas of the GI tract. These defects occur when growth and development of fetal structures are interrupted during the first trimester. This can leave the structure incomplete, resulting in **atresia** (absence or closure of a normal body orifice), malposition, nonclosure, or other abnormalities.

Cleft Lip and Cleft Palate

Cleft lip and cleft palate are two distinct facial defects (Figure 25–3 ➤). Cleft lip with or without cleft palate occurs in 1 out of every 750–1,000 live births. The incidence is higher in Asians (1 in 500) than in Caucasians (1 in 750). The defect is less common in African Americans, with an incidence of 1 out of every 2,000 live births (Patel, Ramaswamy, Grasseschi, et al., 2009).

Cleft lip and palate occur together in approximately 45% of cases, while cleft palate occurs alone approximately 35% of the time, and cleft lip occurs alone approximately 20% of the time (Patel et al., 2009).

Etiology and Pathophysiology

Cleft lip with or without cleft palate results when the maxillary processes fail to fuse with the elevations on the frontal prominence during the sixth week of gestation. Normally union of the upper lip is complete by the seventh week. Fusion of the secondary palate occurs between 5 and 12 weeks of gestation. Failure of the tongue to move downward at the correct time prevents the palatine processes from fusing. Although cleft lip or palate occurs as a feature in many different syndromes, a majority of children with these orofacial defects (70%) do not have an associated syndrome or other birth defect (March of Dimes, 2007; Scapoli, Martinelli, Arlotti, et al., 2008; Wehby & Cassell, 2010).

There is an increased incidence in families with a prior history of cleft lip or palate. The cause is believed to be multifactorial, involving a combination of environmental and genetic influences. When fortification of cereals and breads with folate began in the United States in 1996 as a measure to decrease neural tube defects, the incidence of orofacial clefts also decreased. This may suggest a role for folate in formation of maxillary processes in the fetus (Yazdy, Honein, & Xing, 2007).

Clinical Manifestations

A cleft that involves the lip is apparent at birth. It may be a simple dimple in the vermilion border of the lip or a complete separation extending to the floor of the nose. The defect may be unilateral or bilateral and may occur alone or in combination with a cleft palate defect. Varying degrees of nasal deformity may also be present.

Cleft palate defects are less obvious when they occur without a cleft lip and may not be detected at birth. Clefts of the hard palate form a continuous opening between the mouth and nasal cavity and may be unilateral or bilateral, involving just the soft palate or both the soft and hard palate.

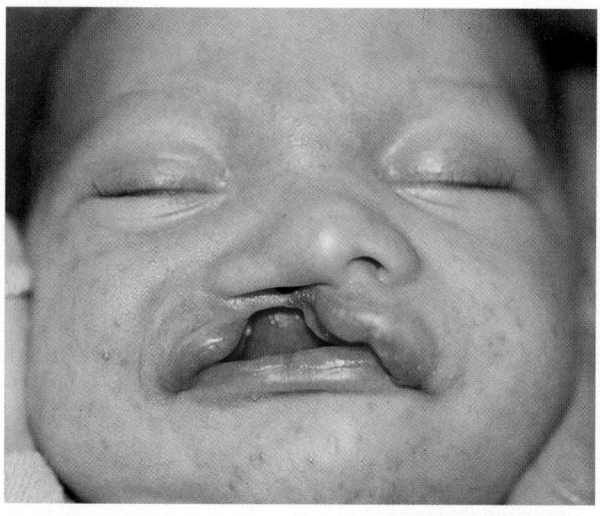

A

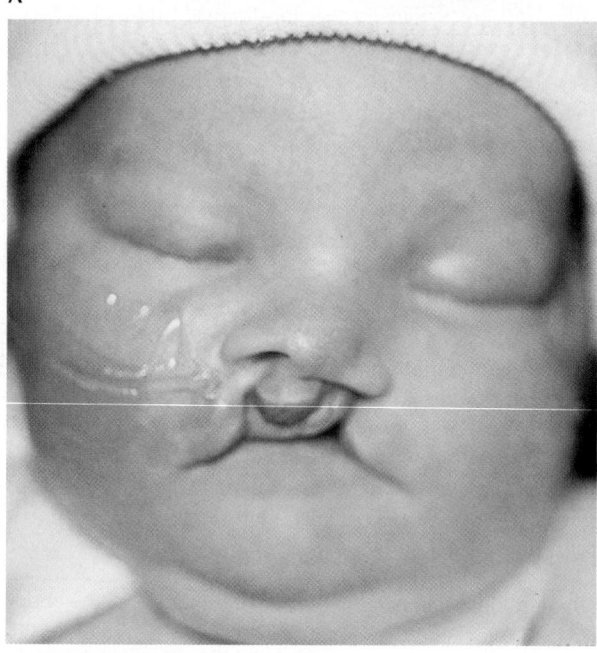

B

FIGURE 25–3 ➤ A, Unilateral cleft lip. B, Bilateral cleft lip.
Courtesy of Dr. Elizabeth Peterson, Spokane, WA.

COLLABORATIVE CARE

A multidisciplinary team is involved in cleft lip and palate management since these children have an increased risk for impairment in speech, hearing, and tooth development (Cassell, Daniels, & Meyer, 2009). Coordinated care by specialists in plastic and oral surgery, audiology, speech, otolaryngology, and orthodontics is necessary

The cleft lip should be repaired during the first 6 months of life (Cassell et al., 2009) (Figure 25–4 ➤). The lip is sutured together using either a diagonal incision or a staggered suture line (z-plasty) (Merritt, 2005). If the defect is severe, the child may need more than one operation to achieve total repair. After surgery, soft elbow immobilizers are used for 2 weeks to prevent the

Discharge teaching should include ways to prevent the infant from touching the suture line such as:

- Bundling an infant in a blanket with arms tucked inside the blanket.
- Using a front-sling baby carrier to immobilize the arms. Front-sling carriers provide the additional benefits of comforting the infant through contact with the parent and of holding the infant upright, which aids in optimal positioning after feedings.

After surgical repair, parents need to be taught how to feed the infant and identify signs of complications (fever, vomiting, respiratory distress). Referral to a home health care agency for support may be helpful. Encourage follow-up visits with health care professionals. The child may need further evaluation of speech development, assessment for presence of ear infections, or a recommendation for plastic surgery.

Evaluation

Expected outcomes of nursing care in the preoperative period include:

- The child does not experience respiratory distress and maintains normal respirations.
- Positive parent–infant bonding is established.
- The child achieves and maintains a normal weight.
- The parent has knowledge of the defect, its correction, and the child's needs.

Expected outcomes of postoperative nursing care are included in the nursing care plan. Additional outcomes include effective pain management, fluid and electrolyte balance, and appropriate home care after surgery.

▲ Health Promotion

The child with cleft lip or cleft palate requires close monitoring and intervention to foster growth and development. Planned assessments of weight, developmental milestones, dental health, hearing, and speech will alert the health care team to problems requiring intervention and maximize the child's potential for normal development.

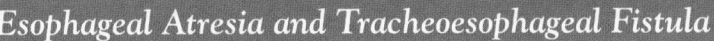

Pathophysiology Illustrated

Esophageal Atresia and Tracheoesophageal Fistula

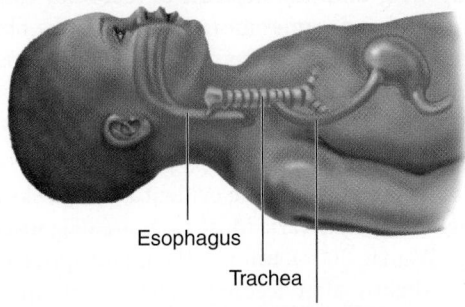

Esophagus

Trachea

Bottom portion of esophagus

FIGURE 25–7 ➤ In the most common type of esophageal atresia and tracheoesophageal fistula, the upper segment of the esophagus ends in a blind pouch connected to the trachea; a fistula connects the lower segment to the trachea.

Esophageal Atresia and Tracheoesophageal Fistula

Esophageal atresia is a malformation that results from failure of the esophagus to develop as a continuous tube during the fourth and fifth weeks of gestation. Esophageal atresia occurs in approximately 1 in 4,000 births, with 90% of those affected also having a tracheoesophageal fistula (Orenstein, Peters, Khan, et al., 2007).

In esophageal atresia, the foregut fails to lengthen, separate, and fuse into two parallel tubes (the esophagus and trachea) during fetal development. Instead, the esophagus may end in a blind pouch or develop as a pouch connected to the trachea by a fistula (tracheoesophageal fistula) (Figure 25–7 ➤). Esophageal atresia is often associated with a maternal history of polyhydramnios. Associated anomalies may occur, including congenital heart defects, gastrointestinal or urinary tract anomalies, and musculoskeletal abnormalities (Orenstein et al., 2007).

Symptoms in the newborn include excessive salivation and drooling, often accompanied by three classic signs for this defect: cyanosis, choking, coughing. Sneezing may also be manifested. During feeding, the infant returns fluid through the nose and mouth. Aspiration places the infant at risk for pneumonia. Depending on the type of defect, the abdomen may become distended because of air trapping.

COLLABORATIVE CARE

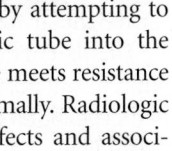

Diagnosis is usually confirmed by attempting to pass a nasogastric or orogastric tube into the stomach. In most cases, the tube meets resistance and can be advanced only minimally. Radiologic examination reveals specific defects and associated anomalies. Careful examination of the lungs is needed. A delay in diagnosis can be fatal because ingested fluid or secretions may enter the lungs and lead to pneumonia (Orenstein et al., 2007).

After diagnosis is confirmed, a nasogastric tube is inserted to suction the upper pouch. Intravenous antibiotics and fluids are begun. Surgery is performed as soon as possible. Surgical correction may be accomplished in several stages. The first stage usually involves ligation of the fistula and insertion of a gastrostomy tube. In the second stage, the two ends of the esophagus are reconnected, if possible. When surgical closure (anastomosis) is not possible, a gastrostomy tube must remain in place for use in feeding. Potential postoperative complications include gastroesophageal reflux, aspiration, and stricture formation. The prognosis is usually good with surgery; however, some conditions are complicated, requiring repeated surgeries and long-term management. In the event that the two ends of the esophagus cannot be reconnected, colonic, jejunal, or gastric segments may be used to lengthen the esophagus (Orenstein et al., 2007).

NURSING MANAGEMENT

The nurse may recognize the signs and symptoms in the immediate newborn period. Assess for difficulty feeding and excessive drooling. Assess for the classic signs of choking, coughing, and cyanosis. Assess for respiratory distress and assess the lung sounds carefully.

Esophageal atresia is a surgical emergency. Preoperatively the infant requires close observation and intervention to maintain a patent airway. Specific interventions include the following:

- Have suction readily available to remove any secretions that accumulate in the nasopharyngeal airway.
- Place the infant with the head of the bed slightly raised to minimize aspiration of secretions into the trachea.
- Use continuous or low intermittent suction to remove secretions from the blind pouch.
- Withhold oral fluids, and provide maintenance intravenous fluids.
- Constantly monitor the infant's vital signs and overall condition.

After surgery, measure gastrostomy drainage, and administer intravenous fluids and antibiotics. Total parenteral nutrition may be needed until gastrostomy or oral feedings are tolerated. Monitoring and assessment of feeding tolerance is ongoing. Feedings are introduced slowly and in small amounts. Assess for respiratory difficulty during reintroduction of feedings. Monitor weight, growth, and developmental achievements.

The parents require emotional support throughout the infant's hospitalization. Clearly explain all procedures. Encourage parents to bond with the infant by stroking and talking to the infant. Eliciting questions and allowing parents to participate in the infant's care, especially feeding (when permitted), can facilitate bonding and help to prepare parents for care of the infant after discharge.

Once enteral feedings have been established, the infant may be discharged from the hospital with a gastrostomy tube in place. Teach the parents about gastrostomy tube care and feeding, signs of infection, and how to prevent postoperative complications (Figure 25–8 ➤). (See Families Want to Know: Teaching the Family About Gastrostomy Tube Feedings.)

The outcomes of nursing care will depend on the extent of the defect and correction. Examples include adequate intake of fluids to promote hydration and growth, absence of respiratory distress, positive parent–infant bonding, healing without infection, and parental use of support and information resources regarding the condition.

Pyloric Stenosis

Pyloric stenosis is a hypertrophic obstruction of the circular muscle of the pyloric canal. Pyloric stenosis occurs in approximately

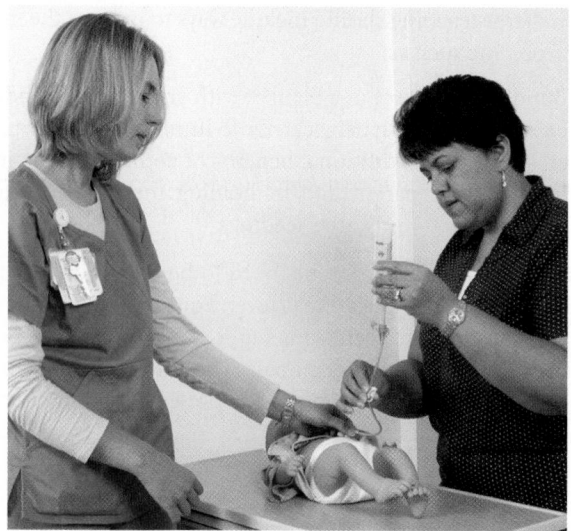

FIGURE 25–8 ➤ The nurse teaches this mother how to administer gastrostomy feedings.

1 in 1,000 live births (Vajnar, 2007). Males are affected more often than females by a 4:1 ratio (Liao, Li, Zhang, et al., 2007). There is an increased incidence in firstborn White males (Wyllie, 2007b).

Etiology and Pathophysiology

The exact cause of pyloric stenosis is unknown, although frequently there is a family history of the disorder. *Hypergastrinemia* (too much gastrin in the blood) is thought to play a role in the development of pyloric stenosis. Studies have indicated a higher incidence of the disorder in infants who received prostaglandin E infusion for patent ductus arteriosus and in infants less than a month old who have received oral erythromycin. Gastroesophageal reflux is frequently also present in premature infants with pyloric stenosis, complicating the differential diagnosis (Joshi, Mahajan, & Kamat, 2006).

Hypertrophy of the circular pylorus muscle results in stenosis of the passage between the stomach and the duodenum, partially obstructing the lumen of the stomach (Figure 25–9 ➤). The lumen becomes inflamed and edematous, which narrows the opening until the obstruction becomes complete. At this time vomiting becomes more forceful. As the obstruction progresses, the infant becomes dehydrated and electrolytes are depleted, resulting in metabolic imbalances.

Clinical Manifestations

Symptoms usually become evident 2 to 8 weeks after birth, although onset may vary. Most cases are diagnosed by 12 weeks of age (Vajnar, 2007). Initially the infant appears well or regurgitates slightly after feedings. The parents may describe the infant as a "good eater" who vomits occasionally. As the obstruction progresses, the vomiting becomes projectile. In **projectile vomiting**, the contents of the stomach may be ejected up to 3 feet from the infant. The vomitus is nonbilious and may become blood tinged because of repeated irritation to the esophagus. The infant generally appears hungry, especially after emesis, is irritable, fails to gain weight, and has fewer and

Families Want to Know
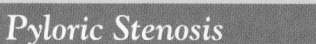
Teaching the Family About Gastrostomy Tube Feedings

The infant or child who has difficulty swallowing, consuming oral feedings, or gaining weight may be a candidate for gastrostomy tube placement. Children with chronic conditions such as failure to thrive, neuromuscular disorders, severe gastroesophageal reflux, and genetic syndromes may need to have a gastrostomy tube placed for long-term enteral feedings (Goldberg, Barton, Xanthopoulos, et al., 2010). See Chapter 11 ∞ for general guidelines related to teaching plans, and the *Clinical Skills Manual.*

General Principles
Preoperatively

■ Assess what the family knows about gastrostomy tube placement and what teaching methods will be most effective in teaching care of the gastrostomy tube and enteral feedings.

■ Show the family pictures or dolls with gastrostomy tubes and explain what the child's abdomen will look like in the immediate postoperative period.

■ Provide the family with a booklet about gastrostomy tubes and enteral feedings.

Postoperatively

■ Show the family the child's gastrostomy tube and reassess their understanding of the tube.

■ When feedings are ordered, demonstrate the first feeding to the parents while explaining each step.

■ Actively involve a family member in the second feeding. With subsequent feedings have a family member feed the child with the nurse watching.

■ Teach the family about:
  • Medication administration
  • Daily care of the tube and the site surrounding the tube
  • How to troubleshoot common complications
  • Phone numbers to call if needed

All family members that are involved in care of the child should practice feeding the child and administering medications to the child prior to discharge. This allows the nurse to assess for understanding of the procedure and gives the family confidence in their ability to care for the child. Some children will need bolus feedings, others may have continuous feedings via a feeding pump, and others may have bolus feedings during the day and continuous feedings at night.

Data from: Borkowski, S. (2005, May). Irritation, redness, and drainage at the site of a pediatric gastrostomy. *Clinical Advisor*, 90–91; Holmes, S. (2004). Enteral feeding and percutaneous endoscopic gastrostomy. *Nursing Standard, 18*(20), 41–43.

---

smaller stools. The infant may become dehydrated and may develop metabolic alkalosis. Loss of gastric secretions results in dehydration and, potentially, metabolic alkalosis. On physical examination, peristaltic waves may be observed across the abdomen and an olive-sized mass in the right upper quadrant may be palpated (Vajnar, 2007).

Pathophysiology Illustrated
Pyloric Stenosis

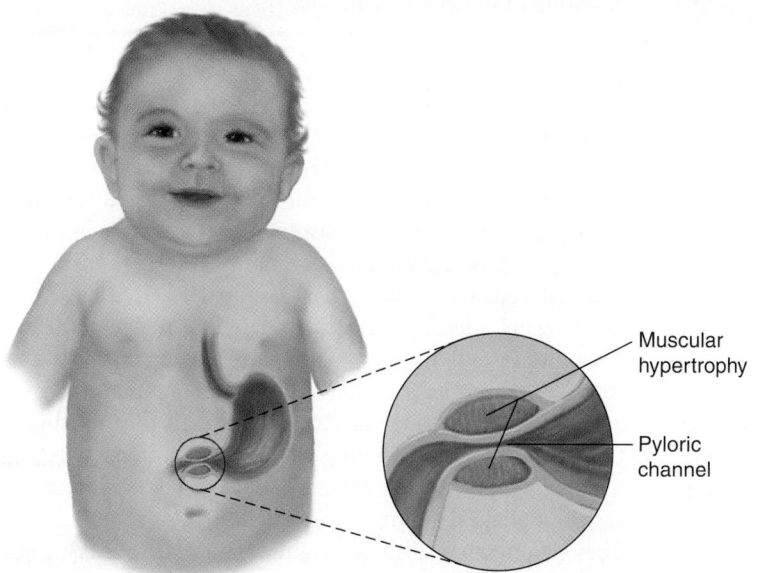

FIGURE 25–9 ➤ In pyloric stenosis, the hypertrophied pyloric muscle causes symptoms of projectile vomiting and visible peristalsis.

Muscular hypertrophy

Pyloric channel

COLLABORATIVE CARE
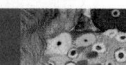

An abdominal ultrasound, to determine the diameter and length of the pyloric muscle, is usually performed to confirm the diagnosis. A thickened pylorus of greater than 4 mm in diameter and length of greater than 14 mm for the pyloric channel are diagnostic of pyloric stenosis (Joshi et al., 2006). An upper gastrointestinal (UGI) study may also be performed, and reveals a narrowing of the pyloric channel, preventing the passage of the contrast medium. Blood tests determine the degree of dehydration, electrolyte imbalance, and anemia (see Chapter 18 ∞); common findings are hypochloremia, hypokalemia, metabolic alkalosis, and hyperbilirubinemia (Vajnar, 2007). Early diagnosis decreases the severity of electrolyte alterations.

Surgery is performed as soon as possible after the infant's fluid and electrolyte balance is restored. Open pyloromyotomy is performed through a periumbilical incision or through a small, transverse upper abdominal incision. Laparoscopic pyloromyotomy is currently used in many cases, and has been shown to be as successful as open pyloromyotomy (Wyllie, 2007b). With both procedures, the pyloric muscle is split to allow the passage of food and fluid.

The prognosis is good. The infant is usually taking fluids within a few hours following surgery and discharged on full-strength formula within 24 hours after surgery.

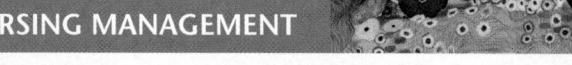

NURSING MANAGEMENT

Nursing Assessment and Diagnosis

Observe the infant's abdomen for the presence of peristaltic waves. Then auscultate bowel sounds, which are usually hyperactive on auscultation. Palpation reveals an olive-shaped mass in the right upper quadrant of the abdomen.

Assess the infant's history of vomiting, vital signs, weight, and nutritional status. Assess skin turgor, fontanels, mucous membranes, urinary output (weigh diapers), and urine specific gravity, to determine whether hydration is adequate. Describe vomiting episodes and estimated emesis amount. Be alert for signs of an electrolyte imbalance, particularly low levels of serum chloride, sodium, and potassium, and an elevated pH. (See Chapter 18 ∞ for a discussion of these electrolyte imbalances.) Assess the parents' level of anxiety related to the child's condition. The child is usually hungry and tries to feed. Crying and general discomfort are frequently observed.

Among the nursing diagnoses that might be appropriate for the child with pyloric stenosis are:

- Deficient Fluid Volume related to inadequate intake and vomiting
- Imbalanced Nutrition: Less than Body Requirements related to vomiting and inability to ingest nutrients
- Sleep Pattern Disturbance related to discomfort and hunger
- Parental Anxiety related to surgery

Planning and Implementation

Nursing care focuses on meeting the infant's fluid and electrolyte needs, minimizing weight loss, promoting rest and comfort, preventing infection, and providing supportive care for parents.

Meet Fluid and Electrolyte Needs

Because projectile vomiting will continue until the obstruction is relieved surgically, withhold oral feedings. Emphasize to the parents the importance of maintaining an NPO status preoperatively. Intravenous fluid therapy is administered to correct fluid and electrolyte imbalances and to maintain adequate hydration. Because gastric fluid is high in potassium, hypokalemia can result. (See Chapter 18 ∞ for a discussion of hypokalemia.) Maintain patency of the nasogastric tube and measure aspirated contents. Inform parents that all diapers will be weighed to measure the infant's output of urine and stool.

Minimize Weight Loss

The infant loses weight because of frequent vomiting. Monitor weight daily both preoperatively and postoperatively. Begin feedings postoperatively according to health care provider orders. Some surgeons prefer an NPO period following pyloromyotomy, with slow, incremental increases in volume and strength of feedings once feeding has resumed, whereas others will implement an earlier postoperative feeding approach.

Promote Rest and Comfort

During the preoperative period the infant is hungry and cries often. The infant is swaddled to maintain warmth and provide comfort. Encourage the parents to hold and cuddle the infant. Provide a pacifier to meet the infant's need to suck.

Postoperatively the infant is uncomfortable because of the surgical incision. Administer analgesics as prescribed to relieve discomfort. Instruct parents to avoid pressure on the incision. When diapering the infant, slide the diaper gently under the buttocks rather than lifting the legs. Swaddling, rocking, and use of a pacifier help to relax the infant. (See Chapter 15 ∞ for a discussion of pain management.)

Prevent Infection

Postoperatively the incision is covered with collodion or Steri-Strips and should be kept clean and dry. Inspect the incision site for redness, swelling, or discharge. Monitor the infant's temperature every 4 hours. Auscultate the lungs to assess for any adventitious sounds.

Provide Supportive Care

The need for hospitalization and surgery creates anxiety for parents. Encourage them to participate in the infant's care and to discuss their fears and concerns. Provide simple and clear explanations about the infant's condition and care. Advise parents that occasional vomiting after surgery may occur.

Discharge Planning and Home Care Teaching

Instruct parents to observe the incision for redness, swelling, or discharge and to notify the physician immediately if these occur or if the infant develops a fever. To reduce the possibility of infection, advise parents to fold the infant's diaper so that it does not touch the incision. Provide instructions about feeding to ensure the infant's intake. See Families Want to Know: Home Care Instructions Following Pyloromyotomy.

Evaluation

Expected outcomes of care include pain control, intake of recommended fluid and food with absence of vomiting, and manifestation of normal growth patterns.

Gastroesophageal Reflux

Gastroesophageal reflux (GER), the return of gastric contents into the esophagus, is the result of relaxation of the lower esophageal sphincter (Suwandhi, Ton, & Schwarz, 2006). GER is one of the most common gastrointestinal disorders in children, affecting approximately 50% of infants ages 0–3 months (International Pediatric Endosurgery Group [IPEG], 2008a). Some "spitting up" after feedings is considered normal in newborn infants, because of the weak cardiac sphincter of the stomach. However, regurgitation that continues and increases in frequency may be caused by GER and requires further investigation.

Regurgitation or vomiting is the most common sign of gastroesophageal reflux in infants (IPEG, 2008a). Children with gastroesophageal reflux are frequently hungry and irritable. They eat often but still lose weight. Infants with reflux are at risk for aspiration and apnea.

Gastroesophageal reflux disease (GERD) is a more serious manifestation of GER. Infants and younger children present with a history of poor weight gain, recurrent vomiting, gener-

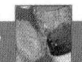
The infant is generally discharged home the day following surgery. Partner with the family to provide home feeding and care instructions. The following information is provided:

■ The infant may be bottle-fed or breastfed.

■ An infant will sometimes vomit after some feedings following surgery—this does not mean the surgical correction was unsuccessful.

■ If the infant vomits, offer a bottle or breast as soon as he or she is interested in feeding again.

■ The infant should be burped after every 1 to 2 ounces during feeding. If breastfeeding, burp the infant every 5 to 10 minutes.

■ After feeding, hold the infant in an upright position for 30 minutes.

■ The infant should not play or be rocked for 30 minutes following feedings.

■ Administer analgesics as prescribed. Inform the health care provider if you believe your infant is not obtaining adequate pain relief.

■ Keep the surgical wound area clean and dry. The bandage or strips may fall off, and this is normal. If not, they will be removed at the follow-up visit.

■ The infant should be sponge bathed only. Tub baths are not allowed until the wound has healed or as instructed by the health care provider.

■ Notify the health care provider if the infant demonstrates any of the following:

  • The infant has redness, drainage, bleeding, or swelling at the surgical site.

  • The infant has a fever of 100.5°F or higher.

  • The infant is inconsolable.

  • The infant vomits the majority of two feedings in a row.

alized irritability, and refusal to feed. Infants may also have a history of arching, respiratory symptoms such as wheezing, and apnea (Gold & Gremse, 2006; IPEG, 2008a; Weill, 2008). Additional symptoms seen in older children and adolescents include heartburn, abdominal/epigastric pain, and regurgitation (Malaty, O'Malley, Abudayyeh, et al., 2008).

COLLABORATIVE CARE

Diagnosis is confirmed by a thorough history of the child's feeding patterns and by diagnostic evaluation. Although a barium swallow is useful in evaluating the cause of vomiting, it lacks specificity in the diagnosis of GER. Esophageal pH monitoring is the preferred test in the diagnosis of GER and the frequency of reflux episodes. Gastric emptying studies are also useful in the diagnosis of GER (IPEG, 2008a).

Treatment depends on the severity of the condition. Generally, feeding modification, thickened feeds, and positioning are effective management for milder cases. A smaller feeding volume may prove beneficial to avoid overdistention of the abdomen and subsequent reflux. The infant should be burped after every 2 ounces (Weill, 2008). Rice cereal is sometimes placed in the infant's bottle to thicken feedings to a consistency similar to nectar. Note that breast milk will not readily thicken with addition of cereal. Prethickened formulas are commercially available. For example, Enfamil AR contains added rice and is

nutritionally balanced (Weill, 2008). These formulas can be administered without enlarging the nipple hole. Formula change to semi-elemental formula, such as Pregestimil, Nutramigen, or Alimentum, may be recommended (Orenstein & McGowan, 2008). Fatty foods and citrus juices are avoided. See Medications Used to Treat Gastroesophageal Reflux on page 768.

Treatment for severe cases of GERD may include surgery to create a valve mechanism by wrapping the greater curvature of the stomach (fundus) around the distal esophagus (fundoplication) (IPEG, 2008a). A gastrostomy tube is frequently inserted during surgery to serve as an access for decompression and as means for feeding if needed (Price, 2007).

Vomiting and feeding disorders can occur throughout childhood as well as in infancy. In older children, a pattern of **chronic vomiting** (low-grade nearly daily emesis) or **cyclic vomiting** (repeated severe vomiting of an episodic nature) can occur. These patterns differ from vomiting seen in colic (Chapter 14 ∞) or gastroesophageal reflux. Chronic vomiting is often associated with upper gastrointestinal tract diseases. Children who experience cyclic vomiting generally have a typical pattern with each episode in relation to time of onset, symptoms, and duration. Episodes of cyclic vomiting are generally triggered by psychological or physiological stress (Cuvellier & Lèpine, 2010). Continuous vomiting of any nature should be evaluated.

NURSING MANAGEMENT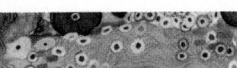

Nursing management focuses on supporting the infant's or child's nutritional intake, promoting interventions to reduce associated complications, and supporting the family. Monitor the infant's weight daily and plot on a growth chart to note progress. Observe for any signs of respiratory distress, and keep the infant's nose and mouth clear of vomitus.

Adequate nutrition must be maintained. Infants receiving oral feedings should be given small, frequent feedings. Elevate the head of the crib to prevent aspiration if vomiting should occur. Parents are encouraged to hold their infant in an upright position for 20 to 30 minutes following feedings. Minimize seated positioning such as in an infant seat since this increases intra-abdominal pressure and promotes reflux (Weill, 2008). If the child has a gastrostomy tube, it is important to maintain skin integrity around the stoma site.

Discharge planning focuses on instructing parents how to feed and position the infant, as well as how to provide comfort and emotional support. Encourage parents to hold and cuddle the infant during all feedings. Providing the infant with a pacifier helps to meet nonnutritive sucking needs. Teach parents how to suction the nose and mouth if vomiting occurs.

Omphalocele and Gastroschisis

Omphaloceles are congenital malformations in which intraabdominal contents herniate through the umbilical cord (Figure 25–10 ►). An omphalocele results when the intestines fail to return to the abdomen when the abdominal wall begins to close by the tenth week of gestation. The size of the sac varies depending on the extent of the protrusion. Large defects may

Medications Used to Treat
Gastroesophageal Reflux

Medication/Action and Indication	Nursing Management

Histamine H-2 Receptor Antagonists
Zantac (ranitidine)
Pepcid (famotidine)
Inhibition of the histamine-2 receptor on the gastric parietal cell, thus blocking gastric acid secretion.
	May be administered with or without food.
	If antacids are prescribed, administer 2 hours before or after H-2 antagonists.
	Teach parents to avoid OTC medications without checking with a health care provider.
	Monitor for side effects:
	    Bradycardia
	    Constipation
	    Nausea
	    Fatigue
	    Confusion
	    Dizziness
	    Headache
	    Irritability
	    Rash
	    Thrombocytopenia

Proton Pump Inhibitors
Prevacid (lansoprazole)
Prilosec (omeprazole)
Blocks the final common pathway of acid production by inhibiting activated proton pumps in the gastric parietal cell canaliculus.
These powerful inhibitors of acid secretion alleviate symptoms and help to heal esophagitis.
	Administer in the morning on an empty stomach.
	Monitor for side effects:
	    Abdominal pain
	    Diarrhea
	    Dizziness
	    Fatigue
	    Headache
	    Hematuria
	    Nausea
	    Proteinuria
	    Rash
	Teach the family to inform their primary health care provider if severe diarrhea occurs.
	Teach the family to inform their primary health care provider if changes in urinary elimination, such as pain or discomfort associated with urination, occur.

Note: Ranitidine is approved for use in infants 1 month of age and older. Famotidine and lansoprazole are approved in children 1 year of age and older. Omeprazole is approved in children 2 years of age and older.

Data from: Bindler, R., & Howry, L. (2005). Pediatric drug guide. Upper Saddle River, NJ: Prentice Hall Health; Gold, B. D., & Gremse, D. A. (2006). Extinguishing the burn: Case studies in pediatric reflux disease. Self Study Supplement to Clinician Reviews; Weill, V. (2008). Gastroesophageal reflux in infancy. Advance for Nurse Practitioners, 16(1), 47–50.

contain intestines, stomach, liver, and the spleen (Zimmerman, 2007). Omphalocele occurs at the base of the umbilical cord. The abdominal contents are covered with peritoneum and amniotic membrane (Khan, 2008). Rupture of the sac results in evisceration of the abdominal contents. Approximately 30% of infants with omphalocele will have an associated chromosomal anomaly, and 30–50% will have congenital heart defects (Lund, Bauer, & Berrios, 2007).

Omphalocele with herniation of intestines into the umbilical cord occurs in 1 in 5,000 births, while omphalocele with herniation of liver and intestines occurs in 1 in 10,000 births (Stoll, 2007).

A related condition is **gastroschisis**, a congenital defect of the ventral abdominal wall, characterized by herniation of abdominal viscera outside the abdominal cavity through a defect in the abdominal wall to the side (most often to the right) of the umbilicus. The most common abdominal organs involved are the small intestine and ascending colon. Unlike the omphalocele, no membrane covers the organs (Figure 25–11 ➤). Gastroschisis occurs in approximately 1–2 in 10,000 births worldwide (Zimmerman, 2007). It is the most common abdominal wall defect in neonates (Lund et al., 2007). Approximately 10–20% of infants with gastroschisis have an associated anomaly, most often intestinal atresias. Anomalies outside of the gastrointestinal tract are uncommon in infants with gastroschisis (Lund et al., 2007). Care of the child with gastroschisis or omphalocele centers on protecting the protruding abdominal organs, correcting the defect, and preventing complications such as hypothermia, infection, and injury to involved organs.

COLLABORATIVE CARE

Both gastroschisis and omphalocele are associated with elevation of maternal serum alpha-fetoprotein (MSAFP). Routine

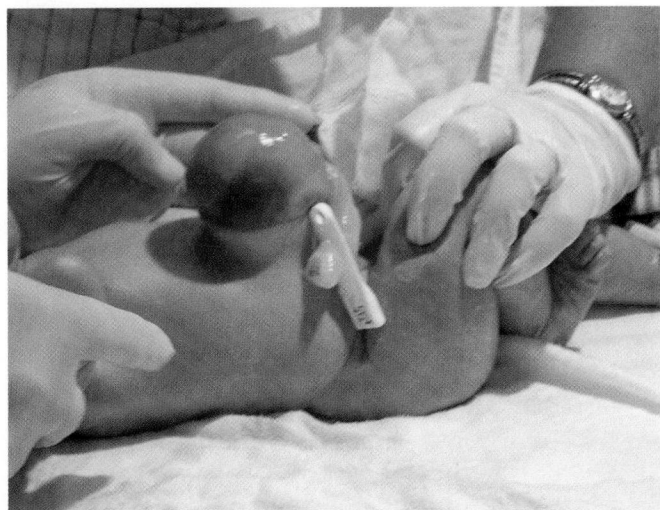

FIGURE 25–10 ➤ In omphalocele, the size of the sac depends on the extent of the protrusion of abdominal contents through the umbilical cord.
Courtesy of Carol Harrigan, RNC, MSN, NNP.

prenatal ultrasonography and determination of MSAFP levels permit early diagnosis and coordination of the team of specialists needed to manage these congenital anomalies including neonatologists and pediatric surgeons (Zimmerman, 2007).

The immediate action upon birth is to protect the sac (in omphalocele) or exposed abdominal contents (in gastroschisis) from injury by placing the infant feet first into a bowel bag (a plastic sterile drape) that extends to the nipple line and is secured with ties. The bowel bag decreases heat loss and allows for visualization of the defect. The child with gastroschisis should first have the exposed abdominal contents covered with moist sterile gauze (Zimmerman, 2007). The child will often be transferred to a neonatal intensive care unit (NICU) with surgical capability for this defect.

Surgical repair of omphalocele and gastroschisis may occur in one or two stages depending on the severity of the defect. One

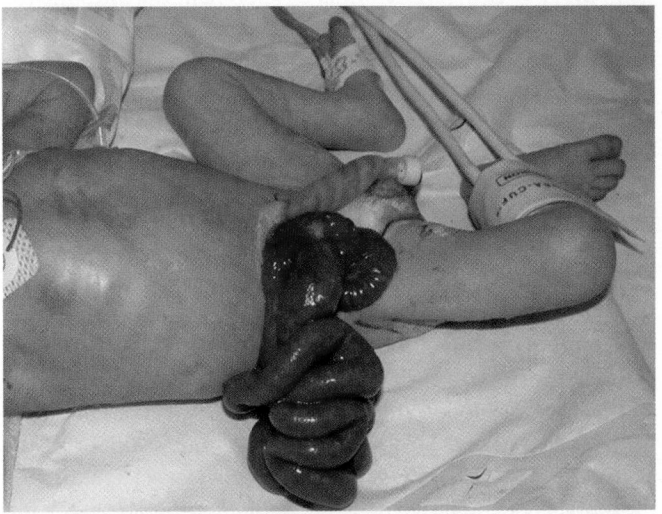

FIGURE 25–11 ➤ The newborn with gastroschisis has abdominal contents located outside the abdominal wall.
Used with permission of the authors and the University of Iowa's Virtual Hospital®, www.vh.org

surgery may be all that is needed to repair a small defect. For larger defects, the first stage of repair may involve nonoperative placement of the abdominal contents or sac into a Silastic silo. Once the abdominal cavity can accommodate the intestinal contents, the child will have surgery to close the abdominal wall (Lund et al., 2007; Zimmerman, 2007).

NURSING MANAGEMENT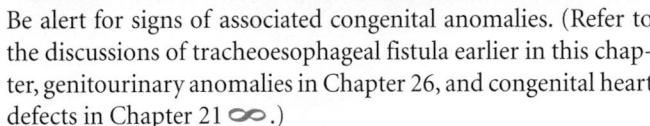

Be alert for signs of associated congenital anomalies. (Refer to the discussions of tracheoesophageal fistula earlier in this chapter, genitourinary anomalies in Chapter 26, and congenital heart defects in Chapter 21 ∞.)

Immediately after birth, follow physician protocol for maintaining the omphalocele sac or for the exposed abdominal contents in gastroschisis, such as with sterile gauze soaked in warm normal saline solution covered with sterile plastic. Monitor vital signs at least hourly, paying close attention to temperature, as the infant can lose heat through the sac. The child should be in a warmer or isolette for maintenance of temperature control. Inspect the area for signs of infection.

Because the infant is NPO preoperatively, maintain fluid and electrolyte balance with intravenous fluids. Postoperative care includes measures to control pain, prevent infection, maintain fluid and electrolyte balance, and ensure adequate nutritional intake. Attainment of bowel motility and function varies and is often delayed for weeks after surgery; parenteral nutrition for the infant is used during this period (Lund et al., 2007).

Throughout the infant's hospitalization, parents need clear, accurate explanations about the infant's condition. To help the parents deal with the crisis of an acutely ill newborn, provide emotional support and encourage parents to express their feelings. When the child has multiple anomalies, parents need ongoing support for the lengthy treatment, numerous hospitalizations, and management of nutritional intake.

Expected outcomes of nursing care depend on the severity of the defect and its correction but may include maintenance of fluid volume balance, healing without infection, maintenance of stable thermoregulatory function, effective pain management, and demonstration of parent–infant bonding and attachment.

Intussusception

Intussusception occurs when one portion of the intestine prolapses and then invaginates or telescopes into another (Figure 25–12 ➤). It is one of the most frequent causes of intestinal obstruction during infancy, second only to pyloric stenosis. Intussusception occurs at a rate of 1.5 to 4 per 1,000 births and is more common in males. Approximately 80% of cases occur in children younger than 2 years (Fagerman & Farber, 2007).

The etiology of intussusception is multifactorial, and direct causes cannot always be identified. Although the exact cause of intussusception is unknown, it is frequently preceded by a viral infection (Waseem & Rosenberg, 2008).

The most common site of intussusception is the ileocecal valve. Telescoping of the intestine obstructs the passage of stool. The walls of the intestine rub together, causing inflammation,

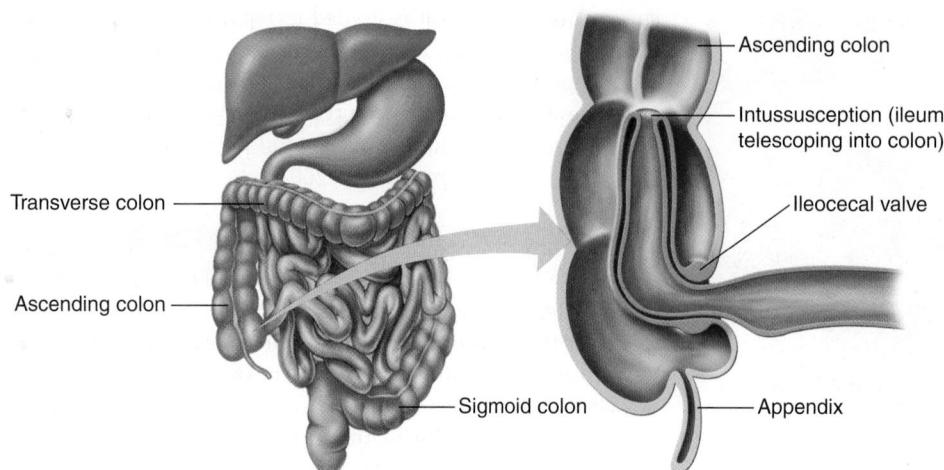

Transverse colon

Ascending colon

Sigmoid colon

Ascending colon

Intussusception (ileum telescoping into colon)

Ileocecal valve

Appendix

FIGURE 25–12 ➤ In infants, intussusception is commonly associated with viral illnesses and gastroenteritis.

edema, and decreased blood flow. This can lead to necrosis and loss of a significant portion of the intestine if not treated promptly (Fagerman & Farber, 2007).

The onset is usually abrupt. A previously healthy infant or child suddenly experiences acute abdominal pain with vomiting and passage of brown stool. There may be periods of comfort between acute episodes of pain. As the condition worsens, painful episodes increase. The stools become red and resemble currant jelly because of the mix of blood and mucus. A palpable mass may be present in the upper right quadrant or mid-upper abdomen.

Diagnosis is made on the basis of the history and confirmed by radiographs and ultrasound of the abdomen. A contrast enema using air or barium can be both diagnostic and therapeutic. In 70–90% of cases, the hydrostatic pressure from the contrast moves the bowel back into place (Fagerman & Farber, 2007).

A nasogastric tube is inserted for gastric decompression. If reduction of the intussusception does not occur with these methods, surgical intervention to reduce the invaginated bowel and remove any necrotic tissue is necessary. Surgery is generally successful in correcting the problem; however, intussusception can recur after hydrostatic reduction or surgical correction.

NURSING MANAGEMENT

Nursing management focuses on maintaining or restoring fluid and electrolyte balance. Intravenous fluids are started immediately. Serum electrolyte monitoring is essential to correct imbalances.

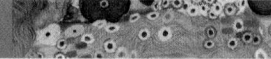
Nursing Alert

The passage of a normal brown stool may indicate that an intussusception has been reduced. Report this finding to the primary care provider immediately since the course of treatment may be altered, especially in the case of a planned surgical reduction.

Postoperative care focuses on monitoring for early signs of infection, managing the child's pain, and maintaining nasogastric tube patency. Assess vital signs, check for abdominal disten-

tion, and assess for return of bowel function. Feeding protocols vary among practitioners. Generally, after normal bowel function returns, clear liquid feeding or breastfeeding can resume. Feedings are then advanced to half-strength milk and other foods as the infant or child tolerates them.

Discharge usually occurs shortly after the infant or child begins taking full feedings. Instruct parents to watch for infection and to call the physician if symptoms recur, a fever develops, or appetite decreases.

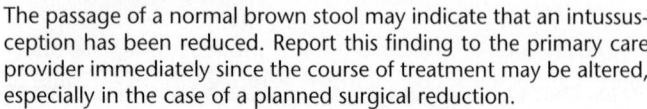
Clinical Tip

Traditionally, the return of bowel sounds postoperatively has been a key indicator of the return of bowel function. Evidence-based research indicates that the best indicators of bowel function in patients undergoing abdominal surgery are passage of flatus and passage of stool (Madsen, Sebolt, Cullen, et al., 2005).

Volvulus

During the 7th–12th weeks of gestation, the small intestine undergoes rapid growth. In normal development the intestine rotates counterclockwise as it settles into its permanent position inside the abdominal cavity. Malrotation of the intestine occurs in approximately 3.9 out of every 10,000 live births (Applegate, 2009). When malrotation of the intestine occurs, the child is at risk for **volvulus**, a twisting of the intestine. Volvulus disrupts blood flow in the intestines and can lead to necrosis of the bowel, short bowel syndrome, and death. Volvulus is considered a surgical emergency. Early diagnosis and treatment is necessary to preserve the bowel and to save the child's life (Markowitz, Dancel, & Shukla, 2008).

Symptoms of volvulus in the infant include bilious vomiting, firm abdomen with distention, irritability secondary to pain, and passage of bloody stools. Confirmation of malrotation of the intestine through GI series or contrast studies supports a diagnosis of volvulus. Emergency exploratory surgery to untwist the bowel is essential (Diana-Zerpa & Shapiro-Stolar, 2007). If a portion of the bowel is necrotic, that portion of the bowel is removed. An ostomy may need to be created, depending on the amount of bowel removed. The child is at risk for developing short bowel syndrome if a significant amount of bowel is removed. See page 789. See the section on ostomies beginning on page 774.

NURSING MANAGEMENT

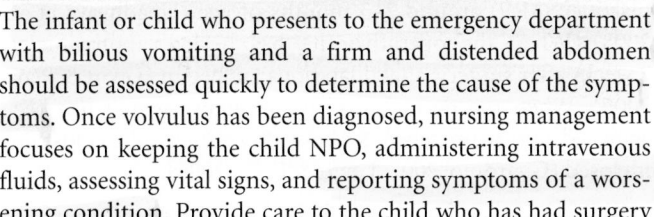

The infant or child who presents to the emergency department with bilious vomiting and a firm and distended abdomen should be assessed quickly to determine the cause of the symptoms. Once volvulus has been diagnosed, nursing management focuses on keeping the child NPO, administering intravenous fluids, assessing vital signs, and reporting symptoms of a worsening condition. Provide care to the child who has had surgery to correct uncomplicated volvulus as described for the child with intussusception.

Hirschsprung Disease

Hirschsprung disease, also known as congenital aganglionic megacolon, is a congenital anomaly in which inadequate motility causes mechanical obstruction of the intestine. The disease occurs in approximately 1 in every 5,000 live births, and is more common in males than females. Hirschsprung disease can occur as a single anomaly or in combination with congenital heart defects and chromosomal abnormalities such as Down syndrome (Kessman, 2006).

Hirschsprung disease is the congenital absence of ganglion cells in the wall of a variable segment of rectum and colon. It is now known that the RET proto-oncogene is a major gene responsible for the disease. The absence of autonomic parasympathetic ganglion cells in the colon prevents peristalsis at that portion of the intestine, resulting in the accumulation of intestinal contents and abdominal distention. In most cases, the area lacking ganglion cells is limited to the rectosigmoid region of the colon (Kessman, 2006).

Clinical manifestations of Hirschsprung disease vary depending on the child's age at onset. In newborns, symptoms include failure to pass meconium within the first 48 hours after birth, abdominal distention, and bilious vomiting (Klar, 2007). If Hirschsprung disease is not treated, the condition can lead to fever, bloody **diarrhea** (frequent watery stools), abdominal distention, and *enterocolitis* (inflammation of the intestines) (Biggs & Dery, 2006).

The older infant or child may have a history of failure to gain weight, malnutrition, chronic progressive **constipation** (difficult and infrequent defecation with passage of hard, dry stool), and recurrent fecal impaction (Kessman, 2006). The child may have a history of pencil thin stools (Biggs & Dery, 2006).

COLLABORATIVE CARE

Diagnosis is made on the basis of the history, bowel patterns, anorectal manometry (reaction of the anal sphincter to distention of the rectum), radiographic contrast studies, and rectal biopsy for presence or absence of ganglion cells. The rectum is small in size on palpation and does not contain stool. Anorectal manometry demonstrates absence of relaxation of the internal sphincter, an expected response to rectal distention. Normally, distention of the rectum produces relaxation of the internal sphincter. Abdominal radiograph and contrast studies reveal a distended small bowel and proximal colon with an empty rectum. Rectal biopsy has proven to be the most reliable test for confirmation of the diagnosis; the absence of ganglionic cells and the presence of hypertrophic nerve trunks confirm the diagnosis (Kessman, 2006).

Treatment in infancy involves surgical removal of the aganglionic bowel through an endorectal pull-through procedure (Mattioli, Prato, Giunta, et al., 2008). In mild cases in otherwise healthy infants, the affected portion of the bowel can be removed in the newborn period. In severe cases or in ill infants, a temporary colostomy is created. Timing of closure of the colostomy and reanastomosis varies among surgeons with the procedure generally being performed sometime between 2 and 6 months of age (Black, 2005; Kessman, 2006). For children not diagnosed in infancy, treatment should be implemented as soon as possible after diagnosis. Whether complete repair is possible in the first surgery, or a colostomy is required, depends on the amount of bowel affected.

The return of normal bowel function depends on the amount of bowel involved. Some fecal incontinence and constipation may persist following surgery. Enterocolitis is a serious complication that can occur before or after surgery, resulting in ischemia and ulceration of the bowel wall. Treatment includes intravenous fluids, antibiotics, and placement of a nasogastric tube for decompression of the abdomen (Kessman, 2006).

NURSING MANAGEMENT

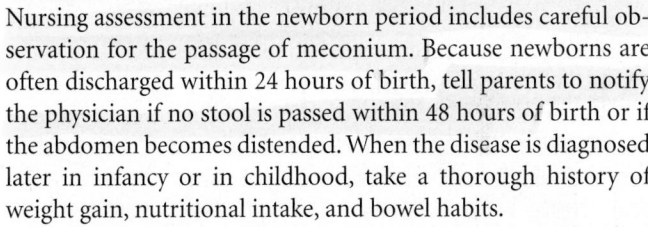

Nursing assessment in the newborn period includes careful observation for the passage of meconium. Because newborns are often discharged within 24 hours of birth, tell parents to notify the physician if no stool is passed within 48 hours of birth or if the abdomen becomes distended. When the disease is diagnosed later in infancy or in childhood, take a thorough history of weight gain, nutritional intake, and bowel habits.

When Hirschsprung disease is diagnosed, nursing care includes monitoring for infection, managing pain, maintaining hydration, measuring abdominal circumference to detect any distention, and providing support to the child and family. Preoperative oral intake varies depending on the surgeon; however, intake is generally restricted to clear fluids the day before surgery. Rectal irrigations may be performed to evacuate the bowel prior to surgery.

Initial postoperative nursing care is the same as for any other infant or child having abdominal surgery: maintain intravenous fluids and nasogastric tube, and monitor intake and output. Administer pain medications as prescribed and assess at least every

Nursing Alert

For the child who has had an endorectal pull-through procedure, it is very important that nothing be placed in the rectum, including thermometers and suppositories. A sign should be placed on the patient's bed to alert all staff caring for the infant. If the child requires rectal dilations, these are delayed for 3 weeks to allow for healing (Klar, 2007).

hour for evidence of pain utilizing a pain scale and documenting assessment. If a colostomy was performed, the stoma should be assessed frequently as well as the return of bowel function. See the section on ostomies on page 774.

Clinical Tip

Following closure of the colostomy in the child who has had a colostomy for several months, the perineal area is not accustomed to contact with stool. Without meticulous skin care, breakdown is very likely. Teach parents to change diapers frequently, clean the perineal area carefully, and apply a protective barrier at each diaper change.

Children occasionally develop constipation, and parents may need guidance to adapt the diet and fluid intake to manage this complication. Because some children develop malabsorption, be alert for signs of poor growth or malnutrition (see Chapter 4 ∞).

Expected outcomes of nursing care include maintenance of fluid and electrolyte balance, adequate nutritional intake to promote growth and development, maintenance of normal bowel patterns, adequate hydration, and maintenance of intact skin.

Anorectal Malformations

Anorectal malformations refer to anomalies of the rectum and distal anus, and the urinary and genital tract and have an incidence of approximately 1 in 3,500–5,000 live births (Upadhyaya, Gangopadhyay, Srivastava, et al., 2008). Anorectal malformations are frequently associated with anomalies of the musculoskeletal system. Chromosomal abnormalities such as trisomy 13, 18, or 21 may coexist, and some babies have VACTERL conditions. VACTERL refers to the presence of three or more of the following anomalies: **v**ertebral anomalies, **a**nal atresia, **c**ongenital heart disease, **t**racheoesophageal fistula and/or esophageal atresia, **r**enal anomalies, and radial **l**imb defects (Stoll, Alembik, Dott, et al., 2007).

The term *imperforate anus* (absence of the anal opening) is frequently used to refer to anorectal malformations and is classified according to the specific defect. Imperforate anus affects males and females equally. Perineal inspection at birth reveals the absent anal opening. Failure to pass meconium within the first 24 hours of birth may be indicative of imperforate anus. Stool in the urine usually indicates the presence of a fistula between the colon and urinary tract. Cloacal malformations in females, in which the urinary tract, vagina, and rectum drain through a common channel, may occur (Levitt & Peña, 2005). Some anorectal malformations may be suspected prenatally on ultrasound, especially in the presence of associated anomalies (Levitt & Peña, 2005). Diagnosis for both defects is usually made at birth or during the newborn assessment of anorectal structures and rectal patency. Ultrasound and lower gastrointestinal radiographic studies are used to confirm the diagnosis and demonstrate the extent of the anomaly.

Medical management depends on the extent of the malformation and presence of associated conditions. Anal stenosis may be treated with dilation alone. An imperforate anal membrane is excised surgically, followed by daily manual dilations. A single

operation, anoplasty, may be used to repair rectoperineal defects (previously known as low defects). Higher defects require a three-stage procedure. A temporary colostomy in the newborn period provides for bowel decompression and for protection of the surgical site when the anomaly is repaired. Reconstructive surgery is generally performed via posterior sagittal anorectoplasty (PSARP) around 2–3 months of age (Upadhyaya et al., 2008). When the operative site has healed, approximately 2 weeks after surgery, anal dilatations are begun (Levitt & Peña, 2005). When the desired size of the anal opening has been achieved, approximately 6–8 weeks after surgery, the colostomy is closed (Guardino, 2007; Levitt & Peña, 2005).

NURSING MANAGEMENT

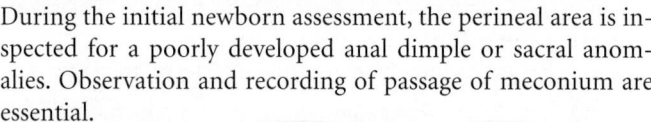

During the initial newborn assessment, the perineal area is inspected for a poorly developed anal dimple or sacral anomalies. Observation and recording of passage of meconium are essential.

Once the diagnosis has been made, intravenous fluids are initiated and a nasogastric tube is inserted to decompress the stomach. Monitor the child's intake and output and cardiorespiratory functioning. Provide emotional support to the parents and give them information about the upcoming surgery.

Postoperative care specific to the child who has had the PSARP procedure centers on protection of the surgical site. A Foley catheter will be in place for 5 days to protect the new anal opening from urine. The colostomy that is still in place protects the surgical site from stool. Provide adequate pain management for the child. Maintain intravenous fluids until the child is able to take liquids by mouth.

Clinical Judgment

Following creation of a new anal opening through the PSARP procedure, the child should have nothing placed in the rectum. What specific procedures should be avoided? What measure will remind others of this contraindication? How can the nurse position the child to avoid pressure on the surgical site?

Nursing care for the child who has had a colostomy takedown is more complex because the bowel has been manipulated during surgery. It is essential to monitor the maintenance of the nasogastric tube to low wall suction until bowel function returns. Provide intravenous fluids or total parenteral nutrition through peripheral or central venous access until the child can tolerate fluids by mouth. Monitor intake and output. The child will frequently have a Foley catheter in place for accurate measurement of urine output.

Care of the operative site may include dressing changes in addition to assessment for signs of infection. As the child begins to pass stool through the anal opening for the first time, skin breakdown is likely. Protect the perineal area with a barrier cream or paste. Provide intravenous pain medication on a regular basis. The nurse is also responsible for administering prescribed antibiotics that protect the child from infection.

The child with associated abnormalities may need several surgeries and interventions to treat all of the conditions present. Partnering with families and the group of health care providers will assist in case management that facilitates the child's health and development. Health promotion and health maintenance that include support of family members, ensuring immunizations, and monitoring developmental status are important.

Discharge Planning and Home Care Teaching

Infants are increasingly discharged shortly after birth, so parents need clear instructions about normal newborn stools and what abnormalities to report so that anorectal defects not obvious at birth are identified early.

If a colostomy is performed in the newborn period, teach parents how to care for the ostomy site (see discussion of ostomies on page 774). Reassure parents that the colostomy will be closed in the future, and help them plan for that hospitalization. Refer them to ostomy support groups in the community or online. Discuss follow-up care and long-term management. Arrange follow-up visits and home care visits to evaluate the child's ostomy site and monitor growth.

After surgery to create the anal opening, teach parents how to take the infant's temperature using the axillary route. Once anal dilatations have begun, the family will be taught how to perform them at home. After the final surgical procedure, discuss feeding regimens and bowel habits necessary to maintain adequate nutrition for growth and development. Advise parents that children with anorectal malformations may have difficulty achieving bowel control. Patience in toilet training is important. When the child reaches an age appropriate for toilet training, encour-

age the family to speak with a health care provider to discuss the child's progress. (See Evidence-Based Practice: Imperforate Anus.)

Expected outcomes of nursing care include adequate fluid intake, normal bowel patterns, parental knowledge of ostomy or other treatment protocols, and eventual success with toilet training.

Hernias

A **hernia** is the protrusion or projection of an organ or a part of an organ through the muscle wall of the cavity that normally contains it. This protrusion may result from the failure of normal openings to close during fetal development or from weakness in the supporting musculature. When intra-abdominal pressure increases (as when the infant cries or strains to pass stool), the weakened area separates, causing a protrusion of underlying organs. Inguinal hernias are the most common type of hernia occurring in children (see Chapter 26 ∞). Other hernias that occur frequently in children are diaphragmatic and umbilical.

Congenital Diaphragmatic Hernia

In a diaphragmatic hernia, abdominal contents protrude into the thoracic cavity through an opening in the diaphragm. Sites of herniation include the substernal space, posterolateral region, and the esophageal hiatus. The cause is a delay or failure in closure of the pleuroperitoneal musculature. The diaphragm, which divides the thoracic and abdominal components, begins to develop in the 4th week of gestation (Coha, 2007).

Evidence-Based Practice
Imperforate Anus

Problem

Despite successful surgery for imperforate anus, the child may have long-term problems with constipation and fecal soiling. Parents may also experience stressors related to their child's condition (Nisell, Öjmyr-Joelsson, Frenckner, et al., 2009). How does a history of imperforate anus affect children and their parents psychosocially?

Evidence

A cross-sectional retrospective study by Nisell, Öjmyr-Joelsson, Frenckner, et al. (2009) examined the psychosocial experiences and potential positive experiences of families who had children born with high or intermediate imperforate anus (IA). Twenty-five mothers and 20 fathers of children with IA participated in the study. Parents of children with juvenile chronic arthritis (JCA) served as the comparison group. Significant findings from the study revealed that mothers of children with IA felt that their social relationships were affected more than mothers of children with JCA. They also reported less respect for their child's will. There were no significant differences in the responses of fathers of children with IA as compared to those of children with JCA. Positive experiences were identified by 48% of mothers and 35% of fathers of children with IA, with no statistical differences when compared to parents of children with JCA. Although 28% of mothers and 25% of fathers had received psychological care in relation to their child's congenital anomaly, this did not correlate with a higher percentage of positive experiences. Positive experiences focused on the development of the child, personal development of the parent, and strengthening of family unity.

Further research by Nisell, Igl, Öjmyr-Joelsson, et al. (2009) examined the psychosocial issues that children with a history of high or intermediate imperforate anus experience. Questionnaires were completed by the same parents utilized in the previous study. While parents of children with IA were more positive in the description of their child's academic adjustment as compared to children with JCA or those with no chronic condition, these parents did indicate that their children were not as socially integrated as children in the other groups. Teachers of these children also completed a questionnaire. Children with IA received lower scores from teachers on questions related to academic performance and adaptive functioning than children with JCA or children with no chronic condition.

Implications

Nurses who care for children with a history of high or intermediate imperforate anus should assess whether the child continues to have difficulty with constipation and soiling. For those children with continued problems related to imperforate anus, the nurse should assess the impact this condition has on the child and the family and provide support as appropriate.

Critical Thinking Application

What age group would be most affected psychosocially by continued problems with fecal soiling related to IA? How can the nurse facilitate coping in the parent and the child?

Intestines and other abdominal structures enter the thoracic cavity through the opening in the diaphragm. The overall incidence of diaphragmatic hernia is 1 in 3,300 live births (Coha, 2007). Associated major anomalies are present in 37–47% of children with congenital diaphragmatic hernia (Colvin, Bower, Dickinson, et al., 2005).

A diaphragmatic hernia is a life-threatening condition with an overall mortality rate of 33% although some individual centers report mortality rates as low as 10% (Mills, Lin, MacNab, et al., 2010). Severe respiratory distress occurs shortly after birth. As the infant cries, abdominal organs extend into the thorax, decreasing the size of the thoracic cavity. The infant becomes dyspneic and cyanotic. Characteristic findings include a barrel-shaped chest and sunken abdomen.

Congenital diaphragmatic hernia is diagnosed in utero by ultrasound in 40–60% of cases (de Buys Roessingh & Dinh-Xuan, 2009). If not identified prenatally the condition is first identified postnatally by physical signs and symptoms; confirmation is made by chest radiologic examination. Magnetic resonance imaging (MRI) is helpful in confirming the diagnosis and in determining the position of organs in the chest and abdomen (Downard, 2008).

The infant is positioned with the head and thorax higher than the abdomen to facilitate downward movement of abdominal organs. A nasogastric tube is inserted to decompress the stomach. Intravenous fluids are administered through an umbilical artery catheter. Immediate respiratory support is essential. Ventilator support is necessary to manage respiratory compromise. Conventional mechanical ventilation, high-frequency oxygen ventilation, and extracorporeal membrane oxygenation (ECMO) are the main methods used for respiratory failure in these children. Nitric oxide, a pulmonary vasodilator, may also be used (Ehrlich & Coran, 2007).

Once the infant's condition is stabilized, the defect is corrected surgically. The chance for a successful repair and survival is affected by the size of the defect. Children who survive will generally continue to have health concerns and should have continued evaluation of pulmonary, nutritional, and neurodevelopmental related problems (Downard, 2008).

NURSING MANAGEMENT

The infant with a diaphragmatic hernia is admitted to the NICU and requires continuous monitoring. Preoperative management centers on providing supportive care to the infant and parents. Place the child on a cardiorespiratory monitor and note the infant's vital signs every 30 minutes. Observe for worsening of respiratory compromise. Maintain intravenous fluid administration. Promote decreased stimulation to keep the infant calm and thus maintain low abdominal pressure. Keep parents informed about the infant's condition, and provide emotional support both before and after surgery.

Postoperative care includes positioning the infant on the affected side to facilitate expansion of the lung on the unaffected side, observing closely for signs of infection, maintaining respiratory support, and carefully monitoring fluid and electrolyte balance. Before discharge, instruct parents in wound care, prevention of infection, and feeding techniques.

Umbilical Hernia

An umbilical hernia results from a weak or imperfectly closed umbilical ring. This condition is common in childhood and occurs more frequently in Black children and low-birth-weight infants (Stoll, 2007).

The hernia appears as a soft swelling covered by skin. Omentum and small intestine herniate or protrude through the opening with coughing, crying, or straining during a bowel movement. It is easily reduced by pushing the bowel back through the fibrous ring. The size of the defect is determined by measuring the diameter of the muscular ring (Stoll, 2007).

Most defects that appear prior to 6 months of age resolve spontaneously by age 1. Surgery is indicated in cases of **strangulation** (closure of the umbilical ring around a portion of the bowel, preventing it from moving back into the abdomen). Surgery is also recommended if the defect does not resolve by 3 to 4 years of age or if the defect becomes larger after 1 to 2 years of age (Stoll, 2007).

Nursing management is generally supportive. Instruct parents not to apply tape, straps, or coins to reduce the hernia as these methods have not proven to be effective and may cause skin breakdown. If surgery is required, it is usually performed in an outpatient surgery unit. Postoperatively, teach parents how to care for the surgical site, to watch for bleeding, and to recognize signs of infection. Reinforce the importance of returning for follow-up evaluation.

■ OSTOMIES

An intestinal **ostomy** is an opening, or **stoma**, into the small or large intestine that diverts fecal matter, providing an outlet when a distal surgical anastomosis, obstruction, or nonfunctioning structure prevents normal elimination (Figure 25–13 ➤). Depending on the integrity and function of anatomic structures, the ostomy may be temporary or permanent. Infants and small children with imperforate anus, necrotizing enterocolitis, Hirschsprung disease, or volvulus may require a temporary or permanent colostomy or ileostomy. Ostomies may also be indi-

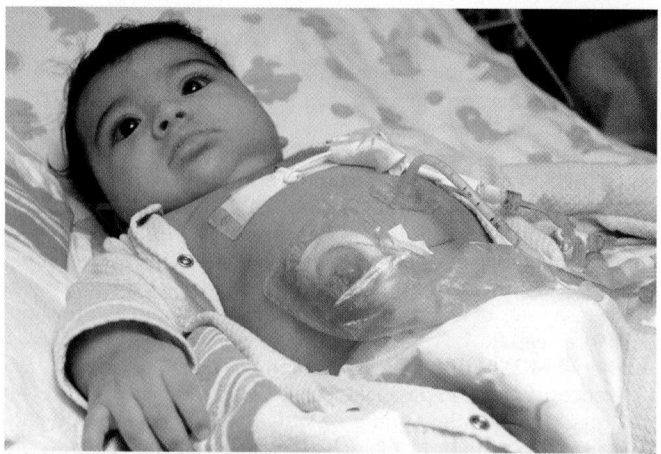

FIGURE 25–13 ➤ This infant has several gastrointestinal problems and requires ostomies both for gastric feedings and for drainage of fecal material. Note the appearance of the healthy stoma.

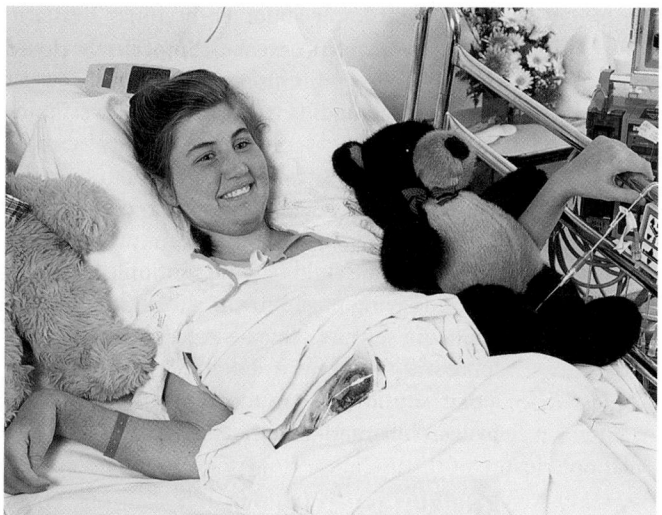

FIGURE 25–14 ➤ Nursing strategies to address altered perceptions of body image and increased feelings of dependence are important when working with adolescents who have ostomies. Support groups or a visit from another teenager who has had an ostomy can facilitate positive coping, as demonstrated by this teenage girl.

cated for children with inflammatory bowel disease, intestinal tumors, or abdominal trauma.

An ostomy may be elective or a surgical emergency. In all cases it affects a child's lifestyle, alters body image, causes anxiety, and increases the risk for alterations in physiologic processes (electrolyte imbalance, increased nutritional requirements). For adolescents, it may also result in dependence at a time when autonomy is a major developmental need (Figure 25–14 ➤).

When assessing the family and child approaching ostomy surgery, it is important to determine their ability to understand and accept the physical changes that will occur. Parents may feel guilt and anger about the ostomy surgery when the child has a genetically transmitted disease, is injured, or has developed an obstruction from necrosis of the bowel. Encourage the parents and child to express their feelings. Correct any misunderstandings. Parents and older children may be referred for counseling and to support groups to help them deal with their feelings. Adolescents often benefit from a visit with an adolescent ostomate (someone who has an ostomy) who can answer questions about living with an ostomy.

NURSING MANAGEMENT

Preoperative Care

Preoperative education focuses on educating the child and family and preparing them for postoperative management. Discuss how the appliance will look, and explain the purpose of the pouch in developmentally appropriate terms. Encourage the parents and child to touch and manipulate all equipment. A younger child can be shown how to place a pouch on a doll. (See Chapter 11 ∞, page 283.) Older children can practice placing a pouch on their skin. These measures help relieve anxiety by providing information and increasing familiarity with the appliance.

Growth & Development   *Ostomy Care*

The preschooler has some manual dexterity and can help with some parts of the procedure for changing an ostomy appliance and cleaning the stoma. Teach the child using a doll or stuffed animal. Many school-age children are able to care for their ostomy independently. Teach them how to prevent leakage around the bag, which could be embarrassing. Adolescents are generally totally independent in their self-care of ostomies. However, they may need support to deal with the fact that they are different from their peers.

In addition to discussion of the appliance, preoperative education should include discussion of pain control and measures that will be used to prevent postoperative complications (turning, coughing, and breathing deeply). Gear the instructions to the child's developmental level. Encourage parental participation to promote compliance.

Postoperative Care

Postoperative care of a child with an ostomy is similar to that for any child who undergoes abdominal surgery. (See the discussion of nursing management for appendicitis and Nursing Care Plan: The Child Undergoing Surgery in Chapter 11 ∞.) Management of the stoma may be done by an "ostomy nurse" or other nurses. Major interventions involve ensuring proper function of the stoma, identifying complications, and instituting daily stoma care. Assess the stoma, quality and amount of fecal matter, skin condition, and adherence of the pouch. Evaluate for the most common complications, which are prolapse, retraction, stenosis, and skin breakdown around the stoma. Evaluate the family's understanding and their ability to care for the ostomy.

Care in the Community

Identify and address home care needs well in advance of discharge. Instructions include skin care, care of the stoma, appliance removal and application, and frequency of appliance changes. Begin teaching immediately after surgery with responsibility for care transferred gradually to the parents and child as they are ready. Discuss diet, activity level, hygiene, clothing, equipment, and financial considerations. Arrange for periodic home visits to see how the family is managing.

Parents and children can be referred to the United Ostomy Associations of America or a local ostomy group for information and support. Make referrals to social services, counseling, and a home health agency, if appropriate.

Expected outcomes of nursing care include successful adjustment to the ostomy, thorough evacuation of the bowel, absence of infection and other complications, intact skin, and formation of a positive self-image in the child.

■ INFLAMMATORY DISORDERS

Inflammatory disorders are reactions of specific tissues of the GI tract to trauma caused by injuries, foreign bodies, chemicals, microorganisms, or surgery. These disorders may be acute or chronic and may involve various segments of the GI tract.

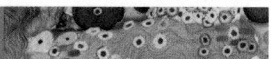 United Ostomy Associations of America Website

Pathophysiology Illustrated
Appendicitis Pain
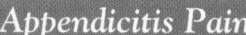

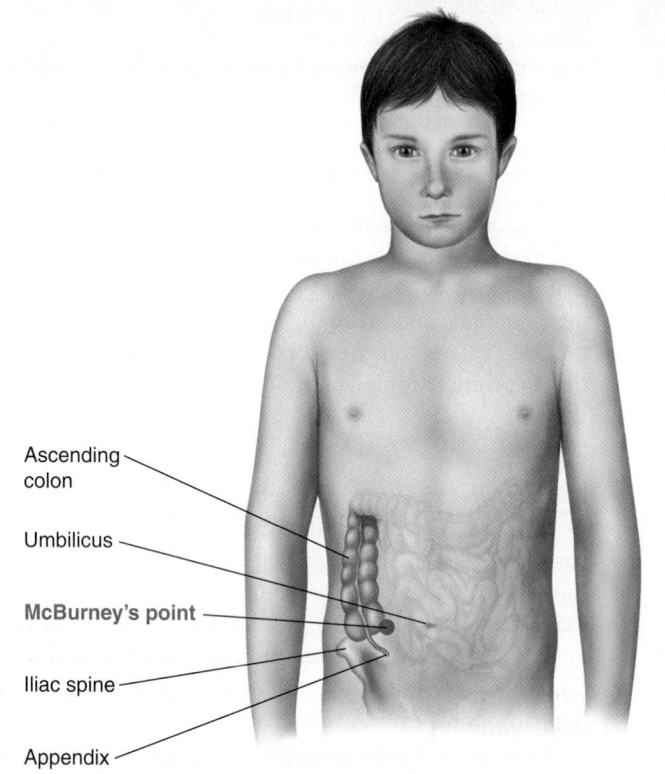

Ascending colon

Umbilicus

McBurney's point

Iliac spine

Appendix

FIGURE 25–15 ➤ Common location of pain in children and adolescents with appendicitis.

Appendicitis

Appendicitis is an inflammation of the vermiform appendix, the small sac near the end of the cecum, and is the most common cause of emergency surgery in children (Wan, Krahn, Ungar, et al., 2009). Each year in the United States, 70,000 children will develop appendicitis. The condition occurs most often in children and adolescents ages 10–19 years. Children younger than 4 years with appendicitis generally present after the appendix has ruptured (Hennelly & Bachur, 2009).

Etiology and Pathophysiology

Appendicitis almost always results from an obstruction in the appendiceal lumen. It can be caused by a fecalith (hard fecal mass), parasitic infestations, stenosis, hyperplasia of lymphoid tissue, or a tumor. Continued secretion of mucus following acute obstruction of the lumen increases pressure, causing ischemia, cellular death, and ulceration.

The appendix may perforate or rupture, resulting in fecal and bacterial contamination of the peritoneum. Peritonitis spreads quickly and if untreated can result in small bowel obstruction, electrolyte imbalances, septicemia, and hypovolemic shock. Early diagnosis and treatment of appendicitis is essential to minimize complications related to rupture (Wan et al., 2008).

Clinical Manifestations

At onset, symptoms include periumbilical cramps, abdominal tenderness, and fever. In adolescent and young adult females, symptoms must be differentiated from those associated with ovulation (mittelschmerz), ruptured ectopic pregnancy, and pelvic inflammatory disease. As the inflammation progresses, pain

in the right lower abdomen becomes constant. Pain is often most intense at McBurney point, halfway between the anterior superior iliac crest and the umbilicus (Figure 25–15 ➤). Symptoms progress to include guarding, rigidity, and rebound tenderness following palpation over the right lower quadrant. Vomiting, diarrhea, or constipation may be present. As appendicitis progresses, the child remains motionless, usually in a side-lying position with knees flexed. If the appendix ruptures, there is usually fever, sudden temporary relief from abdominal pain, guarding and distention of the abdomen, rapid breathing, pallor, chills, and irritability.

COLLABORATIVE CARE
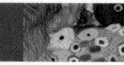

Diagnostic Tests

Diagnosis of appendicitis in young children can be difficult because their pain may be less localized and their symptoms more diffuse than in the older child. Continuing evaluations over several hours are often needed to establish the diagnosis.

The presence of fever and an elevated white blood cell count (above 10,000/mm³) generally occurs in appendicitis. In the opening scenario, Jenna had a WBC count of 22,000/mm³ which was clearly indicative of infection. In addition to these symptoms, a history of mid-abdominal pain migrating to the right lower quadrant, along with rebound tenderness is highly indicative of appendicitis (Bundy, Byerley, Liles, et al., 2007). Abdominal ultrasound and computed tomography (CT) are both useful in the diagnosis of appendicitis. Ultrasound is preferred by some health care providers as the initial screening tool; however, CT scans are more sensitive and should be used in cases where the appendix cannot be seen well on ultrasound or the results are inconclusive (Schwartz, 2008; Zilbert, Stamell, Ezon, et al., 2009).

Clinical Therapy

Treatment involves surgical removal of the appendix (appendectomy) either through laparoscopic or open method (IPEG, 2008b). Preoperatively the child is kept NPO. Intravenous fluids, electrolytes, and antibiotics are administered. Postoperatively the child has an abdominal incision, and intravenous antibiotics may be administered to prevent infection. The child with uncomplicated appendicitis will generally be discharged the next day.

With ruptured appendix, some surgeons prefer to close the wound, whereas others leave the wound open (delayed primary closure), with or without placement of drains. If the wound is left open, it is packed with sterile

Research 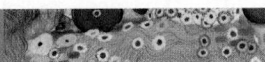 *Ceftriaxone and Metronidazole*

A retrospective review of 250 patients treated for ruptured appendix was conducted to evaluate whether a 5-day course of once-daily ceftriaxone and metronidazole is just as effective as triple antibiotic therapy using ampicillin, gentamicin, and clindamycin, administered 3 to 4 times daily. The once-daily dosing using ceftriaxone and metronidazole was found to provide adequate coverage following surgery for ruptured appendix. Patients were found to have a more rapid reduction in temperature. In addition, since these two drugs are not nephrotoxic, drug levels are not required as with gentamicin. The treatment is also less demanding on nursing staff, laboratory resources, and the patient. It is less expensive since medications are only administered once a day (St. Peter et al., 2006).

saline-soaked gauze. Regardless of whether the wound is left opened or is closed, the child will have a nasogastric tube to decompress the abdomen and will remain NPO until signs of bowel function return. The child will also have a peripheral or temporary central line for administration of intravenous fluids and medications. After surgery for a ruptured appendix, the child will receive antibiotics for several days. A combination of ampicillin, gentamicin, and clindamycin has been the treatment of choice by many surgeons for years, with ampicillin omitted from the regimen in the presence of penicillin allergy. Recent studies support the use of once-daily ceftriaxone and metronidazole as just as effective (St. Peter, Little, Calkins, et al., 2006). The exact regimen continues to vary among surgeons. Morphine is generally given for pain. For the child whose wound was left open, the wound will be closed under sedation in about 5 days.

NURSING MANAGEMENT

Nursing management includes collaborative identification of the child with appendicitis, preoperative and postoperative care, and preventing complications.

Nursing Assessment and Diagnosis

Physiologic Assessment

Preoperatively, a detailed assessment of the child's pain is necessary to differentiate appendicitis from other illnesses (see Chapter 15 ∞). Ask the child to point to the painful area and to describe the pain. Recognize that localizing the pain may be difficult for young children. Note onset, location, and intensity of pain; precipitating factors; and relief measures tried. During abdominal assessment, palpate last to avoid causing additional pain. Assess vital signs to determine baseline values, and monitor every 4 hours thereafter.

Postoperatively, assess fluid volume status every 2 hours. Assess skin turgor, eyes, and mucous membranes for signs of dehydration. Monitor intake and output. Assess for signs of return of bowel function as previously listed. Assess for pain using the appropriate scale. Careful attention should also be paid to the wound site for signs of infection such as increased redness or drainage. Vital signs should be monitored at least every 4 hours. Changes in vital signs, especially temperature, may be indicative of infection.

Psychosocial Assessment

Assessment of the child's coping skills is important. Young children generally have more fears related to the hospitalization and procedures, while older children and adolescents usually focus on what will happen during surgery and on the surgical scar. (See Chapter 11 ∞.) Assess the parents' and child's anxiety about the sudden hospitalization and need for emergency surgery.

Among the nursing diagnoses that might be appropriate for the child with appendicitis are:

• Acute Pain related to inflammation and surgery
• Risk for Deficient Fluid Volume related to fluid volume loss and inadequate fluid volume intake
• Anxiety/Fear related to surgery
• Risk for Infection related to surgical procedure
• Risk for Ineffective Airway Clearance related to decreased mobility and refusal to cough

Planning and Implementation

Nursing management focuses on promoting comfort, maintaining hydration, providing emotional support, supporting respiratory function, providing care of the surgical site, and monitoring for symptoms of infection.

Promote Comfort

Preoperatively, a right side-lying position with knees bent is usually the most comfortable. If the appendix has ruptured, lying on the right side helps the peritoneal cavity drain and facilitates comfort.

Administer analgesics as ordered, and note relief from pain. The child who has an appendectomy for uncomplicated appendicitis will need oral or intravenous pain management for postoperative pain control. Postoperatively the child with a ruptured appendix will require intravenous pain medication frequently and prior to scheduled dressing changes if the wound was left open.

Be alert to the child who does not complain of pain postoperatively following surgery for a ruptured appendix. This child still needs pain medication. While the child may not verbally complain of pain, he or she will cry when approached and will resist or refuse to move in the bed. Proper pain management will facilitate the child's recovery and will help prevent respiratory complications related to immobilization.

Maintain Hydration

An intravenous infusion is initiated preoperatively and continued until bowel function returns after surgery. If the child had a ruptured appendix and has a nasogastric tube for awhile after surgery, accurate assessment of the amount of output from the nasogastric tube is essential. The nurse should be alert to an increase in nasogastric drainage postoperatively, as this drainage should decrease over time. Any concerns should be reported

Clinical Tip

When a child has a nasogastric tube in place, the nurse must keep an accurate measurement of the amount of output from the tube so that adequate fluid replacement can be given. Loss of large amounts of stomach contents without fluid replacement may lead to metabolic alkalosis. Infants are especially at risk for acid-base imbalances.

promptly to the physician. Once bowel function has returned and after the nasogastric tube has been removed, offer clear liquids in small amounts according to physician orders. The child should be monitored closely to make sure he or she does not become nauseated after he or she begins taking oral fluids.

Provide Emotional Support

For many children, this may be their first hospitalization and their first experience with health care personnel beyond their usual health care provider. The nurse must elicit a history, perform a physical examination, coordinate diagnostic tests, and prepare the child for surgery in a short period of time. Emotional support is essential for both child and parents. Good preoperative education can reduce anxiety. Answer any questions the child or parents may have.

Support Respiratory Function

General anesthesia during surgery compromises respiratory function. It is important for the child to turn, cough, and breathe deeply to prevent atelectasis. While the child with uncomplicated appendicitis is usually willing to get out of bed and walk soon after surgery, the child with a ruptured appendix is generally hesitant to move for fear it will hurt. The child may need to be repositioned by family or staff. Adequate pain management is essential. The child will need to get out of bed as soon as his or her condition allows and walk 2–3 times a day to decrease the risk of pulmonary complications and decrease recovery time. Encourage the child to splint the incision area with a pillow during coughing to decrease pain. Incentive spirometry is frequently ordered for the child. Young children may be resistant to this procedure or may be too young to understand the procedure. An effective alternative approach is to give the child bubbles to blow. Praise and rewards such as stickers each time the child completes the task will likely increase compliance with the procedure and decrease the likelihood of complications. Consider Jenna in the opening scenario. What activities would be appropriate to prevent respiratory complications?

Recognize Symptoms of Infection

Assess vital signs and observe the abdominal incision every 4 hours for redness, edema, or drainage. If a drain is present, assess drainage for color, consistency, and amount. The amount of drainage from the wound should decrease gradually as the wound heals. Administer antibiotics as prescribed. The child with an open wound will require wet to dry dressing changes 2–3 times a day, depending on physician orders.

Discharge Planning and Home Care Teaching

For nonrupture the child is discharged once bowel function returns and he or she has a bowel movement. Give parents instructions on reestablishing a nutritious diet slowly and as tolerated. Teach parents to recognize the signs and symptoms of infection and to seek early treatment. If the appendix was ruptured, the child will be hospitalized for several days for intravenous antibiotics. If the wound was left open, it is generally closed after a few days and prior to discharge. Prepare the child and family for this procedure. Sedation or anesthesia is used to decrease the child's anxiety and discomfort.

Normal activities can be resumed fairly quickly, but the child should avoid strenuous activities and contact sports in the immediate postoperative period. Parents should check with the child's physician before allowing the child to resume sports activities. Home tutoring may be needed for a short time so the child can keep up with school work.

Evaluation

Expected outcomes of nursing care include:

- The child's pain is effectively managed.
- The child will not develop a secondary infection.
- The child and parent verbalize understanding of the condition and treatment.
- Effective airway clearance is maintained.
- Adequate hydration is achieved and maintained.
- Restoration of normal nutritional intake will occur.
- The child experiences decreased fear and anxiety associated with the hospitalization and procedures.

Necrotizing Enterocolitis

Necrotizing enterocolitis (NEC) is a potentially life-threatening inflammatory disease of the intestinal tract that occurs primarily in premature infants. It affects from 7–14% of very-low-birth-weight infants, with mortality rates as high as 50% reported (Martin & Walker, 2008). NEC is considered the most common emergency condition of the gastrointestinal tract in newborn infants (Pietz, Achanti, Lilien, et al., 2007). It can be caused by several factors including intestinal ischemia, bacterial or viral infection, and immaturity of the gut (Kliegman & Willoughby, 2005). The disease occurs most often in the distal ileum and proximal colon (McCollough & Sharieff, 2006).

Manifestations generally occur between 3 and 14 days of age, but can occur as early as the first day of life and as late as 3 months of age (Kasson, 2007). The infant may initially show signs of feeding intolerance (increased gastric residuals, vomiting, irritability, and abdominal distention). These signs are caused by inflammation and dilation of the bowel and accumulation of gas in the intestine. Bloody diarrhea may be present because of the hemorrhagic bowel. The condition progresses to lethargy and then episodes of apnea and bradycardia (Bradshaw, 2009).

Diagnosis is made on the basis of characteristic clinical findings and the presence of free peritoneal gas, dilated bowel loops, bowel distention, and bowel wall thickening on abdominal radiographs. Stools and emesis are monitored for occult blood. Laboratory data reveal anemia, leukopenia, leukocytosis, thrombocytopenia, electrolyte imbalance, and metabolic or respiratory acidosis. Blood cultures may be positive for the organism present.

Necrotizing enterocolitis requires prompt intervention. All enteral feedings are discontinued, an orogastric tube is inserted to prevent gastric distention, and intravenous fluids are started. Total parenteral nutrition may be initiated through a central line. Antibiotics are administered prophylactically or to treat sepsis. Radiographs of the abdomen should be performed every 6 hours to see if intestinal perforation has occurred (Kasson, 2007). Perforation or necrosis of the bowel necessitates

Research 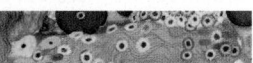 *Necrotizing Enterocolitis Treatment*

Studies continue to demonstrate the effectiveness of supplementation with probiotics, live and beneficial microorganisms that promote normal gut flora, in the prevention of necrotizing enterocolitis. *Lactobacillus acidophilus* and *Bifidobacterium infantis* are examples of organisms that can be administered by special formula (Bradshaw, 2009; Martin & Walker, 2008).

surgical resection of the bowel. An ileostomy or colostomy may be performed.

Long-term complications of necrotizing enterocolitis include short bowel syndrome, strictures, **cholestasis** (disruption of bile flow), impaired nutrition and growth, and delayed development.

Nursing Alert

Cholestasis is a disruption of bile flow. This is the most common problem in survivors of necrotizing enterocolitis. It is a complication of total parenteral nutrition (TPN) and commonly occurs 2 weeks after TPN therapy has been initiated. It is characterized by an elevated bilirubin (greater than 2 mg/dL), hepatomegaly, and elevated serum transaminase. In addition to laboratory assessment, ongoing physical assessment of the child for jaundice is essential.

NURSING MANAGEMENT

Nursing care centers on prevention and early detection of necrotizing enterocolitis to minimize bowel loss, and providing postoperative care. Feedings should be progressed very slowly with frequent assessment of feeding tolerance and abdominal girth. Even minimal changes in circumference can indicate necrotizing enterocolitis; report them to the physician. Maintaining fluid and electrolyte balance is essential. Careful assessment for infection and maintenance of skin integrity is also important. Gradually reestablish feedings once bowel function returns.

Because the symptoms of necrotizing enterocolitis do not generally appear until approximately 5 to 7 days after feedings are begun, parents may not be prepared for the infant's decline. Recovery is slow and can be complicated. Give clear explanations and encourage parents to ask questions and express their fears and concerns. When the infant has a poor prognosis, offer support for the parents of a child with life-threatening illness (see Chapter 13 ∞).

Once the child is discharged, frequent follow-up is needed. Parents need specific education related to feedings, medications, and any other treatments prescribed. The infant requires regular and thorough physical assessments to check weight gain, assess development, and identify signs of complications. If the child had to have an ostomy created, the family must be taught ostomy care (see page 774).

Expected outcomes of nursing care for the child with necrotizing enterocolitis include successful treatment of infection, absence of signs of sepsis, management of fluid and electrolyte status, and provision of adequate nutrition. If surgery is performed, complete healing without infection or other complication is desired. When the child survives, long-term outcomes include normal developmental progression and nutrition to support growth.

Meckel Diverticulum

Meckel diverticulum results when the omphalomesenteric duct, which connects the midgut to the yolk sac during embryonic development, fails to atrophy. Instead, an outpouching of the ileum remains, usually located near the ileocecal valve. The pouch contains gastric or pancreatic tissue, which secretes acid, causing irritation and ulceration. Meckel diverticulum is the most common GI malformation and cause of lower GI bleeding in children and occurs in 2% of the population. Many people are asymptomatic and do not know they have the disorder (Otten & Stoops, 2007).

Clinical manifestations usually appear by 2 years of age. The most common sign is painless dark or bright red rectal bleeding, which results from the obstruction or ulceration. Often blood is passed without stool. Abdominal pain is uncommon, but when it occurs, it may resemble the pain of appendicitis. The child may have symptoms of intussusception, incarcerated hernia, volvulus, or intestinal obstruction. If untreated, diverticulitis may progress to perforation and peritonitis.

Diagnosis is based on the history. Contrast studies are usually not helpful because the diverticulum is often too small to visualize and may not fill with barium. Radionuclide imaging and scanning can usually detect the gastric tissue, confirming the diagnosis.

Treatment is surgical excision of the diverticulum and removal of any involved bowel. The prognosis is good following surgical excision.

NURSING MANAGEMENT

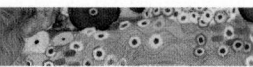

Preoperatively an intravenous infusion is initiated to correct fluid and electrolyte imbalances. Monitor intake and output. Observe for rectal bleeding, and test stools for occult blood. Keep the child on bed rest. Assess vital signs every 2 hours, and monitor for signs of shock. Postoperative care is similar to that for an infant or child undergoing abdominal surgery. (See the earlier discussion of postsurgical nursing management of appendicitis and Nursing Care Plan: The Child Undergoing Surgery in Chapter 11 ∞ .)

At discharge, parents need instructions on caring for the surgical site, preventing infection, providing an adequate diet, and administering prescribed medications.

Inflammatory Bowel Disease
Crohn's Disease and Ulcerative Colitis

Inflammatory bowel disease (IBD) encompasses two distinct chronic disorders, Crohn's disease and ulcerative colitis, that have similar symptoms and treatment (see the accompanying Clinical Manifestations table). Inflammatory bowel disease differs from irritable bowel syndrome, which is discussed in the section on feeding and elimination disorders in Chapter 14 ∞ .

Crohn's disease is a chronic, inflammatory process. It can occur randomly throughout the GI tract; the ileum, colon, and rectum are the most common sites. A distinct feature of Crohn's disease is the development of enteric fistulas between loops of bowel or nearby organs. Mucosal ulcers begin in small locations, and then grow in size and depth into the mucosal wall. Submucosal inflammation can be severe. The etiology is unknown. There is strong evidence to support a genetic association. Crohn's disease is more common in Whites than in Blacks. It is rare in the Asian and Hispanic population (Grossman & Mamula, 2009). It most often develops in adolescents and young adults. Crohn's disease has an incidence of approximately 3–4 in every 100,000 individuals (Hyams, 2007).

The onset of Crohn's disease is subtle. Crampy abdominal pain is usually reported first, followed by diarrhea. Other symptoms include fever, anorexia, growth failure or weight loss, general malaise, and joint pain.

Ulcerative colitis is a chronic recurrent disease of the large intestine and rectal mucosa of unknown etiology. Inflammation is limited to the mucosa, as opposed to Crohn's disease, which extends deep into the bowel wall. Ulcerative colitis can involve the entire length of the bowel with varying degrees of inflammation, ulceration, hemorrhage, and edema. Emotional and other psychosocial factors may influence the presentation and course of the disease. It is more prevalent among persons of Jewish heritage. The disease develops before 20 years of age with peak onset at about 12 years. Ulcerative colitis develops in 15 out of 100,000 individuals in the United States (Hyams, 2007).

The first symptom of ulcerative colitis is usually diarrhea. Lower abdominal pain and cramping are present before and during a bowel movement and are relieved by the passage of stool and flatus. The stool is often mixed with blood and mucus. Weight loss or delayed growth, nutritional deficiencies, and arthralgias often occur as effects of the disease.

COLLABORATIVE CARE

Collaborative care focuses on promoting remission of the disease, promoting optimal nutritional intake, and promoting optimal growth and development.

Diagnostic Tests

Diagnosis centers on evaluating the cause and identifying the extent of involved bowel and differentiating an infectious process (organisms such as *Shigella* and *Salmonella*) from ulcerative colitis. Endoscopy with biopsy is helpful to determine the extent and severity of the inflammatory process. Laboratory and bone age studies help to identify related nutritional, growth, and blood abnormalities.

Anemia is common; an elevated erythrocyte sedimentation rate, elevated C-reactive protein, hypoalbuminemia, and thrombocytosis are other possible findings. Stools are positive for occult blood (Hyams, 2005). Testing for antineutrophil antibodies (pANCA), anti-saccharomyces antibodies (ASCA), and anti-outer membrane porin of *Escherichia coli* (omp C) is helpful in differentiating between ulcerative colitis and Crohn's disease. A positive pANCA is present in approximately 60% of children who have ulcerative colitis and in around 10% of those with Crohn's disease. A positive ASCA or omp C is present in around 60% of those with Crohn's disease (Silbermintz & Markowitz, 2006). An upper GI series with small bowel follow-through is essential in the diagnosis of Crohn's disease. Endoscopy and colonoscopy with biopsy are essential in determining the extent of disease (Hyams, 2005; Silbermintz & Markowitz, 2006).

Clinical Therapy

Crohn's disease and ulcerative colitis have periods of remission and exacerbation. Treatment for both diseases includes pharmacologic interventions (antibiotic, anti-inflammatory, immunosuppressive, and antidiarrheal medications), nutrition therapy, and, in severe cases, surgery. First-line pharmacologic treatment of Crohn's disease involves aminosalicylates. Sulfasalazine inhibits prostaglandin synthesis, thereby decreasing inflammation. Corticosteroids are given orally and as enemas to children with more severe disease. (See Medications Used to Treat Inflammatory Bowel Disease.)

A nutritionist is part of the team treating the child. The goal of nutrition therapy is to provide adequate caloric intake and nutrients necessary for growth. Vitamin, iron, zinc, and folic acid supplementation is frequently required. Total parenteral nutrition is often given to treat nutritional deficiencies and malnutrition, which accompany inflammatory bowel disease. See the *Clinical Skills Manual*. A high-protein, high-carbohydrate, low-fiber diet with normal amounts of fat is recommended.

Clinical Manifestations
Ulcerative Colitis and Crohn's Disease

	Ulcerative Colitis	Crohn's Disease
Type of lesions	Continuous, superficial involvement	Segmental, transmural (through the wall) involvement
Clinical manifestations		
Anal or perianal lesions	Rare	Common
Anorexia	Mild to moderate	Can be severe
Diarrhea	Often severe	Moderate
Growth retardation	Mild	Significant
Pain	Present	Common
Rectal bleeding	Present	Absent
Weight loss	Moderate	Severe
Risk of cancer	Slightly increased	Greatly increased

Medications Used to Treat
Inflammatory Bowel Disease

Medication/Indication	Nursing Management
Aminosalicylates ■ Sulfasalazine ■ Mesalamine Used for anti-inflammatory effect Inhibition of prostaglandins known to cause diarrhea and affect mucosal transport	Do not crush or chew sustained-release tablets. Teach the patient or parents to supplement daily intake of iron. Monitor for side effects: ■ Nausea and vomiting ■ Rash ■ Bloody diarrhea ■ Headache ■ Anorexia
Corticosteroids ■ Prednisone ■ Prednisolone ■ Hydrocortisone enema Used for anti-inflammatory effect	Administer oral medications with meals to reduce gastric irritation. Teach the family to avoid abrupt discontinuation of medication. Teach the family to report delayed wound healing. Monitor for side effects: ■ Nausea ■ Growth suppression ■ Vomiting ■ Hypertension ■ Cushingoid appearance ■ Acne ■ Immunosuppression ■ Altered moods
Immunosuppressants ■ 6-Mercaptopurine (6-MP) ■ Azathioprine ■ Cyclosporine ■ Methotrexate Used for immunosuppressive effect	Monitor for side effects: ■ Nausea ■ Bone marrow suppression ■ Vomiting ■ Infection ■ Anorexia ■ Mucositis ■ Diarrhea Teach the family to avoid exposing the child to persons with infection. Teach the family the importance of good hygiene for the child to avoid infection.
Biological therapies ■ Tumor necrosis factor-α ■ Infliximab (Remicade) ■ Interleukin-10 ■ Thalidomide Prevents TNF-alpha from binding to its receptors (TNF-alpha has been found in stools of patients with Crohn's disease)	Reconstitute IV preparation according to manufacturer directions and administer according to agency protocol. Monitor for side effects: Infusion reactions—fever, chills, chest pain, hypotension, dyspnea, urticaria Discontinue IV infusion if infusion reaction is evident.
Antibiotics ■ Metronidazole ■ Ciprofloxacin Antibacterial against anaerobic bacteria and some gram-negative bacteria in patients with Crohn's disease	Extended-release form should not be chewed or crushed. Administer with food or milk to reduce gastrointestinal distress. Monitor for side effects: ■ Fever ■ Nausea ■ Headache ■ Vomiting ■ Diarrhea ■ Fungal overgrowth

Data from: Aschenbrenner, D. S. (2006). Treatment of pediatric Crohn's disease: A biologic therapy now is approved for use in children. American Journal of Nursing, 106(9), 30; Bindler, R., & Howry, L. (2005). *Pediatric drug guide.* Upper Saddle River, NJ: Prentice Hall Health; Hyams, J. (2005). *Inflammatory bowel disease.* Pediatrics in Review, 26(9), 314–320; Irving, P. M., & Gibson, P. R. (2007). *Infliximab: Getting the most for your money.* Journal of Gastroenterology and Hepatology, 22, 1557–1565; Silbermintz, A., & Markowitz, J. (2006). *Inflammatory bowel disease.* Pediatric Annals, 35(4), 269–274.

If other treatment measures fail to reduce inflammation, surgery is generally indicated. A temporary colostomy or ileostomy is performed to allow the bowel to rest. In Crohn's disease, however, ulcerations tend to recur elsewhere in the GI tract. Biologic therapies such as infliximab (Remicade) have been effective in patients with Crohn's disease who fail to respond to other measures. These therapies have recently been approved for use in children and are emerging as a treatment option in ulcerative colitis (Aschenbrenner, 2006; Irving & Gibson, 2007). In ulcerative colitis, removal of the diseased bowel provides a permanent cure.

NURSING MANAGEMENT

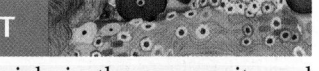

Nursing management occurs mainly in the community and home and focuses on helping the child and family adjust to the emotional impact of a chronic disease, administering medications and diet therapy, monitoring nutritional status, monitoring growth status, and providing appropriate referrals.

Assessment and Diagnosis

Assess for abdominal distention, tenderness, and pain. Monitor bowel sounds and stool pattern; measure abdominal girth.

Nursing diagnoses that apply to the child with inflammatory bowel disease may include:

- Diarrhea related to disease process
- Imbalanced Nutrition: Less than Body Requirements related to bowel inflammation and poor nutritional intake
- Pain (Acute or Chronic) related to inflammatory disease process
- Risk for Deficient Fluid Volume related to loss of fluids through diarrhea
- Disturbed Body Image related to disease process, presence of stoma, and medication side effects

Planning and Implementation

Provide emotional support and counseling to help the child adjust to feeling "different" from peers. Inability to compete with peers and frequent absences from school can affect the child's self-esteem. Collaborate care with parents and assist them in contacting the school district to arrange for tutoring in case extended absences from school become necessary. Encourage the child who is not attending school regularly to maintain contact with friends through telephone calls, cards, and visits.

Body image is a major concern for children and adolescents with inflammatory bowel disease. Corticosteroid therapy causes growth retardation and delayed sexual maturation. Encourage the child to discuss feelings about these side effects. If a permanent colostomy or ileostomy is required, the nurse can assist the child and family to understand the need for surgical treatment. (See the discussion of ostomies earlier in this chapter.) Introduce the child and family to other children who have stomas.

Teach parents about medication administration and diet therapy. Reinforce to both the parents and child the importance of adhering to a strict medication regimen. Emphasize that medications should be continued even when the child is asymptomatic. Discuss the side effects of the drugs and what to do if any of these symptoms occur. (See Families Want to Know: Diet Instructions for Inflammatory Bowel Disease.) Since immune status may be altered by steroid use, have families avoid contact with infectious diseases when the child is taking steroids. Instruct them to report any diseases and fevers the child experiences, and to report the use of steroids to all health care providers. Immunization schedules may need to be altered.

Parents also will require instructions for TPN if it is used, as well as information about care of a central venous catheter, including dressing changes, signs of infection, how to handle infusion pumps and tubing, and how to measure the child's intake and output. Assist parents in obtaining equipment and supplies necessary for the child's care. Have parents demonstrate their

(sidebar, vertical text) Crohn's and Colitis Foundation of America

Families Want to Know
Diet Instructions for Inflammatory Bowel Disease

- Several small feedings are usually better tolerated than three meals daily.
- Limiting fiber intake can help to decrease intestine motility and inflammation. Peel fruits and avoid large quantities of whole grains and nuts.
- If the child is not eating well, offer high-calorie meals. If lactose intolerance is not a problem for the particular child, cream soups, milkshakes, puddings, and custards can be offered.
- Liquid dietary supplements may be helpful to ensure protein and caloric requirements are met.
- Watch for foods that cause intestinal problems for the individual child, and avoid them in the future.
- Avoid having mealtime become a reason for family strife. Seek help of nurses and dietitians if needed.

mastery of care for the central venous catheter and their understanding of TPN techniques during home visits and appointments for health care.

Refer parents to social services and home health care agencies if they are not receiving any of these services. For information about inflammatory bowel disease, refer families to the Crohn's and Colitis Foundation of America.

Evaluation

Expected outcomes of nursing care for the child with inflammatory bowel disease include the following:

- Normal growth and development milestones are achieved.
- The child demonstrates absence of gastrointestinal distress.
- The child and family demonstrate successful management of medications without demonstration of side effects.
- The child remains free from infection due to central line.
- A positive body image is achieved.
- The child demonstrates integration of stress-lowering practices into daily life.

Peptic Ulcer

A peptic ulcer is an erosion of the mucosal tissue in the lower end of the esophagus, in the stomach (usually along the lesser curvature), or in the duodenum (*gastric ulcer* is the term sometimes used when the stomach mucosa is affected). Males are more likely to have peptic ulcers than females; however, peptic ulcers are much less common in children than in adults. African American and Hispanic children are at greater risk for peptic ulcers (Shah & Carroll, 2007).

Ulcers are classified as primary or secondary, depending on their etiology. Primary peptic ulcers occur in healthy children. Secondary (stress) ulcers occur in children with a preexisting illness or injury (often a burn) and in children receiving medications such as salicylates, corticosteroids, and nonsteroidal anti-inflammatory drugs. Diet usually is not a major factor in the development of peptic ulcers in children, although caffeine and alcohol consumption in adolescents may exacerbate the disease. Ulcers in both adults and children are often caused by *Helicobacter pylori*, a gram-negative rod (Shah & Carroll, 2007).

This organism is transmitted by the fecal-oral or oral-oral routes. Infections often occur in several members of a family, especially when the family's water supply is contaminated.

Clinical manifestations vary according to the age of the child and location of the ulcer. The most common symptom is abdominal pain (burning) associated with an empty stomach, which may awaken the child at night. Vomiting and pain after meals, anemia, occult blood in stools, and abdominal distention may also be present.

Diagnosis is based on the history and radiologic studies. *H. pylori* can be diagnosed by culture of the organism taken via gastroscopy, and by measuring urea in the urine and on the breath, since the organism hydrolyzes urea. The goals of medical management are to relieve discomfort and promote healing. When *H. pylori* is the causative agent, antimicrobial agents such as bismuth salts, tetracycline, and metronidazole combination are given. Other drug combinations, such as antacids in liquid form (Maalox, Mylanta) and histamine antagonists (ranitidine, cimetidine, and famotidine), are also used. Antibody titers are measured several times over 6 months to evaluate the effectiveness of therapy. The prognosis is usually good with early intervention.

NURSING MANAGEMENT

Assess the child for abdominal pain, vomiting, and abdominal distention. Assess for family history of *H. pylori* infection. Nursing care centers on interventions to promote adequate nutritional intake, promote healing, and prevent recurrences. Provide a nutritionally sound, age-appropriate diet. Omit foods only if they exacerbate the disorder. Antibiotics must be given as scheduled. Emphasize the importance of continuing drug therapy. The family needs encouragement to continue the medications as ordered and to return for follow-up visits. Children who attend school may prefer to take antacids in the form of tablets. The appropriate form must be completed in order for the child to receive medication at school.

Parents should discuss any additional medications with the primary health care provider before administering to the child. Caution parents to avoid aspirin products, which irritate the gastric mucosa. If an antipyretic or pain medication is needed, acetaminophen should be given. Advise parents to read medication labels if they are unsure of product contents.

Because psychologic stress can contribute to peptic ulcer disease, help the parents and child identify sources of stress in the child's life. Assess coping mechanisms and provide referral for psychologic counseling, if appropriate. Teach relaxation techniques and recommend community classes on yoga or other stress reduction.

■ DISORDERS OF MOTILITY

Fluids are an important part of normal GI functioning. As food passes through the intestines, fluids are reabsorbed and moderately soft stool is formed and evacuated. In disorders such as diarrhea and constipation, fluid production is altered, causing either more or less fluid to be reabsorbed. This can severely alter the characteristics of the stool. Reabsorption of too little water produces diarrhea and can lead to fluid and electrolyte alterations. Reabsorption of too much fluid can cause constipation, which if untreated can lead to bowel obstruction.

Gastroenteritis (Acute Diarrhea)

Gastroenteritis is an inflammation of the stomach and intestines that may be accompanied by vomiting and diarrhea. It can affect any part of the GI tract. It may be an acute problem, caused by viral, bacterial, or parasitic infections, or a chronic problem. Rotavirus is the leading cause of severe gastroenteritis in infants and young children (Cortese & Parashar, 2009) (see Chapter 16 ∞). Children under age 5 years average approximately two episodes of gastroenteritis each year. Infants and small children with gastroenteritis or diarrhea can quickly become dehydrated and are at risk for hypovolemic shock if fluid and electrolyte losses are not replaced (see Chapter 18 ∞). A significant number of infants and young children are hospitalized each year for dehydration secondary to gastroenteritis.

Etiology and Pathophysiology

Diarrhea in children can have many different causes (Table 25–3). The specific etiology is not always identified. The common mechanism is a decrease in the absorptive capacity of the bowel through inflammation, decrease in surface area for absorption, or alteration of parasympathetic innervation. Children in childcare centers and those living in substandard housing with improper sanitation are at increased risk of infectious causes.

TABLE 25–3	Causes of Diarrhea in Children	
Etiology	Bowel Manifestations
Emotional stress (anxiety, fatigue)	Increased motility
Intestinal infection (bacteria [*E. coli, Salmonella, Shigella*], viral [human rotavirus, enteric adenovirus], fungal overgrowth)	Inflammation of mucosa; increased mucus secretion in colon
Food sensitivity (gluten, cow's milk)	Decreased digestion of food
Food intolerance (lactose, introduction of new foods, overfeeding)	Increased motility; increased mucus secretion in colon
Medications (iron, antibiotics)	Irritation and suprainfection
Colon disease (colitis, necrotizing enterocolitis, enterocolitis)	Inflammation and ulceration of intestinal walls; reduced absorption of fluid; increased intestinal motility
Surgical alterations (short bowel syndrome)	Reduced size of colon; decreased absorption surface

Clinical Manifestations

Diarrhea may be mild, moderate, or severe. In mild diarrhea, stools are slightly increased in number and have a more liquid consistency. In moderate diarrhea, the child has several loose or watery stools. Other symptoms include irritability, anorexia, nausea, and vomiting. Moderate diarrhea is usually self-limiting, resolving without treatment within 1 or 2 days. In severe diarrhea, watery stools are continuous. The child exhibits symptoms of fluid and electrolyte imbalance (see Chapter 18 ∞), has cramping, and is extremely irritable and difficult to console.

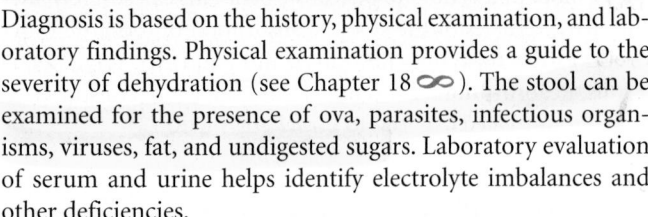

COLLABORATIVE CARE

Diagnosis is based on the history, physical examination, and laboratory findings. Physical examination provides a guide to the severity of dehydration (see Chapter 18 ∞). The stool can be examined for the presence of ova, parasites, infectious organisms, viruses, fat, and undigested sugars. Laboratory evaluation of serum and urine helps identify electrolyte imbalances and other deficiencies.

Medical management depends on the severity of the diarrhea and fluid and electrolyte imbalances. The goal of treatment is to correct the fluid and electrolyte imbalances. For mild and moderate dehydration, oral rehydration therapy is the first intervention. This may be accomplished at home or in the short-stay observation unit in a hospital with solutions such as Pedialyte. Carbonated and very sugary beverages should not be given. Fermentation of sugar in the GI tract causes increased gas, abdominal distention, and an increased frequency of diarrhea. For severe dehydration, rehydration is accomplished by intravenous infusion with a solution chosen to correct the specific imbalances. As soon as possible, introduce clear liquids or breast milk and then progress the child to the regular diet. Foods generally are not withheld for more than 1 to 2 days.

If the diarrhea is caused by bacteria or parasites, antimicrobial therapy may be prescribed. Antiemetics and antidiarrheals are generally not used in young children since they can mask the signs and symptoms of more serious illness.

NURSING MANAGEMENT

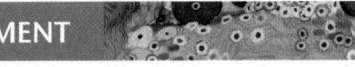

Nursing Assessment and Diagnosis

The nurse may encounter the child and family in the emergency department, urgent care center, clinic, or office. The child may be cared for over several hours at a clinic or urgent care center so that dehydration is treated with intravenous infusion and/or oral rehydration, and then sent home with instructions for parents to care for the child.

If the child is hospitalized, it is important to assess onset, frequency, color, amount, and consistency of stools. If the child is also vomiting, monitor the amount and type of vomitus. Initial and ongoing physical assessment of the child focuses on observing for signs and symptoms of dehydration, which reflect underlying fluid and electrolyte status. Evaluate urinary output and specific gravity. An accurate weight must be obtained on admission and daily thereafter. Monitor vital signs every 2 to

4 hours. A febrile child has increased water loss, contributing to the dehydration. Assess skin integrity, especially in the perineal and rectal areas, and note any breakdown or rashes.

The accompanying Nursing Care Plan lists common nursing diagnoses. Other diagnoses that might also be appropriate include:

- Anxiety (Child and Parent) related to change in health status
- Disturbed Sleep Pattern related to pain
- Imbalanced Nutrition: Less than Body Requirements related to inability to ingest sufficient nutrients

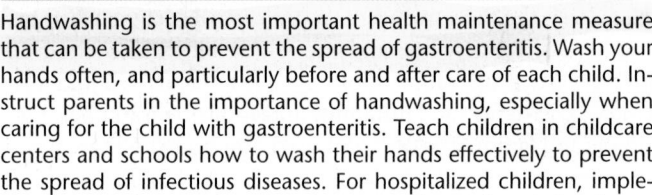

Nursing Alert

Handwashing is the most important health maintenance measure that can be taken to prevent the spread of gastroenteritis. Wash your hands often, and particularly before and after care of each child. Instruct parents in the importance of handwashing, especially when caring for the child with gastroenteritis. Teach children in childcare centers and schools how to wash their hands effectively to prevent the spread of infectious diseases. For hospitalized children, implement contact or enteric precautions according to hospital policy.

Planning and Implementation

Nursing care focuses on providing emotional support, promoting rest and comfort, and ensuring adequate nutrition and hydration. See Nursing Care Plan: The Child with Gastroenteritis for a summary of nursing care.

Provide Emotional Support

The child may have been ill for several days or become suddenly ill a short time before seeking health care. The child and parents are usually anxious, so it is important to allow them to talk and ask questions. The child may require blood tests to help direct rehydration therapy. Most children are cared for at home, although care in a 24-hour monitoring unit may occur. For hospitalized children, use therapeutic play techniques, such as allowing the child to manipulate equipment, to help reduce anxiety (see Chapter 11 ∞). To promote trust, be honest if a procedure will hurt. Encourage the child to express anger, fear, and pain.

Promote Rest and Comfort

Children with gastroenteritis may awaken frequently with periods of vomiting and diarrhea. Provide a quiet, restful environment and cluster nursing care to allow for periods of uninterrupted rest. Darken the room and keep interruptions to a minimum. To reduce the child's anxiety, encourage parents to room in. Place the child's favorite toys and comfort objects within reach. Keep the child's mouth moistened with a wet washcloth, or an occasional ice chip. Provide skin care after each episode of diarrhea. Avoid using commercial baby wipes that contain alcohol as these irritate the skin and cause discomfort for the child.

Ensure Adequate Nutrition and Hydration

Offer liquids throughout the illness, even if an intravenous infusion is in place. Follow guidelines for oral rehydration therapy in Chapter 18 ∞. Small amounts of normal diet for age are provided. Infants are breastfed or given formula. Avoid cow's

NURSING CARE PLAN
The Child with Gastroenteritis

INTERVENTION	RATIONALE	EXPECTED OUTCOME
1. Nursing Diagnosis: Diarrhea related to infectious process		
NIC Priority Intervention: *Diarrhea management:* Prevention and alleviation of diarrhea		**NOC Suggested Outcome:** *Fluid and electrolyte balance:* Balance of water and electrolytes in the intracellular and extracellular compartments of the body
Goal: The child's bowel function will be restored to normal.		
▪ Obtain baseline vital signs and monitor every 2–4 hours.	▪ Fluid and electrolyte imbalances can alter vital body functions.	The child's bowel function returns to normal.
▪ Observe stools for amount, color, consistency, odor, and frequency.	▪ Observation of stools aids in the diagnosis and in monitoring the child's status.	
▪ Test stools for occult blood.	▪ Frequent defecation and some infectious organisms can cause bleeding.	
▪ Monitor results of stool culture and sample for ova and parasites and notify physician of positive results.	▪ Rapid notification of the physician will facilitate treatment.	
▪ Wash hands well before and after contact with the child.	▪ Handwashing helps prevent transmission of microorganisms.	
▪ Isolate the child until the cause of the diarrhea is determined.	▪ Isolation prevents exposure of other patients and staff.	
▪ Assist the child with toileting and hygiene.	▪ The child may be weak, incontinent, physically impaired, or anxious and require assistance to use the bathroom.	
▪ Administer prescribed oral rehydration and intravenous solutions.	▪ These solutions provide necessary fluids and nutrients.	
▪ Notify the physician if diarrhea persists, stool characteristics change, or other symptoms of dehydration electrolyte imbalance occur.	▪ It is important to ensure early intervention.	
2. Nursing Diagnosis: Deficient Fluid Volume related to active fluid volume loss		
NIC Priority Intervention: *Fluid monitoring:* Collection and analysis of patient data to regulate fluid balance		**NOC Suggested Outcome:** *Fluid and electrolyte balance:* Balance of water and electrolytes in the intracellular and extracellular compartments of the body
Goal: The child will become rehydrated and will begin to drink fluids within 24 hours of admission.		
▪ Monitor intake and output. Document time of each voiding. Weigh all diapers.	▪ It is important to determine if output exceeds input. Long periods of time without urine output can be an early indicator of poor renal function.	The child has normal fluid and electrolyte balance as indicated by laboratory evaluation and physical examination. The child should produce 1–2 mL of urine/kg/hr.
▪ Compare admission weight to preadmission weight. Assess weight daily.	▪ The degree of dehydration can be determined by the percentage of weight loss. Daily weights aid in determining progress toward rehydration.	
▪ Assess level of consciousness, skin turgor, mucous membranes, skin color and temperature, capillary refill, eyes, and fontanels every 4 hours.	▪ This assessment will determine degree of hydration and adequacy of interventions.	

(continued)

NURSING CARE PLAN

The Child with Gastroenteritis (continued)

INTERVENTION	RATIONALE	EXPECTED OUTCOME
Assess for vomiting.	Vomiting frequently accompanies diarrhea and contributes to the child's fluid loss.	
Provide oral fluid and electrolyte replacement solution if able to tolerate.	Oral fluids are less invasive than IV fluids. Provides for replacement of essential fluids and electrolytes.	
Provide and maintain IV replacement therapy, as ordered.	Use of IV replacement is based on the degree of dehydration, ongoing losses, insensible water losses, and electrolyte results.	

3. Nursing Diagnosis: Risk for Impaired Skin Integrity related to altered fluid status

NIC Priority Intervention: *Skin surveillance:* Collection and analysis of patient data to maintain skin integrity		**NOC Suggested Outcome:** *Tissue integrity:* Skin and mucous membranes Structural intactness and normal physiologic function of skin and mucous membranes

Goal: The child will remain free of skin breakdown and rashes.

Assess skin of perineum and rectum for signs of skin breakdown or irritation.	Early assessment and intervention can prevent worsening of the condition.	
Provide prevention or restorative care for infants as follows:		
Preventive Care:		
Change diapers every 2 hours or as needed.	Frequent diaper changes minimize skin contact with chemical irritants from stool and urine.	The child's perianal and rectal tissue remains pink and intact.
Wash the diaper area after each soiling.	Washing the diaper area removes traces of stool if present.	
Apply A & D ointment, Aquaphor, or another barrier ointment with each diaper change.	The ointment provides a barrier and protects intact or reddened skin from becoming excoriated.	
Restorative Care:		
Leave the buttocks open to air for a few minutes several times daily, placing absorbent pads under the infant.	Air circulation to the area is promoted.	
Notify the physician if the skin is severely broken or peeling or if a rash is present.	Additional measures such as the use of a barrier cream or paste may be needed to ensure skin healing.	
For toddlers and older children: Tub bathe at least daily (if condition allows) in tepid water. Pat the area dry.	A tub bath helps loosen any fecal matter without scrubbing, which can cause additional irritation to the skin.	
Discourage the wearing of underwear if possible.	This allows air to circulate and prevents accumulation of moisture.	
Apply barrier ointment with each diaper change or as instructed.	Ointment provides a barrier and protects intact or reddened skin from becoming excoriated.	

milk–based formula or regular milk until the diarrhea resolves. The child's diet progresses based on tolerance for feedings. Apple juice and other fruit juices should be avoided since they contain high amounts of carbohydrates which pull circulating fluids into the gut and can prolong the presence of diarrhea.

Discharge Planning and Home Care Teaching

Discharge teaching begins on arrival at the health care facility. Teach the parents about the symptoms of dehydration and what actions to take if diarrhea recurs. Be sure that parents understand the recommended diet progression. Emphasize the necessity of good hygiene practices to prevent the spread of microorganisms that can cause gastroenteritis. If the child attends childcare, have the parent inform the care center about the infection so the staff can be alerted to watch for other cases and can take steps to prevent the spread of infection.

Evaluation

Expected outcomes of nursing care for the child with gastroenteritis are listed in the Nursing Care Plan. Additional outcomes include:

- The child achieves adequate nutritional intake to support growth and development.
- The family describes signs of dehydration and appropriate interventions.
- The family acknowledges the importance of handwashing in decreasing transmission of infectious agents.

Constipation

Constipation is a common complaint in the pediatric population and accounts for 5% of all outpatient visits to the pediatric primary care provider (Tobias, Mason, Lutkenhoff, et al., 2008). Constipation generally appears first in children ages 2–4 years and affects up to one third of children 6–12 years of age each year (Biggs & Dery, 2006). Constipation is more common in school-age males than females, but at other ages it is more common in females. Because stool patterns vary among children, identification of an abnormal pattern is sometimes difficult. Infants usually have several bowel movements a day. For a young child, one bowel movement a day may be normal. As the child grows, however, three to four bowel movements a week may be a normal pattern. The diagnosis of constipation must take into account the child's normal stool patterns.

Etiology and Pathophysiology

Constipation may be caused by an underlying disease, diet, or psychologic factor. It may result from defects in filling, or more commonly emptying, of the rectum. Pathological causes of defective filling include ineffective colonic propulsive activity, caused by hypothyroidism or use of medication, and obstruction, caused by a structural anomaly (stricture or stenosis) or by an aganglionic segment (Hirschsprung disease). If the rectum fails to fill, stasis leads to excessive drying of the stools. Emptying of the rectum depends on the defecation reflex. Lesions of the spinal cord, weakness of the abdominal muscles, and local lesions blocking sphincter relaxation all may impede attempts to defecate.

Constipation during infancy is rare and is most often caused by mismanagement of diet. The transition from formula to cow's milk may cause a transient constipation because the bowel must adjust to the increased protein content of cow's milk.

Constipation in toddlers and preschool-age children is often associated with learning to control body functions. Many children do not like the sensations of a bowel movement and may begin withholding stool, which accumulates in and dilates the rectum until the next urge to defecate. The increasingly hard and painful bowel movement reinforces the child's withholding behavior, and a pattern develops (Biggs & Dery, 2006). See the discussion in this chapter on encopresis.

Constipation in the school-age child, older child, and adolescent is generally related to activity, diet, and toileting habits. The child's diet may be lacking in fiber and contain many starchy foods such as bread and cheese. Constipation may occur due to limited time for toileting. The child may not take time during the day to have a bowel movement or may be hesitant to use an unfamiliar bathroom.

COLLABORATIVE CARE

Collaborative care focuses on determining the underlying pathologic cause of constipation, correcting any structural defect or obstruction, eliminating contributing factors, and assisting the child to establish routine bowel elimination habits.

Diagnostic Tests

Diagnosis is based on a thorough history and physical examination. When digital rectal examination confirms the presence of fecal impaction, further studies are not needed (Biggs & Dery, 2006). If digital rectal examination is contraindicated or the exam does not yield any findings, abdominal radiographs may be useful in identifying fecal impaction. Refer to the section on Hirschsprung disease on page 771 for diagnostic tests used to confirm this diagnosis. When constipation occurs along with growth failure, vomiting, or abdominal pain, further investigation is necessary to rule out other disorders. Tests may include thyroid function tests; measurements of calcium, glucose, and electrolytes; a complete blood count; and urinalysis.

Clinical Therapy

Dietary management is the treatment of choice for constipation that has no underlying pathologic cause. Constipation in young infants can usually be corrected by increasing the amount of fluids or adding 2 ounces of pear or apple juice to daily intake. Increasing physical activity and fluid intake may be effective for some children.

Removing constipating foods (e.g., bananas, rice, and cheese) from the child's diet often decreases the constipation. Increasing the child's intake of high-fiber foods (e.g., whole grain breads, raw fruits and vegetables) and fluids also promotes bowel elimination. A single glycerin suppository or enema may be needed to remove hard stool, followed by dietary and fluid management.

Encouragement from parents and relaxation of bathroom privileges at school promote regularity and return of usual bowel patterns within a short time for school-age children. Children may need to get up earlier to have breakfast to allow time for toileting before going to school.

Constipation may follow surgery, especially in children who are immobilized for several days. Stool softeners and a diet high in fiber and fluids are given to prevent and treat constipation.

Pharmacologic management of severe constipation usually occurs in two stages. The first stage involves disimpaction followed by maintenance therapy (Biggs & Dery, 2006). The evacuation phase is the most difficult for the child and those who are managing the child's constipation.

Consider the most effective means to evacuate the stool while causing the least amount of stress and anxiety to the child. Suppositories and enemas can cause fear in children. Polyethylene glycol electrolyte solution can be administered orally or instilled via a nasogastric tube to promote stool evacuation (Biggs & Dery, 2006). Once the stool has been evacuated, the child may need routine treatment to prevent reaccumulation of stool in the bowel. For children who need daily medication, a lubricant such as mineral oil or an osmotic laxative such as lactulose or polyethylene glycol (MiraLax) is recommended. If only intermittent treatment is required, a stimulant laxative such as bisacodyl might be used (Montgomery & Navarro, 2008). Behavior modification is also an important aspect of treatment for constipation. For example, establish a routine for sitting on the toilet and offer rewards for success (Croffie, 2006).

NURSING MANAGEMENT

Nursing care focuses on teaching parents what constitutes normal bowel patterns in children and the importance of diet in maintaining normal bowel patterns. Assess the child's diet history and obtain a description of bowel patterns from parents. Ask what the family does to treat constipation. Assessment of the child's food likes and dislikes may provide a clue as to the cause of constipation. Regular bowel habits are encouraged by having the child sit on the toilet for 30 minutes after a meal or around the time defecation usually occurs. Providing positive reinforcement during toilet training helps prevent a withholding pattern.

Teach parents dietary measures to promote regularity of bowel movements. Children can be given a high-fiber diet that includes fruits and vegetables. Cut-up fresh fruits, dried fruits, and fruit juice can be offered as snacks. A glycerin suppository, a natural stimulant and lubricant of the bowel, can be used periodically. Caution parents to avoid frequent use of laxatives, stool softeners, and enemas, since overuse can cause bowel dependency. Herbal stimulant laxatives are discouraged for children younger than 12 years. Find out more about any herbs the family commonly uses.

Encopresis

Encopresis is an abnormal elimination pattern characterized by the recurrent soiling or passage of stool at inappropriate times by a child who should have achieved bowel continence. Encopresis is reported to occur in 1–3% of children (Montgomery & Navarro, 2008). Children with primary encopresis have never

Complementary Therapy
Herbal Laxatives

Herbal laxatives are used by some cultures as complementary therapies to treat constipation in children. Examples of herbs and supplements that have been used include psyllium, magnesium, olive oil, glycerol, xantham gum, guar gum, cascara, senna, and castor oil (Culbert & Banez, 2008). Safety and effectiveness of many of these laxatives have not been established in children. Cascara (*Rhamni purshiana*) and senna (*Sannae folum*) are stimulant laxatives that have been approved by the U.S. Food and Drug Administration for use in children older than 2 years of age to treat constipation (Culbert & Banez, 2008; Gardiner & Kemper, 2005). Stimulant laxatives should be used with caution in children, however, as they can lead to dependency as well as abdominal pain. Senna has also been associated with skin problems in children, including diaper rash and blistering (Gardiner & Kemper, 2005).

achieved bowel control. Children with secondary encopresis have been continent of stool for several months.

Encopresis is usually associated with voluntary or involuntary retention of stool in the lower bowel and rectum, leading to constipation, dilation of the lower bowel, and incompetence of the inner sphincter. The retention of stool is usually a result of being "too busy"; the child puts off going to the bathroom because of involvement in interesting activities. The retention of stool leads to constipation that is untreated and chronic. Loose stool leaks around the hard feces, and the child becomes unaware of a need to eliminate. Soiling may occur during the day or night. Bowel movements are irregular, painful, small, and hard. The child may be ridiculed by peers because of his or her offensive body odor. This rejection leads to withdrawal and behavioral problems, often resulting in altered school performance and attendance. The child continues to hold stool because the passage is painful. Parents commonly seek health care, believing that the child has diarrhea or constipation.

The underlying constipation that leads to encopresis may be caused by the stress of environmental changes (e.g., birth of a sibling, moving to a new house, attending a new school), issues of anger and control related to bowel training, diet, a full schedule of activities, or a genetic predisposition.

A thorough history, physical examination, and diagnostic studies (possibly including contrast or barium enema) are necessary to rule out organic causes and anatomic abnormalities. Information about the child's toilet-training habits and parents' attitudes concerning those habits is obtained. A history of eating habits and types of foods eaten is often helpful. Physical examination sometimes reveals a nontender mass in the lower abdomen.

In addition to dietary management and treatment to evacuate the bowel as discussed in the preceding section, behavior modification techniques and psychotherapy may be used. Behavior modification programs that reward and reinforce appropriate toileting habits can be successful. The child should sit on the toilet for several minutes after morning and evening meals. It takes several months for the bowel to be retrained to respond to sphincter stimulation. Psychological-based treatment that involves meetings with both parent and child may be indicated if the child has not responded to other treatment (Reid & Bahar, 2006).

NURSING MANAGEMENT

Prevention of encopresis is the nursing goal. Partner with parents to teach toilet-training techniques, emphasizing the child's developmental readiness (see Chapter 4 ∞). Parents are encouraged to praise the child for successes and avoid punishment and power struggles. Encourage high-fiber diets and regular times for elimination.

Nursing care centers on educating the child and parents about the disorder and its treatment and providing emotional support. Explain the treatment plan, including dietary changes and use of laxatives or stool softeners. Reassure the child that he or she has a healthy body and, with treatment, will achieve normal functioning. The child is monitored for at least 6 months to be certain new patterns have been established.

■ INTESTINAL PARASITIC DISORDERS

Intestinal parasitic disorders occur most frequently in tropical regions. Outbreaks take place where water is not treated, food is incorrectly prepared, or people live in crowded conditions with poor sanitation. In the United States, outbreaks of diseases caused by protozoa or helminths (worms) are increasing. A common cause of infection in the United States is camping and ingesting untreated water. Young children, especially those in childcare, are most at risk of infection. Young children often lack good hygiene practices and are likely to put objects and their hands into their mouths. See Clinical Manifestations: Common Intestinal Parasitic Disorders.

Another common cause of parasitic infection in the young child is related to exposure to pets and wildlife. Pets should be checked for parasites and treated for worms regularly. Sandboxes should be kept covered when not in use so that animals cannot use the sand for defecation. Children should also be taught good hand hygiene after exposure to their pets (Centers for Disease Control and Prevention [CDC], 2008a).

Laboratory examination of stool specimens identifies the causative organism (protozoa, worms, larvae, or ova). Treatment usually involves an anthelmintic. Nursing care centers on preventive teaching. Emphasize the importance of good hygiene practices, especially careful handwashing, after toileting and when handling food. Instruct parents to give prescribed medications as directed even if the child's condition seems to be improved.

■ DISORDERS OF MALABSORPTION

Malabsorption occurs when a child cannot digest or absorb nutrients in the diet. Disorders of malabsorption include celiac disease, lactose intolerance, and short bowel syndrome. Celiac disease and lactose intolerance are discussed in Chapter 14 ∞. Cystic fibrosis, a common cause of malabsorption, is discussed in Chapter 20 ∞.

Short Bowel Syndrome

Short bowel syndrome is a decreased ability to digest and absorb a regular diet because of a shortened intestine. Loss of intestine may result from extensive bowel resection for treatment of necrotizing enterocolitis or inflammatory disorders, or from a congenital bowel anomaly such as gastroschisis, atresia, or intestinal malrotation that led to volvulus.

The extent and location of the involved bowel determine the severity of the disorder. Because specific types of absorption occur primarily in certain parts of the bowel, the section lost determines which vitamins and other nutrients are inadequate. During the first 3 months after bowel resection, watery diarrhea is common. In the transition period, the remaining bowel usually increases its absorptive surface area and partially compensates for the absent intestine. At first, the infant or young child requires nutritional support to provide sufficient nutrients for growth and development. In the initial period, the child only receives TPN. Once the bowel begins to recover, in addition to TPN, feedings by mouth or by tube may be started in small amounts. Feedings by this method stimulate the bowel and prevent atrophy of the mucosa (Goday, 2009). It is essential that the child receive the appropriate nutritional components regardless of the method in which nutrition is delivered.

NURSING MANAGEMENT

Nursing care focuses on meeting the child's nutritional and fluid needs and teaching parents how to care for the child at home. Establishing an adequate nutritional intake and bowel pattern is a lengthy process. TPN is provided initially until a feeding regimen can be established. Oral and enteral feedings are instituted gradually to allow the bowel time to compensate. Provide support to the family and child throughout this period. Teach parents how to prepare and administer total parenteral feedings and care for the central line. See the *Clinical Skills Manual*. Once enteral or tube feedings are begun, teach management of the feeding pump and care of the feeding tube. Ensure regular bowel function and maintain skin integrity. Arrange home visits to monitor the child's growth and development, care of the central line and tube feeding site, and any side effects such as fluid and electrolyte imbalance and diarrhea.

Nursing Alert

The child with short bowel syndrome will receive TPN via a central line. Meticulous care of the central line used for TPN is essential to prevent a central line infection and potential septicemia. Maintaining patency of the central line is also essential as this may be the child's only route for receiving nutrition. It is not uncommon for children with short bowel syndrome to require insertion of multiple central lines over time either due to infection or to occlusion of the line, especially if they require long-term TPN. This is a stress on the child and family who must experience yet another surgical procedure.

■ HEPATIC DISORDERS

The liver is one of the most vital organs in the body. Its primary functions include production of blood clotting factors, fibrinogen, and prothrombin; secretion of bile and *bilirubin* (yellow pigment produced from the breakdown of red blood cells);

Clinical Manifestations
Common Intestinal Parasitic Disorders

Parasitic Infection	Transmission, Life Cycle, Pathogenesis	Clinical Manifestations	Clinical Therapy	Comments
Giardiasis Organism: protozoan *Giardia lamblia* 	Transmission is through person-to-person contact, unfiltered water, improperly prepared infected food, and contact with animals. Cysts are ingested and passed into the duodenum and proximal jejunum, where they begin actively feeding. They are excreted in the stool.	May be asymptomatic. *Infants:* diarrhea, vomiting, anorexia, failure to thrive. *Older children:* abdominal cramps; intermittent loose, foul-smelling, watery, pale, and greasy stools.	Available medications include furazolidone and quinacrine. Furazolidone has fewer side effects than quinacrine but is more expensive. Metronidazole is also effective but is not licensed in the United States for treatment of giardiasis.	Most common intestinal parasitic organism in the United States. Infection may resolve spontaneously in 4–6 weeks without treatment. Parents or caregivers should wear gloves when handling diapers or stool of an infant or child who is infected with parasites.
Enterobiasis (Pinworm) Organism: nematode *Enterobius vermicularis* 	Transmission is from discharged eggs inhaled or carried from hand to mouth. Eggs hatch in the upper intestine and mature in 15–28 days. Larvae then migrate to the cecum. After mating, the female migrates out of the anus and lays up to 17,000 eggs. Movement of worms causes intense itching. Scratching deposits eggs on the hands and under the nails.	Intense perianal itching, irritability, restlessness, and short attention span; in females, can migrate to the vagina and urethra to cause infection. Itching intensifies at night when the female comes to the anal opening to lay eggs.	Available medications include mebendazole, pyrantel pamoate, and piperazine citrate. The child and all household members should be treated at the same time. Treatment may be repeated in 2–3 weeks.	Most common helminthic infection in the United States. Transmission is increased in crowded conditions such as housing developments, schools, and day care centers.
Ascariasis (Type of Roundworm) Organism: nematode *Ascaris lumbricoides* 	Transmission is from discharged eggs carried from hand to mouth. The adult lays eggs in the small intestine. Eggs are excreted in stool, where they incubate for 2–3 weeks. Swallowed eggs hatch in the small intestine. Larvae may penetrate intestinal villi, entering the portal vein and liver, then moving to the lung. Larvae that ascend to the upper respiratory tract are swallowed and proceed to the small intestine, where they repeat the cycle.	Mild infection may be asymptomatic. Severe infection may result in intestinal obstruction, peritonitis, obstructive jaundice, and lung involvement.	Available anthelmintic medications include mebendazole, pyrantel pamoate, or piperazine citrate. Stools should be examined 2 weeks after treatment and monthly for 3 months. Family members and contacts of the child should be treated if indicated. If the child has intestinal obstruction, treatment may include administering piperazine through a nasogastric tube and duodenal suction. Obstructing worms sometimes have to be surgically removed.	Most common in warm climates. Primarily affects children 1–4 years of age.

Clinical Manifestations

Common Intestinal Parasitic Disorders (continued)

Parasitic Infection	Transmission, Life Cycle, Pathogenesis	Clinical Manifestations	Clinical Therapy	Comments
Hookworm disease Organism: nematode *Necator americanus*	Transmission is through direct contact with infected soil containing larvae. Worms live in the small intestine and feed on villi, causing bleeding. Eggs are deposited in the bowel and excreted in feces. Eggs hatch in damp shaded soil. Larvae attach to and penetrate the skin, then enter the bloodstream, migrating to the lungs. Larvae then migrate to the upper respiratory passages and are swallowed.	In healthy individuals, mild infection seldom causes problems. More severe infection may result in anemia and malnutrition. Presence of larvae on the skin may cause burning and itching, followed by redness and papular eruption.	Available medications include mebendazole and pyrantel pamoate. Stools should be examined 2 weeks after treatment and monthly for 3 months. Family members and contacts of the child should be treated if indicated.	Children should wear shoes when outdoors, although other unprotected areas of the skin may still come in contact with larvae.
Strongyloidiasis (Type of Roundworm) Organism: nematode *Strongyloides stercoralis*	Transmission is from the ingestion of discharged larvae in the soil. Life cycle is similar to that of the hookworm, except this roundworm does not attach to the intestinal mucosa, and feeding larvae (rather than eggs) may be deposited in the soil.	Mild infection may be asymptomatic. Severe infection may result in abdominal pain and distention, nausea, vomiting, and diarrhea. Stools may be large and pale, with mucus. Severe infection may lead to a nutritional deficiency.	Available medications include thiabendazole or mebendazole. Treatment may need to be repeated if symptoms recur after treatment. Family members and contacts of the child should be examined and treated if indicated.	Most common in older children and adolescents.
Visceral larva migrans (toxocariasis) Organism: nematode *Toxocara canis* or *T. cati*, commonly found in dogs and cats	Transmission is through the ingestion of eggs in the soil. Ingested eggs hatch in the intestine. Mobile larvae then migrate to the liver and eventually to all major organs (including the brain). Once migration is complete, they encapsulate in dense fibrous tissue.	Most cases are asymptomatic. Affected children may have a low-grade fever and recurrent upper airway diseases. Severe symptoms include hepatomegaly, pulmonary infiltration, and neurologic disturbances. In all cases there is a hypereosinophilia of the blood.	There is no specific treatment. Corticosteroids have been used in severe cases. Thiabendazole has been recommended but efficacy is not established (infection usually resolves spontaneously).	Most common in toddlers. Deworm household pets monthly if indicated. Keep children away from areas contaminated with animal droppings.

Source: Giardia lamblia, *Strongyloidiasis, Hookworm, and Toxocariasis courtesy of the Centers for Disease Control and Prevention, Atlanta, GA. Ascariasis and Enterobiasis from Murray, D. L. (2003). Infectious diseases. In C. D. Rudolph & A. M. Rudolph (Eds.),* Rudolph's pediatrics *(21st ed., pp. 714, 718). Stamford, CT. Appleton & Lange, New York: McGraw-Hill.*

metabolism of fat, protein, and carbohydrates; detoxification of hormones, drugs, and other substances; and storage of vitamins A, D, E, and K and glycogen. Thus, any inflammatory, obstructive, or degenerative disorder that affects liver function can be life threatening. The following discussion focuses on four common liver disorders in children: hyperbilirubinemia, biliary atresia, viral hepatitis, and cirrhosis.

Hyperbilirubinemia

The life span of the red blood cell (RBC) is shorter in newborns than in older children and adults (70 to 90 days versus 120 days). This increased RBC destruction and the fact that the newborn's liver is immature can lead to physiologic jaundice in the newborn (Cohen, 2006). **Hyperbilirubinemia,** an abnormally elevated serum bilirubin level, requires timely assessment and appropriate intervention to prevent central nervous system injury (Smitherman, Stark, & Bhutani, 2006).

Etiology and Pathophysiology

Physiologic jaundice is described as jaundice in the newborn without any other signs of illness (Cohen, 2006). Jaundice occurs in 60% of newborns who are otherwise healthy during the first week of life (Brethauer & Carey, 2010; Smitherman et al., 2006) and 80% of preterm infants (Cohen, 2006). Jaundice is generally noticed when the bilirubin reaches 5–6 mg/dL (Brethauer & Carey, 2010). Symptoms generally resolve by 7–10 days of age without complication (Smitherman et al., 2006).

Clinical Manifestations

Jaundice in the infant is first evident on the face, and then progresses to the trunk and finally to the extremities. Jaundice may be difficult to see in babies with dark skin color. In addition to jaundice, symptoms include lethargy or irritability, and poor feeding (Cohen, 2006).

COLLABORATIVE CARE

Diagnostic Tests

A blood test, performed by heelstick or venipuncture, measures total serum bilirubin (TSB) in the newborn. A transcutaneous bilirubin (TcB) measurement device is a noninvasive method for estimating serum bilirubin in infants. This method for measuring bilirubin is generally within 2–3 mg/dL of the TSB and can be performed instead of the TSB in many cases, especially for those infants in which the TSB is less than 15 mg/dL (American Academy of Pediatrics [AAP], 2004).

Clinical Therapy

Phototherapy most effectively reduces serum bilirubin in newborns with physiologic jaundice. The point at which phototherapy is implemented depends on whether the infant is full or preterm and the age of the infant in hours at the time the bilirubin rises. The goal of phototherapy is to keep the TSB below the exchange transfusion level. The American Academy of Pediatrics (2004) has provided specific guidelines that clinicians can follow in determining the appropriate treatment.

Phototherapy is thought to reduce the amount of indirect, or unconjugated, bilirubin in the baby's bloodstream by promoting excretion via the intestines and kidneys. Phototherapy exposes the infant's skin to blue light, which changes bilirubin into water-soluble forms that can be excreted. The infant may be placed on fiber-optic pads as the sole means of providing phototherapy when mild jaundice exists or in conjunction with overhead phototherapy when bilirubin levels are higher (Cohen, 2006).

Many newborns with hyperbilirubinemia are also mildly dehydrated. When the newborn is breastfed, supplemental breast milk or formula may be given to improve hydration. Supplementation with water or dextrose water is not recommended. If the infant is unable to take adequate fluids and is dehydrated, intravenous fluid should be administered (Moerschel, Cianciaruso, & Tracy, 2008).

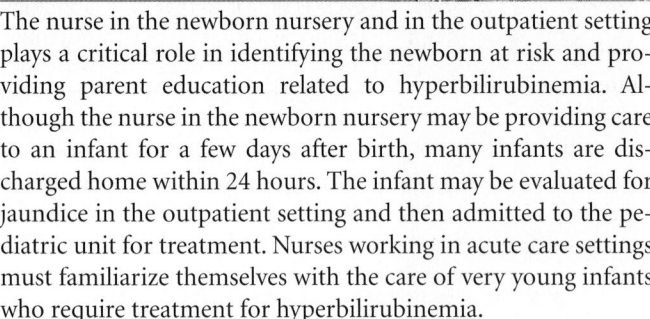

Clinical Tip

The infant's eyes are covered during phototherapy to prevent retinal damage, but eye protection should be removed during feeding and interaction with parents and caregivers (AAP, 2004).

NURSING MANAGEMENT

The nurse in the newborn nursery and in the outpatient setting plays a critical role in identifying the newborn at risk and providing parent education related to hyperbilirubinemia. Although the nurse in the newborn nursery may be providing care to an infant for a few days after birth, many infants are discharged home within 24 hours. The infant may be evaluated for jaundice in the outpatient setting and then admitted to the pediatric unit for treatment. Nurses working in acute care settings must familiarize themselves with the care of very young infants who require treatment for hyperbilirubinemia.

Nursing Assessment and Diagnosis

The newborn should be assessed for jaundice at least every 8–12 hours (Moerschel et al., 2008). If the nurse suspects the presence of jaundice, the infant's primary care provider should be notified and TcB (transcutaneous bilirubin) measurement or TSB (total serum bilirubin) level should be obtained (Cohen, 2006).

Feeding Assessment

The mother who is breastfeeding should nurse her infant at least 8–12 times per day for the first several days (Moerschel et al., 2008). The nurse should be alert to mothers and infants who are having difficulty and require lactation support during the hospital stay and following discharge.

The infant who is breastfed should have 4–6 very wet diapers and 3–4 stools per day by the fourth day of life. Meconium stool should have transitioned to mushy, mustard-colored yellow stools by day 3 to 4. If these parameters are not met, the infant may be at risk for dehydration due to inadequate intake, thus increasing the risk of hyperbilirubinemia (AAP, 2004). Because many mothers and term newborns are discharged within

24 hours after birth, this is important information to teach parents prior to discharge.

Nursing Assessment

Nursing diagnoses that may apply to the newborn with hyperbilirubinemia may include:

- Deficient Fluid Volume related to decreased oral intake and ineffective breast-feeding
- Risk for Impaired Parent/Newborn Attachment related to disruption of parental/newborn interaction due to hospitalization and treatment
- Risk for Imbalanced Body Temperature related to phototherapy
- Risk for Injury related to phototherapy
- Risk for Neurological Impairment related to hyperbilirubinemia

Planning and Implementation

The role of the nurse is to identify the newborn at risk for hyperbilirubinemia, educate parents about newborn jaundice, and care for the newborn and family undergoing treatment for this condition. For the infant undergoing phototherapy, the nurse should monitor the infant frequently, ensuring that the infant is receiving the phototherapy properly. Vital signs should be assessed every 4–8 hours, especially the infant's temperature, which might indicate signs of infection or signs of hypothermia in an infant whose clothing is removed for phototherapy. An accurate measurement of intake and output is essential to make sure the infant is not dehydrated. Assist the family in breast-feeding or bottle-feeding as appropriate.

> **Nursing Alert**
>
> In cases of severe and untreated hyperbilirubinemia, bilirubin encephalopathy can cause serious neurological sequelae. The term *acute bilirubin encephalopathy* is used to describe the acute effects of bilirubin toxicity in the first weeks of life. The term *kernicterus* is used when referring to chronic and permanent brain damage related to bilirubin toxicity (Moerschel et al., 2008).

Discharge Planning and Home Care Teaching

Problems with breastfeeding in the first week of life can contribute to low caloric intake, dehydration, and subsequent risk of neonatal hyperbilirubinemia (AAP, 2004). The nurse assesses adequacy of breastfeeding prior to hospital discharge and coordinates with the newborn's care provider in making appropriate referrals to lactation specialists and support groups in the community when necessary.

For term infants who develop uncomplicated hyperbilirubinemia, home phototherapy may be provided with the use of the fiber-optic pad, also known as a biliblanket (Brethauer & Carey, 2010). Serum bilirubin levels must be monitored regularly at the physician's office or neighborhood laboratory, or by the home health care worker. A visiting or home health care nurse often visits the family to establish the phototherapy and inform parents about the care needed. The nurse partners with other professionals such as staff from a medical supply company (to service equipment), a lactation specialist, and a pediatrician (to coordinate services).

Evaluation

Expected outcomes of nursing interventions include:

- The term or near-term newborn at risk for hyperbilirubinemia is identified prior to discharge and receives appropriate follow-up.
- The infant's parents understand who and when to call if they suspect development of hyperbilirubinemia.
- The infant receives appropriate intervention if hyperbilirubinemia occurs.
- The infant's nutritional and fluid intake are adequate to meet growth and development requirements.
- The infant does not develop neurological sequelae as a result of hyperbilirubinemia.

Biliary Atresia

Biliary atresia results when the extrahepatic bile ducts fail to develop or are closed. The disorder leads to cholestasis, cirrhosis, end-stage liver disease, and death by 2 years of age, if left untreated (Flanigan, 2007; Hartley, Davenport, & Kelly, 2009). Biliary atresia occurs in approximately 1 in 14,000 births in the United States (Wadhwani, Turmelle, Nagy, et al., 2008). It is the most common cause of pathologic jaundice in infants and is the leading indication for pediatric liver transplantation (Hartley et al., 2009; Khalil, Thamara, Perera, et al., 2009).

The cause of biliary atresia is unknown. Absence or blockage of the extrahepatic bile ducts results in blocked bile flow from the liver to the duodenum. This altered bile flow soon causes inflammation and fibrotic changes in the liver. In addition to blockage, the disease can also be caused by hepatocellular dysfunction. Lack of bile acids also interferes with digestion of fat and absorption of fat-soluble vitamins A, D, E, and K, resulting in steatorrhea and nutritional deficiencies. Without treatment the disease is fatal.

Initially the newborn is asymptomatic. Jaundice may not be detected until 2 to 3 weeks after birth. At that point bilirubin levels increase, accompanied by abdominal distention and hepatomegaly (see Appendix D ∞ for bilirubin levels and other liver function tests). As the disease progresses, splenomegaly occurs. The infant experiences easy bruising, prolonged bleeding time, and intense itching. Stools have puttylike consistency and are white or clay colored because of the absence of bile pigments. Excretion of bilirubin and bile salts results in tea-colored urine. Failure to thrive and malnutrition occur as the destructive changes of the disease progress.

Diagnosis is based on the history, physical examination, and laboratory evaluation. Laboratory findings reveal elevated bilirubin levels, elevated serum aminotransferase and alkaline phosphatase values, prolonged prothrombin time, and increased ammonia levels. Percutaneous liver biopsy suggests biliary atresia, and cholangiography and an exploratory laparotomy confirm the diagnosis (Roach & Bruny, 2008).

Treatment involves surgery to attempt correction of the obstruction (hepatoportoenterostomy) and supportive care. In the hepatoportoenterostomy (Kasai procedure), a segment of the intestine is anastomosed to the porta hepatis. The primary purpose of this procedure is to promote bile flow from the liver. Intravenous antibiotics are administered in the postoperative period to prevent cholangitis. Prophylaxis with oral antibiotics is continued for 1–2 years after surgery (Flanigan, 2007).

Additional treatment includes administration of intramuscular vitamin K prior to invasive procedures and surgery to decrease the risk of bleeding afterward; ursodeoxycholic acid (Actigall) to promote bile flow; and vitamins A, D, E, and K to provide supplementation since absorption of these vitamins is impaired. The infant is breastfed or is given Pregestimil or Nutramigen, formulas that contain medium chain triglycerides. As the liver disease worsens, the child may need cholestyramine and antihistamines to help decrease itching. Enteral feedings and TPN may be needed as well (Flanigan, 2007).

While bile flow is achieved with the Kasai procedure in many children with biliary atresia, approximately 70–80% of children having this surgery will eventually need a liver transplant (Roach & Bruny, 2008). Advances in transplantation surgery now make it possible to perform partial liver transplants from living donor resections. This enables transplantation to be performed before the child develops end-stage liver disease (Flanigan, 2007). One-year survival rates of 85% and 86% have been reported in recent studies (Farmer, Venick, McDiarmid, et al., 2007; D'Alessandro, Knechtle, Chin, et al., 2007).

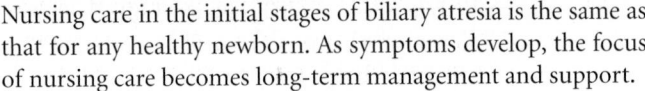

NURSING MANAGEMENT

Nursing care in the initial stages of biliary atresia is the same as that for any healthy newborn. As symptoms develop, the focus of nursing care becomes long-term management and support.

Diagnosis of this potentially fatal disorder can be devastating to parents. Provide emotional support and offer frequent explanations of tests during the initial diagnostic evaluation. As the disease progresses, the infant becomes irritable because of intense itching and the accumulation of toxins. Tepid baths may help to relieve itching and provide comfort. Dry skin by patting rather than rubbing to avoid further skin irritation. Promote rest by grouping nursing activities while the infant is awake. Care following a hepatoportoenterostomy is similar to that for a child undergoing abdominal surgery. (See the earlier discussion of postsurgical nursing management for appendicitis and Nursing Care Plan: The Child Undergoing Surgery in Chapter 11 ∞.) Posttransplant care includes immunosuppressant drugs and close monitoring for vascular complications.

Discharge planning focuses on teaching parents how to care for the child's skin, providing for nutritional needs, administering medications, and monitoring for progressing symptoms of liver disease. When the child has received a transplant, teach parents how to identify signs of rejection (nausea, vomiting, fever, and jaundice), as well as the administration and side effects of immunosuppressant medications. Refer parents to support groups, clergy, or social services if indicated. They will need ongoing visits from a home health care nurse to help them manage the child's complex care. The main expected outcomes of nursing care are the parent's ability to cope with the child's health status and to provide the necessary care. Palliative care may need to be discussed with the family if it becomes evident the child will not survive. See Chapter 13 ∞.

Viral Hepatitis

Hepatitis is an inflammation of the liver caused by a viral infection (Figure 25–16 ➤). It may be acute or chronic. Acute hepatitis is rapid in onset and if untreated may develop into chronic hepatitis. The most frequently diagnosed causative organisms are hepatitis A virus (HAV), hepatitis B virus (HBV), and hepatitis C virus (HCV). A lesser known type is hepatitis D virus (HDV). This type of hepatitis only occurs in individuals who have HBV infection (Holloway & D'Acunto, 2006). Hepatitis E virus (HEV) occurs primarily in developing countries and is rarely seen in the United States (CDC, 2008b). In 2006, the incidence of hepatitis A declined to its lowest rates with only 1.2 cases per 100,000 population reported in the United States. The incidence of hepatitis B has also decreased remarkably over the past several years to a low in 2006 of 1.6 cases per 100,000 population in the United States (Wasley, Grytdal, & Gallagher, 2008). The decline in both of these illnesses is related to routine vaccine administration especially in children.

Etiology and Pathophysiology

Hepatitis A is highly contagious and traditionally has been called infectious hepatitis. Infection occurs primarily through the fecal-oral route. Transmission is by direct person-to-person spread or through ingestion of contaminated water or food (particularly shellfish). Hepatitis A frequently occurs in children in childcare settings where hygiene practices are poor. Food handlers can spread hepatitis A if not aware of their infection; it is a common cause of foodborne illness. The virus can live on surfaces for 1 month. Because the virus is transmitted in the early stages of the disease when individuals are often asymptomatic or only mildly ill, large numbers of people may be exposed before the diagnosis is confirmed (Table 25–4). Most children recover from hepatitis A; however, in rare instances end-stage liver disease can develop (Yazigi & Balistreri, 2007).

Hepatitis B, known traditionally as serum hepatitis, is a serious disease and is the most common type of hepatitis in the United States (McNabb, 2007). Transmission is usually by the parenteral route through the exchange of blood or any body secretion or fluid. Other common transmission routes include sexual activity and transmission from mother to fetus in utero. Adolescents who use intravenous drugs and have unprotected sexual intercourse are at risk for contracting hepatitis B. Major sources for the spread of HBV are healthy chronic carriers. All body fluids of infected individuals are potentially contaminated with the virus.

The hepatitis C virus is transmitted primarily through blood and blood products, and blood banks now test for this virus. Infected children have commonly had repeated transfusions (as in sickle cell disease or hemophilia). Intravenous drug use, body piercing, and multiple sexual partners are also risk factors. Infected mothers may infect their infants before birth or during

Pathophysiology Illustrated
Viral Hepatitis

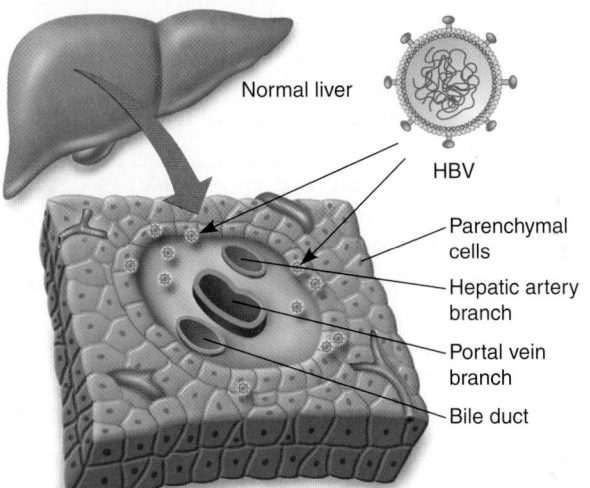

① Virus invades parenchymal cells, causing local degeneration and necrosis

Normal liver

HBV

Parenchymal cells

Hepatic artery branch

Portal vein branch

Bile duct

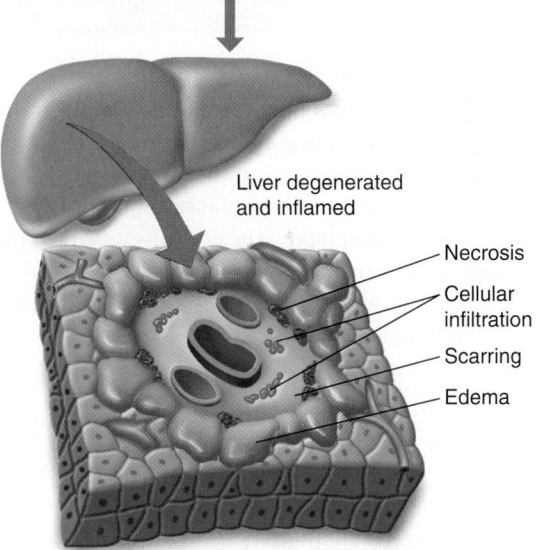

② Infiltration by lymphocytes, macrophages, and other white blood cells causes inflammation that blocks drainage

Liver degenerated and inflamed

Necrosis

Cellular infiltration

Scarring

Edema

③ Structural changes occur in parenchymal cells, resulting in altered liver function:

| Impaired bile excretion | Elevated ALT and alkaline phosphatase levels | Decreased albumin synthesis |

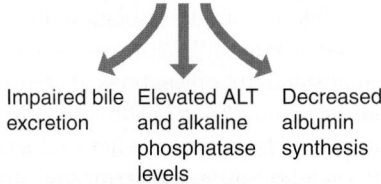

FIGURE 25–16 ➤ The hepatitis virus causes degeneration and necrosis of the liver, which results in abnormal liver function and illness.

breastfeeding. Chronic infection occurs in 70–85% of those individuals infected with hepatitis C (CDC, 2008b). Hepatitis C is now the most common bloodborne infection in the United States (Wasley et al., 2008).

Hepatitis D (delta virus) is a defective virus that can gain entry to a human only in connection with hepatitis B (CDC, 2008b). Hepatitis E infection is primarily transmitted through contaminated water and is most common in developing countries. The only documented cases in the United States have been in individuals who immigrated or visited from a country where the disease is prevalent (Yazigi & Balistreri, 2007).

The liver's response to injury by each virus that causes hepatitis is similar. Initially, invasion of the parenchymal cells by the virus results in local degeneration and necrosis. Subsequent infiltration of the parenchyma by lymphocytes, macrophages, plasma cells, eosinophils, and neutrophils causes inflammation that blocks biliary drainage into the intestine. Impaired bile excretion causes a buildup of bile in the blood, urine, and skin (jaundice). Structural changes in the parenchymal cells account for other altered liver functions.

Clinical Manifestations

Acute hepatitis infection is characterized by two phases, the anicteric (absence of jaundice) phase and the icteric (jaundice) phase. The anicteric phase usually lasts 5 to 7 days. Signs and symptoms include nausea, vomiting, anorexia, malaise, fatigue, right upper quadrant pain, hepatosplenomegaly, and fever. The child becomes irritable, looks ill, and requires rest. In the icteric phase, signs and symptoms include darkening of urine, clay-colored stools, and the characteristic yellowing of the skin and sclera. Many children with hepatitis do not have jaundice, leading to difficulty in disease diagnosis and management. As the jaundice worsens, the child begins to feel better. This phase lasts approximately 4 weeks. Complete recovery with return of normal liver function and laboratory values may take 1 to 3 months.

In some cases, hepatitis becomes chronic. Chronic hepatitis is described as inflammation and necrosis of the liver that lasts for 6 months or longer. A person with chronic hepatitis carries the virus, can transfer it to others, and may develop permanent liver disease (Holloway & D'Acunto, 2006).

COLLABORATIVE CARE

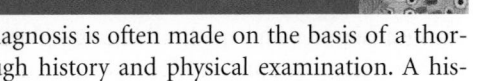

Diagnosis is often made on the basis of a thorough history and physical examination. A history of exposure to persons with the disease is

TABLE 25–4	Comparison of Hepatitis Types			
Type	Immunization Available	Prophylaxis	Primary Transmission	Incubation Period
Hepatitis A	Yes	Immune globulin Hepatitis A vaccine	Fecal-oral	15–19 days
Hepatitis B	Yes	Hepatitis B immune globulin Hepatitis B vaccine	Needlesticks or sharps exposure Intravenous drug use During birth Sexual activity	60–180 days
Hepatitis C	No	None	Needlesticks or sharps exposure Intravenous drug use During birth	14–160 days
Hepatitis D	No	Hepatitis B vaccine	Needlesticks or sharps exposure Intravenous drug use During birth Sexual activity	21–42 days
Hepatitis E	No	None	Fecal-oral	21–63 days

Adapted from: Centers for Disease Control and Prevention. (2008b). Viral hepatitis. Retrieved from http://www.cdc.gov/hepatitis; Yazigi, N., & Balistreri, W. F. (2007). Viral hepatitis. In R. M. Kliegman, R. E. Behrman, H. B. Jenson, & B. F. Stanton (Eds.), Nelson textbook of pediatrics (18th ed., pp. 1680–1690). Philadelphia: Saunders.

significant. Physical examination reveals a tender, enlarged liver, abdominal pain, and flulike symptoms. Laboratory evaluation includes serologic testing (to detect the presence of antigens and antibodies to HAV, HBV, HCV, or HDV) and liver function studies (Holloway & D'Acunto, 2006).

The three goals of medical management are early detection to prevent complications, support and monitoring during the acute phase of the disease, and prevention of the spread of the disease. Management includes bed rest during the flulike phase. If prothrombin times are increased, vitamin K is administered.

The spread of viral infections can be interrupted by elimination of the virus from the infected population, institution of proper hygiene, and passive or active immunization. To date, no antiviral agent has been developed to combat the hepatitis viruses. Prevention depends on breaking the cycle of infection.

Active immunization for hepatitis A, a two-dose series, is recommended for all people at risk of acquiring and transmitting the disease, for children, and for those who wish to acquire immunity to the illness (see Chapter 16 ∞). The CDC recommends that all children receive the first hepatitis A vaccine at 1 year of age (Fiore, Wasley, & Bell, 2006). (Chapter 16 ∞ provides specific information on immunization schedules.)

Immunization for hepatitis B, a three-dose series, is recommended for all children and at-risk adults. The first dose is given within 12 hours of birth to the infant born of a mother who is infected with hepatitis B or to a mother with unknown status (CDC, 2007). Refer to the discussion of immunization in Chapter 16.

Passive immunity to HAV can be achieved with immune globulin from pooled human plasma. It must be administered within 2 weeks of exposure (Fiore et al., 2006). Passive immunity to HBV can be achieved with hepatitis B immune globulin (HBIG). Used for one-time exposure and for infants of mothers who are infected with hepatitis B, it is given within 12 hours of birth.

NURSING MANAGEMENT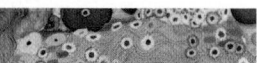

Nursing Assessment and Diagnosis

The nurse usually encounters the child and family in an outpatient setting. In addition to observing the child for characteristic signs of hepatitis (jaundiced skin and sclera), assess for abdominal pain, anorexia, nausea and vomiting, malaise, and arthralgia. For an infant, the hepatitis history of the mother and other family members is important.

Common nursing diagnoses for the child with acute hepatitis might include:

- Risk for Imbalanced Nutrition: Less than Body Requirements related to anorexia, nausea and vomiting
- Fatigue related to disease state
- Risk for Deficient Diversional Activity related to malaise and forced inactivity
- Risk for Body Image Disturbance (Older Child) related to jaundice
- Anxiety (Parent and Child) related to threat to health status

Planning and Implementation

Nursing care involves home and community considerations, as children with hepatitis are seldom admitted to the hospital. The hospitalized child is placed in isolation. Prevention of the disease is integrated into all health care by discussion of immunization and standard precautions. Parents need additional detailed information about health precautions and infection control measures if hepatitis cases have occurred in the family or community. In addition, teach parents the importance of checking with health professionals before administering any medications (even nonprescription medicines), maintaining adequate nutrition, promoting rest and comfort, and providing diversional activities.

Prevent Spread of Infection

Teach the parents and the child infection control measures to help prevent transmission of the virus. For parents, reinforce good hygiene practices, such as washing hands before and after toileting and proper disposal of soiled diapers. Siblings of a child with hepatitis B who have not already been immunized with the hepatitis B vaccine should be vaccinated immediately. Contacts of the child with hepatitis A should receive immune serum globulin and the first immunization in the hepatitis A series. Rifampin may be given in some cases. All health providers should receive the hepatitis B immunization series and use standard precautions at all times. See the *Clinical Skills Manual*.

Clinical Tip

Nurses in childcare centers can provide assessment of the center's procedures and teaching to prevent hepatitis A transmission. Help the center to set standards about:

- Handwashing after each diaper change
- Proper disposal of diapers
- Cleaning diaper-changing surfaces after each diaper change
- Never having food handlers perform diaper changes
- Instructing parents to keep children at home for at least 2 weeks after a diagnosis of hepatitis A
- Informing parents of other children when there is a case of hepatitis A and teaching them the symptoms of the condition

Maintain Adequate Nutrition

Initially, encourage the child to eat favorite foods. Once the anorexia and nausea have resolved, a high-protein, high-carbohydrate, low-fat diet is recommended. Increased protein helps maintain protein stores and prevent muscle wasting. Increased carbohydrates ensure adequate caloric intake and prevent protein depletion. The use of low-fat foods lessens stomach distention. Offer the child small, frequent feedings.

Promote Rest and Comfort

Bed rest is necessary only if the child has severe fatigue and malaise. However, most children voluntarily limit their activities during the initial phase of the disease. Keep the child quiet and comfortable. Offer comfort items such as favorite toys, blankets, and pillows.

Administer Medications

Drug metabolism is altered during hepatitis since the liver cannot detoxify medications readily. As with all liver disorders, medications need to be administered carefully and the child's condition must be monitored for possible drug side effects. Caution parents to check with health professionals before giving any nonprescription medication. For example, acetaminophen is metabolized in the liver, and liver disease can interfere with its breakdown.

Provide Diversional Activities

Hospitalized children with hepatitis are kept in isolation. Non-hospitalized children with hepatitis do not need to be isolated, but they should be kept at home for 2 weeks following the onset of symptoms. Parents who cannot take time off from work may need to arrange home sitters to stay with the child. Offer suggestions for diversional activities during this period. Young children can be given a new toy or favorite activities. Older children and adolescents can be given board games, puzzles, books or magazines, movies, or video games. Phone calls and short visits from friends help school-age children and adolescents maintain contact with peers.

Evaluation

Expected outcomes of nursing care for hepatitis include adequate nutritional intake to meet growth and development needs, participation in quiet, nonfatiguing activities and self-care, positive body image, positive parental coping with stress of the child's condition, and reduced risk of spread of hepatitis to the child's contacts.

Cirrhosis

Cirrhosis is a degenerative disease process that results in fibrotic changes and fatty infiltration in the liver. It can occur in children of any age as the end stage of several liver disorders such as hepatitis and biliary atresia (A-Kader & Balistreri, 2007; Boamah & Balistreri, 2007). The diffuse destruction and regeneration of the hepatic parenchymal cells result in an increase in fibrous connective tissue and disorganization of the liver structure. Progressive scarring that occurs in cirrhosis leads to altered blood flow to the liver, which causes further deterioration of liver function (Boamah & Balistreri, 2007).

Clinical manifestations of cirrhosis vary. Hepatomegaly may be evident on exam. Jaundice occurs as the disease progresses and is an indication of hyperbilirubinemia. Jaundice is sometimes the only sign of hepatic dysfunction so its appearance must be investigated. Pruritus is common in children with cirrhosis although it is not related to the degree of hyperbilirubinemia. Other clinical manifestations of cirrhosis in children include ascites, portal hypertension, encephalopathy, and variceal hemorrhage (Boamah & Balistreri, 2007). Severe end-stage complications signaling hepatic failure can occur at any time and with little warning.

Diagnostic evaluation is based on the child's history of infection or disease with liver involvement. Physical examination may reveal jaundice, skin changes, ascites, and hemodynamic changes. Laboratory evaluation reveals abnormal liver function tests. A liver biopsy may help determine the extent of the parenchymal damage.

Medical management focuses on treating the child's symptoms and achieving optimal nutritional status and growth. See the Clinical Manifestations table on the next page for a summary of treatment for complications of cirrhosis. Liver transplantation is the most common treatment for biliary atresia and metabolic disorders and is the only treatment for end-stage liver disease.

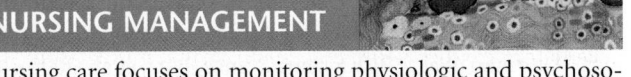

NURSING MANAGEMENT

Nursing care focuses on monitoring physiologic and psychosocial changes to identify early signs of end-stage hepatic failure. Monitor vital signs every 2 to 4 hours. Assess skin for changes

Clinical Manifestations
Cirrhosis Complications

Etiology	Clinical Manifestations	Clinical Therapy
Fluid and electrolyte imbalance	Ascites	Restrict sodium, protein, and fluids. Administer diuretics (e.g., furosemide [Lasix]). Administer intravenous albumin.
Liver dysfunction	Hepatic encephalopathy	Restrict protein. Administer lactulose to control increased ammonia levels. Administer antibiotics. Correct any imbalances that can lead to coma (fluid and electrolyte imbalance).
Esophageal varices	Hemorrhage	Administer blood and blood products. Replace fluid and electrolytes. Administer vitamin B complex and vitamin K. Insert Sengstaken-Blakemore tube in cases of severe bleeding.

including jaundice. Measure weight daily to assess for fluid retention. Measure abdominal girth daily to assess for ascites. Close monitoring of electrolytes and liver function test results helps determine the need for fluid replacement therapy.

Careful administration of medications and monitoring for side effects are necessary because drug metabolism is altered in liver disorders. If ascites is present, provide a low-sodium, low-protein diet and restrict fluids. Remove all water pitchers, glasses, and straws to minimize the child's desire to drink.

Parents of a child with cirrhosis are coping with a life-threatening disorder, and their anxiety and stress are high. The child may be awaiting a liver transplantation that represents the only hope for recovery. Support parents and encourage them to talk about their fears and concerns. Encourage parents to participate in the child's care. Referral to a support group or counseling may be beneficial. See Chapter 13 ∞ for discussion on palliative care.

■ INJURIES TO THE GASTROINTESTINAL SYSTEM

Abdominal Trauma

The majority of abdominal injuries are caused by blunt trauma (86%), with penetrating trauma accounting for the remainder (Pieper, 2007). Falls are the most common cause of abdominal injury in children; however, motor vehicle crashes and pedestrian injuries are the major cause of severe blunt abdominal trauma in children (Potoka & Saladino, 2005). Child abuse involving kicking or punching the abdomen is another cause of blunt abdominal trauma. While not as common as the causes listed previously, abdominal trauma related to child abuse carries a mortality rate of 45–53% (Pariset, Feldman, & Paris, 2010). Penetrating trauma occurs due to impalement on an object, stabbing, or gunshot wounds (Alterman, Daley, Kennedy, et al., 2010). Children are more likely to have abdominal injuries because of their small pliable rib cage and less developed abdominal muscles that provide little protection for major solid organs such as the spleen, liver, and kidneys. In addition, the solid organs in children are larger in proportion to their body size compared to adults, exposing more surface area and making the organ more vulnerable to injury (Alterman et al., 2010; Saxena, Nance, Lutz, et al., 2008).

The kind of injury determines the extent of organ damage. High-velocity blunt trauma, which may occur in motor vehicle crashes, usually involves multiple organs. Solid organs such as

the liver and spleen can be bruised or lacerated. The sudden increase in abdominal pressure that occurs with a lap belt injury causes hollow organs such as the stomach, intestines, and bladder to burst. Sports-related abdominal trauma is often associated with a direct blow to the abdomen, and a single organ is usually injured. Bicycle crashes can result in abdominal injury if the handlebars hit the child in the abdomen (Potoka & Saladino, 2005).

Clinical manifestations of abdominal injury include pain, abdominal distention, muscle guarding, decreased or absent bowel sounds, nausea and vomiting, hypotension, and shock. The external abdomen and back may have penetrating wounds, abrasions, bruising, or markings (e.g., tire tracks or lap belt marks) that provide a clue to injury beneath the skin surface. Ecchymosis and contusions in the lower abdominal area are classic visible signs of seat belt trauma (Eckert, 2005). See Chapter 5 ∞ for techniques of abdominal assessment.

COLLABORATIVE CARE

The injured child is rapidly assessed for airway, breathing, and circulation, and is stabilized before examination of the abdomen is performed. An IV line is inserted for fluid management. A nasogastric tube is inserted to decompress the stomach and to detect the presence of blood. Plain abdominal radiographs may reveal air in the abdomen. An ultrasound can reveal free fluid in the abdomen. A CT scan assesses multiple organs for injury and for the presence of free fluid in the abdomen. Type and crossmatch of blood is also necessary in case the child needs a blood transfusion. In addition, electrolytes and enzyme studies (amylase and lipase) to detect liver, spleen, and pancreas injuries are obtained (Pieper, 2007; Saxena et al., 2008).

Nursing Alert

The child who is restrained in a motor vehicle with only a lap belt is at high risk for abdominal injury in a crash. As the car stops rapidly, the child's body is restrained and flexes around the lap belt. The sudden increase in abdominal pressure causes injury to hollow organs, and sometimes solid organs. Children no longer using car safety seats should sit in a booster seat so that a shoulder restraint is used in addition to the lap belt.

The spleen and the liver are the organs most commonly injured in blunt abdominal trauma. Nonsurgical management is preferred. The spleen plays a major role in immune function; therefore, the organ is salvaged whenever possible to help maintain immune function. Liver lacerations are treated much like spleen lacerations as long as major vessels have not been injured. Nonsurgical management of injury to the spleen in children is successful in 90–98% of cases, while the success rate of nonsurgical management of injuries to the liver in children is 85–90% (Potoka & Saladino, 2005). Exploratory laparotomy is performed to resect hollow organ injuries or to repair liver or spleen lacerations when bleeding is not controlled.

Treatment of an abdominal, liver, or spleen injury takes place in the pediatric intensive care unit (PICU) and focuses on preventing or managing hemorrhage and monitoring for signs of hypovolemic shock. An intravenous infusion is initiated for fluid maintenance and to provide access for blood products. The child is kept NPO. A nasogastric tube is inserted. Blood transfusions and pharmacologic management are used to treat blood loss.

The child is maintained on strict bed rest until bleeding is controlled and the hemoglobin and hematocrit are stable. The length of time the child is hospitalized ranges from 2–5 days depending on the severity of the injury. The length of time for activity restrictions after discharge ranges from 3–6 weeks and also depends on the severity of the injury (Pieper, 2007).

NURSING MANAGEMENT

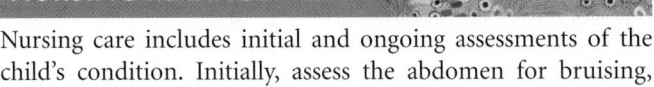

Nursing care includes initial and ongoing assessments of the child's condition. Initially, assess the abdomen for bruising, pain, guarding, rebound tenderness, distention, and absence of bowel sounds (Eckert, 2005). See Chapter 5 ∞ for techniques of abdominal assessment.

Monitor hematocrit and vital signs every hour as warranted to detect hypovolemia (see Chapter 26 ∞). Tachycardia and hypotension may indicate hypovolemia or internal bleeding. Strict monitoring of intake and output will give information to the child's fluid status. Monitor the respiratory status as abdominal injuries may also have thoracic involvement. The child with associated thoracic injuries may not take deep breaths if it is painful.

The child and parents are usually fearful and anxious when the child is admitted with a serious injury. If the injury was preventable, parents may have feelings of guilt or anger. Provide emotional support and avoid judgmental comments or statements that assign blame. Additional nursing care includes maintenance of the nasogastric tube; administration of antibiotics, intravenous fluids, and blood; and monitoring of lab studies as appropriate. Any concerns should be reported to the physician immediately.

Once the child's condition is stabilized, the focus of nursing care shifts to preventive teaching. Parents should be taught safety measures to prevent future injuries. Discuss the use of car safety restraint devices for riding in an automobile (see Chapters 7 through Chapter 9 ∞). If the child's injury was the result of a bicycle fall or crash, discuss the importance of the proper bicycle size and safety measures such as use of a helmet and proper use of hand signals.

Refer to Chapter 17 ∞ for information related to injury to the GI system due to poisoning and ingestion of foreign objects.

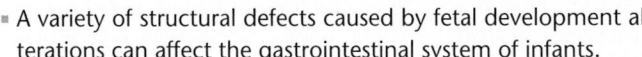

Chapter Highlights

- A variety of structural defects caused by fetal development alterations can affect the gastrointestinal system of infants.
- Cleft lip and palate are structural defects that often involve care by a team of providers such as a plastic surgeon, pediatrician, nurse, audiologist, speech therapist, and orthodontist.
- A variety of defects of the esophagus and trachea can manifest as mild to life-threatening problems in the newborn period.
- Pyloric stenosis is a common cause of projectile vomiting in the newborn period.
- Gastroesophageal reflux is one of the most common gastrointestinal problems in infants and children.
- Abdominal wall defects and anorectal malformations are serious structural defects of infancy.
- Intussusception is one of the most common causes of intestinal obstruction in the pediatric population and primarily occurs in children less than 2 years of age.
- Hirschsprung disease, or aganglionic megacolon, leads to failure to pass normal stools and distention of the abdomen.
- Several of the intestinal problems of childhood necessitate temporary or permanent ostomy placement.
- Hernias can be present in the diaphragmatic area, umbilicus, or inguinal canal.

- The most common inflammatory disorder of the gastrointestinal tract is appendicitis.
- Necrotizing enterocolitis is a potentially life-threatening inflammatory disease of the intestines seen primarily in premature infants after enteral feedings are begun.
- Common inflammatory bowel diseases affecting primarily adolescent and young adult age groups are Crohn's disease and ulcerative colitis.
- Peptic ulcer may be primary (often caused by *H. pylori*) or secondary, in situations of stress, trauma, or other disease.
- Common disorders of motility include diarrhea, constipation, and encopresis.
- Gastroenteritis and parasitic disorders are common causes of gastrointestinal disturbance and distress in children, and may lead to fluid and electrolyte imbalance.
- Short bowel syndrome occurs when surgery is used to treat an intestinal disease and significant sections of the bowel are removed.
- Biliary atresia and hepatitis are the most common liver diseases in young children. Hyperbilirubinemia can occur in newborns.
- Abdominal trauma most often occurs to children involved in motor vehicle accidents.

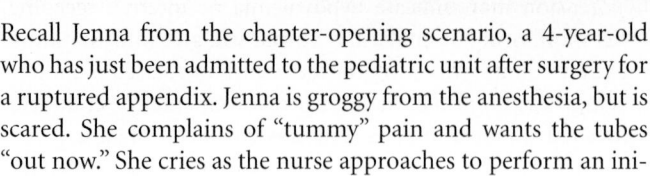

Clinical Reasoning in Action

Recall Jenna from the chapter-opening scenario, a 4-year-old who has just been admitted to the pediatric unit after surgery for a ruptured appendix. Jenna is groggy from the anesthesia, but is scared. She complains of "tummy" pain and wants the tubes "out now." She cries as the nurse approaches to perform an initial assessment.

1. Why was Jenna at increased risk for ruptured appendix compared to a school-age child?
2. Jenna's parents ask why she needs all of the tubes. What information should the nurse include related to the purpose of the nasogastric tube, the Foley catheter, and the PICC line?
3. Considering Jenna's developmental age, how can the nurse help Jenna adapt to the hospitalization experience? (Refer to Chapter 11 ∞.)
4. What interventions are most appropriate with a 4-year-old to decrease the risk of pulmonary complications associated with surgery?

See Pearson Nursing Student Resources for possible responses.

Pearson Nursing Student Resources

Find additional review materials at
nursing.pearsonhighered.com
Prepare for success with NCLEX®-style practice questions, interactive assignments and activities, web links, animations and videos, and more!

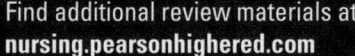

References

A-Kader, H. A., & Balistreri, W. F. (2007). Cholestasis. In R. M. Kliegman, R. E. Behrman, H. B. Jenson, & B. F. Stanton (Eds.), *Nelson textbook of pediatrics* (18th ed., pp. 1168–1675). Philadelphia: Saunders.

Alterman, D. M., Daley, B. J., Kennedy, A. P., Raju, R., & Lee. S. (2010). *Considerations in pediatric trauma.* Retrieved from http://emedicine.medscape.com/article/435031-overview

American Academy of Pediatrics (AAP). (2004). Management of hyperbilirubinemia in the newborn infant 35 or more weeks of gestation. *Pediatrics, 114*(1), 297–316.

Applegate, K. E. (2009). Evidence-based diagnosis of malrotation and volvulus. *Pediatric Radiology, 39*(Suppl. 2), S161–S163.

Aschenbrenner, D. S. (2006). Treatment of pediatric Crohn's disease: A biologic therapy now is approved for use in children. *American Journal of Nursing, 106*(9), 30.

Bates, M. D., & Balistreri, W. F. (2007). Morphogenesis of the liver and biliary system. In R. M. Kliegman, R. E. Behrman, H. B. Jenson, & B. F. Stanton (Eds.), *Nelson textbook of pediatrics* (18th ed., pp. 1657–1661). Philadelphia: Saunders.

Biggs, W. S., & Dery, W. H. (2006). Evaluation and treatment of constipation in infants and children. *American Family Physician, 73*(3), 469–477.

Bindler, R. M., & Howry, L. B. (2005). *Pediatric drugs & nursing implications* (3rd ed.). Upper Saddle River, NJ: Prentice Hall Health.

Black, T. L. (2005). Congenital megacolon. In M. R. Dambro & J. A. Griffith (Eds.), *Griffith's 5-minute clinical consult* (13th ed., p. 260). Philadelphia: Lippincott Williams & Wilkins.

Boamah, L., & Balistreri, W. F. (2007). Manifestations of liver disease. In R. M. Kliegman, R. E. Behrman, H. B. Jenson, & B. F. Stanton (Eds.), *Nelson textbook of pediatrics* (18th ed., pp. 1661–1668). Philadelphia: Saunders.

Borkowski, S. (2005). Clinical challenge. Case 1. Irritation, redness, and drainage at the site of a pediatric gastrostomy. *Clinical Advisor for Nurse Practitioners, 8*(5).

Bradshaw, W. T. (2009). Necrotizing enterocolitis etiology, presentation, management, and outcomes. *Journal of Perinatal and Neonatal Nursing, 23*(1), 87–94.

Brethauer, M., & Carey, L. (2010). Maternal experience with neonatal jaundice. *MCN. The American Journal of Maternal Child Nursing, 35*(1), 8–14.

Bundy, D. G., Byerley, J. S., Liles, E. A., Perrin, E. M., Katznelson, J., & Rice, H. E. (2007). Does this child have appendicitis? *Journal of the American Medical Association, 298*(4), 438–451.

Cassell, C. H., Daniels, J., & Meyer, R. E. (2009). Timeliness of primary cleft lip/palate surgery. *Cleft Palate-Craniofacial Journal, 46*(6), 588–597.

Centers for Disease Control and Prevention (CDC). (2007). *Hepatitis B fact sheet.* Retrieved from http://www.cdc.gov/hepatitis

Centers for Disease Control and Prevention (CDC). (2008a). *What every pet owner should know about roundworms & hookworms.* Retrieved from http://www.cdc.gov/healthypets/Merial_CDCBroch_rsgWEB.pdf

Centers for Disease Control and Prevention (CDC). (2008b). *Viral hepatitis.* Retrieved from http://www.cdc.gov/hepatitis/

Chamley, C. A., Carson, P., Randall, F., & Sandwell, M. (2005). *Developmental anatomy and physiology of children.* St. Louis, MO: Elsevier.

Coha, T. (2007). Congenital lung malformations. In N. T. Browne, L. M. Flanigan, C. A. McComiskey, & P. Pieper, *Nursing care of the pediatric surgical patient* (2nd ed., pp. 237–246). Boston: Jones & Bartlett.

Cohen, S. M. (2006). Jaundice in the full-term newborn. *Pediatric Nursing, 32*(3), 202–208.

Colvin, J., Bower, C., Dickinson, J., & Sokol, J. (2005). Outcomes of congenital diaphragmatic hernia: A population-based study in western Australia. *Pediatrics, 166*(3), 356–363.

Cortese, M. M., & Parashar, U. D. (2009). Prevention of rotavirus gastroenteritis among infants and young children. Recommendations of the Advisory Committee on Immunization Practices (ACIP). *Morbidity and Mortality Weekly Report, 58*(RR2), 1–24.

Croffie, J. M. (2006). Constipation in children. *Indian Journal of Pediatrics, 73*(8), 697–701.

Culbert, T. P., & Banez, G. A. (2008). Integrative approaches to childhood constipation and encopresis. *Pediatric Clinics of North America, 54,* 927–947.

Cuvellier, J., & Lèpine, A. (2010). Childhood periodic syndromes. *Pediatric Neurology, 42,* 1–11.

D'Alessandro, A. M., Knechtle, S. J., Chin, L. T., Fernandez, L. A., Yagci, G., Leverson, G., & Kalayoglu, M. (2007). Liver transplantation in pediatric patients: Twenty years of experience at the University of Wisconsin. *Pediatric Transplantation, 11,* 661–670.

de Buys Roessingh, A. S., & Dinh-Xuan, A. T. (2009). Congenital diaphragmatic hernia: Current status and review of the literature. *European Journal of Pediatrics, 163,* 393–406.

Diana-Zerpa, J. A., & Shapiro-Stolar, T. J. (2007). Malrotation and volvulus. In N. T. Browne, L. M. Flanigan, C. A. McComiskey, & P. Pieper, *Nursing care of the pediatric surgical patient* (2nd ed., pp. 333–342). Boston: Jones & Bartlett.

Downard, C. D. (2008). Congenital diaphragmatic hernia: An ongoing clinical challenge. *Current Opinion in Pediatrics, 20*(3), 300–304.

Eckert, K. (2005). Penetrating and blunt abdominal trauma. *Critical Care Nursing Quarterly, 28,* 41–59.

Ehrlich, P. F., & Coran, A. G. (2007). Diaphragmatic hernia. In R. M. Kliegman, R. E. Behrman, H. B. Jenson, & B. F. Stanton (Eds.), *Nelson textbook of pediatrics* (18th ed., pp. 746–749). Philadelphia: Saunders.

Fagerman, L. E., & Farber, L. D. (2007). Intussusception. In N. T. Browne, L. M. Flanigan, C. A. McComiskey, & P. Pieper, *Nursing care of the pediatric surgical patient* (2nd ed., pp. 343–348). Boston: Jones & Bartlett.

Farmer, D. G., Venick, R. S., McDiarmid, S. V., Ghobrial, R. M., Gordon, S. A., Yersiz, H., et al. (2007). Predictors of outcomes after pediatric liver transplantation: An analysis of more than 800 cases performed at a single institution. *Journal of the American College of Surgeons, 204*(5), 904–916.

Fiore, A. E., Wasley, A., & Bell, B. P. (2006). Prevention of hepatitis A through active or passive immunization. *Morbidity and Mortality Weekly Report, 55*(RR07), 1–23.

Flanigan, L. M. (2007). Biliary atresia and choledochal cyst. In N. T. Browne, L. M. Flanigan, C. A. McComiskey, & P. Pieper, *Nursing care of the pediatric surgical patient* (2nd ed., pp. 379–387). Boston: Jones & Bartlett.

Gardiner, P., & Kemper, K. J. (2005). For GI complaints: Which herbs and supplements spell relief? *Contemporary Pediatrics, 22*(8), 50–55.

Goday, P. S. (2009). Short bowel syndrome: How short is too short? *Clinical Perinatology, 36,* 101–110.

Gold, B. D., & Gremse, D. A. (2006). Extinguishing the burn: Case studies in pediatric reflux disease. *Self Study Supplement to U.S. Pharmacist.*

Goldberg, E., Barton, S., Xanthopoulos, M. S., Stettler, N., & Liacouras, C. A. (2010). A descriptive study of complications of gastrostomy tubes in children. *Journal of Pediatric Nursing, 25*(2), 72–80.

Grossman, A. B. & Mamula, P. (2009). *Crohn disease.* Retrieved from http://emedicine.medscape.com/article/928288-overview

Guardino, K. O. (2007). Anorectal malformations in children. In N. T. Browne, L. M. Flanigan, C. A.

McComiskey, & P. Pieper, *Nursing care of the pediatric surgical patient* (2nd ed., pp. 301–314). Boston: Jones & Bartlett.

Hartley, J. L., Davenport, M., & Kelly, D. A. (2009). Biliary atresia. *Lancet, 374*(14), 1704–1713.

Hennelly, K. E., & Bachur, R. G. (2009). *Pediatrics, appendicitis.* Retrieved from http://emedicine.medscape.com/article/799858-overview

Holloway, M., & D'Acunto, K. (2006, June). An update on the ABC's of viral hepatitis. *Clinical Advisor, 26,* 29–40.

Holmes, S. (2004). Enteral feeding and percutaneous endoscopic gastrostomy. *Nursing Standard, 18*(20), 41–43.

Hyams, J. (2005). Inflammatory bowel disease. *Pediatrics in Review, 26*(9), 314–320.

Hyams, J. (2007). Inflammatory bowel disease. In R. M. Kliegman, R. E. Behrman, H. B. Jenson, & B. F. Stanton (Eds.), *Nelson textbook of pediatrics* (18th ed., pp. 1575–1585). Philadelphia: Saunders.

International Pediatric Endosurgery Group (IPEG). (2008a). IPEG guidelines for the surgical treatment of pediatric gastroesophageal reflux disease (GERD). *Journal of Laparoendoscopic & Advanced Surgical Techniques, 18*(6), x–xiii.

International Pediatric Endosurgery Group (IPEG). (2008b). IPEG guidelines for appendectomy. *Journal of Laparoendoscopic & Advanced Surgical Techniques, 18*(6), vii–ix.

Irving, P. M., & Gibson, P. R. (2007). Infliximab: Getting the most for your money. *Journal of Gastroenterology and Hepatology, 22,* 1557–1565.

Joshi, S., Mahajan, P., & Kamat, D. (2006). Infantile hypertrophic pyloric stenosis. *Consultant for Pediatricians, 5*(2), 106–109.

Kasson, B. R. (2007). Necrotizing enterocolitis. In N. T. Browne, L. M. Flanigan, C. A. McComiskey, & P. Pieper, *Nursing care of the pediatric surgical patient* (2nd ed., pp. 181–193). Boston: Jones & Bartlett.

Kasten, E. F., Schmidt, S. P., Zickler, C. F., Berner, E., Damian, L. A., Christian, G. M., . . . Hicks, T. L. (2008). Team care of the patient with cleft lip and palate. *Current Problems in Pediatric and Adolescent Health, 38,* 138–158.

Kessman, J. (2006). Hirschsprung disease: Diagnosis and management. *American Family Physician, 74*(8), 1319–1322.

Khalil, B. A., Thamara, M., Perera, P. R., & Mirza, D. F. (2009). Clinical practice: Management of biliary atresia. *European Journal of Pediatrics, 169*(4), 395–402.

Khan, A. N. (2008). *Omphalocele.* Retrieved from http://emedicine.medscape.com/article/404182-overview

Klar, M. (2007). Hirschsprung disease. In N. T. Browne, L. M. Flanigan, C. A. McComiskey, & P. Pieper, *Nursing care of the pediatric surgical patient* (2nd ed., pp. 289–300). Boston: Jones & Bartlett.

Kliegman, R. M., & Willoughby, R. E. (2005). Prevention of necrotizing enterocolitis with probiotics. *Pediatrics, 115,* 171–172.

Levitt, M. A., & Peña, A. (2005). Outcomes from the correction of anorectal malformations. *Current Opinion in Pediatrics, 17,* 394–401.

Liao, Z., Li, Z. S., Zhang, W. J., Zou, D. W., Xue, X. C., & Zhang, X. K. (2007). Gastrointestinal: In-

fantile hypertrophic pyloric stenosis. *Journal of Gastroenterology and Hepatology, 22*(10), 1692.

Lund, C. H., Bauer, K., & Berrios, M. (2007). Gastroschisis: Incidence, complications, and clinical management in the neonatal intensive care unit. *Journal of Perinatal & Neonatal Nursing, 21*(1), 63–68.

Madsen, D., Sebolt, T., Cullen, L., Folkedahl, B., Mueller, T., Richardson, C., & Titler, M. (2005). Listening to bowel sounds: An evidence-based practice project: Nurses find that a traditional practice isn't the best indicator of returning gastrointestinal motility in patients who've undergone abdominal surgery. *American Journal of Nursing, 105*(12), 40–49.

Malaty, H. M., O'Malley, K. J., Abudayyeh, S., Graham, D. Y., & Gilger, M. A. (2008). Multidimensional measure for gastroesophageal reflux disease (MM-GERD) symptoms in children: A population-based study. *Acta Pædiatrica, 97,* 1292–1297.

March of Dimes. (2007). *Cleft lip and cleft palate.* Retrieved from http://www.marchofdimes.com/professionals/14332_1210.asp

Markowitz, J. E., Dancel, L. D., & Shukla, P. C. (2008). *Volvulus.* Retrieved from http://emedicine.medscape.com/article/932430-overview

Martin, C. R., & Walker, W. A. (2008). Probiotics: Role in pathophysiology and prevention in necrotizing enterocolitis. *Seminars in Perinatology, 32,* 127–137.

Mattioli, G., Prato, A. P., Giunta, C., Avanzini, S., Rocca, M. D., Montobbio, G., et al. (2008). Outcome of primary endorectal pull-through for the treatment of classic Hirschsprung disease. *Journal of Laparoendoscopic & Advanced Surgical Techniques, 18*(6), 869–874.

McCollough, M., & Sharieff, G. Q. (2006). Abdominal pain in children. *Pediatric Clinics of North America, 53,* 107–137.

McNabb, S. J. N. (2007). Summary of notifiable diseases—United States, 2005. *Morbidity and Mortality Weekly Report, 54*(53), 1–96.

Merritt, L. (2005). Part 2. Physical assessment of the infant with cleft lip and/or palate. *Advances in Neonatal Care, 5*(3), 125–134.

Mills, J. L. A., Lin, Y., MacNab, Y. C., Skarsgard, E. D., & The Canadian Pediatric Surgery Network. (2010). Does overnight birth influence treatment or outcome in congenital diaphragmatic hernia? *Journal of Perinatology, 27*(1), 91–95.

Moerschel, S. K., Cianciaruso, L. B., & Tracy, L. R. (2008). A practical approach to neonatal jaundice. *American Family Physician, 77*(9), 1255–1262.

Montgomery, D. F., & Navarro, F. (2008). Management of constipation and encopresis in children. *Journal of Pediatric Health Care, 22*(3), 199–204.

Nisell, M., Igl, W. I., Öjmyr-Joelsson, M., Frenckner, B., Rydelius, P., & Christensson, K. (2009). Social issues among children with high or intermediate imperforate anus: A proxy perspective. *Journal of Child and Adolescent Psychiatric Nursing, 22*(3), 132–142.

Nisell, M., Öjmyr-Joelsson, M., Frenckner, B., Rydelius, P., & Christensson, K. (2009). Psychosocial experiences of parents of a child with imperforate anus. *Journal for Specialists in Pediatric Nursing, 14*(4), 221–229.

Orenstein, S., Peters, J., Khan, S., Youssef, N., & Hussain, S. (2007). Congenital anomalies: Esophageal atresia and tracheoesophageal fistula. In R. M. Kliegman, R. E. Behrman, H. B. Jenson, & B. F. Stanton (Eds.), *Nelson textbook of pediatrics* (18th ed., pp. 1543–1544). Philadelphia: Saunders.

Orenstein, S. R., & McGowan, J. D. (2008). Efficacy of conservative therapy as taught in the primary care setting for symptoms suggesting infant gastroesophageal reflux. *Journal of Pediatrics, 152*, 310–314.

Otten, M. E., & Stoops, M. M. (2007). Splenectomy, cholecystectomy, and Meckel's diverticulum. In N. T. Browne, L. M. Flanigan, C. A. McComiskey, & P. Pieper, *Nursing care of the pediatric surgical patient* (2nd ed., pp. 357–375). Boston: Jones & Bartlett.

Owens, J. (2008). Parents' experiences of feeding a baby with cleft lip and palate. *British Journal of Midwifery, 16*(12), 778–784.

Pariset, J. M., Feldman, K. W., & Paris, C. (2010). The pace of signs and symptoms of blunt abdominal trauma to children. *Clinical Pediatrics, 49*(1), 24–28.

Patel, P. K., Ramaswamy, R., Grasseschi, M. F., & Morris, D. E. (2009). *Craniofacial, unilateral cleft lip repair.* Retrieved from http://emedicine.medscape.com/article/1279641-overview

Pieper, P. (2007). Pediatric trauma. In N. T. Browne, L. M. Flanigan, C. A. McComiskey, & P. Pieper, *Nursing care of the pediatric surgical patient* (2nd ed., pp. 445–464). Boston: Jones & Bartlett.

Pietz, J., Achanti, B., Lilien, L., Stepka, E. C., & Mehta, S. K. (2007). Prevention of necrotizing enterocolitis in preterm infants: A 20-year experience. *Pediatrics, 119*(1), e164–e170.

Potoka, D. A., & Saladino, R. A. (2005). Blunt abdominal trauma in the pediatric patient. *Clinical Pediatric Emergency Medicine, 6*, 23–31.

Price, F. N. (2007). Gastroesophageal reflux disease: Recognition and management. In N. T. Browne, L. M. Flanigan, C. A. McComiskey, & P. Pieper, *Nursing care of the pediatric surgical patient* (2nd ed., pp. 325–332). Boston: Jones & Bartlett.

Reid, H., & Bahar, R. J. (2006). Treatment of encopresis and chronic constipation in young children: Clinical results from interactive parent-child guidance. *Clinical Pediatrics, 45*(2), 157–164.

Reid, J., Reilly, S., & Kilpatrick, N. (2007). Sucking performance of babies with cleft conditions. *Cleft Palate-Craniofacial Journal, 44*(3), 312–320.

Roach, J. P., & Bruny, J. L. (2008). Advances in the treatment and understanding of biliary atresia. *Current Opinion in Pediatrics, 20*, 315–319.

Rogers, V. E. (2007). Care of the child with an ostomy. In N. T. Browne, L. M. Flanigan, C. A. McComiskey, & P. Pieper, *Nursing care of the pediatric surgical patient* (2nd ed., pp. 105–129). Boston: Jones & Bartlett.

Saxena, A. K., Nance, M. L., Lutz, N., & Stafford, P. W. (2008). *Abdominal trauma.* Retrieved from http://emedicine.medscape.com/article/940726-overview

Scapoli, L., Martinelli, M., Arlotti, M., Palmieri, A., Masiero, E., Pezzetti, F., & Carinci, F. (2008). Genes causing clefting syndromes as candidates for non-syndromic cleft lip with or without cleft palate: A family-based association study. *European Journal of Oral Sciences, 116*, 507–511.

Schwartz, D. (2008). Imaging of suspected appendicitis: Appropriateness of various imaging modalities. *Pediatric Annals, 37*(6), 433–438.

Shah, A., & Carroll, M. (2007). *Peptic ulcer disease.* Retrieved from http://emedicine.medscape.com/article/932308-overview

Silbermintz, A., & Markowitz, J. (2006). Inflammatory bowel disease. *Pediatric Annals, 35*(4), 269–274.

Smitherman, H., Stark, A. R., & Bhutani, V. K. (2006). Early recognition of neonatal hyperbilirubinemia and its emergent management. *Seminars in Fetal and Neonatal Medicine, 11*, 214–224.

St. Peter, S. D., Little, D. C., Calkins, C. M., Murphy, J. P., Andrews, W. S., Holcomb, G. W., III, . . . Ostlie, D. J. (2006). A simple and more cost-effective antibiotic regimen for perforated appendicitis. *Journal of Pediatric Surgery, 41*(5), 1020–1024.

Stoll, B. J. (2007). The umbilicus. In R. M. Kliegman, R. E. Behrman, H. B. Jenson, & B. F. Stanton (Eds.), *Nelson textbook of pediatrics* (18th ed., pp. 775–777). Philadelphia: Saunders.

Stoll, C., Alembik, Y., Dott, B., & Roth, M. P. (2007). Associated malformations in patients with anorectal anomalies. *European Journal of Medical Genetics, 50*(4), 281–290.

Suwandhi, E., Ton, M. N., & Schwarz, S. S. (2006). Gastroesophageal reflux in infancy and childhood. *Pediatric Annals, 35*(4), 259–266.

Tobias, N., Mason, D., Lutkenhoff, M., Stoops, M., & Ferguson, D. (2008). Management principles of organic causes of childhood constipation. *Journal of Pediatric Health Care, 22*(1), 12–23.

Upadhyaya, V. D., Gangopadhyay, A., Srivastava, P., Hasan, Z., & Sharma, S. (2008). Evolution of management of anorectal malformation through the ages. *Internet Journal of Surgery, 17*(1). Retrieved from http://www.ispub.com/journal/the_internet_journal_of_surgery/volume_17_number_1/article/evolution_of_management_of_anorectal_malformation_through_the_ages.html

Vajnar, J. (2007). A common cause of vomiting in infancy. *Journal of the American Academy of Physician Assistants, 20*(1), 58–59.

Wadhwani, S. L., Turmelle, Y. P., Nagy, R., Lowell, J., Dillion, P., & Shepherd, R. W. (2008). Prolonged neonatal jaundice and the diagnosis of biliary atresia. *Pediatrics, 121*(5), e1438–1440.

Wan, M. J., Krahn, M., Ungar, W. J., Edona, C., Sung, L., Medina, L. S., & Doria, A. S. (2009). Acute appendicitis in young children: Cost-effectiveness of US versus CT in diagnosis—A Markov Decision Analytic Model. *Radiology, 250*(2), 378–386.

Warkentin, T. E., & Kelton, J. G. (2005). Thrombocytopenia due to platelet destruction and hypersplenism. In R. Hoffman, E. J. Benz, S. J. Shattil, B. Furie, H. J. Cohen, L. E. Silberstein, & P. McGlave, *Hematology: Basic principles and practice* (4th ed., pp. 2305–2325). St. Louis, MO: Elsevier.

Waseem, M., & Rosenberg, H. K. (2008). Intussusception. *Pediatric Emergency Care, 24*(11), 793–800.

Wasley, A., Grytdal, S., & Gallagher, K. (2008). Surveillance for acute viral hepatitis—United States, 2006. *Morbidity and Mortality Weekly Report, 57*(SS02), 1–24.

Wehby, G. L., & Cassell, C. H. (2010). The impact of orofacial clefts on quality of life and healthcare use and costs. *Oral Diseases, 16*, 3–10.

Weill, V. (2008) Gastroesophageal reflux in infancy. *Advance for Nurse Practitioners, 16*(1), 47–50.

Werlin, S. L. (2007). Exocrine pancreas. In R. M. Kliegman, R. E. Behrman, H. B. Jenson, & B. F. Stanton (Eds.), *Nelson textbook of pediatrics* (18th ed., pp. 1650–1657). Philadelphia: Saunders.

Wyllie, R. (2007a). Normal development, structure, and function. In R. M. Kliegman, R. E. Behrman, H. B. Jenson, & B. F. Stanton (Eds.), *Nelson textbook of pediatrics* (18th ed., pp. 1554–1555). Philadelphia: Saunders.

Wyllie, R. (2007b). Pyloric stenosis and congenital anomalies of the stomach. In R. M. Kliegman, R. E. Behrman, H. B. Jenson, & B. F. Stanton (Eds.), *Nelson textbook of pediatrics* (18th ed., pp. 1555–1558). Philadelphia: Saunders.

Yazdy, M. M., Honein, M. A., & Xing, J. (2007). Reduction in orofacial clefts following folic acid fortification of the U.S. grain supply. *Birth Defects Research (Part A), 79*(1), 16–23.

Yazigi, N., & Balistreri, W. F. (2007). Viral hepatitis. In R. M. Kliegman, R. E. Behrman, H. B. Jenson, & B. F. Stanton (Eds.), *Nelson textbook of pediatrics* (18th ed., pp. 1680–1690). Philadelphia: Saunders.

Zilbert, N. R., Stamell, E. F., Ezon, I., Schlager, A., Ginsburg, H. B., & Nadler, E. P. (2009). Management and outcomes for children with acute appendicitis differ by hospital type: Areas for improvement at public hospitals. *Clinical Pediatrics, 48*(5), 499–504.

Zimmerman, B. T. (2007). Abdominal wall defects. In N. T. Browne, L. M. Flanigan, C. A. McComiskey, & P. Pieper, *Nursing care of the pediatric surgical patient* (2nd ed., pp. 261–271). Boston: Jones & Bartlett.

Alterations in Genitourinary Function

26 chapter

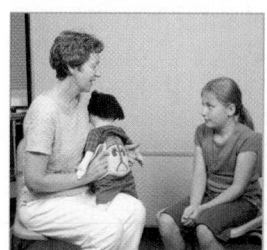

The school nurse phones Mrs. McIntyre to let her know that her daughter Brooke, 9 years old, was referred by the teacher after she had to run to the bathroom a second time during class. Brooke states that it hurts when she urinates and that she feels very tired. She has a temperature of 100°F orally. The nurse is concerned that Brooke may have a urinary tract infection. Mrs. McIntyre arranges to pick her daughter up at school and take her to the pediatric health care facility. Brooke has no prior history of urinary tract infection. History reveals that she recently started taking bubble baths after soccer practice. A urine specimen is obtained by clean catch and the diagnosis of a urinary tract infection is confirmed. Brooke's health care provider writes a prescription for oral trimethoprim-sulfamethoxazole for the infection and Pyridium for pain. When Brooke returns to school the following day, she asks the school nurse why she needs to take medicine. The nurse uses an anatomically correct doll to teach Brooke about the infection.

What should the clinic nurse teach Brooke and her mother about the antibiotic? In addition to pain medication, what methods can Brooke use to provide pain relief? What information should the school nurse include in the teaching?

Learning Outcomes

After reading this chapter, you will be able to do the following:

1. Describe the anatomy and physiology of the genitourinary system and pediatric differences.
2. Discuss the nursing management of a child with a structural defect of the genitourinary system.
3. Develop a nursing care plan for the child with a urinary tract infection.
4. Outline a plan to meet the fluid and dietary restrictions of a child with a renal disorder.
5. Summarize psychosocial issues for the child requiring surgery on the genitourinary tract.
6. Plan nursing care for the child with acute and chronic renal failure.
7. Identify growth and developmental issues for the child with chronic renal failure.
8. Describe nursing education for the adolescent with a sexually transmitted infection.

Key Terms

azotemia / 821
balanitis / 836
chordee / 810
circumcision / 836
cryptorchidism / 837
cystitis / 807
dialysate / 833
disequilibrium syndrome / 834
dysfunctional voiding / 815
end-stage renal disease (ESRD) / 829
enuresis / 814
hydronephrosis / 808
incarceration / 838
nephron / 804
neurogenic bladder / 807
oliguria / 824
osteodystrophy / 824
paraphimosis / 836
phimosis / 836
pyelonephritis / 807
pyeloplasty / 813
renal insufficiency / 813
uremia / 824
uremic frost / 829
urethritis / 839
vesicoureteral reflux / 808

FOCUS ON

The Genitourinary System

ANATOMY AND PHYSIOLOGY

The genitourinary system is made up of the urinary and reproductive organs. The urinary system—kidneys, ureters, bladder, and urethra—excretes wastes and maintains acid-base and fluid and electrolyte balance (Figure 26–1 ➤). The reproductive system consists of internal and external organs that at maturity promote the conception and healthy development of a fetus. Normal renal function requires the following: unimpaired renal blood flow, adequate glomerular ultrafiltration, normal tubular function, and unobstructed urine flow.

The functional unit of the kidney, the **nephron**, contributes to the formation of urine. The nephron is a tubular structure containing the renal corpuscle, proximal convoluted tubule, loop of

Henle, distal convoluted tubule, and collecting duct. The renal corpuscle is composed of the glomerulus (a small group of capillaries) that loops into the Bowman's capsule (Figure 26–2 ➤). The glomerular capillaries serve as the filtration membrane where metabolic wastes and fluids are separated from the blood cells and plasma proteins to form the urine. The kidney maintains the rate of blood flow to keep the glomerular filtration rate fairly constant. The urine flows through the proximal convoluted

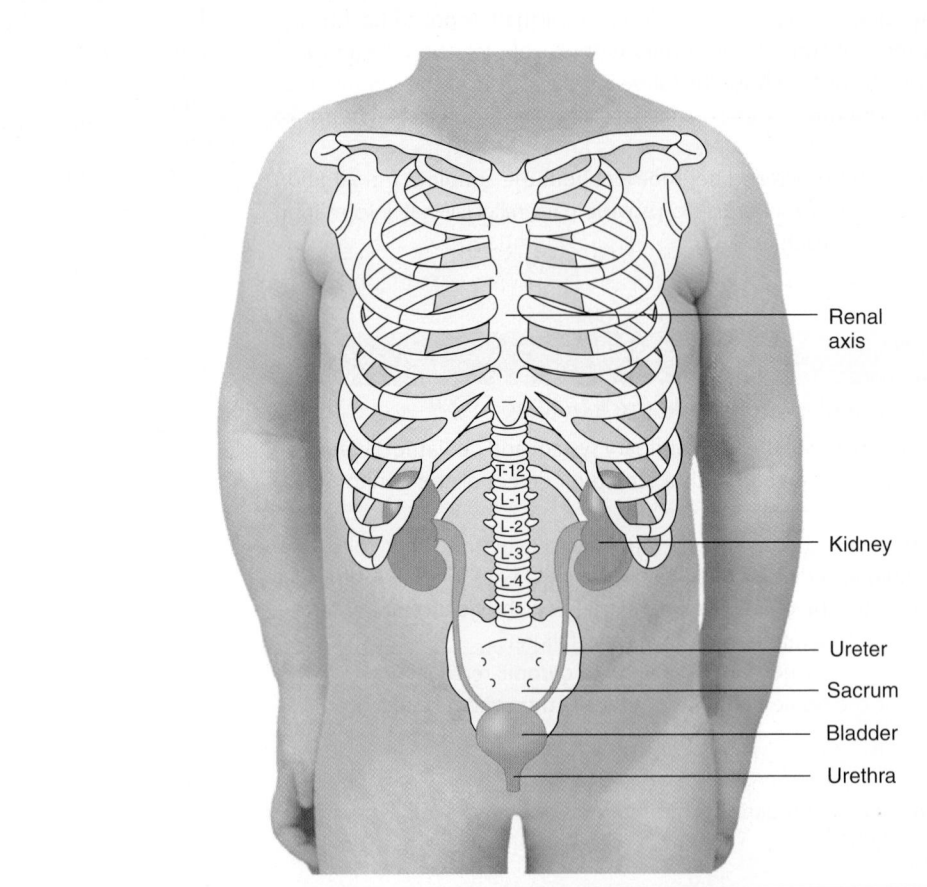

FIGURE 26–1 ➤ The urinary system is composed of the kidneys, ureters, bladder, and urethra. The kidneys are located between the twelfth thoracic (T12) and third lumbar (L3) vertebrae.

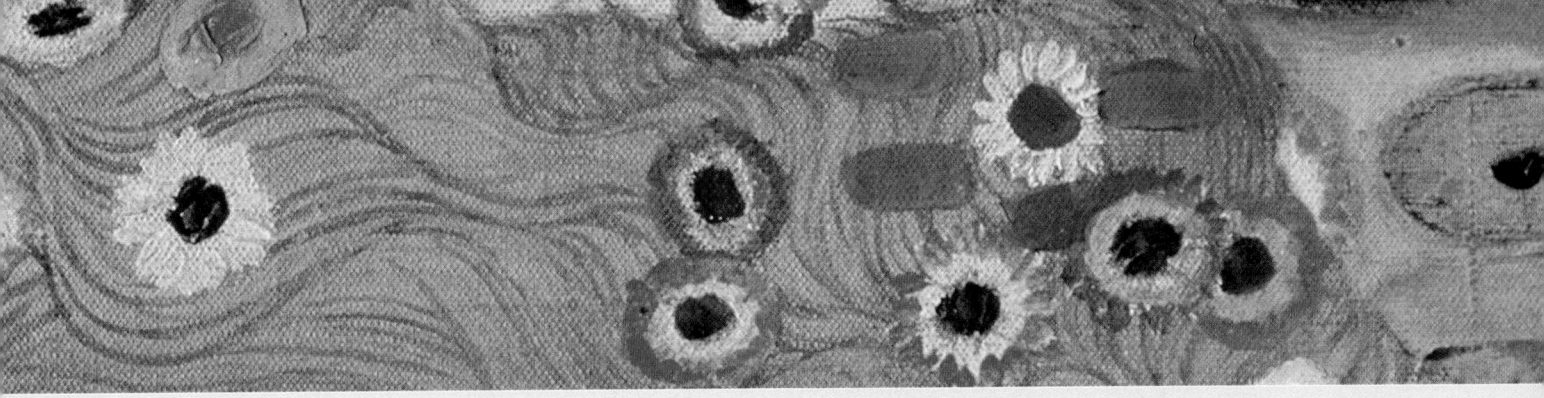

The presence of antidiuretic hormone (ADH) secreted by the posterior pituitary gland causes more water reabsorption, leading to urine concentration. Absence of ADH leads to dilute urine. See Chapter 18 ∞ for more information about fluid and electrolyte physiology.

Urine from the nephron flows into the calyces in the renal pelvis and is funneled into the ureters. The lower end of the ureters connects into the posterior aspect of the bladder. The muscle cells of the ureters move urine to the bladder by peristalsis. Urine collects in the bladder until the internal urethral sphincter relaxes and allows urine to pass into the urethra. Voluntary control of the external urethral sphincter is gained as the child's nervous system matures. Contraction of the bladder during urination compresses the lower end of the ureter and prevents the reflux of urine back into the ureter.

The kidney is essential in activating vitamin D, which is needed for the absorption of calcium and phosphorus from the small intestine. The kidney secretes erythropoietin to stimulate the bone marrow to produce red blood cells. The renin-angiotensin system of the kidney is a hormonal regulator that can increase the systemic blood pressure.

The male reproductive system is composed of the testes and scrotum, penis, prostate, and vas deferens, which drains into the urethra. The testes produce the primary male sex hormone, testosterone. The testes produce sperm after puberty.

The female reproductive system is composed of the ovaries, fallopian tubes, uterus, and vagina. The ovaries produce the primary female sex hormone, estrogen. Beginning between 8 and 12 years of age, the ovaries produce increasing amounts of sex hormones to initiate puberty and sexual maturation. After puberty, the ovaries produce the ovum that may be fertilized by the sperm during its passage through the fallopian tube into the uterus. Complex hormonal factors are involved in puberty, the menstrual cycle, and pregnancy.

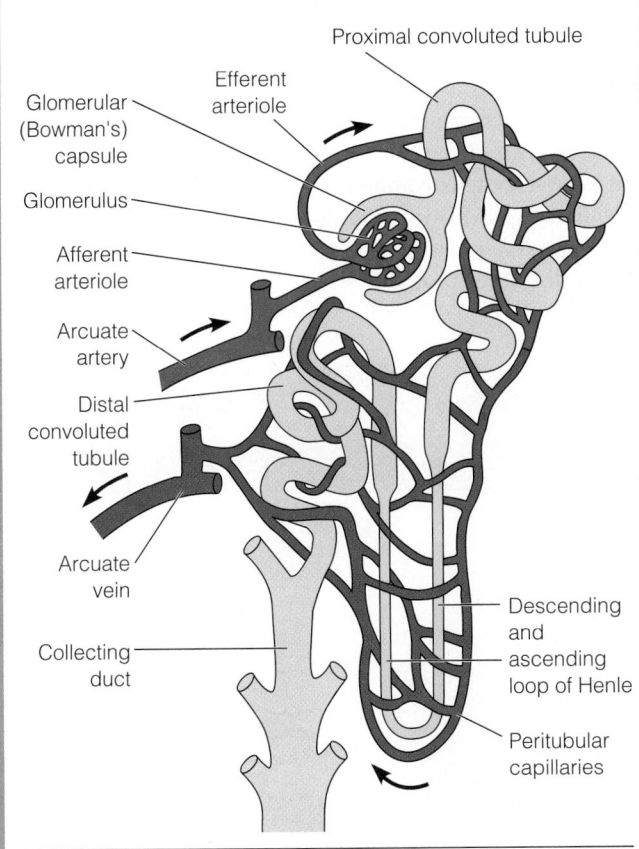

FIGURE 26–2 ➤ The nephron is the structural and functional unit of the kidneys. A nephron holds six glomeruli, Bowman's capsule, proximal tubule, loop of Henle, distal tubule, and the collecting duct.

tubule, the loop of Henle, and into the distal convoluted tubule and collecting duct. Water, electrolytes, and other substances are reabsorbed or secreted in the tubules, including the following (Huether, 2010a):

- **Proximal tubule** Sodium chloride, glucose, potassium, amino acids, bicarbonate, urea, and water are reabsorbed.
- **Loop of Henle** Water and sodium are reabsorbed, leading to urine concentration and secretion of urea.
- **Distal tubule** Sodium chloride, bicarbonate, and water are reabsorbed; potassium, urea, hydrogen ions, and ammonia ions are secreted.
- **Collecting tubule** Water is reabsorbed; sodium, potassium, hydrogen ions, and ammonia ions may be reabsorbed or secreted.

PEDIATRIC DIFFERENCES

Urinary System

All of the nephrons that will make up the mature kidney are present at birth. The kidneys grow and the tubular system matures gradually during childhood, reaching full size by adolescence. Most renal growth occurs during the first 5 years of life. This increase in size is due primarily to enlargement of the nephrons. The kidney's efficiency also increases with age. During the first 2 years of life, the kidneys are less efficient at regulating electrolyte and acid-base balance (see Chapter 18 ∞)

and eliminating some drugs from the body. After the age of 2 years, the kidneys' efficiency markedly increases. Urinary output per kilogram of body weight decreases as the child ages because the kidney becomes more efficient at concentrating urine. The expected output is as follows:

- Infants—2 mL/kg/hr
- Children—0.5 to 1 mL/kg/hr
- Adolescents—40 to 80 mL per hour

Bladder capacity increases with age from 20 to 50 mL at birth to 700 mL in adulthood. A child's bladder capacity (in ounces) can be estimated by adding 2 to the child's age (e.g., a 4-year-old has a bladder capacity of 6 ounces). Stimulation of "stretch receptors" within the bladder wall initiates urination. Simultaneous contraction of the detrusor muscle of the bladder and relaxation of the internal and external sphincters result in emptying of the bladder. Children less than 2 years of age cannot maintain bladder control because of insufficient nerve development (Figure 26–3 ➤).

Reproductive System

The reproductive system in children is functionally immature until puberty. Throughout childhood the genitalia (with the exception of the clitoris in girls) enlarge gradually. The hormonal changes of puberty accelerate anatomic and functional development (see Chapter 5 and Figures 5–40, 5–41, and 5–42 ∞). In girls, the mons pubis becomes more prominent and hair begins to grow. The vagina lengthens, and the epithelial layers thicken. The uterus and ovaries enlarge, and the musculature and vascularization of the uterus also increase. In boys, downy hair begins to appear at the base of the penis, and the scrotum becomes increasingly pendulous as the testes enlarge. The penis increases in length and width.

Use the Assessment Guidelines on page 807 to perform a nursing assessment of the genitourinary system. A list of diagnostic and laboratory tests commonly used to evaluate genitourinary conditions is provided in Table 26–1. See Appendices D and E ∞ for expected laboratory values and further information about specific diagnostic procedures.

As Children Grow

Development of the Genitourinary System

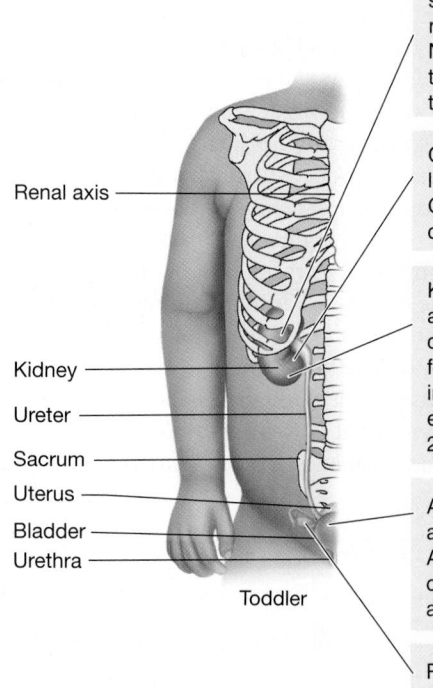
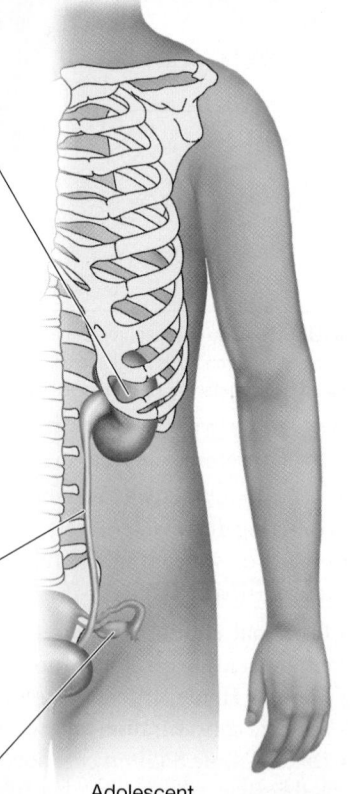

All nephrons are present at birth, the ureters are short, and tubules have a smaller surface area resulting in diminished water reabsorption. Nephrons grow in size, and the kidneys and the tubule system gradually develop during childhood to reach adult size during adolescence.

Glomerular filtration rate is at 30% to 50% of adult levels throughout first year of life (Huether, 2006). Glomerular filtration rate increases during childhood.

Kidneys are less efficient at regulating electrolyte and acid-base balance, and less able to concentrate urine. Diarrhea, infection, and improper feeding may lead to severe acidosis and fluid imbalance. Efficiency of the kidneys in regulating electrolytes and acid-base balance increases after 2 years of age.

Average daily urine output ranges from 15 to 50 mL at birth to 400 mL at 2 months of age (Huether, 2006). Average daily urine output increases during childhood and reaches 700–1500 mL during adolescence (Huether, 2006).

Reproductive system immature.

Reproductive system matures after puberty.

Renal axis
Kidney
Ureter
Sacrum
Uterus
Bladder
Urethra
Toddler
Adolescent

FIGURE 26–3 ➤ Development of the genitourinary system.

Data from: Huether, S. E. (2010b). Alterations of renal and urinary tract function in children. In K. L. McCance & S. E. Huether, Pathophysiology: The biologic basis for disease in adults and children *(6th ed., pp. 1402–1419). Maryland Heights, MO: Mosby Elsevier.*

NURSING MANAGEMENT

The newborn with exposed bladder tissue on the abdomen is assessed for other obvious defects such as epispadias or ambiguous genitalia. The skin surface around the exposed bladder is assessed for excoriation due to leaking urine and covered with plastic wrap for protection from the diaper. The parents are assessed for their response to the infant with a congenital defect and their need for psychosocial support.

Preoperative nursing care centers on preventing infection and trauma to the exposed bladder. The bladder mucosa is covered in sterile plastic wrap to prevent trauma and irritation, and the surrounding area is cleaned daily and protected from leaking urine with a skin sealant.

Postoperatively the wound and pelvis are immobilized to facilitate healing. Internal and external immobilization techniques are used for pelvic closure (see Chapter 29 ∞). Avoid abduction of the infant's legs. Nursing care includes maintaining proper alignment, monitoring peripheral circulation, and providing meticulous wound and skin care.

Monitor renal function by assessing the adequacy of urine output and blood and urine chemistries to detect signs of renal damage. Observe for any signs of obstruction in the drainage tubes such as increased intensity of bladder spasms, decreased urine output, or urine or blood draining from the urethral meatus. Promote comfort and give antibiotics as ordered.

Parents need emotional support to help them cope with the disfiguring nature of the infant's defect and the uncertainty of complete repair. To promote parent–infant bonding, encourage parents to participate in all aspects of the infant's care, including bathing, feeding, and wound care. They may also need guidance in the best way to hold the baby. Discharge teaching should include instructions about dressing changes and diapering, and the need to immediately report any signs of infection or change in renal function. Emphasize the need for routine follow-up visits after surgery to assess urinary function and to ensure that the next stages of surgery for continence control are performed at the appropriate time in the child's development.

Hypospadias and Epispadias

Hypospadias and epispadias are congenital anomalies involving an abnormal location of the urethral meatus (Figure 26–5 ➤). The reported incidence of hypospadias is 1 in 250 male births (Frimberger, Campbell, & Kropp, 2008). The incidence of epispadias is 1 in 40,000 to 1 in 118,000 births. Epispadias occurs twice as often in males as females (Huether, 2010b). With hypospadias, the urethral meatus can be located anywhere along the course of the urethra on the ventral or undersurface of the penile shaft, from the perineum to the tip of the glans. Most cases are mild, with the meatus slightly off center from the tip of the penis; in severe cases, the meatus is located on the scrotum. Hypospadias often occurs in conjunction with congenital chordee. Associated defects may include inguinal hernia, cryptorchidism (undescended testes), and partial absence of the foreskin (Huether, 2010b).

Epispadias and bladder exstrophy are the same condition, but epispadias is the milder expression of the condition (Huether, 2010b). See the section on bladder exstrophy for consistency on page 810. In males with epispadias, the meatal opening is located on the dorsal surface of the penile shaft. The opening may be small or a fissure may extend the entire length of the penis. Females with epispadias have a cleft of the ventral urethra that generally extends to the bladder neck (Huether, 2010b). The remainder of this discussion will focus on hypospadias and males with distal epispadias as the treatment for severe epispadias in males and epispadias in females is similar to the second and third stages of repair of bladder exstrophy (Elder, 2007).

Diagnosis is made by prenatal ultrasound or by examination at birth. The infant should not be circumcised because the foreskin tissue may be used for surgical repair (Pieretti, Pieretti, & Pieretti-Vanmarcke, 2009). The defects are corrected surgically, usually during the first year of life, to minimize psychologic effects when the child is older. Surgery is usually performed in a single operation, often as an outpatient procedure. The goals of surgical repair are:

• Placement of the urethral meatus at the end of the glans penis with satisfactory caliber and configuration for a urinary stream (enabling the child to void in a standing position)

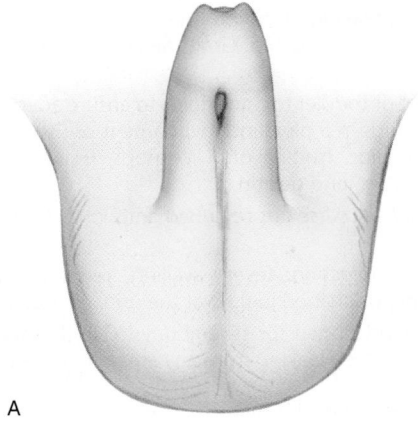
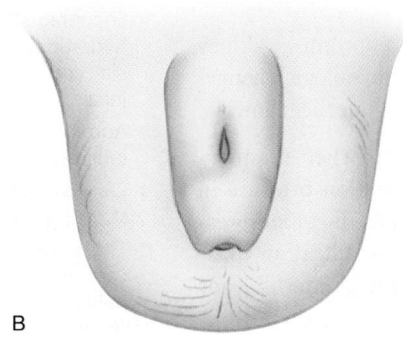

FIGURE 26–5 ➤ Hypospadias and epispadias. A, In hypospadias, the urethral canal is open on the ventral surface of the penis. B, In epispadias, the canal is open on the dorsal surface.

• Release of chordee to straighten the penis (enabling future sexual function)

A caudal nerve block is often used for postoperative pain relief. Anticholinergic medications may be prescribed to relieve bladder spasms.

NURSING MANAGEMENT

It is important to address parents' concerns at the time of birth. Preoperative teaching can relieve some of their anxiety about the future appearance and functioning of the penis.

Postoperative care focuses on protecting the surgical site from injury. The infant or child returns from surgery with the penis wrapped in a simple dressing, and a stent for urinary drainage and to maintain patency of the new opening. Fresh blood may be seen on the dressing and in the stent during the immediate postoperative period, but the urine should become less bloody over a few hours. Plan care to ensure that the stent does not get removed. Refer to the hospital's policy for the appropriate use of immobilizers in this situation.

Encourage fluid intake to maintain adequate urinary output and patency of the stent. Accurate and hourly documentation of intake and output is essential to detect postoperative urinary complications. Notify the physician if there is no urine drainage for 1 hour as this may indicate obstruction.

Pain may be associated with bladder spasms. Anticholinergic medications such as oxybutynin or hyoscyamine may be prescribed. Ibuprofen or acetaminophen may also be given for pain. Antibiotics are often prescribed until the urinary stent falls out.

The child is often discharged the day of surgery. Discharge teaching should include instructions for parents about care of the reconstructed area, double diapering to protect the stent, fluid intake, medication administration, and signs and symptoms of infection (Figure 26–6 ➤). Tell parents when the child needs to see the physician for dressing removal. See Families Want to Know: Caring for the Child After Hypospadias and Epispadias Repair.

Obstructive Uropathy

Obstructive uropathy refers to structural or functional abnormalities of the urinary system that interfere with urine flow and result in urine backflow into the kidneys. The uropathy may be bilateral or unilateral and partial or incomplete. The urinary obstruction may occur anywhere along the urinary tract, including the ureters, renal pelvis, bladder, and urethra. The condition is more common in males than females.

The pressure caused by urine backup compromises kidney function and often causes hydronephrosis. Physiologic changes that may occur as a result of hydronephrosis include the following:

• Cessation of glomerular filtration results when the pressure in the kidney pelvis equals the filtration pressure in the glomerular capillaries. To compensate, the blood pressure increases to increase the glomerular filtration pressure. However, increasing pressure on the glomeruli leads to cell death.

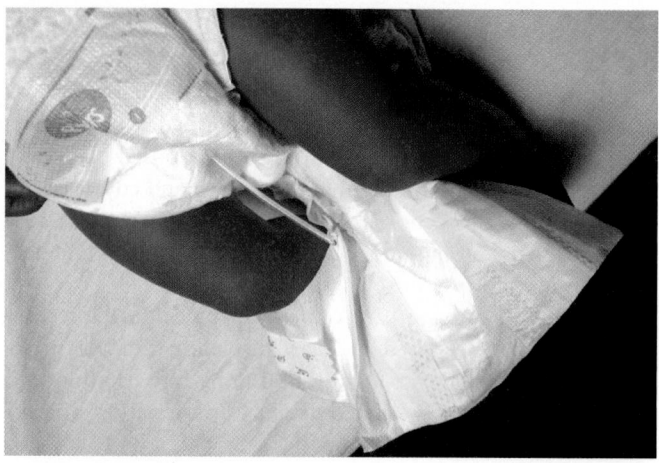

FIGURE 26–6 ➤ A double-diapering technique protects the urinary stent after surgery for hypospadias or epispadias repair. The inner diaper collects stool and the outer diaper collects urine.

• Metabolic acidosis results when the distal nephrons' ability to secrete hydrogen ions is impaired.
• Impairment of the kidney's ability to concentrate urine results in polydipsia and polyuria.
• Obstruction results in urinary stasis, promoting bacterial growth.
• Restriction of urinary outflow causes progressive renal damage and chronic renal failure if untreated.

Obstructive uropathy may be caused by several congenital lesions such as ureteropelvic junction obstruction, posterior

Families Want to Know
Caring for the Child After Hypospadias and Epispadias Repair

Guidelines for the care of children at home following hypospadias or epispadias repair include the following:

■ Use the double-diapering technique to protect the stent (the small tube that drains the urine) or urinary catheter from contamination by stool.

■ Do not bathe the child in the tub until the stent or catheter is removed.

■ Restrict the infant or toddler from activities that put pressure on the surgical site (e.g., playing on riding toys). Avoid holding the infant or child straddled on the hip. Limit the child's activity for 2 weeks.

■ Encourage the infant or toddler to drink fluids to ensure adequate hydration. Provide fluids in a pleasant environment or use a special cup. Offer fruit juice, fruit-flavored ice pops, fruit-flavored juices, flavored ice cubes, and gelatin.

■ Administer the *complete course* of prescribed antibiotics to avoid infection.

■ Observe for signs of infection: fever, swelling, redness, pain, strong-smelling urine, or change in flow of the urinary stream.

■ The urine will be blood tinged for several days. Call the health care provider if urine is seen leaking from any area other than the penis.

urethral valves, and stenosis or hypoplasia of the ureterovesicular junction (Figure 26–7 ➤).

- The ureteropelvic junction (UPJ), the tapered point where the renal pelvis transitions to the ureter, is the most common site of obstruction of the upper urinary tract in infants and children.
- Posterior urethral valves (PUV), abnormal folds of mucosa in the male urethra, are the most common cause of lower urinary tract obstruction in male infants (Hodges, Patel, McLorie, et al., 2009).
- Stenosis of the distal ureter at the ureterovesicular junction leads to dilation of the entire ureter, renal pelvis, and kidney (Huether, 2010b).

Other conditions that can lead to hydronephrosis include prune-belly syndrome, myelomeningocele, and neoplasms. See Box 26–1 for information on prune-belly syndrome. See Clinical Manifestations: Obstructive Lesions of the Urinary System for the differing signs and symptoms of obstructive uropathy by location.

Early diagnosis and treatment is needed to prevent kidney damage and deterioration of renal function. Prenatal ultrasound may detect hydronephrosis and

Pathophysiology Illustrated
Obstruction Sites

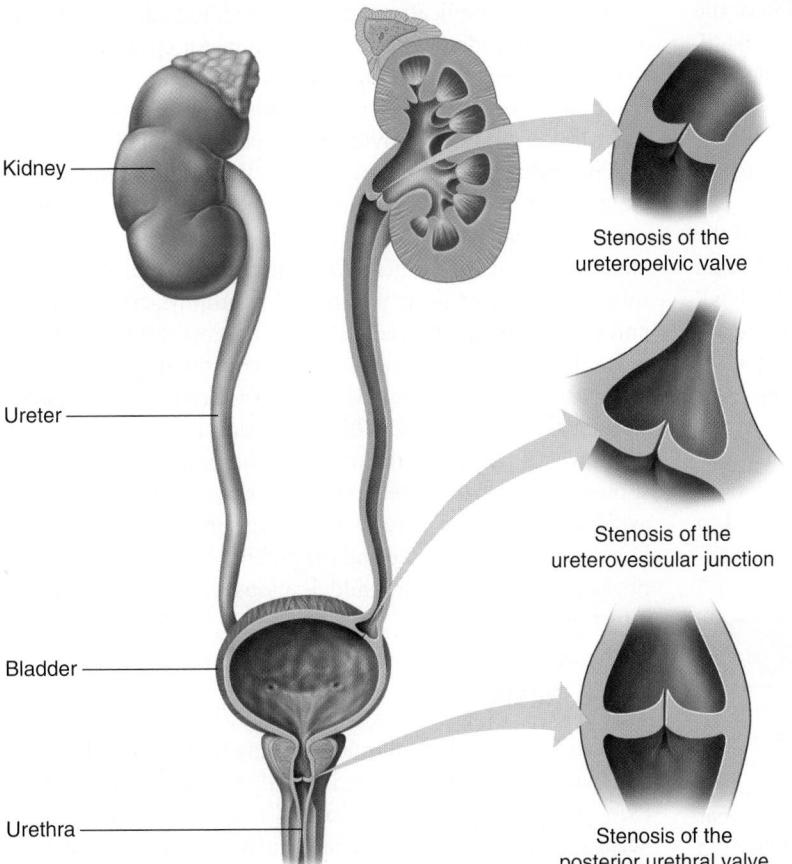

FIGURE 26–7 ➤ The common sites of obstruction in the upper and lower urinary tract. Why would damage from the posterior urethral valves potentially be worse than other obstructions? Upper urinary tract infections are often unilateral. Renal failure is most likely to occur when both kidneys are affected by hydronephrosis.

BOX 26–1 Prune-Belly Syndrome

Prune-belly syndrome, also known as Eagle-Barrett syndrome, is another cause of hydronephrosis. In this congenital defect, the abdominal musculature fails to develop. The skin covering the abdominal wall is thin and resembles a wrinkled prune (Naqvi, Paddack, Kulkarni, et al., 2009). Other characteristics include urinary tract anomalies, poor ureteral peristalsis, enlarged bladder, high risk for recurrent urinary tract infection, vesicoureteral reflux, and bilateral cryptorchidism. Prune-belly syndrome occurs predominantly in males (95%), with an incidence of 1 in 40,000 live births (Elder, 2007).

PUV. Postnatal assessment reveals a distended bladder and signs and symptoms of **renal insufficiency** (decrease in the kidneys' ability to conserve sodium and concentrate the urine). A diuretic-enhanced radionuclide scan and voiding cystourethrogram are performed when UPJ or ureterovesicular obstruction is suspected. See page 807 for diagnostic tests commonly used to identify urinary tract conditions.

The goals of surgical correction or diversion are to lower the pressure within the collecting system, which reduces renal damage, and to prevent stasis, which decreases the risk of infection. Surgical correction may necessitate **pyeloplasty** (removal of an obstructed segment of the ureter and reimplantation into the renal pelvis) or valve repair or reconstruction, depending on the cause of the obstruction. Urinary incontinence resulting from sphincter weakness is a common problem after surgery. Urinary diversion may be performed in conditions such as meningomyelocele and prune-belly syndrome.

NURSING MANAGEMENT

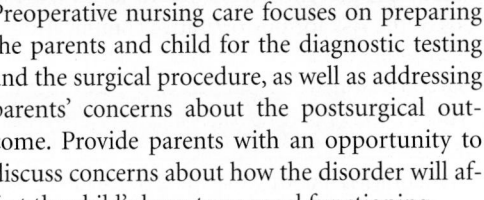

Preoperative nursing care focuses on preparing the parents and child for the diagnostic testing and the surgical procedure, as well as addressing parents' concerns about the postsurgical outcome. Provide parents with an opportunity to discuss concerns about how the disorder will affect the child's long-term renal functioning.

Postoperative care involves monitoring vital signs and intake and output and observing for signs of urine retention, such as decreased output and bladder distention. Administer medications as prescribed, including antibiotics and antispasmodics such as oxybutynin.

Many children are discharged with stents or catheters. Teach parents how to change dressings, double diaper, care for catheters, assess

Clinical Manifestations
Obstructive Lesions of the Urinary System

Obstructive Lesion	Clinical Manifestations
Ureteropelvic junction obstruction	In infants: abdominal mass (enlarged kidney), hypertension, urinary tract infection In children: hematuria, pain, intermittent nausea and vomiting
Posterior urethral valves	In infants: abdominal mass (enlarged kidney), distended bladder, poor urinary stream, urinary tract infection, sepsis, low specific gravity, polyuria, increased creatinine level, failure to thrive In older children: diurnal enuresis, urinary tract infection, dribbling and/or retention of urine, hematuria (Hodges et al., 2009)
Ureterovesicular junction obstruction	Urinary tract infection (recurrent or chronic), hematuria, pain, abdominal mass (enlarged kidney), enuresis

pain and give analgesics, and recognize signs of possible obstruction or infection. Parents should encourage the child to participate in age-appropriate activities. However, children should avoid contact sports because of their potential to injure the bladder.

Vesicoureteral Reflux

In vesicoureteral reflux (VUR), urine flows inappropriately from the bladder into the ureters. Severity ranges from reflux of urine into a nondilated ureter at stage 1 to severe dilation of the ureter, renal pelvis, and calyces at stage 5 (Khoury & Bägli, 2007). The reflux prevents complete emptying of the bladder, and because urine returns to the bladder, it creates a reservoir for bacterial growth (Huether, 2010b; Ključevšek, Ključevšek, Levart, et al., 2010). Bacteria in the urine may be swept up to the kidneys, leading to pyelonephritis.

A renal ultrasound and voiding cystourethrogram reveal the defect and identify severity of reflux (to the ureter and renal pelvis, or causing some dilation of the ureter and renal pelvis). Long-term complications include renal scarring, hypertension, and chronic renal failure (Nelson & Koo, 2008). The goal of treatment is to prevent pyelonephritis and renal scarring. Prophylactic antibiotics may be prescribed to prevent urinary tract infection. Surgical intervention (ureteral reimplantation) may be required depending on the grade of reflux. If a urinary tract infection is present 1 week before surgery, it must be treated to reduce the risk for postoperative complications.

Research *Prophylactic Antibiotics*

A randomized control trial of 218 children, ages 3 months to 18 years, diagnosed with pyelonephritis and mild or moderate vesicoureteral reflux (VUR) evaluated the effect of prophylactic antibiotics on outcomes. Half the children received antibiotics and the remainder did not. Children were seen every 3 months for the year of the study, and each had a urine culture at each visit. Results indicated that the presence of mild or moderate VUR did not increase the incidence of UTI, pyelonephritis, or renal scarring following an acute episode of pyelonephritis. The children who did not receive prophylactic antibiotics had no more infections or renal scarring than the children who did receive antibiotics (Garin, Olavarria, Nieto, et al., 2006).

NURSING MANAGEMENT
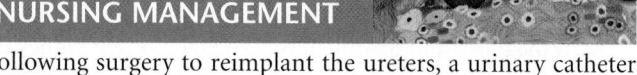

Following surgery to reimplant the ureters, a urinary catheter will be in place. The urine will be bloody initially and clear within 2 to 3 days. Intravenous fluids will be administered at a rate sufficient to maintain adequate urine output. Monitoring urine output is important as clots may cause an obstruction. When urine output is diminished, notify the health care provider and follow orders for irrigating the urinary catheter.

Administer medications as prescribed, including antibiotics and antispasmodics such as oxybutynin. An epidural catheter may have been placed for pain management. Monitor the epidural according to agency protocol. See Chapter 15 ∞. Once this is removed, provide prescribed pain medication.

The child can be discharged when the child has the urinary catheter removed and can void spontaneously. An ultrasound or cystogram may be performed prior to discharge to evaluate the effectiveness of the surgery. Educate the family about the administration of medications including prophylactic antibiotics and antispasmodics if needed. Inform parents of the need for increased fiber in the diet to address the constipating effects of the antispasmodic medication. Guidelines for calling the physician include fever over 38.5°C (101.5°F), abdominal or back pain, or swelling and redness of the incision. The child may take a short shower or tub bath when returning home. The child should avoid active play for 3 weeks following surgery. Provide guidelines for annual follow-up and the potential need to resume prophylactic antibiotics if the child develops recurrent urinary tract infections.

■ ENURESIS

Enuresis is repeated involuntary voiding by a child old enough that bladder control is expected, usually about 5 to 6 years of age. (See Table 26–2 for bladder control milestones.) Enuresis can occur either at night (nocturnal), during the day (diurnal), or both night and day. Enuresis is further categorized as primary and secondary:

• **Primary enuresis**—child has never had a dry night; attributed to maturational delay and small functional bladder; not associated with stress or psychiatric cause.

TABLE 26–2	Milestones in the Development of Bladder Control
Age	Developmental Milestone
1 1/2 years	Child passes urine at regular intervals.
2 years	Child announces when he or she is voiding.
2 1/2 years	Child makes known need to void; can hold urine.
3 years	Child goes to the bathroom by himself or herself; holds urge if preoccupied with play.
2 1/2–3 1/2 years	Child achieves nighttime bladder and bowel control.
4 years	Child shows great interest in going to bathrooms when away from home (shopping centers, movies).
5 years	Child voids approximately seven times a day; prefers privacy; is able to initiate emptying of bladder at any degree of fullness.

- **Secondary enuresis**—child who has been reliably dry for at least 6 months begins bed-wetting; associated with stress, urinary tract infections, diabetes mellitus, and sleep disorders.

Primary nocturnal enuresis is the most common type of enuresis and occurs more frequently in males than females (Elder, 2007). In the United States, approximately 5 to 7 million children over 6 years of age are affected with primary nocturnal enuresis (Ward-Smith & Barry, 2006).

Etiology and Pathophysiology

Enuresis may result from neurologic or congenital structural disorders, illness, or stress. Nocturnal enuresis occurs frequently in children whose parents have a history of bed-wetting. There is a 77% risk if both parents had enuresis, and a 44% risk if one parent had enuresis (Ward-Smith & Barry, 2006).

In most children with primary enuresis, the bladder has a smaller functional capacity, and neuromuscular maturation of the inhibitory fibers is delayed. Minor abnormalities of the bladder neck and urethra are also associated with enuresis. Nocturnal enuresis is also more prevalent in children with obstructive sleep apnea syndrome (Weissbach, Leiberman, Tarasiuk, et al., 2006). Often children with nocturnal enuresis are harder to arouse and may fail to respond to full bladder signals. Some children may produce more urine and exceed the functional bladder capacity due to a lack of circadian rhythm of vasopressin that helps concentrate the urine during sleep (Mercer, 2006). Some children with daytime enuresis may have **dysfunctional voiding**, an abnormality in the storage or emptying phase of urination (Berry, 2005).

Clinical Manifestations

Children with diurnal enuresis may have frequency, urgency, constant dribbling, and involuntary loss of control after voiding. Children with nocturnal enuresis have bed-wetting.

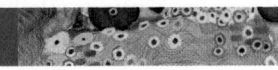

COLLABORATIVE CARE

Diagnostic Tests

Urinalysis on the first voided specimen is performed. The specific gravity provides information about the child's ability to concentrate the urine. Screening for a UTI with a dipstick is performed. A urine culture may reveal that an asymptomatic urinary tract infection is present. Diabetes mellitus, diabetes insipidus, or renal insufficiency should be ruled out in children with both enuresis and polyuria or oliguria. Other diagnostic tests that might be performed include ultrasound of the urinary tract, uroflowmetry, and postvoiding residual urine measurements (Dogan, Akpinar, Gurocak, et al., 2008).

A thorough history can help identify potential causes of enuresis (Box 26–2). Children with enuresis often have a history of constipation (Berry, 2006). Rectal pressure on the posterior bladder wall stimulates the bladder to empty.

The child's lower spine is examined for fistulas, sacral dimples, or tufts of hair that could be signs of occult spina bifida (Chapter 27 ∞). Prolonged hospitalization, family stressors, and preoccupation with school concerns also have been associated with secondary enuresis.

Clinical Therapy

A multitreatment approach is usually most effective. Fluid restriction, bladder training, and enuresis alarms are common approaches (Table 26–3). A spontaneous resolution occurs in 15% of children with enuresis without medical intervention (Ward-Smith & Barry, 2006). Some children with nocturnal enuresis are treated with medications.

- Desmopressin has an antidiuretic effect and is given only on a nighttime basis at the beginning of treatment. Once its effectiveness has been established, it may be used as needed for times when the child is away from home for a short period (e.g., sleepovers or camp) (Berry, 2006).
- Oxybutynin, an anticholinergic medication, has an antispasmodic effect and is used for children with urgency or an overactive detrusor muscle (Vemulakonda & Jones, 2006).
- Imipramine, a tricyclic antidepressant, is often used for nocturnal enuresis. This medication requires close monitoring because of its effects on mood and sleep-arousal patterns and the associated danger of overdoses (Vemulakonda & Jones, 2006).

Relapse often occurs when medications are stopped.

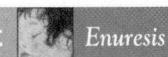

Growth & Development   *Enuresis*

An estimated 15% of 5-year-olds experience primary nocturnal enuresis (Ward-Smith & Barry, 2006). Although wetting episodes decrease as the child gets older, an estimated 4–8% of 12-year-olds and 1–3% of adolescents will continue to have nocturnal enuresis (Berry, 2006). In addition, approximately 3.8% of males and 6% of girls, 7 years of age, have diurnal (daytime) enuresis (Schulman & Berry, 2007).

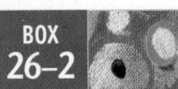

BOX 26–2 Questions to Ask When Taking an Enuresis History

Family History

Is there a family history of renal or urinary structural abnormalities?

Is there a family history of bed-wetting?

Family Management

How serious is the problem for the family?

What happens when the child wets? (Who gets up and changes sheets?)

How is the child treated? Is the child punished or blamed for wetting?

What remedies have been tried?

Toilet Training

Did the child have a difficult time with toilet training?

What method of toilet training did you use? When was toilet training initiated?

What are the child's current voiding and stooling patterns?

How long is the child's longest dry period, and when does it occur?

Does the child have a history of constipation or encopresis?

Stressors

How is the child doing in school? How are relationships with peers?

Are there any changes in the home, such as a new sibling or death in the family?

Are any new or chronic stressors present in the child's life?

How does the problem interfere with play and other activities?

Risk Factors

Diabetes

- Does the child void often or have urgency?
- Is the child frequently thirsty?

Urinary Tract Infection

- Does the child experience burning on urination?
- Has the child had a urinary tract infection before? If so, how many?

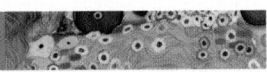

NURSING MANAGEMENT

Nursing Assessment and Diagnoses

Nurses assist in the evaluation of the child with enuresis, obtaining much of the history listed in Box 26–2. A review of the child's elimination patterns and developmental milestones and the parents' methods of toilet training are also essential information. Identify how many bathroom breaks are given during the day at school and if the child uses them. If the child does not use the bathroom at school, identify the reasons. Assess for associated conditions by examining the child's lower spine for fistulas, sacral dimples, or tufts of hair that could be signs of occult spina bifida.

Assess the child's and family's feelings and frustrations about the problem of bed-wetting and their motivation to implement therapies.

Nursing diagnoses that apply to the child with enuresis may include:

- Impaired Urinary Elimination related to inability to control voiding during the day or at night

TABLE 26–3 Nonpharmacological Treatment Approaches for Enuresis

Approach	Description
Fluid restriction	Fluid intake is limited in the evening and before the child goes to bed.
Bladder exercises	The child drinks a large amount and then holds urine as long as he or she can. The child practices stopping voiding midstream. Exercises should continue for at least 6 months.
Timed voiding	The child with diurnal enuresis is instructed to void every 2 hours and to use a double voiding pattern; this trains the bladder to empty completely and avoid overdistention.
Enuresis alarms	A detector strip is attached to the child's pants. The alarm sounds a buzzer that alerts the child when wetting occurs, so the child can get up and finish voiding in the bathroom. This works best for children over 7 years old, and takes 3 to 4 months for success.
Reward system	Set realistic goals for the child and reinforce dry days or nights with stars and stickers on a chart.

- Overflow urinary incontinence related to ignoring urge to void during activities
- Risk for Situational Low Self-Esteem related to embarrassment over lack of bladder control
- Readiness for Enhanced Knowledge (enuresis management) related to motivation of the child

Planning and Implementation

Teach the child and parents about the physiologic development of bladder control and causes and treatment of enuresis. Explore feelings of guilt or blame. Make sure the parents are aware that the child cannot control the wetting. Psychosocial support is an essential part of care since stress is an important cause of secondary enuresis. Provide emotional support to the parents and child, and encourage the child's participation in the treatment plan. Refer the child for counseling or therapy, if appropriate.

Assess the parents' and child's motivation and readiness for interventions. The child needs to be an active participant in the treatment plan for daytime or nighttime wetting. For daytime wetting, the child may need a reminder to go to the bathroom such as a vibrating watch. A discussion with the child's teacher may make it possible for the child to have additional or private bathroom breaks.

Before parents buy an enuresis alarm, suggest that the alarm clock be used in the child's room for several nights to see if the child will arouse. The child may need the parent's help to arouse initially. Find out whether the child shares a room with others who will be disturbed by the alarm. Ask if the child and parents are willing to persist with an enuresis alarm, as it may take months to work. Discuss potential strategies with the family to reduce stressors on the child or to help the child cope with the stressors.

Biofeedback is a complementary therapy that may be used for some cases of enuresis when the child and parents are highly motivated. In the case of bladder sphincter dysfunction, when the pelvic floor muscles contract during voiding, the child may have urgency and frequency associated with daytime or nighttime enuresis. During biofeedback training, the child learns to identify the differences in relaxation and contraction of the bladder muscles, as well as straining. The child then learns to sustain and maintain a relaxed pelvic floor and voluntary sphincter opening (Adams & Vohra, 2009; Liberti, 2005).

Evaluation

Evaluation of nursing care may include:

- The child and family choose one or more interventions that they prefer and persist in using them.
- The child has an increased number of dry nights.

■ RENAL DISORDERS

Nephrotic Syndrome

Nephrotic syndrome does not refer to a specific disease, but rather to a clinical state characterized by edema, massive proteinuria, hypoalbuminemia, hypoproteinemia, hyperlipidemia, and altered immunity. Congenital nephrotic syndrome is a rare disorder of the kidney that manifests shortly after birth with symptoms of edema, proteinuria, and hypoproteinemia. Congenital nephrotic syndrome is generally related to a genetic defect (Jalanko, 2009). Primary nephrotic syndrome results from a disease that affects only the kidney, such as glomerulonephritis. Secondary nephrotic syndrome results from a systemic disease, drugs, or toxins that alter kidney function (Huether, 2010b).

Approximately 85% of children with nephrotic syndrome have a type of primary disease called minimal change nephrotic syndrome (MCNS). It is estimated that 95% of these children respond to steroid therapy (Vogt & Avner, 2007a). MCNS is a common kidney disease in the pediatric population, occurring in 2–16 per 100,000 children (Lahdenkari, Suvanto, Kajantie, et al., 2005) and is more common in males than females (Vogt & Avner, 2007a). MCNS derives its name from the normal or only minimally changed appearance of the glomeruli on light microscopic evaluation. Because MCNS is the most common form of nephrotic syndrome, it is the focus of the following discussion.

Etiology and Pathophysiology

The cause of primary MCNS is not clearly understood but an immune system role is suspected (Vogt & Avner, 2007a). The mechanism of increased glomerular permeability is unknown; however, it may be related to the release of permeability factors from abnormal circulating T cells and the loss of a negative charge in the glomerular capillary wall (Huether, 2010b). In MCNS, increased permeability of the glomerular membrane permits large, negatively charged molecules such as albumin to pass through the membrane and be excreted in the urine. Proteinuria results in decreased oncotic pressure and edema, because fluid remains in the

interstitial spaces instead of being pulled back into the vascular compartment (Vogt & Avner, 2007a). Immunoglobulins are lost, resulting in altered immunity. Loss of protein in the urine, as well as insufficient albumin production by the liver and a decreased albumin concentration as a result of salt and water retention by the kidney, contribute to hypoalbuminemia. Hypercoagulability occurs because of alterations in coagulation factors. The liver, stimulated perhaps by hypoalbuminemia or decreased osmotic pressure, responds by increasing synthesis of lipoprotein, resulting in hyperlipidemia (Huether & Forshee, 2010). Children who develop steroid-resistant nephrotic syndrome are at risk for renal failure (Butani & Ramsamooj, 2009). See Figure 26–8 ➤.

Clinical Manifestations

In most children, edema develops gradually over several weeks. Children may have a history of periorbital edema on waking that resolves during the day as fluid shifts to the abdomen and lower extremities. Other signs include snug fit of clothing and shoes, pallor, hypertension, irritability, anorexia, hematuria, decreased urine output, and nonspecific malaise. The child's urine may be frothy or foamy. Parents often do not seek medical treatment until generalized edema develops on the child's extremities, abdomen, or genitals (Figure 26–9 ➤). Respiratory distress from pleural effusion may occur in some cases.

Massive edema resulting in a dramatic weight gain and abdominal pain, with or without vomiting, may occur, depending on the amount of albumin lost and the amount of sodium ingested. The child becomes malnourished as a result of protein loss in the urine. The skin is pale and shiny with prominent veins, and the hair becomes more brittle. An increased risk of thrombosis is present.

COLLABORATIVE CARE

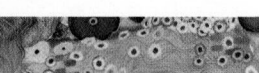

Diagnostic Tests

Diagnosis is based on the history, characteristic symptoms, and laboratory findings. Urinalysis as well as serum albumin, sodium, BUN, cholesterol, and electrolytes are ordered. Urinalysis shows 3+ to 4+ protein. Microscopic hematuria may also be present. Other values that confirm the diagnosis include hypoalbuminemia indicated by serum albumin levels of less than 2.5 g/dL, urinary protein excretion of greater than 40 mg/m^2/hour, and a spot urine protein/creatinine ratio greater than 2.0 (Vogt & Avner, 2007a). Renal ultrasound may be performed to detect structural kidney problems.

Clinical Tip

A protein-to-creatinine (PR/CR) ratio of the first morning void is used to estimate protein excretion in children because of the challenges in obtaining 24-hour urines. Normal PR/CR ratios are less than 0.2 in children 2 years and older and less than 0.5 in children less than 2 years of age (Vogt & Avner, 2007a).

Clinical Therapy

Children may be hospitalized when severe edema or a major infection is present, but are usually treated as outpatients.

Pathophysiology Illustrated
Nephrotic Syndrome

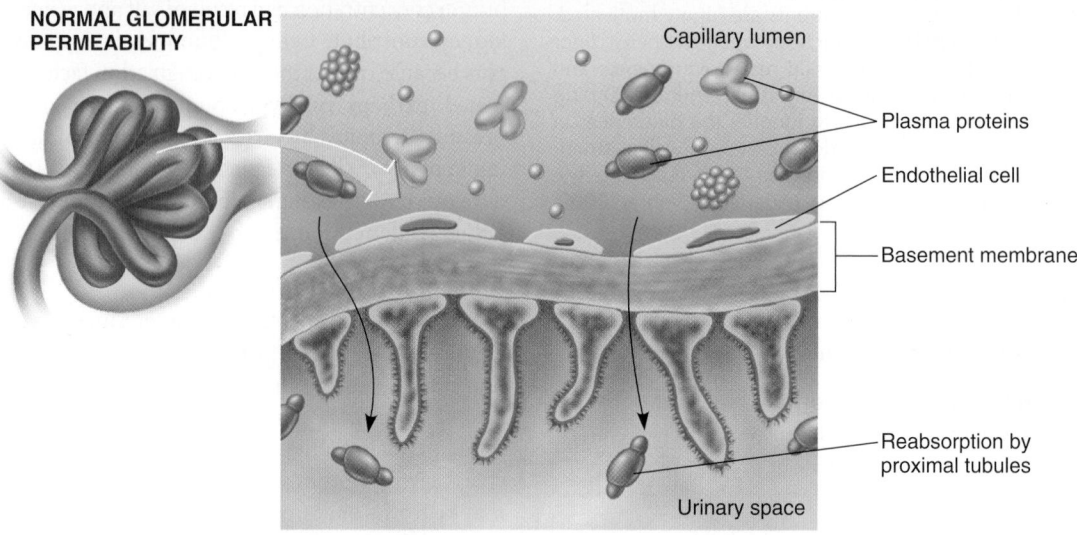

NORMAL GLOMERULAR PERMEABILITY

Capillary lumen

Plasma proteins

Endothelial cell

Basement membrane

Reabsorption by proximal tubules

Urinary space

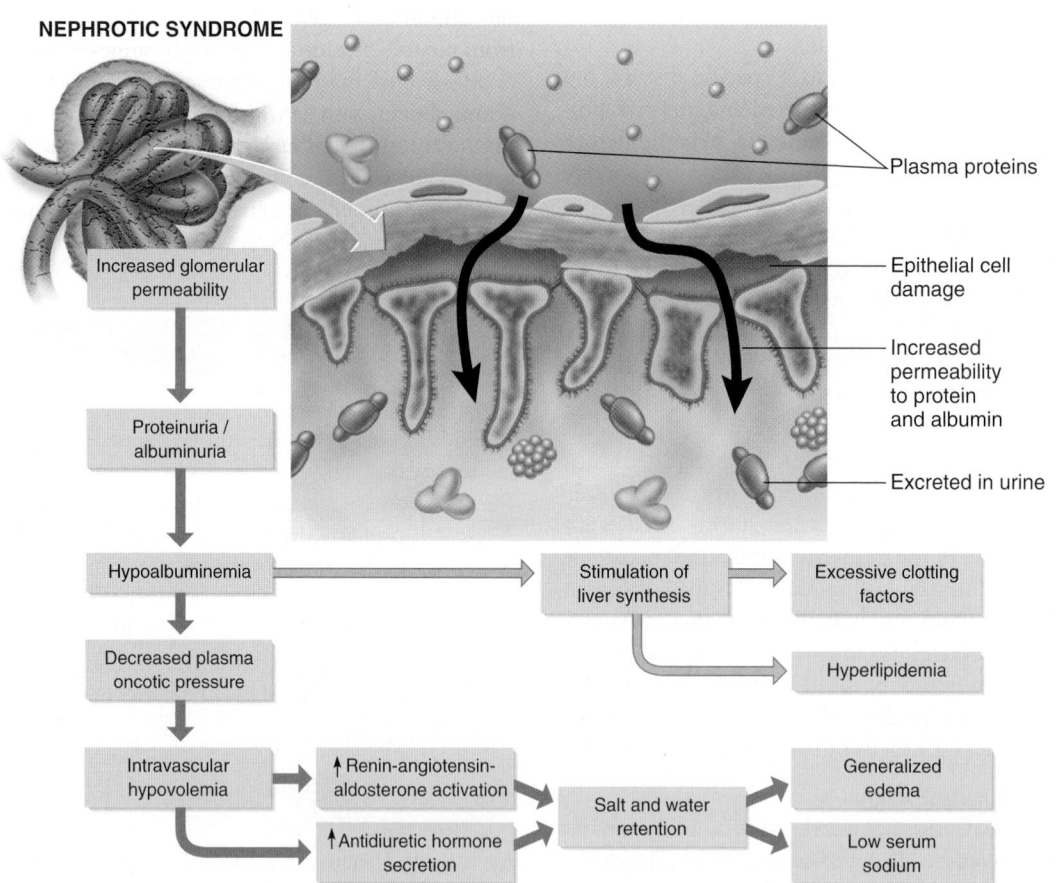

NEPHROTIC SYNDROME

Increased glomerular permeability

Proteinuria / albuminuria

Hypoalbuminemia

Decreased plasma oncotic pressure

Intravascular hypovolemia

↑ Renin-angiotensin-aldosterone activation

↑ Antidiuretic hormone secretion

Salt and water retention

Plasma proteins

Epithelial cell damage

Increased permeability to protein and albumin

Excreted in urine

Stimulation of liver synthesis

Excessive clotting factors

Hyperlipidemia

Generalized edema

Low serum sodium

FIGURE 26–8 ➤ Note the contrast between the normal glomerular anatomy and the changes that exist in nephrotic syndrome permitting protein to be excreted in the urine. The lower albumin blood level stimulates the liver to generate lipids and excessive clotting factors. Edema results from decreased oncotic plasma pressure, renin-angiotensin-aldosterone activation, and antidiuretic hormone secretion.

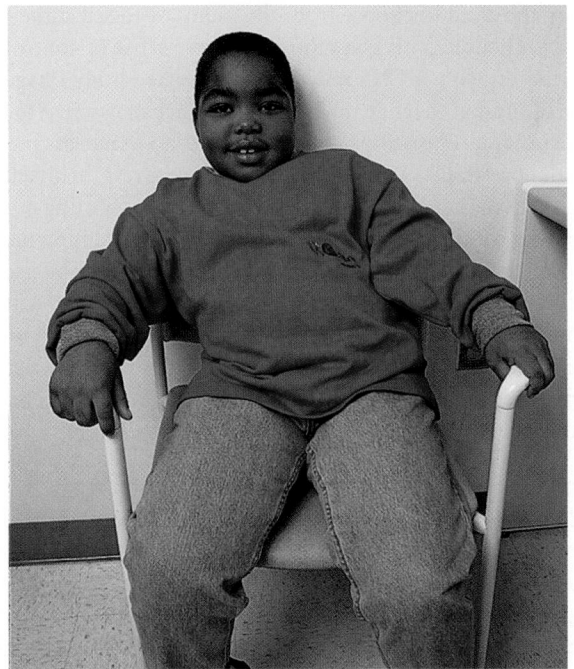

FIGURE 26–9 ➤ This boy has generalized edema, a characteristic finding in nephrotic syndrome.

Clinical therapy focuses on decreasing proteinuria, relieving edema, managing associated symptoms, improving nutrition, and preventing infection. A corticosteroid (such as prednisone) is prescribed to decrease proteinuria. In most children, urine protein levels fall to trace or negative values within 2 to 3 weeks of the start of therapy. Children who respond successfully to therapy continue to take corticosteroids daily for 6 weeks, followed by 6 weeks of alternate-day treatment. The medication is then slowly tapered and discontinued over a 2- to 3-month period. Approximately 90% of children experience complete remission with corticosteroid therapy. Intravenous methylprednisolone may be used in children not responsive to oral steroids (Nachman, Jennette, & Falk, 2008; Vogt & Avner, 2007a). Intravenous administration of albumin followed by furosemide may occasionally be ordered in the child with massive edema who is unresponsive to fluid restriction and parenteral diuretics (Vogt & Avner, 2007a).

Relapses occur in many children with nephrotic syndrome (Vogt & Avner, 2007b). Relapses may become less frequent during adolescence; however, long-term studies have revealed that many adults continue to have relapses (Ruth, Kemper, Leumann, et al., 2005).

Children who have a relapse after drug therapy is discontinued receive repeat therapy. Other medications used include diuretics, antihypertensive agents, and antibiotics. Medications such as cyclophosphamide, cyclosporine, tacrolimus, and mycophenolate may be used to prolong remissions in children with nephrotic syndrome who have frequent relapses (Vogt & Avner, 2007a). Since diuretics can precipitate hypovolemia, hyponatremia, and hypokalemia, electrolyte levels should be carefully monitored.

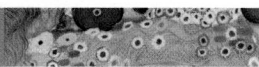

NURSING MANAGEMENT

Goals of nursing focus on managing the child's symptoms, preventing complications, meeting nutritional needs, and addressing the emotional needs of the child and family.

Nursing Assessment and Diagnoses

Nursing assessment focuses on signs of fluid volume excess, complications related to the disorder, and the psychosocial impact of the condition on the child and family.

Physiologic Assessment

Careful assessment of the child's hydration status and edema is essential. Carefully monitor intake and output. Weigh the child daily using the same scale, and measure abdominal girth to monitor changes in edema and ascites (see Figure 18–14 ∞ on page 489). Monitor vital signs every 4 hours to watch for signs of respiratory distress, hypertension, or circulatory overload. Test urine for proteinuria and specific gravity at least once each shift. Assess for hypovolemia during periods of diuresis. Assess for skin breakdown.

Psychosocial Assessment

Children and parents are often fearful or anxious on admission. Because edema often develops gradually, parents may feel guilty if they did not seek medical attention immediately. School-age children with generalized edema are often concerned about their appearance. Careful questioning may be necessary to elicit these concerns. The child hospitalized for a recurrence of nephrotic syndrome may be frustrated or depressed. Assess individual and family coping mechanisms, support systems, and level of stress.

Common nursing diagnoses for the child with MCNS include:

- Risk for Infection related to immunosuppressive therapy
- Risk for Impaired Skin Integrity related to edema and fragile skin
- Excess Fluid Volume related to renal dysfunction and sodium retention
- Imbalanced Nutrition: Less than Body Requirements related to loss of appetite and protein loss in urine

Planning and Implementation

Nursing care is mainly supportive and focuses on administering medications, preventing infection, preventing skin breakdown, meeting nutritional and fluid needs, promoting rest, and providing emotional support to the parents and child.

Administer Medications

It is important to give prescribed medications at the scheduled times. Monitor closely for side effects of corticosteroids such as moon face, increased appetite, increased hair growth, abdominal distention, and mood swings. Monitor for adverse effects of corticosteroids such as hypertension, nausea, and hyperglycemia. Corticosteroids should be tapered rather than abruptly discontinued. An evaluation of fasting blood sugar may be needed during therapy. If the child is receiving albumin intravenously, monitor closely for hypertension or signs of volume overload caused by fluid shifts. If diuretics are used, observe for shock. The child may need to have albumin infused simultaneously with diuretics.

Prevent Infection

Children with MCNS are at risk for infection because of the loss of immunoglobulins in the urine and corticosteroid therapy. Careful hand hygiene is important. Use standard precautions. Strict aseptic technique is essential during invasive procedures. Monitor the child's white blood cell count when cytotoxic drugs are given as bone marrow suppression is a side effect. Monitor vital signs carefully to detect early signs of infection that may be masked by corticosteroid therapy. Decrease the child's social contacts during immunosuppressive treatment, and caution parents and children to avoid exposure to people with respiratory infections and communicable diseases. Emphasize the importance of avoiding shopping malls, sporting arenas, grocery stores, game stores, and other public areas where the risk of exposure to such infections is increased. Immunization schedules may be altered while the child is on steroid therapy. See Chapter 16 ∞ for further discussion of immunizations.

Prevent Skin Breakdown

Meticulous skin care is essential to prevent skin breakdown and potential infection. Assess the skin repeatedly, turn the child frequently, and use therapeutic mattresses (e.g., egg crate, airflow) to help prevent skin breakdown. Keep the skin clean and dry.

Meet Nutritional and Fluid Needs

Keep the child's food preferences in mind when planning menus. Encourage the child to eat by presenting attractive meals with small portions. Socialization during meals may improve the child's appetite. Fluids are not usually restricted except during severe edema.

Nursing Alert

A normal diet for the child's age is recommended. No attempt should be made either to restrict or to increase protein intake. Sodium restriction is recommended while the child is edematous and has protein in the urine (Lane, 2009).

Promote Rest

Provide opportunities for quiet play as tolerated, such as drawing, playing board games, listening to tapes, and watching videos. Adjust the child's daily schedule to allow rest periods after activities. Signs of fatigue may include irritability, mood swings, or withdrawal. Tell the parents and child about the importance of rest. Limiting visitors during the acute phase of the illness may be necessary. Telephone and computer contacts may be encouraged as an alternative to visitors. To provide a sense of control, encourage the child to set his or her own limits on activity.

Provide Emotional Support

Parents and children often need support to cope with this chronic disease. Thoroughly explain the child's disease and treatment regimen to parents. Parental anxiety in combination with the hospitalization may interfere with the child's independence. Help parents promote the child's independence by allowing the child to choose from the menu or to select the daily activity schedule. This gives the child some sense of control.

Children with MCNS may have a distorted body image because of sudden weight gain and edema. They may refuse to look in the mirror, refuse to participate in care, and take less interest in their appearance. Encourage children to express their feelings. Help them maintain a normal appearance by promoting normal grooming routines. Encourage children to wear their own pajamas rather than hospital gowns. Scarves or hats may be used to lessen the child's edematous appearance. Adolescents can be encouraged to write their feelings in a journal as a coping mechanism. These children may have a long-term psychosocial adjustment since they have a chronic condition with concerns about potential relapse.

Discharge Planning and Home Care Teaching

Explain the disease process, prognosis, and treatment plan to parents and school-age children. Make sure parents know how to administer medications and can identify potential side effects. Inform parents about restricting fluid intake until the edema resolves. Instruct parents about the need to monitor urine daily for protein, and have them keep a diary to record the results. Monitoring the child's weight each week may help identify early stages of fluid retention. This helps parents to spot a relapse before edema occurs.

Tutoring may be required for a short period after discharge. However, encourage parents to allow the child to return to normal activities once the acute episode has resolved. Emphasize the importance of avoiding contact with people with infectious diseases, because of the child's reduced immunity. Reinforce to parents that it is important to follow the "no added salt" diet as long as the child is receiving corticosteroid therapy or shows signs of MCNS. Warn them that steroids stimulate appetite, so they need to control the child's food intake and weight gain.

Most children do well with corticosteroid therapy; however, relapses are common. Even children with frequent relapses can experience a spontaneous resolution of MCNS before 30 years of age. Children should have periodic bone density evaluations because of the repeated steroid therapy.

Evaluation

Expected outcomes of nursing care include:

- The child responds to corticosteroid therapy.
- Dietary guidelines of "no added salt" are followed and food intake is controlled during corticosteroid therapy.
- Relapses are identified by parents before generalized edema occurs.
- The child receives the additional recommended immunizations.

A discussion of Wilms tumor can be found in Chapter 24 ∞.

Acute Poststreptococcal Glomerulonephritis

Glomerulonephritis is an inflammation of the glomeruli of the kidneys related to an infection. The incidence of acute poststreptococcal glomerulonephritis (APSGN) is highest in children between 2 and 6 years of age, and the disorder is more common in boys than in girls (Nachman et al., 2008).

Etiology and Pathophysiology

The child with APSGN usually becomes ill after a nephrogenetic strain of group A beta-hemolytic streptococcal infection of the upper respiratory tract or the skin. Often the child contracts a streptococcal infection (e.g., strep throat), recovers, and then develops signs of APSGN after an interval of 10–21 days.

Glomerular damage occurs as a result of an immune complex reaction that localizes on the glomerular capillary wall. Antibody-antigen complexes become lodged in the glomeruli, leading to inflammation and obstruction. Capillaries in the glomeruli are obstructed by damaged tissue cells, and the glomerular filtration rate is reduced. Vascular permeability increases, allowing red blood cells and red cell casts to be excreted. Sodium and water are retained, expanding the intravascular and interstitial compartments and resulting in the characteristic finding of edema. See Figure 26–10 ➤.

Clinical Manifestations

Many children are asymptomatic. In other children, the onset is abrupt with flank or midabdominal pain, irritability, malaise, and fever. Hematuria, proteinuria, **azotemia** (accumulation of nitrogenous wastes in the blood), and hypertension are present in varying degrees. Microscopic hematuria is present in more than 2/3 of cases, while gross hematuria resulting in tea-colored urine occurs in others. Mild periorbital edema occurs early, along with dependent edema of the feet and ankles. Edema may progress in severity (Nachman et al., 2008). Acute hypertension may cause an encephalopathy that includes headache, nausea, vomiting, irritability, lethargy, and seizures. Oliguria may or may not be present (Huether, 2010b).

COLLABORATIVE CARE

Diagnostic Tests

The serum BUN and creatinine concentrations are elevated. Serum protein is decreased due to mild or moderate proteinuria. The white blood cell count and erythrocyte sedimentation rate may be elevated, and serum lipid levels are increased in about 40% of cases. An elevated antistreptolysin O (ASO) titer reflects the presence of antibodies from a recent pharyngeal streptococcal respiratory infection, but the ASO level associated with a recent skin infection is low. The anti-DNase B titer is helpful for detecting antibodies associated with recent skin infections. Most children have a reduced serum complement (C3) level due to the initial infection. Urinalysis reveals hematuria, proteinuria, and red and white cell casts. Anemia is common in the acute phase, usually because extracellular fluid dilutes the serum. The hemoglobin level and hematocrit value may decrease during the late phase as a result of hematuria. Renal biopsy is rarely required unless there is a progressive deterioration in renal function.

Clinical Therapy

Treatment focuses on relief of symptoms and supportive therapy. Bed rest is a key component of the treatment plan during the acute phase. Edema and mild to moderate hypertension should be treated with sodium restriction, diuretics such as furosemide, and antihypertensive medications (Huether, 2010b; Nachman et al., 2008). A course of antibiotics may be given to ensure eradication of the original infectious agent.

Fluid requirements are determined by careful monitoring of urinary output, weight, blood pressure, and serum electrolytes. Initially, only insensible fluid losses are replaced until the status of renal function is known. Dietary restriction of sodium and potassium intake may be necessary; with severe azotemia, protein intake may have to be limited.

The prognosis for most children with APSGN is good. Clinical signs, proteinuria, and hematuria resolve within several weeks. Over 95% of children will recover completely (Huether, 2010b).

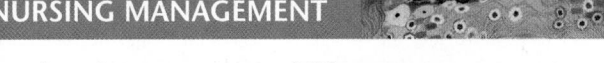

Nursing Alert

Antibiotics are *not* a treatment for acute poststreptococcal glomerulonephritis (APSGN). Instead, antibiotics are prescribed to treat the original infection.

NURSING MANAGEMENT

Nursing Assessment and Diagnoses

As with other renal disorders, care of the child with APSGN requires careful monitoring of vital signs and fluid-electrolyte balance to evaluate renal functioning and to identify complications. Frequently monitor the blood pressure, which can rise as high as 200/120 mmHg. With severe hypertension, assess for signs of central nervous system problems (headache, blurred vision, vomiting, decreased level of consciousness, confusion, and convulsions). Monitor urine for proteinuria, hematuria, and output. Assess edema, which may be periorbital or dependent and shifts as the child's position is changed. Assess for a pulmonary effusion (crackles, dyspnea, and cough).

Nursing diagnoses may include the following:

- Excess Fluid Volume related to decreased glomerular filtration and increased sodium retention
- Risk for Infection related to renal impairment and corticosteroid therapy
- Risk for Impaired Skin Integrity related to tissue edema
- Imbalanced Nutrition: Less than Body Requirements related to loss of appetite and proteinuria
- Effective Therapeutic Regimen Management related to child's medication schedule and treatment regimen after discharge

Planning and Implementation

Nursing care focuses on monitoring fluid status, preventing infection, preventing skin breakdown, meeting nutritional needs, and providing emotional support to the child and family.

Monitor Fluid Status

Monitor vital signs, fluid and electrolyte status, and intake and output. Hypovolemia can occur as a result of fluid shifting from

Pathophysiology Illustrated
Acute Poststreptococcal Glomerulonephritis

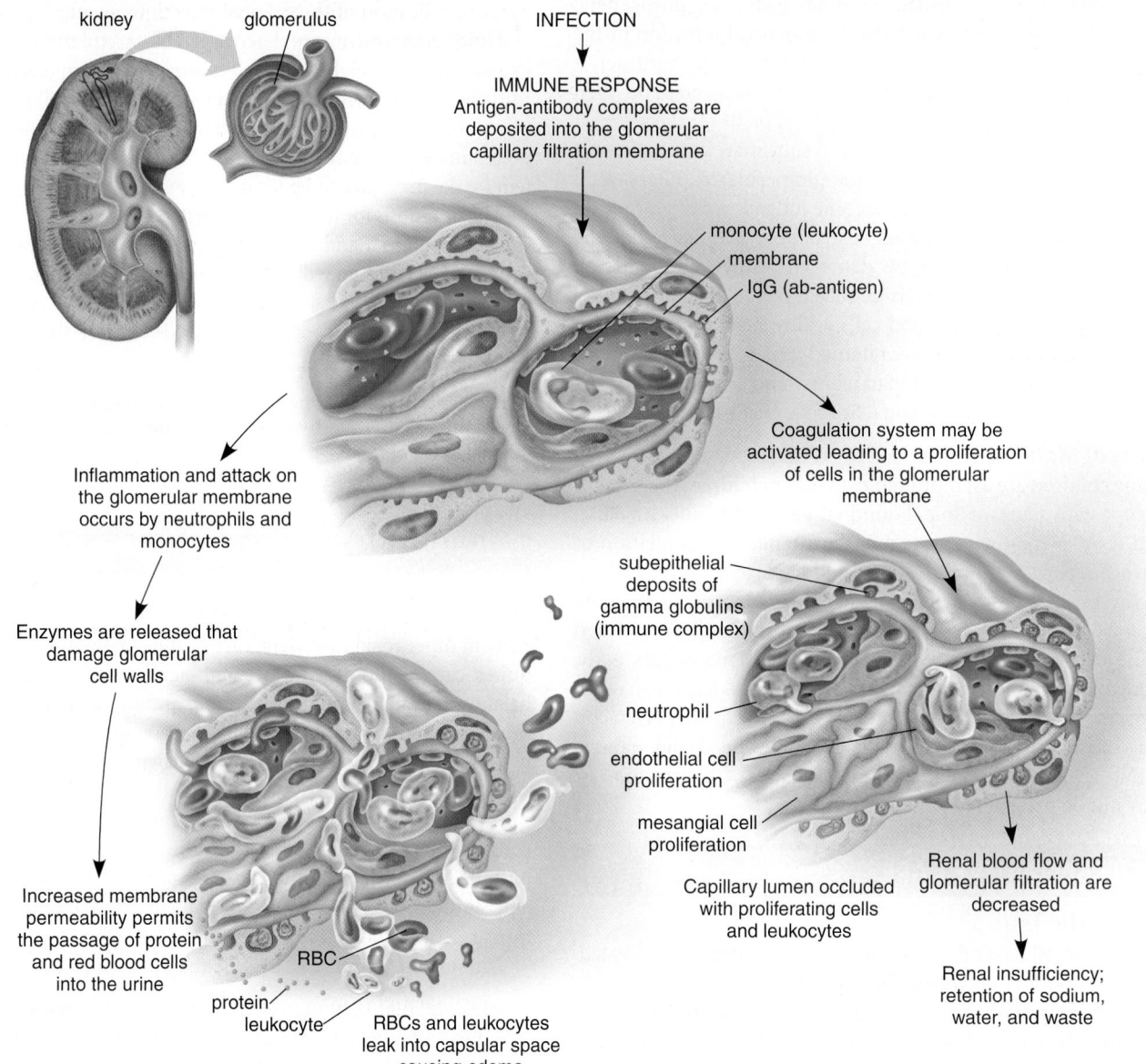

FIGURE 26–10 ➤ Infection from group A beta-hemolytic *Streptococcus* leads to an immune response that causes inflammation and damage to the glomeruli. Protein and red blood cells are allowed to pass through the glomeruli. Blood flow to the glomeruli is reduced due to obstruction with damaged cells. Renal insufficiency results, leading to the retention of sodium, water, and waste.

vascular to interstitial spaces despite the outward clinical signs of excess fluid retention. Monitor the degree of ascites by measuring abdominal girth. Document urine specific gravity. Make sure parents and visitors understand the need to limit fluids to prevent excessive intake.

Prevent Infection

Impaired renal function puts the child at risk for infection. Monitor for signs of infection, including fever, increased malaise, and an elevated white blood cell count. Instruct the family to perform good hand hygiene. Limit visitors, and screen for upper respiratory infections. Screen family members for the presence of streptococcal infection and refer for treatment, if necessary.

Prevent Skin Breakdown

Bed rest is required during the acute phase. Dependent areas or areas prone to pressure are vulnerable to skin breakdown. Turn the child frequently. Make sure the child's bed is free of crumbs or sharp toys. Keep sheets tight and free of wrinkles.

Meet Nutritional Needs

A team approach (including the nurse, renal dietitian, parents, and child) is often needed to meet the child's nutritional needs. In most cases, the child follows a "no added salt" and low-protein diet. Anorexia presents the greatest challenge to meeting daily nutritional requirements during the acute phase of the disease. To increase the child's appetite, encourage parents to bring the child's favorite foods from home, serve foods in age-appropriate quantities, and allow the child to eat with other children or with family members.

Provide Emotional Support

Parents of a child with APSGN often feel guilty. Parents may blame themselves for not responding more quickly to the child's initial symptoms or may believe they could have prevented the development of glomerular damage. Discuss the etiology of the disease and the child's treatment, and correct any misconceptions. Emphasize that it is not possible to predict which of the few children with streptococcal infection will develop APSGN.

Discharge Planning and Home Care Teaching

Children are hospitalized for a few days, but it may take 3 weeks for hypertension and gross hematuria to resolve and longer for the disorder to resolve completely. Discharge planning focuses on teaching parents about the child's medication regimen, potential side effects of medications, dietary restrictions, and signs and symptoms of complications. Teach parents how to take the child's blood pressure and how to test urine for albumin, if ordered. Emphasize that it is important to avoid exposing the child to people with upper respiratory tract infections. Advise parents to allow the child to gradually return to his or her normal routine and activities after discharge, with periods allowed for rest.

Evaluation

Expected outcomes of nursing care are the following:

- The child receives appropriate fluid volume each day and maintains or regains normal urine output.
- The child develops no areas of redness or skin breakdown.
- The child is free of fever and secondary infection.
- The child returns to pre-illness weight and tolerates daily intake that meets nutritional requirements.
- The child's sodium and potassium levels reflect adherence to dietary restrictions.

Hemolytic-Uremic Syndrome

Hemolytic-uremic syndrome (HUS) is the most common cause of acute renal failure in young children, occurring primarily in those under 4 years of age (Huether, 2010b). HUS has a classic triad of signs: (1) hemolytic anemia, (2) thrombocytopenia, and (3) renal insufficiency (Fiorino & Raffaelli, 2006).

HUS is most often caused by *Escherichia coli* strain 0157:H7, which is found in undercooked meat and unpasteurized milk and juices (Fiorino & Raffaelli, 2006; Tan & Silverberg, 2009). The bacteria has also been linked to petting zoos at fairs and festivals (Centers for Disease Control and Prevention [CDC],

2006a). Approximately 10–15% of children with this infection will develop HUS (Fiorino & Raffaelli, 2006).

E. coli strain 0157:H7 produces a toxin that attaches to the glomeruli, collecting ducts, and distal tubules. The toxin damages the lining of the glomerular arterioles, causing the endothelial cells to swell and become occluded with platelets and fibrin clots. This partial occlusion damages the red blood cells, resulting in hemolytic anemia. Platelets cluster in areas of vascular endothelial damage, causing thrombocytopenia. Glomerular filtration is decreased, resulting in hematuria and proteinuria. Oliguria and acute renal failure develop in nearly 50% of affected children with HUS (Huether, 2010b).

An episode of severe gastroenteritis with bloody diarrhea, upper respiratory infection, or UTI precedes the development of HUS by 1 to 2 weeks, followed by 1 to 5 days without symptoms. Signs and symptoms of HUS include hypertension, pallor, bruising, and oliguria. The child may also have fever, anorexia, vomiting and diarrhea, abdominal pain, mild jaundice, and edema or ascites. Neurologic involvement is indicated by irritability, lethargy, and seizures (Huether, 2010b).

The urine is tested for hematuria and proteinuria. Serum chemistries often reveal hyperkalemia and metabolic acidosis as a result of renal failure. A peripheral blood smear with fragments of red blood cells, fibrin fragments, and a decreased platelet count confirms the diagnosis. The hemoglobin is usually less than 8 g/dL and the platelet count is less than 60,000 per mL (Tan & Silverberg, 2009).

Treatment focuses on the complications of acute renal failure and includes fluid restrictions and a high-calorie, high-carbohydrate diet that is low in protein, sodium, potassium, and phosphorus. Enteral nutrition is sometimes needed. The use of antibiotics is controversial; medications may include calcium gluconate or calcium chloride, aluminum hydroxide gel to bind to phosphorus, Kayexalate to remove excess potassium, and antihypertensive agents. Transfusions of fresh packed red blood cells may be ordered to treat severe anemia. Platelets are given if the child is bleeding or if surgery is needed. Transfusions are carefully administered to prevent hypertension caused by hypervolemia. About 40–50% of children with HUS need dialysis and approximately 3–5% of those affected will die (Fiorino & Rafaelli, 2006). Peritoneal dialysis is preferred unless the child has severe colitis and abdominal tenderness. Some children may develop chronic renal failure; however, most regain normal renal function (Huether, 2010b).

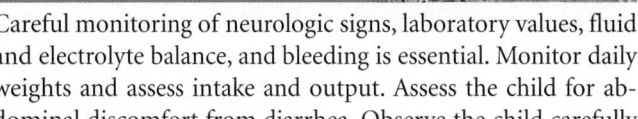

NURSING MANAGEMENT

Careful monitoring of neurologic signs, laboratory values, fluid and electrolyte balance, and bleeding is essential. Monitor daily weights and assess intake and output. Assess the child for abdominal discomfort from diarrhea. Observe the child carefully for signs of progressive renal impairment.

Discharge planning focuses on teaching parents about medications and dietary and fluid restrictions. Follow-up visits are necessary to evaluate the effectiveness of the treatment plan. Teach parents that HUS can be largely prevented by cooking ground beef to 155°F throughout, meaning no rare hamburgers.

Teach them to wash hands carefully when handling raw ground meats, and to make sure utensils and food preparation surfaces touching raw meat do not come into contact with cooked meats.

Polycystic Kidney Disease

Polycystic kidney disease (PKD) is a genetic disorder that has autosomal recessive and autosomal dominant forms. Liver abnormalities are associated with both forms of the disease. The incidence of the autosomal recessive form is 1 per 20,000 births (Salant & Patel, 2008). The autosomal dominant form is one of the most frequently inherited diseases and is the most common inherited renal disorder in the United States, with a prevalence of 1 in 800 live births (Rizk & Chapman, 2008; Watnick & Morrison, 2007). The autosomal dominant PKD results from mutations on the PKD1 locus on chromosome 16 and PKD2 on chromosome 4. The autosomal recessive gene (PKHD1) is located on chromosome 6 (National Kidney and Urologic Diseases Information Clearinghouse, 2009).

In PKD, cellular hyperplasia of the collecting ducts causes them to dilate. Fluid secreted into these ducts enables cyst sacs to form. Initially, cysts are usually less than 2 mm in size and do not obstruct urinary flow. As the child grows, however, the cysts become larger and fibrosis occurs. The cysts slowly replace much of the kidney's mass and reduce kidney function. Tubular atrophy may occur in some children, whereas others have minimal changes in renal function. PKD is associated with liver abnormalities that progress to fibrosis, portal hypertension, and biliary infection, which become more severe with age.

Newborns with autosomal recessive PKD may have enlarged kidneys, detected at birth. Those with the most severe form of the disease die in the neonatal period from pulmonary hypoplasia (Salant & Patel, 2008). Clinical manifestations in infants with autosomal recessive PKD include Potter facies (low-set ears, small jaw, and a flattened nose). Hypertension develops in early infancy and is often severe. Infants may have expected urine output or **oliguria** (urine output less than 0.5 to 1 mL/kg/hr). Respiratory distress and feeding intolerance may develop from the enlarged kidneys (Davis & Avner, 2007). As **uremia** (excess of urea and other nitrogenous waste products in the blood) develops, infants and children develop renal **osteodystrophy** (a complex bone disease process of chronic kidney disease in which there is increased resorption of bone caused by chronic hyperparathyroidism) and progressive developmental delay and growth failure.

Sonogram or renal biopsy confirms the diagnosis. The disease is often diagnosed on prenatal ultrasound. Liver function tests are usually normal initially. A liver biopsy may also be performed. Other family members should be screened for subclinical cases of PKD.

Treatment is supportive. Medications such as diuretics are prescribed for hypertension, and fluid and electrolyte abnormalities are managed. Many children develop end-stage renal disease by 10 years of age. Renal dialysis or transplant prolong survival; however, liver problems may continue to complicate the child's health, even when the renal condition is well controlled. Up to 20–30% of children die by age 15 years (Davis & Avner, 2007).

NURSING MANAGEMENT

Nursing care is the same as that for the child with renal insufficiency and chronic renal failure. Observe the child for signs of progressive renal impairment. Make sure the family schedules and keeps follow-up appointments to assess growth, developmental progress, and the effectiveness of the treatment plan. Family teaching for home management focuses on medications, a diet adequate in protein and calories to support growth, management of acute gastrointestinal illnesses to prevent dehydration, and care for the child with progressive renal insufficiency and a liver disorder. Since the disease is inherited, the family should be referred for genetic counseling.

Renal Failure

Renal failure, which may be acute or chronic, occurs when the kidney is unable to excrete wastes and concentrate urine. Acute renal failure occurs suddenly (over days or weeks) and may be reversible, whereas in chronic renal failure, kidney function diminishes gradually and permanently over months or years.

Both types of renal failure are characterized by azotemia and sometimes oliguria, indicating the kidney's inability to excrete metabolic waste products. The degree of renal impairment is estimated by the glomerular filtration rate (Miller & MacDonald, 2006). Uremia occurs when there is an excess of urea and other nitrogenous waste products in the blood.

Acute Renal Failure

Acute renal failure (ARF) is a sudden loss of adequate renal function in which the kidneys are unable to clear metabolic wastes and to regulate extracellular fluid volume, sodium balance, and acid-base homeostasis. ARF is seen in 2–3% of children cared for in pediatric intensive care units, and up to 8% of infants cared for in neonatal intensive care units (Vogt & Avner, 2007b). Potential causes include hemolytic uremic syndrome, acute glomerulonephritis, sepsis, poisoning, nephrotoxic medications, hypovolemia, obstructive uropathy, and complication of cardiac surgery.

Etiology and Pathophysiology   ARF is a result of decreased perfusion to an otherwise normal kidney in association with a systemic condition. ARF may be caused by prerenal or postrenal factors as well as actual kidney damage (Figure 26–11 ➤).

- Prerenal ARF is a result of decreased perfusion to an otherwise normal kidney in association with a systemic condition. Hypovolemia secondary to dehydration is generally the cause; however, alterations in renal vasculature or cardiac function may also precipitate prerenal ARF. This is the most common type of ARF in infants and young children (Lum, 2007).
- Primary kidney damage (intrinsic factors) may result from infection, diseases such as hemolytic-uremic syndrome or acute glomerulonephritis, cortical necrosis, nephrotoxic drugs, or accidental ingestion of drugs or poisons. The structure most susceptible to damage is the kidney tubule. Injury to the tubule resulting in acute tubular necrosis is the most frequent cause of intrinsic renal failure in children (Lum, 2007).

Pathophysiology Illustrated
Acute Renal Failure

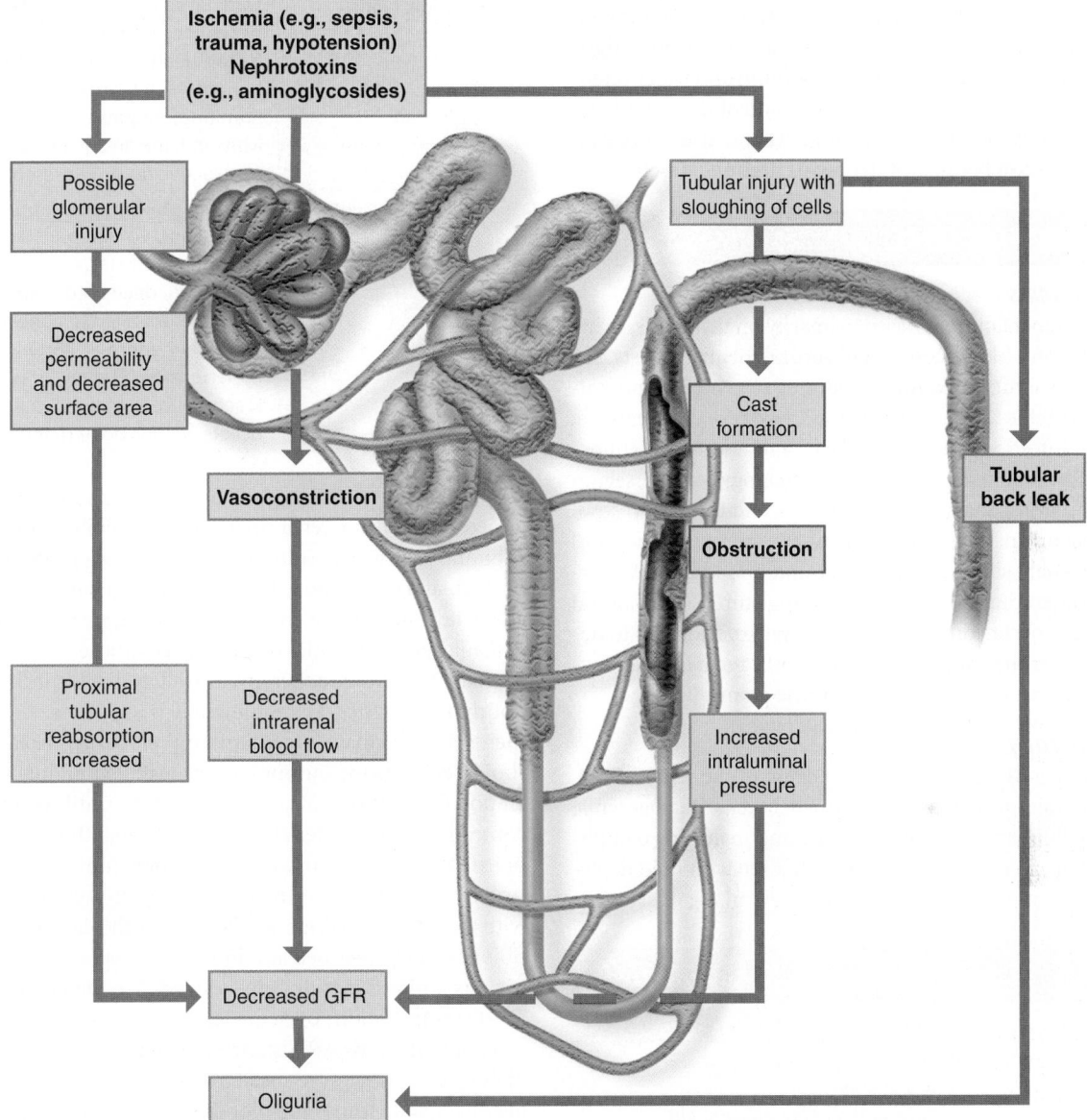

FIGURE 26–11 ➤ The initial kidney injury is usually associated with an acute condition such as sepsis, trauma, and hypotension, or is the result of treatment for an acute condition with nephrotoxic medication. Injury to the kidney can occur because of glomerular injury, vasoconstriction of capillaries, or tubular injury. All consequences of injury lead to decreased glomerular filtration and oliguria.

• Postrenal ARF is caused by obstruction of the urinary flow from both kidneys, such as occurs in posterior urethral valves or a neurogenic bladder. Children may have oliguria, or normal or increased urine output. Renal failure without oliguria usually indicates a less severe renal injury. Children who recover from ARF may have residual kidney damage and compromised renal function.

Clinical Manifestations Characteristically, a healthy child suddenly becomes ill with nonspecific symptoms that indicate a significant illness or injury (e.g., nausea, vomiting, lethargy,

Nursing Alert

Nephrotoxic drugs include the following:

■ Antimicrobials: aminoglycosides, cephalosporins, tetracycline, sulfonamides
■ Radiographic contrast media with iodine (typically used for CT scans)
■ Heavy metals: lead, barium, iron, chromium
■ Nonsteroidal anti-inflammatory drugs (NSAIDs): indomethacin, aspirin, ibuprofen

edema, gross hematuria, oliguria, and hypertension). These symptoms are a result of electrolyte imbalances, uremia, and fluid overload. The child appears pale and lethargic. See the Clinical Manifestations table for more information.

Hyperkalemia is the most life-threatening electrolyte disorder associated with ARF. Hyponatremia affects central nervous system function, resulting in symptoms that range from fatigue to seizures. Edema occurs as a result of sodium and water retention. (Refer to Chapter 18 ∞ for a discussion of these fluid and electrolyte alterations.) Children with ARF are also more susceptible to infection because of depressed immune functioning.

COLLABORATIVE CARE

Diagnostic Tests

Diagnosis of renal failure is based primarily on urinalysis, urine culture, complete blood count, and serum chemistry tests, including BUN, serum creatinine, sodium, potassium, and calcium levels (Table 26–4). These tests may reveal hematuria, proteinuria, infection, anemia, acidosis, and electrolyte abnormalities. Additional tests may include toxicology screens, serum complement levels, antinuclear antibodies, and blood and stool cultures (Boydstun, 2005). The kidneys are normal in size and no signs of renal osteodystrophy are found on radiograph. Various imaging studies to assess kidney structures, renal blood flow, and renal perfusion and function may be performed to determine whether the child has ARF or chronic renal failure. A renal biopsy may be required to examine the glomeruli.

Clinical Therapy

Treatment depends on the underlying cause of the renal failure. The goal is to minimize or prevent permanent renal damage while maintaining fluid and electrolyte balance and managing complications. Initial emergency treatment of children with fluid depletion focuses on rapid fluid replacement at 20 mL/kg of saline or

Clinical Manifestations
Acute Versus Chronic Renal Failure

Type of Renal Failure	Clinical Manifestations
Acute renal failure	Dark urine or gross hematuria, headache, edema, fatigue, crackles, gallop heart rhythm, hypertension, hematuria, lethargy, nausea and vomiting, oliguria Mass in flank area if a cyst, tumor, or obstructive lesion is present
Chronic renal failure	Fatigue, malaise, poor appetite, nausea and vomiting, failure to thrive or short stature Headache, decreased mental alertness or ability to concentrate, secondary enuresis, chronic anemia, hypertension, edema Fractures with minimal trauma, rickets, valgus bone deformity

lactated Ringer's solution given over 5 to 10 minutes and repeated as needed to ensure renal perfusion and stabilize blood pressure. Albumin may also be administered when blood loss is the cause of circulatory depletion. If oliguria persists after restoration of adequate fluid volume, intrinsic renal damage is suspected.

Children with fluid overload, like those with pulmonary edema, need diuretic therapy, as well as dialysis if they respond poorly to diuretics. Once the child is stabilized, fluid requirements are calculated to maintain *zero water balance* (intake should equal urine output and insensible fluid loss). Eliminate all potential sources of potassium intake until hyperkalemia is controlled (see Chapter 18 ∞). Remember that catabolic states or extensive tissue injury may raise potassium levels. Other electrolyte imbalances are treated. Nutrition must be maintained with extra carbohydrate intake during the catabolic state. Antibiotics are prescribed for infection. Nephrotoxic antibiotics such as aminoglycosides are avoided. See Medications Used to Treat Complications of Acute Renal Failure.

Children whose ARF is unresponsive to management require dialysis to correct severe electrolyte imbalances, manage fluid overload, and cleanse the blood of waste products. The clinical situation and age of the child determine whether hemodialysis or peritoneal dialysis is used. Refer to the renal replacement therapy section on page 832.

Prognosis depends on the cause of ARF. When renal failure results from drug toxicity or dehydration, the prognosis is generally good. However, ARF that results from diseases such as hemolytic-uremic syndrome or acute glomerulonephritis may be associated with residual kidney damage.

NURSING MANAGEMENT

Nursing Assessment and Diagnoses

A complete history and physical examination are necessary to identify progression of symptoms and possible causes for renal failure.

TABLE 26–4	Diagnostic Tests for Renal Failure
Diagnostic Tests	Findings in Renal Failure
Urinalysis	
pH	Acidic urine
Osmolarity	Greater than 500: prerenal ARF Less than 350: intrinsic ARF
Specific gravity	High: prerenal ARF Low: intrinsic ARF Normal: postrenal ARF
Protein	Positive
Serum Chemistry*	
Potassium	Elevated
Sodium	Normal, low, or high, depends solely on the amount of water in the body
Calcium	Low
Phosphorus	High
Urea nitrogen	Increased
Creatinine	Increased
pH	Low acidic

*Refer to Appendix D ∞ for normal values for various ages. ARF = acute renal failure.

Clinical Manifestations
Electrolyte Imbalances in Acute and Chronic Renal Failure

Electrolyte Imbalance and Cause	Clinical Manifestations
Hyperkalemia Results from inability to adequately excrete potassium derived from diet and catabolized cells. In metabolic acidosis, potassium also moves from intracellular fluid to extracellular fluid.	▪ Peaked T waves, widening of QRS waves on ECG ▪ Dysrhythmias: ventricular dysrhythmias, heart block, ventricular fibrillation, cardiac arrest ▪ Diarrhea ▪ Muscle weakness
Hyponatremia In the acute oliguric phase, hyponatremia is dilutional, related to the accumulation of fluid in excess of solute.	▪ Change in level of consciousness ▪ Muscle cramps ▪ Anorexia ▪ Abdominal reflexes, depressed deep tendon reflexes ▪ Cheyne-Stokes respirations ▪ Seizures
Hypocalcemia Phosphate retention (hyperphosphatemia) due to impaired renal function depresses the serum calcium concentration. Calcium is deposited in injured cells. Hyperkalemia and metabolic acidosis may mask the common clinical manifestations of severe hypocalcemia.	▪ Muscle tingling ▪ Changes in muscle tone ▪ Seizures ▪ Muscle cramps and twitching ▪ Positive Chvostek sign (contraction of facial muscles after tapping facial nerve just anterior to parotid gland)

Physiologic Assessment

Assess vital signs, level of consciousness, and other neurologic indicators to help identify clinical signs of electrolyte imbalance (see the Clinical Manifestations table). Measure the child's weight on admission to provide a baseline for evaluating changes in fluid status. Monitor urinalysis, urine culture, and blood chemistry studies. Inspect urine for color. Cloudy urine may indicate infection; tea-colored urine suggests hematuria. Assess urine specific gravity as well as intake and output.

Psychosocial Assessment

The unexpected and acute nature of the child's hospitalization creates anxiety for both parents and the child. Assess for feelings of anger, guilt, or fear associated with the hospitalization. Such

Medications Used to Treat
Complications of Acute Renal Failure

Complication	Medication/Action or Indication	Nursing Management
Hyperkalemia (greater than 5.8 mmol/L)	*Kayexalate* Exchanges sodium for potassium	May require up to 4 hours to take effect.
	Calcium gluconate 10%, IV Counteracts potassium-induced increased myocardial irritability	Monitor for ECG changes. Intravenous infiltration may result in tissue necrosis.
	Albuterol Beta-agonist effects cause potassium to be shifted into the cells	Give by aerosol.
Metabolic acidosis	*Sodium bicarbonate or sodium citrate* Helps correct metabolic acidosis by exchanging hydrogen for potassium	*Do not mix with calcium.* Complications include fluid overload, hypertension, and tetany.
Hypocalcemia (less than 2.2 mmol/L)	*Calcium gluconate 10%* Used in presence of tetany; provides ionized calcium to restore nervous tissue function to control serum phosphorus	Administer slowly to prevent bradycardia. Monitor for ECG changes.
Malignant hypertension (blood pressure greater than 95% for age, sex, and height percentile)	*Sodium nitroprusside, nitroglycerin* Relaxes smooth muscle in peripheral arterioles	Administer by continuous intravenous infusion; fall in blood pressure is seen within 10–20 minutes.

feelings are likely if ARF developed as a result of dehydration, a preventable injury, or poisoning. Assess coping mechanisms, family support systems, and level of stress.

Several nursing diagnoses may apply to the child with ARF, including:

- Ineffective Renal Tissue Perfusion related to hypovolemia, sepsis, or drug toxicity
- Excess Fluid Volume related to renal dysfunction and sodium retention
- Imbalanced Nutrition: Less than Body Requirements related to anorexia, nausea, vomiting, and catabolic state
- Risk for Infection related to invasive procedures and monitoring equipment, and diminished immune functioning
- Compromised Family Coping related to sudden hospitalization and uncertain prognosis of child

Planning and Implementation

Nursing care focuses on preventing complications, maintaining fluid balance, administering medications, meeting nutritional needs, preventing infection, and providing emotional support to the child and parents.

Prevent Complications

Careful monitoring of vital signs, intake and output, serum electrolytes, and level of consciousness can alert the nurse to changes that indicate potential complications.

Clinical Tip

The child with renal insufficiency is at greater risk for fluid loss with illness. In cases of acute gastrointestinal illness, these children are at greater risk for dehydration and ARF.

Maintain Fluid Balance

Estimate the child's fluid status by daily monitoring of weight (on the same scale at the same time of day), intake and output, and blood pressure two or three times a day. Also monitor serum chemistry values, especially for sodium. The aim of maintaining fluid balance is to achieve a stable serum sodium concentration and a decrease in body weight by 0.5–1% a day.

If the child has oliguria, limit fluid intake, including parenteral nutrition, to replacement of insensible fluid loss (what is excreted by the lungs, skin, and gastrointestinal tract), which is about one third the daily maintenance requirements in afebrile children. If the child is febrile, fluid administration is increased by 12% for each centigrade degree of temperature elevation.

Administer Medications

Because the kidney's ability to excrete drugs is impaired in ARF, dosages of all medications should be adjusted. The actual dosage of the drug may be reduced or the time interval between doses may be increased. Check drug levels to monitor for drug toxicity. Know the signs of drug toxicity for each medication the child is receiving.

Meet Nutritional Needs

Children are at risk for malnutrition because of their high metabolic rate during ARF. Parenteral or enteral feeding may be used initially to minimize protein catabolism. The diet is tailored to the individual child's need for calories, carbohydrates, fats, and amino acids or protein hydrolysates. Depending on the degree of renal failure, the diet may need to restrict sodium, potassium, and phosphorus. Initiate oral feeding as soon as the child can tolerate it.

Prevent Infection

The child with ARF is extremely susceptible to nosocomial infections because of altered nutritional status, compromised immunity, and numerous invasive procedures. Good hand hygiene and standard precautions are imperative to decrease the risk of infection. Use sterile technique for all invasive procedures and when caring for lines. Drainage from catheter sites should be cultured to check for the presence of infectious organisms. Assess vital signs and lung sounds frequently.

Provide Emotional Support

The sudden onset of ARF presents parents with an unexpected threat to their child's life. Both the child and the parents experience anxiety because of the unexpected hospitalization and the uncertain prognosis. Parents often feel guilty, regardless of the cause of renal failure. This guilt is intensified when renal failure is a result of dehydration or poisoning. Encourage parents to verbalize their fears and help them work through feelings of guilt. Explain procedures and treatment measures to decrease anxiety. Encouraging parents and older siblings to participate in the child's care can increase their sense of control.

Discharge Planning and Home Care Teaching

Encourage parental involvement early in the child's hospitalization. Be sure parents understand the importance of administering medications correctly. Teach family members proper technique for measuring blood pressure so they can monitor the child's blood pressure for hypertension, if ordered. Make sure the parents can identify signs of progressive renal failure (see the following discussion of chronic renal failure).

Diet counseling is a key component of discharge planning and is usually performed by a renal dietitian. Depending on the degree of renal failure, the child's diet may include restrictions on protein, water, sodium, potassium, and phosphorus. The parents should be given written guidelines listing appropriate food choices to assist in menu planning. Ethnic and cultural preferences should be considered in listing menu options.

Continued monitoring of renal function during follow-up examinations is critical as deterioration may occur over time.

Culture *Sodium*

Special effort is often needed to reduce the sodium in the diet of a child eating predominantly Asian cuisine. Sauces and seasonings for foods (soy sauce, mustards, monosodium glutamate, and garlic salt) are sodium rich even though the foods seasoned (rice, vegetables, shrimp, and chicken) are low in sodium. A child eating a diet of predominantly Mexican cuisine may also require significant modification. Individualized counseling and motivation are needed to encourage families to reduce the child's sodium intake and to use spices low in sodium when preparing meals.

Referral to support groups can be helpful for both parents and children. The National Kidney Foundation is a source of numerous publications.

Evaluation

Expected outcomes of nursing care include:

- The child's fluid status is balanced with edema-associated weight loss. Electrolyte and acid-base balance is restored.
- Nutritional needs are met.
- The child acquires no secondary infections.

Chronic Renal Failure

Chronic renal failure (CRF) is a progressive, irreversible reduction in kidney function. The prevalence of CRF is approximately 18 per 1 million children (Vogt & Avner, 2007b).

Etiology and Pathophysiology   In children, CRF usually results from developmental abnormalities of the kidney or obstructed urine flow and reflux, hereditary diseases such as polycystic kidney disease, infections such as hemolytic-uremic syndrome, and glomerulonephritis (Lum, 2007).

The gradual, progressive loss of functioning nephrons ultimately results in **end-stage renal disease (ESRD)**, the most advanced form of CRF. ESRD is characterized by minimal renal function (less than 10% of normal), uremic syndrome, anemia, and abnormal blood values. In ESRD, the kidneys can no longer maintain homeostasis and the child requires dialysis.

The kidneys excrete excess acid in the body and regulate the body's fluid and electrolyte balance. Renal failure disrupts this fluid and electrolyte balance. As renal failure progresses, metabolic acidosis occurs because the kidneys cannot excrete the acids that build up in the body. Retention of excessive sodium and water is a common cause of the elevated blood pressure associated with CRF.

Renal osteodystrophy occurs as the kidneys are unable to produce activated vitamin D and to excrete phosphorus, causing phosphorus levels to rise and serum calcium levels to fall. The parathyroid gland responds by drawing calcium and phosphorus from the bones to maintain the adequate serum calcium and phosphorus levels. Hypocalcemia may occur as the parathyroid glands become less responsive to vitamin D and lower serum calcium levels. Osteodystrophy increases the child's risk for fractures and bone deformities (Miller & MacDonald, 2006).

Growth retardation is caused by disturbances in the metabolism of calcium, phosphorus, and vitamin D; decreased caloric intake; and metabolic acidosis. The kidneys also produce erythropoietin (the growth factor responsible for the production and maturation of red cells); lack of erythropoietin and progressive renal disease are the underlying causes of the anemia of CRF.

Clinical Manifestations   Children with CRF frequently have no symptoms initially. Early renal failure with a glomerular filtration rate (GFR) of 50–75% of normal has few or no clinical signs. As progression continues, renal insufficiency occurs with polyuria as the kidneys cannot concentrate the urine. Symptoms such as pallor, headache, nausea, and fatigue become more classic. Decreased mental alertness and ability to concentrate may be seen. The child may have anemia leading to tachycardia, tachypnea, and dyspnea on exertion. As the disease progresses, the child loses his or her appetite and has complications of renal impairment, including hypertension, pulmonary edema, growth retardation, osteodystrophy, delayed fine and gross motor development, and delayed sexual maturation. Contrast these signs with those of acute renal failure on the Clinical Manifestations table on page 826.

In ESRD, the most advanced form of CRF, renal failure adversely affects all body systems. As the severity of the clinical and biochemical disturbances resulting from progressive renal deterioration increases, uremic symptoms develop. Signs and symptoms of uremic syndrome include nausea and vomiting, progressive anemia, anorexia, dyspnea, malaise, **uremic frost** (urea crystals deposited on the skin), unpleasant (uremic) breath odor, headache, progressive confusion, tremors, pulmonary edema, and congestive heart failure.

COLLABORATIVE CARE

Diagnostic Tests

Laboratory evaluation, including serum electrolytes, phosphate, BUN, creatinine levels, and pH, is used to confirm the diagnosis of chronic kidney disease and the stage of CRF. An early morning urine sample is collected for culture and to calculate the protein-to-creatinine ratio. The child's GFR is calculated from prediction equations using the serum creatinine level and the patient's height and gender. An online GFR calculator is available through the National Kidney Foundation.

Imaging studies are performed to identify renal diseases that could be causing the renal failure. A renal biopsy may sometimes be performed.

Clinical Therapy

CRF is irreversible. However, the course of the disease is variable. Some children progress quickly to renal failure, necessitating dialysis. Other children are managed with a combination of medication and diet therapy for some time before significant renal impairment occurs. Frequent modifications in the treatment plan are often necessary to address the child's changing status.

Dietary management focuses on maximizing caloric intake for growth while limiting phosphorus, potassium, and sodium intake as needed to maintain electrolytes in balance (Vogt & Avner, 2007b). Adequate calcium needs to be part of the meal plan. Enteral or parenteral feedings may be required to achieve optimal protein intake, especially in children under 1 year of age. When CRF is present, extra high-quality protein such as meat, fish, poultry, milk, and eggs is needed to support growth. Optimal protein intake for children is 2.5 g/kg/day (Vogt & Avner, 2007b). Complex carbohydrates should be chosen along with vegetables and fruits that are lower in potassium. Vegetable oils, hard candy, sugar, honey, and jelly may be recommended to add calories to the child's diet.

Medications used in the management of chronic renal failure are discussed in the Medications table on page 830. (See

Complementary Therapy: Herbal Supplements and Children with Chronic Renal Failure.

Children who progress to ESRD require renal replacement therapy. The timetable for dialysis or renal transplantation is different from that of adults; transplantation is the goal so the child has an optimal chance for a more normal childhood. Earlier initiation can prevent some complications of ESRD. In addition to the GFR, nonspecific signs such as uremic syndrome, poorly controlled hypertension, renal osteodystrophy, failure of head circumference measurement to increase normally, developmental delay, and poor growth are used in determining when to initiate therapy. (Refer to the Renal Replacement Therapy section later in this chapter.) Infection is the most common morbidity in children receiving renal replacement therapy (Chavers, Solid, Gilbertson, et al., 2007).

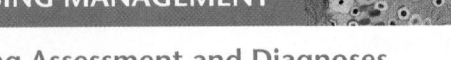

NURSING MANAGEMENT

Nursing Assessment and Diagnoses

Nursing assessment focuses on identifying signs and symptoms of renal failure and associated complications, and assessing the psychosocial effects of renal failure on the child and family.

Physiologic Assessment

The initial and ongoing assessment of the child focuses on identifying complications of renal failure. Observe for signs of edema, poor growth and development, osteodystrophy, and anemia. Assess vital signs, particularly the blood pressure. Observe for signs of electrolyte alterations (see page 827).

Psychosocial Assessment

As renal disease progresses, the number of stressors on the child and family increases. Denial and disbelief are commonly the first reactions. A thorough family assessment can help to identify particular needs of the child and family (see Chapter 2 ∞). The development of ESRD is particularly challenging during childhood and adolescence because of differences in appearance and social, psychological, and physical issues. Nonadherence with treatments can endanger the adolescent's life.

Nursing diagnoses for the child with CRF are similar to those previously listed for ARF. Additional diagnoses might include:

- Delayed Growth and Development related to decreased protein and caloric intake and loss of protein in dialysate

Medications Used to Treat
Children with Chronic Renal Failure

Medication/Action or Indication	Nursing Management
Vitamin and mineral supplement (Nephrocaps) Add vitamins and minerals missing from heavily restricted diet	Only prescribed vitamins should be used; over-the-counter brands may contain elements that are harmful.
Phosphate-binding agents: Calcium carbonate (Tums), calcium acetate (PhosLo), or sevelamer hydrochloride (Renagel) Reduce absorption of phosphorus from the intestines	Ensure that phosphate-binding agent is aluminum-free.
Calcitriol (Rocaltrol) Replace the calcitriol the kidneys are no longer producing to keep calcium balance normal	Monitor serum calcium level. Ensure that calcium supplement is provided.
Epoetin alfa (Epogen, Procrit) Stimulates bone marrow to produce red blood cells, treats anemia due to CRF	Given by IV or subcutaneous injection. Monitor blood pressure as hypertension is an adverse effect. Monitor hematocrit and serum ferritin level according to facility guidelines.
Iron supplementation Treat iron deficiency when epoetin alfa is prescribed	May be administered orally or IV during hemodialysis.
Growth hormone (rhGH) Used to stimulate growth in children with CRF	Record accurate height measurements at regular intervals.
Antihypertensive agents: Angiotensin-converting enzyme (ACE) inhibitor (enalapril, lisinopril) *Loop diuretics* Used with proteinuric kidney disease as it slows the progression to ESRD; used when volume overload is present	Monitor renal function and electrolyte balance.

NURSING CARE PLAN

The Child Receiving Home Peritoneal Dialysis

INTERVENTION	RATIONALE	EXPECTED OUTCOME
1. Nursing Diagnosis: Imbalanced Nutrition: Less than Body Requirements related to poor appetite, feeling of fullness after a small amount, and loss of protein in dialysate		
NIC Priority Intervention: *Nutrition management:* Assistance with or provision of a balanced dietary intake of foods and fluids		**NOC Suggested Outcome:** *Nutrition status:* Food and fluid intake: Amount of food and fluid taken into the body over a 24-hour period
Goal: The child will obtain adequate nutrients each day.		
■ Develop a meal plan in collaboration with a nutritionist to identify the amounts of essential nutrients needed and foods that provide them.	■ Parents need concrete guidelines for food preparation.	The child's intake is adequate for an expected growth pattern to be maintained.
■ Provide small, frequent meals of needed nutrients.	■ The child will feel full with smaller amounts of food because of the dialysate.	
■ Make mealtimes pleasant and avoid battles over the child's intake.	■ The child will be more inclined to eat if there is less stress.	
■ Provide supplements by tube feeding if adequate oral intake is not possible.	■ Adequate nutrition is important for growth and development, and must be supported if oral intake is inadequate.	
2. Nursing Diagnosis: Risk for Infection related to daily invasive procedure		
NIC Priority Intervention: *Infection control:* Minimizing the acquisition and transmission of infectious agents		**NOC Suggested Outcome:** *Infection status:* Presence and extent of infection
Goal: The child will not develop peritonitis.		
■ Wash hands; use sterile gloves and aseptic technique for connection and disconnection of catheters.	■ Aseptic technique reduces the chance of introducing bacteria into the abdomen.	The child does not develop peritonitis.
■ Perform daily catheter site care.	■ Skin around the catheter site will have fewer organisms that could potentially cause infection.	
Goal: If peritonitis occurs, it will be treated appropriately.		
■ Observe for signs of infection (fever, abdominal pain, cloudy dialysate).	■ Early identification of infection will reduce complications.	Hospitalization will not be needed for peritonitis due to early identification and prompt treatment.
■ Report signs of infection to the physician immediately.	■ Rapid intervention may reduce the need for hospitalization.	
3. Nursing Diagnosis: Caregiver Role Strain related to daily dialysis treatments		
NIC Priority Intervention: *Caregiver support:* Provision of necessary information, advocacy, and support to facilitate primary patient care by someone other than a healthcare professional		**NOC Suggested Outcome:** *Caregiver performance:* Direct care: Provision by family care provider of appropriate personal and healthcare for a family member or significant other
Goal: The family copes with daily demands for the child's dialysis treatments.		
■ Discuss the importance of daily, consistent dialysis treatments for the child's overall health status.	■ If parents understand the need for consistent dialysis treatments, they are more likely to adhere to guidelines.	The family adheres to daily dialysis treatment guidelines.
■ Collaborate with the family to identify strategies that could reduce the impact of dialysis on the family's life.	■ When the family participates in planning care, adherence is more likely.	
■ Refer the family to local support groups for emotional support, treatment strategies, and respite care.	■ Support groups may help the family develop effective coping strategies.	

Nursing Alert

Monitor the child receiving hemodialysis for complications that can occur suddenly:

■ Hypotension. Sudden nausea and vomiting, abdominal cramping, tachycardia, and dizziness
■ Rapid fluid and electrolyte exchange. Muscle cramping, nausea and vomiting, and dizziness
■ Disequilibrium syndrome. Restlessness, headache, nausea and vomiting, blurred vision, muscle twitching, and altered level of consciousness

daily nutritional needs. Review ways to reduce the risk of infection, including daily care of the catheter site. Encourage showering rather than tub baths. Activities such as swimming may be discouraged.

Kidney Transplantation

Kidney transplantation provides the only alternative to long-term dialysis for children with ESRD. It can normalize physiology and may let children grow normally. Because delaying transplantation has adverse effects on growth and development, children are given some priority over adults awaiting transplantation. Blood type compatibility between the donor and recipient is essential for a transplant to be successful. A human leukocyte antigen (HLA) system match also improves survival of the graft. A living relative donor kidney has a higher survival rate than a cadaver kidney. Children and their families are carefully screened prior to transplantation in an effort to identify problems that could lead to rejection of the kidney or infection that could be life threatening if the immune system is suppressed.

After transplantation, the child must take immunosuppressive medications such as corticosteroids, azathioprine, cyclosporine, tacrolimus, and polyclonal antibodies, as well as monoclonal antibodies to suppress rejection. See Chapter 22 ∞. Immunosuppression regimens use various combinations and sequences of these drugs to reduce the incidence of acute and chronic rejection. Rejection is a major cause of transplanted kidney loss (Vogler, Wang, Brink, et al., 2007).

Nursing Alert

A large adult kidney is frequently transplanted into the child. This results in increased renal reserve. Clinical signs of rejection may be masked (Vogler et al., 2007). Signs of rejection include fever, increased BUN and serum creatinine levels, pain and tenderness over the abdomen, irritability, and weight gain.

Complications of immunosuppression therapy include opportunistic infection, lymphomas and skin cancer, and hypertension. Nonadherence to therapy is the primary cause of transplanted kidney loss (in 10–15% of pediatric kidney transplant recipients). Nonadherence is highest among families with crises or who do not provide adequate support, and in adolescents who are responsible for taking their medications or have mild cognitive impairment or depression (Feinstein, Keich, Becker-Cohen, et al., 2005). Adherence is higher in adolescents when their parents are

knowledgeable and supportive, and when they promote the adolescent to become competent in self-care. Some primary kidney diseases, such as glomerulonephritis and hemolytic-uremic syndrome, can also recur in the transplanted kidney.

Nursing management includes teaching parents about the transplantation process before it occurs to help prepare them for the experience. Discuss all aspects of the child's care that will have an impact on the family's life, including follow-up appointments, medications, and general health promotion. Monitor adherence to the immunosuppression treatment at each visit in an effort to identify issues early. Teach parents about the signs of acute and chronic rejection and infection, including when and how to notify the child's physician if immediate care is required.

■ STRUCTURAL DEFECTS OF THE REPRODUCTIVE SYSTEM

Phimosis

In **phimosis**, the foreskin over the glans penis cannot be retracted. As a result of natural adhesion, phimosis is a normal finding in uncircumcised infants and young males. Generally the foreskin separates from the glans during childhood, and intermittent erections lead to physiologic foreskin retraction. Obstruction to urine flow may occur when there is narrowing of the preputial opening causing a dribbling stream. **Balanitis** (inflammation or infection of the glans penis) may occur as a result of the obstruction of urine flow.

Paraphimosis, the most serious complication of phimosis, occurs when the foreskin cannot be returned to its normal position over the glans. Blood flow to the penis becomes obstructed with swelling of the glans. Ischemic injury to the glans penis occurs if the constriction is not relieved. Paraphimosis is a medical emergency and requires immediate intervention to preserve the glans penis.

Circumcision, surgical removal of the foreskin, has long been a common practice performed in some countries and cultures during the newborn period. It is performed to prevent phimosis, for ease of proper male hygiene, and to prevent urinary tract infections and penile cancer. See Chapter 5 ∞ for additional information related to circumcision of the newborn.

The procedure removes the skin covering the end of the penis. Circumcision is considered comparatively safe; however, complications such as damage to the urethra and disfigurement to the penis may occur. Betamethasone cream (0.05%) applied twice daily for 4–8 weeks to the outer prepuce is an effective alternative to surgery for phimosis and has few side effects. Often the child is able to achieve foreskin retraction without surgery (Steadman & Ellsworth, 2006).

Nursing Alert

Circumcision is contraindicated in neonates with blood dyscrasias or a family history of bleeding disorder, and in those that are premature. Anomalies such as hypospadias, epispadias, and chordee are other contraindications since the foreskin may be needed for later reconstruction (Steadman & Ellsworth, 2006).

NURSING MANAGEMENT

Nursing initially focuses on educating the parents about cleansing the foreskin and penis of the uncircumcised newborn male. Educate the parents to avoid forcibly retracting the foreskin and prevent complications such as scarring or paraphimosis. Frequent diaper changes help to prevent diaper rash and irritation. When the child is older and the foreskin separates from the penis and easily retracts, teach the parents and the child to pull back the foreskin for cleaning and then to return it to its normal position.

If circumcision is requested by parents of the newborn or it is the method of treatment for phimosis, nursing care focuses on preoperative preparation of the infant, including the advocacy for and assistance in giving the newborn local anesthesia. Postoperatively, the nurse assesses the infant's vital signs and the operative site. Educate the parents to provide proper care for the surgical site, as newborns are discharged within 24 hours of surgery. (See Families Want to Know: Care Following Circumcision.) If a Plastibell device was used in newborn circumcision, parents should receive specific instructions related to care (Davidson, London, & Ladewig, 2008).

If topical steroids are prescribed as treatment, the nurse educates the family to ensure the proper application of the medication along with methods of good hygiene.

Cryptorchidism

Cryptorchidism (undescended testes) occurs when one or both testes fail to descend through the inguinal canal into the scrotum. Normally, the testes descend during the seventh to ninth month of gestation.

Cryptorchidism may be the result of a testosterone deficiency, an absent or defective testis, or a structural problem such as a narrow inguinal canal, short spermatic cord, or adhesions. The disorder occurs in 3–6% of term male infants and in 20–30% of preterm infants (Latendresse, McCance, & Morgan, 2010).

The higher temperature in the abdomen than in the scrotum results in morphologic changes to the testis that begin to occur

Families Want to Know
Care Following Circumcision

Instruct the family to wash hands well before and after each diaper change and to follow these instructions for care following circumcision:

- Cover the head of the penis with a generous amount of petroleum jelly with each diaper change until the redness goes away.
- Pale yellow, sticky drainage may form on the head of the penis and is a normal part of the healing process.
- Squeeze soapy water over the head of the penis once a day, rinse with warm water, and pat dry.
- Contact the health care provider if there is increased redness, bleeding, or swelling of the head of the penis.

Adapted from Davidson, M. R., London, M. L., & Ladewig, P. A. (2008). *Old's maternal-newborn nursing and women's health across the lifespan* (8th ed.). Upper Saddle River, NJ: Pearson/Prentice Hall.

between 6 and 12 months of age. Complications of cryptorchidism include infertility and malignancy (Cakan & Kamat, 2009).

Cryptorchidism is usually detected during the newborn examination when palpation of the scrotum fails to reveal one or both testes. It is not unusual for boys with cryptorchidism to have an inguinal hernia as well. In a majority of cases, the testes descend spontaneously by 3 months of age.

Although diagnosis is made on physical examination, diagnostic studies including ultrasound, CT scan, and MRI are utilized to determine the location of the testes. A diagnostic laparoscope may also be needed to locate the testis. When neither testis can be palpated, hormonal and chromosomal evaluation may be performed to detect an intersex disorder.

If the testes do not descend spontaneously, an orchiopexy is performed around 12 months of age before further damage to the testes occurs (Cakan & Kamat, 2009). The timing for surgery is crucial to preserve fertility and to avoid psychological effects related to fear of castration and body image issues in older children. With an orchiopexy an incision is made at the location of the testis, either in the abdomen or in the inguinal area. Blood vessels are disentangled to allow the testis to reach into the lower scrotum. A second incision is made in the scrotum at the point where the testis is stitched to the inside wall to keep it in place. A protective sealant is often put over the incision that peels off in 3 to 5 days. If the testis is defective or undeveloped, it may be removed surgically to decrease the risk of later malignancies, and a prosthesis may be placed in the scrotum. The goals of surgery are repair of any hernia, enhanced fertility, and psychologic benefit. The orchiopexy also makes it easier to examine the testis for tumors. The risk of testicular cancer is 35 to 50 times greater in men with a history of cryptorchidism (Latendresse et al., 2010).

NURSING MANAGEMENT
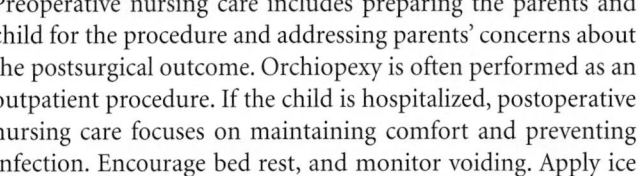

Preoperative nursing care includes preparing the parents and child for the procedure and addressing parents' concerns about the postsurgical outcome. Orchiopexy is often performed as an outpatient procedure. If the child is hospitalized, postoperative nursing care focuses on maintaining comfort and preventing infection. Encourage bed rest, and monitor voiding. Apply ice to the surgical area, and administer prescribed analgesics to relieve pain.

Discharge instructions should include demonstration of proper incision care. The diaper area should be cleaned well with each diaper change to decrease the chance of infection. Sponge bathe the child for 2 days after surgery, after which a tub bath or shower may be taken. No medicine or ointment should be placed over the incision. Teach parents to identify signs of infection such as redness, warmth, swelling, and discharge and to notify the physician if they are discovered. Ibuprofen or acetaminophen may be given for pain. Inform parents to avoid straddling the infant across the hip and to permit no strenuous activity or straddle toy riding for 2 weeks after surgery to promote healing and to prevent injury.

Inguinal Hernia and Hydrocele

An inguinal hernia is a painless inguinal or scrotal swelling of variable size that occurs when abdominal tissue such as bowel extends into the inguinal canal. An inguinal hernia is found in 3.5–5% of full-term infants and 9–11% of preterm infants and occurs more often in boys than girls by a 6:1 ratio (Aiken & Oldham, 2007).

A hydrocele is a fluid-filled mass in the scrotum. The condition is found in 1–2% of male neonates. Most hydroceles resolve spontaneously through reabsorption by 1 year of age (Elder, 2007).

During fetal development, a peritoneal sac precedes the testicle's descent to the scrotum. The lower sac enfolds the testis to become the tunica vaginalis, and the upper sac atrophies before birth. Fluid may become trapped in the tunica vaginalis and cause the hydrocele. When the tunica vaginalis does not atrophy, an abdominal structure may move into it. Inguinal hernias are often associated with abdominal wall defects such as bladder exstrophy and prune-belly syndrome, and are a common occurrence with undescended testes.

Diagnosis is made by physical examination at birth or in early infancy. Palpation of the scrotum reveals a round, smooth, non-tender mass that is noted with either a hernia or hydrocele. Parents may report an intermittent bulge in the groin or swelling in the scrotum. Swelling associated with a hernia may become more apparent with straining and reduced in size when quiet or asleep.

Outpatient surgery is performed at an early age (usually after 3 months of age to reduce anesthesia risks) to avoid **incarceration** (hernia cannot be reduced and circulation to trapped tissue is impaired), which is a medical emergency. A nerve block may be given in the operating room to reduce postoperative pain. The prognosis is generally excellent.

With incarceration, the child has an acute onset of pain, abdominal distention, vomiting, and an irreducible mass. Other findings may include an edematous, erythematosus scrotum accompanied by abdominal distention, poor feeding, and bloody stools (Aiken & Oldham, 2007). Efforts are made to reduce the hernia before surgery by sedating the child and applying firm manual pressure on the affected side. If the hernia is reduced, surgery is often performed within 48 hours. If the hernia cannot be reduced, emergency surgery is performed (Hartmann, 2008).

NURSING MANAGEMENT

Nursing care for hydrocele and inguinal hernia includes explaining the disorder and its treatment and providing preoperative and postoperative teaching and support. The incision is covered with a protective sealant rather than a dressing. Provide pain medication as ordered. Inform parents that the scrotum may be edematous and may appear bruised after surgery. Incision care involves careful cleaning of the diaper area.

Testicular Torsion

Testicular torsion is an emergency condition in which the testis suddenly rotates on its spermatic cord, cutting off its blood supply. The arteries and veins in the spermatic cord become twisted and interrupt the blood supply, leading to vascular engorgement and ischemia. Testicular torsion occurs in an estimated 1 in 4,000 males before 25 years of age (Bradway & Rodgers, 2009; DuFour, 2008). Approximately two thirds of cases occur in boys between the ages of 12 and 18 (DuFour, 2008). Often the testicles are positioned transversely in the scrotum secondary to a congenital anomaly known as a bell clapper deformity. In this deformity, the tunica vaginalis has an inappropriately high attachment to the testes, allowing them to rotate freely and twist spontaneously on the spermatic cord. Approximately 12% of males have this deformity (Rupp & Zwanger, 2010). Bilateral testicular torsion can occur in neonates but is considered rare (Baglaj & Carachi, 2007).

Manifestations include severe pain and erythema in the scrotum, nausea and vomiting, abdominal pain, and scrotal swelling that is not relieved by rest or scrotal support. The testes are tender on palpation and become edematous. The cremasteric reflex is absent. Symptoms generally start when the child is sleeping or inactive, but they can occur after trauma, sexual activity, or exercise. The affected testis is positioned higher in the scrotum than the unaffected testis because of the shortened vascular pedicle. Color Doppler ultrasonography is frequently used to confirm the diagnosis. Urinalysis is useful in differentiating testicular torsion from epididymitis. Males with testicular torsion will generally have a normal urinalysis (Bradway & Rodgers, 2009; DuFour, 2008).

Testicular torsion is a surgical emergency. Treatment must be implemented within 6 hours to prevent ischemia and necrosis (Bradway & Rodgers, 2009). During surgery (orchiopexy), the testis is untwisted and stitched to the side of the scrotum in the correct position. The procedure is usually performed bilaterally to prevent future torsion in the other testis. If the testicle does not regain blood flow or is already necrotic it is removed via orchiectomy (Bradway & Rodgers, 2009; Leung & Kao, 2008).

NURSING MANAGEMENT

Nursing management involves psychological support for the child and family related to the need for emergency surgery and concern about the child's future fertility. Reassure parents that as only one testis is usually involved, fertility should not be affected. The child often goes home within a few hours of surgery; thus, the child and family need to be taught about proper care of the incision and pain management. Explain to parents that the child should not lift heavy objects for 4 weeks or participate in strenuous activity for 2 weeks after surgery to promote healing. Teach the adolescent testicular self-examination.

■ SEXUALLY TRANSMITTED INFECTIONS

Sexually transmitted infections (STIs) are a major national public health concern, and they pose a significant health risk to children and adolescents. The Centers for Disease Control and Prevention (CDC) reports that approximately 19 million new cases of STIs occur each year, with young people ages 15 to 24 years accounting for almost half the infections (CDC, 2009). Children and adolescents can become infected with sexually transmitted organisms through sexual experimentation, sexual play, molestation, and sexual abuse.

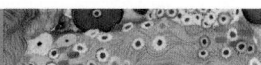

Nursing Alert

When a child younger than 10 years is found to have gonorrhea or other sexually transmitted infection, consider the possibility of sexual abuse. When anorectal symptoms are found, suspect molestation (see Chapter 18 ∞).

Results from the CDC National 2007 Youth Risk Behavior Survey revealed that 47.8% of high school students had engaged in sexual intercourse and 38.5% of sexually active adolescents had not used a condom at last sexual intercourse (CDC, 2008). Adolescents are considered an at-risk population because of their inexperience and lack of knowledge about STIs. They may disregard the importance of using barrier protection, may have multiple sexual partners, may have sex frequently, and often do not seek medical treatment until symptoms are well advanced.

Frequently diagnosed STIs include chlamydia, genital herpes (herpes simplex type 2), gonorrhea, genital warts (human papillomavirus), trichomoniasis, and syphilis. Refer to the Clinical Manifestations: Common Sexually Transmitted Infections table for more information.

State and local health departments are responsible for controlling the spread of STIs through health promotion programs, staff training, reporting systems, diagnosis, treatment, patient counseling, and the notification of sex partners. To reduce all sexually transmitted infections, the CDC recommends abstinence from sexual contact, or a long-term mutually monogamous relationship with a partner who has been tested for STIs and is known to be uninfected (CDC, 2006c). A new vaccine has been approved for adolescents to prevent human papillomavirus. See Chapter 16 ∞ .

Human immunodeficiency virus is discussed in Chapter 22, and hepatitis B, another infection that can be transmitted sexually, is discussed in Chapter 25 ∞ .

NURSING MANAGEMENT

Nursing Assessment and Diagnoses

Nursing assessment focuses on identifying signs and symptoms indicative of sexually transmitted infections, assessing for the potential for asymptomatic sexually transmitted infections, and assessing the psychosocial impact on the child or adolescent with a sexually transmitted infection.

The nurse usually encounters the child or adolescent and family in the emergency department, outpatient clinic, or nursing unit. Since adolescents are often afraid of the consequences of reporting symptoms, good assessment and communication skills are important considerations for the nurse, particularly when asking questions about sexual activity, partners, and the possibility of abuse. Essential to communication is maintaining a warm, encouraging, nonjudgmental approach and conveying acceptance when discussing sexual health issues with the child or adolescent. In order to achieve the adolescent's cooperation, confidentiality must be ensured. Offer support to the adolescent and encourage the seeking of parental guidance and involvement.

Clinical Tip

Key areas to discuss when obtaining a sexual history include information related to partners, pregnancy prevention, protection from sexually transmitted infections, sexual practices, and past history of STIs (CDC, 2006c).

Assess the child or adolescent for manifestations as described in the Clinical Manifestations table. When a child or adolescent is diagnosed with one STI, it is essential to screen for the presence of other STIs, as these diseases may coexist. Adolescents who are symptomatic may postpone care due to feeling uncomfortable about genital examinations. Given that many adolescents have

Clinical Manifestations

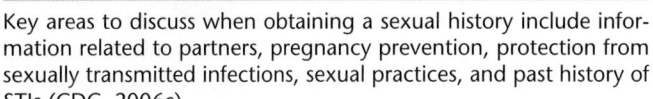

Common Sexually Transmitted Infections

Sexually Transmitted Infection	Clinical Manifestations and Complications	Clinical Therapy and Patient Education
Chlamydia *Chlamydia trachomatis*	Adolescent females: yellow mucopurulent endocervical discharge, dysuria, pelvic pain, mild abdominal pain, vaginal spotting, cervicitis, salpingitis, pelvic inflammatory disease (PID); 75% are asymptomatic (Grimshaw-Mulcahy, 2006). Adolescent males: **urethritis** (an infection of the urethra), mucoid gray or clear discharge, dysuria, proctitis, epididymitis; 50% are asymptomatic (Grimshaw-Mulcahy, 2006). Complications associated with chlamydia in females include PID and infertility. Chlamydia is a leading cause of early pneumonia and conjunctivitis in newborns.	Diagnosis is by culture or a nucleic acid-amplified test on the urine. Recommended medication therapy includes doxycycline, or erythromycin for 7 days, or single-dose azithromycin. Persons who are HIV positive with chlamydia receive the same treatment as those who are HIV negative. All sexual partners should be evaluated, tested, and treated. Infected persons should abstain from sexual intercourse until they and their sex partners have completed treatment to prevent reinfection. Encourage use of condoms. All sexually active female adolescents should be screened at least annually for chlamydia.

(continued)

Clinical Manifestations

Common Sexually Transmitted Infections (continued)

Sexually Transmitted Infection	Clinical Manifestations and Complications	Clinical Therapy and Patient Education
Genital herpes *Herpes simplex virus 1* (HSV-1) or 2 (HSV-2)	Most infected with HSV-2 are not aware of their infection. Presentation can be variable and ranges from no symptoms to systemic involvement. Common symptoms include dull pain, itching, and small lesions or pimples on genitalia, buttocks, or thighs. Two types of lesions develop, either fluid-filled blisters on an erythematous base or more commonly, painful papules and ulcers. Ulcers can appear between vaginal folds, in posterior cervix, on glans penis, on shaft of penis, in rectum, or in anus. Ulcers heal within 2–4 weeks. Lymph nodes closest to lesions are frequently enlarged. Disease frequently recurs four to five times a year with episodes lasting 5–10 days. Triggers include stress, menses, or trauma.	Diagnosis is confirmed by virology and type-specific serologic tests. There is no permanent cure. Recommended drug therapy is acyclovir given for 7–10 days. Antiviral medications can shorten and prevent outbreaks during the period of time the person takes the medication. Daily suppressive therapy for herpes can reduce transmission to partners. A cesarean delivery is usually performed for pregnant women who are infected. Discourage oral sex if ulcers are present in mouth, on lips, in vagina, or on penis. Discourage anal sex when lesions are active. Encourage use of condoms, although they may not prevent transmission. Emphasize that the patient remains contagious, even after lesions are healed.
Gonorrhea *Neisseria gonorrhoeae*	Symptoms and severity vary from mild to severe and are different for males and females. In females, areas that can be infected include urethra, cervix, fallopian tubes, and Bartholin and Skene glands. In males, areas include urethra, prostate, seminal vesicles, epididymis, and Littre and Cowper glands. Females with gonorrhea may be asymptomatic. The classic sign is discharge from the vagina and urethra; however, infections involving the conjunctiva, pharynx, and anus area are also seen. Prepubescent girls: heavy, thick green or creamy vaginal discharge, vulvovaginitis. Pubescent girls: purulent vaginal discharge, cervicitis, fallopian tube and pelvic inflammatory disease involvement can lead to sterility. Prepubescent and adolescent boys: yellow purulent urethral discharge, erythematous meatus, frequency, dysuria, and painful or swollen testicles. Although many men with gonorrhea may have no symptoms at all, some men have signs or symptoms that appear 2 to 5 days after infection; symptoms can take as long as 30 days to appear. Signs and symptoms of rectal infection in both genders include discharge, anal itching, soreness, bleeding, or painful bowel movements. However, they may be asymptomatic. Infections in the throat may cause a sore throat but are usually asymptomatic. Transmission to the neonate during vaginal delivery can cause blindness, joint infection, or sepsis. Gonorrhea is a common cause of PID.	Diagnosed by culture of vaginal or urethral discharge or nucleic acid-amplified test on the urine. Recommended drug therapy includes a single dose of ceftriaxone IM or cefixime orally in one dose. Sexual partners should be treated if the adolescent has had sexual contact within 60 days of onset of symptoms. Encourage use of condoms or abstinence. Emphasize the importance of taking all of the medication prescribed to cure gonorrhea. The individual and all sex partners must avoid sex until they have completed their treatment for gonorrhea.

Clinical Manifestations
Common Sexually Transmitted Infections (continued)

Sexually Transmitted Infection	Clinical Manifestations and Complications	Clinical Therapy and Patient Education
Human papillomavirus (HPV)	The most common STI in adolescents in the United States (Forhan, Gottlieb, Sternberg, et al., 2009). Warts are small, flat, and fleshy-colored with a cauliflower appearance. Adolescent females: warts clustered or alone on the vulva, perineal area, vagina, or cervix; itching, bleeding, burning, irritation. A subclinical infection may be detected through a Pap smear. HPV can lead to cervical cancer. Adolescent males: may be asymptomatic; warts on the penis, near base of penis on scrotal skin, or near anus.	Diagnosis is based upon physical findings or biopsy. The Pap smear may be abnormal. No cure exists. Treatment for external genital warts may include cryotherapy, topical podophyllin resin, imiquimod 5% cream, podofilox 9.5% solution, or gel. Encourage abstinence or condom use, but condoms are not sufficient to prevent contact transmission. The disorder is transmissible even after treatment. HPV vaccine (see Chapter 16 ∞).
Trichomoniasis *Trichomonas vaginalis*	Adolescent females: pale yellow to gray-green discharge that may be frothy or have a fishy odor, dysuria, vulvar pruritus, occasional abdominal pain; symptoms worsen during menses, more commonly have symptoms than males. Adolescent males: most common site is the urethra; mucoid or purulent urethral discharge, pruritus, dysuria; however, males are usually asymptomatic.	Diagnosis is by culture. Treatment includes metronidazole or tinidazole orally as a single dose or metronidazole orally twice a day for 7 days. Both partners should be treated at the same time to eliminate the parasite. Avoid drinking alcohol during and for several days after treatment if a single dose is used. Sexual contact should be avoided until both partners are cured. No follow-up test is needed if symptoms resolve after treatment.
Syphilis *Treponema pallidum*	Appearance of classic signs and symptoms of syphilis depends on stage of disease. *Primary stage*: manifests as an ulcer on labia, within vagina, on penis, in anus, or on lips or tongue that appears at invasion site approximately 2 weeks to 3 months after infection. Ulcer has an indurated border and smooth base (chancre), and it is painless. Lymphadenopathy is usually present. Ulcer spontaneously heals within 5 weeks. *Second stage*: appears up to 10 weeks after initial infection with fever, malaise, lymphadenopathy, patchy alopecia, and diffuse rash. Rash can be macular, papular, papulosquamous, or bullous, and appearance on the palms and soles is classic. Flat mucous patches called condylomata latum appear on genitals. *Latent stage*: asymptomatic, follows the second stage by about 6 weeks. It can last for several years or be lifelong. *Tertiary stage*: occurs more than 2 years after onset and manifests as changes to the cardiovascular system, bone, skin, or viscera. *Neurosyphilis*: an infection of the central nervous system, can occur during any stage.	Diagnosis is by serologic tests or direct fluorescent antibody tests of lesion exudates. Due to the risk of fetal death, every pregnant woman should have a blood test for syphilis. Syphilis is easy to cure in its early stages. Recommended drug therapy includes single IM injection of benzathine penicillin G. For children allergic to penicillin, erythromycin PO is prescribed for 15 days. Saline compresses and a topical antibiotic are often used to treat lesions on the skin. Treat all sexual contacts within the past 90 days to 1 year of diagnosis, depending on stage when diagnosed. During syphilis treatment, abstain from sexual contact with new partners until the syphilis sores are completely healed. Encourage abstinence or the use of condoms plus spermicidal foams, cream, or jelly to prevent infection.

Source: Data from American Academy of Pediatrics. (2009). Red book: Report of the Committee on Infectious Disease (28th ed.). Elk Grove Village, IL: Author; Centers for Disease Control and Prevention. (2006b). HPV and HPV vaccine information for health care providers; Centers for Disease Control and Prevention (CDC). (2006c). Sexually transmitted diseases treatment guidelines, 2006. Morbidity and Mortality Weekly Report, 55(RR-11), 1–94. Centers for Disease Control and Prevention (CDC). (2007a). Update to CDC's Sexually transmitted diseases treatment guidelines, 2006: Fluoroquinolones no longer recommended for treatment of gonococcal infections. Morbidity and Mortality Weekly Report, 56(14), 332–336; Centers for Disease Control and Prevention (CDC). (2007b). Updated recommended treatment regimens for gonococcal infections and associated conditions—United States, April 2007; Forhan, S. E., Gottlieb, S. L., Sternberg, M. R., Xu, F., Datta, S. D., McQuillan, G. M., et al. (2009). Prevalence of sexually transmitted infections among female adolescents aged 14 to 19 in the United States. Pediatrics, 124(6), 1505–1512; Grimshaw-Mulcahy, L. J. (2006, March). Chlamydia: Diagnosing the hidden STD. Clinical Advisor, 32–41.

subclinical cases or are asymptomatic, routine screening of sexually active adolescents is recommended.

Nursing diagnoses that may apply to the child or adolescent with a sexually transmitted infection include:

- Anxiety related to presence of sexually transmitted infection
- Pain related to genital irritation
- Deficient Knowledge (Sexually Transmitted Infections) related to cause, transmission, treatments, and prevention
- Disturbed Body Image related to genital lesions, presence of genital infection

Planning and Implementation

The nurse focuses on identifying adolescents at risk for STIs, providing appropriate education, and preventing transmission and complications.

When counseling the adolescent, reinforce the importance of treating all sexual partners and modifying high-risk sexual behaviors. Partner notification is essential in order to provide treatment if the partner is infected, and to reduce the risk of reinfection. Encourage sexually active adolescents to receive hepatitis B immunization if not already obtained.

Care in the Community

Education includes promoting abstinence, which means avoiding *any* type of sexual contact with a partner. (See Families Want to Know: Preventing STIs and Their Consequences.) The nurse, in partnership with schools and community organizations, is active in sexual health promotion.

Work with sexually active adolescents to identify methods of reducing the risk of contracting STIs. Suggestions include the use of latex condoms (though the possibility of STI transmission still exists even with the use of latex condoms), voiding immediately after sexual intercourse, and appropriate genital hygiene with soap and water. Assist adolescents to avoid sexual partners who are at higher risk for STIs, such as intravenous drug users and those who have multiple sexual partners. Emphasize to the adolescent that even with applying these measures, there is no guaranteed protection against STIs except when using abstinence. Explain to the adolescent that some STIs, such as chlamydia, are asymptomatic.

Additional teaching includes dispelling myths of how STIs are spread. Instruct the child or adolescent that STIs are not contracted from sharing bath towels, clothing, and drinking glasses, or from sitting on toilet seats. Inform the female taking contraceptives that birth control offers no protection against STIs.

Evaluation

Expected outcomes for the child or adolescent with a sexually transmitted infection are:

- The child or adolescent remains free from pain.
- An understanding of the transmission, prevention, and treatment of sexually transmitted infections is demonstrated by the adolescent.
- The adolescent has a positive body image.
- Reduced anxiety is displayed by the child or adolescent.

Families Want to Know
Preventing STIs and Their Consequences

Collaborate with the child and family to promote the following recommendations in preventing STIs and their consequences:

- Abstinence is the best method to prevent STIs.
- Limit the number of sexual contacts; practice mutual monogamy.
- Always use condoms and spermicidal gels or foams for vaginal and anal intercourse.
- Refrain from oral sex if the partner has active sores in the mouth, vagina, anus, or penis.
- Reduce high-risk sexual behaviors. Use of recreational drugs and alcohol can increase sexual risk taking.
- Seek care as soon as symptoms are noticed and make sure your partner gets treatment.
- Seek annual screening for STIs.

Pelvic Inflammatory Disease (PID)

Pelvic inflammatory disease (PID) is a serious infection of the upper genital tract caused by the ascending spread of organisms in the cervix and vagina. An estimated 85% of cases of PID are caused by complications of sexually transmitted infections, primarily gonorrhea and chlamydia (Abatangelo, Okereke, Parham-Foster, et al., 2010).

The infection ascends into the uterus and fallopian tubes during the menses when the cervix mucosal plug is open and retrograde menstrual blood can flow into the fallopian tubes. Signs and symptoms of PID may include fever, mild or dull bilateral lower abdominal pain, dysmenorrhea that is worse or longer lasting than usual, dysuria, vaginal discharge, pain with sexual activity, and prolonged or increased menstrual bleeding. Most cases are mild.

No specific laboratory test exists for PID. During a pelvic examination, uterine or adnexal tenderness or tenderness with cervical motion is present. Other criteria that help support the diagnosis of PID include an elevated erythrocyte sedimentation rate, elevated C-reactive protein level, white blood cells seen on microscopic examination of vaginal secretions, and documented cervical infection with gonorrhea or chlamydia (CDC, 2006c). A transvaginal sonogram may reveal thickened and fluid-filled fallopian tubes with or without free pelvic fluid. A pregnancy test, HIV test, and cultures for STIs should be performed.

Parenteral antibiotic therapy is often used for the first 24 hours before converting to oral antibiotics for the remaining 14 days of treatment. Common intravenous antibiotics used include a combination of cefotetan or cefoxitin plus doxycycline. If doxycycline is contraindicated, clindamycin plus gentamicin may be substituted (CDC, 2006c). Oral regimens include ceftriaxone or cefoxitin, plus doxycycline with or without metronidazole (CDC, 2007b). Follow-up physical examination is performed in 72 hours to ensure treatment adherence and to detect improvement in symptoms and reduced tenderness of the uterus, adnexae, and cervix. Rehospitalization and IV antibiotics are initiated if no improvement is noted.

NURSING MANAGEMENT

A sexual history should be obtained from all adolescent females to identify the risk for sexually transmitted infection and PID. Risk factors for adolescents include those who have an STI, multiple sexual partners, lack of consistent condom use, use of douching, smoking, alcohol use, and the exchange of sex for money or drugs (Abatangelo et al., 2010; Reyes, Kumar, & Abbuhl, 2009).

Administer medications intravenously for the first 24 hours, making arrangements for the adolescent to return for a second dose 12 hours after the first. Provide education for the ongoing treatment with oral antibiotics, ensuring that the adolescent understands the importance of taking all medications on schedule for the full 14 days. Provide signs of adverse effects and actions to take if they occur.

Determine if the adolescent's parents have been informed about the illness, and assist the adolescent to discuss the health problem with the parents. If parents are unaware of the health problem, discuss the importance of telling the parents so that they can help identify any problems that develop during treatment.

Provide counseling about methods to reduce the risk for re-infection with a sexually transmitted infection. Provide information about the potential consequences of infertility, ectopic pregnancy, and chronic abdominal pain for this infection and the increased risk for these consequences with subsequent infections. Encourage regular health visits with screening for sexually transmitted infections, as future chlamydia and gonorrhea infections may be asymptomatic.

Chapter Highlights

- Functions of the urinary system include excretion of wastes, maintenance of acid-base and fluid and electrolyte balance, regulation of blood pressure, production of erythropoietin, and regulation of calcium metabolism.
- Bladder capacity increases with growth, from 20 to 50 mL in newborns to 700 mL in adults.
- Urinary tract infections are common infections in children. Factors placing the child at risk for a UTI include urinary stasis, infrequent voiding, irritated perineum, constipation, masturbation, sexual abuse, and sexual activity in adolescent females.
- Structural defects of the urinary system—including bladder exstrophy, hypospadias and epispadias, obstructive uropathy, vesicoureteral reflux, and posterior ureteral valves—generally require surgical treatment.
- Bladder exstrophy is a congenital defect in which the abdominal wall does not fuse during fetal development, leading to exposure of the bladder wall, a separation of the rectus muscles, and widening of the symphysis pubis.
- Surgical correction of hypospadias and epispadias generally occurs during the first year of life to minimize psychological effects on the child.
- Obstruction of the urinary tract interferes with urine flow and results in hydronephrosis or urine backflow into the kidneys. This results in significant damage to the kidney and is a common cause of renal failure in children.
- Vesicoureteral reflux may result from a structural anomaly in which the ureters insert in an abnormal position into the bladder. Urinary tract infections are often a complication of this disorder.
- Prune-belly (Eagle-Barrett) syndrome is a rare congenital disorder in which the skin covering the abdominal wall is thin and resembles a wrinkled prune. Anomalies associated with this syndrome include urinary tract anomalies, enlarged bladder, vesicoureteral reflux, and bilateral cryptorchidism.
- Nocturnal enuresis often occurs in children whose parents have a history of enuresis. Very few children have a structural or neurological cause. Higher rates of enuresis have been noted in children with obstructive sleep apnea.
- Minimal change nephrotic syndrome is characterized by edema that develops over several weeks, weight gain, hypertension, irritability, hematuria, malaise, anorexia, and foamy or frothy urine.
- Acute poststreptococcal glomerulonephritis results from a beta-hemolytic group A streptococcal infection of the respiratory tract or skin. Most children have a complete recovery of kidney function.
- Hemolytic-uremic syndrome is often associated with ingestion of *E. coli* strain 0157:H7, which produces a toxin that attacks the kidneys. The child develops hemolytic anemia, thrombocytopenia, and acute renal failure that can progress to chronic renal failure.
- Polycystic kidney disease is a genetic disorder with both autosomal recessive and autosomal dominant forms that lead to chronic renal failure. It may be detected prenatally or in young children by ultrasound.
- Acute renal failure occurs when kidney function diminishes abruptly and is often reversible. It may occur as a complication of trauma, sepsis, cardiac surgery, or drug toxicity. It is also seen in critically ill neonates with asphyxia, sepsis, or shock.
- Chronic renal failure is progressive and irreversible reduced function of the kidneys, eventually resulting in end-stage renal disease. It often results from developmental abnormalities of the kidneys or urinary tract.
- Children with end-stage renal disease are treated with renal replacement therapy, including hemodialysis, peritoneal dialysis, or kidney transplant.
- Structural defects of the male reproductive system include phimosis, cryptorchidism, inguinal hernia and hydrocele, and testicular torsion.

■ Nursing care of sexually transmitted infections includes identifying the cause and organism, providing appropriate treatment, preventing transmission and complications, and educating the child, adolescent, and family.

■ Pelvic inflammatory disease (PID) is an infection of the upper genital tract (uterus and fallopian tubes) caused by the ascending spread of organisms (usually chlamydia or gonorrhea) in the cervix and vagina.

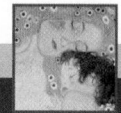

Clinical Reasoning in Action

Recall Brooke from the opening scenario. She is an active 9-year-old who is involved in many activities at school. Her recent urinary tract infection forced her to leave class to run to the bathroom. She was given a prescription for oral antibiotics.

1. What developmental considerations should the nurse incorporate when teaching Brooke about prevention of future UTIs?

2. What desired outcomes should the nurse include in the teaching plan?

3. What are the potential problems that Brooke could encounter if she does not take the medication as prescribed?

4. If Brooke has another urinary tract infection in the next few months, what diagnostic procedures might be used to rule out other potential causes?

See Pearson Nursing Student Resources for possible responses.

Pearson Nursing Student Resources

Find additional review materials at
nursing.pearsonhighered.com
Prepare for success with NCLEX®-style practice questions, interactive assignments and activities, web links, animations and videos, and more!

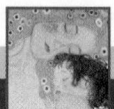

References

Abatangelo, L., Okereke, L., Parham-Foster, C., Parrish, C., Scaglione, L., Zotte, D., & Leslie-Faith, M. T. (2010). If pelvic inflammatory disease is suspected empiric treatment should be initiated. *Journal of the American Academy of Nurse Practitioners, 22,* 117–122.

Adams, D., & Vohra, S. (2009). Complementary, holistic, and integrative medicine: Nocturnal enuresis. *Pediatrics in Review, 30,* 396–400.

Aiken, J. J., & Oldham, K. T. (2007). Inguinal hernias. In R. M. Kliegman, R. E. Behrman, H. B. Jenson, & B. F. Stanton (Eds.), *Nelson textbook of pediatrics* (18th ed., pp. 1644–1650). Philadelphia: Saunders.

Aldridge, M. D. (2008). How do families adjust to having a child with chronic kidney failure? A systematic review. *Nephrology Nursing Journal, 35*(2), 157–162.

American Academy of Pediatrics. (2009). *Red book: Report of the Committee on Infectious Disease* (28th ed.). Elk Grove Village, IL: Author.

Anacleto, F. E., Resontoc, L. P., & Padilla, G. H. (2009). Bedside diagnosis of outpatient childhood urinary tract infection using three-media dipslide culture test. *Pediatric Nephrology, 24,* 1539–1543.

Baglaj, M., & Carachi, R. (2007). Neonatal bilateral testicular torsion: A plea for emergency exploration. *Journal of Urology, 177,* 2296–2299.

Bakr, A., Amr, M., Sarhan, A., Hammad, A., Ragab, M., El-Refaey, A., & El-Mougy, A. (2007). Psychiatric disorders in children with chronic renal failure. *Pediatric Nephrology, 22,* 128–131.

Berry, A. (2005). Helping children with dysfunctional voiding. *Urologic Nursing, 25*(3), 193–200.

Berry, A. K. (2006). Helping children with nocturnal enuresis. *American Journal of Nursing, 106*(8), 56–63.

Boydstun, I. I. (2005). Acute renal failure. *Adolescent Medicine Clinics, 16*(1), 1–9.

Bradway, C., & Rodgers, J. (2009). Evaluation and management of genitourinary emergencies. *Nurse Practitioner, 34*(5), 37–43.

Butani, L., & Ramsamooj, R. (2009). Experience with tacrolimus in children with steroid-resistant nephrotic syndrome. *Pediatric Nephrology, 24,* 1517–1523.

Cakan, N., & Kamat, D. (2009). Cryptorchidism: Primary care evaluation and management. *Consultant for Pediatricians, 8*(2), 46–50.

Centers for Disease Control and Prevention (CDC). (2006a). Outbreaks of *Escherichia coli* 0157:H7 associated with petting zoos—North Carolina, Florida, and Arizona, 2004 and 2005. *Journal of the American Medical Association, 295*(4), 378–380.

Centers for Disease Control and Prevention (CDC). (2006b). *HPV and HPV vaccine information for health care providers.* Retrieved from http://www.cdc.gov/std/HPV/hpv-vacc-hcp-3-pages.pdf

Centers for Disease Control and Prevention (CDC). (2006c). Sexually transmitted diseases treatment guidelines, 2006. *Morbidity and Mortality Weekly Report, 55*(RR-11), 1–94.

Centers for Disease Control and Prevention (CDC). (2007a). Update to CDC's *Sexually transmitted diseases treatment guidelines, 2006:* Fluoroquinolones no longer recommended for treatment of gonococcal infections. *Morbidity and Mortality Weekly Report, 56*(14), 332–336.

Centers for Disease Control and Prevention (CDC). (2007b). *Updated recommended treatment regimens for gonococcal infections and associated conditions—United States, April 2007.* Retrieved from http://www.cdc.gov/std/treatment/2006/updated-regimens.htm

Centers for Disease Control and Prevention (CDC). (2008). Youth risk behavioral surveillance—United States 2007. *Morbidity and Mortality Weekly Report, 57*(SS-4).

Centers for Disease Control and Prevention (CDC). (2009). *Trends in reportable sexually transmitted diseases in the United States, 2007: National surveillance data for chlamydia, gonorrhea, and syphilis.* Retrieved from http://www.cdc.gov/STD/stats07/trends.htm

Chavers, B. M., Solid, T. A., Gilbertson, D. T., & Collins, A. J. (2007). Infection-related hospitalization rates in pediatric *versus* adult patients with end-stage renal disease in the United States. *Journal of the American Society of Nephrology, 18,* 952–959.

Craig, J., Simpson, J., Williams, G. J., Lowe, A., Reynolds, G. J., Graham, J., et al. (2009). Antibiotic prophylaxis and recurrent urinary tract infection in children. *New England Journal of Medicine, 361*(18), 1748–1759.

Davidson, M. R., London, M. L., & Ladewig, P. A. (2008). *Olds' maternal-newborn nursing and women's health across the lifespan* (8th ed.). Upper Saddle River, NJ: Pearson/Prentice Hall.

Davis, I. D., & Avner, E. D. (2007). Conditions particularly associated with hematuria. In R. M. Kliegman, R. E. Behrman, H. B. Jenson, & B. F. Stanton (Eds.), *Nelson textbook of pediatrics* (18th ed., pp. 2168–2188). Philadelphia: Saunders.

Dogan, H. S., Akpinar, B., Gurocak, S., Akata, D., Bakkaloglu, M., & Tekgul, S. (2008). Non-invasive evaluation of voiding function in asymptomatic primary school children. *Pediatric Nephrology, 23,* 1115–1122.

DuFour, J. L. (2008). Testicular torsion: Respond quickly to urologic emergency. *Advance for Nurse Practitioners, 16*(6), 65–66.

Dulczak, S., & Kirk, J. (2005). Overview of the evaluation, diagnosis, and management of urinary tract infections in infants and children. *Urologic Nursing, 25*(3), 185–191.

Elder, J. S. (2007). Urologic disorders in infants and children. In R. M. Kliegman, R. E. Behrman, H. B. Jenson, & B. F. Stanton (Eds.), *Nelson textbook of pediatrics* (18th ed., pp. 2221–2271). Philadelphia: Saunders.

Feinstein, S., Keich, R., Becker-Cohen, R., Rinat, C., Schwartz, S. B., & Frishberg, Y. (2005). Is non-compliance among adolescent renal transplant recipients inevitable? *Pediatrics, 115*(4), 969–973.

Fiorino, E. K., & Raffaelli, R. M. (2006). Hemolytic-uremic syndrome. *Pediatrics in Review, 27*(10), 398–399.

Forhan, S. E., Gottlieb, S. L., Sternberg, M. R., Xu, F., Datta, S. D., McQuillan, G. M., et al. (2009). Prevalence of sexually transmitted infections among female adolescents aged 14 to 19 in the United States. *Pediatrics, 124*(6), 1505–1512.

Frimberger, D., Campbell, J., & Kropp, B. P. (2008). Hypospadias outcome in the first 3 years after completing a pediatric urology fellowship. *Journal of Pediatric Urology, 4,* 270–274.

Garin, E. H., Olavarria, F., Nieto, V. G., Valenciano, B., Campos, A., & Young, L. (2006). Clinical significance of primary vesicoureteral reflux and urinary antibiotic prophylaxis after acute pyelonephritis: A multicenter, randomized controlled study. *Pediatrics, 117*(3), 626–632.

Grimshaw-Mulcahy, L. J. (2006, March). Chlamydia: Diagnosing the hidden STD. *Clinical Advisor,* 32–41.

Hartmann, R. W. (2008). Congenital complete inguinal-scrotal hernia. *Consultant for Pediatricians, 7*(12), 526–527.

Hellerstein, S. (2009). *Urinary tract infection.* Retrieved from http://emedicine.medscape.com/article/969643-overview

Hodges, S., Patel, B., McLorie, G., & Atala, A. (2009). Posterior urethral valves. *Scientific World Journal, 9,* 1119–1126.

Huether, S. E. (2010a). Structure and function of the renal and urologic systems. In K. L. McCance & S. E. Huether, *Pathophysiology: The biologic basis for disease in adults and children* (6th ed., pp. 1355–1364). Maryland Heights, MO: Mosby Elsevier.

Huether, S. E. (2010b). Alterations of renal and urinary tract function in children. In K. L. McCance & S. E. Huether, *Pathophysiology: The biologic basis for disease in adults and children* (6th ed., pp. 1402–1419). Maryland Heights, MO: Mosby Elsevier.

Huether, S. E., & Forshee, B. A. (2010). Alterations of renal and urinary tract function. In K. L. McCance & S. E. Huether, *Pathophysiology: The biologic basis for disease in adults and children* (6th ed., pp. 1365–1401). Maryland Heights, MO: Mosby Elsevier.

Jalanko, H. (2009). Congenital nephrotic syndrome. *Pediatric Nephrology, 24,* 2121–2128.

Khoury, A., & Bägli, D. J. (2007). Reflux and megaureter. In A. J. Wein, L. R. Kavoussi, A. C. Novick, A. W. Partin, & C. A. Peters, *Campbell-Walsh urology* (9th ed., pp. 3423–3481). Philadelphia: Elsevier Saunders.

Ključevšek, D., Ključevšek, T., Levart, T. K., Novljan, G., & Kenda, R. B. (2010). Catheter-free methods for vesicoureteric reflux detection: Our experience and a critical appraisal of existing data. *Pediatric Nephrology, 25*(7), 1201–1206.

Kozlowski, L. J. (2008). The acute pain service nurse practitioner: A case study in the postoperative care of the child with bladder exstrophy. *Journal of Pediatric Health Care, 22,* 351–359.

Lahdenkari, A., Suvanto, M., Kajantie, E., Koskimies, O., Kestila, M., & Jalanko, H. (2005). Clinical features and outcome of childhood minimal change nephrotic syndrome: Is genetics involved? *Pediatric Nephrology, 20,* 1073–1080.

Lane, J. C. (2009). *Nephrotic syndrome.* Retrieved from http://emedicine.medscape.com/article/982920-treatment

Latendresse, G. A., McCance, K. L., & Morgan, K. (2010). Alterations of the reproductive systems. In K. L. McCance & S. E. Huether, *Pathophysiology: The biologic basis for disease in adults and children* (6th ed., pp. 816–922). Maryland Heights, MO: Mosby Elsevier.

Leung, A. K. C., & Kao, C. P. (2008). A collage of genital lesions, Part 2. *Consultant for Pediatricians, 7*(9), 369–370.

Liberti, J. (2005). Biofeedback therapy in pediatric urology. *Urologic Nursing, 25*(3), 206–210.

Lum, G. (2007). Kidney & urinary tract. In W. W. Hay, M. L. Leven, J. M. Sondheimer, & R. R. Deterding, *Current pediatric diagnosis and treatment* (18th ed., pp. 684–707). New York: McGraw-Hill.

Mercer, R. (2006, May). Enuresis in the older child. *Nursing Spectrum, 21.*

Miller, D., & MacDonald, D. (2006). Management of pediatric patients with chronic kidney disease. *Pediatric Nursing, 32*(2), 128–134.

Nachman, P. H., Jennette, J. C., & Falk, R. J. (2008). Primary glomerular disease. In B. M. Brenner, *Brenner & Rector's the kidney* (8th ed., pp. 987–1066). Philadelphia: Saunders Elsevier.

Naqvi, M., Paddack, J., Kulkarni, A., Akangire, G., & Subhani, M. (2009). What's your diagnosis? Sharpen your physical diagnostic skills. *Consultant for Pediatricians, 8*(9), 333–335.

National Kidney and Urologic Diseases Information Clearinghouse. (2009). *Financial help for treatment of kidney failure.* NIH Publication No. 09–4765. Retrieved from http://kidney.niddk.nih.gov/kudiseases/pubs/pdf/Financial-Help-Kidney.pdf

National Kidney Foundation. (2007). *Use of herbal supplements in chronic kidney disease.* Retrieved from http://www.kidney.org/atoz/atozPrint.cfm?id=123

Nelson, C. P., & Koo, H. P. (2008). *Vesicoureteral reflux.* Retrieved from http://emedicine.medscape.com/article/1016439-overview

Pieretti, R. V., Pieretti, A., & Pieretti-Vanmarcke, R. (2009). Circumcised hypospadias. *Pediatric Surgery International, 25,* 53–55.

Raszka, W. V., & Khan, O. (2005). Pyelonephritis. *Pediatrics in Review, 26*(10), 364–369.

Razzaq, S. (2006). Hemolytic uremic syndrome: An emerging health risk. *American Family Physician, 74*(6), 991–996.

Reyes, I., Kumar, R., & Abbuhl, S. (2009). *Pelvic inflammatory disease.* Retrieved from http://emedicine.medscape.com/article/796092-overview

Riaño-Galán, I., Málaga, S., Rajmil, L., Ariceta, G., Navarro, M., Loris, C., & Vallo, A. (2009). Quality of life of adolescents with end-stage renal disease and kidney transplant. *Pediatric Nephrology, 24,* 1561–1568.

Rizk, D., & Chapman, A. (2008). Treatment of autosomal polycystic kidney disease (ADPKD): The new horizon for children with ADPKD. *Pediatric Nephrology, 23,* 1029–1036.

Robbins, C., & Shew, M. L. (2009). UTIs in adolescents: Common infections, uncommon challenges. *Contemporary Pediatrics, 26*(7), 48–54.

Rupp, T. J., & Zwanger, M. (2010). *Testicular torsion.* Retrieved from http://emedicine.medscape.com/article/778086-overview

Ruth, E. M., Kemper, M. J., Leumann, E. P., Laube, G. F., & Neuhaus, T. J. (2005). Children with steroid-sensitive nephrotic syndrome come of age: Long-term outcome. *Journal of Pediatrics, 147*(2), 202–207.

Salant, D. S., & Patel, P. S. (2008). Polycystic kidney disease and other inherited tubular disorders. In A. S. Fauci, E. Braunwald, D. L. Kasper, S. L. Hauser, D. L. Longo, J. L. Jameson, & J. Loscalzo, *Harrison's principles of internal medicine* (17th ed., pp. 1797–1806). New York: McGraw-Hill.

Schulman, S. L., & Berry, A. K. (2007, January). A simple, step-wise approach to the child with daytime wetting. *Contemporary Urology,* 19–29.

Steadman, B., & Ellsworth, P. (2006). To circ or not to circ: Indications, risks, and alternatives to circumcision in the pediatric population with phimosis. *Urologic Nursing, 26*(3), 181–194.

Tan, A. J., & Silverberg, M. A. (2009). *Hemolytic uremic syndrome.* Retrieved from http://emedicine.medscape.com/article/779218-overview

Terrill, C. J. (2007). Nutrition and the pediatric patient with CKD. *Nephrology Nursing Journal, 34*(1), 89–92.

United States Renal Data System. (2008). *2008 Annual data report.* Retrieved from http://www.usrds.org/atlas.htm

Vemulakonda, V. M., & Jones, E. A. (2006). Primer: Diagnosis and management of uncomplicated daytime wetting in children. *Nature Clinical Practice Urology, 3*(10), 551–559.

Vogler, C., Wang, Y., Brink, D., Wood, E., Belsha, C., & Walker, P. D. (2007). Renal pathology in the pediatric transplant patient. *Advances in Anatomic Pathology, 14*(3), 202–216.

Vogt, B. A., & Avner, E. D. (2007a). Conditions particularly associated with proteinuria. In R. M. Kliegman, R. E. Behrman, H. B. Jenson, & B. F. Stanton (Eds.), *Nelson textbook of pediatrics* (18th ed., pp. 2188–2195). Philadelphia: Saunders.

Vogt, B. A., & Avner, E. D. (2007b). Toxic neuropathies: Renal failure. In R. M. Kliegman, R. E. Behrman, H. B. Jenson, & B. F. Stanton (Eds.), *Nelson textbook of pediatrics* (18th ed., pp. 2204–2219). Philadelphia: Saunders.

Warady, B. A., & Chada, V. (2007). Chronic kidney disease in children: The global perspective. *Pediatric Nephrology, 22*(12), 1999–2009.

Ward-Smith, P., & Barry, D. (2006). The challenge of treating enuresis. *Urologic Nursing, 26*(3), 222–224.

Watnick, S., & Morrison, G. (2007). Nephrology. In S. J. McPhee, M. A. Papadakis, & L. M. Tierny, Jr., *Current medical diagnosis and treatment* (46th ed.). New York: McGraw-Hill.

Weissbach, A., Leiberman, A., Tarasiuk, A., Goldbart, A., & Tal, A. (2006). Adenotonsillectomy improves enuresis in children with obstructive sleep apnea syndrome. *Pediatric Otorhinolaryngology, 70,* 1351–1356.

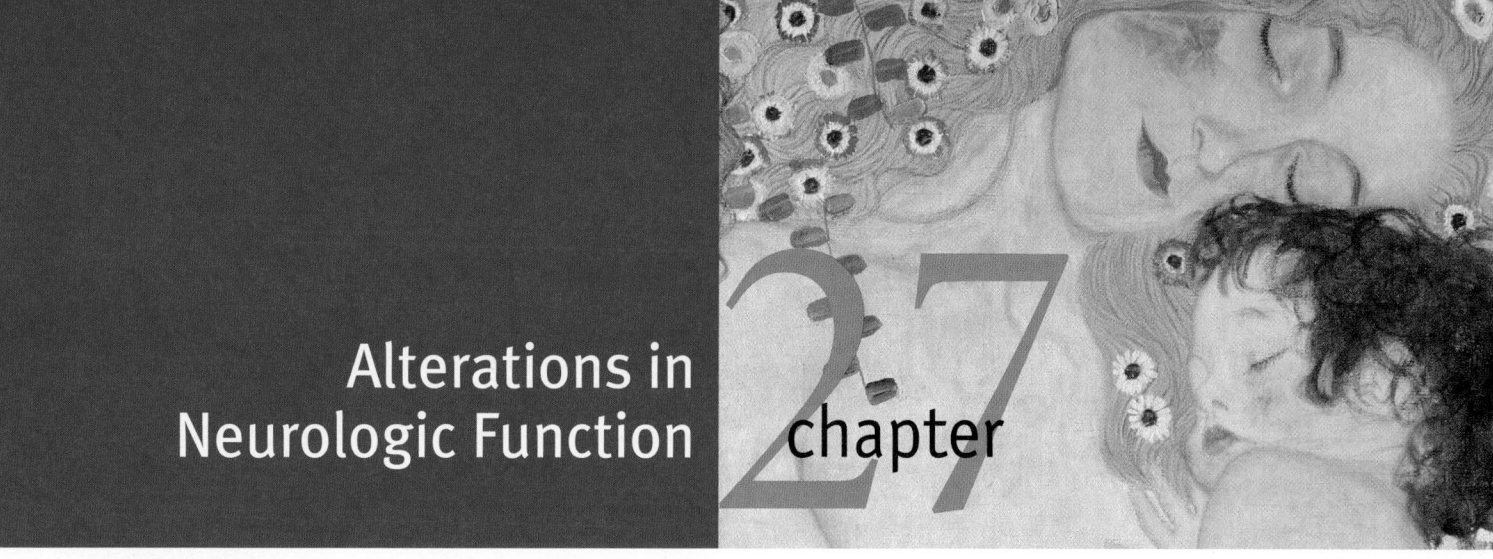

Alterations in Neurologic Function

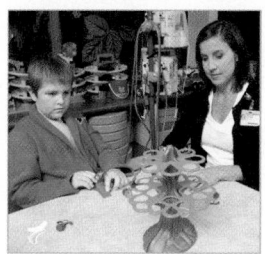

Andy, 8 years old, had a severe headache and fever. After seeing his primary care physician, Andy was sent to the emergency department to be evaluated for meningitis. Andy had a lumbar puncture in the emergency department that revealed white cells in his spinal fluid. The spinal fluid was sent to the lab for culture and sensitivities. An intravenous line was inserted and antibiotics were initiated as soon as the culture was obtained.

On admission to the hospital, Andy was lethargic and irritable, and he complained of a severe headache. No petechial lesions or signs of increased intracranial pressure were identified. His temperature was 40°C (104°F). Andy reported a pain level of 8 in his head and neck. An opioid pain medication and acetaminophen were prescribed.

Andy's initial antibiotic was changed to match the culture sensitivities when the results became available 2 days later. After 24 hours on the appropriate antibiotic, he was no longer considered infectious. Four days have passed, and Andy is beginning to feel like getting up and visiting the playroom for short periods.

What is the nurse's role in the acute care of the child with meningitis? What support does the family need to cope with this serious infection and provide supportive care for the child? What are some potential long-term consequences of this condition?

Learning Outcomes

After reading this chapter, you will be able to do the following:

1. Describe the anatomy and physiology of the neurologic system and pediatric differences.
2. Choose the appropriate assessment guidelines and tools to examine infants and children with altered levels of consciousness and other neurologic conditions.
3. Differentiate between the signs of a seizure and status epilepticus in infants and children, and plan appropriate nursing care for each condition.
4. Differentiate between signs of bacterial meningitis, viral meningitis, encephalitis, Reye syndrome, and Guillain-Barré syndrome in infants and children.
5. Plan family-centered nursing care for the child with myelomeningocele and hydrocephalus.
6. Plan family-centered nursing care for the child with cerebral palsy in a community setting.
7. Contrast the initial nursing management for mild and severe traumatic brain injury.
8. Discuss initiatives to prevent drowning in children.

Key Terms

areflexia / 869
assistive technology / 888
aura / 856
automatisms / 856
autonomic dysreflexia / 897
cerebral edema / 863
cerebral perfusion
  pressure / 852
clonic / 856
coma / 852
consciousness / 852
Cushing triad / 852
diplegia / 883
encephalopathy / 868
febrile seizures / 856
focal / 856
fontanels / 850
herniation / 853
intracranial pressure / 852
microcephaly / 872
myelination / 851
myelomeningocele / 872
neural tube / 850
nuchal rigidity / 864
opisthotonic position / 864
papilledema / 853
paresthesia / 857
postictal period / 856
posturing / 852
sequelae / 866
status epilepticus / 856
stupor / 852
tonic / 856

The Neurologic System

ANATOMY AND PHYSIOLOGY

The brain, spinal cord, and nerves are the major structures of the nervous system (Figure 27–1 ➤). The brain is protected by the skull and covered by three layers of tissue called the meninges—the dura mater, arachnoid, and pia mater. Cerebrospinal fluid circulates within the ventricles of the brain and around the brain and spinal cord.

The brain is a complex organ that controls, regulates, or co-ordinates many body functions. See Table 27–1 for the primary functions of the brain's structures. Stimuli are received from the environment, and the brain enables response for adaptation, survival, and maintenance of body functions. The 12 cranial nerves arise from the brainstem and have many important sensory and motor functions (Table 27–2).

The spinal cord, covered by the vertebrae, transmits impulses to and from the brain, conveying sensory information and relaying impulses that stimulate motor responses. Spinal nerves send and receive information to specific body locations. Nerve impulses are transmitted by chemical substances (e.g., norepinephrine, acetylcholine, dopamine, histamine, and serotonin)

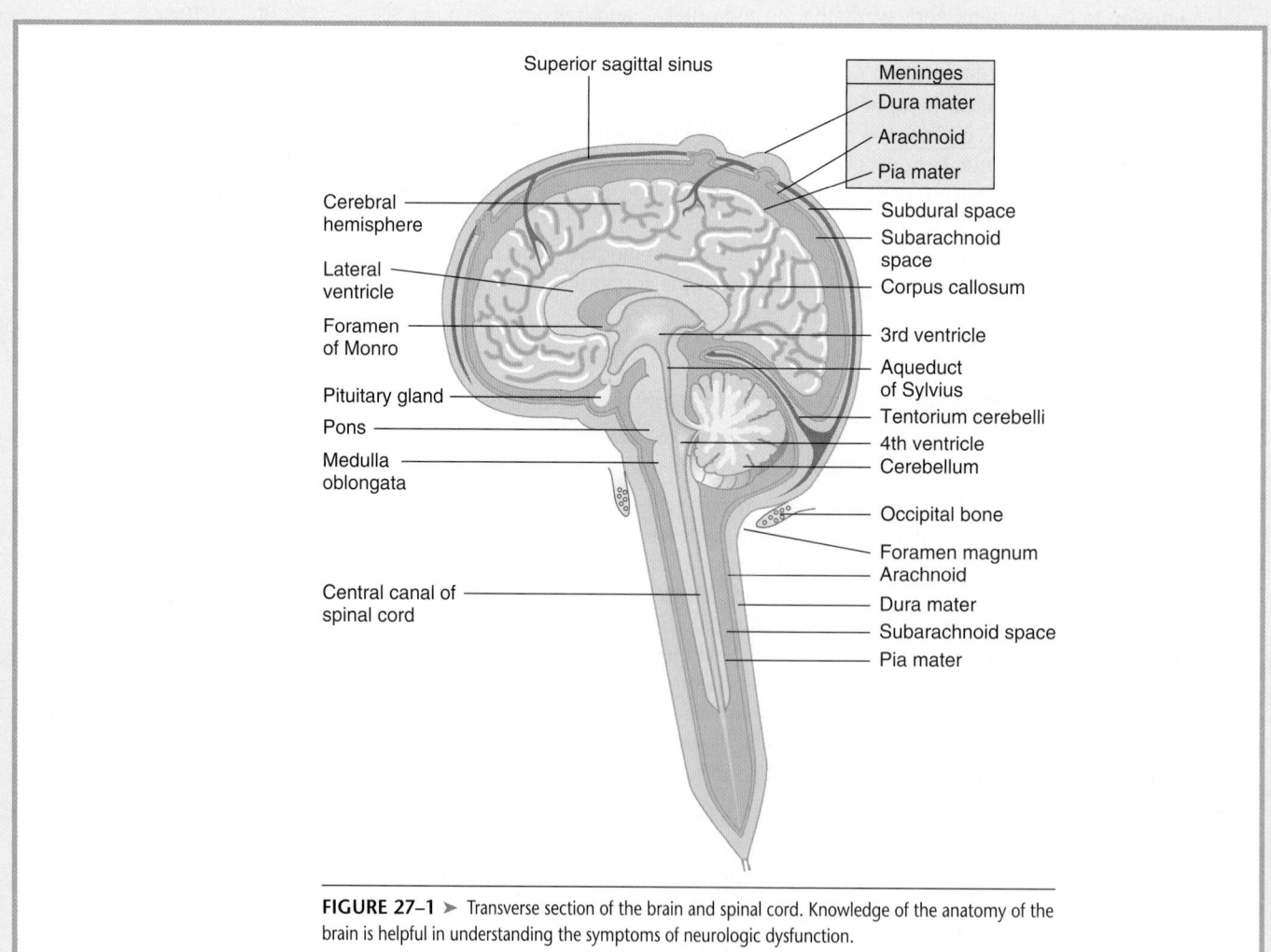

FIGURE 27–1 ➤ Transverse section of the brain and spinal cord. Knowledge of the anatomy of the brain is helpful in understanding the symptoms of neurologic dysfunction.

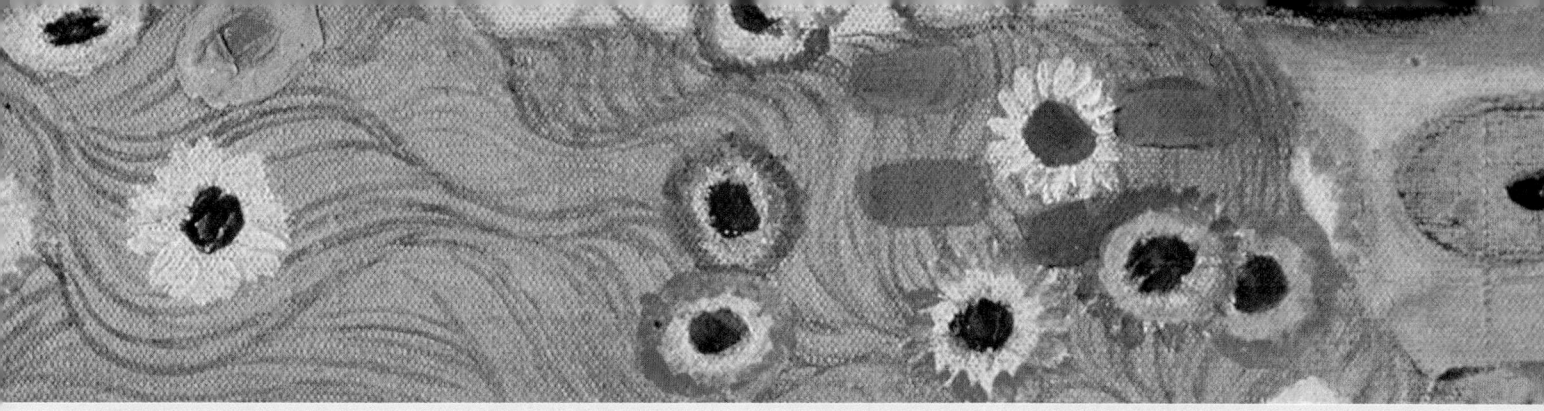

TABLE 27–1 The Brain Structures and Their Primary Functions

Brain Structure	Functions and Control
Cerebrum	Higher mental functions, general movement, perception, and integration of all functions in lobes below
Frontal lobe	Voluntary skeletal muscle movement, fine repetitive motion, eye movements, motor aspects of speech
Parietal lobe	Interpretation of sensations (taste, visual, smell, hearing, temperature, pressure, pain, texture, two-point discrimination); recognition of body parts, proprioception
Occipital lobe	Vision center and interpretation of vision
Temporal lobe	Hearing or the perception, reception, and interpretation of sounds, long-term memory
Insula (corpus callosum)	Coordination of activities between the two hemispheres of the cerebrum
Limbic system	Mediation of certain primitive behavior responses, visceral emotional responses, feeding behaviors, biologic rhythms, and sense of smell
Thalamus	Interpretation of most sensations except smell; relay center for sensory motor information
Hypothalamus	Maintenance of temperature, autonomic nervous system function, endocrine function, wakefulness; regulation of emotional expression
Cerebellum	Conscious and reflexive control of muscle tone, maintenance of balance and posture
Brainstem	Location of the descending and ascending motor and sensory pathways; connects the cerebrum, cerebellum, and spinal cord; origin of the 12 cranial nerves

TABLE 27–2 The Cranial Nerves and Their Functions

Cranial Nerves	Function
Olfactory (I)	Reception and interpretation of smell
Optic (II)	Visual acuity, visual fields
Oculomotor (III)	Many eye movements, raise the eyelids, pupil constriction
Trochlear (IV)	Inward and downward eye movement
Trigeminal (V)	Opening and closing the jaw, chewing; eyelid and corneal sensation; sensation of the face, mouth and nose mucosa, tongue, and ear
Abducens (VI)	Lateral eye movement
Facial (VII)	Facial expression, eye closure, and lip speech sounds; taste sensation on anterior two thirds of tongue; pharyngeal sensation
Acoustic (VIII)	Sense of hearing and equilibrium
Glossopharyngeal (IX)	Muscles for swallowing and guttural speech; gag reflex; taste sensation of posterior one third of tongue, nasopharyngeal sensation
Vagus (X)	Sensation behind ear and in a portion of the external ear canal; involuntary control of the heart and lungs
Spinal accessory (XI)	Shrug the shoulders and turn the head
Hypoglossal (XII)	Tongue movement; swallowing, tongue speech sounds

and electrical conduction enabling the impulse to travel through the synapses from neuron to neuron.

The peripheral nerves transmit impulses from the nerve pathways to the cerebral cortex through simple spinal reflex arcs. The upper motor neurons consist of the fibers originating in the anterior horn of the spinal cord that travel to the brainstem and the nerve cells in the cerebral cortex. The lower motor neurons consist of the peripheral nerves and branches that transmit impulses to the anterior horn of the spinal cord.

The autonomic nervous system maintains a steady state of the internal body organs' and glands' involuntary functions. It is divided into the sympathetic nervous system, which mobilizes the body to respond in times of need or stress; and into the parasympathetic nervous system, which works to conserve and restore energy.

Pediatric Differences

The brain and spinal cord are formed early in gestation from the neural plate, which evolves into the neural groove and neural folds. By the fourth week of gestation the neural folds close to form the **neural tube**, embryonic origin of the central nervous system (CNS). The neural folds close first in the cervical region and then in both the cranial and caudal directions. The brain forms in the cranial end, and the spinal cord forms in the remainder of the neural tube (Boss & Huether, 2010). Any insult (such as inadequate folic acid) or critical event (teratogen, infection, substance abuse, or trauma) during this early gestational period can result in a neural tube defect such as spina bifida.

The anatomic and physiologic differences between the nervous systems of children and adults help explain why children and adults have different neurologic problems (Figure 27–2 ➤). For example, the brain and spinal cord are protected by the skeletal structures of the skull and vertebrae. In infants, however, the cranial bones and vertebrae are not completely ossified. The infant's brain and spinal cord are thus at greater risk for injury. The bones of the skull are separated but held together with bands of connective tissue to allow for normal brain growth. **Fontanels** are spaces of connective tissue covering the brain at the junction of skull bones that gradually close and ossify. The posterior fontanel closes at 3 months of age, and the anterior fontanel closes by 18 to 24 months of age. (See

---

As Children Grow

Anatomic Differences in the Structures of the Nervous System Between Children and Adults

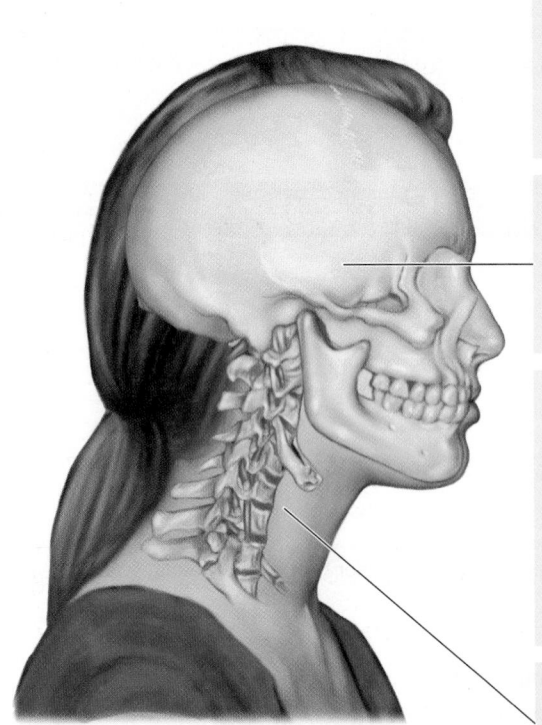
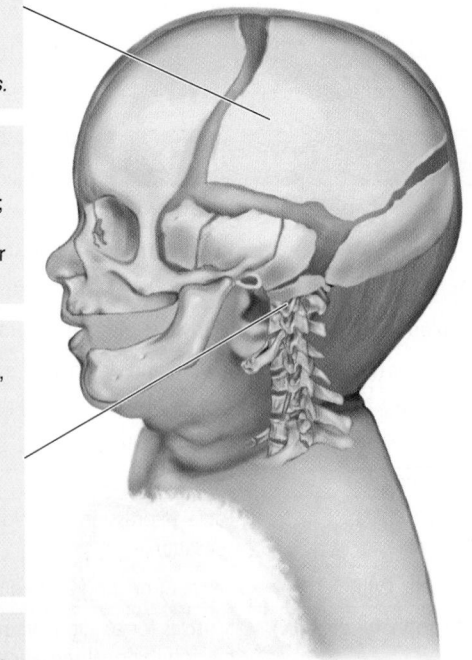

Top heavy, head is large in proportion to body; neck muscles poorly developed; thin cranial bones not well developed; unfused sutures; skull expands until age 2 years. *Prone to brain injury and skull fracture with falls.*

Head size proportional to body; neck muscles well developed, can reduce risk for brain injuries; sutures are ossified by age 12 years; no expansion of skull after 5 years.

Excessive spinal mobility; immature muscles, joint capsule, and ligaments of cervical spine; wedge-shaped, cartilaginous vertebral bodies; incomplete ossification of vertebral bodies. *Greater risk for high cervical spine injury at C1-C2 level or vertebral compression fractures with falls.*

Well developed muscles and ligaments reduce spinal mobility; vertebral bodies completely formed and ossified.

FIGURE 27–2 ➤ The skull and brain grow and develop rapidly during early childhood. Infants and young children are at higher risk for injury to the brain and spinal cord because of developing anatomic structures.

Figure 5–11 in Chapter 5 ∞.) The suture lines between the skull bones interlock as early as 6 months of age; by 12 years of age the sutures are completely ossified and cannot be separated (Boss & Huether, 2010).

A full-term newborn has a complete but immature nervous system. The infant is born with all of the nerve cells that will exist throughout life, but maturation of these nerve cells continues after birth. The number of glial cells and dendrites, which enable receipt of nerve impulses, continues to increase until approximately 4 years of age. Brain growth results in increasing head circumference in infants and toddlers, and continues until the child is 12 to 15 years of age.

Myelination, the progressive covering of axons with layers of myelin or a lipid protein sheath, is also incomplete at birth. Lack of myelination is associated with the presence of primitive reflexes in infants (see Table 5–17 ∞). As the myelination progresses, the primitive reflexes disappear. The myelination process proceeds in a cephalocaudal direction, and it accounts for the progressive acquisition of fine and gross motor skills and coordination during early childhood; it is ultimately responsible for the speed and accuracy of nerve impulses.

The brain depends upon a continuous blood flow to meet its high demands for oxygen. Through an autoregulatory process, the cerebral blood vessels dilate to maintain the cerebral blood flow in response to physiologic changes such as decreased cardiac output, increased intracranial pressure, or constriction of the neck's blood vessels due to positioning. Brain cells become damaged in a very short time when blood flow and oxygenation are not maintained. Because the nervous system helps to control and coordinate many body functions, alterations in neurologic function can have widespread effects on the body's metabolism.

Use the Assessment Guidelines below to perform a nursing assessment of the neurologic system. A list of diagnostic and laboratory tests used to evaluate neurologic system function is provided in Table 27–3. See Appendix D ∞ for laboratory values and Appendix E ∞ for nursing management associated with diagnostic procedures.

TABLE 27–3	Diagnostic Procedures/Laboratory Tests Used to Evaluate Neurologic Conditions*
Diagnostic Procedures	Laboratory Tests
Computed tomography (CT) Electroencephalogram (EEG) Intracranial pressure (ICP) monitoring Lumbar puncture Magnetic resonance imaging (MRI) Positron emission tomography (PET) scan Radiograph (X-ray) Ultrasonography	Arterial blood gases Complete blood count Cultures Toxicology screening

*See Appendices D and E ∞ for information about these diagnostic procedures and expected laboratory values.

Assessment Guidelines for the Child with a Neurologic Condition

Assessment Focus	Assessment Guidelines
Level of consciousness	▪ Is the infant or child lethargic or hard to arouse? ▪ Is the infant or child irritable or difficult to console? ▪ Note that the Glasgow Coma Scale provides a numerical score for future comparison. See Table 27–5.
Cranial nerves	▪ Assess the cranial nerves (Table 5–16 ∞). See also Table 27–6 for methods to indirectly assess cranial nerves in the unconscious child.
Fontanels and sutures	▪ Palpate fontanels and suture lines on the scalp of the infant.
Cognitive function	▪ Are the child's verbal skills developmentally appropriate for age? ▪ Does the child follow directions appropriately?
Pupils	▪ Check the pupils for size and reaction to light and accommodation. See Figure 27–3.
Vital signs	▪ Assess heart rate, respiratory rate, and blood pressure. ▪ Monitor for an increased systolic blood pressure, a widened pulse pressure, bradycardia, and irregular respirations (late signs of increased intracranial pressure).
Posture and movement	▪ Inspect the infant's posture and movement by using the primitive reflexes. See Table 5–17 ∞. ▪ Observe the child's play or other spontaneous activity to assess strength as well as symmetry and smoothness of movements. ▪ Are the child's motor skills developmentally appropriate for age? Were motor skills acquired at the appropriate age? Has the child lost a previously acquired skill? ▪ Evaluate muscle strength and tone, comparing side to side. Is any weakness or spasticity present? ▪ Test the child's coordination for smoothness and symmetry of response. ▪ Assess deep tendon reflexes for smoothness and symmetry of response. See Table 5–19 ∞.
Neck stiffness	▪ Assess for neck stiffness (nuchal rigidity).
Pain	▪ Assess level of pain when present.
Family history	▪ Is there a family history of headaches, seizures, neurofibromatosis, or other neurologic conditions?

■ ALTERED STATES OF CONSCIOUSNESS

Level of consciousness (LOC) is perhaps the most important indicator of neurologic dysfunction. **Consciousness**, the responsiveness of the mind to sensory stimuli, has two components: *alertness*, or the ability to react to stimuli, and *cognitive power*, or the ability to process the data and respond either verbally or physically. *Unconsciousness* is depressed cerebral function, or the brain's inability to respond to stimuli. Altered LOC can be further categorized as:

- **Confusion.** Disorientation to time, place, or person; loss of clear thinking. Answers to simple questions may be correct, but complex question responses may be inaccurate.
- **Delirium.** State characterized by confusion, fear, irritability, agitation, and mental or motor excitement.
- **Lethargy.** Deep sleep; limited speech and movement; aroused with moderate stimulation, but falls asleep easily once stimulation is removed.
- **Stupor.** Deep sleep, responds only to vigorous stimulation and returns to the unresponsive state when the stimulus is removed. For example, the child may react to a needlestick but not a milder stimulus such as touching the skin.
- **Coma.** Unconsciousness; the child cannot be aroused even by painful stimuli.
- **Persistent Vegetative State.** Permanent loss of function of the cerebral cortex with reflexive responses only (eyes following objects, response to pain, hand grasping, facial grimacing, groaning or other sounds).

Etiology and Pathophysiology

Infection of the brain and meninges is the most common cause of an altered LOC in children (Avner, 2006). Other causes include trauma, hypoxia, poisoning, seizures, alcohol or substance abuse, endocrine or metabolic disturbances (e.g., diabetic ketoacidosis), electrolyte or acid-base imbalance, brain tumor, stroke, or a congenital structural defect. Any of these pathologic processes can also cause increased **intracranial pressure** (ICP), the force exerted by brain tissue, cerebrospinal fluid, and blood within the cranial vault. Decreased **cerebral perfusion pressure**, the amount of pressure needed to ensure that adequate oxygen and nutrients will be delivered to the brain, often results when the arterial blood flow to the brain is reduced due to increased ICP. Discovering the cause of the decreased LOC is essential so that immediate treatment can begin, to prevent possible secondary effects of the illness or injury.

Clinical Manifestations

Decline in a child's level of consciousness often follows a sequential pattern of deterioration. Initial changes may be subtle: a slight disorientation to time, place, and person. The child may become restless or fussy, and actions that normally calm or soothe the child only increase irritability. As responsiveness decreases, the child may become drowsy but still respond to loud verbal commands and withdraw from painful stimuli. Keeping the child awake is sometimes difficult. Then response to pain progresses from purposeful to nonpurposeful. The child may exhibit flexor (decorticate) or extensor (decerebrate) **posturing**,

TABLE 27–4	Signs of Increased Intracranial Pressure	
Timing of Signs	Signs
Early signs	Headache Visual disturbances, diplopia Nausea and vomiting Dizziness or vertigo Slight change in vital signs Pupils not as reactive or equal Sunsetting eyes (sclera visible above iris), cranial nerve VI palsy Seizures Slight change in level of consciousness, restlessness *Infant has above signs plus:* Irritability Bulging fontanel Wide sutures, increased head circumference Dilated scalp veins High-pitched, catlike cry
Late signs	Significant decrease in level of consciousness **Cushing triad** • Increased systolic blood pressure and widened pulse pressure • Bradycardia • Irregular respirations Fixed and dilated pupils

abnormal positions assumed after severe injury or damage to the brain. The speed of deterioration varies between children, and with the condition causing alteration in consciousness. In some cases, the changes are rapid and stages may be skipped, such as when the child has a serious brain injury.

Clinical manifestations of increased ICP are provided in Table 27–4.

COLLABORATIVE CARE

Diagnostic Tests

The Glasgow Coma Scale is used to quantify the level of consciousness, thus enabling future comparison of improvement or deterioration in the child's condition. Pediatric criteria take into account the child's developmental age for each category of the test (Table 27–5).

Laboratory tests include a complete blood cell count, blood chemistry, clotting factors, and blood culture; toxicology assessments of both blood and urine; and urinalysis with culture. A lumbar puncture may be performed to assess the cerebrospinal fluid for protein, glucose, or blood cells. An electroencephalogram (EEG) identifies damaged or nonfunctioning areas of the brain. Computed tomography (CT) or magnetic resonance imaging (MRI) is used to detect any lesions, structural abnormalities, vascular malformations, or edema. Skull radiographic studies are used to detect fractures or bony malformations.

TABLE 27-5		Glasgow Coma Scale for Assessment of Coma in Infants and Children	
Category	Score	Infant and Young Child Criteria	Older Child and Adult Criteria
Eye opening	4	Spontaneous opening	Spontaneous
	3	To loud noise	To verbal stimuli
	2	To pain	To pain
	1	No response	No response
Verbal response	5	Smiles, coos, cries to appropriate stimuli	Oriented to time, place, and person; uses appropriate words and phrases
	4	Irritable; cries	Confused
	3	Inappropriate crying	Inappropriate words or verbal response
	2	Grunts, moans	Incomprehensible words
	1	No response	No response
Motor response	6	Spontaneous movement	Obeys commands
	5	Withdraws to touch	Localizes pain
	4	Withdraws to pain	Withdraws to pain
	3	Flexor posturing	Flexor posturing
	2	Extensor posturing	Extensor posturing
	1	No response	No response

Add the score from each category to get the total. The maximum score is 15, indicating the best level of neurologic functioning. The minimum is 3, indicating total neurologic unresponsiveness.

Reprinted with permission from Jankowitz, B. T., & Adelson, P. D. (2006). Pediatric traumatic brain injury: Past, present, and future. Developmental Neuroscience, 28, 264–275. Copyright © S. Karger AG, Basel.

Nursing Alert

Before a lumbar puncture is performed, assess the child for severe increased ICP that could lead to **herniation** (protrusion of brain contents into the brainstem area) as cerebrospinal fluid is removed. In addition to checking for the signs of increased ICP listed in Table 27–4, an ophthalmoscopic examination of the retina is performed to determine if **papilledema**, swelling of the optic disc, is present. The lumbar puncture should be postponed if signs of severe increased ICP are present.

Clinical Therapy

Clinical therapy focuses on early diagnosis of the cause of an altered LOC and intervention to prevent further insult to the central nervous system. The child is treated with oxygen, and assisted ventilation is provided when gas exchange is inadequate. Metabolic, acid-base, or electrolyte imbalances are corrected. Antibiotics are initiated for suspected infection.

Efforts to maintain the cerebral perfusion pressure are important so that adequate oxygen and nutrients are supplied to brain tissue. In cases of hypovolemia, intravenous fluids are given. In cases of poor perfusion and fluid overload, a vasopressor medication such as dopamine is administered to increase cardiac output and perfusion of the brain. If the ICP is markedly increased and is caused by an obstruction leading to the accumulation of cerebrospinal fluid, a ventricular tap can be performed to decrease the pressure and temporarily relieve a life-threatening condition.

NURSING MANAGEMENT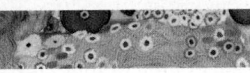

Nursing Assessment and Diagnosis

Initially assess the child's physiologic status, focusing on the child's responsiveness to the environment or stimuli, ability to maintain the airway, vital signs, and breathing patterns. A baseline neurologic assessment should be performed, using the

Growth & Development *Glasgow Coma Scale Assessment*

Following are developmentally appropriate cues in the Glasgow Coma Scale Assessment:

- Eye opening. Note whether eye opening is spontaneous or occurs in response to stimuli.
- Verbal response. Crying in an infant is a positive response. The 2-year-old child who says "no" to each command is also responding in an age-appropriate way.

- Motor response. Motor score is probably the most critical aspect of this test, since the child cannot control reflexes. A fearful toddler may refuse to open his or her eyes or talk to strangers, but the child's reflexes should automatically respond to appropriate stimuli. Ask the child to reach for a finger puppet or doll rather than your hand. This makes the child feel less threatened, and the toy can be a reward.

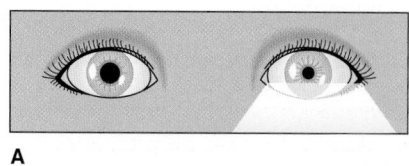

A

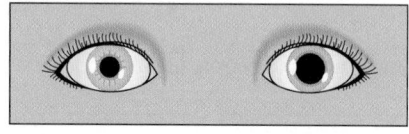

B

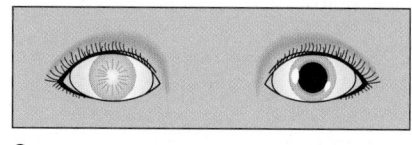

C

FIGURE 27–3 ➤ Pupil findings in various neurologic conditions with altered consciousness. A, A unilateral dilated and reactive pupil is associated with an intracranial mass. B, A fixed and dilated pupil may be a sign of impending brainstem herniation. C, Bilateral fixed and dilated pupils are associated with brainstem herniation from increased intracranial pressure.

guidelines on page 851. Perform routine neurologic checks. Evaluate pupil size and reactivity, eye movements, and motor function (see Figure 27–3 ➤). Monitor vital signs. Increased systolic blood pressure, a wide pulse pressure, and bradycardia indicate increased intracranial pressure. Observe for other signs of increased ICP listed in Table 27–4. Repeated assessments should be performed and compared with baseline findings. The Glasgow Coma Scale may be used to assess the injured child at specified intervals.

Assess the child's cranial nerves (see Table 5–16 ∞). The child's responses may differ significantly when stress and anxiety are reduced, so encourage the parents to take part in the examination to reduce the child's anxiety. In the unconscious child, cranial nerve assessment and interpretation are more challenging (Table 27–6).

Assess the child's airway. The presence of a cough or gag reflex indicates that the child is able to protect the airway from aspiration. Assess the child's respiratory effort and color. Monitor pulse oximetry and arterial blood gas measurements. Adequate air exchange to keep oxygen and carbon dioxide levels within normal ranges and maintaining acid-base balance are critical to reduce the risk of hypoxemia and increased ICP. If the child cannot maintain an adequate respiratory effort, mechanical ventilation will be necessary.

Clinical Judgment

Some signs of the intact neurologic status of an infant, age newborn to 2 months old, are a cry with a loud and energetic quality, a strong suck, and suck-swallowing coordination. What is one additional sign?

Nursing diagnoses that might be appropriate for the child with an altered LOC include:

- Ineffective Breathing Pattern related to neuromuscular dysfunction associated with increased intracranial pressure
- Risk for Aspiration related to poor control of secretions with decreased level of consciousness
- Risk for Impaired Skin Integrity related to agitation and skin rubbing against sheets
- Impaired Verbal Communication related to physiologic condition of decreased level of consciousness
- Interrupted Family Processes related to care of a child with an acquired disability

Planning and Implementation

Hospital-Based Care

Nursing care of the child with altered LOC or increased ICP focuses on maintaining airway patency, monitoring neurologic status, performing routine care, providing sensory stimulation, and providing emotional support to parents. Nursing care for the child with increased ICP is described on page 892.

Ensure that the child's airway is clear at all times. If the child is having difficulty managing secretions or does not have a gag reflex, intubation is performed. A tracheostomy may be performed for long-term airway management. Frequent suctioning

TABLE 27–6	Assessment of Cranial Nerves in the Unconscious Child	
Cranial Nerves	Reflex	Assessment Procedure and Normal Findings[a]
II, III	Pupillary	Shine a light source in the eye. *Rapid, concentrically constricting pupils indicate intact cranial nerves II, III.*
II, IV, VI	Oculocephalic	Should be performed with eyes held open (doll's eyes) and head turned from side to side. *Eyes gazing straight up or lagging slightly behind head motion indicate intact cranial nerves.* Precaution: Cervical spine injury must be ruled out before this assessment is performed.
III, VIII	Oculovestibular	Place the head in a midline and slightly elevated position. Inject ice water into the ear canal. *Eyes deviating toward the irrigated ear indicate intact cranial nerves III, VIII.* Precautions: Cervical spine injury must be ruled out before this assessment is performed. Tympanic membrane must be intact; otherwise, brain may be filled with bacteria-laden fluid. *Note:* This assessment is usually performed by a physician.
V, VII	Corneal	Cornea is gently swabbed with a sterile cotton swab. *A blink indicates intact cranial nerves V, VII.*
IX, X	Gag	Pharynx is irritated with tongue depressor or cotton swab. *Gagging response indicates intact cranial nerves IX, X.*

[a]Italic indicates normal findings.

may be required. Keep suction apparatus with catheters, oxygen, resuscitation bag and mask, and extra tracheostomy tubes (if applicable) at the bedside. Perform pulse oximetry or arterial blood gas analysis at regular intervals to ensure that gas exchange is adequate. Assisted ventilation may be required. (See the *Clinical Skills Manual.*)

Anticipate that seizures may occur. Pad the side rails to protect the child from injury.

Perform routine nursing care. If the corneal reflex is absent, place artificial tears in the eyes and cover them with gauze, taping over so they remain closed. Perform routine mouth care by brushing the teeth and using swabs with water.

Provide adequate nutrition. Nutrients may initially be supplied intravenously, although a nasogastric or transpyloric tube may be inserted if the child is unconscious or not alert enough to take food by mouth. A gastrostomy tube may be inserted if it is anticipated that enteral feeds will be needed for longer than 3 months. (See the *Clinical Skills Manual.*)

Prevent complications associated with immobility (muscle atrophy, contractures, and skin breakdown) as described in the clinical tip below. Support physical therapy efforts with extra passive range of motion exercises.

Clinical Tip

Regarding care of the child who is immobile:

- Keep the body in proper alignment with splints or rolls made of towels or blankets.
- Perform passive or gentle range of motion exercises three or four times per day according to physician's orders.
- Maintain skin integrity:
  - Change position every 2 hours.
  - Place the child on an air or foam mattress, or use sheepskin under the child.
  - Massage the child gently using lotion.
  - Cover skin exposed to rubbing with transparent film.
- Sequential compression devices may be used in some cases to prevent deep vein thrombosis.

Provide sensory stimulation. Because the child with a severely altered LOC may be able to hear, talking to him or her may be beneficial. Listening to music or tapes of family members talking or reading can soothe a child who has an altered LOC when family members cannot be present. Explain all procedures and actions to the family and the child, even though the child's state of consciousness is altered.

When the child becomes more alert, gradually and repeatedly orient the child to time, place, and person, depending on his or her age and level of understanding. Encourage parents to bring objects or toys from home to make the environment more familiar and promote a feeling of security.

Provide emotional support to the child and family. Explain the child's condition in simple terms. Encourage parents to take part in the child's care and therapy as much as possible. If the child's usual functioning has been permanently impaired, refer the family to the appropriate psychologic and social services for emotional support. (See Chapter 13 ∞ for nursing care of

families coping with a child's life-threatening illness.) Give family members opportunities to express their feelings.

Discharge Planning and Home Care Teaching

The child's transition from the hospital to home, a long-term care facility, or inpatient rehabilitation center must be well planned. If long-term care is needed, identify a case manager or social worker who can help with planning the child's care, including home health nursing, adaptation of the home, and purchase of special equipment.

Care in the Community

Home care nurses play a vital role in the care of the child with an acquired neurologic dysfunction and prolonged altered LOC. Teach the family how to care for the child with severe neurologic dysfunction and to perform routine procedures such as maintaining the airway, providing skin care, feeding, positioning, performing exercises, and offering stimulation. Regular follow-up visits are needed to assess the child's progress and to modify the treatment plan.

The child should be linked with community rehabilitation services through an early intervention program or school-based program. The case manager should help the family have an individualized education plan (IEP) developed for the child (see Chapter 12 ∞).

Evaluation

Expected outcomes of nursing care include the following:

- The child's airway is maintained and the brain is adequately oxygenated.
- Complications of immobility are prevented.
- The family provides appropriate care to the child with prolonged altered consciousness to reduce the potential number of long-term disabilities.

SEIZURE DISORDERS

Seizures are periods of abnormal electrical discharges in the brain that cause involuntary movement, as well as behavior and sensory alterations. One in 20 children will have a seizure (with or without fever) by age 18 years, but many children who have one seizure will never experience a second (Fisher, 2007).

Epilepsy is a chronic disorder characterized by recurrent, unprovoked seizures secondary to an underlying brain abnormality. Approximately 45,000 children under age 15 years

Culture *Seizures*

Seizures may have a special meaning to different cultural groups. For example, the Hmong believe the child is experiencing quag dab peg, or "the spirit catches you and you fall down." Traditional Hmong view the condition as serious, but take pride in the child who has the condition, as they have a link to the spirit world. In 1997, Anne Fadiman wrote a compelling story about the cultural conflict between a Hmong family and health care providers over the treatment of their daughter's seizures, *The Spirit Catches You and You Fall Down* (Spector, 2009).

develop epilepsy each year (Epilepsy Foundation, 2009). Approximately 30% of epilepsy cases occur by age 4 years (Boss & Huether, 2010).

Etiology and Pathophysiology

When an excessive number of neurons in the brain become overexcited, they discharge abnormally, leading to seizures. Seizures may result from a CNS structural defect or a disorder that affects CNS functioning, such as brain injury, infection, electrolyte disturbance, toxins, and brain tumor. Genetic factors may predispose the child for seizures. Some seizures have no known cause. See the Clinical Manifestations table for the etiology of various types of seizures.

Partial, or **focal**, seizures are caused by abnormal electrical activity in one hemisphere or a specific area of the cerebral cortex, most often the temporal, frontal, or parietal lobes. The seizure may spread regionally and the symptoms are related to the region of the cortex affected.

Generalized seizures are the result of diffuse electrical activity that begins in both brain hemispheres simultaneously, spreading throughout the cortex into the brainstem. The child's movements and spasms are bilateral and symmetric.

Febrile seizures are generalized seizures that occur in children in connection with a fever (39°C or 102°F or higher) and associated acute illness. No evidence of intracranial infection or other defined cause is found. It is believed that the sensitivity of the young child's developing brain to fever is the mechanism for the seizure. Febrile seizures commonly occur between 6 months and 5 years, with a peak incidence between 18 and 24 months of age (Blumstein & Friedman, 2007). The higher the fever, the greater the risk for a febrile seizure, especially in a child with a positive family history. Children who have one febrile seizure have a 30–40% greater chance of having future febrile seizures (Leung & Robson, 2007).

Status epilepticus occurs when the child has a continuous seizure or recurrent seizures, lasting more than 20 minutes without return to baseline neurologic condition. Approximately 10% of children develop this condition after a diagnosis

of epilepsy (Goldstein, 2008). The prolonged length of the seizure potentially compromises the airway during the tonic phase. Additionally, the basal metabolic rate rises during the peak of seizure activity, increasing the demand for oxygen and glucose.

Clinical Manifestations

The symptoms of a seizure depend on its type and duration. Seizures are classified into two types: *partial (focal) seizures* and *generalized seizures*. The characteristics of the various types of partial and generalized seizures are presented in the clinical manifestations table below.

Partial seizures often start with an aura or an abrupt, unprovoked alteration in behavior. Children may have a partial seizure that progresses to a generalized seizure.

Generalized tonic-clonic seizures are the most common seizure type in children (Blumstein & Friedman, 2007). The **tonic** phase is characterized by unconsciousness and continuous muscular contraction. The **clonic** phase is characterized by alternating muscular contraction and relaxation. During the **postictal period** following seizure activity, the level of consciousness is decreased. The length of the postictal period varies among children. Some children have an **aura** (a visual, auditory, taste, or motor sensation that gives warning of an impending seizure or migraine headache). Once the pattern of an aura is recognized, the child may have time to avoid injury by getting to the floor. During a status epilepticus episode the child may become pale or cyanotic as a result of hypoxia or hypoglycemia.

Febrile seizures involve generalized tonic-clonic movements with the eyes rolling back, generally lasting 1 to 2 minutes. A brief postictal period follows.

Growth & Development *Signs of Newborn Seizure*

The only evidence of seizures in neonates may be lip smacking, eye deviations, or apneic episodes (Blumstein & Friedman, 2007).

Clinical Manifestations
Types of Seizures

Type of Seizure and Cause	Clinical Manifestations
Partial Seizures *Complex partial seizures* (psychomotor seizures) Lesions, cysts, or tumors Perinatal trauma Focal sclerosis (i.e., scarring of the mediotemporal lobe from prolonged febrile seizures) Vascular anomalies (i.e., arteriovenous malformations, a congenital malformed tangle of blood vessels in the brain) Brain trauma	*Onset:* 3 years of age to adolescence Consciousness is impaired immediately; lasts 30 seconds up to 5 minutes; postseizure amnesia or confusion May have abnormal motor activity, twitching, loss of tone, tingling or numbness; may progress to a generalized seizure Aura frequently present, unusual taste or odor Feelings of anxiety, fear, or déjà vu (sensation that event occurred before) Abdominal pain Posturing Staring into space, mental confusion **Automatisms** (unusual body movements without purpose)—lip smacking, lip chewing, sucking

Clinical Manifestations
Types of Seizures (continued)

Type of Seizure and Cause	Clinical Manifestations
Simple partial seizures (focal seizures) Focal damage (e.g., with cerebral palsy) Tumors or lesions Arteriovenous malformation Brain abscesses	*Onset:* any age No loss of consciousness; lasts less than 30 seconds; no postseizure confusion No aura Motor responses may involve one extremity, part of extremity, or ipsilateral extremities with eyes and head turning in opposite direction Sensory responses involve **paresthesia** (decreased sensation or tingling); auditory, olfactory, or visual sensations; autonomic (sweating, pupil dilation) or psychic symptoms Motor and sensory involvement may be combined and progress to generalized seizure Jacksonian march (rare in children): tonic contractions of either fingers of one hand, toes of one foot, or one side of face become clonic or tonic-clonic movements that spread to adjacent muscles of the affected extremity or same side of body
Generalized Seizures *Tonic-clonic seizures* (grand mal seizures) Cerebral damage from perinatal trauma, brain trauma, tumors, structural lesions, metabolic and neuromuscular degenerative disorders Genetic link Many are idiopathic	*Onset:* any age, rare before 6 months of age, strong familial incidence Abrupt onset seizure, 1- to 2-minute loss of consciousness, postseizure confusion (few minutes to hours) May or may not have aura As all muscles contract (tonic phase) the body becomes stiff and rigid, followed by rhythmic jerking motions (clonic phase) Drooling or foaming at mouth as secretions are not swallowed Eyes roll upward or deviate to one side; pupils dilated Abdominal or chest wall rigidity with leg, head, and neck extended, and arms flexed or contracted Cry or grunt as air is forced out when diaphragm and chest muscles contract Urinary or bowel incontinence as muscles become flaccid during clonic phase Characterized by sleepiness, arousal difficulty; hypertension; diaphoresis; headache, nausea, vomiting; poor coordination, decreased muscle tone; confusion, amnesia; slurred speech; visual disturbances; combativeness
Absence seizures (petit mal, or lapse seizures) Hyperventilation Genetic predisposition	*Onset:* age 3–12 years with remission in adolescence More prevalent in females May go on to develop other generalized seizures Hyperventilation or flashing lights may trigger a seizure No aura; brief loss of consciousness, usually lasts 5–10 seconds, rarely exceeds 30 seconds; no postseizure confusion, lethargy, or sleepiness, but amnesia regarding the seizure Frequent attacks (50–100 per day), may cluster, interfere with learning; episodes may be confused with daydreaming or inattentiveness Child may continue simple movements such as walking or looking, but ceases activities such as reading; slight decrease or loss of muscle tone (head may droop, objects may be dropped)
Juvenile myoclonic seizures Genetic disorder with possible locus on chromosome 6p11, 15q14, 6q24, or 10q35 (Boss & Huether, 2010)	*Onset:* more prevalent in adolescents No loss of consciousness, child recovers in seconds, no postictal period Most often occur upon falling asleep or awakening Quick involuntary muscle jerks of the neck, shoulders, and arms Child usually has normal intelligence
Infantile spasms (myoclonic epilepsy of infancy, salaam seizures) ARX and CDKL5 gene mutations (Boss & Huether, 2010) Tuberous sclerosis Brain insult	*Onset:* begin at age 4 to 8 months Occur in clusters, 5 to 150 per day, may be worse when waking or falling asleep Episodes of abrupt flexor (jackknife seizures), extensor or mixed jerks occurring in flurries Seizures increase in intensity and severity over time, leading to a loss in developmental milestones and disability
Lennox-Gastaut syndrome Epilepsy syndrome	Onset: between 1 and 5 years; usually in males Includes a variety of generalized seizures, e.g., tonic-clonic, drop attacks, absence, myoclonic activities Associated with intellectual disability (mental retardation), delayed development, and personality disorders

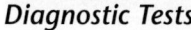

COLLABORATIVE CARE

Diagnostic Tests

After the child's first seizure, a thorough history should be taken from the parent, primary caretaker, or witnesses to the event. Details include a description and length of the seizure, presence or absence of an aura, and whether the child lost consciousness. This information helps to identify the type of seizure according to the International Classification of Epileptic Seizures.

Based on the history and physical findings, diagnostic tests ordered may include a complete blood cell count, blood chemistry, urine culture, and lumbar puncture. A lead level and tests for inborn errors of metabolism may be considered. Radiologic tests such as CT scanning or MRI and angiography may be performed to identify a cerebral lesion or metabolic disorder in the brain. An EEG is often performed at a follow-up visit between seizures. If the child is taking any anticonvulsants, the serum drug blood level is monitored regularly.

Clinical Therapy

Many seizures are self-limiting and require no emergency intervention. When the seizure is prolonged, emergency therapy includes airway management, supplemental oxygen, intravenous benzodiazepines, and careful monitoring of vital signs. Serum electrolytes, glucose, and blood gases may be monitored. Monitor for continued motor activity, which may be less intense after benzodiazepines are given. The postictal period ranges from 30 minutes to 2 hours. When the child's seizure does not stop as expected with emergency intervention, treatment for status epilepticus is initiated (Table 27–7).

Children with febrile seizures are usually not treated with an anticonvulsant because the seizure is usually over before arrival at the emergency department. Acetaminophen is given to lower the temperature. Long-term anticonvulsants are not recommended for simple febrile seizures because of their adverse effects (Leung & Robson, 2007).

Most seizure disorders are treated with anticonvulsants. A single medication (monotherapy) is preferred for seizure control to minimize the side effects such as sleepiness, decreased attention and memory, difficulty with speech, ataxia, and diplopia. Monotherapy works for 60–70% of children with new-onset epilepsy (Wolf & McGoldrick, 2006). An alternate antiepileptic may be used if seizure control is not achieved with the first medication or if unacceptable side effects occur. Some children require multiple medications for seizure control. See Medications Used to Treat Seizures. Serum drug levels are monitored to achieve therapeutic levels or identify if toxicity is possible. Therapeutic ranges of medications may be exceeded to control seizures when tolerated by the child.

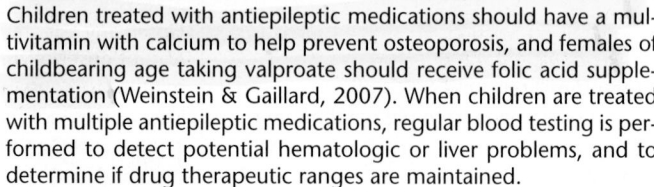

Nursing Alert

Children treated with antiepileptic medications should have a multivitamin with calcium to help prevent osteoporosis, and females of childbearing age taking valproate should receive folic acid supplementation (Weinstein & Gaillard, 2007). When children are treated with multiple antiepileptic medications, regular blood testing is performed to detect potential hematologic or liver problems, and to determine if drug therapeutic ranges are maintained.

Surgery to remove a section of the brain with a localized seizure focus may occasionally be performed when seizures are not responsive to medication and the child has a poor quality of life (Major & Thiele, 2007). A vagal nerve stimulator, a pacemaker-like device that transmits electrical impulses to the vagus nerve, is another option for children with partial intractable seizures (Major & Thiele, 2007).

A ketogenic diet (high-fat, adequate protein for growth, and very low carbohydrate) is occasionally used for children with intractable seizures. This diet is customized to help the child maintain an ideal body weight, maximize ketosis, and achieve optimal seizure control. Family motivation must be high to maintain the rigid diet because improved seizure control is directly related to diet compliance for a year or longer (Figure 27–4 ➤). Diet side effects include dyslipidemia, constipation, kidney stones, and slowed growth. Constipation is treated with medium chain

TABLE 27–7	Management of Status Epilepticus
Type of Care	Clinical Therapy
Emergency assessment and management	• Maintain a patent airway. Muscle rigidity may compromise the airway. Keep suction equipment at the bedside in case secretions are excessive. • Give oxygen by mask, as increased metabolic demands deplete oxygen stores. • Monitor vital signs and circulation with a pulse oximeter and cardiorespiratory monitor. • Perform a neurologic assessment.
Ongoing urgent care	• Establish an intravenous line for fluids and medications. • Administer glucose if the child is hypoglycemic; the physical stress of the seizure may result in declining glucose levels. • Insert a nasogastric tube. • Protect the child from injury. • Manage thermoregulation.
Medications	• Administer benzodiazepines such as diazepam, lorazepam, or midazolam. If there is no response, the dose may be repeated. Phenytoin or phenobarbital may be necessary if seizure activity continues. Cumulative doses of drugs may produce apnea, so be prepared to assist ventilations.

Medications Used to Treat
Seizures

Medication and Action	Nursing Management
Benzodiazepines (Diazepam, Lorazepam) CNS depressant; anticonvulsant properties	▪ Administer IV push medication very slowly into the IV port closest to the child's body. ▪ Monitor for hypotension, tachycardia, and respiratory depression.
Phenobarbital Limits spread of seizure activity by increasing threshold for motor cortex stimuli	▪ Administer IV push medication very slowly into the IV port closest to the child's body. ▪ Monitor the child's vital signs frequently when given IV. ▪ May crush tablets and mix with food or fluid.
Phenytoin (Dilantin) Reduces voltage, frequency, and spread of electrical discharges within motor cortex to inhibit seizure activity	▪ Educate family to provide an adequate intake of vitamin D, folic acid, and calcium. ▪ Inform parents of side effects of acne, gingival hyperplasia, and hirsutism. ▪ Encourage frequent dental care.
Carbamazepine (Tegretol) Action similar to phenytoin	▪ Give with food to enhance absorption. ▪ Do not administer suspension simultaneously with another liquid medication to prevent formation of a precipitate. ▪ Causes photosensitivity reactions.
Valproic acid (Depacon, Depakote) Anticonvulsant, unknown mechanism of action	▪ Do not use carbonated beverage to dilute syrup. Tablets and capsules should not be chewed. Give with food to decrease gastrointestinal irritation. ▪ Do not use drug in combination with aspirin, sedatives, and allergy medications. ▪ Monitor platelet count and bleeding times.
Ethosuximide (Zarontin) Depresses motor cortex and increases CNS threshold to stimuli	▪ Monitor for weight loss or anorexia. ▪ Give with food if gastrointestinal upset occurs.
Felbamate (Felbatol) Blocks repetitive firing of neurons and increases seizure threshold	▪ Monitor weight for gain or loss. ▪ Monitor regularly for hematologic and liver problems.
Gabapentin (Neurontin) Gamma-aminobutyric acid (GABA) neurotransmitter analog	▪ Monitor vision, concentration, and coordination as medication may cause impairments. ▪ Do not take medication within 2 hours of an antacid.
Lamotrigine (Lamictal) Inhibits release of glutamate (neurotransmitter) in brain tissue	▪ Educate family about photosensitivity side effect. ▪ Monitor for adverse effects if used with valproic acid.
Tiagabine (Gabitril filmtabs) GABA inhibitor	▪ Give with food. Avoid using with over-the-counter medications that cause drowsiness. ▪ Monitor for signs of CNS depression.
Topiramate (Topamax) GABA inhibitor	▪ Monitor for metabolic acidosis. ▪ Increase fluid intake to reduce risk of kidney stones. ▪ Monitor for adverse effects of psychomotor, speech, and language slowing.
Levetiracetam (Keppra) Anticonvulsant, unknown mechanism of action	▪ Do not engage in hazardous activities such as driving any motorized vehicle (e.g., ATV or car) until effect of drug is known. ▪ Do not abruptly discontinue the medication.
Oxcarbazepine (Trileptal) May block voltage-sensitive sodium channels to stabilize hyperexcited neural membranes	▪ Monitor for hyponatremia. ▪ Use barrier contraception as the drug interferes with hormonal contraception methods.
Vigabatrin GABA inhibitor	▪ Monitor vision, can cause blindness. ▪ Not approved for use in children in the United States.
Zonisamide (Zonegran) Facilitates dopaminergic and serotonergic neurotransmission	▪ Increase fluid intake to reduce risk of kidney stones. ▪ Report dizziness, excess drowsiness, lack of coordination, or double vision.

Data from: Wilson, B. A., Shannon, M. T., & Shield, K. M. (2009). Nurse's drug guide 2009. Upper Saddle River, NJ: Prentice Hall Health; Blumstein, M. D., & Friedman, M. J. (2007). Childhood seizures. Emergency Medical Clinics of North America, 25, 1061–1086; Wolf, S. M., & McGoldrick, P. E. (2006). Recognition and management of seizures. Pediatric Annals, 35(5), 332–344.

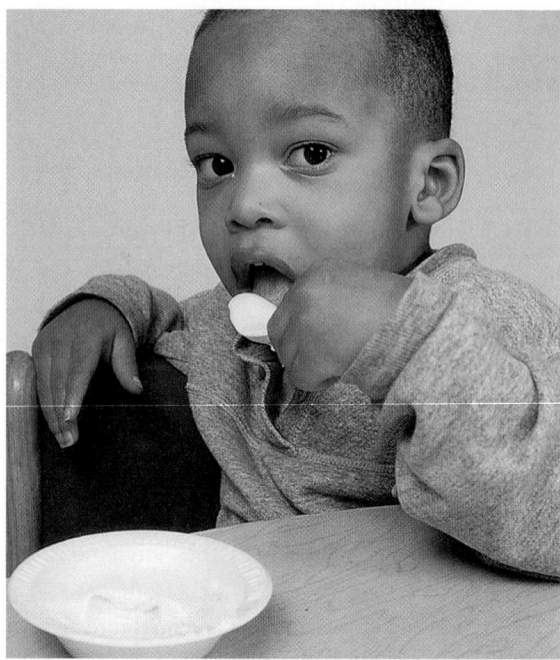

FIGURE 27–4 ➤ The family must make an effort to make the high-fat diet appealing to the child on a ketogenic diet, despite their personal feelings about eating large amounts of food such as mayonnaise, as this child is doing.

triglycerides (MCT) oil and increased fluids. Kidney stones are treated by increasing fluids and alkalinizing the urine. About 10–15% of children who initiate the ketogenic diet are seizure-free after 1 year and 30% have greater than a 90% reduction in seizures, even after discontinuing the diet (Freeman, Kossoff, & Hartman, 2007). Many families discontinue the diet because it is too difficult or not seen as effective. A modified Atkins diet with a restriction of carbohydrates to 10 to 20 grams per day without reducing calories or protein is an alternative diet associated with reduced seizures (Freeman et al., 2007).

A trial of antiepileptic medication withdrawal is often attempted for children who have been seizure-free for 2 to 5 years. Approximately 70% of children remain seizure-free without medications (Wolf & McGoldrick, 2006).

NURSING MANAGEMENT

Assessment and Diagnosis

Assess and monitor the child's physiologic status. Observe the specific seizure activity, LOC, vital signs, and signs of hypoxia. During the postictal period, monitor the child's vital signs, perform neurologic checks, and keep the environment safe. Remember that the child's decreased LOC may be the result of the postictal state. Once the child is stable, a more definitive assessment can be made.

Collect and analyze historical information about the seizure activity. See Box 27–1.

Assess the family's adaptation to the seizure disorder, including how well the family is coping with the uncertainty of when the next seizure will occur.

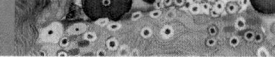

BOX 27–1 History Questions to ask about Seizures

Just before the seizure:
- What was the child doing?
- Did the child complain of feeling ill (headache, nausea, vomiting, muscle pain, fever) or feeling "funny"?
- Did the child suffer any trauma?
- Did the child get into any medications or poisons?

During the seizure:
- What movements of the arms and legs were seen? On one or both sides of the body or in one extremity only?
- Did the child exhibit any chewing or other type of automatic behavior?
- Were the pupils dilated or the eyes deviated to one side?
- Did the child's color change (pale, red, blue)?
- Was the child incontinent of urine or stool?
- Was the child aware of surroundings or able to respond to questions?
- How long did the episode last? Was the child lethargic, weak, or uncoordinated when waking up? Did the child have loss of memory or confusion?

Common nursing diagnoses for the child with a seizure disorder include:

- Ineffective Breathing Pattern related to neuromuscular dysfunction during the tonic phase of a seizure
- Ineffective Airway Clearance related to inability to control or manage secretions during the seizure
- Risk for Trauma related to fall with onset of seizure activity
- Chronic Low Self-Esteem related to refractory seizures and loss of bowel and bladder control during seizure activity
- Anxiety related to unpredictable nature of seizure disorder
- Ineffective Therapeutic Regimen Management related to poor adherence with medications

Planning and Implementation

Nursing care focuses on maintaining airway patency, ensuring safety, administering medications, and providing emotional support. Both acute care and long-term management are involved.

Maintain Airway Patency

Place nothing in the child's mouth during a seizure because loose teeth may be knocked out and aspirated. Position the child on his or her side so secretions can drain. Monitor the child to ensure adequate oxygenation: the child's color should be pink, the heart rate should be at a normal or slightly elevated rate for age, and the pulse oximetry reading (SpO_2) should be greater than 95%. Oxygen is usually administered when the pulse oximetry reading falls below 95%.

Ensure Safety

Protect the child from self-harm during violent seizures (Figure 27–5 ➤). If the child is in bed, pad the side rails to prevent injury. The child with frequent, recurrent seizures should wear a helmet to protect the head during falls. All children with seizure disorders should wear some form of medical alert identification.

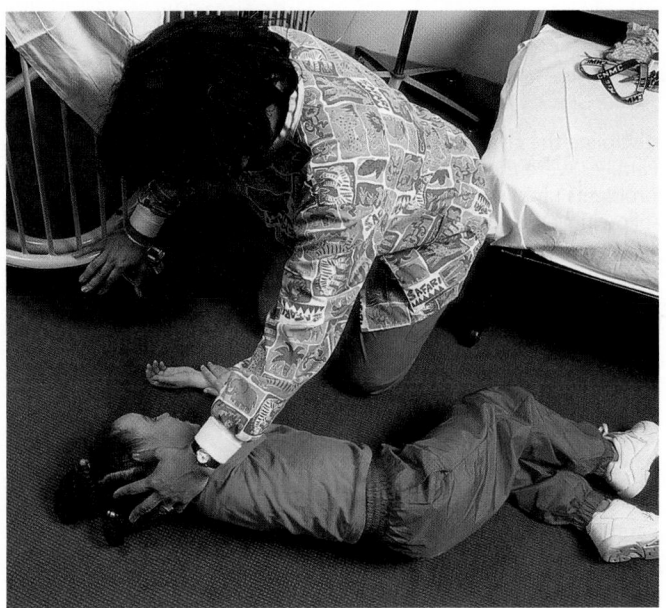

FIGURE 27–5 ➤ A child who has a seizure when standing should be gently assisted to the floor and placed in a side-lying position. Clear the area of any objects that might cause harm to the child. Do not insert anything into the child's mouth.

Administer Medications

Take special precautions when administering intravenous medications (diazepam, lorazepam, or fosphenytoin) for the emergency management of status epilepticus. Give these IV push medications very slowly over several minutes to minimize the risk of respiratory or circulatory collapse.

Medications for the ongoing management of seizures are given orally. When a child is NPO (nothing by mouth) because of illness or on the day of surgery, seizure medications are usually given with a swallow of water. Obtain medication orders in these cases.

Clinical Tip

When the child on a ketogenic diet is hospitalized, limit glucose and dextrose from all sources, including intravenous fluids, elixirs, suspensions, and syrups. Alternatively obtain medications in pill form, crush them, and mix with an allowable food approved by the pharmacy.

Provide Emotional Support

Seizures are frightening to the child and family because of the loss of control of body movements and possible loss of consciousness. Parents often feel guilty about the child's seizure disorder and need guidance to treat the child as normally as possible. Refer the child and family to support groups and counseling services if indicated. See Evidence-Based Practice: Supporting Children with Epilepsy and Their Parents.

Discharge Planning and Home Care Teaching

Encourage parents to express their fears and anxieties. Answer their questions honestly, and refer them to organizations such as the Epilepsy Foundation of America and Internet resources,

where they can get more information about the child's disorder. Be sure parents know how to administer medications and keep the child safe. Discuss with them whom to call with questions and when to return for follow-up.

The parents of children with recurrent febrile seizures should be taught how to properly administer antipyretics. Parents need to know, however, that antipyretics may not prevent a future febrile seizure associated with an acute illness. The potential toxicity of an anticonvulsant in a child with febrile seizures is often considered greater than the risk of the seizures, and parents can be reassured that complications from febrile seizures are rare.

Care in the Community

Educate the child and parents about medication regimens. Explain the purpose of each drug, its schedule for administration, and the importance of giving all doses. Provide information about the side effects of medications ordered, and alert parents to the signs of toxic reactions or undermedication. Explain how to use rectal diazepam (Diastat) for acute management of a seizure, if prescribed. Ensure that information is shared directly with the older child so that he or she can begin taking more responsibility for self-care and gain a sense of self-control. Regular dental care is also important because of the effect of phenytoin (Dilantin) on the gingiva. Explain the importance of follow-up visits to health care providers so that medication blood levels and the effectiveness of the child's medications can be monitored. Monitor the child's growth as the dosage needs to be adjusted to keep the medication within its therapeutic range as the child grows.

Clinical Tip

The blood for serum drug levels is ideally obtained just prior to a dose so that it can be representative of the child's lowest serum level.

Adolescent females need to be educated about the potential teratogenicity of some anticonvulsants, such as valproic acid and carbamazepine, that are associated with neural tube defects and heart defects. Contraception should be used when the adolescent is sexually active. When pregnancy is desired, anticonvulsants with a lower risk for birth defects may be prescribed.

Clinical Tip

Some antiepileptic medications, such as phenobarbital, primidone, phenytoin, carbamazepine, and oxcarbazepine, cause a drug interaction with low-estrogen oral contraceptive pills that can lead to contraceptive failure. Effective contraception may require the use of medroxyprogesterone depot injections or an intrauterine device (Thomas, 2006).

Teach families about safety guidelines for the child. Families of children with severe seizure disorders need to develop an emergency care plan so that emergency personnel know about their needs for care in advance (see Chapter 10 ∞). A medical alert tag should be worn. See Families Want to Know: Safety for the Child with a Seizure Disorder.

Evidence-Based Practice

Supporting Children with Epilepsy and Their Parents

Problem

Children with epilepsy and their parents need information and support to improve their adjustment to living with epilepsy.

Evidence

One qualitative study used focus groups to identify information needs of 11 children (7 to 15 years of age) and 15 parents. Children reported frustration because health care providers talked with their parents and did not explain seizures in a way the children understood. They recognized that they were different from other children because of their diet, need to take medication at school, or limitations in some physical activities. Parents described challenges in being their child's advocate, trying to get information about the treatment plan and expected course of the child's disorder, and wishing for coordinated care, such as a health care home (see Chapter 6 ∞). Parents were concerned about the different medications prescribed and became confused when medications or dosages were adjusted. Parents also worried about the physical and emotional health of their children (McNelis, Buelow, Myers, et al., 2007).

A study using structured telephone interviews with parents of 224 children (4 to 14 years) having epilepsy focused on identifying family factors associated with behavior problems in children. At the onset of seizures, 32% of children had behavior problems, most commonly attention and social problems, along with anxiety and depression. Parents were interviewed about the family environment, specifically family mastery (family emotion, a sense of control over events, family organization, and cooperation among family members) and family esteem/communication, as well as their perceived worry and need for information and support. Families with a disorganized family environment and low parent confidence in ability to discipline the child had greater child behavior problems at baseline. Families were more likely to have a child with greater internalizing problems (anxiety and depression) if difficulties were found with the following tasks: family mastery, disciplining the child, and encouraging child autonomy. These families also had a continuing need for information and support, and experienced greater worry 24 months after seizure onset than families whose child had less anxiety and depression. The children of families that gained confidence in child discipline over the 24-month study period had fewer internalizing problems. Parents requested support in the form of discussions about the child's future, the child's mental health, fears about the child's seizures, and having the child talk with other children who have seizures (Austin, 2004).

Implications

Parents often have no prior experience with epilepsy, and studies reveal that parents and children often do not have their concerns and needs well addressed by health care providers. Assess for child behavior problems and parenting behaviors, and provide education and support at the time of new-onset seizures. Parents need guidance related to parenting their children and understanding that discipline is important for all children. Referral to support groups is one way to provide ongoing support and education that can improve the child's and family's coping with a seizure disorder.

Critical Thinking Application

Refer to Chapters 8 and 9 ∞ for guidelines about child discipline methods, and develop a series of questions to identify how parents discipline their child with epilepsy. Identify some strategies to help the parents implement effective age-appropriate discipline for children 3 to 6 years of age.

Assist the family to work with school administrators to develop an individualized health plan so the child can receive needed medications and care during school hours. Teachers and school administrators should know what to do if the child has a seizure and what information to report about the seizure. Parents may want to provide a towel and change of clothing for the child to use if incontinence occurs along with the seizures.

Physical activity and exercise are important for all children. Encourage participation in sports when adequate supervision is

Families Want to Know

Safety for the Child with a Seizure Disorder

Children with epilepsy have more injuries of all sorts, including burns and falls. These children are also at increased risk for death due to drowning. Planning for safety includes the following:

- Children who bathe alone should use the shower. The child should not be left alone in a bathtub with a water level.
- A buddy and lifeguard should always be present when the child swims.
- A life vest should always be worn when boating.
- A child with frequent seizures should wear a helmet to protect the head in case of a fall.
- The child should not play or stand around open flames or outdoor grills.
- The child should avoid areas where fall risks are increased.

provided. Children with well-controlled seizures may participate in most team sports, and activities like bicycle riding. Activities such as rope climbing, rock or mountain climbing, tree climbing, snow skiing, scuba diving, and sky diving are more dangerous if seizures are not well controlled. Swimming and water sports require one-to-one supervision.

The child may be afraid of having a seizure in front of friends. Reassure the child and family that taking medications regularly should control seizures. Children need to be able to explain to peers what a seizure is and what to do if they are present when one occurs. However, adolescents are often hesitant to reveal a seizure disorder to peers because of embarrassment over being different. A support group may be valuable to help relieve those feelings. Summer camps for children with seizures can be a safe and comfortable place for the child to enjoy outdoor activities. Encourage parents to boost the child's self-image by emphasizing what the child can do, rather than focusing on contraindicated activities. Depending on state laws, most adolescents can drive after they have been seizure-free for at least 2 years.

Evaluation

Expected outcomes of nursing management include the following:

- The child achieves good seizure control with medication, ketogenic diet, or surgical intervention.

- Injuries associated with seizures are prevented through the use of effective safety measures.
- The child's self-esteem is enhanced through participation in well-supervised sports and activities.

■ INFECTIOUS DISEASES

Bacterial Meningitis

Meningitis, an inflammation of the meninges, can be caused by either bacterial or viral agents. Bacterial meningitis is more serious than viral meningitis and is sometimes fatal. Newborns and infants are at greatest risk for bacterial meningitis. Infants and children who develop meningitis have the potential for acute complications and long-term morbidity.

Etiology and Pathophysiology

Meningitis may occur secondary to other infections such as otitis media, sinusitis, pharyngitis, cellulitis, pneumonia, tuberculosis, or septic arthritis; brain trauma; or a neurosurgical procedure. Two organisms, meningococcus and pneumococcus, cause 95% of cases in children in the United States. *Haemophilus influenzae* type b remains a common causative organism in developing countries. *Group B Streptococcus* is most likely to cause meningitis in newborns (Mann & Jackson, 2008). (See Chapter 16 ∞ for more information about these infectious organisms.) Risk factors for meningitis include immunosuppression, a ventriculoperitoneal shunt, cochlear implant, CNS trauma, or a recent sinus or ear infection (Mann & Jackson, 2008).

In many cases, bacteria in the blood spread to the CNS and enter the subarachnoid space. An inflammatory response then follows (Figure 27–6 ➤). Bacterial toxins cause the brain to become inflamed and edematous, leading to **cerebral edema** (the increase in intracellular and extracellular fluid in the brain that results from anoxia, vasodilation, or vascular stasis) and increased ICP. If the infection spreads to the ventricles, they can become obstructed, causing hydrocephalus. The infection may

Pathophysiology Illustrated
Central Nervous System Infection

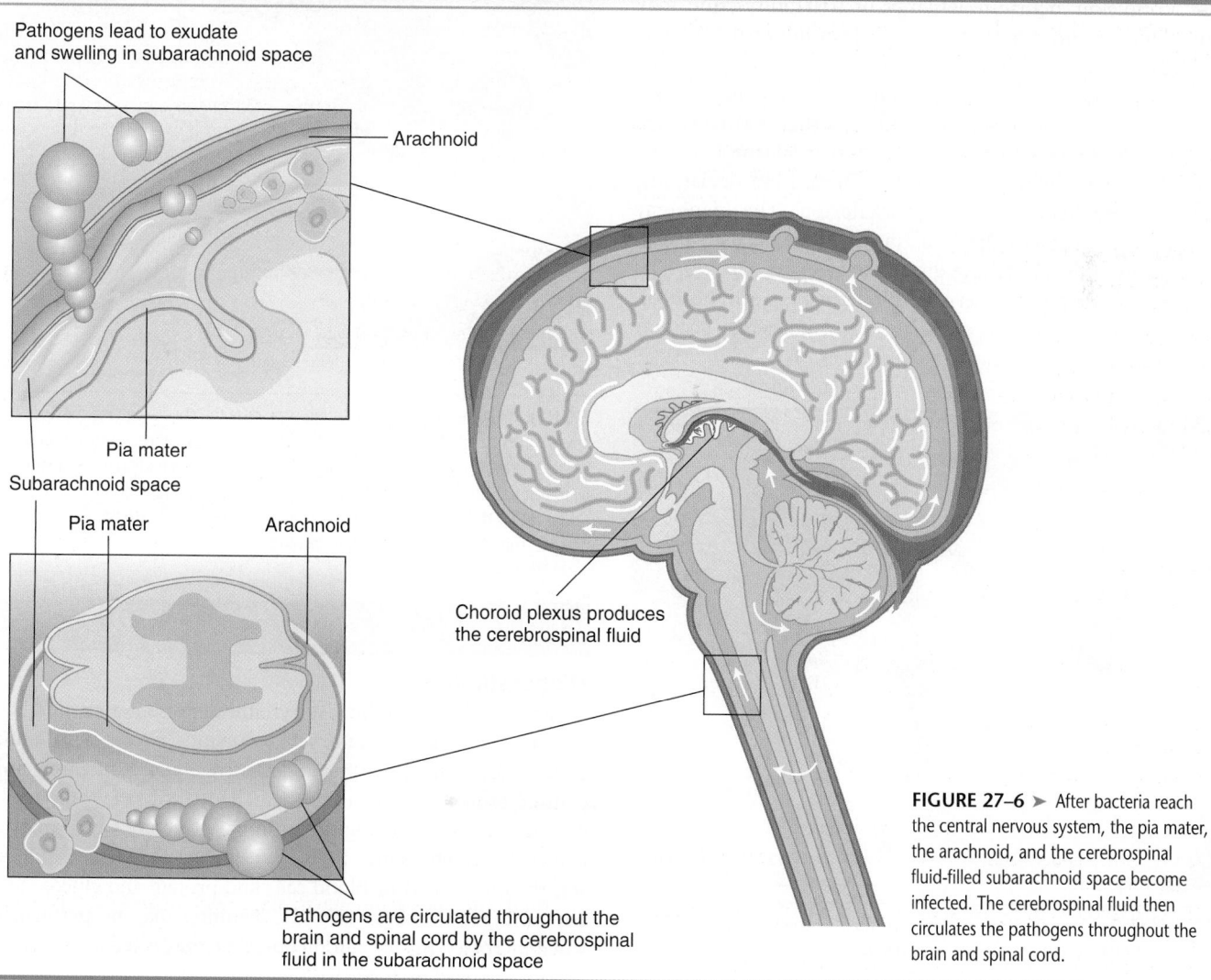

Pathogens lead to exudate and swelling in subarachnoid space

Arachnoid

Pia mater

Subarachnoid space

Pia mater   Arachnoid

Choroid plexus produces the cerebrospinal fluid

Pathogens are circulated throughout the brain and spinal cord by the cerebrospinal fluid in the subarachnoid space

FIGURE 27–6 ➤ After bacteria reach the central nervous system, the pia mater, the arachnoid, and the cerebrospinal fluid-filled subarachnoid space become infected. The cerebrospinal fluid then circulates the pathogens throughout the brain and spinal cord.

trigger the syndrome of inappropriate antidiuretic hormone (SIADH) (see Chapter 30 ∞).

Health Promotion

Haemophilus influenzae type b was the most common cause of bacterial meningitis in children prior to the use of the Hib conjugate vaccine. It is now rare, with a rate of 0.11 cases per 100,000 children less than age 5 years (Centers for Disease Control and Prevention, 2009). Immunization of infants with the pneumococcal vaccine is reducing the incidence of meningitis caused by specific serotypes of *Streptococcus pneumoniae* included in the vaccine (Mann & Jackson, 2008).

Clinical Manifestations

Symptoms are variable and depend on the child's age, the pathogen, and the length of the illness before diagnosis. Onset may be sudden or may develop over 1 to 2 days. Symptoms in the young infant may include fever, change in feeding pattern, vomiting, or diarrhea. The anterior fontanel may be bulging or flat. The infant may be alert, restless, lethargic, or irritable. However, rocking or cuddling, which normally calms a fussy infant, only irritates the infant with meningitis.

Older children are usually febrile, have altered consciousness (confusion, delirium, lethargy, or irritability), and may have vomiting and complaints of muscle or joint pain. A hemorrhagic, petechial rash, changing to purpura or large necrotic patches, may be seen in meningococcal meningitis (see Chapter 16 ∞ , page 414). The child also displays other symptoms consistent with meningeal irritation: headache (most often frontal), photophobia, esotropia (inward eye deviation), and **nuchal rigidity** (resistance to neck flexion). The infant may assume an **opisthotonic position**, in which the head and neck are hyperextended, to relieve discomfort (Figure 27–7 ➤). The child may have a positive Kernig or Brudzinski sign, or both, on examination (Figure 27–8 ➤). Seizures and apnea may occur as the condition progresses.

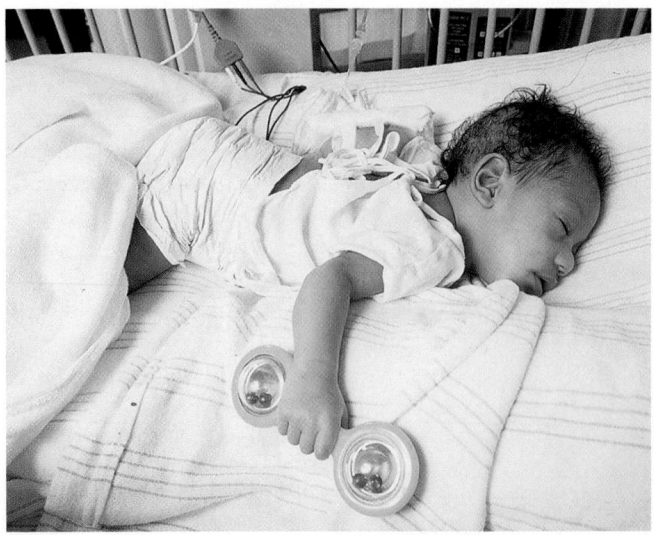

FIGURE 27–7 ➤ The child with bacterial meningitis assumes an opisthotonic position, with the neck and the head hyperextended, to relieve discomfort.

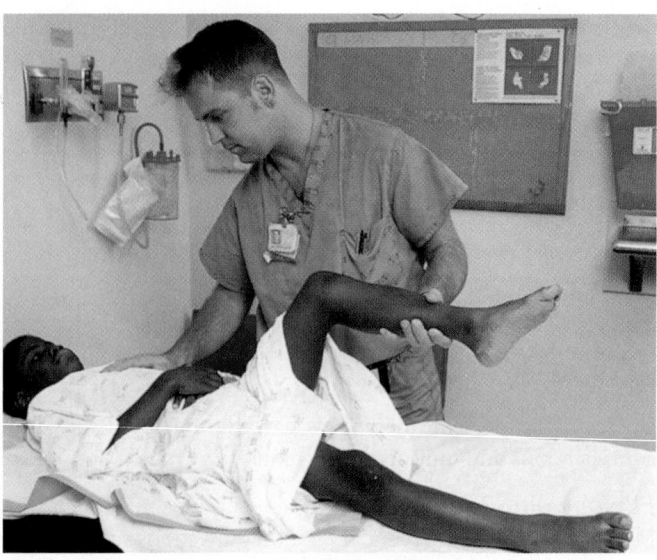

A

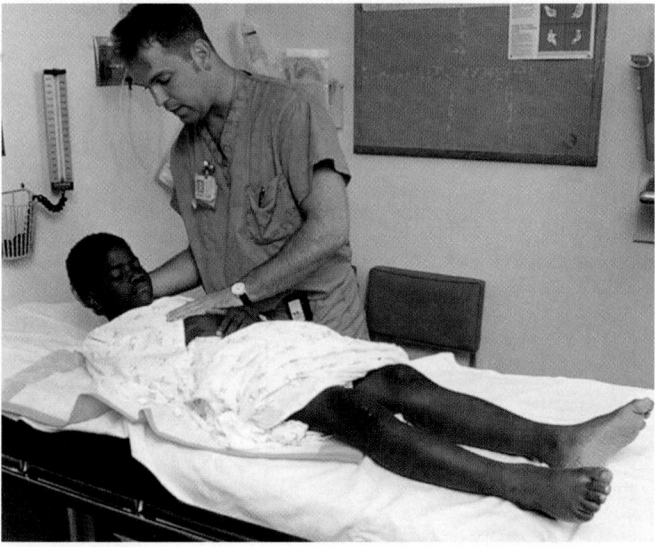

B

FIGURE 27–8 ➤ A, To test for Kernig sign, raise the child's leg with the knee flexed. Then extend the child's leg at the knee. If any resistance is noted or pain is felt, the result is a positive Kernig sign. This is a common finding in meningitis. B, To test Brudzinski sign, flex the child's head while in a supine position. If this action makes the knees or hips flex involuntarily, a positive Brudzinski sign is present. This is a common finding in meningitis.

COLLABORATIVE CARE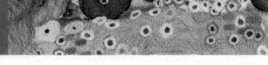

Diagnostic Tests

Diagnosis is based on the history, clinical presentation, and laboratory findings. Laboratory tests include a complete blood count, blood cultures, serum electrolytes and osmolality, and clotting factors. Blood cultures usually identify the responsible organism causing meningitis. A lumbar puncture, performed to culture the cerebrospinal fluid (CSF), measure pressure, and assess the fluid for white blood cells and protein and glucose levels, confirms the diagnosis. CT scanning may be performed when increased ICP or a brain abscess is suspected.

Clinical Therapy

Antibiotics are usually administered as soon as diagnostic tests are obtained. Antibiotics commonly used to treat bacterial meningitis include ampicillin, ceftriaxone, cefotaxime, penicillin G, and vancomycin. Antibiotics are often changed once culture and sensitivity results are known, since many organisms have resistance to certain antibiotics. These medications are administered intravenously for 7 to 21 days, depending on the organism and the child's clinical response. Corticosteroids (dexamethasone) are often given to infants and children to reduce the risk of death and severe hearing loss. Invasive monitoring of ICP may be initiated (Mann & Jackson, 2008).

If the child is in shock, aggressive fluid resuscitation is performed to maintain an adequate cerebral perfusion pressure. Intravenous fluids may initially be restricted to two-thirds maintenance as careful monitoring for increased ICP and for fluid retention associated with SIADH (see Chapter 30 ∞) is initiated. If cerebral edema is present, fluids are usually restricted and medications (e.g., mannitol) are administered.

Depending on the causative organism, the disease may need to be reported to the local health department. Contacts who have not been previously immunized with the meningococcal vaccine may need to take prophylactic antibiotics, such as rifampin or ciprofloxacin.

Some infants and children who have had bacterial meningitis suffer neurologic damage despite early, aggressive management. Complications may include severe hearing loss, seizures, hydrocephalus, subdural effusion, diabetes insipidus, SIADH, developmental delay, learning problems, and behavior problems.

NURSING MANAGEMENT

Nursing Assessment and Diagnosis

Frequently assess the child's physiologic status, including vital signs and level of consciousness, and compare to the baseline neurologic assessment to identify changes in the child's condition. Measure the infant's head circumference frequently because of the potential for development of hydrocephalus. Be alert for signs of a change in the child's condition and response to treatment. Monitor the child's ability to control secretions and to drink sufficient fluids. Monitor intake and output. Assess for any sensory deficits. Identify parents' concerns about this potentially life-threatening condition.

Several nursing diagnoses that may apply to the child with bacterial meningitis are listed in the accompanying Nursing Care Plan. Additional nursing diagnoses might include:

- Risk for Aspiration related to altered level of consciousness and poor secretion control
- Risk for Deficient Fluid Volume related to poor oral fluid intake
- Anticipatory Grieving (Parent) related to the child's potentially life-threatening condition
- Caregiver Role Strain related to a hospitalized child and other family responsibilities

Planning and Implementation

The accompanying Nursing Care Plan summarizes care for the child with bacterial meningitis. Nursing care begins with emergency treatment and continues as the child's condition stabilizes. Monitor respiratory and neurologic status, maintain hydration, administer medications, and prevent complications. Promote comfort with reduced stimulation (dim lights, quiet room) and by placing the child in a side-lying position. Isolate the child according to hospital protocol until the causative organism is identified and at least 24 hours of effective treatment has occurred.

Monitor the child's response to antibiotic therapy. Observe for signs of gastrointestinal bleeding, which is a potential complication of corticosteroid use.

Nursing Alert

Monitor the serum sodium concentration and urine specific gravity because these children are at risk for SIADH. Maintenance and replacement fluids are usually given to children with bacterial meningitis. If SIADH occurs, moderate fluid restriction with an isotonic solution is ordered until serum sodium levels return to normal.

Respond to parents' concerns about their child's condition, explaining all measures to increase the child's comfort and to treat the illness. Identify ways parents can help meet the child's comfort needs. Parents may also need help figuring out how to meet the needs of other children at home while spending time with the hospitalized child. Ensure that the parents and close family contacts receive prophylaxis, if prescribed.

Discharge Planning and Home Care Teaching

Identify and address home care needs well in advance of discharge. Follow-up visits are important to monitor for complications and sequelae. Help parents deal with any physical disabilities resulting from the child's illness and any emotional, social, and financial repercussions of the child's condition. Teach parents what to do if the child has a seizure.

Infants and toddlers with neurologic sequelae should be referred to an early intervention program. Refer parents to the appropriate social service agencies for support and assistance. If the child has a hearing loss, referral to an otolaryngologist and speech and language specialist should be made. Encourage early identification of other neurologic sequelae, such as learning problems. Children with hearing, learning, or attention deficit disorders need an individualized education plan (see Chapter 12 ∞), and parents may need help planning for the child's special educational needs.

Prevention is a major role for nurses. Encourage parents to get their infants and children fully immunized with the *Haemophilus influenzae*, pneumococcal, and meningococcal vaccines.

Evaluation

Expected outcomes of nursing care are provided in the accompanying Nursing Care Plan.

NURSING CARE PLAN

The Child with Bacterial Meningitis

INTERVENTION	RATIONALE	EXPECTED OUTCOME
1. Nursing Diagnosis: Impaired Gas Exchange related to decreased level of consciousness		
NIC Priority Intervention: *Respiratory monitoring:* Collection and analysis of patient data to ensure airway patency and adequate gas exchange		**NOC Suggested Outcome:** *Respiratory status: Ventilation:* Movement of air in and out of the lungs
Goal: The child's respiratory failure does not progress to respiratory arrest.		
▪ Place the child on a cardiorespiratory monitor with a 20-second alarm.	▪ The alarm on the monitor alerts staff that the child is having bradycardia or an apneic episode.	The child's respiratory failure is managed with assessment and prompt treatment.
▪ Have resuscitation equipment, including oxygen, resuscitation bag with mask, and suction apparatus, at the bedside.	▪ Equipment is readily available in case of respiratory arrest.	
▪ Stimulate the child if apneic; if no response, begin assisted ventilations and call for the resuscitation team.	▪ Stimulation may encourage spontaneous respirations; if not, ventilation is necessary. Calling for the resuscitation team ensures help in managing the child in a timely manner.	
▪ Monitor heart rate and perform compressions if necessary.	▪ The child with apnea may have bradycardia resulting from cardiac hypoxia.	
2. Nursing Diagnosis: Risk for Injury related to infection of cerebrospinal fluid and potential sequelae		
NIC Priority Intervention: *Health screening:* Detecting health risks or problems by means of history, examination, and other procedures		**NOC Suggested Outcome:** *Immune status:* Adequacy of natural and acquired appropriately targeted resistance to internal and external antigens
Goal: The child will suffer minimal CNS injury secondary to infection.		
▪ Administer antibiotics and corticosteroids as prescribed.	▪ Antibiotics help eradicate the pathogen and prevent cerebral edema. Corticosteroids diminish inflammatory response and reduce the chance of neurologic **sequelae** (abnormal conditions resulting from a disease, treatment, or injury).	The child's condition improves significantly within 48–72 hours (fever decreases and no signs of neurologic sequelae are detected).
▪ Note return of fever, nuchal rigidity, or irritability. Monitor vital signs, and assess for signs of increased ICP. Measure head circumference once or twice daily. Note changes in responsiveness. Notify the physician immediately if any signs are detected.	▪ Watching for common sequelae, such as subdural effusion or hydrocephalus, ensures prompt treatment.	
Goal: The child will not develop cerebral edema as a result of water retention.		
▪ Monitor for SIADH and watch for signs of increased ICP.	▪ SIADH can be either avoided or quickly managed if recognized early.	Cerebral edema does not develop. If SIADH or increased ICP occurs, the condition is treated promptly so effects are minimized.
▪ Perform strict intake and output measurements. Determine urine specific gravity. Check electrolytes and osmolality of both serum and urine. Weigh the child daily. Restrict fluids and give sodium chloride as prescribed.	▪ Low urine output with a high specific gravity is a sign of fluid retention and SIADH. The child is maintained with restricted fluids and provided sodium supplements to reduce the possibility for cerebral edema.	

NURSING CARE PLAN

The Child with Bacterial Meningitis (continued)

INTERVENTION	RATIONALE	EXPECTED OUTCOME
Goal: The child will be free of injury resulting from disseminated intravascular coagulation (DIC).		
■ Be aware of needlesticks that continue to bleed and lesions that continue to ooze. Monitor clotting times.	■ Prompt recognition leads to management of the coagulopathy.	The child does not sustain injury from DIC.
■ Administer blood products, vitamin K, or heparin as ordered.	■ Prompt recognition allows for early initial treatment of DIC. The child may bleed to death if treatment is delayed.	
Goal: The child with any degree of hearing loss will be identified.		
■ Arrange for hearing assessment prior to discharge.	■ Hearing loss is a common complication. Early intervention is needed to promote growth and development.	The child with identified hearing loss is referred to an appropriate specialist or program for intervention.
3. Nursing Diagnosis: Acute Pain related to meningeal irritation		
NIC Priority Intervention: *Pain management:* Alleviation of pain or reduction in pain to a level of comfort acceptable to patient		**NOC Suggested Outcome:** *Comfort level:* Feelings of physical and psychologic ease
Goal: The child will be as comfortable as possible.		
■ Assess pain with age-appropriate pain scales.	■ Pain scales provide the ability to quantify pain for future comparison.	The child is calm and expresses increased comfort.
■ Minimize tactile stimulation.	■ Sensory stimulation increases discomfort.	
■ Allow the child to assume a comfortable position.	■ The child determines the most comfortable position. Opisthotonic position may be the most comfortable.	
■ Keep the lights dim and maintain a quiet environment.	■ Dim lights reduce the discomfort from photophobia. Noise can disturb the child.	
■ Provide pain medication as prescribed.	■ Pain medication is appropriate for acute discomfort associated with the illness.	
4. Nursing Diagnosis: Risk for Infection (Family and Close Contacts) related to pathogens in the cerebrospinal fluid		
NIC Priority Intervention: *Infection control:* Minimizing the acquisition and transmission of infectious agents		**NOC Suggested Outcome:** *Infection status:* Presence and extent of infection
Goal: Caretakers or family members will have no apparent evidence of infection.		
■ Explain rationale and dose schedule for taking rifampin or ciprofloxacin.	■ Rifampin and ciprofloxacin provide prophylaxis for many bacterial pathogens responsible for meningitis.	Family members and other close contacts verbalize the schedule for rifampin or ciprofloxacin therapy.

Viral (Aseptic) Meningitis

Viral meningitis is an inflammatory response of the meninges to a viral organism, characterized by an increased number of blood cells and protein in the CSF. In the United States, an enterovirus most often causes viral meningitis (Mann & Jackson, 2008).

Generally, the child with viral meningitis appears less ill than the child with bacterial meningitis. The child may be irritable or lethargic and usually has a fever. Other symptoms include general malaise, headache, photophobia, gastrointestinal distress, upper respiratory symptoms, and a maculopapular rash. The child may also show signs of meningeal irritation such as stiff neck, back pain, and positive Kernig and Brudzinski signs (see Figure 27–8). The infant may have a tense anterior fontanel. Seizures are rare. Symptoms usually resolve spontaneously within 3 to 10 days.

The child with fever and meningeal signs is hospitalized. Blood, urine, and CSF analyses and cultures are performed. Polymerase chain reaction testing helps detect viral meningitis.

Until the diagnosis of viral meningitis is confirmed, the child is treated aggressively, as if he or she has bacterial meningitis. Treatment is supportive of symptoms.

NURSING MANAGEMENT

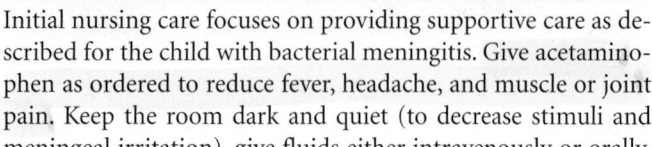

Initial nursing care focuses on providing supportive care as described for the child with bacterial meningitis. Give acetaminophen as ordered to reduce fever, headache, and muscle or joint pain. Keep the room dark and quiet (to decrease stimuli and meningeal irritation), give fluids either intravenously or orally, and promote comfort with proper positioning.

The child and family need information about the disease. Explain medical and nursing procedures in terms that the child and family can understand. Keep parents informed about the child's progress. Once the diagnosis of viral meningitis is made, immediately begin discharge planning and teaching for home care. Explain that recovery may take several weeks but that complete recovery is expected.

Encephalitis

Encephalitis is an acute inflammation of the brain often caused by a virus that is transmitted by a mosquito, such as West Nile virus and western equine virus. Inflammation of the meninges is also common. Epidemics occur most commonly in warm weather seasons. The encephalitis may occur as a direct or primary infection when the virus successfully gets past the blood-brain barrier. Children may have significant neurologic sequelae.

Signs and symptoms include fever, irritability, severe headache, and bulging fontanel, followed by altered mental status. The child may have flaccid or spastic paralysis. Meningeal irritation signs such as nuchal rigidity, photophobia, and positive Kernig and Brudzinski signs are common. Focal or generalized seizures may occur. Altered mental status may progress to coma over hours or days.

Diagnosis is based on history and laboratory findings. Information about insect bites or travel to areas where cases of encephalitis are present should be obtained (e.g., West Nile virus or eastern equine encephalitis). CSF culture and analysis, blood serologic tests, and nasopharyngeal and stool specimens are evaluated in an attempt to identify pathogens causing the symptoms. Testing for virus-specific immunoglobulin M antibodies with enzyme-linked immunosorbent assay (ELISA) is performed after 5 days of acute illness. A CT scan and MRI may be performed. An EEG may help assess seizure activity and help localize the area of the brain affected.

The child with encephalitis is at risk for seizures, respiratory failure, and increased ICP, and treatment is supportive. Children with encephalitis may recover completely, but many are left with serious neurologic deficits.

NURSING MANAGEMENT

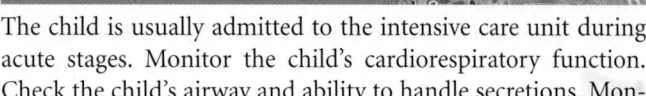

The child is usually admitted to the intensive care unit during acute stages. Monitor the child's cardiorespiratory function. Check the child's airway and ability to handle secretions. Monitor respiratory status by observing color, pulse oximetry readings, and arterial blood gas values. Provide seizure precautions, and have appropriate equipment for managing seizures at the bedside. Provide support to the parents and family as they cope with the life-threatening nature of this condition.

When the child's level of consciousness begins to improve, he or she may at first be confused and disoriented. Orient the child to the hospital environment. Encourage parents to take an active role in the child's physical and emotional care during recovery, for example, bringing favorite stuffed animals or music from home. Engage in therapeutic play (refer to Chapter 11 ∞ for techniques). Give the child age-appropriate toys to encourage a return to normal behavior.

Provide the parents with instructions about home care. Plan follow-up visits so the child can be evaluated for neurologic sequelae. Ensure that children are referred for physical, occupational, and speech therapies as needed. Refer parents to home care, social services, family counseling, and support groups.

Reye Syndrome

Reye syndrome is an acute **encephalopathy**, a cerebral dysfunction caused by a toxic, injury, inflammatory, or anoxic insult that may result in permanent tissue damage, although the dysfunction may improve over time. In the 1980s, an association was reported between the use of aspirin for influenza or varicella and the subsequent development of Reye syndrome. The condition is now rare since most parents give children acetaminophen or ibuprofen rather than aspirin for viral illnesses and flulike symptoms. The mortality rate due to Reye syndrome is high.

Nursing Alert

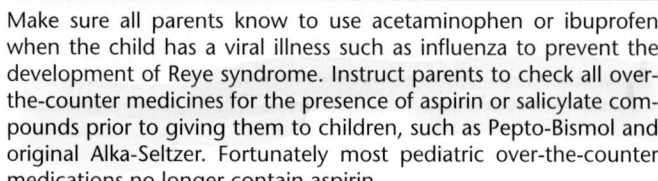

Make sure all parents know to use acetaminophen or ibuprofen when the child has a viral illness such as influenza to prevent the development of Reye syndrome. Instruct parents to check all over-the-counter medicines for the presence of aspirin or salicylate compounds prior to giving them to children, such as Pepto-Bismol and original Alka-Seltzer. Fortunately most pediatric over-the-counter medications no longer contain aspirin.

Reye syndrome is classified as a secondary mitochondrial hepatopathy, caused by a drug toxic to the liver, toxin, metal, or metabolite caused by a poorly functioning organ. In the case of Reye syndrome, an interaction between a viral illness and aspirin occurs in a susceptible individual (Carey & Balistreri, 2007). The disorder is characterized by cerebral edema, hypoglycemia, and an enlarged, fatty, poorly functioning liver due to an elevated level of short chain fatty acid and hyperammonemia.

Reye syndrome begins with nausea and vomiting, mental status changes, seizures, and progressive unresponsiveness. The condition has five stages that indicate increasing signs of cerebral edema and neurologic dysfunction, resulting in a final stage with coma, seizures, flaccidity, loss of deep tendon reflexes, and respiratory arrest.

The diagnosis of Reye syndrome is based on an abrupt change in the child's level of consciousness and diagnostic laboratory tests that have no other identifiable cause. CSF analysis usually reveals white blood cells. Radiographic imaging reveals cerebral edema. Liver enzyme and ammonia levels are elevated, blood glucose levels are below normal, and prothrombin time is prolonged. A liver biopsy is sometimes performed to confirm the diagnosis.

The child with Reye syndrome is cared for in a pediatric intensive care unit. The goal of medical management is to provide supportive treatment and to prevent the secondary effects of cerebral edema and metabolic injury associated with the elevated short-chain fatty acids and ammonia levels. Mechanical ventilation is often needed once the child is comatose. Perform arterial and venous blood pressure monitoring. The child is monitored for signs of increased ICP secondary to cerebral edema. Hypoglycemia is treated with intravenous glucose. Electrolytes, blood chemistry, and blood pH are monitored.

NURSING MANAGEMENT

Nursing care focuses on monitoring the child's physical status, providing emotional support, and teaching parents about disease prevention. Check the child's respiratory and neurologic status frequently, and note any signs of improvement or deterioration. Refer to the discussion of nursing management of altered states of consciousness on page 853 for specific nursing interventions. Look for changes in laboratory values that indicate acidosis, an elevation of ammonia levels, or hypoglycemia. Monitor the child's intake and output. Correct imbalances by administering fluids, electrolytes, or medications as ordered. Prevent complications associated with immobility.

If the child survives and is discharged, follow-up care to identify neurologic sequelae is important. Developmental and neurologic deficits may occur and are more severe in children under 2 years of age. Arrange for home nursing visits or frequent office visits during the recovery period so that developmental and neurologic status can be monitored. Inform parents about community resources that can help them deal with the child's recovery.

Guillain-Barré Syndrome (Postinfectious Polyneuritis)

Guillain-Barré syndrome is an acute inflammatory demyelination of many spinal nerve roots. This condition may lead to deteriorating motor function and paralysis that progresses in an ascending pattern, as well as paresthesia and **areflexia** (absent reflexes to pain and other stimulation).

Guillain-Barré syndrome is thought to be caused by an autoimmune response to an infectious organism, usually within 1 to 3 weeks of a gastrointestinal or respiratory illness. Associated organisms are *Campylobacter jejuni*, *Cytomegalovirus*, Epstein-Barr virus, influenza, and *Mycoplasma pneumoniae*. It has also been associated with immunizations for influenza and rabies (Sarnat, 2007). The immune reaction is focused on the peripheral nerve myelin sheath that is attacked by macrophages. Demyelination and blocked transmission of nerve impulses to the muscles results. The damaged peripheral nerves then begin to atrophy.

Infants have an onset of rapidly progressive severe hypotonia, possible respiratory distress, irritability, and feeding difficulties.

Older children have rapidly progressive symmetric weakness and muscle pain with varying degrees of distal paresthesia and numbness in the legs. This ascending weakness spreads to the upper extremities, trunk, chest, neck, face, and head. Deep tendon reflexes may be diminished or absent. The child may develop acute ataxia or an inability to walk. Difficulty swallowing and facial weakness are signs of impending respiratory failure. Respiratory effort may be inadequate for proper ventilation. Cranial nerves may be affected, causing Bell palsy, for example. A dysfunctional autonomic nervous system may cause such symptoms as an unstable blood pressure and cardiac rate, postural hypotension, or profound bradycardia (Sarnat, 2007).

Diagnostic criteria of Guillain-Barré syndrome include progressive motor weakness (minimal weakness of the legs to total paralysis of all extremities), and areflexia of varying degrees. CSF analysis reveals twice the limit of normal protein levels, normal glucose level, and fewer than 10 white blood cells per cubic millimeter, a positive indicator of the condition (Sarnat, 2007). Bacterial and viral cultures are usually negative. Electroconduction tests such as electromyography show acute muscle denervation.

Clinical therapy for Guillain-Barré syndrome is intravenous immune globulin (IVIG) for several days if the child is unable to ambulate. Guidelines for administration of IVIG can be found in Chapter 22 ∞. Responses to IVIG are dramatic, often occurring within days. Alternate treatment is a plasma exchange to remove autoantibodies (Cirillo, 2008). If the condition progresses rapidly, respiratory support with intubation may be needed. Physical therapy and supportive care are initiated to promote early ambulation. The condition is rarely fatal.

NURSING MANAGEMENT

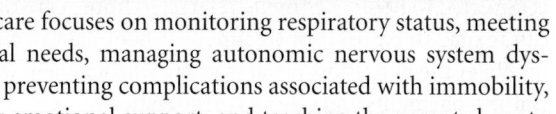

Nursing care focuses on monitoring respiratory status, meeting nutritional needs, managing autonomic nervous system dysfunction, preventing complications associated with immobility, providing emotional support, and teaching the parents how to care for the child after discharge.

Monitor Cardiorespiratory Status

Place the child on a cardiorespiratory monitor to continuously assess the child's cardiorespiratory status, especially in the early phase of illness. Look for signs indicating the need for endotracheal intubation and mechanical ventilation (e.g., dyspnea, inability to handle secretions, inadequate respiratory effort, and color changes).

Manage Autonomic Nervous System Dysfunction

Monitor the child's vital signs closely for episodes of tachycardia, bradycardia, and hypotension. Blood pressure fluctuations and autonomic instability have been linked to asystole (Sarnat, 2007). Observe frequently for decreased responsiveness. Intervene promptly if these or other signs of autonomic nervous system dysfunction are noted.

Meet Nutritional Needs

Assess whether the child is having difficulty swallowing. If the child has no gag reflex, maintain nutritional needs with intravenous supplements or nasogastric tube feedings.

Prevent Complications

Prevent complications associated with immobility (see the Clinical Tip on page 855). Ensure good postural alignment, and turn the child every 2 hours. Maintaining skin integrity is also important.

Evaluate the child's muscle tone, strength, and symmetry. When the child's condition begins to improve, recovery of lost strength is the priority. Active exercise is emphasized in physical therapy. Encourage family members to participate in the child's care, especially during the recovery phase. They can help with the activities of daily living and reinforce what the child has learned in physical therapy.

Provide Emotional Support

Explain the progression of Guillain-Barré syndrome to the parents and the child during the initial stages. Witnessing a rapid deterioration in their child's physical status can be frightening; therefore, preparation is essential to reduce their anxieties. Be honest when discussing the child's recovery and prognosis.

Have parents bring in the child's favorite toys, dolls, or books to make him or her feel more secure. Playing with or reading to the child can also be comforting.

Discharge Planning and Home Care Teaching

Home care needs should be identified and addressed well in advance of discharge. Support the parents as they prepare for the child's return home, especially when the return to full strength is expected to be slow. Provide referral to home care nurses who can manage all aspects of treatment, rehabilitation, and follow-up. Refer the parents to social workers who can help with financial arrangements and school considerations.

Care in the Community

Help the child to adjust to any residual effects of Guillain-Barré syndrome. Help the child practice exercises learned in physical therapy sessions, and encourage the child to perform activities of daily living, such as brushing the teeth or combing the hair. Refer the child to outpatient rehabilitation programs to promote recovery.

To promote a positive self-image, praise any effort the child makes to be self-sufficient. The child may be frustrated and angry. Allow the child to express these feelings in an appropriate way, either during play or in conversation.

▧ HEADACHES

Up to 75% of children experience a headache by age 15 years. Migraine headaches occur in 1% of children by age 7 years, and 5% of children by age 15 years. Approximately 20% of children in the United States have chronic headaches (Rubin, Suecoff, &

Knupp, 2006). Headaches may be associated with school absence, decreased extracurricular activity, and poor academic achievement.

Headaches have both benign (migraine, inflammatory, and tension) and structural causes.

- Migraine headaches may be triggered by stress; foods containing nitrates, glutamate, caffeine, tyramine, and salt; menses; oral contraceptives; fatigue; and hunger. Another family member often has similar headaches, so there may be a genetic predisposition.
- Tension headaches may be associated with stresses due to school, insecurity, or conflict in the family.
- Medication overuse (rebound) headaches are associated with the frequent use of medications for headaches, more than 2 to 3 times a week. Medications involved include acetaminophen, nonsteroidal anti-inflammatories (NSAIDs), decongestants, opioids, benzodiazepines, and ergotamines (Gladstein & Mack, 2005).

Signs and symptoms of headaches in children and adolescents vary by cause. See Clinical Manifestations: Headaches.

Clinical Tip ◣

Some children experience an *aura* warning of an impending migraine headache, such as seeing spots or a shimmery film that gets larger or feeling numbness or tingling. In the case of migraines, the adolescent can take medication in an effort to abort the headache. In epilepsy, the aura may warn the child to avoid injury by getting to the floor.

Diagnosis involves taking a detailed history of the headache characteristics, including the following questions:

- How long has the child been having headaches? How often do they occur?
- Is there a family history of headaches?
- Where does the head hurt? Does it involve the neck and shoulders?
- What other symptoms occur—an aura, light sensitivity, nausea, vomiting?
- Does anything trigger the headache?
- What home treatment is provided? What relieves the headache?

Complementary Therapy
Self-Hypnosis for Headaches

Relaxation and cognitive behavioral therapies have been demonstrated to reduce the severity and frequency of headaches in children and adolescents. In a recent study, 178 youth (mean age of 11 years) were taught to perform self-hypnosis over 3 to 4 visits. These children reported an average decrease in the frequency of headaches from 4.7 per week to 1.4 per week, and headaches were reported to be less intense and less prolonged (Kohen & Zajak, 2007).

Clinical Manifestations
Headaches

Type of Headache and Cause	Clinical Manifestations	Clinical Therapy
Migraine—vascular, acute recurrent	▪ Unilateral or bilateral pulsatile throbbing pain in frontal or temporal region lasting for 1 to 72 hours ▪ Pain may be aggravated by routine physical activities ▪ Sensitivity to light and sound ▪ Nausea and vomiting ▪ May have a visual or sensory aura preceding the headache ▪ Relief with sleep	▪ Ibuprofen, acetaminophen, or naproxen ▪ Medications to abort migraine (sumatriptan nasal spray) for adolescents ▪ Noise and light avoidance during acute headache ▪ Headache diary to identify food or other triggers ▪ Avoidance of identified food triggers and caffeine ▪ Relaxation techniques and biofeedback
Tension—muscular contraction, acute recurrent or chronic nonprogressive	▪ Bilateral dull, achy pain in band around head, in neck, and in shoulders that may last for hours or days ▪ Pain not aggravated by increased physical activity ▪ Unlikely to have nausea and vomiting, sensitivity to light or sound, vertigo, or visual disturbances	▪ Relaxation techniques and rest ▪ Analgesic and anti-inflammatory medications ▪ Ice pack
Medication overuse—acute recurrent	▪ Dull, bilateral, or unilateral pain in frontal area ▪ Occur 5 times a week or 15 times a month ▪ Can vary in character, location, and severity from time to time ▪ Usually increase in frequency and severity over time, paralleling the increase in medication use ▪ Recur with the abortive therapy or when medication wears off	▪ Withdrawal of all medications for headaches (caffeine, acetaminophen, NSAIDs, and triptans) (Kossoff & Mankad, 2006) ▪ Substitution of medications that do not cause rebound may be used if headaches do not decrease in a month ▪ Clonidine may be used to treat withdrawal symptoms
Inflammatory—sinusitis or dental abscess, acute localized	▪ Facial pain or tenderness over affected sinus ▪ Dull, constant pressure ▪ Severity of pain varies with head position ▪ Fever	▪ Analgesic, antipyretic, and anti-inflammatory medications ▪ Antibiotic medications ▪ Cold or heat application
Structural—space-occupying lesion, hemorrhage, increased intracranial pressure, chronic progressive	▪ Severe pain that increases in frequency and severity, often in occipital or frontal location; increases with coughing, sneezing, or straining ▪ Pain awakens child or is present when awakening ▪ Vomiting that is persistent or preceded by recurrent headache ▪ Abnormal neurologic signs (e.g., double vision, papilledema, strabismus, weakness, ataxia)	▪ Surgery ▪ Analgesic medications

Source: Data from: Lewis, D. W. (2007). Pediatric migraine. *Pediatrics in Review, 28*(2), 43–52; Fisher, P. G. (2005). Help for headaches: A strategy for your busy practice. *Contemporary Pediatrics, 22*(11), 34–40.

The child is assessed for neurologic signs such as altered LOC, abnormal cranial nerves, papilledema, and motor or sensory deficits. Vital signs are also assessed. Radiologic studies (CT scan or MRI) are used if a structural problem or pathologic condition is suspected.

Clinical therapy includes relaxation techniques, analgesics, and anti-inflammatory medications. Food elimination diet trials are often used to identify foods that trigger headaches, but they are often unsuccessful. Medications to abort migraines (sumatriptan nasal spray) may be prescribed for adolescents who have an aura. Some adolescents with frequent migraines that interfere with usual activities may be treated with a daily medication, such as cyproheptadine, beta-blockers, calcium channel blockers, tricyclic antidepressants, or anticonvulsants (valproic acid, topiramate, and gabapentin) (Lewis, 2007).

NURSING MANAGEMENT

Nursing management involves assessing the child for potential neurologic signs associated with headaches and assisting the child and family to identify strategies for relieving the headaches. Encourage the child to keep a calendar or diary of headaches, including the events and stresses occurring at the time as well as foods eaten.

Clinical Tip

The foods most commonly identified as migraine headache triggers are cheese, chocolate, and citrus fruits. Other potential triggers include processed meats, yogurt, monosodium glutamate, aspartame, and alcoholic beverages (Gunner, Smith, & Ferguson, 2008).

Make sure the child learns to take the prescribed medications appropriately. Emphasize the need to avoid using nonprescribed over-the-counter pain medications to reduce the risk for developing medication overuse headaches.

Teach the child relaxation techniques (breathing control training, mental imagery, progressive muscle relaxation, and biofeedback) to manage stress and the pain associated with the headaches. Encourage the child to maintain a healthy lifestyle with regular sleep and awakening times, healthy eating, regular exercise, and adequate hydration.

See Chapter 24 ∞ for care of the child with a brain tumor.

■ STRUCTURAL DEFECTS

Microcephaly

Microcephaly indicates a small brain with a head circumference that is more than 3 standard deviations below the mean for age and sex. The brain's architecture is grossly normal, but very small. It may have genetic or environmental causes (e.g., fetal or postnatal insult, intrauterine infection) (Puruggananan, 2006). Children with microcephaly have cognitive impairments. See Chapter 28 ∞ for care of the child with intellectual disability.

Hydrocephalus

Hydrocephalus is the body's response to an imbalance between the production and absorption of CSF. The condition is often congenital and associated with other CNS malformations. The overall incidence is estimated to be 1 per 500 children (National Institute of Neurological Disorders and Stroke, 2008). It is commonly associated with **myelomeningocele**, a spinal fluid-filled meningeal sac that contains a portion of the spinal cord and nerves protruding through a vertebral defect. See page 876 for care of the child with myelomeningocele.

Etiology and Pathophysiology

CSF is produced at a consistent rate of 500 mL per day (Duffy, 2010). When the amount of CSF absorbed is less than the amount produced, the ventricles enlarge. Hydrocephalus may be either communicating or noncommunicating, and congenital or acquired.

In communicating hydrocephalus, the CSF flows freely among normal channels and pathways, but absorption of the CSF in the subarachnoid space and the arachnoid villi is impaired. It may be acquired from postinfectious meningitis or from intraventricular hemorrhage in a preterm infant, or it may be caused by a congenital malformation in the subarachnoid spaces.

Noncommunicating hydrocephalus is responsible for most cases in children. It results from a blockage in the ventricular system that prevents CSF from entering the subarachnoid space, resulting in enlargement of the ventricles (Figure 27–9 ➤). Potential causes include infection, hemorrhage, tumor, surgery, or structural deformity. Congenital structural defects causing non-

Pathophysiology Illustrated

Hydrocephalus

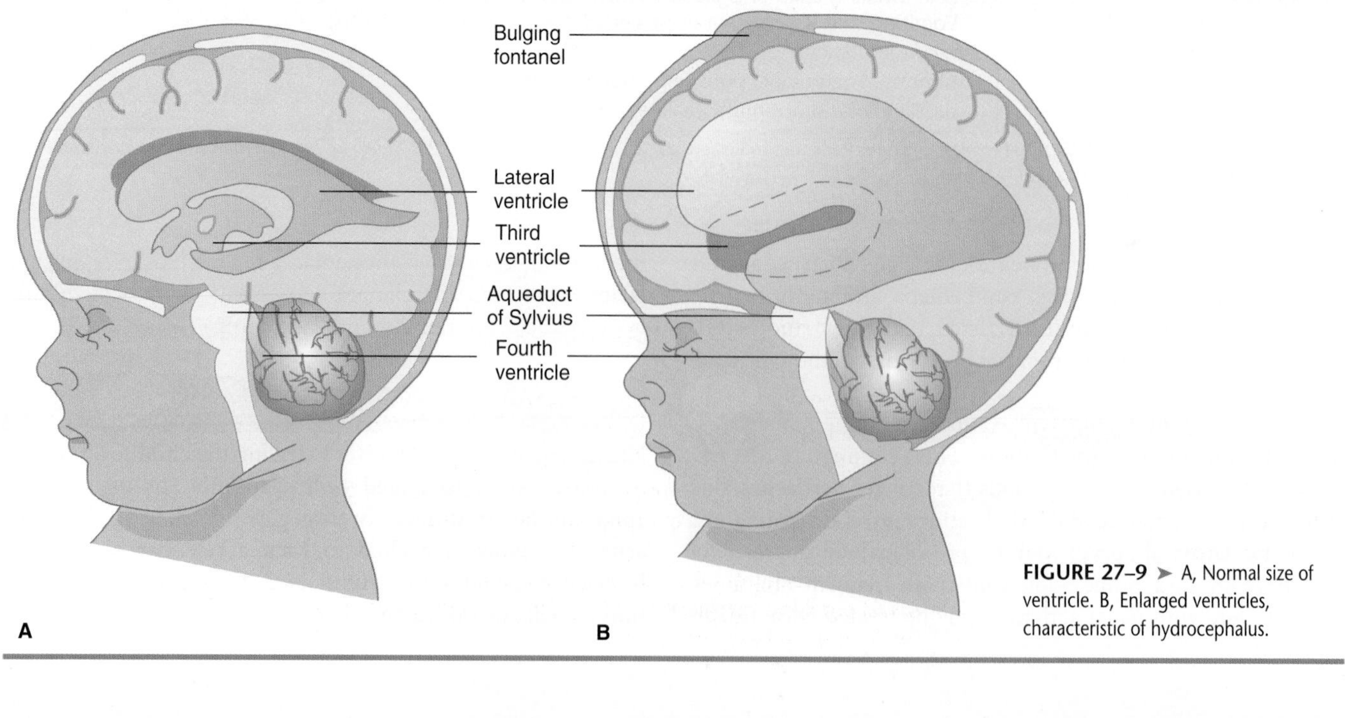

A

B

FIGURE 27–9 ➤ A, Normal size of ventricle. B, Enlarged ventricles, characteristic of hydrocephalus.

communicating hydrocephalus include the Chiari II malformation (found in most children with myelomeningocele), aqueduct of Sylvius stenosis (obstruction of CSF flow through the aqueduct, a recessive X-linked condition), and the Dandy-Walker syndrome (hydrocephalus, a posterior fossa cyst, and hypoplasia of the cerebellum).

Clinical Manifestations

The signs and symptoms of hydrocephalus vary with the age of the child. See Clinical Manifestations: Hydrocephalus. The predominant sign in infants is a rapidly increasing head circumference (Figure 27–10 ➤). Older children show signs of increased ICP (see Table 27–4).

COLLABORATIVE CARE

Diagnostic Tests

The diagnosis of hydrocephalus may be made prenatally by ultrasound or based on clinical manifestations and neuroimaging studies after birth. Daily measurements of the infant's head circumference are performed in any infant at risk of developing hydrocephalus. In the infant whose fontanel is still open, ultrasonography or echoencephalography may be used to confirm the diagnosis. In older children with signs of increased ICP, CT scanning and MRI diagnose hydrocephalus and in some cases reveal the anatomic cause. CT and MRI are also used to evaluate shunt failure.

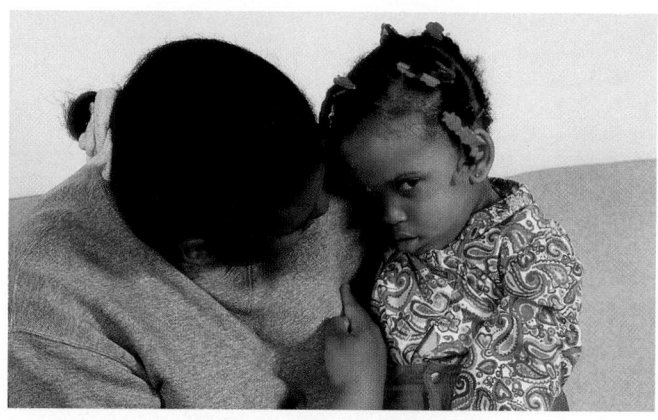

FIGURE 27–10 ➤ In communicating hydrocephalus, an excessive amount of cerebrospinal fluid accumulates in the subarachnoid space, producing the characteristic head enlargement with prominent forehead seen in this child.

Clinical Therapy

Clinical therapy for hydrocephalus involves removing the obstruction (e.g., surgical removal of a tumor) or creating a new pathway to divert excess CSF. A catheter or shunt is placed in the ventricle and passes the CSF to the peritoneal cavity, atrium of the heart, or pleural spaces. Ventriculoperitoneal shunts (Figure 27–11 ➤) are commonly used, although a ventriculoatrial shunt may be used in older children. Shunt systems consist of four parts: a ventricular catheter, a pumping chamber or reservoir, a one-way pressure valve, and a distal catheter. Initial

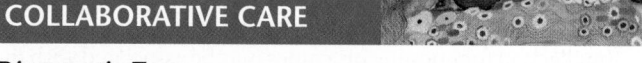

Clinical Manifestations
Hydrocephalus

Causes	Clinical Manifestations
Congenital Structural Defect in Infancy Dandy-Walker syndrome Chiari II malformation Intraventricular hemorrhage	*Early Signs* Rapidly increasing head circumference; tense, bulging fontanel, split sutures Bossing (protrusion) of frontal area, face is disproportionate for skull size Difficulty holding head up Macewen or "cracked-pot" sign with percussion Prominent, distended scalp veins, translucent scalp skin, splitting sutures, bulging anterior fontanel Increased tone or hyperreflexia, Babinski sign Irritability or lethargy, poor feeding Decline in level of consciousness *Late Signs* Apnea Sunsetting eyes Difficulty swallowing or feeding; vomiting Shrill, high-pitched cry Cardiopulmonary depression (severe cases)
Acquired Hydrocephalus in Older Child After Closure of Sutures Postinfectious Tumor Hemorrhage	Signs of increased intracranial pressure Headache upon arising with nausea and vomiting Fussiness, sleepiness, confusion, apathy, or altered level of consciousness Personality change, loss of interest in daily activities Poor judgment or verbal incoherence, worsening school performance, memory loss Ataxia, spasticity, or other alterations in motor development Visual problems (papilledema, blurred vision, double vision) No increase in head circumference

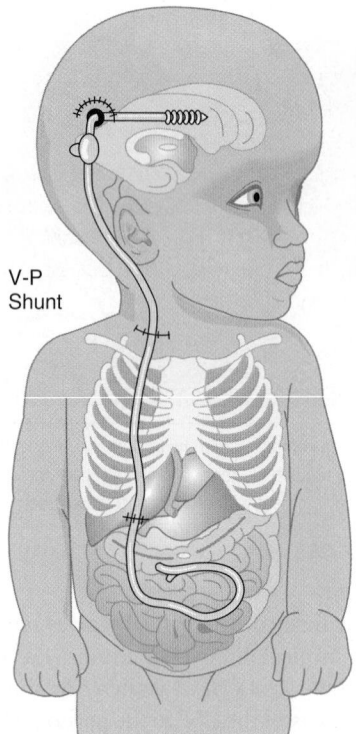

V-P
Shunt

FIGURE 27–11 ➤ A ventriculoperitoneal shunt, commonly used to treat children with hydrocephalus, is usually placed at 3–4 months of age.

shunt placement is usually performed early in infancy. Tubing of adequate length is now inserted to accommodate the child's growth and reduce the need for future surgery. Children with ventriculoatrial shunts receive perioperative intravenous and intraventricular antibiotics to reduce the risk for infection (Duffy, 2010). An alternative surgical approach for some cases of noncommunicating hydrocephalus is endoscopic third ventriculostomy. During this procedure a small perforation is made in the floor of the third ventricle to create a pathway for CSF to bypass an obstruction in the aqueduct of Sylvius (Chiafery, 2006).

Nursing Alert

The Chiari syndrome may occur with the Chiari II malformation and involves a downward displacement of the cerebellum, brainstem, and fourth ventricle and herniation through the foramen magnum into the cervical spaces. This displacement can cause sudden death, respiratory difficulty, swallowing difficulties, and the need for assisted ventilation. Rapid surgical decompression may be needed to reduce brainstem compression and to prevent death if the ventriculoperitoneal shunt does not resolve the problem (Warner, 2007).

Mechanical complications of a shunt may include blockage at either the proximal or the distal end of the catheter, kinking of the tubing, or valve breakdown. Infants or children with shunt failure show signs and symptoms of recurrent hydrocephalus and increased ICP. Shunt materials and systems continue to be refined in an attempt to reduce mechanical problems.

Clinical Tip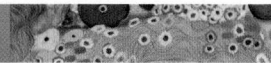

Technology advances have resulted in programmable shunts that enable adjustment of pressure, resulting in a reduction in the number of shunt revisions. These shunts are sensitive to magnets, so they must be checked and reprogrammed to the correct pressure level after an MRI diagnostic procedure (Duffy, 2010).

The most serious complication is shunt infection, occurring at a rate of 8%, most often within a few months of placement (Duffy, 2010). The infection may be confirmed by culture of the CSF obtained from the reservoir located in the burr hole (the hole in the skull through which the shunt is placed). In most cases the shunt is removed, an external drainage device is placed, and intravenous antibiotics are prescribed. A new shunt is inserted when the CSF cultures are sterile.

Intellectual functioning outcomes may be associated with the cause of the hydrocephalus and the age at diagnosis. Approximately one third of infants with hydrocephalus have an intelligence quotient (IQ) in the normal range. The greater risk for cognitive impairment is in children diagnosed in utero or at birth. Children with comorbid conditions, such as spina bifida, epilepsy, and cerebral palsy, also are at greater risk for cognitive impairment. Reading comprehension is a specific learning disability associated with hydrocephalus. Additionally, 60% of children have motor delays or disability (Duffy, 2010).

NURSING MANAGEMENT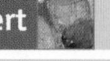

Nursing Assessment and Diagnosis

It is important for nurses to become familiar with the clinical manifestations of hydrocephalus to ensure prompt identification and treatment. Measure head circumference of all infants at each well-child visit to detect the condition at an early stage.

Assess the child with a ventriculoperitoneal shunt for signs and symptoms of shunt failure and infection. Measure the infant's head circumference daily when shunt failure is suspected. Report any abnormalities to the physician immediately.

Nursing Alert

In infants under age 1 year, important signs and symptoms of shunt failure include unusual irritability, bulging fontanel, separation of sutures, increasing head circumference, vomiting, diminished appetite, sleep pattern disturbance, and fever. In older children, observe for signs of increased ICP, such as headache, nausea and vomiting, and decreased LOC. The symptoms may be subtle, and symptom-free periods may occur (Lee & DiPatri, 2008).

Nursing diagnoses that might be appropriate for the child with hydrocephalus include:

- Risk for Infection related to surgical procedure
- Impaired Physical Mobility (Level 2) related to decreased muscle neck mass to lift the increased weight of head

- Risk for Caregiver Role Strain related to care of a child with a chronic condition or life-threatening illness
- Risk for Delayed Growth and Development related to repeated shunt infections and hospitalizations
- Risk for Injury related to potential shunt failure

Planning and Implementation

Hospital-Based Care

Nursing care focuses on providing preoperative and postoperative care and providing emotional support.

Provide Preoperative Care. Position the child carefully; do not stretch or strain the neck muscles, since they must support the large head. Holding the child may be difficult because of the additional weight of the head. Provide good skin care. Reduce the chances for skin breakdown by placing sheepskin or a lamb's wool blanket under the head. Prevent any other complications associated with immobility (see page 855). Attend to the child's special nutritional needs. Because the infant is prone to vomiting, frequent small feedings and frequent burping are beneficial.

Provide Postoperative Care. After surgery, the child is usually placed in a flat position to prevent rapid CSF drainage. The head of the bed is gradually elevated over 1 to 2 days. Take vital signs every 2 to 4 hours. Maintain aseptic technique when performing incision care. Monitor the child carefully for any signs of shunt malfunction, increased ICP, or infection.

Support the parents and explain the child's condition and all procedures to be performed. Encourage parents and family to help with the child's care in the hospital when appropriate. Be sympathetic and understanding, and allow parents to express their concerns. If hydrocephalus occurs during early infancy, the parents will be anxious about the impact of the chronic condition and subsequent surgical procedures. If hydrocephalus is secondary to neoplasm, however, the parents' anxieties are compounded by their child's life-threatening illness. Assure parents that most children with shunts lead normal lives; they attend school and interact with others the same way as their peers.

Discharge Planning and Home Care Teaching

Identify and address home care needs well in advance of discharge. Teach parents to care for the surgical site until healed. Teach parents about the signs and symptoms of shunt failure and infection. See Families Want to Know: Signs of Shunt Mal-

Families Want to Know

Signs of Shunt Malfunction or Infection

Parents should seek immediate medical attention if the infant or child experiences any of the following signs of shunt malfunction or infection:

- Headache, progressive or worsening
- Drowsiness or inappropriate sleepiness during the day, irritability
- Nausea, vomiting
- Personality changes or changes in school performance
- Fever
- Redness or swelling along the shunt tract

function or Infection. Provide contact information for the pediatrician and the neurosurgeon; ensure that parents know they should contact a physician immediately if they suspect a problem. Make sure that parents educate other caregivers and teachers about these signs so that needed care is not delayed.

Inform parents that the child may develop a seizure disorder, and indicate how to care for the child if a seizure occurs. Refer families to the appropriate home care, social services, and support groups such as the Hydrocephalus Association. See the companion website for resources.

Care in the Community

Infants and children need frequent monitoring to ensure proper shunt functioning. Head circumference is measured at each health visit to monitor growth. Assess the child for visual problems and cognitive, speech, and motor developmental delays. Refer the child and family to an early intervention program to promote developmental progress. School-age children may need to have an individualized education plan developed (see Chapter 12 ∞).

Clinical Tip

After the shunt placement, the head circumference may decrease by 1 to 2 cm as the pressure is relieved. Head growth due to brain development may then be noted in 2 to 4 months. If head growth resumes sooner than that, shunt failure may be present (Duffy, 2010).

Encourage parents to promote an optimal health status by promoting good nutrition and reducing exposure to infections. Teach parents alternate positions for burping infants with an enlarged head and to use an infant seat for positioning after feeding to reduce regurgitation. Parents needing childcare for children less than age 2 years should seek a setting with fewer children, such as family or home-based childcare, if possible, to decrease exposure to infection. Encourage the use of good hand hygiene by all caregivers.

Health Promotion

Teach parents to protect the infant from injury by using a rear-facing car safety seat. These infants have poor head control due to an enlarged head, and the forward-facing position increases their risk of cervical spine injury and death in a car crash. Support the child's head and body position with towel rolls to maintain proper positioning.

As the child grows, encourage parents to avoid becoming overprotective and to allow the child to develop normally. Helmets should only be worn for sports and activities that require a helmet. Contact sports with a high potential for head and abdominal impact are often restricted.

Evaluation

Expected outcomes of nursing care include the following:

- The child develops adequate neck muscle control to interact with the environment.

- Shunt infections and malfunctions are rapidly identified by the parents and medical attention is sought quickly.
- The child's potential for growth and development is maximized by care and a stimulating environment.

Neural Tube Defects

The neural tube is the tissue that ultimately develops the CNS, including the brain and spinal cord. The incidence of neural tube defects is 1 per 3,000 pregnancies in the United States (Boss & Huether, 2010). Types of neural tube defects include the following:

- **Anencephaly.** The brain does not develop above the brainstem.
- **Encephalocele.** A protrusion of meningeal tissue or meningeal-covered brain is observed through a defect in the skull.
- **Spina Bifida Occulta.** The posterior vertebral arches fail to fuse, most commonly at the fifth lumbar or first sacral vertebrae. The spinal cord and meninges lie entirely within the vertebral canal and the condition is usually not visible externally. A tuft of hair, a dermoid cyst, or hemangioma may be found over the site.
- **Spina Bifida Cystica.** There is a defect in closure of the posterior vertebral arch with protrusion through the bony spine.
- **Meningocele.** A spinal fluid-filled meningeal sac filled with CSF protrudes through a vertebral defect, associated with no abnormalities of the spinal cord. The sac covering the defect may be translucent or membranous. The spinal cord and spinal root are in normal position, and the child usually has no neurologic defects. Surgery is performed on the newborn to close the lesion.
- **Myelomeningocele (spina bifida).** A spinal fluid-filled meningeal sac contains a portion of the meninges; spinal cord or nerve roots protrude through a vertebral defect. Fluid leakage may also occur as the lesion is poorly covered with imperfect tissue.

Myelomeningocele or Spina Bifida

Myelomeningocele (often called spina bifida) refers to a failure of the neural tube to close within the first 4 weeks of gestation, resulting in a defect in one or more vertebrae through which a cystic sac with CSF and spinal cord contents can protrude. The malformation can occur anywhere along the vertebral column, and it is most common at the lumbar or sacral portion of the spine. The incidence is 0.5 to 1 per 1,000 pregnancies, making it one of the most common developmental disorders of the CNS (Boss & Huether, 2010).

Etiology and Pathophysiology

The cause of spina bifida is unknown, although environmental factors such as chemicals (excessive use of alcohol), medications (e.g., valproic acid and carbamazepine used for seizures, isotretinoin for acne), genetic factors, and maternal health conditions (insulin-dependent diabetes mellitus, gestational diabetes, folic acid deficiency, and maternal obesity) have been implicated. The

Research — *Folate Fortification of Foods*

Mandatory fortification of all enriched grain products with folate was initiated in 1998. The most recent data analysis of birth certificates from 2003 to 2005 revealed a 6.9% reduction in the prevalence of spina bifida in infants born to mothers of all races and ethnic groups. Reduction in prevalence was higher (19.8%) among non-Hispanic Black infants than for Hispanic and non-Hispanic White infants (Boulet, Gambrell, Shin, et al., 2009).

increased incidence of the condition in families indicates a possible genetic influence.

Bowel and bladder control is affected in children with defects in the thoracic and lumbar regions. Renal damage may result from neurologic impairment and urinary retention. Hydrocephalus is present in 85% of children with myelomeningocele. Seizures and visual-perceptual problems may also occur.

The Arnold-Chiari II malformation commonly occurs with myelomeningocele. It involves downward displacement of the cerebellum, cerebellar tonsils, brainstem, and fourth ventricle. Altered function of the cranial nerves often occurs. This condition is potentially life-threatening when the cerebellum and brainstem are compressed through the foramen magnum of the skull (Boss & Huether, 2010).

Clinical Manifestations

A sac-like protrusion on the infant's back indicates meningocele or myelomeningocele (Figure 27–12 ➤). The clinical manifestations (weakness, paralysis, and sensory loss) are related to the location of the defect: the higher the defect, the greater the neurologic dysfunction as described here:

- Thoracic or lumbar 1–2 level—paralysis of the legs, weakness, and sensory loss in the trunk and lower body region are found.
- Lumbar 3 level—can flex hips and extend the knees; the ankles and toes are paralyzed.
- Lumbar 4–5 level—can flex hips and extend the knees; weak or absent ankle extension, toe flexion, and hip extension.
- Sacral level—mild weakness in ankles and toes; bladder and bowel function may be affected.

Sensory loss is more pronounced on the back of the legs and the feet. The loss of lower extremity motor and sensory functioning may not be symmetric. The range of potential problems for the child with spina bifida is listed in the accompanying clinical manifestations table.

COLLABORATIVE CARE

Diagnostic Tests

Diagnosis is usually made prenatally, but after birth the lesion is examined and the neurologic status is evaluated. Radiologic imaging by ultrasonography, CT scan, MRI, and flat films of the spinal column can pinpoint the bony defect. Subsequent testing is performed to evaluate bowel and bladder function, neurologic and motor function, and cognitive function.

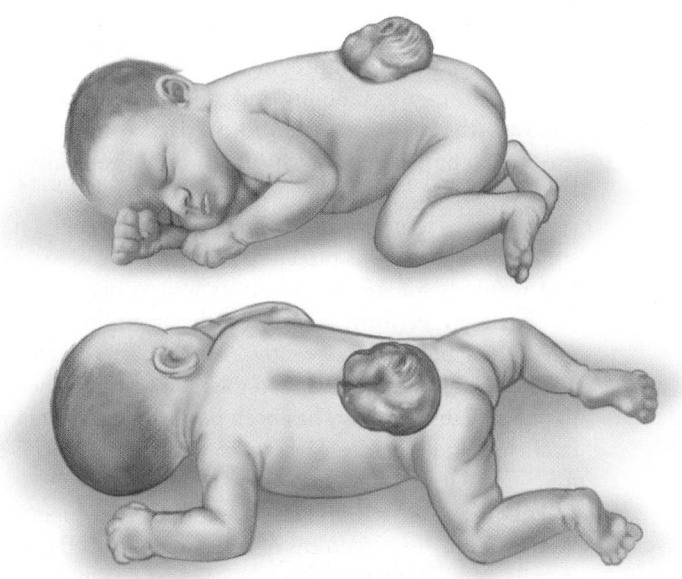

FIGURE 27–12 ➤ Lumbosacral myelomeningocele is caused by a neural tube defect that results in incomplete closure of the vertebral column. As shown here, the meninges (and sometimes the spinal cord) protrude as a sac-like structure.

Clinical Therapy

During birth, efforts are made to prevent injury to the lesion or traction on the spinal cord. Surgery to close and repair the lesion usually occurs within 24 to 48 hours of the infant's birth to reduce infection. Depending upon the size of

Clinical Manifestations
Myelomeningocele

Cause	Clinical Manifestations
Interruption of the spinal cord at site of the spinal defect	Loss of motor and sensory function of the abdomen and lower extremities, dependent upon defect level Scoliosis or kyphosis Incontinence of urine or urinary retention Incontinence of feces or constipation Sensory loss around anus and genitalia
Muscle imbalance	Hip abnormalities, hip dysplasia Foot deformities (e.g., clubfoot)
Chiari II malformation	*Infants:* Difficulty swallowing Apnea, respiratory difficulty, inspiratory stridor Weak or poor cry Sustained backward arching of head (opisthotonic) *Older children:* Choking, hoarseness, vocal cord paralysis Disordered breathing during sleep Stiffness or spasticity of arms and hands Loss of feeling or sensation
Brain and spinal cord abnormalities	Hydrocephalus Learning problems, attention deficit disorder Problems with perceptual motor skills Memory and organization problems Problems with numerical reasoning

the defect, the excision may be extensive. In rare cases, uteromyelomeningocele repairs are performed on the fetus.

Braces are used to support joint position and mobility. Assistive devices such as walkers, crutches, and wheelchairs are used to enhance mobility. To minimize the risk for osteoporosis, the diet should ensure adequate calcium and vitamin D, and weight-bearing activities should be encouraged.

Interventions for a neurogenic bladder are initiated early to prevent kidney damage and to maintain bladder function and promote urinary continence. Clean intermittent catheterization is performed on a regular schedule (every 3 to 4 hours) (see the *Clinical Skills Manual*). A Mitrofanoff procedure that creates a reservoir for urine and a stoma for catheterizing the bladder from the abdominal wall to improve access for catheterization is a surgical option to improve continence in older children (Figure 27–13 ➤).

Dietary fiber, stool softeners, and glycerin or bisacodyl suppositories are prescribed for bowel evacuation and to promote continence. Surgery to create a channel between the skin and bowel (Malone antegrade continence enema) is often performed in older children. This procedure enables a child or adolescent to infuse an enema into the ascending and transverse colon to promote bowel evacuation (Doolin, 2006).

Prognosis depends on the type of defect, the level of the lesion, and other complicating factors. Children often need multiple surgeries and invasive procedures. For example, acquired scoliosis in an adolescent may be a sign of a tethered cord, hydromyelia (expansion of the central canal of the spinal cord with increased CSF accumulation), or shunt failure. Surgery to address these problems may improve the scoliosis (Rowe & Jadhav, 2008). A team of physicians, nurses, and therapists from the neurosurgery, orthopedic, urology, and physical medicine departments work with the child and family to form a comprehensive care plan.

NURSING MANAGEMENT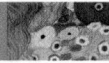

Nursing Assessment

Monitor the newborn for integrity of the sac and CSF leakage. Assess the extremities for deformities. Frequently assess the vital signs and stay alert for signs of infection. Following surgery, observe the wound healing. Note any signs of infection and CSF leakage. Measure the head

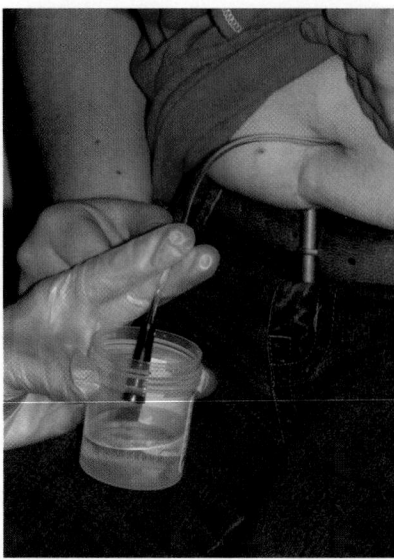

FIGURE 27–13 ➤ This child has had a Mitrofanoff procedure to make it easier to perform self-catheterization and maintain modesty. Clean intermittent self-catheterization is performed, and the catheters can be reused until they become brittle. Catheters should be washed with soap and water, rinsed, and stored in a plastic bag.

circumference prior to and daily after surgery to assess for potential hydrocephalus. Assess intake and output.

Nursing Alert

More than half of children with myelomeningocele develop a latex allergy, and the risk increases as the child ages (Liptak, 2007). Always use nonlatex materials when providing care to the child in all settings. If the child has had an allergic reaction, the child should carry an epinephrine auto-injector and nonlatex gloves and other nonlatex equipment for an emergency. The child should also wear a medical alert tag. See Chapter 22 ∞ for information on latex allergy. The Spina Bifida Association maintains an updated list of products containing latex and potential substitutes. See the companion website for more information.

The child with myelomeningocele may be hospitalized for surgery to correct deformities. Assess the child's responsiveness and level of pain. Assess neurologic status for any deterioration in function that could be associated with shunt failure or problems with the spinal cord. Assess the range of motion of joints and mobility status. Assess intake and output.

Examples of nursing diagnoses for the child with myelomeningocele include:

- Impaired Physical Mobility related to neuromuscular impairment
- Risk for Latex Allergy Response related to multiple surgical procedures
- Risk for Disproportionate Growth related to caloric intake in excess of needs due to limited mobility
- Impaired Skin Integrity associated with the use of braces and a wheelchair
- Risk for Infection related to urinary retention

Planning and Implementation

Nursing care focuses on providing preoperative and postoperative care, promoting mobility, and providing emotional support.

Cover the sac on the newborn's back with a sterile saline dressing to protect its integrity and monitor for leakage of CSF. Place the infant in a prone position with hips slightly flexed and legs abducted to minimize tension on the sac. Maintain this position using towel rolls placed between the knees. Assess the infant regularly for motor deficits as well as bladder and bowel involvement. Perform urinary catheterization on a regular schedule if needed. Frequently assess the vital signs and stay alert for signs of infection. Feed the infant with the head turned to one side until surgery has been performed. The infant is difficult to handle before surgery, so tactile stimulation such as touching, patting, and cuddling may be comforting.

Following surgery, monitor the infant's vital signs carefully. Watch closely for symptoms of infection, especially meningitis, increasing head circumference, and pain. The infant should be placed in prone or side-lying position for sleep until healing has occurred (despite guidelines to put infants to sleep on their backs), and then supine position for sleep may be used. Keep the diaper away from the incision site.

Gentle range of motion exercises should be started as soon as possible to prevent muscle contractures and atrophy. Use caution when performing range of motion because these children have brittle bones that fracture easily. Splints may be used to maintain extremity alignment.

Support the parents by keeping them informed about their child's status. Allow them to express their frustrations and anger. As soon as parents are able to cope with the child's condition, encourage them to become involved in the child's care in the hospital.

The child with myelomeningocele may be hospitalized for surgery numerous times to correct deformities. Monitor the child's level of pain and provide pain management (see Chapter 15 ∞). As the child may have decreased pain sensation in lower extremities, careful assessment is needed. Assess dressing sites for bleeding and drainage. Monitor the distal extremities for swelling and circulation.

Discharge Planning and Home Care Teaching

Identify and address home care needs well in advance of discharge. Help parents obtain special devices such as splints, wedges, and rolls, if needed, to prevent complications. Instruct parents how to position, handle, and feed the infant, and to perform range of motion exercises. Teach parents to begin a bowel management program and to perform intermittent clean catheterization and establish a schedule for catheterization every 3 to 4 hours.

Growth & Development 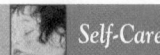 *Self-Care*

Treat older children according to their intellectual level, not their motor development. Encourage them to take responsibility for self-care, such as self-catheterization, and recognize their need to control their body functions. Promote interaction with peers in the hospital and participation in activities. If children are hospitalized for an extended time, arrange schooling.

Teach parents the signs and symptoms of increased ICP, hydrocephalus, shunt infection or malfunction, and urinary tract infection. Home care nursing or a case manager should be arranged, if necessary. The home care nurse reinforces the skills learned in the hospital and the case manager coordinates the numerous health care professionals working with the child and family. Refer parents to resource groups such as the Spina Bifida Association of America.

Care in the Community

To reduce complications and promote optimal development, children with myelomeningocele need comprehensive care, including health promotion, planned and coordinated by a knowledgeable team of health care professionals. This care may be provided in partnership with the primary care physician.

Parents need to teach the child to perform intermittent self-catheterization at an appropriate age, so the child can be more independent when attending school. If the child has had a Mitrofanoff procedure performed, monitor for any signs that the stoma is becoming stenosed. It is important to report stenosis so that dilatation can occur and possibly prevent the need for surgical revision of the stoma (Gray, Blackinton, & White, 2006). When the child begins school, an individualized health plan should be developed to ensure that the child has access to the restroom and assistance as needed for toileting, as well as accommodations for mobility challenges. School nurses should be prepared to assist children with catheterization (Katrancha, 2008).

Clinical Tip

The child who has clean intermittent catheterization performed usually has bacteria in the urine, but this is not treated unless the child becomes symptomatic. Symptoms of a urinary tract infection that should be treated include foul odor or discharge, a change in mood or personality, or fatigue (Gray et al., 2006).

Good nutrition planning is important to prevent obesity and to reduce constipation and complications such as fecal impaction. Bowel training is initiated to control bowel evacuation at appropriate times and places. A high-fiber diet helps ensure adequate stool. At a convenient time, a glycerin or bisacodyl suppository can be given. Consistency in time of day for bowel evacuation is important. Several resources to help with a bowel management program are available through the Spina Bifida Association.

Promote safety and independent mobility with proper use of braces, walkers, crutches, canes, and in some cases custom-designed wheelchairs and car safety seats (Figure 27–14 ►). For other safety guidelines, see Families Want to Know: Safety for the Child with Spina Bifida.

Parents are faced with the long-term financial issues of caring for the child who needs regular new adaptive equipment to match growth, as well as other medical supplies. At least 75% of children born with spina bifida generally survive to at least the early adult years (Nehring & Faux, 2006). Parents thus need to learn how to act as the child's case manager, or to work effectively with the person in this role.

Research — *Bowel Management Challenges*

A qualitative descriptive study involving seven parents of children with spina bifida focused on finding an effective bowel management program. Parents described their frustration with finding a bowel management program that was effective for their child to prevent embarrassment when accidents occurred. They were concerned about the child's self-image because of incontinence, malodor, or fecal soiling. Additionally parents felt that health care providers did not view bowel management with the same priority that parents did (Sawin & Thompson, 2009).

Craniosynostosis

Craniosynostosis is the premature closing of the cranial sutures during the first 18 to 20 months of life. This condition occurs in up to 1 in 1,800 to 2,200 live births, and boys are affected twice as often as girls. Chromosome abnormalities and autosomal dominant conditions such as Apert syndrome and Crouzon syndrome are responsible for up to 40% of cases (Boss & Huether, 2010). Some cases not associated with a syndrome are believed to be familial pattern with autosomal dominant inheritance (Koh & Gries, 2007).

Closure of the cranial sutures usually takes place at predetermined times during the child's development. Problems arise if one or more sutures close early. One theory is that abnormal development occurs at the base of the skull that places exaggerated forces on the dura that act to disrupt cranial suture development (Kinsman & Johnston, 2007). Bone growth continues in a direction parallel to the prematurely fused suture line, which leads to compensatory overgrowth at normal suture lines. Sagittal synostosis (scaphocephaly) accounts for 50% of cases (Koh & Gries, 2007). Bicoronal synostosis is associated with Alpert or Crouzon syndromes. (Figure 27–15A and B ►).

Diagnosis is often made at birth by clinical appearance and palpation of a bony ridge along a skull suture line. Skull radiographs, CT scan, and MRI confirm the diagnosis. Surgical approaches include a spring-mediated cranioplasty, or reconstructive skull remodeling is performed to promote brain development and vision and to improve cosmetic appearance

Families Want to Know
Safety for the Child with Spina Bifida

Due to the loss of sensation in the lower extremities, the child may not immediately recognize injuries. Several actions routinely taken by the child and family will reduce the risk for injury.

■ Daily, check all skin surfaces and pressure points associated with sitting, braces, and shoes for abrasions, scrapes, reddened areas, and other lesions. Stop using the braces or shoes until the skin heals or redness disappears.

■ Keep all skin surfaces clean and dry. Wear socks without wrinkles under braces.

■ Use a gel-filled cushion and teach the child to shift his or her position hourly when in the wheelchair to avoid pressure sores.

■ Avoid burns to the lower extremities by checking the temperature of bath water and car safety seats in a hot car.

■ Use safe ambulation techniques with walkers, canes, and crutches.

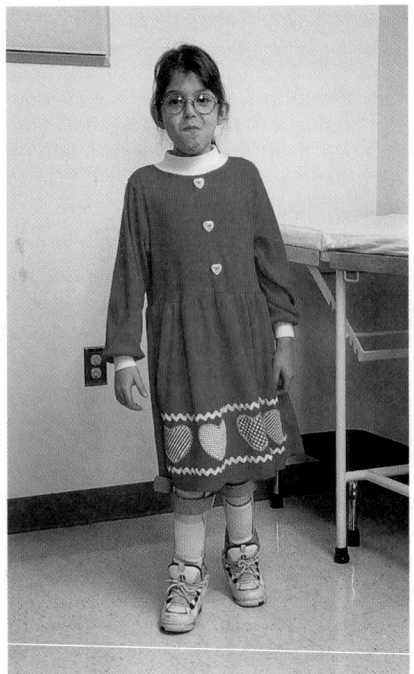

A

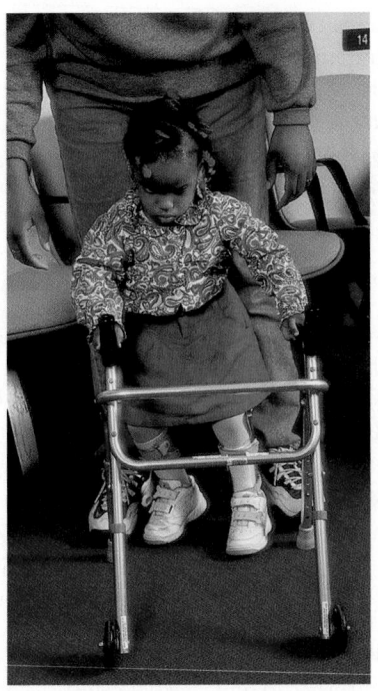

B

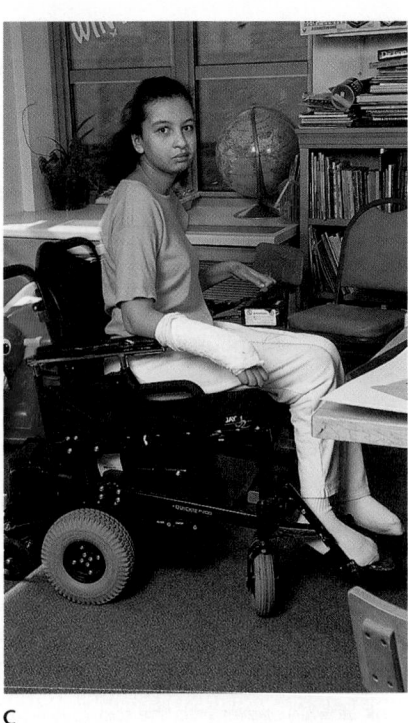

C

FIGURE 27–14 ➤ Help determine the best assistive device for the child to gain the most independence for mobilizing and to promote development. The child may change devices in different settings to promote optimal independence. A and B, Braces and walkers may be best for young children to promote an upright posture that encourages a normal interaction with the environment. C, A motorized wheelchair can assist the child with a significant neurologic impairment to achieve independence and mobility.

(Koh & Gries, 2007). Many children need multiple procedures. Hydrocephalus is a potential complication.

After surgery, it is important for the incision to remain dry and intact. The nurse should also observe the child for symptoms of increased ICP (see Table 27–4). Explain to parents that surgery will improve the child's appearance. Most children with craniosynostosis not associated with a syndrome have good surgical outcomes, and their brains develop normally.

Positional Plagiocephaly

Positional *plagiocephaly* (flattening of the occipital area of the skull) is seen increasingly in healthy infants put to sleep on their backs to prevent sudden infant death syndrome (Jorganic, Lynch, Littlefield, et al., 2009). See Figure 27–15C. The sutures do not close prematurely, but when the infant's sleep position does not change, the weight of the head flattens the skull. The flattened area may make the skull asymmetric when the infant has a

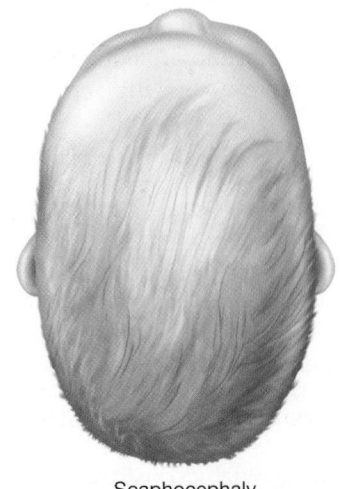

A   Scaphocephaly

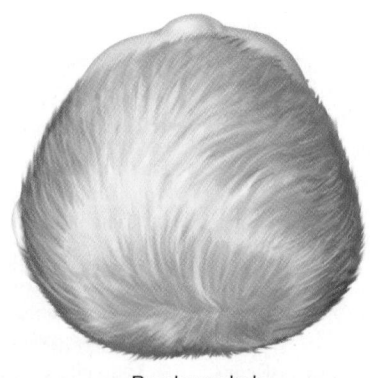

B   Brachycephaly

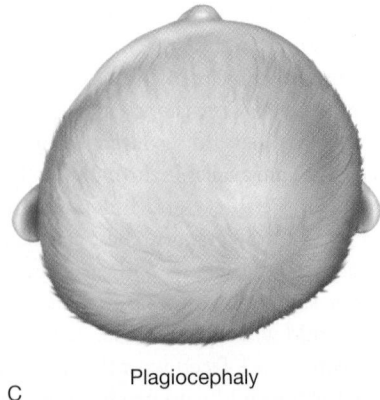

C   Plagiocephaly

FIGURE 27–15 ➤ In craniosynostosis, the head shape is dependent upon which sutures are involved. A, Scaphocephaly or dolichocephaly accounts for 50% of cases (Koh & Gries, 2007). Premature closure of the sagittal suture causes a long, narrow skull and flattened parietal bones with a prominent occiput, a broad forehead, and small or absent anterior fontanel. B, Brachycephaly or bicoronal synostosis is associated with Crouzon syndrome. The head shape is shortened anterior to posterior and the occiput is flattened. The infant may have hypertelorism and underdeveloped eye orbits with prominent eyes. C, Positional plagiocephaly is often asymmetric flattening of the occiput due to preferred position when supine or torticollis.

positional preference, such as with congenital torticollis. It is speculated that infants develop a positional preference because of the location of the crib in the room that encourages looking toward the door and the parent's holding preference for bottle-feeding. Additionally, infants often do not have enough supervised tummy-time to promote neck muscle development (van Vlimmeren, van der Graaf, Boere-Boonekamp, et al., 2007).

A helmet device to correct severe cases of positional plagiocephaly or brachycephaly is most effective in infants under 12 months of age and when treatment is initiated at 6 months of age because the skull bones are more malleable. The helmet is worn for 23 hours a day for 3 months. Remolding of the head shape continues after that treatment period because the infant spends more time awake and upright. Younger infants may be successfully treated with positioning strategies.

Clinical Tip

Encourage parents to try to reduce the infant's preference for lying supine in one position. One strategy is to rotate the crib every day so the infant must turn his or her head in a different direction to look at who comes into the room. Rotate the arm used for formula-feeding the infant. When the child is alert and can be continuously supervised, place the infant in prone position on the floor for short periods to promote neck muscle strength and interaction with nearby objects.

■ NEONATAL ABSTINENCE SYNDROME

Illicit substances that may cause neonatal abstinence syndrome when used by the mother during pregnancy include opiates (heroin, meperidine, methadone), CNS stimulants (cocaine, propoxyphene, amphetamines), and CNS depressants (barbiturates, alcohol, and marijuana). It is estimated that 5.1% of women 15 to 44 years of age used illicit drugs during pregnancy, but the rate varies by age group: 7.1% among women ages 18 to 25 years and 3% among women ages 26 to 44 years (Substance Abuse and Mental Health Services Administration, 2009). Binge alcohol use during the first trimester of pregnancy was reported by 10.3% of pregnant women ages 15 to 44 years (Substance Abuse and Mental Health Services Administration, 2009). See Chapter 28 ∞ for information about fetal alcohol syndrome.

Illicit substances readily cross the placenta, enter the fetal circulation, and have the same effects on the fetus that they do in the mother. Fetal death, low birth weight, small head circumference, prematurity, congenital anomalies, and impaired development may result (Rayburn, 2007). The mother's repeated use of narcotics or other substances leads to tolerance and physical dependence in the fetus. If the mother is still actively using drugs at the time of birth, the neonate has signs of abrupt withdrawal from the illicit substance shortly after birth.

Signs of opioid withdrawal include hypertonia, irritability, excitability, jitteriness, tremors, tachypnea, sneezing, stuffy nose, high-pitched cry, diarrhea, regurgitation, poor feeding, apnea, and seizures (Sweeney, 2009). Withdrawal symptoms for opiates usually appear 24 to 48 hours after birth, barbiturate withdrawal

symptoms appear between 4 and 14 days after birth, and cocaine or amphetamine withdrawal symptoms appear up to 7 days after birth. Mothers, however, may use multiple substances. Long-term issues for children with cocaine exposure in utero include potential difficulties with hyperactivity, distractibility, and attention problems (Bada, Das, Bauer, et al., 2007).

Diagnosis is based on the history of maternal substance abuse and physical signs in the infant. EEG abnormalities may be noted. Urine testing provides information on drug use immediately prior to labor, and meconium screening provides information on drug use by the mother for the last half of the pregnancy. The infant's hair may also be tested. If urine is positive, compare the results with medications used during labor and delivery. Chain of custody for specimens may be needed.

Behavioral and neurologic functioning may also be assessed with diagnostic tools such as the Brazelton Neonatal Behavioral Assessment scale. This tool evaluates infants on habituation (ability to respond to and then inhibit response to discrete stimuli when asleep), general arousal level, orientation, quality of movement and tone, autonomic stability, reflexes, and responsiveness when aroused (Olsson, 2007).

Treatment is generally supportive. Infants with cocaine exposure need to have reduced environmental stimuli and swaddling. Medications such as phenobarbital, diazepam, methadone, clonidine, and paregoric may be prescribed to alleviate symptoms of drug withdrawal. If the mother is still using illicit drugs, breastfeeding is discouraged since the drugs cross over into milk.

NURSING MANAGEMENT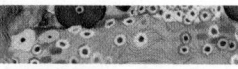

Prevention and early identification of the infant with neonatal abstinence syndrome is an important nursing role. Providing information for all parents about the risks and effects of various abused substances increases the chance that they will avoid these substances in future pregnancies.

Crying and poor feeding should increase the nurse's suspicion of neonatal abstinence syndrome. Observe the newborn closely for poor sucking, seizures, vomiting and diarrhea, dehydration, and an increased metabolic rate. Many withdrawal symptoms are identical to symptoms of infection, bowel obstruction, electrolyte disorder, hydrocephalus, and intracranial anomaly, so consider the possibility that the infant could have both neonatal abstinence syndrome and another condition.

Clinical Tip

Several techniques are used to calm and soothe the newborn with neonatal abstinence syndrome:

■ Keep the infant in a quiet environment, away from beeping monitors and paging speakers.

■ Keep the lighting subdued and minimize stimulation to promote rest and sleep.

■ Comfort and pacify the infant with swaddling and a pacifier for sucking needs. Rocking along with soothing music may be calming. Infant massage may also be beneficial in some infants.

Provide frequent, small, high-calorie feedings. Formula with 24 calories per ounce may be recommended. Patience is needed when feeding these infants because of poor sucking and swallowing coordination. Teach parents to use a calm approach and soothing voice when feeding. Newborns may initially feed better in the side-lying position while swaddled. Hold the infant with the spine flexed to decrease extensor tone.

Administer prescribed medications, if ordered for drug withdrawal, and monitor the infant's response. Keep in mind, however, that many infants are managed without drugs. Protect the newborn's skin as jitteriness may lead to greater skin surface rubbing against sheets and cause scratches and abrasions.

Assess the strengths, safety, and competence of the mother and other potential caregivers. Determine if the mother is still using illicit drugs and identify other family supports that may help provide the care and safety needed by the newborn. Begin working with the mother and other family members to demonstrate strategies for promoting parent–infant interaction, minimizing stimulation, and promoting feeding. Make plans for careful follow-up by health professionals (social services, physicians, and nurses) so that the infant's safety is ensured and the growth and development are monitored and promoted. In some cases, referral to child abuse protective services may be made.

Long-term follow-up care of the child should be planned to ensure regular developmental testing and assessment for catch-up growth and neurobehavioral problems.

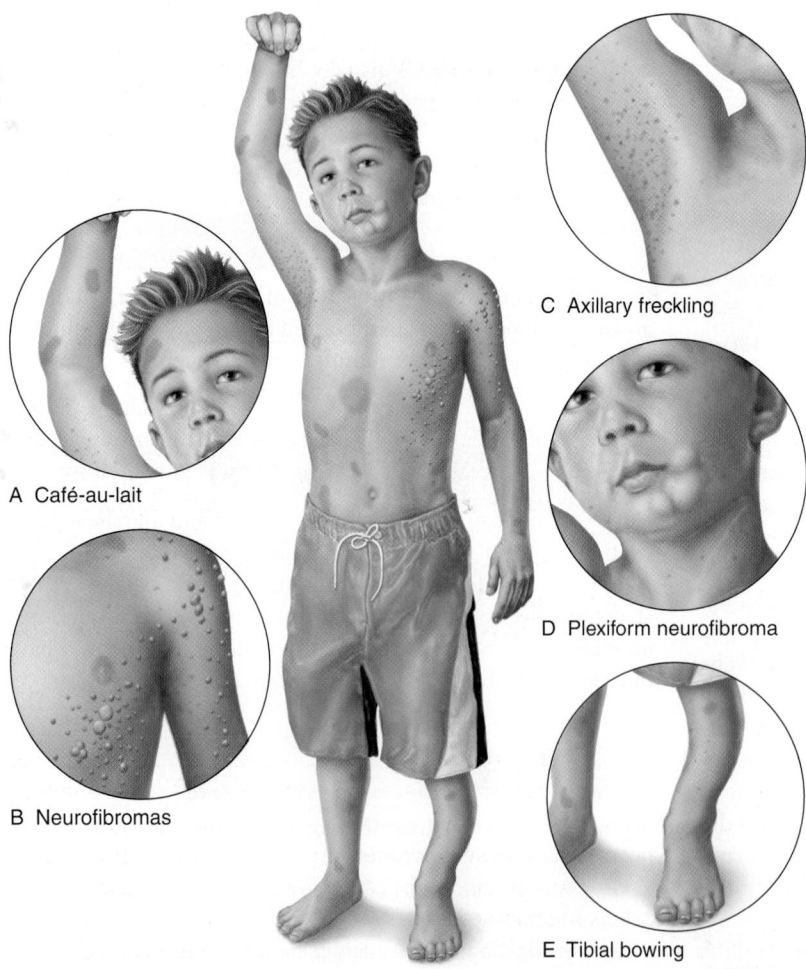

A Café-au-lait

B Neurofibromas

C Axillary freckling

D Plexiform neurofibroma

E Tibial bowing

FIGURE 27–16 ➤ Physical signs of neurofibromatosis 1 become more apparent during adolescence. Café-au-lait spots enlarge, axillary freckling appears, and multiple neurofibromas develop. Some children develop plexiform neurofibromas.

■ NEUROFIBROMATOSIS

Neurofibromatosis 1 (NF1), or von Recklinghausen disease, is an autosomal dominant genetic disorder in which tumors grow along nerves. Skin pigmentation changes and bone deformities also occur. The incidence of the disorder is 1 per 3,500 live births (Black & Wilson, 2009). The NF1 gene is located on chromosome 17. Approximately 30–50% of cases result from new mutations (National Institute of Neurological Disorders and Stroke, 2009).

Neurofibromas (tumors) develop from cells of the nerve sheath, usually along the peripheral nerves or at nerve endings. The neurofibroma may be an isolated growth, or extend along the length of a nerve and include nerve branches (plexiform neurofibroma). Dermal neurofibromas, which usually begin to appear around the time of puberty, may reside in the skin or project above the skin surface. Tumors may also develop in the brain, along a cranial nerve, or along spinal nerve roots. Children with NF1 may be at risk for leukemia, rhabdomyosarcoma, and pheochromocytoma (Theos & Korf, 2006).

The disorder is characterized by six or more café-au-lait spots (darker than the surrounding skin) 5 mm or larger seen at birth or by 2 years of age. The spots grow to 15 mm or larger by adulthood. Freckling in the axillary and inguinal areas is common. Lisch nodules, tan or brown benign tumors on the iris of the eye, are a diagnostic sign. Tumors begin to grow on or under the skin beginning during puberty. Pain may occur when a tumor compresses a nerve or grows in the spinal cord. Scoliosis and thinning or bowing of the tibia may also occur. See Figure 27–16 ➤.

Vision deficits or blindness is found in 20% of children due to a tumor along the optic pathway. Precocious puberty or delayed puberty and menarche may occur when the optic tumor invades the hypothalamus. Hypertension may develop in association with renal vascular stenosis or a pheochromocytoma, a tumor of the adrenal gland (see Chapter 30 ∞). Other manifestations include hyperactivity, learning disabilities, speech problems, and seizures.

Diagnosis is made in infancy or early childhood by characteristic physical findings and a positive family history. Radiology imaging (MRI of the brain and radiographs of the spine and other bones) is performed when problems are detected. Ophthalmic examinations should be performed at least annually during childhood to detect optic tumors, to monitor Lisch nodules, and to detect vision deficits.

Clinical therapy focuses on monitoring the child's growth, development, blood pressure, spine for scoliosis, timing of sexual development, and development of neurofibromas. Genetic counseling is offered. When neurofibromas are disfiguring or cause problems because of their location, surgery may be performed to remove the tumor. Most children and adults with mild symptoms can live a normal, productive life.

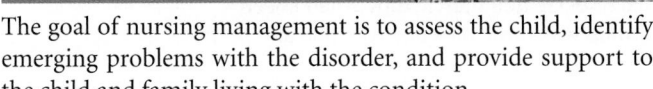

NURSING MANAGEMENT

The goal of nursing management is to assess the child, identify emerging problems with the disorder, and provide support to the child and family living with the condition.

Nurses assess the child to identify signs of neurofibromatosis. Vital signs with blood pressure are monitored for hypertension. Screen vision to detect any vision impairment. Monitor growth and development to detect any unusual patterns, identifying signs of early or late pubertal development. Perform scoliosis screening on a frequent basis. Note any evidence of tibial bowing or thinning. School performance should be monitored as learning disabilities and hyperactivity are known problems. Pay attention to any mass that is rapidly enlarging or causing new pain.

Provide psychological support to the child and family. In children with moderate to severe conditions, the tumor development during adolescence will cause cosmetic problems leading to problems with self-image and self-esteem. Adolescents may fear the response of peers to the tumors and isolate themselves. Identify peers or refer the adolescent to support groups. Focus on the child's strengths and encourage continuing development of those strengths. See the companion website for more information.

■ CEREBRAL PALSY

Cerebral palsy (CP) is a group of permanent disorders of movement and posture development that cause activity limitation. It results from a nonprogressive disturbance that occurred in the fetal or infant brain. CP is primarily a motor disorder, but the child may also have sensory, perceptual, cognitive, communicative, and behavioral problems (Rosenbaum, Paneth, Leviton, et al., 2007). CP occurs in 1.5 to 2 cases per 1,000 live births (Jones, Morgan, & Shelton, 2007a). Four types of motor dysfunction are seen with cerebral palsy—spastic, dyskinetic, ataxic, and mixed—related to the location of brain insult.

Etiology and Pathophysiology

Most CP cases are caused by brain insult (complications of prematurity; prenatal, perinatal, and genetic factors; or fetal viral infection). The rate of CP increases with decreasing gestational age and in premature infants with intraventricular hemorrhage (Rais-Bahrami & Short, 2007). An estimated 6–7% of CP cases are associated with birth asphyxia (Nield, Nanda, Someshwar, et al., 2007). After birth, risk factors for CP include neonatal sepsis and hyperbilirubinemia, as well as CNS infection, and brain injury or anoxic insult in children under 2 years.

Clinical Manifestations

Cerebral palsy is characterized by abnormal muscle tone and lack of coordination with spasticity found in the majority of cases. Characteristics include:

- Hypotonia—floppiness, increased range of motion, diminished reflex response
- Rigidity—hypertonia with tense, tight muscles
- Spasticity—hypertonia with uncoordinated, awkward, stiff movements; scissoring or crossing of the legs; exaggerated reflex reactions; found in majority of cases
- Athetosis—constant involuntary writhing motions, more severe distally
- Ataxia—irregularity in muscle coordination or action
- Hemiplegia—involvement of one side of the body; upper extremities more dysfunctional than lower extremities
- **Diplegia**—involvement of all extremities; lower extremities more affected than upper; usually spastic
- Quadriplegia—involvement of all extremities; arms in flexion and legs in extension

Children have a variety of symptoms depending on their ages. See the clinical manifestations table on page 884 for symptoms by type of CNS injury. The wide variability in symptoms are related to the area of the brain involved and the degree of anoxia. Children with CP usually have delayed developmental milestones. Other common problems include intellectual disability; epilepsy; visual defects such as strabismus, nystagmus, or refractory errors; hearing loss; language delay; or seizures. Feeding and speech may be difficult because of oral motor involvement.

COLLABORATIVE CARE

Diagnostic Tests

Diagnosis is usually based on clinical findings. Many children with delayed developmental milestones or neuromuscular abnormalities at 1 year of age continue to show gradual improvement in function. CP must be distinguished from other neurologic conditions, and signs may be subtle. Suspicious historical findings include a premature infant (less than 1500 g birth weight or less than 28 weeks' gestation), maternal intrauterine infection, multiple birth, or an anoxic event (Pellegrino, 2007).

Ultrasonography can be used to detect fetal and neonatal abnormalities of the brain, such as intraventricular hemorrhage. Neuromotor tests are used to evaluate the presence of normal movement patterns and absence of primitive reflexes and abnormal tone. Once CP is suspected, CT scans and MRI provide information about anatomic structures and help identify the cause of CP. Positron emission tomography (PET) or single-photon emission computed tomography (SPECT) may provide information about brain metabolic functioning (Pellegrino, 2007).

Clinical Therapy

Some children who are delayed in meeting developmental milestones or have neuromuscular abnormalities at age 1 year show

Clinical Manifestations
Cerebral Palsy by Type of Insult

Classification and Type of Insult	Clinical Manifestations
Spastic Cerebral cortex or pyramidal tract injury 75% of cases	Persistent hypertonia, rigidity Exaggerated deep tendon reflexes Persistent primitive reflexes Leads to contractures and abnormal curvature of the spine
Dyskinetic Extrapyramidal, basal ganglia injury 10–15% of cases	Abnormalities of muscle tone that affect the body Inconsistent muscle tone, may change hour to hour or day to day, may have rigid muscle tone when awake and normal or decreased muscle tone when asleep Tremors, impaired voluntary muscle control, difficulty with fine and purposeful motor movements Exaggerated posturing
Ataxic Cerebellar (extrapyramidal) injury 5–10% of cases	Abnormalities of voluntary movement involving balance and position of the trunk and limbs Difficulty controlling hand and arm movements during reaching Increased or decreased muscle tone Hypotonia in infancy Muscle instability and wide-based unsteady gait
Mixed Injuries to multiple areas	No dominant motor pattern Unique compensatory movements and posture to maintain control over specific neuromotor deficits Combination of characteristics from other types

gradual improvement in function. Half of the infants suspected to be at risk for CP at age 1 year are unimpaired neurologically by age 2 years (Nehring, 2010).

Clinical therapy focuses on helping the child develop to his or her maximum level of independence. Referrals are made for physical, occupational, and speech therapy, as well as special education to improve motor function and ability. Braces and splints, serial casting, and positioning devices (prone wedges, standers, and sidelyers) are used to promote range of motion, skeletal alignment, stability, and control of involuntary movements, and to prevent contractures. Physical therapy and occupational therapy promote optimal independent functioning.

Surgical interventions may be required to improve function by balancing muscle power and stabilizing uncontrollable joints (e.g., an Achilles tendon lengthening to increase the ankle range of motion or releasing the hamstrings to correct knee flexion contractures). A dorsal rhizotomy may be performed for spastic diplegia to cut the afferent fibers that contribute to spasticity; however, some muscle weakness may result from the procedure (Pelligrino, 2007).

Medications are given to control seizures, to control spasms (skeletal muscle relaxants, baclofen, and benzodiazepines), and to minimize gastrointestinal side effects (cimetidine or ranitidine). Benzodiazepines affect brain control of muscle tone to help control spasticity. Dantrolene is a calcium channel blocker that inhibits muscle contraction. Baclofen is administered orally or by intrathecal pump to decrease spasticity (Figure 27–17 ➤). Botulinum toxin injection into specific muscles is a relatively new therapy used to help control spasticity.

The prognosis for infants and children with cerebral palsy depends on the level of physical involvement and on the presence of cognitive, visual, or hearing deficits. Early intervention

programs can significantly improve performance. Many children with hemiplegia or ataxia show some improvement with maturation and are able to ambulate. Others need assistance with mobility and activities of daily living.

NURSING MANAGEMENT

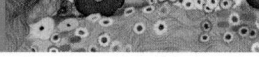

Nursing Assessment and Diagnosis

Be alert for children whose histories indicate an increased risk for CP. Assess all children at each health care visit for developmental delays. Note any orthopedic, visual, auditory, or intellectual deficits. Assess for newborn reflexes (see Chapter 5 ∞), which may persist beyond the normal age in a child with CP, such as a persistent tonic neck reflex beyond age 6 months. Iden-

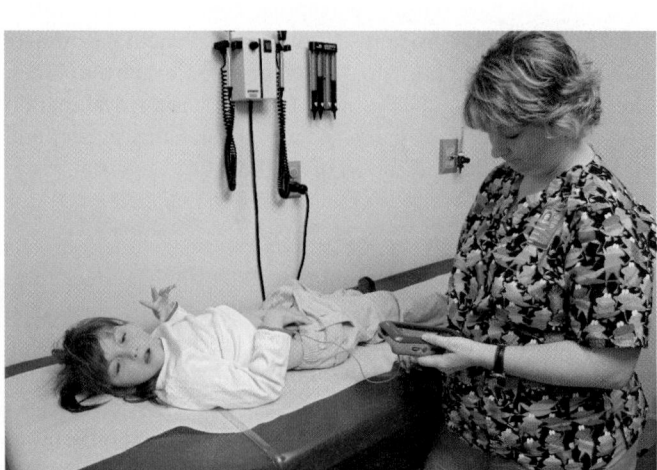

FIGURE 27–17 ➤ Child having a baclofen pump filled.

tify infants that appear to have an abnormal muscle tone or abnormal posture (e.g., head lag beyond age 6 months, arched back, poor trunk control and balance, toe or heel walking) (Jones et al., 2007a). Asymmetric or abnormal crawling by using two or three extremities or hand dominance prior to age 18 months indicates a motor problem. A simple screening test involves placing a clean cloth on the infant's face. Infants normally use two hands to remove it, but the infant at risk for CP uses one hand or does not remove the cloth. Record dietary intake as well as height and weight percentiles for children who are suspected to have or are diagnosed with the condition.

Nursing diagnoses for the child with CP vary, depending on the type of CP, the child's symptoms and age, and the family situation. The accompanying Nursing Care Plan includes several diagnoses that might be appropriate. Additional nursing diagnoses might include:

- Risk for Constipation related to low intake of fiber and fluids and insufficient physical activity
- Impaired Tissue Integrity related to decreased physical mobility and limited self-care ability
- Impaired Verbal Communication related to hearing and/or speech impairment
- Impaired Home Maintenance related to child's developmental disability and inadequate support system
- Chronic Pain related to spasticity and stretching exercises to prevent contractures
- Delayed Growth and Development related to lack of muscle strength or limited social interaction

Planning and Implementation

The accompanying Nursing Care Plan summarizes care for the child with CP. Since the condition varies in severity and manifestations, interventions need to be adapted to the child and family. Nursing care focuses on providing adequate nutrition, maintaining skin integrity, promoting physical mobility, promoting safety, promoting growth and development, teaching parents how to care for the child, and providing emotional support.

Provide Adequate Nutrition

Children with CP require high-calorie diets or supplements to the diet because of feeding difficulties associated with spasticity. Many children have difficulty chewing and swallowing. Give the child small amounts of soft foods at a time. Utensils with large, padded handles may be easier for the child to use. Make sure the child gets sufficient fluids as the child may not be able to communicate thirst. Children with severe CP may need a gastrostomy tube to obtain adequate nutrition. Adequate fiber is needed to prevent constipation, and some children need a bowel management program to treat chronic constipation.

Maintain Skin Integrity

Take special care to protect the bony prominences from skin breakdown. Monitor the skin under splints and braces for redness. If the skin is red, the braces or splints should be removed and not worn until the redness is gone. (See Families Want to Know: Safety for the Child with Spina Bifida on page 879.)

Proper body alignment should be maintained at all times. Support the child with pillows, towels, and bolsters whether the child is in bed or in a chair. Support the head and body of a floppy infant. A child with spasticity may have scissored, extended legs, and a child with athetoid movements may be difficult to carry and transport. Assist the family to find a car safety seat adapted for the child's needs.

Promote Physical Mobility

Range of motion exercises are essential to maintain joint flexibility and to prevent contractures. Consult with the physical

---

Complementary Therapy
Hippotherapy

The child with CP may benefit from massage therapy or hippotherapy (horse riding). Riding a horse benefits the child's body posture and promotes balance and muscle functioning (Jones, Morgan, & Shelton, 2007b).

NURSING CARE PLAN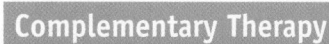
The Child with Cerebral Palsy

INTERVENTION	RATIONALE	EXPECTED OUTCOME
1. Nursing Diagnosis: Impaired Physical Mobility related to decreased muscle strength and control		
NIC Priority Intervention: *Exercise therapy, joint mobility:* Use of active and passive body movement to maintain joint flexibility		**NOC Suggested Outcome:** *Joint movement—active:* Range of motion of joints with self-initiated movement
Goal: The child will attain maximum physical abilities possible.		
▪ Perform developmental assessment and record age when milestones are achieved (e.g., reaching for objects, sitting).	▪ Delayed developmental milestones are common with CP. As one milestone is achieved, interventions are revised to focus on the next skill.	The child reaches maximum physical mobility and all developmental milestones.

(continued)

NURSING CARE PLAN

The Child with Cerebral Palsy (continued)

INTERVENTION	RATIONALE	EXPECTED OUTCOME
■ Plan activities to use gross and fine motor skills (e.g., holding eating utensils, toys positioned to encourage reaching). Allow time for the child to complete activities.	■ Many activities of daily living and play activities promote physical development. The child may perform tasks more slowly than most children.	
■ Perform range of motion exercises every 4 hours for the child unable to move body parts. Position the child to promote tendon stretching (e.g., foot plantar flexion, legs extended at the knees and hips).	■ Exercises and positioning promote mobility and increased circulation, and decrease the risk of contractures.	
■ Arrange for and encourage parents to keep appointments with a rehabilitation therapist.	■ A regularly reevaluated and revised rehabilitation program helps to promote development.	
■ Teach the family to maintain appropriate brace wear.	■ Adaptive devices are often necessary to maximize physical mobility.	

2. Nursing Diagnosis: Disturbed Sensory Perception (Visual or Auditory) related to cerebral damage

NIC Priority Intervention: *Communication enhancement: Visual deficit:* Assistance with accepting or learning alternative methods for living with diminished vision		**NOC Suggested Outcome:** *Sensory function: Vision:* Extent to which visual images are sensed, with and without assistive devices

Goal: The child will receive and benefit from varied forms of sensory and perceptual input.

■ Encourage regular vision examinations. Promote the use of glasses or contact lenses when needed.	■ Corrective lenses enhance sensory input. Regular vision assessment may identify lens prescription changes.	The child receives adequate visual sensory/perceptual input to foster developmental progress.

3. Nursing Diagnosis: Imbalanced Nutrition: Less than Body Requirements related to difficulty in chewing and swallowing and high metabolic needs

NIC Priority Intervention: *Nutrition management:* Assistance with or provision of a balanced dietary intake of foods and fluids		**NOC Suggested Outcome:** *Nutritional status: Nutrient intake:* Adequacy of nutrients taken into body

Goal: The child will receive nutrients needed for normal growth.

■ Monitor height and weight and plot on a growth grid. Perform hydration status assessment.	■ Insufficient intake can lead to impaired growth and dehydration.	The child shows normal growth patterns for height, weight, and other physical parameters.
■ Teach the family techniques to promote caloric and nutrient intake and to prevent aspiration: • *Position the child upright for feedings.* • *Place foods far back in the mouth to overcome tongue thrust.* • *Use soft and blended foods. Allow extra time for chewing and swallowing.* • *Obtain adaptive handles for utensils and encourage self-feeding skills.*	■ Aspiration pneumonia is a risk for the child with poor swallowing. ■ Special techniques can facilitate food intake. Adaptive handles may help the child better manage feeding self.	
■ Teach care of a gastrostomy tube and tube-feeding technique as appropriate.	■ Tube-feeding may be needed for the child to get adequate intake.	

NURSING CARE PLAN

The Child with Cerebral Palsy (continued)

INTERVENTION	RATIONALE	EXPECTED OUTCOME
4. Nursing Diagnosis: Ineffective Therapeutic Regimen Management (Family) related to excessive demands made on family with child's complex care needs		
NIC Priority Intervention: *Family mobilization:* Utilization of family strengths to influence patient's health in a positive direction		**NOC Suggested Outcome:** *Family functioning:* Ability of the family to meet the needs of its members through developmental transitions
Goal: The family will adapt to growth and development needs of the child with CP.		
■ Allow chances for parents to verbalize the impact of CP on the family. Provide referral to other parents and support groups.	■ The family needs to explore the emotional and social impact of the child's care so they can integrate and grow from the experience.	The child demonstrates appropriate growth and developmental progress. The family successfully supports all of its members.
■ Explore community services for rehabilitation, respite care, childcare, and early intervention programs. Refer family as appropriate.	■ Diverse services are available and will be needed due to the multiple impacts of CP on the child.	
■ During visits, review the child's achievements and praise the family for care provided.	■ The child's achievements are positive reinforcement of the family's efforts.	
■ Teach the family skills needed to manage the child's care (e.g., medication administration, muscle stretching, seizure management).	■ Complex skills must be learned before they can be performed efficiently.	
■ Teach case management techniques.	■ The child requires care by many specialists, and many parents become case managers to coordinate care.	
■ Involve siblings in the care for the child with CP. Review with parents the needs of all children in the family.	■ Siblings of the child with CP may feel left out because of the care provided. Special efforts help to meet the developmental needs of all family members.	
5. Nursing Diagnosis: Deficient Diversional Activity (Child) related to poor social skills		
NIC Priority Intervention: *Recreation therapy:* Purposeful use of recreation to promote relaxation and enhancement of social skills		**NOC Suggested Outcome:** *Play participation:* Use of activities as needed for enjoyment, entertainment, and development by children
Goal: The child will engage in activities that maximize growth and development.		
■ Refer the family to an early intervention program. Encourage contact with other children.	■ The child needs a variety of activities and contact with other children and adults to maximize development.	The child engages in activities to maximize development.
■ Work with the school to develop an IEP that encourages interaction with peers and a variety of activities that support development.	■ The education system is obligated to work with families to provide methods to enhance learning, including social interactions.	
■ Investigate recreational programs for children with disabilities and share information with the parents.	■ Recreational programs for children with disabilities may provide social experiences and physical activity.	

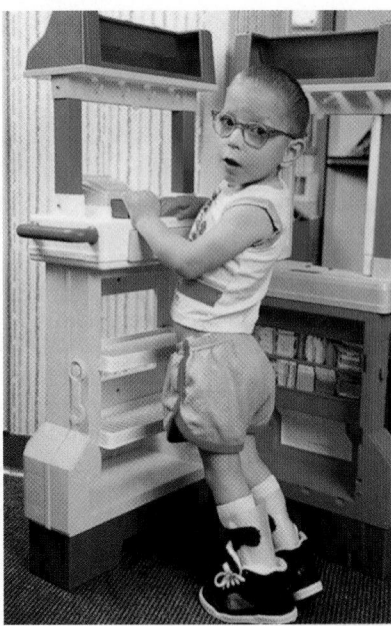

FIGURE 27–18 ➤ A child with cerebral palsy has abnormal muscle tone and lack of physical coordination. Encourage the parents to find ways for the child to interact with the environment to promote development.

therapists who work with the child and help with recommended exercises. Refer parents to the appropriate resources for help getting adaptive devices (Figure 27–18 ➤). Teach parents to position the child to foster flexion rather than extension so that the child can more easily interact with the environment (for example, by bringing objects closer to the face). Encourage parents to bring in the child's *adaptive appliances* (braces, positioning devices) for use during the hospitalization; however, secure them as the family may have difficulty replacing them if lost.

Promote Safety

Safety belts should be used for children in strollers and wheelchairs. Determine if an adaptive car safety seat is needed so the child can be safely transported. A child with chronic seizures should wear a helmet to protect against further injury.

Promote Growth and Development

Remember that as many as 60% of children with CP are physically but not intellectually disabled (Nehring, 2010). Use terminology appropriate for the child's developmental level. Help the child develop a positive self-image to ensure emotional health and social growth. Children with a hearing impairment may need referral to learn American Sign Language or other communication methods. Provide audio and visual activities for the child who is quadriplegic.

Adaptive and assistive technology may be needed to promote mobility and communication. **Assistive technology** is any item, equipment, or product customized for use to promote the functional capabilities and independence of an individual with disabilities. Examples include computers, adaptive utensils, and customized wheelchairs.

Foster Parental Knowledge

Teach parents about the disorder and arrange sessions to teach them about all of the child's special needs. Teach administration, desired effects, and side effects of medications prescribed for seizures. Make sure parents are aware of the need for dental care for children because of the enamel defects and malocclusion that commonly occur in children with CP, and the gum hyperplasia that occurs with some anticonvulsants.

Provide Emotional Support

Refer parents to individual and family counseling, if appropriate. Listen to the parents' concerns and encourage them to express their feelings and ask questions. Explain what they can expect from future treatment. Work with other health care professionals to help families adjust to this chronic disease.

Care in the Community

Children with CP need continuous support in the community. A case manager such as the parent or nurse is often needed to coordinate care. Parents may need financial assistance to provide for the child's needs and to obtain appliances such as braces, wheelchairs, or adaptive utensils. Children need new adaptive devices, ongoing developmental assessment and care planning, and possibly surgery as they grow. Although the brain lesion does not change, it manifests differently as the child grows. For example, once the child begins to walk, the extensor tone may cause Achilles cord tightening. Braces may decrease deformities, but surgery may eventually be needed. Technology offers many new strategies to promote communication and self-care.

Monitor the child's growth. When the child is unable to ambulate, use a scale that accommodates a wheelchair when weighing. Height measurements may be inaccurate and tools to assess ulnar length may be more accurate for a height measurement (Jones et al., 2007b). Schedule regular vision and hearing screening during health promotion visits, and give immunizations according to the recommended schedule. Educate parents about the possible risk for a seizure associated with the vaccines.

Early intervention programs can help parents learn to meet their child's special needs, including physical, occupational, and speech therapy, as well as educational needs. The child often needs an IEP to maximize learning potential (see Chapter 12 ∞). The nurse can help parents meet the needs of the child with CP in preschools, schools, offices, clinics, and other settings. In addition, the nurse makes referrals as appropriate to support groups, as well as organizations such as the United Cerebral Palsy Association and Shriners Hospitals. Recreational activities may be identified through the local United Cerebral Palsy chapter.

An individualized transition plan developed during adolescence assists the family and adolescent with CP to develop plans for adult living. Vocational training options can be explored. See Chapter 12 ∞.

Evaluation

Expected outcomes of nursing care for the child with CP are provided in the Nursing Care Plan.

INJURIES OF THE NEUROLOGIC SYSTEM

Traumatic Brain Injury

A traumatic brain injury (TBI) can be defined as any trauma to the head that causes a change in level of consciousness or an anatomic abnormality of the brain. Traumatic brain injury is the leading cause of death and disability among children. On an annual basis in children under 15 years, there are 435,000 emergency department visits, 37,000 hospitalizations, and 2,685 deaths (Centers for Disease Control and Prevention, 2008). Up to 90% of deaths of injured children are associated with TBI (Atabaki, 2007). Inflicted TBI occurs at an estimated rate of 25 to 31 cases per 100,000 infants under age 1 year (Barr, Rivera, Barr, et al., 2009).

Etiology and Pathophysiology

TBI may be caused by blunt (e.g., head struck by an object, shaking) or penetrating (e.g., bullet) mechanisms. Infants have thinner and more pliable skulls, putting them at even greater risk for skull fractures and intracranial injury (Atabaki, 2007). Children under age 2 years have a higher risk for intracranial injury after TBI.

The injury impact transfers energy through the skull and meninges to the brain. The primary injury occurs on impact, when the initial cellular damage takes place. The injury may result from a direct blow to the head (coup injury) or from movement of the brain within the skull (contrecoup injury), such as from shaken baby syndrome (Figure 27–19 ➤). At the time of impact, scalp injuries, skull fractures, contusions, and hematomas of brain tissue may occur.

Growth & Development — *Brain Injury Causes by Age Group*

Mechanisms of injury are related to developmental stages and exposures, such as the following (Keenan & Bratton, 2006):

- Infants—shaken baby syndrome, child abuse, falls, and motor vehicle crashes. See Chapter 17 ∞ for more details on child abuse.
- Toddlers and preschoolers—falls down stairs, out a window, or from climbing; motor vehicle–related injuries as passengers or pedestrians.
- School-age children—motor vehicle crashes, either as passengers or pedestrians; bicycle crashes; and inline skating, scooter, or skateboard mishaps.
- Adolescents—motor vehicle crashes (often alcohol or drugs are involved), struck by an object, sports-related injuries, and firearm injuries.

The secondary injury is the biochemical and cellular response to the primary injury. Impaired cerebral blood flow can lead to ischemia and brain damage. Brain cells are further damaged by the release of amino acids and an inflammatory response that increases the permeability of the blood-brain barrier. Cerebral edema results in increased ICP. The brain injury is further compounded by decreased cerebral perfusion pressure, limiting the blood flow that delivers oxygen and nutrients and removes accumulated toxins from cell death.

Coup/Contrecoup Injury Animation

Pathophysiology Illustrated
Brain Injury

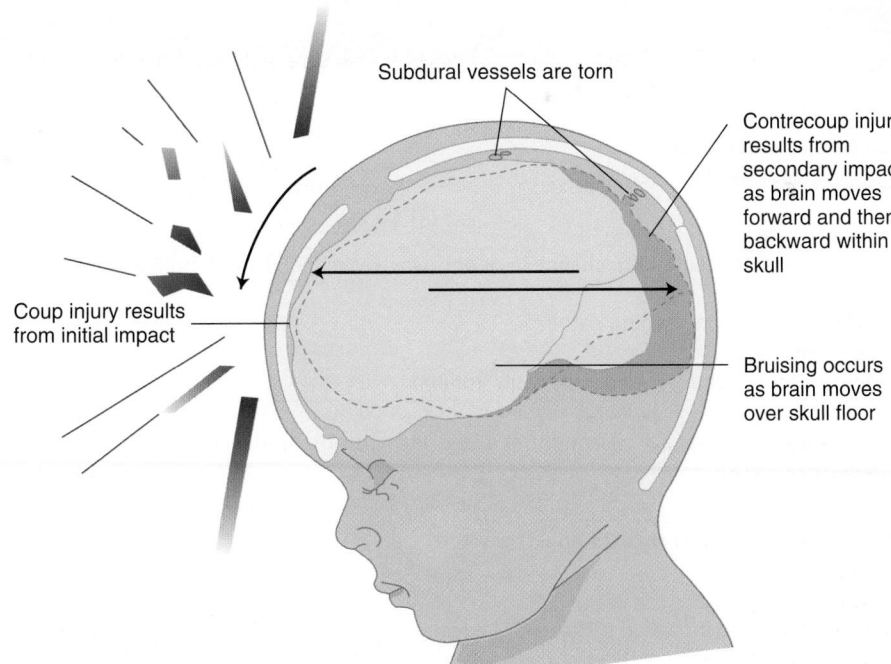

Subdural vessels are torn

Contrecoup injury results from secondary impact as brain moves forward and then backward within skull

Coup injury results from initial impact

Bruising occurs as brain moves over skull floor

FIGURE 27–19 ➤ Brain injury can result from a direct blow to the head (coup injury) or the acceleration-deceleration movement of the brain (contrecoup injury). The inertial forces resulting when the head and skull stop moving allow the brain tissue to continue moving within the skull. This results in tearing of nerves, fibers, and blood vessels.

Clinical Manifestations

The signs and symptoms of brain injuries in children depend on the pathologic features and severity of the injury. The child with a mild brain injury may remain conscious or have brief loss of consciousness (seconds to a few minutes). The child with a moderate brain injury loses consciousness for 5 to 10 minutes. A child with a severe brain injury is usually unconscious for more than 10 minutes and may rapidly show signs of increased ICP. See the Clinical Manifestations table below.

Unconsciousness may result from increased ICP, cerebral edema, intracranial hematomas, hemorrhage, or parenchymal damage to both cerebral cortices or the brainstem. See Clinical Manifestations: Intracranial Hematomas on the next page. Post-traumatic seizures are common.

Nursing Alert

Shaken baby syndrome or shaken impact syndrome should be suspected in any infant who arrives in the emergency department with seizures, failure to thrive, respiratory irregularities, or coma. The infant has a large head and relatively weak neck muscles. A frustrated adult can shake an infant and cause coup and contrecoup injuries that tear nerve fibers as the brain moves back and forth in the skull. Lethargy, vomiting, and increasing irritability may be additional presenting signs. Infants with TBI associated with shaken baby syndrome are more likely to have clinical findings of retinal hemorrhages, subdural hematomas, posterior rib fractures, and metaphyseal fractures (Salehi-Had, Brandt, Rosas, et al., 2006).

Vital signs are important indicators of brain injury. Changes in respiratory effort or periods of apnea can occur secondary to shock, injury to the spinal cord above C4, or damage to or pressure on the medulla. Heart rate and blood pressure are indices of brainstem function. Tachycardia can be a sign of blood loss, shock, hypoxia, anxiety, or pain. Cushing triad is associated with significantly increased ICP, and impending herniation or compromised blood flow to the brainstem. It is characterized by hypertension, increased systolic pressure with wide pulse pressure, bradycardia, and irregular respirations. Refer to page 852 for more information about altered states of consciousness and increased ICP.

Reflexes may be hyporesponsive, hyperresponsive, or nonexistent. The child may assume a flexor, extensor, or flaccid posture (see Figure 27–20 ➤).

COLLABORATIVE CARE

Diagnostic Tests

Identifying the severity of a brain injury involves history, observation, neurologic examination, and diagnostic testing. Obtain information about how the injury occurred, the child's initial responses and current responses, any loss of consciousness or confused behavior, and the child's memory of the event. For example, if the injury resulted from a fall, what was the distance fallen, what surface did the head strike, and where on the head was the primary impact? Did the child have a seizure or vomit?

Laboratory tests include a complete blood cell count, blood chemistry, toxicology screening, and urinalysis. Radiographs detect fractures of the skull and cervical vertebrae. A CT scan detects fractures, intracranial hemorrhage, swelling, and diffuse axonal injury (tearing of nerve fibers throughout the brain). An MRI scan is used during recovery to determine the extent of brain damage. PET scans measure the blood flow in the brain. A fracture indicates a more serious injury. Many children with brain injuries have multiple other injuries. Even though cervical spine injuries are rare, children with a moderate or severe brain

Clinical Manifestations

Traumatic Brain Injury by Severity

Type of Brain Injury	Clinical Manifestations
Concussion or mild brain injury	Low-grade headache that won't go away Slowness in thinking, acting, speaking, reading Memory problems Loss of balance, unsteady walking Difficulty paying attention or concentrating, change in performance at school, lack of motivation or interest in favorite toys Feeling tired all the time, change in sleeping pattern Change in eating patterns Increased sensitivity to lights, sounds, distractions; easily irritated
Moderate brain injury	Glasgow Coma Scale score of 9 to 12 Posttraumatic amnesia for 1 to 24 hours Loss of consciousness
Severe brain injury	Glasgow Coma Scale score of 8 or less Amnesia after the event lasting longer than 24 hours Coma Increased intracranial pressure Unconsciousness may result from increased ICP, cerebral edema, intracranial hematomas, hemorrhage, or parenchymal damage to both cerebral cortices or the brainstem. See Clinical Manifestations: Intracranial Hematomas. Posttraumatic seizures are common.

Clinical Manifestations
Intracranial Hematomas

Type of Hematoma	Clinical Manifestations
Subdural Hematoma Results from severe brain trauma, including shaken child syndrome More common in infants less than age 1 year Inertial forces cause laceration of the bridging veins; a venous hematoma forms beneath the dura and presses directly on the brain	▪ Symptoms may occur 48–72 hours after the injury ▪ Change in level of consciousness (confusion, agitation, or lethargy) ▪ Nausea or vomiting ▪ Headache ▪ Retinal hemorrhages in both eyes ▪ Pupil on side of injury may be fixed and dilated ▪ Seizures
Epidural Hematoma Rare in children, especially those less than 4 years of age Results from blunt trauma (most often falls), assaults, or baseball to temporal area; may have linear skull fracture Arterial or venous bleeding occurs between the skull and the dura	▪ Minimal or absent symptoms from initial impact ▪ Delayed onset followed by rapid deterioration in mental status and signs of increased ICP ▪ Headache or full fontanel ▪ Paresis of cranial nerves III and VI ▪ Papilledema ▪ Fixed and dilated pupil
Intracerebral Hematoma Result of deep contusion or intracerebral laceration (secondary to foreign body, bony penetration, or impalement) Causes diffuse bleeding in parenchyma; there may be a hematoma with associated small areas of bleeding	▪ Symptoms depend upon the size and location of the hematoma; may change if size increases due to uncontrolled bleeding ▪ Altered consciousness

injury should have a potential cervical spine injury ruled out by radiologic imaging.

Clinical Therapy

The initial management of a child with moderate to severe TBI is based on the child's physiologic status (see page 894 for mild TBI or concussion). The airway must be clear and stable. Hypoxia and hypercapnia can cause vasodilation and increased ICP and must be prevented. If indicated, the child is intubated. Mechanical ventilation with supplemental oxygen at the child's normal respiratory rate is often used for the first 24 hours after injury to maintain the oxygenation level. (See the *Clinical Skills*

Manual.) Sedation and paralytic agents may be used to reduce the child's resistance to mechanical ventilation and to lower the ICP (Mansfield, 2007).

Nursing Alert

In the child with moderate head injury, the oxygen saturation should be maintained at higher than 95% to prevent vasodilation and increased ICP. For the severely injured child who is intubated, monitor arterial blood gas results. The PaO_2 of 70–100 mmHg indicates satisfactory management of oxygenation.

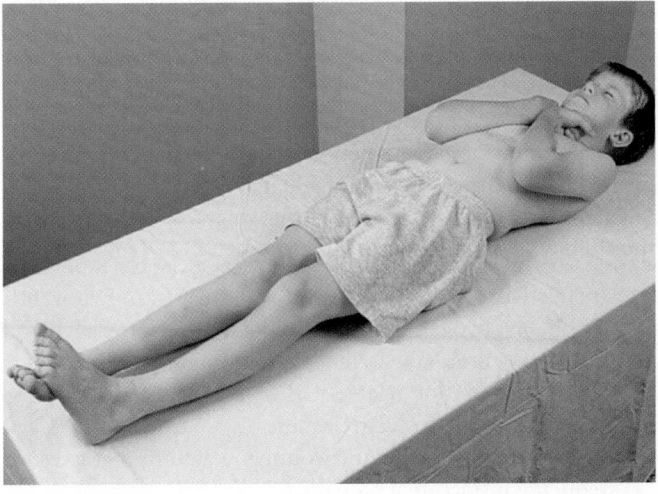

A

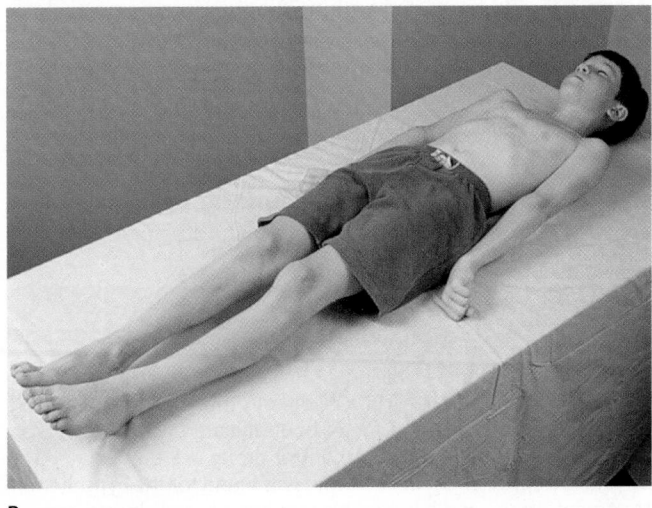

B

FIGURE 27–20 ➤ A, Flexor (decorticate) posturing, characterized by rigid flexion, is associated with lesions above the brainstem in the corticospinal tracts. B, Extensor (decerebrate) posturing, distinguished by rigid extension, is associated with lesions of the brainstem.

Shock is treated aggressively with fluid boluses. Maintaining the child's blood pressure within the normal range helps keep the brain adequately perfused. This ensures that the brain gets adequate oxygen and nutrients and that the accumulated neurotoxins are removed. If shock is present, fluid administration is focused on maintaining the blood pressure. Only after the child is hemodynamically stable will fluids be restricted, if necessary.

If increased ICP is present, cerebral perfusion is reduced and ischemia occurs. If it is not relieved, brain contents begin shifting in the cranium, potentially leading to herniation. Invasive ICP monitoring (catheter into the ventricle or a bolt into the subarachnoid space) may be initiated in the child with severe TBI, especially if the child is sedated. The goal is to maintain the ICP at 15 to 20 mmHg (Saiki, 2009). Mannitol or a hypertonic saline (3–23.4%) is often used for control of increased ICP (Rangel-Castillo, Gopinath, & Robertson, 2008). Pain and sedation management promote comfort and help control the ICP. Corticosteroids are not recommended for reducing ICP. The environment is kept as quiet as possible.

Invasive procedures may be necessary to reduce increased ICP, such as burr holes or surgery to remove an intracranial hematoma. A ventricular catheter may be placed to drain CSF and to monitor pressure. The child may be placed in a chemically induced coma to reduce brain activity during this acute care phase. In some cases, the intracranial pressure cannot be controlled and death occurs. See Chapter 13 ∞ for brain death criteria.

Intracranial hematomas are space-occupying lesions that expand rapidly or slowly, depending on whether they are arterial or venous in origin. They must be located quickly. Some lesions require rapid surgical evacuation to minimize the secondary effects of the injury.

If the child has no cervical spine injury, the head of the bed is elevated up to 30 degrees. The child's head is kept in the midline to promote venous (jugular) drainage from the brain. Hip flexion is avoided. A urinary catheter is inserted to monitor output, and electrolytes should be checked frequently. Enteral nutrition support should be started within 72 hours using a postpyloric feeding tube to reduce the risk for aspiration.

Aggressive support continues until the child regains consciousness and rehabilitation can be initiated, or until the child dies. Physical therapists, occupational therapists, and speech therapists are members of the rehabilitation team. Moderate and severe TBI may result in a permanent disability, such as epilepsy, motor and cognitive impairments, learning problems,

Research — *Hypothermia*

A random control trial involving 225 children studied the use of hypothermia to treat severe TBI. Children in the experimental group had hypothermia of 32.5°C for 24 hours initiated within 8 hours after injury, and children in the control group were maintained at 37°C. No improvement in outcomes was found for the hypothermia treatment group, and it is possible that hypothermia increases mortality (Hutchinson, Ward, Lacroix, et al., 2008).

hearing and vision impairment, communication problems, and behavioral or emotional problems. Difficulties with learning skills are common, such as with short-term memory, attention span, goal setting, problem solving, and sequencing multistep actions (Catroppa & Anderson, 2009).

Clinical Tip

Beliefs that young age and brain development are protective or that brain plasticity allows better recovery after brain injury are changing as research findings emerge. Studies of children with severe TBI are identifying that the immature brain is more vulnerable to diffuse injury. Skills that are not well established are more likely to be disrupted than well-established skills. Functional recovery may be restricted to the younger child's fewer existing skills (Kirkwood, Yeates, & Wilson, 2006).

NURSING MANAGEMENT

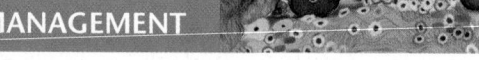

Nursing Assessment and Diagnosis

Assess the child's neurologic status frequently using the guidelines on page 851, and compare the child's status to baseline findings, noting improvement, stability, or deterioration. Evaluate the child's level of consciousness using the Glasgow Coma Scale (see Table 27–5). When the child has a decreased level of consciousness shortly after a brain injury, consider if a posttraumatic seizure occurred and if the child is still in the postictal state. Assess the cranial nerves (Table 5–16 and Table 27–6), and pupils for size and reactivity. Monitor vital signs closely. Note any abnormal posturing.

If a ventricular catheter or bolt is inserted, monitor the actual pressure readings. Changes in these signs may indicate hypoxia, decreased perfusion, shock, or increased ICP. The cause of any deterioration must be quickly determined and appropriate interventions taken.

Observe for physiologic and behavioral signs of pain. Assume that the child with increased ICP is in pain, even when unresponsive. (See Chapter 15 ∞.)

In the child who is moderately injured, observe breathing patterns and check color and level of consciousness. Check the pulse oximeter; the oxygen saturation should remain over 95%. Report any sign of decreased oxygenation or signs and symptoms of increased ICP to the physician immediately (see Table 27–4).

Examples of nursing diagnoses that might be appropriate for the child with TBI include:

- Ineffective Cerebral Tissue Perfusion related to hypoventilation, hypovolemia, and/or reduction of arterial blood flow to the brain due to increased intracranial pressure
- Risk for Aspiration related to decreased level of consciousness and loss of protective reflexes
- Risk for Imbalanced Fluid Volume related to therapies for reducing intracranial pressure
- Compromised Family Coping related to life-threatening injury to child

Planning and Implementation

Hospital-Based Care

The child with a severe TBI is initially cared for in the pediatric intensive care unit. Nursing care focuses on maintaining cerebral perfusion and minimizing increases in ICP, preventing complications, and providing emotional support.

Maintain cardiopulmonary function. Some children need mechanical ventilation to protect the airway and maintain oxygenation. Keep suction equipment at the bedside in case aspiration occurs. Avoid suctioning unless essential for airway maintenance because it increases ICP.

Reduce physiologic stresses on the body that could increase ICP. The nurse should minimize unpleasant stimuli when possible, keep the environment quiet, and avoid jarring the bed. Pain management and temperature control are important. Position the child to avoid excessive flexion of the hips and neck that could slow venous circulation. Monitor the effect of nursing procedures on the level of ICP and determine if the child responds better when procedures are clustered rather than spread over time. Encourage parents to talk to the child and provide comforting touch.

Clinical Tip

For each degree of Centigrade temperature increase, the metabolic rate increases by 10–13%. In addition, fever causes vasodilation of cerebral blood vessels and may increase ICP. Temperature management is essential for a better neurologic outcome (Rangel-Castillo et al., 2008).

Administer medications as ordered. Diuretics may be prescribed to remove excess fluid from the body and the brain if the cerebral perfusion pressure is adequate. Sedatives may be given to decrease the metabolic demands on the brain. Pain medication is provided to promote comfort.

Provide oral care to keep mucous membranes moist and intact, but use care when the gag reflex is absent. Pad and cushion bony prominences, provide skin care, and change the child's position frequently. The eyes should be protected from corneal irritation with ophthalmic ointment and patching. Enteral feeding may be used initially, slowly progressing to oral foods as tolerated. Fluids are given to meet daily fluid requirements. Stool softeners and suppositories should be used as needed to prevent constipation. The side rails of the bed should be padded to protect the child if a seizure occurs.

Promote recovery and prevent physical deformities. Perform passive range of motion exercises to prevent contractures. Splints may be used to maintain joints in functional positions. Work with physical, occupational, and speech therapists to assist with exercises and help teach parents the techniques so they can work with the child in the hospital and at home.

After the child survives the critical injury and is moved to a pediatric care unit, begin promoting general awareness when the child is ready using toys, books, music, or games based on the child's age and ability. Encourage parents to bring in favorite toys, stuffed animals, and recordings of the child's favorite music or of family members talking. Assist the family to provide stimulation but to also provide quiet when the child displays agitation.

Provide emotional support to the family in collaboration with the social workers, physicians, psychologists, rehabilitation therapists, and members of the clergy. All providers caring for the child can help the family adapt to having a child with a new disability.

Sometimes, despite all efforts, the child dies due to the consequences of the brain injury. Provide support for the family while brain death testing is performed. See Chapter 13 ∞ for information to support the family when termination of life support and organ donation are discussed.

Discharge Planning and Home Care Teaching

Children with severe TBI may be transferred to an inpatient rehabilitation unit. Other children may have outpatient rehabilitation prescribed; thus, home care needs should be identified and addressed well in advance of discharge. For children with disabilities, determine what adaptations and assistive technology are needed in the home, such as a wheelchair, walker, braces, or special bed. A case manager is often identified to coordinate services and resources during rehabilitation. Social services intervention may be needed when brain injury results from child abuse or shaken baby syndrome.

Give parents information about home care for children with moderate or severe TBI and possible behaviors to expect from the child. See the next page for parent education for the child with a mild TBI or concussion.

Care in the Community

Home care nursing may be important for the child with an acquired neurologic dysfunction and prolonged altered consciousness. The home care nurse can take over the case management for the child who is disabled and make sure the environment is safe. The nurse can teach the family to meet the child's needs, monitor the intake of fluids and foods, as well as position the child and perform range of motion exercises to reduce contractures. Regular follow-up visits are needed to assess the child's recovery and to modify the treatment plan.

Even though the child looks normal within days of a mild or moderate brain injury, parents and teachers need to be aware that brain healing takes up to 6 weeks. Typical behavior during this healing period may include any of the following behaviors: tiring easily, memory loss or forgetfulness, easy distractibility, difficulty concentrating, difficulty following directions, irritability or short temper, and needing help starting and finishing tasks. The child should not be returned to a full school schedule too quickly to prevent fatigue and frustration. Neuropsychiatric and educational assessment should be initiated if recovery is

Law & Ethics   *Disability Benefits for TBI*

A child with a TBI that results in severe functional limitations expected to last for a continuous 12-month period or longer may qualify for Social Security Supplemental Security Income (SSI) benefits.

Brain Injury Resources

prolonged. Education accommodations are often different from those needed by children with other types of learning disabilities. An IEP is often needed. See Chapter 12 ∞.

Strategies to assist the child with a mild brain injury to return to school over the first few weeks include the following (Kirkwood et al., 2006):

- Provide extra assistance to help the child make up missed work.
- Provide rest periods and breaks during the school day.
- Reduce the homework and class workload.
- Reduce the number of tests to no more than one per day, and do not set a time limit for taking the test.
- Seat the child to minimize distractions.

The child or adolescent facing long-term rehabilitation needs support to adjust to the disability and to find the strength to maximize his or her abilities. Identify recreational opportunities for the child with disabilities to promote exercise and self-esteem. The adolescent may need to gain vocational skills and learn to live independently. Refer parents to the Brain Injury Association and other organizations for more information.

Prevention of brain injury is another important role of the nurse. Encourage parents to obtain, and require children to use, protective helmets for bicycling, skateboarding, inline skating, and other sports. Parents should be encouraged to wear a helmet themselves as role models. Encourage parents to monitor playgrounds for appropriate use of wood chips or cushioning tiles to reduce the severity of injuries associated with falls.

Evaluation

Examples of expected outcomes of nursing care for the child with traumatic brain injury include the following:

- Cerebral perfusion pressure is maintained at an adequate rate to sustain brain oxygenation.
- Muscle function is maintained and physical deformities are prevented with range of motion exercises and splinting during the recovery stages of the brain injury.
- Parents are supported through the child's acute recovery phase and learn to provide care the child will need at home.
- The child's school performance is monitored and appropriate educational resources are provided to support the child's learning.

Specific Head Injuries

Scalp Injuries

Injuries to the scalp, which can be caused by falls, blunt trauma, or penetration of a foreign body, are usually benign. Although bleeding may be extensive, hypovolemia or shock is uncommon unless the patient is an infant.

Lacerations should be irrigated with copious amounts of sterile normal saline solution and inspected for bony fragments or depressions, CSF leakage with a dural tear, or debris. If the injury is simple, the laceration can be sutured or stapled, and the child discharged from the emergency department. If not, a neurosurgeon should be consulted.

Concussion (Mild TBI)

A concussion usually results from a direct blow to the head, face, or neck that causes an alteration in mental status (e.g., amnesia, dizziness, memory or orientation impairment, unsteady gait), but not necessarily loss of consciousness (Kirkwood et al., 2006). It is secondary to stretching, compression, or shearing of nerve fibers. The injury is metabolic rather than gross structural damage or focal injury. Concussions are categorized by three levels of severity (Table 27–8).

On assessment, injured athletes may be confused about their assignment, be unsure about the game or score, move clumsily, answer questions slowly, show behavior or personality change, or forget events before or after the injury. Postconcussive symptoms reported by children and injured athletes include headache, nausea, dizziness or balance problems, blurry vision, sensitivity to light or noise, sluggishness, problems with concentration or memory, or fatigue (Lovell, 2009). These symptoms usually disappear within several weeks but may last up to 6 months. Tell parents and teachers to expect the child to have altered behavior, and encourage them to help the child who is aware of differences to maintain self-esteem.

Pediatric concussive syndrome, which is believed to be caused by an injury to the brainstem, is seen in children who are less than 3 years old. The child seems stunned at the time of injury, but does not lose consciousness. Later, however, the child becomes pale, clammy, and lethargic, and may vomit. These children may be placed in a short-stay unit for observation and usually recover within 24 hours. Postconcussive cognitive deficits do not become apparent until at least 24 hours after injury (Adirim, 2007).

No standard practice exists for evaluation of children with mild TBI or concussion (Adirim, 2007). Brain imaging studies may not be ordered unless signs of severe injury are present. Treatment is supportive. Children are observed in the emergency department for several hours before being sent home with parents instructed to watch them closely for decreased responsiveness. Any child who is unconscious for more than 5 minutes or has amnesia of the event may be admitted to the hospital to rule out other injury. Neuropsychiatric testing may be required before permitting an athlete to return to play.

Children who have had one brain injury are at greater risk for a subsequent brain injury (Swaine, Tremblay, Platt, et al., 2007). Young athletes suffering a second concussion before complete recovery from the first may develop *second impact syndrome*. This syndrome results in acute brain swelling, neurologic or cognitive deficits, and sometimes death from the cumulative ef-

TABLE 27–8	Levels of Concussion Severity
Grade 1	Transient confusion, no loss of consciousness, no posttraumatic amnesia, and duration of mental status abnormalities of less than 15 minutes
Grade 2	Transient confusion with posttraumatic amnesia, no loss of consciousness, and duration of mental status abnormalities of 15 minutes or longer
Grade 3	Any loss of consciousness, seconds or minutes

Data from Adirim, T. A. (2007). Concussions in sports and recreation. Clinical Pediatric Emergency Medicine, 8, 2–6.

fect of these concussions. Recommendations should be followed for the management of sports-related concussions to reduce the risk of disability and death. Removal from sports participation ranges from 7 days to the entire season, depending on the severity of concussion and neurologic symptoms. The athlete should be allowed to return to full game play only when symptom-free after a gradual increase in activities (Kirkwood et al., 2006).

Skull Fractures

A fracture to any of the eight cranial bones is caused by a considerable force to the head. Any area of the skull with swelling or a hematoma should be evaluated for possible fracture. Diagnosis is made by visual inspection, palpation, radiologic study, or CT scan. Treatment should always include neurosurgical consultation. Management of skull fractures depends on the type and extent of the injury (Table 27–9).

The child may have focal symptoms depending on the area of injury. Altered LOC ranges from confusion and disorientation to stupor. Treatment involves hospitalization for observation and to rule out other injuries. Surgical treatment may sometimes be necessary. Sequelae are focal and specific to the area of the brain injured.

Penetrating Injuries

Gunshot wounds to the head can damage tissue, bone, and blood vessels. Low-velocity bullets enter and ricochet within the cranial vault, destroying brain tissue and blood vessels. Although the child may be conscious just after the injury, the LOC quickly deteriorates because of the edema surrounding the penetration tract. High-velocity bullets, however, cause immediate, severe damage on impact. CT scans evaluate gunshot trauma and pinpoint the location of bullet and bone fragments as well as parenchymal damage. Surgery is performed to debride the tract, evacuate any hematomas, and remove accessible bone or bullet

particles. Children with gunshot wounds to the head have a high mortality. Those who survive may suffer multiple focal deficits and seizures.

Impalement injuries may occur in children in association with darts, dog bites, or other sharp objects. All objects must be left in place and removed in the operating room by a neurosurgeon. The child with an impalement injury is at high risk for focal injury and infection. After surgery, children with this type of injury are managed as with other postoperative head injuries, with attention focused on LOC, increased ICP, and infection control.

Spinal Cord Injury

The incidence of spinal cord injury in children is estimated to be 2 cases per 100,000 children (Vitale, Goss, Matsumoto, et al., 2006). Children account for about 2–5% of all spinal cord injuries. Most of these injuries occur in the cervical area (Slotkin, Lu, & Wood, 2007). Motor vehicle crashes and falls are the leading cause of spinal cord injuries. Adolescents comprise approximately 50% of the pediatric population with a spinal cord injury, and their injuries usually are associated with recreation and sports, such as football and diving into shallow water (Slotkin et al., 2007).

The mechanism of injury determines the type of lesion that occurs (Figure 27–21 ➤). Hyperflexion injuries (e.g., extreme bending around a lap belt) produce tears or avulsions and fractures of vertebral bodies, as well as subluxation and dislocation. Rotation may cause joint dislocations or unstable spinal fractures. Extension may result in the so-called hangman's fracture, ligament tears, or avulsion fractures of vertebral bodies, as well as central or posterior spinal cord syndrome. Compression fractures may result from a hyperflexion injury or from football injuries, diving, or falls.

TABLE 27–9 Types of Skull Fractures	
Injury	Clinical Therapy
Linear Fracture Results from impact to large area of the skull. Usually no symptoms. May have overlying hematoma or soft-tissue swelling. Most common type of fracture.	If fracture is on temporal bone or crosses sagittal suture line, a CT scan is performed to detect potential epidural hematoma. Consider the possibility of intentional injury. No treatment is commonly needed.
Depressed Fracture Break in skull itself or an area shattered into many fragments. Pieces of bone may be depressed into brain tissue with hematoma forming on top.	Plain radiographic film or CT scan. Surgery to elevate bone fragments when depression is greater than 5 mm. Tetanus prophylaxis is given as needed. Many are associated with intracranial injury and posttraumatic epilepsy.
Compound Fracture Combination of a full-thickness scalp laceration and depressed skull fracture with the bone exposed. It is considered a penetrating fracture if the dura is torn.	Visual diagnosis along with radiographic studies. Surgical debridement, a search for foreign bodies, and copious irrigation are performed. Parenteral antibiotics and tetanus prophylaxis are provided as needed.
Basilar Fracture Fracture at the base of the skull that may involve the frontal, ethmoid, sphenoid, temporal, or occipital bones. A dural tear may be present.	Diagnosis is confirmed by signs of blood behind the tympanic membranes, CSF leakage from the nose or ears, periorbital ecchymosis (raccoon eyes), or bruising of the mastoid (Battle sign). CT imaging locates the fracture site. Antibiotics are prescribed. Surgical repair of the site of the CSF leak is performed if the leak persists after 7 to 10 days. Transient or permanent cranial nerve injuries occur (e.g., hearing loss).

Data from: Dias, M. S. (2004). Traumatic brain and spinal cord injury. Pediatric Clinics of North America, 51, 271–303; Atabaki, S. M. (2007). Pediatric head injury. Pediatrics in Review, 28(6), 215–223.

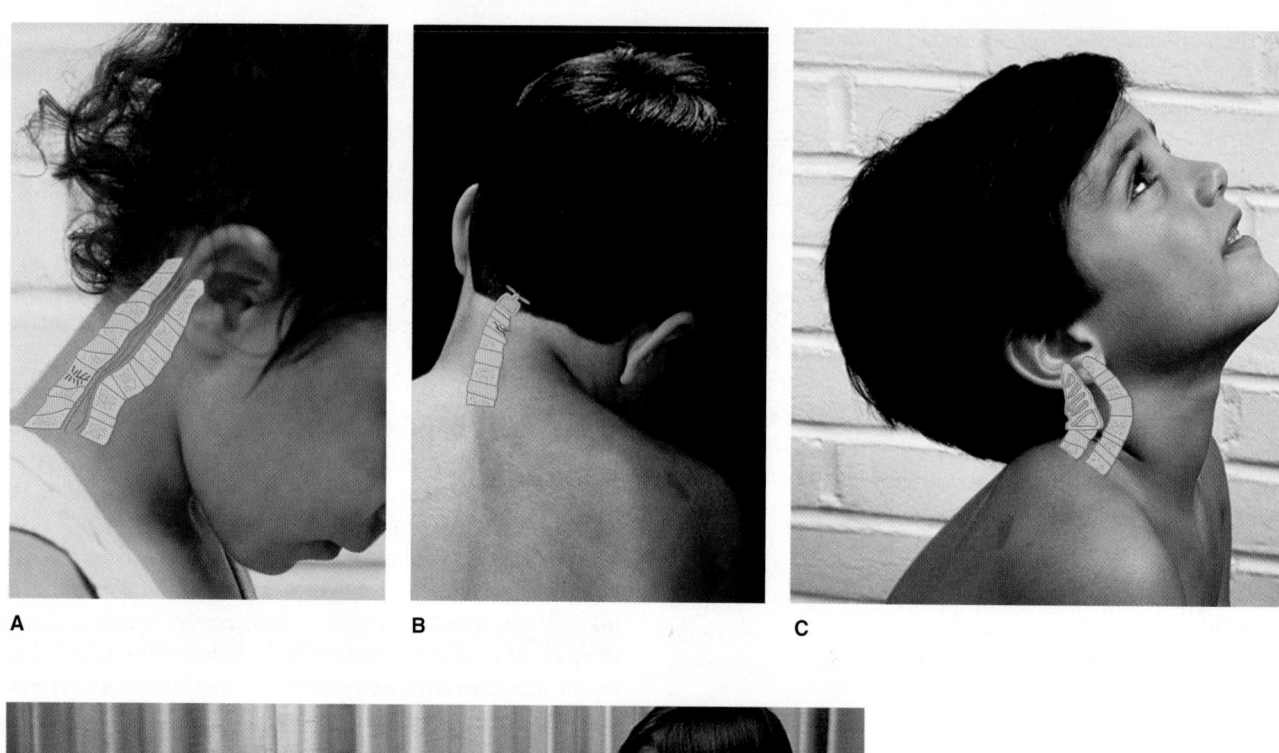

A B C

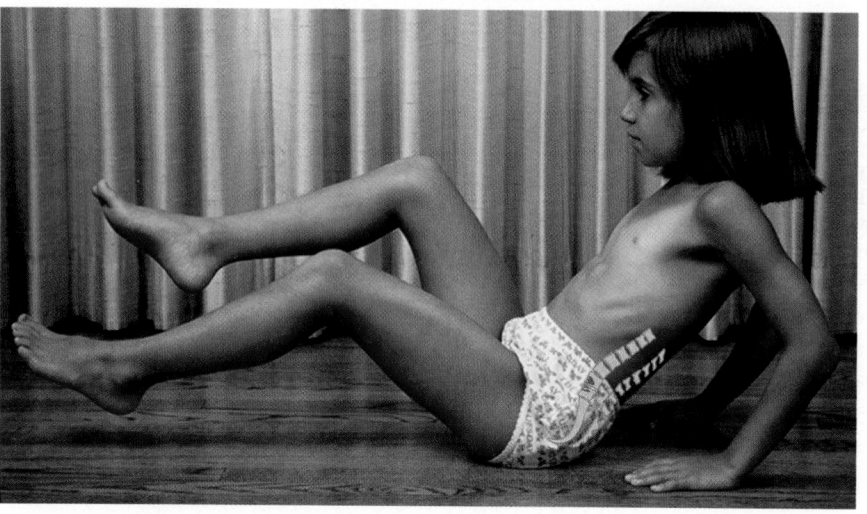

D

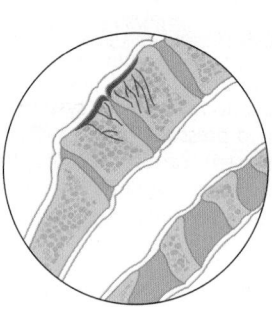

FIGURE 27–21 ➤ Mechanics of injury to the spinal cord. A, Hyperflexion. B, Lateral flexion. C, Extension. D, Compression.

Children are prone to specific kinds of spinal cord injuries because of the extreme mobility and flexibility of their spinal column. Table 27–10 describes the spinal cord injuries most common in children.

Spinal cord injuries are classified as complete or incomplete. Complete lesions are irreversible and involve a loss of sensory, motor, and autonomic function below the level of the injury. Incomplete lesions involve varying degrees of sensory, motor, and autonomic function below the level of injury. Hypotension, loss of bladder and bowel control, and loss of environmental thermoregulatory function are associated with autonomic nervous system dysfunction. The higher the level of spinal cord injury, the more severe the neurologic damage.

At the time of injury, the child is flaccid and areflexic below the lesion. Children can experience spinal shock, in which the child has flaccidity and loss of reflexes, but some return of func-

tion occurs within the first 72 hours of injury. As neurologic recovery begins, spinal reflex activity returns and increasing spasticity is seen below the level of the lesion.

The child can also experience neurogenic shock in which there is loss of vasomotor tone and autonomic nervous system innervation of the heart, resulting in hypotension, bradycardia,

Growth & Development *Vertebral Development*

The vertebrae are incompletely ossified in children under 9 years. The vertebral facet joints are more shallow and horizontal, allowing the vertebrae to glide during injury. The ligaments and joint capsules are more elastic and can stretch more than in adults without tearing. In young children the vertebral column can lengthen up to 2 inches, but the spinal cord can only lengthen by 0.25 inches without tearing (Slotkin et al., 2007).

TABLE 27–10	Spinal Cord Injuries in Children
Spine Region	Injury Characteristics
Cervical region	• Site of 60% of spinal injuries in children through 10 years • Injury above C3 segment causes respiratory arrest and death without ventilator support; many injuries above this level are fatal • Diaphragm function is present when injury is at C5 level • Quadriplegia with some function of upper extremities when injury is at C6–C7 level • Loss of sphincter function, loss of sensation below sternum
Thoracic region	• Site of 20% of injuries, usually between 8 and 14 years • Full control of upper extremities including hands • Poor trunk balance
Thoracolumbar region	• Full control of muscles in abdomen and upper back • Good trunk balance
Lumbar region	• Most injuries occur at the L2 to L4 levels, probably as a result of improperly placed lap belts • Below L3 may have functioning of muscles of upper leg, loss of ankle and foot control

and peripheral vasodilation (see Chapter 21 ∞). Priapism (prolonged penile erection) may be present. Respiratory compromise may occur due to paralysis of the diaphragm.

Nursing Alert

Autonomic dysreflexia is a medical emergency in which overactivity of the autonomic nervous system causes an abrupt onset of an elevated blood pressure, bradycardia in adolescents (tachycardia in younger children), cardiac arrhythmias, severe headaches, blurred vision, profuse sweating, piloerection, and flushing of the skin. It is most often seen in children with spinal cord injury higher than T6. The young child may have irritability or lethargy. This response can be triggered by a full bladder, kidney stone, urinary tract infection, or full rectum. Treatment involves positioning the patient upright, loosening tight clothing, emptying the bladder, or eliminating any precipitating stimulus. The child's blood pressure and heart rate should be assessed every 2 to 5 minutes. Antihypertensive medications are given if hypertension is sustained. Prevention of autonomic dysreflexia involves an effective bowel and bladder program (Somani, 2009).

Diagnosis is made by observation, neurologic examination, and radiologic studies of the cervical, thoracic, and lumbar spine to determine if a vertebral or compression fracture is present. The child's immobilized position is unchanged until radiographs are read by a radiologist and the spine is declared uninjured. In addition, CT scanning, MRI, fluoroscopy, or myelography may be performed. Up to 30–40% of children who have a spinal cord injury do not have evidence of bony radiographic abnormality (Slotkin et al., 2007). If profound or progressive paralysis occurs immediately or within 48 hours, an MRI can detect the injury to ligaments and soft tissues.

Spinal injuries are managed aggressively as the spinal injury extends upward 1 to 2 levels during the immediate hours and days after the injury (Hayes & Arriola, 2005). The child with a spinal cord injury may be placed in skeletal traction or a halo device. Surgery to reduce and internally fixate the fracture is performed for unstable fractures and dislocations. Decompression of the spinal cord and nerve roots may be performed if the tran-

section is not complete or if compression by a clot, herniated disk, or other lesion is present and can be relieved.

To decrease neurologic sequelae, methylprednisolone may be administered in high doses to children with motor deficits within 8 hours of injury for up to 48 hours. However, research evidence has not confirmed its benefit on neurologic outcomes (Mathison, Kadom, & Krug, 2008). If administered, gastrointestinal prophylaxis is provided to reduce the risk for an ulcer. Atropine and norepinephrine may be given to manage spinal shock. Pain is managed.

Complications of spinal cord injury include:

• Impaired respiratory function due to a paralyzed diaphragm or diminished vital capacity
• Scoliosis if severe compression injury occurs before the skeleton is mature
• Hip instability due to poor acetabular development
• Pathologic fractures of the long bones due to immobilization hypercalcemia
• Pressure sores
• Deep vein thrombosis
• Autonomic dysreflexia

Spasticity, muscle atrophy, increased risk of respiratory problems, weight gain, osteoporosis, and other skeletal problems are long-term issues for many children. An interdisciplinary approach is required to manage the rehabilitation and long-term care needs of the child and family. The goal of rehabilitation is to promote independence in daily activities, as well as mobility, strength, power, and endurance.

NURSING MANAGEMENT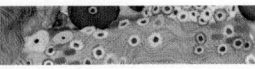

Hospital-Based Care

Nursing care focuses on monitoring vital signs, meeting nutritional needs, maintaining skin integrity, promoting independent functioning, encouraging therapeutic play, providing emotional support, and promoting rehabilitation.

Monitor vital signs and be alert for any changes, especially those that may signify increased respiratory difficulty or neurogenic shock (hypotension, bradycardia, and peripheral vasodilation), increased ICP (see Table 27–4), or autonomic dysreflexia. Monitor intake and output. Monitor bladder and bowel function.

Assess the cranial nerves as they may be affected by swelling around a cervical spinal cord injury. Note the return of reflexes and change from flaccid tone to spasticity. Identify any changes in level of sensation or motor function. Carefully check the immobilizing device, if present, to ensure that the spine remains stable.

Ensure adequate nutrition. A child with complete paralysis may require a gastrostomy tube. When the child begins to eat, feed soft foods slowly as the child may have some swallowing difficulties.

Prevent skin breakdown. See Chapter 31 ∞. Observe surgical sites for signs of infection or inflammation. Provide regular traction pin site care according to institutional guidelines.

Promote independent functioning by reinforcing the exercises and skills learned in physical and occupational therapy. Use supports, boots, footboards, splints, and braces as recommended by the therapists to prevent contractures (Figure 27–22 ➤). If hand mobility is limited, explore options for independence. Encourage the child to be as independent as possible in a wheelchair. An important mobility goal is to achieve wheelchair transfer and to perform self-care. Identify adaptive equipment that make these goals possible.

Achieving bowel and bladder control may be difficult, so intermittent urinary catheterizations may be necessary. (See the *Clinical Skills Manual.*) Anticipate that constipation will occur and initiate bowel training with a diet high in fiber and the use of stool softeners.

Therapeutic play appropriate for the child's developmental level is an important part of the healing process. Provide as many normal activities for the child as possible, but do not give the child tasks that he or she will have difficulty completing. Child-life teachers or tutors can help the child keep up with school work. Television, videotapes, and music can offer diversion for prolonged hospitalization. Children with paraplegia can learn to use their arms and hands to play interactive games. Devices can also be adapted so that the child can play computer games or manipulate the television or radio.

Support the child emotionally. Encourage the child to meet small, short-term goals, including those that involve self-care. Encourage the child to express fears and frustrations.

Be compassionate and understanding. Encourage siblings to visit, answer their questions honestly, and help them to discuss their feelings. Involve the parents and siblings in the child's care as much as possible. When appropriate, encourage the family to help with activities of daily living.

Discharge Planning and Home Care Teaching

Many children are discharged to inpatient rehabilitation facilities. Assist with arrangements for the transfer. Work closely with the child, parents, and other members of the health care team concerning placement. Home care needs, reintegration into educational programs, and safety issues should be identified and addressed well in advance of discharge from the rehabilitation facility. Refer families to social services, family counseling, and support groups, if indicated.

Submersion Injury and Drowning

Drowning is the process resulting in primary respiratory impairment from submersion/immersion in a liquid medium that results in death. *Submersion injury* is the term used when the child survives. Children between 1 and 4 years and males 15 to 24 years have the highest risk for drowning (Meyer, Theodorou, & Berg, 2006). Drowning is a leading cause of injury-related deaths in children. Most drownings occur in fresh water such as ponds and residential swimming pools.

A child can drown in as little water as it takes to cover the nose and mouth. The events preceding drowning follow a sequential pattern. The child trapped in water panics, struggles, tries to move using swimming motions, and holds his or her breath. The child aspirates a small amount of water from the oropharynx, causing a laryngospasm and hypoxia. Because of increasing panic and hypoxia, the child swallows more water, and may vomit and aspirate stomach contents. As the laryngospasm passes, reflex inspiration occurs. Inhaled water and aspirated stomach contents affect lung compliance and impair alveolar gas exchange.

Severe hypoxia leads to brain ischemia, cerebral edema and increased ICP, and secondary cerebral injuries, and may result in death. Many children who survive have neurologic impairment

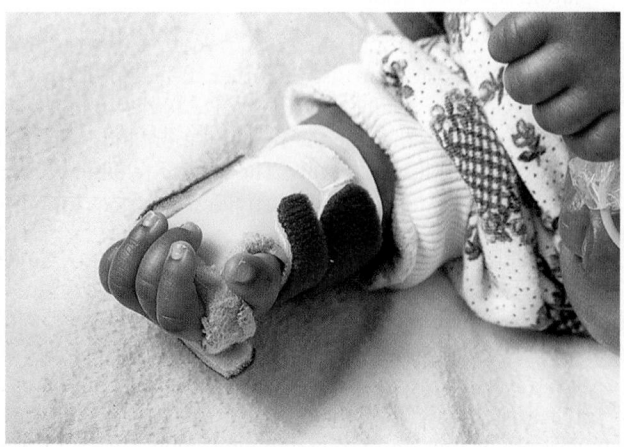

FIGURE 27–22 ➤ Splints are often used to prevent contractures, thus maintaining optimal functioning of the child's hands or feet.

Growth & Development | *Drowning Age and Location*

Approximately 40–50% of children injured in submersion incidents are under 4 years of age, with peak incidence between ages 1 and 2 years. The majority (78%) of infant drownings are in bathtubs. The most common drowning locations for children 1 to 4 years are artificial pools (56%). Among children 5 years and older, 63% of drownings occur in natural bodies of fresh water (Zuckerbraun & Saladino, 2005).

If a young child is submerged in cold water, the resulting hypothermia may trigger the diving reflex. This reflex slows the heart and decreases oxygen need in the tissues, potentially delaying damage to the brain and heart (Wagner, 2009). See Chapter 31 ∞ for information on hypothermia.

that affects functional recovery even after successful cardiopulmonary resuscitation (CPR).

The child with submersion injury exhibits a wide variety of signs and symptoms depending on the length of time underwater, the temperature of the water, the response to the episode, and the initial treatment performed at the scene. Children submerged less than 5 to 10 minutes and resuscitated at the scene have few symptoms and often fully recover without neurologic impairment. Signs and symptoms of the rescued child may be decreased LOC ranging from stupor to total unresponsiveness, apnea or irregular respirations, gastric distention, and seizures. The child submerged for longer periods will likely die or have severe neurologic impairment, except in some rare cases of submersion in icy water (Meyer et al., 2006).

Immediate CPR performed at the scene is associated with the best outcomes (Figure 27–23 ➤). The child should be transported to the hospital even if the child begins breathing spontaneously. If the child is severely hypothermic (less than 30°C), active and passive rewarming actions are used during resuscitation.

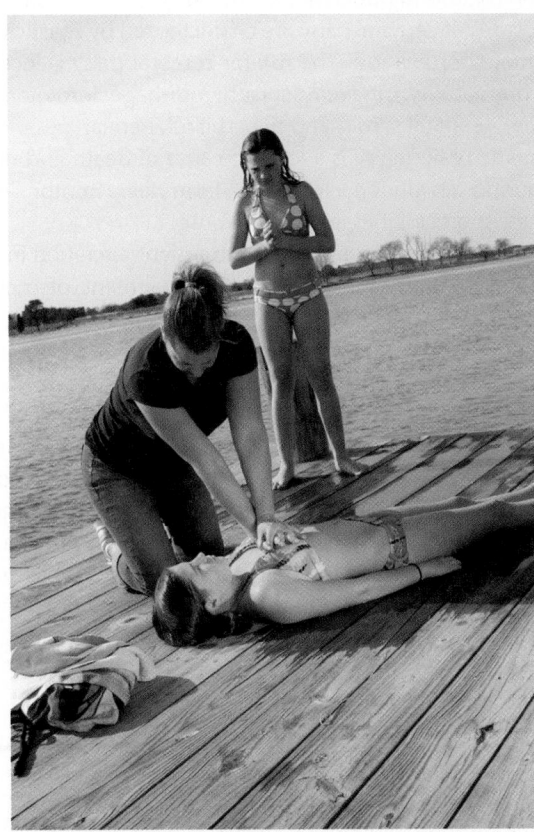

FIGURE 27–23 ➤ The best chance of survival after a submersion injury is immediate CPR. Another bystander has run to call 911.

All surviving drowning victims should be admitted to the hospital for at least 24 hours or observed in a short-stay observation unit for several hours, even when asymptomatic. Many life-threatening complications, including respiratory distress and cerebral edema, may not become evident for at least 12 hours after the incident.

The child may need mechanical ventilation to keep the alveoli open, to promote adequate oxygenation, and to prevent respiratory acidosis. After hypovolemia is corrected, fluids may be restricted and diuretics may be used to help reduce cerebral edema. Vasopressor medication may be used to maintain a normal blood pressure. Predictors of good outcome are spontaneous purposeful movements and normal brainstem function in the first 24 hours after submersion (Meyer et al., 2006).

NURSING MANAGEMENT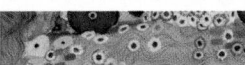

Nursing care of the child who survives a drowning incident focuses on monitoring the child's neurologic and cardiopulmonary status and providing emotional support to the family.

Monitor the child's responsiveness, spontaneous respiratory efforts, oxygenation, and pulse. Perform frequent neurologic assessments. Attach a cardiorespiratory monitor and pulse oximeter for continuous assessment information about the child's oxygenation status.

Implement the nursing interventions for a child with altered states of consciousness as described on page 853. If cerebral edema develops, implement nursing interventions as described on page 892.

Provide emotional support to the family. Be nonjudgmental and allow parents to express their feelings. Reassure parents who exhibit guilt reactions that their child is receiving all possible medical treatment. Parents often face an unknown prognosis. See Chapter 13 ∞. Encourage them to seek assistance from social workers, members of the clergy, close friends, and relatives. Arrange for appropriate referrals. If the child's prognosis is poor, an ethical consult may be offered to educate the family about options for decision making regarding sustaining or terminating life support.

Identify and address home care needs well in advance of discharge. Assist with arrangements for the child with minor deficits. Assign a case manager to the child with significant neurologic impairments so that long-term care options can be explored. Inpatient or outpatient rehabilitation options should be matched to the child's needs and family resources.

Drowning can be prevented by education, legislation, and changes in the environment. Pool owners should erect climb-proof 5-foot fences around all *four* sides of the pool to reduce access to the pool by young children. Local ordinances may require such fences. Pool owners should learn CPR so that immediate resuscitation can begin if a child is found submerged. Adolescents should learn the dangers of mixing alcohol and swimming. Five- and 10-gallon buckets should be kept empty when not in use. Emphasize the importance of closely supervising children when near or in the water, whether at pools, at the beach, or in the bathtub.

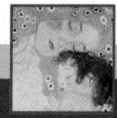

Chapter Highlights

- The nervous system is complete with all nerve cells at birth. Myelination continues throughout childhood.
- Altered level of consciousness is caused by infection, trauma, hypoxia, poisoning, seizures, alcohol or substance abuse, endocrine or metabolic disturbances (e.g., diabetic ketoacidosis), electrolyte or acid-base imbalance, intracranial space-occupying lesion, stroke, and a congenital structural defect.
- Emergency care for the child with a prolonged generalized seizure includes airway management, supplemental oxygen, intravenous benzodiazepines, and careful monitoring of vital signs and motor activity. Carefully document the duration of the seizure or series of seizures to detect status epilepticus.
- Neurologic damage from bacterial meningitis often occurs in infants and young children despite early, aggressive management. Complications may include sensorineural hearing loss, seizures, hydrocephalus, subdural effusion, diabetes insipidus, SIADH, developmental delay, learning problems, and behavior problems.
- Encephalitis is an acute inflammation of the brain often caused by a virus that is transmitted by a mosquito, such as West Nile virus and western equine virus. Presenting signs include a severe headache, fever, irritability, and altered mental status.
- Reye syndrome is an encephalopathy with a high mortality rate that is associated with aspirin use for a mild viral illness. Because most parents give children acetaminophen or ibuprofen rather than aspirin for flulike symptoms and varicella, Reye syndrome has become rare.
- Guillain-Barré syndrome is a disorder of deteriorating motor function and paralysis that progresses in an ascending pattern, paresthesia, and areflexia. It may be caused by an autoimmune response to an infectious organism, usually within 1 to 3 weeks of a gastrointestinal or respiratory illness.
- More than 75% of children experience a headache by age 15 years. Types of benign headache include migraines, inflammatory (sinusitis), and tension.
- Microcephaly is a small brain that may be caused by genetic transmission, fetal or postnatal insult, or intrauterine infection.
- Hydrocephalus is caused by the blockage of cerebrospinal fluid flow through normal channels and pathways or the impaired absorption of cerebrospinal fluid in the subarachnoid space and the arachnoid villi. It can be associated with a congenital condition or acquired from meningitis or intraventricular hemorrhage, tumor, or structural deformity.
- The more common types of neural tube defects include anencephaly (no development of the brain above the brainstem), encephalocele (protrusion of meningeal or skin-covered brain through the skull), and myelomeningocele or spina bifida.
- Myelomeningocele or spina bifida is a malformation of the vertebrae and spinal canal with a protrusion of a meningeal sac filled with a portion of the spinal cord. It is the most common developmental disorder of the CNS.
- Positional plagiocephaly, a flattened occiput, is seen increasingly when infants who are placed on their backs to prevent sudden infant death syndrome do not change the position of the head. The weight of the infant head sometimes flattens the skull. Strategies to encourage the child to change the position of the head may help reduce its occurrence.
- Hypertonia, tremors, extensor leg posture, and poor sucking and feeding difficulties in the newborn may be related to the direct effect of cocaine on the developing central nervous system. Irritability, jitteriness, high-pitched cry, and excessive sucking may also be seen with withdrawal from other illicit substances.
- Neurofibromatosis 1 is characterized by multiple café-au-lait spots, darker than the surrounding skin, that are 5 mm or larger in infants but grow to 15 mm in diameter during adolescence. Multiple benign tumors grow on or under the skin beginning during puberty.
- Most cases of cerebral palsy are characterized by spasticity and a lack of coordination. The risk for cerebral palsy is increased with prematurity, intraventricular hemorrhage, intrauterine infection, neonatal sepsis, and hyperbilirubinemia.
- Traumatic brain injury is a leading cause of death and disability during childhood. It results from falls, motor vehicle crashes, sports injuries, and child abuse.
- Concussions are associated with a transient alteration in mental status (amnesia, dizziness, and impairment of memory, orientation, and balance) resulting from the stretching, compression, and shearing of nerve fibers after an impact injury to the head.
- Spinal cord injuries, although relatively rare in children, often result from significant forces such as from motor vehicle crashes. Because of the child's larger and heavier head and weaker neck muscles, cervical spine injuries are more common.
- Children who have the best outcomes following drowning include those submerged less than 5 minutes who receive immediate cardiopulmonary resuscitation.

Clinical Reasoning in Action

Recall 8-year-old Andy with meningitis at the beginning of the chapter. Andy has a cochlear implant that increases his risk for development of meningitis. During the first days of Andy's hospital stay, he is irritable and resists moving because his head and neck hurt. Pain medication is provided to increase his comfort. His IV fluids are carefully managed for the first few days until it is known that the syndrome of antidiuretic hormone will not develop. Although he remains responsive during the initial days in the hospital, he naps a lot. On day 2, Andy has a generalized seizure that is effectively treated with lorazepam. Since Andy may have developed a seizure disorder due to meningitis, seizure precautions are initiated. As the infection begins to resolve, Andy begins feeling better and seeks opportunities for diversion.

1. Describe the pathophysiology that could account for Andy's infection and seizure.
2. Identify age-appropriate diversions for Andy during his hospital stay.
3. Describe the neurologic nursing assessments that should be performed on Andy at regular intervals during his initial days in the hospital.
4. Develop a nursing care plan for Andy that takes into account his treatment, pain, and lethargy. Be sure to address hydration, seizure precautions, and family education.

See Pearson Nursing Student Resources for possible responses.

Pearson Nursing Student Resources
Find additional review materials at
nursing.pearsonhighered.com
Prepare for success with NCLEX®-style practice questions, interactive assignments and activities, Web links, animations and videos, and more!

References

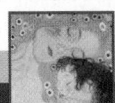

Adirim, T. A. (2007). Concussions in sports and recreation. *Clinical Pediatric Emergency Medicine, 8*, 2–6.

Atabaki, S. M. (2007). Pediatric head injury. *Pediatrics in Review, 28*(6), 215–223.

Austin, J. K. (2004). Behavioral issues involving children and adolescents with epilepsy and the impact of their families: Recent research data. *Epilepsy and Behavior, 5*(Suppl. 3), S33–41.

Avner, J. R. (2006). Altered states of consciousness. *Pediatrics in Review, 27*(9), 331–337.

Bada, H. S., Das, A., Bauer, C. R., Shankaran, S., Lester, B., LaGasse, L., et al. (2007). Impact of prenatal cocaine exposure on child behavior problems through school age. *Pediatrics, 119*(2), e348–e359.

Barr, R. G., Rivera, F. P., Barr, M., Cummings, P., Taylor, J., Lengua, L. J., & Meredith-Benitz, E. (2009). Effectiveness of educational materials designed to change knowledge and behaviors regarding crying and shaken-baby syndrome in mothers of newborns: A randomized, controlled trial. *Pediatrics, 123*(3), 972–980.

Black, J. S., & Wilson, B. (2009). Neurofibromatosis type 1. *Consultant for Pediatricians, 8*(12), 433.

Blumstein, M. D., & Friedman, M. J. (2007). Childhood seizures. *Emergency Clinics of North America, 25*, 1061–1086.

Boss, B. J., & Huether, S. E. (2010). Alterations in neurologic function in children. In K. L. McCance, S. E. Huether, V. L. Brashers, & N. S. Rote, *Pathophysiology: The biologic basis for disease in adults and children* (6th ed., pp. 665–695). St. Louis, MO: Mosby Elsevier.

Boulet, S. I., Gambrell, D., Shin, M., & Honein, M. A. (2009). Racial/ethnic differences in birth prevalence of spina bifida—United States, 1995–2005. *Morbidity and Mortality Report, 57*(53), 1409–1413.

Carey, R. G., & Balistreri, W. F. (2007). Mitochondrial hepatopathies. In R. M. Kliegman, R. E. Behrman, H. B. Jenson, & B. F. Stanton (Eds.), *Nelson textbook of pediatrics* (18th ed., pp. 1696–1698). Philadelphia: Elsevier Saunders.

Catroppa, C., & Anderson, V. (2009). Neurodevelopmental outcomes in pediatric traumatic brain injury. *Future Neurology, 4*(6), 811–821.

Centers for Disease Control and Prevention. (2008). *Traumatic brain injury.* Retrieved from http://www.cdc.gov/TraumaticBrainInjury/tbi_concussion.html

Centers for Disease Control and Prevention. (2009). Invasive Haemophilus influenza type B disease in five young children—Minnesota, 2008. *Morbidity and Mortality Weekly Report, 58*(03), 58–60.

Chiafery, M. (2006). Care and management of the child with shunted hydrocephalus. *Pediatric Nursing, 32*(3), 222–225.

Cirillo, M. L. (2008). Neuromuscular emergencies. *Clinical Pediatric Emergency Medicine, 9*, 88–95.

Dias, M. S. (2004). Acute traumatic brain and spinal cord injury. *Pediatric Clinics of North America, 51*, 271–303.

Doolin, E. (2006). Bowel management for patients with myelodysplasia. *Surgical Clinics of North America, 86*, 505–514.

Duffy, L. V. (2010). Hydrocephalus. In P. J. Allen, J. A. Vessey, & N. A. Shapiro (Eds.), *Primary care of the child with a chronic condition* (5th ed., pp. 546–561). St. Louis, MO: Mosby Elsevier.

Epilepsy Foundation. (2009). *Epilepsy and seizure statistics.* Retrieved from http://www.epilepsy foundation.org/about/statistics.cfm

Fisher, P. G. (2005). Help for headaches: A strategy for your busy practice. *Contemporary Pediatrics, 22*(11), 34–40.

Fisher, P. G. (2007). First and second seizure: What to know and do. *Contemporary Pediatrics, 24*(4), 80–89.

Freeman, J. M., Kossoff, E. H., & Hartman, A. L. (2007). The ketogenic diet: One decade later. *Pediatrics, 119*(3), 535–543.

Gladstein, J., & Mack, K. J. (2005). Chronic daily headaches in adolescents. *Pediatric Annals, 34*(6), 472–479.

Goldstein, J. (2008). Status epilepticus in the pediatric emergency department. *Clinical Pediatric Emergency Medicine, 9,* 96–100.

Gray, E. H., Blackinton, J., & White, G. M. (2006). Stoma care in the school setting. *Journal of School Nursing, 22*(2), 74–80.

Gunner, K. B., Smith, H. D., & Ferguson, L. E. (2008). Practice guideline for diagnosis and management of migraine headaches in children and adolescents: Part two. *Journal of Pediatric Health Care, 22*(1), 52–59.

Hayes, J. S., & Arriola, T. (2005). Pediatric spinal injuries. *Pediatric Nursing, 31*(6), 464–467.

Hutchinson, J. S., Ward, R. E., Lacroix, J., Hébert, P. C., Barnes, M. A., Bohn, D. J., et al. (2008). Hypothermia therapy after traumatic brain injury in children. *New England Journal of Medicine, 358*(23), 2447–2456.

Jankowitz, B. T., & Adelson, P. D. (2006). Pediatric traumatic brain injury: Past, present, and future. *Developmental Neuroscience, 28,* 264–275.

Jones, M. W., Morgan, E., & Shelton, J. E. (2007a). Cerebral palsy: Introduction and diagnosis (Part 1). *Journal of Pediatric Health Care, 21*(3), 146–152.

Jones, M. W., Morgan, E., & Shelton, J. E. (2007b). Primary care of the child with cerebral palsy: A review of systems (Part II). *Journal of Pediatric Health Care, 21*(4), 226–237.

Jorganic, J. L., Lynch, J. M., Littlefield, T. R., & Verelli, B. C. (2009). Risk factors associated with deformational plagiocephaly. *Pediatrics, 124*(6), e1126–e1133.

Katrancha, E. D. (2008). Clean intermittent catheterization in the school setting. *Journal of School Nursing, 24*(4), 197–204.

Keenan, H. T., & Bratton, S. L. (2006). Epidemiology and outcomes of pediatric traumatic brain injury. *Developmental Neuroscience, 28,* 256–263.

Kinsman, S. L., & Johnston, M. V. (2007). Congenital anomalies of the central nervous system. In R. M. Kliegman, R. E. Behrman, H. B. Jenson, & B. F. Stanton (Eds.), *Nelson textbook of pediatrics* (18th ed., pp. 2443–2456). Philadelphia: Saunders Elsevier.

Kirkwood, M. W., Yeates, K. O., & Wilson, P. E. (2006). Pediatric sports-related concussion: A review of the clinical management of an oft-neglected population. *Pediatrics, 117*(4), 1359–1371.

Koh, J. L., & Gries, H. (2007). Perioperative management of pediatric patients with craniosynostosis. *Anesthesiology Clinics, 25,* 465–481.

Kohen, D. P., & Zajak, R. (2007). Self-hypnosis training for headaches in children and adolescents, *Journal of Pediatrics, 150*(6), 635–639.

Kossoff, E. H., & Mankad, D. N. (2006). Medication-overuse headache in children: Is initial preventive therapy necessary? *Journal of Child Neurology, 21*(1), 45–48.

Lee, P., & DiPatri, A. J. (2008). Evaluation of suspected cerebrospinal fluid shunt complications in children. *Clinical Pediatric Emergency Medicine, 9,* 76–82.

Leung, A. K. C., & Robson, W. L. M. (2007). Febrile seizures. *Journal of Pediatric Health Care, 21*(4), 250–255.

Lewis, D. W. (2007). Pediatric migraine. *Pediatrics in Review, 28*(2), 43–52.

Liptak, G. S. (2007). Neural tube defects. In M. L. Batshaw (Ed.), *Children with disabilities* (6th ed., pp. 419–438). Baltimore: Paul H. Brooks.

Lovell, M. (2009). The management of sports-related concussion: Current status and future trends. *Clinical Sports Medicine, 28,* 95–111.

Major, P., & Thiele, E. A. (2007). Seizures in children: Laboratory diagnosis and management. *Pediatrics in Review, 28*(11), 405–413.

Mann, K., & Jackson, A. (2008). Meningitis. *Pediatrics in Review, 29*(12), 417–429.

Mansfield, R. T. (2007). Severe traumatic brain injuries in children. *Clinical Pediatric Emergency Medicine, 8,* 156–164.

Mathison, D. J., Kadom, N., & Krug, S. E. (2008). Spinal cord injury in the pediatric patient. *Clinical Pediatric Emergency Medicine, 9,* 106–123.

McNelis, A., Buelow, J., Myers, J., & Johnson, E. A. (2007). Concerns and needs of children with epilepsy and their parents. *Clinical Nurse Specialist, 21*(4), 195–202.

Meyer, R. J., Theodorou, A. A., & Berg, R. A. (2006). Childhood drowning. *Pediatrics in Review, 27*(5), 163–168.

National Institute of Neurological Disorders and Stroke. (2008). *Hydrocephalus fact sheet.* Retrieved from http://www.ninds.nih.gov/ disorders/hydrocephalus/detail_hydrocephalus .htm

National Institute of Neurological Disorders and Stroke. (2009). *Neurofibromatosis fact sheet.* Retrieved from http://www.ninds.nih.gov/ disorders/neurofibromatosis/detail_ neurofibromatosis.htm#137783162

Nehring, W. M. (2010). Cerebral palsy. In P. J. Allen, J. A. Vessey, & N. A. Shapiro (Eds.), *Primary care of the child with a chronic condition* (5th ed., pp. 326–346). St. Louis, MO: Mosby.

Nehring, W. M., & Faux, S. A. (2006). Transitional and health issues of adults with neural tube defects. *Journal of Nursing Scholarship, 38*(1), 63–70.

Nield, L. S., Nanda, S., Someshwar, J., Dalcanto, F. C., Someshwar, S., Collins, J. J., & Jaynes, M. (2007, June). Cerebral palsy: A multisystem review. *Consultant for Pediatricians, 6*(6), 337–343.

Olsson, J. (2007). The newborn. In R. M. Kliegman, R. E. Behrman, H. B. Jenson, & B. F. Stanton (Eds.), *Nelson textbook of pediatrics* (18th ed., pp. 41–42). Philadelphia: Elsevier Saunders.

Pellegrino, L. (2007). Cerebral palsy. In M. L. Batshaw, L. Pellegrino, & N. J. Roizen (Eds.), *Children with disabilities* (6th ed., pp. 387–408). Baltimore: Paul H. Brooks.

Purugganan, O. H. (2006). Abnormalities in head size. *Pediatrics in Review, 27*(12), 473–476.

Rais-Bahrami, K., & Short, B. L. (2007). Premature and small-for-dates infants. In M. L. Batshaw, L. Pellegrino, & N. J. Roizen (Eds.), *Children with disabilities* (6th ed., pp. 107–122). Baltimore: Paul H. Brooks.

Rangel-Castillo, L., Gopinath, S., & Robertson, C. S. (2008). Management of intracranial hypertension. *Neurologic Clinics, 26,* 521–541.

Rayburn, W. R. (2007). Maternal and fetal effects from substance use. *Clinics in Perinatology, 34,* 559–571.

Rosenbaum, P., Paneth, N., Leviton, A., Goldstein, M., Bax, M., Damiano, D., et al. (2007). A report: The definition and classification of cerebral palsy, April 2006. *Developmental Medicine and Child Neurology, 49,* 8–14.

Rowe, D. E., & Jadhav, A. L. (2008). Care of the adolescent with spina bifida. *Pediatric Clinics of North America, 55,* 1359–1374.

Rubin, D. H., Suecoff, S. A., & Knupp, K. G. (2006). Headaches in children. *Pediatric Annals, 35*(5), 345–353.

Saiki, R. L. (2009). Current and evolving management of traumatic brain injury. *Critical Care Clinics of North America, 21,* 549–559.

Salehi-Had, H., Brandt, J. D., Rosas, A. J., & Rogers, K. K. (2006). Findings in older children with abusive head injury: Does shaken-child syndrome exist? *Pediatrics, 117*(5), e1039–e1044.

Sarnat, H. B. (2007). Neuromuscular disorders. In R. M. Kliegman, R. E. Behrman, H. B. Jenson, & B. F. Stanton (Eds.), *Nelson textbook of pediatrics* (18th ed., pp. 2531–2567). Philadelphia: Elsevier Saunders.

Sawin, K. J., & Thompson, N. M. (2009). The experience of finding an effective bowel management program for children with spina bifida: The parent's perspective. *Journal of Pediatric Nursing, 24*(4), 280–291.

Slotkin, J. R., Lu, Y., & Wood, K. B. (2007). Thoracolumbar spinal trauma in children. *Neurosurgery Clinics of North America, 18,* 621–630.

Somani, B. K. (2009). Autonomic dysreflexia: A medical emergency with spinal cord injury. *International Journal of Clinical Practice, 63*(3), 350–352.

Spector, R. E. (2009). *Cultural diversity in health and illness* (7th ed., pp. 3–4). Upper Saddle River, NJ: Pearson.

Substance Abuse and Mental Health Services Administration, Office of Applied Statistics. (2009). *Results from the 2008 National Survey on Drug Use and Health: National Findings* (NSDUH Series H-36, HHS Publication No. SMA 09-4434). Rockville, MD: Department of Health and Human Services.

Swaine, B. R., Tremblay, C., Platt, R. W., Grimard, G., Zhang, X., & Pleiss, I. B. (2007). Previous head injury is a risk factor for subsequent head injury in children: A longitudinal cohort study. *Pediatrics, 119*(4), 749–758.

Sweeney, N. M. F. (2009). Neonatology. In J. W. Custer & R. E. Rau (Eds.), *The Harriet Lane handbook* (18th ed., pp. 481–505). Philadelphia: Elsevier Mosby.

Theos, A., & Korf, B. R. (2006). Pathophysiology of neurofibromatosis type 1. *Annals of Internal Medicine, 144*(11), 842–849.

Thomas, S. (2006). Management of epilepsy and pregnancy. *Journal of Postgraduate Medicine, 52*(1), 57–63.

Van Vlimmeren, L. A., van der Graaf, Y., Boere-Boonekamp, M. M., L'Hoir, M. P., Helders, P. J. M., & Englebert, R. H. H. (2007). Risk factors for deformational plagiocephaly at birth and at 7 weeks of age: A prospective cohort study. *Pediatrics, 119*(2), e408–e418.

Vitale, M .G., Goss, J. M., Matsumoto, H., & Roye, D. P. (2006). Epidemiology of pediatric spinal cord injury in the United States, years 1997 and 2000. *Journal of Pediatric Orthopedics, 26*(6), 745–749.

Wagner, C. (2009). Pediatric submersion injuries. *Air Medical Journal, 28*(3), 116–119.

Warner, W. C. (2007). Myelomeningocele. In S. T. Canale & J. H. Beaty, *Campbell's operative orthopedics* (11th ed., pp. 1450–1474). Philadelphia: Mosby Elsevier.

Weinstein, S. L., & Gaillard, W. D. (2007). Epilepsy. In M. L. Barshaw, L. Pellegrino, & N. J. Roizen (Eds.), *Children with disabilities* (6th ed., pp. 439–460). Baltimore: Paul H. Brooks.

Wilson, B. A., Shannon, M. T., & Shield, K. M. (2009). *Nurse's drug guide 2009*. Upper Saddle River, NJ: Prentice Hall Health.

Wolf, S. M., & McGoldrick, P. E. (2006). Recognition and management of pediatric seizures. *Pediatric Annals, 35*(5), 332–344.

Zuckerbraun, N. S., & Saladino, R. A. (2005). Pediatric drowning: Current management strategies for immediate care. *Clinical Pediatric Emergency Medicine, 6*, 49–56.

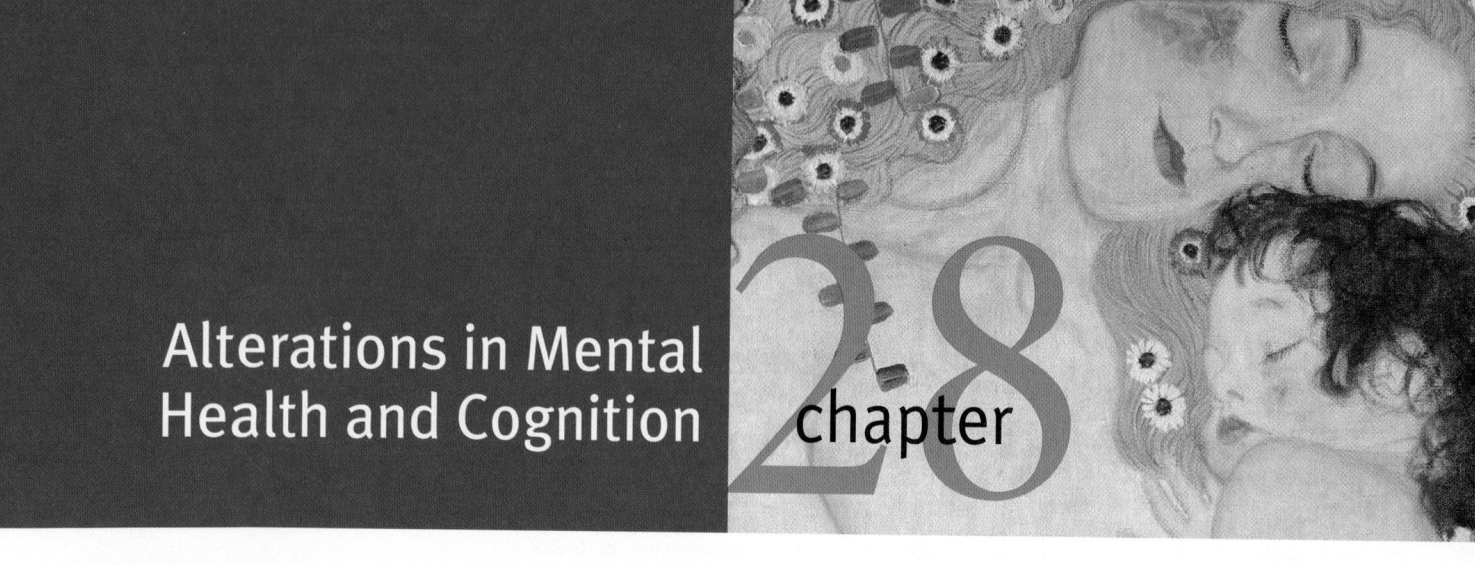

Alterations in Mental Health and Cognition

chapter 28

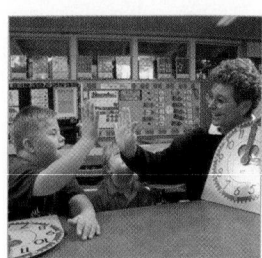

Jeremiah, a 7-year-old boy with Down syndrome, enjoys attending his special education classroom. Jeremiah is the youngest of four children and was born after an unplanned pregnancy to a mother and father in their forties. Their youngest child at that time was 12 years of age. Although they accepted that they would have another child, Jeremiah's parents learned after an amniocentesis during the pregnancy that their son had Down syndrome. His parents progressed through stages of shock, denial, anger, and sadness. Thanks to a strong support system, they soon learned more about Down syndrome, resolved their grief, and grew to love their infant son. The siblings loved their new brother and seemed to have little trouble accepting the fact that he was different from their original expectations.

During infancy, Jeremiah developed gastroesophageal reflux and frequent otitis media. Since his parents had health care insurance, they were able to seek assistance as needed. When he was almost a year of age, the family enrolled Jeremiah in an early intervention program. He was about 4 months behind in developmental milestone achievement, but through the intervention program he quickly gained fine and gross motor skills. He eventually progressed from the early intervention program to preschool, and recently began attending a special education classroom. How can the school nurse work with the family to review Jeremiah's transition to school and provide information about obtaining and wearing an alert identification bracelet? What special concerns should be addressed related to Jeremiah's entry to school and his general health status?

Key Terms

adaptive functioning / 934
affect / 932
agoraphobia / 926
anhedonia / 921
behavior modification / 909
cognitive therapy / 907
coprolalia / 932
copropraxia / 932
developmental disability / 934
echolalia / 911
evidence-based practice / 907
learning disabilities / 933
intellectual disability / 934
pervasive developmental disorders (PDDs) / 911
play therapy / 907
stereotypy / 911

Learning Outcomes

After reading this chapter, you will be able to do the following:

1. Define mental health and describe major mental health alterations in childhood.
2. Contrast pediatric differences and issues related to mental health and cognition.
3. Discuss the clinical manifestations of the major mental health alterations of childhood and adolescence.
4. Plan for the nursing management of children and adolescents with mental health alterations in the hospital and community settings.
5. Describe characteristics of common cognitive alterations of childhood.
6. Use evidence-based practice to plan nursing management for children with cognitive alterations.
7. Establish and evaluate expected outcomes of care for the child with a cognitive alteration.

FOCUS ON Mental Health and Cognition

PEDIATRIC DIFFERENCES IN MENTAL HEALTH AND COGNITION

Some mental health and cognitive conditions in children originate from a genetic or physiologic cause, for example, intellectual disability (previously called *mental retardation*) and childhood schizophrenia. Often the family and surrounding environments in which children live influence their characteristics and contribute to dysfunctions such as anxiety, depression, and posttraumatic stress disorder. A unique and challenging interplay of genetics and environment influence mental health and cognitive conditions, making diagnosis and treatment challenging.

Children differ from adults both in mental health care needs and in the types and progression of mental health disruptions. During childhood, the necessity for bonding and attachment to significant adults forms the foundation of the child's healthy mental development. Therefore, young children rely on adults for establishment of mental health. The child's unique genetic makeup couples with these environmental factors, thereby contributing to a state of mental health. Cognitive disorders are also a result of a unique interplay of genetic and environmental causes. The brain develops from the fetal neural tube early in development, with much critical embryology occurring in the fourth to sixth week of gestation, at which point many women are unaware that they are pregnant. During this time, the brain is not protected by the blood-brain barrier and is at risk for injury from the fetal environment. Environmental conditions such as maternal alcohol ingestion or intake of certain medications can influence the developing fetus's brain.

In addition, children with mental health alterations sometimes display different clinical manifestations for mental illness than adults; therefore, diagnosis is difficult and challenging. For example, a child with a tic syndrome may be mistakenly diagnosed as hyperactive, and the treatment therefore would not be appropriate to the underlying condition.

At birth the brain makes up about 25% of body weight; this percentage decreases to about 2% of weight by adulthood. Most of the brain structure is present at birth, but during the first 5 years of life the brain continues to develop and mature as the young child gains fine and gross motor, social, and language skills. Development and differentiation occur during childhood spurts with fine motor skills improvement and during adolescent years when perception, motor function, and advanced thinking processes further develop (Chamley, Carson, Randall, et al., 2005). The child remains vulnerable to external forces during periods of brain growth and development. The influence of drugs, poor nutrition, traumatic brain injury, and absence of emotional nurturance are all examples of factors that can interfere with healthy brain and cognitive development.

Examples of diagnostic and laboratory tests used for mental health and cognition include magnetic resonance imaging (MRI), radiograph (x-ray), electroencephalogram, positron emission tomography (PET) scan, neuropsychological testing, and toxicology screening (see Appendix E ∞). Use the Assessment Guidelines on the next page to perform a nursing assessment.

The purpose of this chapter is to provide the knowledge and tools that can help you to provide appropriate care for children with alterations in mental health or cognition. Much of the care for mental health alterations is provided by psychiatric–mental health specialists, so the nurse collaborates with these specialists to identify problems, support and carry out therapy, provide education for the family, and refer the family to appropriate resources. Children with mental health or cognitive disorders are sometimes hospitalized, visit well-child clinics, and attend schools. Nurses in all settings must gain the skills to provide care for these children. See Chapter 14 ∞ for a description of eating disorders.

Cognitive conditions are commonly managed by the family and the school personnel. The nurse collaborates with families and school personnel to plan and evaluate care for the child with cognitive conditions such as intellectual disability. A thorough knowledge of development is a prerequisite to understanding both mental health disruptions and cognitive conditions since developmental status is often altered in both mental health and cognitive conditions.

Most mental health conditions are treated in community settings, and nurses in these settings play an active role in the treatment and support of the child and family. Nurses may function as case managers, assisting a family to deal with all areas of the child's care. Occasionally a child is hospitalized for treatment of a significant mental health disruption, or is hospitalized for treatment of another health problem and requires continued mental health services.

Assessment Guidelines for the Child with an Alteration in Mental Health or Cognition

Assessment Focus	Assessment Guidelines
History	▪ Describe prenatal care and problems. Was there any trauma at birth? ▪ Is there a diagnosed mental health disorder in the child or other family members? ▪ Is there a history of any neurological injuries or diseases? ▪ What medications is the child taking? ▪ Ask the child, without family present, about use of drugs and alcohol, and about sexual activity.
Growth	▪ Is growth progressing along the same channel or growth percentile? ▪ What was the growth pattern of siblings?
Development	▪ Perform regular developmental screening to identify any variations from expected developmental milestones. Further testing is required if screening suggests any abnormalities. ▪ What is the progression of skills reported by the family? ▪ Are there any unusual capabilities or deficits? ▪ Inquire about progression in school and extracurricular activities.
Social skills	▪ Describe the relationship between the child and significant adults. Is close attachment evident? Are there signs of attachment disorders such as lack of eye contact, smiles, or response to others in the environment? ▪ Describe the school-age child's daily schedule, including family and peer activities. Does the child have friends and engage in several activities with them on a regular basis? Does the child generally interact well with others? Has the child recently had a change in school performance? ▪ Have the teen describe daily activities and friends. Is there a combination of peer and family influence on personal decision making?
Affect	▪ Describe facial expression and response to the nurse. ▪ Observe body size, position, and posture. ▪ Are interaction behaviors typical for the setting and age of the child? ▪ Does the child display interest in surroundings? ▪ Is the child dressed in an appropriate manner? Does the child establish eye contact?
Appearance	▪ Is the child's clothing appropriate for age, setting, and developmental level?
Behaviors	▪ Describe level of consciousness and interaction with surroundings. ▪ Inquire about recent reported changes in behavior (e.g., sleep, eating patterns, communication with others, school performance, friendships, risky activities). ▪ Are problem behaviors identified by the child or parent? ▪ Are there particular events that were associated with problem behaviors?
Life events	▪ Has the child or family experienced recent stress or trauma? ▪ Have there been any changes in family structure? ▪ Evaluate chronic health conditions in family members.

▪ MENTAL HEALTH ALTERATIONS

Mental health is foundational to a sense of personal well-being, physical health, relationships, and learning (Simpson, Cohen, Pastor, et al., 2008). A variety of conditions cause mental health alterations in children and adolescents. Overall, about 1 in 4–5 children and adolescents has a mental health disorder, and 1 in 10 has a disorder that profoundly interferes with daily functioning; mental health disorders affect 15 million children and adolescents (Melnyk, Baker, Walsh, et al., 2007). However, less than 35% of children with mental health alterations receive mental health services (Mark & Buck, 2006; Storch & Elder, 2009).

Nurses are leaders in the field of pediatric mental health care. The National Association of Pediatric Nurse Practitioners (NAPNAP) advocates for mental health screening and early interventions. Key components of care include a life span approach, culturally competent care, integration of mental health practices into school settings, integration of families into care, and application of evidence-based practice (Melnyk et al.,

2007). Many professionals, such as teachers, school counselors, psychologists, and others, work in the field of mental health. The nurse collaborates with these health care professionals to provide comprehensive mental health care for children and adolescents.

Some general clinical manifestations, therapies, and nursing management issues are discussed in the following text. A number of specific conditions, such as developmental and behavioral disorders, attention deficit hyperactivity disorder, mood disorders, anxiety disorders, suicide, tic disorders, and schizophrenia, are described in subsequent sections, along with information about their management.

Clinical Manifestations

The manifestations of mental health alterations in children are varied, but most can be identified through careful developmental and behavioral screening. Children with mental health conditions often do not display usual developmental milestones at the times predicted, may have social interaction problems with family members or other people, or may have demonstrated a change in performance from former developmental achievement. Functional patterns of living such as the ability to feed and care for self, regulation of sleep and nutritional intake, and ability to self-regulate during activities may be lacking. Repetitive actions, behavioral instability and outbursts, and withdrawal are other important signs of mental health disruption. Manifestations are described in more detail with each condition described in this chapter.

COLLABORATIVE CARE

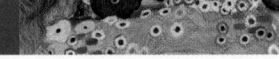

Diagnostic Tests

Diagnostic tests frequently involve screening for conditions such as depression, suicide, and anxiety. Developmental screening is often pertinent. Blood results may be used to verify some conditions and to establish substance use that may manifest as a mental health disorder. Brain imaging may be useful in some cases. In addition, a thorough physical assessment is essential.

Clinical Therapy

The primary treatment goal in the management of children and adolescents with mental health disorders is to assist the child and family to achieve and maintain an optimal level of functioning through interventions designed to reduce the impact of stressors. Therapeutic interventions and communication are based on the principle that feelings motivate behaviors. Parents and others who are close to the child often fall into the habit of reacting to the child's behaviors rather than trying to find out what feelings may be precipitating the undesirable actions. Although behaviors may be considered in treatment, feelings and life experiences are often explored to provide insight and to lead to behavior change. Medication may be used to enhance and support other therapy, or may be the major therapeutic measure.

Treatment Modes **Evidence-based practice** (EBP) refers to a body of scientific knowledge and its relationship to health care services (see further discussion in Chapter 1 ∞). While the research basis for care in all areas of pediatric health is generally scant, there is even less scientific basis to support interventions in mental health services. Nurses must apply evidence-based practice to enhance mental health care when possible, and participate in research and outcomes measurement so that additional strong evidence can be gathered on the best approaches to care (Kazak, Hoagwood, Weisz, et al., 2010).

Three basic treatment modes based on evidence-based practice are used: individual, family, and group therapy. The choice of treatment mode must take into account the child's age and developmental stage, as well as the family situation and access to care. Most therapists incorporate several intervention strategies simultaneously within these modes. Different strategies are more or less effective and appropriate for children and adolescents in various stages of development. A thorough understanding of developmental needs, expectations, and abilities is therefore essential for mental health professionals. Treatment modes and therapeutic strategies commonly used with children and adolescents are described in the following text.

Individual Therapy Individual therapy involves only the child and the therapist. Treatment of specific emotional problems or disorders may involve various techniques such as play therapy, psychodrama, art therapy, and **cognitive therapy** (a technique used to help a person recognize automatic negative thinking). Individual therapy may be short term (four to six sessions) or long term (lasting for several years).

Family Therapy Family therapy involves the exploration of a particular emotional problem and its manifestations among the family members. Family therapy is based on the idea that an individual's emotional symptoms or problems are an expression of emotional symptoms or problems in the family. The focus is on the relationships among the family members, rather than the psychologic conflict within each individual member.

Group Therapy Group therapy involves an ongoing or limited number of sessions in which several individuals participate. The emphasis is on the interpersonal styles of relating to one another in the group. Group therapy is particularly effective with adolescents because of the importance of the peer group at this age. An advantage of group therapy is that stimuli and feedback come from multiple sources (the group members) instead of just one person (the therapist).

Therapeutic Strategies

Play Therapy Play is often called the language or work of the child. From a developmental perspective, children progressively learn to express feelings and needs through action, fantasy, and finally language. The special quality of play buffers children against the pressures and demands of daily life. Play facilitates mastery of developmental stages by strengthening physical and neurologic processes. Play also assists in cognitive learning, setting the stage for problem solving and creativity.

Play therapy is a technique that reveals problems on a fantasy level through the use of toys, dolls, clay, art, and other creative objects. It is often used with preschool and school-age children who are experiencing anxiety, stress, and other specific nonpsychotic mental disorders. Play therapy encourages the child to act out feelings such as anger, hostility, sadness, and fear. It also provides the opportunity for the therapist to help the child understand, on a conscious or unconscious level, personal responses and behavior in a safe, supportive environment.

Clinical Tip

Play therapy, a technique used with children who have psychosocial disorders, is different from therapeutic play, which may be used with many hospitalized children (see Chapter 11 ∞). Although some techniques overlap, only a specialist is qualified to provide play therapy. However, anyone with a basic knowledge of development can plan therapeutic play approaches.

Art Therapy Children who may be apprehensive about playing can sometimes be encouraged to participate in art therapy, using brief drawing exercises. This technique is appropriate for children of all ages, including adolescents. The drawings can help the therapist gain information about the child, the family, and the interactions between the child and family. However, children's drawings should never be used solely to form a definitive diagnosis.

Drawing as a means for communication with children has been used for many years. Art can be viewed as a window or doorway through which a child's emotions and experiences can be viewed (Kortesluoma, Punamaki, & Nikkonen, 2008). This makes it an effective assessment technique with children too young to express certain situations verbally. In addition, it allows them expression of feelings, and thus becomes an intervention. Following a drawing session with a discussion in which the child explains a piece of art is especially helpful.

Art is also versatile and can be accomplished in practically any setting. One nurse described the use of drawings with children living in shelters after Hurricane Katrina (Looman, 2006). According to the author, art increased the amount of information a child could communicate and enhanced management of experienced trauma. It was a familiar activity that provided a comfortable space in which children could explore the occurrences and feelings about losing their homes, pets, or family and friends.

Nurses who work with children in any setting should consider the use of drawings. Provide a table and drawing materials for children waiting for a health care examination, bring art materials to the child in the hospital, and consider the activity with children who have experienced trauma.

When used in conjunction with a thorough history and appropriate psychologic testing information, art therapy can guide the child's treatment. These drawing exercises provide an opportunity to help in the healing process. The therapist can assist the child to release feelings of anger, pain, or fear onto paper, where they can be examined objectively. Figures 28–1 to 28–4 ➤ present examples of this technique.

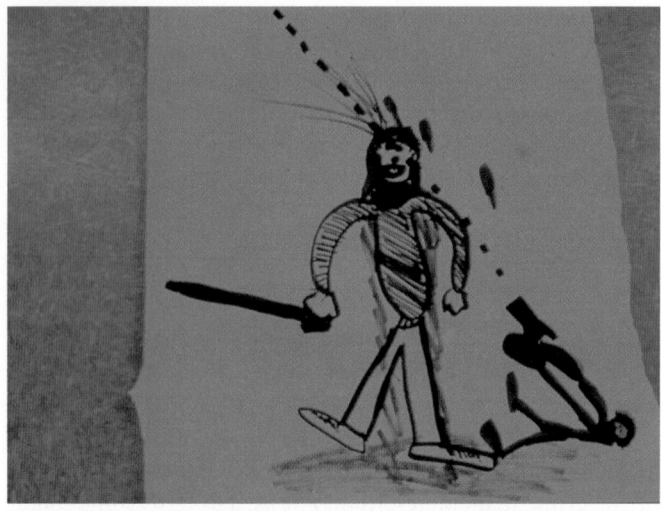

FIGURE 28–2 ➤ "Self-Portrait." Drawn by a 15-year-old boy who was admitted through the emergency department after a failed suicide attempt by hanging. He had a psychiatric diagnosis of depression and polysubstance abuse (including inhalants and alcohol) and insisted that he was a member of a satanic cult in his hometown. Most of his drawings depicted a preoccupation with violence and suicide. The boy said he always felt a "darkness" like a shadow that followed him around and wanted him dead. His family history was significant for depression and suicide on both his mother's and his father's side. His father also had a lengthy history of polysubstance abuse and alcoholism. The boy was discharged to a long-term residential treatment facility for adolescents.

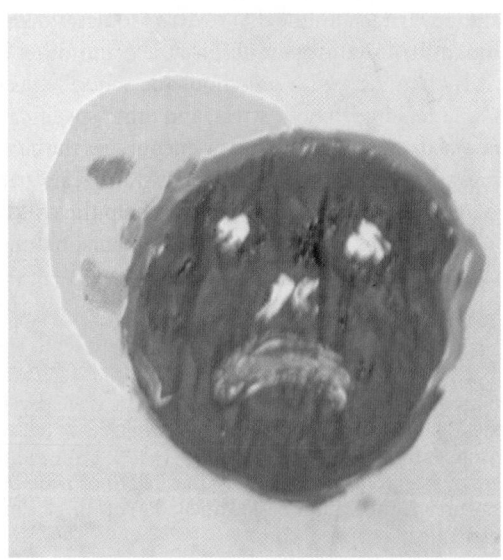

FIGURE 28–1 ➤ "Me." Drawn by a 14-year-old girl with major depression, anxiety, and school phobia who had experienced multiple losses over several years. Her mother had severe chronic lung problems and diabetes, and the girl had stopped attending school for fear that something would happen to her mother. This drawing represents the girl's obvious feelings of sadness and depression but also indicates a glimmer of hope (represented by the yellow mask coming from behind the dark mask of depression).

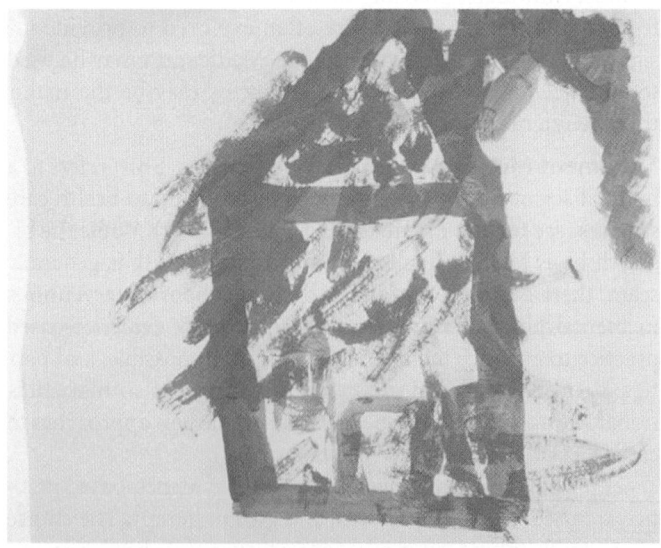

FIGURE 28–3 ➤ "An Activity." Drawn by an 8-year-old boy who was initially admitted to the medical-surgical floor of a pediatric hospital for dehydration resulting from vomiting and diarrhea. Psychiatric evaluation was ordered for extreme anxiety. These drawings, completed during the initial interview, led to further investigation, which revealed that the child had started a house fire in which his grandmother was killed. The family's home and all their belongings were lost. No one had known that the child had set the fire. Further sessions indicated that he had been setting neighborhood garage fires and watching them burn from a distance.

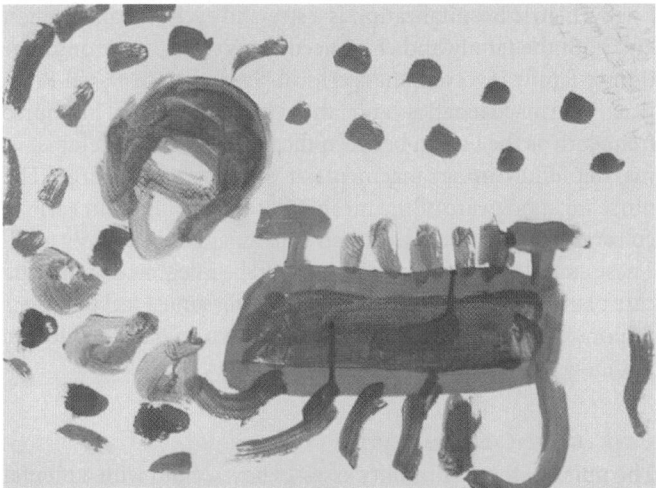

FIGURE 28–4 ➤ "A Family Activity." By the same boy who drew Figure 28–3. This drawing depicts a recurring incident of physical and emotional abuse by his mother's live-in boyfriend. It shows the family bathtub with feces and blood smeared on the floor and walls. The boy reported that when either he or his 3-year-old brother had a toileting accident the boyfriend would make them go into the bathroom and stand in the bathtub while he smeared the feces on the walls. He would then hit the children and make them clean up the mess. The boy had previously been removed from the mother's custody for neglect. He was transferred from the medical-surgical area to the inpatient children's psychiatric unit, where he received a diagnosis of depression, overanxious disorder, and child abuse (physical and emotional). Charges were filed against the mother's boyfriend and custody of both children was temporarily revoked.

Cognitive and Behavior Therapy (CBT)   A combination of cognitive and behavioral therapy is useful in treating many mental health conditions in children.

Cognitive therapy teaches application of thinking patterns to change reactions to situations that cause anxiety or other undesirable conditions. The child is taught how his or her brain and body are working; this understanding assists the child in having control over an experience.

Behavior modification is a therapeutic technique that uses stimulus and response conditioning to alter inappropriate behaviors. It reinforces desirable behaviors by helping the child to replace maladaptive behaviors with more appropriate ones. This technique is based on the assumption that any learned behavior can be unlearned. Thus, if parents, nurses, teachers, and other adults consistently reinforce desirable behaviors, the child will eventually alter or discontinue undesirable behaviors. Behavior modification may include (1) removing the child from the home to a more structured environment, such as a hospital, for a brief time, and (2) instructing the parents, teachers, and other appropriate adults to be agents of behavioral change. Several ongoing sessions may be required with the adults involved, using role-play and other techniques. Consistency is the most important principle in the successful use of behavior modification.

Visualization and Guided Imagery   The techniques of visualization and guided imagery begin with specific directions for progressive relaxation according to the child's ability. These forms of therapy use the child's imagination and positive thinking to reduce stress and anxiety, decrease the experience of pain or discomfort, and

promote healing. The techniques are especially useful in the management of anxiety disorders and chronic pain. It is not easy for every child to use his or her imagination in this way, so the technique may not work or be appropriate for every child.

Hypnosis   Hypnosis involves varying degrees of suggestibility and deep relaxation effects. This technique is useful for children and adolescents because they can usually be hypnotized more easily than adults. Hypnosis is especially helpful in treating physical symptoms with a psychologic component, anxiety, and phobias, as well as managing severe physical symptoms or discomfort (pain or nausea) associated with a physiologic disorder or its treatment (e.g., cancer or juvenile rheumatoid arthritis).

NURSING MANAGEMENT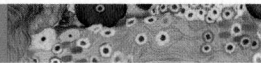

Nursing Assessment and Diagnosis

Ongoing assessment of all children and their families for mental health risk should be performed from the beginning of life and throughout childhood and adolescence (National Association of Pediatric Nurse Practitioners, 2007). When a potential mental health condition exists, the child should receive further assessment from a mental health specialist. Nursing assessment focuses on child behaviors, family interactions, lifestyle routines, developmental progression, and history of treatment for mental health or cognitive conditions. During all health visits, mental health screening should be integrated into care so that disruptions can be identified. See Chapter 6 ∞ for specific questions to ask during health promotion and health maintenance visits. A resource commonly used to identify diagnostic criteria for known mental health conditions is the *Diagnostic and Statistical Manual of Mental Disorders;* the current edition is the *DSM-IV-TR* (American Psychiatric Association, 2000) and its criteria for several conditions are listed throughout this chapter. A new and revised edition of the *DSM* is in preparation and is expected to be published in 2013.

Once a mental health problem is identified, the nurse assesses the child for related issues and conditions. Mental health is linked to development, so developmental screening tests are administered. Mental health status can influence activity level, physiological parameters, and risk for certain conditions. Therefore, height and weight, review of systems, vital signs, nutrition, physical activity, and medication/substance use history are important to perform. Family interactions, stressors, and methods of coping are assessed (see Chapter 2 ∞ for further details on family assessment).

Many nursing diagnoses can be formulated based on particular mental health conditions and child situations. Some examples include:

- Impaired Adjustment related to multiple stressors
- Anxiety related to situational or maturational crises
- Ineffective Coping related to inadequate social support
- Dysfunctional Grieving related to difficulty expressing loss of significant other
- Ineffective Role Performance related to inadequate support system and inadequate linkage with healthcare system

Planning and Implementation

Care in the Hospital

Although most mental health disorders are managed effectively with therapy and/or medication on an outpatient basis, some necessitate admission to an inpatient psychiatric setting. In addition, you may encounter the child with a mental health disorder during hospitalization for a concurrent physiologic problem that requires hospitalization. If a child is hospitalized for a concurrent problem, the child's current level of mental health functioning needs to be assessed in relation to the mental health disorder.

Nursing care includes carrying out the prescribed treatment plan and administering psychotropic medications. The child's medication regimen should be evaluated for administration schedule, dosage, side effects, and effectiveness. Inform the therapist of the child's hospitalization if the child has been hospitalized for a concurrent condition, and consult with the therapist regarding appropriate approaches for the child.

An important nursing intervention is to ensure the child's safety. Actions begin in the emergency department if a child is admitted for a mental health crisis. Remove or lock potentially dangerous material in the room such as medications, tubing, and a sharps container. The parent, guardian, or health professional should remain with the child at all times. Inform the family member of the need to stay with the child and how to immediately notify the nurse if the adult needs to leave or if the child's condition changes. Part of the initial care is to evaluate risk by asking if the child has tried to hurt him- or herself or been thinking about that. Ask about recent stresses, thoughts of hurting someone else, and why the child thinks he or she has been brought to the emergency department. If the child is admitted to the psychiatric unit, follow unit policies for ensuring safety for children who are at risk of hurting themselves or others.

Psychiatric hospitalization is a stressful event for all families, and both the family and child need supportive care. Continuation of family involvement is critical. See Evidence-Based Practice: Pharmacogenetics and the Nursing Role. The nurse frequently is the liaison between the family and the therapist in making follow-up arrangements at the time of discharge. The nurse must be aware of the meaning of mental illness in various cultural groups and the treatments that may be commonly used. These complementary therapies should be integrated within the care plan when considered safe, and families must feel that their responses and approaches to the child with a mental disorder are not judged by health professionals.

Care in the Community

The nurse in the community assesses how a child with a mental health disorder is functioning in each part of the microsystem (see Chapter 4 ∞), such as home, childcare, school, and with friends. The family's view of mental health and illness is important to understand. Risk and protective factors of the child and family are assessed (see Chapter 17 ∞). The nurse conducts therapy sessions and performs ongoing evaluation and updates of the child's level of functioning. Changes in the child and family stressors and coping mechanisms are identified, and pharmacologic interventions are evaluated.

Since many children do not receive adequate mental health services, nurses need to be knowledgeable about resources for mental health care and facilitate their use by the child and family. The nurse in the community often acts as a partner to inform other health professionals such as psychiatrists, psychologists, school counselors, teachers, and hospital nurses about the child's mental health status.

Evidence-Based Practice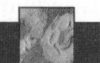
Pharmacogenetics and the Nursing Role

Problem

Great variability is seen in the response to psychotropic medicines used to treat mental health disorders such as depression. Children and adolescents show even more variability than adults so close monitoring is essential. New technologies provide information about individual responses to medications, but nurses may be unaware of these applications.

Evidence

The fields of genetics and genomics are growing rapidly (see Chapter 3 ∞). Currently, pharmacogenetic testing is being used so that clinicians can select the best psychotropic medications for particular patients. For example, a genetic test for a gene that codes for high manufacture of a body enzyme that breaks down a particular medication predicts that the patient will not respond well to that particular medication. Another psychotropic can be chosen to enhance response. On the other hand, if the patient is a slow metabolizer of the medication, an increased risk of toxicity results (Prows & Saldana, 2009).

Implications

The nurse in a setting where children and adolescents are treated for psychiatric disorders has an important role in applying new knowledge related to pharmocogenetics and pharmacogenomics. First,

the nurse also needs to take a careful history of other medications, over-the-counter products, and herbal remedies since many of these substances compete with psychotropic medications for metabolism in the body. When a DNA test is recommended prior to beginning medication, families need to understand the reason for the test. They will also need explanations about the test results and how they relate to the specific medication that has been prescribed. It is important that all children and adolescents receiving psychotropic medications be closely monitored for responses and side effects. The nurse is integral to the ongoing evaluation of the prescribed therapy (Theoktisto, 2009).

Critical Thinking Application

What questions do you think a family is likely to ask when they learn that a genetic test is recommended before prescribing medication to an adolescent experiencing a mental health disruption such as severe depression? Where will you find the information about pharmacogenetics and pharmacogenomics that will provide necessary background for you and the family? How can pharmacogenetic testing enhance the treatment of individuals by both leading to a therapeutic response in a short time and avoiding serious side effects? What is the nursing role in history taking and in monitoring for the child or adolescent on psychotropic medication?

Mental health is defined in different ways by various cultural groups. For most it is a sense of well-being, peace, and productive use of the mind. In many cultures, care of the "spirit" is believed necessary to promote mental health. An identity with one's community and spiritual wholeness may be promoted by storytelling, singing, and rites of passage. An array of therapies are used to support and restore mental health. Use of certain objects such as herbs may be considered important to preserve mental health. For example, lemon balm and lavender are used by some people to promote relaxation. Other therapies may include healers, family and community support, relaxation or meditation, teas and other nutritional products, and exorcism. Find out how individuals and cultural groups define mental health and how they believe health is maintained. Be alert to learn if mental disorders are viewed as a negative stigma or are openly accepted and discussed. Ask about what the family believes will help to enhance the child's mental health, and integrate these practices into the plan of care whenever it is safe to do so.

Evaluation

Desired outcomes for mental health care depend on the particular condition and the child's situation. Some examples are:

- The child demonstrates the ability to self-restrain compulsive or impulsive behaviors.
- The child successfully adapts to changes in family structure and roles.
- The child verbalizes feelings of productivity and self-worth.
- The family is able to identify and use available social support.
- The child and family demonstrate the ability to draw upon spiritual beliefs for comfort.

■ DEVELOPMENTAL AND BEHAVIORAL DISORDERS

Autistic Spectrum Disorders (or Pervasive Developmental Disorders)

It is estimated that 12–16% of children have a developmental or behavioral disorder. One of the most common sets of disorders is pervasive developmental disorders. **Pervasive developmental disorders (PDDs)** begin in early childhood and are characterized by impaired social interactions and communication, with restricted interests, activities, and behaviors (Centers for Disease Control and Prevention [CDC], 2006a). The disorders are also called autistic spectrum disorders (ASDs) and are classified into five types:

- Autistic disorder
- Asperger syndrome
- Rett disorder
- Childhood disintegrative disorder
- Pervasive developmental disorder not otherwise specified

About 4–12 children in 1,000 have autistic spectrum disorder, and about 1 in 150 children have autistic disorder (commonly called simply autism) (CDC 2007a, 2009a). This incidence represents a large increase from formerly described levels. Before 1985, about 0.4–0.5 children in 1,000 were diagnosed with autistic disorder. It is unclear whether there is a true increase in cases or simply improved techniques in making the diagnosis, as well as an enlarged diagnostic category that includes more children (Johnson, Myers, & Council on Children with Disabilities, 2007). The disorder is more common in males than females. Peak age at diagnosis is 6–11 years, but symptoms often begin at 18–24 months of age (Johnson et al., 2007).

Etiology and Pathophysiology

The etiology of autistic spectrum disorders is unknown. Genetic transmission, immune responses, and neuroanatomy are all being investigated as causes. Neurotransmitters such as dopamine, serotonin, and opioids are abnormal in some children and are a focus of research. Brain size and head circumference may be enlarged in the young child with the disorder, so malfunction of the cortex and connectivity among brain regions may be abnormal (Williams & Minshew, 2007). Fetal alcohol syndrome, fragile X syndrome, phenylketonuria, Down syndrome, and tuberous sclerosis are all associated with a higher-than-normal incidence of autism (Johnson et al., 2007). Advanced parental age, rubella infection in pregnancy, and teratogens have been associated with ASDs. Despite concern expressed in earlier medical and lay press, there has been no demonstrated relationship of either measles-mumps-rubella vaccine or thimerosal (mercury-based preservative in some vaccines) with the incidence of ASDs (see Chapter 16 ∞ for further information on immunizations) (American Academy of Pediatrics, 2010a).

Clinical Manifestations

The essential features typically become apparent by the time a child is 3 years of age. A primary finding is impairment in social interactions. Social interactions are always complex and involve perceptions of the other person as well as social behaviors. The child with autism does not learn the common characteristics of these social interchanges. As a result, the child may be unable to converse normally, may fail to initiate conversations, and may have impaired observations of nonverbal behavior.

Children with autism may manifest disturbances in the rate or sequence of development. These children are unable to relate to people or to respond to social and emotional cues. In addition, they engage in **stereotypy**, or rigid and obsessive behavior. Characteristically these repetitive behaviors in affected children include head banging, twirling in circles, biting themselves, and flapping their hands or arms. Frequently a child's behavior is self-stimulating or self-destructive. Responses to sensory stimuli are frequently abnormal and include an extreme aversion to touch, loud noises, and bright lights. Emotional lability is common (Figure 28–5 ➤).

Communication difficulties or delays in speech and language are common and are often the first symptoms that lead to diagnosis. Absence of babbling and other communication by 1 year, absence of two-word phrases by 2 years, and deterioration of previous language skills are characteristic (Johnson et al., 2007). Children with autism may eventually learn to talk, in some cases well, but their speech is likely to show certain abnormalities: using "you" in place of "I"; engaging in **echolalia** (a compulsive parroting of what is heard); repeating questions rather than

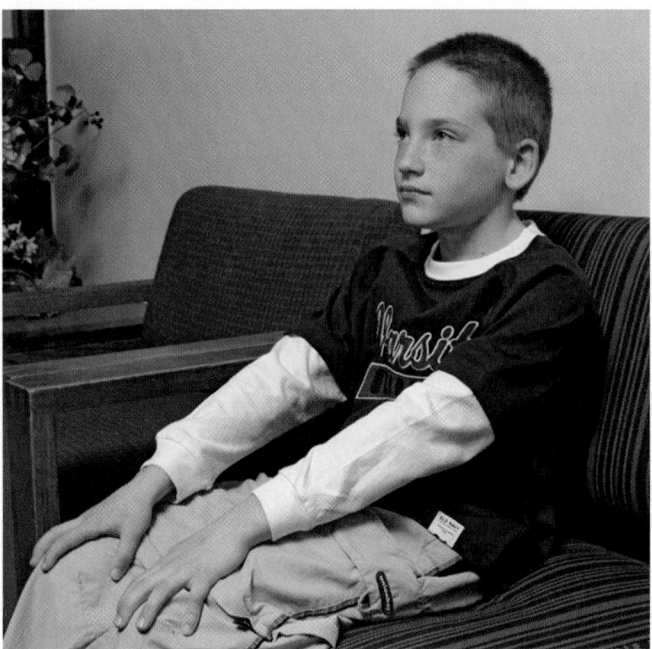

FIGURE 28–5 ➤ This child with autism sits stiffly in the chair and engages in rhythmic rocking behavior. He has a disengaged appearance and does not readily interact with other children or adults who are in his environment.

answering them; and having fascination with rhythmic, repetitive songs and verses.

Behaviors of children with autism show several differences from others. They have great difficulty dealing with new situations, and show agitation and withdrawal when routines are changed. They do not commonly explore objects but have stereotyped behaviors. They may line up objects, play with the same objects over and over, and have certain rituals that must be performed. They often become upset if these normal routines are disrupted. Rituals may involve eating only certain types or colors of foods or eating in specific patterns. Children with autism may manifest disturbances in the rate or sequence of development. They are frequently cognitively impaired but can demonstrate a wide range of intellectual ability and functioning. Cognitive impairment may become manifested early in life by slow developmental progression, particularly in social skills. Some children are impaired in particular areas of development while others are above normal. Head circumference growth is abnormal in some children, mainly in the first year of life (Dawson, Munson, Webb, et al., 2007).

The specific clinical manifestation differences among the types of autistic spectrum disorder are listed in the Clinical Manifestations: Autistic Spectrum Disorders (Pervasive Developmental Disorders) table on the next page.

COLLABORATIVE CARE

The first step in identification of children at risk of ASD is surveillance at each health care visit. Since diagnosis and treatment are often delayed, the American Academy of Pediatrics has identified a multistage process for surveillance and screening:

1. Perform surveillance at early health care visits to identify if a sibling has ASD, parents or other caregivers are concerned about the developmental progression of the child, or the provider notes abnormalities in child behavior.
2. The health care provider determines if the child appears to be at risk for ASD.
3. The health care provider evaluates the risks. If risk exists, the provider administers an age-appropriate and ASD-specific screening tool.
4. If no risk exists, an ASD-specific tool is administered at the 18- and 24-month visits.
5. Select the appropriate screening tool for the age and risk profile of the child.
6. If screening is negative for a child with some risk, provide information to parents and evaluate again in 1 month. If screening is positive, refer for comprehensive ASD evaluation, including audiology, and begin early intervention programs (Johnson et al., 2007).

Several screening tests are available for use in health maintenance visits if autistic disorder is suspected. Additional testing is performed to rule out other causes of the child's behavior. Tests may include neuroimaging (computed tomography [CT] scan or magnetic resonance imaging [MRI]), lead screening, metabolic studies, DNA analysis, and electroencephalogram. Diagnosis is based on the presence of specific criteria, as described in the *DSM-IV-TR*. See Table 28–1 for the autistic disorder and the *DSM-IV-TR* for specific criteria for other autistic syndrome disorders. See Chapters 5 ∞ and 27 ∞ for further descriptions related to assessment of the neurological system.

Early intervention assists in maximizing the child's potential by improving developmental skills and decreasing severity of symptoms, as well as establishing helpful support for parents (Rogers & Vismara, 2008). Treatment centers on teaching children how to focus and learn, managing behavior to reward appropriate behaviors, encouraging positive or adaptive coping skills, and facilitating effective communication. Speech therapy is an essential part of treatment (Weber & Newmark, 2007). The goals of treatment are to reduce rigidity or stereotypy (repetitive, obsessive, machinelike movements) and other maladaptive behaviors. Some children must be physically restrained from aggressive or self-destructive behaviors.

Medications are used with some children to treat associated behavioral disorders but are not effective in treatment of autistic syndrome itself. Medications used for associated conditions may include stimulants, selective serotonin reuptake inhibitors (SSRIs), and mood stabilizers. Some families choose to use complementary therapies to assist their child who has autism.

NURSING MANAGEMENT

Nursing Assessment and Diagnosis

The nurse may encounter the child with autism during routine well-child visits, or when parents seek care for a suspected hearing impairment, speech difficulty, or developmental delay. Early and frequent developmental screening of all children can help in referral for thorough assessment and identification of cases. Par-

Clinical Manifestations

Autistic Spectrum Disorders (Pervasive Developmental Disorders)

Disorder	Clinical Manifestations	Clinical Therapy
Autistic disorder	Impaired social, communicative, and behavioral development, usually noted in the first year of life.	Early intervention is key to maximal performance. Interventions focus on improving behaviors and communication skills, providing physical and occupational therapy, structuring play interactions with other children, and educating parents about the child's needs.
Asperger syndrome	Impaired social interactions with normal language development for age; pitch, tone, and other speech characteristics may be abnormal. Verbal skills involving spelling and vocabulary are high, but concept formation, language flexibility, and comprehension are low. Intellectual functioning may be at a high level, particularly in certain areas, while social skills are limited.	Social interactions are the focus of therapy.
Rett disorder	Early development appears normal and symptoms emerge at 6–18 months. Ataxia, hand-wringing, intermittent hyperventilation, dementia, and growth retardation show progressive increase. Appears only in females and is an X-linked dominant disorder; mutations occur in the gene MeCP2, affecting methyl-CpG-binding protein 2, which is important in brain development.	Early intervention in areas of abnormal behaviors.
Childhood disintegrative disorder	First 2–5 years of development appear normal, followed by deterioration in many areas of functioning. Regression in toileting and other skills may occur. Behaviors finally stabilize at some point without further deterioration.	Focus on areas of developmental function that show abnormality. Individualized education plans are needed in school to deal with communication, play, physical therapy, and teaching management skills to parents.
Pervasive developmental disorder not otherwise specified	Severe social impairment without meeting *DSM* criteria for other types of autistic spectrum disorder.	Behavioral therapy focuses on building social skills.

TABLE 28–1 *DSM-IV-TR* Diagnostic Criteria for Autistic Disorder

A. A total of six or more items from 1, 2, and 3, with at least two from 1, and one each from 2 and 3:
    1. Qualitative impairment in social interaction, as manifested by at least two of the following:
        a. Marked impairment in the use of multiple nonverbal behaviors such as eye-to-eye gaze, facial expression, body posture, and gestures to regulate social interaction
        b. Failure to develop peer relationships appropriate to developmental level
        c. A lack of spontaneous seeking to share enjoyment, interests, or achievements with other people
        d. Lack of social or emotional reciprocity
    2. Qualitative impairments in communication as manifested by at least one of the following:
        a. Delay in, or total lack of, the development of spoken language (not accompanied by an attempt to compensate through alternative modes of communication such as gesture or mime)
        b. In individuals with adequate speech, marked impairment in the ability to initiate or sustain a conversation with others
        c. Stereotyped and repetitive use of language or idiosyncratic language
        d. Lack of varied, spontaneous make-believe play or social imitative play appropriate to developmental level
    3. Restricted repetitive and stereotyped patterns of behavior, interests, and activities, as manifested by at least one of the following:
        a. Encompassing preoccupation with one or more stereotyped and restricted patterns of interest that is abnormal either in intensity or in focus
        b. Apparently inflexible adherence to specific, nonfunctional routines or rituals
        c. Stereotyped and repetitive motor mannerisms (e.g., hand or finger flapping or twisting, or complex whole-body movements)
        d. Persistent preoccupation with parts of objects
B. Delays or abnormal functioning in at least one of the following areas, with onset prior to age 3 years:
    (1) social interaction, (2) language as used in social communication, or (3) symbolic or imaginative play.
C. The disturbance is not better accounted for by Rett's syndrome or childhood disintegrative disorder.

Reprinted with permission from the Diagnostic and Statistical Manual of Mental Disorders, *Fourth Edition, Text Revision. Copyright © 2000 American Psychiatric Association.*

Complementary Therapy
Autism Treatments

Some parents who have a child with autism choose to use complementary and alternative medicine (CAM). A popular treatment approach includes dietary therapy with vitamin A, vitamin C, vitamin B$_6$, magnesium, omega-3 fatty acids, and use of gluten-free or casein-free diets. Complementary drug therapy includes secretin, a pancreatic gastrointestinal peptide, and Pepcid or other antacids. Some parents believe that detoxification by limiting certain dietary intake or using Epsom salt baths can be helpful. Music therapy has been used to improve social interactions, and massage to enhance response to touch and communication. Additional therapies include homeopathy, craniosacral therapy, Reiki, hyperbaric chambers, and biofeedback. Chelation therapy is not approved but has been used by some physicians and families as a treatment for autism. The rationale is that autism is related to collection of heavy metals such as mercury in the body. Chelation is a treatment with serious potential side effects (see Chapter 17 ∞ for further information about chelation for treatment of lead poisoning). The report of a death of a young boy being treated for autism with chelation reinforces the danger of using untested therapies (Beauchamp, Willis, Betz, et al., 2006; CDC, 2010a; Weber & Newmark, 2007).

Nurses can help parents to evaluate studies on complementary care and encourage them to initiate only one treatment at a time to measure any effectiveness seen. Ask about therapies being used and discuss safeguards to avoid any undesired side effects. Read about new studies on complementary therapies and evaluate the rationale, efficacy, side effects, and other pertinent information in order to assist families.

---

ents may report abnormal interaction such as lack of eye contact, disinterest in cuddling, minimal facial responsiveness, and failure to talk. Be alert to parental observations that the baby or young child does not look at them or provide other developmental or behavioral cues.

Nursing Alert

"Red flags" that should be recognized as characteristic of autism include no babbling or communication gestures by 12 months, no single words by 16 months, no spontaneous two-word phrases by 24 months, and loss of language or social skill previously achieved (Johnson et al., 2007).

Assessment at every health care visit focuses on language development, response to others, and hearing acuity (see Chapters 5 and 19 ∞).

Carefully evaluate the child for history of developmental milestones and refer for abnormalities. Perform developmental screening that considers several areas of development including motor activity, social skills, and language. Recall that the child may have normal performance in one area such as motor skills and delayed development in another area such as language skills. Likewise, language may be normal for age but social interactions may be quite delayed. Include questioning about adaptive skills such as toilet training and feeding patterns. Inquire about school performance since some areas may be normal while others are delayed. Observe the child in play situations and evaluate the use of creative and exploratory play versus more repetitive patterns.

Perform hearing and vision screening if possible to rule out sensory problems.

When a child with a diagnosis of autistic disorder is hospitalized for a concurrent problem, obtain a history from the parents regarding the child's routines, rituals, and likes and dislikes, as well as ways to promote interaction and cooperation. The child may carry a special toy or object to play with during times of stress. Ask about the child's behaviors as well as observing them on admission. Obtain a history of acute and chronic illnesses and injuries. Ask about eating patterns and food restrictions. Inquire about CAM in a nonjudgmental and supportive manner.

Nursing diagnoses must be tailored to fit the individual needs of the child. Examples of diagnoses that may be appropriate for children with autistic syndromes include the following:

- Impaired Verbal Communication related to altered perceptions
- Impaired Social Interaction related to developmental disability
- Disturbed Thought Processes related to mental disorder
- Risk for Injury related to cognitive impairment
- Risk for Caregiver Role Strain related to chronicity and demands of child's condition
- Disabled Family Coping: Compromised related to having a child with prolonged disability

Planning and Implementation

Nursing care focuses on stabilizing environmental stimuli, providing supportive care, enhancing communication, maintaining a safe environment, giving the parents anticipatory guidance, and providing emotional support.

Stabilize Environmental Stimuli

Children with autism interpret and respond to the environment differently from other individuals. Sounds that are not distressing to the average person may be interpreted by children with autism as louder, more frightening, and overwhelming. The child needs to be oriented to new settings such as a classroom or the hospital room and may adjust best to a small classroom or a hospital room with only one other child. Encourage parents to bring the child's favorite objects from home, and try to keep these objects in the same places, because the child does not cope well with changes in the environment.

Provide Supportive Care

Developing a trusting relationship with the child who has autism is often difficult. Adjust communication techniques and teaching to the child's developmental level. Ask parents about the child's usual home routines, and maintain these routines as much as possible when the child is out of the home. Because self-care abilities are often limited, the child may need assistance to meet basic needs. School programs and individualized education plans (see Chapter 10 ∞) can help the child to learn self-care skills. When possible, schedule daily care and routine procedures at consistent times to maintain predictability. Encourage parents to remain with the hospitalized child and to participate in daily care planning. Parents are integral parts of the treatment team when the child's learning goals are established in early intervention or school programs. Identify rituals for naptime and bedtime, and maintain them to promote rest and sleep. Integrate patterns that facilitate intake of nutritious foods at mealtimes.

Enhance Communication

Because children with autism have impaired communication, nursing care focuses on utilizing and improving communication with the child. Speech is used when possible; short, direct sentences are most effective. If the child responds well to visual cues, then pictures, computers, and other visual aids may form an important part of interaction. Sign language is used with some children.

Maintain a Safe Environment

Monitor children with autism at all times, including bathtime and bedtime. Close supervision is needed to ensure that the child does not obtain any harmful objects or engage in dangerous behaviors. For the child who engages in head banging or other abusive behaviors, bicycle helmets and hand mitts can be the least restrictive method to provide safety. They enable the child to participate in activities and engage in a social environment to the degree possible.

Provide Anticipatory Guidance

Approximately half of all children with autistic disorder require lifelong supervision and support, especially if the disorder is accompanied by intellectual disability (Johnson et al., 2007). Some children may grow up to lead independent lives, although they will have social limitations with impaired interpersonal relationships. Encourage parents to promote the child's development through behavior modification and specialized educational programs. The overall goal is to provide the child with the guidance, education, and support necessary for optimal functioning.

Care in the Community

Families need support to cope with the challenges of caring for the child with autism. Help them to identify resources for childcare, such as special toddler programs and preschools, and parent support groups. They may need specialized transportation services for the child or other social supports. The child will need an individualized education and health plan; the school nurse is instrumental in team management to establish these plans (Lobar, Fritts, Arbide, et al., 2008). The parent or primary caretaker often has difficulty obtaining respite care and may need assistance to find suitable resources. Siblings of the child with autism may need help to explain the disorder to their friends or teachers.

Genetic counseling should be offered to the family. Information on immunizations is necessary, because parents may have heard about a potential connection between immunization and the disorder. They should be encouraged to have the child immunized on the recommended schedule. Parents may have questions about where to find information on complementary and alternative therapies.

Parents can also be referred to the Autism Society of America, the American Academy of Pediatrics, and the Centers for Disease Control and Prevention for information.

Evaluation

Expected outcomes of nursing care for the child with autism are for the child to demonstrate performance of self-care to maximum potential, consistent developmental progression, and communication strategies that enable socialization. The family should demonstrate successful management of the child's symptoms and maintain a safe environment.

Attention Deficit Disorder and Attention Deficit Hyperactivity Disorder

Attention deficit disorder (ADD) is a variation in central nervous system processing characterized by developmentally inappropriate behaviors involving inattention. When hyperactivity and impulsivity accompany inattention, the disorder is called attention deficit hyperactivity disorder (ADHD). The latter is the more common condition and affects from 6–9% of all school-age children (Froehlich, Lanphear, Epstein, et al., 2007). Boys are affected almost four times more often than girls. The condition also affects adolescents and adults. Children with the disorder often continue to manifest at least some of the symptoms as they grow into adulthood.

Etiology and Pathophysiology

Although a variety of physical and neurologic disorders are associated with ADHD, children with identifiable causes represent a small proportion of this population. Examples of known associations include exposure to high levels of lead or mercury in childhood, severe nutritional deficiencies, and prenatal exposure to alcohol or tobacco smoke (American Academy of Pediatrics, 2010b). Other prenatal factors associated with a higher incidence of ADHD include preterm labor, impaired placenta functioning, and impaired oxygenation. Seizures and serious head injury are other potential associations. Genetic factors may be important, as well as family dynamics and environmental characteristics. ADHD occurs more commonly within families, and investigations are ongoing to identify candidate genes. It is likely that gene-environment interactions are implicated in the condition (Plomp, Van Engeland, & Durston, 2009; Wallis, Russell, & Muenke, 2008).

The pathophysiology of ADD/ADHD is not totally understood. However, some children exhibit a deficit in the catecholamines dopamine and norepinephrine, lowering the threshold for stimuli input. The disorder is marked by brain maturation delay in the areas of self-regulation. Increased input from stimuli and decreased self-regulation cause the hallmark inability to inhibit stimuli and motor activity. Slow brain maturity has been demonstrated on imaging studies. The cortex is particularly affected and may explain the school and concentration challenges of the condition (National Institutes of Health, 2007).

Clinical Manifestations

Children with ADD and ADHD have problems related to decreased attention span, impulsiveness, or increased motor activity (Figure 28–6 ➤). Symptoms can range from mild to severe. The child has difficulty completing tasks, fidgets constantly, is frequently loud, and interrupts others. Sleep disturbances are

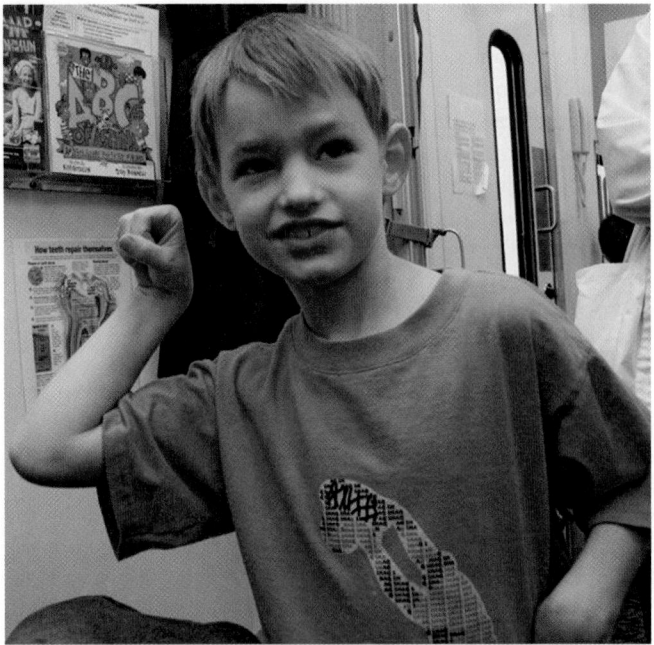

FIGURE 28–6 ➤ This child with ADHD was challenged by a visit to a health care facility for dental care. He found it difficult to remain in the chair for the examination, and once it was over, he rapidly ran from one piece of equipment to another in the facility. He asked what things were for but did not wait for answers. His engaging personality emerged as he posed briefly for a picture. Such behaviors can be exhausting for parents to manage and may create safety hazards in the health care setting.

common. Because of these behaviors, the child often has difficulty developing and maintaining social relationships and may be shunned or teased by other children.

Typically, girls with ADHD show less aggression and impulsiveness than boys, but far more anxiety, mood swings, social withdrawal, rejection, and cognitive and language problems. Girls tend to be older at the time of diagnosis. Children are frequently diagnosed with the disorder soon after beginning school, when demands increase for attentive behavior.

COLLABORATIVE CARE

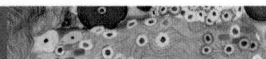

Diagnostic Tests

Diagnosis begins with a careful history of the child, including family history, birth history, growth and developmental milestones, behaviors such as sleep and eating patterns, progression and patterns in school, social and environmental conditions, and reports from parents and teachers. A physical examination should be performed to rule out neurological diseases and other health problems. The mental health specialist then tests the child and administers questionnaires to the parent and teacher. It is important to identify other conditions that may either mimic as ADD/ADHD or exist in conjunction with the disorders. These might include depression, anxiety, learning disorder, conduct disorder, or oppositional defiant disorder.

Children are usually brought for evaluation when behaviors escalate to the point of interfering with the daily functioning of

teachers or parents. When children have learning disabilities or anxiety disorders, the problem is commonly misdiagnosed as ADHD without further evaluation of the child's symptoms. Obtaining an accurate diagnosis by a pediatric mental health specialist is vital. Specific diagnostic criteria (Table 28–2) must be applied to all children with the potential diagnosis of ADD or ADHD. Behaviors both at home and at school or childcare must be evaluated, because abnormal patterns in two settings are needed for diagnosis. The diagnosis of ADD may be difficult due to the absence of hyperactivity behaviors. A variety of tests are available for use by the trained professional in establishing the diagnosis (Table 28–3).

Clinical Therapy

Based on the findings, desired outcomes are established for the child's performance and management of the disorder. Treatment is established to meet the desired behavioral outcomes, and includes a combination of approaches, such as environmental changes, behavior therapy, and pharmacotherapy. It is expected that treatment will be long term.

Children often benefit from environmental changes. Decreasing stimulation, for example, by turning off television, keeping the environment quiet, and maintaining an orderly and clutter-free desk or study area without distraction, may help the child to stay focused on the task at hand. Another relatively simple change is appropriate classroom placement, preferably in a small class with a teacher who can provide close supervision and a structured daily routine. Consistent limits and expectations should be set for the child. Children living in chaotic homes and communities may function better if the environment can be simplified. When aggressive behaviors occur, therapeutic approaches such as play and group therapy may be useful.

Behavior therapy involves rewarding the child for desired behaviors and applying consequences for undesirable behaviors. Children may be rewarded by praise or earn points toward a movie or other desired outing for staying seated during meals or quietly listening in a classroom. Cues are established so that a child can subtly be reminded when impulsive or hyperactive behaviors are escalating. All adults who are in close contact with the child, such as parents and teachers, must be informed and involved in the established behavioral program.

Children with moderate to severe ADD/ADHD are frequently treated with pharmacotherapy. Methylphenidate (Ritalin, Concerta) is most often prescribed, with alternatives of dextroamphetamine (Dexedrine or Adderall) and the nonstimulant medication atomoxetine. A skin patch that releases medication over a 9-hour period is available, facilitating ease of administration (May & Kratochvil, 2010).

Guidelines have been issued that recommend thorough evaluation of children before a stimulant or other medication is prescribed, in order to rule out any cardiac condition that could be affected by medication use. They include:

- Patient and family history of conditions associated with sudden cardiac death
- All medications and health supplements

TABLE 28–2	*DSM-IV-TR* Diagnostic Criteria for Attention Deficit Hyperactivity Disorder

A. Either 1 or 2:

    1. Inattention: Six (or more) of the following symptoms of inattention have persisted for at least 6 months to a degree that is maladaptive and inconsistent with developmental level:

        a. Often fails to give close attention to details or makes careless mistakes in school work, work, and other activities

        b. Often has difficulty sustaining attention in tasks or play activities

        c. Often does not seem to listen when spoken to directly

        d. Often does not follow through on instructions and fails to finish school work, chores, or duties in the workplace (not due to oppositional behavior or failure to understand instructions)

        e. Often has difficulty organizing tasks and activities

        f. Often avoids, dislikes, or is reluctant to engage in tasks that require sustained mental effort (such as school work or homework)

        g. Often loses things necessary for tasks or activities (e.g., toys, school assignments, pencils, books, or tools)

        h. Is often easily distracted by extraneous stimuli

        i. Is often forgetful in daily activities

    2. Hyperactivity-impulsivity: Six (or more) of the following symptoms of hyperactivity-impulsivity have persisted for at least 6 months to a degree that is maladaptive and inconsistent with developmental level:

Hyperactivity

        a. Often fidgets with hands or feet or squirms in seat

        b. Often leaves seat in classroom or in other situations in which remaining seated is expected

        c. Often runs about or climbs excessively in situations in which it is inappropriate (in adolescents or adults, may be limited to subjective feelings of restlessness)

        d. Often has difficulty playing or engaging in leisure activities quietly

        e. Is often "on the go" or acts as if "driven by a motor"

        f. Often talks excessively

Impulsivity

        g. Often blurts out answers before questions have been completed

        h. Often has difficulty awaiting turn

        i. Often interrupts or intrudes on others (e.g., butts into conversations or games)

B. Some hyperactive-impulsive or inattentive symptoms that caused impairment were present before age 7 years.

C. Some impairment from the symptoms is present in two or more settings (e.g., at school [or work] and at home).

D. There must be clear evidence of clinically significant impairment in social, academic, or occupational functioning.

E. The symptoms do not occur exclusively during the course of a pervasive developmental disorder, schizophrenia, or other psychotic disorder and are not better accounted for by another mental disorder (e.g., mood disorder, anxiety disorder, dissociative disorder, or a personality disorder).

Reprinted with permission from the Diagnostic and Statistical Manual of Mental Disorders, *Fourth Edition, Text Revision. Copyright © 2000 American Psychiatric Association.*

TABLE 28–3	Screening Tests for ADD/ADHD

Test	Source
Vanderbilt Parent and Teacher Scales	Wolraich, M. L. (1998). *Journal of Abnormal Child Psychology, 26,* 141; Wolraich, M. L. (2003). *Journal of Pediatric Psychology, 28,* 559.
Connors' Parent and Teacher Rating Scales—Revised—Long Form	Connors, C. K. (1998). *Journal of Abnormal Child Psychology, 26,* 257, 279.
Swanson, Nolan, and Pelham Questionnaire II Teacher and Parent Rating Scale (SNAP-IV)	Swanson, J. M. (1992). *School-based assessments and interventions for ADD students.* Irvine, CA: KC Publications.
Disruptive Behavior Disorder Scale	Pelham, W. E. (1992). *Journal of the American Academy of Child and Adolescent Psychiatry, 31,* 210.
ADHD Rating Scale	DuPaul, G. J. (1991). *American Academy of Child and Adolescent Psychiatry, 20,* 245.
Revised Behavioral Problems Checklist	Quay, H. C., & Peterson, D. R. (1987). *Manual for the Revised Behavioral Problem Checklist.* Coral Gables, FL: University of Miami.

Data from: Brown, R. T., Amler, R. W., Freeman, W. S., et al. (2005). Treatment of attention-deficit/hyperactivity disorder: Overview of the evidence. Pediatrics, 115, *749–757; Vierhile, A., Robb, A., & Ryan-Krause, P. (2009). Attention-deficit hyperactivity disorder in children and adolescents: Closing diagnostic, communication, and treatment gaps.* Journal of Pediatric Health Care, 23(1S), S5–S19.

Medications Used to Treat
ADHD

Medication	Action and Indication	Nursing Implications
Methylphenidate	A derivative of piperidine that acts like amphetamine. May work in ADHD treatment by enhancing catecholamine effects in the nervous system, improving attention span and task performance. Schedule II drug in Schedule of Controlled Substances.	Available in short-acting forms as Ritalin, Methylin, and Focalin. Also in intermediate-acting forms of Ritalin SR, Metadate ER, and Methylin ER. Available in long-acting forms of Concerta, Metadate CD, and Ritalin LA. Transdermal 9-hour patches are also available.
		The variety of available forms makes it important to read labels carefully and inform families about proper administration of the child's specific type of drug. Periodic growth measurements are needed. Behavior and school performance are monitored.
Amphetamine preparations	Synthetic sympathomimetic amine with stimulant effect on CNS. Increases release of norepinephrine and dopamine by blocking their reuptake. Schedule II drug in Schedule of Controlled Substances.	Available in short-acting forms of Dexedrine, DextroStat, and Adderall. Intermediate-acting forms include Adderall and Dexedrine Spansules. A long-acting form is Adderall-XR. Read labels and instruct in proper administration. Monitor vital signs and growth measurements periodically.
Atomoxetine	This is the first nonstimulant drug for treatment of ADHD. It inhibits norepinephrine reuptake, decreases hyperactivity and impulsivity of ADHD, and may assist with improving mood and decreasing anxiety.	Available in capsules at a variety of dosages. Recommended starting dose for children is 0.5 mg/kg/day. Has been shown to have long-lasting effect of 1 day or longer. Side effects are uncommon and transient, with dyspepsia or vomiting, fatigue, decreased appetite, and dizziness most common. Have the child change position slowly if dizziness occurs; caution teen not to drive until effects of drug are clear. Perform periodic growth measurements.

Adapted from Ganem, 2008.

- Physical examination, especially of the cardiovascular system
- Electrocardiogram
- Pediatric cardiology consult if any abnormalities are identified

(Vetter, Elia, Erickson, et al., 2008)

See Medications Used to Treat ADHD.

A variety of other treatments have been attempted for ADHD, and are commonly used by families. Chiropractic manipulation,

Complementary Therapy
ADD and ADHD

A variety of complementary approaches, in addition to or instead of traditional behavioral therapy and medication, have been tried in children with ADD or ADHD. Chiropractic manipulation, biofeedback, visual or auditory therapy, and dietary interventions have been used. Dietary therapies include elimination of dietary components such as highly processed foods, sugar, aspartame, or yeast; use of supplements such as omega-3 or omega-6 fatty acids, iron, magnesium, zinc, and vitamin B_6; and herbs such as Pycnogenol, melatonin, echinacea, St. John's wort, and ginkgo biloba. Ask parents about alternative therapies used and investigate what is known about them in order to share this information with parents (Brulotte, Bukutu, & Vohra, 2009; Rucklidge, Johnstone, & Kaplan, 2009).

biofeedback, and dietary interventions (both elimination diets and supplement use) are examples of common complementary or alternative therapies.

Although ADHD was once thought to be a disorder of childhood that gradually improved with age, it is now believed that symptoms continue into adulthood and that careful management in childhood assists in lessening problems of social functioning later in life.

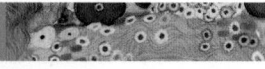

NURSING MANAGEMENT

Nursing Assessment and Diagnosis

The nurse often encounters the family who is concerned about the child's behavior before a diagnosis has been made. Ask about family and birth history and have the parents describe the child's behaviors. Perform developmental testing and look specifically for attention span and physical activity. Refer the family to their pediatric health care home for further assessment. A complete patient and family history, physical examination, and electrocardiogram are needed prior to beginning medication (Vetter et al., 2008).

The nurse may encounter the child with ADHD in the hospital when parents bring the child for treatment of an injury (e.g., fracture) or other problem. Explore the parent's report of the child's attention span in detail. Usually within a few minutes in an unstructured setting or waiting area, the child with ADHD becomes restless and searches for distraction. Gather information about the child's activity level and impulsiveness. Be alert for information that reveals a serious problem, such as hurting animals or other children. Obtain information about distractibility, attention deficit in activities of daily living, characteristic ways of reacting, and the extent of impulsiveness when the child is receiving medication. Find out how the family manages at home and what treatments are being applied.

Examples of nursing diagnoses that may be appropriate for a child with ADHD include the following:

- Impaired Verbal Communication related to altered perceptions
- Impaired Social Interaction related to chronic episodes of impulsive behavior
- Chronic Low Self-Esteem related to behaviors associated with ADD/ADHD
- Risk for Injury related to high level of impulsiveness and excitability
- Risk for Caregiver Role Strain related to management of the child with unpredictable moods and high energy

Planning and Implementation

Prevention of symptoms of ADHD can focus on limiting television exposure for young children and encouraging daily vigorous physical activity for all children.

Nursing care of the hospitalized child with ADD/ADHD focuses on administering medications, managing the child's environment, implementing behavioral management plans, providing emotional support to the child and family, promoting self-esteem, and ensuring ongoing care. Care in the community includes the same components along with guiding parents to appropriate resources when needed.

Administer Medications

Stimulant and nonstimulant medications increase the child's attention span and decrease distractibility. Be alert for the common side effects of these medications, including anorexia, insomnia, and tachycardia. Administering medication early in the day helps to alleviate insomnia. Anorexia can be managed by giving medication at mealtimes. Baseline cardiac examinations are needed, as well as periodic reevaluation. Careful monitoring of weight, height, and blood pressure is necessary. Instruct families about the abuse potential of stimulant drugs and teach them to keep the medications locked and to administer them only as directed.

Minimize Environmental Distractions

The child may need to be placed in an environment with minimal distractions. When hospitalized, this may mean a room with only one other child. Potentially harmful equipment should be kept out of reach. Television and video game time needs to be monitored and limited. Use shades to darken the room during naps or at bedtime and minimize noise. Teach parents to minimize distractions at home during periods when the

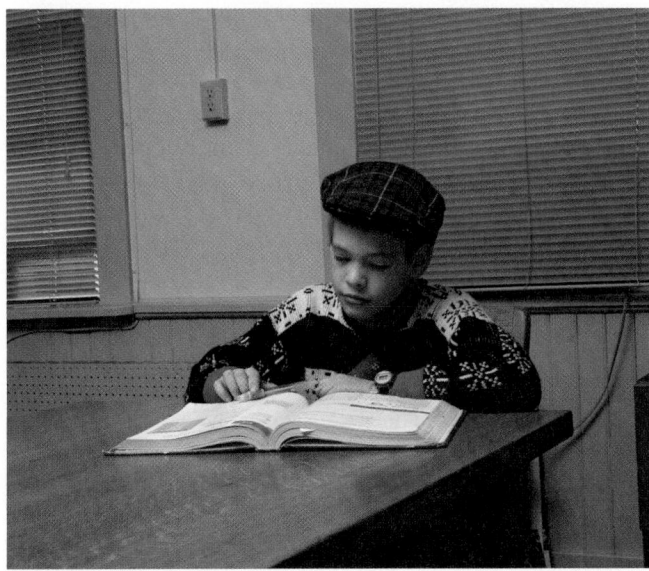

FIGURE 28–7 ➤ Managing the environment to provide quiet places with minimal distractions is often necessary for the child with ADHD. This boy reads and does homework in a room with few pictures, no music, and only the book with homework on the table. He is also assisted by structure such as a scheduled time for homework, with short breaks to walk around every 10–15 minutes.

child needs to concentrate; for example, when doing school work (Figure 28–7 ➤). Visits to areas such as shopping malls and playgrounds may need to be limited. Plenty of daily exercise and minimal use of television/video games may assist the child in being able to concentrate when needed for school and other tasks.

Implement Behavioral Management Plans

Behavior modification programs can help to reduce specific impulsive behaviors—for example, setting up a reward program for the child who has taken medication as ordered or completed a homework assignment. The rewards may be daily as well as weekly or monthly, depending on the child's age. For example, one completed homework assignment might be rewarded with 30 minutes of basketball or a bike ride; assignments completed for a week might be rewarded with participation in an activity of the child's choice on the weekend.

If punishment is necessary, the behavior should be corrected while simultaneously supporting the child as a person. Punishment is generally withdrawal of a privilege, and should follow the offense quickly because the child may not otherwise connect the punishment with the behavior.

Provide Emotional Support

Children with ADD/ADHD offer a special challenge to parents, teachers, and health care providers. Parents must cope simultaneously with managing the difficult needs and demands of a child who is hard to handle, obtaining appropriate evaluation and treatment, and understanding and accepting the diagnosis, even when the child exhibits different behaviors with different people. Family support is essential. Educate both the parents and the child about the importance of appropriate expectations and consequences of behaviors. Teach skills that will help as the child grows older: making lists of tasks to accomplish; having routines for eating, sleeping, recreation, and school work; minimizing stimuli in the environment when completing work; and asking teachers and friends to identify when behavior is inappropriate. When the child is hospitalized for another condition, the time may provide a brief respite from constant care by the parent. The activity, impulsivity, and general high energy of children with ADHD can fatigue parents. They may wish to spend a few hours each day at home or a nearby residence for families when the child is hospitalized. Ask them how they manage at home and offer ideas for respite care.

Promote Self-Esteem

Help the child to understand the disorder at an appropriate developmental level, and facilitate a trusting relationship with health care providers. Assist the child with social skills through the use of role-play, small-group play, and modeling. Promote the child's self-esteem by emphasizing the positive aspects of behavior and treating instances of negative behavior as learning opportunities. Help the child to develop ego strengths (the conscious ability to screen outside stimuli and to control internal demands), which will result in better impulse control and thus increase self-esteem over time. Encourage skills at which the child excels and consider the use of support groups for children in school. Praise the hospitalized child for lying still for a procedure, taking a medication on time, or helping a staff member to carry toys around to other children.

Care in the Community

Most children with ADD/ADHD are only hospitalized when needing care for another condition. Parents need support to understand the diagnosis and to learn how to manage the child. Explain the diagnosis and what is known about attention deficit disorders. Provide written materials, Internet sites, and an opportunity to ask questions.

Emphasize the importance of a stable environment, at home as well as at school. At home, the child may have difficulty staying on task. Parents need to consider the child's age and developmental appropriateness of tasks, give clear and simple instructions, and provide frequent reminders to ensure completion. Routines in the evening can promote good sleep patterns.

The nurse can serve as a liaison to teachers and school personnel, or as the case manager for the child. An individualized education plan may be needed (see Chapter 10 ∞), with clear

expected outcomes stated for the child's behaviors. Individualized education plans or periods of instruction free from the distractions of the entire class may enable the child to improve school performance. Parents may have difficulty understanding the need for these approaches because the child often tests with above-average intelligence. Reinforce the importance of providing a structured environment free from unnecessary external stimuli. Be sure that parents understand behavioral approaches that will help the child, how to administer prescribed medications, and the importance of returning for health care visits to monitor for side effects. Medication should be locked safely away at home to keep it away from other children and prevent illegal use of this controlled substance. An individualized school health plan may be needed for medication management. See Families Want to Know: School Suggestions for Children with ADD/ADHD.

Parents may have heard about ADD/ADHD in the media and can have many questions about its cause and management. Providing information about complementary and alternative treatments is a nursing role. The National Institutes of Health sponsors the National Center for Complementary and Alternative Medicine (NCCAM) and is a reliable source for parents and professionals.

Families Want to Know
School Suggestions for Children with ADD/ADHD

Parents can work with teachers to provide for a school environment that fosters attention and learning. Some ideas that may be helpful include:

- Have the child sit near the front of the class.
- Plan a reminder that is apparent to the teacher and student but not to other children when the child needs to concentrate on attention. This might be an object placed on the student's desk or a light hand placed on the shoulder or arm.
- Give instructions orally and in written form and repeat them more than once.
- Provide opportunities to take notes. Make lists of assignments and mark them off when accomplished. Have a planned time to go through the child's backpack daily so notices are seen and homework is completed and in a uniform location.
- Use computers for making lists and taking notes. The child may need to listen in class, record the teacher, and take notes later from the recording.
- If the child has well-developed fine or gross motor skills, integrate motor movement into learning situations whenever possible.
- Provide quiet places with minimal distraction for examinations. Offer additional time.
- Allow time for organizing clothing, the child's desk, and other areas.
- Go over assignments and tests with the child in person to explain areas that are understood and those that need attention.
- Find the child's areas of excellence and allow for performance in these ways. Some children are talented in dance, others in art or extemporaneous speech.
- Never call the child names, make fun of behavior or performance, or call him or her "hyperactive" in front of other children, teachers, or parents.

Culture *Mental Health and Stigma*

Many families who have a child with ADHD or another mental health disorder are embarrassed and feel shame because of the diagnosis, especially in certain cultural groups, and in very structured and highly achieving families. When taking histories from family members, it is best to be sensitive to the stigma some may feel. Ask questions in a private setting and ask about the family's feelings regarding a mental health disorder. Is there someone in their family who they can talk to about the diagnosis? Provide information in a nonjudgmental manner and provide support if appropriate from other families with similar experiences.

As the child grows older, provide explanations about the disorder and information about techniques that will assist in dealing with problems. Emphasize the importance of doing homework or other tasks requiring concentration in a quiet environment without background noise from a television or radio. Encourage children with ADHD to keep assignment notebooks and use checklists to help them accomplish specific tasks.

Evaluation

Expected outcomes of nursing care for the child with ADD or ADHD include the following:

- Parents and child demonstrate understanding of the disorder.
- The family accurately and safely manages medication administration.
- The child demonstrates an increase in attentiveness and decrease in hyperactivity, impulsivity, and sleep disturbance.
- The child displays formation of a positive self-image.
- The child manifests formation of healthy social interactions with peers and family.
- The child achieves educational performance to maximum potential.

■ MOOD DISORDERS

Depression

Depression is psychological distress of body, mood, and thoughts that can range from mild to severe. Only in recent years has depression in children been recognized as a clinical condition. Many children referred to child guidance centers and mental health professionals because of behavioral difficulties or poor achievement actually suffer from depression. The incidence of major depression is estimated to be about 3% in childhood and about 14% in adolescence, with 3–8% of adolescents experiencing major depressive disorder (Hamrin & Magorno, 2010). A history of substance abuse and anxiety disorder increases risk. Family stress and experiencing abuse also increase risk, and cultural variations in rates exist (Hamrin & Magorno, 2010).

Growth & Development *Symptoms of Depression*

Symptoms of depression in children vary according to their developmental levels. *Infants* may fail to eat and grow, while *toddlers* may show regressive behaviors in toileting and other activities. *Preschoolers* have less symbolic and other play activities, and demonstrate self-destructive play themes. They may whine and show irritability, show disinterest, and lack confidence. *School-age children* may show a decrease in academic performance, increased or decreased activity, somatic complaints, and loss of friends. The older school-age child may talk of running away or show signs of boredom and low self-esteem. *Adolescents* can have a wide array of symptoms such as anxiety, decreased social contact, poor school performance, lack of prior involvement in activities, poor self-care, sleep and eating disturbances, difficulty with parents and teachers, suicidal thoughts, or focus on violence. Sadness and **anhedonia** (inability to experience pleasure) are common at all ages (National Institute of Mental Health, 2010).

Etiology and Pathophysiology

Theories have been proposed to explain the cause of depression in children and adolescents. Depression may be biologic in origin or a result of learned helplessness, cognitive distortion, social skills deficit, or family dysfunction. The physiological theory focuses on monoamine neurotransmission. These amines include indolamine, serotonin, norepinephrine, and dopamine; decreased levels are sometimes found in depression. Magnetic resonance imaging has suggested brain changes in individuals who are depressed, which may indicate a biological basis (National Institute of Mental Health, 2009).

Parental depression is a strong predictor of childhood depression. Abuse and neglect, family conflict, parental death, and low socioeconomic status predispose children to depression. Other psychiatric diagnoses are common in children with depression; these include conditions such as ADHD, anxiety disorder, bipolar disease, or substance abuse (Lack & Green, 2009).

Clinical Manifestations

Characteristic findings of major depression in children and adolescents include declining school performance; withdrawal from social activities; sleep disturbance (either too much or too little); appetite disturbance (too much or too little); multiple somatic complaints, especially headaches and stomachaches; decreased energy; difficulty concentrating and making decisions; low self-esteem; and feelings of hopelessness. There is much variation among children at different ages in the symptoms displayed, and they often have some but not all of the major criteria. Symptoms vary according to children's developmental levels.

COLLABORATIVE CARE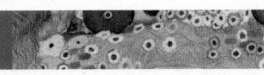

All children should be screened for depression (U.S. Preventive Services Task Force, 2009). Once depression or major depressive disorder is diagnosed, comprehensive assessment of the child should occur, in order to rule out physical illness that can be linked to depressive symptoms. These may include diabetes, cancer, obesity, and some other conditions (U.S. Preventive Services

Task Force, 2009). Initial psychiatric assessment is performed by a child psychologist or child psychiatrist. A variety of scales and techniques are used; however, little guidance is available relating to evaluation of children under 6 years of age. Examples of useful tools are the Children's Depression Inventory (Revised) (CDI), the Revised Children's Manifest Anxiety Scale, the Beck Depression Inventory, the Preschool Feelings Checklist, the Reynolds Child Depression Scale, the Reynolds Adolescent Depression Scale, the Patient Health Questionnaire-Adolescent Version (PHQ-A), the Guideline for Adolescent Preventative Services Questionnaire, the Hopelessness Scale for Children, and the Center of Epidemiologic Studies Depression Scale for Children (CES-D). The child is assessed for various mental health problems since comorbidities or combination with other disorders is common (Garzon, 2007; Hamrin & Magorno, 2010).

Treatment may include psychotherapy and psychotropic medication, a combination that is more effective than either approach alone (Cheung, Zuckerbrot, Jensen, et al., 2007). Often a combination of individual, family, and group therapy provides the greatest benefits for young children and adolescents. Involving parents, other family members, school personnel, and friends in the treatment plan is essential. Group therapy is an effective treatment measure for adolescents because of the importance of peer group relationships during the teenage years. Cognitive behavioral therapy (CBT) may be used with adolescents, and play therapy may be used with younger children. CBT focuses on thoughts and behaviors, leading to understanding of negative thoughts and increasing activities that provide pleasure (Cheung et al., 2007; Zuckerbrot, Cheung, Jensen, et al., 2007). Supportive interactions with health care providers and active problem solving are approaches that improve outcomes in adolescents.

Antidepressant medications, most commonly the selective serotonin reuptake inhibitors (SSRIs); tricyclic antidepressants (TCAs) such as imipramine (Tofranil) and desipramine (Norpramin); and amitriptyline (Elavil) may be prescribed. The only antidepressant approved to treat major depressive disorders in pediatric patients is fluoxetine HCl (Prozac), but others are used by clinicians when the child does not respond to Prozac. See Medications Used to Treat Depression below.

Nursing Alert

Sudden cardiac death has occurred in several children on tricyclic antidepressants (TCAs). Because of this risk, serum levels should be monitored and electrocardiograms (ECGs) are performed. Specific ECG changes along with a resting heart rate above 100, systolic blood pressure above 130 mmHg, and diastolic blood pressure above 85 mmHg necessitate immediate report to the prescriber. A narrow margin exists between the therapeutic and lethal dose in children. Additionally, TCAs have not shown efficacy in treating depression in children, and so the risk outweighs the benefit (Hirsch & Carlson, 2007).

The SSRIs act to block reuptake of serotonin in the synapse, so that serotonin levels (which influence mood) increase. Although the SSRIs are generally considered safer than some other types of antidepressants, their use in children has been limited, so side effects must be monitored. The major serious side effect of the SSRIs is serotonin syndrome, a condition characterized by agitation, muscle twitching, gastric upset, chills, fever, confusion, and dizziness. Generally the child is started with a low dose, which is increased slowly to minimize the chance of side effects. There have been reports of children who developed suicidal thoughts and committed suicide while taking SSRIs. Because of these reports and the lack of efficacy evidence, children and adolescents taking SSRIs must be closely monitored by a psychiatric–mental health specialist (Bridge, Iyengar, Salary, et al., 2007; Cheung et al., 2007; U.S. Preventive Services Task Force, 2009). The U.S. Food and Drug Administration (FDA) recommends that a patient medication guide be provided to each patient explaining the risks of the drug and precautions to take; information and instructions are also on the drug label.

NURSING MANAGEMENT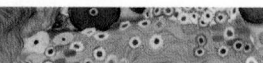

Nursing Assessment and Diagnosis

A thorough history and physical examination, including observation of behavior, are obtained at the time of admission. Assess the child for common risk factors for depression (Table 28–4).

Several nursing diagnoses that may be appropriate for the child or adolescent hospitalized with depression are included in the accompanying Nursing Care Plan. Other diagnoses may include the following:

- Imbalanced Nutrition: More than Body Requirements related to eating in response to internal cues other than hunger

Medications Used to Treat

Depression

Selective Serotonin Reuptake Inhibitor (SSRI) Drugs Used to Treat Depression

Medication	Starting Dose	Usual Effective Dose	Selected Side Effects
Fluoxetine (Prozac)	10 mg/day	20 mg/day	Restlessness, headaches, akathisia
Sertraline (Zoloft)	25 mg/day	50 mg/day	Dry mouth, gastric upset
Paroxetine (Paxil)	10 mg/day	20 mg/day	Dry mouth, weight gain
Fluvoxamine (Luvox)	50 mg/day	150 mg/day	Dry mouth, gastric upset
Citalopram (Celexa)	10 mg/day	20 mg/day	Dry mouth, nausea, sleep disturbance

Data from: Cheung, Zuckerbrot, Jensen, et al. (2007); Custer & Rau (2009).
Note: Drugs are started at low starting doses and titrated upward as needed to achieve therapeutic goals. Although a variety of SSRIs are used in treatment of children and adolescents, the only FDA-approved medication for major depressive disorder in this age group is Prozac, and the only FDA-approved medications for OCD in the pediatric age group are Prozac, Zoloft, Luvox, and Anafranil.

TABLE 28–4	Risk Factors for Child and Adolescent Depression	
Child	Family	School and Social Situations
• Frequent feelings of sadness, sleep problems, or loss of interest in activities • Increase in risk taking and impulsivity • Previous suicide attempt • Alcohol or substance abuse • Diagnosed psychotic disorder • Chronic illness and frequent hospitalization	• Parental neglect, abuse, or loss • Dysfunctional family relationships • Family history of depression, suicide, substance abuse, alcoholism, or other psychopathology	• Academic pressures and underachievement • Stressful social relationships • Declining participation in social events

• Powerlessness related to sense of helplessness
• Chronic Low Self-Esteem related to negative self-evaluation

Planning and Implementation

Nursing care of the child or adolescent hospitalized for depression includes administering medications and other therapy, and providing supportive care. Monitor vital signs of youth receiving antidepressant medications. Watch for common side effects of the agent(s) used. Carefully monitor for serious side effects of TCAs and SSRIs and be aware that lower doses are used at initiation with doses increasing slowly to the desired level. Frequent face-to-face follow-up visits are needed. When dosages are altered, all behavior and ideation changes must be closely monitored. Monitor cardiovascular status, including hypertension and tachycardia; observe motor movement; and record dietary intake. Help parents to evaluate inpatient settings to be certain the care provided will best meet the needs of the child or adolescent. (See Families Want to Know: Selecting a Facility for the Child with Mental Illness.) Refer to the Nursing Care Plan for specific nursing interventions for the child or adolescent hospitalized with depression.

Discharge Planning and Home Care Teaching

When the child has been hospitalized and is returning home, teach parents to recognize signs and symptoms of worsening depression. Parents should also be taught dosages and side effects of any prescribed medications. Review data in the patient medication guide provided by the pharmacy for any medications. Caution parents not to alter the dose or discontinue the drug without the guidance and monitoring of the prescriber. Instruct the family to remove guns, ammunition, and other potentially harmful items from the home. Have the family immediately seek emergency care if they are concerned about the child's safety or worsening condition. Refer the family to appropriate health care professionals and to support groups for family members dealing with depression.

Care in the Community

Most children with depression are cared for in the community. Maintain regular contact with family members through their health care visits to outpatient agencies and by making home visits. Monitor the child's affect, activity, and food intake. School teachers and counselors often are aware of the child's ability to perform in the school setting. Have the family schedule after-school care so young children are not left at home alone for ex-

tended periods. Assist the family in finding support for financial and emotional needs related to managing the child's depression.

Expected outcomes for nursing care of the child with depression are found in the accompanying Nursing Care Plan.

Bipolar Disorder (Manic Depression)

Bipolar disorder is a mental illness in which extreme changes in affect and energy are manifested. Moods most often alter between *mania* (high energy and euphoria) and depression. Children often present with irritability, hyperactivity, risk taking, or going without sleep. About 1% of children and adults suffer from bipolar illness, with a high rate of onset from 15 to 19 years, although occurrence as young as preschool age can occur. There is a high rate of attempted suicide as well as other disorders such as ADHD, anxiety, and substance abuse, all of which complicate diagnosis (Apps, Winkler, & Jandrisevits, 2008; Lack & Green, 2009).

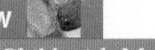

Families Want to Know
Selecting a Facility for the Child with Mental Illness

Families need guidelines to assist them in obtaining care and evaluating service facilities for a child with a mental disorder. They can be referred to the National Alliance on Mental Illness (http://www.nami.org) and Mental Health America (http://www.nmha.org). Provide local numbers for suicide prevention and the National Suicide Prevention Lifeline Crisis Line (1-800-273-TALK or -8255).

When hospitalization is needed, provide information from the American Association of Children's Residential Treatment Centers (http://www.aacrc-dc.org). Nurses can provide questions for the families to ask:

■ What is the staff to youth ratio?
■ What are the guidelines for chemical and physical restraint?
■ Are children isolated alone when behaviors are inappropriate?
■ Are children constantly monitored visually when in restraint or when potentially dangerous to self or others?
■ Does the child have a full physical and psychological evaluation by a specialist within 24 hours of entry to the facility?
■ What professionals review the plan of care and how often?
■ To whom can the family speak for regular updates on the child?
■ How often can the family visit?
■ What services will be covered by insurance?
■ What subjective feelings does the family member have when visiting the unit and facility?
■ What services will be offered on an ongoing basis upon discharge?

NURSING CARE PLAN

The Child or Adolescent Hospitalized with Depression

INTERVENTION	RATIONALE	EXPECTED OUTCOME
1. Nursing Diagnosis: Hopelessness related to long-term stress		
NIC Priority Intervention: *Hope instillation:* Facilitation of the development of a positive outlook		**NOC Suggested Outcome:** *Hope:* Presence of internal state of optimism that is personally satisfying and life supporting
Goal: The child or adolescent will discuss feelings of hopelessness.		
▪ Encourage open expression of feelings. Explore hopeless, sad, or lonely feelings. Maintain an accepting and nonjudgmental attitude regarding feelings expressed by the child. Point out the connection between feelings and behavior. Assess the child or adolescent to identify the precipitating event when feelings of sadness arose.	▪ Expressing feelings may help to relieve sadness, loneliness, despair, and hopelessness.	By discharge, the child or adolescent expresses an interest in the future.
▪ Encourage the child or adolescent to take part in self-care and unit activities. Use routines to establish feelings of control.	▪ An active role in self-care and treatment helps the child or adolescent to feel more in control.	
▪ Medicate as ordered and document results.	▪ Antidepressants modify mood to a more hopeful outlook.	
2. Nursing Diagnosis: Ineffective Individual Coping related to inadequate social support or disturbance in pattern of appraisal of threat		
NIC Priority Intervention: *Coping enhancement:* Assisting a patient to adapt to perceived stressors, changes, or threats which interfere with meeting life demands and roles		**NOC Suggested Outcome:** *Coping:* Actions to manage stressors that tax an individual's resources
Goal: The child or adolescent will use effective coping skills.		
▪ Teach positive, effective coping strategies such as guided imagery and relaxation. Assist the child or adolescent to focus on strengths rather than weaknesses.	▪ Therapeutic techniques can help the child or adolescent to replace negative thoughts and images with more positive and effective beliefs and images. These interventions foster resilience.	The child or adolescent verbalizes and demonstrates the ability to cope appropriately for his or her age.
▪ Assist the child or adolescent to identify friends, family members, and others who are positive and supportive.	▪ This process helps the child or adolescent to become aware that people can be caring and supportive (thus validating self-esteem).	
3. Nursing Diagnosis: Impaired Social Interaction related to self-concept disturbance		
NIC Priority Intervention: *Socialization enhancement:* Facilitation of ability to interact with others		**NOC Suggested Outcome:** *Social interaction skills:* An individual's use of effective interaction behaviors
Goal: The child or adolescent will participate in and initiate activities and conversation.		
▪ Assist the child or adolescent to identify topics and activities of interest.	▪ The more the child or adolescent focuses on areas of interest, the less he or she will focus on internal anxiety and depression.	By discharge, the child or adolescent initiates conversation and activities with staff and peers.
▪ Encourage interaction with peers and staff.	▪ Each positive interaction reinforces feelings of success. Each success reinforces the desire for future social interaction.	
▪ Facilitate visits from family and friends.	▪ Visits from family and friends reinforce positive and rewarding relationships.	

NURSING CARE PLAN

The Child or Adolescent Hospitalized with Depression (continued)

INTERVENTION	RATIONALE	EXPECTED OUTCOME
▪ Provide guidance to the family regarding interaction that promotes self-esteem.	▪ The family's existing interaction style is often negative.	

4. Nursing Diagnosis: Imbalanced Nutrition: Less than Body Requirements related to loss of appetite secondary to depression

NIC Priority Intervention: *Nutrition management:* Assistance with or provision of a balanced dietary intake of foods and fluids		NOC Suggested Outcome: *Nutritional status:* Amount of food and fluid taken into the body over a 24-hour period

Goal: The child or adolescent's daily intake will be adequate to maintain optimal nutritional status.

▪ Offer nutritious finger foods, sandwiches, and high-calorie liquid supplements frequently throughout the day.	▪ Convenient easy-to-eat foods encourage the child or adolescent to eat and maintain nutritional status.	The child or adolescent's daily intake will be adequate to maintain optimal nutritional status by discharge.
▪ Offer easy-to-carry drinks that are high in vitamins, minerals, and calories.	▪ These are a convenient method for meeting hydration and electrolyte needs.	
▪ Encourage daily vigorous physical activity of at least 30 minutes.	▪ Physical activity stimulates appetite.	

Bipolar disorder is classified into four types:

- Bipolar I—includes a severe manic episode that requires hospitalization or causes functional impairment in life
- Bipolar II—at least one episode of mild to moderate mania (hypomania) and one of depression
- Cyclothymic disorder—manifests as multiple mild manic and depressive episodes
- Bipolar not otherwise specified—rapid mood fluctuations, mania without depressive episodes, or chronic depression with hypomania episodes

(Roberts, 2007)

When parents or close relatives are affected, the child is more likely to have the disorder. Anxiety and ADHD sometimes precede the disorder. Genetics and environment likely interact to create the condition in youth. Brain imaging shows abnormalities of the frontal and prefrontal cortex, the hippocampus, the basal ganglia, and the left amygdala, which is the center for experiencing fear (National Institute of Mental Health, 2009).

The manic phase of bipolar illness is characterized by hyperactivity and high energy, irritability, explosive outbursts, aggression, and sometimes hallucinations. In the depressive phase, the child is sad, has alterations in sleep and eating patterns, feels worthless, is lacking in energy, and is socially withdrawn, similar to any depressive illness. Mania may be the persistent symptom in children, or rapid cycles of mania and depression can occur throughout the day (Lack & Green, 2009).

Diagnosis and treatment of bipolar disorder should be performed by mental health specialists. Use of alcohol or illegal drugs should be ruled out as a cause of symptoms, even in chil-

dren. Since the manic phase is often manifested by hyperactivity, the child may incorrectly be treated with stimulants (see discussion of ADHD earlier in this chapter), thus worsening the disease. Irritability, elation, labile moods, and sleep disturbance are common in children (Apps et al., 2008; DelBello, Adler, & Strakowski, 2006; Lack & Green, 2009).

The treatment of bipolar disease involves a variety of drugs used to stabilize mood. Examples include lithium, divalproex, carbamazepine, olanzapine, oxcarbazepine, lamotrigine, quetiapine, and risperidone; only lithium is approved by the FDA for use in those from 12–18 years (Apps et al., 2008). However, other drugs are prescribed by clinicians with careful monitoring performed. Early treatment is key to preventing chronic, serious mental illness.

Nurses are instrumental in identifying children with the disorder, referring to mental health specialists, providing information to families, and monitoring the drugs and psychotherapy for the child. All of the medications used for treatment have side effects that require follow-up and regular monitoring. Assist parents to find resources for health care since medications and other treatments may be costly. Parents and children need information about the disorder since it may recur several times during life. Parents need resources and assistance to deal with the effects of the disorder on the family.

■ ANXIETY AND RELATED DISORDERS

Anxiety disorders affects youth as well as adults. Some of the more common types seen in children and adolescents are described in the following text, with detailed nursing management described after the last condition, posttraumatic stress disorder.

Generalized Anxiety Disorder

Anxiety is a subjective feeling of uncertainty and helplessness, usually accompanied by central nervous system (CNS) signs, including restlessness, trembling, perspiration, and rapid pulse. Anxiety is second to only substance abuse (see Chapter 17 ∞) in incidence for mental disorders and it is a common mental disorder among children. From 20–28% of youth experience some type of anxiety disorder. Although all children experience anxiety at certain times, those with anxiety disorder are excessively worried about many things, are difficult to reassure, and are not able to distract themselves from the worry. Many youth have accompanying physical complaints such as headache or stomachache, and comorbid diagnoses such as depression and substance use are common (Keeley & Storch, 2009).

Diagnosis is performed by a mental health specialist; treatment is usually cognitive behavior therapy (CBT) and may include medication. CBT can include child or family interventions that focus on relaxation, recognition of feelings, and self-talking (learned words or phrases said to oneself to aid in management of distress). Medications that have been reported to be successful in children include SSRIs and benzodiazepines (Keeley & Storch, 2009).

Separation Anxiety Disorder

Separation anxiety disorder is characterized by an extreme state of uneasiness when in unfamiliar surroundings and often by refusal to visit friends' homes or attend school for at least 2 weeks. It is a common type of anxiety disorder manifested by children (Beesdo, Knappe, & Pine, 2009; Kendall, Compton, Walkup, et al., 2010). Approximately 75% of children with separation anxiety disorder refuse to attend school (see School Phobia, to follow). This disorder occurs in approximately 4–5% of children and in twice as many girls as boys. The peak age for occurrence is 7 to 9 years. It may be sporadic and recurrent. It may be acute in onset (preceded by a traumatic event) or slow to develop over time (Keeley & Storch, 2009).

Children with separation anxiety disorder tend to be perfectionistic, overly compliant, and eager to please. They appear to cling to the parent or caretaker. They may use physical complaints such as headaches, abdominal pain, nausea, and vomiting in an attempt to avoid being away from the parent. Depression frequently accompanies separation anxiety disorder. The resulting avoidant behaviors can interfere with personal growth and development, academic achievement, and social functioning.

Diagnosis is made by a mental health specialist. Treatment includes CBT with both the child and parents. Parents learn about

Growth & Development *Separation Anxiety*

The separation anxiety experienced by a 2-year-old differs from the psychiatric disorder in age appropriateness, duration, and severity. Separation anxiety disorder affects children of preschool age or older, lasts for at least 2 weeks, and is characterized by excessive anxiety. In contrast, the separation anxiety experienced by the toddler directly follows a separation from a familiar caretaker, lasts only for a short time after the separation, and is a normal characteristic response in toddlers.

the disorder and how to structure the setting so that the child is expected to attend school. Consistency in expectations is needed since if the child is permitted to stay home some days or has missed school and other activities for longer periods, treatment is more difficult. The child learns what situations cause anxiety and how to handle it. Both parents and the child work out the expectations for behavior for the child with the mental health therapist; school personnel need to be included in the treatment plan. Medication has occasionally been used if CBT is not helpful.

Panic Disorder

Panic disorder is the presence of recurrent, unexpected panic attacks. These attacks are periods of intense fear and discomfort in the absence of real danger. The lifetime risk of panic disorder ranges from 1–5% (Keeley & Storch, 2009). Predictive factors for panic attacks in adolescence include a history of separation or other anxiety disorder earlier in life, and history of parental panic attack.

Examples of the physical symptoms experienced are palpitations, sweating, chills, hot flashes, shaking, shortness of breath, choking, chest pain, nausea, and dizziness. The person describes feelings of danger or doom. There may be accompanying agoraphobia in some people. **Agoraphobia** is an anxiety of being in places or situations from which escape may be difficult or embarrassing, or in which help may not be available. The attacks may be continuous or episodic, but generally are chronic in nature.

Diagnosis is made by a mental health specialist. Similar to anxiety, treatment may involve individual and family interventions using CBT, and the use of SSRI medication in some cases.

Obsessive-Compulsive Disorder

Individuals with obsessive-compulsive disorder (OCD) may be mildly or severely affected. From 1–4% of children are affected, and about 80% of adults with OCD were affected in childhood (Keeley & Storch, 2009). Affected children have recurrent obsessive thoughts, commonly about contamination, harm, sex, or moral concerns. These obsessions are handled through a series of compulsive behaviors that interfere with daily life. Examples of behaviors are excessive handwashing, counting objects, and hoarding substances. These practices may take 1 or more hours each day. Children with OCD differ from adults in several ways. Children have more aggressive obsessions such as fears of catastrophe, more commonly hoard objects, and are more likely to have religious obsessions. The presence of comorbidity with other mental health disorders is common.

The basal ganglia of the brain are affected and a genetic link is observed. A neurochemical cause may be related to abnormal serotonin metabolism. MRI changes in the basal ganglia and certain cortical regions have been noted. Poststreptococcal autoimmune disorder may be a cause in some cases (D'Alessandro, 2009).

Diagnosis is made by a mental health specialist. The disorder may have been present for some time before diagnosis as parents tend to overlook or deny the symptoms, and children may hide the behaviors. Treatment may involve CBT, where the feared occurrence is presented and the person learns that no harm will occur. Involvement of the family in treatment is important so

Research   *PANDAS*

Pediatric autoimmune neuropsychiatric disorders associated with streptococcal infections (PANDAS) are characterized by obsessive-compulsive and/or tic disorders, childhood onsets, association with group A beta-hemolytic streptococcal infections, and neurological abnormalities. It is believed that in certain children, the strep infection leads to a neural autoimmune response, resulting in the psychiatric disorder. Research continues to identify possible mechanisms, results, and treatments for the cause of OCD (D'Alessandro, 2009; Gabbay, Coffey, Babb, et al., 2008).

that members learn how to handle the child's ritualistic behaviors. Medications such as clomipramine and the SSRIs are effective in most children and adolescents. Nurses identify potential cases, refer for mental health evaluation, and provide teaching and support for families.

School Phobia (Social Phobia)

School phobia (also known as social phobia, school avoidance, or school refusal) is a persistent, irrational, or excessive fear of negative evaluation or embarrassment in social situations and therefore of attending school. The child may fear being harmed or losing control. Social and school phobia can occur in children as young as 5 years of age, often emerges at 11 or 12 years, and can occur in children up to 16 years; about 7% of children manifest the phobia (Keeley & Storch, 2009).

Children with social phobia may fear asking for directions, ordering food at a restaurant, and speaking in the classroom. Children commonly report that teachers and peers "pick on" them. Somatic complaints are similar to those in children with separation anxiety disorder. Symptoms may be present only on school days and not on weekends or holidays, especially when school phobia is manifested. The social withdrawal that occurs in this disorder further impairs the child since social interactions are needed for normal developmental progression.

Diagnosis is made by a mental health specialist. A variety of instruments are available for assessing social phobia. Treatment includes the family and child, and establishes firm limits for behavioral expectations and consequences. CBT is used, including education of the youth about the condition, body awareness of symptoms, and methods of managing feelings. SSRI medications may sometimes be needed to lessen anxiety in social situations so the child can experience success in these interactions (Bothe & Olness, 2007).

Conversion Reaction

Conversion reaction is a disorder in which a disturbance or loss of sensory, motor, or other physical functions suggests neurologic or other somatic disease. The disturbance or loss cannot be explained by any known pathophysiologic mechanism. Instead, psychologic factors are involved. About 3% of the population experiences conversion reactions at some time. Adolescence and early adulthood are common times for the onset to occur, with onset rare before 10 years or after 35 years (Oyama, Paltoo, & Greengold, 2007).

Conversion reactions develop in response to a catastrophic event such as threat, loss, or harm. Clinical manifestations include altered sensations such as blindness or deafness; paralysis or ataxia, including inability to stand or walk and loss of ability to speak (aphonia); involuntary movements, such as pseudoepileptic convulsions; and constant complaints of pain with no physical basis (psychogenic pain). Children under 10 years usually present with gait abnormalities or seizures. The onset of conversion symptoms is usually dramatic and sudden. Symptoms often appear to be neurologic, but on careful examination obvious discrepancies are found. The person is usually calm about the symptoms even though they are serious. Often the child or family members appear indifferent or unconcerned over what health care providers consider an overwhelming physical disability.

Children suspected of having a conversion reaction require a complete physical and neurologic evaluation to rule out any possible physiologic basis for the symptoms. Individual and family therapy is usually necessary to identify the source of the psychologic conflict, pain, or need resulting in the conversion symptoms. Pharmacological approaches may also be used.

Posttraumatic Stress Disorders

Acute stress disorder can occur after any life-threatening event and is manifested in the first month after exposure to the event. Symptoms include repeatedly reliving the traumatic experience, anxiety, and increased arousal. Similarly, *posttraumatic stress disorder* (PTSD) victims have experienced or witnessed a life-threatening event; however, the symptoms of distress continue for more than 1 month and cause impairment in functioning (Hamblen, Norris, Pietruszkiewicz, et al., 2009; Kassam-Adams, Marsac, & Cirilli, 2010). Estimates of the incidence of PTSD are hard to obtain. It is assumed that about 40% of youth have an episode of trauma that could lead to PTSD and that 6% have symptoms of the disorder. While 20% of children may experience PTSD after traumatic events, the prevalence rises to 90% when the trauma is severe (CDC, 2006b).

Etiology and Pathophysiology

Examples of traumatic events that are associated with posttraumatic stress include sexual or other child abuse, rape, car crash, fire, hurricane, bombings, witnessing violence, and having an experience in war. The treatment of PTSD is discussed in this section; consult Chapter 17 ∞ for further examples of the types of violence that affect children and methods for reducing youth exposure to violent, traumatic events.

The disorder involves both a traumatic event and the child's reaction to this event. It is believed that brain changes occur in trauma, leading to neurobiological alterations that cause dysfunction of memory. Overreactivity of the amygdala, underreactivity of the prefrontal cortex, and increased dopamine in the medial prefrontal cortex are observed. Those with other psychiatric disorders, a family history of psychiatric illness, and severe or lengthy trauma all possess risk factors.

Clinical Manifestations

The very young child with PTSD may show regression in behavior, sleep disturbance, or demonstration of anxiety. Children may be unable to remember the true sequence of the traumatic event, reenact the event in play and drawings, and search for warning signs of future trauma. Adolescents commonly exhibit impulsive or aggressive behaviors. Children of any age have feelings of fear, terror, and helplessness, and may relive the event frequently in thoughts and nightmares. There is a state of hypervigilance and exaggerated startle response, such as to touch or loud noises. The child feels detached from others and alone. Even if the child appears to have adapted and functions normally immediately after the traumatic event, several weeks or even months later, the symptoms of PTSD can begin to appear (National Center for PTSD, 2008).

COLLABORATIVE CARE

The diagnosis is made by a mental health specialist. A history of traumatic events with normal childhood developmental behaviors before the event is characteristic. A variety of instruments are available to screen for symptoms characteristic of the disorder.

Counseling by a mental health specialist is the main therapy for PTSD. CBT is the treatment of choice, with both the child and family members included (Figure 28–8 ➤). Young children show significant improvement in symptoms after a course of CBT (Legerstee, Tulen, Dierchx, et al., 2010; Scheeringa, Salloum, Arnberger, et al., 2007; Smith, Yule, Perrin, et al., 2007). A variety of antidepressants and SSRIs can be used for pharmacologic treatment, with the medication tailored to the specific symptoms that are most distressing and have been resistant to CBT.

NURSING MANAGEMENT

Nursing management for PTSD and other anxiety disorders focuses on partnering with other health professionals and families

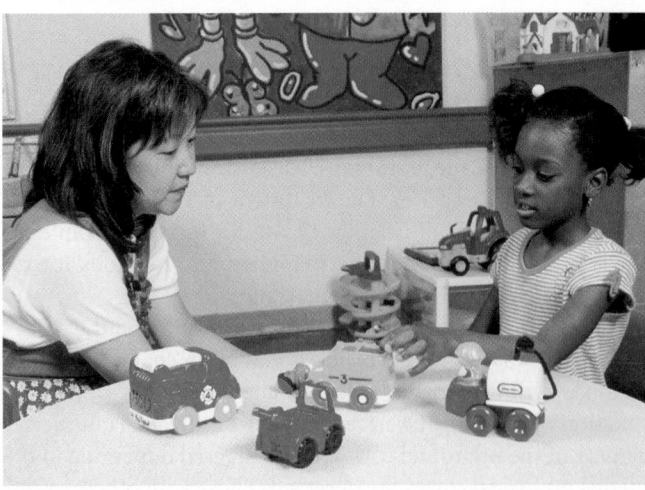

FIGURE 28–8 ➤ A psychologist uses play therapy to help Cassandra, a young girl who is experiencing PTSD. The child was in a car crash and physically recovered but has experienced nightmares about the event. She also developed a fear of leaving home. The therapist allows Cassandra to play with cars and talk about the event. She uses cognitive-behavior therapy to suggest ways of handling the thoughts and fears. This helps Cassandra to gain control over the event so that it is not so frightening and does not interfere with her functioning in daily life.

to relieve the child's anxiety and return him or her to a normal and developmentally appropriate level of functioning.

Nursing Assessment and Diagnosis

Nurses often help to identify PTSD victims and others with anxiety disorders so that care can be obtained. Ask about traumatic events in the past and how the child reacted. Inquire about recent changes in the child's behavior. Include school attendance, complaints of physical illness, sleep patterns, and rituals in behavior. Youth who run away from home and present at homeless shelters are often suffering from PTSD; assessment for the condition should be part of the initial history (Thompson, Maccio, Desselle, et al., 2007). Based on the data gathered, the child's symptoms, and the mental health diagnosis, the nurse determines nursing diagnoses. Some examples include:

- Anxiety related to unconscious conflict
- Ineffective Coping related to perceived high degree of threat
- Powerlessness related to chronic mental illness
- Disturbed Sleep Pattern related to anxiety
- Post-Trauma Syndrome related to motor vehicle or other accidents

Planning and Implementation

Nursing care for anxiety disorders focuses on cognitive and behavioral therapies to enhance coping skills. Mental health nurses may conduct group therapy sessions both in inpatient and community settings (Figure 28–9A and B ➤). Group sessions for children often provide a forum for discussion of fears, an opportunity to enhance skills of working together, and an opportunity to learn coping skills. Being a member of a group with other children experiencing anxiety or trauma can remove the stigma and allow the child the freedom to explore the behavior and its causes. Several of the techniques described in the chapter beginning, such as drawing pictures and discussing them or telling stories, are used by mental health nurses in child therapy groups.

Children need to learn relaxation techniques. Nurses may teach such techniques or recommend that the child consider participation in yoga or guided imagery classes. Inquire about

Complementary Therapy
Complementary and Alternative Practice for Mental Health

- Medications—for example, St. John's wort, kava, ginseng, ginkgo biloba, lemon balm
- Diet—for example, omega-3 fatty acids, vitamin and mineral supplements, removal of food dyes
- Self-hypnotic relaxation—to reduce pain and anxiety
- Acupuncture—to reduce anxiety and depression
- Massage therapy—to reduce anxiety, anger, and grief
- Reflexology (manual stimulation of specific points on the foot)—to reduce anxiety
- Guided imagery—to reduce anxiety
- Biofeedback (use of machines to watch muscle or skin responses)—to reduce anxiety

Data from Soh & Walter, 2008.

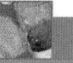

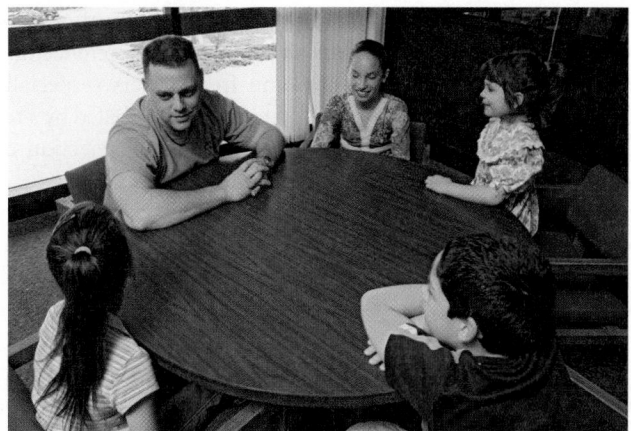

A

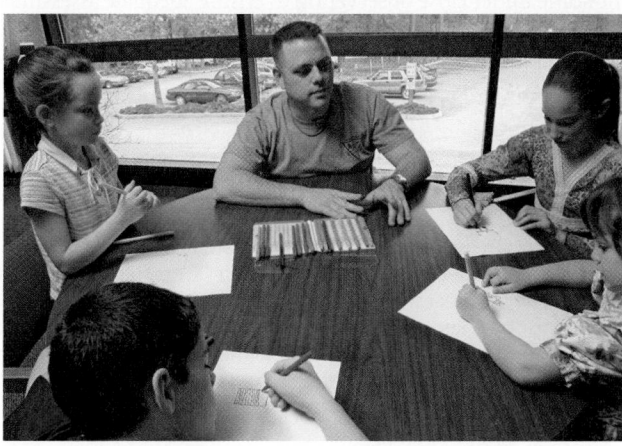

B

FIGURE 28–9 ➤ A, This nurse conducts a group therapy session for children who have experienced traumatic events and have resulting anxiety disorders. He is clearly engaged, has a positive rapport, and fosters exchanges among the children. B, Playing games and drawing are frequent techniques used in the group, followed by discussion of events and feelings. The children learn from the nurse and each other ways in which they can handle anxiety.

measure of the success of therapy. The community or school nurse can relay this information.

Nurses often administer medications to children being treated for PTSD or other disorders. Be alert for side effects and ensure the family knows how to safely administer the drugs. They should be kept securely locked away. Have the child return for follow-up as needed since some medications may take several weeks to achieve effects, and close monitoring is essential. The child should have a medication alert tag for drugs being taken.

Evaluation

The outcomes of nursing care for the child with anxiety disorder center on return to normal developmental activities, engagement in social relationships, learned coping skills for dealing with stress, and maintenance of safety.

■ SUICIDE

Suicide is the third leading cause of death in adolescents between 15 and 19 years of age. Although suicide rates decreased in individuals between 10 and 24 years of age during 1990–2003, since then suicide rates have increased, with about 7.32 per 100,000 (CDC, 2007c). Suicide accounts for about 12% of deaths in teens, and about 4,500 deaths annually in the United States. About 9.7% of teens report at least one suicide attempt, 17% report suicidal thoughts in the previous year, and 8% attempted suicide within the previous year (CDC, 2007b).

Males die as a result of suicide four times more often than females. This statistic is reversed for suicide attempts, perhaps because boys use lethal methods such as guns, hanging, and

alternative therapies that the child and family are using or have an interest in beginning, and refer as needed.

Parents or other significant people should be included in the treatment program. Nurses often teach them basic information about the child's diagnosis and therapy. They should be in at least some therapy sessions with the child. Provide resources that they need to get relief from worry about the child, guilt about causing an accident that triggered the child's symptoms, or other feelings related to the diagnosis. (See Families Want to Know: Talking with Children About Traumatic Events.)

Insurance companies may provide limited payment for mental health services. Help the family to see the importance of recommended therapy and assist them to find resources for care, if needed.

School personnel may need to know about the child's treatment. Collaborate with families to provide needed information. Some schools have counselors that can be instrumental in carrying out treatment plans at school and acting as a resource in that setting. School personnel may be asked to provide feedback about the child's attendance, performance, and social skills as a

Some ethnic groups have a high rate of suicide. For example, Native Americans and Alaska Natives have a rate of suicide at 1.5 times the national average; suicide is the second leading cause of death in these ethnic groups (CDC, 2007b). The historic pain experienced by these ethnic groups and lack of opportunities for many youth may be some of the reasons for a high suicide rate. Hispanic females have a higher rate of suicide than other gender and ethnic groups. White males have traditionally had the highest rates of suicide, but recently Blacks have had greatly increasing numbers of suicides (CDC, 2006b). *Healthy People 2020* goals focus on eliminating such health disparities by finding the causes, decreasing rates of suicide, educating about risk factors, and establishing prevention programs (U.S. Department of Health and Human Services, 2010).

jumping more often than girls, who more commonly use drug overdose and wrist cutting.

It is not unusual for health care professionals and parents to label suicide attempts by children and adolescents as accidents. Up to half of childhood suicides may be recorded as accidents; suicide data for children under age 10 years are not maintained. Adults may have difficulty believing that young children, in particular, would have any reason to want to end their lives. Accurate identification and treatment are needed for youth at risk of suicide. All suicide attempts must be taken seriously and mental health treatment begun immediately (Shain & American Academy of Pediatrics, 2007).

Many risk factors for suicide exist in children and adolescents (Table 28–5). The most common precursor to adolescent suicide is depression (see previous discussion). Common signs or symptoms of an underlying depression that could lead to suicide include boredom, restlessness, problems with concentration, ir-

TABLE 28–5 Risk and Protective Factors for Suicide in Children and Adolescents

Risk Factors	Protective Factors
• History of previous attempted suicide	• Emotional well-being
• Friend's suicide or attempted suicide	• Satisfactory school performance
• School problems or changes in grades	• Participation in sports or other group events
• Pregnancy	• Weight satisfaction
• Drug use or abuse	• Parent/family connectedness
• Problems with a romantic relationship	• Family issues
• Minority sexual practice	• School connectedness
• Loneliness, withdrawal	• Safe school
• Feelings of anxiety	• Safe neighborhood
• History of chronic family problems	• Caring adult presence at school or elsewhere
• Chronic illness	• Availability of school counseling
• Physical, emotional, or sexual abuse	• School policies on fighting, bullying
• History of suicide in a family member	
• History of depression	
• Chronic low self-esteem	
• Change in behavior	
• Change in weight	
• Sleep disturbance	
• Giving away special possessions	
• Access to firearms and ammunition	

ritability, lethargy, intentional misbehavior, preoccupation with one's own body or health, discomfort with sexual preference, and excessive dependence on or isolation from others (especially adults or caregivers). The depression may be exacerbated by a recent psychosocial stress such as loss or perceived rejection or ridicule. A previous attempt is also a common risk factor.

The child or adolescent found to be at high risk for suicide may be admitted to a mental health unit for care or cared for in a community mental health facility. Treatment may include individual, group, or family therapy. Negotiating a no-suicide contract is one method that may be used with a suicidal youth. In the contract, the child agrees not to attempt suicide during a specified time period. When a suicide attempt is made, the child or adolescent may be hospitalized for 24 hours, kept in a short-term monitoring unit, or sent home under close observation to ensure adequate assessment and monitoring. It is important to provide crisis intervention at the time of the suicide attempt to minimize the opportunity for repeat attempts and begin a therapeutic treatment plan.

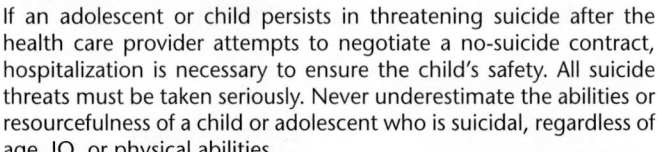

Nursing Alert

If an adolescent or child persists in threatening suicide after the health care provider attempts to negotiate a no-suicide contract, hospitalization is necessary to ensure the child's safety. All suicide threats must be taken seriously. Never underestimate the abilities or resourcefulness of a child or adolescent who is suicidal, regardless of age, IQ, or physical abilities.

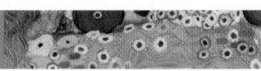

NURSING MANAGEMENT

Nursing Assessment and Diagnosis

The major nursing role is in prevention of suicide. All children and adolescents in health promotion visits and emergency departments should be evaluated for risk. Health promotion visits are an opportunity to be alert for children with depression, substance abuse, recent stresses, and changes in behavior. Inquire about sleep patterns, feelings of sadness, and use of alcohol and other substances. Gather a family history of mental health disorders, suicide attempts, and stresses. Ask about how often the youth talks with or has meals with the family. Be aware of the risk of self-inflicted accidental strangulation.

Most suicides are committed with firearms, which are usually obtained from the home. Ask at each health care visit if the family has firearms. Encourage parents to keep them unloaded, with ammunition and firearms locked in separate locations. Be sure that children and adolescents do not have access to the keys for the locked firearms.

Some nursing diagnoses possible for the child at risk of suicide include:

- Risk for Suicide related to hopelessness and substance abuse
- Risk for Self-Directed Violence related to history of suicide attempts, present suicidal ideation, and recent failure in school
- Readiness for Enhanced Family Coping related to recent teen attempted suicide

A tragic cause of unintentional strangulation death in children results from the "choking game." About 25 children annually die in the United States from this practice, with a mean age of 13 years. When the blood supply to the brain is interrupted and then rushes back, some people report a feeling of euphoria or a "high." Children and adolescents may seek the experience for the feelings it creates and may even become addicted to it. Unfortunately, some children become accidentally strangled and die from the experience. Methods that children use to cut off oxygen include using their hands to apply pressure to the carotids in the neck, or tying belts, cords, towels, and other items to the neck and then around doorways or other solid objects. Some children perform these rituals with others who then rescue them so that they begin breathing; many of the injuries occur when children are alone since there is no one to perform a rescue. Teachers, parents, and other adults typically have not heard of or are unaware that children are performing these rituals. Adults can watch for signs such as conjunctival hemorrhage, headaches, bruising in the neck area, periods of disorientation, hoarseness, and finding items tied to doors and other solid objects. Parents can also be alert if the history of a family computer has shown the child's entry to a website that describes the practice. Nurses in schools and other settings should educate children about the dangers of this strangulation and should provide materials for teachers and parents to inform them of the risk (CDC, 2008b, 2010b).

Planning and Implementation

Care in the Hospital

Many children at risk of suicide or who have just attempted to commit suicide will be admitted to the hospital for a period of monitoring. Therapy is begun and medications can be given under close supervision.

Nursing care centers on taking appropriate precautions to ensure the safety of a child or adolescent at risk of suicide. The child and the environment of the hospital or other setting are monitored for any object that could be used for self-harm. All potentially harmful objects, such as shoestrings, belts, pantyhose, hair ribbons, and medications (including all over-the-counter preparations), are removed. All personal care items (including toothbrush and shampoo) are kept locked at the nursing station and monitored constantly when used by the child.

Children or adolescents who are considered at high risk for suicidal behaviors are attended by a nursing staff member at all times, including while using the bathroom and sleeping. It may be necessary for the child to dress in a plain hospital gown, be kept in a visually monitored seclusion room, or (if seriously impaired and self-abusive) be medicated for restraint for a period of time. Restraints are used only when ordered by the physician and interdisciplinary team caring for the youth. Physical restraint is only a short-term approach to provide immediate safety, if necessary. Chemical (medication) restraint may be needed to prevent self-injury by the person who is suicidal. See page 923 for information to help families find services and evaluate facilities when choosing care for their child who is suicidal. Documentation of safety precautions and patient behavior is needed.

Hospitalization continues as long as the child's behavior is self-destructive. Children are referred for intensive individual and family therapy to begin in the hospital and continue after discharge.

Care in the Community

Encourage parents to keep follow-up clinic appointments, to watch for self-destructive behaviors, and to administer any prescribed medications according to the treatment schedule. Arrange home visits and other community resources for families. Fewer than one half of adolescents who attempt suicide are referred for mental health evaluation and follow-up, so nurses are instrumental in referrals and in encouraging the care that youth need.

Education in all school settings is appropriate to assist children in knowing about resources of help when needed and in identifying peers at risk. Mental health services of all types should be available in and embedded in schools since that is the setting where youth spend much of their time (U.S. Department of Health and Human Services, 2010). Be alert for children and adolescents at risk for suicide in any setting. Assess children and adolescents in schools, outpatient settings, and emergency departments for the possibility of suicidal behavior. Report threats of suicide and depressive behavior. Recognize that when one suicide has occurred, there may be an increased risk for friends of the victim. Teach students to report to teachers, nurses, or counselors about friends who have threatened suicide or seem depressed or display behaviors different from usual. Nurses often plan with mental health specialists to implement suicide prevention programs in schools and communities (U.S. Department of Health and Human Services, 2010). Provide supportive services to family and friends when suicide occurs. Consult websites and refer parents as appropriate.

Evaluation

Some desired outcomes related to suicide risk include:

- The family develops coping strategies to support the suicidal member.
- The child or adolescent takes actions to decrease sadness and increase interest in life events.
- The child or adolescent remains safe with no further suicide attempts or ideation.

■ TIC DISORDERS AND TOURETTE SYNDROME

Tics are sudden, rapid, recurrent, nonrhythmic, and brief motor movements or vocalizations. They may involve movement of the head or upper body, blinking of eyes, or a variety of verbal noises. They may be worse during periods of stress or tiredness. About 10–20% of children have mild motor tics at some time that gradually disappear with no intervention. Mid-adolescence is the most common age for tics to appear. When the tics are severe or last over 1 year, they are considered chronic and may require attention from a mental health provider.

Severe motor tics accompanied by verbal utterances are known as Tourette syndrome. The syndrome is seen in 3 out of every 1,000 children and is often accompanied by other diagnoses such as attention deficit and learning disabilities. Children with

Tourette syndrome may exhibit **coprolalia**, the involuntary utterance of obscenities, profanities, and racial slurs; or **copropraxia**, the involuntary use of obscene gestures (CDC, 2009b).

There is an underlying genetic cause for tic disorders since about 75% have a family history. Boys are more affected than girls, suggesting an autosomal dominant transfer. The direct pathophysiology of the disorder is unknown, but dopamine, serotonin, and other neurotransmitter and neuropeptide levels are disrupted. Comorbidity commonly involves obsessive-compulsive disorder and ADHD (National Institute of Neurological Disorders and Stroke, 2010).

Careful diagnosis and identification of the disruptive effects of tics are the first steps. Education and reassurance may assist some children with tics. Relaxation and management of stresses in school and other settings may be helpful. The disorders have been treated with medications in some cases (National Institute of Neurological Disorders and Stroke, 2010).

Nursing care involves supporting parents and encouraging normal developmental progression for the child. Stress should be minimized and relaxation techniques taught. Administer medications and teach families about desired and side effects. If the child's verbal utterances are disruptive in the classroom, partner with families and the school to arrange for home tutors for a while if needed. The nurse can teach school personnel and other children about the disorder so that they understand the child's behaviors.

■ TRICHOTILLOMANIA

Trichotillomania, or chronic self hair pulling, can affect children and adolescents. Head hair is most commonly pulled, leaving patches of baldness, but eyebrows, eyelashes, and pubic and other body hair may be involved. Incidence is greatest in middle childhood but it can occur earlier or later. Hair pulling may occur in brief periods of stress or over longer periods during sedentary activities.

Trichotillomania is classified as an impulse control disorder. It has similarities to both obsessive-compulsive disorder and to Tourette syndrome, both described earlier in this chapter (Guynn & Gulley, 2009). Behavioral therapy, hypnosis, and SSRI medication therapy are generally used in treatment. Group therapy may be an effective support mechanism that decreases guilt and feelings of isolation regarding the disorder.

People affected by the disorder usually feel shame and guilt. They try to hide the disorder and may not seek help for an extended period. The nurse should be alert for the disorder when head or body hair is missing, someone is wearing a wig, or eyebrows are heavily penciled. An appropriate way to question the child is to say, "Some people pull out their hair. I notice that you have no eyebrows or eyelashes. Is pulling them out something you do?"

Refer the child or adolescent to a health care professional. Try to establish a trusting atmosphere that fosters communication about the disorder. Encourage participation in the treatment plan. Ensure follow-up for care so effectiveness of treatment can be measured.

■ SCHIZOPHRENIA

Schizophrenia, a psychotic disorder that is rare in young children, occurs in 1 in 10,000 children. Although the condition can manifest in childhood, it is more common in adolescence (Addington & Rapoport, 2009; Mayo Clinic, 2009).

The cause of schizophrenia is unknown, but genetic predisposition and neurotransmitter dysfunction are suspected causes (Mayo Clinic, 2009). The brain is altered in the disease, with progressively enlarged ventricles and nervous system arousal. Impaired glucose metabolism is often present. Onset is usually slow with increasing intensity over time. Most often the child demonstrates restlessness, poor appetite, and social withdrawal over a period of several weeks to months. Behavioral problems, slowed development, and minor neurologic symptoms may occur.

The clinical manifestations of schizophrenia are the same in children as in adults. Characteristic behaviors of the individual with schizophrenia include social withdrawal, impaired social relationships, flat **affect** (outward appearance of feeling or emotion), difficulty completing normal daily activities, regression, loose associations (thought characterized by speech in which ideas shift from one subject to another that is unrelated), poor judgment and problem solving, anxiety, delusions, and hallucinations. Motor abnormalities may include rocking and arm flapping. Onset of symptoms may be triggered by an important loss (death of a significant other, parent, child, or friend).

Prompt diagnosis can lead to early treatment and more positive outcomes. Physical examination, laboratory tests, and psychological examination should be completed by a mental health specialist. Clinical therapy for childhood schizophrenia is multifaceted, including individual psychotherapy, family therapy, social and academic skill training, and various psychotropic medications (antipsychotics such as haloperidol [Haldol], dozapine, olanzapine, and risperidone; antianxiety agents such as lorazepam [Ativan]; and antidepressants such as imipramine [Tofranil]). Drugs are only moderately effective at controlling hallucinations and delusions, responses vary considerably among individuals, and children may have different responses than adults. Side effects will determine what drugs are used and their duration. Antipsychotic medication is continued for at least 4 to 6 weeks before effectiveness can be determined. Medications often must be continued for several months or years after recovery from an acute schizophrenic episode, although medication-free trials may be attempted in children who have shown an absence of symptoms for 6 to 12 months.

Episodes of acute schizophrenia often require inpatient hospitalization on a psychiatric unit for thorough diagnosis and beginning management. Treatment may include an intensive school-based program in a structured, supervised setting with specially trained professionals. The goal of initial treatment is to reduce or control psychotic episodes and provide a safe, structured environment for the child or adolescent, enabling the child to live each day at an optimal level of functioning. Outpatient care is provided following initial diagnosis and establishment of the treatment regimen.

Most children require long-term treatment, including intermittent periods of hospitalization. Children or adolescents whose symptoms are difficult to control and who present a safety risk to themselves or others may require long-term residential treatment. Earlier age at diagnosis and delay in treatment lead to a poorer prognosis.

Nursing Management

The nurse may encounter the child or adolescent with schizophrenia during hospitalization for an acute episode, for treatment of another problem, or while working with the individual in the community. Nursing care centers on providing for the child's physical safety and psychologic care, as well as normal growth and development.

Family education and involvement in the treatment plan are essential. The family is taught to monitor the child's symptoms and progression. Educating the child and parents about the risk of recurrence and methods to alleviate side effects of prescribed medications may increase compliance with the treatment plan. The nurse performs assessments of the child for common medication side effects. Growth measurements, neurological assessment, and laboratory studies are needed.

The family is assisted in establishing educational plans for the child and for integration within the school system. The nurse communicates with school personnel to ensure understanding of the child's condition and ongoing management of the individualized education plan.

■ COGNITIVE ALTERATIONS

A wide array of cognitive conditions occur in childhood. Some are mild and not diagnosed until a child has difficulty in school, whereas others may be associated with physical signs that are visible at birth.

Learning Disabilities

Learning disabilities are a common problem of young children, affecting about 5–10% of school-age children. About 8% of children with low birth weight and 5% of those with normal birth weight are diagnosed with learning disabilities; the incidence is highest in those children with special health care needs (Altarac & Saroha, 2007; Centers for Disease Control and Prevention, 2008a). Involved are neurological conditions in which the brain cannot receive or process information in the normal manner. Often the impairment is only in one or two types of learning, making diagnosis difficult. Common types of learning disorders are listed in the Clinical Manifestations: Learning Disabilities table. Children may have difficulty in processing visual information, which may be manifested in reading, writing, and mathematics performance. Others may have more difficulty with oral information, leading to problems in language development and reading.

The causes of learning disorders are complex. Sometimes they are related to low birth weight or problems during the perinatal period. The disabilities should be diagnosed by a learning specialist such as a psychologist with specialty training. A series

Clinical Manifestations
Learning Disabilities

Disorder	Clinical Manifestations
Dyslexia	Difficulty with writing, reading, and spelling
Dyscalculia	Mathematics and computation problems
Dysgraphia	Difficulty with writing, spelling, and composition
Dyspraxia	Problems with manual dexterity and coordination

of cognitive and developmental tests are most commonly used. Brain scanning with MRI is showing promise for diagnostic clues in the future. There may be a genetic component since their occurrence is more common when other family members are affected. Treatments involve learning how to compensate for the difficulties by using capabilities that are intact. Some children need to have all material written for them, and others need to have oral presentations. Specific learning goals are established with the assistance of learning specialists. Children with learning disabilities should have individualized education plans (IEPs) established with realistic goals for school performance (see Chapter 10 ∞ for further information about IEPs).

Nursing Management

Nurses play a major role in the identification of children with learning disabilities. You may be in contact with families during health promotion visits or other settings when parents relay concerns about the child's performance or difficulty in some aspect of school. Ask about a family history of learning problems and evaluate the child's history for prematurity, low birth weight, head injury, seizure activity, and other chronic health conditions. Assess the young child for the following developmental milestones which can indicate learning disability:

- Delay in developmental tasks such as tying shoes, buttoning, or hopping
- Delay in expressive or receptive speech
- Delay in naming objects or reading
- Delay in fine and gross motor milestones
- Difficulty following simple instructions

(National Joint Committee on Learning Disabilities, 2006)

When a child may have a learning disability, refer the family to the school or other testing resource. Partner with the family to plan for the child's learning needs. Help the family to work closely with the child, provide a setting at home to maximize potential for learning, and build healthy self-esteem in the child. Assist the family to work with the school to establish annual goals for the child. A multidisciplinary team commonly works within the school, and includes teachers, therapists, and the family to plan for the child's learning needs. Most children with learning disabilities can learn to perform well in their areas of strength and compensate for areas of difficulty. Early intervention is key to success and building positive self-image regarding abilities.

Intellectual Disability (Mental Retardation)

Intellectual disability is now the preferred term for what was previously called *mental retardation.* **Intellectual disability** is defined as significant limitation in intellectual functioning and adaptive behavior. It is manifested in differences in conceptual, social, and practical adaptive skills, beginning before the age of 18 years (American Association on Intellectual and Developmental Disabilities, 2008). Later events that lead to limitations in function are commonly referred to as brain injury. Intellectual functioning is generally characterized by an IQ below 70 to 75 with significant impairments in **adaptive functioning** (the ability of an individual to meet the standards expected for the cultural group). The child with intellectual disability has adaptive deficits in at least two areas such as communication, self-care, home living, social/interpersonal skills, use of community resources, self-direction, functional academic skills, work, leisure, health, or safety. A low IQ score by itself does not necessarily correlate with impairment in the ability to carry out adaptive skills. The child should be evaluated within the contexts of the individual cultural and community environment. The IQ score and the level of adaptive skills together determine the degree of severity of intellectual disability.

Intellectual disability is one type of **developmental disability,** any of a variety of chronic conditions that are characterized by mental or physical impairments. Other examples include pervasive developmental disorder, cerebral palsy (see Chapter 27 ∞), and sensory loss (see Chapter 19 ∞). A developmental disability begins by the age of 21 years, and lasts throughout life (CDC, n.d.).

Etiology and Pathophysiology

Intellectual disability occurs in 12 per 1,000 children, a decrease from 15.5 per 1,000 one decade ago (CDC, n.d.). Its causes can be grouped into three general categories: prenatal errors in the development of the CNS, prenatal or postnatal changes in the biologic environment of the person, and external forces leading to CNS damage. Prematurity, intrauterine growth retardation, environmental hazards, and many other conditions can lead to intellectual disability. In each instance, the precipitating factor causes a change in the form, function, and adaptation of the central nervous system. Table 28–6 provides examples of common causes of intellectual disability for each category.

Three common conditions from prenatal life that are associated with intellectual disability are Down syndrome, fragile X syndrome, and fetal alcohol syndrome. They will be discussed

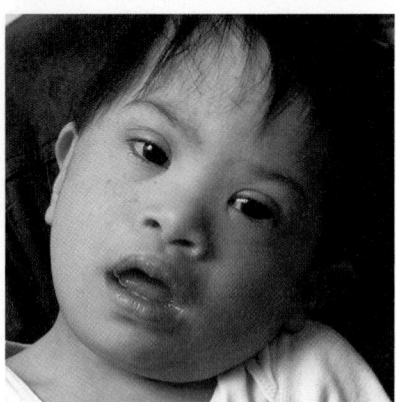

FIGURE 28–10 ➤ A child with Down syndrome.

in greater detail in this section, followed by nursing management for children with intellectual disability from any cause. In the United States, about 1 in 800 infants, or 5,500 infants each year, are born with Down syndrome (American Academy of Pediatrics, 2009; CDC, 2006a; van Riper, 2007). See Figure 28–10 ➤. The syndrome is caused by an extra chromosome; the child has 47 rather than 46 chromosomes (see discussion of genetic transmission in Chapter 4 ∞). The most common chromosome affected is 21, so that the child often has trisomy 21, or three copies instead of two of chromosome 21. In addition to intellectual disability and physical signs, the child with Down syndrome is at higher risk of developing other conditions such as cardiac defects, hearing loss, strabismus, gastrointestinal problems, orthodontic conditions, thyroid disease, dermatologic conditions, and leukemia (Barnhart & Connolly, 2007; Fonatsch, 2010). Jeremiah, who was described in the opening scenario, was born with Down syndrome. He had gastrointestinal (GI) reflux and otitis media frequently as a young child.

Fragile X syndrome is caused by a single recessive gene abnormality on the X chromosome. A permutation to the X chromosome may occur in males or females. When a father or mother passes the faulty X chromosome to a daughter, it may remain as a permutation or may change into a true mutation. The daughter has two X chromosomes and therefore does not manifest this recessive disorder; however, she can give the mutated X chromosome to her son, who becomes affected with fragile X. The mutation of fragile X is on gene FMRP-1, which instructs cells to make a protein necessary for normal brain development. The faulty gene creates a deficiency in the FMR1 protein that

TABLE 28–6	Common Conditions Associated with Intellectual Disability	
Prenatal Conditions	Biologic Environment	External Forces
Down syndrome	Inborn errors of metabolism (e.g., phenylketonuria, hypothyroidism)	Traumatic brain injury (e.g., accident)
Fragile X syndrome		Poison ingestion (acute or chronic)
Fetal alcohol syndrome		Hypoxia/anoxic insult
Maternal infection (e.g., rubella, cytomegalovirus)		Infection (e.g., meningitis)
		Environmental deprivation

Fetal alcohol syndrome is more common in groups with higher intake of alcohol. Because several Native American tribes have a high rate of alcoholism, the federal government and some tribes have joined to lower that risk among this ethnic group. On some reservations, such as the Yakama Nation in Washington State, alcoholic beverages are not sold and educational programs are in place.

leads to brain changes. The condition is often associated with other conditions such as ADHD, anxiety, and autism (Hay, 2008; Roberts, Mankowski, Sideris, et al., 2009).

Fetal alcohol syndrome (FAS) is caused by the effect of ethyl alcohol on the developing fetus (Figure 28–11 ➤). The term *fetal alcohol spectrum disorder (FASD)* describes the wide range of effects from the condition, which can range from FAS to a milder condition called fetal alcohol effects (FAE) (Ismail, Buckley, Budacki, et al., 2010). Alcohol ingestion by the pregnant woman can influence development of many body organs, and its effects can range from mild to severe. Despite many years of education, alcohol use remains a leading cause of intellectual disability, affecting 0.3 to 1.5 of 1,000 births in the United States, or 8,000 to 12,000 infants annually (CDC, 2010c).

Chapter 30 ∞ discusses phenylketonuria and hypothyroidism, two common biochemical causes of intellectual disability. Other causes involve traumatic brain injury and infections of the central nervous system (see Chapter 27 ∞).

Clinical Manifestations

Mild intellectual disability was originally described as an intelligence quotient (IQ) between 50 and 70, moderate disability as IQ of 35 to 50, severe disability as IQ of 20 to 35, and profound disability as IQ below 20. Although an IQ below 70 is generally considered indicative of intellectual disability, the functional assessment of the child is now considered to be a more accurate identification of the child's performance and needs. Children who are intellectually disabled manifest delays in all areas of development, including motor movement, language, and adaptive behavior. They usually achieve developmental milestones more slowly than the average child. These developmental delays may be the first indication to parents and care providers of the child's condition.

Intellectual disability is sometimes accompanied by sensory impairment, speech problems, motor and orthopedic disabilities, and seizure disorders. Of children with the disability, 10–30% manifest one such disorder. Table 28–7 lists several physical characteristics associated with Down syndrome, fragile X syndrome, and fetal alcohol syndrome.

COLLABORATIVE CARE

Diagnostic Tests

Intellectual disability is diagnosed and initial treatment is planned in a multistep process, and by involving a multidisciplinary team that involves a developmental specialist, physician, geneticist, nurse, teacher, language therapist, and rehabilitation specialists. See Table 28–8 for a description of the *DSM-IV-TR* for intellectual disability.

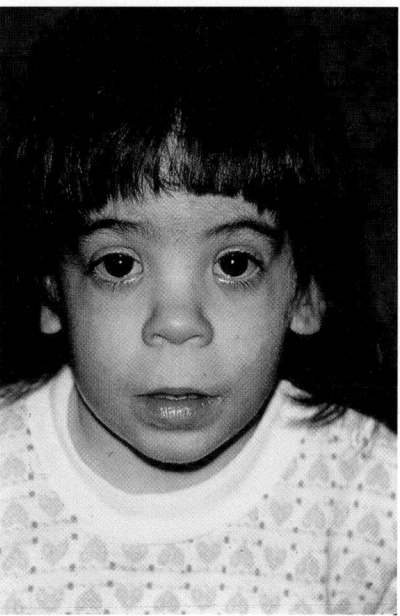

FIGURE 28–11 ➤ A child with fetal alcohol syndrome.
Used with permission from Dr. Sterling Clarren, Seattle, WA. Clarren, S. K., & Smith, D. W. © 1978. The fetal alcohol syndrome. New England Journal of Medicine, 298, 1063–1067. Massachusetts Medical Society. All rights reserved.

First, a comprehensive history and evaluation of the child's physical characteristics, developmental level, and intellectual and adaptive functioning is carried out. Laboratory tests such as chromosome analysis, blood enzyme levels, lead levels, or cranial imaging provide valuable information in some circumstances. A three-generation family history is performed (American Academy of Pediatrics, 2007).

Developmental screening using a test such as the Denver II (see Chapter 6 ∞) can help to identify children who may be at risk. Tests of intellectual and adaptive functioning are performed when disability is suspected. A neurologic examination may indicate asymmetry of movement or strength, irritability or lethargy, or abnormal pitch to an infant's cry. Because intellectual disability may be accompanied by physical abnormalities, it is important to observe the child for facial symmetry, distance between the eyes, level of the ears, hair growth, and palmar creases. These abnormalities may be cues to other health problems.

Clinical Therapy

Based on the results of the evaluation, a multidisciplinary team plans the support needed to maximize the child's potential for development. Management focuses on early intervention to improve the degree of adaptive functioning. Simultaneous

The Education for All Handicapped Children Act, P.L. 94–142, provides free appropriate education to all children with disabilities between 2 and 21 years of age. Amendments to this act in 1986 (P.L. 99–457) encouraged states to provide early intervention services for infants and toddlers with developmental delay by providing federal funding.

TABLE 28–7   Characteristics of Three Common Conditions Associated with Intellectual Disability

Down Syndrome	Fragile X Syndrome	Fetal Alcohol Syndrome
Small head (microcephaly)	Long face	Flat midface
Flattened forehead	Prominent jaw	Low nasal bridge
Wide, short neck	Large ears	Long philtrum with narrow upper lip
Epicanthal eye folds	Frequent otitis media	Short upturned nose
White spots on eye iris (Brushfield spots)	Large testicles	Poor coordination
Congenital cataracts	Epicanthal eye folds	Failure to thrive
Flat nose	Strabismus	Skeletal and joint abnormalities
Small, low-set ears	High-arched palate	Hearing loss
Protruding tongue	Scoliosis	
Short broad hands	Pliable joints	
Simian line on palm		
Wide space between first and second toes		
Hearing loss		
Increased incidence of diabetes, congenital heart defect, and leukemia		
Hypotonia		

treatment of associated physical, emotional, and behavioral problems is provided. Depending on the child's condition, special education programs and physical or occupational therapy may be necessary (Figure 28–12 ➤).

The child may require supportive care and assistance with activities of daily living (ADLs). The plans for intervention change as the child grows and family situations evolve. Some schools and community agencies offer transitional classes when children who are intellectually disabled reach adolescence and young adulthood. These services help to teach self-care skills that may enable some youth to live in group homes or other community settings. Families receive help in planning for the child's future as parents look toward retirement. Information is

TABLE 28–8   *DSM-IV-TR* Diagnostic Criteria for Intellectual Disability (Mental Retardation)

A. Significantly subaverage intellectual functioning: an IQ of approximately 70 or below on an individually administered IQ test (for infants, a clinical judgment of significantly subaverage intellectual functioning)

B. Concurrent deficits or impairments in present adaptive functioning (i.e., the person's effectiveness in meeting the standards expected for his or her age by his or her cultural group) in at least two of the following areas: communication, self-care, home living, social/interpersonal skills, use of community resources, self-direction, functional academic skills, work, leisure, health, and safety

C. The onset is before age 18 years

Reprinted with permission from the Diagnostic and Statistical Manual of Mental Disorders, *Fourth Edition, Text Revision. Copyright © 2000 American Psychiatric Association.*

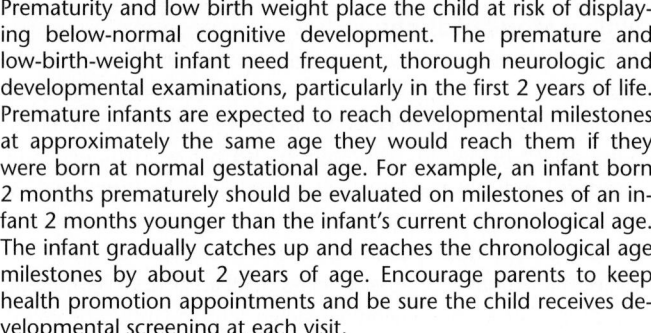

Nursing Alert

Prematurity and low birth weight place the child at risk of displaying below-normal cognitive development. The premature and low-birth-weight infant need frequent, thorough neurologic and developmental examinations, particularly in the first 2 years of life. Premature infants are expected to reach developmental milestones at approximately the same age they would reach them if they were born at normal gestational age. For example, an infant born 2 months prematurely should be evaluated on milestones of an infant 2 months younger than the infant's current chronological age. The infant gradually catches up and reaches the chronological age milestones by about 2 years of age. Encourage parents to keep health promotion appointments and be sure the child receives developmental screening at each visit.

provided on living options, health insurance, work opportunities, and other needs. This can also provide respite services for parents and other family members who have spent much time with the child for many years.

NURSING MANAGEMENT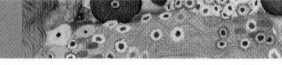

Nursing Assessment and Diagnosis

Nurses can help to identify children with intellectual disability through history taking, observation, and developmental screening during early childhood. The history should provide information about the mental and adaptive functioning of birth parents and other family members because intellectual disability may cluster in some families, and conditions such as fragile X syndrome are genetic in origin. The pregnancy and birth history can provide important information relating to alcohol and

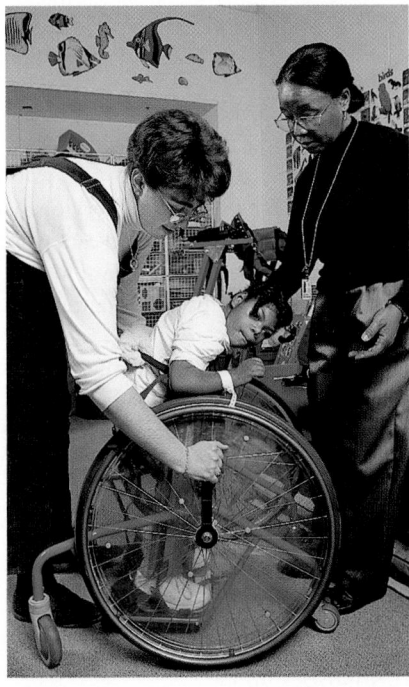
A

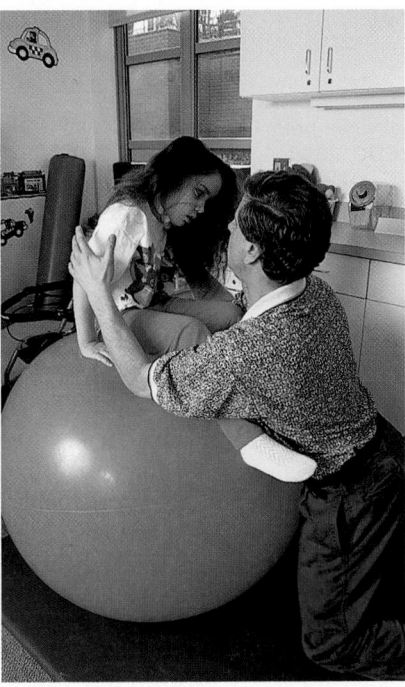
B

FIGURE 28–12 ➤ Physical therapy is an important component of medical management for many children who have intellectual disabilities. A, This girl with severe intellectual disability uses a wheelchair. She is being positioned in a mobile prone stander, which enables her to interact in a different manner with her therapists and the environment. B, Physical therapists also provide outpatient care in the community to children with varying degrees of disability.

drug use by the mother during pregnancy. Be alert for a history of difficult pregnancy and problems during delivery.

When genetic conditions in the family predispose family members to intellectual disability, careful assessment of the child is needed. Children from deprived environments or those at risk because of environmental factors such as lead poisoning (see Chapter 17 ∞) are more likely to manifest disability.

Many children with intellectual disability are not diagnosed with the condition until they reach school age, particularly if the condition is mild or moderate. Early intervention, however, can help to enhance the child's functioning later. During home visits, during clinic appointments, in childcare centers, and during hospitalization, be alert for signs of developmental delays, multiple (more than three) physical anomalies associated with a specific condition (see Table 28–7), or neurologic alterations. Developmental assessment should be part of each health care visit.

Once the diagnosis of intellectual disability has been made, assess the adaptive functioning of the child and family. A functional assessment of the child should be performed, including toileting, dressing, and feeding skills. Assess the child's language, sensory, and psychomotor functioning. Assess the home and community for safety hazards. Observe how the family is managing with the child. Assess the availability of services such as support groups for parents and special education opportunities for children. Evaluate the coping skills of family members.

Clinical Judgment

Jeremiah, described in the opening scenario, has recently been enrolled in a school program. Think ahead to his needs as an adolescent. What information will his family need to provide a healthy and safe experience for him regarding drinking, sexuality, and other adolescent issues? Where will you find information to assist Jeremiah and his family when he reaches adolescence?

Several nursing diagnoses may be appropriate for the child with intellectual disability, depending on the degree, cause, and outcome of the condition. Diagnoses that relate to impairments in adaptive functioning and family impact include the following:

- Delayed Growth and Development related to neonatal disease or condition
- Imbalanced Nutrition: Less than Body Requirements related to inability to ingest sufficient food
- Self-Care Deficit: Dressing, Toileting, Bathing related to developmental disability
- Impaired Verbal Communication related to developmental disability
- Risk for Injury related to lack of understanding of environmental hazards
- Compromised Family Coping related to the child's developmental variations

Planning and Implementation

Prevention is important for some types of intellectual disability. All pregnant women or those who may become pregnant should stop ingestion of alcohol and nonprescription drugs. Encourage regular prenatal visits; this helps to prevent premature births, which have a higher association with intellectual disability than birth at term.

Nearly all children with intellectual disability are cared for in the community; however, they may have conditions that require periodic hospitalization or frequent health care visits. When needed, nursing care focuses on providing emotional support and information to family members, assisting the child with adaptive functioning, and fostering parental management of the child's activities. When possible, the nurse uses preventive teaching to lower the risk of intellectual disability.

Nursing Alert

Fetal alcohol syndrome (FAS) is a preventable cause of intellectual disability. About 12–15% of women consume alcohol while pregnant, and 2% engage in frequent or binge drinking (CDC, 2010c). This indicates that all women must receive clear messages about the dangers of drinking while pregnant. Teach all pregnant women that total abstention from alcohol for the entire length of pregnancy is the only completely effective method of preventing FAS. Include this in teaching to all adolescent girls, so they are aware of how alcohol can harm their infant if they become pregnant. Emphasize that the most dangerous time may be early in pregnancy before women commonly know they are pregnant (Monsen, 2009).

Provide Emotional Support and Information

Family members need empathy and support both at the time of diagnosis and in the ensuing years. Parents may be in an acute or chronic state of grief over the loss of what they imagined to be the perfect child. Encourage them to verbalize their feelings. Introducing them to parents of other children with intellectual disabilities may provide assistance and support as they learn how to manage the child's needs. Discuss the availability of respite care to provide parents with a break from caretaking. Other family members such as grandparents and siblings may also be experiencing grief or guilt and should be given an opportunity to talk about their feelings.

Clinical Tip

To determine the impact of the child with intellectual disability on the family, ask parents to describe (1) family activities that include the child, (2) strategies that parents and siblings use to deal with community attitudes about the child, and (3) in the case of a child with other disabilities, methods of managing the child's care and planning for future care needs.

Parents need honest information and answers to their questions about the child's condition. Reinforce information provided by genetic counselors and other health care professionals. Parents need to be informed about community resources designed to assist children with intellectual disability. Such resources include the Zero to Three Project, special education preschools and schools, county health services, and respite care. Ask parents if they have questions about IEPs. Refer parents to Internet sources, and help them to interpret information received and analyze its strengths and limitations. Review federal and state laws and services that might be helpful to the family. Examples include the following:

- The Administration on Developmental Disabilities (ADD) is the U.S. organization that ensures that the Developmental Disabilities (DD) Act goals are met. The DD Act implements the Developmental Disabilities and Bill of Rights Act of 2000 and seeks to enhance life through training activities, educating the community, eliminating barriers, and influencing policy (Administration for Children & Families, 2008).

- State Councils on Developmental Disabilities (SCDD) are present in each state to increase integration of children with developmental disabilities.
- Public Law (P.L.) 94–142 of 1975 mandated that all children, including those with handicaps, be provided with public education and related services.
- Public Law (P.L.) 99–457 of 1986 expanded the services of P.L. 94–142 to include children from birth to 5 years who need special education. Its focus is the importance of fostering development and enhancing the capacity of families to meet the needs of children.
- Public Law (P.L.) 101–336 of 1990 is known as the Americans with Disabilities Act (ADA). It prohibits discrimination and ensures equal opportunity for persons with disabilities in employment, state and local government services, public accommodations, commercial facilities, and transportation.
- The Individuals with Disabilities Education Act (IDEA) Amendments of 1997 strengthened the academic expectations and accountability for children with disabilities.

Maintain a Safe Environment

Children with intellectual disabilities require close supervision because they may lack an understanding of common hazards. Ensure safety in the hospital environment. Assist parents to provide safety at home and school and to teach their child necessary skills such as pedestrian safety. Consider both physical and emotional safety. The child with intellectual disability may be trusting of others and sometimes is at risk for physical or sexual abuse.

Provide Assistance with Adaptive Functioning

Encourage parents' efforts to maximize the child's areas of strength and identify needs related to adaptive behaviors. Refer them to resources to assist in the areas of adaptive functioning in which the child has impairment, such as communication, self-care activities, or social skills. During hospitalization, support parents' efforts to maintain the child's skills in toileting, dressing, and self-care by planning interventions to use the skills being taught at home.

Care in the Community

The child with intellectual disability needs ongoing care throughout childhood, and adaptation of interventions as development occurs and the family's needs evolve. Parents often act as case managers for the child's care. Assist parents as necessary to acquire the skills required to coordinate the child's plan of care. Evaluate the child's needs regularly and assist parents with the treatment plan as necessary. Assist with plans for education and for services such as physical or speech therapy. Most children with intellectual disability have an individualized education plan designed to meet their specific learning needs. Parents, nurses, and others such as teachers and language therapists are part of the team that establishes this plan. Promote optimal development and socialization. As the child reaches adolescence, education is directed toward a vocation, issues of sexuality, and the goal of independent living, when appropriate.

Specific guidelines for care are available for the child with Down syndrome. These guidelines suggest times for evaluation of hearing, growth, cardiac function, and other areas designed for early identification and treatment of associated disorders (American Academy of Pediatrics, 2007; Van Cleve, Cannon, & Cohen, 2006; Van Cleve & Cohen, 2006). There are specific growth grids for children with Down syndrome, and specific topics to suggest for anticipatory guidance during health care visits.

Evaluation

The expected outcomes of nursing care depend on the child's needs and developmental level. Early in the diagnostic phase, desired outcomes may involve the family's understanding of the diagnosis and the child's special needs. Later outcomes may focus on the child's communication of self-help skills. Outcomes related to cognitive performance and adaptive skills may be developed during childhood.

▲ Health Promotion

Health promotion visits are important for all children with disabilities. Nurses must carefully assess nutrition, physical activity, and oral care. Can the child feed self and make healthy food choices? Is regular oral care performed? Is it difficult to maintain regular physical activity? Other mental health comorbidities such as ADHD or depression may emerge, so mental health evaluation is performed at each health promotion visit. Preventive care such as safety teaching and administration of immunizations is integrated to ensure health maintenance.

Chapter Highlights

- Major treatment modes for children with mental health disorders include individual therapy, family therapy, and group therapy.
- Therapeutic strategies for treatment of children and adolescents with mental health disorders include play therapy, art therapy, behavior therapy, visualization, and hypnosis.
- Families often attempt to treat mental health conditions with use of alternative and complementary therapy; nurses can provide information to assist families in evaluating the results of these therapies.
- Nurses are involved in conducting mental health assessments, preventing disorders when possible, participating in evidence-based interventions to treat disorders, and evaluating success of treatments.
- Autistic spectrum disorder is the major type of pervasive developmental disorder, and is manifested by abnormal behavior, social interaction, and communication.
- Attention deficit disorder (ADD) and attention deficit hyperactivity disorder (ADHD) are characterized by developmentally inappropriate behaviors involving inattention, and sometimes hyperactivity.
- ADD and ADHD must be diagnosed using recommended criteria and are commonly treated with a combination of behavioral, environmental, and medication therapies.
- Schizophrenia is a psychotic disorder manifested by social withdrawal, delusions, and hallucinations.
- Mood disorders in childhood and adolescence are commonly manifested as depression or manic depression (bipolar disorder).
- Several anxiety disorders occur in children and adolescents, most notably generalized anxiety, separation anxiety, panic, obsessive-compulsive disorder, school (social) phobia, conversion reaction, and posttraumatic stress disorder.

- Behavioral therapy and selective serotonin reuptake inhibitors (SSRIs) are used in treatment of anxiety disorders; their use in children must be closely monitored.
- Posttraumatic stress disorder may occur as victims relive the terror of traumatic events.
- Suicide is a frequent cause of death among youth.
- Nurses are key health professionals in identifying youth at risk of suicide, instituting suicide prevention programs, and counseling family and friends of suicide victims.
- Children may experience tic disorders that impair development and social interactions; medications are helpful in treatment of these disorders.
- Childhood schizophrenia presents a crisis for families and may require inpatient hospitalization for youth affected.
- Nurses play a role in identifying children with potential learning disabilities, referring for diagnosis, and partnering with the family to provide a positive learning environment for the child.
- Intellectual disability is defined as subaverage intellectual and adaptive functioning, and is caused by chromosomal, genetic, or environmental factors.
- Nurses identify children with possible intellectual disability by careful evaluation of development.
- A multidisciplinary team plans the care for children with intellectual disability and periodically evaluates the child's progress and the family's needs.
- Nurses play a vital role in maintaining the mental health of children, preventing mental health problems, identifying children at risk of mental health disorders, and providing care or referring families for mental health services.

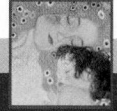

Clinical Reasoning in Action

Recall the opening scenario. Jeremiah is a 7-year-old child who has Down syndrome. He has been relatively healthy after some GI and ear problems in early childhood. His early intervention programs and now his entrance into school have provided a strong and nurturing environment for learning.

1. How will you decide if the physical growth and psychological development that Jeremiah is demonstrating are what would be expected for a child with his condition? What regular physical assessments are needed, due to some common accompanying health problems seen in children with Down syndrome?

2. Based on his history of frequent otitis media, what assessments will you perform now? See Chapter 19 ∞ for ideas.

3. What is the genetic basis for Down syndrome? Why are older parents more at risk for having a child with the syndrome?

4. Find evidence-based practice guidelines to help you plan some physical activities that Jeremiah is likely to enjoy. How will you integrate them into his family and school life?

5. Jeremiah's parents are requesting information about what plans they should make for his care when they start planning for retirement. How can you assist them in locating resources to assist with the future care that Jeremiah will need as he grows into teen years and young adulthood?

See Pearson Nursing Student Resources for possible responses.

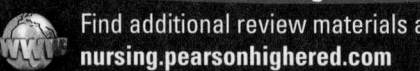

References

Addington, A. M., & Rapoport, J. L. (2009). The genetics of childhood onset schizophrenia: When madness strikes the prepubescent. *Current Psychiatric Reports, 11*(2), 156–161.

Administration for Children and Families (2008). Americans with Disabilities Act: Questions and Answers. Retrieved from http://www.ada.gov/q%26aeng02.htm

Altarac, M., & Saroha, E. (2007). Lifetime prevalence of learning disabilities among US children. *Pediatrics, 119*, S77–S83.

American Academy of Pediatrics. (2007). Policy statement: Health supervision for children with Down syndrome. *Pediatrics, 120*(3), 663–664.

American Academy of Pediatrics. (2009). *Down syndrome.* Retrieved from http://www.healthychildren.org

American Academy of Pediatrics. (2010a). *Vaccines and side effects: The facts.* Retrieved from http://www.healthychildren.org

American Academy of Pediatrics. (2010b). *Causes of ADHD.* Retrieved from http://www.healthychildren.org

American Association on Intellectual and Developmental Disabilities. (2008). *Frequently asked questions on intellectual disability and the AAIDD*

definition. Retrieved from http://www.aamr.org/content_185.cfm

American Psychiatric Association. (2000). *Diagnostic and statistical manual of mental disorders* (4th ed., text revision). Washington, DC: Author.

Anderson, E. R., & Mayes, L. C. (2010). Race/ethnicity and internalizing disorders in youth: A review. *Clinical Psychology Review, 30*, 338–348.

Apps, J., Winkler, J., & Jandrisevits, M. D. (2008). Bipolar disorders: Symptoms and treatment in children and adolescents. *Pediatric Nursing, 34*, 84–88.

Barnhart, R. C., & Connolly, B. (2007). Aging and Down syndrome: Implications for physical therapy. *Physical Therapy, 87*(10), 1399–1406.

Beauchamp, R. A., Willis, T. M., Betz, T. G., Villanacci, J., Rozin, L., Brown, M. J., et al. (2006). Deaths associated with hypocalcemia from chelation therapy—Texas, Pennsylvania, and Oregon, 2003–2005. *Morbidity and Mortality Weekly Report, 55*, 204–207.

Beesdo, K., Knappe, S., & Pine, D. S. (2009). Anxiety and anxiety disorders in children and adolescents: Developmental issues and implications for DSM-V. *Psychiatric Clinics of North America, 32*(3), 483–524.

Bothe, D., & Olness, K. (2007). Worried sick: Anxiety among youth. Part 2. *Contemporary Pediatrics, 24*(8), 82–89.

Bridge, J. A., Iyengar, S., Salary, C. B., Barbe, R. P., Birmaher, B., Pincus, H. A., et al. (2007). Clinical response and risk for reported suicidal ideation and suicide attempts in pediatric antidepressant treatment. *Journal of the American Medical Association, 297*, 1683–1696.

Brulotte, J., Bukutu, C., & Vohra, S. (2009). Complementary, holistic, and integrative medicine: Fish oils and neurodevelopmental disorders. *Pediatrics in Review, 30*(4), e29–33.

Centers for Disease Control and Prevention (CDC). (n.d.). *Intellectual disabilities among children.* Retrieved from http://www.cdc.gov

Centers for Disease Control and Prevention (CDC). (2006a). Improved national prevalence estimates for 18 selected major birth defects—United States, 1999–2001. *Morbidity and Mortality Weekly Report, 54*, 1301–1305.

Centers for Disease Control and Prevention (CDC). (2006b). Youth Risk Behavior Surveillance—United States, 2005. *Morbidity and Mortality Weekly Report, 55*(SS-5), 1–112.

Centers for Disease Control and Prevention (CDC). (2007a). Prevalence of autism spectrum disorders—Autism and developmental disorders monitoring network. *Morbidity and Mortality Weekly Report, 56*(SS-1), 1–40.

Centers for Disease Control and Prevention (CDC). (2007b). *Suicide.* Atlanta: Author.

Centers for Disease Control and Prevention (CDC). (2007c). Suicide trends among youths and young adults aged 10–24 years—United States, 1990–2004. *Morbidity and Mortality Weekly Report, 56,* 905–908.

Centers for Disease Control and Prevention. (2008a). QuickStats: Percentage of children ages 6–17 years with learning disability (LD) and attention deficit hyperactivity disorder (ADHD), by birthweight—National Health Interview Survey, United States, 2004–2006. *Morbidity and Mortality Weekly Report, 57*(34), 947.

Centers for Disease Control and Prevention (CDC). (2008b). Unintentional strangulation deaths from the "choking game" among youths ages 6–19 years—United States 1995–2007. *Morbidity and Mortality Weekly Report, 57*(06), 141–146.

Centers for Disease Control and Prevention (CDC). (2009a). Prevalence of autistic spectrum disorders—Autism and developmental disabilities monitoring network, United States, 2006. *Morbidity and Mortality Weekly Report, 58*(SS10), 1–20.

Centers for Disease Control and Prevention (CDC). (2009b). Prevalence of diagnosed Tourette syndrome in persons aged 6–17 years—United States, 2007. *Morbidity and Mortality Weekly Report, 58*(21), 581–585.

Centers for Disease Control and Prevention (CDC). (2010a). *Autistic syndrome disorders treatment.* Retrieved from http://www.cdc.gov/ncbddd/autism/treatment.html

Centers for Disease Control and Prevention (CDC). (2010b). *The choking game: Risky youth behavior.* Retrieved from http://www.cdc.gov

Centers for Disease Control and Prevention (CDC). (2010c). *Fetal alcohol spectrum disorders (FASDs).* Retrieved from http://www.cdc.gov

Chamley, C. A., Carson, P., Randall, D., & Sandwell, M. (2005). *Developmental anatomy and physiology of children.* New York: Elsevier.

Cheung, A. H., Zuckerbrot, R. A., Jensen, P. S., Ghalib, K., Laraque, D., Stein, R. E. L., & GLAD-PC Steering Group. (2007). Guidelines for adolescent depression in primary care (GLAD-PC): II. Treatment and ongoing management. *Pediatrics, 120,* e1313–1326.

Custer, J. W., & Rau, R. E. (2009). *The Harriet Lane Handbook* (18th ed.). St. Louis: Mosby.

D'Alessandro, T. M. (2009). Factors influencing the onset of childhood obsessive compulsive disorder. *Pediatric Nursing, 35*(1), 43–46.

Dawson, G., Munson, J., Webb, S. J., Nalty, T., Abbott, R., & Toth, K. (2007). Rate of head growth decelerates and symptoms worsen in the second year of life in autism. *Biological Psychiatry, 61*(4), 458–464.

DelBello, M. P., Adler, C. M., & Strakowski, S. M. (2006). The neurophysiology of childhood and adolescent bipolar disorder. *CNS Spectrum, 11,* 298–311.

Fonatsch, C. (2010). The role of chromosome 21 in hematology and oncology. *Genes and Chromosomes in Cancer, 49*(6), 497–508.

Froehlich, T. E., Lanphear, B. P., Epstein, J. N., Barbaresi, W. J., Katusic, S. K., & Kahn, R. S. (2007). Prevalence, recognition, and treatment of attention-deficit/hyperactivity disorder in a national sample of US children. *Archives of Pediatrics and Adolescent Medicine, 161,* 857–864.

Gabbay, V., Coffey, B. J., Babb, J. S., Meyer, L., Wachtel, C., Anam, S., & Rabinovitz, B. (2008). Pediatric autoimmune neuropsychiatric disorders associated with streptococcus: Comparison of diagnosis and treatment in the community and at a specialty unit. *Pediatrics, 122,* 273–278.

Ganem, J. A. (2008). Treating children with ADHD. *Clinicians CME.* Retrieved from http://www.jobsoneducation.com/cliniciansCME/index.asp?page=courses/105821/disclaimer.htm&lsn_id=105821

Garzon, D. L. (2007, February). Childhood depression. *Advance for Nurse Practitioners,* 35–44.

Guynn, C., & Gulley, T. (2009, November). Trichotillomania. *Consultant for Pediatricians,* 408.

Hamblen, J. L., Norris, F. H., Pietruszkiewicz, S., Gibson, L. E., Naturale, A., & Louis, C. (2009). Cognitive behavioral therapy for postdisaster distress: a community based treatment program for survivors of Hurricane Katrina. *Administration and Policy in Mental Health 36*(3), 206–214.

Hamrin, V., & Magorno, M. (2010). Assessment of adolescents for depression in the pediatric primary care setting. *Pediatric Nursing 36*(2), 103–111.

Hay, D. A. (2008). Fragile X – a challenge to models of the mind and to best clinical practice. *Cortex 44*(6), 626–627.

Hirsch, A. J., & Carlson, J. S. (2007). Prescription practices and empirical efficacy of psychopharmacologic treatments for pediatric major depressive disorder. *Journal of Child and Adolescent Psychiatric Nursing, 20,* 222–233.

Ismail, S., Buckley, S., Budacki, R., Jabbar, A., & Gallicano, G. I. (2010). Screening, diagnosing and prevention of fetal alcohol syndrome: Is this syndrome treatable? *Developmental Neuroscience, 32*(2), 91–100.

Johnson, C. P., Myers, S. M., & Council on Children with Disabilities. (2007). Identification and evaluation of children with autism spectrum disorders. *Pediatrics, 120,* 1183–1215.

Kassam-Adams, N., Marsac, M. L., & Cirilli, C. (2010). Posttraumatic stress disorder symptom structure in injured children: Functional impairment and depression symptoms in a confirmatory factor analysis. *Journal of the American Academy of Child and Adolescent Psychiatry, 49*(6), 616–625.

Kazak, A. E., Hoagwood, K., Weisz, J. R., Kratochwill, T. R., Vargas, L. A., & Banez, G. A. (2010). A meta-systems approach to evidence-based practice for children and adolescents. *American Psychologist, 65*(2), 85–97.

Keeley, M. L., & Storch, E. A. (2009). Anxiety disorders in youth. *Journal of Pediatric Nursing, 24*(1), 26–40.

Kendall, P. C., Compton, S. N., Walkup, J. T., Birmaher, B., Albano, A. M., Sherill, J., et al. (2010).

Clinical characteristics of anxiety disordered youth. *Journal of Anxiety Disorders, 24,* 360–365.

Kortesluoma, R. L., Punamaki, R. L., & Nikkonen, M. (2008). Hospitalized children drawing their pain: The contents and cognitive and emotional characteristics of pain drawings. *Journal of Child Health Care, 12*(4), 284–300.

Lack, C. W., & Green, A. L. (2009). Mood disorders in children and adolescents. *Journal of Pediatric Nursing, 24*(1), 13–25.

Legerstee, J. S., Tulen, J. H., Dierckx, B., Treffers, P. D., Verhulst, F. C., & Utens, E. M. (2010). CBT for childhood anxiety disorders: Differential changes in selective attention between treatment responders and non-responders. *Journal of Child Psychology and Psychiatry, 51*(2), 162–172.

Lobar, S. L., Fritts, M. K., Arbide, Z., & Russell, D. (2008). The role of the nurse practitioner in an individualized education plan and coordination of care for the child with Asperger's syndrome. *Journal of Pediatric Health Care, 22,* 111–119.

Looman, W. S. (2006). A developmental approach to understanding drawings and narratives from children displaced by Hurricane Katrina. *Journal of Pediatric Health Care, 20,* 158–166.

Mark, T. L., & Buck, J. A. (2006). Characteristics of U.S. youths with serious emotional disturbance: Data from the National Health Interview Survey. *Psychiatric Services, 57,* 1573–1578.

May, D. E., & Kratochvil, C. J. (2010). Attention-deficit hyperactivity disorder: Recent advances in paediatric pharmacotherapy. *Drugs, 70*(1), 15–40.

Mayo Clinic. (2009). *Childhood schizophrenia.* Retrieved from http://www.mayoclinic.com/health/childhood-schizophrenia/DS00868

Melnyk, B., Baker, D., Walsh, E. H., Hornor, G., Pachler, M., Sheppard, M. T., et al. (2007). NAP-NAP position statement on integration of mental health care in pediatric primary care settings. *Journal of Pediatric Health Care, 21*(5), 29A–30A.

Monsen, R. B. (2009). Prevention is best for fetal alcohol syndrome. *Journal of Pediatric Nursing, 24*(1), 60–61.

National Association of Pediatric Nurse Practitioners. (2007). NAPNAP position statement on integration of mental health care in pediatric primary care settings. *Journal of Pediatric Health Care, 21,* 19A–30A.

National Center for PTSD. (2008). *PTSD in children and adolescents.* Retrieved from http://ncptsd.va.gov/ncmain/ncdocs/fact_shts/fs_children.html

National Institute of Mental Health. (2009). *What affects a child's risk of getting bipolar disorder?* Retrieved from http://www.nimh.nih.gov/health/publications/bipolar-disorder-in-children-and-teens-a-parents-guide/what-affects-a-childs-risk-of-getting-bipolar-disorder.shtml

National Institute of Mental Health. (2010). *Depression in children and adolescents.* Retrieved from http://www.nimh.nih.gov/health/topics/depression/depression-in-children-and-adolescents.shtml

National Institute of Neurological Disorders and Stroke. (2010). *Tourette syndrome fact sheet.* Retrieved from http://www.ninds.nih.gov/disorders/tourette/detail_tourette.htm

National Institutes of Health. (2007). *Brain matures a few years late in ADHD, but follows normal pattern* [News release]. Retrieved from http://www.nih.gov/news/pr/nov2007/nimh-12.htm

National Joint Committee on Learning Disabilities. (2006). *Learning disabilities and young children.* Retrieved from http://www.ncld.org

Oyama, O., Paltoo, C., & Greengold, J. (2007). Somatoform disorders. *American Family Physician 76*(9), 1333–1338.

Plomp, E., Van Engeland, H., & Durston, S. (2009). Understanding genes, environment and their interaction in attention-deficit hyperactivity disorder: Is there a role for neuroimaging? *Neuroscience, 164*(1), 230–240.

Prows, C. A., & Saldana, S. N. (2009). Nurses' genetic/genomics competencies when medication therapy is guided by pharmacogenetic testing: Children with mental health disorders as an exemplar. *Journal of Pediatric Nursing, 24*(3), 179–188.

Roberts, J. E., Mankowski, J. B., Sideris, J., Goldman, B. D., Hatton, D. D., Mirrett, P. L., Baranek, G. T., et al. (2009). Trajectories and predictors of the development of very young boys with fragile X syndrome. *Journal of Pediatric Psychology, 34*(8), 827–836.

Roberts, M. (2007). *The many faces and facets of BP.* Retrieved from http://www.nami.org/Content/Contentgroups/bp_and_Schizophrenia_Digest/The_Many_Faces_and_Facets_ofBP.htm

Rogers, S. J., & Vismara, L. A. (2008). Evidence-based comprehensive treatments for early autism. *Journal of Clinical Child and Adolescent Psychology, 37*, 8–38.

Rucklidge, J. J., Johnstone, J., & Kaplan, B. J. (2009). Nutrient supplementation approaches in the treatment of ADHD. *Expert Review of Neurotherapeutics, 9*(4), 461–476.

Scheeringa, M. S., Salloum, A., Arnberger, R. A., Weems, C. F., Amaya-Jackson, L., & Cohen, J. A. (2007). Feasibility and effectiveness of cognitive-behavioral therapy for posttraumatic stress disorder in preschool children: Two case reports. *Journal of Traumatic Stress, 20*, 631–636.

Shain, B. N., & American Academy of Pediatrics Committee on Adolescence. (2007). Suicide and suicide attempts in adolescents. *Pediatrics, 120*(3), 669–676.

Simpson, G. A., Cohen, R. A., Pastor, P. N., & Reuben, C. A. (2008). *Use of mental health services in the past 12 months by children ages 4–17 years: United States 2005–2006* (NCHS Data Brief No. 8). Hyattsville, MD: National Center for Health Statistics.

Smith, P., Yule, W., Perrin, S., Tranah, T., Dalfleish, T., & Clark, D. M. (2007). Cognitive-behavioral therapy for PTSD in children and adolescents: A preliminary randomized controlled trial. *Journal of the American Academy of Child and Adolescent Psychiatry, 46*, 1051–1061.

Soh, N. L., & Walter, G. (2008). Complementary and alternative medicine (CAM) treatments and pediatric psychopharmacology. *Journal of the American Academy of Child and Adolescent Psychiatry 47*(4), 364–368.

Storch, E. A., & Elder, J. H. (2009). Introduction to the special series on child and adolescent mental health. *Journal of Pediatric Nursing, 24*(1), 1–2.

Theoktisto, K. M. (2009). Pharmacokinetic considerations in the treatment of pediatric behavioral issues. *Pediatric Nursing, 35*(6), 369–375.

Thompson, S. J., Maccio, E. M., Desselle, S. K., & Zittel-Palamara, K. (2007). Predictors of posttraumatic stress symptoms among runaway youth utilizing two service sectors. *Journal of Traumatic Stress, 20*, 553–563.

U.S. Department of Health and Human Services (2010). Healthy People 2020. Retrieved from http://www.healthypeople.gov/hp2020/

U.S. Department of Veterans Affairs. (2008). *PTSD in children and adolescents.* Retrieved from http://www.ptsd.va.gov/professional/pages/ptsd_in_children_and_adolescents_overview_for_professionals.asp

U.S. Preventive Services Task Force. (2009). *Screening and treatment for major depressive disorder in children and adolescents: Recommendation statement* (AHRQ Publication No. 09-05130-EF-2). Rockville, MD: Association for Healthcare Research and Quality.

Van Cleve, S. N., Cannon, S., & Cohen, W. I. (2006). Part II: Clinical practice guidelines for adolescents and young adults with Down syndrome: 12 to 21 years. *Journal of Pediatric Health Care, 20*, 198–205.

Van Cleve, S. N., & Cohen, W. I. (2006). Part I: Clinical practice guidelines for children with Down syndrome from birth to 12 years. *Journal of Pediatric Health Care, 20*, 47–54.

van Riper, M. (2007). Families of children with Down syndrome: Responding to "a change of plans" with resilience. *Journal of Pediatric Nursing, 22*, 116–127.

Vetter, V. L., Elia, J., Erickson, C., Berger, S., Blum, N., Uzark, K., & Webb, C. L. (2008). Cardiovascular monitoring of children and adolescents with heart disease receiving stimulant drugs: A scientific statement from the American Heart Association Council on Cardiovascular Disease in the Young Congenital Cardiac Defects Committee and the Council on Cardiovascular Nursing. *Circulation, 117*, 2407–2423.

Wallis, D., Russell, H. F., & Muenke, M. (2008). Review: Genetics of attention deficit/hyperactivity disorder. *Journal of Pediatric Psychology, 33*(10), 1085–1099.

Weber, W., & Newmark, S. (2007). Complementary and alternative medical therapies for attention-deficit/hyperactivity disorder and autism. *Pediatric Clinics of North America, 54*, 983–1006.

Williams, D. L., & Minshew, N. J. (2007). Understanding autism and related disorders: What has imaging taught us? *Neuroimaging Clinics of North America, 17*, 495–509.

Zuckerbrot, R. A., Cheung, A. H., Jensen, P. S., Stein, R. E. K., Laraque, D., & GLAD-PC Steering Group. (2007). Guidelines for adolescent depression in primary care (GLAD-PC): I. Identification, assessment, and initial management. *Pediatrics, 119*, 101–108.

Alterations in Musculoskeletal Function

chapter 29

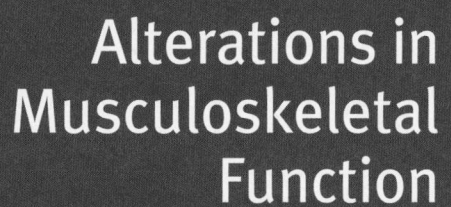

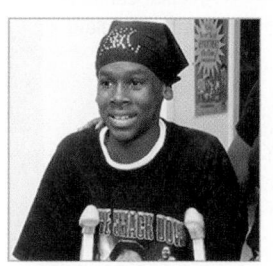

Douglass was admitted to the clinic today for application of a short leg cast. He broke his left lower fibula nearly a week ago when he was on a trampoline with three friends, trying to see who could jump the highest. Douglass slipped and his lateral leg hit the frame on the side. His friends helped him off the trampoline and called his mother, who transported Douglass to the emergency department.

His mother states that Douglass is now 12 years old and in middle school. He has been going to a friend's house nearly every day after school and spending time on activities such as the trampoline and inline skating, as well as watching television and playing video games. She felt this was safer than Douglass being at home alone during her work hours, but is now starting to wonder whether to allow him to engage in activities with his friend. In the emergency department after the accident, a splint was used to provide support for a few days and allow the swelling to decrease before today's cast application. Douglass has been non–weight bearing on his leg and has been using crutches.

What teaching does Douglass need to keep the cast intact and to ensure his safety? What special adaptations will be needed in his home and school? How can the clinic nurse partner with the school nurse to provide for Douglass's transition back to school? Is there any way his injury could have been avoided? The information in this chapter will discuss issues such as these and help you to provide effective care for children like Douglass who have musculoskeletal disorders.

Key Terms

Learning Outcomes

After reading this chapter, you will be able to do the following:

1. Describe pediatric variations in the musculoskeletal system.
2. Plan nursing care for children with structural deformities of the foot, hip, and spine.
3. Recognize signs and symptoms of infectious musculoskeletal disorders and refer for appropriate care.
4. Collaborate with families and other health care providers to plan care for children with musculoskeletal disorders that are chronic or require long-term care.
5. Plan nursing interventions to promote safety and developmental progression in children who require braces, casts, traction, and surgery.
6. Provide nursing care for fractures and other sports injuries, including teaching for injury prevention and evidence-based nursing interventions for the child who has sustained a fracture or other sports injury.

The Musculoskeletal System

ANATOMY AND PHYSIOLOGY

The musculoskeletal system is composed of the bones and muscles; joints, the supporting structures that facilitate movement; and tendons and ligaments that connect parts of the system. Cartilage is the connective tissue precursor to bone, and remains in some structures such as ears and ribs throughout life. Bone formation is a dynamic system at any age, but particularly so in children and adolescents. Children depend on a functioning musculoskeletal system to enable support and movement, which in turn ensures that exposure to various stimuli and normal development can occur.

Bones are composed of osseous or dense connective tissue; they contain an exterior shell or cortex, and an inner, primarily protein, matrix (Figure 29–1 ➤). The cells covering the cortex are called lining cells or compact bone, and protect the bone from penetration by circulating blood cells and other components of circulation; this covering is called the **periosteum**. The inner matrix is composed of a series of interconnected plates called cancellous, trabecular, or spongy bone. Spaces between these plates are called bone marrow, and this is the area where **hematopoiesis** (production and development of blood cells) occurs. In addition to the lining cells found on the bone exterior, other types of cells include **osteoblasts**, which synthesize and lay down bone and then attract calcium and phosphates to strengthen the bone; **osteoclasts**, which resorb bone in the constant process of bone formation and breakdown; and **osteocytes**, which are special osteoblasts that sense and respond to bone pressure and bending to direct the process of bone remodeling. The process of bone growth and remodeling is influenced by factors such as pressure (via physical activity), hormones (parathyroid hormone, glucocorticoids, insulin-like growth factor, calcitonin), and external factors (dietary intake of calcium and phosphorus, bisphosphonate drugs, gallium, and so on).

The 206 bones of the human body include several types:

- *Long bones* such as the fibula, tibia, femur, humerus, and ulna; most childhood growth occurs in these bones
- *Short bones* such as those in the wrist and ankle
- *Flat bones* such as the skull, sternum, and ribs; the ribs retain large components of cartilage even when mature
- *Irregular bones* which have a variety of shapes and sizes, such as vertebrae, pelvis bones, and scapula

Muscles are collections of cells that can contract, causing the accompanying skeleton to move. Muscle fibers require a supply of blood and nerves, and vary from small to quite large in size. Muscle cells develop in response to the stimulation of activity. Types of muscle cells include:

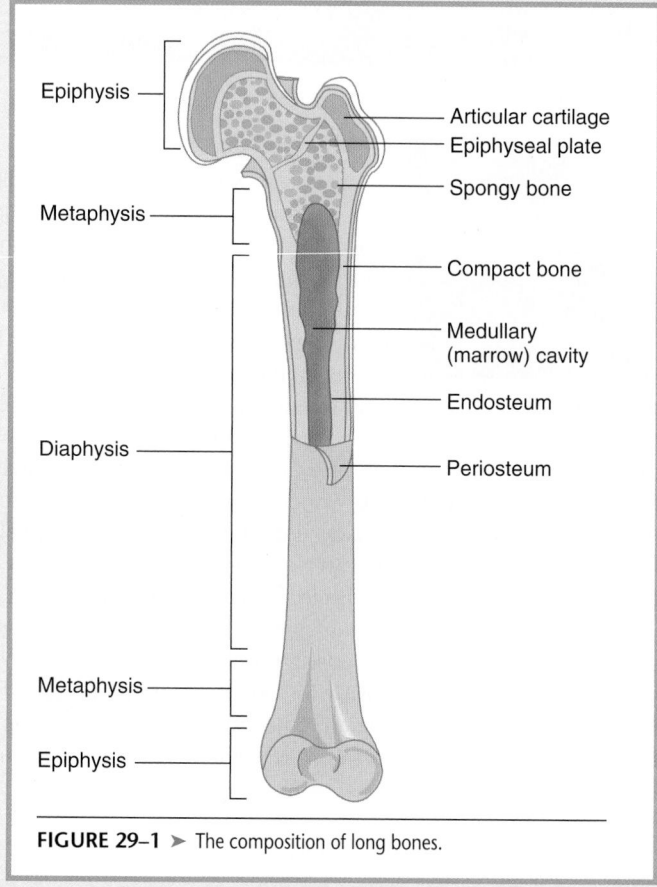

FIGURE 29–1 ➤ The composition of long bones.

- *Skeletal* (striated) or *voluntary* muscles that involve the biceps, triceps, deltoid, gluteus maximus, and others
- *Smooth* (short-fibered) or *involuntary* muscles such as those in the gastrointestinal tract, lungs, and pupils of the eye
- *Cardiac* (striated, special-function) muscles that ensure the heart's constant contraction and relaxation

Muscles enable parts of the body to flex and extend, abduct and adduct, and carry out other motions (Figure 29–2 ➤). As one muscle flexes, the opposing muscle must extend to allow the movement.

Several other structures enable the musculoskeletal system to function. The **joints** are articulations or connections between bones. Fibrous joints provide for little movement (those in the skull are an example), cartilaginous joints allow for slight movement (vertebral joints are a good example), and synovial joints are movable within certain limits (knee, hip, elbow, and shoulder are examples). Joints are complex in structure and function,

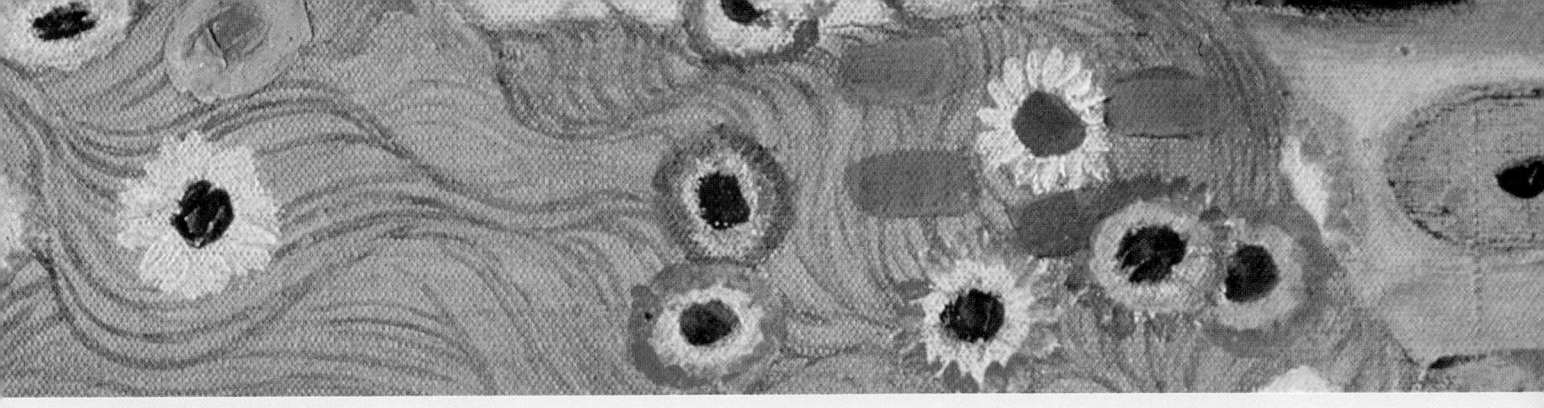

Varus
An abnormal position of limb that involves bending inward toward the midline of the body

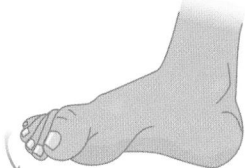

Valgus
An abnormal position of a limb that involves bending outward away from the midline of the body

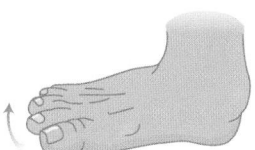

Supination
Lying on the back or placing the hand so that palm faces upward

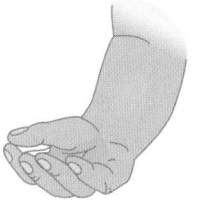

Pronation
Lying on the stomach or placing the hand so the palm faces downward

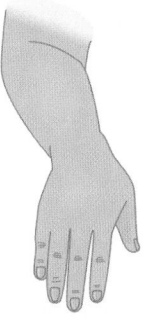

Adduction
Lateral movement of limbs toward the midline of the body

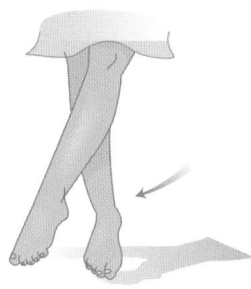

Abduction
Lateral movement of limbs away from the midline of the body

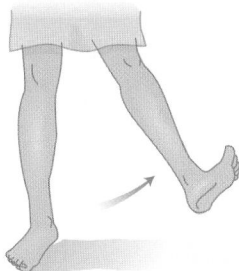

Flexion
A decrease in angle between bones forming a joint

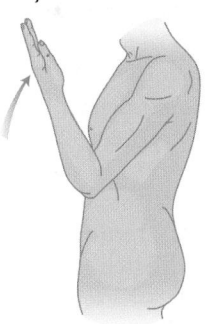

Extension
A movement that brings a limb into a straight position

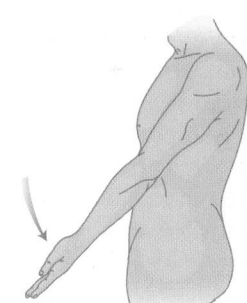

Inversion
Turning inward, usually more than normal

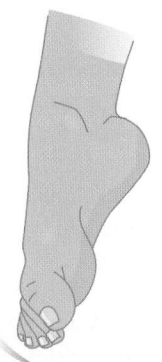

Eversion
Turning outward

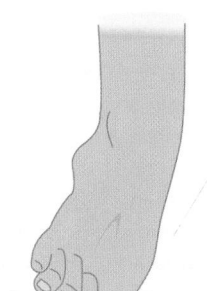

Internal rotation
Rotation of a body part towards the midline of the body

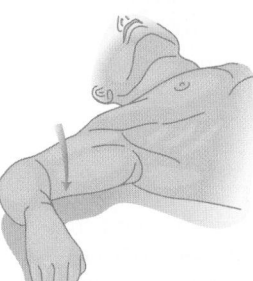

External rotation
Rotation of a body segment away from the midline of the body

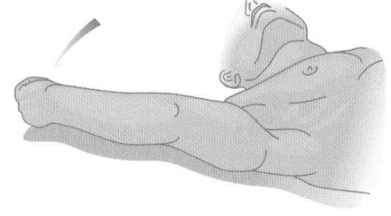

FIGURE 29–2 ➤ Musculoskeletal positions and joint motions.

containing the fibrous end of the bone, synovial membrane and fluid, other sacs called bursae, and ligaments. **Ligaments** are tough fibers that bind the ends of bones together. **Tendons** are fibrous bands that connect bone to its accompanying muscles, allowing the bone to move when a muscle contracts or relaxes.

PEDIATRIC DIFFERENCES

Bones

Several differences exist between the bones of children and those of adults. Although primary centers of **ossification** (bone formation) are nearly complete at birth, a fibrous membrane still exists between the cranial bones (fontanels). The posterior fontanel closes between 2 and 3 months of age. The anterior fontanel does not close until approximately 18 months of age, allowing for growth of the brain and skull. Most growth of the skull occurs by 2 years of age, with the skull reaching full size by 16 years.

Secondary ossification occurs as the long bones grow. Cartilage cells at the epiphyses (an area enriched with blood cells) are replaced by osteoblasts (immature bone cells), which push the end of the bone away from the shaft and engineer the deposition of calcium within the newly formed bone. Calcium intake during childhood and adolescence is essential to provide adequate bone density that will prevent osteoporosis and fractures in adulthood. See Chapter 14 ∞ for a discussion of inadequate calcium intake during school age and adolescence. Because growth takes place at the epiphyseal plates, injuries to this portion of a long bone are of particular concern in young children. The rapid bone growth of childhood facilitates healing after fractures, but may also lead to "growing pains," as muscles are pulled when bones grow quickly. The ends of the long bones (epiphyses) remain cartilaginous, allowing growth, until approximately age 20 years, when skeletal maturation is complete. At this time, the epiphyseal plate closes, cartilage at the site is replaced by bone, and only an epiphyseal line remains (Figure 29–3 ➤).

Children and adolescents may sustain injury to the musculoskeletal system from falls, car crashes, and sports. Fractures are one type of common injury. The long bones of children are porous and less dense than those of adults. For this reason, children's bones can bend, buckle, or break as a result of a simple fall. In addition to the structural differences between the bones of children and adults, there are functional differences in the skeletal system of children. Before birth, the thoracic and sacral regions of the spine are convex curves. As the infant learns to hold up the head, the cervical region becomes concave. When the child learns to stand, the lumbar region also becomes concave. Failure of the spine to assume these final curves results in an abnormal curvature of the spine (kyphosis or lordosis).

Muscles, Tendons, and Ligaments

The muscular system, unlike the skeletal system, is almost completely formed at birth, with any remaining increase achieved in the first year of life. As a child grows, muscles do not increase in number, but rather in length and circumference. Muscle fibers reach maximum diameter in girls at about 10 years of age, and in boys at 14 years. Muscle strength continues to increase until about 25–30 years of age.

As Children Grow
Musculoskeletal System

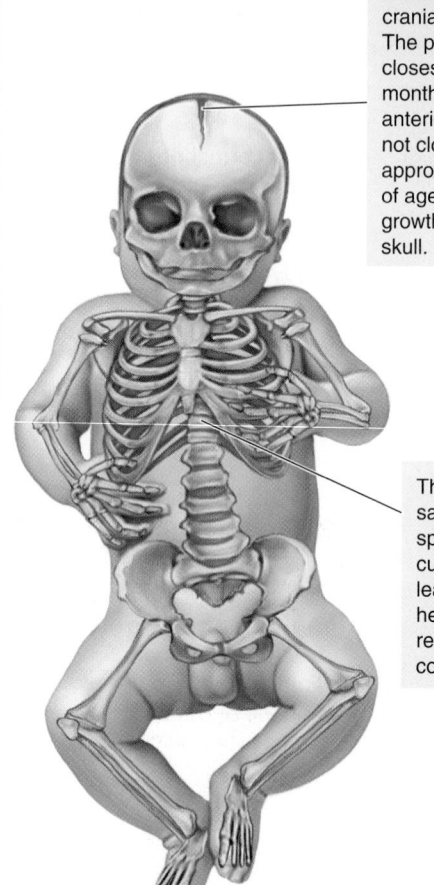

A fibrous membrane still exists between the cranial bones (fontanels). The posterior fontanel closes between 2 and 3 months of age. The anterior fontanel does not close until approximately 18 months of age, allowing for growth of the brain and skull.

The thoracic and sacral regions of the spine are convex curves. As the infant learns to hold up the head, the cervical region becomes concave.

FIGURE 29–3 ➤ Skeletal and muscle development throughout childhood.

Until puberty, both ligaments and tendons are stronger than bone. When these structural differences are not recognized, a childhood fracture is sometimes mistaken for a sprain. A **sprain** is a tearing of ligaments, the structural support connecting bones, usually caused when a joint is twisted or otherwise traumatized. Tendons, which connect bones to muscles, grow in length and fibrous tissue as mechanical pressure is placed on them.

Use the Assessment Guidelines on page 948 to perform a nursing assessment of the musculoskeletal system. Many diagnostic and laboratory tests are used for the musculoskeletal system. Examples can be found in Table 29–1; see Appendices D and E ∞ for more information about these tests and procedures.

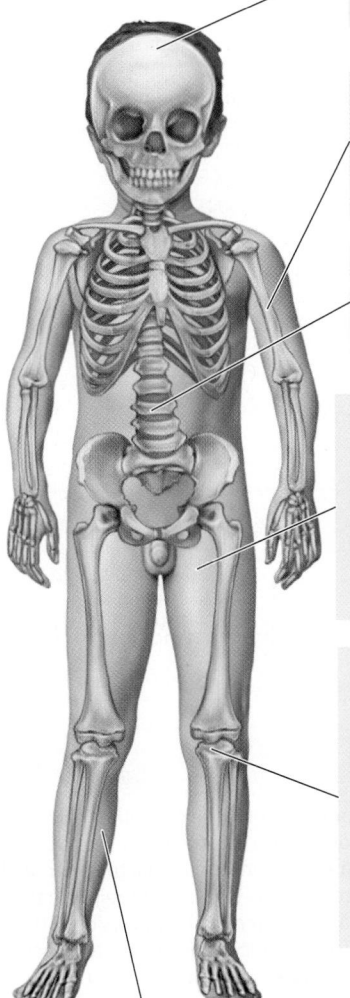

Most growth of the skull occurs by 2 years of age, with the skull reaching full size by 16 years.

The long bones of children are porous and less dense than those of adults, leading to higher rates of fracture.

When the child learns to stand, the lumbar region becomes concave in shape.

As a child grows, muscles do not increase in number, but rather in length and circumference. Muscle fibers reach maximum diameter in girls at about 10 years of age, and in boys at 14 years.

During childhood, cartilage cells at the epiphyses (an area enriched with blood cells) are replaced by osteoblasts (immature bone cells), which push the end of the bone away from the shaft and engineer the deposition of calcium within the newly formed bone.

The rapid bone growth of childhood facilitates healing after fractures, but may also lead to "growing pains" as muscles are pulled when bones grow quickly.

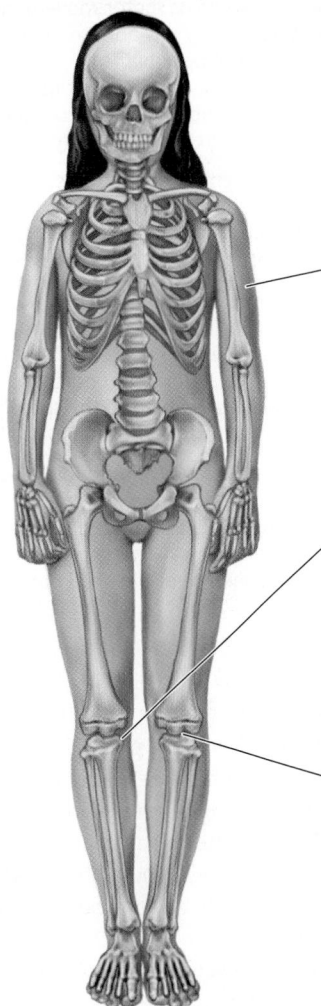

Muscle strength continues to increase until about 25–30 years of age.

The ends of long bones (epiphyses) remain cartilaginous, allowing growth, until approximately age 20 years, when skeletal maturation is complete. At this time the epiphyseal plate closes, cartilage at the site is replaced by bone, and only an epiphyseal line remains.

Until puberty, both ligaments and tendons are stronger than bone. As the child ages and cartilage is replaced by bone, the resulting bone is stronger than ligaments or tendons. Rates of fractures decrease while injuries to ligaments and tendons increase.

TABLE 29–1	Diagnostic and Laboratory Procedures/Tests for the Musculoskeletal System	
Diagnostic Procedures		**Laboratory Tests**
Arthrogram		Alkaline phosphatase (ALP)
Bone scan		C-reactive protein (CRP)
Computed tomography (CT)		Erythrocyte sedimentation
Dual energy x-ray absorptiometry (DEXA)		rate (ESR or sed rate)
Electromyelogram		Rheumatoid factor (RF)
Evoked potential		
Magnetic resonance imaging (MRI)		
Radiograph (x-ray)		
Ultrasound		

Assessment Guidelines for the Child with a Musculoskeletal System Alteration

Assessment Focus	Assessment Guidelines
Muscles	▪ Is muscle mass symmetrical? ▪ Are fine and gross motor movements in line with developmental expectations? ▪ Can you identify any abnormal signs such as asymmetry of movement, tenderness, masses, weakness, hypotonia, or hypertonia? ▪ Can the school-age child get up from a lying or sitting position in the usual manner? ▪ Can you describe the child's usual daily physical activity? ▪ Has there been a loss of ability to perform developmental milestones?
Joints	▪ Are movements smooth and symmetrical? ▪ Are there any signs of tenderness, decreased range of motion, inflammation, crepitus/grinding, or masses? ▪ Do the hips of newborns and infants manifest symmetrical full range of motion? ▪ Were there recent events of trauma such as in sports or a fall?
Bones	▪ Are any masses noted? ▪ Are arms and legs the same length? ▪ Is there a recent decrease or change in mobility, such as limping? ▪ Are bones in alignment, or are abnormalities noted such as bowlegs or knock-knees? ▪ Upon spinal screening, is the spine properly aligned? (See the screening procedure in this chapter.) ▪ In what sports does the child participate? Is recommended protective gear worn?
Tendons and ligaments	▪ Do all joints move through full range of motion? ▪ Is there any pain upon joint motion or palpation? ▪ Are there feelings of grinding or crepitus as the joint moves? ▪ Has there been a recent sports or other injury? ▪ In what sports does the child participate?

The musculoskeletal system helps the body to protect its vital organs, support weight, control motion, store minerals, and supply red blood cells. Bones provide a rigid framework for the body, muscles provide for active movement, and tendons and ligaments hold the bones and muscles together. Alterations in musculoskeletal functioning thus can have a significant impact on a child's growth and development.

Musculoskeletal disorders may be congenital, such as clubfoot, or acquired, such as osteomyelitis. They may require short- or long-term management, and may be treated on an outpatient basis or require hospitalization. Many musculoskeletal disorders require surgical correction, casting, or braces. This chapter provides a discussion of many of the musculoskeletal disorders of childhood and adolescence. Additional conditions related to this system are fully described in other chapters; for example, bone tumors are presented in Chapter 24, cerebral palsy in Chapter 27, and juvenile rheumatoid arthritis in Chapter 22 ∞.

▪ DISORDERS OF THE FEET AND LEGS

Metatarsus Adductus

Metatarsus adductus, the most common congenital foot deformity, is characterized by an inward turning of the forefoot at the tarsometatarsal joints (Figure 29–4 ➤). Often referred to as "intoeing," metatarsus adductus affects male and female infants equally and occurs in approximately 1 in 1,000 births, with more common incidence among siblings, twins, and multiple births. It occurs more often in certain neurological conditions such as cerebral palsy (Hagmann, Dreher, & Wenz, 2009; Hutchinson, 2010; Sankar, Weiss, & Skaggs, 2009). The condi-

tion is most likely caused by both intrauterine positioning and genetic factors.

Nursing Alert

Metatarsus adductus is a major cause of intoeing. Other causes can occur, especially as children get older. If intoeing is first observed when the child walks (12–18 months), internal tibial torsion may be the cause. This generally improves with walking. Intoeing that persists until 2–4 years may be related to femoral anteversion. Stretching exercises, ballet, and ice skating may help to decrease anteversion. Skewfoot or S-shaped foot may be corrected by casting or surgery (Hutchinson, 2010).

Foot radiographs may be taken and physical assessment of the foot is performed. Treatment depends on the degree of foot flexibility. If the foot can be readily maneuvered past the neutral position, simple exercises may correct the problem (see Families Want to Know: Stretching Exercises for Metatarsus

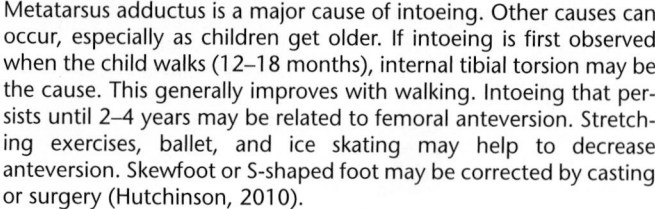

Families Want to Know
Stretching Exercises for Metatarsus Adductus

▪ Hold the infant's foot securely by the heel. Maintain the heel in this position.
▪ Move the forefoot outward away from the body with the other hand.
▪ Hold the foot in this position for 5 seconds.
▪ Repeat five times during each diaper change.

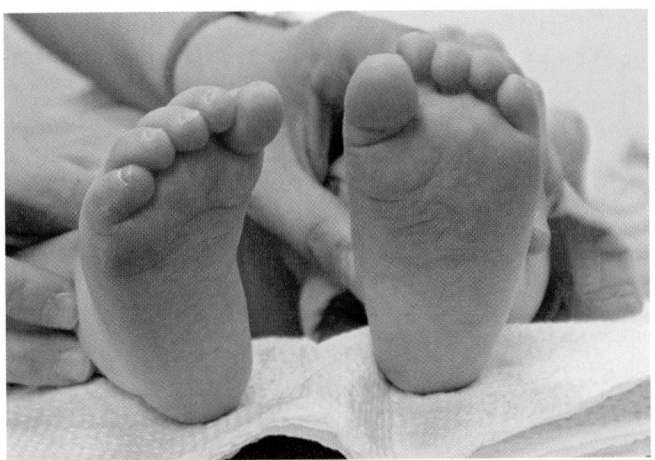

FIGURE 29–4 ➤ Metatarsus adductus is characterized by convexity (curvature) of the lateral border of the foot. The child's right foot shows the disorder. Note that the forefoot turns inward and appears out of alignment with the remainder of the foot.

Adductus). Most cases will resolve spontaneously by the time the infant is about 3 months of age. Serial casting is the treatment of choice for curvature angles greater than 15 degrees, or in cases that do not improve. The infant's feet are placed in a position as close to neutral as possible and are held secure with casts. Casts are changed weekly until the desired correction is achieved. Braces and orthopedic shoes may also be used to maintain correction after casting.

Nursing Management

Reassure parents that the child's condition can be corrected. If the child's deformity is mild, teach parents simple stretching exercises that can be performed at each diaper change. If casting is necessary, provide cast care as outlined in Box 29–1 and teach parents how to care for the child in a cast at home. If metatarsus adductus persists into childhood without correction, the challenge is to find shoes that accommodate the unusual shape of the foot.

BOX 29–1 **Nursing Care of the Child in a Plaster Cast**

- A plaster cast takes anywhere from 24–48 hours to dry. When handling the cast, be gentle and use the palms of your hands, as fingertips can indent plaster and create pressure areas.
- After the cast is applied, elevate the extremity on a pillow above the level of the heart. Elevation helps to reduce swelling and increases venous return.
- If the cast is applied after surgery, there may be drainage or bleeding through the cast material. Circle the stain and note the date and time on the cast to provide a means of assessing the amount of fluid lost.
- Assess the distal pulses, and check the fingers and toes for color, warmth, capillary refill, and edema. Assess sensation as well as movement. Any deviation from normal may indicate nerve damage or decreased blood supply.
- During the first 24 hours, the casted extremity should be checked every 15–30 minutes for 2 hours, then every 1–2 hours thereafter. The skin should be warm. It should blanch when slight pressure is applied and then return to its normal color within 3 seconds **(1)**. For the next 2 days, the casted extremity should be assessed at least every 4 hours.
- Check the edges of the cast for roughness or crumbling. If necessary, pull the inner stockinette over the edge of the cast and tape.
- The rough edges of the cast may also be alleviated by "petaling." This is done by securing tape or padding to the inside of the cast and pulling it over the edge, covering the jagged or broken pieces of plaster, and securing it to the outer surface of the cast **(2, 3, 4)**. Moleskin may be used on the cast as well.
- Keep the cast as clean and dry as possible. Cover the cast with a plastic bag or plastic wrap when the child bathes or showers.

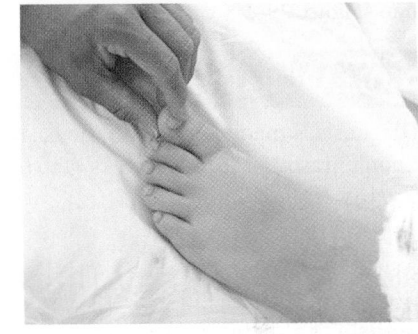

(1)

- The skin under the cast may itch; however, do not use powders or lotions near the edges or under the cast as they can cause skin irritation.
- Be sure that children do not put small objects between the casts and their extremities either during play or to scratch the skin to alleviate itchiness; these actions can cause skin irritation as well as neurovascular compromise and the objects may inadvertently be dropped into the cast.

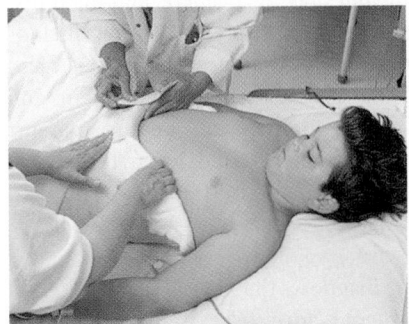

(2)

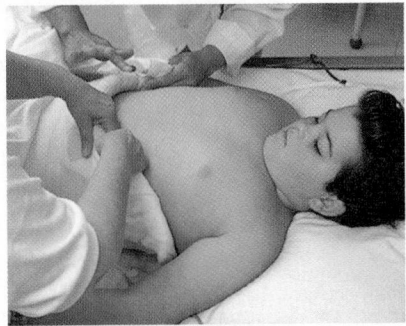

(3)

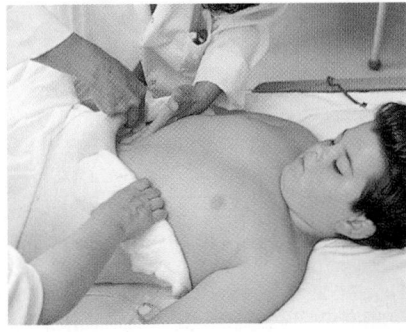

(4)

Clubfoot

Clubfoot, or equinovarus, is a congenital abnormality in which the foot of the newborn is not in the usual position. It occurs in approximately 1 in 1,000 births, affects boys nearly twice as often as girls, and is bilateral in about half of the cases (Gurnett, Boehm, Connolly, et al., 2008).

Etiology and Pathophysiology

The exact cause of clubfoot is unknown; however, several possible etiologies have been proposed. Some authorities believe abnormal intrauterine positioning causes the deformity. Neuromuscular or vascular problems are suspected as causes by others. Yet other experts believe there is a genetic component, either at the chromosomal level or by the arrest of normal fetal development. A strong family history of clubfoot is present in nearly 15% of cases of the deformity (Paton, Fox, Foster, et al., 2010).

Clinical Manifestations

A true clubfoot (talipes equinovarus) involves three areas of deformity: the midfoot is directed downward (**equinus**), the hindfoot turns inward (**varus**), and the forefoot curls toward the heel (adduction) and turns upward in partial supination. Most children have a combination of findings, with muscles, tendons, and bones involved. The condition may range from mild to severe involvement, with the latter often associated with additional malformations in the newborn such as meningomyelocele. The foot is small with a shortened Achilles tendon. Muscles in the lower leg are atrophied, but leg lengths are generally normal (Figure 29–5 ➤).

COLLABORATIVE CARE

Diagnosis is made at birth on the basis of visual inspection, or may be made upon ultrasound at 16–20 weeks' gestation. Radiographs after birth confirm the severity of the condition.

Pathophysiology Illustrated
Bilateral Clubfoot Deformity

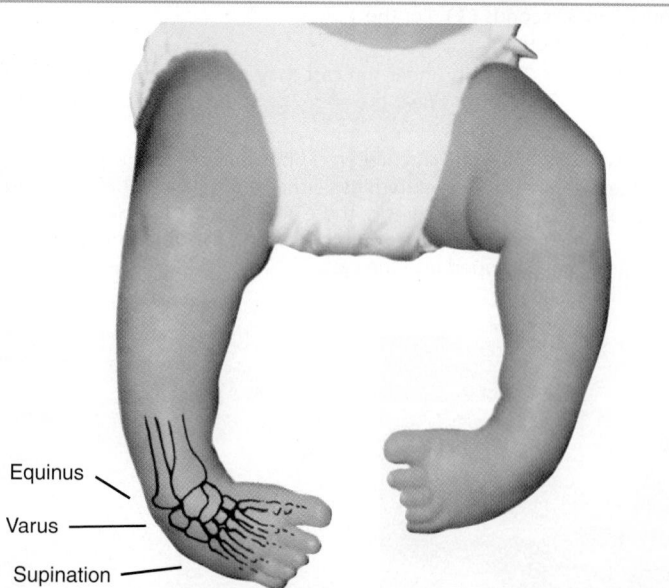

Equinus
Varus
Supination

FIGURE 29–5 ➤ Parents of a child with clubfoot will have many questions. Can the condition be treated? Will the child be able to walk normally after surgery? Will parents need help caring for the infant? How much will surgery and other care cost? Will any subsequent children have a clubfoot?
Modified from Staheli, L. T. (1992). Fundamentals of pediatric orthopedics (p. 5.10). New York: Raven Press.

Early treatment is essential to achieve successful correction and reduce the chance of complications. Serial casting is the treatment of choice. Casting should begin as soon as possible after birth. Timing is critical, because the short bones of the foot, which are primarily cartilaginous at birth, begin to ossify shortly thereafter. The foot is manipulated to achieve maximum correction, first of the varus deformity and then of the equinus deformity. A long leg cast is applied to hold the foot in the desired position, and the cast is changed weekly for approximately 4 to 6 weeks until maximum correction is achieved. If the deformity has been corrected, the child wears an open-toed shoe connected to a bar to retain the position (Gurnett et al., 2008). If the deformity has not been corrected, surgical intervention may be implemented.

The age at which a child undergoes clubfoot surgery varies among surgeons. However, if surgery is needed, it usually occurs when children are between 3 and 12 months of age. The one-stage posteromedial release procedure, which involves realignment of the bones of the foot and release of the constricting soft tissue, is commonly performed. The foot is held in the proper position by one or more stainless steel pins. A cast is then applied with the knee flexed to prevent damage to the pin and to discourage weight bearing (Figure 29–6 ➤). Casting continues for 6 to 12 weeks. The child may then need to wear a brace or corrective shoes, depending on the severity of the deformity and the surgeon's preference. Alternatively, the Ponseti technique uses a simple Achilles tenotomy following serial manipulation and casting, followed by use of a foot-abduction brace. This technique has a good record of success (Gottschalk, Karol, & Jeans, 2010).

NURSING MANAGEMENT

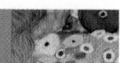

Nursing Assessment and Diagnosis

Nursing assessment, which begins at birth and continues throughout the child's subsequent outpatient casting visits and hospitalization for surgery, includes taking a genetic and birth history, performing a physical examination (including position and appearance of the foot), and assessing the child's motor development and family's coping mechanisms. Because parents will need to bring the child for frequent cast changes, assess access to transportation and other arrangements that are necessary to facilitate these visits.

Nursing diagnoses that may apply to the child with a clubfoot deformity are as follows:

- Impaired Physical Mobility related to prescribed movement restriction of cast

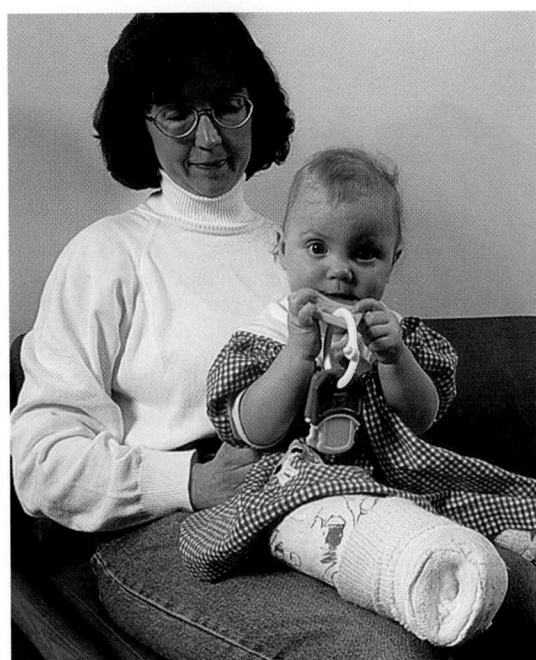

FIGURE 29–6 ➤ This girl has a long leg cast, which was applied after surgery to correct her clubfoot.

- Risk for Impaired Skin Integrity related to cast
- Risk for Impaired Parenting related to birth of a child with a physical defect
- Health-Seeking Behaviors (Parental) related to lack of information about deformity, treatment, and home care

Planning and Implementation

Nursing management involves providing emotional support, educating the family about home care of the child in a cast and the importance of keeping appointments at the outpatient facility for cast changes, preparing the family for the child's hospitalization if surgery is to occur, and providing postsurgical care.

Provide Emotional Support

Clubfoot is a condition that affects both the child and the family. The child's foot deformity is upsetting to parents, and they need emotional support to allay their fears. Helping parents understand the condition and its treatment is essential.

Encourage parents to hold and cuddle the child and to take an active role in the child's care to help promote bonding. Explain that, with treatment, the child will grow and develop normally.

Provide Cast and Brace Care

Routine cast care is outlined in Box 29–1 on page 949 and is important to ensure skin and neurovascular integrity. Provide support information to the parents during the casting treatment. After serial casting is complete, or following surgery, the child may progress to wearing a brace or special shoe for 6 to 12 months. Braces should fit snugly but should not interfere with neurovascular function. Before the child begins to wear a brace, check the skin for any areas of redness or breakdown. Provide parents with guidelines for brace wear as outlined in the following text. Emphasize that proper skin care is essential. If

skin redness develops, arrange to have the fit of the brace evaluated and modified, if necessary.

Clinical Tip

When an infant is receiving serial casting for clubfoot, recommend that the parent soak the cast off the night before a scheduled cast change. The baby can be placed in a warm bath, during which the cast will start to disintegrate and can be unrolled. This avoids exposure of the baby to the loud sound of the cast cutter, and allows for the infant's leg to be washed and out of the cast overnight. Parents can also be encouraged to bring a bottle to the clinic. If the baby is hungry and feeding, the foot is more easily kept still for the cast application.

Provide Postsurgical Care

Routine postoperative care after surgical correction includes neurovascular status checks every 2 hours for the first 24 hours and observing for any swelling around the cast edges. Apply ice bags to the foot, and keep the ankle and foot elevated on a pillow for 24 hours to promote healing and help with venous return. Check for drainage or bleeding. Administer pain medication routinely for 24 to 48 hours. Popliteal or epidural blocks may be placed during surgery and used in the immediate postsurgical period for pain control (Figure 29–7 ➤). The nurse monitors these blocks for effectiveness and any undesired effects (see Chapter 15 ∞ for detailed instructions on pain management). See the *Clinical Skills Manual* for details on monitoring nerve blocks.

Discharge Planning and Home Care Teaching

Parents should be given written instructions for care of the child with a cast (see Families Want to Know: Care of the Child with a Cast). In addition, assist them in the following ways.

- Demonstrate the use of a sponge bath to protect the cast from water breakdown. Have parents contact the health care provider if the cast gets wet with water or urine.
- Discuss several options for clothing that accommodate a cast, for example, one-piece snap suits or sweatpants.

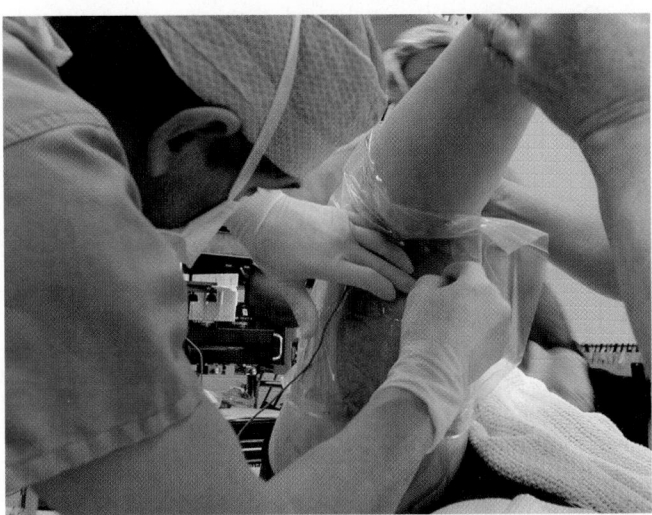

FIGURE 29–7 ➤ The insertion of a popliteal block during surgery. The site will be wrapped and the tubing connected to an infusion pump. The nurse will monitor the infusion and pain control after surgery.
Courtesy of Shriners Hospital, Spokane, WA.

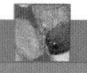
Skin Care

■ Check the skin around the cast edges for irritation, rubbing, or blistering. The skin should be clean and dry.

■ Cleanse the skin just under the cast edges and between the toes or fingers with a cotton-tipped applicator and rubbing alcohol. Avoid using lotions, oils, and powders near the cast as they may cause caking.

■ Avoid poking sharp objects down inside the cast as this may result in sores.

Cast Care

■ Keep the cast dry. Protect plaster with a cast shoe, thick sock, or sling.

■ Allow a new, wet cast to air-dry for 24 hours. Raise it on pillows just above heart level to prevent edema.

■ Begin walking on a leg cast only when the physician gives permission.

■ Be alert for possible complications.

■ Verify toes or fingers are pink, not blue or white.

■ Keep skin warm; the tips of the toes should blanch when pinched.

Notify the Health Care Provider if Any of the Following Occur

Unusual odor beneath the cast

Burning, tingling, or numbness in the casted arm or leg

Drainage through the cast

Swelling or inability to move the fingers or toes

Slippage of the cast (change in amount of fingers or toes that are visible)

Cracked, soft, or loose cast

Sudden, unexplained fever

Unusual fussiness or irritability in an infant or child

Blue or white fingers or toes

Pain that is not relieved by any comfort measures (e.g., repositioning or pain medication)

Note: Courtesy of Shriners Hospital for Children, Spokane, WA.

• Discuss potential safety hazards that may result from awkward positioning. Be sure the child is properly situated in a car safety seat for the trip home.

• Suggest that parents make an effort to place toys within the child's reach, because movements of a child in a cast may be slowed.

Once the child progresses to use of special shoes or a brace, provide teaching on brace care for the family. See Families Want to Know: Guidelines for Brace Wear.

Nursing Alert

Advise parents that umbrella strollers may not be sturdy enough to support an infant's casted leg. Some infant swings do not provide a foot rest; its absence can contribute to cast slippage or breakdown. Observe the child in the family's car seat to be sure the casted leg is adequately supported. A pillow may need to be placed under the leg for support.

■ Braces should be as comfortable as possible and the child should have adequate mobility while wearing the brace.

■ Have the child begin wearing the brace for periods of 1–2 hours and then progress to 2–4 hours.

■ Check the skin at 1- to 2-hour intervals initially, then every 4 hours once the skin has been clear for several days. If redness is apparent, leave the brace off and allow the skin to clear. If breakdown has occurred, the brace cannot be replaced until healing is complete. (See Chapter 31 ∞ for a discussion of pressure ulcers.)

■ Always have the child wear a clean white sock, t-shirt, or other thin white liner beneath the brace. Be sure the liner is wrinkle-free under the brace. Avoid using powders or lotions that can cause skin to break down. Toughen any sensitive areas using alcohol wipes 3–4 times daily.

■ Reapply the brace when the skin returns to its normal color.

■ Return to the physician or orthotic specialist if discomfort or red areas persist or if the brace needs adjustment or repair or is outgrown.

■ Check the brace daily for rough edges.

Evaluation

Expected outcomes of nursing care include maintenance of skin integrity, recovery without complications after surgery, normal developmental progression of the child, and demonstrated knowledge by parents for care of braces or casts, as needed.

Genu Varum and Genu Valgum

Genu varum (bowlegs) is a deformity in which the knees are widely separated while the ankles are close together and the lower legs are turned inward (varus). In genu valgum (knock-knees), the knees are close together and the lower legs are directed outward (valgus). Chapter 5 ∞ discusses the assessment of bowlegs and knock-knees in children (Figure 29–8 ➤).

At certain stages of a child's development, the appearance of bowlegs or knock-knees is normal. Until 2 to 3 years, the knees are normally bowed, showing varus alignment, and by 4 to 5 years, some knock-knee or valgus alignment commonly emerges. Persistent genu varum or genu valgum should be evaluated. Two pathologic causes of genu varum are Blount's disease and rickets. **Blount's disease** is characterized by abnormal growth on the medial side of the proximal tibia, which causes an increasing varus deformity. It is believed to be due to increasing compression forces across the medial knee and is more common in overweight, Black, and female children (Hosalkar, Gholve, & Wells, 2007). **Rickets** is a result of inadequate bone mineralization, usually caused by a deficiency of calcium, vitamin D, or both (see Chapter 14 ∞ for a description of the association between rickets and diet). Since the bones are decalcified or softened, long bones such as those in the legs may bend into a bowed position. Occasionally rickets is congenital and is caused by an X-linked autosomal dominant or recessive gene with the chromosome location Xp22.31-p21.3. It results in an enzyme deficiency of alkaline phosphatase which in turn leads to excessive

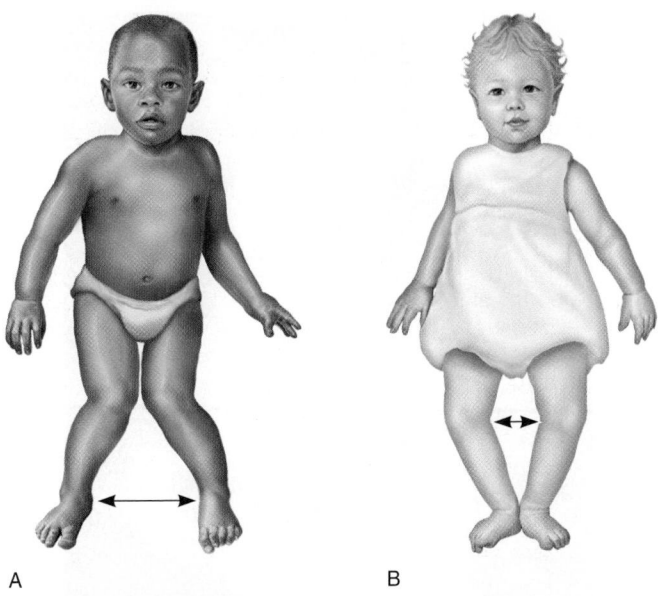

A   B

FIGURE 29–8 ➤ A, Genu valgum or knock-knees. Note that the ankles are far apart when the knees are together. B, Genu varum or bowlegs. The legs are bowed so that the knees are far apart as the child stands.

inhibitors of bone mineralization. This type of rickets is rare and is called familial hypophosphatemic rickets (FHR).

Measurements, radiographs, arthrography (joint radiographs), MRI, and CT imaging may be used for accurate diagnosis. Braces are often used to correct mild deformities that could worsen as the child grows. Braces for bowlegs are worn at night; those for knock-knees are worn both day and night. Duration of brace wear is determined by the severity of the deformity, which is usually evaluated by radiographs. If the deformity continues to worsen, surgical intervention is necessary. Surgery is common in the treatment of Blount disease. An **osteotomy** (cutting of the bone) is performed and the tibiofemoral angle is surgically corrected. The child is then placed in a cast for approximately 6 to 10 weeks, or until full healing has occurred.

Nursing Management

Reassure parents that bowlegs and knock-knees are usually a normal part of a child's growth and development. These conditions often resolve in time and require no treatment other than monitoring.

Nursing care focuses on educating the parents and child about the condition and its treatment. Provide the child and family with guidelines for brace wear and maintenance (see page 952).

■ DISORDERS OF THE HIP

Developmental Dysplasia of the Hip

Developmental dysplasia of the hip (DDH) refers to a variety of conditions in which the femoral head and the acetabulum are improperly aligned. These conditions include hip instability, **dislocation** (displacement of the bone from its normal articulation with the joint), **subluxation** (in this instance, a partial dislocation), and acetabular **dysplasia** (abnormal cellular or structural development leading to instability) (Sewell,

Rosendahl, & Eastwood, 2009). In the past, DDH was referred to as congenital dislocated hip (CDH). The disorder's revised name emphasizes that many cases of dislocation, subluxation, and dysplasia occur well after the neonatal period and involve more than a simple dislocation.

DDH is present in 1–3% of newborns. The condition affects girls four times as often as boys. It can be unilateral or bilateral (Sewell et al., 2009).

Etiology and Pathophysiology

Although the exact cause of DDH is unknown, genetic factors appear to play a role. DDH is 20 to 50 times more common in first-degree relatives of an infant with the condition than in the general population. If one child of a set of identical twins has DDH, the other twin is affected 30–40% of the time. Some types of DDH are linked to early gestational events at 12 and 18 weeks' gestation, as the lower limbs rotate and surrounding muscles develop. However, milder cases may be influenced by mechanical forces in the last month of pregnancy such as breech position or large fetal size, and some cases develop after birth as the hip assumes an extended rather than flexed position (Kleposki, Abel, & Sehgal, 2010; Sewell et al., 2009).

The left hip is involved more often than the right hip as a result of intrauterine positioning of the left side of the fetus against the mother's sacrum. Maternal estrogen may cause laxity of the hip joint and capsule, leading to joint instability, especially in females who respond to these estrogen levels. Cultural factors may also be associated with DDH.

Clinical Manifestations

Common signs and symptoms of DDH include limited abduction of the affected hip, asymmetry of the gluteal and thigh fat folds, and telescoping or pistoning of the thigh (Figure 29–9 ➤). The older child with untreated DDH walks with a significant limp, which results from telescoping of the femoral head into the pelvis. The longer the disorder goes untreated, the more pronounced the clinical manifestations become, and the worse the prognosis.

COLLABORATIVE CARE

From 60–80% of hip abnormalities noted in infants resolve by 2 months of age, so practitioners use care and caution in diagnosing DDH; only 15–25% of infants have known risk factors for the disorder. Therefore, the American Academy of Pediatrics

Culture   *Variations in DDH Rates*

Infants who are positioned on cradle boards or traditionally swaddled, as in some Native American cultures, have a high incidence of developmental dysplasia of the hip (DDH). Eastern European children, who are commonly swaddled, also have a high incidence of DDH. In both of these cases, the legs are maintained in an adducted position. The condition occurs less commonly in infants carried on the mothers' hips since the infants' legs are maintained in the abducted position. The disorder is rarely seen in Chinese and African children (hip carrying is common in these groups) (Hosalkar, Horn, Friedman, et al., 2007).

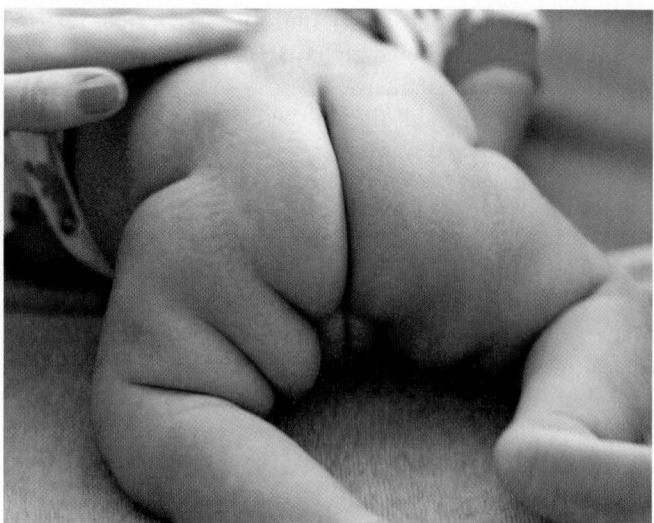

FIGURE 29–9 ➤ The asymmetry of the gluteal and thigh fat folds is easy to see in this child with developmental dysplasia of the hip.

and the Pediatric Orthopaedic Society of North America recommend that all infants and young children should be screened for DDH until walking is well established at about 1 year of age (Schwend, Schoenecker, Richards, et al., 2007; U.S. Preventive Services Task Force, 2006a, 2006b). Physical examination reveals Allis sign (one knee lower than the other when the knees are flexed) and positive Ortolani–Barlow maneuver in babies under 8 to 12 weeks. Refer to Chapter 5 ∞ for a discussion of the assessment of hip dysplasia in newborns and infants. Radiographs are generally not reliable until approximately 4 months of age, because the pelvis in a newborn is still primarily cartilaginous. Before 4 months, ultrasonography may be useful for diagnosis. After that age, radiographs are used for diagnosis. Family history of DDH and a female born in the breech position necessitate careful evaluation (Schwend et al., 2007; U.S. Department of Health and Human Services, 2006).

Treatment plans vary according to the child's age. For infants younger than 6 months, the Pavlik harness is the most commonly used method for hip reduction (Figure 29–10 ➤). The Pavlik harness is a dynamic splint, that is, a splint that allows movement. It ensures hip flexion and abduction and does not allow hip extension or adduction. For infants older than 6 months, surgery with closed reduction is performed (positioning the head of the femur into the acetabulum without an incision of the skin), followed by the application of a spica cast. In children over 18 months of age, open or closed reduction surgery and casting are usually necessary and later bracing may also be required (Figure 29–11 ➤).

Early screening, detection, and treatment enable the majority of affected children to attain normal hip function.

NURSING MANAGEMENT

Nursing Assessment and Diagnosis

Assessment for DDH begins at delivery and continues through all health promotion visits during the first 2 years of life. The specific family history or birth data may indicate a high-risk

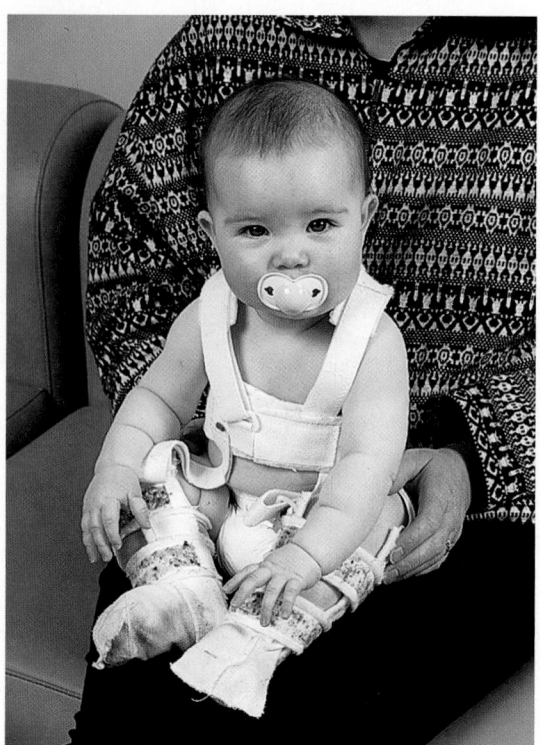

FIGURE 29–10 ➤ The most common treatment for DDH in a child under 3 months of age is a Pavlik harness. A shirt should be worn under the harness to prevent skin irritation (it was omitted for clarity in this photograph).

infant, as does oligohydramnios, large-for-gestational-age infant, or breech birth. Instructions for performing the physical examination to assess the infant for DDH are provided in Chapter 5 ∞. Further assessments are determined by the

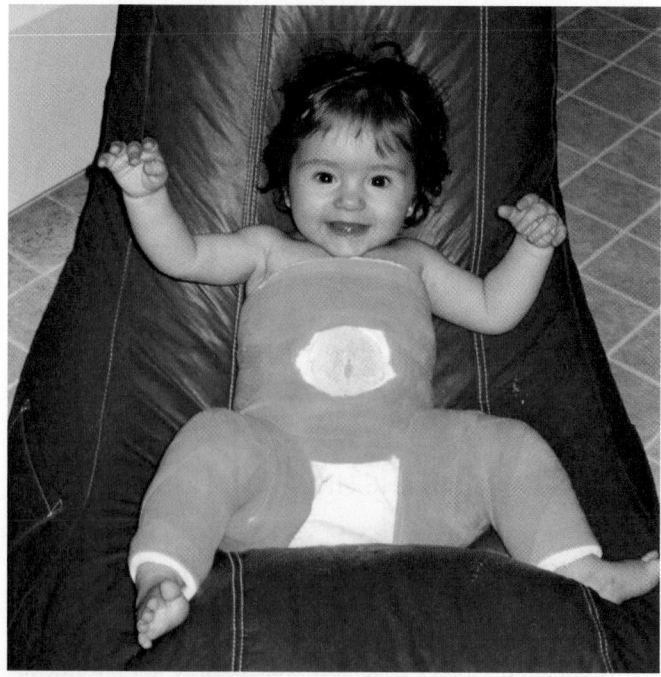

FIGURE 29–11 ➤ The infant treated for DDH is often in a spica cast after surgery.

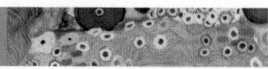
Courtesy of Michael Berkman, MD Web Corporation. http://mdwebcorp.com

treatment provided. Skin assessments are performed on the child in traction or a cast, every few minutes at first and progressing to once or twice daily at home. Respiratory and circulatory assessments are included when the child is immobilized. Ongoing assessments of the child's growth and development are needed.

Clinical Tip

Weigh the child in a cast once the cast is dry so a baseline casted weight can be used for comparison during the weeks and months while the cast remains in place.

The following nursing diagnoses may apply to the child with DDH:

- Impaired Physical Mobility related to prescribed movement restriction (Pavlik harness, traction, spica cast, brace)
- Risk for Impaired Skin Integrity related to irritation from harness straps or skin traction
- Risk for Altered Urinary Elimination or Constipation related to immobility caused by treatment
- Risk for Imbalanced Nutrition related to decreased appetite
- Risk for Delayed Growth and Development related to limited mobility and potential decreased exposure to stimulation
- Health-Seeking Behavior (Parental) related to lack of information about disease process and treatment

Planning and Implementation

The infant with DDH is often cared for at home and in outpatient facilities. If surgery is performed, the child is hospitalized for surgery and the immediate postoperative period. Nursing care varies according to the medical treatment and the child's age. Management includes providing cast care; preventing complications resulting from immobility; promoting normal growth and development; and teaching parents how to care for a child in a cast, traction, or a Pavlik harness at home. Because treatment may interfere with the child's normal movement, the treatment plan should take into consideration the child's age and developmental stage.

Provide Cast Care

The principles of routine cast care presented in Box 29–1 apply to the care of spica casts. Special techniques should be used to help keep the cast clean and dry in children who are not toilet trained. Female and male urinals can be used for older children. Use a plastic lining to protect the cast edges during elimination for older children and use a small disposable diaper to cover the perineum in babies, tucking edges beneath the cast. Be sure to change the diaper frequently to prevent soiling of the cast.

Control Pain

If the child has surgery to correct DDH, pain control in the immediate postoperative period is needed. Assess the child's pain frequently in a method appropriate for age (see Chapter 15 ∞). Administer intravenous and oral pain medications as prescribed.

Use methods such as holding, rocking, and gentle music to calm the child. An ice bag placed on top of the cast at the operative site may be helpful; use caution to avoid leakage of the melted ice onto the cast. Encourage parents to be present and provide care when possible.

If pain is not controlled or if it increases over time, compression at the surgical site may be occurring. Promptly report this to the physician. Pain in the infant may be manifested by a combination of physiological and behavioral changes.

Prevent Complications Resulting from Immobility

Immobilization from traction or a cast can cause alterations in physiologic functioning. Take the following actions to prevent complications:

- Assess breathing patterns and lung sounds frequently for congestion or respiratory compromise.
- Perform skin and neurovascular assessments approximately every 2 hours.
- Use adequate padding and skin wrapping to avoid placing pressure on the popliteal space. Such pressure could lead to nerve damage.
- Change the child's position every 2 to 3 hours while awake to help avoid areas of pressure and promote increased circulation. The child with a cast can be placed either prone or supine or positioned on the floor and supported with pillows.
- Prevent skin irritation and breakdown in the child with a cast. Use moleskin to provide protection from rough edges. Place tape around the perineal opening of the cast to prevent soiling.
- Increase fluids and fiber in the child's diet, as a change in bowel or bladder status is commonly associated with immobility.
- If prescription allows, release the child from external traction for meals and daily care. The time out of external traction should not exceed 1 hour per day. Encourage parents to hold and cuddle the child at this time to promote comfort and bonding.

Clinical Tip

Neurovascular assessment involves evaluation of temperature, movement, color, capillary refill, pulses, and sensation. Even if the child is not old enough to respond to questions about sensation, usually brushing the hands or sheets along the toes elicits a movement from the child and indicates sensation. Report any abnormalities immediately. Keep limbs aligned during traction. For the child in a spica cast, elevate the lower body on pillows immediately after surgery to decrease edema under the cast at the operative site.

Promote Normal Growth and Development

Engage the child in activities that stimulate the upper extremities and all five senses. Provide stimulating toys such as stacking blocks, brightly colored mobiles, soft balls, or musical toys. Position toys within the child's reach and interact with the child as much as possible.

Use caution in selecting toys appropriate for the child's developmental age. If the child is in a cast, be sure that toys or parts cannot be swallowed or stuck inside the cast. Place a t-shirt over the cast so that the edges are securely covered and it is difficult for the child to place something under them. Provide toys that are large and soft, use diversion such as play and music to occupy the child's attention, and assess the child frequently.

Discharge Planning and Home Care Teaching

Parents must learn how to care for a child in traction or a spica cast at home. The active participation of family members in the daily care of the child while hospitalized gradually increases their confidence in their ability to provide care at home. Home care needs should be identified and addressed well in advance of discharge. Before discharge, be sure the parents have the following information:

- Instructions about general cast care (see pages 949 and 952), positioning, bathing, toileting, and age-appropriate diversional activities.
- Importance of performing and reporting changes in neurovascular assessment.
- Instructions regarding the bar between the legs of a spica cast. It is not to be used for holding or lifting the child; it is only for positioning the legs properly. Using the bar to lift can cause the cast to fracture, weaken, or disintegrate.
- Appropriate referrals for periodic assessment by a visiting nurse or home health nurse.
- Family resources to care for the child.

Before discharge, have parents demonstrate how to dress and feed a child in a spica cast. Ensure that safe travel arrangements have been made for the day of discharge. Help parents to obtain an appropriate car safety seat in advance of discharge. Encourage parents to let the child interact with other children at home, and to provide the child in a cast with similar opportunities for play and social activities.

Care in the Community

Have parents of an infant in a Pavlik harness demonstrate proper application of the harness and care of the infant while in the harness. Teach family members about the daily care (bathing, dressing, and feeding) of the infant. Ideally, the harness is worn 23 hours per day and is removed only for skin checks and bathing. The hips and buttocks should be supported carefully when the infant is out of the harness. Demonstrate how to feed the infant in an upright position to maintain abduction and how to change a diaper without removing the harness. (See Families Want to Know: Guidelines for Pavlik Harness Application.)

Instruct the parents of an infant with a harness or a child in a cast to look for any reddened or irritated areas near the harness or cast edges and to check toes frequently for proper circulation. Frequent repositioning reduces the risk of pressure sores or circulatory compromise. The infant should wear an undershirt and socks under the harness to prevent rubbing of the skin.

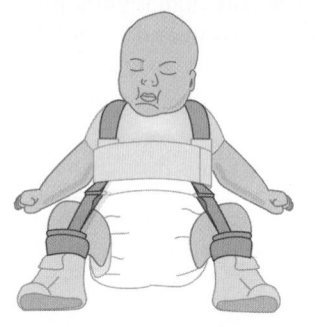 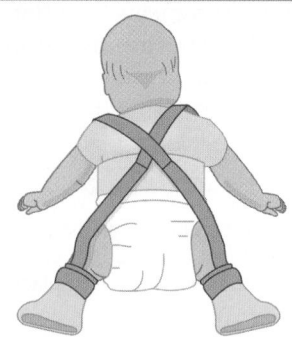

1. Position the chest halter at the nipple line and fasten with Velcro.
2. Position the legs and feet in the stirrups, being sure the hips are flexed and abducted. Fasten with Velcro.
3. Connect the chest halter and leg straps in front.
4. Connect the chest halter and leg straps in back.

All the straps are marked at the first fitting with indelible ink so they can be reattached easily after the harness is rinsed and dried.

Safety precautions are important as the child will not have normal mobility. Parents will need to use a specially designed car seat that accommodates the child with abducted hips (see Families Want to Know: Transporting the Child with Orthopedic Devices). Strollers and cribs should provide sufficient room to protect the legs from injury and to prevent hip adduction.

The American Academy of Pediatrics has established the following guidelines for transporting children with special health care needs:

■ Placement in the rear seat is preferable.

■ If the front seat must be used, the front passenger air bag should be disconnected. The National Highway and Traffic Safety Administration provides information and assistance (1-888-327-4236 or http://www.nhtsa.dot.gov).

■ Use only car seat transport systems approved for use with children with special needs.

■ Install and use seats as instructed. Never alter a car safety seat to transport a child.

■ When reasonable, a child should be moved from a wheelchair or other special device to the vehicle safety seat.

■ Pieces of medical equipment required during transportation (such as monitors or oxygen) or that are being transported with the child (such as wheelchair or walker) should be secured to the floor of the vehicle.

■ If the child is transported by school bus, state and federal recommendations for school bus transportation of children with special needs should be followed.

■ Keep a cellular phone and emergency equipment in the vehicle.

Note: Data adapted from American Academy of Pediatrics, Committee on Injury and Poison Prevention. (1999 and 2006). *Children with special health care needs.* Retrieved from http://www.aap.org/healthtopics/specialneeds .cfm; *Parenting corner: Questions and answers: Transporting children with special health care needs.* Retrieved from http://www.aap.org/publiced/BR_ SpNeedsCarSeats.htm

Evaluation

Expected outcomes for nursing care of the child with developmental dysplasia of the hip include the following:

- Skin integrity is maintained.
- The infant shows no complications related to immobility.
- Parents have adequate knowledge of the condition, treatment, and necessary home care.
- A safe environment is maintained for the child.
- The child attains normal mobility by the end of the treatment period.

Legg-Calvé-Perthes Disease

Legg-Calvé-Perthes disease (also called Perthes disease) is a self-limiting condition characterized by avascular necrosis of the femoral head. The disease occurs in approximately 1 in 12,000 children, with a predominance of cases in males. It usually occurs between the ages of 2 and 12 years, with an average age of 7 years at onset. The disease is bilateral in 20% of cases (Hosalkar et al., 2007).

Etiology and Pathophysiology

The necrosis associated with Legg-Calvé-Perthes disease results from an interruption of the blood supply to the femoral epiphysis. How and why this occurs is not completely understood, but several predisposing factors have been identified. A coagulation system disorder may cause repeated vascular interruptions to the proximal femur. Disturbed blood supply to the epiphyseal plate of the femoral bone is noted, leading to flattening and necrosis of the femoral head (Kleposki et al., 2010). About 10% of children with Perthes have a positive family history; the condition is five times more common in males, and it occurs most often in White males with short stature (Kleposki et al., 2010). Trauma may cause a subchondral fracture and resultant synovitis, which in turn causes pressure that occludes the blood supply. Children with Legg-Calvé-Perthes disease often have delayed skeletal maturation, increased thyroid levels, and low somatomedin C (insulin-like growth factor). It is more common in those with low birth weight, increased parental age, and exposure to environmental tobacco smoke. Some cultural variations occur.

Clinical Manifestations

Legg-Calvé-Perthes disease progresses through four distinct stages after the original insult (usually unidentified) occurs, over a period of 1 to 4 years. Early symptoms of the disease include a mild pain in the hip or anterior thigh and a limp, which are aggra-

Culture *Incidence of Legg-Calvé-Perthes Disease*

Legg-Calvé-Perthes disease is most common among White, Japanese, and Chinese children. It is less common among Blacks and Native Americans. This suggests a genetic link to the disease, as does the more frequent occurrence in certain families. However, the cause is not known so the reason for ethnic variation in incidence is not certain (Hosalkar et al., 2007).

Clinical Manifestations
Legg-Calvé-Perthes Disease

Stage	Clinical Manifestations
Prenecrosis	An insult causes loss of blood supply to the femoral head.
I—Necrosis	Avascular stage (3–6 months); the child is asymptomatic, bone radiographs are normal, and the head of the femur is structurally intact but avascular.
II—Revascularization	Period of 1–4 years characterized by pain and limitation of movement. Bone radiographs show new bone deposition and dead bone resorption. Fracture and deformity of the head of the femur can occur.
III—Bone healing	Reossification takes place; pain decreases.
IV—Remodeling	The disease process is over, pain is absent, and improvement in joint function occurs.

vated by increased activity and relieved by rest. The child favors the affected hip and limits hip movement to avoid discomfort. See Clinical Manifestations: Legg-Calvé-Perthes Disease.

As the disease progresses, range of motion becomes limited and weakness and muscle wasting develop. The affected thigh is 2 to 3 cm smaller than the unaffected thigh. Prolonged hip irritability may produce muscle spasms and pain increases. Gradually, revascularization begins and pain decreases.

COLLABORATIVE CARE

Diagnostic Tests

Because the child's initial symptoms are so mild, parents often do not seek medical attention until symptoms have been present for several months. Diagnosis is made using standard anteroposterior and frog-leg radiographs. As previously noted, radiographs taken early in the course of the disease may be normal or show vague widening of the cartilage space. Bone scans and MRI may show the disease process earlier than radiographs. Laboratory studies of the blood, such as white blood cell (WBC) count, help to rule out inflammatory synovitis of the hip. Protein C, protein S, and APC-R (resistance to activated protein C) laboratory tests may be performed to evaluate if a coagulation abnormality is present (Burns, Dunn, Brady, et al., 2009).

Clinical Therapy

Medical management and prognosis depend on the degree of femoral involvement and the clinician's decision. Early detection is important. The desired outcome is a pain-free hip that functions properly. To promote healing and prevent deformity, the femoral head must be contained within the hip socket to maintain its sphericity. Observation and examination over time are most commonly used with physical rehabilitation, and occasionally traction or casting. The Toronto brace is an example of

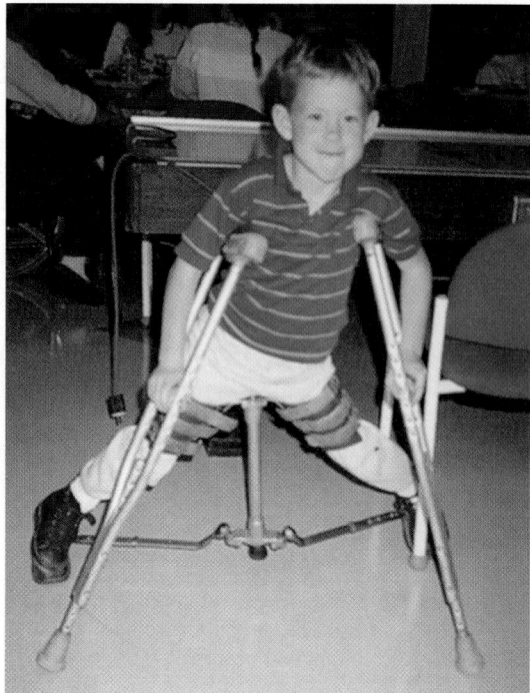

FIGURE 29–12 ➤ Although the Toronto brace may seem formidable for a child to wear, you can see by this photograph that, as usual, children adapt quite well to it.

a treatment that allows mobility without pressure on the head of the femur. Severe disease may be treated by surgery to release adductor muscles, treat the acetabulum or femur, and restore range of motion (Figure 29–12 ➤). Prognosis is best if the child is young and has a mild form of the disorder (Fabry, 2010). Children with untreated disease or those diagnosed late in the disease process may develop osteoarthritis, hip dysfunction, or leg length discrepancy.

NURSING MANAGEMENT

Nursing Assessment and Diagnosis

Legg-Calvé-Perthes disease should be suspected in any child, especially a boy age 2 to 12 years, who complains of hip discomfort accompanied by a limp. The school nurse may be the first person to observe the child with symptoms of the disease. The child may complain of pain and have to rest during physical education classes. In this case, immediate referral should be made to the health care provider. Question the child who has an apparent limp about pain, and assess the child's range of motion. Ask if the child previously injured the hip.

Nursing diagnoses, which center on altered activities and compliance, may include the following:

- Impaired Physical Mobility related to restriction of treatment
- Risk for Injury related to potential complications resulting from noncompliance with the treatment regimen
- Impaired Adjustment related to duration of treatment or nonadherence to recommended therapy
- Deficient Diversional Activity related to forced inactivity

Planning and Implementation

Children with Legg-Calvé-Perthes disease often receive all of their treatment at home. Helping the child and family comply with the prescribed treatment plan may be challenging, because children develop the disease at an age when they are usually very active. The child, who may have little pain, often finds immobilization and physical rehabilitation recommendations difficult.

Promote Normal Growth and Development

Parents should be given suggestions to help redirect the child's energy within the limitations in mobility imposed by treatment. A return to school promotes a feeling of normalcy. Coordinate the return to school by facilitating the child's use of an elevator or ramp as needed in that setting. Collaborate with the family to provide instruction for school personnel and other children to foster understanding of the child's condition and treatment. Activities that involve peers also help the child achieve developmental milestones. Help the child adjust to wearing a brace or cast if that is the treatment used.

Care in the Community

Both the child and the family should be aware that treatment generally takes more than 2 years. Emphasize the importance of following the treatment plan to ensure adequate hip containment and proper healing. Teach the family how to care for a child with special devices or following surgery. Follow-up visits should be arranged at regular intervals, and home care visits may be helpful for some families.

Evaluation

Expected outcomes of nursing care are elimination of hip pain and discomfort, normal development during the period of immobilization, and parent and child knowledge of treatment regimen.

Slipped Capital Femoral Epiphysis

Slipped capital femoral epiphysis (SCFE) occurs when the femoral head is displaced from the femoral neck. This condition is seen in approximately 10 out of every 100,000 adolescents, commonly during the growth spurt between the ages of 12 and 15 years in boys and 10 and 13 years in girls. Boys are more often affected than girls. White and Black children are affected more often than other ethnic groups, as are children who are overweight and those with sports injuries or other trauma, a history of radiation therapy, or endocrine disease (Gholve, Cameron, & Millis, 2009; Shank, Thiel, & Klingele, 2010).

Pathophysiology Illustrated

Slipped Epiphysis

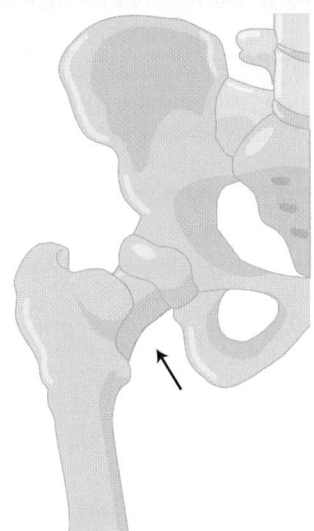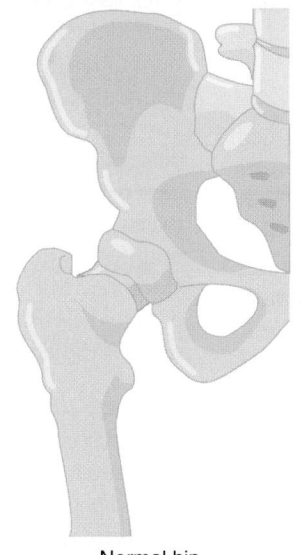

Slipped epiphysis   Normal hip

FIGURE 29–13 ➤ In slipped capital femoral epiphysis, the femoral head is displaced from the femoral neck at the proximal epiphyseal plate.

Etiology and Pathophysiology

The cause of SCFE is unknown. Predisposing factors include obesity, a recent growth spurt, and endocrine disorders such as hypothyroidism and hypogonadism. Slippage of the femoral head occurs at the proximal epiphyseal plate, and the femur displaces from the epiphysis (Figure 29–13 ➤). Slippage is usually gradual (chronic), but may also result from acute trauma. The synovial membrane becomes inflamed, edematous, and painful. If untreated, callous formation occurs, resulting in a deformed hip with limited range of motion.

Clinical Manifestations

Symptoms include limp; knee, thigh, groin, or hip pain; and loss of hip motion. Out-toeing, decreased internal rotation, and external rotation with flexion of the leg are symptomatic (Kleposki et al., 2010). The condition is categorized as acute, chronic, or acute-on-chronic. Acute SCFE has a sudden onset of less than 3 weeks' duration. The child has sudden, severe pain and cannot bear weight. An acute slip may be associated with traumatic injury. Chronic SCFE has a duration of longer than 3 weeks. It presents with persistent hip pain, which is generally aching or mild and can be referred to the thigh, knee, or both. A limp and decreased range

 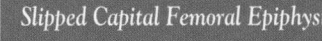
of motion may also occur. Acute-on-chronic SCFE is an additional slippage in a child with a chronic condition. The child with a chronic slip sustains a traumatic incident that causes further slippage of the femoral head, causing sudden, severe pain. The youth may be able to walk (stable SCFE) or unable to bear weight (unstable SCFE) (Aronsson, Loder, Breur, et al., 2006).

COLLABORATIVE CARE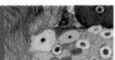

A complete history provides information about risk factors and development of the condition. Radiographs are used to confirm the diagnosis. A bone scan, ultrasound, CT, and MRI are sometimes performed to verify the extent of injury.

The goal of medical management is to stabilize the femoral head while keeping displacement to a minimum and retaining as much hip function as possible. Surgical treatment is usually necessary; this involves fixation of the epiphysis with screws or pins. If the condition is stable, a single screw into the hip in an outpatient procedure is sufficient for stabilization; if unstable, surgery may involve two or three pins placed into the epiphysis to stabilize the femoral head (Aronsson et al., 2006). Medical treatment, which is occasionally used, includes a regimen of no weight bearing, bed rest, a spica cast, and Buck or Russell traction (see traction description later in the chapter).

The prognosis is related to the severity of the deformity and the occurrence of complications, such as avascular necrosis of the femoral head or **chondrolysis** (the breaking down and absorption of cartilage).

NURSING MANAGEMENT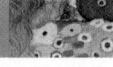

Nursing Assessment and Diagnosis

The child usually presents with hip pain or referred pain to the groin, thigh, or knee, and limited mobility. A thorough history is needed to assess for injury as a cause. Assess the child's range of motion, pain, and limp, if apparent. Refer the child for treatment immediately if SCFE is suspected. This condition is considered an emergency, and the child must be treated immediately to keep weight off the affected joint (Kleposki et al., 2010).

Nursing diagnoses that may apply to the child with SCFE are as follows:

- Impaired Physical Mobility related to treatment
- Acute Pain related to hip injury
- Risk for Disturbed Body Image related to treatment

- Risk for Delayed Growth and Development related to mobility restrictions
- Risk for Imbalanced Nutrition: More than Body Requirements related to immobility
- Ineffective Tissue Perfusion: Peripheral related to traction, casting, and other treatments

Planning and Implementation

Weight control interventions for the child or adolescent with overweight or obesity is an important preventive measure. Nursing management for the child with a diagnosis of SCFE involves caring for the child in traction or after surgery, administering medications and other pain control interventions, maintaining mobility within the limits imposed by treatment, providing adequate nutrition, educating the child and family about the disorder, providing emotional support, and promoting compliance with the treatment plan.

Encourage Appropriate Nutritional Intake and Physical Activity

A growing adolescent needs adequate amounts of proteins, carbohydrates, and calcium to promote skeletal healing. Provide written instructions about nutritional requirements necessary to promote bone healing and maintain an ideal body weight. If a child is overweight, encourage weight loss by decreasing percent of fat in the diet, as well as controlling caloric intake if it is excessive (see Chapter 14 ∞). This decreases pressure on the femoral epiphysis and can also lead to a more positive self-image. Incorporate upper body exercises into treatment, both to assist in weight control and to build muscle. Physical therapy is useful to facilitate a program of upper body exercise and teach safe ways of increasing the total amount of physical activity.

Provide Emotional Support

Because the onset of SCFE is usually unexpected, the child and family may find themselves facing surgery with little warning. Explain the treatment plan simply and thoroughly. Reassure the child and family that with proper compliance, treatment should be successful.

Discharge Planning and Home Care Teaching

Assist the family to plan for the child's return to school. If attendance is not possible for a period of time due to traction or surgery, arrange for tutors and computer communication with school as needed. Follow-up visits are necessary until the child's epiphyseal plates close. It is not uncommon for SCFE to occur in the other hip. Make sure the child and family are aware of symptoms such as decreased range of motion or pain that could indicate onset of the disorder in the other hip. Tell parents to contact their health care provider immediately if these symptoms occur.

Evaluation

Expected outcomes of nursing care for the child with SCFE include maintenance of normal weight and recommended nutritional intake, absence of complications of immobility, successful adaptation to school following treatment, and family recognition of the need for ongoing monitoring for complications.

■ DISORDERS OF THE SPINE

Scoliosis

Scoliosis is a lateral S- or C-shaped curvature of the spine that is often associated with a rotational deformity of the spine and ribs. Many individuals exhibit some degree of spinal curvature, but curvatures of more than 10 degrees are considered abnormal. Curves are either idiopathic or compensatory, the latter occurring as the spine curves to compensate for a structural deformity such as leg length discrepancy. Idiopathic scoliosis occurs most often in girls, especially during the growth spurt between the ages of 10 and 13 years. From 1–3% of adolescents manifest with idiopathic scoliosis of greater than 10 degrees (Mooney, Mayer, & Woodbridge, 2007). Early onset of idiopathic scoliosis occurs before 10 years of age and comprises 15% of cases (Spiegel, Hosalkar, & Dormans, 2007).

Etiology and Pathophysiology

The cause of scoliosis is complex. Structural scoliosis may be congenital, idiopathic, or acquired (associated with neuromuscular disorders such as muscular dystrophy or myelodysplasia, or secondary to spinal cord injuries).

In idiopathic structural scoliosis (the most common type), the spine for unknown reasons begins to curve laterally, with vertebral rotation. The most common curve is a right thoracic and left lumbar deformity. As the curve progresses, structural changes occur. The ribs on the concave side (inside of the curve) are forced closer together, while the ribs on the convex side separate widely, causing narrowing of the thoracic cage and formation of the rib hump. The lateral curvature affects the vertebral structure. Disk spaces are narrowed on the concave side and spread wider on the convex side, resulting in an asymmetric vertebral canal (Figure 29–14 ➤).

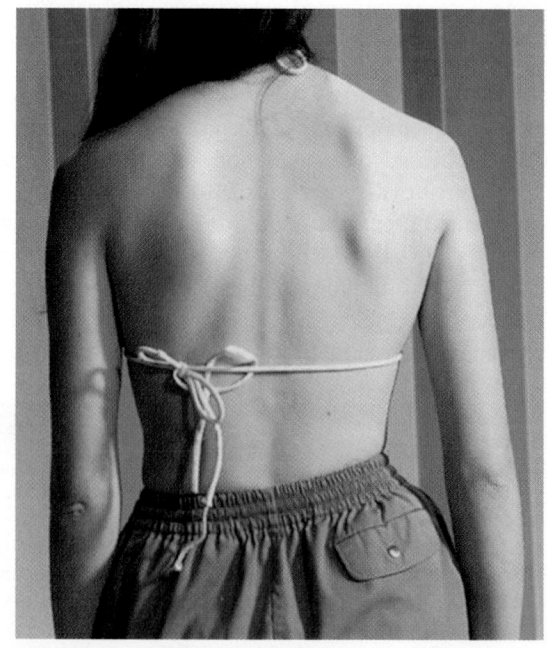

FIGURE 29–14 ➤ A child may have varying degrees of scoliosis. For mild forms, treatment will focus on strengthening and stretching. Moderate forms will require bracing. Severe forms may necessitate surgery and fusion. Clothes that fit at an angle, such as this teenage girl's shorts, and anatomic asymmetry of the back provide clues for early detection.

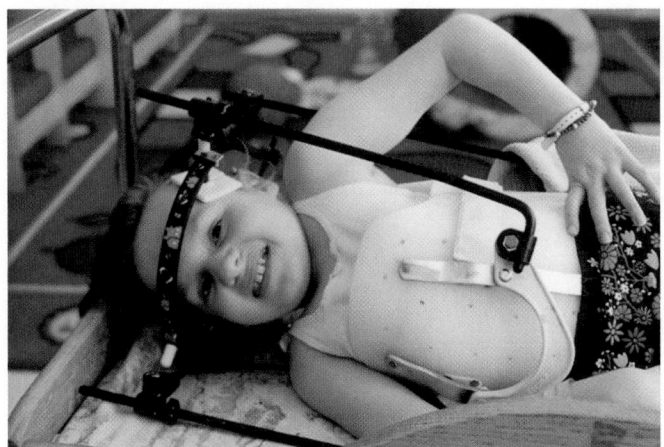

FIGURE 29–15 ➤ In severe scoliosis, the child may wear a halo brace, shown here, to hold the body in position after surgery.

Scoliosis can also occur in congenital diseases involving the spinal structure and in the musculoskeletal changes seen in conditions such as myelomeningocele, cerebral palsy (see Chapter 27 ∞), or muscular dystrophy. It can also be acquired after injury to the spinal cord. The child in Figure 29–15 ➤ acquired scoliosis after chemotherapy and radiation to the chest during treatment for cancer.

Clinical Manifestations

The classic signs of scoliosis include truncal asymmetry, uneven shoulder and hip height, a one-sided rib hump, and a prominent scapula. However, the child does not generally complain of pain or discomfort. If diagnosis does not occur before the curvature reaches about 40 degrees, some compensatory problems may develop. Hip and back pain can result, and lung compromise can lead to fatigue or dyspnea with exertion.

COLLABORATIVE CARE

A complete medical history for previous conditions and treatments is performed. Family history of scoliosis is obtained. Observation and radiographic examination are used to diagnose scoliosis. Additional diagnostic studies include MRI, CT scan, and bone scan, which are used to assess the degree of curvature.

Early detection is essential to successful treatment. The goal of medical management is to limit or stop progression of the curvature. Adequate treatment and follow-up maximize the child's chances for proper spinal alignment. The treatment regimen chosen depends on the degree and progression of the curvature and the reaction of the child and family to medical management.

Treatment of children with mild scoliosis (curvatures of 10 to 20 degrees) consists of physical rehabilitation to improve posture and muscle tone and to maintain, or possibly increase, flexibility of the spine. Emphasis is placed on bending strength toward the outside of the curve while stretching the inside of the curve. These exercises do not influence the course of condition progression, however, and the child should be evaluated by a physician at 3-month intervals, with radiographic evaluation every 6 months.

Medical management of moderate scoliosis (used commonly for curvatures of 20 to 40 degrees) includes either regular monitoring of the curve progression or bracing, most commonly with a Boston brace. The goal of wearing a brace is to maintain the existing spinal curvature with no increase. Brace wear begins immediately after diagnosis. To achieve maximum effectiveness, the brace should be worn 23 hours per day. Brace treatment is lengthy and requires a high degree of compliance, which can be difficult for adolescents who view body image or sports involvement as important.

Children with severe scoliosis (curvatures of 40 to 50 degrees or more) commonly require surgery, which involves spinal fusion. The majority of spinal fusions are performed using instrumentation of the spinal cord. These treatments stabilize the spine well during surgery, may be accompanied by bone grafting to the spine, and require no long-term therapy or postoperative casting. Following surgery with wires or instrumentation, the child is on bed rest during a recovery period and then is sometimes fitted with anteroposterior plastic shells (also called thoracolumbar sacral orthotics) that are worn for several months to provide stability for the spine. The wires will remain in the back forever. Occasionally in severe cases, halo traction is used postoperatively to provide support for the unstable spine (see Figure 29–15).

Several new treatments are being explored for scoliosis treatment, including implants to allow for expansion of the thorax to accommodate lung function, spinal implants known as growing rods, and spinal stapling. Genetic testing is also being explored to predict outcomes and assist with selection of therapy (Cruz & Smith, 2010).

NURSING MANAGEMENT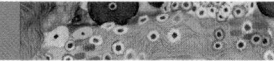

Nursing Assessment and Diagnosis

School nurses often screen children for scoliosis, generally in the fifth and seventh grades. Several states mandate this screening, but it is not required in all states (U.S. Preventive Services Task Force, 2006b). When abnormalities are noted, the child is referred to an orthopedic center for further evaluation. Children should be examined every 6 to 9 months thereafter. If scoliosis is detected, the child's brothers and sisters should be examined and observed closely. (See Table 29–2.)

Once scoliosis has been identified, the nurse's focus becomes education and follow-up. Any child with scoliosis should have a comprehensive neurologic, cardiac, and respiratory examination, since the rib cage deformity can influence the functioning of these systems.

The following nursing diagnoses may apply to the child with scoliosis who is not undergoing surgery:

- Risk for Impaired Adjustment to the Exercise Program related to duration and intensity of exercise
- Impaired Physical Mobility related to brace
- Risk for Impaired Skin Integrity related to brace
- Ineffective Breathing Pattern related to rib cage deformity
- Health-Seeking Behaviors (Child and Parent) related to unfamiliarity with disease process
- Risk for Disturbed Body Image related to condition and treatment

Common nursing diagnoses for the child who is having surgery can be found in the accompanying Nursing Care Plan.

TABLE 29–2 **Visual Screening for Scoliosis**			
From the Front	From the Back	While the Adolescent Holds Hands Together and Bends Over Slightly	While the Adolescent Holds Hands Together and Bends Over Toward the Floor
Is the head midline? • Are the shoulders at the same height? • Is there the same amount of space between the arms and body on each side?	Is the head midline? • Are the shoulders at the same height? • Are the scapulae equally prominent and at the same height? • Is the spine straight? • Is there the same amount of space between the arms and body on each side? • Are the hips at the same height?	Are the scapular humps even?	Are the flank humps even? • Is the spine straight? • Is there a marked roundness when viewed from the side (evidence of kyphosis)?

Planning and Implementation

An important aspect of nursing care is patient education. Patient compliance is critical to the success of treatment. Children and their families need to understand the condition and the stages of treatment, particularly adolescents who are undergoing treatment for scoliosis. Children or adolescents facing surgery require education, reassurance, and support. Teach about pain control and the PCA (patient-controlled analgesia) pump. Often the child donates some of his or her own blood prior to surgery, and the family may also donate so the child's or a family member's blood is transfused in surgery. The adolescent will benefit from learning about deep breathing, positioning, surgical incision, and all other aspects of postoperative care. The ac-

companying Nursing Care Plan summarizes nursing care for the child undergoing surgery for scoliosis.

Promote Understanding and Acceptance of the Treatment Plan

Provide instructions about exercises that will help to decrease the severity of the spinal curvature. Demonstrate the exercises, and explain their purpose (e.g., to strengthen back muscles). Help the child adjust to wearing a brace. Adolescents, in particular, may be reluctant to wear an external device such as a brace. To promote a sense of control, allow the adolescent to choose when to exercise and when to be out of the brace, within the treatment guidelines. Provide reassurance and encouragement

NURSING CARE PLAN

The Child Undergoing Surgery for Scoliosis

INTERVENTION	RATIONALE	EXPECTED OUTCOME
1. Nursing Diagnosis: Deficient Knowledge (Child and Parents) related to lack of information about surgery		
NIC Priority Intervention: *Teaching, disease process and preoperative:* Assisting the patient to understand information and mentally prepare for surgery and postoperative recovery		**NOC Suggested Outcome:** *Knowledge:* Extent of understanding conveyed about scoliosis treatment
Goal: The child and parents will verbalize understanding of the disease, its treatment, and the surgical procedure.		
▪ Teach the child and family about the course of the disease, its signs and symptoms, and treatment. Provide appropriate handouts. Encourage the child and parents to ask questions.	▪ Understanding and involvement increase motivation and compliance while reducing fear.	The child and family accurately verbalize knowledge about the disease and its treatment. The child and family ask appropriate questions about postoperative care.
▪ Begin preoperative teaching at the time of admission. Orient the child to hospital and postoperative procedures. Before surgery, have the child demonstrate log-rolling, range of motion exercises, and the use of an incentive spirometer. Discuss pain management.	▪ Preoperative teaching and familiarity with hospital procedures reduce the stress related to surgery and postoperative complications.	

NURSING CARE PLAN

The Child Undergoing Surgery for Scoliosis (continued)

INTERVENTION	RATIONALE	EXPECTED OUTCOME

2. Nursing Diagnosis: Ineffective Breathing Pattern related to hypoventilation syndrome

NIC Priority Intervention: *Airway management and respiratory monitoring:* Facilitation of patency of air passages and analysis of patient data		NOC Suggested Outcome: *Respiratory status: Ventilation:* Movement of air in and out of the lungs

Goal: The child will show no signs of respiratory compromise.

■ Monitor respiratory status, especially after the administration of analgesics. Apply a pulse oximeter.	■ Evaluation of the child's respiratory condition anticipates and avoids complications. Analgesics such as morphine may increase or potentiate respiratory compromise.	The child has no respiratory complications.
■ Administer oxygen if ordered.	■ Oxygen increases peripheral oxygen saturation to 95–100%.	
■ Have the child use an incentive spirometer.	■ Spirometry increases lung expansion and aeration of the alveoli.	
■ Monitor intake and output.	■ Good hydration promotes loose secretions and helps prevent infection.	
■ Reposition the child at least every 2 hours.	■ Repositioning ensures inflation of the lung fields.	

3. Nursing Diagnosis: Risk for Injury related to neurovascular deficit secondary to instrumentation

NIC Priority Intervention: *Injury prevention:* Instituting special precautions with patient at risk		NOC Suggested Outcome: *Risk control:* Actions to eliminate or reduce modifiable health risks

Goal: The child's neurovascular system will remain intact as evidenced by circulation, sensation, and motor checks. The child will feel no numbness or tingling.

■ Monitor the child's color, circulation, capillary refill, warmth, sensation, and motion in all extremities. Perform neurovascular checks every 2 hours for the first 24 hours and then every 4 hours for the next 48 hours. Record presence of pedal and distal tibial pulses every hour for 48 hours. Report changes and abnormal findings immediately.	■ When the spinal column is manipulated during surgery, altered neurovascular status, thrombus formation, and paralysis are possible complications. ■ Postoperative complications include loss of bowel or bladder control, weakness or paralysis, and impaired vision or sensation.	The child exhibits only temporary alteration (pale skin, faint pulse, and edema occur, but then resolve within the initial postoperative phase). The child returns to the preoperative baseline state by discharge.
■ Have the child wear antiembolism stockings until ambulatory. The stockings may be removed for 1 hour 2–3 times daily.	■ Antiembolism stockings prevent blood clots and promote venous return. Thrombus formation is a postoperative risk.	
■ Check for any pain, swelling, or a positive Homans sign in the legs. Record any evidence of edema.	■ Swelling may indicate a tight dressing and tissue damage. A positive Homans sign and pain may indicate thrombus formation.	
■ Monitor input and output.	■ Abnormalities may indicate a fluid shift problem.	
■ Encourage and assist the child with range of motion exercises, both passive and active.	■ Activity promotes mobility and reduces the risk of thrombus formation.	

(continued)

NURSING CARE PLAN

The Child Undergoing Surgery for Scoliosis (continued)

INTERVENTION	RATIONALE	EXPECTED OUTCOME
4. Nursing Diagnosis: Pain related to spinal fusion with instrumentation		
NIC Priority Intervention: *Pain management:* Alleviation of pain or a reduction of pain to a level of comfort acceptable to the patient		**NOC Suggested Outcome:** *Pain level:* Amount of reported or demonstrated pain
Goal: The child will verbalize an adequate level of comfort or show absence of pain behavior within 1 hour of a specific nursing intervention.		
▪ Assess the level of pain and initiate pain management strategies as soon as possible. Use patient-controlled analgesics if ordered.	▪ Adequate pain management allows for faster healing and a more cooperative patient. Patient-controlled analgesics may be effective.	The child experiences pain relief early in the postoperative period.
▪ Administer pain medication around the clock to help ensure pain relief, especially during the first 48 hours. Monitor epidural blocks and patient-controlled analgesia or other methods used for pain control.	▪ Medicating around the clock helps to maintain comfort. Monitoring ensures patient safety.	
▪ Use nonpharmacologic pain management techniques, such as imagery, relaxation, touch, music, application of heat and cold, and reduced environmental stimulation to supplement medications (see Chapter 15 ∞).	▪ Alternative treatments also interrupt the pain stimulus and provide relief. Nonpharmacologic methods can be an effective adjunct to pain management.	
▪ Document pain assessment, interventions, and the child's reactions.	▪ Proper documentation guides the selection of the most effective means of pain control.	
▪ Reassure the child that some discomfort is expected and that a variety of measures can be tried to reduce discomfort.	▪ Realistic expectations decrease anxiety and give the child a sense of control.	
5. Nursing Diagnosis: Impaired Physical Mobility related to movement restrictions and pain		
NIC Priority Intervention: *Positioning and ambulation:* Moving the patient to provide comfort and promote healing, assist with walking		**NOC Suggested Outcome:** *Ambulation:* Ability to walk from place to place
Goal: The child will maintain proper body alignment and progress with activity as ordered by the physician. If no anteroposterior shell bracing is required, the child will have active mobility by the third to fifth postoperative day.		
▪ Reposition the child every 2 hours using the log-roll technique. Support the back, feet, and knees with pillows.	▪ Proper positioning prevents twisting or turning the spine.	The child is as mobile as appropriate for condition within 3–5 days after surgery.
▪ Have the child perform passive and active range of motion exercises every 2 hours for 48 hours and then every 4 hours while awake. Have the child dangle his or her legs at bedside by the second to fourth postoperative day or as ordered by the surgeon. Begin ambulation generally by the third to fifth postoperative day. Note any complaints of dizziness, or pallor. Proceed slowly.	▪ Exercises help maintain strength, circulation, and muscle tone. If the spine is stable and the physician has ordered no external support, the child may progress to full ambulation as tolerated. If the spine is not stable, great care must be taken until external supportive devices are used.	

and promote interaction with peers. Suggest that the adolescent work with a peer support person who is being treated for scoliosis or has had the condition in the past. Provide information about fashionable clothing that can be worn with the brace.

Discharge Planning and Home Care Teaching
Home care needs should be identified and addressed well in advance of discharge after spinal surgery. The child must learn to adapt to a new set of body mechanics. Show the child how to do simple tasks without bending or twisting the torso. Have the child demonstrate the ability to perform activities of daily living before discharge from the hospital. Collaborate with physical therapy/rehabilitation to plan for the youth's needs related to safe and effective movement with the brace.

Activities for the child who has had spinal surgery are commonly limited for a period of time. Restrictions usually should be followed for 6 to 8 months, depending on the type of surgery and the surgeon (see Families Want to Know: Postoperative Activities After Spinal Surgery). Emphasize to both the child and the family the importance of compliance, and give them written discharge instructions. Follow-up visits are important. The child should be examined 4 to 6 weeks after discharge, then every 3 to 4 months for 1 year, and every 1 to 2 years thereafter.

Several organizations provide information and assistance to families of children with scoliosis. Referrals can be made as appropriate.

Evaluation
Expected outcomes of nursing care for the child with scoliosis treated by brace are maintenance of intact skin and compliance with prescribed therapy. Expected outcomes after surgical correction are listed in the accompanying Nursing Care Plan.

Torticollis, Kyphosis, and Lordosis
Torticollis is tilt of the head caused by rotation of the cervical spine. The cause is generally an injury sustained to the sternocleidomastoid muscle at the time of birth or to a cervical spine abnormality. Stretching exercises or surgical lengthening of the sternocleidomastoid muscle are usual treatments. Occasionally the cause of torticollis is visual impairment, leading to constant turning in one direction to see with the better eye.

Kyphosis (hunchback) and lordosis (swayback) are two other types of spinal curvature that may occur in children. The type of kyphosis seen in adolescence is most commonly Scheuermann disease, an abnormality in ossification of anterior vertebral bodies; it differs from the degenerative kyphosis sometimes seen in the elderly. Postural lordosis is a characteristic finding in toddlers, but should disappear by the school-age years.

Nurses can perform thorough musculoskeletal assessments of children (see Chapter 5 ∞) and refer any children with abnormalities for further evaluation. Clinical therapy depends on the cause and degree of the curvature, and the age of the child at onset. See Clinical Manifestations: Treatment of Kyphosis and Lordosis.

■ ADDITIONAL DISORDERS OF THE BONES AND JOINTS

Osteoporosis and Osteopenia
Osteoporosis, a condition in which there is decreased density and mass of bone, promotes the risk of fractures, and is commonly associated with aging. However, children can have **osteoporosis** (also known as metabolic bone disease or a bone mineral density more than 2.5 standard deviations below the norm) related to imbalanced nutrition or other pathological conditions. Osteoporosis is preceded by **osteopenia** or low bone mass, which is between 1 and 2.5 standard deviations below the norm (Bowman & Russell, 2006).

Etiology and Pathophysiology
Very-low-birth-weight infants who are premature often have osteopenia of prematurity because much of bone mass is usually acquired in the latter weeks of pregnancy. In addition, they may have other health problems after birth and be unable to ingest enough nutrients to meet metabolic needs for bone growth. Premature infants are often less active than other infants, which decreases the amount of mechanical loading on their bones, a factor known to increase bone resorption and decrease bone mass (Bachrach, 2007; Litmanovitz, Dolfin, Arnon, et al., 2007).

Children who have decreased mechanical loading may show signs of osteoporosis. Children with spina bifida or cerebral palsy that interferes with ambulation have limited pressure on

Clinical Manifestations

Treatment of Kyphosis and Lordosis

Condition	Clinical Manifestations	Clinical Therapy
Kyphosis Excessive convex curvature of the cervical thoracic spine. (Scheuermann kyphosis is a common type.)	*Clinical manifestations:* Visible hunchback or rounded shoulders, shortness of breath or fatigue, pain, abdominal creases and light hamstrings in severe cases. *Diagnostic tests:* Spinal curvature is assessed by having the child bend 90 degrees at the waist and noting roundness at the scapular area from the side. Sharp angulation is visible. Diagnosis is confirmed by radiograph.	*Medical therapy:* Exercises are prescribed for a mild condition; bracing is commonly used; spinal fusion surgery is performed in severe cases. *Nursing management:* Provide support. Encourage exercises and diligent brace wear. Help the child to deal with the psychologic stress of altered body image.
Lordosis Excessive concave curvature of the lumbar spine with an angle of more than 60 degrees; most common in prepubescent girls and Blacks.	*Clinical manifestations:* Presence of swayback, prominent buttocks, hip flexion contractures, tight hamstrings. *Diagnostic tests:* Spinal curvature is assessed by looking at the standing child from the side. Lumbar lordosis is confirmed by visualizing the spine on standing, lateral radiograph.	*Medical therapy:* Treatment focuses on exercises and postural awareness. Bracing and surgery are rarely prescribed. *Nursing management:* Provide support. Reassure the child and family that the condition is often outgrown as the child matures. Encourage physical conditioning exercises and follow-up examinations on a yearly basis.

bones, and bone mass in affected extremities and the spine have lower mass. Some other conditions are associated with lower bone mass, including Turner syndrome, growth hormone deficiency, osteogenesis imperfecta, juvenile rheumatoid arthritis, and diabetes. Children who are treated for disorders or injuries with casting and bracing are also at high risk of osteoporosis due to immobilization. Children treated for some types of cancer have increased rates of osteoporosis. See Figure 29–16 ➤ for other effects of immobility on body systems.

Adolescence is a period when adequate intakes of calcium and vitamin D are needed to maximize bone formation and prevent osteoporosis later in life. Adolescents, particularly females, often do not meet the recommended dietary allowance (RDA) for these nutrients and are at risk for osteoporosis even though it may not be manifested for years. Other lifestyle patterns of youth that decrease bone formation are smoking, alcohol use, and keeping weight at a very low level. Those with anorexia nervosa are clearly at risk for osteoporosis.

Clinical Manifestations

Osteoporosis is a silent disease, as is its precursor osteopenia; those who have the disorders are often without signs or symptoms for years. The problem may become apparent when a baby or child has a fracture and radiologic studies make the problem evident.

COLLABORATIVE CARE

Bone mineral content and density are measured by single-photon absorptiometry (SPA), dual-photon absorptiometry

(DPA), and dual energy x-ray absorptiometry (DEXA). Although uncommonly used, serum studies such as bone-specific alkaline phosphatase, phosphorus, and type-I collagen can be used to measure osteoblastic and osteoclastic activity. Over 90% of the body's calcium is stored in bone, so serum calcium is not reflective of bone density.

Premature newborns at risk for osteopenia of prematurity need collaborative management by neonatologists, neonatal nutritionists, and neonatal nurses. Breast milk is enhanced by adding special fortifiers; premature formula should be used rather than regular baby formula. When babies need enteral or parenteral feedings, calcium to phosphorus ratios are carefully balanced to enhance osteoblastic activity. Extremity range of motion for very-low-birth-weight newborns can decrease bone loss in the period after birth. Up to 8 weeks of assisted range of motion exercise decreases loss of bone strength and enhances bone health in low-birth-weight premature infants (Litmanovitz et al., 2007).

For older children at risk of developing osteoporosis, calcium and vitamin D intake is encouraged and oral supplements may be given. Standing therapy for those who are nonambulatory can provide mechanical weight and enhance bone density. Bisphosphonates, calcitonin, fluoride, and parathyroid hormone may be used to treat children and adolescents with osteoporosis (Kamboj, 2007). When a cast or other immobilizing device is removed from a child, a gradually increasing program of exercise in collaboration with physical rehabilitation professionals promotes bone strengthening and lowered risk for fractures or related sequelae.

Pathophysiology Illustrated

Effects of Immobility

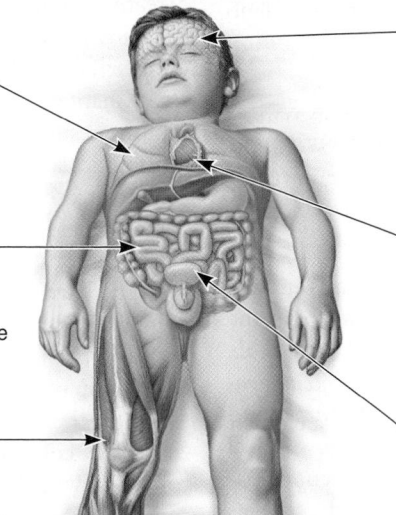

Respiratory System
- Decreased lung expansion and impaired gas exchange
- Retained secretions, ineffective cough, and increased risk of infection

Cognitive and Nervous System
- Sensory deprivation
- Confusion, anxiety, stress, disturbed sleep
- Delayed development
- Disturbed sleep patterns
- Disturbed self concept and body image

Nutrition and Gastrointestinal System
- Decreased intestinal tone and motility leading to constipation
- Decreased metabolic rate
- Anorexia, nausea, negative nitrogen balance

Cardiovascular System
- Increased cardiac workload
- Orthostatic hypotension
- Pooling of blood and thrombus formation

Musculoskeletal System
- Decreased muscle strength and tone
- Lack of coordination, altered gait, and increased risk of falls
- Decreased range of motion and joint flexibility
- Pain and activity intolerance
- Osteopenia and osteoporosis

Urinary System
- Decreased bladder tone and stasis of urine
- Increased risk of urinary tract infection and renal calculi

Integumentary System
- Pressure ulcers
- Pain
- Infection

FIGURE 29–16 ➤ The effects of immobility on the body involve all systems.

NURSING MANAGEMENT

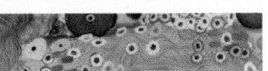

Nursing Assessment and Diagnosis

Nurses identify newborns, children, and adolescents at risk of developing low bone mass and density. This is accomplished by identifying diseases putting the child at risk. Ask about exercise and activity patterns, and physical therapy for children who are nonambulatory. Dietary intake is measured periodically for all youth at health promotion visits, and RDAs for calcium, phosphorus, and vitamin D are compared to intake.

Nursing diagnoses that may apply to the child with osteoporosis include the following:

- Imbalanced Nutrition related to inability to consume essential nutrients
- Risk for Injury to Bones related to decreased bone mass and density
- Ineffective Health Maintenance related to inadequate dietary intake

Planning and Implementation

Perform dietary analysis of children at risk (see Chapter 14 ∞ for detailed methods for diet assessment). Refer children at risk to nutritionists and physicians for further education and diag-

nosis. Suggest referrals to physical rehabilitation to recommend weight-bearing exercise. Administer nutritional supplements when prescribed and teach families how to give these medications. Collaborate with families to provide therapy that stimulates weight bearing for children who are nonambulatory. Teach parents how to recognize fractures in children who may not have normal sensation and are unable to report them. Edema, unusual shape of a limb, fussiness of the child, and falls should be promptly reported.

When osteoporosis is due to immobility, many other symptoms occur as well. Be alert for these problems and integrate physical activity in care as much as possible to minimize their effects.

Evaluation

Expected outcomes of nursing care for the child with a potential for osteoporosis include adequate intake of recommended amounts of nutrients, absence of fractures, and normal findings on studies of bone mineral content and density.

Osteomyelitis

Osteomyelitis is an infection of the bone, most often one of the long bones of the lower extremity. It may be acute or chronic and may spread into surrounding tissues. Although osteomyelitis may occur at any age, it is most common in children

Osteomyelitis in a newborn is of great concern, because before 18 months of age the blood vessels cross the growth plates. This creates a higher risk of epiphyseal involvement with resultant limb length discrepancy.

between the ages of 1 and 12 years. Boys are affected two to three times as often as girls, primarily because they have a greater incidence of trauma. Overall incidence is 1 in 5,000 youth (Copley, 2009; Kocher, Lee, Dolan, et al., 2006).

Etiology and Pathophysiology

Osteomyelitis is caused by a microorganism, which is usually bacterial but can be viral or fungal. *Staphylococcus aureus* is the most common causative pathogen, followed by *Escherichia coli*, group B streptococci, *Streptococcus aureus*, *Streptococcus pyogenes*, *Pseudomonas aeruginosa*, *Haemophilus influenzae*, and *Kingella kingae* (Copley, 2009). Trauma to the bone or surgical interventions commonly are the initial causes of infection. Osteomyelitis may follow another infection in the body, such as upper respiratory infection.

The infecting organism spreads through the bloodstream or via a penetrating injury to the bone, where it becomes established. Most infections in children begin in the metaphysis (see Figure 29–1), which has a sluggish blood supply. Eventually the infection may penetrate the bone cortex and periosteum. Inflammation and abscess formation can lead to interruption of the blood supply to the underlying bone, involvement of the surrounding soft tissue, and, if the infection is left untreated, necrosis.

Clinical Manifestations

Symptoms include constant pain, edema, decreased mobility of the infected joint, and fever. Redness over the area may occur. The child may refuse to walk or may limp. Because the onset of acute osteomyelitis is generally rapid, it is sometimes misdiagnosed as a sports injury.

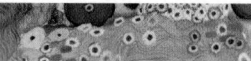

COLLABORATIVE CARE

A history suggestive of osteomyelitis includes an upper respiratory infection or blunt trauma followed by pain at the area of a growth plate. Laboratory evaluation shows leukocytosis and an elevated erythrocyte sedimentation rate (ESR) and C-reactive protein. The degree of ESR elevation is directly related to the severity of the infection. Radiographs and bone scans may identify the area of involvement. A needle aspiration of the site or a blood culture can confirm the diagnosis and provide a culture of the causative organism. Other studies may include enzyme-linked immunosorbent assay (ELISA) for Lyme antibody titer, antistreptolysin-O for recent streptococcus infections, or purified protein derivative (PPD) for exposure to tuberculosis (Ratliff, 2007).

In children with extensive orthopedic surgery, or in those with immunosuppression, a short course of prophylactic antibiotic may be administered after surgery to prevent infection.

Medical management for infection begins with the intravenous administration of a broad spectrum antibiotic, even before culture results are available. Since *S. aureus* is a common cause of infection, the antibiotic should be effective against this organism. Treatment is influenced by the possibility of methicillin-resistant *S. aureus* (MRSA), so beginning antibiotics are usually vancomycin or clindamycin, drugs that are effective against MRSA (see Chapter 16 ∞ for further discussion of MRSA). Once the culture results are obtained, the antibiotic may be altered. Oral antibiotics are given once an adequate response has occurred. However, extended intravenous home therapy may be used. Antibiotic therapy continues for about 3 to 6 weeks. When an adequate response is not obtained within 2 to 3 days, the area may be aspirated again, or surgical drainage may be carried out. Intravenous fluids may be administered to ensure adequate hydration.

Prompt diagnosis and treatment usually result in complete resolution of the infection. The prognosis is related to the initiation of therapy—the earlier treatment begins, the better the outcome. Long-term unfavorable outcomes include disruption of the growth plate, which can interrupt growth and damage the joints from septic arthritis, and recurrent infection.

NURSING MANAGEMENT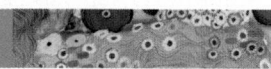

Nursing Assessment and Diagnosis

A thorough history, including information about the onset of symptoms and a history of recent infections or puncture wounds, is essential. Ask about immunization status, especially tetanus. Assess the affected area for signs of redness, edema, pain, and decreased range of motion. Measure vital signs since increased temperature and pulse may provide clues about worsening infection.

Nursing diagnoses that may apply to the child with osteomyelitis are as follows:

- Acute Pain related to biologic injury
- Impaired Physical Mobility related to discomfort
- Risk for Infection (Sepsis) related to spread of infection
- Risk for Imbalanced Nutrition: Less than Body Requirements related to loss of appetite
- Health-Seeking Behaviors (Child and Parent) related to lack of information about disease process

Planning and Implementation

Nursing management focuses on performing cultures and obtaining blood samples, administering antibiotics, protecting the child from the spread of infection, and encouraging a well-balanced diet with generous amounts of fluid. Standard precautions should be used, with transmission-based precautions for any drainage from the site of infection.

Obtain Cultures and Blood Work

When osteomyelitis is suspected, blood cultures and cultures of any open wound must be performed before the first dose of antibiotic. Obtain continuing blood samples as needed to monitor ESR and C-reactive protein.

When a child has a possible diagnosis of osteomyelitis, ensure that all cultures (e.g., blood, wound) are taken before antibiotic therapy begins. However, the cause of infection is not always identified from culture, so ESR and C-reactive protein are followed carefully in these cases to identify if treatment is successful.

Administer Fluids and Medications

Administer intravenous fluids as ordered to maintain the child's hydration status. Antibiotics are administered intravenously at first, then orally. Monitor the intravenous site and provide care for the central line, if used (refer to the *Clinical Skills Manual*). In the early stages of the infection, analgesics are prescribed to relieve the associated pain and joint tenderness.

Protect from the Spread of Infection

Strict aseptic technique and transmission-based precautions should be used during all dressing changes. Children and family members should avoid direct contact with any dressings or drainage. Teach good hygiene practices, including hand hygiene, to maintain infection control. Take vital signs and evaluate the child frequently for symptoms indicating the spread of infection (e.g., increasing pain, difficulty breathing, increased pulse rate, fever).

Encourage a Well-Balanced Diet

Educate both the child and the parents about healthy dietary choices that promote the healing process. Providing a high-protein diet and extra vitamin C will contribute to this process. Encourage increased fluid intake to provide adequate hydration and circulation.

Discharge Planning and Home Care Teaching

Emphasize the importance of completing the full course of antibiotic therapy, especially for children who have undergone surgical drainage of an abscess or lesion. Some children may be discharged on intravenous antibiotics, in which case the family needs instruction for home administration, as well as referral to a home health agency. Explain that failure to follow the prescribed antibiotic therapy may result in chronic infection. Emphasize the importance of returning for blood analysis to monitor progression of healing.

If the child is homebound for a period of time during treatment, assist the family in planning for completion of school tasks.

- Contact the school and ask that work be sent home.
- Arrange for a tutor if needed.
- Facilitate computer communication between the child, teacher, and other students.
- Help family members to plan for help at home to monitor the child when they are at work or performing other tasks.
- Refer to financial resources as appropriate for the services the child needs.
- Suggest activities that the child can do at home to foster developmental progression.

Consider the child's age and developmental level to provide suggestions for the family if the child will be immobilized at home. If the child is homebound for the treatment period, assist the family in planning for completion of school tasks.

Evaluation

Expected outcomes of nursing care for the child with osteomyelitis include the following:

- The child shows response to treatment and further absence of signs of infection or sepsis.
- The child completes the prescribed course of antibiotics.
- The family remains free of infection.
- The child ingests adequate intake of fluids and nutrients during the treatment period.
- The child reports absence of pain.
- The child is able to return to normal activities of daily living.

Skeletal Tuberculosis and Septic Arthritis

Skeletal tuberculosis (Figure 29–17 ➤) and septic arthritis are two infections that, although infrequent, may affect children and adolescents. See Clinical Manifestations: Treatment of Skeletal Tuberculosis and Septic Arthritis on page 970 for clinical manifestations, diagnostic tests, and medical and nursing management for these infections.

Achondroplasia

Dwarfism is a genetic condition usually resulting in an adult height of 58 inches or less. The most common cause of dwarfism

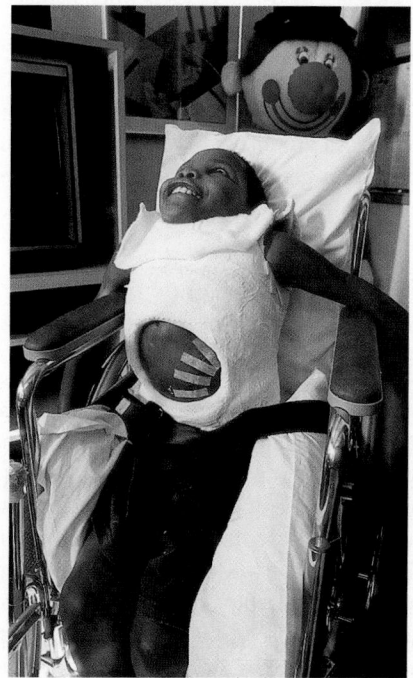

FIGURE 29–17 ➤ This boy from Kenya had surgery to correct severe kyphosis and scoliosis, caused by tuberculosis of the spine. A Risser cast has been applied to maintain stability of the spine and thoracic cage during healing. Notice the area cut out of the cast to allow for auscultation of the abdomen, as well as to facilitate the child's comfort and adequate intake of food.

Clinical Manifestations
Treatment of Skeletal Tuberculosis and Septic Arthritis

Condition	Clinical Manifestations	Diagnostic Tests and Clinical Therapy	Nursing Implications
Skeletal Tuberculosis Rare mycobacterial infection that can be destructive. The spine is the most frequent site of infection (Pott's disease), with joints and other sites sometimes affected.	Depending on the site, pain, limp, severe muscle spasms, kyphosis, muscle atrophy, "doughy" swelling of joints, decreased joint motion, changes in reflexes, and low-grade fever.	*Diagnostic tests:* Diagnostic studies include tuberculosis skin test, complete blood count (CBC), synovial fluid analysis, and radiographs of affected limb or joint. *Clinical therapy:* Antibiotic therapy (using a combination of drugs) for 6–9 months is the treatment of choice. The affected site is immobilized. Disease may become resistant to these drugs, and additional drug therapy may be necessary.	Educate the child and family about the disorder, and stress the importance of complying with long-term antibiotic therapy. Test all members of the family for tuberculosis. Report the disease to the local health department. Facilitate the immobilization and physical therapy of the child at home.
Septic Arthritis Joint infection of the synovial space most often caused by *Haemophilus influenzae, Staphylococcus,* and *Streptococcus.*	Fever, pain, local inflammation, joint tenderness, swelling, and loss of spontaneous movement.	*Diagnostic tests:* CBC with differential ESR, blood cultures. Diagnosis is made based on joint aspiration findings. Results are commonly 100,000 WBCs, 75% neutrophils, and ESR over 44 mm/hr. Radiographic changes may not be evident until later in the disease process.	Educate the child and family about the disorder and emphasize the importance of proper antibiotic therapy.
The most common site of infection is the knee, followed by the hip, ankle, and elbow. Most common in children over 3 years of age.	The infant may be irritable, cries when handled, and refuses food.	*Clinical therapy:* This is a medical emergency requiring prompt treatment to avoid permanent disability. Treatment involves joint aspiration, open drainage, and irrigation, followed by intravenous antibiotic therapy for 3–4 weeks and then oral antibiotics. If the full course of antibiotic treatment is not completed, the child risks recurrent infection and further degeneration of the infected joint.	Carefully position the painful joint. Administer antibiotics as ordered. Use transmission-based precautions. Encourage fluids to ensure adequate hydration. Support and rest the joint; provide activities that do not require joint movement.

is achondroplasia, which causes short arms and legs. The torso and head are approximately normal size, but decreased growth of long bones causes short stature. This is known as disproportionate short stature. Achondroplasia is caused by an abnormal gene of chromosome 4 and occurs in 1 in 26,000 births (March of Dimes, 2007). The gene is coded to produce proteins called fibroblast growth factor receptors. When fewer receptors are produced, the cells cannot respond normally to signals from growth factors. Achondroplasia may occur as a new genetic mutation with no previous family history or can occur when one or both parents also have the condition. There are other less common forms of dwarfism, with about 200 identified types.

Children with achondroplasia have short legs and arms; short fingers with a separation between the middle and ring fingers;

and a large, prominent forehead. Hydrocephalus sometimes occurs in children with achondroplasia (see Chapter 27 ∞ for a description of hydrocephalus). Most children with the disorder inherit the gene from one parent. Since only one faulty gene must be present for manifestation of the disorder, it is a dominant characteristic. When a child inherits two copies of the gene from two affected parents, a fatal form of achondroplasia occurs that is characterized by a small thorax, respiratory failure, and death in infancy.

Children with the disorder are diagnosed prenatally, at birth, or shortly after. When there is a family history, genetic testing before or after birth identifies the presence of the faulty gene. Characteristics common in the growth disorder include frequent otitis media, dental malocclusion, short fingers, bowing of legs, marked lordosis and kyphosis, and sleep apnea (Shirley & Ain, 2009). The child may be slow at meeting gross motor developmental milestones.

There is currently no treatment for the disorder, although gene therapy and human growth hormone therapy are being explored as possible treatments for the future. Some children and adults with dwarfism have undergone limb lengthening procedures. Other orthopedic intervention may be needed to treat back pain or bone problems. For those children who develop hydrocephalus, insertion of a shunt to divert excess fluid may be needed. Treatment of conditions such as otitis media and malocclusion of teeth is provided.

Nursing Management

Nurses play an important role in helping families when a child is diagnosed with achondroplasia. If a parent has the condition or there is a positive family history of dwarfism, prenatal genetic counseling should be offered. Explain findings of testing and provide assistance with decision making about pregnancy if needed. Nurses assist parents who have a child with achondroplasia to adjust to the diagnosis, particularly if the parents have had no previous experience with the condition. They may feel guilt and anxiety, so contact with other families who have children with achondroplasia can be a supportive intervention.

Nurses help the child with achondroplasia to develop a positive self-concept during childhood. Many resources are available that provide suggestions about how to foster a positive self-concept, adjust the home to facilitate the child with achondroplasia, and assist the child with adjustments in school settings. Partner with school nurses to ensure the child's successful inclusion in school facilities and establishment of an individualized education plan. Although some families decide to explore limb lengthening procedures, most organizations state that focus should be placed on development of a healthy self-image rather than encouraging limb lengthening.

Nurses provide careful assessments of children throughout childhood. Head circumference is especially important in early childhood to identify hydrocephalus if it should occur. Carefully evaluate growth with specialized growth grids for achondroplasia, evaluate dental health at each visit, and perform developmental assessment with special emphasis on gross motor skills. Suggest activities such as swimming and biking that provide activity with little stress on bones. Provide resources that assist the family with planning for car safety seats, methods of adjusting the home, and partnering with the school to provide a supportive atmosphere for the child. Some helpful organizations include Little People of America, Dwarf Athletic Association of America, Human Growth Foundation, Magic Foundation for Children's Growth and Related Adult Disorders, and March of Dimes. Refer for care for otitis media and provide postoperative care if ear tubes are inserted (see Chapter 19 ∞). Refer to dentists and orthodontists and encourage regular dental care.

Marfan Syndrome

Marfan syndrome is another example of an autosomal dominant disorder. About 1 in 5,000 children are affected with the syndrome, which manifests with several conditions of connective tissue (Ha, Seo, Lee, et al., 2007; von Kodolitsch & Robinson, 2007). The most common problems are cardiac (mitral valve prolapse, aortic regurgitation, abnormal aortic root dimensions), skeletal (pectus excavatum, long arms and digits, scoliosis, elongated head, high arched palate), ocular (lens subluxation), and respiratory (pneumothorax) (Mayo Clinic, 2007). A woman with Marfan syndrome has an increased risk of complications during pregnancy, primarily due to the extra requirements placed on the heart. The average age for diagnosis is 3 years, and a heart murmur is the usual finding. Careful assessment identifies additional characteristics of the condition along with a positive family history.

Diagnosis is made after a complete family history, a detailed physical examination, an eye examination, a thorough heart examination, radiographs of the chest, and MRI or CT. Diagnosis in children is often difficult because many features of Marfan syndrome are not apparent until adolescence (Mayo Clinic, 2007).

Clinical Judgment

Both achondroplasia and Marfan syndrome are autosomal dominant disorders. Does the child need one or two affected genes to manifest the disorders? If one parent has the disorder, what is the chance that a pregnancy will result in an affected child? Are there carriers who do not manifest the disease? (See Chapter 3 ∞ for further information about autosomal dominant inheritance.)

There is no treatment for the syndrome, which causes abnormal formation of fibrillin matrix in connective tissue. However, early diagnosis can be successful in treating the cardiac abnormalities with medication or surgery to prevent dissection of the aorta, the major cause of death. Surgery may be needed to correct scoliosis, pectus excavatum, or pneumothorax. Careful monitoring throughout life is needed to prevent and treat abnormalities associated with the disorder.

Nursing management of Marfan syndrome begins with identification of infants and children with symptoms of the disorder. Once diagnosed, collaboration with a cardiologist, ophthalmologist, and orthopedist is needed throughout life. The child may require surgery for one or more conditions, may require antibiotics during elective procedures or dental care if the mitral valve is affected, and needs an echocardiogram and other cardiac studies regularly. The nurse may need to explain the disorder to the family and provide referrals for genetic counseling. The child needs support during childhood to learn about the disorder and to manage the medication and monitoring required. Ongoing health care is needed throughout life to assess for and treat related conditions.

Osteogenesis Imperfecta

Osteogenesis imperfecta (OI), also known as brittle bone disease, is a connective tissue disorder that primarily affects the bones. Children with this condition have fragile bones that are more likely to fracture. The major type of osteogenesis imperfecta occurs in 1 in 30,000 live births and affects boys and girls equally. The underlying disorder is a biochemical defect in the production of collagen. The disease is genetically transmitted, generally in an autosomal dominant inheritance pattern, although some types are transmitted in a recessive pattern. The most common types are caused by mutations on the COLIA1 or COLIA2 genes on chromosomes 17 and 7 (Online Mendelian Inheritance in Man, 2008).

Clinical manifestations include multiple and frequent fractures; blue sclerae; thin, soft skin; increased joint flexibility; enlargement of the anterior fontanel; weak muscles; soft, pliable, brittle bones; and short stature. Most children with OI are short in height and may have decreased range of motion in several joints. Conductive hearing loss can occur by adolescence or young adulthood (Pillion & Shapiro, 2008).

The disease is classified into four types (Martin & Shapiro, 2007). In type I disease, the most common form, children have fragile bones, blue sclerae, weakened tooth dentin, and hearing loss that manifests in adolescence. In type II disease, the ribs and skeleton are extensively involved; most children with this form of the disease die in utero or shortly after birth. Type III disease is identified in the newborn period or in infancy when the child sustains numerous fractures and manifests blue sclerae. Severe bone fragility and kyphoscoliosis are observed. Most children with type III disease die in childhood as a result of cardiorespiratory failure. Type IV disease is characterized by fractures without other symptoms of the disease. Bowing of the legs and other structural deformities can occur; however, the incidence of fractures decreases beginning in puberty.

Improved knowledge about the genetic transmission of this disease means that some cases of osteogenesis imperfecta can be identified before birth using ultrasound or collagen analysis of chorionic villus cells. In many cases, however, diagnosis of osteogenesis imperfecta is made only when the child has a delay in walking or sustains a fracture. Radiographic evaluation may detect both old and new fractures, and can lead to an erroneous diagnosis of child abuse.

Tests such as DEXA can be used to measure bone density. Serum alkaline phosphatase may be elevated; other measures of bone metabolism such as serum osteocalcin, procollagen 1 C-terminal peptide, collagen 1 teleopeptide, and urine deoxypyridinoline may be performed occasionally to measure effects of experimental medication. There is no cure for osteogenesis imperfecta. Medical management consists primarily of fracture care and prevention of deformities. The goal is to maximize the child's independence and mobility while minimizing the risk of fractures. Treatment includes physical therapy; casting, bracing, or splinting; surgical stabilization; nutritional management with high vitamin D and calcium; and bisphosphonate medication such as pamidronate. Hematologic stem cell transplant has been used successfully in some children with severe osteogenesis imperfecta and is under further research (Undale, Westendorf, Yaszemski, et al., 2009).

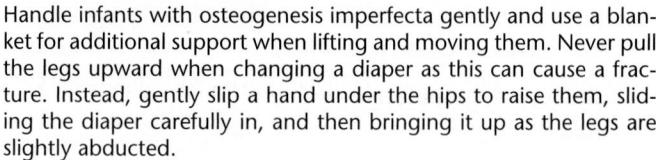

Research *Pamidronate*

Pamidronate is a bone resorption inhibitor that is being used experimentally in children with osteogenesis imperfecta. Low-dose medication is given intravenously every 6 months, and appears to significantly reduce bone fractures and pain. Density of lumbar bones was improved in children receiving the medication. Recently, another bisphosphonate that can be administered orally is showing promise in the treatment of OI (Salehpour & Tavakkoli, 2010).

Nursing Management

Nursing care is primarily supportive and focuses on educating the parents and child about the disease and its treatment. The family may have been suspected of child abuse before the disease was diagnosed, and they should be given an explanation about the similar presenting symptoms of these cases. Ask about the child's favorite activities since these will need to be integrated into plans for physical activity and developmental progression. Perform careful growth measures and developmental screening.

To prevent fractures, children with osteogenesis imperfecta must be handled gently. The trunk and extremities should be supported when the child is moved. Tasks such as bathing and diapering may cause fractures and should be performed carefully.

Nursing Alert

Handle infants with osteogenesis imperfecta gently and use a blanket for additional support when lifting and moving them. Never pull the legs upward when changing a diaper as this can cause a fracture. Instead, gently slip a hand under the hips to raise them, sliding the diaper carefully in, and then bringing it up as the legs are slightly abducted.

Children with osteogenesis imperfecta commonly have several or many fractures during childhood. The period of immobility and casting causes further bone breakdown due to decreased weight bearing, further increasing the chance of fracture. The child should have a well-balanced diet with additional vitamin C, vitamin D, and calcium to encourage healing and bone growth. Calories should be limited to maintain weight at recommended levels since immobility can lead to overweight and the child is generally short for age. Partner with parents if the child is receiving experimental bisphosphonate medication, so that doses are properly administered and serum/urine samples are obtained for monitoring.

When the child needs a fracture stabilized in surgery, or is having rods inserted to strengthen bones, surgical care management is important. Assess the child's vital signs and growth measurements. Obtain accurate weight before surgery and again after with the cast in place. Administer fluids and use pain control techniques such as medication and other comfort measures. Be alert for signs of infection such as osteomyelitis, or respiratory or urinary tract infection. Begin fluids and perform dietary teaching before discharge to promote intake that fosters healing. Follow activity orders precisely to minimize safety hazards for the child. Partner with physical and occupational therapists to plan for the child's return home and to school and to ensure the family can perform range of motion exercises and other therapies. Ensure that the family has an approved car safety seat to transport the child.

Emphasize the importance of maintaining normal patterns of growth and development. Toddlers should be helped to explore and interact safely in their environment. Socialization is essential during the school-age and adolescent years. Encourage exercise, such as swimming, to improve muscle tone and prevent obesity. Independent functioning is promoted by the use of adaptive equipment and motorized wheelchairs. Maintenance of function can depend on proper rehabilitation services. The nurse can arrange and manage such services for the family.

The Osteogenesis Imperfecta Foundation provides information about the disease and can put families in touch with others who have the disease. Parents should receive genetic counseling. For parents who have a child with type II or III OI, the terminal nature of the condition necessitates psychological support, linkage to potential resources, and assistance with managing other tasks of family life (see Chapter 13 ∞ for management of end-of-life care). The siblings and extended family will need support to understand the disease and deal with their feelings and the affected child.

Expected outcomes include minimal fractures with optimal healing, normal range of motion, maintenance of a healthy diet and recommended weight, achievement of developmental milestones, family support, and adequate resources to provide necessary treatments for the child.

■ MUSCULAR DYSTROPHIES

The muscular dystrophies are a group of inherited diseases characterized by muscle fiber degeneration and muscle wasting. These disorders can begin early or late in life, and onset can be at birth or gradual. They are all terminal disorders but the progression can vary from a few to many years.

Many types of muscular dystrophies affect children and adults. The most common form of childhood muscular dystrophy is Duchenne muscular dystrophy (pseudohypertrophy), which occurs in 2.2 to 5.5 of 10,000 live male births (Kemper & Wake, 2007). **Pseudohypertrophy** refers to enlargement of the muscles as a result of their infiltration with fatty tissue. The gene for Duchenne muscular dystrophy was identified in 1987; it is carried in the Xp21.2 region of the chromosome and is either absent or deleted in affected children. This area codes for a protein called dystrophin, which is needed as a muscle membrane stabilizer. In the absence of dystrophin, a cascade of cellular events occurs, leading to necrosis in the fibers and their replacement by connective tissue. Since this is an X-linked disorder, it is seen only in males. There is similar incidence in various ethnic groups.

Becker muscular dystrophy is also X-linked and affects 1 in 30,000 males (Becker Muscular Dystrophy, n.d.). Although the gene mutation is similar to Duchenne, it is milder in form. Other rare muscular dystrophies manifest in infancy, later childhood, or adolescence. There are a variety of genetic mutations ranging from X-linked to autosomal.

Clinical manifestations vary with type of disease. With Duchenne muscular dystrophy, muscle weakness begins in the lower extremities in early childhood. Children with Duchenne muscular dystrophy compensate for weak lower extremities by using the upper extremity muscles to raise themselves to a standing position (Gowers maneuver) (Figure 29–18 ➤). The parents may notice the child tripping, toe walking, and displaying enlargement of the calf muscles. By the middle teen years, the child's condition has usually progressed so that walking is not possible. The disease continues to rise, potentially causing conditions such as scoliosis, other musculoskeletal conditions, cardiomyopathy, and respiratory difficulty. Fractures may occur when the child falls. Becker muscular dystrophy is similar but emerges later and more slowly.

The dystrophies of infancy are manifested by generalized weakness and hypotonia. The infant may have difficulty with sucking and swallowing. Ocular problems may be present. Adolescent onset disease is generally milder and slower to progress. Some individuals may live into middle adulthood. See Clinical Manifestations: Muscular Dystrophies of Childhood on page 975.

Biochemical examinations such as serum enzyme assay, muscle biopsy, and electromyography confirm the diagnosis. Serum creatine kinase (CK) is elevated early in the disease. Dystrophin, the muscle protein that is deficient in muscular dystrophy, can be measured by muscle biopsy. Genetic testing establishes the specific abnormality and type of disease present. Testing of newborns may be offered to families who have one child with the disease since this helps some families to adapt and prepare for the care the child will need. Respiratory function is measured periodically with pulmonary function tests and overnight pulse oximetry (Kravitz, 2009).

There is no effective treatment for childhood muscular dystrophy. Research is being directed at several techniques to repair mutations by gene therapy and stem cell therapy, override the genetic error in order to produce dystrophin, and apply stem cell therapy (Ciafaloni & Moxley, 2008; Kuehn, 2007). The steroids prednisone and deflazacort may prolong muscle function, preserving walking for a longer period. Rehabilitative therapy can maximize independence and physical activity to decrease hazards of immobility. Children and families can benefit from mental health support due to the progressive and terminal nature of the disease.

Progressive weakness and muscle deformity result in chronic disability (Figure 29–19 ➤). The goal of medical management is to provide support and prevent complications such as infection or spinal deformities. Respiratory infections are vigorously treated with deep breathing, coughing, nebulizer treatments, and antibiotics; comprehensive and regular cardiac evaluations are recommended. The team approach to managing the child with muscular dystrophy ensures a comprehensive management plan. Team members should include physicians (pediatrician, orthopedic surgeon, neurologist), nurses, physical and occupational therapists, a nutritionist, a psychologist or mental health therapist, and a social worker.

Nursing Management

Nursing care focuses on promoting independence and mobility and providing psychosocial support that helps the child and family deal with this progressive, incapacitating disease. Nearly all body systems become involved in the care required, and emotional care is important for the child and family.

Monitor all vital signs as well as cardiac and respiratory functioning. Assess urinary function and frequency of bowel movements. Periodically measure strength and range of motion. Assess mobility via ambulation or assisted device. Perform periodic developmental and nutritional assessments, and provide parents with suggestions for encouraging the child's development. Meet with teachers to evaluate the child's learning needs and functioning in the classroom.

Osteogenesis Imperfecta Foundation Website

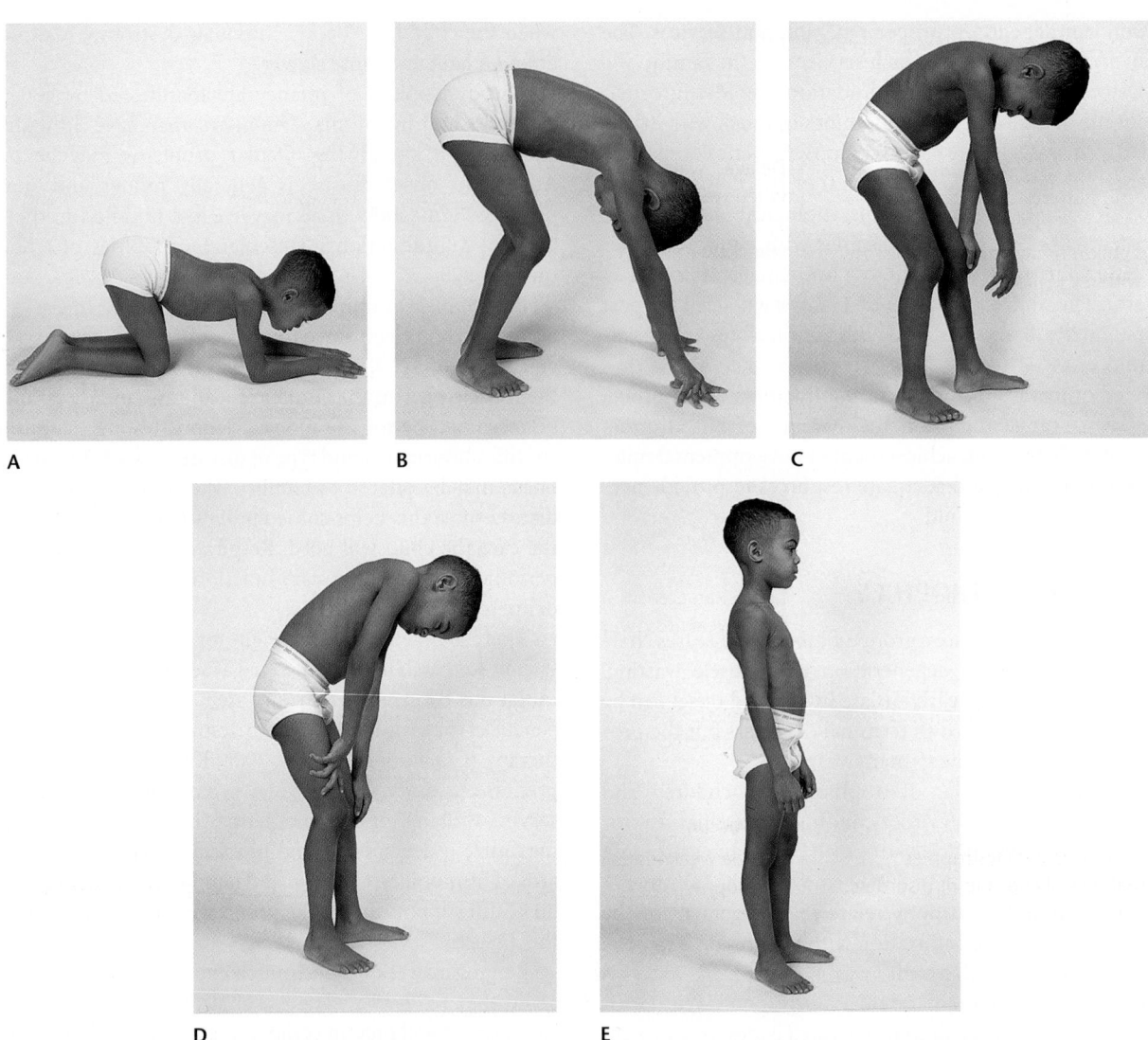

FIGURE 29–18 ➤ Since the leg muscles of children with muscular dystrophy are weak, these children must perform the Gowers maneuver to raise themselves to a standing position. A and B, The child first maneuvers to a position supported by arms and legs. C, The child next pushes off the floor and rests one hand on the knee. D and E, The child then pushes himself upright.

Law & Ethics *Muscular Dystrophy Care*

The child with muscular dystrophy has a shortened life span. Parents provide intensive care and require support both physically and emotionally as the child's condition progresses. The child continues to develop in many ways, especially cognitively, as the years pass. Therefore, the needs for explanation and ability to understand the diagnosis change for the child over time. Such a complex chronic disease requires that an interdisciplinary group form a team with collaboration on a regular basis. The child, family, and a variety of health, social, and educational professionals should all be part of the team. The plan of care will include physical, emotional, cognitive, and palliative care; it will evolve and change as the child grows older. Nurses are essential members of the team and may work with families as team managers to assist with planning and foster collaboration among health professionals.

Encourage the child to be independent for as long as possible. Concentrate on what the child can accomplish, and do not ask the child to complete tasks that may prove frustrating. Establish an individualized education plan with the school district. Reading books to the child, listening to tapes, and watching television offer stimulation during hospitalization. Exercise as tolerated contributes to muscle strength. Physical therapy helps the child ambulate and prevents joint contractures. It is important to provide good back support and proper posture by keeping the child's body in alignment when using a wheelchair.

Maintain the function of body systems by administering oxygen and respiratory therapy as prescribed. Soft foods, gavage, or enteral tube feedings may be needed to promote nutrition. Maintain bowel function with fluids, high-fiber foods, and medications as needed. Monitor and ensure adequate fluid intake and output. Assess for signs of infection. Perform range of motion and provide for physical activity to level of ability. Splints may be needed to maintain extremities in proper position.

Clinical Manifestations
Muscular Dystrophies of Childhood

Type of Dystrophy	Clinical Manifestations	Clinical Therapy
Duchenne Muscular Dystrophy X-linked recessive disorder seen in boys (on Xp21 gene); however, 30–50% of affected children have no family history. Onset: within the first 3–4 years of life.	Delayed walking; frequent falls; easily tired when walking, running, or climbing stairs; toe walking, hypertrophied calves; waddling gait; lordosis; positive Gowers maneuver; intellectual disability frequently seen.	Supportive care; physical therapy and braces to help maintain mobility and prevent contractures. Most children need to use a wheelchair by 12 years of age; death usually occurs during adolescence from respiratory or cardiac failure.
Becker Muscular Dystrophy X-linked recessive disorder. Onset: usually after 5 years.	Symptoms are similar to those of Duchenne muscular dystrophy, but milder and delayed; child is mobile until late teens; normal intelligence; congestive heart failure; contractures.	Supportive care, same as for Duchenne muscular dystrophy. Slow progression; death usually occurs by 30–50 years of age.
Fascioscapulohumeral Muscular Dystrophy Autosomal dominant disorder (on 4q35 chromosome). Onset: later childhood and adolescence.	Face, shoulder girdle, lower limbs affected; unable to raise arms over head; lordosis; cannot close eyes, whistle, smile, or drink from a straw because of inability to move face; characteristic appearance includes facial weakness, winging of the scapula, thin arms, well-developed forearms.	Physical therapy. Slow progression; confined to wheelchair as older adult, but usually attains normal life span.
Emery-Dreifuss Muscular Dystrophy X-linked recessive disorder (on Xq28 gene). Onset: childhood.	Early onset of contractures followed by weakness; Achilles tendon, elbow, and spine affected; muscle weakness in upper body follows, with lower body weakness occurring later, cardiac conduction defect may occur.	Physical therapy. Surgery. Pacemaker insertion.
Congenital Muscular Dystrophies Autosomal recessive group of disorders. Onset: present at birth.	Muscle weaknesses present at birth, motor development delay, contractures and joint deformities, hypotonia.	Correction of skeletal deformity (orthosis or surgery). Usually nonprogressive.

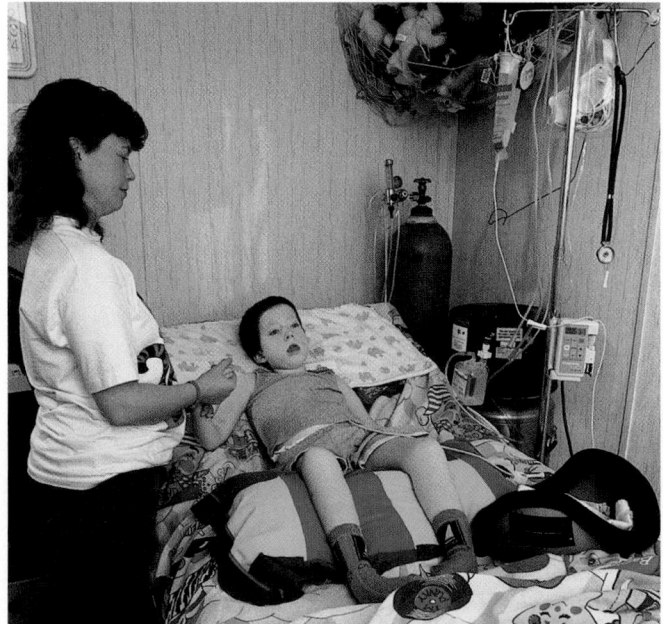

FIGURE 29–19 ➤ This young boy with muscular dystrophy needs to receive tube feedings and home nursing care. He attends school when possible and is able to use an adapted computer.

Families may be challenged by the care the child needs. Assist them to find resources to manage this care as well as provide a nurturing environment for other children and family members. Refer the family to financial resources and for respite care as needed. Parents may exhibit feelings of guilt and hopelessness. Encourage parents to express their feelings. Genetic counseling is recommended for the entire family, and it is especially important

Complementary Therapy
Muscular Dystrophy

Many families who have a child with muscular dystrophy will use different types of complementary care. The nurse always assesses for such approaches, provides information as needed by the family, makes recommendations for complementary therapies that may be helpful, and cautions against those that could be harmful due to interactions with medications or other problems. Common complementary care used in muscular dystrophy includes dietary enhancement. This enhancement includes vitamins A, C, E, D, and B-complex; minerals such as calcium, magnesium, zinc, and selenium; probiotic supplement; omega-3 fatty acids; herbal remedies such as green and rhodioloa rosea teas; muscular and immunologic enzymes such as coenzyme Q10, N-acetyl cysteine, acetyl-L-carnitine, creatine, and L-theanine; melatonin to promote sleep; and massage to assist with reduction of muscle spasms (University of Maryland Medical Center, 2007).

to identify women who are carriers of one of the X-linked disorders. Siblings may feel neglected because their brother or sister is receiving so much attention. They may also be concerned that they will develop the disease. Encourage the parents to involve siblings in the child's care to reassure them of their importance. Provide ongoing support during hospitalizations, management of home care, and the child's changes in condition. Perform continual assessments of the child's condition, the family management plan, and use of complementary therapies. End-of-life care should be integrated when needed into the nursing care plan (see Chapter 13 ∞). Refer family members to resource and support groups such as the Muscular Dystrophy Association and the National Institute of Arthritis and Musculoskeletal and Skin Diseases (NIAMS).

Desired outcomes of care involve maximum independence and maintenance of activities of daily living with needed assistance.

■ INJURIES TO THE MUSCULOSKELETAL SYSTEM

Musculoskeletal injuries are classified according to the mechanism, location, and force of injury. Strains, sprains, dislocations, and fractures are the most common musculoskeletal injuries in children, and athletic participation, car crashes, and other accidents are frequent causes (see Evidence-Based Practice: Backpack Use and Pain). Distinguishing among these injuries is often difficult. See the clinical manifestations table on the next page. A detailed discussion of fractures follows.

Fractures

A fracture is a break in a bone that occurs when more stress is placed on the bone than the bone can withstand. Fractures, which may occur at any age, occur frequently in children because their bones are less dense and more porous than those of adults. Refer back to Douglass in the opening scenario who sustained a fracture during recreation with friends.

Stress fractures are becoming more common in adolescents, especially among those who limit their intake of calories and calcium in an attempt to remain lean for sports such as distance running or gymnastics. These fractures may present with chronic pain that changes in intensity. Be alert to this possibility when teenagers' diets and athletic activities place them at risk.

The risk of bone fractures is significantly increased with higher cola consumption and television viewing time and with lower levels of physical activity and lower milk intake (Manias, McCabe, & Bishop, 2006). Teach healthy diet and activity patterns to youth and their families to decrease these health risks.

Etiology and Pathophysiology

Fractures in children may result from direct trauma to a bone (falls, sports injuries, abuse, motor vehicle crashes) or bone diseases (osteogenesis imperfecta) that result in weakening of the bone. Trauma may be caused by an acute injury, direct and forceful impact, or overuse such as in chronic and repetitive activities. Children with osteoporosis and osteopenia are more prone to fractures (see description of these conditions earlier in the chapter). Child abuse is a cause of fracture and should be suspected when the type of fracture is uncommon at a given age. For example, femur fractures are most common at 2 to 3 years and in adolescence; a femur fracture in an infant is suggestive of the possibility of abuse (see Chapter 17 ∞).

Clinical Manifestations

Signs and symptoms of fractures vary depending on the location, type, and nature of the causative injury. Fractures are generally characterized by pain, abnormal positioning, edema, immobility or decreased range of motion, ecchymosis, guarding, and crepitus. Childhood fractures most often involve the clavicle, tibia, ulna, and femur, with distal forearm fractures of

Problem

Many children wear backpacks that are heavy and are carried for large parts of the day. Lower back, neck, and shoulder pain seem to be increasing in children (Shilt & Barnett, 2007) and a possible connection with backpacks has been suggested.

Evidence

Several studies have investigated the relationships between backpack use and complaints of pain. One study found that carrying a backpack over one shoulder, having heavier backpacks, and carrying the pack lower rather than higher were associated with greater back and shoulder pressure (Macias, Murthy, Chambers, et al., 2008). Another study found that younger students and females are more prone to injury from heavy backpacks. These researchers recommended that 10% of body weight should be the safe cutoff for backpack weight (Bauer & Freivalds, 2009; Moore, White, & Moore, 2007).

Implications

A clear association between backpack use and weight and complaints of pain is evident, especially among females. Therefore,

nurses should ask about backpack use at health promotion visits and advise on how to wear them. The American Academy of Pediatrics lists recommendations for backpack use:

- Have wide, padded shoulder straps and wear the pack on both shoulders, close to the body.
- Use a padded back and waist strap.
- Wear the backpack over both shoulders and evenly distribute its weight.
- Be sure the backpack is lightweight (no more than 10–20% of the youth's weight) or consider a rolling pack if it is heavy.
- Practice back strengthening exercises and learn to bend at the knees.

Critical Thinking Application

How will you partner with youth who are in sports after school to plan how to carry school items and sports gear safely? What exercises can you plan to help strengthen the back and thighs for carrying a pack? What children are most at risk for back pain from heavy backpacks?

Clinical Manifestations
Strains, Sprains, and Dislocations

Condition	Clinical Manifestations	Clinical Therapy
Strain ■ Stretching or tearing of either a muscle or a tendon, usually from overuse (e.g., back strain resulting from improper or overly heavy lifting, shoulder and elbow tears from baseball).	■ Vary according to the type and severity of the strain. Pain can be acute or chronic.	■ Rest and support of the injured part until the muscle or tendon heals and normal activity can occur.
Sprain ■ Stretching or tearing of a ligament, usually caused by a fall, sports injury, or motor vehicle crash (e.g., anterior cruciate ligament [ACL] tear requiring reconstruction).	■ Edema, joint immobility, and pain.	■ For the first 24–36 hours: Rest Ice Compression Elevation ■ After the first 24–36 hours, mobility is gradually increased.
Dislocation ■ Complete displacement of an articular joint surface, usually associated with a fall, sports injury, or motor vehicle crash. Although almost any joint may be dislocated, most dislocations occur in the shoulder, knee, and hip.	■ Pain and tenderness, swelling and obvious deformity, and instability of the joint.	■ Varies according to the site and severity of the injury, and consists of: • Shoulder: Open or closed reduction followed by the application of a sling. • Knee: Closed reduction with gentle traction, then immobilization with a splint. • Hip (posterior): Immediate closed reduction or possibly open reduction, traction, or hip spica cast. • Hip (anterior): Immediate closed reduction, extension traction, and hip spica cast.

the radius or ulna the most common type. Fractures to the pelvis are often associated with motor vehicle crashes. Stress fractures are most common in the tibia, fibula, metatarsals, and calcaneus (Custer & Rau, 2009). Epiphyseal (growth plate) injuries are dangerous in children as they can interfere with future bone growth at the site. Types of fractures are described using the Salter-Harris classification system (Figure 29–20 ➤).

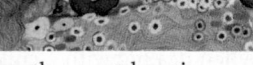

COLLABORATIVE CARE

Radiographs are useful for determining the exact location and type of fracture. However, in very young children the higher amounts of collagen and cartilage make diagnosis by radiograph challenging. Examination and palpation of the area by a skilled clinician is essential.

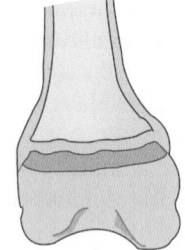 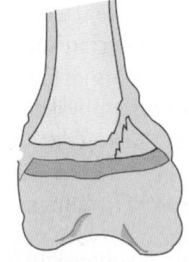 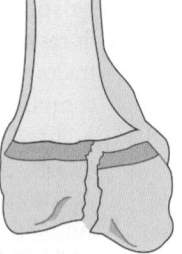 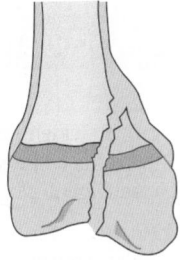 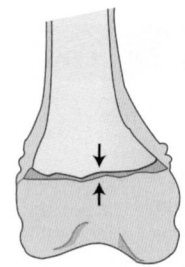

Type I
Common
Growth plate undisturbed
Growth disturbances rare

Type II
Most common
Growth disturbances rare

Type III
Less common
Serious threat to growth
and joint

Type IV
Serious threat to growth

Type V
Rare
Crush injury causes cell death in
growth plate, resulting in
arrested growth and limited
bone length
If growth plate is partially
destroyed, angular deformities
may result

FIGURE 29–20 ➤ The Salter-Harris classification system is based on the angle of the fracture in relation to the epiphysis. Additional types of fractures include *incomplete*, in which the break occurs in only one side of the cortex; *oblique*, in which the fracture slants across the long axis of the bone; *compression*, in which two bones are jammed together (usually occurs in the spinal area); and *compacted*, in which one bone fragment is wedged into another.

Emergency care focuses on accurate diagnosis, pain management, and establishment of a treatment plan. Medical treatment consists of two basic steps: reduction to realign displaced or fragmented bones, and immobilization so that healing can occur.

A closed reduction aligns the bone by manual manipulation or traction. Sedation and additional pain management techniques are used during closed reduction. An open reduction requires surgical alignment of the bone, often using pins, plates, wires, or screws. For open fractures, surgery must also be performed for debridement, to remove dead tissue and clean the wound. Casting is the most common external method of immobilization. Casts may be placed on extremities (short or long leg or arm cast) or the upper body to immobilize the spine, or may be applied from chest to legs to stabilize the pelvis or hips (spica cast). Leg casts may be walking or nonwalking casts. Cast material is either plaster or a synthetic fabric. Other external methods of stabilization include traction and splinting. Pins may be inserted to stabilize the fracture, and can be used with or without casts or traction. A combination of treatments may be needed in the child with multiple fractures following a car crash or other trauma.

Healing of fractures is influenced by factors including age, size of the involved bone, and fracture site. The healing process progresses from cartilaginous callous formation to bone remodeling and bone callous formation (Figure 29–21 ➤). Fractures heal more quickly in children than in adults. Immobilization is essential for the bone healing process to take place. If a fracture is properly reduced, complications should be minimal (Table 29–3).

NURSING MANAGEMENT

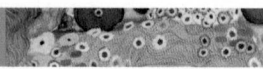

Nursing Assessment and Diagnosis

When dealing with a child who is injured, be alert to the signs and symptoms of fractures and soft-tissue injuries before moving the child. Try to identify the cause of the injury by asking the child, parents, or other family members what happened. Evaluate pain, edema, and any abnormal positioning of the injured area. When a child is admitted to the emergency department or hospital, nursing assessment includes the extent of the injury, the degree of pain, and the child's vital signs (respiratory status, pulse, blood pressure).

Nursing Alert

It is uncommon for children to have repeated fractures. If they occur, make further assessments for their cause. The child may suffer from osteogenesis imperfecta. If attention deficit hyperactivity disorder (ADHD) is present or if the child has a mental health problem, excessive risky behavior may be the cause of fractures. When children are found on radiograph to have several old and healing fractures, or multiple fractures of the same or different bones, they may be victims of physical abuse, particularly if the caretaker's explanation of fracture does not match the clinical picture. An example could be the parent who claims the child fell from a chair, but there is a severe arm fracture and skull fracture. See Chapter 17 ∞ for a description of child abuse and Chapter 28 ∞ for a discussion of ADHD.

The following nursing diagnoses may apply to the child with a fracture:

- Acute Pain related to injury
- Risk for Impaired Skin Integrity related to treatment
- Risk for Infection related to open fracture or trauma
- Impaired Physical Mobility related to treatment
- Health-Seeking Behaviors related to lack of information about treatment and expected outcome

Planning and Implementation

Nurses may be in community settings when children experience a fracture, and need to provide emergency care and arrange for transport. Emergency personnel are informed of the assessment data to provide for safe care. In addition, nurses are aware that repeated fractures in the same child can be a sign of other health care conditions. Nursing care focuses on care of the child before and after fracture reduction, encouraging mobility as ordered, maintaining skin integrity, preventing infection, and teaching the parents and child how to care for the fracture. If conscious sedation or pain blocks are used, nursing care for these procedures is needed. When caring for a child who has undergone fracture reduction, it is important to be aware of the signs of complications. Notify the physician immediately if these signs occur. The major serious complication is **compartment syndrome**, or a condition of increased pressure in a limited space such as the soft tissue of an extremity, which compromises circulation and nervous innervation. (See Clinical Manifestations: Compartment Syndrome.)

Clinical Tip

When in doubt about the nature of an injury, apply a splint and raise the body part above heart level. Splinting immobilizes the site, prevents further damage, and decreases pain. Be sure to immobilize both the joint above and below the injury. Raising the body part helps to minimize edema and increase comfort.

TABLE 29–3	Complications of Fracture Reduction
Complication	Clinical Therapy
Infection Acute (may occur with open fractures) Chronic (osteomyelitis)	Debridement, drainage, culture, and treatment with antibiotics
Neurovascular injury resulting from physical nerve damage	Nerve repair
Vascular injury	Vascular repair, amputation, tendon lengthening
Malunion (undesired healed alignment of bone) or delayed union	Corrective osteotomy; prolonged immobilization
Nonunion	Surgical intervention; internal fixation
Leg length discrepancy	Shoe lift

Clinical Manifestations
Compartment Syndrome

Clinical manifestations begin about 30 minutes after tissue ischemia starts. Major manifestations are:

- Paresthesia (tingling, burning, loss of two-point discrimination)
- Pain (unrelieved by medication, characterized by crying in the young child)
- Pressure (skin is tense or discolored, cast appears tight)
- Pallor (pale, gray, or white skin tone)
- Paralysis (weakness or inability to move extremity)
- Pulselessness (weak or absent pulse)

Check extremities for:

- Color
- Temperature
- Capillary refill
- Peripheral pulses
- Edema
- Sensation
- Motor ability
- Pain

Document results and report changes or abnormal results immediately (Custer & Rau, 2009).

Maintain Proper Alignment

Immobilization is used to maintain proper alignment of the fracture. Casts and traction are methods used for immobilizing an injured child. Cast care guidelines are included in Box 29–1 on page 949.

Different types of traction are used, depending on the location and type of fracture (Table 29–4). Nursing care for the child in traction is described in Box 29–2.

Monitor Neurovascular Status

Neurovascular assessment is used for early detection of compartment syndrome, which may occur with a crush injury or when a fracture is reduced. Swelling associated with inflammation reduces blood flow to the affected area, and casting causes further constriction of blood flow. Monitor the child's sensation to touch, temperature, movement, strength of the pulse, and capillary refill time in the extremity distal to the injury. Monitor every 15 minutes after the cast is applied for at least 2 hours and then every 1 to 2 hours, depending on the care facility's policy and the child's condition. Keep the cast elevated above heart level to minimize edema.

Promote Mobility

The amount of mobility the child is allowed is ordered by the physician, and restrictions depend on the extent and site of the fracture. Fractures of the hip or pelvis may involve body casts, and providing wheeled carts makes mobility possible. Children with leg fractures can sometimes bear weight on the cast; but if they cannot bear weight, they move around with crutches, walkers, or wheelchairs. See the *Clinical Skills Manual* for information on crutch walking.

Discharge Planning and Home Care Teaching

Most fractures can be easily managed at home. Activities are generally limited for approximately 8 weeks. Teach the parents and child cast care, activity restrictions, and how to identify problems that should be reported (see page 952). Help parents to identify any modifications that may be needed at home and school. The child who has to manage steps at home or school may need special training with crutches or a temporary ramp. Refer parents to home health nurses or home teaching services, if indicated. Provide pertinent teaching to prevent future injuries.

Sports Injuries

Sports injuries are the most common type of injury in youth from 13 to 19 years. Football, cycling, and basketball are the sports most commonly associated with injury (Simon, Bublitz, & Hambidge, 2006). Fractures, described previously, are common sports injuries of young athletes and may be treated on an outpatient basis or may require surgery and hospitalization (Deakin, Crosby, Moran, et. al., 2007). However, a variety of other injuries that affect the musculoskeletal system are common in sports. Children and adolescents have characteristics that put them at risk for injury. These include:

- Vulnerability of growth plates to injury, especially the distal tibia and fibula
- Increased joint mobility from lax tendons and ligaments, leading to injury of the knee, ankle, and hip
- More porous bones that lead to fractures and to more common injury to underlying organs
- Lack of experience in the sport and inadequate training
- Lack of acceptance of protective gear
- Impatience with taking the time to heal after injury

Some common sports injuries are listed in Table 29–5. Treatment for sprains, strains, dislocations, and fractures was previously described. (Head and neck injuries are discussed in Chapter 27 ∞ and dental emergencies in Chapter 19 ∞.) A few general approaches to minimize and treat injuries for youth athletes follow.

Athletes can benefit from teaching that enhances performance of their sports and also minimizes the chance of injury. They should receive instruction in correct techniques from a person qualified to coach and supervise children. Encourage youth to gradually increase time and intensity at a sport, rather than immediately playing a new sport for long periods of time. Have parents inquire about the coach's experience and also verify that the coaching staff is prepared in emergency care.

The nurse should be alert for sports injuries during contact with children and adolescents in health promotion visits. Ask about sports participation for all youth, but especially when there are complaints of sore muscles, edema of body parts, and bruises. Perform neurovascular assessment of extremities, including color, temperature, capillary refill time, edema, pulses, sensation, and pain. Phrase questions so that you identify sports such as skateboarding or snowboarding, which may not be performed under supervision or in organized sports programs. Youth may not consider these "sports."

Pathophysiology Illustrated
Process of Bone Healing

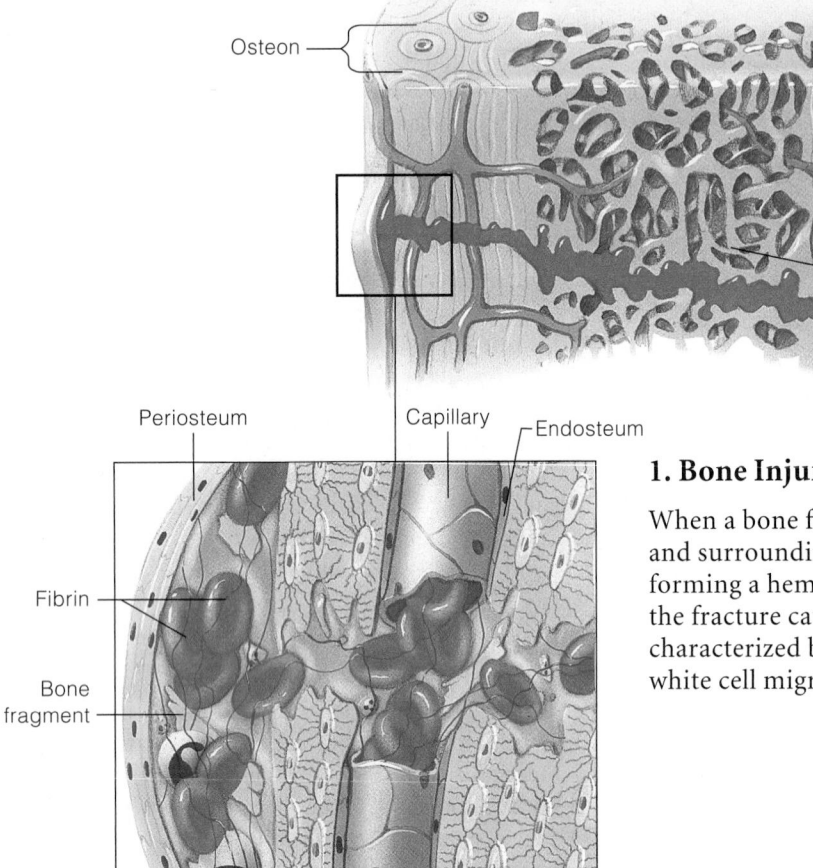

Osteon — Lamellae

Blood vessel in central canal

Blood vessel in perforating canal

Compact bone

Trabecular bone

Periosteum

Hematoma in fracture

Periosteum · Capillary · Endosteum

Fibrin

Bone fragment

Osteocyte

1. Bone Injury

When a bone fractures, blood vessels within the bone and surrounding soft tissues tear and begin to bleed, forming a hematoma. Necrotic bone tissue adjacent to the fracture causes an intense inflammatory response characterized by vasodilation, exudate formation, and white cell migration to the fracture site.

2. Fibrocartilaginous Callus Formation

Clotting factors within the hematoma form a fibrin meshwork. Within 48 hours, fibroblasts and new capillaries growing into the fracture form granulation tissue that gradually replaces the hematoma. Phagocytes begin to remove cell debris.

Osteoblasts, bone-forming cells, proliferate and migrate into the fracture site, forming a fibrocartilaginous callus. The osteoblasts build a web of collagen fibers from both sides of the fracture site that eventually unites to connect bone fragments, thus splinting the bone. Chondroblasts lay down patches of cartilage that provide a base for bone growth.

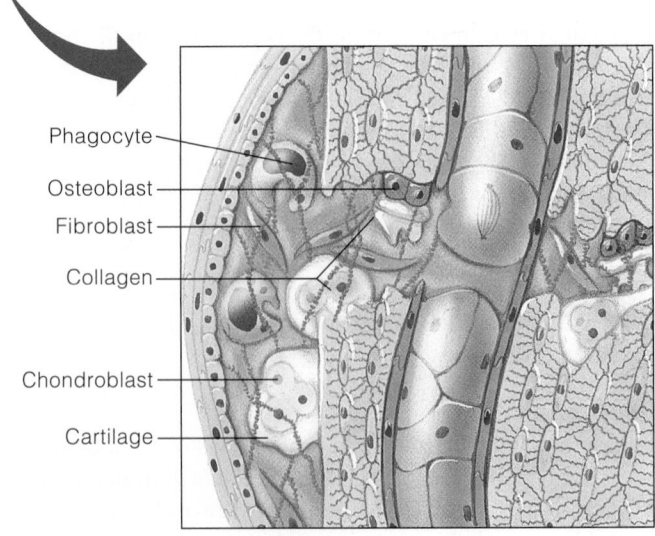

Phagocyte

Osteoblast

Fibroblast

Collagen

Chondroblast

Cartilage

FIGURE 29–21 ➤ Any injury to the bone brings about a multistep process of bone formation that lasts about 3 months.

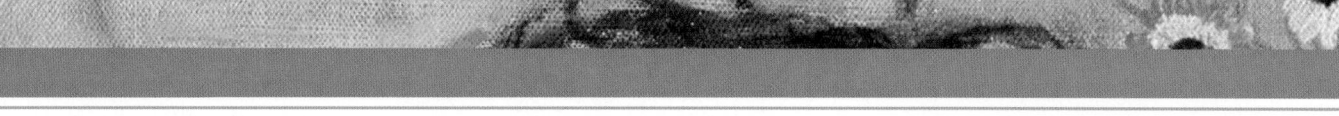

4. Bone Remodeling

Osteoblasts continue to form new woven bone, which is in turn organized into the lamellar structures of compact bone. Osteoclasts resorb excess callus as it is replaced by mature bone.

As the bone heals and is subjected to the mechanical stress of everyday use, osteoblasts and osteoclasts respond by remodeling the repair site along the lines of force. This ensures that the repaired section of bone eventually resembles the structure of the uninjured part.

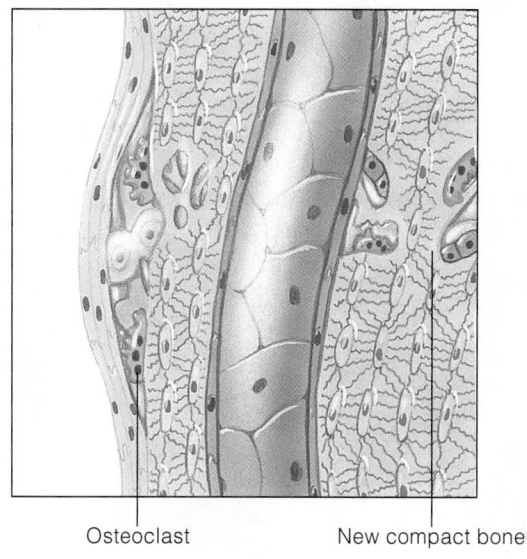

Osteoclast   New compact bone

3. Bony Callus Formation

Osteoblasts continue to proliferate and synthesize collagen fibers and bone matrix, which are gradually mineralized with calcium and mineral salts to form a spongey mass of woven bone. The trabeculae of woven bone bridge the fracture. Osteoclasts migrate to the repair site and begin removing excess bone in the callus. Bony callus formation usually continues for 2 to 3 months.

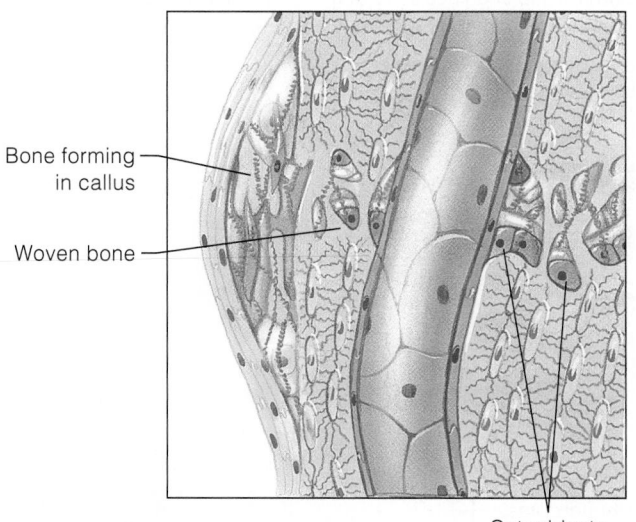

Bone forming in callus

Woven bone

Osteoblasts

| TABLE 29–4 | **Types of Traction** |

Type

Skin Traction

Pull is applied to the skin surface, which puts traction directly on the bones and muscles. Traction is attached to the skin with adhesive materials or straps, or foam boots, belts, or halters.

Dunlop Traction (can be either skeletal or skin)

Used for fracture of the humerus. The arm, which is flexed, is suspended horizontally with straps placed on both the upper and lower portions for pull from both sides.

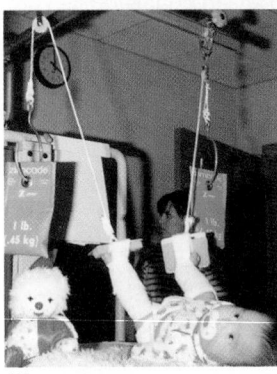 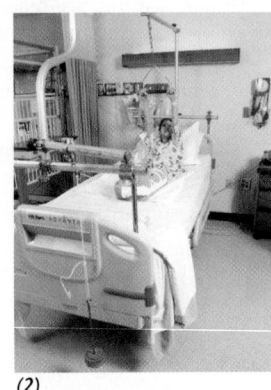

(1)   *(2)*

Bryant Traction (1)

Used specifically for the child under 3 years of age and weighing less than 17.5 kg (35 lb), who has developmental dysplasia of the hip or a fractured femur. This bilateral traction is applied to the child's legs and kept in place by wrapping the legs from foot to thigh with elastic bandages. The hips are flexed at a 90-degree angle, with knees extended. This position is maintained by attaching the traction appliance to weights and pulleys, which are suspended above the crib. The buttocks do not rest on the mattress, but are slightly elevated off the bed.

Buck Traction (2)

Used for knee immobilization, to correct contractures or deformities, or for short-term immobilization of a fracture. It keeps the leg in an extended position, without hip flexion. Traction is applied to the extremity in one direction (straight line) with a single pulley system.

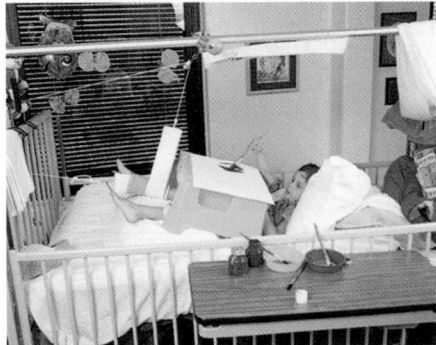

(3)

Russell Traction (3)

Used for fractures of the femur and lower leg. Traction is placed on the lower leg while the knee is suspended in a padded sling. The hips and knees, which are slightly flexed, are immobilized. One force is applied by a double pulley to the foot, and another force is applied upward using a sling under the knee and an overhead pulley.

Skeletal Traction

Pull is directly applied to the bone by pins, wires, tongs, or other apparatus that have been surgically placed through the distal end of the bone.

Skeletal Cervical Traction

Used for cervical spine injuries to reduce fractures and dislocations; Crutchfield, Gardner-Wells, or Vinke tongs are placed in the skull with burr holes. Weights are attached to the apparatus with a rope and pulley system to the hyperextended head.

Halo Traction

Used to immobilize the head and neck after cervical injury or dislocation. Also used for positioning and immobilization after cervical injury.

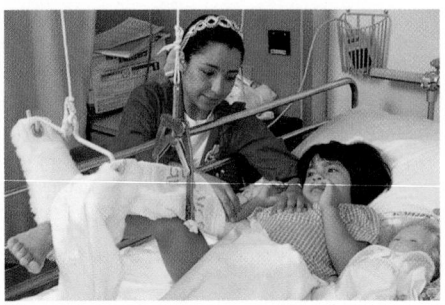

(4)

90-90 Traction (4)

Used for fractures of the femur or tibia. A skeletal pin or wire is surgically placed through the distal part of the femur, while the lower part of the extremity is in a boot cast. Traction ropes and pulleys are applied at the pin site and on the boot cast to maintain the flexion of both the hip and knee at 90 degrees. This traction can also be used for treatment of an upper extremity fracture.

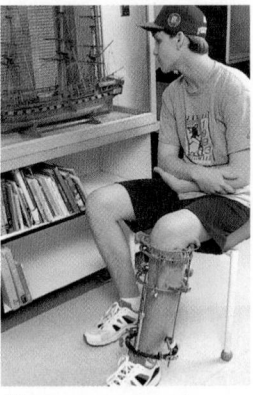

(5)

External Fixators (5)

These devices can be used in the treatment of simple fractures, both open and closed; complex fractures with extensive soft-tissue involvement; correction of bony or soft-tissue deformities; pseudoarthroses; and limb length discrepancy. They are attached to the extremity by percutaneous transfixing of pins or wires to the bone.

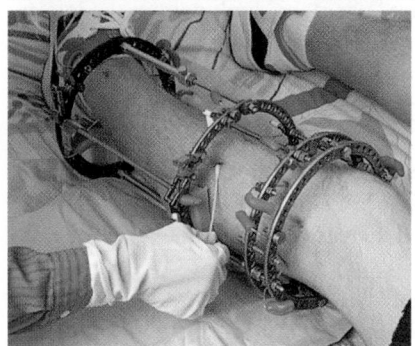

BOX 29-2 Nursing Care of the Child with Traction or External Fixator

1. Assess the child in traction by first checking the equipment. Make sure that the equipment is in the proper position. Observe both the body appliance and the attached weights and pulleys. Make certain that the child's body is in proper alignment.
2. Assess the skin under the straps and pin insertion sites for any signs of redness, edema, or skin breakdown.
3. Assess the extremity by checking neurovascular status frequently (check warmth, color, distal pulses, capillary refill time, movement, and sensation).
4. Provide pin care when ordered using sterile technique. Clean the area surrounding the pin with cotton-tipped applicators saturated with normal saline or half-strength hydrogen peroxide. Clean the area again with sterile water or more saline. Apply an antibacterial ointment, if ordered, using another cotton-tipped applicator.
5. When external skin traction is used, remove the traction device and perform skin care every 4 hours.
6. Place a sheepskin pad under the child's extremity if prescriptions permit.

Teach the importance of warming up for 10–15 minutes before participation and cooling down for a corresponding period at the end of an activity. Encourage wearing recommended safety gear for the sport including equipment such as a well-fitted protective helmet, face masks, eye protection, mouth guards, elbow and wrist guards, gloves, knee pads, and shin pads. Parents may need assistance to learn recommended equipment, and to obtain resources for its purchase. Frequent updates are needed as the child grows. Teach the child not to ignore pain.

▲ Health Promotion

When a child has a fracture from sports or other activities, ask details about how the injury occurred. If protective gear is recommended and was not worn, reinforce the need for protection. Suggest financial resources to assist with purchase of protective gear as necessary.

Injuries such as muscle strains should be treated promptly. They involve several steps:

- Resting the injury for 24–48 hours, applying ice for 20 minutes four times daily, applying compression with an elastic wrap to provide comfort and decrease edema, and elevating the part affected above heart level (RICE treatment)
- Gradually increasing motion to the part
- Adding flexibility and resistance or strengthening exercises
- Returning gradually to the sport, usually in 2–3 weeks after injury

Partner with the child, family, and other health professionals to plan for activity whenever an injury has occurred. Praise the family and youth for physical activity, which is an important part of a healthy lifestyle. Provide community resources to foster sports participation.

Amputations

Amputation—the complete absence of a body extremity—can be either congenital or acquired. Approximately two thirds of

TABLE 29-5	Common Sports Injuries
Sport	Types of Injuries
Baseball/Basketball	• Hand and finger fractures and sprains • Contusions and sprains of upper or lower extremities; wrists, elbows, knees, and ankles are common sites • Injury to body parts when hit by a ball (i.e., broken teeth; face, head, eye, and chest injuries)
Football	• Head and neck injury such as skull or cervical vertebrae fracture • Pulled muscles or dislocations in shoulders and legs
Gymnastics	• Wrist and elbow fractures and strains • Tendonitis in elbows and ankles/legs
Hockey (ice and inline)	• Dental injury • Leg fractures • Head and neck injuries
Soccer	• Head and neck injuries • Strains and fractures of legs
Wrestling	• Fractures and dislocations of upper and lower extremities

amputations in children are congenital and one third are acquired. Congenital amputations can be caused by constrictive amniotic bands, drugs, or irradiation. Acquired amputations are generally associated with trauma such as lawn mower injury and car crashes, or the result of a disease or disorder.

The child with an absent limb should be fitted with a prosthesis as soon as feasible, to foster a positive body image, independence, and self-confidence and to ensure that the child's motor skills develop as normally as possible. The prosthetic device should be reevaluated as the child progresses physically and developmentally. Frequent stump reconstructions are often necessary in children with traumatic amputations, because as children grow, so do their bones, and the skin tends to adhere to the bone. Bone may need to be cut and soft tissue added to keep the stump rounded. Joint fusions or stump lengthenings may also be needed to allow for the effective use of a prosthesis. Several prosthetic revisions are needed as the child grows and develops.

Nursing Management

Nursing care focuses on providing emotional support regarding altered body image, managing pain, maintaining skin integrity, and encouraging maximal independent functioning.

Recovering from the loss of a limb is one of the most difficult challenges facing a child. Emphasize what the child can do rather than what he or she cannot do. Good listening skills are important.

The child who has had surgery or a traumatic injury experiences pain. Many of the techniques discussed in Chapter 15 ∞

are useful interventions. After surgery, an epidural may be the treatment of choice. Oral analgesics are used during the period of adaptation to a prosthesis if tenderness is present. Children often regularly experience "phantom" limb pain in the lost extremity. A pain management referral may be helpful to integrate treatment into the plan of care.

The child usually begins by wearing the prosthetic device for 1 to 2 hours at a time. Check the skin for any redness or breakdown. If such conditions develop, leave the prosthesis off and allow the skin to clear before reapplying. Have the prosthesis adjusted if necessary, and increase wearing time as tolerated by the child.

Children with amputated limbs quickly learn how to accommodate to the prosthetic device. Make use of physical therapy programs that are specifically designed to help the child perform activities of daily living.

Answer any questions the family has about how to care for the prosthetic device and how to perform skin checks. Encourage parents to allow the child to participate in peer activities that are physically and emotionally challenging. Sporting activities that enable the child to participate using modified equipment are a good way to build self-confidence and motivation. For example, ski centers may offer programs that teach children with physical disabilities how to ski. The Special Olympics is another motivating option for some children. Assess the need for counseling and offer referrals as appropriate.

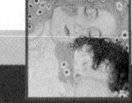

Chapter Highlights

- Children may develop musculoskeletal conditions as a result of congenital conditions, developmental variations, or trauma.
- Talipes equinovarus (clubfoot) is a common unilateral or bilateral variation in newborns that is treated by casting, traction, and/or surgery.
- Genu varum and genu valgum are normal variations at certain times in development that may need treatment if they persist.
- The nurse may identify developmental dysplasia of the hip (DDH) during newborn assessments and must refer the child for care to a specialist.
- Mild DDH may be treated by a harness, but more severe cases may require surgery for the child to walk normally.
- Legg-Calvé-Perthes is a reversible disease most commonly seen in school-age boys, and causes necrosis of the femoral head.
- Slipped capital femoral epiphysis is treated by casting, traction, or more commonly surgery with pinning to stabilize the epiphysis.
- Scoliosis is a lateral curvature of the spine, and nurses commonly screen adolescents to identify the disorder.
- Scoliosis may require exercises, bracing, or surgery with instrumentation and spinal fusion.

- Osteoporosis can occur in premature infants, in children with conditions that lead to immobility and decreased weight bearing, and in youth with inadequate calcium or vitamin D intake.
- Osteomyelitis most commonly follows another infection and requires prompt treatment to prevent sepsis and serious injury to the bone.
- The child with osteogenesis imperfecta (brittle bone disease) requires careful handling by the nurse and parents to prevent fractures while fostering developmental progression.
- Muscular dystrophies are inherited diseases characterized by muscle wasting and degeneration.
- Children can experience a variety of fractures due to sports, car crashes, and other injuries.
- Many sports injuries experienced by youth can be avoided by proper equipment and training.
- Casts, braces, and traction are common interventions for musculoskeletal disorders; nursing interventions minimize development of problems related to these treatments.

Clinical Reasoning in Action

Recall the opening scenario. Douglass, 12 years old, has a fractured fibula from a fall while jumping on a trampoline. He talks openly in the office about how much fun he has at his friend's house after school and shares that he hopes his mother will still let him go there. He is also nervous about returning to his busy school with a cast and crutches.

Douglass has normal vital signs and neurovascular checks of the lower extremities. He ambulates well with crutches but appears slow and careful. Douglass admits that he has been pretty "crazy" at his friend's house and takes chances on the trampoline that he should not take. He is worried that his friends at school will make fun of him now that he has a cast and crutches.

1. Douglass's fracture did not disrupt the growth plate. What is the type of his fracture according to the Salter-Harris classification? If his growth plate had been disturbed, what are some possible long-term outcomes?

2. What is Douglass's developmental stage according to Erikson? Can that explain his risk-taking behaviors at his friend's house? Douglass's mother is worried about whether she should allow her son to continue going to his friend's house. What questions can you help her to ask the friend's parents about supervision, activities allowed, and plans for emergencies?

3. List two nursing diagnoses dealing with the physical systems and two focusing on psychosocial systems for Douglass.

4. What evidence-based nursing interventions can you establish for each nursing diagnosis?

See Pearson Nursing Student Resources for possible responses.

Pearson Nursing Student Resources

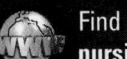

Find additional review materials at
nursing.pearsonhighered.com
Prepare for success with NCLEX®-style practice questions, interactive assignments and activities, web links, animations and videos, and more!

References

American Academy of Pediatrics, Section on Cardiology and Cardiac Surgery. (2005). Cardiac health supervision for individuals affected with Duchenne or Becker muscular dystrophy. *Pediatrics, 116,* 1569–1573.

Aronsson, D. D., Loder, R. T., Breur, G. J., & Weinstein, S. L. (2006). Slipped capital femoral epiphysis: Current concepts. *Journal of the American Academy of Orthopedic Surgeons, 14,* 666–679.

Bachrach, L. K. (2007). Consensus and controversy regarding osteoporosis in the pediatric population. *Endocrine Practice, 13,* 513–520.

Bauer, D. H., & Freivalds, A. (2009). Backpack load limit recommendations for middle school students based on physiological and psychophysical measurements. *Work, 32*(3), 339–350.

Beck, J., Weinberg, J., Hamnegard, C. H., Spahija, J., Olofson, J., Grimby, G. Y., & Sindery, C. (2006). Diaphragmatic function in advanced Duchenne muscular dystrophy. *Neuromuscular Disorders, 16,* 161–167.

Becker Muscular Dystrophy. (n.d.). *Becker muscular dystrophy.* Retrieved from http://www.beckermusculardystrophy.org

Bowman, B. A., & Russell, R. M. (Eds.). (2006). *Present knowledge of nutrition* (9th ed.). Washington, DC: International Life Sciences Institute.

Burns, C. E., Dunn, A. M., Brady, M. A., Starr, N. B., & Blosser, C. G. (2009). *Pediatric primary care* (4th ed.). Philadelphia: Elsevier Saunders.

Chan, G., & Chen, C. T. (2009). Musculoskeletal effects of obesity. *Current Opinions in Pediatrics, 21*(1), 65–70.

Ciafaloni, E., & Moxley, R. T. (2008). Treatment options for Duchenne muscular dystrophy. *Current Treatment Options in Neurology, 10*(2), 86–93.

Copley, L. A. (2009). Pediatric musculoskeletal infection: Trends and antibiotic recommendations. *Journal of the American Academy of Orthopedic Surgeons, 17*(10), 618–626.

Cruz, A. I., & Smith, B. G. (2010). Update on scoliosis in children and adolescents. *Contemporary Pediatrics, 27*(1), (retrieved online – no pgs yet)

Custer, J. W., & Rau, R. E. (Eds.). (2009). *The Harriet Lane handbook.* Philadelphia: Mosby Elsevier.

Deakin, D. E., Crosby, J. M., Moran, C. G., & Chell, J. (2007). Childhood fractures requiring inpatient management. *Injury, 38,* 1241–1246.

Fabry, G. (2010). The hip from birth to adolescence. *European Journal of Pediatrics, 169,* 143–148.

Gholve, P. A., Cameron, D. B., & Millis, M. B. (2009). Slipped capital femoral epiphysis update. *Current Opinion in Pediatrics, 21,* 39–45.

Gottschalk, H. P., Karol, L. A., & Jeans, K. A. (2010). Gait analysis of children treated for moderate clubfoot with physical therapy versus the Ponseti cast technique. *Journal of Pediatric Orthopedics, 30*(3), 235–239.

Grottkau, B. E., Epps, H. R., & Di Scala, C. (2005). Compartment syndrome in children and adolescents. *Journal of Pediatric Surgery, 40,* 678–682.

Gurnett, C. A., Boehm, S., Connolly, A., Reimschisel, T., & Dobbs, M. B. (2008). Impact of congenital talipes equinovarus etiology on treatment outcomes. *Developmental Medicine & Child Neurology, 50,* 498–502.

Ha, H. I., Seo, J. B., Lee, S. H., Kang, J. W., Goo, H. W., Lim, T. H., & Shin, M. J. (2007). Imaging of Marfan syndrome: Multisystemic manifestations. *Radiographics, 27,* 989–1004.

Hagmann, S., Dreher, T., & Wenz, W. (2009). Skewfoot. *Foot and Ankle Clinics, 14*(3), 409–434.

Hosalkar, H. S., Gholve, P. A., & Wells, L. (2007). Torsional and angular deformities. In R. M. Kliegman, R. E. Behrman, H. B. Jenson, & B. F. Stanton (Eds.), *Nelson textbook of pediatrics* (18th ed., pp. 2784–2790). Philadelphia: Saunders Elsevier.

Hosalkar, H. S., Horn, B. D., Friedman, J. E., & Dormans, J. P. (2007). The hip. In R. M. Kliegman, R. E. Behrman, H. B. Jenson, & B. F. Stanton (Eds.), *Nelson textbook of pediatrics* (18th ed., pp. 2800–2811). Philadelphia: Saunders Elsevier.

Hutchinson, B. (2010). Pediatric metatarsus adductus and skewfoot deformity. *Clinical Podiatric Medicine & Surgery, 27*(1), 93–104.

Kamboj, M. K. (2007). Metabolic bone disease in adolescents: Recognition, evaluation, treatment and prevention. *Adolescent Medicine: State of the Art Reviews, 18*(1), 24–46.

Kemper, A. R., & Wake, M. A. (2007). Duchenne muscular dystrophy: Issues in expanding newborn screening. *Current Opinion in Pediatrics, 19,* 700–704.

Kleposki, R. W., Abel, K., & Sehgal, K. (2010, June). Common pediatric hip diseases in primary care. *Clinical Advisor,* 21–26.

Kocher, M. S., Lee, B., Dolan, M., Weinberg, J., & Shulman, S. T. (2006). Pediatric orthopedic infections: Early detection and treatment. *Pediatric Annals, 35,* 112–122.

Kravitz, R. M. (2009). Airway clearance in Duchenne muscular dystrophy. *Pediatrics 123,* S231–S235.

Kuehn, B. M. (2007). Studies point way to new therapeutic prospects for muscular dystrophy. *Journal of the American Medical Association, 298,* 1385–1386.

Litmanovitz, I., Dolfin, T., Arnon, S., Regev, R. H., Nemet, D., & Eliakim, A. (2007). Assisted exercise and bone strength in preterm infants. *Calcified Tissue International, 80,* 39–43.

Macias, B. R., Murthy, G., Chambers, H., & Hargens, A. R. (2008). Asymmetric loads and pain associated with backpack carrying by children. *Journal of Pediatric Orthopedics, 28*(5), 512–517.

Manias, K., McCabe, D., & Bishop, N. (2006). Fractures and recurrent fractures in children: Varying effects of environment factors as well as bone size and mass. *Bone, 39,* 652–657.

March of Dimes. (2007). *Achondroplasia.* Retrieved from http://www.marchofdimes.com

Martin, E., & Shapiro, J. R. (2007). Osteogenesis imperfecta: Epidemiology and pathophysiology. *Current Osteoporosis Reports, 5*(3), 91–97.

Mayo Clinic. (2007). *Marfan syndrome.* Retrieved from http://www.mayoclinic.com/health/marfan-syndrome/DS00540/DSECTION=6

Mooney, V., Mayer, J., & Woodbridge, D. (2007, September). Adolescent scoliosis: Exercise therapy may help correct the condition. *Consultant for Pediatricians,* 509–515.

Moore, M. J., White, G. L., & Moore, D. L. (2007). Association of relative backpack weight with reported pain, pain sites, medical utilization, and lost school time in children and adolescents. *Journal of School Health, 77,* 232–239.

Murray, A. W., & Wilson, N. I. (2008). Changing incidence of slipped capital femoral epiphysis: A relationship with obesity. *Journal of Bone and Joint Surgery, 90*(1), 92–94.

Online Mendelian Inheritance in Man. (2008). *Osteogenesis imperfecta.* Retrieved from http://www.ncbi.nlm.nih.gov/entrez/dispomin/cgi?id=166200

Paton, R. W., Fox, A. E., Foster, P., & Hehily, M. (2010). Incidence and etiology of equino-varus with recent population changes. *Acute Orthopaedica Belgium, 76*(1), 86–89.

Pillion, J. P., & Shapiro, J. (2008). Audiological findings in osteogenesis imperfecta. *Journal of the American Academy of Audiology, 19*(8), 595–601.

Ratliff, C. R. (2007). Osteomyelitis. *Advance for Nurse Practitioners, 15*(7), 25–30.

Salehpour, S., & Tavakkoli, S. (2010). Cyclic pamidronate therapy in children with osteogenesis imperfecta. *Journal of Pediatric Endocrinology and Metabolism, 23*(102), 73–80.

Sankar, W. N., Weiss, J., & Skaggs, D. C. (2009). Orthopaedic conditions in the newborn. *Journal of the American Academy of Orthopaedic Surgeons, 17*(2), 112–122.

Sapountzi-Krepia, D., Psychogiou, M., Peterson, D., Zafari, B., Iordanopoulou, E., Michailidou, F., & Christodoulou, A. (2006). The experience of brace treatment in children/adolescents with scoliosis. *Scoliosis, 22,* 8.

Schwend, R. M., Schoenecker, P., Richards, B. S., Flynn, J. M., & Vitale, J. (2007). Screening the newborn for developmental dysplasia of the hip. *Journal of Pediatric Orthopaedics, 27,* 607–610.

Sewell, M. D., Rosendahl, K., & Eastwood, D. M. (2009). Developmental dysplasia of the hip. *British Medical Journal, 339,* b4464. doi:10.1136/bmj.b4454

Shank, C. F., Thiel, E. J., & Klingele, K. E. (2010). Valgus slipped capital femoral epiphysis: Prevalence, presentation, and treatment options. *Journal of Pediatric Orthopedics, 30*(2), 140–146.

Shilt, J. S., & Barnett, T. M. (2007, May). Back pain in children: Keys to evaluation and treatment. *Consultant for Pediatricians,* 281–290.

Shirley, E. D., & Ain, M. C. (2009). Achondroplasia: Manifestations and treatment. *Journal of the American Academy of Orthopedic Surgery, 17*(4), 231–241.

Simon, T. D., Bublitz, C., & Hambidge, S. J. (2006). Emergency department visits among pediatric patients for sports-related injury: Basic epidemiology and impact of race-ethnicity and insurance status. *Pediatric Emergency Care, 22,* 309–315.

Spiegel, D. A., Hosalkar, H. S., & Dormans, J. P. (2007). The spine. In R. M. Kliegman, R. E. Behrman, H. B. Jenson, & B. F. Stanton (Eds.), *Nelson textbook of pediatrics* (18th ed., pp. 2811–2822). Philadelphia: Saunders Elsevier.

Undale, A. H., Westendorf, J. J., Yaszemski, M. J., & Khosla, S. (2009). Mesenchymal stem cells for bone repair and metabolic bone diseases. *Mayo Clinic Proceedings, 84*(10), 893–902.

University of Maryland Medical Center. (2007). *Muscular dystrophy.* Retrieved from http://www.umm.edu/altmed/ConsConditions/MuscularDystrophycc.html

U.S. Department of Health and Human Services. (2006). *Screening for developmental dysplasia of the hip: Recommendation statement* (AHRQ Publication No. 05(06)-0585-A). Rockville, MD: Agency for Healthcare Quality and Research.

U.S. Preventive Services Task Force. (2006a). Screening for developmental dysplasia of the hip: Recommendation statement. *American Family Physician, 73,* 1192–1198.

U.S. Preventive Services Task Force. (2006b). *The guide to clinical preventive services.* Agency for Healthcare Research and Quality. Retrieved from http://www.preventiveservices.ahrq.gov

Von Kodolitsch, Y., & Robinson, P. N. (2007). Marfan syndrome: An update of genetics, medical and surgical treatment. *Heart, 93,* 755–760.

Alterations in Endocrine and Metabolic Function

chapter 30

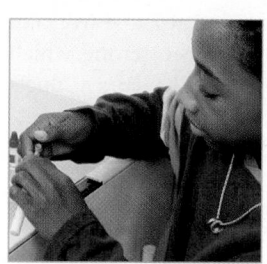

Anthony Maxwell, 12 years old, has just been diagnosed with type 1 diabetes. His parents sought medical attention from their family physician after Anthony complained of being constantly thirsty and hungry for over a week. Despite his vigorous appetite, he has lost 5 pounds since his last recorded weight. The family recalls that Anthony had a viral illness 3 months ago but recovered from the illness without difficulty. His mother says that Anthony has seemed lethargic for the last several days.

Anthony and his family must now learn to manage his diabetes using a combination of diet, exercise, and insulin therapy. Monitoring his serum glucose level is important in determining how much insulin he will require every day. Anthony's meals and activities will be coordinated with his insulin doses. During his short hospitalization and follow-up sessions, the nurse educates Anthony and his family regarding the cause, long-term implications, and management of diabetes. What are the key components of the teaching plan for Anthony and his family related to management of type 1 diabetes? How can Anthony be involved in his care while hospitalized?

Key Terms

Learning Outcomes

After reading this chapter, you will be able to do the following:

1. Describe the anatomy and physiology of the endocrine system and pediatric differences.
2. Identify the function of important hormones of the endocrine system.
3. Summarize signs and symptoms that may indicate a disorder of the endocrine system.
4. Identify all conditions for which short stature is a sign.
5. Develop a nursing care plan for each type of acquired metabolic disorder.
6. Develop a family education plan for the child who needs lifelong cortisol replacement.
7. Distinguish between the nursing care of the child with type 1 and type 2 diabetes.
8. Describe collaborative management for the child with type 1 and type 2 diabetes.
9. Plan care for the child with an inherited metabolic disorder.

FOCUS ON

The Endocrine System

ANATOMY AND PHYSIOLOGY

The endocrine system controls the cellular activity that regulates growth and body metabolism through the release of hormones. **Hormones** are chemical messengers secreted by various glands that exert controlling effects on the cells of the body. Overlapping with all body systems, the general functions of the endocrine system include the following:

- Differentiation of the reproductive and central nervous systems in the fetus
- Regulation of the pace of growth and development in concert with the central nervous system throughout childhood and adolescence
- Coordination of the male and female reproductive systems, enabling sexual reproduction
- Maintenance of an optimal level of hormones for body functioning
- Maintenance of homeostasis, a healthy internal environment, in the presence of a constantly changing external environment

The endocrine and nervous systems interact to regulate responses within the body and with the external environment.

The hypothalamic-pituitary axis (or system) produces a number of releasing and inhibiting hormones that regulate the function of many endocrine glands, including the thyroid, adrenal, and male and female reproductive glands. The hypothalamus synthesizes many hormones, and the pituitary gland works by stimulating or inhibiting the release of these hormones. The pituitary gland also secretes certain hormones. Hormones originating from this axis regulate growth. Other endocrine glands include the parathyroid glands and the islets of Langerhans in the pancreas (Figure 30–1 ➤). All of these glands secrete hormones into the bloodstream, which carries them to target organs or tissues. Most hormones exert their influence through interaction with receptors in the target cells of specific tissues (Table 30–1).

Hormone secretion regulation occurs through a *negative feedback* mechanism that maintains an optimal internal body environment (Figure 30–2 ➤). Negative feedback occurs when an endocrine gland or secretory tissue receives a message that the target cells have received an adequate amount of hormone. In response, further secretion is inhibited. Secretion is resumed only when the secretory tissue receives another message indicating that levels of the hormone are low.

PEDIATRIC DIFFERENCES

The endocrine system is responsible for sexual differentiation during fetal development. As the embryo develops, the initial re-productive structures are the same (a pair of gonads, two pairs of ducts, and the genital tubercle). Beginning at 7 to 8 weeks of gestation, the male embryo begins secreting testosterone, which causes the gonads to differentiate into testes. The pairs of ducts develop into the vas deferens. The female embryo begins secreting estrogen, causing the gonads to differentiate into ovaries,

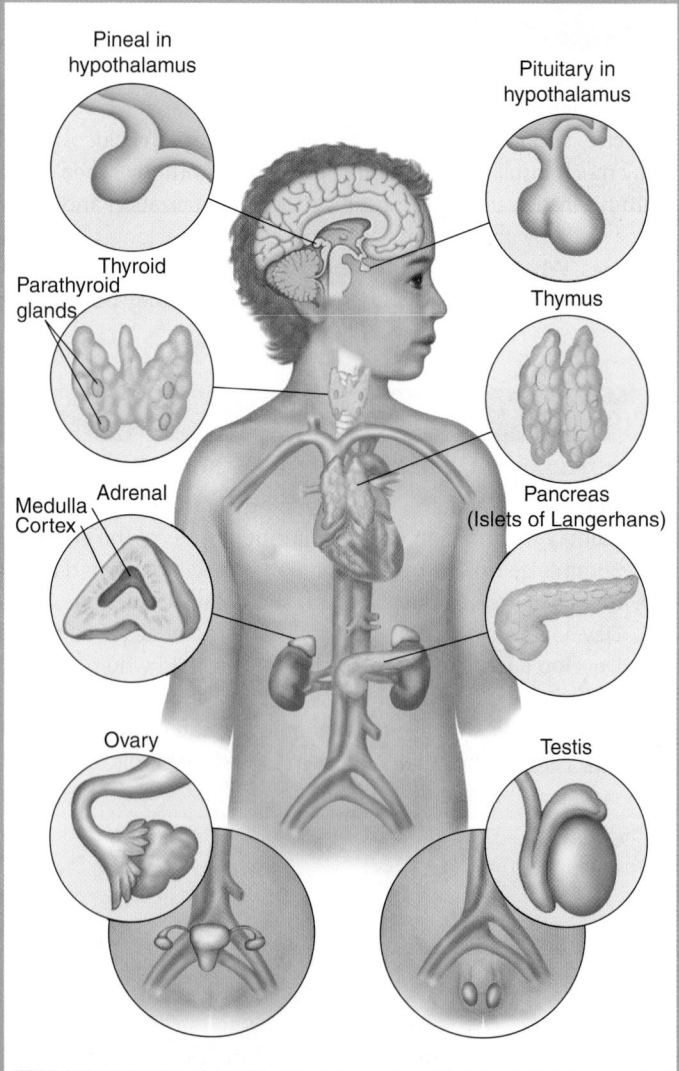

FIGURE 30–1 ➤ Major organs and glands of the endocrine system.

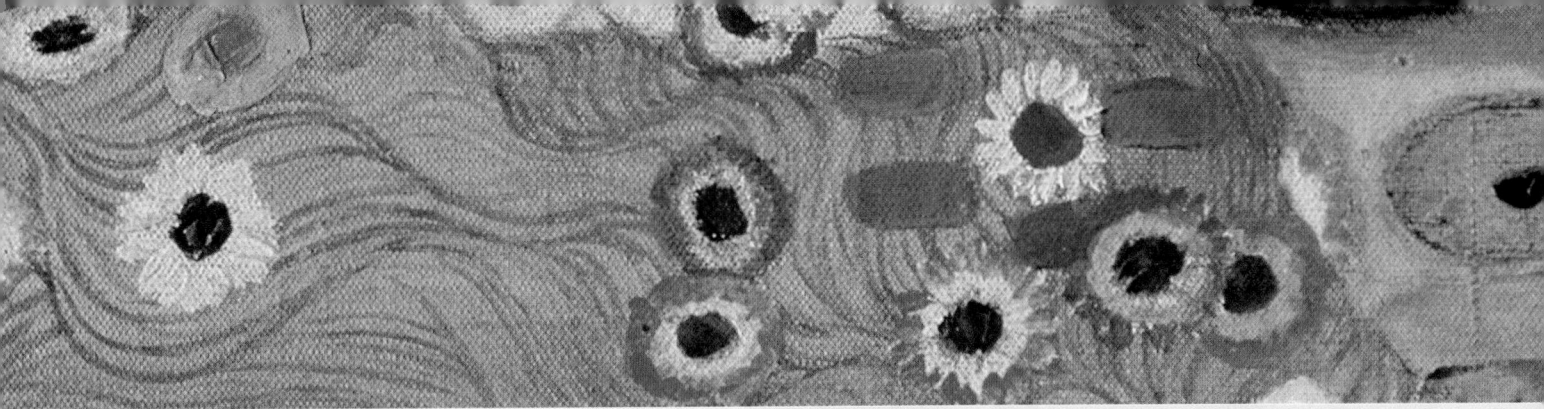

TABLE 30–1 Endocrine Glands and Their Functions

Gland/Hormone	Function
Anterior Pituitary	
Growth hormone (somatotropin)	Regulates metabolic process related to growth
Thyroid-stimulating hormone (TSH)	Stimulates thyroid hormone secretion
Adrenocorticotropic hormone (ACTH) (corticotrophin)	Stimulates secretion of glucocorticoids and androgens
Follicle-stimulating hormone (FSH) (a gonadotropin)	Stimulates secretion of estrogen; stimulates follicle maturation in ovaries; also critical for sperm production in males
Luteinizing hormone (LH) and interstitial cell-stimulating hormone (ICSH) (male analogue) (a gonadotropin)	Stimulates secretion of androgens in males and progesterone in females
Prolactin-releasing hormone	Stimulates secretion of prolactin that stimulates the secretion of milk during lactation
Melanocyte-stimulating hormone (MSH)	Stimulates skin pigmentation
Posterior Pituitary	
Antidiuretic hormone (ADH) (vasopressin)	Promotes water reabsorption back into the blood, decreasing urine output
Oxytocin	Stimulates uterine contractions and breast milk letdown reflex
Beta endorphins	May regulate body temperature, food and water intake
Thyroid	
Thyroxine (T_4) and triiodothyronine (T_3)	Regulates metabolic rate of all cells, body heat production; protein, fat, and carbohydrate catabolism in all cells
Thyrocalcitonin	Stimulates bone ossification and development
Parathyroid	
Parathyroid hormone	Regulates serum calcium levels and excretion of phosphorus
Adrenal	
Aldosterone	Increases sodium ion reabsorption, and increases potassium and hydrogen ion excretion in the kidneys
Androgens	Stimulates bone development and secondary sexual characteristics
Cortisol	Stimulates anti-inflammatory reactions, protects from stress
Epinephrine	Activates sympathetic nervous system; stimulates increase in blood pressure and blood glucose levels
Pancreas (Islets of Langerhans)	
Insulin	Facilitates cellular glucose utilization
Glucagon	Increases blood glucose when low by stimulating glycogenolysis
Somatostatin	Inhibits insulin and glucagon secretion; may prevent excess insulin secretion
Ovaries	
Estrogen	Stimulates development of breasts and ova
Progesterone	Stimulates breast glandular development; acts to maintain pregnancy
Testes	
Testosterone	Stimulates production of sperm, development of secondary sexual characteristics, and closure of epiphysis

while the ducts develop into the uterus and the fallopian tubes. The genital tubercle also differentiates and develops the male and female external genitalia.

The endocrine system is also responsible for stimulating growth and development during childhood and adolescence. Growth hormone, produced by the anterior pituitary gland, is secreted in pulses when the child is in stage 4 sleep, stimulates the growth of muscles, and improves bone mineralization (Grimberg & De León, 2005). Multiple hormones in the endocrine system, including the growth hormone, thyroid hormone, adrenal and gonadal androgens, and estrogen, are responsible for skeletal growth and maturation, including the

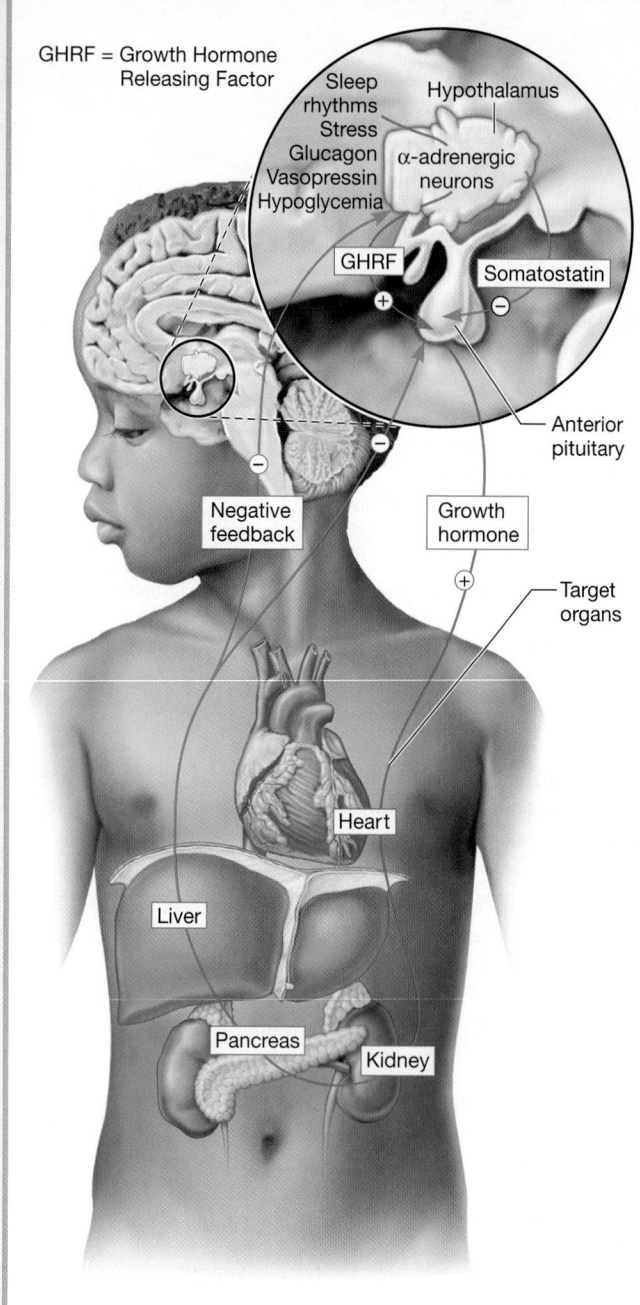

GHRF = Growth Hormone
Releasing Factor

Sleep rhythms
Stress
Glucagon
Vasopressin
Hypoglycemia

Hypothalamus

α-adrenergic
neurons

GHRF

Somatostatin

Anterior
pituitary

Negative
feedback

Growth
hormone

Target
organs

Heart

Liver

Pancreas

Kidney

FIGURE 30–2 ➤ Feedback mechanism in hormonal stimulation of the gonads during puberty.

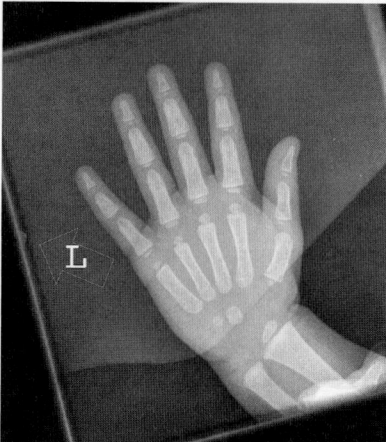

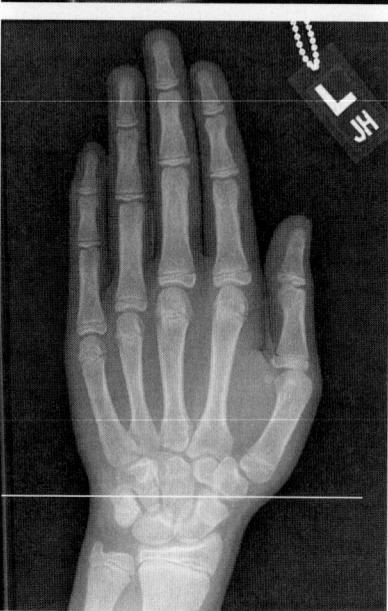

FIGURE 30–3 ➤ The radiographs of the hand and wrist of a 3-year-old and 13-year-old girl reveal significant differences in skeletal maturation that are closely tied to physiologic maturation. The 3-year-old has many bones in the hand and wrist that have not fully developed. The secretion of estrogen during puberty has resulted in the development and calcification of secondary ossification centers of most of the bones in the hand and wrist of the 13-year-old.

Courtesy, Dorothy Bulas, M.D., Children's National Medical Center.

appearance of secondary ossification centers in the bones (Carroll, 2010). Estrogen secretion associated with puberty is a dominant stimulator of increased skeletal maturity that can be detected by examining the child's **bone age** (stage of bone ossification) (Figure 30–3 ➤) (Lee & Kulin, 2005).

During childhood, the production of sex hormones (estrogen, progesterone, and testosterone) is low. **Puberty** (sexual maturation, lasting an average of 4.5 years) occurs when the gonads begin to secrete increased amounts of the sex hormones estrogen and androgens. At the average age of 9 years in girls and 11 years in boys, the hypothalamus produces increased amounts of gonadotropin-releasing hormone (GnRH). This hormone stimulates the anterior pituitary gland to secrete luteinizing hormone (LH) and follicle-stimulating hormone (FSH). In boys, LH stimulates testosterone production and FSH stimulates sperm production. In girls, LH and FSH stimulate development and maturation of the ova and ovulation. These hormones in turn stimulate the gonads to secrete more sex hormones, resulting in the development of primary and secondary sex characteristics. They also stimulate the genitalia to grow to adult proportions. At about 6 years of age, the adrenal glands may begin an increased secretion of adrenal hormones (**adrenarche**) (Lee, 2005). These

Puberty often begins at an earlier age in children of both sexes who have higher weights than average. Delayed puberty is more likely to occur in children who exercise excessively or who have a low body mass index, such as with anorexia nervosa (Pinyerd & Zipf, 2005).

adrenal hormones lead to the development of increased testicular size, axillary hair and pubic hair, early changes in body growth, and adult body odor. Pubertal development usually follows a specific sequence (accelerated growth, breast development, adrenarche, and menarche) (Pinyerd & Zipf, 2005). See Figures 5–40, 5–41, and 5–42 ∞ for the development of secondary sexual characteristics in males and females.

Menarche, the onset of menstruation, occurs in most girls between 11 and 13 years of age, and is a significant sign of sexual maturity. Menstruation is controlled by several hormones (FSH, LH, estrogen, and progesterone). For 1 to 2 years, cycles are anovulatory of variable duration. In contrast, males begin producing sperm once testicular and penile growth has occurred, around 13.5 to 14 years (Pinyerd & Zipf, 2005).

TABLE 30–2	**Diagnostic Tests and Laboratory Procedures for the Endocrine System**
Diagnostic Procedures	Laboratory Tests
ACTH stimulation test Adrenal (ACTH) suppression test Bone age Computed tomography (CT) Fluid deprivation test Karyotype Magnetic resonance imaging (MRI) Thyroid radioactive iodine uptake (RAIU) scan	Fasting plasma glucose Hemoglobin A_{1c} Hormone levels Insulin-like growth factor (IGF-1) and IGFBP-3 Newborn metabolic screening Provocative growth hormone testing Thyroid antibodies

See Appendices D and E ∞ for more information about these tests and procedures.

Use the Assessment Guidelines for the Child with an Endocrine Condition to perform a nursing assessment. Examples of diagnostic and laboratory tests used to evaluate endocrine conditions are provided in Table 30–2.

Assessment Guidelines for the Child with an Endocrine Condition

Assessment Focus	Assessment Guideline
Growth	▪ Carefully measure weight, length, or height, and plot on the appropriate growth chart. ▪ Compare measurements at different ages to assess the growth pattern over time and to assess the growth velocity.
Blood pressure/pulse	▪ Assess blood pressure and pulse and compare to expected norms for age. See Appendix D ∞.
Facial characteristics	▪ Inspect the face for unusual features such as a protuberant tongue, protuberant eyes, moon face, and hirsutism.
Neck	▪ Palpate the neck for an enlarged thyroid or goiter. Assess for webbing.
Muscles	▪ Assess strength and muscle tone. Assess for the presence of cramps or tremors.
Genitalia and secondary sexual characteristics	▪ Assess external genitalia for signs of ambiguous genitalia, or inappropriate size for age. ▪ Determine the child's stage of development for each characteristic (breast and pubic hair for girls, genital and pubic hair for boys) by comparing to the images in Figures 5–40, 5–41, and 5–42 ∞. ▪ Assess the sexual maturity rating with information in Figure 5–43 ∞. Compare the stage of development to the age of the boy or girl to determine early or delayed onset of puberty.
Body odor	▪ Assess body odor for unusual smell (e.g., sweet, musty, cheesy, sweaty feet).
Skin	▪ Assess skin color, noting areas of unusual pigmentation.
Mental status	▪ Note affect. Assess for anxiety, irritability, or lethargy.
Family history	▪ Assess for family history of metabolic or endocrine disorders. Is there a history of early or delayed puberty, early or delayed growth? What is the height of parents? Are there family members with short stature?

Endocrine disturbances result in alterations in metabolism, growth and development, and behavior that may have significant implications for children. If not diagnosed and treated early, these conditions can result in delays in growth and development, intellectual disability (previously called mental retardation), and, occasionally, death. However, treatment, which usually consists of supplementa-

tion of missing hormones, adjustment of hormone levels, or dietary measures, allows most children to live a normal life.

Inborn errors of metabolism—inherited biochemical abnormalities of the urea cycle and amino acid and organic acid metabolism—often have a significant impact on the endocrine system's ability to support growth and development. Some chromosomal abnormalities also result in disturbances in growth and sexual development.

■ DISORDERS OF PITUITARY FUNCTION

Growth Hormone Deficiency

Growth hormone deficiency is a disorder caused by decreased activity of the pituitary gland. Because most children with this disorder secrete inadequate amounts of growth hormone, the term *growth hormone deficiency* is often preferred to *hypopituitarism*. The disorder is diagnosed earlier in males than females since males are generally referred sooner for evaluation of short stature (Grimberg, Stewart, & Wajnrajch, 2008).

Etiology and Pathophysiology

The release of growth hormone from the anterior pituitary gland is controlled by the hypothalamus, which secretes releasing and inhibitory factors (somatostatin). Growth hormone (GH) stimulates linear growth and bone mineral density, as well as the growth of all body tissues. Growth hormone also stimulates the synthesis of proteins in the liver, among them the somatomedins or insulin-like growth factors, which promote glucose utilization by the cells and cell proliferation.

Infarction of the pituitary gland (such as that related to sickle cell disease), central nervous system infection, disease, tumors of the pituitary gland or hypothalamus (primarily craniopharyngiomas and gliomas), other brain tumors, cranial irradiation, brain trauma, chemotherapy, and psychosocial deprivation may cause growth hormone deficiency by interfering with the production or release of growth hormone. Other major causes of short stature include familial short stature, hypothyroidism, Turner syndrome, **constitutional growth delay** (a late pubertal growth spurt caused by delayed pubertal hormone secretion), chronic renal failure, Cushing syndrome, Down syndrome, inborn error of metabolism, and severe cardiac, pulmonary, or gastrointestinal disease. Psychosocial dwarfism is a syndrome of emotional deprivation that causes transient growth hormone deficiency that is reversed by placing the child in a nurturing environment (Sirotnak, 2008).

Clinical Manifestations

Children with growth hormone deficiency have normal birth weights and lengths. By the age of 1 year, however, they are below the 3rd percentile on the growth chart. The child characteristically grows at a rate of less than 5 cm (2 in.) per year. Other characteristic findings in infants include hypoglycemic seizures, hyponatremia, neonatal jaundice, pale optic discs, micropenis, and undescended testicles. Children with growth hormone deficiency tend to appear "cherubic" and exhibit youthful facial features, higher pitched voices, delayed dentition, "ripply" abdominal fat, decreased muscle mass, delayed skeletal maturation, and delayed sexual maturation.

COLLABORATIVE CARE

Diagnostic Tests

Any child whose height is 2 to 3 standard deviations below the mean height for age or whose measurement is falling off the normal growth chart should be evaluated for short stature

TABLE 30–3 Diagnostic Tests for Short Stature

Test	Purpose Related to Short Stature
IGF-1 and IGFBP-3	Screens for growth hormone deficiency
MRI of the pituitary gland	Detects pituitary malformation or tumor
Provocative growth hormone testing	Tests for growth hormone deficiency
Bone age	Identifies other potential causes of delayed growth
Karyotype (girls)	Detects Turner syndrome (see page 1021)
Thyroid function studies	Detects hypothyroidism (see page 997)
ACTH and cortisol levels	Detects other pituitary hormonal deficiencies
Urine creatinine, pH, specific gravity, urea nitrogen, electrolytes	Detects chronic renal failure (see Chapter 26 ∞)
Complete blood count and erythrocyte sedimentation rate	Screens for inflammatory bowel disease with anemia
Antigliadin antibodies	Screens for celiac disease

Source: Data from: Parks, J. S., & Felner, E. I. (2007a). Hormones of the hypothalamus and pituitary. In R. M. Kliegman, R. E. Behrman, H. B. Jenson, & B. F. Stanton, Nelson textbook of pediatrics (18th ed., pp. 2291–2293). Philadelphia: Saunders Elsevier; Parks, J. S., & Felner, E. I. (2007b). Hypopituitarism. In R. M. Kliegman, R. E. Behrman, H. B. Jenson, & B. F. Stanton, Nelson textbook of pediatrics (18th ed., pp. 2293–2299). Philadelphia: Saunders Elsevier; Grimberg, A., & De León, D. D. (2005). Disorders in growth. In T. M. Moshang, Pediatric endocrinology: The requisites in pediatrics (pp. 127–167). St. Louis, MO: Elsevier Mosby.

(Table 30–3). A child whose screening tests reveal low levels of insulin-like growth factors requires further evaluation by a pediatric endocrinologist. A careful history, physical examination, assessment of pubertal development and unusual facies, and radiologic studies are necessary to rule out familial short stature and constitutional growth delay, which are normal variants, and skeletal dysplasias or psychosocial short stature, which requires further evaluation.

Radiographic imaging of the hand or wrist bone is used to evaluate the stage of bone ossification, and thus the child's bone age. Using standardized norms for bone ossification, it can be determined if the child's chronologic age and bone age match. Significantly delayed (less than the child's age) or advanced (greater than the child's age) bone age may be indicative of the possibility of a systemic chronic disease or hormone abnormality requiring investigation. Provocative growth hormone testing, in which various medications (arginine, clonidine, glucagon, insulin, L-dopa) are administered to stimulate release of growth hormone, is a diagnostic test that may be used to confirm growth hormone deficiency.

Clinical Therapy

For growth hormone deficiency, replacement therapy with growth hormone (GH) is administered to promote growth and development. Most indications for growth hormone replacement require daily or alternate day subcutaneous injections; however, outcomes are improved with frequent dosing (Lee & Menon, 2005).

The child usually experiences increased growth velocity for the first year of treatment, followed by a gradual decrease in growth for subsequent months or years. Growth should progress at least at the normal growth rate for age while maintained on growth hormone treatment. Replacement therapy is continued until either the child achieves an acceptable height or growth velocity drops to less than 2 cm (1 in.) per year. Additionally, a bone age of greater than 14 years in girls and 16 years in boys is criteria to stop treatment (Parks & Felner, 2007b). Close monitoring of growth and endocrinology visits every 3 to 4 months are needed. If growth is slower than anticipated, improper preparation and administration of growth hormone and adherence to therapy must be considered before the dosage is increased (Parks & Felner, 2007b).

Nursing Management

Nursing care consists of monitoring growth, teaching the child and family about the disorder and its treatment, and providing emotional support. Carefully measure the child's height and weight and plot them on a growth chart.

Teach the parents and child about growth hormone replacement therapy, preparation and administration of subcutaneous injections, rotating injection sites, potential side effects, and actions to take if noticed. Provide the parents with ideas about how to minimize the child's stress associated with daily injections. Give parents educational resources, such as information from the MAGIC Foundation and the Human Growth Foundation. Replacement therapy is expensive, costing $20,000 or more per year (Lee, Davis, Clark, et al., 2006) and may not be covered by insurance; therefore, parents may require financial assistance that is sometimes available from the growth hormone manufacturers.

Clinical Tip

Encourage the parents to promote optimal nutrition and adequate caloric and iron intake in the child prior to starting and during growth hormone treatment. Lack of adequate nutrition may affect the child's growth response (Zadik, Sinai, Zung, et al., 2005).

Children with growth hormone deficiencies, especially those due to tumors and trauma from radiation or surgery, may have academic problems because of acquired learning disabilities. Before the child enters school, or returns to school after treatment for a tumor, a comprehensive evaluation should be performed to identify potential problems.

The best results occur when treatment is begun at an early age, before the psychologic effects of short stature become apparent and when attainment of near normal height can be reached. People often treat children who are short on the basis of their size rather than their age, and such children experience social prejudice about height. Teasing is a common problem. The teenage years may be particularly stressful because of adolescents' characteristic preoccupation with body image.

Encourage parents and teachers to treat the child in an age-appropriate manner. The child should dress in clothing that reflects chronologic age. Emphasize the child's strengths, support independence, and encourage participation in age-appropriate activities to aid in the development of a positive self-image. Suggest that the child take part in sports in which ability does not depend on size (e.g., swimming, gymnastics, wrestling, ice skating, and martial arts). Identifying positive role models, people of short stature who accomplish their goals, also promotes a positive image. Refer the child for counseling, if appropriate.

Growth Hormone Excess (Hyperpituitarism)

Hyperpituitarism, a disorder in which excessive secretion of growth hormone increases the growth rate, is rare in children. If combined with precocious puberty, a tumor of the hypothalamus may be present. Affected children can grow to 7 or 8 feet in height when oversecretion occurs before closure of the epiphyseal plates. If the disorder occurs after closure of the epiphyseal plates, **acromegaly** occurs. In acromegaly, abnormal growth of the hands and feet occurs, as well as a protruding brow and lower jaw; the nasal bone enlarges; and spacing between the teeth increases.

Because tall stature is valued in our society, assessment of children (particularly males) with accelerated linear growth is often delayed. Any child whose predicted height exceeds that consistent with parental height should be evaluated for possible growth problems and underlying pathologic conditions.

A complete history is obtained, and physical examination and laboratory testing are performed. Increased levels of IGF-1 establish the diagnosis of growth hormone excess. Radiologic examination for bone age is obtained to determine if the epiphyseal plates have begun to fuse. Radiologic studies are used to detect a tumor. Thorough evaluation is required to differentiate growth hormone excess from familial tall stature.

Treatment depends on the cause of the excessive growth and may involve surgical removal of a tumor or pituitary gland (hypophysectomy), radiation therapy, or radioactive implants. High doses of sex steroids are given to close the epiphyseal plates. The child may need lifelong pituitary hormone replacement following surgery.

Nursing Management

Early identification of the child with excessive growth rate is essential. Monitor growth trends and refer children whose height growth rate exceeds expected development for further evaluation and treatment to retard the accelerated growth rate. Nursing care focuses on educating the parents and child about the disorder and its treatment, providing emotional support, and, if surgery is required, providing preoperative and postoperative teaching and care (refer to Chapter 11 ∞).

Tall stature, like short stature, can be stressful for children. Children who are tall are often treated as if they were older than their chronologic age. Tall adolescents may have problems with self-image, and girls in particular may worry about their appearance.

Nursing care focuses on teaching the parents and child about the disorder and its treatment, providing emotional support, and, if surgery is required, providing preoperative and postoperative teaching and care.

Diabetes Insipidus

Diabetes insipidus is a disorder of the posterior pituitary gland characterized by excessive thirst and excretion of large amounts of dilute urine. Two forms of diabetes insipidus can occur: central (neurogenic) antidiuretic hormone (ADH) deficiency and familial nephrogenic diabetes insipidus. Both disorders involve ADH, a hormone secreted by the posterior pituitary gland. In normal circumstances, thirst is the regulator for ADH release (Kache & Ferry, 2005). The most important function of ADH is to bind to the collecting ducts of the kidney and promote reabsorption of water back into the circulation.

Etiology and Pathophysiology

ADH facilitates concentration of the urine by stimulating reabsorption of water from the distal tubule of the kidney. When ADH is inadequate, the tubules do not resorb water, leading to **polyuria** (passage of a large volume of urine in a given period). Therefore, the body is unable to conserve water, resulting in severe dehydration.

Diabetes insipidus can occur at any age and results from inadequate production or secretion of ADH or arginine-vasopressin (central or neurogenic diabetes insipidus) or inability of the renal collecting tubules to respond to the ADH (nephrogenic diabetes insipidus). Brain tumors and their treatment are the most common cause of central diabetes insipidus (Kache & Ferry, 2005). Other causes of central diabetes insipidus include brain trauma, central nervous system infection, and neurosurgery. Genetic nephrogenic diabetes insipidus is not as common as the acquired type, but its presentation is more severe. Transient nephrogenic diabetes insipidus may be caused by drug toxicity or an adverse drug reaction (Breault & Majzoub, 2007).

Clinical Manifestations

Polyuria and **polydipsia** (excessive thirst) are the cardinal signs of diabetes insipidus. Polydipsia is the body's attempt to preserve fluid balance. Additional manifestations observed in children with diabetes insipidus include hypernatremia, dilute urine, and dehydration. See the clinical manifestations table below.

Although the onset of symptoms is usually sudden, diagnosis is often delayed. Children who can quench their thirst may not complain to parents about symptoms. In infants, symptoms may include vomiting, polyuria, poor skin turgor, and irritability (Kache & Ferry, 2005).

In all forms of diabetes insipidus, the urine cannot be concentrated, no matter how dehydrated the child becomes. A dehydration episode usually leads to the diagnosis. Serum sodium concentration and osmolality increase rapidly to pathologic levels. Seizures may occur in response to extreme electrolyte imbalances. Often an unconscious child is admitted to the emergency department with dehydration and hypernatremia. The diagnosis is confirmed if the urine osmolality is less than 300 mOsm/kg and the serum osmolality is greater than 300 mOsm/kg (Breault & Majzoub, 2007).

Clinical Tip

A fluid deprivation test may be performed to further establish the diagnosis of diabetes insipidus. During the fluid deprivation test, advise parents that the child will be frustrated and irritable from thirst. No one should drink in front of the child during the testing period. Monitor the child's vital signs, intake, and output carefully. The test is stopped if the child loses 5% of body weight and develops a fever and hypotension (Kache & Ferry, 2005).

COLLABORATIVE CARE

Diagnostic Tests

Initial testing involves serum electrolyte concentrations and a urinalysis including specific gravity and osmolality. Urine osmolality is decreased (less than 300 mOsm/kg), urine specific gravity is decreased (less than 1.005), serum sodium is elevated, and the urine to serum osmolality ratio is less than 1 (Kache & Ferry, 2005). An MRI may be ordered to visualize the pituitary gland to detect a tumor. Diagnosis is confirmed by measuring the plasma arginine vasopressin (AVP) level before and during a fluid deprivation test, which is usually conducted in the hospital or in a carefully controlled outpatient setting for up to

Clinical Manifestations
Diabetes Insipidus

Cause	Clinical Manifestations	Clinical Therapy
Central Diabetes Insipidus ADH deficiency Familial or idiopathic	Polyuria, polydipsia Nocturia, enuresis Thirsty at night, irritable if fluids withheld Constipation, fever, dehydration	Desmopressin acetate
Nephrogenic Diabetes Insipidus Inherited or acquired Decreased responsiveness of kidneys to ADH	Polyuria, polydipsia Hypernatremia in neonatal period Dehydration, fever, vomiting Mental status changes	Diuretics High fluid intake Salt- and protein-restricted diet

8 hours. Fluid intake is prohibited during the procedure. Weight, urine output, specific gravity, and osmolality are measured every 2 hours. The specific gravity remains low (less than 1.005) even after dehydration. A dose of aqueous vasopressin is given after several hours. The response of a decreased urine output and increased urine concentration confirms the diagnosis of central diabetes insipidus. No response to vasopressin is seen in cases of nephrogenic diabetes insipidus. Many children with central diabetes insipidus have deficiencies of other anterior pituitary hormones, so testing for those deficiencies will also be conducted.

Clinical Therapy

Children who can access water and who have an intact thirst mechanism can maintain serum sodium and osmolality status; however, medications decrease polyuria and polydipsia. Fluid management may be the safest and preferred treatment. Infants may be given dilute formula (1/10th strength) to provide needed calories and water (Kache & Ferry, 2005).

Central ADH deficiency is treated by subcutaneous, intranasal, or oral desmopressin acetate (DDAVP). The medication reduces urinary output, enabling the child to live a more normal life with a decrease in thirst, urinary output, and nocturia. The dose of DDAVP must be titered for sufficient coverage of metabolic needs while not high enough to cause water overload (Raine, Donaldson, Gregory, et al., 2006a).

Nephrogenic diabetes insipidus is treated with thiazide diuretics, which promote sodium excretion and stimulate the proximal tubule to reabsorb water. Prostaglandin inhibitors (indomethacin) may also be prescribed to have an additive effect on decreased water excretion. The child is allowed liberal fluid intake. The child's sodium and potassium levels must be carefully monitored to prevent hypernatremia and hypokalemia (Kache & Ferry, 2005; Raine et al., 2006a) (see Chapter 18 ∞).

Nursing Alert

When the child with diabetes insipidus has an acute illness, the child's physician should be notified immediately. Dehydration and hypernatremia may develop rapidly, and hypernatremia can cause intellectual disability, seizures, and cerebral calcification. Intravenous fluids will be needed to prevent or treat dehydration. See Chapter 16 ∞. Serum sodium and serum osmolality must be carefully monitored.

Nursing Management

Nursing care centers on administering medications and teaching parents how to manage the condition and recognize signs of altered fluid status. Educate parents about making fluids available to the child as needed, administering DDAVP, obtaining and recording daily weights, measuring intake and output, and recognizing signs of inadequate fluid intake (see Chapter 18 ∞). The child should consume fluids equal to the amount of output (sometimes as much as 75 mL/kg) (Ferry, 2005). Parents may need to weigh diapers to monitor urine output in infants. Cold fluids are often preferred and help relieve thirst. The child's fluid intake will need to be adjusted to prevent dehydration during an illness. Children often wake to drink fluids at night, but infants will need to have fluids provided. Many infants have coexisting brain damage and need nasogastric or gastrostomy feeding to maintain adequate hydration and nutrition. However, care should be taken to avoid the intake of excessive fluid as the child will not be able to excrete the excess water load with DDAVP treatment.

The child with chronic diabetes insipidus should always wear medical alert identification to indicate the presence of the disorder. Collaborate with the parents and school officials to make arrangements to provide the child unrestricted access to toilet facilities and water.

Syndrome of Inappropriate Antidiuretic Hormone

Syndrome of inappropriate antidiuretic hormone (SIADH) results from an excessive amount of serum ADH. It is seen in children with central nervous system infections, brain tumors, and brain trauma; in children with pulmonary disorders such as pneumonia, asthma, or cystic fibrosis; and in children receiving positive pressure ventilation. Some medications including diuretics and chemotherapy have been associated with SIADH.

Failure of normal feedback mechanisms from the hypothalamus, pituitary gland, and kidney results in excessive secretion of ADH, leading to water reabsorption despite the presence of a low serum osmolality. ADH secretion causes increased permeability of the distal renal tubules and collecting ducts, resulting in water reabsorption, increased intravascular volume, and decreased urine output (Ferry, 2005). Elevated ADH also causes suppression of the renin-angiotensin mechanism and sodium excretion. The outcome is **water intoxication** (an abnormal proportion of water to sodium in the extracellular fluid), hyponatremia, and cerebral edema (Ferry & Pascual-y-Baralt, 2009).

Signs of SIADH include elevated blood pressure, distended jugular veins, crackles in lung fields, weight gain without edema, fluid and electrolyte imbalance, and concentrated urine with decreased urine output. As serum sodium levels continue to fall, lethargy, confusion, headache, altered level of consciousness, seizures, and coma occur due to cerebral edema.

Laboratory findings include a high urine osmolality (greater than 100 mOsm/kg), low serum osmolality (less than 280 mOsm/kg), low serum sodium (less than 135 mM), and significantly decreased blood urea nitrogen (BUN; less than 10/dL) (Ferry & Pascual-y-Baralt, 2009).

Treatment includes fluid management, medications, and treatment of the underlying condition when possible. Fluids are restricted to prevent further dilution of the blood. Medications include diuretics, demeclocycline to block action of ADH at the renal collecting tubules, and hypertonic saline IV fluids. Oral urea has recently been evaluated for treatment with promising results (Huang, Feldman, Schwartz, et al., 2006). After the acute phase, a daily fluid allowance is calculated to two-thirds maintenance to prevent excess water intake and potential complications such as congestive heart failure or pulmonary edema. See Chapter 18 ∞ for calculation of the maintenance fluid amount for the child.

Nursing Management

Nursing care focuses on maintenance of fluid and electrolyte balance and prevention of complications associated with the disorder. Monitor changes in level of consciousness, headache, and seizure activity. Monitor vital signs, intake and output, serum sodium, urine osmolality, and specific gravity. Weigh the child daily to assess for weight gain, which may indicate a sign of water intoxication. Assess nutritional intake status and appetite.

Educate the parents about the child's fluid restrictions and the hidden sources of water and fluids in foods to help avoid excessive fluid intake. Parents need to understand the importance of weighing the child daily and reporting weight gain that could indicate fluid retention. Depending on the cause of the disorder, lifelong medication may be required. If the child is prescribed demeclocycline, emphasize to the family the importance of follow-up care since the drug has nephrotoxic side effects. The child should wear medical alert identification identifying the disorder and treatment.

Precocious Puberty

Puberty normally occurs between 8 and 13 years of age in girls and between 9 1/2 and 14 years of age in boys. Precocious puberty is defined as the appearance of any secondary sexual characteristics before 8 years of age in girls (breast development or pubic hair) and 9 years of age in boys (pubic hair) (Pinyerd & Zipf, 2005). Precocious puberty is not as common in males as in females, and warrants a thorough evaluation due to the likelihood of a central nervous system tumor (Kaplowitz, 2006a).

Central precocious puberty or true precocious puberty occurs when the hypothalamus is prematurely activated to secrete gonadotropin-releasing hormone, and it is usually considered idiopathic (deVries, Shtaif, Phillip, et al., 2009). Other potential causes include tumors of the ovary, adrenal gland, and pituitary gland, and a rare genetic condition known as McCune-Albright syndrome (Keefe, 2007).

Clinical Tip

Hormone levels vary throughout the day, making it difficult to get a measurement of the child's peak hormone level. Provocative testing is used to measure hormone levels when an endocrine condition is suspected. A medication known to stimulate the secretion of the hormone being tested is administered and serial blood samples are collected to measure the child's response.

Culture ⟶ *Onset of Puberty*

Differences exist by race in the onset of puberty and secondary sexual characteristics. Black girls begin puberty one half to one year earlier than White girls (Kaplowitz, 2006b). Menstruation begins at an average age of 12.1 years in Black girls and at an average age of 12.8 years in White girls. Additionally, the mean age of thelarche (breast development) is around 9 years of age in Black girls and 10 years of age in White girls (Nelson, 2007).

Isolated signs of premature sexual development such as premature **thelarche** (breast development), premature menarche (vaginal bleeding without other signs of sexual development), and premature adrenarche (development of pubic and axillary sexual hair) before 8 years of age in girls and 9 years in boys often need no treatment.

Children with precocious puberty have an advanced bone age (premature skeletal maturation) and may appear unusually tall for their age. Their growth ceases prematurely, however, as the hormones stimulate early closure of the epiphyseal plates, potentially resulting in short stature without treatment. Behavior changes may include mood swings and emotional lability.

Serum diagnostic studies include luteinizing hormone (LH), follicle-stimulating hormone (FSH), testosterone, or estradiol. Provocative testing includes gonadotropin-releasing hormone (GnRH) stimulation to confirm the diagnosis. Radiologic imaging of the brain, as well as a bone age, may be performed.

Central nervous system (CNS) tumors require surgery, radiation, and/or chemotherapy. Treatment may be initiated immediately to slow or stop the progression of sexual development in children younger than the expected age of puberty. A gonadotropin-releasing hormone analogue (GnRHa) is administered, usually leuprolide acetate (Lupron) injections once a month or nafarelin acetate (Synarel) intranasally twice a day. Treatment often continues until a more normal age for puberty is reached (e.g., 11 years in girls and 12 years in boys). Simple monitoring of growth patterns may be the only intervention for children closer to the lower expected age for puberty to begin.

Nursing Management

Nursing care centers on teaching the child and parents about the condition and its treatment, promoting growth, and providing emotional support. Inform the child in age-appropriate terms that physiologic changes are normal but occurring at an earlier than usual age. Reassure the child that friends will experience the same stages of development eventually. Emphasize to the family that the child's social, cognitive, and emotional development matches his or her age, even though the physical development is advanced.

Children with precocious puberty often become self-conscious as body changes occur. Provide the child opportunities to express concerns and discuss issues related to body changes. The child may need to practice role-playing as a coping mechanism to manage teasing by other children. Encourage the family to dress the child in a manner appropriate to his or her chronologic age, even though the child may look older. Provide privacy during physical examinations. Advise parents that they may need to discuss issues of sexuality with the child at an earlier age than normal. Refer the child and family for counseling if appropriate.

Teach the family proper medication administration and adherence to treatment regimen. Determine the family's ability to financially manage the cost of treatment. Assistance in covering the cost of therapy may be available through pharmaceutical companies and third-party payers.

■ DISORDERS OF THYROID FUNCTION

Hypothyroidism

Hypothyroidism is a disorder in which levels of active thyroid hormones are decreased. This disorder may be congenital or acquired. Congenital hypothyroidism occurs in approximately 1 in 4,000 live births and is twice as common in girls as in boys. In comparison to White infants, it is less prevalent in Black infants but more prevalent in Hispanic and Native American infants (LaFranchi, 2007).

Etiology and Pathophysiology

Thyroid hormones are important for growth and development and for metabolizing nutrients and energy. When these hormones are not available to stimulate other hormones or specific target cells, growth is delayed and intellectual disability develops.

Congenital hypothyroidism is usually caused by thyroid *dysgenesis* (defective/underdeveloped). A small percentage of cases are caused by an inborn error of thyroxine synthesis. Some children have a transient form of congenital hypothyroidism due to transplacental transfer of maternal thyroid-blocking antibodies or antithyroid medications (LaFranchi, 2007).

Acquired hypothyroidism usually results from chronic lymphocytic thyroiditis (Hashimoto's thyroiditis, autoimmune thyroiditis). The thyroid is infiltrated by lymphocytes that cause an autoimmune reaction and an enlarged thyroid. Acquired hypothyroidism may also be related to polyglandular autoimmune syndromes, systemic disease, thyroidectomy, radiation, or exposure to drugs or substances such as lithium that interfere with thyroid hormone synthesis (LaFranchi, 2007).

Clinical Manifestations

Infants with congenital hypothyroidism have few clinical signs of the disorder in the first weeks of life. In untreated infants, the characteristic cretinoid features (thickened protuberant tongue, thick lips, dull appearance) appear during the first few months of life (Figure 30–4 ➤). Other signs include prolonged hypotonia, cool extremities, mottling, umbilical hernia, difficulty feeding, lethargy, constipation, and a hoarse cry (Péter & Muzsnai, 2009). Intellectual disability (cretinism) is irreversible if the disorder is not treated beginning in early infancy.

Children with acquired hypothyroidism have many of the same signs as adults: decreased appetite; dry, cool skin; thinning hair or hair loss; depressed deep tendon reflexes; bradycardia; constipation; sensitivity to cold temperatures; abnormal menses; and a **goiter** (a nontender enlarged thyroid gland). Manifestations unique to children include change in past normal growth patterns with a weight increase, decreased height velocity, delayed bone and dental age, muscle hypertrophy with muscle weakness, and delayed or precocious puberty.

COLLABORATIVE CARE

Diagnostic Tests

Congenital hypothyroidism is usually detected during newborn screening of thyroxine (T_4) and TSH levels, which is mandatory in all 50 states. Newborn screening has greatly reduced the incidence of intellectual disability associated with this disorder

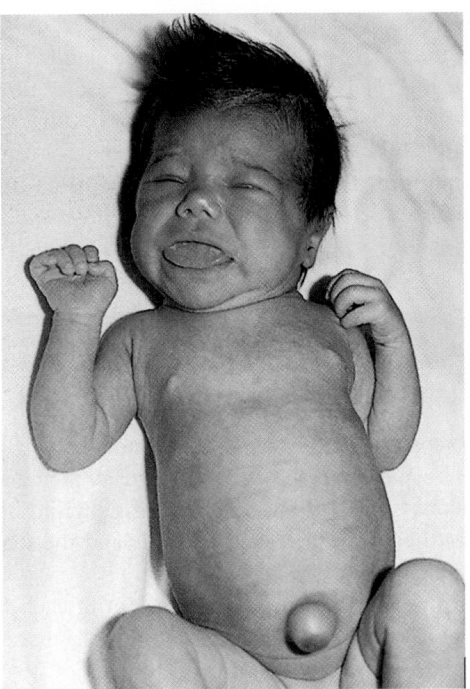

FIGURE 30–4 ➤ Child with congenital hypothyroidism.
From Zitelli, B. J., & Davis, H. W. (Eds.). (2007). Atlas of pediatric physical diagnosis (5th ed., p. 357). Philadelphia: Mosby-Elsevier.

(Péter & Muzsnai, 2009). A decreased T_4, normal T_3, and elevated thyroid-stimulating hormone level indicate hypothyroidism. An elevated TSH level indicates that the disease originated in the thyroid, not the pituitary. Two tests are frequently performed so that the disorder is identified early, before the newborn leaves the hospital and at the first health care visit at 1 to 2 weeks of age. Rapid response from the laboratory testing the samples is important to reduce the time to diagnosis and the effects of hypothyroidism on the infant's development.

Clinical Therapy

If the T_4 level is below normal and the TSH level is increased, the synthetic thyroid hormone levothyroxine (Synthroid) is prescribed. The dose is increased gradually as the child grows to ensure a **euthyroid** (normal thyroid) state. A pediatric endocrinologist monitors treatment. Periodic evaluation of T_4 and TSH serum levels, bone age, and growth parameters is necessary to assess for signs of excess or inadequate thyroid hormone. A trial without medication may be attempted when the child is about 3 years of age if the child has not required increasing doses of levothyroxine to maintain the TSH level. If after 6 weeks the TSH level is elevated, lifelong medication will be needed (Rossi, Caplin, & Alter, 2005).

Nursing Alert

Slipped capital femoral epiphysis has been associated with hypothyroidism and growth hormone deficiency. Any child receiving growth hormone treatment who complains of hip pain or knee pain, or who manifests a limp must be evaluated for this disorder (Darendeliler, Karagiannis, & Wilton, 2007). See Chapter 29 ∞ for further information on this condition.

To ensure an adequate growth rate and prevent intellectual disability, the hormone must be taken throughout life. Children with congenital hypothyroidism that is diagnosed before 3 months of age have the best prognosis for optimal mental development. Children with acquired hypothyroidism usually have normal growth following a period of catch-up growth. Many adolescents with Hashimoto thyroiditis have a spontaneous remission.

NURSING MANAGEMENT

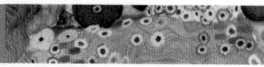

Nursing Assessment and Diagnosis

Routine neonatal screening is performed before discharge from the hospital and is often repeated at the infant's first health visit to evaluate levels of circulating thyroid hormones. Emphasize the importance of these visits and the screening to be performed.

Record the length or height and weight at each follow-up visit and plot on a growth curve. The child is assessed for signs of inadequate growth to determine if the dose of thyroid hormone needs to be adjusted and to monitor compliance with medication. Conduct developmental screening to detect delays in developmental milestones.

Among the nursing diagnoses that might be appropriate for the child with hypothyroidism are:

- Imbalanced Nutrition: Less than Body Requirements related to loss of appetite
- Risk for Delayed Development related to delayed initiation of thyroid replacement therapy
- Risk for Disproportionate Growth related to poor adherence to thyroid hormone therapy
- Constipation related to decreased bowel motility
- Fatigue related to inadequate dose of thyroid medication

Planning and Implementation

Nursing care focuses on teaching the parents and child about the disorder and its treatment and monitoring the child's growth rate. Explain how to administer thyroid hormone, which is only available in tablet form (e.g., tablets can be crushed and mixed in a small amount of formula or applesauce, as long as it can be ensured that the child gets all of the medication). Advise parents that the child may experience temporary sleep disturbances or behavioral changes in response to therapy. Teach the parents how to assess for an increased pulse rate, which could indicate the presence of too much thyroid hormone, and advise them to report problems such as fatigue, which could indicate an improper drug dose that needs to be adjusted.

Caution parents to dress the child appropriately for the season to prevent hypothermia. Modify the child's diet by increasing the amount of fruits and bulk if constipation is a problem.

Reassure the family that the child has the best chance of normal development when the hormone replacement therapy is given as prescribed. Reinforce the importance of follow-up visits to assess growth rate and response to therapy and to regulate drug dosages as the child grows. Periodic assessments of educational achievement are needed. Even with good control, adolescents have persistent visual-spatial deficits, and memory and attention problems. Parents should be informed that in most cases therapy will be lifelong and it is needed to promote the child's mental development. When the cause is genetic, make a referral for genetic counseling.

Evaluation

Expected outcomes of nursing care of the child with hypothyroidism include:

- The child maintains adequate growth of height and weight, following a percentile curve throughout childhood.
- The child's diet contains adequate fruits and bulk to prevent constipation.
- The child's cognitive development is appropriate for age.

Hyperthyroidism

Hyperthyroidism occurs when thyroid hormone levels are increased, resulting in excessive levels of circulating thyroid hormones. Hyperthyroidism is rare in children and adolescents, occurring in only .02% of children, primarily in adolescents ages 11–15. The disorder is almost always due to Graves disease (LaFranchi, 2007).

Etiology and Pathophysiology

Graves disease is an autoimmune disorder. Immunoglobulins produced by the B lymphocytes stimulate oversecretion of thyroid hormones, resulting in the clinical symptoms. It has a high familial incidence.

Other less common causes of hyperthyroidism result from thyroiditis and thyroid-secreting hormone tumors, including thyroid adenomas and carcinomas, as well as pituitary adenomas. Congenital hyperthyroidism can occur in infants of mothers with Graves disease because of transplacental transfer of immunoglobulins.

Clinical Manifestations

Signs and symptoms are caused by hyperactivity of the sympathetic nervous system. Characteristic findings include an enlarged, nontender thyroid gland (goiter), prominent eyes (**exophthalmos**) (Figure 30–5 ➤), eyelid lag, tachycardia, nervousness, restlessness or irritability, increased appetite with weight loss, emotional lability, heat intolerance, diaphoresis, insomnia, tremor, and muscle weakness. The thyroid gland may be slightly enlarged or grow to three to four times its normal size; feel warm, soft, and fleshy; and have an auditory bruit on auscultation. Onset is subtle, and the condition often goes unrecognized for 1 to 2 years.

Children with Graves disease usually have difficulty concentrating, behavioral problems, and declining performance in school. They become easily frustrated in the classroom and overheated and fatigued during physical education class. It is difficult for them to relax or sleep. These symptoms usually prompt parents to seek medical treatment for them.

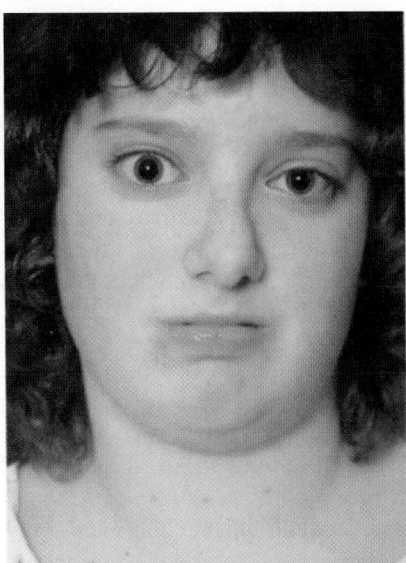

FIGURE 30–5 ➤ Exophthalmos and an enlarged thyroid in an adolescent with Graves disease.
From Zitelli, B. J., & Davis, H. W. (Eds.). (2007). Atlas of pediatric physical diagnosis (5th ed., p. 357). Philadelphia: Mosby-Elsevier.

The most serious complication of hyperthyroidism is severe **thyrotoxicosis**, also called thyroid crisis or thyroid storm. It is a life-threatening emergency resulting from extreme hyperthyroidism, in which elevated circulating levels of thyroid hormone result in a hypermetabolic state. Symptoms include muscle weakness, tremor, diarrhea, excessive sweating, and palpitations, and can progress to coma or cardiac failure (Amer, 2005).

COLLABORATIVE CARE

Diagnostic Tests

Diagnostic studies include laboratory evaluation of serum TSH, T_3 (triiodothyronine) and T_4 levels, and a thyroid scan. T_3 and T_4 levels are markedly elevated while the TSH level is decreased. Serum studies are also performed to detect thyroid antibodies (anti-TG and anti-TPO).

Clinical Therapy

The goal of clinical therapy is to inhibit excessive secretion of thyroid hormones. Treatment may include drug therapy, radiation therapy, or surgery. Drug therapy is most often the initial treatment, but compliance is often a problem because of drug side effects. Methimazole (Tapazole) and propylthiouracil (PTU) are administered to inhibit thyroid (T_3 and T_4) secretion (Amer, 2005). PTU therapy can cause temporary side effects, including skin rashes, urticaria, and lymphadenopathy. If rash, fever, or sore throat develops, a health care professional should perform hematologic studies. Treatment continues for 2 years or longer until remission occurs. An estimated 25% achieve remission within 2 years, and 50% achieve it within 5 years (Amer, 2005). Symptoms usually improve within weeks of starting treatment. Adjunct therapy with beta-adrenergic blocking agents such as propranolol (Inderal) may be administered to relieve symptoms of tremors, tachycardia, lid lag, and excessive sweating (LaFranchi, 2007).

If drug therapy is ineffective, radiation therapy using oral radioactive iodine is the next treatment choice. Thyroidectomy (removal of most of the thyroid) provides an immediate cure, avoiding radiation and possible long-term complications of radioactive iodine. However, destruction or removal of the thyroid gland often results in permanent hypothyroidism, necessitating lifelong hormone replacement therapy (Kaguelidou, Carel, & Leger, 2009). Manipulation of the parathyroid gland during surgery may result in excess release of parathyroid hormone, leading to hypercalcemia. Monitoring of serum calcium levels following a thyroidectomy is essential.

NURSING MANAGEMENT

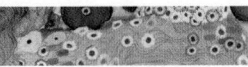

Nursing Assessment and Diagnosis

Assess the child's vital signs, as blood pressure and pulse may be elevated. Keep a record of food intake. Accurate measurement and recording of height and weight are important to establish baselines and identify patterns of growth. Observe the child's behavior, activity, and level of fatigue.

Common nursing diagnoses for the child with hyperthyroidism include:

- Ineffective Thermoregulation (Elevated) related to illness and excessive activity of the sympathetic nervous system
- Imbalanced Nutrition: Less than Body Requirements related to high metabolic needs
- Disturbed Body Image related to changes caused by illness (prominent eyes, excessive perspiration, and tremors)
- Fatigue related to hypermetabolic state and sleep deprivation

Planning and Implementation

Nursing care focuses on teaching the child and parents about the disorder and its treatment, promoting rest, providing emotional support, and, if the child needs surgery, providing preoperative and postoperative teaching and care. Promote increased caloric intake by providing five or six moderate meals per day. Encourage the child and family to express their feelings and concerns about the disorder, especially when deciding among the three treatment options or during the period when medication dosage adjustments are frequently needed. Pointing out even slight improvements in the child's condition may increase the child's adherence with therapy.

Children with hyperthyroidism are easily fatigued. Rest periods should be scheduled at school and home, and physical activities should be kept to a minimum until symptoms resolve. Encourage parents to provide a cool environment and allow the child to wear fewer clothes until symptoms subside.

Children who have partial or total removal of the thyroid gland receive antithyroid drugs, such as iodine, for approximately 2 weeks before surgery to reduce the vascularity and size of the thyroid gland and to decrease the risk of thyroid storm.

Teach the child and parents about drug therapy and instruct parents to watch for side effects of antithyroid drugs, including fever, urticaria, and lymphadenopathy. Provide preoperative teaching (see Chapter 11 ∞), as young children may be fearful about having their throat "cut."

Postoperatively, elevate the head of the bed to 30 degrees to promote a patent airway. A tracheostomy kit, suction supplies, and IV calcium gluconate should be immediately available for emergency treatment of hypocalcemia and respiratory distress. If thyroidectomy is performed, thyrotoxicosis does not immediately resolve because the half-life is 7 to 8 days. Antithyroid medications should be slowly tapered (Boger & Perrier, 2004).

Teach the family about the need for lifelong thyroid hormone replacement if radiation or surgery is performed. Encourage the family to adjust food intake to prevent obesity as the child's metabolic rate declines and weight gain may occur. The child should wear medical alert identification. Make sure the child is monitored regularly to ensure that the T_4 level is adequate to sustain growth.

Evaluation

Expected outcomes of nursing care for the child with hyperthyroidism include:

- The child achieves balanced thermoregulation.
- The child participates in daily activities without experiencing fatigue.
- The child demonstrates a positive body image.

■ DISORDERS OF THE PARATHYROID

Children usually have four parathyroid glands located posterior to the thyroid gland. Their primary function is to work in conjunction with vitamin D to regulate total body calcium. Ionized calcium influences release of parathyroid hormone, which acts on both bone and the kidney to maintain normal serum levels. The hormone also acts on the kidney to increase vitamin D synthesis, which assists in calcium balance. It is related as well to magnesium and phosphorus balance; low magnesium levels stimulate parathyroid hormone release and the hormone leads to lowered phosphate serum levels.

Hyperparathyroidism

Primary hyperparathyroidism, rare during childhood, is most often the result of a tumor (adenoma) that secretes the hormone without proper regulation (Doyle & DiGeorge, 2007). Secondary hyperparathyroidism is due to disease outside of the parathyroid gland, leading to excessive secretion of parathyroid hormone. This is commonly seen in chronic renal failure when the kidneys are unable to reabsorb calcium, causing low serum calcium levels and stimulating continual secretion of parathyroid hormone to maintain normal serum calcium levels (Molina, 2006). See Chapter 26 ∞ for further discussion of renal failure.

At any age, symptoms of primary hyperparathyroidism may include bone pain, nephrolithiasis (kidney stones), and pathologic bone fractures. Hypercalcemia may cause symptoms of muscle weakness, peptic ulcer disease, fatigue, volume depletion, and subtle mental disturbance. Abdominal pain may be present and may indicate pancreatitis (Potts, 2008).

There is often a delay between development of symptoms and diagnosis. Elevated serum calcium and parathyroid hormone (PTH) levels are diagnostic. Radiographic images may reveal signs of rickets. For primary hyperparathyroidism, unilateral surgical parathyroid exploration is performed to remove the affected gland and biopsy the other gland on the same side (George, Acharya, Bandgar, et al., 2010). Treatment of secondary hyperparathyroidism focuses on prevention of hypercalcemia utilizing vitamin D replacement and phosphorus binders.

Nursing Management

Nursing care centers on fluid management and electrolyte monitoring. In children who require surgery, assess for respiratory distress and a potential airway obstruction due to edema and a potential hematoma around the tracheal space. Monitor for signs of infection.

Following surgery, educate the child and parents to recognize signs of hypocalcemia and to provide appropriate amounts of calcium supplementation. After diagnosis or after surgical intervention, follow-up is important to monitor serum calcium and phosphorus levels.

Hypoparathyroidism

Primary hypoparathyroidism is rare, but it may result from congenital disorders (parathyroid aplasia, DiGeorge syndrome), surgical removal of the parathyroid glands, disease processes that destroy the parathyroid glands (Wilson disease, hemochromatosis), or medications (i.e., aluminum, asparagine, doxorubicin, cytosine, arabinoside). The primary result is hypocalcemia and hyperphosphatemia. Hypoparathyroidism can also be idiopathic.

> **Nursing Alert**
>
> Dilute intravenous calcium per hospital protocol. Infiltration of IV calcium can cause extravasation and tissue sloughing. Always check the patency of the IV prior to administration. Monitor ECG during administration. Evaluate for hypocalcemia and hypercalcemia after administration.

Infants may display hyperirritability, muscle rigidity, seizures, vomiting, abdominal distention, apneic episodes, or intermittent cyanosis or twitching. Muscle pain and cramps may progress to numbness, stiffness, and tingling of the hands and feet. A positive **Chvostek sign** (spasm of facial muscles after tapping facial nerve) reveals hyperreflexia. Life-threatening tetany and convulsions may occur with severe hypocalcemia (Doyle & DiGeorge, 2007).

Serum calcium and PTH levels are low and serum phosphorus is elevated. Radiographs often demonstrate increased bone density. A 12-lead ECG may demonstrate a prolonged QT interval. In emergencies, intravenous calcium and calcitriol are administered to treat seizures, tetany, life-threatening hypotension, and cardiac arrhythmias. Oral calcitriol and calcium are prescribed. Foods with high phosphorus content (dairy products and eggs) are limited (Doyle & DiGeorge, 2007).

Nursing Management

Assess and stabilize the airway, breathing, and circulation. In the acute care setting, children should be placed on a cardiorespiratory monitor. Maintain seizure precautions until normal serum calcium levels are attained. Obtain intravenous access and administer calcium supplementation as ordered.

Partner with the family to ensure their understanding of the need for calcium supplementation and reduced intake of phosphorus. Teach the family that periodic monitoring of calcium levels is important. Inform the family that hypoparathyroidism may require lifelong therapy.

■ DISORDERS OF ADRENAL FUNCTION

Cushing Disease

Cushing disease, also called adrenocortical hyperfunction, is characterized by a group of symptoms resulting from excess levels of glucocorticoids (especially cortisol) in the bloodstream. It is rare in children and the true incidence is unknown. During infancy, most cases of endogenous Cushing disease are due to a functioning adrenocortical tumor. The tumor is usually a malignant carcinoma; however, it may be a benign adenoma (White, 2007). Other causes include hyperplasia of one or both adrenal glands and benign tumors of the adrenal glands. The increased secretion of cortisol alters metabolism.

The initial sign in most children is gradual excessive weight gain followed by linear growth retardation, hypertension, and mental and behavioral problems. It generally takes 2 to 5 years for the child to develop the characteristic "cushingoid" appearance, which includes a moon face (chubby cheeks and a double chin) and fat pads over the shoulders and back (buffalo hump).

Clinical Tip

The most common reasons for cushingoid features in children are excessive doses of corticosteroids and prolonged use of corticosteroids as treatment for other diseases. Cushingoid features may develop in a shorter time than occurs with Cushing disease. See Figure 24–10 ∞. Corticosteroids suppress adrenal function when given long term. These children may have Cushing syndrome.

See the clinical manifestations table for signs of Cushing disease.

Diagnosis is based on characteristic physical findings and laboratory values, including increased 24-hour urinary levels of free cortisol and 17-hydroxycorticosteroid (17-OHCs), and elevated nighttime salivary cortisol level. The child has chronic hyperglycemia and an elevated hemoglobin A_{1c}. See Appendix D ∞ for expected laboratory values.

The adrenal suppression test with an 11 p.m. dose of dexamethasone reveals that adrenal cortisol output is not suppressed overnight as would occur normally in children. Computed tomography (CT) and magnetic resonance imaging (MRI) detect tumors in the adrenal and pituitary glands.

Surgical removal of the pituitary adenoma is the current treatment of choice when this is the cause of Cushing disease. Replacement glucocorticoid therapy may be needed for several months after surgery. Irradiation of the pituitary is performed when surgical removal of the adenoma does not substantially reduce cortisol levels. Alternatively, medications may be given for management of hypercortisolism by interrupting adrenal steroid synthesis.

Nursing Alert

Signs of acute adrenal insufficiency may include increased irritability, headache, confusion, restlessness, nausea and vomiting, diarrhea, abdominal pain, dehydration, fever, loss of appetite, and lethargy. If untreated, the child will go into shock. In newborns, the symptoms include failure to thrive, weakness, vomiting, and dehydration. Hyponatremia and hyperkalemia are key signs.

Lifelong glucocorticoid and mineralocorticoid replacement is required when both adrenal glands are removed. The prognosis for children with malignant adrenal tumors is poor.

Nursing Management

Nursing assessment includes monitoring the child's vital signs, fluid status, nutritional status, and weight. Additional assessment includes monitoring muscle strength and endurance during hospital play activities. Postoperative assessment includes

Clinical Manifestations

Cushing Disease

Etiology	Clinical Manifestations	Nursing Management
Catabolism of protein	Muscle weakness and wasting, capillary weakness and bruising, growth failure with delayed bone age, fatigue	Plan periods of rest for the child. Cluster nursing care. Assess skin for bruising. Assess and plot growth and development.
Decreased absorption of calcium from the intestines	Demineralization of bones, osteoporosis	Monitor serum calcium levels.
Increased appetite	Weight gain primarily on the trunk; striae on the abdomen, buttocks, thighs	Assist in meal planning. Refer to a nutritionist.
Salt retention	Increased blood volume and hypertension	Teach the family to monitor and record the child's blood pressure.

monitoring the child's vital signs and fluid and nutritional status, and assessing muscle strength and endurance during hospital play activities.

Teach the child and family about the disorder and its treatment. For children undergoing surgery, provide preoperative and postoperative teaching and care. Answer any questions the child and family may have and explain all laboratory and diagnostic tests. Explain to parents that the child's cushingoid appearance is reversible with treatment. Refer to Chapter 24 ∞ for general nursing care of the child with cancer. Provide nutritional guidance or refer the child and parents to a nutritionist to promote maintenance of an appropriate weight.

For children who need cortisol replacement therapy because both adrenal glands were surgically removed, administering the drug early in the morning mimics the normal diurnal pattern of cortisol secretion. Cortisol replacement in the postoperative period must be explained carefully to parents. Hydrocortisone (Cortef, Solu-Cortef, cortisone acetate) comes in tablet or injectable form. Parents may need to crush the tablet and mix with a small amount of applesauce, but the entire dose of medication must be taken. The oral preparations of cortisone have a bitter taste and can cause gastric irritation. Giving the dose at mealtimes and using antacids between meals helps reduce these side effects. Teach parents how and when to administer the injectable form—usually when the child is vomiting, has diarrhea, or cannot take the oral medication. Failure to give medication when the child is ill may lead to severe illness and cardiovascular collapse. See Families Want to Know: Hydrocortisone Administration.

Teach parents to be alert to signs of acute adrenal insufficiency during the withdrawal of corticosteroid therapy, and to inform all health care providers of the child's condition and medication. The child should wear medical alert identification at all times.

Congenital Adrenal Hyperplasia

Congenital adrenal hyperplasia, sometimes called adrenogenital syndrome, adrenocortical hyperplasia, or congenital adrenogenital hyperplasia, is an autosomal recessive disorder that causes a deficiency of one of the enzymes necessary for the synthesis of cortisol and aldosterone.

Families Want to Know
Hydrocortisone Administration

Teach the family the following tips regarding hydrocortisone administration:

- Always give the medication on time since the prescribed schedule follows the body's normal cortisol release pattern.
- Never abruptly discontinue the medication.
- If the child has vomiting or diarrhea and is unable to take the medication by mouth, administer the injections to replace oral doses as instructed and notify the physician immediately. Higher doses of hydrocortisone are needed when the child is ill.
- Always have injectable hydrocortisone available at home, at school, and everywhere the child travels. An emergency kit should be available at all times to supply cortisol to the child during acute illnesses and stressful situations.

Etiology and Pathophysiology

More than 90% of children with congenital adrenal hyperplasia have partial or complete 21-hydroxylase enzyme deficiency that results in inadequate production of aldosterone and cortisol. This form has an autosomal recessive inheritance pattern, and the defective gene CYP21 is located on the short arm of chromosome 6. About 5–8% of children have deficiency of 11β-hydroxylase. Mutations on defective gene CPY11B1 of chromosome 8 result in inadequate cortisol and excess levels of other steroids and testosterone synthesis (Henwood & Katz, 2005). The remaining 2–5% of cases involve deficiencies of other enzymes. Congenital adrenal hyperplasia occurs in 1 in 10,000–15,000 live births (Kwon & Tsai, 2007).

Of the two classic forms of the disorder, 75% are salt losing, caused by aldosterone deficiency, and 25% are non–salt losing with **virilization** (the production of masculine secondary sexual characteristics in females). In all forms, increased secretion of ACTH occurs in response to diminished cortisol levels (Kwon & Tsai, 2007).

During fetal development, the lack of cortisol triggers the pituitary to continue secretion of ACTH. This stimulates overproduction of the adrenal androgens. Virilization of the female external genitalia begins in week 10 of gestation. If untreated after birth, the overproduction of androgens results in accelerated height, early closure of the epiphyseal plates, and premature sexual development with both pubic and axillary hair.

Clinical Manifestations

Congenital adrenal hyperplasia is the most common cause of **pseudohermaphroditism** (ambiguous genitalia) in newborn girls. The female infant is born with an enlarged clitoris and partial or complete labial fusions. The vagina usually has a common opening with the urethra (Figure 30–6 ►). Females who are severely virilized may be mistaken for males with cryptorchidism, hypospadias, or micropenis. The uterus, ovaries, and fallopian tubes are normal. The male infant may look normal at birth or may have a slightly enlarged penis and hyperpigmented scrotum. The male may have tall stature and an adult-sized penis by

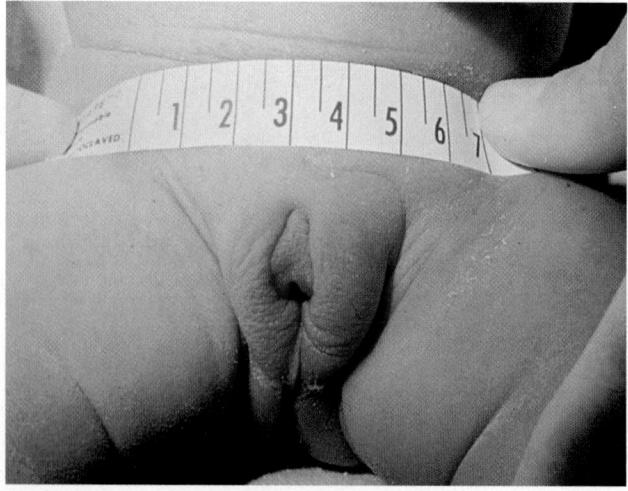

FIGURE 30–6 ► Newborn girl with ambiguous genitalia.
Courtesy of Patrick C. Walsh, MD.

school age, but the testes are appropriately sized for age. Partial enzyme deficiency produces less obvious symptoms. Precocious puberty, tall stature for age, acne, and excessive muscle development may be noted in both males and females as the child grows. Females may have irregular periods. Due to early epiphyseal fusion, adult stature is shorter.

Signs of adrenal insufficiency may be the first indication of the disorder. Recurrent vomiting, dehydration, metabolic acidosis, hypotension, and hypoglycemia are characteristic signs of the salt-wasting form of the disorder. Hypertension with hypokalemic alkalosis is alternately found in children with 11-hydroxylase deficiency.

COLLABORATIVE CARE

Diagnostic Tests

Diagnosis in infants and children is usually confirmed by laboratory evaluation of serum 17-hydroxyprogesterone (17-OHP) level. Routine newborn screening for congenital adrenal hyperplasia is performed in all 50 states (National Newborn Screening and Genetics Resource Center, 2009). Prenatal diagnosis is available. In instances of ambiguous genitalia, a **karyotype** (a microscopic chromosome study in which the 46 chromosomes of the child are lined up in pairs from largest to smallest to detect errors in chromosome number, shape, and size) determines the infant's gender. Ultrasonography may be used to visualize pelvic structures.

In the salt-wasting form of the disorder, the child may have hyponatremia, hyperkalemia, acidosis, hypoglycemia, a high urine sodium level, and low serum and urinary aldosterone levels. Serum concentrations of testosterone in girls and androstenedione in boys and girls are elevated in affected infants. Measurement of ACTH and 17-OHP levels reveal high readings, while serum cortisol is inappropriately low in comparison to ACTH (White, 2007). Diagnosis may be delayed in the non-salt-losing form until 3 to 7 years.

Clinical Therapy

The goal of treatment is to suppress adrenal secretion of androgens by replacing deficient hormones. Antenatal steroids (dexamethasone) have been shown to reduce the severity of genital masculinization in females with congenital adrenal hyperplasia. Continued use of dexamethasone in the postnatal period has been shown to be effective as well (Kulshreshtha, Khadgawat, Eunice, et al., in press). Treatment of affected children is accomplished by the lifelong use of oral glucocorticoids (dexamethasone, prednisone, or hydrocortisone). The glucocorticoid replacement reduces secretion of ACTH, which had overstimulated the adrenal cortex. As a result, excessive adrenal androgen production is suppressed. The dose is individualized by monitoring growth parameters, bone age, and hormone levels. If the infant has the salt-wasting form of the disorder, salt is added to the infant's formula and a mineralocorticoid (Florinef) is given to replace the missing hormone. Hormone dosage must be *doubled* or *tripled* during acute illnesses or injury and for surgery. Adrenalectomy may be recommended in cases when medical therapy is ineffective (White, 2007).

Reconstructive surgery of the enlarged clitoris is often performed on girls during the first year of life; however, some centers support waiting until adolescence, allowing the patient to participate in the decision for surgery.

NURSING MANAGEMENT
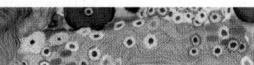

Nursing Assessment and Diagnosis

Assess the infant and child for signs of dehydration, electrolyte imbalance, and hypovolemic shock in the salt-wasting form of the disease. Monitor the airway, breathing, circulation, and responsiveness. Assess vital signs and assess peripheral perfusion (capillary refill, distal pulses, color and temperature of the extremities) frequently to detect early changes in condition such as hypovolemia.

Assess the parents' emotional response to a child with ambiguous genitalia and a chronic condition. Explore their values and beliefs regarding gender roles and sexuality while awaiting results of the karyotype.

Nursing diagnoses for the child with congenital adrenal hyperplasia might include:

- Impaired Parenting related to a child with undetermined gender identity
- Caregiver Role Strain related to care of a child with a chronic, potentially life-threatening condition
- Risk for Deficient Fluid Volume related to failure of regulatory mechanisms and excess excretion of salt by the kidneys
- Risk for Disproportionate Growth related to accelerated growth and premature closure of epiphyseal plates

Planning and Implementation

Nursing care of the newborn with congenital adrenal hyperplasia focuses on teaching parents about the disorder and its treatment, providing emotional support, and preoperative and postoperative teaching for parents of infants undergoing reconstructive surgery. The administration of glucocorticoids and mineralocorticoids must be carefully controlled.

It is often difficult for parents to accept that their infant, whose genitalia look male, is really female. Reassure parents that with medication and surgery the genitalia assume a female appearance and all organs necessary for future childbearing are usually functional. Several surgeries may be performed before 2 years of age and then during adolescence to dilate the vagina. Because of the risk for adrenal insufficiency, the child will most likely be hospitalized for surgery rather than having outpatient surgery.

Nurses can assist parents in educating the child's siblings, grandparents, other family members, and childcare workers about the condition. In the newborn nursery, the infant should be referred to as "your beautiful infant," not "your son" or "your daughter," until gender identity is confirmed.

Inform parents that genetic counseling should be provided for the child during adolescence. Parents considering a future pregnancy should also be informed that prenatal testing may detect congenital adrenal hyperplasia in the fetus. Refer the family for counseling, if indicated.

Care in the Community

Teach parents about the special problems that develop in the salt-wasting form of the disease during acute illness. Explain the medication regimen and help the family develop an emergency care plan. The child should wear medical alert identification. Teach parents how to administer intramuscular injections of hydrocortisone (see page 1002). If injectable hydrocortisone is not available, the child needs urgent treatment in an emergency department. The child may become dehydrated quickly and need intravenous fluid and electrolyte replacement in addition to higher doses of hydrocortisone.

An individualized health plan should be developed to inform the school nurse and teachers about the special care needed if the child becomes ill at school. Injectable hydrocortisone should be kept at the school for emergency use.

Evaluation

Expected outcomes of nursing care for congenital adrenal hyperplasia include:

- Parents learn to give glucocorticoids appropriately when the child is ill and prevent episodes of adrenal crisis.
- Families effectively cope with the virilized appearance of the child's genitalia and bond with the child.

Adrenal Insufficiency (Addison Disease)

Adrenal insufficiency, also known as Addison disease, is a rare disorder in childhood characterized by a deficiency of glucocorticoids (cortisone), mineralocorticoids (aldosterone), and adrenal androgens. The lack of glucocorticoids affects the body's ability to handle stress. The majority of cases are caused by an autoimmune process, but it also may be acquired after infection, metabolic disease, and metastatic disease (Antal & Zhou, 2009).

Adrenal insufficiency usually develops slowly as the adrenal glands deteriorate. The early signs may not be noticed but include weakness with fatigue, lethargy and emotional lability, anorexia and salt craving, and poor weight gain or weight loss. Skin changes include hyperpigmentation at pressure points, lip borders, gingival margins, nipples, palms, soles, body creases, and scarred areas of the body, and generalized bronzing of the skin or freckling without tan lines, even in winter months. Additional signs include abdominal pain, nausea, vomiting, diarrhea, and symptomatic hypoglycemia. If the child experiences a stressful period (illness, injury, or surgery), acute adrenal insufficiency may occur. Signs of an adrenal crisis include weakness, fever, abdominal pain, hypoglycemia with seizures, hypotension, dehydration, shock, and coma.

Serum cortisol and urinary 17-hydroxycorticoid levels are measured in the early morning. Low levels of serum cortisol are associated with adrenal insufficiency. The ACTH stimulation test is used to detect adrenal gland reserve. Electrolyte values generally reveal low serum sodium, elevated serum potassium, and low fasting blood glucose levels. Computed tomography may be used to visualize the adrenal glands.

Treatment involves replacement of the deficient hormones. Oral hydrocortisone is given in the lowest therapeutic dose to control symptoms and promote normal growth. Fludrocortisone acetate (Florinef) replaces the missing mineralocorticoid in children with aldosterone deficiency. Adrenal crisis is treated by aggressive fluid resuscitation, intravenous glucose, and intravenous hydrocortisone. The precipitating illness or injury is then treated along with adequate doses of glucocorticoid, and maintenance doses of mineralocorticoid. Children will also need increased doses of steroids during periods of increased physiologic stress, such as surgical procedures, illnesses, and injuries. In these cases, the dose of hydrocortisone should be doubled or tripled and continued for 24–48 hours or for as long as the stress lasts before resuming the maintenance dose. Injectable hydrocortisone should always be available in case the child is vomiting or unable to take oral fluids (Antal & Zhou, 2009).

Nursing Management

Nursing management focuses on educating the child and parents about the disorder, providing emotional support, and caring for the child during acute episodes. See the earlier discussion of congenital adrenal hyperplasia for further details.

Pheochromocytoma

Pheochromocytoma is a tumor of the adrenal gland, but it may be extra-adrenal with no anatomic connection. In most cases, these tumors are benign and curable. They can occur in a familial pattern (autosomal dominant trait) with a 3:2 male to female ratio. Most tumors diagnosed in children are identified between the ages of 6 and 14 years; however, this only accounts for 10% of these tumors as most are identified during adult years (White, 2007). Pheochromocytomas may also be associated with neurofibromatosis. See Chapter 27 ∞.

The tumor causes an excessive release of the catecholamines epinephrine and norepinephrine, leading to hypertension. Clinical manifestations include episodes of severe hypertension, palpitations, profuse sweating, and headache. Because release of catecholamines (norepinephrine and epinephrine) from the tumor is not continuous, these symptoms occur intermittently (Cook, 2009).

Diagnosis is based on 24-hour urine studies to detect the presence of increased urinary catecholamines and vanillylmandelic acid (VMA) levels. Radiologic imaging with CT, positron emission tomography (PET) scan, MRI, and ultrasound studies are required to locate the tumor in preparation for surgery. Most are located on the adrenal gland, but they may also be located in the chest, abdomen, pelvis, head, and neck (Karagiannis, Mikhailidis, Athyros, et al., 2007).

The treatment of choice is curative surgical removal of all identified tumors; however, the procedure may precipitate a pheochromocytoma crisis, so preventive treatment is provided. Alpha- and beta-adrenergic blocking agents to control hypertension, tachycardia, and catecholamine release are given for 10 to 14 days before surgery (Karagiannis et al., 2007). Plasma catecholamines are used to measure the effectiveness of the preoperative adrenergic blockade. Postoperatively, for several days, a 24-hour urine collection is measured for catecholamines to determine if all tumor sites were removed. With successful removal of all tumor sites, the prognosis is generally good. Follow-up is important to assess for recurrence.

Nursing Management

Nursing care is mainly supportive. Provide preoperative and postoperative teaching and care (see Chapter 13 ∞). Preoperatively, monitor vital signs and observe for signs of complications associated with pheochromocytoma crisis. Administer antihypertensives and watch for any signs of hyperglycemia (see page 1017). Postoperatively, the child may be managed initially in an intensive care unit. Monitor blood pressure and glucose levels. Hypoglycemia and hypotension may occur following the withdrawal of excessive amounts of catecholamines. Observe for changes in neurologic status, respiratory distress, and signs of shock. Lifelong follow-up care with screening for hypertension and increased urinary catecholamine levels is required as symptoms recur if the child has other tumors not yet detected that activate at a later age (White, 2007).

■ DISORDERS OF PANCREATIC FUNCTION

Diabetes Mellitus

Diabetes mellitus, the most common metabolic disease in children, is a disorder of hyperglycemia resulting from defects in insulin secretion, insulin action, or both, leading to abnormalities in carbohydrate, protein, and fat metabolism (American Diabetes Association, 2008a). There are two main types of diabetes. Most children have immune-mediated type 1 diabetes, formerly called insulin-dependent diabetes mellitus or juvenile diabetes. However, a disturbingly large number of children are being diagnosed with type 2 diabetes, formerly called noninsulin-dependent diabetes (Alemzadeh & Wyatt, 2007).

Type 1 Diabetes

In the United States, approximately 1 in every 400–600 children and adolescents have type 1 diabetes (American Diabetes Association, 2008b). Peak incidence of onset in childhood is from 7–15 years of age; however, type 1 diabetes can present at any age (Alemzadeh & Wyatt, 2007). Caucasians experience a higher incidence of type 1 diabetes than other racial groups. Boys and girls are equally affected.

Etiology and Pathophysiology Type 1 diabetes results from destruction of pancreatic islet beta cells, which fail to secrete insulin. The body becomes dependent on exogenous sources of insulin. Type 1 diabetes is a multifactorial disease caused by autoimmune destruction of insulin-producing pancreatic beta cells in individuals who are genetically predisposed (American Diabetes Association, 2008a). Type 1 diabetes has familial tendencies but does not show any specific pattern of inheritance. Inheritance of the DR3 and DR4 markers on the human leukocyte antigen (HLA) complex on chromosome 6 increases the likelihood of developing type 1 diabetes. If the child inherits one marker, the child's risk is two to three times higher. If both markers are inherited, the child's risk is 7 to 10 times higher (Alemzadeh & Wyatt, 2007). However, the child inherits a susceptibility to the disease rather than the disease itself. It is believed that an event such as a virus triggers the inflammatory process, resulting in development of islet cell serum antibodies. These antibodies can be detected in the blood months to years before development of the clinical symptoms (Cooke & Plotnick, 2008a).

Insulin helps transport glucose into the cells so that the body can use it as an energy source. It also prevents the outflow of glucose from the liver to the general circulation. It is hypothesized that type 1 diabetes may be caused by a genetic component, environmental influences, or an autoimmune response that damages the pancreatic beta cells (Alemzadeh & Wyatt, 2007). Environmental factors such as enteroviruses or toxins are believed to lead to an autoimmune destruction of the beta cells in the islets of Langerhans (Figure 30–7 ➤). Antigens are generated that lead to production of antibodies that indicate ongoing destruction of the islet cells. As the destruction continues, insulin secretion decreases. It is estimated that at least 80% of the beta cells are destroyed before the onset of clinical symptoms of diabetes (Cooke & Plotnick, 2008a).

As the secretion of insulin decreases, the blood glucose level rises and the glucose level inside the cells decreases. When the renal threshold for glucose (180 mg/dL) is exceeded, **glycosuria** (abnormal amount of glucose in the urine) occurs as a result of osmotic diuresis (Alemzadeh & Wyatt, 2007). Fluids follow the highly osmotic glucose, and water is excreted in large volumes (polyuria).

When glucose is unavailable to the cells for metabolism, free fatty acids provide an alternate source of energy. The liver metabolizes fatty acids at an increased rate, producing acetyl coenzyme A (CoA). The by-products of acetyl CoA metabolism (ketone bodies) accumulate in the body, resulting in a state of metabolic acidosis, or ketoacidosis. (Refer to Chapter 18 ∞ for discussion of metabolic acidosis.)

Clinical Manifestations The classic signs of type 1 diabetes are polyuria, polydipsia, and **polyphagia** (excessive appetite) with significant weight loss. See the accompanying Clinical Manifestations: Diabetes by Type table. Other signs include unexplained fatigue or lethargy, headaches, and stomachaches. Enuresis may also occur in a previously toilet-trained child. Adolescent girls may have vaginitis caused by *Candida*, which thrives in the hyperglycemic tissues. Symptoms develop gradually and insidiously but have usually been present less than a month when diagnosed. Approximately 29% of patients with new-onset type 1 diabetes are ill with diabetic ketoacidosis (DKA), a type of metabolic acidosis (Rewers, Klingensmith, Davis, et al., 2008). See page 1015 for more information on DKA. See Box 30–1 for information about cystic fibrosis–related diabetes.

COLLABORATIVE CARE

Diagnostic Tests

Diagnosis is based on the presence of classic symptoms, a hemoglobin A_{1c} greater than or equal to 6.5% and one of the following plasma glucose levels (American Diabetes Association, 2010a, p. S13):

- Fasting plasma glucose greater than or equal to 126 mg/dL (7 mmol/L), no caloric intake for at least 8 hours

Pathophysiology Illustrated
Mechanism of Diabetes Mellitus

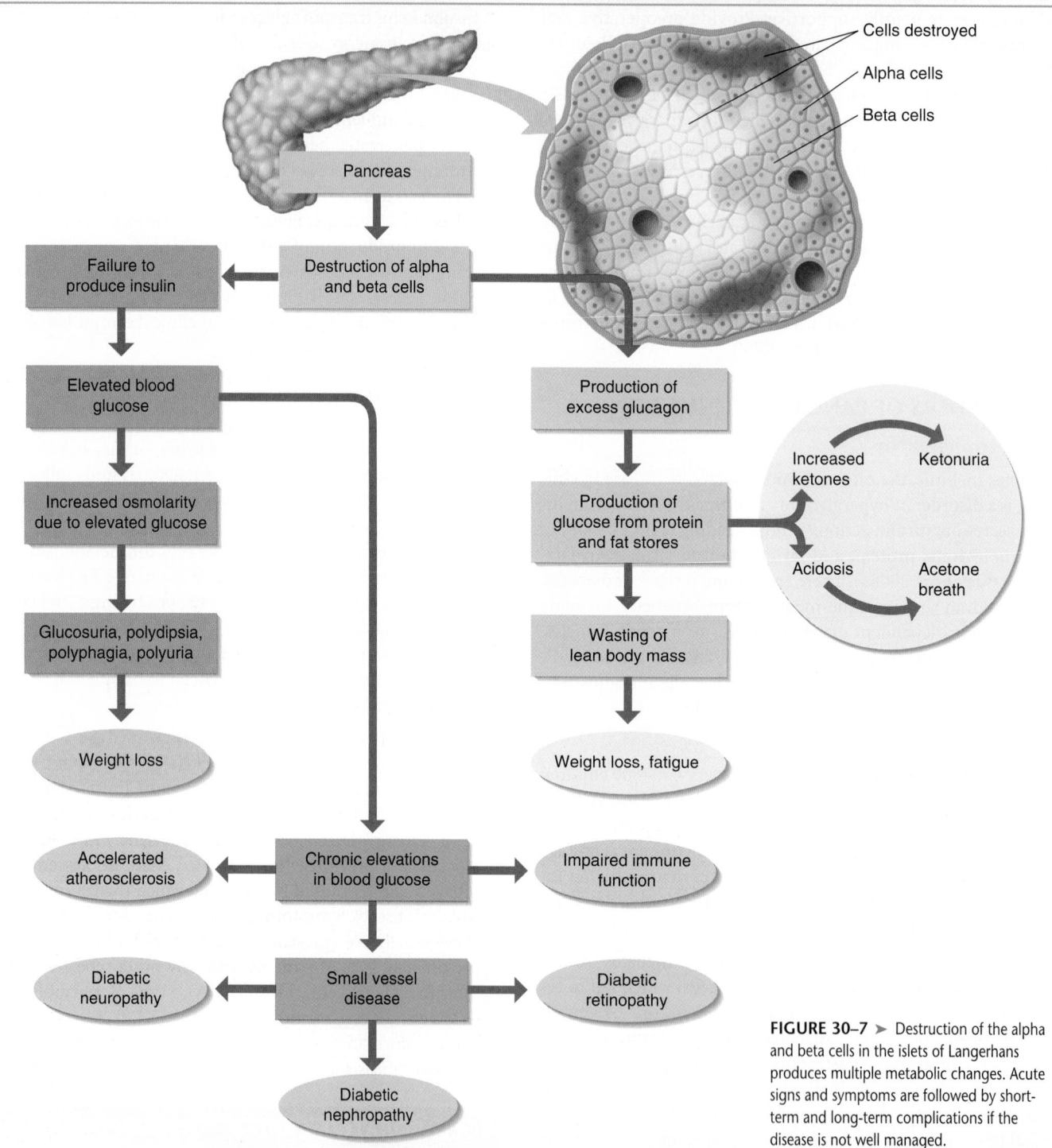

FIGURE 30–7 ➤ Destruction of the alpha and beta cells in the islets of Langerhans produces multiple metabolic changes. Acute signs and symptoms are followed by short-term and long-term complications if the disease is not well managed.

- Two-hour plasma glucose greater than or equal to 200 mg/dL (11.1 mmol/L) during an oral glucose tolerance test
- Random plasma glucose concentration greater than or equal to 200 mg/dL (11.1 mmol/L)

When an asymptomatic child's screening test reveals an elevated glucose level, confirmation of a second fasting plasma glucose level should be performed. An oral glucose tolerance test is rarely required. Other laboratory tests for known autoantibodies can indicate an autoimmune attack against the insulin-producing beta cells of the pancreas, and may be helpful in some cases to distinguish between type 1 and type 2 diabetes. Plasma c-peptide levels and fasting insulin levels will be low in type 1 diabetes (Berry, Urban, & Grey, 2006a).

Clinical Manifestations
Diabetes by Type

Cause	Clinical Manifestations	Clinical Therapy
Type 1—immune-mediated, insulin deficiency due to pancreatic beta-cell destruction	Polyuria, polydipsia May have polyphagia Weight loss Ketoacidosis on initial presentation in approximately 30% of cases, at continued risk for ketoacidosis Short duration of symptoms Ketosis Initial period of decreased insulin requirement, then need insulin for survival	Blood glucose monitoring Insulin Dietary management, balancing carbohydrate intake to insulin Exercise
Type 2—insulin resistance with relative insulin secretory defect	Obese, little or no weight loss, or may have significant recent weight loss Acanthosis nigricans Long duration of symptoms Polyuria, polydipsia, may be mild or absent Glycosuria without ketonuria in 33% of cases on initial presentation Ketoacidosis may be present Lipid disorders Hypertension Androgen-mediated problems such as acne, hirsutism, menstrual disturbances, polycystic ovary disease Fatigue due to insulin resistance	Diet with decreased calories and low-fat foods Decrease sedentary activity time or increase routine physical activity Blood glucose monitoring Oral medication (metformin) to improve insulin sensitivity May need insulin initially

Clinical Therapy

Clinical therapy for type 1 diabetes focuses on glycemic control by combining insulin, nutrition management to support growth and maintain blood glucose at near normal levels, an exercise regimen, and psychosocial support.

Insulin Therapy   Multiple approaches to insulin therapy for children and adolescents are available, and an approach that works for the child and family should be selected.

Children often need several daily injections of insulin before meals and at bedtime to maintain an optimal blood glucose level. Several forms of insulin are available as identified in the accompanying Medications table.

BOX 30–1   Cystic Fibrosis–Related Diabetes

Cystic fibrosis–related diabetes (CFRD) has features similar to those of types 1 and 2 diabetes; however, it is considered a separate condition. In cystic fibrosis, the pancreas does not produce sufficient insulin (as in type 1 diabetes), which is referred to as **insulin deficiency**. Another mechanism of CFRD is **insulin resistance**, an impairment in insulin receptors on cell membranes, leading to inability to transfer sufficient amounts of glucose into cells, requiring higher levels of insulin for metabolism. Insulin deficiency and insulin resistance combined can lead to the development of diabetes more frequently in patients with cystic fibrosis than in the general population (Cystic Fibrosis Foundation, 2009).

Clinical Tip

Insulin is usually provided in prepackaged doses of 100 units/mL. Diluted insulin prepared by a pharmacist may be used for infants and toddlers who require a small insulin dosage. Insulin cartridges, disposable pens, and other devices are available, making insulin easy to carry by adolescents for frequent insulin injections during the day.

Basal-bolus insulin regimens have resulted in improved glycemic control in the pediatric population (American Diabetes Association, 2010a). Insulin can be administered by an insulin pump or by multiple daily injections. When multiple injections are used, basal insulin is administered once a day using a very long-acting insulin. A bolus of rapid-acting insulin is administered with each meal and snack based on the carbohydrate grams consumed and the blood glucose level. This means that a child may get 6 to 7 injections a day. Stress, infection, and illness may either increase or decrease insulin needs. If basal-bolus therapy for type 1 diabetes is to be effective, the child and family need to do each of the following:

- Monitor the blood glucose appropriately to establish insulin requirements. For example, test glucose before and 2 hours following meals, as well as once a week at midnight and 3 a.m.
- Count carbohydrates consumed
- Anticipate exercise in the daily routine.

Medications Used to Treat
Type 1 Diabetes Mellitus and Average Insulin Action Times (Subcutaneous Route)

Type	Onset	Peak	Duration	Action
Rapid Acting Insulin lispro, insulin glulisine, or insulin aspart	10–30 min	0.5–1.5 hr	3–5 hr	Insulin is an endogenous hormone, secreted by the beta cells of the pancreas. It lowers the blood glucose level by stimulating glucose passage across cell membranes and uptake into the cells. It also promotes the conversion of glucose to glycogen and inhibits hepatic glucose production from glycogen.
Short Acting Regular	0.5–1 hr	2–5 hr	5–8 hr	
Very Long Acting Glargine or detemir	1–2 hr	None	Up to 24 hr	

Source: Data from: Fleury-Milfort, E. (2008). Insulin replacement therapy: Minimizing complications and side effects. Advance for Nurse Practitioners, 16 (11), 32–39; Wright, E. E. (2009). Overview of insulin replacement therapy. Journal of Family Practice, 58 (8), S3–S9; Miles, H. L., & Acerini, C. L. (2008). Insulin analog preparations and their use in children and adolescents with type 1 diabetes mellitus. Pediatric Drugs, 10 (3), 163–176.

Clinical Tip

Advantages of rapid-acting insulin in therapy to achieve tight glucose control include:

- Decreased number of nocturnal hypoglycemic episodes
- Matching the insulin to the actual food intake of an infant or toddler (very helpful when their food intake is unpredictable)
- Flexibility in timing and amounts of meals and snacks to address variable appetites

Continuous subcutaneous insulin infusion (CSII) pump therapy is increasingly used by children and adolescents as the technology makes it possible to more closely match the plasma insulin levels in children who do not have diabetes. CSII pump therapy has been used successfully in children of all ages and has been found to improve glycemic control in the pediatric population (Berhe, Postellon, Wilson, et al., 2006; Nimri, Weintrob, Benzaquen, et al., 2006). Advantages and disadvantages of an insulin pump are outlined in Table 30–4.

The goal of insulin therapy is to maintain blood glucose levels as near normal as possible, while avoiding episodes of severe hypoglycemia. Glycemic goals for children younger than 6 years are generally less tight since they lack the cognitive capacity to recognize and respond to hypoglycemic symptoms (Berhe et al., 2006).

Insulin therapy is evaluated every 3 months with a hemoglobin A_{1c} (HbA$_{1c}$) level, an objective measurement of glycemic control. It represents the amount of glucose that binds to the hemoglobin molecule, predicting average glucose concentration over the prior 2 months (Cooke & Plotnick, 2008a). See Table 30–5 for the HbA$_{1c}$ goals for children of different ages. It is also important to determine if the HbA$_{1c}$ matches recorded blood sugars.

Nutrition Therapy The goal of nutrition therapy is to provide adequate calories for the child's normal growth and development. An evaluation of the child's food intake, metabolic status, and lifestyle is necessary before establishing a nutrition plan. Daily caloric requirements are individualized for each child according to need. To facilitate adherence to the nutritional plan, an individualized approach with considerations of the child and family's culture, lifestyle, and financial means should be incorporated. Careful instruction by a nutritionist is essential in the management of diabetes.

Carbohydrate counting provides flexibility in meal planning and is simple for children and adolescents to use. One carbohydrate choice equals 15 grams of carbohydrates. The number of carbohydrate choices needed at meals and snacks vary depending on the child's individualized nutrition plan. Generally, one unit of insulin covers 15 grams of carbohydrates, making insulin dosage calculation for meal coverage relatively easy; however, a different ratio of insulin to carbohydrates may be calculated for individual children. If additional carbohydrates are eaten at a meal or snack, the number of insulin units can be adjusted, providing further flexibility. A high-fiber diet is also recommended for improved control of blood glucose.

Exercise Program Physical activity is associated with increased insulin sensitivity. Regular exercise and fitness improves glucose control, reduces cardiovascular risk factors, contributes to weight loss, and improves overall well-being. Blood lipid levels are also positively affected. However, the child must have an adequate caloric intake to prevent hypoglycemia. Excessive exercise associated with sports requires careful planning and management.

Complications Complications of type 1 diabetes (retinopathy, heart disease, renal failure, and peripheral vascular disease) result from long-term hyperglycemic effects on the blood vessels. Without careful management, children with diabetes may develop renal failure and loss of vision in adulthood. Intensive therapy is expected to reduce the risk for or delay the development of these complications. Risk may be further reduced if the adolescent does not begin smoking and if the blood pressure is controlled.

TABLE 30–4 Advantages and Disadvantages of an Insulin Infusion Pump	
Advantages	Disadvantages
• Delivers a continuous infusion of insulin to match the basal rate needed plus an insulin bolus at mealtime to more closely simulate normal pancreatic function • Helps maintain blood glucose control between meals • Decreases HbA_{1c} level • Improves glycemic control • Improves growth in children • Reduces number of injections • New pumps calculate bolus insulin dose to carbohydrates consumed • Allows child to eat with less adherence to a schedule and have a more flexible lifestyle • Reduces number of injection sites, so variation in absorption decreases • Fewer incidents of diabetic ketoacidosis	• Requires highly motivated child and supportive parents and health care professionals • Requires willingness to live connected to a device (can be disconnected for short periods by removing or clamping the catheter; however, DKA can occur within hours of interruption of insulin flow) • The site must be changed every 2–4 days, at least 1 inch from the last site; involves changing syringe, catheter, and skin setup • Infections can occur at the injection site • Must still monitor blood glucose levels and carbohydrates consumed • Weight gain is common when blood glucose control improves • Cost • Risk of DKA secondary to pump failure

Source: Data from: Eugster, E. A., Francis, G., & Lawson-Wilkins Drug and Therapeutics Committee. (2006). Position statement: Continuous subcutaneous insulin infusion in very young children with type 1 diabetes. Pediatrics, 118(4), 1244–1249; Nimri, R., Weintrob, H. B., Benzaquen, H., Ofan, R., Fayman, G., & Phillip, M. (2006). Insulin pump therapy in youth with type 1 diabetes: A retrospective paired study. Pediatrics, 117(6), 2126–2131; Wood, J. R., Moreland, E. C., Volkening, L. K., Svoren, B. M., Butler, D. A., & Laffel, L. M. B. (2006). Durability of insulin pump use in pediatric patients with type 1 diabetes. Diabetes Care, 29(11), 2355–2360.

TABLE 30–5 Goals for Blood Glucose and Hemoglobin A_{1c} by Age of the Child			
	Blood Glucose Goals		
Age	Before Meals	Bedtime/Overnight	Hemoglobin A_{1c}
Children under 6 years	100 to 180 mg/dL	110 to 200 mg/dL	Less than 8.5% (but greater than 7.5%)
Children 6 to 12 years	90 to 180 mg/dL	100 to 180 mg/dL	Less than 8%
Adolescents 13 to 19 years	90 to 130 mg/dL	90 to 150 mg/dL	Less than 7.5%

Data from: American Diabetes Association. (2010a). Standards of medical care in diabetes—2010. Diabetes Care, 33(Suppl. 1), S11–S61.

NURSING MANAGEMENT

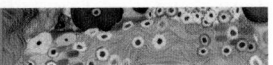

Nursing Assessment and Diagnosis

Nursing assessment focuses on a physiologic assessment of the child, but also on collecting the environmental, developmental, and psychosocial information that is needed to develop a nursing care plan for the family's management of a chronic illness.

Physiologic Assessment

Children are generally admitted to the hospital at the time of diagnosis. Assess the child's physiologic status, focusing on vital signs and level of consciousness. Assess hydration by checking mucous membranes, skin turgor, and urine output. Blood initially is collected hourly to monitor blood gases, glucose, and electrolytes. The frequency of blood collections will depend on whether the child is in diabetic ketoacidosis and the time of the diagnosis. Once the child is stable, assess dietary and caloric intake and the ability of the child or family to manage care.

Psychosocial Assessment

Parents may feel guilty at the time of diagnosis if they waited to seek care until the child began to experience symptoms of diabetic ketoacidosis. Assess coping mechanisms, family strengths and resources, ability to manage the disease, and educational needs of both the child and parents. Identify family stressors that will cause challenges in long-term diabetes management. Examples of questions to use in assessing the family's strengths and limitations in the child's disease management include:

- Do both parents or the single parent work? What hours?
- Besides the parent(s), who is involved in the child's care?
- What is the child's usual daily schedule? Does the schedule vary on the weekend or any other days of the week?
- Does the child have health insurance? What coverage exists for diabetes education, treatment, and home management?
- Does the child have any cognitive, behavioral, motor, or visual problems coexisting with this condition?
- What other family stressors coexist with the diagnosis?

Developmental Assessment

Assess the child's developmental level, particularly fine motor skills and cognitive level. The child will need to learn how to obtain and read a blood glucose sample or inject insulin. Children can usually perform some of these tasks with supervision by 6 to 8 years of age.

Adolescents often perceive type 1 diabetes as a disability and may deny having the disease so they can be like their peers when eating and exercising. Talk with the adolescent and assess problem-solving skills associated with daily condition management, and the ability to manage special circumstances such as illness or changes in exercise. Self-management is the eventual goal, and the child's responsibilities are gradually increased.

Several diagnoses that may apply to the child newly diagnosed with type 1 diabetes are provided in the accompanying Nursing Care Plan. Additional diagnoses that may be appropriate include the following:

- Risk for Deficient Fluid Volume related to active fluid loss associated with hyperglycemia
- Ineffective Breathing Pattern related to neuromuscular dysfunction associated with metabolic acidosis
- Ineffective Coping related to inability to admit impact of disease on lifestyle

Planning and Implementation

Nursing care focuses on teaching the child and parents about the disease and its management, planning dietary intake, providing emotional support, and planning strategies for daily management in the community. Refer to the accompanying Nursing Care Plan, which summarizes nursing care for the child who is hospitalized with newly diagnosed type 1 diabetes. Some hospitals have developed clinical pathways to streamline and standardize diabetes care.

Provide Education

The nurse is an important member of the management team and is usually responsible for educating the child and family. The majority of teaching may be performed by an advanced practice nurse or a certified diabetes nurse educator in the clinic setting, since children may be hospitalized only briefly following diagnosis. Other members of the management team include the physician, nutritionist, and social worker.

The timing and amount of information provided are especially important in the first days following diagnosis. Both the child and parents are very tired, and they are often in a state of shock and disbelief. Information presented during this period needs to be repeated. This time should be used to assess learning needs and to answer the family's questions. Initial teaching focuses on the survival skills necessary for home management, including insulin administration, blood glucose testing, record keeping, meal planning, and the recognition and treatment of both hypoglycemia and hyperglycemia (Habich, 2006).

Explain the goals of insulin therapy. Teach the parents and child (if appropriate) how to draw up and administer insulin and to perform blood glucose tests. Rotating the injection sites is important to decrease the chances of *lipoatrophy*, loss of subcutaneous tissue, or hypertrophy, in which collagen is replaced by fat cells (Figure 30–8 ➤). The absorption rate of insulin varies by the site used. Insulin is usually absorbed most rapidly from the abdomen; however, insulin absorption is increased in the extremities with exercise. An understanding of the different types of insulin and their actions is essential.

Once the child and parents demonstrate understanding of this information, teach guidelines for recognizing and managing episodes of hyperglycemia during acute illness and using an in-

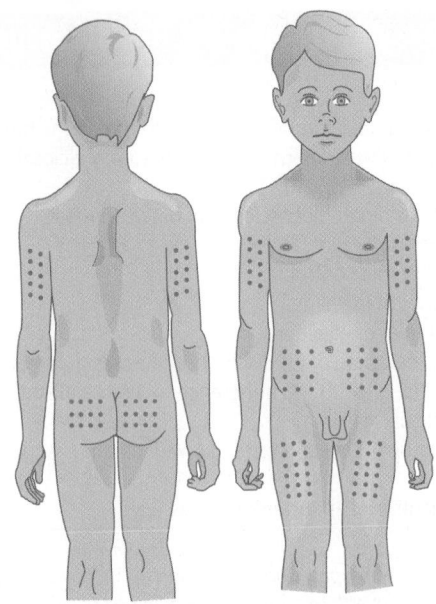

FIGURE 30–8 ➤ Insulin injection sites. Give all morning insulin in one site (e.g., arms) and all evening insulin in another (e.g., legs) because of different rates of absorption from these sites. Space injections about 1/2 inch (1.25 cm) apart.

sulin correction scale. A correction scale indicates specific insulin dosages appropriate for a particular blood glucose level. The family also needs to learn "sick day" care guidelines to prevent diabetic ketoacidosis. (See Families Want to Know: Teaching About Sick Day Guidelines.)

Caution parents to check the blood glucose level of a toddler who is extremely sleepy or irritable, as these can be signs of either hypoglycemia or hyperglycemia.

Support Nutrition Adherence

While no specific meal plan is recommended for children with diabetes, 50% of their calories should be carbohydrates, 10–20% of their calories should be protein, and 30% of their calories should be fat (American Academy of Pediatrics, 2009). The child

---

Families Want to Know
Teaching About Sick Day Guidelines

When the child with diabetes is sick, parents need to be extra attentive to the child's glycemic control. The following recommendations should be followed (Doyle & Grey, 2010):

- Seek medical attention for fever or other signs of infection.
- Monitor the blood glucose levels more often than routine (every 1 to 4 hours).
- Test urine ketones when the blood glucose level is greater than 200 mg/dL.
- The usual dose of insulin may be increased for high blood glucose levels.
- Do not skip doses of insulin.
- Maintain hydration. A large fluid intake is essential if the child cannot eat as usual. Fluids should have carbohydrates to maintain the child's usual caloric intake. If the child cannot consume adequate amounts of fluids, seek medical attention.

NURSING CARE PLAN

The Child Hospitalized with Newly Diagnosed Type 1 Diabetes Mellitus

INTERVENTION	RATIONALE	EXPECTED OUTCOME
1. Nursing Diagnosis: Deficient Knowledge (Survival Skills) related to lack of exposure to diabetic management in the newly diagnosed child		
NIC Priority Intervention: *Teaching, individual:* Planning, implementing, and evaluating a teaching program designed to address a patient's particular need		**NOC Suggested Outcome:** *Knowledge:* Extent of understanding conveyed about diabetic treatment regimen
Goal: The child and parents will acquire survival skills for home management.		
▪ Assess the child's developmental level and select an educational approach and self-care activities to match.	▪ Learning goals for the child must match knowledge and skill expectations appropriate for developmental stage.	The child and parents demonstrate proper technique for blood glucose monitoring, urine testing for ketones, drawing up and injecting insulin doses, survival food guidelines, and record keeping.
▪ Teach blood glucose monitoring, drawing up and injecting insulin, urine testing for ketones, record keeping, survival food guidelines, and when to call the health care provider.	▪ Diabetic management survival skills are needed for initial home management until more extensive education can be completed that permits more independent management.	
▪ Use demonstration/return demonstration until the child and family are comfortable with procedures.	▪ Return demonstration permits evaluation, positive reinforcement, and guidance for modification of techniques.	
Goal: The child and parents will recognize signs and symptoms of hypoglycemia and hyperglycemia.		
▪ Teach signs and symptoms of hypoglycemic and hyperglycemic reactions.	▪ Recognition of and treatment of poor glucose control will prevent progression of symptoms.	The child and family can describe symptoms of hypoglycemia and hyperglycemia.
▪ Teach the child to test blood glucose when feeling different than usual, and record the reading and symptoms felt.	▪ The child learns his or her specific symptoms of hyper- and hypoglycemia.	
2. Nursing Diagnosis: Risk for Injury (Complication) related to potential episodes of hypoglycemia and diabetic ketoacidosis		
NIC Priority Intervention: *Risk identification:* Analysis of potential risk factors, determination of health risks, and prioritization of risk reduction strategies for an individual or group		**NOC Suggested Outcome:** *Risk control:* Actions to eliminate or reduce actual, personal, and modifiable health threats
Goal: The child will experience few episodes of hypoglycemia during hospitalization.		
▪ Assess the child at least every 2 hours for signs of hypoglycemia. If signs are present, check blood glucose to verify and administer a source of quick sugar.	▪ Hypoglycemia commonly occurs during hospitalization because of change in diet, lack of food intake, or illness.	The child, family, and staff manage episodes of hypoglycemia without a crisis developing.
▪ When the child is NPO for a special procedure, verify with the physician when food, fluids, and insulin are to be given, or if an intravenous infusion with dextrose is to be given.	▪ Giving insulin without food intake can lead to hypoglycemia. Intravenous dextrose and insulin can be used when the child must be NPO.	
▪ Have glucose paste or 50% dextrose solution readily available.	▪ Dextrose is used for emergency intravenous treatment of severe hypoglycemia. Glucose paste is used for oral treatment.	

(continued)

NURSING CARE PLAN

The Child Hospitalized with Newly Diagnosed Type 1 Diabetes Mellitus (continued)

INTERVENTION	RATIONALE	EXPECTED OUTCOME
Goal: The child's condition is treated slowly to gradually reverse hyperglycemia and ketoacidosis and to prevent cerebral edema.		
■ Assess the child's mental status for improvement or deterioration.	■ Improvement in mental status may indicate successful treatment. Deterioration may indicate onset of cerebral edema.	The child's hyperglycemia and ketoacidosis resolve without additional complications.
■ Check blood glucose and urine ketones frequently to confirm reduction in blood glucose level and ketosis, and to identify the insulin dose for administration.	■ Frequent blood glucose and ketone level determination helps assess progress in treating ketoacidosis.	
■ Monitor and control IV fluid intake. Measure output.	■ The child with ketoacidosis will be dehydrated. IV fluid intake needs to be carefully controlled to prevent cerebral edema.	
■ Have insulin doses checked by a second nurse.	■ Doses are frequently small, increasing the possibility of error.	
Goal: The child and parents will demonstrate emergency management of hypoglycemia.		
■ Identify sources of glucose to give in case of hypoglycemic reaction. Tell the child and parent to carry glucose tablets or paste with them at all times.	■ Access to sources of glucose and its rapid administration are important for emergency care.	The child and family can identify several glucose sources for emergencies. The child and family have a source of glucose with them at each visit.
Goal: The child and parents will demonstrate management of sick days.		
■ Teach the child and family to test blood glucose and urine for ketones with acute symptoms and notify the health care provider.	■ When the child is ill, hyperglycemia needs special management to prevent progression to ketoacidosis.	The child's hyperglycemic episodes do not progress to ketoacidosis.
3. Nursing Diagnosis: Imbalanced Nutrition: Less than Body Requirements related to glycosuria		
NIC Priority Intervention: *Nutrition management:* Assistance with or provision of a balanced dietary intake of foods and fluids		**NOC Suggested Outcome:** *Nutritional status:* Extent to which nutrients are available to meet metabolic needs
Goal: The child will eat a well-balanced diet and maintain normal height and weight proportions.		
■ Encourage and serve meals and snacks with consistent carbohydrates at the same time each day.	■ A consistent diet keeps blood glucose levels stable during the initial disease management stages.	The child regains weight lost and demonstrates normal growth and stable blood glucose levels.
■ Provide a calorie nonrestricted diet.	■ This enables weight lost during the onset of diabetes to be regained.	
Goal: The child and parents will state understanding of dietary management of diabetes mellitus.		
■ Make an appointment with a nutritionist who can assess the child's favorite foods and promote their integration into the child's diet. Reinforce the dietary information taught.	■ The nutritionist can develop dietary recommendations that fit the specific needs of the child and include favorite foods, thereby increasing compliance with the diet.	The child and parents describe nutritional needs of the child and select the dietary management best suited to the family's and child's eating habits.
■ Provide sample menus and teach the use of carbohydrate counting.	■ This information assists the family and adolescent with diet planning.	

needs adequate calories to reach or maintain a desirable body weight. The Food Guide Pyramid (see Chapter 14 ∞) may be used to teach the child and family the correct portions and which foods are considered carbohydrates, fats, and proteins. A variety of simple and complex carbohydrates should be eaten. An increased ratio of polyunsaturated fats should be eaten to reduce serum lipid levels.

Eating at consistent intervals is important for glycemic control, whether counting carbohydrates or following a conventional meal plan (three meals and three snacks a day). Although the child with diabetes is not restricted from eating any food, the child and parents need to learn about the relationship between foods eaten and insulin needed. Meal plans also need to be adjusted for exercise. Nonnutritive sweeteners such as aspartame and saccharin may be used in moderation. The child and family should learn how to read food labels. The meal plan should be customized, with the assistance of a nutritionist, to the child's age, cultural and family food preferences, and activity level.

Provide Emotional Support

The diagnosis of type 1 diabetes often comes as a shock to the family. If there is a familial history, parents may feel guilty about having caused the disease. The diagnosis of a chronic disease that requires daily management can be difficult to accept. Give parents information about diabetes education programs, refer them to support groups with other parents of children with diabetes, and help them to learn the role they can play in managing the disease.

Support for the child depends on his or her age and developmental stage. Encourage the child to express feelings about the disease and its management. The adolescent may benefit from contact with other adolescents who have diabetes. See Evidence-Based Practice: Adolescent Diabetes and Quality of Life.

Discharge Planning and Home Care Teaching

Home care needs should be identified and addressed before discharge. Initial survival skills described earlier are taught with the plans for ongoing outpatient education.

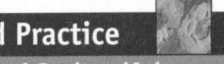

Evidence-Based Practice
Adolescent Diabetes and Quality of Life

Problem

A number of factors are associated with how adolescents with diabetes view their quality of life.

Evidence

A study involving 115 adolescents with diabetes (ages 11 to 18 years) examined their perception of parental involvement, care, and control in relation to health-related quality of life and metabolic control. Their perceptions were compared to 9,345 healthy adolescents and 291 adolescents with physical disabilities. Adolescents with diabetes reported a higher level of parental control than both healthy adolescents and adolescents with disabilities, and this higher level of control was significantly associated with a lower health-related quality of life. Adolescents with diabetes reported a significantly higher health-related quality of life score when they perceived a higher degree of parental care and involvement, and a lower degree of parental control and overprotection. Their HbA$_{1c}$ level was not significantly related to perceptions of parental care, control, or involvement, potentially due to the challenges of maintaining metabolic control during puberty (Graue, Wentzel-Larsen, Hanestad, et al., 2005).

Another study examined responses of 39 adolescents between the ages of 13 and 17 years who completed the Diabetes Quality of Life for Youths questionnaire. Of the 22 domains listed on the questionnaire, only 3 were cited as important: family, friends, and school. Functional health of the participants was perceived as similar to their peers, and 74% of the adolescents had attended a diabetes camp at least once. The study confirmed not only the importance of family to adolescents with diabetes, but the importance of peers as well, whether it be at school or summer camp (Cheung, Cureton, & Canham, 2006).

An additional study measured how monitoring and discussing health-related quality of life (HRQoL) improved psychosocial well-being in adolescents with type 1 diabetes. Ninety-one adolescents between the ages of 13 and 17 with type 1 diabetes participated in the study and were randomly assigned to the HRQoL intervention group or the control group. During a 12-month period, all partici-

pants had 3 scheduled visits for routine diabetes care at 3-month intervals. The intervention group completed the Pediatric Quality of Life Inventory on a computer at each visit prior to being seen by the health care provider. The results were discussed with the adolescent during the visit. Over the 12-month period, mean scores for psychosocial health, behavior, mental health, and family activities improved in the intervention group except for those adolescents with the highest hemoglobin A$_{1c}$ values. Adolescents in the intervention group demonstrated higher self-esteem at follow-up visits and were more satisfied with care than those in the control group (de Wit, Delemarre-van de Waal, Bokma, et al., 2008).

Implications

Developmental tasks of adolescents focus on development of self-concept and self-esteem. Adolescents with type 1 diabetes must also cope with the increasing responsibility for complex self-management, including insulin administration, blood glucose testing, exercise, and nutrition. Self-esteem and self-concept often become linked with the disease as peers react to the differences noted. Life satisfaction, perceived control, and worries associated with having diabetes are important considerations when counseling the teenager and family about the management of diabetes. Additionally, it is important to know that adolescents value parental involvement and care rather than perceiving it as a reason for conflict. Parental involvement and supervision is important in helping adolescents transition successfully to self-management of their disease. Peers are also very important to adolescents with diabetes. Continued involvement in school activities and summer camps provide excellent avenues for friendship and promote a positive quality of life. Additionally, monitoring and discussing quality of life issues with adolescents can lead to improved psychosocial health.

Critical Thinking Application

What questions can be used to explore an adolescent's perceptions of family involvement, care, and control? How can you address quality of life issues in adolescents with diabetes? What questions can be used to determine the adolescent's satisfaction with peer relationships?

Make every effort to incorporate the diabetic regimen (insulin administration, food plan, blood glucose monitoring, and exercise) into the family's present lifestyle. The fewer changes the family has to make, the greater the chance of adherence.

The family and child that is newly diagnosed with diabetes should be made aware of the "honeymoon phase." This is a period during new-onset diabetes when the child has some residual beta-cell function, which reduces exogenous insulin requirements. The child and family may assume this is an indication that the diabetes "is better." However, the insulin requirement does eventually return. The duration of this phase varies among individuals.

Make sure the parents inform all health care providers that the child has diabetes. Special planning is needed for diagnostic procedures and surgery that require the child to have food withheld for several hours to prevent the child from experiencing hypoglycemia or hyperglycemia. Provide written materials and refer parents to books and other materials they can use in teaching the child about diabetes. The Juvenile Diabetes Research Foundation and the American Diabetes Association are good sources of information.

Care in the Community

During follow-up visits, ask the child or parents about signs indicating problems of diabetic control. Questions to ask that could help identify problems in diabetic control include:

- Is the child hungry at meals? Between meals?
- How much fluid is the child drinking?
- Has the child been going to the bathroom frequently or had episodes of bed-wetting?
- Does the child have dry skin?
- Are there sores on the feet? Do scratches or scrapes take a long time to heal?
- Has the child had any skin infections?
- Does the child have changes in mood (depression, unexplained sadness, irritability) or energy level from day to day or throughout the day?
- Have there been any changes in vision?

Record growth measurements and vital signs in the child's chart. Review the child's typical dietary intake and exercise regimens. Assess the child's sexual development using the Tanner staging guidelines (see Chapter 5 ∞). Puberty may be delayed if diabetic control is inadequate. Evaluation for the potential complications of diabetes should be performed annually, including blood for lipid levels, blood pressure, liver and renal function, urine for albumin, an ophthalmologic examination for retinopathy, and a neurologic examination of the extremities for neuropathies.

▲ Health Promotion

Encourage regular physical activity and educate the child to modify insulin dosage or food intake for extra physical activity periods. Encourage the child to participate in sports when interested and learn how to balance exercise, food intake, and insulin dosage.

Research *Adolescent Diet and Diabetes*

The dietary intake of 132 adolescents with type 1 diabetes was compared with that of 131 adolescents without diabetes. Both groups had a mean age of 12 years and were comparable by sex, race, ethnicity, and stage of pubertal development. Using a 24-hour recall method, there was no difference in the number of calories consumed by the two groups. The adolescents with diabetes consumed a greater percentage (and more grams) of fat and protein and a smaller percentage of carbohydrates than adolescents without diabetes. Of concern is the greater amount of saturated fat consumed by adolescents with diabetes that may contribute to cardiovascular disease in the future (Helgeson, Viccaro, Becker, et al., 2006).

Learning Self-Management

Education is ongoing, especially for children who develop diabetes at a young age. As they grow and assume more responsibility for their care, they need to learn more about the pathophysiology of the disease and the rationale for its management. Teach parents to be alert to signs of maladaptation, such as helpless, demanding, or whining behaviors, and any evidence of poor coping. Additional behaviors may include skipping blood glucose testing and losing or damaging equipment. Toddlers with diabetes present an additional challenge for parents, since they are generally picky eaters, but must eat enough for the insulin dose. Referral for counseling may be appropriate for some families.

Continually work with the child to help him or her assume responsibility for self-care, and with parents to promote the child's self-care (Figures 30–9 ➤ and 30–10 ➤). The child's developmental stage and cognitive level influence his or her readiness

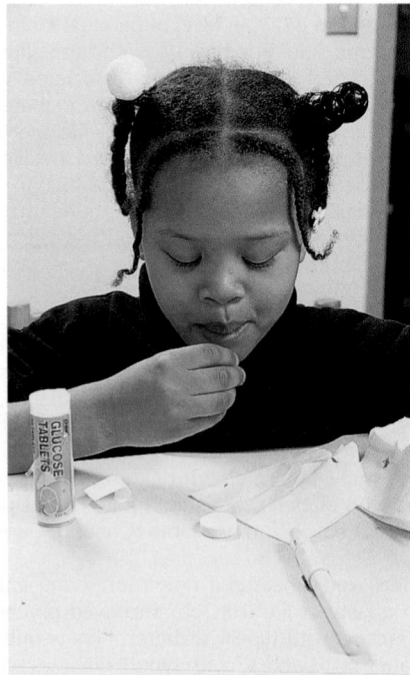

FIGURE 30–9 ➤ This girl is old enough to understand the need to take glucose tablets or another form of a rapidly absorbed sugar when her blood glucose level is low.

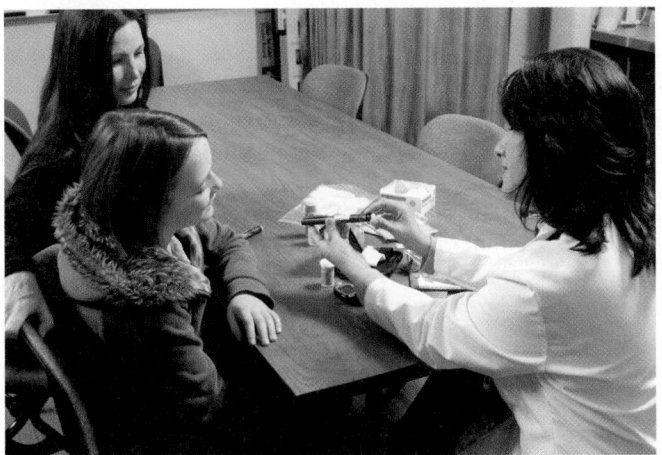

FIGURE 30–10 ➤ The mother and child are being taught how to use an insulin pen.

to take on responsibility for self-care (Figure 30–11 ➤). Summer camps and other programs for children with diabetes are often helpful in providing education and support.

The preschool child's need for autonomy and control can be met by allowing the child to choose snacks, pick which finger to stick for glucose testing, and help parents to gather necessary supplies. School-age children can learn to test blood glucose, administer insulin, and keep records. They should be taught how to select foods and portion sizes appropriate for dietary management and how to plan food intake for an exercise program. School-age children need to learn to recognize the signs of hypoglycemia and hyperglycemia, and understand the importance of carrying a rapidly absorbed sugar product.

Although adolescents understand explanations about the potential complications of diabetes, they are present-time oriented, and may rebel against the daily regimen of insulin injections, the food plan, and the exercise plan. Successful self-care depends in part on the adolescent's adjustment to the chronic nature of the disease and feelings of being different from peers.

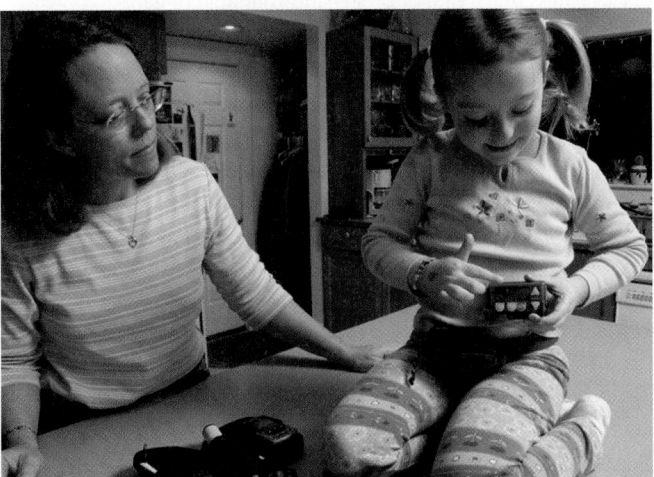

FIGURE 30–11 ➤ This young girl is learning to check her insulin pump, which she carries in a pouch around her waist.

Although the adolescent is able to manage self-care, the desire to be like peers may interfere with treatment adherence. Talk with the adolescent to assess his or her mood and to evaluate his or her motivation to manage the meal plan, exercise regimen, blood glucose monitoring, and insulin therapy. Discuss how carbohydrate counting and insulin dose adjustment may provide the flexibility to participate in activities with peers. Collaborate with the adolescent in preparation to assume care, and assist parents in accepting the growing independence from adult supervision. A discussion of the hazards associated with having diabetes and the use of alcohol, drugs, and tobacco should occur. At every subsequent health care visit, the adolescent should be asked about alcohol intake.

The child with diabetes should be treated as any other child without a chronic condition, including limit setting and consistent discipline for unacceptable behavior. Children with type 1 diabetes may learn maladaptive behaviors, using their disease to obtain something they want. The child with type 1 diabetes may develop circulatory and neurologic changes over time. Emphasize the importance of good foot care from an early age; for example, wearing clean cotton socks; changing socks and shoes when they are damp; washing, drying, and powdering feet; and keeping toenails short.

Explain to parents that the child should wear some type of medical alert identification. Help them have an individualized health plan developed (see Chapter 12 ∞) to ensure that school administrators and teachers can identify the signs of hypoglycemia or hyperglycemia and provide emergency management.

Clinical Tip

The child with diabetes needs an individualized diabetes medical management plan (DMMP) for management of diabetes while in school or childcare. Information that should be included in the DMMP includes when blood glucose testing should be performed, insulin administration and storage, meals and snacks needed, symptoms and management of hypoglycemia and hyperglycemia, participation in physical activity, need for ketone monitoring, and emergency lockdown/evacuation instructions. Parents need to ensure that the school or childcare provider has all essential equipment and supplies for the child's management as well as phone numbers for the parents and the child's health care provider for diabetes (American Diabetes Association, 2010b).

Evaluation

Expected outcomes of nursing care for children with type 1 diabetes can be found in the Nursing Care Plan on pages 1011–1012.

Diabetic Ketoacidosis

Diabetic ketoacidosis (DKA) is the common and potentially life-threatening condition that occurs primarily in children with type 1 diabetes. Potential causes of DKA include missed insulin doses or incorrect administration of insulin, an illness, trauma, or surgery. DKA may be present in children with new-onset diabetes.

Insulin deficiency is accompanied by a compensatory increase in hormones (epinephrine, norepinephrine, cortisol, growth hormone, and glucagon) that are released when inadequate glucose is delivered to the cells. The muscle cells break down protein into amino acids that are then converted to glucose by the liver, leading to hyperglycemia. The adipose tissue releases fatty acids that are transformed by the liver into ketone bodies. Their accumulation leads to ketoacidosis. The hyperglycemia causes an osmotic diuresis resulting in dehydration, acidosis, and hyperosmolarity. The rising ketones lead to metabolic acidosis. DKA is associated with severe metabolic, electrolyte, and fluid imbalances. See Chapter 18 ∞.

Characteristic signs of DKA include polyuria, polydipsia, weight loss, abdominal pain, nausea and vomiting, tachycardia, signs of dehydration, flushed ears and cheeks, Kussmaul respirations, acetone breath, altered level of consciousness, and hypotension. Hyperglycemia, glycosuria, and ketonuria are also present. In response to metabolic acidosis, children complain of abdominal or chest pain, nausea, and vomiting. The disorder may progress to electrolyte disturbances, arrhythmias, altered consciousness, shock, and death if untreated.

DKA is present with the following findings: blood glucose level greater than 200 mg/dL serum ketones, acidosis (pH less than or equal to 7.3 and bicarbonate less than 15 mEq/L), glycosuria, and ketonuria (Cooke & Plotnick, 2008b). Electrolyte disorders also occur (hyperkalemia, hyperchloremia, hyponatremia, hypophosphatemia, hypocalcemia, and hypomagnesemia). The BUN and creatinine are elevated due to dehydration. Medical management includes isotonic intravenous fluids and electrolytes for dehydration and acidosis. Short-acting insulin (0.1 unit/kg per hour) is administered by continuous infusion pump to decrease the serum glucose level at a rate not to exceed 100 mg/dL/hr. Faster reduction of hyperglycemia and serum osmolality increases the risk for cerebral edema. When glucose is lowered too rapidly, water is freed and attracted to the glucose. Bicarbonate is not routinely used for treatment of DKA as it places the child at increased risk for hypokalemia, acidosis, and cerebral edema (Cooke & Plotnick, 2008b). As insulin is administered, potassium shifts to the cells, resulting in hypokalemia. Potassium supplementation is given only after confirmation of renal function.

Cerebral edema is the most common cause of DKA-related deaths. Mannitol is kept on standby for treatment of neurological symptoms secondary to cerebral edema (Cooke & Plotnik, 2008b). See Chapter 27 ∞ for information about cerebral edema.

Clinical Tip

Insulin binds to IV tubing. Run 50 to 100 mL of insulin through the new IV tubing to saturate all the binding sites. This ensures that the full dose of insulin reaches the child from the outset.

Nursing Management

Continuously monitor the child's vital signs, respiratory status, perfusion, and mental status. Assess for changes in neurologic status, respiratory pattern, blood pressure, and heart rate. Monitor for cardiac arrhythmias associated with hypokalemia. As-

sess for signs of dehydration, including dry skin and mucous membranes and depressed fontanels in infants. Monitor blood glucose levels hourly or as indicated. Frequently monitor the electrolytes and acid-base status, as well as urine glucose and ketone levels as indicated. Intake and output are monitored hourly.

Intravenous fluids are given in boluses of 10 to 20 mL/kg rapidly over 5 minutes if the child is in hypovolemic shock. Adequate fluids are given to reverse the fluid deficit. The insulin infusion must be carefully titrated to control the gradual reduction in hyperglycemia. The child is tapered off intravenous insulin and transitions to subcutaneous insulin when clinically stable. Oral feedings are reintroduced when the child is alert and the glucose level is stabilized.

The prevention of future episodes of DKA is important. Increased attention to blood glucose and urine ketone monitoring is especially important when the child has significant stressors such as an illness. It is important for the child and family to understand that insulin is required even when the child is not eating to counter the hormones secreted in response to the stressor. The parents and child need to learn strategies to keep hyperglycemic episodes from progressing to DKA. The child's urine should be tested for ketones every 4–6 hours if the blood glucose reading is 240 mg/dL or greater, or if the child is sick (American Diabetes Association, 2008c). If the child has an elevated blood glucose and moderate or large amounts of ketones, treatment with extra insulin and fluids can be initiated. See Families Want to Know: Preventing DKA.

Families Want to Know
Preventing DKA

When to Monitor for DKA

- Abdominal pain
- Nausea and vomiting that persists for over 6 hours
- More than five diarrheal stools in 1 day
- A 1- or 2-day history of polyuria and polydipsia
- Has illness (e.g., viral or other) and is unable to eat

Recognizing Signs of DKA

- Change in mental status
- Temperature over 102°F (38.9°C) for 12 hours
- Blood glucose 400 mg/dL on two separate readings
- Moderate to large ketones present in urine
- Fruity breath odor
- Evidence of a bacterial infection (e.g., fever, drainage, dysuria, or other evidence of a urinary tract infection)
- Difficulty breathing
- Decreased urine output

Data from: Bismuth, E., & Laffel, L. (2007). Can we prevent diabetes ketoacidosis in children? *Pediatric Diabetes, 8*(6), 24–33; Doyle, E. A., & Grey, M. (2010). Diabetes mellitus (types 1 and 2). In P. J. Allen, J. A. Vessey, & N. A. Schapiro (Eds.), *Primary care of the child with a chronic condition* (5th ed., pp. 427–446). St. Louis, MO: Mosby; Masharani, U. (2008). Diabetes mellitus and hypoglycemia. In S. J. McPhee, M. A. Papadakis, L. M. Tierney, Jr., R. Gonzales, & R. Zeiger, *Current medical diagnosis and treatment 2008*. Retrieved from McGraw-Hill's Access Medicine http://www.accessmedicine.com

Hypoglycemia in the Child with Diabetes

Hypoglycemia can develop within minutes in children with type 1 diabetes mellitus. The symptoms outlined in the clinical manifestations table below may occur when blood glucose levels drop or fall below 70 mg/dL. Children are at risk of hypoglycemia due to their rapid growth rates, unpredictable eating habits, and physical activity. Severe hypoglycemia episodes may occur at night in children who are treated with two to three injections per day. Other common causes include an error in insulin dosage, errors in injection technique, inadequate calories because of missed meals, or exercise without a corresponding increase in caloric intake. Severe hypoglycemia can cause seizures.

Hypoglycemia can be diagnosed on the basis of the sudden onset of signs and symptoms. See the accompanying clinical manifestations table. Give glucose immediately but only in the form of a low-fat carbohydrate-containing snack or drink, sugar gel, glucose tablets, or glucose paste. If the child becomes unconscious, administer glucagon or if unavailable, administer sugar gel or glucose paste squeezed onto the gums. In the hospital setting, administer an intravenous infusion of dextrose to prevent progression of symptoms. Since the effects of dextrose and glucagon are temporary, additional snacks or a meal is provided. The child should be continually observed for several hours after treatment.

Clinical Judgment

Symptoms such as confusion and behavior changes can be present in both hyperglycemia and hypoglycemia. When blood glucose monitoring equipment is immediately available, the nurse should check the child's blood glucose level prior to initiating treatment. What action should the nurse take if blood glucose monitoring equipment is not readily available?

Nursing Management

Teach parents and children to recognize the signs of hypoglycemia and take appropriate action. (See Families Want to Know: Treating Hypoglycemic Episodes.) Teach parents to give an intramuscular (IM) or subcutaneous (SQ) dose of **glucagon** (a hormone produced by the pancreas that helps release stored glucose from the liver) for severe cases of hypoglycemia. Reinforce the importance of balancing dietary intake, insulin, and exercise every day.

Clinical Manifestations
Hypoglycemia and Hyperglycemia

Cause	Clinical Manifestations	Clinical Therapy
Hypoglycemia ■ Insulin dose too high for food eaten ■ Insulin injection into muscle ■ Too much exercise for insulin dose ■ Too long between meals/snacks ■ Too few carbohydrates eaten ■ Illness, stress	*Rapid onset* Irritability, nervousness, tremors, shaky feeling, difficulty concentrating or speaking, behavior change, confusion, repeating something over and over Unconsciousness, seizure, shallow breathing, tachycardia Pallor, sweating Moist mucous membranes, hunger Headache, dizziness, blurred vision, double vision, photophobia Numb lips or mouth	If conscious, give 15 grams of carbohydrate. Wait 15 minutes and recheck blood glucose level. Give another 15 grams of carbohydrate if blood glucose level is 70 mg/dL or below. Recheck the blood glucose level in 15 minutes. If unconscious, give glucagon by injection.
Hyperglycemia ■ Insulin dose too low for food eaten ■ Illness or injury, stress ■ Too many carbohydrates eaten ■ Meals/snacks too close together ■ Insulin injected just under skin or injected into hypertrophied areas ■ Decreased activity	*Gradual onset* Lethargy, sleepiness, slowed responses, or confusion Deep, rapid breathing Flushed skin, dry skin Dry mucous membranes, thirst, hunger, dehydration Weakness, fatigue Headache, abdominal pain, nausea, vomiting Blurred vision Shock	Give additional insulin at usual injection time. Give correction scale insulin doses for specific blood glucose levels when ill or injured. Give extra injections if hyperglycemia and moderate to large ketones. Increase fluids.

■ If the child shows signs of hypoglycemia (pallor, sweating, tremors, dizziness, numb lips or mouth, confusion, irritability, altered mental status), test the blood glucose level.

■ Assist the child to perform the test, as skills needed to get an accurate reading deteriorate with altered mental status.

■ If the blood glucose reading is less than or equal to 70 mg/dL, give glucose rapidly. Use one of the following to give 15 grams of rapid-acting glucose to raise the blood sugar level:
  • 1/2 cup fruit juice
  • 1/2 cup of regular cola or soda
  • 1 small box raisins
  • 3 to 4 glucose tablets

■ Wait 15 minutes and recheck the blood glucose level. Repeat the glucose if it is still less than or equal to 70 mg/dL. Recheck the blood glucose level in another 15 minutes.

■ Once blood sugar has returned to at least 80 mg/dL, give a more substantial snack such as cheese and crackers if the next meal will be more than 30 minutes later or an activity or exercise is planned.

■ If the child is unconscious, spread glucose paste on the gums or administer IM or SQ glucagon.

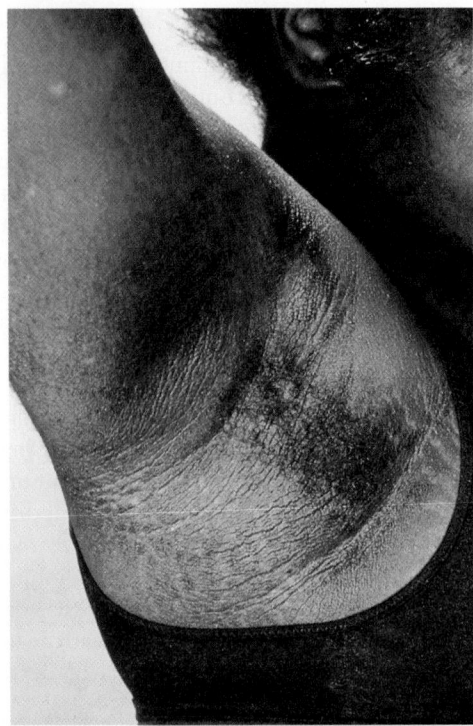

FIGURE 30–12 ➤ Acanthosis nigricans.
Courtesy of Audrey Austin, M.D., Children's National Medical Center, Washington, DC.

Type 2 Diabetes

Type 2 diabetes is a disease associated with insulin resistance (an alteration of the insulin receptor that signals the presence of insulin in the interior of cells). Significant risk factors for type 2 diabetes include obesity, low levels of physical activity, a diet high in fat, race, and family history of diabetes (Alemzadeh & Wyatt, 2007; Berry et al., 2006a). Several genes on chromosomes 1q, 12q, 20q, and 7q are associated with the predisposition for development of type 2 diabetes (Vivian, 2006). Most children are diagnosed between the ages of 8 and 19 years (Berry et al., 2006a).

The increasing number of children being diagnosed with type 2 diabetes has caused significant concern in the health care community. An estimated 8–45% of children older than 10 years of age with a new diagnosis of diabetes have type 2 (Berry, Urban, & Grey, 2006b). The true incidence in children is unknown as many children are undiagnosed.

Etiology and Pathophysiology   Type 2 diabetes is a complex metabolic disorder with insulin resistance being the central abnormality. In response to the increased body weight, the visceral fat produces a cytokine hormone (tumor necrosis factor) that desensitizes cellular insulin receptor within cells to insulin. The pancreatic cells produce more insulin in an attempt to overcome the insulin resistance and facilitate glucose transfer. This results in **hyperinsulinemia** (elevated insulin levels in the blood). The child maintains a balance between hyperinsulinemia and insulin resistance and a normal glycemic state. As insulin resistance worsens, the islet of Langerhans beta cells fail in their ability to hypersecrete insulin. This leads to impaired glucose tolerance, and overt diabetes develops. The onset of puberty and increased secretion of the growth hormone is believed to be a contributing factor in the development of insulin resistance (Vivian, 2006).

Clinical Manifestations   Signs and symptoms of type 2 diabetes vary upon initial presentation from those for type 1. See the clinical manifestations table on page 1007. Onset is more insidious, and a history of polydipsia and polyuria is absent or mild (Berry et al., 2006a). **Acanthosis nigricans**, hyperpigmentation and thickening of the skin with velvety irregularities in the skin folds of the back of the neck and medial aspect of the thighs and axillae, is a common finding and is associated with insulin resistance. The finding is present in 60–90% of children with type 2 diabetes (Adams & Lammon, 2007) (Figure 30–12 ➤). The child is usually obese, with a high waist circumference. The child may present with diabetic ketoacidosis at the time of diagnosis (Rewers et al., 2008).

COLLABORATIVE CARE

Diagnostic Tests

Blood glucose levels of 200 mg/dL or greater without fasting, or a fasting glucose 126 mg/dL or greater are diagnostic of diabetes.

Children of African American, Native American, Hispanic, Alaska Native, and Asian/Pacific Islander origins are at greater risk for developing type 2 diabetes (Adams & Lammon, 2007; Berry et al., 2006b). Particularly affected are members of some Native American tribes that historically have had a high level of exercise and hunter-gatherer diets. In some groups, such as the Pima Indians of the Southwest, 22.3–50.9 per 1,000 children are reported to have type 2 diabetes mellitus (Adams & Lammon, 2007).

Hemoglobin A_{1c} provides an indicator of average glucose concentration over the prior 2 months (Cooke & Plotnick, 2008a). Urine is tested and ketones are found in about 50% of children. Islet cell autoantibodies, fasting insulin levels, glutamic acid decarboxylase autoantibody test (GAD-65), and C-peptide levels are used to differentiate between type 1 and type 2 diabetes. The child with type 2 diabetes has elevated insulin and C-peptide levels whereas these levels are normally low in the child with type 1 diabetes. Islet cell and GAD-65 autoantibodies are rarely found in the child with type 2 diabetes (Berry et al., 2006a). A fasting lipid profile is obtained since dyslipidemia (primarily elevated LDL-C and triglycerides) is usually present. High blood pressure for age, gender, and height percentile is also seen (see Appendix B).

Clinical Therapy

The multiple goals for managing the child with type 2 diabetes include the following: normalizing the blood glucose and HbA_{1c} levels, decreasing weight, increasing exercise, normalizing lipid profile and blood pressure, and preventing complications. Nutrition education and weight loss is the major therapy. The child needs to have gradual sustained weight loss, metabolic control of blood glucose levels, exercise, and emotional support.

If the child or adolescent presents with severe hyperglycemia or diabetic ketoacidosis, insulin will be required to gain initial glycemic control. Once metabolic control is achieved, oral medication (metformin) is initiated as the child is weaned off insulin. Metformin is used when diet and exercise efforts are inadequate to control hyperglycemia. Metformin improves the sensitivity of target cells to insulin, slows the gastrointestinal absorption of glucose, and reduces the hepatic and renal glucose production. It can be used when there is normal liver and kidney function and no ketosis. The dosage may be gradually increased to improve metabolic control. If additional medication is needed, sulfonylurea or meglitinides may be used; however, they are not approved for use in children in the United States due to liver toxicity (Alemzadeh & Wyatt, 2007). Insulin may only be needed for periods of increased stress, but the adolescent may ultimately require insulin for glycemic control if weight and exercise goals are not met.

NURSING MANAGEMENT

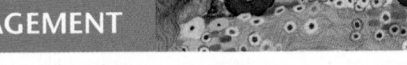

Nursing Assessment and Diagnosis

Because the child with type 2 diabetes often does not have an acute onset, assess any child with a body mass index (BMI) greater than the 85th percentile for age and gender for signs of insulin resistance (acanthosis nigricans, hypertension, and dyslipidemia). Family history of diabetes in a child who is overweight is a reason to begin screening for the condition. Once the child has been diagnosed, monitor the child's blood glucose levels and blood pressure. Assess the child's diet and activity patterns to determine appropriate changes for disease management. Consider evaluating the siblings for diabetes.

Nursing diagnoses that may apply to the child with type 2 diabetes include:

- Imbalanced Nutrition, More than Body Requirements related to high fat food intake and inadequate exercise
- Activity Intolerance related to sedentary lifestyle and disease state (insulin resistance)
- Ineffective Therapeutic Regimen Management (Family and Individual) related to family conflict over changing eating patterns
- Situational Low Self-Esteem related to situational crisis associated with diagnosis of new-onset chronic illness

Clinical Tip

Both the American Diabetes Association and the American Academy of Pediatrics recommend diabetes screening for children over 10 years of age when the child has a BMI greater than the 85th percentile for age and gender and at least two additional risk factors (Cox & Polvado, 2008; Vivian, 2006):

■ Family history of type 2 diabetes in a first- or second-degree relative

■ Member of a high-risk racial or ethnic group, such as Native American, African American, Hispanic, Asian American, or Pacific Islander

■ Signs of insulin resistance or associated condition such as acanthosis nigricans, hypertension, dyslipidemia, or polycystic ovary syndrome

Planning and Implementation

The child with type 2 diabetes may be hospitalized at the time of diagnosis because of ketoacidosis. However, the nurse in an inpatient setting is more likely to encounter this child when hospitalized for another condition or during health care visits in clinics or schools. Nursing care focuses on managing the child's blood glucose levels and hypertension during the hospitalization, assessing growth and dietary intake, evaluating goals for weight loss and exercise programs, and reviewing the child's knowledge about diabetes and strategies for management at home.

Clinical Tip

The American Diabetes Association considers a fasting glucose level of 100–125 mg/dL (5.6–6.9 mmol/L) to be an *impaired fasting glucose* (IFG), and a 2-hour postload glucose level of 140–199 mg/dL (7.8–11.0 mmol/L) to be an *impaired glucose tolerance* (IGT). Individuals with IFG or IGT are considered at increased risk to develop diabetes. A hemoglobin A_{1c} value of 5.7–6.4% is an additional risk factor for the development of diabetes (American Diabetes Association, 2010a).

Care in the Community

Since the child is usually diagnosed and managed on an outpatient basis, nursing care focuses on teaching the child and parents about the disease and its management, managing dietary intake, providing emotional support, and planning strategies for daily management in the community.

Educate the child and family about the disease and lifestyle changes required for effective management of the condition.

Focus on the need to increase activity with routine exercise of at least 30 to 60 minutes daily and by decreasing sedentary activity time, such as computer and television viewing time to no more than 2 hours daily. Customize the activity strategy for each child with motivation to develop a regular routine.

Work with the family to substitute alternatives to high-calorie and high-fat foods with a meal plan sensitive to the family's resources and ethnic preferences. Suggestions include limiting fast food and using fruits and vegetables as snacks rather than foods high in fat and sugar. Assess the child's height, weight, and BMI on each visit, and plot on the appropriate growth curve for age and gender. A gradual sustained weight loss or decrease in BMI is the goal. If the child is experiencing a growth height spurt, maintenance of weight rather than weight loss is the goal. Encourage the entire family to make dietary changes, especially since other family members are also at risk for the condition. The nutritional patterns in the family are a key part of treatment.

Clinical Tip

Early intervention is needed to reduce the incidence of type 2 diabetes in a child who is at risk, as well as potential complications, such as hypertension. Identify children at risk by carefully analyzing the family history, height, weight, and blood pressure measurements. Plot the growth measurements on the growth chart to identify the child who is overweight or at risk for overweight. Compare the blood pressure reading to the table of values for age, sex, and height to identify the risk for hypertension. Plan further interventions based upon the findings (Bindler & Bruya, 2006).

Teach the child and family to perform home blood glucose testing to monitor glycemic control. This will let the child and family know that efforts to manage the disease are successful. Check HbA$_{1c}$ levels at each visit to determine the average blood glucose level for the past 3 months. When dietary control and exercise are not successful in reducing blood glucose levels, teach the child and family about the prescribed oral medication.

Give the child and family opportunities to talk about the impact of the disease on their lives. Identify resources for information about strategies that have worked for other families. Identify local support groups and peer groups for the family and child. Suggest weekly activities, summer camps, and other ongoing programs to provide necessary support and motivation.

Make sure the child gets annual evaluations for potential complications of diabetes. The tests to be performed include blood for lipid levels, blood pressure, liver and renal function, urine for albumin, an eye exam for retinopathy, and a neurologic exam of the extremities for neuropathies. The child with type 2 diabetes has the same risk for developing long-term vascular complications as the child with type 1 diabetes when hyperglycemia is poorly controlled.

Evaluation

Examples of expected outcomes of nursing care include:

• The child decreases sedentary activity time to under 2 hours a day.

• The child's intake of fruits and vegetables increases to 5 to 8 daily, and total fat intake decreases to less than 30% of total calories.

• The child's body mass index slowly and consistently decreases.

■ DISORDERS OF GONADAL FUNCTION

Gynecomastia

Gynecomastia is a proliferation of glandular breast tissue in males occurring in approximately 50–60% of adolescent boys (Johnson & Murad, 2009). It is sometimes confused with subcutaneous fat pads in obese males. Gynecomastia occurs when the ratio of estrogen to testosterone is greater than the usual male ratio. It is also associated with Klinefelter syndrome and drugs that increase the circulating concentration of prolactin such as marijuana, tricyclic antidepressants, and calcium channel blockers. The condition disappears in 1 to 2 years, and the amount of breast tissue varies among boys. If gynecomastia is severe and is causing distress to the adolescent, a referral to a plastic surgeon for possible reduction is indicated (Raine, Donaldson, Gregory, et al., 2006c).

Nursing care focuses on reassuring the boy and his parents that gynecomastia is common and transient. Because of the body image concerns common during adolescence, embarrassment is a frequent problem. Recommend clothing styles and other methods to camouflage the enlarged breasts.

Amenorrhea

Amenorrhea, or lack of menstruation, may be primary or secondary. Criteria for primary amenorrhea include absence of menarche by age 14.5 years in association with no growth or development of secondary sexual characteristics, or absence of menses by age 16 when secondary sexual characteristics and growth are present.

Secondary amenorrhea is the cessation of menstrual periods 6 months or 3 cycles after menstruation has begun; it is characterized by an absence of spontaneous bleeding for at least 120 days. Pregnancy is the most common cause of secondary amenorrhea in adolescents. It is common for adolescents to have irregular menstrual cycles and duration of the menstrual period for 1 to 2 years after menarche. A large number of cycles are anovulatory for the first 2 years after menarche.

Primary amenorrhea is most often caused by structural defects of the reproductive system; chromosomal abnormalities (such as Turner syndrome); or hypothalamic or pituitary tumors, thyroid dysfunction, or polycystic ovary syndrome. No underlying pathologic condition is found in some adolescents. Primary or secondary amenorrhea may be found in competitive athletes and in youth with anorexia nervosa (see Chapter 14 ∞).

A thorough history (including sexual activity), physical examination, and laboratory evaluation are required to determine the cause of amenorrhea. The history focuses on asking questions about recent excessive weight loss or gain; excessive physical activity or sports training; chronic illness; use of illegal drugs, birth control pills, or phenothiazines; emotional prob-

Growth & Development *Female Athletes and Inadequate Nutrition*

Girls competing in sports such as gymnastics, ballet, and long-distance running feel the need to maintain a low weight and specific body type. Reduced adipose tissue leads to a reduction in leptin, and subsequently a reduction in gonadotropin-releasing hormone and low serum estrogen levels (Bloomfield, 2006). Amenorrhea or oligomenorrhea and bone demineralization often result. This, in turn, may increase the girl's risk of fractures and osteoporosis in young adulthood (Landry, 2007) (see Chapter 29 ∞).

Complementary Therapy

Dysmenorrhea

Nonpharmacologic methods that may be useful in the treatment of dysmenorrhea include heat, transcutaneous nerve stimulation, distraction, acupuncture, rest, exercise, and topical heat therapy. Increasing the intake of dietary omega-3 fatty acids, use of herbal supplements, and use of fennel essential oil may help to relieve symptoms. Intake of vitamin B_1, vitamin E, calcium, and magnesium may also help relieve symptoms of dysmenorrhea (Doty & Attaran, 2006; Harel, 2006).

lems; and age of the mother at menarche. A family history helps to identify other female family members with similar issues. The physical examination focuses on evaluating the adolescent's stage of sexual development and assessing for hirsutism (see Chapter 5 ∞). A vaginal exam is performed to determine vaginal patency and if the vaginal mucosa is estrogenized. A pregnancy test is performed. Bone age and hormone levels are evaluated (estrogen, LH, FSH, and prolactin).

Treatment of amenorrhea depends on the specific cause. The most common approach is to prescribe birth control pills containing both estrogen and progesterone. Athletic teenagers are encouraged to eat a well-balanced, high-calorie diet. Calcium supplements may be ordered. Estrogen with progesterone in low doses may be prescribed for athletes to reduce the risk for osteoporosis. Nursing management centers on patient education and emotional support. The goal is to maintain normal growth and development.

Dysmenorrhea

Dysmenorrhea (menstrual pain or cramping) is a common complaint of adolescent girls. Primary dysmenorrhea occurs in the absence of pathologic disorders. Dysmenorrhea accounts for more hours of missed school by females than any other cause. Approximately 15% of adolescent females report that dysmenorrhea affects their activities of daily living (Doty & Attaran, 2006).

Primary dysmenorrhea is usually caused by an increased secretion of prostaglandins that are produced during the ovulatory cycle. Prostaglandin causes smooth muscle contraction in the uterus, leading to ischemia and pain.

Dysmenorrhea usually occurs prior to the beginning of the menstrual period and ends on the second day of the period. The cramping pain in the lower abdomen and pelvic region ranges from mild to severe and varies with the individual. Pain may also radiate to the back or thighs. Other symptoms may include nausea, headache, backache, vomiting, diarrhea, fatigue, and urinary frequency.

Secondary dysmenorrhea is defined as painful menstruation associated with pelvic abnormalities and is seen in approximately 10% of adolescent females and young women with dysmenorrhea. It is most commonly caused by endometriosis in this population (Harel, 2006).

The treatment of choice is nonsteroidal anti-inflammatory drugs (NSAIDs) such as ibuprofen and naproxen sodium. These drugs inhibit prostaglandin synthesis, which leads to a re-

duction in uterine activity and pain. Oral contraceptives may be prescribed to prevent ovulation and to decrease prostaglandin production.

Nursing Management

Nursing care centers on providing patient education and emotional support. Instruct the adolescent with chronic dysmenorrhea to keep a calendar and begin taking NSAIDs 1 day before the onset of the menstrual period. The medications should be taken with food to minimize side effects.

■ DISORDERS RELATED TO SEX CHROMOSOME ABNORMALITIES

Turner Syndrome

Turner syndrome is the most common sex chromosome abnormality in females. Affected girls have a missing or partial absence of one X chromosome. It occurs in approximately 1 in 2,000 live female births (Simpson, 2009). Approximately 99% of fetuses with the disorder are spontaneously aborted, generally during the first trimester of pregnancy (Doswell, Visootsak, Brady, et al., 2006). In the absence of one X chromosome, the oocytes in the ovaries disappear and are nearly all gone by age 2 years. Other specific clinical manifestations are related to specific missing genes.

Characteristic clinical findings in the newborn include lymphedema of the hands and feet, a webbed neck, a low hairline, low-set ears, cubitus valgus (increased angle at the elbow), and widely separated nipples. Other characteristic signs include high arched palates, small mandibles, and short fourth metacarpals. During childhood, short stature becomes apparent (less than 5th percentile). During adolescence, there is a lack of breast development, pubertal delay, and amenorrhea (Malaisamy, Cakan, & Kamat, 2008; Simpson, 2009) (Figure 30–13 ➤).

Growth usually proceeds at a normal rate for the first 2 to 3 years of life and then slows. Breast tissue, which begins to bud at about 10 to 12 years, fails to develop fully. Only in rare instances does a girl with Turner syndrome menstruate spontaneously or become able to conceive. Without treatment, final height is approximately 20 cm (8 in.) lower than the expected mean adult female height (Malaisamy et al., 2008).

Among the conditions that may be associated with Turner syndrome are congenital heart defects such as coarctation of aorta or bicuspid aortic valve, hypertension, structural abnormalities of the kidney, autoimmune thyroiditis, celiac disease,

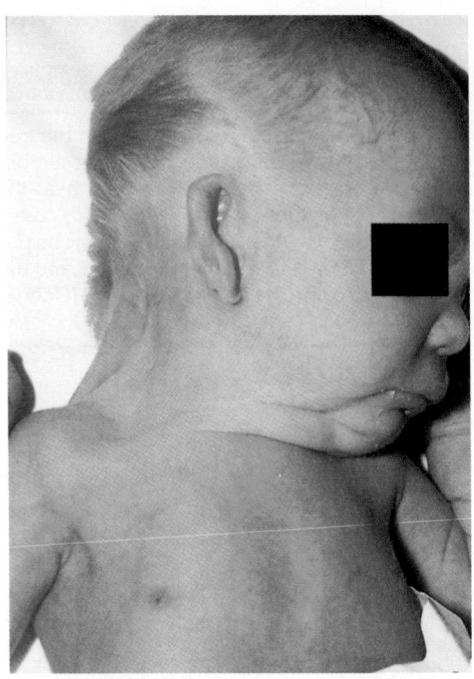

FIGURE 30–13 ➤ What characteristic physical manifestations of Turner syndrome can you identify in this girl?

From Zitelli, B. J., & Davis, H. W. (Eds.). (2007). Atlas of pediatric physical diagnosis (5th ed., p. 14). Philadelphia: Mosby-Elsevier.

hearing loss, orthodontic anomalies, strabismus, congenital hip dysplasia, and scoliosis (Morgan, 2007).

The condition is diagnosed definitively by a karyotype, which reveals the classic 45,X chromosome pattern or a combination 45,X/46,XX pattern (Morgan, 2007). Turner syndrome may be suspected prenatally based on results of maternal serum screening and ultrasound. The diagnosis must be confirmed by chorionic villus testing or amniocentesis (Loscalzo, Bondy, & Biesecker, 2006). In addition, the child should be evaluated for other disorders associated with Turner syndrome such as congenital heart and renal defects.

Management involves carefully monitoring the child's growth. A growth chart made especially for girls with Turner syndrome is available from the Turner Syndrome Society of the United States. Growth hormone therapy is prescribed to promote growth during childhood. Therapy begins as early as 12–24 months of age and continues until the child has reached a bone age of 14 years (Morgan, 2007). Anabolic steroids, preferably oxandrolone, may be used in combination with growth hormone therapy to augment growth (Malaisamy et al., 2008). Supplemental estrogen therapy is usually begun during the preteen years and continued throughout life. This treatment produces pubertal changes such as breast development and pubic hair. Estrogen therapy also helps to preserve bone mineral density (Morgan, 2007).

Nursing Management

Nursing assessment is focused on monitoring growth rates and observing for signs of cardiac, renal, gastrointestinal, vision, hearing, musculoskeletal, or thyroid dysfunction. Carefully measure the child's height and plot on the growth curve. Teach

the family the correct administration of growth hormone and potential side effects.

The lack of growth and sexual development associated with Turner syndrome presents problems not only for physical growth but also for psychosocial development. The girl's perception of her body and how she differs from peers affects self-image, self-consciousness, and self-esteem. In the United States, cultural values place importance on attaining normal to tall stature. Children who are short tend to be treated according to their size rather than their age. Emphasis is also placed on sexual maturity. Encourage parents to treat the child by her chronological age rather than size. The nurse can help the child adapt to the condition and gain self-esteem. Be an active listener and reinforce abilities and skills that the girl exhibits. Encourage parents to provide support. The Turner Syndrome Society can provide additional information about the disorder for parents and adolescents.

Klinefelter Syndrome

Klinefelter syndrome is a common genetic condition that occurs in boys who have an extra X chromosome (usually 47,XXY). It occurs in approximately 1 in 650 males. Klinefelter syndrome is associated with hypogonadism (decreased secretory activity of the gonad), infertility in males, and tall stature (Boada, Janusz, Hutaff-Lee, et al., 2009).

Klinefelter syndrome is frequently diagnosed when the onset of puberty is delayed or an abnormal progression is evident. Testicular size is decreased at all ages. Less facial and body hair may develop. Gynecomastia is a characteristic finding. Other physical features include fifth finger *clinodactyly* (bending or curving), hypotonia, and *hypertelorism* (increased distance between the eyes (Zeger, Zinn, Lahlou, et al., 2008).

Klinefelter syndrome may also be diagnosed during the school-age years when the child is having difficulty at school. Speech and reading delays are common (Zeger et al., 2008). In addition, boys with Klinefelter syndrome may have auditory processing problems that are frustrating to the child. Intelligence quotient (IQ) scores may be similar to those of siblings, but academic difficulty is common because of problems with memory, data retrieval skills, and verbal processing (Misra & Lee, 2005).

Chromosomal analysis revealing one or more extra X chromosomes confirms the diagnosis. The goal of treatment is to stimulate masculinization and the development of secondary sex characteristics when adolescence is delayed. Testosterone replacement is begun when the boy is 11 or 12 years of age. A testosterone preparation is given by intramuscular injection every 3 to 4 weeks to maintain serum testosterone levels within the normal range. The dose is increased gradually every 6–9 months until a maintenance dose is achieved in adults (Rapaport, 2007). Hormone treatment helps improve psychologic well-being and social functioning (Misra & Lee, 2005). It also helps to promote normal body proportions and prevent gynecomastia.

Nursing Management

Nursing care consists of educating the parents and child about the syndrome, evaluating the child's and family's coping mechanisms, assisting with school problems, and reinforcing the child's strengths. Encourage parents to channel their son's energy into areas that will provide opportunities for success and productive experiences. Emphasize the importance of rewarding the boy's successes in school, sports, or hobbies. Make genetic counseling available to adolescents, if indicated, because sexual functioning and fertility may be impaired.

■ INBORN ERRORS OF METABOLISM

Inborn errors of metabolism are inherited biochemical abnormalities of the urea cycle, amino acid, and organic acid metabolism. Therefore, protein, carbohydrate, fat, electrolyte, blood, and respiratory metabolism can be affected. Individually they are rare disorders; however, as a group they are a significant health problem in infancy.

The biochemical defect usually causes an abnormal chemical by-product to accumulate in the blood, urine, or tissues or results in a decreased amount of normal enzymes. Most disorders are associated with protein intolerance with symptoms developing shortly after formula or breast milk feedings are begun.

Clinical manifestations usually occur within days or weeks of birth. Signs and symptoms may include lethargy and poor feeding, persistent vomiting, abnormal muscle tone and seizures, apnea and tachycardia, and an unusual urine or body odor (musty, sweet odor of maple syrup or burnt sugar, or cheesy or sweaty feet).

Newborn screening has been demonstrated to save lives and to prevent serious disability. The American College of Medical Genetics recommends newborn screening for 29 disorders (Barbouth, Morales, & Villalba, 2009). In most states, newborn screening programs lead to the detection of several conditions before symptoms develop.

In some cases, disorders associated with inborn errors of metabolism are not detected until signs and symptoms are present. Initial laboratory tests include measurement of serum glucose, electrolytes, blood gases, and serum ammonia. Test results make it possible to classify the disorder by the presence of hypoglycemia, metabolic acidosis, hyperammonemia, or liver dysfunction. Further diagnostic laboratory tests are then performed on newborns with positive results.

Treatment, when available, focuses on replacing or reducing the amount of the substance causing the biochemical abnormality.

Four of the more common inborn errors of metabolism—phenylketonuria, galactosemia, fatty acid oxidation defects, and

Law & Ethics — *Newborn Screening*

Although all states have laws related to newborn screening, there is no federal mandate related to this. Each state sets guidelines for newborn screening. The ability of states to implement and expand their newborn screening programs is dependent in part on federal funding. The Newborn Screening Saves Lives Act was signed into law in April 2008. This law increases the ability of states to screen newborns, to provide health care services and treatment to newborns and children, and to provide counseling and education to parents and health care professionals (Barbouth et al., 2009).

maple syrup urine disease—are presented in this section. Congenital hypothyroidism and congenital adrenal hyperplasia, which are also considered inborn errors of metabolism, were discussed earlier in this chapter.

Phenylketonuria

Phenylketonuria (PKU) is an autosomal recessive inherited disorder of amino acid metabolism that affects the body's use of protein. It is caused by a mutation of the phenylalanine hydroxylase gene. The incidence is approximately 1 in 15,000 live births per year in the United States (Arnold, 2009). The defect results in an accumulation of phenylalanine in the blood or phenylalanine metabolites in the urine. If untreated, this disease leads to irreversible brain damage and severe intellectual disability. Phenylalanine levels above 20 mg/dL are indicative of classic PKU (Widaman, 2009).

Children with PKU have a deficiency of the liver enzyme phenylalanine hydroxylase that normally breaks down the essential amino acid phenylalanine into tyrosine. As a result, phenylalanine accumulates in the blood, causing a musty or mousy body and urine odor, irritability, vomiting, hyperactivity, hypertonia, hyperreflexive deep tendon reflexes, seizures, and an eczema-like rash (Rezvani, 2007).

Infants appear normal at birth except for lighter skin complexion than their nonaffected siblings. If diagnosis is delayed, intellectual disability may be severe. Microcephaly, prominent maxilla and widely spaced teeth, enamel hypoplasia, and growth retardation are other common findings in untreated children (Rezvani, 2007).

Screening for PKU is required by state law in all 50 states. For best results, the newborn should have begun formula or breast milk feeding before specimen collection. Early hospital discharge places newborns at risk for false negative screening tests if screened within 24 hours of birth. Screening needs to occur no sooner than 48 hours after birth, or the test should be repeated at 1 to 2 weeks of age. If the test shows elevated levels of plasma phenylalanine, a repeat quantitative test is performed. If the second test is positive, the family is referred to an outpatient treatment center. Serum phenylalanine should be measured periodically throughout life.

PKU is treated using special formulas and a diet low in phenylalanine to keep plasma phenylalanine levels between 2 and 6 mg/dL (Arnold, 2009). The diet must also meet the child's needs for optimal growth. Breastfeeding is possible if phenylalanine levels are monitored. High-protein foods (meats and dairy products) and aspartame are avoided because they contain large amounts of phenylalanine. Elemental medical foods (modified protein hydrolysates in which the phenylalanine has been removed) are used instead. The low-phenylalanine diet should be maintained throughout life to avoid declines in IQ and neuropsychological abilities (White, Waisbren, & van Spronsen, 2010). The low-phenylalanine diet is especially important for adolescent females and women prior to conception and during pregnancy to prevent congenital anomalies (microcephaly, intellectual disability, and congenital heart defects) in the fetus (March of Dimes, 2008; Widaman, 2009).

Nursing Management

Nursing care is mainly supportive and focuses on teaching parents about the disorder and its management. The low-phenylalanine diet is a rigid, strict diet that excludes many foods. Educate the family about sources of phenylalanine, and refer the family to a nutritionist to establish an appropriate meal plan. Parents and children need a great deal of support to promote compliance. The formula and elemental medical food costs are relatively high. The formula is usually reimbursed by insurance, but negotiations with health plans may help parents obtain some support for medical foods. Refer parents of an affected child who are considering a future pregnancy and adolescents with the disorder for genetic counseling.

Galactosemia

Galactosemia, a disorder of carbohydrate metabolism, has an autosomal recessive inheritance pattern. It occurs in approximately 1 in 50,000 live births (March of Dimes, 2008).

Galactosemia results from a deficiency of the liver enzyme galactose 1-phosphate uridyltransferase (GALT), one of three enzymes needed to convert galactose to glucose. The lack of enzyme leads to an accumulation of galactose metabolites in the eyes, liver, kidney, and brain, rapidly damaging the organs and causing life-threatening problems. Children become susceptible to *E. coli* sepsis (Kishnani & Chen, 2007).

Early signs include poor sucking, failure to gain weight due to vomiting followed by diarrhea, hypoglycemia, and an enlarged liver. Later signs include intellectual disability, jaundice, ascites, sepsis, lethargy, seizures, hypotonia, cataracts, and coma. Babies may die within 1 month of birth without treatment, usually due to sepsis. If the infant is not diagnosed with galactosemia at birth, cirrhosis of the liver and intellectual disability progress and become irreversible (Kishnani & Chen, 2007).

Routine newborn screening for galactosemia is performed in all U.S. newborn screening programs (March of Dimes, 2008). Infants who are not screened at birth are identified once they become symptomatic. The diagnosis is based upon history, physical examination, and laboratory tests (galactose, AST, and ALT are abnormally high). Urine specimens are checked for reducing substances (the Clinitest is positive and the Clinistix is negative) in several specimens while the infant is receiving human milk or formula with lactose.

Treatment involves placing infants on a lactose- or galactose-free formula. Improvement in the infant's condition is generally seen within 24 hours. A galactose-free diet (no milk or cheese products, including foods with dry milk products) is prescribed when the infant is ready for solids. These dietary restrictions are lifelong (March of Dimes, 2008). Despite compliance with the diet, complications (learning disabilities, speech defects, ovarian failure, and neurologic syndromes) develop in many children (Kishnani & Chen, 2007).

Nursing Management

Nursing management focuses on educating the parents and child about the disorder and required diet, assessing coping abilities, and providing emotional support. Refer the family to a nutritionist for diet counseling. Families must learn to screen foods for added milk solids and to avoid medications, such as antibiotics, that have lactose fillers. Calcium supplementation may be needed. Advise parents that several galactose-free cheeses are sold commercially. Because the disorder is inherited, refer the family for genetic counseling.

Defects in Fatty Acid Oxidation

Mitochondrial oxidation of fatty acids is an energy-producing pathway that becomes essential during periods of starvation, when the body fuel converts from carbohydrate to fat. Gene defects can occur in nearly every stage in the fatty acid oxidation pathway, resulting in many subclasses of fatty acid oxidation defects. All of these defects are autosomal recessive traits and occur in both males and females (Stanley & Bennett, 2007).

Screening has revealed that fatty acid oxidation disorders are among the most common inborn errors of metabolism. If undiagnosed, these disorders can lead to serious complications affecting the brain and other organs. Symptoms can progress to coma and then death (March of Dimes, 2006).

The most common presentation is an acute-onset life-threatening coma and hypoglycemia induced by a period of fasting. Other manifestations often include cardiomyopathy, hepatomegaly, and muscle weakness. Infants and children can be asymptomatic except for times during fasting or stress.

Diagnosis can occur during routine newborn screening when laboratories use mass spectrometry. Most cases are identified during an acute presentation of symptoms when laboratory evaluation may include blood gases, electrolytes, hepatic profile, plasma lactate, plasma amino acids, urine organic acids, acylcarnitine profile, quantitative carnitine levels, and urine for ketones. Hypoglycemia is usually present and ketone levels are unusually low (Thomas & Van Hove, 2007). Liver function tests demonstrate elevated transaminases, urea, and ammonia. Plasma and tissue concentrations of total carnitine are reduced. Skin biopsies are often obtained for fibroblast analysis. Physical examination may reveal hepatomegaly due to fatty infiltration.

Treatment includes the prevention of hypoglycemia by avoiding fasting, ensuring that no more than 8–12 hours passes before food is eaten. Carnitine supplementation may be required in some disorders as it is useful in preventing low blood sugar and assists in removing metabolic waste from cells (Thomas & Van Hove, 2007).

Nursing Management

Nursing management involves educating parents about the importance of frequent feedings and avoidance of fasting. These children should not go longer than 8 to 12 hours without food. Infants should be fed around the clock every 2 to 4 hours. If the infant or child is unable to sustain oral intake during an acute illness, he or she must be referred to the hospital for intravenous dextrose supplementation. Even simple infections such as an ear infection or influenza can become life threatening for these children. Several snacks and meals of low-fat and high-carbohydrate foods (i.e., cereal, pasta) are recommended throughout the day. Genetic counseling should be offered to the family. If one child in the family is diagnosed with the disorder, the siblings should also be tested, even if they are asymptomatic.

Maple Syrup Urine Disease

Maple syrup urine disease (MSUD) is a disorder of amino acid metabolism that has an autosomal recessive inheritance pattern. It is rare, occurring in approximately 1 in 180,000 newborns, but occurs as often as 1 in 176 newborns among some Pennsylvania Mennonites (Bodamer & Lee, 2008).

In MSUD, three essential amino acids (leucine, isoleucine, and valine) cannot be metabolized because of absent or defective enzyme branched-chain alpha-ketoacid dehydrogenase (Simon et al., 2006). All three amino acids are essential to form normal structures such as the hair, skin, and muscle. Leucine has the potential to accumulate in the brain and cause cerebral edema, progressive neurologic impairment, and death (Bodamer & Lee, 2008).

Within 4 to 7 days of life, the newborn develops symptoms of poor appetite, lethargy, vomiting, variable muscle tone, irritability, seizures, high-pitched cry, severe ketoacidosis, and a sweet odor of maple syrup in body fluids. The symptoms may quickly progress to coma and death if not treated (Bodamer & Lee, 2008; March of Dimes, 2006).

Most but not all states require newborn screening for this condition. Diagnosis is made with laboratory tests of the urine for positive ketones and blood tests for elevated leucine, isoleucine, alloisoleucine (a stereoisomer of isoleucine not normally found in blood), and valine.

Treatment during the acute stage involves removal of the branched-chain amino acids and their metabolites from the tissues and body fluids. Some critically ill infants may require dialysis to remove these compounds because renal clearance is poor. Lifelong treatment includes specially designed medical formulas and foods rich in amino acids, calories, vitamins, minerals, and other nutrients as prescribed; these special medical foods have the three amino acids removed. The child needs special low-protein foods that are adequate for growth with enough calories to support twice the child's basal metabolic rate. Daily urine testing is required to determine if ketones are being excreted, an indication that the body is in a catabolic state. A liver transplant has been performed in a few affected children who were subsequently able to tolerate a normal diet (Rezvani & Rosenblatt, 2007). The long-term prognosis of affected children is guarded as severe ketoacidosis, cerebral edema, or death may occur during any stressful situation, including infection or surgery.

Nursing Management

Nursing care includes educating the family about the disorder and special dietary requirements. The parents need to learn how to mix the child's special formula with a natural protein source, amino acid supplements, and water. The child needs formula even when ill; provide a sick day plan to prevent ketoacidosis. The child should be permitted moderate exercise only to prevent increases in leucine levels. Help families identify sources of information or support groups who can share recipes and tips for managing the child's condition. See the companion website for resources.

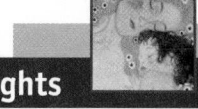

Chapter Highlights

- Puberty is the process of sexual maturation that occurs when the gonads secrete increased amounts of the sex hormones estrogen and testosterone, resulting in the development of primary and secondary sexual characteristics.

- The anterior pituitary gland is considered to be the "master gland" of the body because of its role in the production of hormones that regulate the secretion of other hormones.

- Children with hypopituitarism have short stature as a result of growth hormone deficiency. Treatment with growth hormone early in life enables these children to potentially attain genetically appropriate heights.

- An excessive secretion of growth hormone or hyperpituitarism may cause children to have tall stature, growing up to 7 or 8 feet in height if no intervention is provided before the epiphyseal plates close.

- In diabetes insipidus, the urine cannot be concentrated, no matter how dehydrated the child becomes. Diagnosis rarely occurs until the child experiences hypernatremic dehydration.

- Syndrome of inappropriate antidiuretic hormone (SIADH) results from an excessive amount of serum antidiuretic hormone (ADH) leading to water intoxication and hyponatremia.

- Precocious puberty is defined as the appearance of any secondary sexual characteristics before 8 years in girls and 9 years in boys. If no treatment is provided, the hormones will stimu-late closure of the epiphyseal plates and the child will have short stature as an adult.

- Untreated or ineffectively treated congenital hypothyroidism results in impaired growth and intellectual disability.

- Signs of hyperthyroidism include an enlarged, nontender thyroid gland (goiter), prominent eyes, eyelid lag, tachycardia, nervousness, restlessness or irritability, increased appetite with weight loss, emotional lability, heat intolerance, increased sweating, insomnia, tremor, and muscle weakness.

- During infancy and childhood, most cases of Cushing disease are due to a malignant adrenal tumor. It generally takes 2 to 5 years for the child to develop the characteristic cushingoid appearance.

- Congenital adrenal hyperplasia has two forms, salt losing or non-salt losing with virilization. The salt-losing form accounts for 75% of cases and is caused by aldosterone deficiency and overproduction of androgen. The non-salt-losing form accounts for the other 25% of cases.

- Adrenal insufficiency, though rare in children, is characterized by weakness with fatigue, anorexia and salt craving, poor weight gain or weight loss, hyperpigmentation at pressure points, generalized bronzing of the skin, abdominal pain, nausea and vomiting, and diarrhea.

- Congenital adrenal hyperplasia is the most common cause of pseudohermaphroditism (ambiguous genitalia) in newborn girls.
- Pheochromocytoma is a rare benign tumor of the adrenal gland that causes labile hypertension and intermittent signs associated with epinephrine and norepinephrine secretion.
- Diabetes mellitus type 1 is the most common metabolic disease in children and one of the most common chronic diseases in school-age children. It is a disorder of carbohydrate, protein, and fat metabolism.
- Treatment of the child with diabetic ketoacidosis includes intravenous fluids and electrolytes for dehydration and acidosis. Insulin is given by continuous infusion pump to decrease the serum glucose level at a slow but steady rate to prevent the development of cerebral edema.
- Common causes of hypoglycemia in children with type 1 diabetes include an error in insulin dosage, inadequate calories because of missed meals, or exercise without a corresponding increase in caloric intake.
- Type 2 diabetes mellitus is a condition that results from insulin resistance and affects 8–45% of children over 10 years of age. Children most commonly affected are obese, and many have family members with the same type of diabetes.
- Secondary amenorrhea is the cessation of spontaneous menstrual periods for at least 120 days and occurs 6 months or three cycles after menarche.
- Turner syndrome is diagnosed definitively by a karyotype, which reveals the classic 45,X chromosome pattern or 46,XX pattern with one misshapen X chromosome.

- Signs of Klinefelter syndrome include gynecomastia, delayed onset of puberty with an abnormal progression, decreased testicular size, and less facial and body hair than normal.
- Inborn errors of metabolism—inherited biochemical abnormalities of the urea cycle and amino acid and organic acid metabolism—often have a significant impact on the endocrine system's ability to support growth and development. These disorders include phenylketonuria, galactosemia, defects in fatty acid oxygenation, and maple syrup urine disease.
- Children with phenylketonuria (PKU) have a deficiency of the liver enzyme phenylalanine hydroxylase that normally breaks down the essential amino acid phenylalanine into tyrosine. It is treated with special formula and engineered foods.
- Galactosemia results from a deficiency of a liver enzyme needed to convert galactose to glucose. This leads to an accumulation of galactose metabolites in the eyes, liver, kidney, and brain, rapidly damaging the organs and causing life-threatening problems.
- In the inborn error of metabolism involving a defect in fatty acid oxygenation, the most common presentation is an acute-onset life-threatening coma and hypoglycemia induced by a period of fasting.
- Maple syrup urine disease is a rare inherited enzyme deficiency that results in ketoacidosis unless special formula, engineered foods, and extra calories are eaten.

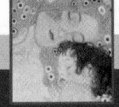

Clinical Reasoning in Action

Recall Anthony, the 12-year-old in the opening scenario, who is newly diagnosed with type 1 diabetes. His glucose is now stabilized and he is receiving basal-bolus insulin therapy. Anthony is learning to check his own serum glucose and demonstrates the correct technique. He states that he is afraid of giving himself a "shot" and becomes anxious when he receives injections. Anthony will soon be discharged from the hospital and will receive further diabetes education on an outpatient basis. Anthony's parents are eager to learn about caring for him, but express concerns now that he will not be able to participate in sports activities as he has in the past.

1. Considering Anthony's age and developmental level, how will the nurse explain type 1 diabetes to Anthony?
2. How will the nurse address Anthony's reluctance to self-administer his insulin? What are some potential causes of Anthony's reluctance?
3. What skills must Anthony's parents demonstrate prior to his discharge from the hospital?
4. What will the nurse explain to Anthony and his parents regarding activity, exercise, and participation in sports?

See Pearson Nursing Student Resources for possible responses.

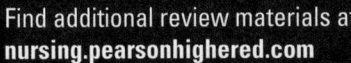

Pearson Nursing Student Resources

Find additional review materials at
nursing.pearsonhighered.com

Prepare for success with NCLEX®-style practice questions, interactive assignments and activities, web links, animations and videos, and more!

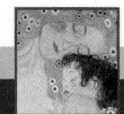

References

Adams, M. H., & Lammon, C. A. B. (2007). The presence of family history and the development of type 2 diabetes mellitus risk factors in rural children. *Journal of School Nursing, 23*(5), 259–266.

Alemzadeh, R., & Wyatt, D. T. (2007). Diabetes mellitus in children. In R. M. Kliegman, R. E. Behrman, H. B. Jenson, & B. F. Stanton (Eds.), *Nelson textbook of pediatrics* (18th ed., pp. 2402–2431). Philadelphia: Saunders Elsevier.

Amer, K. S. (2005). Advances in assessment, diagnosis, and treatment of hyperthyroidism in children. *Journal of Pediatric Nursing, 20*(2), 119–126.

American Academy of Pediatrics. (2009). *Pediatric nutrition handbook* (6th ed., pp. 673–699). Elk Grove Village, IL: Author.

American Diabetes Association. (2008a). Diagnosis and classification of diabetes mellitus. *Diabetes Care, 31*(Supp. 1), S55–S60.

American Diabetes Association. (2008b). Diabetes care in the school and day care setting. *Diabetes Care, 31*(Suppl. 1), S79–S86.

American Diabetes Association. (2008c). *Ketoacidosis.* Retrieved from http://www.diabetes.org/ type-1-diabetes/ketoacidosis.jsp

American Diabetes Association. (2010a). Standards of medical care in diabetes—2010. *Diabetes Care, 33*(Suppl. 1), S11–S61.

American Diabetes Association. (2010b). Diabetes care in the school and day care setting. *Diabetes Care, 33*(Suppl. 1), S70–S74.

Antal, Z., & Zhou, P. (2009). Addison disease. *Pediatrics in Review, 30*(12), 491–493.

Arnold, G. L. (2009). *Phenylketonuria.* Retrieved from http://emedicine.medscape.com/article/ 947781-overview

Barbouth, D., Morales, A., & Villalba, R. (2009). Expanded newborn screening: An update for pediatricians. *Pediatric Annals, 38*(8), 431–438.

Berhe, T., Postellon, D., Wilson, B., & Stone, R. (2006). Feasibility and safety of insulin pump therapy in children aged 2 to 7 years with type 1 diabetes: A retrospective study. *Pediatrics, 117*(6), 2132–2137.

Berry, D., Urban, A., & Grey, M. (2006a). Management of type 2 diabetes in youth (Part 2). *Journal of Pediatric Health Care, 20*(2), 88–97.

Berry, D., Urban, A., & Grey, M. (2006b). Understanding the development and prevention of type 2 diabetes in youth (Part 1). *Journal of Pediatric Health Care, 20*(1), 3–10.

Bindler, R. M., & Bruya, M. A. (2006). Evidence for identifying children at risk for being overweight, cardiovascular disease, and type 2 diabetes in primary care. *Journal of Pediatric Health Care, 20*(2), 82–87.

Bismuth, E., & Laffel, L. (2007). Can we prevent diabetes ketoacidosis in children? *Pediatric Diabetes, 8*(6), 24–33.

Boada, R., Janusz, J., Hutaff-Lee, C., & Tartaglia, N. (2009). The cognitive phenotype in Klinefelter syndrome: A review of the literature *including* genetic and hormonal factors. *Developmental Disabilities Research Reviews, 15,* 284–294.

Bloomfield, D. (2006). Secondary amenorrhea. *Pediatrics in Review, 27*(3), 113–115.

Bodamer, O. A., & Lee, B. (2008). *Maple syrup urine disease.* Retrieved from http://emedicine .medscape.com/article/946234-overview

Boger, M. S., & Perrier, N. D. (2004). Advantages and disadvantages of surgical therapy and optional extent of thyroidectomy for the treatment of hyperthyroidism. *Surgical Clinics of North America, 84,* 849–874.

Breault, D. T., & Majzoub, J. A. (2007). Diabetes insipidus. In R. M. Kliegman, R. E. Behrman, H. B. Jenson, & B. F. Stanton (Eds.), *Nelson textbook of pediatrics* (18th ed., pp. 2299–2301). Philadelphia: Saunders Elsevier.

Carroll, K. L. (2010). Alterations of musculoskeletal function in children. In K. L. McCance & S. E. Huether, *Pathophysiology: The biologic basis for disease in adults and children* (6th ed., pp. 1618–1643) Maryland Heights, MO: Mosby Elsevier.

Cheung, R., Cureton, V. Y., & Canham, D. L. (2006). Quality of life in adolescents with type 1 diabetes who participate in diabetes camp. *Journal of School Nursing, 22,* 53–58.

Cook, L. K. (2009). Pheochromocytoma. *American Journal of Nursing, 109*(2), 50–53.

Cooke, D. W., & Plotnick, L. (2008a). Type 1 Diabetes Mellitus in pediatrics. *Pediatrics in Review, 29,* 374–385.

Cooke, D. W., & Plotnick, L. (2008b). Management of diabetic ketoacidosis in children and adolescents. *Pediatrics in Review, 29,* 431–436.

Cox, D., & Polvado, K. (2008). Type 2 diabetes in children and adolescents. *Advance for Nurse Practitioners, 16*(11), 43–45.

Cystic Fibrosis Foundation. (2009). *Cystic fibrosis-related diabetes.* Retrieved from http://www.cff .org/LivingWithCF/StayingHealthy/Diet/ Diabetes/

Darendeliler, F., Karagiannis, G., & Wilton, P. (2007). Headache, idiopathic intracranial hypertension and slipped capital femoral epiphysis during growth hormone treatment: A safety update from the KIGS database. *Hormone Research, 68*(Suppl. 5), 41–47.

deVries, L., Shtaif, B., Phillip, M., & Gat-Yablonski, G. (2009). Kisspeptin serum levels in girls with central precocious puberty. *Clinical Endocrinology, 71,* 524–528.

deWit, M., Delemarre-van de Waal, H. A., Bokma, J. A., & Hass, K. (2008). Monitoring and discussing health-related quality of life in adolescents with type 1 diabetes improve psychosocial well-being. *Diabetes Care, 31*(8), 1521–1526.

Doswell, B. H., Visootsak, J., Brady, A. N., & Graham, J. M. (2006). Turner syndrome: An update and review for the primary physician. *Clinical Pediatrics, 45,* 301–313.

Doty, E., & Attaran, M. (2006). Managing primary dysmenorrhea. *Journal of Pediatric & Adolescent Gynecology, 19,* 341–344.

Doyle, D. A., & DiGeorge, A. M. (2007). Disorders of the parathyroid. In R. M. Kliegman, R. E. Behrman, H. B. Jenson, & B. F. Stanton (Eds.), *Nelson textbook of pediatrics* (18th ed., pp. 2340–2348). Philadelphia: Saunders Elsevier.

Doyle, E. A., & Grey, M. (2010). Diabetes mellitus (Types 1 and 2). In P. J. Allen, J. A. Vessey, & N. A. Schapiro (Eds.), *Primary care of the child with a chronic condition* (5th ed., pp. 427–446). St. Louis, MO: Mosby.

Eugster, E. A., Francis, G., & Lawson-Wilkins Drug and Therapeutics Committee. (2006). Position statement: Continuous subcutaneous insulin infusion in very young children with type 1 diabetes. *Pediatrics, 118*(4), 1244–1249.

Ferry, R. J. (2005). Salt wasting and the syndrome of inappropriate antidiuretic hormone. In T. M. Moshange, *Pediatric endocrinology: The requisites for pediatrics* (pp. 269–274). St. Louis, MO: Elsevier Mosby.

Ferry, R. J., & Pascual-y-Baralt, J. F. (2009). *Syndrome of inappropriate antidiuretic hormone secretion.* Retrieved from http://emedicine.medscape.com/ article/924829-overview

Fleury-Milfort, E. (2008). Insulin replacement therapy: Minimizing complications and side effects. *Advance for Nurse Practitioners, 16*(11), 32–39.

George, J., Acharya, S. V., Bandgar, T. R., Menon, P. S., & Shah, N. S. (2010). Primary hyperparathyroidism in children and adolescents. *Indian Journal of Pediatrics, 77*(2), 175–178.

Graue, M., Wentzel-Larsen, T., Hanestad, B. R., & Sovik, O. (2005). Health-related quality of life and metabolic control in adolescents with diabetes: The role of parental care, control, and involvement. *Journal of Pediatric Nursing, 20*(5), 373.

Grimberg, A., & De León, D. D. (2005). Disorders of growth. In T. M. Moshange, *Pediatric endocrinology: The requisites for pediatrics* (pp. 127–167). St. Louis, MO: Elsevier Mosby.

Grimberg, A., Stewart, E., & Wajnrajch, M. P. (2008). Gender of pediatric recombinant human growth hormone recipients in the United States and globally. *Journal of Clinical Endocrinology and Metabolism, 93*(6), 2050–2056.

Habich, M. (2006). Establishing a standard for pediatric inpatient diabetes education. *Pediatric Nursing, 32*(2), 113–115.

Harel, Z. (2006). Dysmenorrhea in adolescents and young adults: Etiology and management. *Journal of Pediatric and Adolescent Gynecology, 19,* 363–371.

Helgeson, V. S., Viccaro, L., Becker, D., Escobar, O., & Siminerio, L. (2006). Diet of adolescents with and without diabetes. *Diabetes Care, 29*(5), 982–987.

Henwood, M. J., & Katz, L. E. L. (2005). Disorders of the adrenal gland. In T. M. Moshange, *Pediatric endocrinology: The requisites for pediatrics* (pp. 193–213). St. Louis, MO: Elsevier Mosby.

Huang, E. A., Feldman, B. J., Schwartz, I. D., Geller, D. H., Rosenthal, S. M., & Gitelman, S. E. (2006). Oral urea for the treatment of chronic syndrome of inappropriate antidiuresis in children. *Journal of Pediatrics, 148*, 128–131.

Johnson, R. E., & Murad, M. H. (2009). Gynecomastia: Pathophysiology, evaluation, and management. *Mayo Clinic Proceedings, 84*(11), 1010–1015.

Kache, S., & Ferry, R. J. (2005). Diabetes insipidus. In T. M. Moshange, *Pediatric endocrinology: The requisites for pediatrics* (pp. 257–267). St. Louis, MO: Elsevier Mosby.

Kaguelidou, F., Carel, J. C., & Leger, J. (2009). Graves' disease in childhood: Advances in management with antithyroid drug therapy. *Hormone Research, 71*, 310–317.

Kaplowitz, P. B. (2006a). Precocious puberty: Making the distinction between common normal variants and more serious problems. *Contemporary Pediatrics, 23*(8), 55–57.

Kaplowitz, P. B. (2006b). Pubertal development in girls: Secular trends. *Current Opinion in Obstetrics and Gynecology, 18*(5), 487–491.

Karagiannis, A., Mikhailidis, D. P., Athyros, V. G., & Harsoulis, F. (2007). Pheochromocytoma: An update on genetics and management. *Endocrine-Related Cancer, 14*, 935–956.

Keefe, S. (2007, February). Precocious puberty. *Advance for Nurses*, 41–42.

Kishnani, P. S., & Chen, Y. (2007). Defects in galactose metabolism. In R. M. Kliegman, R. E. Behrman, H. B. Jenson, & B. F. Stanton (Eds.), *Nelson textbook of pediatrics* (18th ed., pp. 609–610). Philadelphia: Saunders Elsevier.

Kulshreshtha, B., Khadgawat, R., Eunice, M., & Ammini, A. C. (in press). Congenital adrenal hyperplasia: Results of medical therapy on appearance of external genitalia. *Journal of Pediatric Urology*.

Kwon, K. T., & Tsai, V. W. (2007). Metabolic emergencies. *Emergency Medicine Clinics of North America, 25*(4), 1041–1060.

LaFranchi, S. (2007). Disorders of the thyroid gland. In R. M. Kliegman, R. E. Behrman, H. B. Jenson, & B. F. Stanton (Eds.), *Nelson textbook of pediatrics* (18th ed., pp. 2316–2340). Philadelphia: Saunders Elsevier.

Landry, G. L. (2007). Female athletes: Menstrual problems and the risk of osteopenia. In R. M. Kliegman, R. E. Behrman, H. B. Jenson, & B. F. Stanton (Eds.), *Nelson textbook of pediatrics* (18th ed., p. 2865). Philadelphia: Saunders Elsevier.

Lee, J. M., & Menon, R. K. (2005). Growth hormone for short children without growth deficiency: Issues and practices. *Contemporary Pediatrics, 22*(10), 46–53.

Lee, J. M., Davis, M. M., Clark, S. J., Hofer, T. P., & Kemper, A. R. (2006). Estimated cost effectiveness of growth hormone therapy for idiopathic short stature. *Archives of Pediatrics and Adolescent Medicine, 160*, 263–269.

Lee, P. A. (2005). Early pubertal development. In T. M. Moshange, *Pediatric endocrinology: The requisites for pediatrics* (pp. 73–86). St. Louis, MO: Elsevier Mosby.

Lee, P. A., & Kulin, H.E. (2005). Normal pubertal development. In T. M. Moshange, *Pediatric endocrinology: The requisites for pediatrics* (pp. 63–71). St. Louis, MO: Elsevier Mosby.

Loscalzo, M. L., Bondy, C. A., & Biesecker, B. (2006). Issues in prenatal counseling and diagnosis in Turner syndrome. *International Congress Series, 1298*, 26–29.

Malaisamy, A., Cakan, N., & Kamat, D. M. (2008). Genetic disorders: What is this disorder—And what is the prognosis? Two Girls with short stature. *Consultant for Pediatricians, 7*(7), 277–284.

March of Dimes. (2006). *Quick reference: Recommended newborn screening tests: 29 disorders*. Retrieved from http://www.marchofdimes.com/professionals/14332_15455.asp

March of Dimes. (2008). *Newborn screening tests*. Retrieved from http://www.marchofdimes.com/professionals/14332_1200.asp

Masharani, U. (2008). Diabetes mellitus and hypoglycemia. In S. J. McPhee, M. A. Papadakis, L. M. Tierney, Jr., R. Gonzales, & R. Zeiger, *Current medical diagnosis and treatment 2008*. Retrieved from McGraw-Hill's Access Medicine. http://www.accessmedicine.com

Miles, H. L., & Acerini, C. L. (2008). Insulin analog preparations and their use in children and adolescents with type 1 diabetes mellitus. *Pediatric Drugs, 10*(3), 163–176.

Misra, M., & Lee, M. M. (2005). Delayed puberty. In T. M. Moshange, *Pediatric endocrinology: The requisites for pediatrics* (pp. 87–101). St. Louis, MO: Elsevier Mosby.

Molina, P. E. (2006). Parathyroid gland & Ca^{2+} & Po^{4-} regulation. In *Endocrine physiology* (2nd ed.). Retrieved from McGraw-Hill's Access Medicine. http://www.accessmedicine.com

Morgan, T. (2007). Turner syndrome: Diagnosis and management. *American Family Physician, 76*(3), 406–410.

National Newborn Screening and Genetics Resource Center. (2009). *National newborn screening status report*. Retrieved from http://genes-r-us.uthscsa.edu/nbsdisorders.pdf

Nelson, R. (2007). Little women. *American Journal of Nursing, 107*(12), 25–26.

Nimri, R., Weintrob, H. B., Benzaquen, H., Ofan, R., Fayman, G., & Phillip, M. (2006). Insulin pump therapy in youth with type 1 diabetes: A retrospective paired study. *Pediatrics, 117*(6), 2126–2131.

Parks, J. S., & Felner, E. I. (2007a). Hormones of the hypothalamus and pituitary. In R. M. Kliegman, R. E. Behrman, H. B. Jenson, & B. F. Stanton (Eds.), *Nelson textbook of pediatrics* (18th ed., pp. 2291–2293). Philadelphia: Saunders Elsevier.

Parks, J. S., & Felner, E. I. (2007b). Hypopituitarism. In R. M. Kliegman, R. E. Behrman, H. B. Jenson, & B. F. Stanton (Eds.), *Nelson textbook of pediatrics* (18th ed., pp. 2293–2299). Philadelphia: Saunders Elsevier.

Péter, F., & Muzsnai, O. (2009). Congenital disorders of the thyroid: Hypo/hyper. *Endocrinology Metabolism Clinics of North America, 38*, 491–507.

Pinyerd, B., & Zipf, W. B. (2005). Puberty—Timing is everything. *Journal of Pediatric Nursing, 20*(2), 75–82.

Potts, J. T. (2008). Diseases of the parathyroid gland and other hyper- and hypocalcemic disorders. In A. S. Fauci, E. Braunwald, D. L. Kasper, S. L. Hauser, D. L. Longo, J. L. Jameson, & J. Loscalzo (Eds.), *Harrison's principles of internal medicine* (17th ed). Retrieved from http://www.accessmedicine.com

Raine, J. E., Donaldson, M. D. C., Gregory, J. W., Savage, M. O., & Hintz, R. L. (2006a). Salt and water balance. In J. E. Raine, M. D. C. Donaldson, J. W. Gregory, M. O. Savage, & R. L. Hintz, *Practical endocrinology and diabetes in children* (2nd ed., pp. 147–155). Malden, MA: Blackwell.

Raine, J. E., Donaldson, M. D. C., Gregory, J. W., Savage, M. O., & Hintz, R. L. (2006c). Puberty. In J. E. Raine, M. D. C. Donaldson, J. W. Gregory, M. O. Savage, & R. L. Hintz, *Practical endocrinology and diabetes in children* (2nd ed., pp. 69–90). Malden, MA: Blackwell.

Rapaport, R. (2007). Hypofunction of the testes. In R. M. Kliegman, R. E. Behrman, H. B. Jenson, & B. F. Stanton (Eds.), *Nelson textbook of pediatrics* (18th ed., pp. 2379–2384). Philadelphia: Saunders Elsevier.

Rewers, A., Klingensmith, G., Davis, C., Petitti, D. B., Pihoker, C., Rodriquez, B., et al. (2008). Presence of diabetic ketoacidosis at diagnosis of diabetes mellitus in youth: The Search for Diabetes in Youth Study.

Rezvani, I. (2007). Defects in metabolisim of amino acids. In R. M. Kliegman, R. E. Behrman, H. B. Jenson, & B. F. Stanton (Eds.), *Nelson textbook of pediatrics* (18th ed., pp. 529–532). Philadelphia: Saunders Elsevier.

Rezvani, I., & Rosenblatt, D. S. (2007). Valine, leucine, isoleucine and related organic acidemias. In R. M. Kliegman, R. E. Behrman, H. B. Jenson, & B. F. Stanton (Eds.), *Nelson textbook of pediatrics* (18th ed., pp. 540–549). Philadelphia: Saunders Elsevier.

Rossi, W. C., Caplin, N., & Alter, C. A. (2005). Thyroid disorders in children. In T. M. Moshange, *Pediatric endocrinology: The requisites for pediatrics* (pp. 171–190). St. Louis, MO: Elsevier Mosby.

Simon, E., Flaschker, N., Schadewaldt, P., Langenbeck, U., & Wendel, U. (2006). Variant maple syrup urine disease (MSUD)—The entire spectrum. *Journal of Inherited Metabolic Disease, 29*, 716–724.

Simpson, T. (2009). Short stature in a 6-year-old female. *Pediatric Nursing, 35*(1), 64, 68.

Sirotnak, A. P. (2008). *Child abuse and neglect: Psychosocial dwarfism*. Retrieved from http://emedicine.medscape.com/article/913843-overview

Stanley, C. A., & Bennett, M. J. (2007). Disorders of mitochondrial fatty acid β-oxidation. In R. M. Kliegman, R. E. Behrman, H. B. Jenson, & B. F. Stanton (Eds.), *Nelson textbook of pediatrics* (18th ed., pp. 567–573). Philadelphia: Saunders Elsevier.

Thomas, J. A., & Van Hove, J. L. K. (2007). Inborn errors of metabolism. In W. W. Hay, M. J. Levin, J. M. Sondheimer, & R. R. Deterding, *Current pediatric diagnosis and treatment* (18th ed.). Access Medicine: McGraw-Hill Companies.

Vivian, E. M. (2006). Type 2 diabetes in children and adolescents—The next epidemic? *Current Medical Residents Opinion, 22*(2), 297–306.

White, D. A., Waisbren, S., & van Spronsen, F. J. (2010). The psychology and neuropathology of phenylketonuria. *Molecular Genetics and Metabolism, 99*, s1–s2.

White, P. C. (2007). Disorders of the adrenal glands. In R. M. Kliegman, R. E. Behrman, H. B. Jenson, & B. F. Stanton (Eds.), *Nelson textbook of pediatrics* (18th ed., pp. 2349–2374). Philadelphia: Saunders Elsevier.

Widaman, K. F. (2009). Phenylketonuria in children and mothers: Genes, environments, behavior. *Current Directions in Psychological Science, 18*(1), 48–52.

Wood, J. R., Moreland, E. C., Volkening, L. K., Svoren, B. M., Butler, D. A., & Laffel, L. M. B. (2006). Durability of insulin pump use in pediatric patients with type 1 diabetes. *Diabetes Care, 29*(11), 2355–2360.

Wright, E. E. (2009). Overview of insulin replacement therapy. *Journal of Family Practice, 58*(80), S3–S9.

Zadik, Z., Sinai, T., Zung, A., & Reifen, R. (2005). Effect of nutrition on growth in short stature before and during growth-hormone therapy. *Pediatrics, 116*(1), 68–72.

Zeger, M. P. D., Zinn, A. R., Lahlou, N., Ramos, P., Kowal, K., Samango-Sprouse, C., & Ross, J. L. (2008). Effect of ascertainment and genetic features on the phenotype of Klinefelter syndrome. *Journal of Pediatrics, 152*, 716–722.

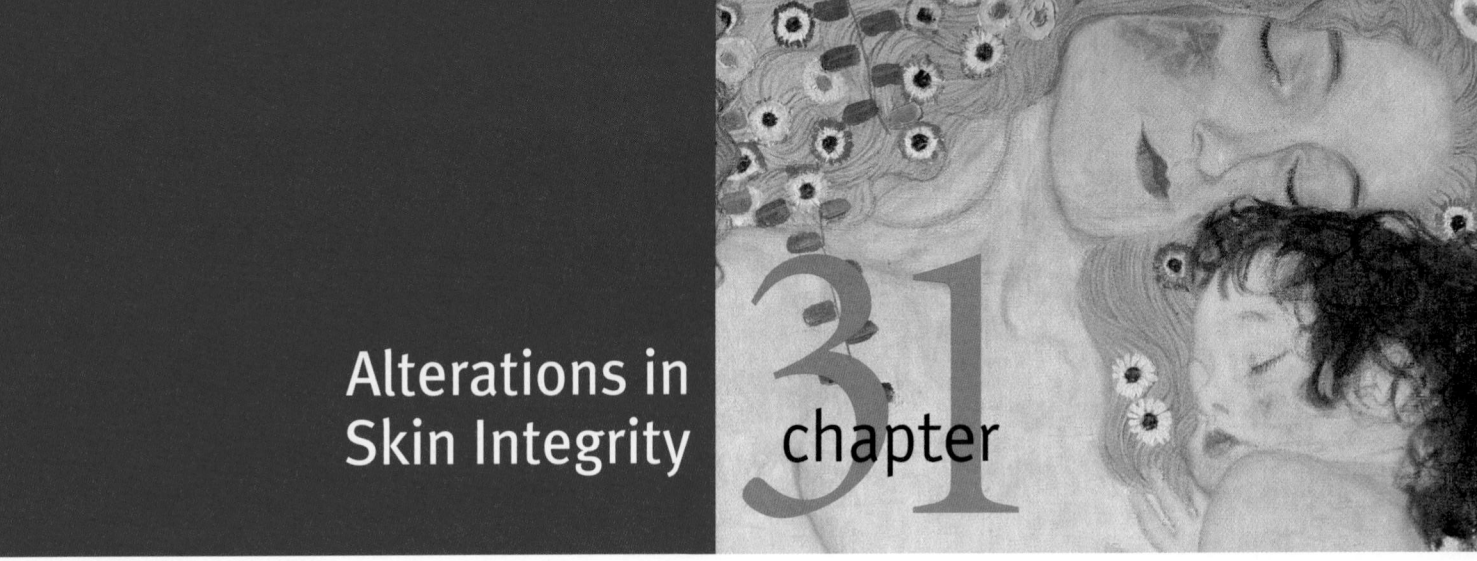

Alterations in Skin Integrity

31 chapter

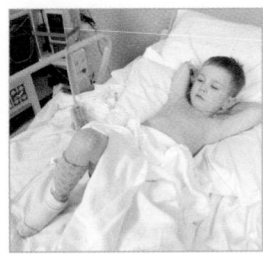

Joshua, 6 years old, was admitted to the hospital with a burn to his lower leg. He was playing with matches and his pants leg caught on fire. Fortunately his father heard his cries, and he quickly put out the flames. Joshua received emergency care to stop the burning process, and then went to the operating room for wound debridement. His pain was initially managed with IV morphine. By Joshua's second day of hospitalization, it was determined that most of his burn injury was deep partial thickness. It was not known at that time if a skin graft would be needed. A burn dressing and a vacuum-assisted closure device were applied to his leg to promote healing. Joshua was discharged home with the vacuum-assisted closure device after 4 days, with twice weekly dressing changes scheduled in the hospital's burn clinic.

It is now 3 days later, and Joshua has come to the clinic for his first burn dressing change. It is performed in the sedation suite, in case additional debridement is needed. Joshua's mother stays with him while the sedation is administered and then goes to the waiting room. Joshua's dressing change and sedation experience are uneventful. When the dressing is removed, granulation tissue is seen and no odor or purulent drainage that might indicate infection is present. The dressing and vacuum-assisted closure device are reapplied.

After the dressing change, some time is spent talking with Joshua's mother. She reports that Joshua has been eating the recommended high-protein, high-calorie diet to promote wound healing. Joshua's mother wonders how long it will take to determine if a skin graft will be needed.

What is the nurse's role in providing care to the child with a burn injury? What other members of the health care team are important to promote an optimal recovery?

Key Terms

autograft / 1059
circumferential / 1058
comedones / 1034
cryotherapy / 1040
debridement / 1033
dermatophytoses / 1041
dermis / 1032
epidermis / 1031
epithelialization / 1033
eschar / 1058
escharotomy / 1058
frostbite / 1066
hypertrophic scar / 1035
intertriginous / 1037
involution / 1053
keloid / 1035
kerion / 1042
lichenification / 1033
melanin / 1032
phototoxic / 1049
stratum corneum / 1031
telangiectasia / 1034
urticaria / 1043
xerosis / 1044

Learning Outcomes

After reading this chapter, you will be able to do the following:

1. Describe important pediatric differences in the anatomy and physiology of the child's skin.
2. Classify the characteristics of skin lesions caused by irritants, drug reactions, mites, infection, and injury.
3. Differentiate between the stages of wound healing.
4. Compare the skin conditions that have a hereditary cause or predisposition.
5. Plan the nursing care for a child with alterations in skin integrity, including dermatitis, infectious disorders, and infestations.
6. Prepare an education plan for adolescents with acne to promote self-care.
7. Summarize the process to measure the extent of burns and burn severity in children.
8. Plan the nursing care for the child with a full-thickness burn injury.
9. Evaluate prevention strategies to reduce the risk of injury from burns, bites, and stings.

FOCUS ON

The Integumentary System

ANATOMY AND PHYSIOLOGY

The skin is the largest organ in the body and performs several essential functions. The skin protects underlying tissues from invasion by microorganisms and from trauma. The nerves in the skin enable the perception of touch, pain, pressure, heat, and cold. The skin also assists the body to conserve heat by constricting blood vessels. Dilation of blood vessels and the secretion of sweat by the eccrine sweat glands enable the body to release excess heat. The sweat glands, secreting a solution of water, electrolytes, and urea, also help to rid the body of toxins. The skin supplements the body's intake of vitamin D by synthesizing this vitamin from ultraviolet light.

The skin has three distinct layers: the epidermis, the dermis, and the subcutaneous fatty layer that separates the skin from the underlying tissue (Figure 31–1 ➤). The **epidermis** is the thin, rapidly growing, outermost layer of skin. Skin is continually shed by the **stratum corneum**, the superficial layer of the epidermis. The thickness of the epidermis varies by location on the body (e.g., 0.3 mm on the eyelids and 1.5 mm on the soles of the feet) (Nicol & Huether, 2010a). The epidermis contains the melanocytes that synthesize and secrete melanin when the skin is exposed to ultraviolet light. The Langerhans cells within the

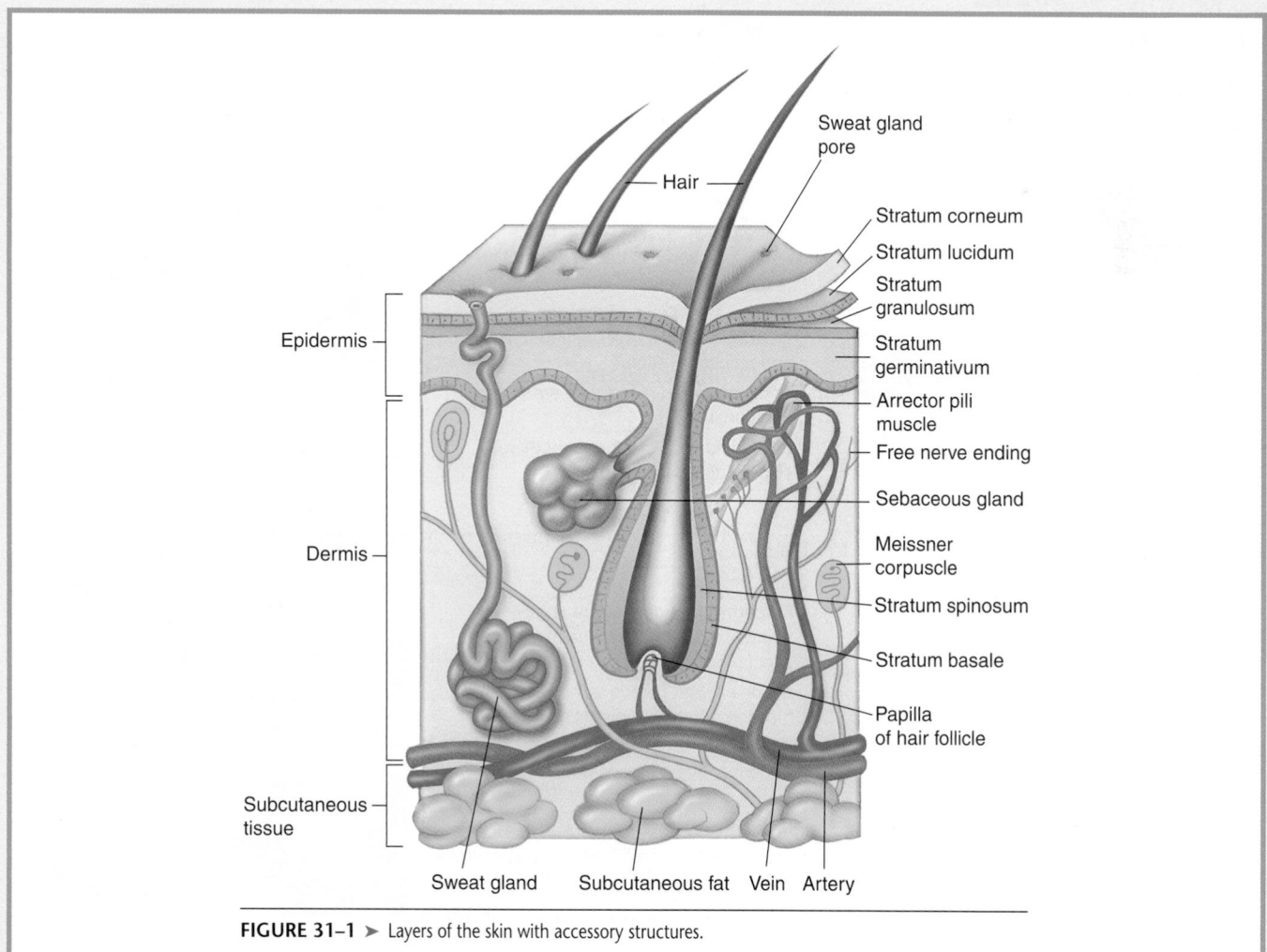

FIGURE 31–1 ➤ Layers of the skin with accessory structures.

epidermis initiate the skin's immune response when exposed to environmental antigens.

The **dermis**, the middle layer of the skin, is mostly composed of connective tissue, which allows the skin to stretch and contract with movement. Nerves, muscles, hair follicles, sebaceous and sweat glands, lymph channels, and blood vessels are all contained within the dermis. Mast cells located within the dermis play a role in the skin's hypersensitivity reactions.

The third skin layer, the subcutaneous layer, connects the dermis to the muscle below. This layer of fat cells helps insulate the body from cold temperatures. The sebaceous glands appear all over the body except on the palms of the hands and soles of the feet, and are connected with hair follicles in most cases. Sebum, a lipid substance produced and secreted into the hair follicle or directly onto the skin, lubricates the skin and hair.

Eccrine sweat glands, located in the dermis, open onto the skin's surface. They secrete sweat, an odorless, watery fluid containing sodium, chloride, urea, and other body wastes. As the body temperature elevates, an increased production of sweat evaporates and cools the body.

Apocrine sweat glands are primarily located in the axillary and genital areas, and their secretions contain more lipids and proteins. Decomposition of the fluid secreted by these glands leads to body odor.

PEDIATRIC DIFFERENCES

The newborn's skin is the largest organ of the body, but it is 40–60% thinner than adult skin (Lund & Kuller, 2007). With thinner skin and less subcutaneous fat, the infant loses heat more rapidly, has greater difficulty regulating body temperature, and becomes more easily chilled than an older child or an adult. The thinner skin also increases the potential absorption of topical medications. The infant's skin contains more water than an adult's and has loosely attached cells. As the infant grows, the skin toughens and becomes less hydrated, making it less susceptible to bacteria (Figure 31–2 ➤).

Melanin, a peptide synthesized by an enzyme in melanocytes, influences skin color. Melanin production is low at birth and during the newborn period, accounting for the lighter skin in newborns of all races. Newborns and young infants are therefore more susceptible to damage from the sun and ultraviolet light.

Sebaceous glands and eccrine sweat glands are functional at birth in a term infant, although somewhat immaturely. The apocrine glands do not function until puberty.

Use the assessment guidelines on page 1033 to perform a nursing assessment of the integumentary system. A list of diagnostic and laboratory tests used to evaluate skin conditions is provided in Table 31–1.

As Children Grow
Integumentary System Changes

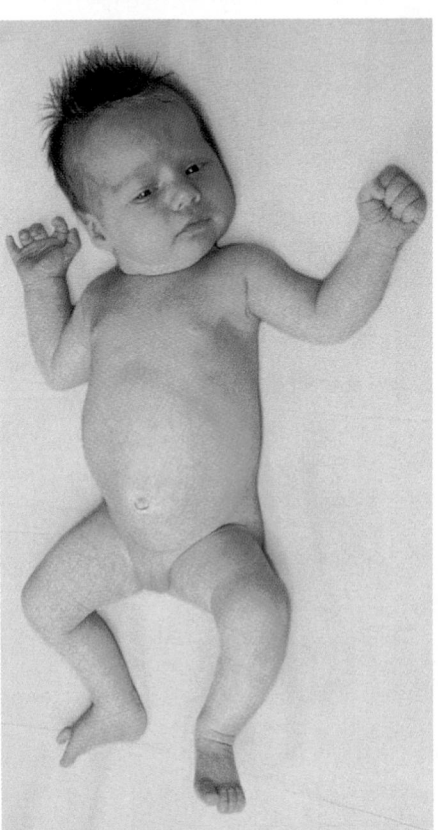

Newborns
Skin is very thin
Epidermis is loosely bound to the dermis, friction can cause separation of the layers with blistering
Eccrine sweat glands function, produce sweat in response to heat and emotional stimuli
Apocrine sweat glands are small and nonfunctional
Less melanin is present at birth so skin is lighter colored

Adolescents
Skin thickens
Epidermis and dermis are tightly bound, increasing resistance to infection and irritation
Eccrine sweat glands achieve full function, after puberty males sweat more than females
Apocrine sweat glands mature during puberty
Melanin is at adult levels, determining skin color and serving as a shield against ultraviolet radiation

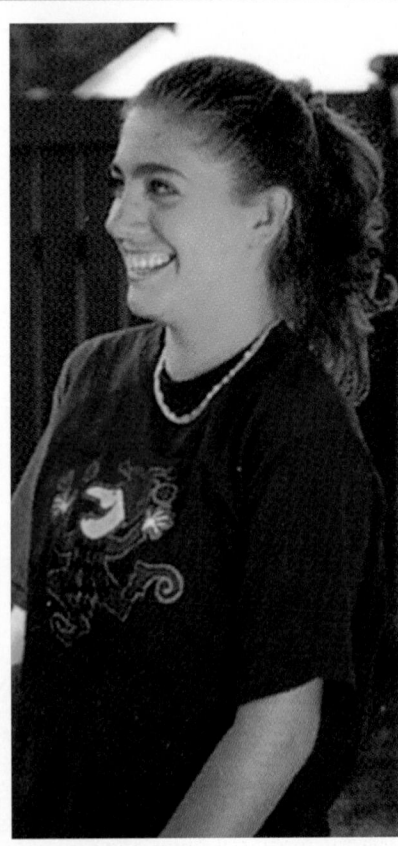

FIGURE 31–2 ➤ The structures of the skin mature during childhood, reaching adult function at puberty.

TABLE 31-1	Diagnostic Tests and Procedures for Integument Evaluation	
Diagnostic Procedures		**Laboratory Tests**
Culture of wound or skin drainage Tissue biopsy Computed tomography (CT) Radiograph Ultrasound		Complete blood count Immunoglobulin E Potassium hydroxide on skin scrapings

See Appendices D and E ⟶ for more information about these tests and procedures.

Assessment Guidelines for the Child with a Skin Condition

Assessment Focus	Assessment Guidelines*
Skin characteristics	▪ Inspect the skin for color, elevations, and imperfections. ▪ Palpate the skin for texture, moisture, temperature, turgor, and edema.
Hair	▪ Inspect the scalp hair for color, distribution, and cleanliness. Inspect for nits (lice eggs) that adhere to the hair. ▪ Inspect for areas of hair loss or broken hairs.
Lesions	▪ Describe skin lesions according to the characteristics listed in Figure 5–10 ⟶ and Table 31–2. Note erythema, signs of scratching (excoriation), or secondary infection. ▪ Identify the location or distribution of lesions on the body (e.g., generalized, diaper area, flexor surfaces). ▪ Palpate lesions for induration and temperature. ▪ Measure the size of lesions (length, width, and height when appropriate).
Pain	▪ Assess level of pain when present.
Temperature	▪ Assess the body temperature.
Family history	▪ Identify family members with allergies or chronic skin conditions.

*See Chapter 5 ⟶ for examination techniques.

■ SKIN LESIONS

Skin lesions vary in size, shape, color, and texture characteristics. The two major types of skin lesions are primary lesions and secondary lesions. Primary lesions arise from previously healthy skin and include macules, patches, papules, nodules, tumors, vesicles, pustules, bullae, and wheals (see Figure 5–10 ⟶). Secondary lesions result from changes in primary lesions. They include crusts, scales, **lichenification** (thickening of the skin with increased visibility of normal skin furrows), scars, keloids, excoriation, fissures, erosion, and ulcers (Table 31–2). It is important for the nurse to be able to identify and describe the primary and secondary skin lesions and understand their underlying cause and treatment.

Complementary Therapy
Oils and Gels

Some skin conditions have complementary therapies for which scientific studies have demonstrated a benefit. Evening primrose oil given orally is used for atopic eczema. Aloe vera gel used topically is effective for superficial burns and abrasions (National Center for Complementary and Alternative Medicine, 2008b).

■ WOUND HEALING

Wound healing occurs in three overlapping phases: inflammation, reconstruction, and maturation, so the wound fills in, seals, and finally shrinks (Rote & Huether, 2010). See Figure 31–3 ➤.

Inflammation, the initial response at the injury site, usually lasts 3 days after injury (Bookout, 2008). Vasodilation occurs shortly after injury, allowing leukocytes, phagocytes, and lymphocytes to travel to the injury site. Plasma leaks from blood vessels due to capillary permeability and the increased blood flow. The wound is sealed with a blood clot containing fibrin and trapped cells, preventing bacterial invasion and joining the wound edges. Bacteria, dead cells, and other inflammatory products are drained by lymphatic vessels.

Reconstruction or **epithelialization** (the process by which epithelial cells grow into the wound from surrounding healthy tissue), the second phase, may last from 3 to 21 days (Bookout, 2008). Capillary budding to reestablish the blood flow and natural **debridement** (enzyme action by macrophages and neutrophils to clean the lesion and dissolve the clot or scab) occur. The wound contracts. Fibroblasts multiply, producing collagen and granulation tissue to fill the wound to skin level. A fine layer of epithelial cells forms over the site. Many dressings are used during wound healing (Table 31–3).

Maturation or remodeling, the third phase, involves continued collagen production for scar formation. As the scar flattens

TABLE 31–2 Common Secondary Skin Lesions and Associated Conditions

Lesion Name	Description	Example
Burrow	A narrow, raised irregular channel caused by a parasite	Scabies
Comedones	Plugs of sebaceous and keratin material in hair follicles	Acne
Crust	Dried residue of serum, pus, or blood	Impetigo
Erosion	Loss of superficial epidermis; moist but does not bleed	Ruptured chickenpox vesicle
Excoriation	Abrasion or scratch mark	Scratched insect bite
Fissure	Linear crack in skin	Tinea pedis (athlete's foot)
Lichenification	Thickening of skin with increased visibility of normal skin furrows	Eczema (atopic dermatitis)
Scale	Thin flake of exfoliated epidermis	Dandruff, psoriasis
Scar	Replacement of destroyed tissue with fibrous tissue	Healed surgical incision
Telangiectasia	Dilated, superficial blood vessels	Birthmark
Ulcer	Deeper loss of skin surface; bleeding or scarring may ensue	Chancre

Pathophysiology Illustrated
Wound Healing

Inflammation

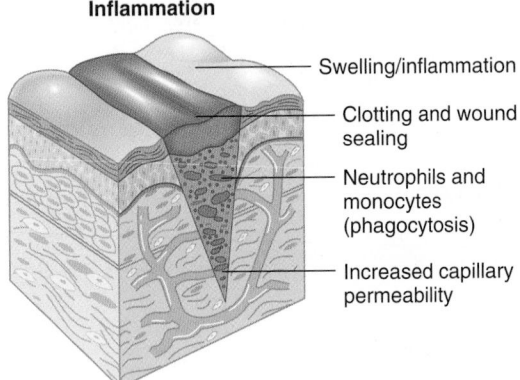

- Swelling/inflammation
- Clotting and wound sealing
- Neutrophils and monocytes (phagocytosis)
- Increased capillary permeability

Inflammation (3–5 days)
Increased blood flow to area carrying plasma with leukocytes, phagocytes, and lymphocytes to the site
Increased capillary permeability, causing swelling
Phagocytosis
Dilute toxins, produced by bacteria and dying cells, removed by lymphatic system
Clot formation that seals the wound with fibrin and trapped cells and platelets

Reconstruction

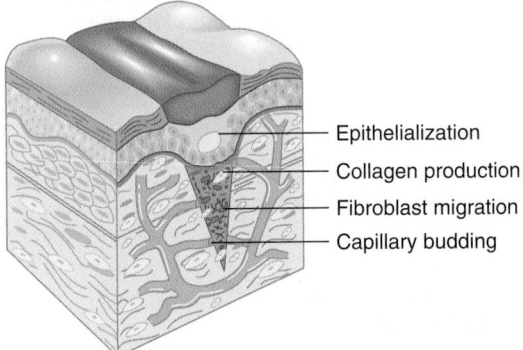

- Epithelialization
- Collagen production
- Fibroblast migration
- Capillary budding

Reconstruction (4 days to 2 weeks)
Debridement or cleanup of the site, fibrinolytic enzymes dissolve the fibrin clots
Regeneration of destroyed cells if injury is minor
Collagen production for scar formation occurs when tissue is too injured to regenerate
Epithelialization with granulation tissue that includes capillary budding and becomes scar tissue
Wound contraction, inward movement of the wound edge

Maturation

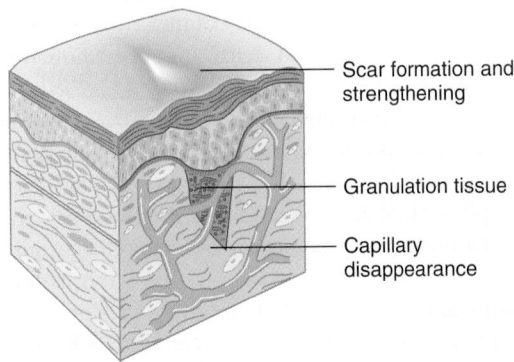

- Scar formation and strengthening
- Granulation tissue
- Capillary disappearance

Maturation (Months to 2 Years)
Remodeling of the site as scar tissue forms
Scar formation and strengthening
Capillary disappearance from scar tissue

FIGURE 31–3 ➤ Wound healing occurs in three phases: inflammation, reconstruction, and scar maturation.

Note: From Rote, N. S., & Huether, S. E. (2010). Innate immunity: Inflammation. In K. L. McCance & S. E. Huether, Pathophysiology: The biologic basis for disease in adults and children (6th ed., pp. 183–216). St. Louis, MO: Elsevier Mosby.

TABLE 31–3	Dressings Used During Wound Healing
Category	Uses and Characteristics
Alginates/hydrofibers	Used with moderate to heavy exudate Absorb wound exudate and form a gel-like covering over the wound to maintain a moist wound environment Require a secondary dressing
Foam	Used for wounds with heavy exudates and packing deep wounds Used during the inflammatory phase following debridement, when drainage is at its peak Keeps the exudates off the wound to decrease the maceration of surrounding tissue Can be left in place 3–4 days
Hydrocolloids	Used for granulating and epithelializing wounds with low or moderate amounts of exudates Occlusive and adhesive React with wound exudate to form a gel-like covering to protect the wound bed and maintain a moist environment
Hydrogels	Used for wounds with little or no exudates Increase the moisture content and help to clean and debride necrotic tissue Do not adhere to wound, so removal is pain-free Usually changed 3 times a week
Transparent films	Used to protect wound from bacterial contamination Semipermeable, waterproof Help maintain a moist environment Permit evaluation of wound without removal Changed up to 3 times a week

Data from: Wound Care Information Network. (2010). Wound product category and index. Retrieved from http://wound101.com/prodindx.htm

and fades, it gradually strengthens and devascularizes. The scar will only be about 80% as strong as the original tissue (Bookout, 2008). Maturation can take months to years, depending on the extent of the injury. Formation of a **keloid**, a scar that extends beyond the original boundaries of the wound, is caused by an imbalance between collagen synthesis and collagen breakdown. The cause is unknown, but there is a familial tendency. A **hypertrophic scar** is one that is raised but stays within the original boundaries of the wound.

■ DERMATITIS

Many skin inflammations occur in early childhood. Most are easily treated and do not have long-term consequences. Dermatitis is a condition in which the skin changes in response to external stimuli. The most common types of acute dermatitis in infants, children, and adolescents are contact dermatitis, diaper dermatitis, and seborrheic dermatitis. See page 1044 for atopic dermatitis (eczema). Because these skin disorders can cause an emotional response in the family and child, be supportive and reassure them that the child is not infectious.

Contact Dermatitis

Contact dermatitis is an inflammation of the skin that occurs in response to direct contact with an allergen or irritant. Irritant contact dermatitis is more common.

An external irritant causes an inflammatory response, but not an immune response. Common irritants include soaps, detergents, fabric softeners, bleaches, lotions, urine, and stool. An irritant can affect the skin any time that adequate concentration and contact duration occur. Sweating and friction enhance the absorption of the allergen or irritant. A discrete area of redness corresponds to the exposure location. The rash usually develops within a few hours of contact, peaks within 24 hours, and quickly resolves with removal of the irritant.

Clinical Tip

Phytophotodermatitis can result when the child has skin contact with a chemical (psoralen) that sensitizes the skin to sunlight. Psoralen is found in lemons, limes, figs, mangos, celery, carrots, parsley, and some weeds and grasses. Following sun exposure, painful erythema and blistering develop at the site of the exposure, followed by hyperpigmentation. The hyperpigmentation fades over several months (Wallace, 2007).

Allergic contact dermatitis is a delayed hypersensitivity reaction. An antigen is absorbed from the skin's surface during the initial sensitization phase, and an immune memory is created. After a repeated exposure or a long-term exposure, dermatitis develops. Common allergens include poison ivy, poison oak, lanolin, rubber, leather, nickel, fragrances, and latex. Children may have both irritant and allergic reactions to latex, found in many types of hospital equipment and supplies, as well as in products in the home and community. See Chapter 22 ∞ to review the immune response to allergens and for information about latex allergy.

Allergic contact dermatitis is characterized by erythema, edema, pruritus, vesicles, or bullae that rupture, ooze, and crust. The rash is usually limited to the area of contact. Symptoms develop several hours after exposure, after the immunologic response has been activated. Symptoms can last up to 3 to 4 weeks without treatment.

TABLE 31–4	Distribution of Lesions by Type of Allergen
Distribution of Lesion	Allergen
Face, eyelids	Cosmetics, hair and skin care products, nail cosmetics, eyeglasses
Ear lobes, neck	Nickel, fragrances
Lips, mouth	Oral hygiene products, bubble gum, lipstick
Trunk	Snaps, buckles, moisturizers, sunscreen, cleansers
Feet	Rubber or leather chemical in shoes

Data from: Nijhawan, R. I., Matiz, C., & Jacob, S. E. (2009). Contact dermatitis: From basics to allergodromes. Pediatric Annals, 38(2), 99–108; Timm-Knudson, V. L., Johnson, J. S., Ortiz, K. J., & Yiannias, J. A. (2006). Allergic contact dermatitis to preservatives. Dermatologic Nursing, 18(2), 130–136.

A patient history and the distribution of the lesions provide clues about the source and identity of the irritant or allergen. See Table 31–4. Patch testing may be used to identify the allergen.

Treatment involves removal and future avoidance of the offending agent (e.g., clothes, plant, soap). Calamine lotion can be applied to the affected skin. Cool compresses with aluminum acetate (Burow's solution) promote drying and relieve itching. Oatmeal or Aveeno may be added to the bathwater to relieve itching. Antihistamines may be given for a sedative effect when the child is too irritable to sleep. Acute allergic contact dermatitis is managed with medium potency topical corticosteroids when less than 10% of the body surface area is affected; however, they should not be applied to open lesions. The topical corticosteroids are applied to the affected area twice a day for 2 to 3 weeks. Stopping the treatment too soon can cause rebound dermatitis. Reactions to poison ivy covering more than 10% of the body surface area may require treatment with oral corticosteroids for 7 to 14 days and a tapered dose for 7 to 10 additional days.

Nursing Management

Patient education for home care management focuses on care of the skin and prevention of future exposures. Teach parents how to apply topical corticosteroids and to keep using the ointment for 2 to 3 weeks even when the skin shows signs of healing. If oatmeal or Aveeno soaks are used to relieve itching, caution parents that the tub will be slippery, and to pat the child dry to leave the product film in place. Alternatively encourage the use of Burow's solution compresses to relieve itching. Familiarize parents with the symptoms of infection in the affected area (i.e., increased redness, oozing, fever) and tell them when to return for follow-up care. See Families Want to Know: Exposure to Poison Ivy or Poison Oak.

Teach parents to avoid exposure to allergens or irritants. Advise parents to wash all clothes before the first wearing and to rinse clothes an extra time to remove all the soap. Mild soap should be used to clean the skin. Place a barrier between the irritant (e.g., metal, shoe leather) and the skin. If a nickel allergy exists, avoid use of nickel jewelry and belt buckles.

Families Want to Know

Exposure to Poison Ivy or Poison Oak

- The rash is caused by contact with the sap of the plant, either directly or indirectly (clothing, a pet, or other person). Avoid hugging a pet exposed to poison ivy until it has been bathed. Once a rash has developed, it is not contagious.
- React quickly to wash off sap with Zanfel (a product that removes poison ivy sap), or with soap and lukewarm water, within 10 minutes if possible. Be sure to scrub under the nails.
- Do not rub fingers exposed to poison ivy against broken skin or in the eyes.
- Launder clothing worn during exposure, and wash hands after handling exposed clothing.
- Search the yard and remove all plants. Wear vinyl gloves to handle plants (cloth and rubber gloves allow sap to penetrate). Do not burn the plants removed; put them in a trash bag for disposal. A person with a sensitivity may inhale the smoke and develop airway inflammation.
- For children with sensitivity to poison ivy, an over-the-counter barrier cream such as IvyBlock can help prevent skin penetration of plant oil.

Diaper Dermatitis

Diaper dermatitis, a common cause of irritant contact dermatitis, occurs in approximately one third of young children. It is most common in infants from 9 to 12 months of age (Montoya, 2008). The irritants, urine and feces, interact with the skin to cause dermatitis. The urine increases the wetness and pH of the skin, increasing abrasion and its permeability to irritants and microbes. Fecal organisms provide more irritants. Urine metabolizes to ammonia, also a skin irritant.

Candida albicans, a secondary infection, is a common complication of diaper dermatitis or antibiotic therapy for another condition. It is frequently the underlying cause of severe diaper rash. Diaper candidiasis often occurs simultaneously with oral candidiasis (see page 1040).

The rash is characterized by glazed red plaques over skin in contact with the diaper area. Usually the perineum, genitals, and buttocks are affected, and the skin folds are spared. In severe cases, the infant develops a rash that is fiery red, raised, and confluent. Pustules with tenderness may also be present. If a *Candida albicans* secondary infection occurs, the rash has bright red scaly plaques with sharp margins in the skin folds. Small papules and pustules may be seen, along with satellite lesions (Figure 31–4 ➤).

Mild diaper dermatitis is treated with a water-impermeable barrier or protective sealant such as zinc oxide, Aquaphor, Desitin, or Balmex after every diaper change. In some cases, a combination product (e.g., karaya powder or Stomahesive protective powder) may be effective. An antifungal topical medication (e.g., nystatin or miconazole) is applied to the skin before the barrier ointment for *Candida albicans* infections, and continued for several days after the rash clears. Topical corticosteroids are not recommended for diaper dermatitis because occlusion in the diaper area increases corticosteroid systemic absorption (Montoya, 2008).

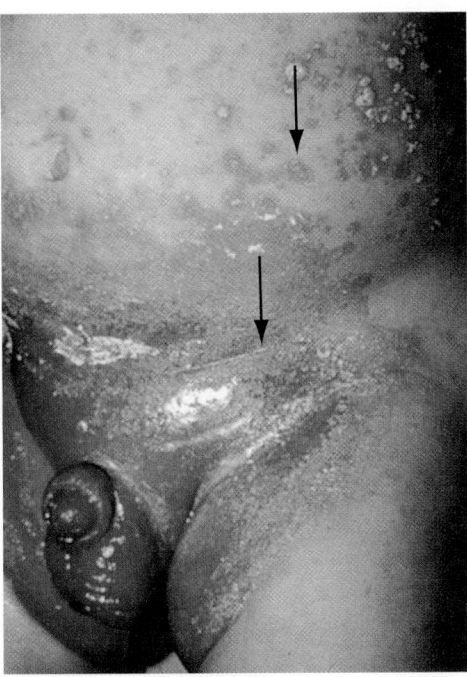

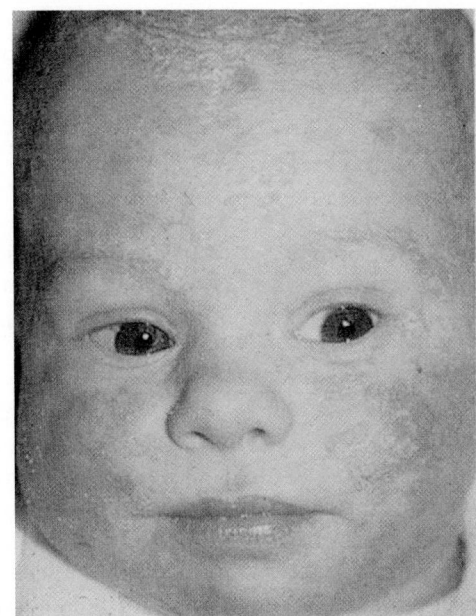

FIGURE 31–5 ➤ Seborrheic dermatitis.

FIGURE 31–4 ➤ Diaper dermatitis with *Candida albicans* secondary infection. Note the inflammation in the skin fold and satellite lesions above the diaper area. *Courtesy of the Centers for Disease Control and Prevention, Atlanta, GA.*

Nursing Management

Severe diaper dermatitis can be a major source of stress for parents who must care for a child in constant discomfort. Instruct parents to change the diaper as soon as the infant is wet, or at least every 2 hours during the day and once during the night.

Encourage parents to use superabsorbent disposable diapers, which tend to reduce the frequency and severity of diaper dermatitis. When wet, these diapers form a gel that keeps the skin drier than cloth diapers; however, diapers should still be changed every 2 to 3 hours. Tell parents to avoid using tight diapers and waterproof pants. Use of A & D ointment, zinc oxide, or other barrier products helps protect the skin from urine and stool. Mineral oil may help to remove pastes so fresh medication can be applied.

Advise parents to wash the perianal area with warm water or a waterless cleanser (Aquanil HC lotion or Cetaphil) only after a bowel movement. Soaps remove lipids and are a skin irritant. Pat the skin dry; do not rub. Advise parents to use soft paper towels with water or baby wipes without alcohol or fragrance at other times. Talcum powder is abrasive and should not be used. Exposing the diaper area to air helps aid healing; for example, parents could allow the child to go without a diaper while lying on an absorbent pad or cloth. Watch for signs of infection if a diaper rash is present since the damaged skin can allow infectious organisms to grow.

Seborrheic Dermatitis

Seborrheic dermatitis is a recurrent inflammatory skin condition thought to be caused by an overgrowth of a yeast, *Malassezia furfur* (formerly *Pityrosporum ovale*). The condition is thought to be influenced by hormones. The rash is found over the areas of the body where the sebaceous glands are most plentiful: scalp (cradle cap), forehead, and postauricular and periorbital areas. It may also occur on the skin of the eyelids, inguinal area, or nasolabial folds. The condition is frequently seen in infants up to 3 months of age and in adolescents.

Common symptoms are pruritus and a mildly erythematous, adherent, waxy scaling of the scalp (or "dandruff"). Yellow-red patches with greasy scaling may be present, typically on the scalp and nasolabial folds on the face, behind the ears, on the upper chest, and sometimes on the **intertriginous** (skin folds of the neck, axillae, antecubital fossa) areas (Figure 31–5 ➤). The rash itches less than atopic dermatitis.

Prevention for young infants consists of daily shampooing. Once seborrhea develops, an emollient (e.g., white petroleum or baby oil) is left on the scalp for about 20 minutes to soften the crusts. The scales are removed by brushing with the fingertips or a soft toothbrush. The hair is then shampooed and rinsed thoroughly. A shampoo containing tar may be used in infants if baby shampoo is not effective (O'Connor, McLaughlin, & Ham, 2008).

Lesions on the body can be treated with shampoos containing selenium sulfide or salicylic acid. Use baby shampoo to wash lesions on the eyelids and eyelashes. Treatments are continued for several days after the lesions disappear. Topical corticosteroids are used to treat seborrhea, but they should not be used around the eyes. Topical calcineurin inhibitors (e.g., tacrolimus and pimecrolimus) are also effective for adolescents (Poindexter, Burkhart, & Morrell, 2009).

Nursing Management

Teach new parents to wash the infant's hair regularly with each bath. Reassure parents that gentle cleansing will not harm the infant's "soft spot." Demonstrate bathing to show them the proper technique, if necessary. Follow-up is seldom necessary, as the condition resolves with treatment. Advise adolescents that emotional distress may trigger future flare-ups and to initiate treatment promptly when symptoms begin.

■ BACTERIAL INFECTIONS

Impetigo

Impetigo, the most common bacterial skin condition, is a highly contagious, superficial (epidermal) infection. The most common sites are the face and around the mouth, the hands, the neck, and the extremities.

Minor skin injuries, insect bites, and dermatitis provide the portal for the infectious agent. *Staphylococcus aureus* and group A beta-hemolytic streptococcus are usually responsible. *Staphylococcus aureus* colonizes on the skin and mucous membranes, particularly in the nose and throat. This infection occurs more commonly in children in close physical contact with others, such as in childcare settings, or who have poor hygiene.

Impetigo lesions begin as a papule that turns into a vesicle at the injury site. The vesicle ruptures and forms an erosion, and serous fluid forms the characteristic honey-colored crusts. Pruritus and regional lymphadenopathy may be present. The rash may spread to the face and extremities by self-inoculation (Figure 31–6 ➤). In bullous impetigo, vesicles stimulated by a toxin enlarge and coalesce to form bullae with sharp margins and no surrounding erythema. A thin honey-colored crust forms when the bullae rupture. When the crust is removed a moist, erythematous lesion with a collar of skin around the erosion is seen. The lesions form more commonly in moist skinfold areas.

Impetigo is diagnosed by appearance of lesions, or a Gram stain and bacterial culture. Local treatment involves removal of the crusts and application of a topical antibiotic. Crusts are soaked in warm water and gently scrubbed off with an antiseptic soap. A topical bactericidal ointment may be applied, such as mupirocin (3 times a day for 5 to 7 days) or retapamulin (twice a day for 5 days) (Bell, 2007). The infection is communicable for 24 hours after topical treatment is begun. In communities with high rates of bacteria resistance, oral antibiotics (e.g., dicloxa-

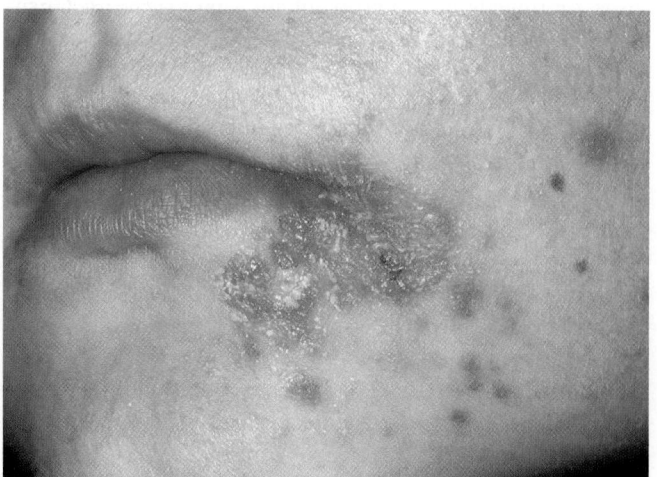

FIGURE 31–6 ➤ Characteristic honey-colored crusts of impetigo.
Dr. P. Marazzi/Photo Researchers, Inc.

cillin, or a macrolide) may be the initial treatment. Bullous impetigo is treated with systemic antibiotics. A bacterial culture is needed if the treatment response is poor.

> **Clinical Tip**
>
> If the child has a history of recurrent impetigo, determine if a person in contact with the child is a nasal carrier of *Staphylococcus aureus*. The carrier can be effectively treated with topical mupirocin ointment applied to the nares two times daily for 5 days (Zajac & Jacobson, 2009).

Nursing Management

Advise parents that they must continue oral or topical medications for the full number of days prescribed. If the child's lesions do not start to improve within 24 hours with the care previously described, the health care provider should be contacted. A culture may be needed.

Tell the parents to observe all close contacts and family members for lesions. The child who is infected should not share towels or toiletries with others. All linens and clothing used by the child should be washed separately with detergent in hot water. Keep fingernails short and clean to prevent the spread of infection by scratching. Inform the childcare center about the infection, so staff can sanitize toys and surfaces. The child can return to the childcare center after 24 hours of treatment. Athletes should not return to practice or compete until the treatment is determined to be effective.

Community-Acquired Methicillin-Resistant *Staphylococcus aureus*

Community-acquired methicillin-resistant *Staphylococcus aureus* (CA-MRSA) is an organism that causes an aggressive skin and soft-tissue infection in healthy children. CA-MRSA is colonized on the skin, the mucous membranes, and nares of healthy individuals who are carriers. Transmission may occur by droplet during respiratory infection, by contaminated hands, or by contact with contaminated surfaces. Risk factors include participation in team sports, close skin-to-skin contact, cuts or abrasions on the skin, contact with contaminated surfaces, poor hygiene, crowded living conditions, childcare center attendance, and recurrent skin infections (Hinckley & Allen, 2008).

Clinical manifestations include furuncles (abscesses). Swelling, warmth, purulent drainage, fever, and pain may be present. The lesion may invade deeper tissues.

Diagnosis is made by culturing the drainage from an incised abscess. Treatment involves incision and drainage followed by a systemic antibiotic to which CA-MRSA is susceptible, such as clindamycin, oxacillin, and dicloxacillin.

Nursing Management

Make sure parents and adolescents understand the importance of taking the full course of the prescribed antibiotic. Educate parents to prevent the spread of CA-MRSA by using good hand hygiene and clean disposable gloves to change the dressing. Dispose of used dressings in a plastic bag that can be tightly closed or sealed. Encourage parents to disinfect surfaces that come into contact with the wound or wound drainage. Use hot water to wash linens and clothing used by the child, and dry clothes in a hot dryer.

Nurses have a major role in prevention of CA-MRSA infections. Encourage good hand hygiene. Reduce exposure to infection by covering wounds and bandages. Athletes should shower with soap and water after practices and competitions. Towels and personal items should not be shared. Shared athletic equipment should be cleaned regularly. Encourage athletes to care for wounds and report those that are potentially infected.

Folliculitis

Folliculitis is a superficial inflammation of the pilosebaceous hair follicle caused by infection, trauma, or irritation. The causative organism is usually *Staphylococcus aureus*. The condition is common in children and teenagers because of increased sweat production. Folliculitis may be associated with *Pseudomonas aeruginosa* exposure in a poorly chlorinated pool or hot tub.

Symptoms include pain or pruritus, localized swelling, and the formation of tiny dome-shaped, yellowish pustules and red papules at follicular openings with surrounding erythema. Individual lesions may become deeper and form an abscess (furuncle). Lesions are usually seen in clusters on the face, scalp, trunk, and extremities, or in areas covered by bathing suits (if associated with pool or hot tub use). Some children have fever, aching, and flu-like symptoms.

Treatment of inflamed follicles consists of washing the affected area with a topical antibacterial cleanser (e.g., chlorhexidine) and water. A benzoyl peroxide gel or wash or another drying agent will also help clear the infection. Ruptured lesions heal with hyperpigmentation and no scarring. Complications are rare. If lesions do not resolve within a week, the child may need systemic antibiotics (e.g., ciprofloxacin) and, if the infection is deep, incision and drainage.

Nursing Management

Nursing management focuses on educating the parents and child about prevention. Advise children to shower daily and after exercise, to cleanse with an antibacterial soap, and to wear loose cotton clothing. Talk with parents about the importance of maintaining the correct pH level and chlorine concentration in swimming pools and hot tubs. Bathing suits of affected children should be laundered and well dried before the next use.

Cellulitis

Cellulitis is an acute inflammation of the dermis and underlying connective tissue. The condition usually occurs on the face and extremities as a result of trauma or a compromised skin barrier.

The child often has a history of trauma, impetigo, folliculitis, or recent otitis media. Common causative organisms are *Staphylococcus aureus*, *Streptococcus pyogenes*, and *Streptococcus pneumoniae*. The condition may also result from a nearby abscess or sinusitis.

Characteristic signs and symptoms include red or lilac, tender, warm, edematous skin that may have an ill-defined, nonelevated border (Figure 31–7 ➤). Onset is rapid, and the child

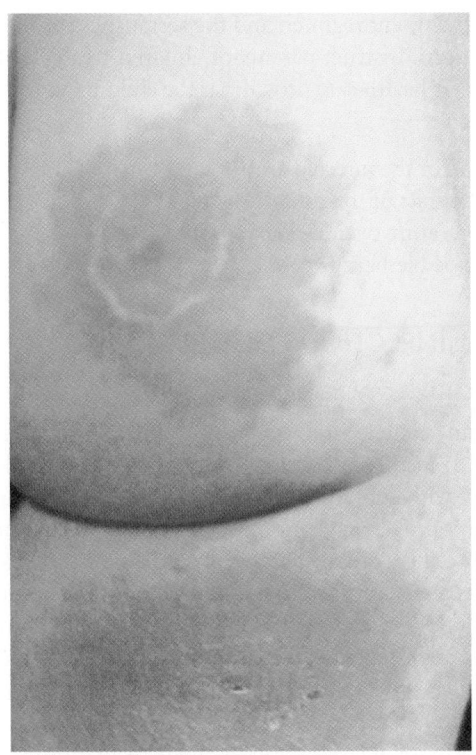

FIGURE 31–7 ➤ Characteristic appearance of cellulitis.
Used with permission from Ben-Amitai, D., & Ashkenazi, S. (1993). Common bacterial skin infections in children. Pediatric Annals, 22(4), 226. *Photograph courtesy of Dr. Aryeh Metzker.*

appears ill. Other symptoms include fever, chills, malaise, and enlarged, tender lymph nodes. Lymphangitis may be present. In some cases, a rapidly progressive lesion may result in septicemia.

Diagnostic tests include blood work and cultures. Blood studies may show an increase in white blood cells. Cultures are taken by needle aspiration, if possible, to identify the causative organisms. Cultures of the blood and spinal fluid are taken if the child has a toxic (very ill) appearance.

Children with severe cases or a large affected surface area are hospitalized and treated with systemic antibiotics and analgesics to prevent sepsis. If the face is involved, intravenous (IV) antibiotic therapy is administered to avoid serious complications. Children with cellulitis on the trunk, limbs, or perianal area may be treated on an outpatient basis with oral antibiotics. Recovery begins within 48 hours, but therapy should continue for at least 10 days (Morelli, 2007b). Periorbital cellulitis is discussed in Chapter 19 ∞ .

Nursing Management

Assessment centers on recognition of infection, documentation of location and related symptoms, and monitoring of vital signs. Because of the risk of sepsis, the child is monitored carefully. Administer prescribed oral or IV antibiotics as scheduled. Supportive care includes warm compresses to the affected area four times daily, elevation of the affected limb, and bed rest. Outpatient follow-up is crucial to ensure response to therapy.

Advise parents about possible complications, such as abscess formation. Reinforce to parents the importance of compliance with the treatment regimen and the seriousness of the possible complications. Instruct parents of children treated at home to contact their health care provider if the child has any of the following signs:

- Spread of the infected area in the 24- to 48-hour period after the start of treatment
- Temperature over 38.3°C (101°F)
- Increased lethargy

■ VIRAL INFECTIOUS DISORDERS

Molluscum Contagiosum

Molluscum contagiosum is a skin infection caused by a poxvirus. Transmission occurs by direct contact, sexual contact, or contact with contaminated objects. Spread can occur by autoinoculation. The incubation period is 2 to 7 weeks but may be up to 6 months (American Academy of Pediatrics, 2009).

Lesions are pearl-like, flesh-colored smooth papules about 3 to 5 mm in size with a central depression. A plug of infectious material can be expressed when punctured. Lesions most commonly appear on the face, trunk, and extremities. Adolescents who are sexually active may have lesions in the genital and pubic areas. Up to 20 lesions appear singly or in groups, but children with impaired immunity or atopic eczema may have more lesions. Inflammation of the lesion may occur prior to clearance, giving the appearance of erythematous nodules. The lesions often disappear spontaneously in 6 to 12 months, but the condition can continue for several years.

In mild cases, the condition resolves spontaneously without intervention. In other cases, treatment involves destruction of the lesions, using curettage, **cryotherapy** (freezing each lesion with liquid nitrogen), or cantharidin application. Topical anesthesia is needed for curettage. Scarring may result from clinical therapy. Secondary infections are treated with topical or oral antibiotics.

Nursing Management

Nursing education focuses on reducing disease transmission. Children who are infected should avoid public swimming pools, hot tubs, and other joint bathing situations because the virus is more easily transmitted when the skin is wet. Towels and sponges should not be shared. The skin should be washed daily with gentle fragrance-free cleansers, followed by application of a hypoallergenic moisturizer or emollient to the entire skin surface. Teach parents to recognize potential secondary infections.

When intervention such as curettage or cryotherapy is performed, inform the child about what will happen, and then pro-

Culture | *Treatment for Molluscum Contagiosum*

The parents and child with darker skin need to be informed about the potential for hyperpigmentation resulting from treatment for molluscum contagiosum with liquid nitrogen or canthacur, a blistering medication (Richards, 2006). Other options that do not result in hyperpigmentation should be explored if the parents and child desire treatment.

vide distraction during the procedure to reduce anxiety. Ensure that the child has adequate topical anesthetic to minimize any pain from the intervention. If cantharidin is applied, teach the parents to wash it off 2 to 6 hours after treatment or when a blister is noted (Nelson & Morrell, 2007).

Warts (Papillomavirus)

Several types of human papillomavirus infect epithelial cells and cause warts. Various types of warts are found in children: common warts that appear on any skin surface and plantar warts found on the feet. The human papillomavirus is commonly transmitted by direct skin-to-skin or mucous membrane contact. The virus also survives on surfaces, and transmission can occur with contact, such as plantar warts from locker room floors. The incubation period may be 2 to 6 months; however, a latency period may exist in some cases. Children with immune compromise are more susceptible and often have numerous warts.

Common warts appear as skin-colored, rough, scaly papules and nodules on exposed skin surfaces. Individual and multiple warts may be seen, or large plaques may form if autoinoculation occurs. Warts usually cause no pain or itching unless in skin surface areas or creases that become irritated. Plantar warts appear as papules and plaques on the bottom of feet that grow inward and cause pain. Small black dots result from thrombosed vessels on the surface of the warts caused by weight bearing.

No intervention may be recommended as warts often resolve spontaneously over a couple of years and clinical therapy may be traumatic for children. Duct tape left in place for 6 consecutive days, followed by cleaning and pumice abrasion, and repeated each week for 2 months is often effective and painless (Morelli, 2007c). If warts cause pain or a social stigma, clinical therapy may be initiated. Treatment may involve cryotherapy, application of caustic substances or peeling agents, electrocautery, and laser therapy. Treatment is not always successful and may result in scarring. Immunologic medications (oral and topical) are being investigated for use in treating warts.

Nursing Management

Educate the parents and child about how warts are spread by picking at or chewing on them. Teach the parents and child about the application of peeling agents and caustic substances when prescribed for home use. If the reaction to the substance is painful, encourage the parents to reduce the frequency of the treatment until the pain subsides and then to resume the original treatment schedule. Successful treatment may take several months, and the parents and child may need encouragement to continue the therapy and remain optimistic.

Other viral skin conditions are described in Chapter 16 ∞.

■ FUNGAL INFECTIONS

Oral Candidiasis (Thrush)

Thrush is a fungal infection that occurs as an acute condition in newborns (usually acquired during birth from the vaginal canal of a mother who is infected). Children who regularly use a corticosteroid inhaler or have received antibiotics disturbing nor-

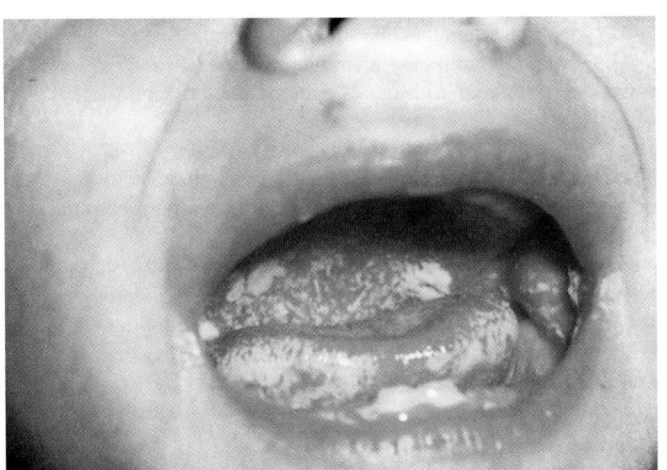

FIGURE 31–8 ➤ Thrush, an acute pseudomembranous form of oral candidiasis, is a common fungal infection in infants and children.
Used with permission from Zitelli, B. J., & Davis, H. W. (Eds.). (1997). Atlas of pediatric physical diagnosis (3rd ed., p. 104, fig. 4–50a). St. Louis, MO: Mosby.

mal flora are also at risk. It may occur as a chronic condition in young children who have an immune disorder.

Oral thrush is characterized by white patches that look like coagulated milk on the oral mucosa (Figure 31–8 ➤). Milk residue can be removed from the oral mucosa with gentle swabbing, but attempts to remove thrush lesions may cause bleeding. The infant may refuse to nurse or feed because of discomfort and pain. The infant may also have diaper dermatitis superinfection with candidiasis. Fever is usually not present.

Treatment involves oral nystatin suspension or clotrimazole, which is applied to the mouth and tongue after feedings. Fluconazole or itraconazole may be used for immunocompromised patients with oropharyngeal thrush. If infection is severe, occurs in the esophagus, or invades other body systems, oral fluconazole or IV amphotericin B may be prescribed for a minimum of 21 days.

Nursing Management

Educate parents to give the oral medication to infants, using a swab to apply the suspension to the buccal mucosa and tongue surfaces. Then allow the infant to swallow the remaining suspension. Teach older children to swish the solution around in the mouth before swallowing it.

To prevent a reinfection, educate parents about sterilizing bottle nipples and pacifiers. The breasts of mothers breastfeeding may become infected through contact with the infant's mouth and should be treated. Teach children with asthma to rinse the mouth well with water after using a corticosteroid inhaler to prevent candidiasis. If a spacer is used, it should also be rinsed with water after use. A commercial antiseptic spray may be used on toys that cannot be autoclaved, but follow directions carefully so the child does not ingest any harmful residue.

Dermatophytoses (Ringworm)

Dermatophytoses are fungal infections that affect the skin, hair, or nails. Children of all ages may be affected. Dermatophytoses may spread from person to person, from animal to person, or indirectly by contact with an infected person's clothing or linens. The

most common infections are tinea capitis, tinea corporis, tinea cruris, and tinea pedis. See the clinical manifestations table for common organisms, signs and symptoms, and clinical therapy.

Diagnosis may be confirmed through microscopic examination of the hair and scalp scrapings using a potassium hydroxide (KOH) wet mount to reveal rows and chains of spores within the hair shaft. A fungal culture can also be taken, using a swab and throat culture tube. A Wood's lamp is also useful in identifying some forms of tinea. For example, a *Microsporum* infection fluoresces a brilliant green under the Wood's lamp, but *Trichophyton tonsurans*, the most common cause of tinea capitis, does not fluoresce (American Academy of Pediatrics, 2009, p. 662). See the Clinical Manifestations table on the next page for clinical therapy for different dermatophytosis lesions.

Nursing Management

All members of the family and household pets should be assessed for fungal lesions. Since person-to-person transmission is common, avoid contact with the child's hair, hair accessories, brushes, and hats. In some cases, the family may have an asymptomatic carrier, so all family members should be treated. Teach parents and older children or teenagers that fungi are found in soil and are transmitted through direct contact with infected persons and animals.

Advise parents to give oral griseofulvin with fatty foods such as whole milk or peanut butter to enhance absorption. To prevent recurrence of the infection, the medications must be used for the entire prescribed period, even if the lesions are gone. Advise parents about the possibility of the "id" reaction so they will continue to give the medication.

For children with *tinea cruris*, encourage loose-fitting undergarments to promote dryness. With *tinea pedis*, keep the feet clean and dry and the nails clipped short. Encourage the use of 100% cotton socks that pull moisture away from the skin. Encourage children to wear shower shoes in public showers and locker rooms.

Inform parents of children with tinea capitis that hair regrowth is slow and may take 6 to 12 months. In some cases hair loss is permanent, which can be particularly stressful for older children or adolescents. Provide emotional support.

Clinical Manifestations
Dermatophytoses

Infection Site and Clinical Manifestations	Clinical Therapy
Tinea capitis (scalp) Scaly pustular bald areas with indistinct margins; may appear as seborrhea, with yellow, greasy scales; erythema or lesion lighter than skin color (see Figure 31–9A ➤). Broken hairs; dotted stubbed appearance where weakened hair has broken off. Mild itching. **Kerion**—large purulent tender boggy mass on scalp with drainage.	Griseofulvin orally for 8–12 weeks, OR terbinafine orally for 4–6 weeks in children over age 4 years, with treatment continued 2 weeks after lesion resolves. Selenium sulfide shampoo 2–3 times weekly leaving the shampoo on the scalp for 10 minutes before rinsing. Encourage family members to use the shampoo 2–3 times a week to reduce the number of fungus spores in the household. Kerion treatment may require the addition of oral corticosteroids to oral antifungal agents.
Tinea corporis (trunk) Pink, scaly circular patch with an expanding border, may be scaly or erythematous throughout; slightly raised borders with a clearing center (see Figure 31–9B). Usually acquired from contact with infected humans, animals, and contaminated surfaces (American Academy of Pediatrics, 2009, p. 663).	Topical cream (e.g., clotrimazole, miconazole, tolnaftate, naftifine, terbinafine) twice a day for 4–6 weeks. Topical corticosteroids are not used. Selenium sulfide shampoo 2–3 times a week on the child's body to help reduce the number of spores. Family members may also use the shampoo. An oral antifungal agent is prescribed for extensive lesions or no response to topical therapy.
Tinea cruris ("jock itch") Scaly, erythematous annular lesions on groin and upper thighs; may have elevated lesions, papules, or vesicles. May spread to abdomen and buttocks, usually spares the penis and scrotum.	Topical antifungal agent such as clotrimazole, miconazole, tolnaftate, naftifine, or terbinafine twice daily for 4–6 weeks. Topical corticosteroids are not used. Wash body area with selenium sulfide shampoo. Decrease moisture and occlusion in area.
Tinea pedis ("athlete's foot") Vesicles or erosions on instep or between toes (fissures, red scaly); dry scaly patches or plaques with erythema on plantar and lateral surfaces of foot. Peeling maceration and fissures in lateral toe web spaces indicate secondary bacterial involvement. Pruritus.	Broad-spectrum topical antifungal agent with antibacterial properties, e.g., econazole, clotrimazole, or miconazole 1 to 2 times a day. Allow feet to air-dry. Use 100% cotton socks, change twice daily; put socks on before other clothing to reduce transmission of fungus.

Data from: American Academy of Pediatrics. (2009). Red book 2009: Report of the Committee on Infectious Diseases (18th ed., pp. 661–666). Elk Grove Village, IL: Author. No Permission Needed

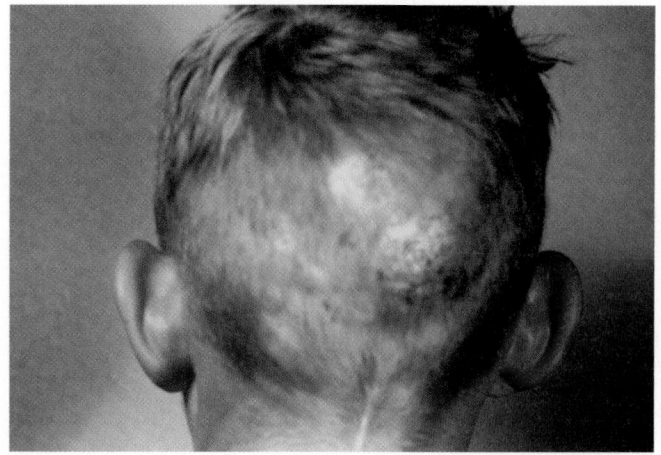

A

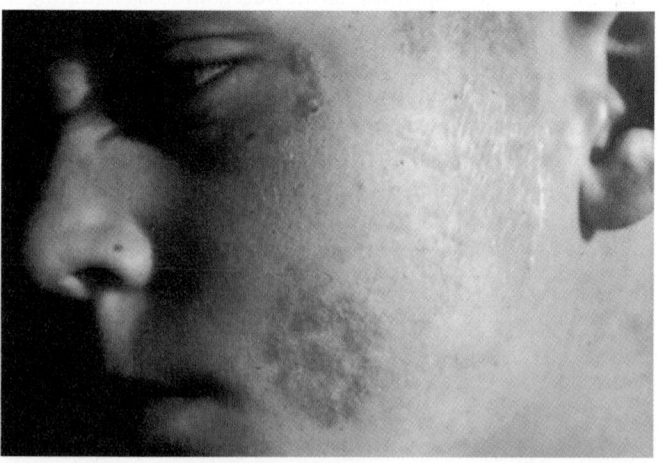

B

FIGURE 31–9 ➤ A, Tinea capitis. B, Tinea corporis.

Photographs courtesy of the Centers for Disease Control and Prevention, Atlanta, GA.

▪ DRUG REACTIONS

Adverse reactions to over-the-counter or prescription medications are relatively common. Children with drug allergies usually have reactions after ingestion (e.g., aspirin, antibiotics, sedatives), injection (e.g., penicillin), or topical application. Drug sensitivities may result from variations in an individual's ability to tolerate a particular drug or drug concentration, or from allergic responses. (See Chapter 22 ∞ for a description of allergic reactions.)

Reactions may occur after 1 or 2 doses when the child has previously taken the drug, but it may take up to 7 days for sensitivity to occur to a drug not previously administered. The most common reactions in children are erythematous macules and papules or **urticaria**, pruritic skin eruption with well-defined erythematous margins and pale centers. Drugs most likely to cause maculopapular eruptions, urticaria, and pruritus include the following: sulfonamides, anticonvulsants, antibiotics (penicillins, cephalosporins, erythromycin, vancomycin), and nonsteroidal anti-inflammatory drugs (NSAIDs). Be alert to the possibility of serious drug reactions that may become a medical emergency. See the clinical manifestations table.

The treatment of choice for most drug sensitivity reactions is discontinuation of the causative drug. In some cases, a drug may be continued with careful monitoring when a sensitivity reaction occurs because it is the best treatment choice. Supportive measures should be taken to decrease the intensity of the reaction. An antihistamine may be used to block the release of histamine, which causes the rash. Topical corticosteroids, cool compresses, and baths may also be prescribed for pruritus. The child with Stevens-Johnson syndrome or toxic epidermal necrosis must be hospitalized and treated on a burn unit.

Nursing Management

Teach parents to be alert for the signs of drug sensitivity reactions. Obtain a careful history of the child's past reactions to medications before starting new therapies. If a reaction occurs, discontinue the medication until the physician is notified. See nursing care of the child with burns on page 1055 for cases of severe drug reactions.

Nursing Alert

Children with a true drug allergy (having a past serious systemic reaction) should never be treated with that drug again. Prominently mark the child's records so that all allergies are easily identified. The child should wear a medical alert bracelet.

Clinical Manifestations
Drug Reactions

Type of Reaction and Associated Drugs	Clinical Manifestations
Allergic drug reaction Most commonly caused by sulfonamides, tetracyclines, NSAIDs, oral contraceptives, barbiturates, and phenolphthalein.	Erythematous, pruritic macules and papules; urticaria that moves from one body part to another. A fixed drug reaction (lesion occurs in same site as earlier drug reaction) is unusual; may commonly involve the face, genitals, and sacrum; may heal with hyperpigmentation.
Erythema multiforme minor Hypersensitivity reaction to anticonvulsants, penicillins, salicylates, sulfa antibiotics, barbiturates, and phenytoin; infectious agents (e.g., herpes simplex virus).	Skin lesions may be preceded by fever, malaise, and upper respiratory symptoms. Widespread pruritic macules progress to target lesions (papules, vesicles, or bullae in a pale ring with an erythematous border), and then to plaques. May progress to blisters and bullous lesions. Lesions common on palms and soles, elbows, extensor surface of forearms and legs; few mucosal lesions.
Stevens-Johnson syndrome (SJS) and toxic epidermal necrolysis (TEN) Potentially life-threatening hypersensitivity reaction or autoimmune response to penicillins, sulfonamides, anticonvulsants, or NSAIDs, or reaction to infectious disease such as *Mycoplasma pneumoniae*. Believed to be forms of the same disease and the most severe form of erythema multiforme.	Prodromal infection for 1–7 days with cough, coryza, sore throat, fever, malaise, headache, muscle aches, and joint pain. Vomiting and diarrhea may be seen. Widespread blistering, erosions, and ulcerations of mucous membranes followed by crusting and conjunctivitis; precedes skin rash by 1 to 2 days. Target lesions, bullae, and erosions (similar to partial-thickness burns) may spread to cover up to 10% of the skin surface in SJS, 10–30% in overlapping SJS and TEN, and more than 30% in TEN; full-thickness epidermis peels off in sheets easily with light pressure. Corneal blistering can lead to scarring and blindness. Respiratory and gastrointestinal tracts may have mucosal sloughing. Causes hypopigmentation in children with dark skin, but hyperpigmentation in children with light skin. Hyperpigmentation fades over time. Signs of sepsis.

Data from Nicol, N. H., & Huether, S. E. (2010b). Alterations of the integument in children. In K. L. McCance, S. E. Huether, V. L. Brashers, & N. S. Rote, Pathophysiology: The biologic basis for disease in adults and children (6th ed., pp. 1680–1694). St. Louis, MO: Mosby Elsevier; Aber, C., Connelly, E. A., & Schachner, L. A. (2007). Fever and rash in a child: When to worry? Pediatric Annals, 36(1), 30–38; Morelli, J. G. (2007d). Vesiculobullous disorders. In R. M. Kliegman, R. E. Behrman, H. B. Jensen, & B. F. Stanton, Nelson textbook of pediatrics (18th ed., 2685–2693). St. Louis, MO: Elsevier Mosby.

CHRONIC SKIN CONDITIONS

Atopic Dermatitis (Eczema)

Atopic eczema (atopic dermatitis) is a chronic, relapsing, superficial inflammatory skin disorder characterized by intense pruritus. The condition affects up to 20% of infants, children, and adolescents (Shaw, Burkhart, & Morrell, 2009). Up to 60% of children who develop the condition do so during the first year of life (Gonzalez, Unwala, & Connelly, 2008). Children with atopic eczema may have or develop other allergic conditions such as asthma and food allergy.

Etiology and Pathophysiology

Although the etiology of eczema is unknown, a complex interaction of genetic predisposition, environmental exposure, infectious agents, defects in the skin barrier function, and immunologic responses contributes to its development (Akdis, Akdis, Bieber, et al., 2006). An allergic form of eczema begins in early childhood and occurs in 70–85% of affected children. Most children have T-cell activation and increased IgE levels. The onset of the nonallergic form of eczema occurs at a later age (Peterson & Chan, 2006). Atopic eczema triggers include stress, temperature and humidity changes, allergens (foods before age 3 years and inhalants at later ages), and irritants (e.g., detergents and abrasive clothing) (Akdis et al., 2006).

Children with eczema have **xerosis**, generally dry skin that is more likely to crack and fissure. The barrier function of the skin is impaired, leading to increased water loss from the epidermis and decreased elasticity. Chronically dry skin allows irritants to penetrate and makes the child more susceptible to infection.

Clinical Manifestations

Acute atopic dermatitis is characterized by papulovesicular and erythematous lesions with exudate, crusts, and pruritus (Figure 31–10 ➤). Excoriation from scratching is common. Some patches may weep. Chronic eczema characteristics include darkened, thickened skin with prominent skin lines (lichenification), excoriation, dryness, and scaling. Inflammation usually occurs on the face, neck, and extensor surfaces in

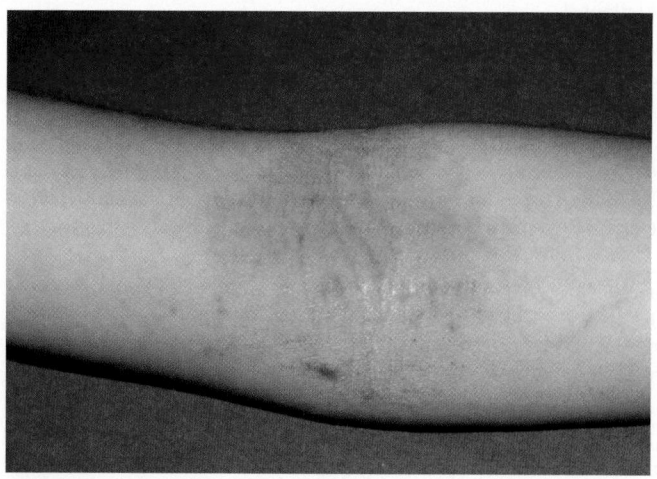

FIGURE 31–10 ➤ Chronic atopic eczema.
Dr. P. Marazzi/Photo Researchers, Inc.

infants, but flexor surfaces (antecubital and popliteal areas) are often involved in children over age 2 years. The diaper area is usually spared in infants because the skin is damp, and the diaper protects the area from scratching. The itching interferes with sleep and causes irritability. The child may move so much due to itching discomfort that a perception of hyperactivity may occur. Erythema and warmth may indicate a secondary bacterial infection. Some children have repeated atopic eczema flares or chronic eczema into adulthood.

COLLABORATIVE CARE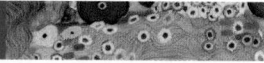

Diagnostic Tests

Eczema is distinguished from other forms of dermatitis by its history and clinical manifestations. No laboratory tests are diagnostic. Diagnostic criteria for eczema include an itching skin condition with three of the following factors (Ong & Boguniewicz, 2007):

- History of flexural dermatitis (knees, ankles, neck, or cheeks) if less than 4 years old
- History of asthma or hay fever in a child, or in a first-degree relative if less than 4 years old
- History of dry skin in past year
- Skin rash occurring before 2 years of age
- Visible flexural dermatitis; dermatitis on cheeks, forehead, and outer limbs if less than 4 years old

Clinical Therapy

Atopic eczema has no cure, so the goals of treatment are to hydrate and lubricate the skin, reduce pruritus, minimize inflammatory changes, and try to determine what triggers flares. The skin is lubricated by applying occlusive topical emollients within 3 minutes of leaving the water after bathing. This traps moisture in the skin and promotes flexibility of the skin without cracking. Moisturizing ointments and creams should be applied 3 to 4 times a day, or whenever the skin feels dry.

Topical corticosteroids reduce inflammation and help control the flare. Ointments are preferred over creams because of their occlusive effect, which ensures a stronger barrier and absorption into the skin. Many different preparations and strength categories of topical corticosteroids are available to treat acute flares. Mid-strength corticosteroids are used twice daily for 2 weeks and must be applied before the skin moisturizer is used. Lower strength corticosteroids are used for thinner skin areas, such as the face, diaper area, and skin folds. When the inflammation resolves, topical corticosteroids are tapered in frequency of application and potency and then discontinued. Prolonged use of large amounts of steroids through the skin can lead to adrenal suppression. Oral corticosteroids may be used for an acute exacerbation; however, there is often a rebound effect in which the rash returns after the medication is discontinued. See Medications Used to Treat Atopic Dermatitis.

Children with atopic eczema often have *Staphylococcus aureus* colonization, which can trigger an immune cascade that increases pruritus. Topical antibiotics are used to treat excoriated, open lesions and those that appear infected. Oral antibiotics such as cephalosporin for 5 days may be used to treat superin-

Medications Used to Treat

Atopic Dermatitis

Medications and Action	Nursing Management
Antihistamines (e.g., diphenhydramine, hydroxyzine), oral Control of itching, and sedation.	Encourage nighttime use for acute flares when itching interferes with sleep. If given during the day, they may cause sleepiness and interfere with learning.
Antibiotics (topical and oral) Antimicrobial action to treat cutaneous skin superinfections.	Educate parents about potential hypersensitivity reaction symptoms.
Corticosteroids (topical and oral) Anti-inflammatory, suppression of the hypothalamic pituitary-adrenal axis.	Educate parents to avoid using topical corticosteroids around the eyes, due to the potential for development of glaucoma or cataracts with exposure to the medication. Do not use on healthy skin. Avoid the use of occlusive dressings that can increase absorption.
Calcineurin inhibitors (tacrolimus, pimecrolimus, topical) T-lymphocyte activation is inhibited, as well as the release of cytokines and inflammatory mediators from anti-IgE-activated skin mast cells and basophils.	Inform the child and parents to expect a sensation of burning, redness, and itching for the first few days of therapy; symptoms generally decrease after a few days of treatment. Sunscreens should be used because of potential increased risk for skin cancer with sun exposure.

fections. In some cases a longer course of an antibiotic is needed for chronic recurrent infections (Tofte, 2007). Superinfections with herpes simplex may be treated with acyclovir.

Topical calcineurin inhibitors (tacrolimus and pimecrolimus) help suppress T-cell activation and are increasingly used as a second-line treatment for some children, but they may be too expensive for some families. The medication has been approved by the U.S. Food and Drug Administration (FDA) for children over 2 years of age for short-term or intermittent treatment of moderate or severe atopic eczema who do not respond to other topical therapy. However, the FDA issued a warning of increased risk for cancer among children younger than age 2 years in association with these medications, limiting wider use of the medications (U.S. Food and Drug Administration, 2006).

Oral immunomodulating agents (e.g., azathioprine, cyclosporine, or mycophenolate) or phototherapy may be used when atopic eczema does not respond to other therapies (Krakowski, Eichenfield, & Dohil, 2008).

Antihistamine agents such as diphenhydramine (Benadryl) or hydroxyzine (Vistaril and Atarax) have a limited effect on itching, but the sedative effect may help promote sleep.

Complementary Therapy

Probiotics

Probiotics, the bacteria found in some yogurts and fermented foods, may be an effective supplemental therapy for atopic eczema. Some small studies have found a relationship between a daily serving of *Lactobacillus acidophilus* (e.g., in yogurt and yogurt drinks with active cultures) and a reduced severity of atopic eczema. These probiotics should not be used in children who are immunocompromised or have short gut syndrome due to a risk of bacteremia (Schuerman & Vezeau, 2007).

The relationship between food allergies and eczema continues to be studied. Food allergies associated with atopic eczema may include milk, eggs, wheat, soy, fish, peanuts, and nuts. Skin testing for food allergy may be performed when severe atopic eczema does not respond to treatment. A food challenge should follow to identify eczema triggers before imposing dietary restrictions (Forbes, Saltzman, & Spergel, 2009). See Chapter 22 ∞ for more information on food allergies.

NURSING MANAGEMENT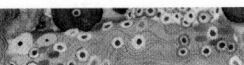

Nursing Assessment and Diagnosis

Take a thorough history, including any family history of allergy, environmental or dietary factors, past exacerbations, and what makes the eczema flare. Note distribution and type of lesions, presence of weeping, or signs of infection.

Clinical Judgment

What are the signs and symptoms that help distinguish between an atopic eczema flare and a secondary infection?

Identify the impact that the skin disorder is having on the child and family. How is the family managing the daily care routine? Do the child, siblings, or other family members have disturbed sleep because of the child scratching? What concerns does the child have about his or her appearance? Is the child's self-esteem disturbed? What other stresses has the child's skin disorder placed on the family? Does the family have concerns about medication use?

Common nursing diagnoses that may be appropriate for the child with atopic dermatitis include:

- Impaired Tissue Integrity related to chemical irritants and mechanical factors (abrasive clothing)

- Disturbed Sleep Pattern related to prolonged physical discomfort (itching)
- Risk for Infection related to breaks in skin barrier
- Chronic Low Self-Esteem related to chronic illness and peer reaction to visible skin lesions
- Ineffective Therapeutic Regimen Management (Families) related to excessive demands made on the family to keep the condition under control

Planning and Implementation

Nursing management focuses on education and emotional support. Atopic dermatitis can be controlled, but there is no cure. Advise parents that the lesions are not contagious and will not usually result in scarring. Help parents and adolescents deal with the frustration of the acute flares of the condition by reinforcing that remissions do occur even with consistent home care. See Families Want to Know: Atopic Eczema Skin Care.

Clinical Tip

Teach parents and adolescents how to apply topical ointments or creams. Apply a thin layer over the entire area and rub in the medication gently and completely. Treatment should continue until the skin clears. Help ensure that parents receive adequate amounts of topical corticosteroids for effective treatment. It takes about 6 g to cover the entire body of a 6-month-old infant, 10 g to cover the entire body of a 2-year-old, 13 g for a 5-year-old, and 18 g for a 10-year-old (Findlay, 2007). Fortunately most children do not have atopic eczema over the entire body, and the ointment is used only where there is a flare. For calcineurin inhibitors, a pea-size amount should cover a 2-inch circle.

To reduce pruritus, aggressively treat flares and control the environment. A humidifier counteracts dryness of the surrounding air, minimizing loss of skin moisture. Air conditioning limits unnecessary sweating that can exacerbate inflamed areas.

Research — *Bleach Bath*

A recent study investigated the effectiveness of soaking in a bath with a dilute bleach concentration (1/2 cup in a 40-gallon bathtub) for 5 to 10 minutes twice a week. A total of 31 children 6 months to 17 years of age were randomly assigned to either soak in the bleach bath and have intranasal mupirocin treatment or soak in plain bathwater and have white petrolatum nasal treatment. The eczema severity scores decreased significantly for all body sites except the unexposed head and neck in the group with dilute bleach baths and nasal mupirocin treatment (Huang, Abrams, Tlougan, et al., 2009).

The child, parents, and siblings may be tired because of lost sleep when the child scratches during the night during a flare. School performance may be affected if the child has sleep deprivation or if the child has physical discomfort that interferes with learning. If an oral antihistamine has been ordered, make sure the parents understand when to give the medication to maximize its effectiveness to produce a full night of sleep.

Atopic dermatitis produces visible changes that can affect a child's self-confidence and self-esteem. Identify activities that the child can participate in to improve self-esteem. Because humidity and sweating can make atopic dermatitis worse, encourage the child to shower after a sporting event or strenuous activity. Needed medications and emollients can then be applied.

Help parents and children deal with the frustration of the flare by reinforcing that remissions do occur with good home care. Provide encouragement and positive reinforcement for improvements in the child's skin during health care visits. Eczema that is difficult to manage is more stressful and has a more profound effect on the child's and family's quality of life. A daily massage using emollients may help improve the penetration of medications and reduce redness, scaling, lichenification, excoriation, and pruritus. This may improve the child's disposition and comfort.

Families Want to Know
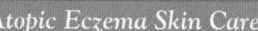
Atopic Eczema Skin Care

- Help the parents select an unscented emollient ointment or cream (Eucerin, Aveeno, Vanicream, Cetaphil, SBR Lipocream, or white petroleum) that fits into the family's budget. White petrolatum is inexpensive, safe, and easily applied. Lotions have a high water and alcohol content that will further dry the skin (Tofte, 2007).
- Daily bathing hydrates the skin. Salt or baking soda added to the bath water may help if water stings the child's open lesions. Dilute bleach may be used to reduce *Staphylococcus aureus* colonization.
- Let the child soak in warm water for several minutes once or twice a day. Use mild, unscented cleanser only on dirty areas. Rinse well. Immediately apply the emollient to wet skin, within 3 minutes of leaving the water, covering the entire body. If the child bathes only once a day, emollients should be applied twice a day.
- When the child has a flare, bathe the child twice a day and apply the topical corticosteroids or calcineurin inhibitor medication on affected areas. Emollients are applied on top of medications, as well as over the rest of the body.
- Wet wraps may be used for 5 to 7 days during acute flares to enhance the penetration of medications and to add moisture to the

skin. The child is bathed as usual, and topical corticosteroids and emollients are applied to the skin. The child puts on a warm damp layer (e.g., a form-fitting T-shirt) over the treated skin, and this is covered with a dry layer, such as pajamas. The child is kept warm until the layers dry. Wet wraps are not used for more than 5 to 7 days because of a potential risk of superinfection (Krakowski et al., 2008).
- In areas with low humidity, apply emollients to the skin more frequently. Corticosteroids should be applied no more than twice a day.
- Encourage the child to wear loose cotton clothing rather than wool or other irritating fabrics. Avoid the use of harsh detergents that may irritate the skin when laundering clothing.
- Keep the child's fingernails trimmed and place clean cotton gloves or socks over the infant's or child's hands to decrease scratching and reduce the chance of secondary infection.
- Emphasize the importance of following the treatment plan to promote healing of existing lesions and to reduce the risk of secondary infections.

Medications Used To Treat
Head Lice

Name of Medication/Preparation	Nursing Management
First-Line Pesticide Treatment Permethrin 1% Crème Rinse—Nix	Apply after shampooing and towel drying the hair. Leave on 10 minutes and rinse.
Pyrethrin shampoo (0.17–0.33%) or piperonyl butoxide (2–4%)—RID, A-200, R&C, Triple X, Pronto, Tisit, Licide	Apply to dry hair and scalp. Lather, leave on 10 minutes, and rinse with cool water. Repeat 7 to 10 days later. Wet hair dilutes the product and may contribute to treatment failure.
Ulesfia 5% benzyl alcohol lotion FDA-approved non-neurotoxic treatment, lice die by suffocation, approved for children age 6 months and older.	Apply to dry hair, saturating hair and scalp. Rinse after 10 minutes. Repeat in 7 days. Protect the eyes during use. Available by prescription.
Second-Line Pesticide Treatment Malathion 0.5% lotion or gel Organophosphate that causes paralysis and death of lice. Approved for children over age 6 years.	Apply to dry hair. Leave on 4 minutes and rinse. No retreatment needed. Is flammable, do not expose child to electric heat sources.
Lindane 1% shampoo or lotion Causes paralysis of lice and interferes with their ability to feed. Least effective chemical treatment due to resistance.	Apply to dry scalp and hair until soaked and allowed to dry naturally. Leave on for 8 to 12 hours and then rinse. Repeat 7 to 9 days later.
Non-FDA Approved Trimethoprim/sulfamethoxazole, oral Ivermectin—antiparasitic, oral	Drug in bloodstream is ingested by louse, destroys bacterial flora in louse intestine. Does not treat the nits.

Data from: Diamantis, S. A., Morrell, D. S., & Burkhart, C. N. (2009). Pediatric infestations. Pediatric Annals, *38(6), 326–332; U.S. Food and Drug Administration Center for Drug Evaluation and Research. (2009).* Ulesfia. *Retrieved from http://www.accessdata.fda.gov/scripts/cder/drugsatfda/index.cfm?fuseaction=Search.DrugDetails*

Infestation with lice can be upsetting for both the child and family. Emphasize to the family that anyone can get lice. Thorough interventions and education are essential for effective treatment. All family members and contacts of the child should be examined for infestation and should be treated as necessary. Tell parents that children infested with lice should return to childcare or school the day after the first pediculicide treatment is completed. Teach the child not to share clothing, headwear, or combs.

Explain to parents that most of the shampoo and rinses prescribed are pesticides and must be used for the time specified and as directed. An extra bottle of shampoo may be needed if the child has extra long hair. Keep these products out of the eyes and mouth of the child during their use because they will irritate mucous membranes. Parents should not use a creme rinse, combination shampoo/conditioner, or conditioner before using lice medicine. The hair should not be washed again for 1–2 days after the lice medicine is removed.

To remove nits, use a small-toothed comb, tweezers, and a basin filled with water or isopropyl alcohol to dip and clean the comb and tweezers. Comb 1-inch sections from the scalp outward and pin these out of the way when done. Nits adhere to the hair shaft and must be manually pulled down the shaft with the comb, tweezers, or fingernails. All nits should be removed. Have blunt-nosed scissors available to cut a hair shaft below the level of the nit when the nit cannot be removed. Put the child under a bright light and use distractions such as a video to keep the child occupied during the procedure. An alternative therapy for boys is to cut off the hair in a close buzz cut. A shorter haircut for girls may also help with nit removal.

Although lice can survive for only about 3 days away from a human host, nits may hatch 8 to 10 days later. For this reason, the child's bedding and clothing should be changed daily, laundered in hot water with detergent, and dried in a hot dryer for 20 minutes. Nonessential bedding and clothing can be stored in

Research — Lice

A recent study was conducted at multiple centers with 812 children with live lice. All children had been unsuccessfully treated for lice with topical insecticides in the prior 2 to 6 weeks. Children in the study were randomly assigned to treatment for lice at the study site with either malathion application to the hair or oral ivermectin on days 1 and 8. Of the children receiving ivermectin, 95.2% were lice-free on day 15, versus 85.0% receiving malathion. Oral ivermectin was significantly superior to malathion in these difficult-to-treat lice infestations, and could be an alternative therapy to malathion (Chosidow, Giraudeau, Cottrell, et al., 2010).

Complementary Therapy
Hot Air Treatment

Hot air with high volume and a comb-like device at the end of the hose has been found to be effective in the treatment of lice. While the hot air is blowing, the hair is slowly combed, taking about 30 minutes to treat the entire scalp. The mortality rate for eggs and lice is nearly 100% without the use of any medications. The specially developed hot air machine, the LouseBuster, can be used in schools and other health care settings (Goates, Atkin, Wilding, et al., 2006; LouseBuster, 2010).

a tightly sealed bag for 2 to 3 weeks and then washed. Hair accessories, brushes, and combs should be discarded or soaked in hot soapy water (54.4°C [130°F]) for 10 minutes. Vacuum furniture and carpets and treat them with a hot iron when possible. It is not recommended that the family use an insecticide in the home to kill the lice on carpets, furniture, and other items with which young children and pets come into contact. Seal toys and other personal items that cannot be washed or dry cleaned in a plastic bag for 2 weeks.

Scabies

Scabies is a highly contagious infestation caused by the mite *Sarcoptes scabiei*. It is spread by skin-to-skin contact and through sexual contact. Children of all ages and both sexes can be affected.

The female mite burrows into the upper layer of the epidermis (stratum corneum) to lay eggs that hatch in approximately 3 to 4 days. The larvae proceed toward the surface of the skin, emerge, mature, mate, and dig new burrows. The cycle repeats every 14 to 17 days. A delayed type IV hypersensitivity reaction to the mites, debris, and feces occurs within 4 to 6 weeks of infestation (Diamantis et al., 2009). Because the mite usually takes at least 45 minutes to burrow into the skin, transient contact is unlikely to cause infestation.

Symptoms include a rash with various types of lesions (papules, vesicles, pustules, and nodules), severe pruritus that worsens at night, and restlessness. Lesions are usually located in the web spaces of the fingers and toes, in the umbilicus, and around the axillae, wrists, elbows, inner thighs, and waist (Figure 31–13 ➤). Infants may have lesions on the palms, soles, and scalp. The burrow lesions may appear as a threadlike, grayish line on the skin surface 1 to 10 cm in length, which may end in a pinpoint vesicle. Lesions may be obliterated by the child's scratching and secondary infection.

Diagnosis is confirmed by examining scrapings from a burrow under the microscope, which reveals actively moving mites, fecal pellets, eggs, or nits. Treatment involves application of a scabicide, such as 5% permethrin lotion or lindane, over the entire body from the neck down, with special attention to the hands, fingers, feet, and toes, and under the nails. Application of the scabicide is preceded by a soap and water bath. When the skin is cool and dry, apply the lotion. The lotion is left in place for 8 to 12 hours and then rinsed off (Diamantis et al., 2009). The treatment may need to be repeated. All close contacts, members of the household, and childcare contacts should be treated at the same time, even if they have no symptoms. Treatment failure is usually due to inadequate treatment or reinfestation by an untreated contact. Secondary infection is treated with antibiotics after culture to identify sensitivities. Itching may persist for 6 weeks after treatment and may be treated with an oral antihistamine (e.g., Benadryl, Atarax).

Nursing Management

Educate parents about the proper application of the scabicide. Make sure parents understand the importance of keeping the medication on the skin for the full 8 to 12 hours. The child should have scabicide reapplied to the hands if hands are washed

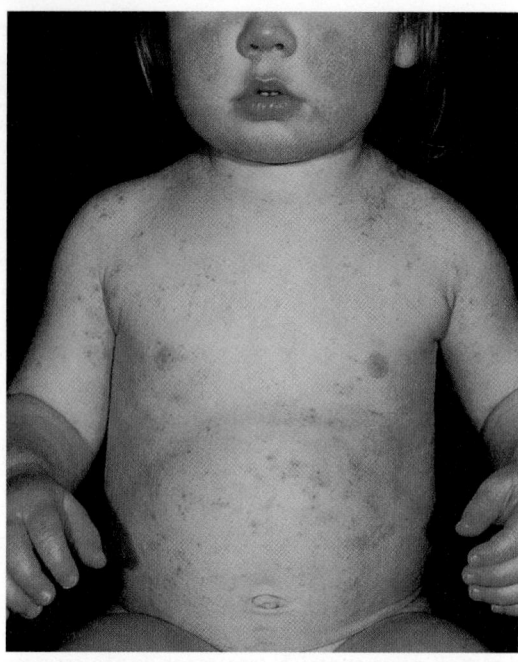

FIGURE 31–13 ➤ Diffuse scabies in an infant. The lesions are most numerous around the axillae, chest, and abdomen.
Used with permission from Habif, T. P. (1990). Clinical dermatology: A color guide to diagnosis and therapy (2nd ed., p. 298). St. Louis, MO: Mosby-Year Book.

or if the child sucks the fingers or thumb. Mitts or socks over the hands of young children may reduce the chance of ingesting the scabicide by placing the fingers in the mouth.

Advise parents that scabies is transmitted by close contact and is very contagious. All clothing, bedding, and pillowcases used by the child should be changed daily, washed with hot water, and put in a hot dryer for 40 minutes. Nonwashable toys and other items should be sealed in plastic bags for 2 weeks.

Treat all household contacts simultaneously. Visiting family members should not touch the affected child until treatment is completed. If they do, they should wash their hands well. Inform the parents about signs of secondary infections and that itching and nodules may persist for weeks after effective treatment. Encourage the use of emollients as the treatment dries the skin.

Scabies, like pediculosis, can be embarrassing or upsetting for the child and family. Educate the child and parents about the condition, its spread, and treatment measures to prevent recurrence.

■ INFANTILE HEMANGIOMAS

Vascular tumors or hemangiomas occur in 1–3% of all newborns; however, by the age of 1 year, approximately 10% of infants are affected. An increased incidence has been noted in females, preterm infants, and low-birth-weight infants who are fair-skinned; and the face is the most common site of hemangiomas (Haggstrom, Drolet, Baselga, et al., 2007). The risk for a hemangioma is greater in children of women who had chorionic villus sampling during pregnancy (Christinson-Lagay & Fishman, 2006).

Vascular tumors are neoplasms of endothelial cells and increased numbers of small blood vessels that undergo rapid growth and proliferation during the first 6 to 10 months of life and may lead to ulceration. This phase is followed by a slow **involution** (process of decreasing in size) that may take years. Hemangiomas may be superficial (located in the epidermis), deep (located in the dermis or subcutaneous tissue), or mixed superficial and deep. When multiple hemangiomas are found, some may be in major organs, such as the liver. Complications caused by the rapid growth and pressure against or obstruction of vital structures (e.g., airway, eye, or ear canal) may occur. A large facial hemangioma may be associated with PHACE syndrome (*P*osterior fossa malformation, large facial *H*emangioma, *A*rterial anomalies, *C*ardiac defects, and *E*ye abnormalities) (Metry, Siegel, Cordisco, et al., 2008).

Infantile hemangiomas begin as barely visible telangiectasias (dilated superficial blood vessels) or red macules that begin to grow rapidly and become bright red and compressible. Some lesions ulcerate with rapid growth. Superficial hemangiomas are bright red vascular cutaneous plaques that resemble strawberries. Deep hemangiomas appear as bluish tumors covered with normal-appearing epidermis. Mixed hemangiomas have features of both superficial and deep tumors. The lesions, appearing any place on the body, are minimally compressible and have no bruit or thrill. As the hemangioma involutes, signs of tissue atrophy, wrinkles, telangiectasias, and hypopigmentation may be noted.

Initial diagnosis is by physical examination and monitoring the growth of the vascular tumor. When a vital organ could become obstructed, ultrasound, computed tomography, or magnetic resonance imaging may be performed.

Some hemangiomas are monitored and receive no treatment. Hemangiomas in problem areas are often treated by high doses of systemic corticosteroids during the proliferation phase to slow the growth. Injections of corticosteroids into small localized hemangiomas are sometimes performed (Truong, Chang, Berk, et al., 2010). A course of several pulsed dye laser treatments is used for many superficial hemangiomas during the proliferative phase. Topical anesthesia and eye protection should be provided (Stier, Glick, & Hirsch, 2008). The hemangioma will darken to a purple shade for 1 to 2 weeks followed by gradual lightening of the treated skin surface without scarring. Children with darker skin have a longer interval between treatments. Surgical removal of an ulcerated hemangioma may be considered if the scarring outcome would be acceptable (Christinson-Lagay & Fishman, 2006).

Clinical Tip

A port-wine stain on one side of the face in the distribution of the ophthalmic and maxillary branches of the trigeminal nerve may indicate the presence of Sturge-Weber syndrome, an intracranial vascular anomaly. Children with Sturge-Weber syndrome are at high risk for glaucoma and may develop epilepsy, intellectual disability, attention deficit hyperactivity disorder, and stroke-like episodes (Stier et al., 2008). Regular ophthalmic examinations should be scheduled.

Nursing Management

Assess the distribution of the hemangioma and consider the potential for complications as it goes through a rapid growth stage.

Monitor the child for signs of any complications, such as ulceration or stridor potentially caused by compression on the airway. Assess the parents' response to the infant's appearance and how they are managing interactions with friends and family about the infant's changing appearance. Take photos of the infant at each visit so that parents have a record of improvements once therapy is initiated.

Teach the parents about the type of vascular lesion and potential treatment options. When corticosteroids are prescribed, teach the parents about administration, the need to take the full course as prescribed, and potential side effects. Inform parents that a rapidly growing hemangioma may ulcerate. Teach them what signs to expect and how to protect the skin until a physician is seen.

Talk with parents about comments made about the infant's appearance and provide some possible responses that parents can make. To promote attachment, help the parents see the infant's positive characteristics, such as responsiveness and smiling. Show photos of other children with similar lesions who have completed therapy to show that improvements in appearance are gradual, but possible.

Prepare parents for the changes in the child's appearance with pulsed dye laser therapy. Some swelling may occur after the treatment, so the application of ice packs for 10 minutes every hour during the first day may help. Teach parents to protect the skin surface from trauma after pulsed dye laser treatments and to keep the infant's nails short to prevent scratching. Cleanse the area treated with water and pat it dry. Inform parents to avoid sun exposure for several weeks after the treatments, and to use sunscreen in the future.

■ INJURIES TO THE SKIN

Pressure Ulcers

An increasing number of children with disabilities who are cared for in hospital, community, and home care settings are at risk for skin breakdown and pressure ulcers. Children at greatest risk are those with limited mobility, the inability to change positions, sensory deficits, or incontinence (Table 31–5). Another risk is skin rubbing against bedding as occurs with high activity. A reported rate in pediatric critical care settings was 27%, while other hospital settings may have a rate of 1–13% (Noonan, Quigley, & Curley, 2006).

TABLE 31–5	Sites and Potential Causes of Pressure Ulcers
Sites	Potential Causes
Occipital region of scalp, ear	Inability to lift head
Sacrum and buttocks	Confinement to bed or wheelchair
Legs and feet	Leg braces, casts
Spine and neck	Scoliosis brace
Knees and elbows	Rubbing against bed sheet
Sternum, iliac crest	Ventilated in prone position

Soft tissues and capillary beds may be compressed between a bony prominence and another surface. Tissue ischemia occurs when high pressure is maintained over a short period of time or low pressure is maintained over a prolonged time (Butler, 2006). The cells are deprived of oxygen and nutrients, and metabolic waste products accumulate, injuring the soft tissue. Without appropriate intervention, the injury progresses rapidly and a pressure ulcer forms.

The earliest sign of skin damage is an area of redness that does not go away within 30 minutes of removing the pressure or skin irritant. Children with dark skin may have persistent red, blue, or purple discoloration. Pressure ulcers are staged to describe the extent of injury (Figure 31–14 ➤). Secondary infection may occur.

The Braden Q Scale (for children under age 5 years) and the Braden Scale can be used to assess the child's risk for pressure ulcers. For early stages of skin damage, treat by removing pressure from the affected site until the skin has healed. Children who use leg braces for alignment and mobility are often put in wheelchairs. Children who use wheelchairs are often put on bed rest on a pressure-reducing surface. Frequent repositioning is needed. A transparent film may be applied to affected red skin to minimize friction. Pressure ulcers are treated with dressings that do not ad-

Growth & Development — *Pressure Sites*

The site of greatest pressure in infants and young children is the occiput. Older children have increased pressure on the sacral and occipital areas.

here to the wounds, such as hydrocolloids, gels or hydrogels, and alginates. See the companion website for the Braden scales.

Nursing Management

Carefully inspect the dependent skin surfaces of all infants and children confined to bed at least three times in each 24-hour period using the appropriate Braden scale. Evaluate the risk for skin damage based on factors that can contribute to skin breakdown. Identify the size (length, width, and depth) and character of the skin lesion. Note and describe any signs of infection, the appearance of wound edges, type of tissue at the wound base, and drainage.

Develop protocols for pressure ulcer prevention so that children at high risk are identified. Initiate appropriate interventions such as increased ambulation, frequent position changes, pressure-reducing surfaces, and moisture barriers. If the child is

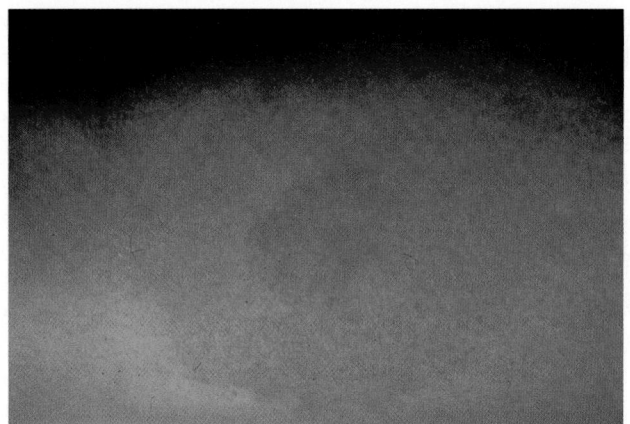

A

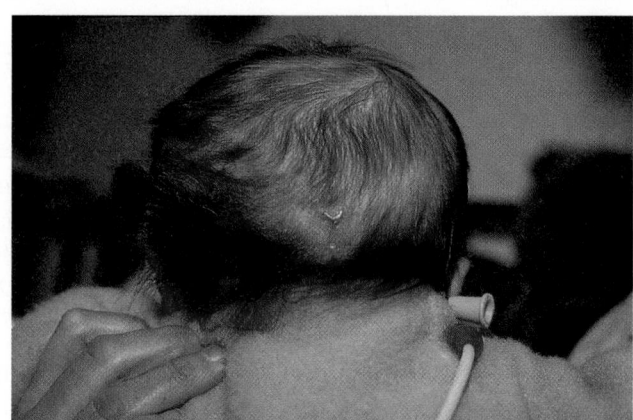

B

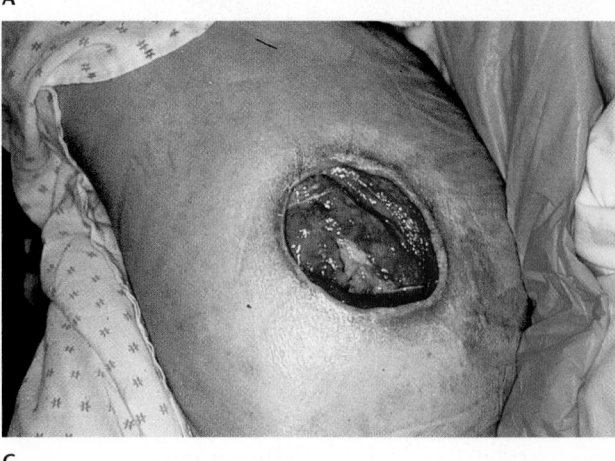

C

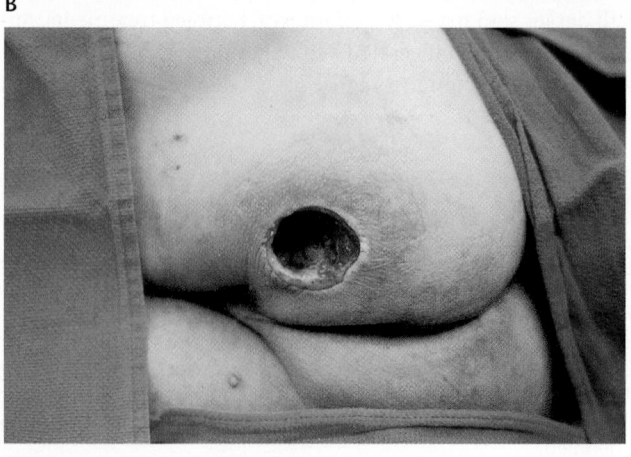

D

FIGURE 31–14 ➤ A, Stage 1, nonblanchable erythema of intact skin; skin color or temperature may be different from surrounding skin. B, Stage 2, blister or abrasion, partial-thickness loss with damage through the epidermis; no slough or eschar is present. C, Stage 3, full-thickness loss with exposure of subcutaneous tissue. D, Stage 4, full-thickness loss with exposure of muscle, tendon, or bone.

Courtesy of Sandra Quigley, Children's Hospital, Boston, MA.

Problem

Infants and children, especially those with chronic conditions, are at risk for pressure ulcers. What information about the rate of pressure ulcers and factors that increase their risk of development is important for prevention and nursing management?

Evidence

In a large children's hospital, approximately 6% of 252 child patients were found to be at high risk for a pressure ulcer using the Braden Q Scale and 1.6% had a pressure ulcer. Thirteen children had pressure-related injuries associated with pulse oximetry or other medical devices (Noonan et al., 2006). Pilot testing of the Starkid Skin Scale for skin integrity assessment was conducted in a large pediatric hospital. Skin breakdown was found in 80 (23%) of 347 children, and approximately 75% were described as Stage 1. Affected children were more likely to be younger and smaller, and to have more medical devices, more episodes of diarrhea, and a lower score on the assessment scale (Suddaby, Barnett, & Facteau, 2005). The Braden Scale was used to assess 155 children, aged birth to 17 years, in four German pediatric hospitals to identify the prevalence of pressure ulcers. A total of 43 children (27.7%) were found to have one or more pressure ulcers, most being Grade 1. However, 7 children

(4.5%) had pressure ulcers of Grade 2 or higher. Many of the pressure ulcers were associated with splints, cables, and tubes used in the child's care (Schlüer, Cignacco, Müller, et al., 2009).

Implications

Factors that increase a child's risk for pressure ulcers include the following: friction from casts and orthotic devices, excessive motion, inability to move independently, diminished or no sensation, moisture on the skin from soiling, and sedation and care in a critical care unit with medical devices. This information can be used to develop prevention guidelines, such as a turning schedule; skin inspection under braces, orthotics, and medical devices; rotation of pulse oximetry sensor sites; and positioning and taping devices (e.g., endotracheal and nasogastric tubes) to reduce pressure against the skin.

Critical Thinking Application

Use the Braden Scale or Braden Q Scale (for children under 5 years) to assess the risk of a child with an acute illness and one with a chronic illness for pressure ulcers. Then perform a complete assessment of these children to identify any skin breakdown. Develop a nursing care plan for the high-risk child to prevent and treat skin breakdown.

---

incontinent, change the diaper frequently. Ensure an adequate intake of fluids, proteins, and vitamins to keep the skin healthy. (See Evidence-Based Practice: Pressure Ulcers in Children.)

Moist wounds heal more rapidly than dry wounds. Cell migration across the moist wound bed more effectively fights infection and removes cellular debris (Butler, 2006). Provide wound care and dressing changes according to agency guidelines. These guidelines may include saline irrigation, debridement, and a dressing appropriate for the wound condition. (See the *Clinical Skills Manual.*) Gauze wraps to hold the dressing in place help prevent skin damage caused by adhesives.

Teach parents of children with braces to inspect the skin under the braces every day for irritation (redness or blisters). Help the child to use a mirror with a long handle to inspect skin on the bottom and sides of the feet, behind the knees, and on the lower legs. Check all edges of the braces for roughness or breakage that can pinch or scrape the skin. If any skin irritation is seen and redness does not go away within 30 minutes, do not put the brace back on until the skin heals. Inform the child's physician so that treatment can be started immediately. To prevent braces from rubbing on bare skin, have the child wear cotton socks under the braces and make sure the shoes are large enough to accommodate the brace, socks, and the foot (Figure 31–15 ➤). Advise parents to return to a prosthetist regularly for brace refitting as the child grows.

Children who use a wheelchair are at risk for skin breakdown on the buttocks and lower back from the pressure of sitting for hours. A wheelchair gel or foam cushion can distribute and shift the child's weight when sitting in the chair. Teach the child to change position by doing wheelchair push-ups or by shifting the weight (leaning to the side or forward) for several minutes every 10 to 15 minutes. Make sure the child wears a safety belt when sitting in the wheelchair. Teach school personnel about the

child's recommended protocol so they can provide opportunities in school to change positions and reinforce the routine.

Burns

Burns are a common cause of pediatric injury, and the third highest cause of death in children (Gauglitz, Herndon, & Jeschke, 2008). An average of 120,856 children and adolescents

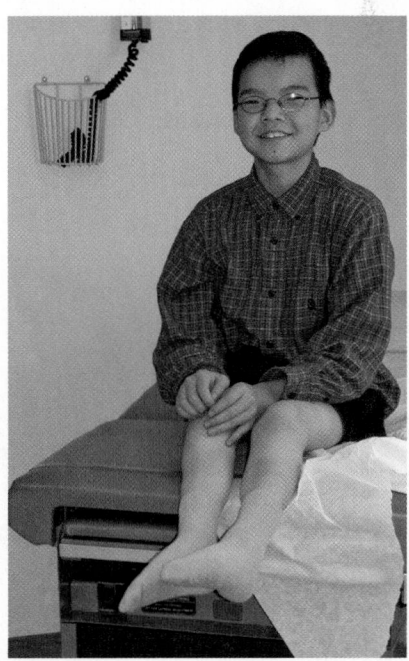

FIGURE 31–15 ➤ Sam has meningomyelocele. He wears socks under his braces to help prevent them from rubbing directly against his skin. He uses crutches and a wheelchair for mobility. What other measures should Sam and his parents take to prevent skin breakdown?

under age 21 years are treated in emergency departments each year. Children less than 6 years of age and boys experience the most burn injuries. The majority of burn injuries occur in the home (D'Souza, Nelson, & McKenzie, 2009).

There are four main types of burns: thermal, chemical, electrical, and radioactive. Thermal burns, the most common in children, result from flames, scalds (such as hot water or grease), or contact with hot objects (such as a woodstove or curling iron). Chemical burns occur when children touch or ingest caustic agents. Electrical burns are caused by direct or alternating current in electrical wires, appliances, or high-voltage wires. Radiation burns result from exposure to radioactive substances or sunlight. Burns are a common form of child abuse, accounting for up to 25% of all cases (Mahindra, Guillen, & Glick, 2009). See Chapter 17 ∞ for a description of child abuse.

Etiology and Pathophysiology

Children at different developmental stages are at risk for different types of burns.

- Infants are most often injured by thermal burns (scalding liquids, house fires).
- Toddlers are at risk for thermal burns (pulling hot liquids or grease onto themselves) (Figure 31–16 ➤), electrical burns (biting electrical cords) (Figure 31–17 ➤), contact burns, and chemical burns (ingesting cleaning agents and other substances) associated with exploring the environment.
- Preschool-age children are most often injured by scalding or contact with hot appliances (curling irons, ovens).
- School-age children are at risk for thermal burns (playing with matches, fireworks, scald burns from spilled beverages heated in the microwave oven), electrical burns (climbing high-voltage towers, climbing trees, contact with electrical wires), and chemical burns (combustion experiments) associated with their curiosity and interest in experimentation.
- Adolescents also experience thermal, chemical, and electrical burns.

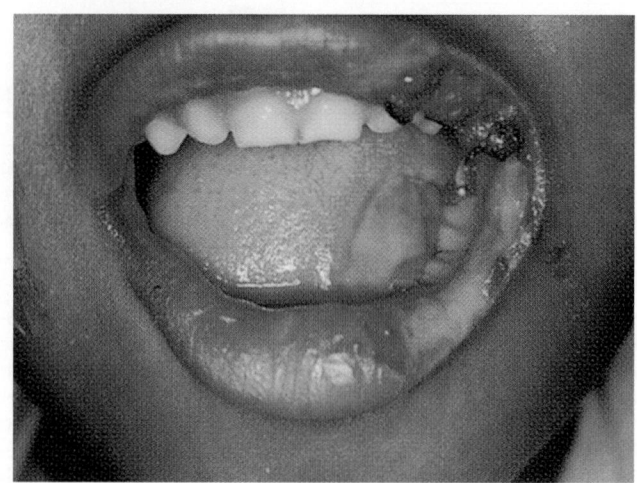

FIGURE 31–17 ➤ Electrical burn caused by biting on an electrical cord. The burn is caused when the current arcs through the lips, often causing a full-thickness injury through the mucosa, muscle, nerves, and blood vessels. The labial artery may be injured and cause significant bleeding once the eschar falls off after 2 to 3 weeks.
Courtesy of Dr. Lezley McIveen, Department of Dentistry, Children's National Medical Center, Washington, DC.

Immediately after the burn, intense vasoconstriction occurs in response to substances released by the injured cells. Ischemia resulting from vasoconstriction may increase the depth of the burn injury. Then vasoactive hormones are released that increase capillary permeability. This permits fluid and plasma to shift into the interstitial spaces, causing edema and decreased volume circulating in the blood vessels. Capillary integrity is not restored for 18 to 36 hours after the burn injury. The child loses increased water and heat through the injured epidermis. The child's metabolic rate and need for calories increase in the attempt to maintain body temperature. The depth of the burn depends upon the temperature and duration of the heat application, and on the ability of tissues to dissipate the transferred energy.

Nursing Alert

A full-thickness burn can occur after immersion in water for only 5 seconds if the temperature is 60°C (140°F), and after 15 seconds if the temperature is 56°C (133°F). Coffee and other hot beverages are served at temperatures high enough to cause a serious scald burn injury (Burn Foundation, 2010). Set hot water heaters to 48°C (120°F) to help prevent scald burns. Do not hold young children in the lap while drinking hot beverages.

Clinical Manifestations

Burns are classified by depth of penetration into the skin (Figure 31–18 ➤). Burn depth may be defined as partial thickness or full thickness. Partial-thickness burns, in which the injured tissue can regenerate and heal, may be either first or second degree. Full-thickness burns, in which the injured tissue cannot regenerate, are also known as third-degree burns. Signs of infection may include purulent drainage, swelling, erythema, discoloration of wound margins, and pain in the uninjured skin around the wound.

Animation: Burns

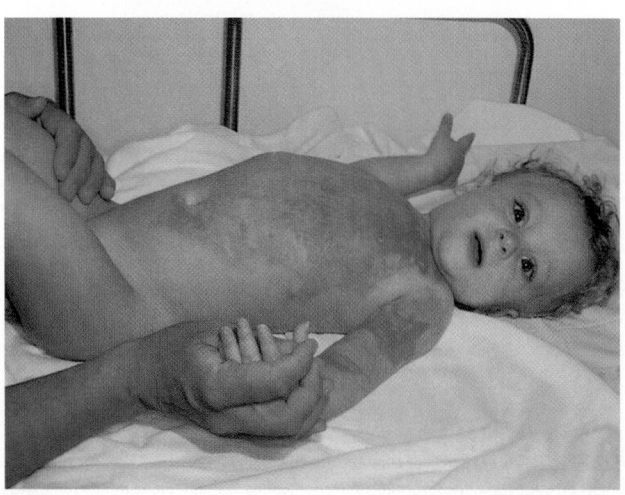

FIGURE 31–16 ➤ Thermal (scald) burns are the most common burn injury in infancy.

Pathophysiology Illustrated

Classification of Burns

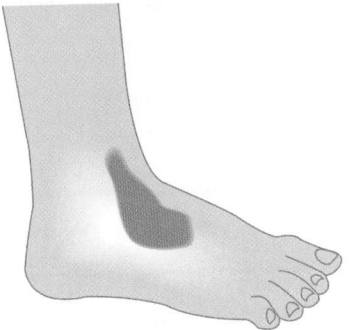

Superficial Partial Thickness (First Degree)
Damages only outer layer of skin; burn is painful and red; heals in a few days (e.g., sunburn)

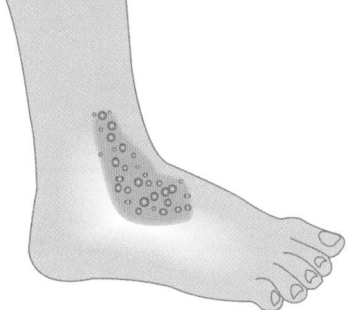

Partial Thickness (Second Degree)
Involves epidermis and upper layers of dermis; may have sparing of sweat gland and sebaceous glands; heals in 10–14 days

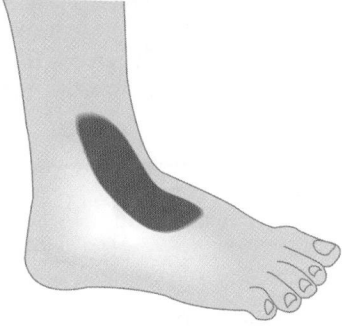

Full Thickness (Third Degree)
Involves all of epidermis and dermis; may also involve underlying tissue; nerve endings usually destroyed; requires skin grafting

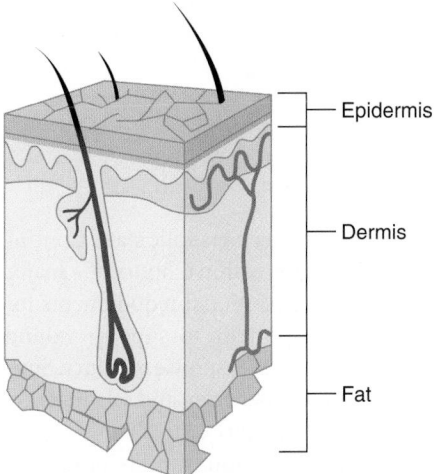

— Epidermis

— Dermis

— Fat

Erythema, blanches on pressure, no bullae, peeling after a few days due to premature cell death

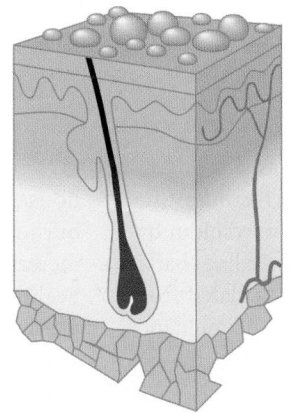

Blisters or bullae, erythema, blanches on pressure, pain and sensitivity to cold air, minimal scar formation

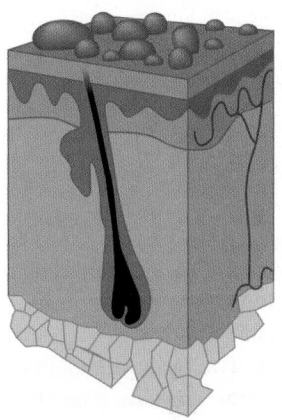

Skin may appear brown, black, deep cherry red, white to gray, waxy or translucent, usually no pain, injured area may appear sunken

FIGURE 31–18 ➤ Burn characteristics by depth of injury.

COLLABORATIVE CARE

Diagnostic Tests

Burn severity is determined by the depth of the burn injury, percentage of body surface area (BSA) affected, and involvement of specific body parts. A Lund and Browder chart with BSA distributions for various body parts at different ages is used to calculate the area affected by the burn injury (Figure 31–19 ➤). The palm of a child's hand (without fingers and thumb) is 1% of his or her body surface area and can be used to make a quick estimate of the burn size. Reassessment of the extent of burn injury is performed 24 to 48 hours after the injury. Criteria for major burns that should be cared for in a specialized burn center include (American College of Surgeons, 2006, p. 79):

- A partial-thickness burn greater than 10% BSA
- Burns involving the hands, face, feet, genitalia, perineum, and major joints
- Full-thickness burns
- Electrical burns, including lightning injury
- Inhalation injury

Clinical Therapy

Initial Treatment   The first step is to ensure that the child has an airway, is breathing, and has a pulse. Then remove jewelry and clothing and apply moist soaks or ice (if a small surface area is affected) to stop the burning process and to relieve pain. If a chemical causes the burns, remove the clothing and wash with large amounts of water or an appropriate neutralizing agent. A tetanus vaccine booster is given if more than 5 years have passed since the last vaccine, or when the child has not completed the full vaccine series.

Treatment of Major Burns   The goals of treatment include decreasing burn fluid losses, preventing infection, controlling pain, promoting nutrition, and salvaging all viable tissue. Fluid

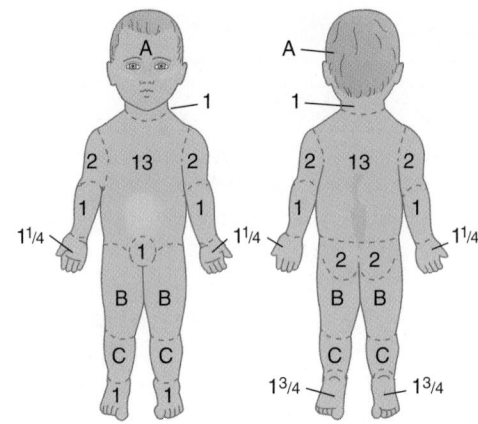

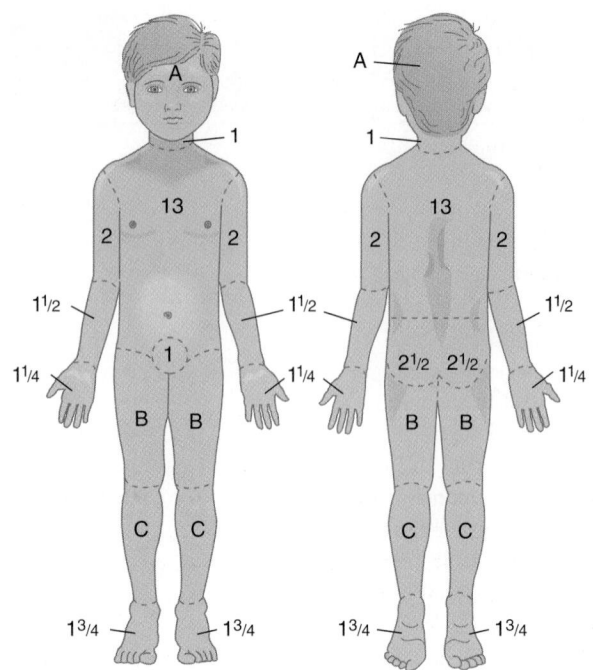

Relative Percentages of Areas Affected by Growth

Area	Age in years					
	0	1	5	10	11	Adult
A = ¹/₂ of head	9¹/₂	8¹/₂	6¹/₂	5¹/₂	4¹/₂	3¹/₂
B = ¹/₂ of one thigh	2³/₄	3¹/₄	4	4¹/₂	4¹/₂	4³/₄
C = ¹/₂ of one lower leg	2¹/₂	2¹/₂	2³/₄	3	3¹/₄	3¹/₂

FIGURE 31–19 ➤ Lund and Browder chart for determining percentage of body surface areas in pediatric burn injuries. A, Infant. B, Child of 5 years.
Note: From Artz, C. P., & Moncrief, J. A. (1969). The treatment of burns (2nd ed.). Philadelphia: Saunders. Adapted.

replacement is necessary to maintain the cardiovascular and renal systems. Fluid shifts from the vasculature to the interstitial spaces (third spacing) soon after the burn and can result in hypovolemic shock. Fluid replacement for the first 24 hours after the injury is based on a fluid volume formula calculated from the child's body weight, affected BSA, and normal maintenance needs. Two examples of this calculation are the Parkland and Galveston formulas (Gauglitz et al., 2008):

- Parkland Formula: 3–4 mL × body weight (kg) × percentage of total BSA burned = total 24-hour fluid requirement in mL. Maintenance fluids must be added to the amount of fluid calculated with this formula.
- Shriners Burn Hospitals—Galveston Formula: 5000 mL/m² burned area + 2000 mL/m² of total BSA = total 24-hour fluid requirement in mL.

Lactated Ringer's or normal saline solution is the preferred fluid. Half of the total volume calculated for the 24-hour period is infused over the first 8 hours, starting at the time of the burn rather than arrival time in the emergency department. The remainder is distributed evenly over the next 16 hours. Urine output is used to monitor end organ perfusion. When the urine output reaches 1 mL/kg/hour in children weighing less than 30 kg, fluid resuscitation ends and the fluid rate is reduced (Hazinski, Mondozzi, & Baker, 2010). Efforts are also focused on maintaining the child's temperature because heat is lost rapidly through burned skin.

Fever is a normal, expected outcome of any significant burn injury, but it is not always a sign of infection. Treatment may include acetaminophen, ice packs, cooling blankets, or cool hydrotherapy sessions. Infection is a frequent complication, and wounds are cultured to identify specific organisms for antibiotic therapy.

A serious burn injury causes a hypermetabolic state. Continuous enteral feedings are often begun within 6 hours of a major burn injury to support the child's nutritional requirements for increased calories and additional protein, to support wound healing, and to support the body's stress response to injury. Supplemental vitamins C and E, zinc, copper, iron, and selenium are given to promote wound healing (Gauglitz et al., 2008).

Aggressive pain management with intravenous opioids is needed around the clock and for all procedures. The burns can cause a significant emotional stress that increases the perception of pain. See Chapter 15 ∞ for more information on pain management. Cimetidine or other H₂ blockers may be ordered to prevent a burn stress ulcer.

Special consideration is needed when burns involve certain areas of the body:

- Deep partial-thickness and full-thickness burns develop **eschar** (the tough leathery scab that forms over severely burned areas) with no elasticity. When the burn is **circumferential** (around an entire extremity or the torso), blood flow can become restricted as a result of edema, leading to tissue hypoxia. An **escharotomy** (incision into the constricting tissue) may be necessary to restore peripheral circulation.
- Facial burns usually cause significant edema. Care must be taken to ensure airway patency. An ophthalmologist should be consulted for burns to the eye to assess damage and prescribe treatment. If the lips are burned, an infant may be unable to suck.
- Burns of the hands require careful management to maintain function. Special splinting and physical therapy are usually necessary.

• Perineal burns are at higher risk for infection because of frequent contamination with urine and stool. Frequent dressing changes are required. A urinary catheter is usually inserted but is removed once hydration status is stable to minimize the risk of urinary tract infection.

Wound Management Burn wound care has several goals: (1) to remove necrotic tissue and speed wound debridement, (2) to maintain moist wound conditions and adequate circulation, (3) to conserve body heat and fluids, (4) to protect the wound from infection, and (5) to control scarring and prevent scar contracture. Several treatment regimens are used to achieve these goals.

When the child has an extensive burn, the entire body is bathed to initiate debridement (removal of dead tissue to speed the healing process). Sedation and anesthesiology support may be ordered for pain management during debridement. The dead tissues are carefully cut away when preparing the wound for grafting.

Various options are used for wound management after debridement. Traditional burn care for a partial-thickness injury involves the application of antibacterial agents, such as silver sulfadiazine (Silvadene), mafenide acetate (Sulfamylon), or bacitracin after initial cleansing. Dressings are added to cover the burned area and are changed once or twice daily.

Newer silver-based antimicrobial dressings (e.g., Aquacel, Acticoat) have been developed that provide a sustained-release delivery of silver valued for its antimicrobial activity (Figure 31–20 ➤). As these dressings absorb exudate from the wound they can be left in place for many days (Duffy, McLaughlin, & Eichelberger, 2006). When the dressing is removed, a layer of eschar may also be debrided. These dressing changes are often painful, so pain management is needed.

Hydrotherapy may be used to cleanse extensive wounds before debridement, to increase vasodilation and circulation, and to speed healing. Hydrotherapy and debridement may be performed with the child in a shower rather than a tub to reduce infection risk. The water loosens exudate, topical medications, and dead tissue. Tap water and an antimicrobial soap are often used for debridement. Gentle washing is necessary to protect new epithelial cells. In addition, the dressings that adhere to the skin may be soaked to help loosen them. Superficial partial-thickness burns re-epithelialize within 3 weeks.

Skin grafting is necessary with any deep partial-thickness and full-thickness burn. Often a biologic dressing (e.g., Integra or Biobrane) or allograft (cadaver skin from a skin bank) is used to cover deep burns to improve the condition of a deep second- or third-degree burn until an **autograft** (use of healthy skin taken from an uninjured area of the child's body) can be performed. This covering is effective in decreasing infection risk and pain, protecting against fluid loss, and promoting revascularization. The biologic dressing or graft is placed after the wound is debrided in the operating room to reveal healthy, bleeding tissue. This forms a protective barrier over the wound surface to decrease infection risk and to protect against fluid loss. An autograft is permanent. The donor site (where the autograft was harvested) is a new wound, causing pain and requiring close monitoring for signs of infection.

Vacuum-assisted wound closure is sometimes used for management of partial-thickness burns, graft sites, and other complex wounds. Once the burn site is debrided, a foam dressing is applied and sealed with adhesive. The vacuum then places controlled negative pressure over all the tissues covered. It works by increasing local blood perfusion, reducing edema, decreasing the amount of bacterial colonization, drawing wound edges together, and ultimately reducing the time needed for wound healing (Horn & Beebe, 2009; Preston, 2008). Children may be sent home and return to the hospital every few days for dressing changes, as occurred with Joshua in the chapter-opening scenario.

During the rehabilitation stage, pressure garments, also known as Jobst garments, are used to reduce development of hypertrophic scarring and contractures (Figure 31–21 ➤). Such garments are worn 23 hours a day for 6 to 8 months to shorten the time of scar maturation and to reduce the thickness of scars.

Severe morbidity is likely to occur with major burns. Significant scarring may occur regardless of autografting and the use of pressure garments. Contractures and loss of function are also possible. Children with major burns require comprehensive follow-up, sometimes involving repeated hospitalizations for surgery to release burn contractures or perform new grafting, or cosmetic surgery for scar revision.

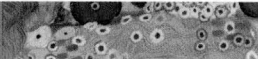

NURSING MANAGEMENT

Nursing Assessment and Diagnosis

Nursing assessment first focuses on the potential for life-threatening injuries that need immediate care. After the child's condition has been stabilized, the history, physical assessment, and psychosocial assessment are performed.

Emergency Assessment

Emergency assessment is based on the ABCs of basic life support (airway, breathing, and circulation). Assessment of the airway is necessary, especially when there are signs of smoke inhalation or burns to the face and neck. It is important to identify other potential injuries when the mechanism of injury includes a fall or explosion. Identify signs of respiratory distress and any potential bleeding source. A weak, thready pulse; tachycardia; and pallor

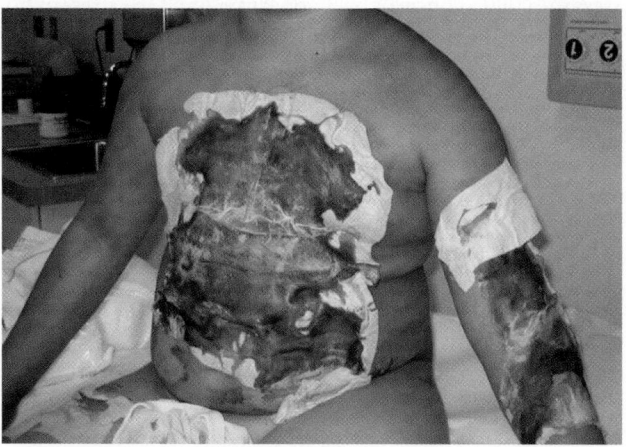

FIGURE 31–20 ➤ Child with a scald burn treated with an Aquacel AG® dressing, one of the newer silver-embedded dressings. Note the absorbed exudate that is visible through the burn dressing.
Courtesy of Martin Eichelberger, MD, and Lisa Ring, RN, PNP, Children's National Medical Center.

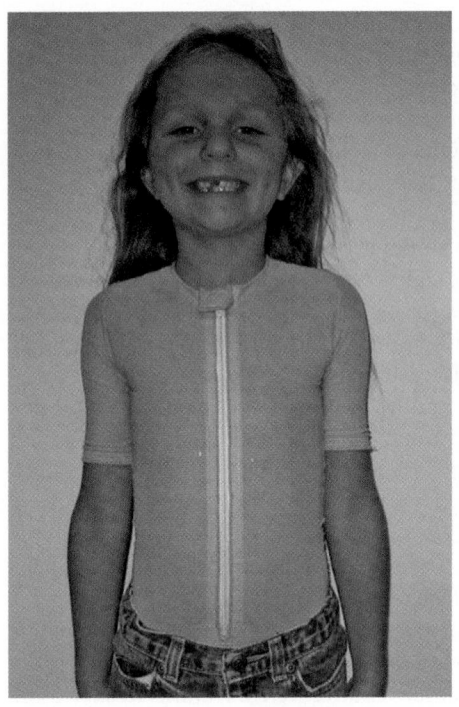

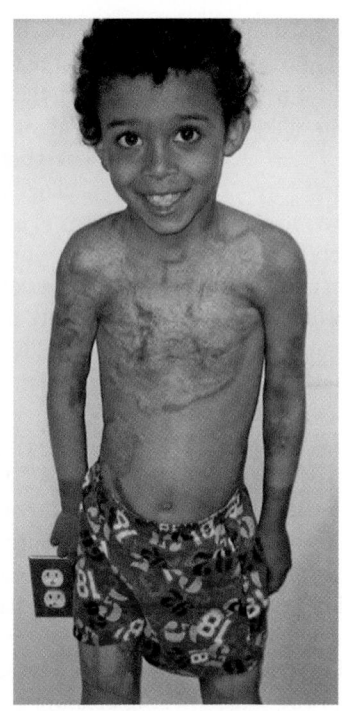

A

B

FIGURE 31–21 ➤ A, Pressure garment used to reduce hypertrophic scarring from a burn on the chest. B, Hypertrophic scar on the chest.
Courtesy of Martin Eichelberger, MD, and Lisa Ring, RN, PNP, Children's National Medical Center.

are important signs of early shock that may provide clues to an internal injury.

History

Obtain information about the type of burn (e.g., thermal, electrical, chemical) and a complete history. When taking a burn history, carefully document the type of injury, time of injury, people present at the time of the injury, first aid administered, and history of other unusual injuries or emergency department visits. If a burn injury was preventable, parents may be emotionally stressed by feelings of guilt. Take care to avoid sounding accusatory when questioning parents about the injury. Be alert for the potential of child abuse when the history does not match the burn injury. Child neglect can be a factor in the burn of an inadequately supervised child.

Nursing Alert

Signs of child abuse include glove and sock line burns, burns that spare flexor surfaces such as on the perineum or popliteal area, contact burns from cigarettes or irons, and zebra burn lines from contact with a hot grate (Figure 31–22 ➤). Photographs are often taken to document these burn injuries.

Physical Assessment

Assess the extent of burn injury (depth and BSA affected). Frequently monitor the vital signs, including pain. Weigh the child daily.

Monitor the child's circulatory and respiratory status to identify signs of hypovolemia in the first 24 hours or fluid overload as capillary integrity is restored. Perform a head-to-toe assessment at the beginning of every shift followed by system-specific assessments, depending on clinical findings and changes in the child's

status. For example, frequently assess edema, eschar, and distal pulses in a burned extremity to monitor peripheral circulation. Monitor electrolytes as well as intake and output carefully. A urinary catheter may be inserted to enable close monitoring of urine output. Be alert to signs of infection such as purulent drainage, odor, and edematous, red, or discolored wound margins.

Nursing Alert

If a burn is circumferential, assess for an increase in cyanosis, deep tissue pain, and capillary refill time, and a decreased pulse distal to the burn. If these signs are detected, notify the physician immediately.

Psychosocial Assessment

Assess the child's concerns over appearance and the stress of hospitalization. Determine if the child has memories or nightmares about the burn and arrange psychologic support as needed. Identify any family stressors that may need to be addressed during the child's care.

Common nursing diagnoses for the child with a major burn injury are included in the accompanying Nursing Care Plan: The Child with a Major Burn Injury. Additional nursing diagnoses for the child with a major burn might include:

- Hyperthermia related to increased metabolic rate and trauma
- Acute Pain related to physical injury agents
- Ineffective Peripheral Tissue Perfusion related to mechanical reduction of blood flow (edema) to an extremity with a circumferential burn
- Disturbed Body Image related to burn injury
- Anxiety related to situational crisis and threat of death or disfigurement

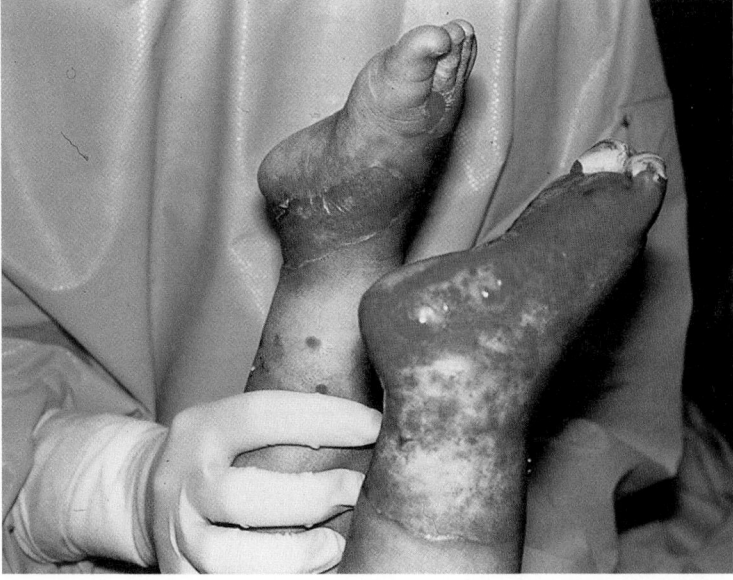
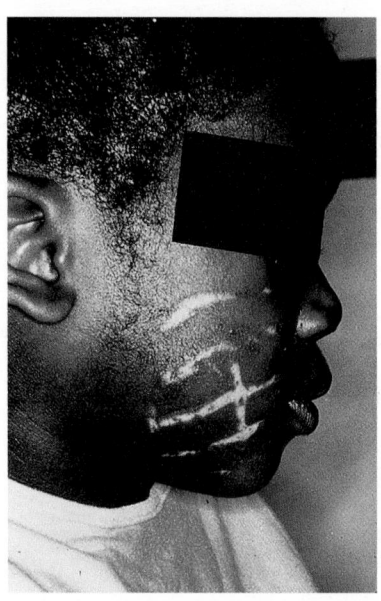

A   **B**

FIGURE 31–22 ➤ Burn injuries associated with child abuse. A, Burns of the hands or feet that are distributed like gloves or stockings indicate dipping in hot water. B, Zebra burns from a grate.

(A) Used with permission of the American Academy of Pediatrics, "Visual Diagnosis of Child Abuse Slide Kit." (B) Courtesy of the Kempe Children's Center, Denver, CO.

Planning and Implementation

Nursing care focuses on performing burn care, preventing complications, and providing emotional support. Care of the child with a burn injury involves various treatments designed to promote healing and prevent complications. These include dressing changes, hydrotherapy, antibiotic therapy, pain management, physical therapy, play therapy, psychological support, and possibly skin graft care. See the Nursing Care Plan for some important aspects of burn care.

Pain Management

Assess the child's pain frequently and provide pain management throughout the day and night. (See Chapter 15 ∞.) Cover burns as air movement and temperature change irritate exposed nerve endings and cause pain. Perception of procedural pain may be intensified as the child has ongoing background pain from the injury (Connor-Ballard, 2009). Ensure that the child receives adequate pain management and sedation for debridement and dressing changes to reduce anxiety associated with care. Provide diversion to help the child focus on a pleasant activity rather than pain.

Fluid and Nutrition Support

Administer IV fluids at the rate prescribed for resuscitation for the first 24 hours. Enteral feeding may be needed initially by the child with extensive burns until the child is able to eat. Once the child is able to eat, provide a diet high in protein and calories. Identify food items that the child likes, and encourage the family to bring food in that the child may prefer to eat. Provide small frequent feedings to increase the number of calories consumed each day.

Wound Care

The burned area is debrided and cleaned, often with a chemical enzyme cleanser. Then an antibacterial/antimicrobial medica-

tion or dressing is applied. Topical medications are often covered with a dressing. At each dressing change, the wound needs to be assessed for appearance, exudate, odor, appearance of surrounding tissue, and presence of granulation tissue. (See the *Clinical Skills Manual*.)

A semipermeable wound membrane may be applied to a debrided superficial partial-thickness burn. These membranes protect the burned tissue from trauma, prevent fluid loss, create a moist environment for healing, and provide a physical barrier to bacteria. Monitor the burn under the semipermeable membrane carefully for signs of infection, which could deepen the burn wound. When the burn heals, the wound membrane loosens, permitting it to be trimmed.

Allografts or autografts may be placed in the operating room after debridement to prepare the burned tissue for the graft. Following the grafting procedure, wet dressings with antibiotic solution are used for several days, followed by other dry dressings with antibiotics. Splints may be required to promote healing when the skin over a joint is burned. The child may be on bed rest for several days following an autograft to protect the graft until it has a vascular supply. Donor sites are treated as separate wounds.

Provide Emotional Support

Children with burns have received a profound insult to their body and their self-image. Fear and anxiety about disfigurement and scarring are common, especially among adolescents. The shock and pain of the injury cause increased stress, as do the unfamiliar surroundings and presence of health care providers.

An attitude of genuine interest and concern by the nurse is essential. Continuity of care providers is important in developing a trusting relationship with the child and family. Encourage the child and parents to voice concerns, and show understanding and support. Make appropriate referrals to social workers,

NURSING CARE PLAN

The Child with a Major Burn Injury

INTERVENTION	RATIONALE	EXPECTED OUTCOME
1. Nursing Diagnosis: Risk for Infection related to trauma and destruction of skin barrier		
NIC Priority Intervention: *Infection protection:* Prevention and early detection of infection in a patient at risk		**NOC Suggested Outcome:** *Risk control:* Actions to eliminate or reduce actual, personal, and modifiable health threats
Goal: The child will be free of infection during the healing process.		
■ Take vital signs frequently.	■ Increased temperature is an early sign of infection, but it is also a common response to burn injury.	The child either stays free of secondary infection, or has infection diagnosed and treated early.
■ Use standard precautions (gown, gloves, mask) when wounds of a major burn are exposed. Do not allow visitors who have an infectious disease.	■ These precautions reduce the risk of wound contamination.	
■ Clip hair around burns.	■ Hair harbors bacteria and can irritate the wound.	
■ Keep the burn dressing clean and intact.	■ A clean and intact dressing reduces the number of bacteria introduced to the burned site.	
■ Do not place the IV in any burned area.	■ Avoiding the burned area reduces the risk of wound contamination.	
■ Administer oral or IV antibiotics for diagnosed infections as prescribed.	■ Antibiotics administered as prescribed help to clear the infection quickly.	
2. Nursing Diagnosis: Risk for Imbalanced Fluid Volume related to loss of fluids through wounds and to subsequent excess fluid intake		
NIC Priority Intervention: *Fluid management:* Promotion of fluid balance and prevention of complications resulting from abnormal or undesired fluid levels		**NOC Suggested Outcome:** *Fluid balance:* Balance of water in the intracellular and extracellular compartments of the body
Goal: The child will maintain adequate urine output.		
■ Monitor vital signs, central venous pressure, capillary refill time, and pulses.	■ The child is initially at risk for hypovolemic shock and needs fluid resuscitation (see Chapter 21 ∞).	The child maintains normal urine output, and burn site edema is not excessive.
■ Administer IV and oral fluids as ordered.	■ Careful calculation of fluid needs and ensuring proper intake helps keep the child properly hydrated.	
■ Monitor intake and output.	■ The child is at risk for fluid overload during hydration, and for edema in the burned tissues.	
■ Weigh the child daily using the same scale and amount of clothing.	■ Significant weight loss or gain can help determine fluid imbalances.	
■ Insert a urinary catheter if prescribed.	■ A catheter helps maintain accurate output measurement during the critical care stage.	
■ Monitor for hyponatremia and hypercalcemia (see Chapter 18 ∞).	■ Sodium is lost with burn fluid and potassium is lost from damaged cells, causing electrolyte imbalances.	

NURSING CARE PLAN

The Child with a Major Burn Injury (continued)

INTERVENTION	RATIONALE	EXPECTED OUTCOME
3. Nursing Diagnosis: Impaired Physical Mobility related to joint stiffness due to burns		
NIC Priority Intervention: *Exercise therapy, joint mobility:* Use of active or passive body movement to maintain or restore joint flexibility		**NOC Suggested Outcome:** *Joint movement (active):* Range of motion of joints with self-initiated movement
Goal: The child will maintain maximum range of motion.		
■ Arrange physical and occupational therapy twice daily for stretching and range of motion exercises. Splint as ordered.	■ Positioning in alignment and range of motion exercises help to prevent contractures.	The child maintains maximum range of motion without contractures.
■ Encourage activities to promote range of motion (toss a bean bag, mimic animal movements).	■ Fun activities help the child with diversion and provide movement.	
4. Nursing Diagnosis: Imbalanced Nutrition: Less than Body Requirements related to high metabolic needs		
NIC Priority Intervention: *Nutrition management:* Assistance with or provision of balanced dietary intake of foods and fluids		**NOC Suggested Outcome:** *Nutritional status:* Extent to which nutrients are available to meet metabolic needs
Goal: The child will maintain weight and demonstrate adequate serum albumin and hydration.		
■ Provide an opportunity to choose meals. Offer a variety of high-protein and high-calorie foods. Provide snacks.	■ A variety of food encourages intake. General malaise and anorexia lead to poor healing.	The child maintains weight, adequate hydration, and normal serum albumin.
■ Encourage the child to have meals with other children.	■ Socialization improves intake.	
■ Provide a multivitamin supplement.	■ Vitamin C aids zinc absorption; zinc aids in healing.	
■ Provide enteral feedings as needed.	■ A child with a burn greater than 10% of BSA needs assistance to meet nutrition requirements.	
■ Weigh the child daily.	■ Daily weight checks provide an objective evaluation.	

chaplains, and child-life specialists to ensure that the child and family receive necessary services.

Therapeutic play is encouraged for children, even if they can only observe initially. It serves several purposes for the child with a major burn:

- It provides an outlet for frustration, independence, and creativity.
- It promotes activities that challenge range of motion.
- It normalizes the child's daily routine.
- It encourages the child, who sees the progress other children make day by day.

Families are at risk for emotional stress. The family needs information and frequent updates. This promotes trust between the family and the health care team. Warn them to expect edema and changes in the child's body with the injury response. Parents often feel guilty and responsible for the child's injury. Help parents focus on recovery rather than past actions. Fear usually re-

sults from lack of knowledge about the severity of the burn and the child's status, especially in the early stages of burn care and admission to the intensive care unit. Involve parents in their child's care, learning how to change dressings, assessing for infection and dehydration, and performing range of motion exercises to aid in the child's recovery.

Research *Burns and Stress*

A study of 52 children between 12 and 48 months of age admitted to a burn hospital evaluated for evidence of an acute stress response within 1 month of the burn injury. An acute stress response was found in 29% of the children. These children had symptoms that included reliving the injury, hyperarousal, and appearing detached or emotionally numb. Risk factors associated with the child's acute stress response included size of the burn, pulse rate, pain, and parents' stress symptoms. The child's pain was related to the parents' acute stress response (Stoddard, Saxe, Ronfeldt, et al., 2006).

Prevent Complications

The health care team works to prevent complications such as infection, sepsis, pneumonia, and renal failure, as well as possible irreversible loss of function of the burned area. Standard precautions are often used to reduce the child's risk for infection, and identified infections need to be treated early to reduce the risk for sepsis or pneumonia.

Significant scarring may occur regardless of autografting. Contractures and loss of function are also possible.

Discharge Planning and Home Care Teaching

Identify and address home care needs well in advance of discharge. Discharge planning may include instructing parents in nutrition and diet needs, safety in the home, protection of the burned surface, signs of infection and actions to take, use of pressure garments, and range of motion exercises to prevent contractures.

Provide support and encouragement to parents as they learn how to care for the child with burns. Many burn centers use silver-embedded burn dressings to reduce the frequency of dressing changes needed, and perform the dressing changes in a clinic setting or sedation suite because parents find it so difficult to change the dressings knowing that they will inflict pain on their child. If parents do choose to perform dressing changes, provide pain medication and guidelines for how far in advance of the dressing change the medication should be given. Specific guidelines for dressing changes should be outlined so that parents and health care team members have the same focus. Parents should first observe care being performed and then provide repeat demonstrations until competent.

Care in the Community

Care of the child with a burn requires long-term therapy and rehabilitation. Long-term care commonly occurs in the home, with frequent visits to health care professionals. Children with extensive burns or with burns in locations where scarring may limit function must often wear a pressure (e.g., Jobst) garment for months, and sometimes a face mask if the face was burned (see Figure 31–21A). The garment is removed only for bathing and laundry of the garment. The pressure garment may present a threat to the child's body image, but it is an important way to decrease scarring. Help families understand the need for the special garment and masks and how to clean and care for them.

Clinical Tip

Moisturizing creams can be used after healing to relieve residual drying. The healed skin is very sensitive to sunburn, so cover the area or use a sunscreen. Sunscreen also helps prevent hyperpigmentation after burn healing.

Continued physical therapy and occupational therapy are often needed to increase strength and dexterity in performing self-care skills and to prevent contractures. Emphasis is placed on returning to normal activities of daily living as soon as possible, such as returning to school. Some children have home tutors or computer connections to school for a time to ensure opportunities for learning while decreasing their risk of exposure to infection.

School reentry is often a traumatic experience, especially for older children and adolescents, because of the fear of rejection, decreased self-esteem, and impaired body image. The child's primary nurse, social worker, and child-life specialist may visit the school of a child with a burn injury before the child returns to school—bringing photographs of the child, pressure garments, or other items—to inform classmates and allow them to explore their feelings about the child's burn injury. Some communities may offer support groups for families and children with burn injuries. Referral to these groups may be beneficial.

A major role of nurses in the community is prevention. Provide burn prevention information to parents at each health promotion visit. Become involved with a Safe Kids coalition or with local firefighters to help educate families and caregivers about ways to prevent scald burns and house fires. Examples of prevention messages include the following:

- Maintain appropriate temperature settings for hot water heaters.
- Keep the handles of pots on the stove turned toward the wall and dishes with hot liquids out of the toddler's reach.
- Keep infants and toddlers off the lap when drinking hot beverages or eating soup.
- Keep matches, lighters, and flammable materials away from children.
- Install smoke detectors and replace the batteries annually.

Management of Minor Burns

Many children with minor burns are cared for at home after an initial visit to the emergency department or urgent care clinic. Discuss home remedies for minor burn care. (See Families Want to Know: Caring for Minor Burns.) For superficial burns covering a small area, use moist soaks to stop the burning process and to relieve pain. Any open blisters are debrided, and a thin layer of an antibiotic medication (e.g., silver sulfadiazine) is spread over the burn. Do not place this medication close to the eyes or mouth. Bacitracin is often used for burns on the face. The burn is then covered with one or two layers of gauze. Acetaminophen with codeine may be prescribed for burn dressing changes at home. Burn dressings should be changed twice daily. This involves cleaning the burn and reapplying antibiotic cream.

Educate the parents about increasing the child's fluid intake to compensate for loss of fluid through damaged skin. A high-calorie, high-protein diet is necessary to meet the increased nutritional requirements of healing. Infection is a common complication. Educate the parents to observe for signs of infection (inflammation extending under the dressing, bad odor, excessive exudates, and fever), and notify the physician immediately if noticed. The child should be seen within 48 hours of initial treatment to monitor progress. Reinforce to parents the importance of follow-up appointments.

Sunburn

Sunburn is a burn injury to the outer layer of skin caused by excess sun exposure, or sun exposure after taking phototoxic drugs (e.g., acne medication, sulfonamides, tetracycline, non-

- Place the burn under cool, running water to stop the burning process and to help reduce pain. Do not use ice as it can cause more damage to the injured skin.
- Do not use butter or margarine on the burn as it may introduce bacteria into the wound.
- Remove all clothing and jewelry from the burned area.
- Topical application of the gel from the leaf of an aloe vera plant may help promote healing (National Center for Complementary and Alternative Medicine, 2008a).
- Apply a topical antibiotic such as bacitracin to the burned area on the face.

steroidal anti-inflammatory drugs, and birth control pills). Young children have less melanin to protect their skin against harmful ultraviolet rays. More than half of a person's lifetime sun exposure occurs before 20 years of age (Land & Small, 2008). Much of this sun exposure occurs between peak sun hours of 10 a.m. and 3 p.m.

Erythema, pain, skin tenderness, swelling, blistering, and itching usually develop 3 to 5 hours after exposure to ultraviolet (UV) B rays. UVA rays cause deeper skin damage (Bell, 2008). Increased vasodilation and vascular permeability result in the extravasation of fluid to the tissues and white blood cell migration to the damaged skin. The erythema peaks in 12 to 24 hours and subsides after 72 hours. Systemic complaints include malaise, insomnia (because of skin tenderness), fatigue, headaches, and chilling (because of rapid heat loss).

Treatment is generally supportive. Pain can be relieved by cool water compresses, ice packs, local anesthetic sprays or creams, and emollients. Extra fluids should be provided. Some health care providers prescribe low-potency topical corticosteroids for unblistered skin and NSAIDs for pain relief and to reduce inflammation (Land & Small, 2008).

Nursing Management

Educate parents and children about preventing sunburn. (See Families Want to Know: Preventing Sunburn.) Advise them that repeated blistering sunburns may lead to permanent skin damage, skin cancer, cataracts, and premature aging of the skin.

Hypothermia

Hypothermia is a condition in which the core body temperature falls below 35°C (95°F). This occurs when the heat loss exceeds what the body can produce. Hypothermia is a life-threatening emergency that can occur in any season and any geographic location. Infants and young children are at risk because of immature temperature regulatory mechanisms, thinner skin, limited subcutaneous fat, and high skin surface area to body mass ratio. Adolescent risk is increased by behaviors such as drug and alcohol use or engaging in outdoor activities without proper equipment or clothing.

Primary hypothermia results from environmental exposure, and heat is lost through radiation, conduction, convection, and evaporation. Shivering, an initial response, is the body's attempt to rewarm the blood before it returns to the body's core. As the core body temperature falls, the body tries to conserve the core temperature, using vasoconstriction to shunt blood to the body core for rewarming. Increased muscle tone and an increased metabolic rate occur. Hypothermia leads to increased blood viscosity, slows blood through the capillaries, and facilitates blood coagulation.

Symptoms of mild hypothermia (32° to 35°C [90° to 95°F]) include fatigue, slurred speech, poor coordination, confusion and poor judgment, inappropriate behavior, shivering, tachycardia, and tachypnea. Symptoms of moderate hypothermia include depressed respirations, slow pulse, low blood pressure, pale or cyanotic color, shivering, and dilated pupils. Lethargy, mental impairment, irrational thinking, hallucinations, and coma develop as the central nervous system becomes depressed. Profound hypothermia (below 28°C [84°F]) is characterized by apnea, no shivering, low blood pressure, ventricular fibrillation, dilated and unresponsive pupils, and coma.

Clinical therapy focuses on resuscitation, if necessary, and gradual core body rewarming. The child who has profound hypothermia should receive cardiopulmonary resuscitation until the body temperature returns to normal because the hypothermia may have preserved vital organs. Aggressive techniques for rewarming in moderate to profound cases may include humidified, warm oxygen, warmed intravenous fluids, and warm packs to the core circulation areas (axillae, groin, and neck). Peritoneal lavage and dialysis may be used in some cases of profound hypothermia. Hypoglycemia is a common complication and is treated with IV glucose. For mild hypothermia, rewarming techniques include external heat lamps, immersion in warm water, and an electric blanket.

Nursing Management

Monitor vital signs and urine output during active rewarming and assess for cold-related injuries. See the following section on frostbite.

Prevention is a primary nursing goal. Educate parents to layer children's clothing in cold climates, recognize signs of hypothermia, and decrease time of cold exposure. Teach parents how to treat mild hypothermia. Teach school-age children and adolescents who go on camping and hunting trips how to recognize and manage hypothermia in themselves and others. Teach preventive techniques such as to avoid riding snowmobiles or walking on ice that is not known to be thick enough to support the weight.

If a child becomes hypothermic during an outing such as a camping trip, a warm person should get into a sleeping bag (or under the blankets) next to the child after any wet or heavy clothing is removed. This action will warm the child and prevent further heat loss. First aid for hypothermia includes moving the child to a dry area and removing any wet clothing. Replace with warm, dry clothing, and encourage the child to drink a warm, high-calorie liquid, if able.

Frostbite

Frostbite is a cold injury that results from overexposure of the skin cells to temperatures low enough to cause crystal formation. Frostbite develops in tissues exposed to temperatures below freezing for more than an hour when environmental protection is inadequate. Areas of the body at high risk for frostbite include the hands, feet, cheeks, nose, and ears.

With cold exposure, the skin initially responds with vasoconstriction and vasodilation. As ice crystals develop in the extracellular fluid, water moves out and dehydrates the cells. As the cold injury progresses, circulation to the area is impaired, and cell death results from ischemia. Vascular stasis leads to thrombosis. In severe cases, gangrene may develop (Nicol & Huether, 2010a).

Clinical manifestations depend on the severity and depth of the cellular damage after rewarming (Nicol & Huether, 2010a).

- **Superficial skin affected.** Numb, central white area surrounded by redness and edema, no blistering.
- **Full-thickness skin affected.** Erythema, vesicle formation with clear or pink fluid, surrounded by edema and redness.
- **Full-thickness and subcutaneous skin affected.** Local edema, grayish blue color, hemorrhagic vesicles, tissue necrosis.
- **Deeper cold injury.** Deep cyanosis, no vesicles or local edema, necrosis of subcutaneous tissue or lower, possibly involving the muscles or tendons. Gangrene develops.

With superficial injury, the skin appears pale and is numb. Rapid rewarming causes a flush and the sensation of tingling, burning, or prickling in the affected area. With deeper injury, the skin may appear mottled and cyanotic followed by erythema, swelling, and burning pain with rewarming. Vesicles and bullae develop in 24 to 48 hours that slowly heal. The extent of injury usually is not initially apparent.

If frostbite is suspected, get the child to a warmer environment for rewarming. Because the frostbitten area is numb, extreme caution is needed to protect it from any trauma. Do not rub or massage the area. Slowly rewarm the affected area to decrease the chance of cellular damage. Immerse the affected part in water warmed to 40° to 42°C (104° to 107.6°F) until it is thawed. Analgesics are needed because thawing causes significant pain. The affected skin is gently cleaned with saline during healing and covered loosely with sterile dressings. Wound care may be similar to that provided to a child with burns. Amputation may be needed when circulation is not restored.

Nursing Management

As with hypothermia, the prevention is a nursing goal. Teach parents to layer the children's clothing for warmth and to pack extra blankets and clothing if cold temperatures are expected during outdoor activities. Hats covering the ears should be worn. Teach adolescents how to avoid frostbite during hunting and other cold weather expeditions. Wet clothing should be changed quickly.

Early care is instrumental in minimizing permanent injury. Severe frostbite requires hospitalization, fluid management, dressing changes, and careful attention to diet. Provide emo-

Nursing Alert

Frostbite can occur if a chemical cold pack (found in many first aid kits) is left in contact with the skin for too long. When a chemical cold pack is used, cover it with a few layers of clothing or a towel and monitor the skin under the pack frequently. Remove the chemical cold pack if the skin starts to looks white or has decreased sensation. Remove the cold pack periodically to allow the skin to rewarm.

tional support to the child and family while they wait to learn the full extent of the injury and disability.

Animal Bites

Approximately 42% (150,000) of nonfatal dog bites that are treated in emergency departments each year in the United States occur among children under 14 years of age. The injury rates are highest among boys 5 to 9 years of age (Howell & Powell, 2007). In many cases the child knows the dog, and most bites happen in the home or a familiar place. Bites are often associated with the child's inappropriate behavior, such as teasing, rough play, or interfering with feeding or the care of puppies. Other animals that may bite include cats, birds, turtles, and wild animals such as bats, squirrels, and raccoons.

Assessment includes noting the location and number of puncture wounds, abrasions, lacerations, and crushing injuries; redness or swelling at entry sites; redness extending out from the site (possible cellulitis); and any drainage related to the bite. Examination for damage to nerves, muscles, tendons, and blood vessels is also performed. Dog bites tend to be crush injuries and gashes, rather than clean, sharp lacerations. Cat bites tend to be puncture wounds. Radiographic films are needed for bites to the head and neck or any bites that may have penetrated bone to identify additional injuries.

To decrease infection, initial treatment involves wound irrigation, removal of devitalized tissue, and a clean dressing. Sedation and pain management may be needed for some children. Small wounds may be closed with adhesive strips rather than suturing because of the potential for infection. Severe bites sometimes require surgical closure or reconstruction. Wounds over joints should be immobilized and elevated. Cat bites often result in puncture wounds, 50% of which become infected (American Academy of Pediatrics, 2009, p. 187). Puncture wounds should not be irrigated or sutured. Cat bites can result in septic arthritis and osteomyelitis if a bone or joint is punctured. Antibiotics are prescribed for many injuries.

Dog bites should be reported, and the dog should be confined and observed for 10 days for signs of rabies. Cat bites are also dangerous because cats less often have rabies immunization. If the animal develops rabies during that interval, human rabies immune globulin (HRIG) is administered immediately, followed by a rabies vaccine injection on days 3, 7, 14, and 28 following the first injection. No delay in administering rabies vaccine occurs when the child is bitten by a wild animal in which rabies cannot be excluded. (See Chapter 16 ∞ for rabies information.)

Nursing Management

If a child is bitten by an animal, take a complete and accurate history that includes the following information: extent of the injury, circumstances surrounding the attack, present location of the animal, and attempts to assess the animal's health.

Wound care is important. To decrease infection in nonpuncture wounds, high-pressure wound irrigation with large quantities of sterile saline or lactated Ringer's solution is performed rather than scrubbing. One method of high-pressure irrigation involves the use of an 18-gauge needle attached to a 60-cc syringe filled with saline. Apply a clean dressing and elevate the affected body part to reduce bleeding. Check the child's immunization record to determine whether a tetanus booster is necessary. Debridement of puncture wounds may be performed in the operating room.

As children with bites are often cared for at home, teach the parents about the normal healing process, proper wound care, and the signs and symptoms of infection that indicate a need to return for care.

Educate parents about preventing animal and human bites and the importance of teaching children appropriate behavior around other children and animals. Parents and children need to understand that any dog may bite at any time. See Families Want to Know: Preventing Animal Bites.

Human Bites

Human bites are more common than most people realize. They may occur among toddlers and young children, and adolescents also receive human bites in association with an altercation. Because the mouth harbors many bacteria, infection is fairly

Families Want to Know
Preventing Animal Bites

- Never leave a young child alone with an animal.
- Do not buy or adopt a pet unless you are confident of your child's ability to respect it.
- Spay or neuter the pet to reduce aggression.
- Teach children the following rules:
  - Avoid all unfamiliar animals and report them to a parent.
  - Avoid contact with all wild animals.
  - Do not touch an animal when it is eating, sleeping, or nursing puppies.
  - Do not try to separate fighting dogs.
  - Never overexcite an animal, even in play. Do not roughhouse or play games that stimulate aggressive behavior. Do not tease or throw objects at an animal.
  - Never put your face close to an animal. Seek permission before hugging or petting an animal.
  - If approached by a dog, stay calm, stand still, talk softly, and back away slowly until the dog loses interest; don't run or scream.
  - If attacked, stand still like a tree. If knocked down, curl into a ball and protect the face and neck.
- If an animal (wild or unknown) is sick or acting strangely, notify the health department.

common. Assess the risk for hepatitis B and HIV infection. Antibiotics may be prescribed to prevent systemic complications. Initial treatment includes irrigation with sterile saline and debridement. Instruct parents about how to care for the wound. Follow-up is important to watch for infection. When human bites occur in a childcare or school setting, inform parents about the bite so they can discuss potential risks and follow-up care with a health care provider.

Insect Bites and Stings

Insect bites and stings occur frequently in children and usually are not a cause for concern. Exceptions include bites or stings by insects that carry parasites or communicable diseases (ticks, mosquitoes), those of venomous insects (spiders), and those that produce an allergic reaction. Up to 3% of the population is sensitized to bee stings and has a generalized response to stings, but the rate is much lower in children (Järvinen, 2009). (For a discussion of communicable diseases carried by ticks and mosquitoes, e.g., Lyme disease and Rocky Mountain spotted fever, see Chapter 16 ∞.)

See the Clinical Manifestations: Insect Bites and Stings table for signs of bites and stings and their treatment.

Nursing Management

The goal of nursing care is prevention. Become familiar with the harmful insects in your area, so you can identify them and recognize their effects. Teach children to avoid spiders and other biting or stinging insects. Many commercial repellents are available. Most products contain DEET (diethyltoluamide), picaridin, or oil of lemon eucalyptus and are effective against many insects including mosquitoes, fleas, ticks, and chiggers. However, DEET does not repel stinging insects. The repellent should be reapplied if washed off by sweating or getting wet. Wash DEET off the skin with soap and water once the child is back indoors. Caution parents to avoid overuse of products containing DEET, especially with infants and small children. Do not apply to young children's hands, as they may rub it into the eyes and mouth.

Warn parents against using heavily perfumed shampoos, powders, soaps, or lotions, or dressing children in bright clothing when outdoors, as these may attract insects. Teach children to stay calm when a bee or wasp approaches and to slowly walk away without swatting. Avoid eating sweet foods and beverages outdoors as these will attract bees and wasps. Pour beverages into a cup or use a straw rather than drinking directly from a can to prevent stings to the mouth and lips by unseen bees.

Household pets may be a source of fleas or ticks. Use preventive treatments against fleas and ticks if pets are allowed prolonged contact with children.

When a known allergy to *Hymenoptera* (bees or wasps) has occurred, the child should wear a medical alert identification and carry an emergency kit with epinephrine (EpiPen). Teach parents and school personnel how to administer the EpiPen, and then to call 911 for emergency care and transport.

Snake Bites

Venomous snakes are found in most areas of the United States. During warm months, snakes are active and likely to bite if disturbed. Fortunately, many bites are dry, delivering no venom. Attempts to identify the snake causing the bite should be made to determine if it is venomous.

Rattlesnake, copperhead, and cottonmouth venom is composed of proteolytic enzymes, glycoproteins, and vasoactive substances that cause local and systemic symptoms. Coral snake venom causes neuromuscular paralysis (Holve, 2009). The amount and toxicity of the venom injected has an impact on the consequences of the snakebite. Because children usually receive a higher amount of venom relative to body mass, their response may be greater than an adult's.

Puncture marks, white wheal, and burning sensation appear at the site of the bite. Pain, erythema, bruising, and edema rapidly develop and extend from the site for up to 24 hours. The swelling may progress without treatment to involve the entire extremity. Swelling may put the child at risk for compartment syndrome. Systemic signs include dizziness, tachycardia, nausea, vomiting, diarrhea, diaphoresis, chills, and muscle fasciculation. Signs of a severe response may include hypotension, altered consciousness, bleeding from multiple sites (disseminated intravascular coagulation), pulmonary edema, and renal failure.

Clinical therapy involves immobilization of the extremity and a cold compress to slow the spread of the venom. Laboratory studies include complete blood count, platelet count, coagulation studies, electrolytes, and renal function. The Poison Control Cen-

Clinical Manifestations

Insect Bites and Stings

Type	Clinical Manifestations	Clinical Therapy
Mosquitoes and Fleas Local inflammation results from sensitization to mosquito salivary proteins. 	Local reactions: ■ Discrete, red papules and edema at the bite site with itching; minimal discomfort. ■ Pruritic wheals and bullae tend to develop with repeat exposure. Rare systemic reactions with generalized urticaria, angioedema, nausea, vomiting, wheezing, and other signs of anaphylaxis.	■ Apply cold compresses or ice to the site. ■ Antihistamine medication may be given. ■ Systemic reactions need emergency medical treatment.

Clinical Manifestations
Insect Bites and Stings (continued)

Type	Clinical Manifestations	Clinical Therapy
Bee or Wasp Sting Hymenoptera Venoms contain enzymes that affect vascular tone and permeability.	Local reactions: ■ Mild, local pain. ■ Erythema and edema. Systemic reactions: • Cutaneous—generalized urticaria, flushing, angioedema, pruritus. • Respiratory—wheezing, throat tightening, dysphagia, hoarseness, cough. • Circulatory—dizziness, hypotension, loss of consciousness. • Gastrointestinal—abdominal pain, vomiting, diarrhea.	■ Remove stinger as soon as possible. ■ Use ice or cold compresses and elevate extremity. ■ Massage a dash of meat tenderizer (papain powder) and a drop of water into the skin for 5 minutes to relieve the pain. ■ Antihistamine medication may be given. ■ Treat systemic reactions with glucocorticoids and antihistamines or epinephrine. ■ Carry epinephrine auto-injector. ■ Venom immunotherapy is given for systemic reactions.
Fire Ants Venom is hemolytic and neurotoxic, causing a histamine-like response.	Local reactions: ■ A black center at the point of the bite, or a trail of lesions across the skin. ■ Initial wheal becomes a vesicle in a few hours; in 24 hours, the fluid is cloudy, and the vesicle has a red halo. ■ Pruritus, erythema, edema, induration. ■ Systemic and anaphylactic reactions can occur.	■ Apply ice or cold compresses. ■ Antihistamine medication may be given. ■ Elevate extremity. ■ Provide same therapy for systemic reactions as for bee stings.
Black Widow Spider Venom is neurotoxic.	■ Stinging sensation at time of bite. ■ Localized edema and erythema, two fang marks, dull crampy ache around site, petechiae branching from site. ■ Systemic reaction in 1–3 hours, symptoms peak in 3–12 hours, diminish in 72 hours. ■ Muscle rigidity of chest and/or abdomen. ■ Severe muscle cramping, sweating, nausea, vomiting, restlessness. ■ Hypertension and arrhythmias. ■ Oliguria.	■ Apply ice. ■ Benzodiazepine medication may be prescribed for muscle spasms. ■ Opioids may be prescribed for pain management. ■ Antihistamine medication may be given. ■ Hydrocortisone may decrease the inflammatory response. ■ Antivenom IV is used in severe reactions after a negative skin test for hypersensitivity to horse serum.
Brown Recluse Spider Venom contains proteolytic enzymes and sphingomyelinase D, a cytotoxic factor.	■ Within 2 hours, sinking blue macule with a halo of inflammation at bite site, pain. ■ Systemic symptoms include fever, chills, nausea and vomiting, and hemolysis. ■ A hemorrhagic blister forms in 1 to 2 days with a necrotic ulcer seen when it breaks. Most ulcers are 1 to 2 cm in diameter, but some progress to 15 cm in diameter with full-thickness injury.	■ Apply ice or cold compresses. ■ Cleanse the wound and provide good wound care. ■ Analgesics are given for pain management. ■ Oral anti-inflammatory agent may be prescribed. ■ Antibiotics are given for secondary infection. ■ Excision and skin grafting are performed in cases of severe necrosis.

Data from: Järvinen, K. M. (2009). Allergic reactions to stinging and biting insects and arachnids. Pediatric Annals, 38(4), 199–209; Holve, S. (2009). Venomous spiders, snakes, and scorpions in the United States. Pediatric Annals, 38(4), 210–217.

ter is contacted to obtain treatment guidelines. Specific antivenom is usually administered within 4 to 6 hours. CroFab, a newer antivenom used for cottonmouth, copperhead, and rattlesnake bites, is available and has a lower rate of severe hypersensitivity reactions than antivenoms made from horse serum (Holve, 2009). Children at risk for a severe hypersensitivity reaction are pretreated with IV antihistamines and corticosteroids (Holve, 2009). The use of NSAIDs is avoided because of coagulopathies (Reuter-Rice, 2008). Acetaminophen and codeine may be prescribed for pain management. The child's immunization record is reviewed to determine if a tetanus toxoid booster is needed. Antibiotics are not administered unless an infection develops.

Nursing Management

Nursing care involves assessing the child for initial and progressive signs of the venom's effect. Monitor the child's vital signs and the distal extremity's neurovascular status. Measure the circumference of the affected extremity for future comparison. Clean the wound with germicidal soap and water. Keep the child quiet and calm to slow the circulation. Help the child identify the snake from pictures of snakes common to the area; however, keep in mind that other venomous snakes may be kept as exotic pets.

The antivenom is diluted in saline and slowly administered intravenously as ordered. Help locate additional antivenom if the hospital does not have an adequate supply. Monitor the child for progressive signs of venom effect, and for antivenom hypersensitivity. Provide skin care for the swollen and tense skin to prevent abrasions and to prevent additional injury. Monitor the site for necrosis and secondary infection. Provide emotional support to the child and family.

As children with bites are often cared for at home, teach the parents about the normal healing process, proper wound care, and the signs and symptoms of infection. Teach children and their family to avoid future snakebites. When in areas where snakes may live, the child should wear protective clothing such as leather boots, avoid reaching into areas where snakes may hide, and avoid any actions that may provoke a snake.

Contusions

Contusions are soft-tissue injuries that have a variety of causes. Often it is difficult to assess whether an injury has caused underlying tissue damage. An injury does not have to break the skin to result in internal damage. Radiographic examination may be necessary to rule out broken bones or further tissue damage. Signs and symptoms that indicate a need for treatment include swelling that does not subside within 72 hours, intense pain, inability to move the injured part, and infection.

Elevate the injured extremity and apply ice as soon as possible after injury. This can reduce inflammation and swelling in the area.

Foreign Bodies

Many skin injuries result from penetration of foreign particles. Common substances include gravel from abrasions, bee stingers, and splinters. Treatment of superficial foreign bodies involves irrigating the wound to try to forcibly dislodge the debris. A deeply embedded foreign body is best removed under medical supervision to avoid permanent injury or scarring.

Lacerations

Lacerations are caused by cuts or tears to the skin. In many cases, the cut is minor and can be managed at home with gentle cleansing, antibiotic ointment, and a bandage. More extensive lacerations and those on the face or over joints often need closing to promote healing and reduce scarring. Laceration repair is performed after wound cleansing and appropriate local analgesia to control pain. Sutures or dermal adhesive may be used. Sutures are usually removed about 7 days later.

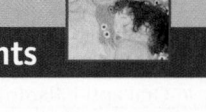

Chapter Highlights

- Functions of the skin include perception of pain, heat, and cold; protective barrier against microorganisms, ultraviolet radiation, and loss of body fluids; temperature regulation; vitamin D synthesis; and excretion.
- Wound healing has three overlapping phases: inflammation, proliferation (reconstruction), and remodeling (maturation).
- Contact dermatitis is a skin inflammation that occurs following direct contact with an allergen, causing an immune response, or with an irritant, resulting in no immune response.
- Superabsorbent disposable diapers reduce the frequency and severity of diaper dermatitis because, when wet, a gel forms inside the diaper keeping moisture away from the skin.

- Seborrheic dermatitis is an inflammatory skin condition due to an overgrowth of *Malassezia furfur* yeast in areas of sebaceous gland activity. Lesions are commonly found on the scalp, forehead, and postauricular and periorbital areas.
- The classic impetigo lesion begins as a vesicle surrounded by edema and redness. The vesicle fluid turns cloudy and ruptures, leaving a honey-colored crust on an ulcerated base.
- Folliculitis, a superficial inflammation of the pilosebaceous follicle, may be associated with *Pseudomonas* exposure in a poorly chlorinated pool or hot tub.

- Children with cellulitis appear ill with fever, chills, malaise, and enlarged lymph nodes. The infected site is red or lilac in color, warm, edematous, and tender with an indistinct border.
- Viral skin infections include molluscum contagiosum and warts (papillomavirus).
- Oral thrush (candidiasis) is characterized by white patches that resemble coagulated milk on the oral mucosa and may bleed when removed.
- Children being treated for tinea capitis may develop an "id" hypersensitivity reaction rash to the fungal antigen, and this is not an allergic reaction to the medication.
- Drug reactions vary in severity from a simple allergic reaction and erythema multiforme minor to potential life-threatening conditions such as erythema multiforme major (Stevens-Johnson syndrome and toxic epidermal necrolysis).
- Treatment of atopic eczema involves hydration and lubrication of the skin by bathing followed by emollients to trap in skin moisture. Topical corticosteroids are used to treat skin flares and then discontinued.
- Acne medications, tretinoin or isotretinoin, are phototoxic, resulting in sunburn with even minimal exposure. Protection with sunscreen or protective clothing is important to prevent significant sunburn.
- Psoriasis is a chronic skin condition with pruritic, thick, silvery, scaly erythematous plaques having irregular borders surrounded by normal skin.
- Treatment for lice includes a pediculicide applied to the hair, and combing the hair with a fine-toothed comb to remove all the nits. A second treatment is needed in 7 days.
- Scabies is a mite infestation in which the female mite burrows under the skin to lay eggs which causes irritation and intense itching.
- Hemangiomas undergo a period of rapid growth during infancy before involuting. The rapid growth may cause significant complications, such as pressure on the airway, eye, or ear canal.

- Children at greatest risk for pressure ulcers are those with limited mobility, sensory deficits, or the inability to change positions. Tissue ischemia occurs when the soft tissues and capillary beds are compressed between a bony prominence and another surface.
- Of the four main types of burns (thermal, chemical, electrical, and radioactive), thermal burns are most common in children. Infants, toddlers, and preschool-age children most commonly suffer scald burns. Other types of thermal burns include flames and contact with a hot object.
- Initial treatment for a child with a significant burn injury includes emergency assessment of the airway, breathing, and circulation; and stopping the burning process by removing jewelry and clothing, and applying moist soaks or ice.
- More than half of a person's lifetime exposure to the sun occurs before 20 years of age. Repeated blistering sunburns during childhood increase the risk for development of melanoma.
- Children are at greater risk for hypothermia because of their thinner skin, limited subcutaneous fat, and high surface area to body mass ratio. Body heat is lost more quickly in water or when clothing is wet.
- Frostbite occurs when ice crystallizes in the tissues, causing cellular dehydration and ischemic damage.
- Children at highest risk for dog bites are those 5 to 9 years old. Most children know the dog that bites them.
- Insects and spiders with venomous bites include bees, fire ants, black widow spiders, and brown recluse spiders.
- Venomous snakes living in the wild in the United States include rattlesnakes, copperheads, water moccasins, and coral snakes. Initial treatment includes immobilization of the extremity and cold compresses to slow the spread of the venom.

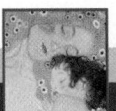

Clinical Reasoning in Action

Recall Joshua, 6 years old, who was admitted to and discharged from the hospital with a deep partial-thickness burn caused by flames associated with playing with matches. He is making his second visit to the burn clinic for a burn dressing change 5 days after discharge. Because no debridement is expected on this visit, he will not go to the sedation suite. Joshua is given pain medication in the burn clinic to help cover the discomfort of the burn dressing change. He is anxious about the dressing change and worries that it will hurt.

Finding activities to keep Joshua occupied is already becoming a challenge to his mother. She is concerned about how to keep Joshua occupied now that he is feeling better. She and Joshua's father are worried about how they will prevent future injuries since Joshua is so energetic and curious. Joshua's mother has had no difficulty identifying high-calorie foods for

him to eat, but she is not sure if Joshua is getting enough extra protein to promote the wound healing.

1. What signs of wound infection must you observe for?
2. What nursing support may help the child deal with a painful and disfiguring injury? What are some developmentally appropriate complementary therapies for pain management that can be used during the burn dressing changes?
3. What suggestions can you make to help the family review needed injury prevention strategies to protect Joshua from future injuries?
4. What are some foods or strategies that Joshua's mother can use at home to provide the high-protein and high-calorie diet needed for healing?

See Pearson Nursing Student Resources for possible responses.

Pearson Nursing Student Resources

Find additional review materials at
nursing.pearsonhighered.com
Prepare for success with NCLEX®-style practice questions,
interactive assignments and activities, web links, animations and
videos, and more!

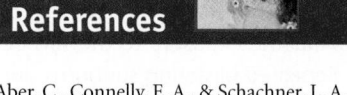

References

Aber, C., Connelly, E. A., & Schachner, L. A. (2007). Fever and rash in a child: When to worry? *Pediatric Annals, 36*(1), 30–38.

Akdis, C. A., Akdis, M., Bieber, T., Bindslev-Jensen, C., Bogunlewicz, M., Eigenmann, P., et al. (2006). Diagnosis and treatment of atopic dermatitis in children and adults: European Academy of Allergology and Clinical Immunology/American Academy of Allergy, Asthma and Immunology/ PRACTALL consensus report. *Journal of Allergy and Clinical Immunology, 118*(1), 152–169.

American Academy of Pediatrics, Committee on Infectious Diseases. (2009). *Red book: Report of the Committee on Infectious Diseases* (28th ed.). Elk Grove Village, IL: Author.

American College of Surgeons, Committee on Trauma. (2006). *Resources for optimal care of the injured patient 2006.* Chicago: Author.

Bell, E. A. (2007). New topical offers a choice in impetigo treatment. *Infectious Diseases in Children, 20*(10), 12.

Bell, E. A. (2008). An update on sunscreen. *Infectious Diseases in Children, 21*(6), 14–15.

Bookout, K. (2008). Wound care product primer for the nurse practitioner: Part I. *Journal of Pediatric Health Care, 22*(1), 60–63.

Burn Foundation. (2010). *Safety facts on scald burns.* Retrieved from http://www.burnfoundation.org/programs/resource.cfm?c=1&a=3

Butler, C. T. (2006). Pediatric skin care: Guidelines for assessment, prevention, and treatment. *Pediatric Nursing, 32*(5), 443–450.

Christinson-Lagay, E. R., & Fishman, S. J. (2006). Vascular anomalies. *Surgical Clinics of North America, 86,* 393–425.

Chosidow, O., Giraudeau, B., Cottrell, J., Izri, A., Hofmann, R., Mann, S. G., & Burgess, I. (2010). Oral ivermectin versus malathion lotion for difficult-to-treat head lice. *New England Journal of Medicine, 362*(10), 896–905.

Connor-Ballard, P. A. (2009). Understanding and managing burn pain: Part 1. *American Journal of Nursing, 109*(4), 48–56.

Diamantis, S. A., Morrell, D. S., & Burkhart, C. N. (2009). Pediatric infestations. *Pediatric Annals, 38*(6), 326–332.

D'Souza, A. L., Nelson, N. G., & McKenzie, L. B. (2009). Pediatric Burn Injuries Treated in US Emergency Departments Between 1990 and 2006. *Pediatrics, 124*(5), 1424–1430.

Duffy, B. J., McLaughlin, P. M., & Eichelberger, M. R. (2006). Assessment, triage, and early management of burns in children. *Pediatric Emergency Medicine, 7,* 82–93.

Findlay, J. (2007). Treating atopic dermatitis. *Contemporary Pediatrics, 24*(6 Suppl.), 4–12.

Forbes, L. R., Saltzman, R. W., & Spergel, J. M. (2009). Food allergies and atopic dermatitis: Differentiating myth from reality. *Pediatric Annals, 38*(2), 84–90.

Gauglitz, G. G., Herndon, D. N., & Jeschke, M. G. (2008). Emergency treatment of severely burned pediatric patients: Current therapeutic strategies. *Pediatric Health, 2*(6), 761–775.

Goates, B. M., Atkin, S. J., Wilding, K. G., Birch, K. G., Cottam, M. R., et al. (2006). An effective nonchemical treatment for head lice: A lot of hot air. *Pediatrics, 118*(5), 1962–1970.

Gonzalez, M. E., Unwala, R., & Connelly, E. A. (2008). A red scaly baby. *Contemporary Pediatrics, 25*(6), 28–33.

Groff, B. M. B., Tromberg, J. S., & Wilson, B. B. (2009). Adolescent acne: Effective therapy for a serious condition. *Consultant for Pediatricians, 8*(6, suppl.), S5–S14.

Haggstrom, A. N., Drolet, B. A., Baselga, E., Chamlin, S. L., Garzon, M. C., Horii, K. A., et al. (2007). Prospective study of infantile hemangiomas: Demographic, prenatal, and perinatal characteristics. *Journal of Pediatrics, 150*(3), 291–294.

Hazinski, M. F., Mondozzi, M. A., & Baker, R. A. U. (2010). Shock, multiple organ dysfunction syndrome, and burns in children. In K. L. McCance, S. E. Huether, V. L. Brashers, & N. S. Rote, *Pathophysiology: The biologic basis for disease in adults and children* (6th ed., pp. 1727–1754). St. Louis, MO: Mosby Elsevier.

Hinckley, J., & Allen, P. J. (2008). Community-associated MRSA in the pediatric primary care setting. *Pediatric Nursing, 34*(1), 64–71.

Holve, S. (2009). Venomous spiders, snakes, and scorpions in the United States. *Pediatric Annals, 38*(4), 210–217.

Horn, P. L., & Beebe, A. C. (2009). Lawn mower injuries in pediatric patients. *Journal of Trauma Nursing, 16*(3), 136–141.

Howell, J. F., & Powell, S. T. (2007). Companion animals and human health risk: Animal bites and rabies. *Topics in Advanced Practice Nursing eJournal, 7*(2).

Huang, J. T., Abrams, M., Tlougan, B., Rademaker, A., & Paller, A. S. (2009). Treatment of *Staphylococcus aureus* colonization in atopic dermatitis decreases disease severity. *Pediatrics, 123*(5), e808–e814.

Järvinen, K. M. (2009). Allergic reactions to stinging and biting insects and arachnids. *Pediatric Annals, 38*(4), 199–209.

Keri, J. E. (2006). Acne: Improving skin and self-esteem. *Pediatric Annals, 35*(3), 174–179.

Krakowski, A. C., Eichenfield, L. F., & Dohil, M. A. (2008). Management of atopic dermatitis in the pediatric population. *Pediatrics, 122*(4), 812–824.

Kumar, J., Kimura, L., & Kamat, R. (2009). Snakebite envenomation. *Consultant for Pediatricians, 8*(9), 340, 343.

Land, V., & Small, L. (2008). The evidence on how to best treat sunburn in children: A common treatment dilemma. *Pediatric Nursing, 34*(4), 343–348.

Leung, A. K. C., Fong, J. H. S., & Pinto-Rojas, A. (2005). Pediculosis capitis. *Journal of Pediatric Health Care, 19*(6), 369–378.

LouseBuster. (2010). Retrieved from http://www.lousebuster.com

Lund, C. H., & Kuller, J. M. (2007). Integumentary system. In C. Kenner & J. W. Lott, *Comprehensive neonatal care: An interdisciplinary approach* (4th ed., 65–91). Philadelphia: Saunders Elsevier.

Mahindra, P., Guillen, C., & Glick, S. A. (2009). A 5-year-old girl with scarring. *Pediatric Annals, 38*(7), 359–364.

Meadows-Oliver, M. (2009). Tinea capitis: Diagnostic criteria and treatment options. *Pediatric Nursing, 35*(1), 53–57.

Merritt, B., Burkhart, C. N., & Morrell, D. S. (2009). Use of isotretinoin for acne vulgaris. *Pediatric Annals, 38*(6), 311–320.

Metry, D. W., Siegel, D. H., Cordisco, M. R., Pope, E., Prendiville, J., Drolet, B. A., et al. (2008). A comparison of disease severity among affected male versus female patients with PHACE syndrome. *Journal of the American Academy of Dermatology, 58*(1), 81–87.

Montoya, C. (2008). Diaper dermatitis: Smart and effective management. *American Journal for Nurse Practitioners, 12*(9), 11–20.

Morelli, J. G. (2007a). Acne. In R. M. Kliegman, R. E. Behrman, H. B. Jensen, & B. F. Stanton (Eds.), *Nelson textbook of pediatrics* (18th ed., 2759–2764). Philadelphia: Elsevier Saunders.

Morelli, J. G. (2007b). Cutaneous bacterial infections. In R. M. Kliegman, R. E. Behrman, H. B. Jensen, & B. F. Stanton (Eds.), *Nelson textbook of pediatrics* (18th ed., 2759–2764). Philadelphia: Elsevier Saunders.

Morelli, J. G. (2007c). Cutaneous viral infections. In R. M. Kliegman, R. E. Behrman, H. B. Jensen, & B. F. Stanton (Eds.), *Nelson textbook of pediatrics* (18th ed., 2751–2754). Philadelphia: Elsevier Saunders.

Morelli, J. G. (2007d). Vesiculobullous disorders. In R. M. Kliegman, R. E. Behrman, H. B. Jensen, & B. F. Stanton (Eds.), *Nelson textbook of pediatrics* (18th ed., 2685–2693). St. Louis, MO: Elsevier Mosby.

Muhrer, J. C. (2009). Melanoma: Current incidence, diagnosis, and preventive strategies. *Journal for Nurse Practitioners, 5*(1), 35–46.

National Center for Complementary and Alternative Medicine. (2008a). *Aloe vera*. Retrieved from http://nccam.nih.gov/health/aloevera/

National Center for Complementary and Alternative Medicine. (2008b). *Herbs at a glance*. Retrieved from http://nccam.nih.gov/health

Nelson, K. C., & Morrell, D. S. (2007). Spreading bumps: Molluscum contagiosum in the pediatric population. *Pediatric Annals, 36*(12), 814–818.

Nestor, M. S. (2007). The use of photodynamic therapy for treatment of acne vulgaris. *Dermatologic Clinics, 25*, 47–57.

Nicol, N. H., & Huether, S. E. (2010a). Structure, function, and disorders of the integument. In K. L. McCance, S. E. Huether, V. L. Brashers, & N. S. Rote, *Pathophysiology: The biologic basis for disease in adults and children* (6th ed., pp. 1644–1679). St. Louis, MO: Mosby Elsevier.

Nicol, N. H., & Huether, S. E. (2010b). Alterations of the integument in children. In K. L. McCance, S. E. Huether, V. L. Brashers, & N. S. Rote, *Pathophysiology: The biologic basis for disease in adults and children* (6th ed., pp. 1680–1694). St. Louis, MO: Mosby Elsevier.

Nijhawan, R. I., Matiz, C., & Jacob, S. E. (2009). Contact dermatitis: From basics to allergodromes. *Pediatric Annals, 38*(2), 99–108.

Noonan, C., Quigley, S., & Curley, M. A. Q. (2006). Skin integrity in hospitalized infants and children: A prevalence survey. *Journal of Pediatric Nursing, 21*(6), 445–453.

O'Connor, N. R., McLaughlin, M. R., & Ham, P. (2008). Newborn skin: Part 1. Common rashes. *American Family Physician, 77*(1), 47–52.

Ong, P. Y., & Boguniewicz, M. (2007). Atopic dermatitis and contact dermatitis in the emergency department. *Clinical Pediatric Emergency Medicine, 8*, 81–86.

Paller, A. S., Siegfried, E. C., Langley, R. G., Gottlieb, A. B., Pariser, D., Landells, I., et al. (2008). Etanercept treatment for children and adolescents with plaque psoriasis. *New England Journal of Medicine, 358*(3), 241–251.

Peterson, J. D., & Chan, L. S. (2006). A comprehensive management guide for atopic dermatitis. *Dermatologic Nursing, 18*(6), 531–542.

Poindexter, G. B., Burkhart, C. N., & Morrell, D. S. (2009). Therapies for pediatric seborrheic dermatitis. *Pediatric Annals, 38*(6), 333–338.

Preston, G. (2008). An overview of topical negative pressure therapy in wound care. *Nursing Standard, 23*(7), 62–66.

Reuter-Rice, K. (2008). Bites that bleed: Crotalid envenomation. *Journal of Pediatric Health Care, 22*(4), 258–261.

Richards, C. A. (2006, April). Treatment tips for common dermatologic problems in ethnic patients. *Infectious Diseases in Children*, 66–67.

Rote, N. S., & Huether, S. E. (2010). Innate immunity: Inflammation. In K. L. McCance, S. E. Huether, V. L. Brashers, & N. S. Rote, *Pathophysiology: The biologic basis for disease in adults and children* (6th ed., pp. 183–216). St. Louis, MO: Elsevier Mosby.

Schlüer, A. B., Cignacco, E., Müller, M., & Halfes, R. J. (2009). The prevalence of pressure ulcers in four paediatric institutions. *Journal of Clinical Nursing, 18*, 3244–3252.

Schuerman, G., & Vezeau, T. (2007). All bugs aren't bad: Probiotics in the treatment of atopic dermatitis. *American Journal for Nurse Practitioners, 11*(4), 28–35.

Shaw, M. G., Burkhart, C. N., & Morrell, D. S. (2009). Systemic therapies for pediatric atopic dermatitis: A review for the primary care physician. *Pediatric Annals, 38*(7), 380–387.

Shy, R. (2007). Tinea corporis and tinea capitis. *Pediatrics in Review, 28*(5), 164–173.

Silverberg, N. B., Silverberg, J. I., & Silverberg, A. I. (2005). Eradicating acne vulgaris of puberty: What makes for optimal therapy? *Contemporary Pediatrics, 22*(10 Suppl.), 12–22.

Stier, M. F., Glick, S. A., & Hirsch, R. J. (2008). Laser treatment of pediatric vascular lesions: Port wine stains and hemangiomas. *Journal of American Academy of Dermatology, 58*(2), 261–285.

Stoddard, F. J., Saxe, G., Ronfeldt, H., Drake, J. E., Burns, J., Edgren, C., & Sheridan, R. (2006). Acute stress symptoms in young children with burns. *Journal of American Academy of Child and Adolescent Psychiatry, 45*(1), 87–93.

Suddaby, E. C., Barnett, S., & Facteau, L. (2005). Skin breakdown in acute care pediatrics. *Pediatric Nursing, 31*(2), 132–138, 148.

Sullivan-Whalen, M., & Gilleaudeau, P. (2007). Psoriasis: Hope for the future. *Nursing Clinics of North America, 42*, 467–484.

Timm-Knudson, V. L., Johnson, J. S., Ortiz, K. J., & Yiannias, J. A. (2006). Allergic contact dermatitis to preservatives. *Dermatologic Nursing, 18*(2), 130–136.

Tofte, S. (2007). Atopic dermatitis. *Nursing Clinics of North America, 42*, 407–419.

Truong, M. T., Chang, K. W., Berk, D. R., Heerema-McKenney, A., & Bruckner, A. L. (2010). Propranolol for the treatment of a life-threatening subglottic and mediastinal infantile hemangioma. *Journal of Pediatrics, 156*(2), 335–338.

U.S. Food and Drug Administration (FDA). (2006). *Pimecrolimus (marketed as Elidel Cream) information*. Retrieved from http://www.fda.gov/Drugs/DrugSafety/PostmarketDrugSafetyInformationforPatientsandProviders/ucm153524.htm

U.S. Food and Drug Administration Center for Drug Evaluation and Research. (2009). *Ulesfia*. Retrieved from http://www.accessdata.fda.gov/scripts/cder/drugsatfda/index.cfm?fuseaction=Search.DrugDetails

Wallace, G. (2007). Child with "bruising." *Consultant for Pediatricians, 6*(12), 659–660.

Wong, L., & Rogers, M. (2006). Psoriasis: Varied presentations, individualized treatment. *Contemporary Pediatrics, 23*(1), 33–39.

Wound Care Information Network. (2010). *Wound product category and index*. Retrieved from http://wound101.com/prodindx.htm

Zaenglein, A. L., & Thiboutot, D. M. (2006). Expert committee recommendations for acne management. *Pediatrics, 118*(3), 1188–1199.

Zajac, L., & Jacobson, A. (2009). Impetigo: Taking on a common skin infection. *Clinical Advisor, 12*(7), 30–34.

Appendix A

Physical Growth Charts

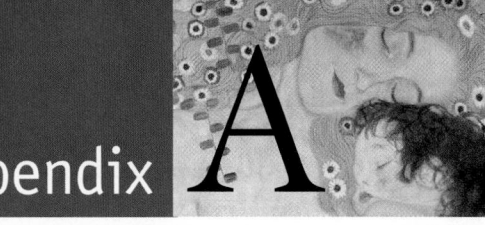

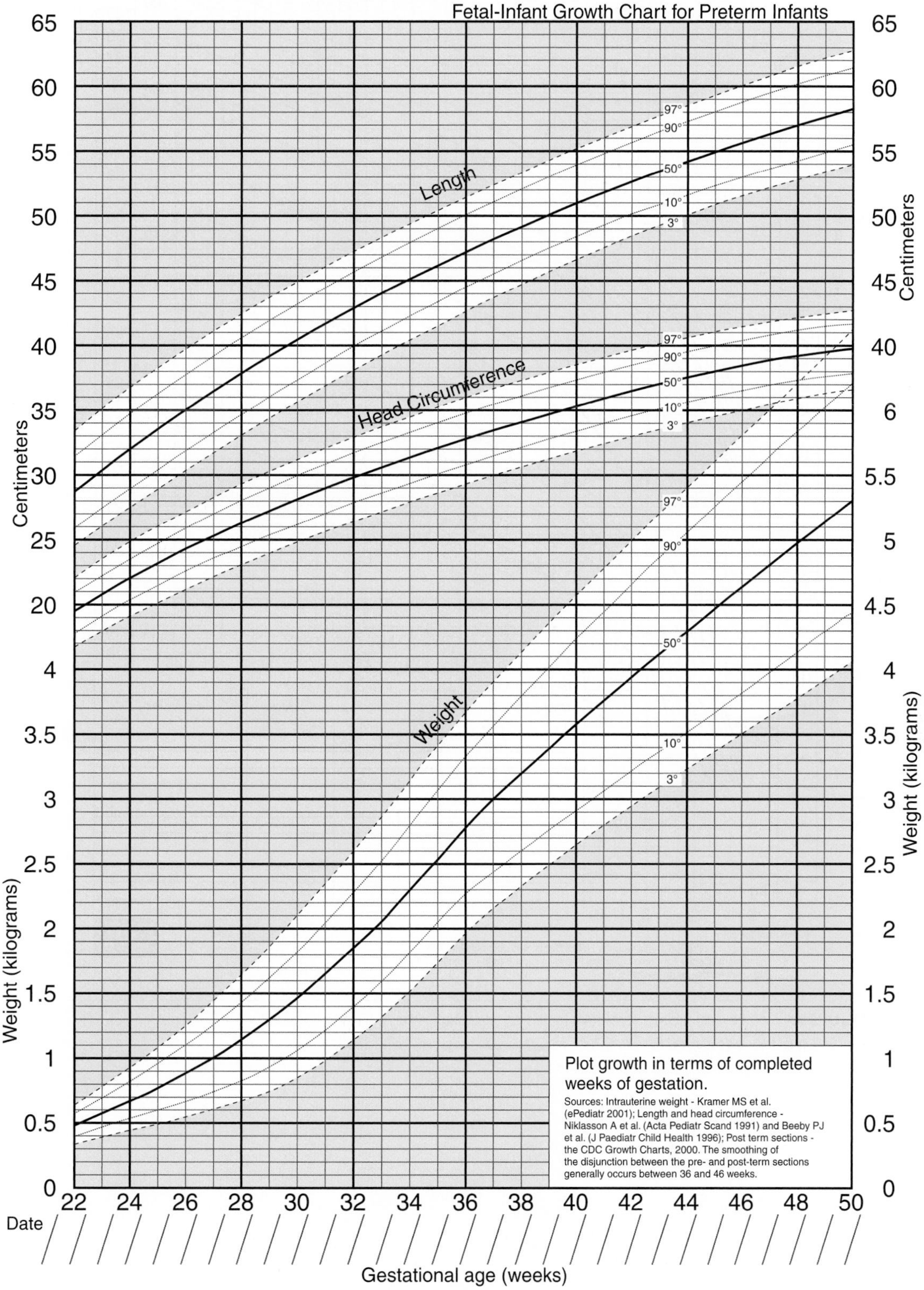

Fetal-Infant Growth Chart for Preterm Infants
Length
Head Circumference
Weight
97°
90°
50°
10°
3°
Centimeters
Weight (kilograms)
65
60
55
50
45
40
35
30
25
20
6
5.5
5
4.5
4
3.5
3
2.5
2
1.5
1
0.5
0
22
24
26
28
30
32
34
36
38
40
42
44
46
48
50
Date
Gestational age (weeks)
Plot growth in terms of completed weeks of gestation.
Sources: Intrauterine weight - Kramer MS et al. (ePediatr 2001); Length and head circumference - Niklasson A et al. (Acta Pediatr Scand 1991) and Beeby PJ et al. (J Paediatr Child Health 1996); Post term sections - the CDC Growth Charts, 2000. The smoothing of the disjunction between the pre- and post-term sections generally occurs between 36 and 46 weeks.

FIGURE A–1 ➤ Fetal-infant growth chart for preterm infants.

From: Fenton, T. R. (2003). A new growth chart for preterm babies: Babson and Benda's chart updated with recent data and new format. BMC Pediatrics, 3*(1), 13.*

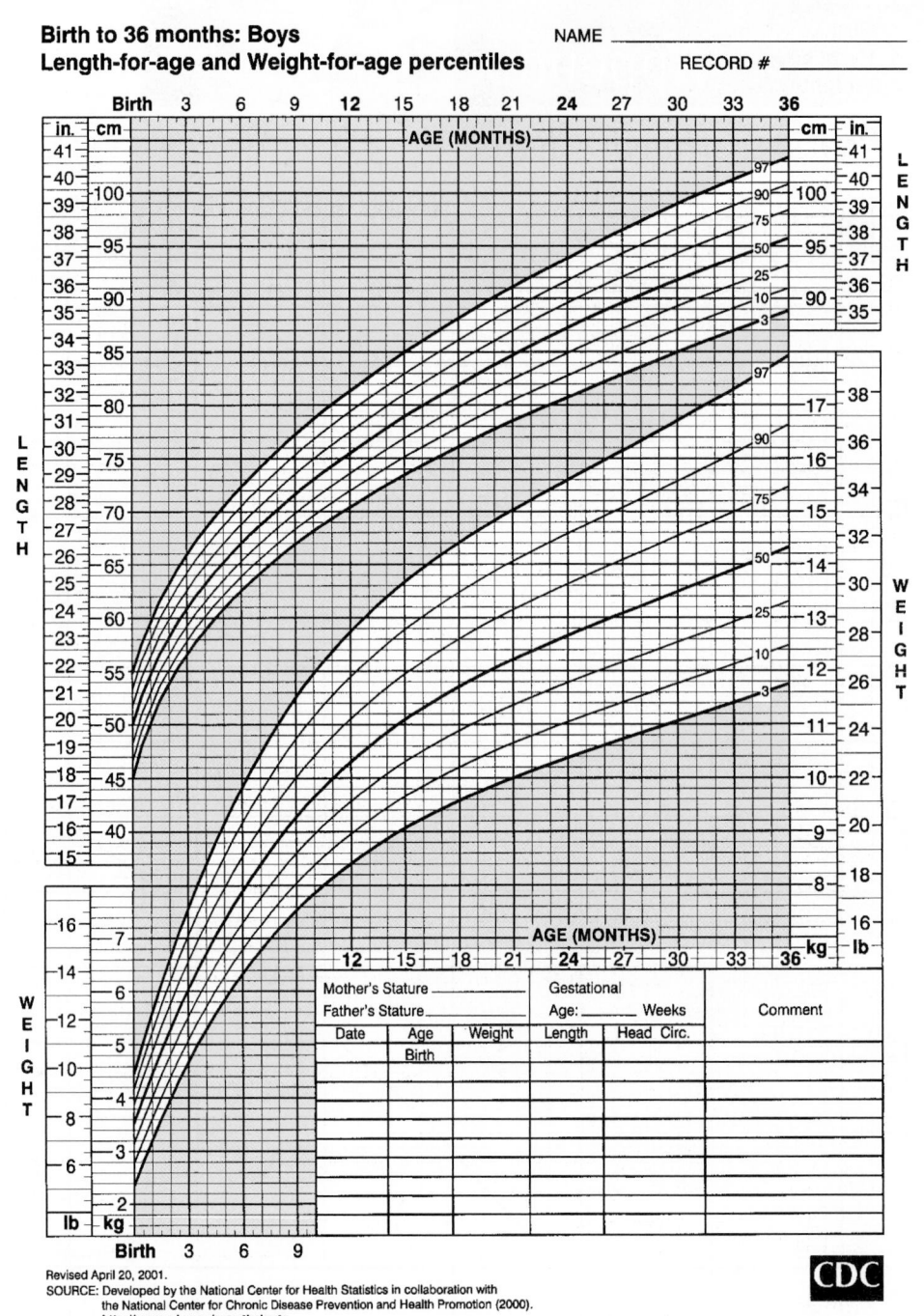

FIGURE A–2 ➤ Physical growth percentiles for length and weight—boys: birth to 36 months.

From Centers for Disease Control and Prevention, 2001. http://www.cdc.gov/growthcharts

Birth to 36 months: Boys
Head circumference-for-age and
Weight-for-length percentiles

NAME _____

RECORD # _____

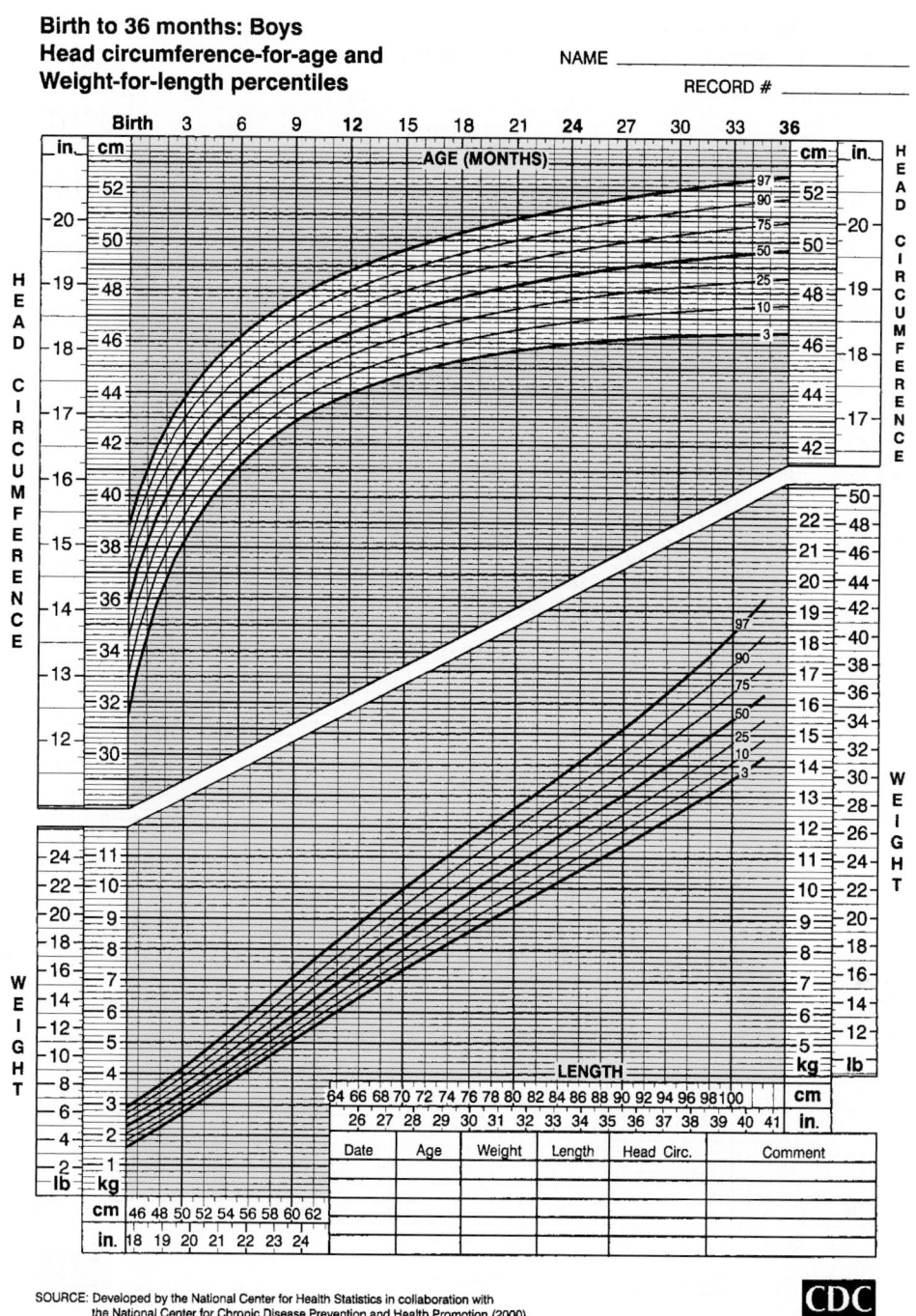

SOURCE: Developed by the National Center for Health Statistics in collaboration with
the National Center for Chronic Disease Prevention and Health Promotion (2000).
http://www.cdc.gov/growthcharts

CDC

FIGURE A–3 ➤ Physical growth percentiles for head circumference, weight for length—boys: birth to 36 months.

From Centers for Disease Control and Prevention, 2001. http://www.cdc.gov/growthcharts

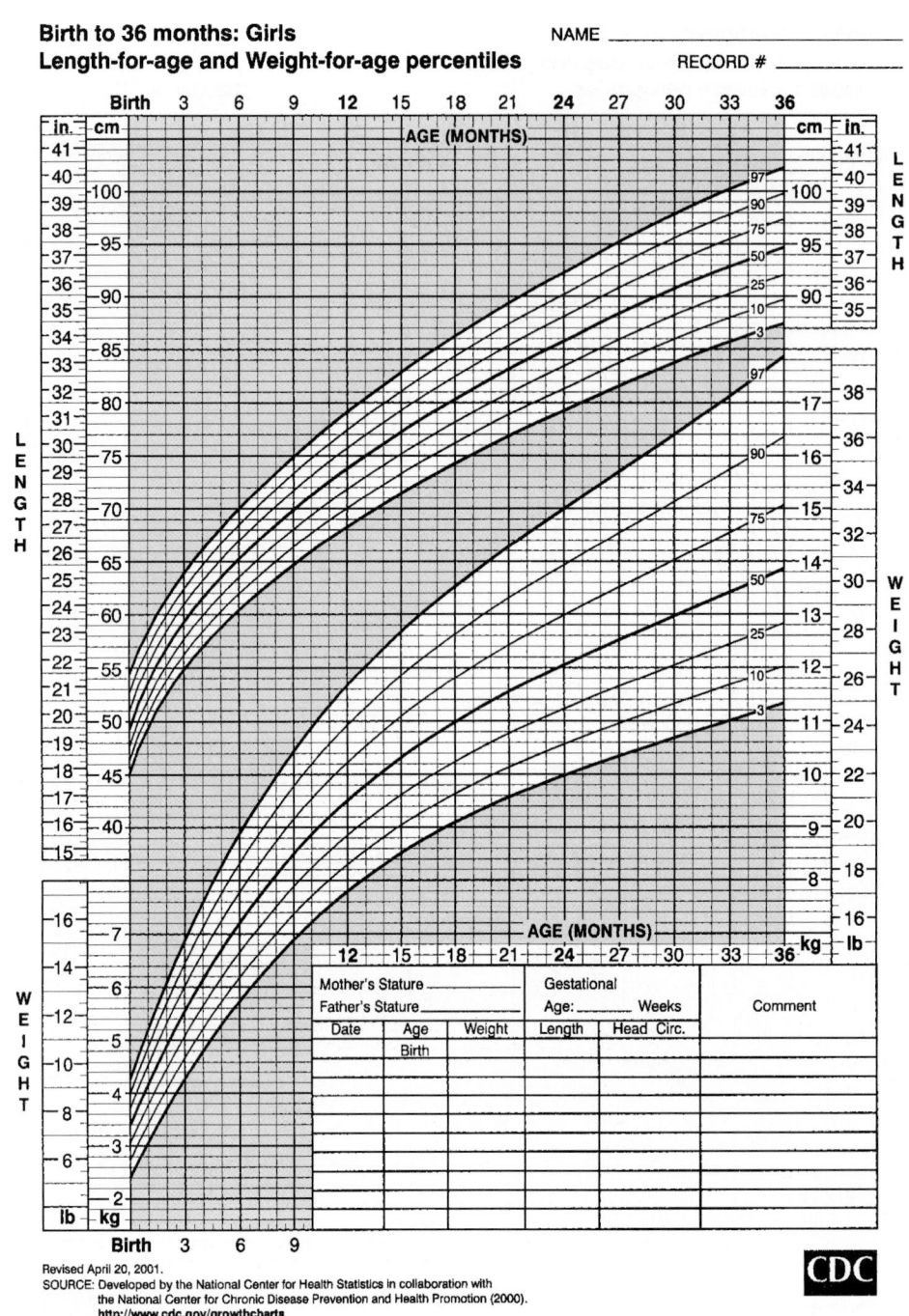

FIGURE A–4 ➤ Physical growth percentiles for length and weight—girls: birth to 36 months.

From Centers for Disease Control and Prevention, 2001. http://www.cdc.gov/growthcharts

Birth to 36 months: Girls
Head circumference-for-age and
Weight-for-length percentiles

NAME _____

RECORD # _____

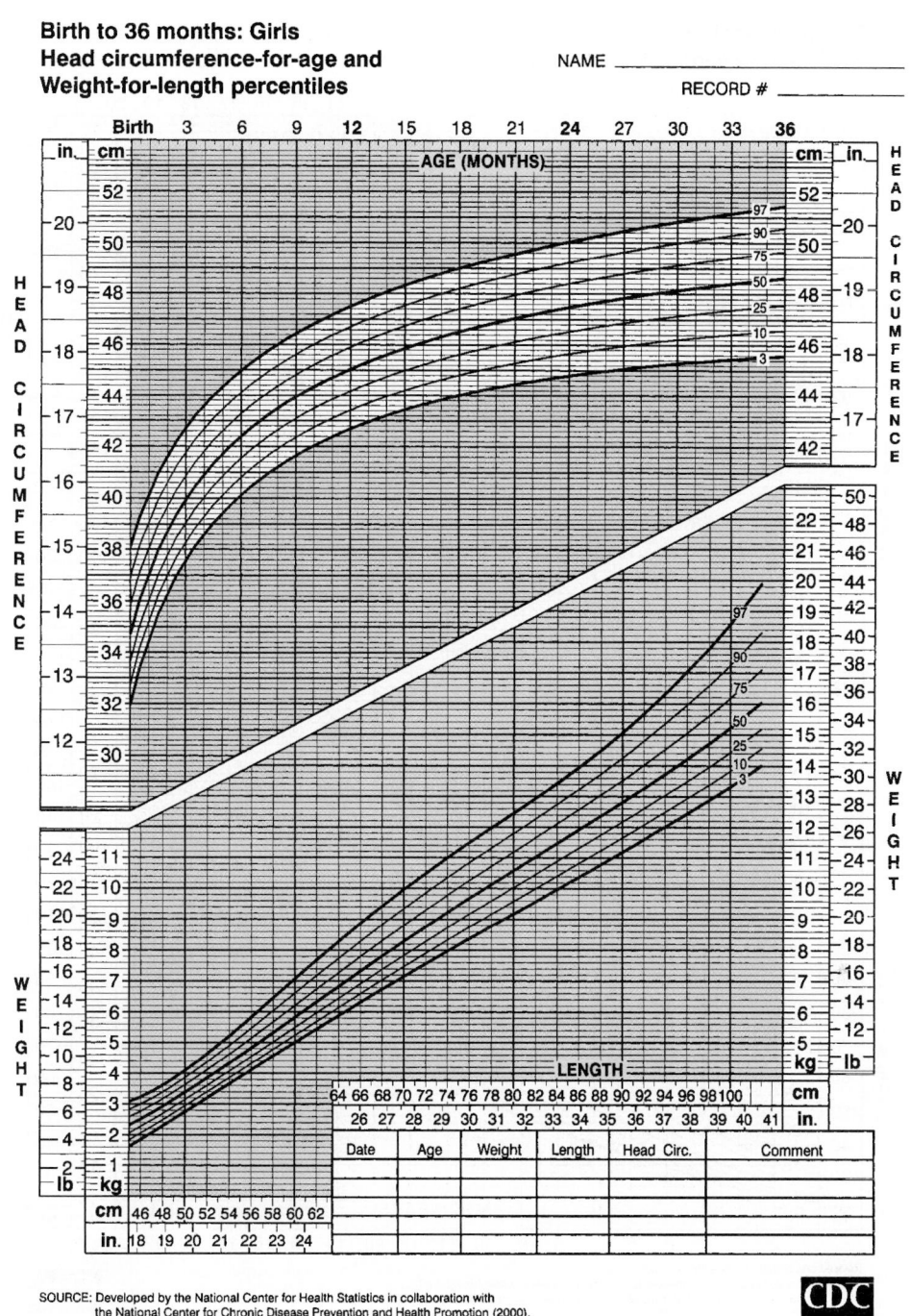

SOURCE: Developed by the National Center for Health Statistics in collaboration with
the National Center for Chronic Disease Prevention and Health Promotion (2000).
http://www.cdc.gov/growthcharts

CDC

FIGURE A–5 ➤ Physical growth percentiles for head circumference, weight for length—girls: birth to 36 months.
From Centers for Disease Control and Prevention, 2001. http://www.cdc.gov/growthcharts

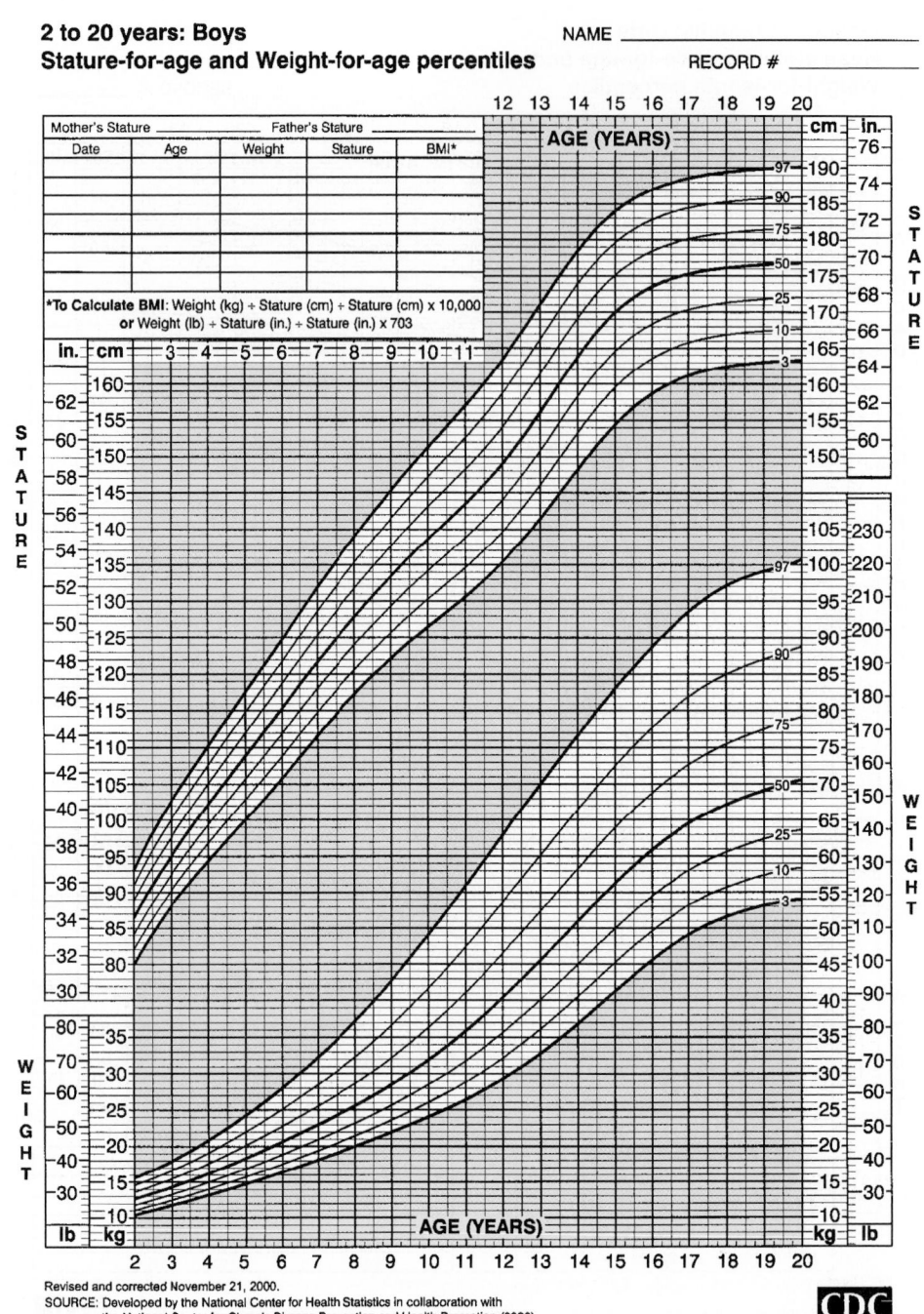

FIGURE A–6 ➤ Physical growth percentiles for stature and weight according to age—boys: 2 to 20 years.

From Centers for Disease Control and Prevention, 2001. http://www.cdc.gov/growthcharts

2 to 20 years: Boys
Body Mass Index-for-age percentiles

NAME _____

RECORD # _____

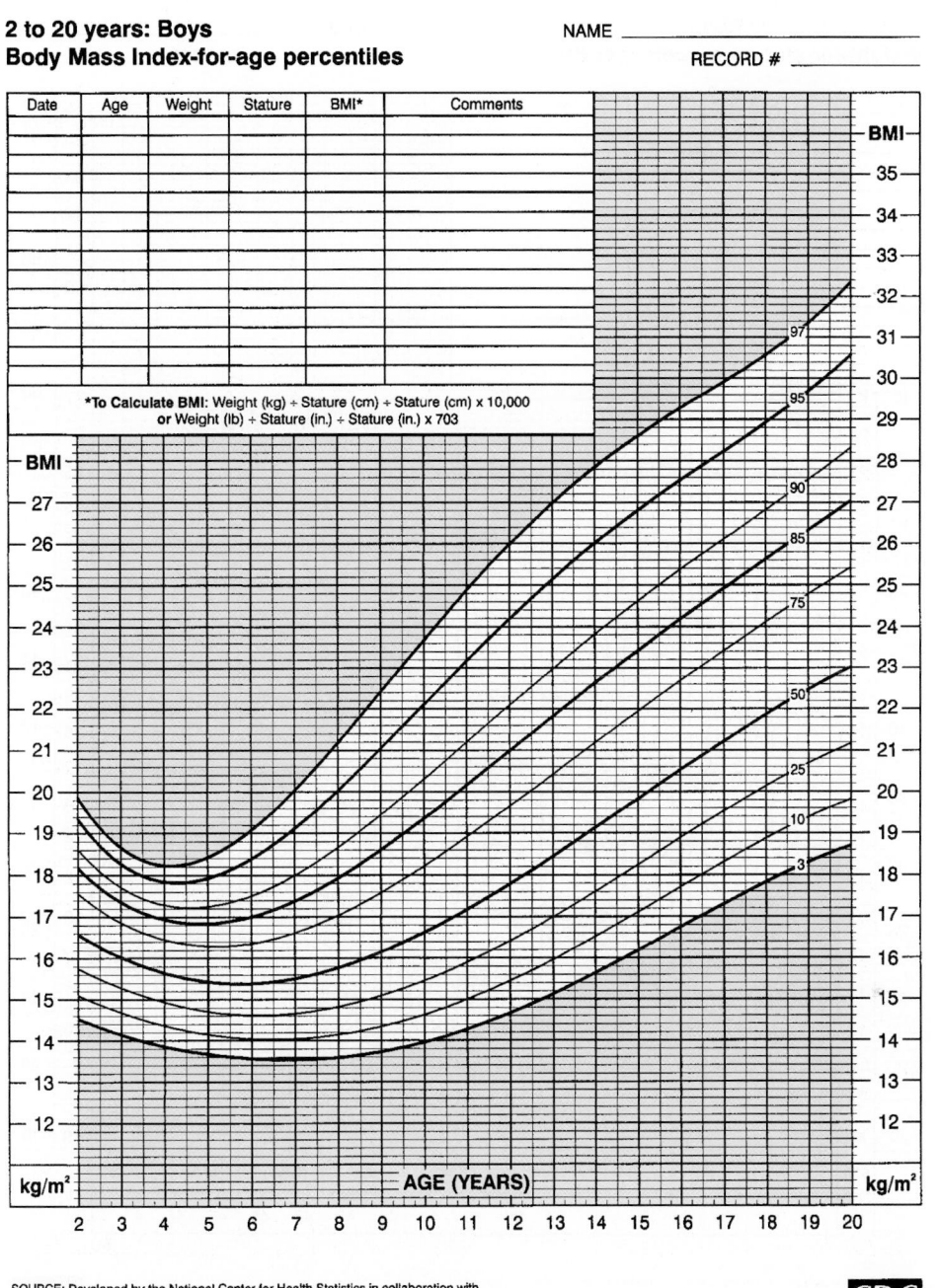

*To Calculate BMI: Weight (kg) ÷ Stature (cm) ÷ Stature (cm) x 10,000
or Weight (lb) ÷ Stature (in.) ÷ Stature (in.) x 703

AGE (YEARS)

SOURCE: Developed by the National Center for Health Statistics in collaboration with
the National Center for Chronic Disease Prevention and Health Promotion (2000).
http://www.cdc.gov/growthcharts

CDC

FIGURE A–7 ➤ Physical growth percentiles for body mass index according to age—boys: 2 to 20 years.
From Centers for Disease Control and Prevention, 2001. http://www.cdc.gov/growthcharts

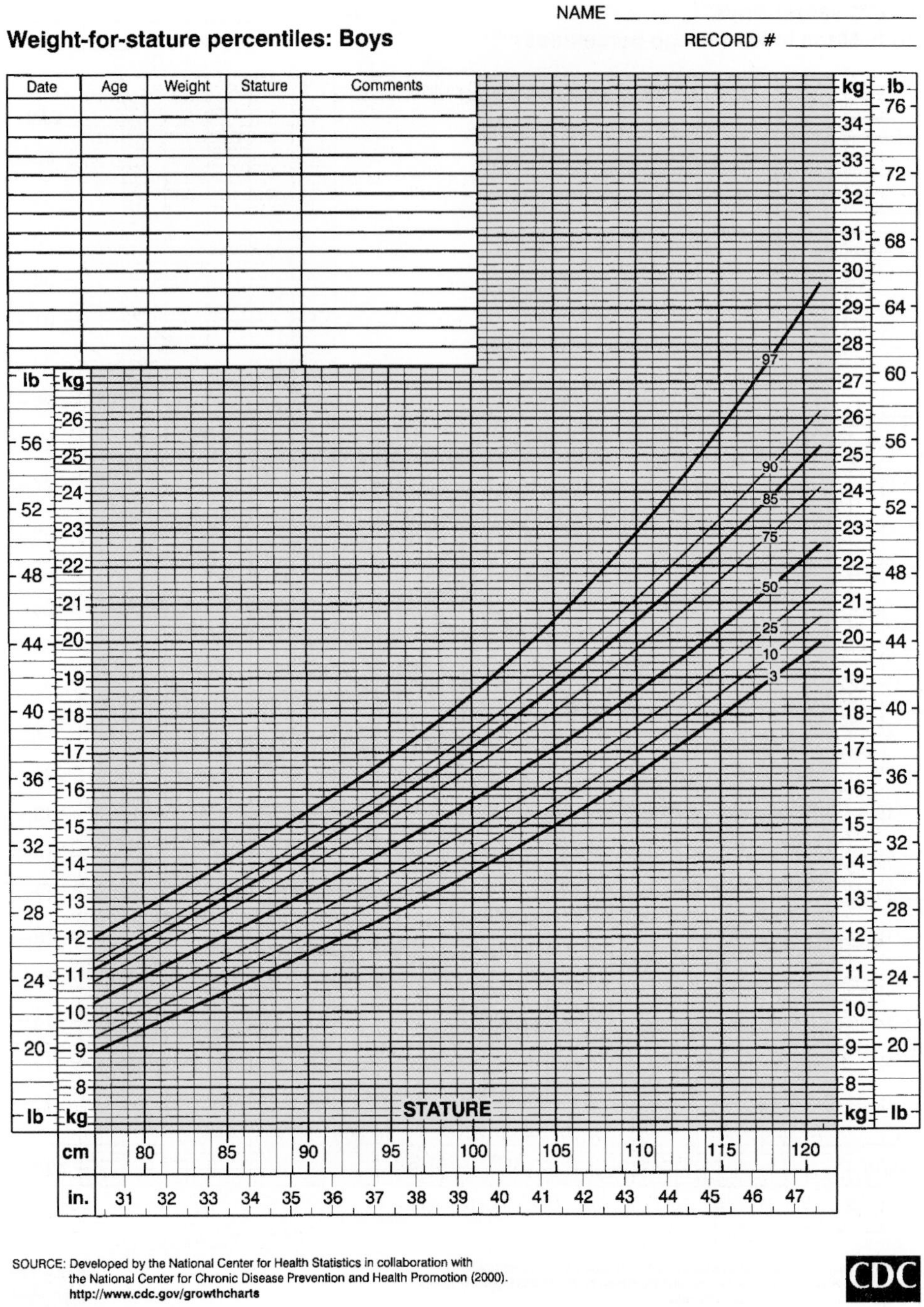
NAME
Weight-for-stature percentiles: Boys
RECORD #
Date
Age
Weight
Stature
Comments
kg
lb
97
90
85
75
50
25
10
3
STATURE
cm
in.
SOURCE: Developed by the National Center for Health Statistics in collaboration with the National Center for Chronic Disease Prevention and Health Promotion (2000). http://www.cdc.gov/growthcharts
CDC

FIGURE A–8 ➤ Physical growth percentiles for weight for stature—boys: 2 to 20 years.
From Centers for Disease Control and Prevention, 2001. http://www.cdc.gov/growthcharts

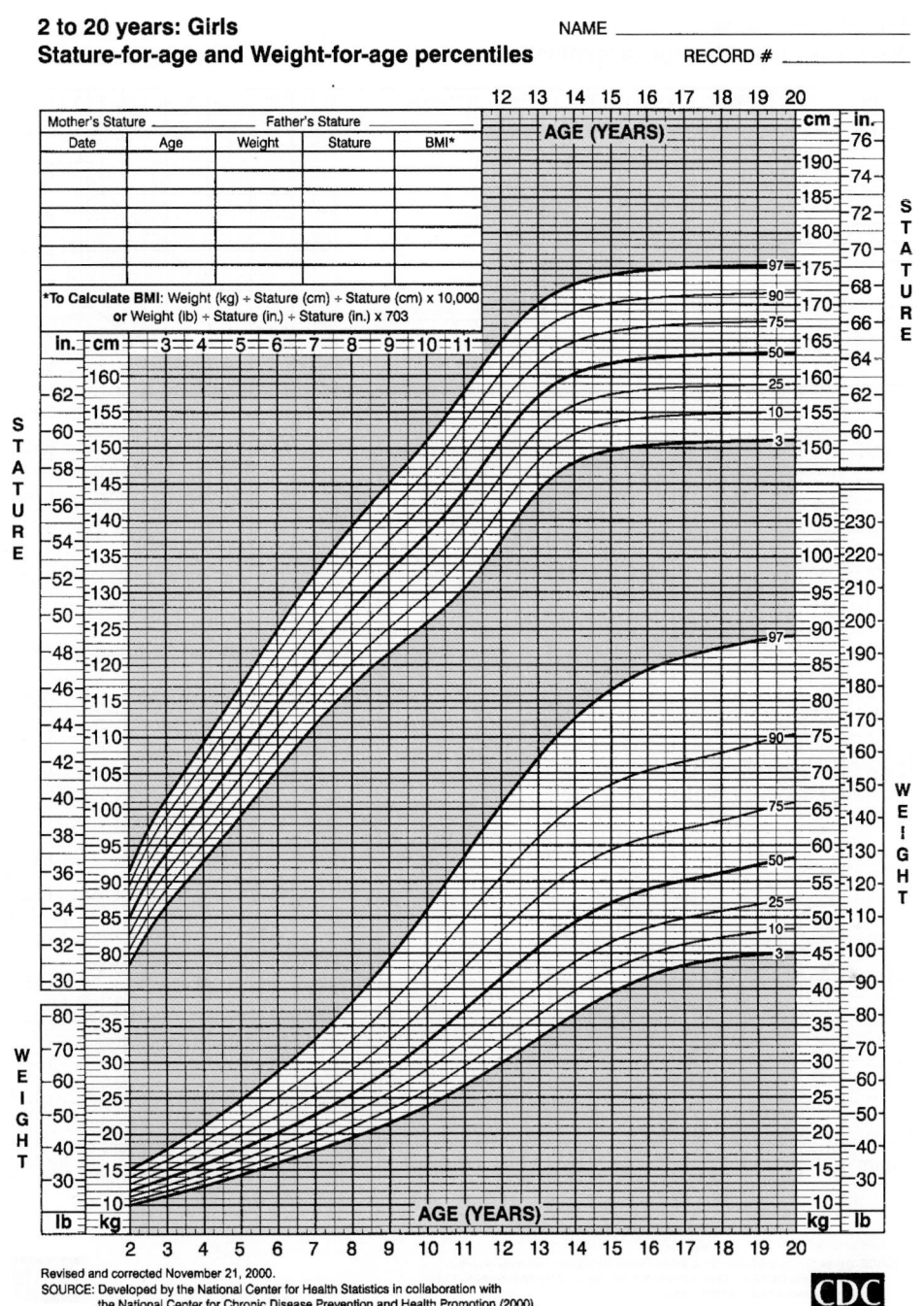

2 to 20 years: Girls
Stature-for-age and Weight-for-age percentiles

NAME _____

RECORD # _____

Revised and corrected November 21, 2000.
SOURCE: Developed by the National Center for Health Statistics in collaboration with
the National Center for Chronic Disease Prevention and Health Promotion (2000).
http://www.cdc.gov/growthcharts

FIGURE A–9 ➤ Physical growth percentiles for stature and weight according to age—girls: 2 to 20 years.

From Centers for Disease Control and Prevention, 2001. http://www.cdc.gov/growthcharts

2 to 20 years: Girls
Body Mass Index-for-age percentiles

NAME _____

RECORD # _____

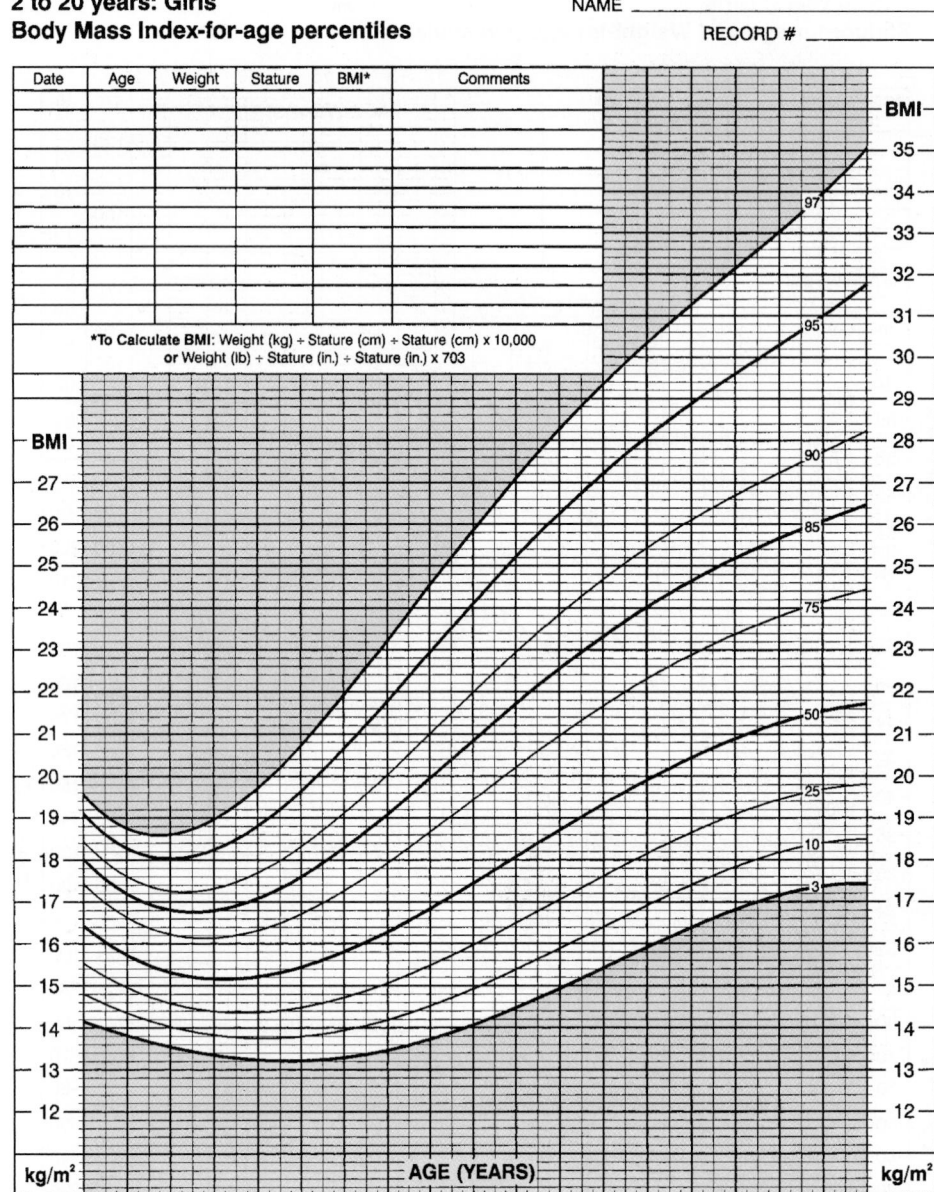

*To Calculate BMI: Weight (kg) ÷ Stature (cm) ÷ Stature (cm) x 10,000
or Weight (lb) ÷ Stature (in.) ÷ Stature (in.) x 703

SOURCE: Developed by the National Center for Health Statistics in collaboration with
the National Center for Chronic Disease Prevention and Health Promotion (2000).
http://www.cdc.gov/growthcharts

CDC

FIGURE A–10 ➤ Physical growth percentiles for body mass index according to age—girls: 2 to 20 years.
From Centers for Disease Control and Prevention, 2001. http://www.cdc.gov/growthcharts

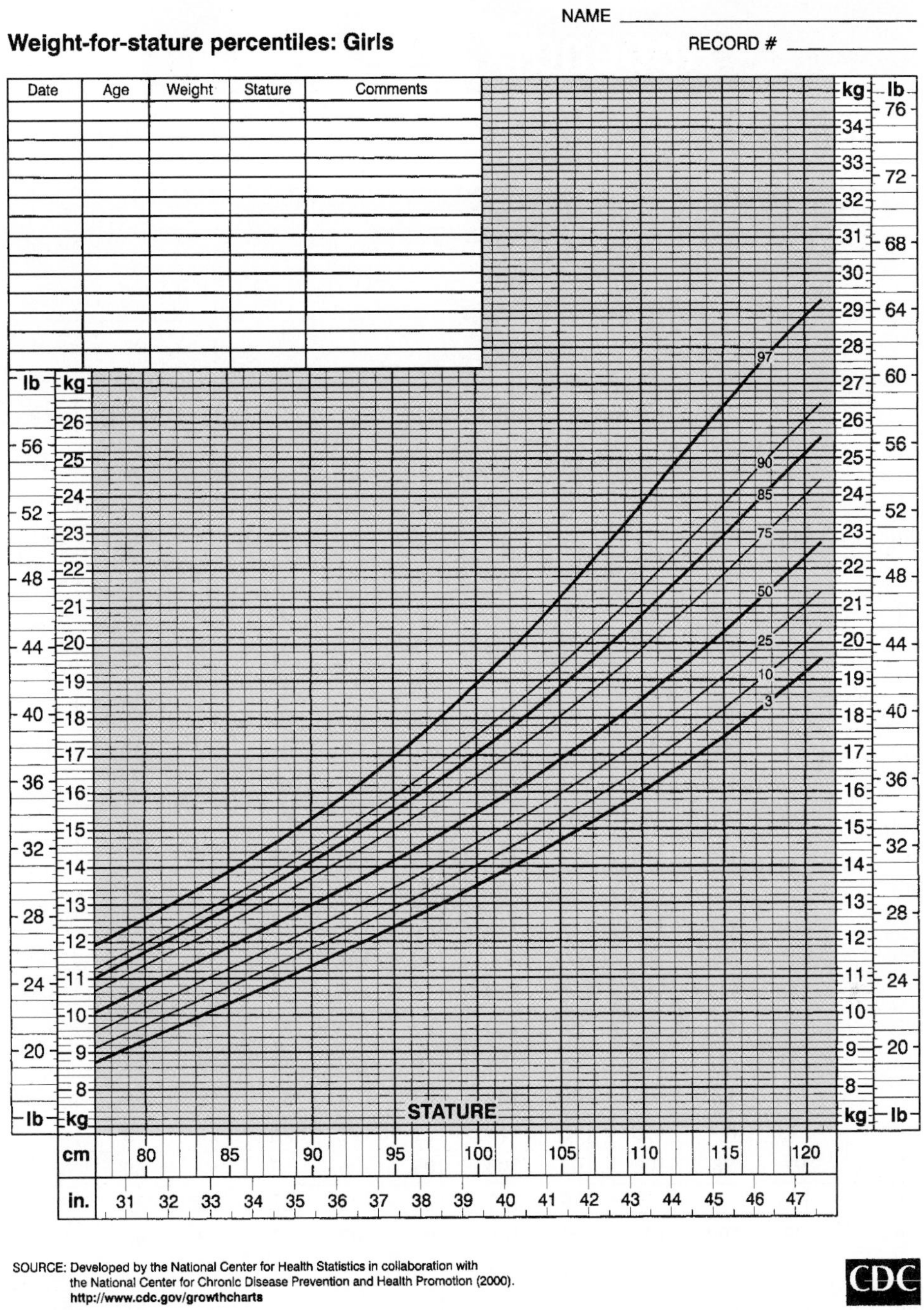
NAME
Weight-for-stature percentiles: Girls
RECORD #
Date
Age
Weight
Stature
Comments
STATURE
cm
in.
kg
lb
97
90
85
75
50
25
10
3
SOURCE: Developed by the National Center for Health Statistics in collaboration with the National Center for Chronic Disease Prevention and Health Promotion (2000).
http://www.cdc.gov/growthcharts
CDC

FIGURE A–11 ➤ Physical growth percentiles for weight for stature—girls: 2 to 20 years.

From Centers for Disease Control and Prevention, 2001. http://www.cdc.gov/growthcharts

Appendix B
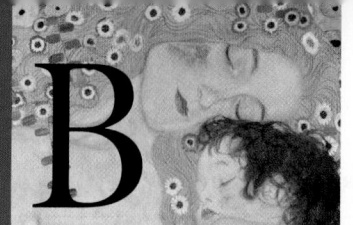

Blood Pressure Tables

TABLE B–1 Blood Pressure Levels for Boys by Age and Height Percentile. Use the child's height percentile for the age and sex from the standard growth charts found in Appendix A∞. A blood pressure value at the 50th percentile for the child's age, sex, and height percentile is considered the midpoint of the normal range. A reading above the 95th percentile indicates hypertension.

AGE (YEAR)	BP PERCENTILE	SYSTOLIC BP (mmHg) PERCENTILE OF HEIGHT							DIASTOLIC BP (mmHg) PERCENTILE OF HEIGHT						
		5TH	10TH	25TH	50TH	75TH	90TH	95TH	5TH	10TH	25TH	50TH	75TH	90TH	95TH
1	50th	80	81	83	85	87	88	89	34	35	36	37	38	39	39
	95th	98	99	101	103	104	106	106	54	54	55	56	57	58	58
2	50th	84	85	87	88	90	92	92	39	40	41	42	43	44	44
	95th	101	102	104	106	108	109	110	59	59	60	61	62	63	63
3	50th	86	87	89	91	93	94	95	44	44	45	46	47	48	48
	95th	104	105	107	109	110	112	113	63	63	64	65	66	67	67
4	50th	88	89	91	93	95	96	97	47	48	49	50	51	51	52
	95th	106	107	109	111	112	114	115	66	67	68	69	70	71	71
5	50th	90	91	93	95	96	98	98	50	51	52	53	54	55	55
	95th	108	109	110	112	114	115	116	69	70	71	72	73	74	74
6	50th	91	92	94	96	98	99	100	53	53	54	55	56	57	57
	95th	109	110	112	114	115	117	117	72	72	73	74	75	76	76
7	50th	92	94	95	97	99	100	101	55	55	56	57	58	59	59
	95th	110	111	113	115	117	118	119	74	74	75	76	77	78	78
8	50th	94	95	97	99	100	102	102	56	57	58	59	60	60	61
	95th	111	112	114	116	118	119	120	75	76	77	78	79	79	80
9	50th	95	96	98	100	102	103	104	57	58	59	60	61	61	62
	95th	113	114	116	118	119	121	121	76	77	78	79	80	81	81
10	50th	97	98	100	102	103	105	106	58	59	60	61	61	62	63
	95th	115	116	117	119	121	122	123	77	78	79	80	81	81	82
11	50th	99	100	102	104	105	107	107	59	59	60	61	62	63	63
	95th	117	118	119	121	123	124	125	78	78	79	80	81	82	82
12	50th	101	102	104	106	108	109	110	59	60	61	62	63	63	64
	95th	119	120	122	123	125	127	127	78	79	80	81	82	82	83
13	50th	104	105	106	108	110	111	112	60	60	61	62	63	64	64
	95th	121	122	124	126	128	129	130	79	79	80	81	82	83	83
14	50th	106	107	109	111	113	114	115	60	61	62	63	64	65	65
	95th	124	125	127	128	130	132	132	80	80	81	82	83	84	84
15	50th	109	110	112	113	115	117	117	61	62	63	64	65	66	66
	95th	126	127	129	131	133	134	135	81	81	82	83	84	85	85
16	50th	111	112	114	116	118	119	120	63	63	64	65	66	67	67
	95th	129	130	132	134	135	137	137	82	83	83	84	85	86	87
17	50th	114	115	116	118	120	121	122	65	66	66	67	68	69	70
	95th	131	132	134	136	138	139	140	84	85	86	87	87	88	89

BP, blood pressure.

National Heart, Lung, and Blood Institute. (2004). Blood pressure tables for children and adolescents from the fourth report on the diagnosis, evaluation, and treatment of high blood pressure in children and adolescents. Retrieved from http://www.nhlbi.nih.gov/guidelines/hypertension/child_tbl.htm

TABLE B–2	Blood Pressure Levels for Girls by Age and Height Percentile. Use the child's height percentile for the age and sex from the standard growth charts found in Appendix A ∞. A blood pressure value at the 50th percentile for the child's age, sex, and height percentile is considered the midpoint of the normal range. A reading above the 95th percentile indicates hypertension.

		SYSTOLIC BP (mmHg)							DIASTOLIC BP (mmHg)						
		PERCENTILE OF HEIGHT							PERCENTILE OF HEIGHT						
AGE (YEAR)	BP PERCENTILE	5TH	10TH	25TH	50TH	75TH	90TH	95TH	5TH	10TH	25TH	50TH	75TH	90TH	95TH
1	50th	83	84	85	86	88	89	90	38	39	39	40	41	41	42
	95th	100	101	102	104	105	106	107	56	57	57	58	59	59	60
2	50th	85	85	87	88	89	91	91	43	44	44	45	46	46	47
	95th	102	103	104	105	107	108	109	61	62	62	63	64	65	65
3	50th	86	87	88	89	91	92	93	47	48	48	49	50	50	51
	95th	104	104	105	107	108	109	110	65	66	66	67	68	68	69
4	50th	88	88	90	91	92	94	94	50	50	51	52	52	53	54
	95th	105	106	107	108	110	111	112	68	68	69	70	71	71	72
5	50th	89	90	91	93	94	95	96	52	53	53	54	55	55	56
	95th	107	107	108	110	111	112	113	70	71	71	72	73	73	74
6	50th	91	92	93	94	96	97	98	54	54	55	56	56	57	58
	95th	108	109	110	111	113	114	115	72	72	73	74	74	75	76
7	50th	93	93	95	96	97	99	99	55	56	56	57	58	58	59
	95th	110	111	112	113	115	116	116	73	74	74	75	76	76	77
8	50th	95	95	96	98	99	100	101	57	57	57	58	59	60	60
	95th	112	112	114	115	116	118	118	75	75	75	76	77	78	78
9	50th	96	97	98	100	101	102	103	58	58	58	59	60	61	61
	95th	114	114	115	117	118	119	120	76	76	76	77	78	79	79
10	50th	98	99	100	102	103	104	105	59	59	59	60	61	62	62
	95th	116	116	117	119	120	121	122	77	77	77	78	79	80	80
11	50th	100	101	102	103	105	106	107	60	60	60	61	62	63	63
	95th	118	118	119	121	122	123	124	78	78	78	79	80	81	81
12	50th	102	103	104	105	107	108	109	61	61	61	62	63	64	64
	95th	119	120	121	123	124	125	126	79	79	79	80	81	82	82
13	50th	104	105	106	107	109	110	110	62	62	62	63	64	65	65
	95th	121	122	123	124	126	127	128	80	80	80	81	82	83	83
14	50th	106	106	107	109	110	111	112	63	63	63	64	65	66	66
	95th	123	123	125	126	127	129	129	81	81	81	82	83	84	84
15	50th	107	108	109	110	111	113	113	64	64	64	65	66	67	67
	95th	124	125	126	127	129	130	131	82	82	82	83	84	85	85
16	50th	108	108	110	111	112	114	114	64	64	65	66	66	67	68
	95th	125	126	127	128	130	131	132	82	82	83	84	85	85	86
17	50th	108	109	110	111	113	114	115	64	65	65	66	67	67	68
	95th	125	126	127	129	130	131	132	82	83	83	84	85	85	86

BP, blood pressure.

National Heart, Lung, and Blood Institute. (2004). Blood pressure tables for children and adolescents from the fourth report on the diagnosis, evaluation, and treatment of high blood pressure in children and adolescents. *Retrieved from http://www.nhlbi.nih.gov/guidelines/hypertension/child_tbl.htm*

Appendix C

Recommended Dietary Allowances

TABLE C–1 Dietary Reference Intakes for Infants, Children, and Adolescents

	AGE	VITAMIN A (mcg/d)	VITAMIN D (mcg/d)	VITAMIN E (mg/d α-tocopherol)	VITAMIN K (mcg/d)	VITAMIN C (mg/d)	THIAMIN (mg/d)	RIBOFLAVIN (mg/d)	NIACIN (mg/d)	VITAMIN B$_6$ (mg/d)	
Infants	0–6 months	400*	10*	4*	2.0*	40*	0.2*	0.3*	~0.2*	0.1*	
	7–12 months	500*	10*	5*	2.5*	50*	0.3*	0.4*	~0.4*	0.3*	
Children	1–3 years	300	10*	6	30*	15	0.5	0.5	6	0.5	
	4–8 years	400	10*	7	55*	25	0.6	0.6	8	0.6	
Males	9–13 years	600	10*	11	60*	45	0.9	0.9	12	1.0	
	14–18 years	900	10*	15	75*	75	1.2	1.3	16	1.3	
Females	9–13 years	600	10*	11	60*	45	0.9	0.9	12	1.0	
	14–18 years	700	10*	15	75*	65	1.0	1.0	14	1.2	

*Values are Adequate Intakes (AIs) rather than Recommended Dietary Allowances (RDAs). All other values on the chart are RDAs. See Chapter 14 ∞ for a discussion of nutrient requirements.

Note: Data from Otten, J. J., Hellwig, J. P., & Meyers, L. D. (Eds.). (2006). Dietary Reference Intakes: The essential guide to nutrient requirements. Washington, DC: National Academies Press; Wagner, C. L., Greer, F. R., & Section on Breastfeeding and Committee on Nutrition. (2008). Prevention of rickets and vitamin D deficiency in infants, children, and adolescents. Pediatrics, 122(5), 1142–1152.

TABLE C–2 Recommended Dietary Allowances

	AGE	PROTEIN	CARBOHYDRATE	POLYUNSATURATED FATTY ACIDS n-6	POLYUNSATURATED FATTY ACIDS n-3	TOTAL FAT	FIBER
Infants	0–6 months	1.52 g/kg/d or 9.1 g/d*	60 g/d*	4.4 g/d	0.5 g/d	31 g/d	NE
	7–12 months	1.5 g/kg/d	95 g/d*	4.6 g/d	0.5 g/d	30 g/d	NE
Children	1–3 years	1.1 g/kg/d or 13 g/d	130 g/d	7 g/d (linoleic)	0.7 g/d (α-linolenic)	NE	19 g/d
	4–8 years	0.95 g/kg/d or 19 g/d	130 g/d	10 g/d (linoleic)	0.9 g/d (α-linolenic)	NE	25 g/d
Males	9–13 years	0.95 g/kg/d or 34 g/d	130 g/d	12 g/d (linoleic)	1.2 g/d (α-linolenic)	NE	31 g/d
	14–18 years	0.85 g/kg/d or 52 g/d	130 g/d	16 g/d (linoleic)	1.6 g/d (α-linolenic)	NE	38 g/d
Females	9–13 years	0.95 g/kg/d or 34 g/d	130 g/d	10 g/d (linoleic)	1.0 g/d (α-linolenic)	NE	26 g/d
	14–18 years	0.85 g/kg/d or 46 g/d	130 g/d	11 g/d (linoleic)	1.1 g/d (α-linolenic)	NE	26 g/d

*Values are Adequate Intakes (AIs) rather than Recommended Dietary Allowances (RDAs). All other values on the chart are RDAs.
NE = not established.
All data from Institute of Medicine. (2002). Dietary Reference Intakes. Washington, DC: National Academies Press. http://www.nap.edu/iom

FOLATE (mcg/d)	VITAMIN B$_{12}$ (mcg/d)	CALCIUM (mg/d)	PHOSPHORUS (mg/d)	MAGNESIUM (mg/d)	IRON (mg/d)	ZINC (mg/d)	IODINE (mcg/d)	SELENIUM (mcg/d)
65*	0.4*	210*	100*	30*	0.27*	2.0*	110*	15*
80*	0.5*	270*	275*	75*	11	3	130*	20*
150	0.9	500*	460	80	7	3	90	20
200	1.2	800*	500	130	10	5	90	30
300	1.8	1300*	1250	240	8	8	120	40
400	2.4	1300*	1250	240	11	11	150	55
300	1.8	1300*	1250	410	8	8	120	40
400	2.4	1300*	1250	360	15	9	150	55

Appendix D

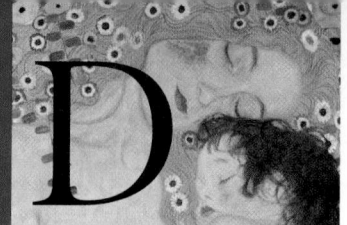

Normal Laboratory Values

All laboratory value intervals listed are approximate. Consult your local laboratory for guidelines as to normal values for the specific testing procedures used.

Normal Blood Chemistry Value Intervals

Albumin (S)[1]

1 month–1 year:	2.8–4.8 g/dL
1–18 years:	3.2–4.7 g/dL

Alkaline Phosphatase (S)[1]

Age	Male Units/L	Female Units/L
1–30 days	75–316	48–406
1–3 years	104–345	108–317
4–6 years	93–309	96–297
7–9 years	86–315	69–325
10–12 years	42–362	51–332
13–15 years	74–390	50–162
16–18 years	52–171	47–119

Alpha-fetoprotein (AFP) (S)[1]

Newborns:	50–100,000 ng/mL
1–3 months:	40–1000 ng/mL

Bilirubin (S)[1]

Conjugated	Newborns: Less than 0.6 mg/dL
Total	Birth–5 days: Less than 11.7 mg/dL

Blood Gases

Carbon Dioxide, Partial Pressure (P_{CO_2}) (B)[1]

Infants:	27–41 mmHg (3.6–5.5 kPa)
Children:	32–48 mmHg (4.3–6.4 kPa)

Oxygen, Partial Pressure (P_{O_2}) (B)[1]
Greater than 1 day: 83–108 mmHg (11–14.4 kPa)

Bicarbonate, Actual (P)[3]
22–29 mmol/L

pH (B)[1]

0–6 months:	7.18–7.51
6–12 months:	7.27–7.49

Base Excess (B)[1]

Infants:	−7 to −1 mmol/L
Children:	−4 to +2 mmol/L
Thereafter:	−3 to +3 mmol/L

Oxygen Saturation (B)[1]

Newborns:	85–90%
Thereafter:	95–99%

Cholesterol (S)[2]

Total Cholesterol

Borderline:	170–199 mg/dL
Elevated:	Greater than 200 mg/dL

High-Density Lipoprotein
Greater than 35 mg/dL

Low-Density Lipoprotein

Borderline:	110–129 mg/dL
Elevated:	130 mg/dL and higher

Triglycerides
Less than 150 mg/dL

Coagulation Values[4]

Fibrinogen	175–400 mg/dL
International normalized ratio (INR)	2–3
Partial thromboplastin time, activated (aPTT)	22–34 seconds
Prothrombin time (PT)	11–15 seconds

C-Reactive Protein (CRP) (P, S)[1]
0.68–8.2 mg/L

Creatinine (S, P)[1]

1–7 days:	0.7–1.2 mg/dL (0.06–0.11 micromol/L)
7 days–1 year:	0.2–0.5 mg/dL (0.02–0.04 micromol/L)
1–9 years:	0.2–0.8 mg/dL (0.02–0.07 micromol/L)
10–18 years:	0.5–1.1 mg/dL (0.04–0.1 micromol/L)

Electrolytes[1]

Calcium (S, P)

Newborns:	7.9–10.7 mg/dL
Thereafter:	8.7–10.7 mg/dL

Chloride (S, P)
96–110 mmol/L

Glucose (S, P)
70–126 mg/dL (3.9–7 mmol/L)

Magnesium (P, S)
1.6–2.4 mg/dL (0.66–0.99 mmol/L)

Osmolality (S)
280–300 mOsm/kg

Phosphorus, Inorganic (S, P)
2.5–6.5 mg/dL (0.81–2.1 mmol)

Potassium (S, P)
3.3–4.6 mmol/L

Sodium (P, S)
134–143 mmol/L

KEY for type of Specimen: S = serum; B = whole blood; P = plasma

Urea Nitrogen (S, P)

1–13 years:	5–17 mg/dL (1.8–6 mmol/L)
14–19 years:	8–21 mg/dL (2.9–7.5 mmol/L)

Hematology Values (B)

Values for children 2 to 12 years

Hematocrit (HCT)[1]

31.7–39.8%

Hemoglobin (HGB)[1]

10.2–13.4 g/dL

Mean Corpuscular Hemoglobin (MCH)[1]

23.7–29.5 picograms

Mean Corpuscular Hemoglobin Concentration (MCHC)[1]

31.8–34.9%

Mean Corpuscular Volume (MCV)[1]

71.3–87.6 micrometer[3]

Red Blood Cell (RBC)[1]

$3.89–5.03 \times 10^{12}$/L

White Blood Cell (WBC)[1]

$4.86–11.40 \times 10^9$/L

Differential[1]

Neutrophils	34.3–76.9%
Eosinophils	0–4.8%
Basophils	0–1%
Lymphocytes	1–50.6%
Atypical lymphocytes	2–4%
Monocytes	3.5–13.9%

Platelet Count[3]

$150–400 \times 10^9$/L

Reticulocyte Count[1]

0.8–2.8%

Erythrocyte Sedimentation Rate (Micro)[4]

1–13 mm/hr

Hemoglobin A$_{1c}$ (B)[1]

Normal: 4–7%

Hemoglobin F (B)[4]

0–2% Fetal hemoglobin

Growth Hormone (P, S)[1]

0–6.9 years:	Less than 13.7 mcg/L
7–10.9 years:	Less than 16.5 mcg/L
11–14.9 years:	Less than 14.5 mcg/L
15–18.9 years:	Less than 13.5 mcg/L

Iron-Related Values

Ferritin (P, S)[1]

1–5 years:	6–24 ng/mL
6–9 years:	10–55 ng/mL
10–19 years:	Males 23–70 ng/mL
	Females 6–40 ng/mL

Iron (S, P)[1]

5–11 am: 20–105 mcg/dL (3.6–18.8 micromol/L)

Iron-Binding Capacity (S, P)[1]

1–5 years:	268–441 mcg/dL (48–79 micromol/L)
6–9 years:	240–508 mcg/dL (43–91 micromol/L)
10–19 years:	290–570 mcg/dL (52–102 micromol/L)

Lead (B)[3]

Less than 10 mcg/dL (0.48 mmol/L)

Phenylalanine (P)[3]

Less than 2 mg/dL (120 micromole/L)

Thyroid Hormones

Thyroid-Stimulating Hormone (TSH) (P, S)[1]

Age	Males	Females
1–30 days	0.52–16 mUnit/mL	0.72–13.1 mUnit/mL
1 month–5 years	0.55–7.1 mUnit/mL	0.46–8.1 mUnit/mL
6–18 years	0.37–6 mUnit/mL	0.36–5.8 mUnit/mL

Thyroxine (T$_4$) (S, P)[1]

1–3 days:	8–20 mcg/dL
Under 1 year:	5–15 mcg/dL
Over 1 year:	4.5–11 mcg/dL

Thyroxine, "Free" (Free T$_4$) (S, P)[1]

1–3 days:	2–5 ng/dL
3–30 days:	0.9–2.2 ng/mL
Thereafter:	0.8–2 ng/mL

Thyroxine-Binding Globulin (TBG) (P)[1]

0–6 years:	16.2–33.8 mg/L
7–12 years:	15–29.2 mg/L
13–18 years:	13.4–28.7 mg/L

Triiodothyronine (T$_3$) (S)[1]

0–11 years:	90–260 ng/dL
12–18 years:	100–210 ng/dL

Normal Value Ranges: Urine

Albumin[4]

Less than 1 mg/dL

Catecholamines (Norepinephrine, Epinephrine)[1]

Values in mmol/mol creatinine

Age	Norepinephrine	Epinephrine
Less than 1 year	0.017–0.207	0–0.232
1–4 years	0.017–0.194	0–0.051
4–10 years	0.018–0.072	0.003–0.057
10–18 years	0.003–0.07	0.001–0.027

Creatinine[1]

3–8 years:	0.11–0.68 g/24 hr
9–12 years:	0.17–1.41 g/24 hr
13–17 years:	0.29–1.87 g/24 hr
Adults:	0.63–2.5 g/24 hr

Osmolality[4]

500–800 mOsm/kg water

Should be higher than serum osmolality

Protein[4]

Less than 150 mg/24 hr

Specific Gravity

1.01–1.03

Normal Value Ranges: Sweat

Electrolytes[1]

Sodium and chloride: under 40 mmol/L

Normal Value Ranges: Cerebrospinal Fluid

Protein[1]

Under 1 month: 15–153 mg/dL
Over 1 month: 15–48 mg/dL

Glucose[1]

All ages: 41–84 mg/dL (60–80% of blood glucose)

References

[1]Adapted from: Soldin, S. J., Brugnara, C., & Wong, E. C. (2007). *Pediatric reference ranges* (6th ed.). Washington, DC: AACC Press.

[2]Data from: Daniels, S. R., Greer, F. R., & Committee on Nutrition. (2008). Lipid screening and cardiovascular health in childhood. *Pediatrics, 122*(1), 198–208.

[3]Data from: Kliegman, R. M., Behrman, R. E., Jenson, H. B., & Stanton, B. F. (2007). *Nelson textbook of pediatrics* (18th ed.). Philadelphia: Saunders Elsevier.

[4]Data from: Corbett, J. V. (2008). *Laboratory tests and diagnostic procedures with nursing diagnoses* (7th ed.). Upper Saddle River, NJ: Pearson Prentice Hall.

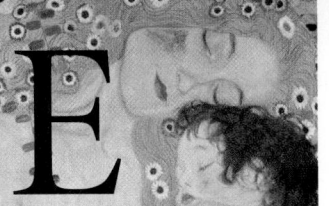

Diagnostic Tests and Procedures

Procedure, Description, and Purpose	Nursing Management
ACTH Stimulation Test A drug, metyrapone, is administered to block the production of cortisol. In persons with pituitary insufficiency, the ACTH level does not increase as expected.	• Phenytoin and estrogen compounds interfere with the test results. • Contact the laboratory for timing of the blood specimens to be collected.
Adrenal Suppression Test Dexamethasone, a potent corticosteroid, is administered to suppress the pituitary and ACTH production. In cases of Cushing syndrome, high levels of serum cortisol continue to be produced.	• Administer dexamethasone as prescribed. • Contact the laboratory for timing of the blood specimens to be collected. A plastic tube is used rather than glass.
Arteriography/Angiogram A contrast dye is injected to allow visualization of blood vessels. Useful in evaluating patency of blood vessels and blood flow to parts of the body and in identifying abnormal vasculature.	• Obtain history of hypersensitivity to iodine, seafood, or radiographic contrast dye. Antihistamines and/or steroids may be ordered if allergy is suspected. • Tell the child to expect a warm, flushing feeling that could last a few minutes. • Ensure that the child remains still during procedures so that pictures are clear. • During and after the test, monitor vital signs; assess for vasovagal and allergic reactions.
Arthrogram After a local anesthetic, a needle is inserted into a joint (e.g., knee or shoulder). Samples of joint fluid may be aspirated, and then dye is injected into the joint cavity. The joint is moved to spread the dye. Radiographs are taken with the joint in various positions to detect joint damage.	• Prepare the child and family for the procedure. • Local anesthesia is often used with general anesthesia for very young children. Support the child when the local anesthetic is inserted. • Rest, ice on the joint, elevation, and an analgesic may be needed for discomfort after the procedure.
Barium or Contrast Enema Barium or barium and air are administered via a tube through the rectum to the colon. The large intestine is visualized to detect any abnormalities. Fluoroscopy is used to monitor the process and radiographs are taken.	• Give parents preprocedure instructions regarding diet, laxatives, and/or enemas. • Prepare the child and parents for the procedure and to expect the sensation of fluid entering the rectum. Tell the child of the need to not have a bowel movement until told it is okay to do so. • Ensure that the child holds still while the radiographs are taken.
Biopsy Removal and examination of tissue from the body organs or skin to detect malignancies or the presence of disease. Biopsies can be obtained in several ways: • Surgical excision at tissue site • Needle aspiration at tissue site, with or without ultrasound • Needle insertion into skin • Brush method, scraping cells and tissue with stiff bristles as is done with a Pap smear • Punch, using an instrument to excise a small area of tissue	• Prepare necessary instruments and specimen containers. Assist with preparation of the biopsy site. • Monitor the child receiving sedation and analgesia according to protocol. • Ensure that the child remains still during the procedure. • Apply a dressing if appropriate to the site after the procedure. • Label specimens accurately and arrange for specimen transport as recommended. • Teach the family to care for the wound and to monitor the site for infection.
Bone Marrow Aspiration Marrow is removed from pelvic or iliac crest bones through a needle with a syringe used for aspiration. The test is diagnostic for leukemia, metastatic tumors, and some anemias. Marrow may also be harvested for transplant.	• The child is usually given anesthesia, or sedation and analgesia. Follow monitoring guidelines during and after the procedure. • The site is prepped with a cleansing agent according to agency protocol. • Positioning is determined by the site used (e.g., side-lying for the iliac crest). • After the procedure, maintain the child on bed rest for at least 1 hour. • Mild analgesics are provided for pain at the harvest site.
Bronchoscopy A flexible, fiber-optic bronchoscope is used to visualize the trachea and bronchi to identify and extract foreign objects in the airway, or for a biopsy.	• Maintain NPO status preprocedure according to agency guidelines. • The child will often be sedated for the procedure, so monitor the child according to agency guidelines. • Monitor vital signs per protocol after the procedure. Resume oral feedings as prescribed.

Procedure, Description, and Purpose	Nursing Management
Cardiac Catheterization A radiopaque catheter is passed through a large vein or artery in an arm or leg to the heart. It is then threaded to the heart chambers or coronary arteries, or both, guided by fluoroscopy. The procedure enables precise measurement of oxygen saturation within the heart's chambers and great arteries and pressure gradients in the pulmonary vessels or heart chambers. This helps assess for: • Congenital heart defects • Cardiac valvular disease • Coronary artery disease • Evaluation of artificial valves Other purposes of cardiac catheterization include heart muscle biopsy, tissue sampling for heart transplant rejection, or radiofrequency ablation for a heart rhythm disturbance.	• Preparation includes discontinuation of anticoagulant therapy a week prior to the test and no food or fluid 6–8 hours preprocedure. Have the child void. • Prepare the child about the equipment to be used and sensations that will be felt. • Obtain history of hypersensitivity to iodine, seafood, or radiographic contrast dye. Antihistamines and/or steroids may be ordered if allergy is suspected. Assess for allergic reaction during the procedure. • An IV is started for sedation administration, and to provide access for emergency drugs if needed. • ECG leads are applied to the chest to monitor heart activity. Vital signs and heart rhythm are monitored according to agency protocol. • See Chapter 21 ∞ for nursing management after the procedure.
Computed Tomography (CT) The CT scan is a radiographic procedure that examines body sections from different angles, producing a three-dimensional cross section of any body structure. It may be performed with or without contrast dye. CT is used to screen for head, liver, abdominal, and renal lesions; tumors; edema; abscesses; and bone destruction; and to locate foreign objects in soft tissue, such as the eye.	• Depending upon the body system evaluated, the infant or child may be NPO and require bowel evacuation prior to the study. • If contrast dye is to be used, obtain a history about any hypersensitivity to iodine, seafood, or radiographic contrast dye. If allergy is suspected, antihistamines and/or steroids may be ordered prior to the procedure. Assess for allergic reaction during the procedure. • Prepare the child for the procedure by describing the equipment, noises and other expected sensations, and how the child can help during the procedure. • If sedation is ordered for infants and small children to keep them still, monitor them according to protocol. • If contrast dye is used, encourage fluids after the procedure.
Cultures Cultures are taken to isolate and identify microorganisms causing infection, and often to identify the specific antibiotics to which the organisms are sensitive. Cultures commonly used with children include blood, throat, sputum, stool, wound, urine, and cerebrospinal fluid.	• Collect culture specimens before administering new antimicrobials to prevent false results. List any antimicrobials given on the laboratory slip. • Send all specimens immediately to the laboratory, or refrigerate the specimen. • Use strict aseptic technique to handle the specimen. Keep lids on sterile specimen containers.
Cystoscopy A flexible fiber-optic scope is inserted through the urethra into the bladder to inspect the interior urethra and bladder for inflammation, tumors, stones, or structural abnormalities. The procedure may be done simultaneously with a voiding cystourethrogram (see page 1097).	• Keep infants and children NPO prior to the study if sedation will be used. • Administer sedation as prescribed and monitor the child according to protocol. • Encourage fluids after the procedure to detect problems with voiding. • Inform the child and parents that dysuria and frequency may occur for a short time following the procedure.
Dual Energy X-ray Absorptiometry (DEXA) DEXA is a radiographic procedure emitting two photon energy beams used to measure bone mineral density in children at risk for glucocorticoid-induced osteoporosis.	• Identify factors increasing a child's risk for osteoporosis or skeletal problems. • Explain the procedure and equipment to be used to the child and parents. • Inform the child of the need to not move, and let the child know the test does not cause pain.
Echocardiography An ultrasound study of the heart is used to identify the heart size, structure, pattern of movement, hemodynamics, blood flow, and blood flow disturbances. The ultrasound probe (transducer) is held over the chest (transthoracic) or inserted through the esophagus (transesophageal) to send an ultrasound beam to the tissues. The reflected sound waves are then transformed into scans, graphs, or sounds (Doppler).	• Explain the procedure to the parents and child. Inform the child of the need to hold still for the procedure. • Inform the child that a gel will be applied to the skin and a transducer will move over the area, but that the test causes no pain.
Electrocardiography (ECG or EKG) and Ambulatory Electrocardiography An ECG records the electrical impulses of the heart via electrodes and a galvanometer (ECG machine). Eight electrodes are placed on the chest and an electrode is placed on each extremity. The lead selector is turned to read the 12 standard leads. A Holter monitor may be attached to capture ambulatory ECG readings over a 24-hour period. An ECG is used to detect cardiac arrhythmias, to identify electrolyte imbalances, or to monitor ECG changes during an exercise or stress test.	• Obtain a list of current medications and when they were last taken. • Inform the child that patches will be applied to the skin and wires will be attached, and that the test causes no pain. • Ask the child to hold still for a brief time. A pacifier or bottle may help the infant be still. • Encourage the child with a Holter monitor to engage in usual activities, but no swimming or bathing in a tub or shower is allowed until the electrodes are removed. • Ask the parents of the child wearing a Holter monitor to keep a diary of any events or emotional stress that causes symptoms. A daily schedule of sleep, eating, exercise, and other activities may be requested.

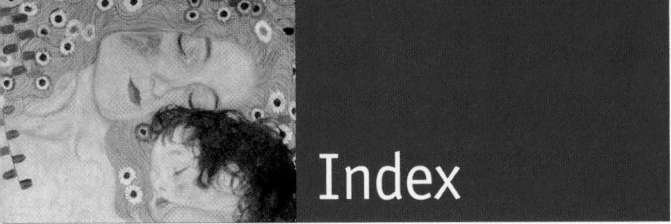

Index

Page numbers followed by italic f indicate figures and those indicated by italic t or b indicate tables or boxes